THE AMERICAN PSYCHIATRIC PUBLISHING

Textbook of PSYCHOSOMATIC MEDICINE

Psychiatric Care of the Medically Ill

SECOND EDITION

Editorial Board

THE AMERICAN PSYCHIATRIC PUBLISHING

Textbook of PSYCHOSOMATIC MEDICINE

Psychiatric Care of the Medically Ill

SECOND EDITION

Edited by

James L. Levenson, M.D.

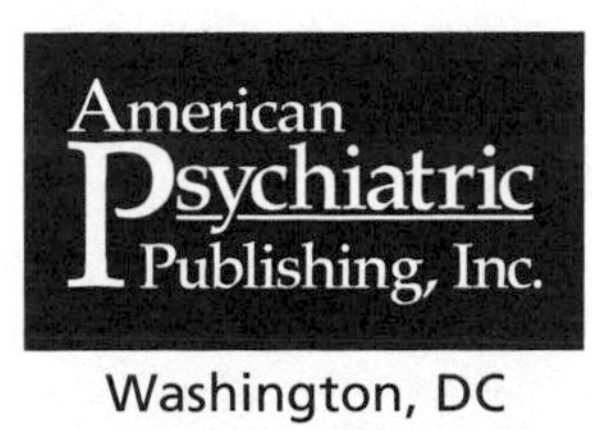

Washington, DC
London, England

Note: The authors have worked to ensure that all information in this book is accurate at the time of publication and consistent with general psychiatric and medical standards, and that information concerning drug dosages, schedules, and routes of administration is accurate at the time of publication and consistent with standards set by the U.S. Food and Drug Administration and the general medical community. As medical research and practice continue to advance, however, therapeutic standards may change. Moreover, specific situations may require a specific therapeutic response not included in this book. For these reasons and because human and mechanical errors sometimes occur, we recommend that readers follow the advice of physicians directly involved in their care or the care of a member of their family.

Books published by American Psychiatric Publishing, Inc., represent the views and opinions of the individual authors and do not necessarily represent the policies and opinions of APPI or the American Psychiatric Association.

If you would like to buy between 25 and 99 copies of this or any other APPI title, you are eligible for a 20% discount; please contact APPI Customer Service at appi@psych.org or 800-368-5777. If you wish to buy 100 or more copies of the same title, please e-mail us at bulksales@psych.org for a price quote.

Manufactured in the United States of America on acid-free paper
14 13 12 11 10 5 4 3 2 1
Second Edition

Typeset in ITC Legacy Serif and Adobe Frutiger.

American Psychiatric Publishing, Inc.
1000 Wilson Boulevard
Arlington, VA 22209-3901
www.appi.org

Library of Congress Cataloging-in-Publication Data
The American Psychiatric Publishing textbook of psychosomatic medicine: psychiatric care of the medically ill / edited by James L. Levenson. – 2nd ed.
p. ; cm.
Textbook of psychosomatic medicine
Includes bibliographical references and index.
ISBN 978-1-58562-379-2 (hardcover : alk. paper) 1. Medicine, Psychosomatic—Textbooks. I. Levenson, James L. II. Title: Textbook of psychosomatic medicine.
[DNLM: 1. Psychophysiologic Disorders. 2. Psychosomatic Medicine—methods. WM 90]
RC49.A417 2011
616.08—dc22

2010038366

British Library Cataloguing in Publication Data
A CIP record is available from the British Library.

Contents

PART III

Specialties and Subspecialties

PART IV
Treatment

Contributors

Susan E. Abbey, M.D., F.R.C.P.C.
Director, Program in Medical Psychiatry, and Director, Psychosocial Team, Multi-Organ Transplant Program, University Health Network; Associate Professor, Department of Psychiatry, Faculty of Medicine, University of Toronto, Toronto, Ontario, Canada

Yesne Alici, M.D.
Attending Psychiatrist, Geriatric Services Unit, Central Regional Hospital, Butner, North Carolina

Andrew A. Angelino, M.D.
Associate Professor, Department of Psychiatry and Behavioral Sciences, Johns Hopkins University School of Medicine, Baltimore, Maryland

David J. Axelrod, M.D., J.D.
Assistant Professor, Internal Medicine, Jefferson Medical College; Clinical Director, Thomas Jefferson University Hospital Sickle Cell Program, Philadelphia, Pennsylvania

Rosemary Basson, M.D.
Department of Psychiatry, University of British Columbia, Vancouver, British Columbia, Canada

Madeleine Becker, M.D., M.A.
Assistant Professor, Department of Psychiatry and Human Behavior, Thomas Jefferson University, Philadelphia, Pennsylvania

Charles H. Bombardier, Ph.D.
Professor and Head, Division of Clinical and Neuropsychology, Department of Rehabilitation Medicine, University of Washington, Seattle

John Michael Bostwick, M.D.
Professor of Psychiatry, Mayo Clinic College of Medicine, Rochester, Minnesota

William Breitbart, M.D.
Chief, Psychiatry Service, Department of Psychiatry and Behavioral Sciences, and Attending Psychiatrist, Pain and Palliative Care Service, Department of Medicine, Memorial Sloan-Kettering Cancer Center; Professor of Clinical Psychiatry, Department of Psychiatry, Weill Medical College of Cornell University, New York, New York

Rebecca W. Brendel, M.D., J.D.
Assistant Psychiatrist, Massachusetts General Hospital; Assistant Professor of Psychiatry, Harvard Medical School, Boston, Massachusetts

Brenda Bursch, Ph.D.
Professor, Clinical Psychiatry and Biobehavioral Sciences, and Pediatrics, David Geffen School of Medicine at UCLA, Los Angeles, California

Alan J. Carson, M.B.Ch.B., M.Phil., M.D., F.R.C.Psych.
Consultant Neuropsychiatrist and Part-Time Senior Lecturer, Department of Clinical Neurosciences, Western General Hospital, University of Edinburgh, Edinburgh, United Kingdom

Harvey Max Chochinov, M.D., Ph.D., F.R.S.C.
Director and Canada Research Chair in Palliative Medicine, Manitoba Palliative Care Research Unit, CancerCare Manitoba; Distinguished Professor of Psychiatry and Family Medicine, Departments of Psychiatry and Family Medicine, University of Manitoba, Winnipeg, Manitoba, Canada

Michael R. Clark, M.D., M.P.H., M.B.A.
Associate Professor and Director, Adolf Meyer Chronic Pain Treatment Services, Department of Psychiatry and Behavioral Sciences, The Johns Hopkins Medical Institutions, Baltimore, Maryland

Kathy L. Coffman, M.D.
Staff Psychiatrist, Psychiatry and Surgery; and Program Director, Psychosomatic Medicine Fellowship, Cleveland Clinic, Cleveland, Ohio

Lewis M. Cohen, M.D.
Professor of Psychiatry, Tufts University School of Medicine, Boston, Massachusetts; Director of Renal Palliative Care Initiative, Baystate Medical Center, Springfield, Massachusetts

Catherine C. Crone, M.D.
Associate Professor of Psychiatry, George Washington University Medical Center, Washington, D.C.; Vice Chair, Department of Psychiatry, Inova Fairfax Hospital, Falls Church, Virginia; Clinical Professor of Psychiatry, Virginia Commonwealth University School of Medicine, Northern Virginia Branch, Fairfax, Virginia

Daniel Cukor, Ph.D.
Assistant Professor of Psychiatry, SUNY Downstate Medical Center, Brooklyn, New York

Niccolo D. Della Penna, M.D.
Instructor, Department of Psychiatry and Behavioral Sciences, Johns Hopkins University School of Medicine, Baltimore, Maryland

Michael J. Devlin, M.D.
Professor of Clinical Psychiatry, Columbia University College of Physicians and Surgeons; Clinical Co-Director, Eating Disorders Research Unit, New York State Psychiatric Institute, New York, New York

Mary Amanda Dew, Ph.D.
Professor of Psychiatry, Psychology, and Epidemiology; Director of Quality of Life Research, Artificial Heart Program, Western Psychiatric Institute and Clinics, University of Pittsburgh Medical Center, Pittsburgh, Pennsylvania

Chris Dickens, M.B.B.S., Ph.D.
Senior Lecturer in Psychological Medicine, Department of Psychiatry, Manchester Royal Infirmary, Manchester, United Kingdom

Andrea F. DiMartini, M.D.
Associate Professor of Psychiatry and of Surgery, Western Psychiatric Institute; Consultation Liaison to the Liver Transplant Program, Starzl Transplant Institute, University of Pittsburgh Medical Center, Pittsburgh, Pennsylvania

Christopher R. Dobbelstein, M.D.
Clinical Assistant Professor of Psychiatry, Western Psychiatric Institute and Clinic, University of Pittsburgh Medical Center, Pittsburgh, Pennsylvania

Ilyse Dobrow DiMarco, Ph.D.
Director of Eating Disorders and Weight Management Program, The American Institute for Cognitive Therapy, New York, New York

Steven A. Epstein, M.D.
Professor and Chair, Department of Psychiatry, Georgetown University Hospital and School of Medicine, Washington, D.C.

Jesse R. Fann, M.D., M.P.H.
Associate Professor, Department of Psychiatry and Behavioral Sciences, and Adjunct Associate Professor, Departments of Rehabilitation Medicine and Epidemiology, University of Washington, Seattle; Affiliate Investigator, Fred Hutchinson Cancer Research Center; and Director, Psychiatry and Psychology Service, Seattle Cancer Care Alliance, Seattle, Washington

Charles V. Ford, M.D.
Professor, Department of Psychiatry and Behavioral Neurobiology, University of Alabama at Birmingham, Birmingham, Alabama

Andrew Francis, Ph.D., M.D.
Professor of Psychiatry, Department of Psychiatry and Behavioral Sciences, Stony Brook University Medical Center, Health Sciences Center, Stony Brook, New York

Oliver Freudenreich, M.D.
Assistant Professor of Psychiatry, Division of Psychiatry and Medicine, Department of Psychiatry, Massachusetts General Hospital, Boston, Massachusetts

Gregory L. Fricchione, M.D.
Professor of Psychiatry, Division of Psychiatry and Medicine, Department of Psychiatry, Massachusetts General Hospital, Boston, Massachusetts

Ann Goebel-Fabbri, Ph.D.
Psychologist, Behavioral and Mental Health Unit, Joslin Diabetes Center; and Instructor in Psychiatry, Department of Psychiatry, Harvard Medical School, Boston, Massachusetts

Mark S. Groves, M.D.
Assistant Clinical Professor of Psychiatry and Neurology, Albert Einstein College of Medicine; Attending Psychiatrist, Departments of Psychiatry and Neurology, Beth Israel Medical Center, New York, New York

Madhulika A. Gupta, M.D., F.R.C.P.C.
Professor, Department of Psychiatry, Schulich School of Medicine and Dentistry, University of Western Ontario, London, Ontario, Canada

Elspeth Guthrie, M.B., Ch.B., M.R.C.Psych., M.Sc., M.D.
Honorary Professor of Psychological Medicine and Medical Psychotherapy, University of Manchester; Consultant in Psychological Medicine, Manchester Royal Infirmary, Manchester, United Kingdom

Daniel Hicks, M.D.
Associate Professor and Director of Psychosomatic Medicine, Department of Psychiatry, Georgetown University Hospital and School of Medicine, Washington, D.C.

Michael R. Irwin, M.D.
Distinguished Professor of Psychiatry and Biobehavioral Sciences, UCLA David Geffen School of Medicine; Norman Cousins Chair for Psychoneuroimmunology, UCLA Semel Institute for Neuroscience and Human Behavior; and Director, Cousins Center for Psychoneuroimmunology, Los Angeles, California

Joel P. Jahraus, M.D.
Executive Director, Park Nicollet Melrose Institute, Minneapolis, Minnesota; Adjunct Clinical Professor, University of Minnesota Medical School, Minneapolis, Minnesota

Richard Kennedy, M.D., Ph.D.
Postdoctoral Fellow, Section on Statistical Genetics, Department of Biostatistics, University of Alabama-Birmingham, Birmingham, Alabama

Paul L. Kimmel, M.D.
Senior Advisor, Division of Kidney, Urologic, and Hematologic Diseases, National Institute of Diabetes, Digestive, and Kidney Diseases, National Institutes of Health, Bethesda, Maryland

Lois E. Krahn, M.D.
Professor of Psychiatry, Mayo Clinic College of Medicine; Chair, Department of Psychiatry and Psychology, Mayo Clinic, Scottsdale, Arizona

Elisabeth J. Shakin Kunkel, M.D.
Professor, Department of Psychiatry and Human Behavior, Thomas Jefferson University, Philadelphia, Pennsylvania

Maeve Leonard, M.B., M.R.C.Psych.
Clinical and Research Tutor in Psychiatry, Graduate Entry Medical School, University of Limerick, Limerick, Ireland

James L. Levenson, M.D.
Professor of Psychiatry, Medicine, and Surgery, Virginia Commonwealth University School of Medicine, Richmond, Virginia

Madeline Li, M.D., Ph.D., F.R.C.P.C.
Assistant Professor, Department of Psychiatry, University of Toronto; Psychiatrist, Department of Psychosocial Oncology and Palliative Care, Princess Margaret Hospital, University Health Network, Toronto, Ontario, Canada

Antonio Lobo, M.D., Ph.D.
Professor and Chairman, Department of Medicine and Psychiatry, Universidad de Zaragoza; and Chief, Psychosomatics and Consultation-Liaison Psychiatry Service, Hospital Clínico Universitario, Zaragoza, Spain

Constantine G. Lyketsos, M.D., M.H.S.
The Elizabeth Plank Althouse Professor and Chairman, Department of Psychiatry, Johns Hopkins Bayview Medical Center; Vice Chairman, Department of Psychiatry and Behavioral Sciences, The Johns Hopkins Hospital; Co-Director, Division of Geriatric Psychiatry and Neuropsychiatry, and Director, Memory and Alzheimer's Treatment Center, The Johns Hopkins University and Hospital, Baltimore, Maryland

Dimitri D. Markov, M.D.
Assistant Professor, Departments of Psychiatry and Human Behavior and of Medicine, Thomas Jefferson University, Philadelphia, Pennsylvania

Elaine Martin, M.D.
Fellow in Psychosomatic Medicine, Department of Psychiatry and Human Behavior, Thomas Jefferson University, Philadelphia, Pennsylvania

Mary Jane Massie, M.D.
Professor of Clinical Psychiatry, Weill Medical College of Cornell University; Attending Psychiatrist, Memorial Sloan-Kettering Cancer Center, New York, New York

David J. Meagher, M.D., M.R.C.Psych., M.Sc.
Professor of Psychiatry, University of Limerick Medical School, Castletroy, Limerick, Ireland

Franklin G. Miller, Ph.D.
Bioethicist, Department of Bioethics, Clinical Center, Bethesda, Maryland

Kimberley Miller, M.D., F.R.C.P.C.
Lecturer, University of Toronto; Attending Psychiatrist, Princess Margaret Hospital, Toronto, Ontario, Canada

Gail Musen, Ph.D.
Assistant Investigator, Behavioral and Mental Health Unit, Joslin Diabetes Center; and Instructor in Psychiatry, Department of Psychiatry, Harvard Medical School, Boston, Massachusetts

Philip R. Muskin, M.D.
Chief, Consultation-Liaison Psychiatry, Columbia University Medical Center; Professor of Clinical Psychiatry, Columbia University College of Physicians and Surgeons; Faculty, Columbia University Psychoanalytic Center for Training and Research, New York, New York

Shamim H. Nejad, M.D.
Instructor in Psychiatry, Department of Psychiatry, Massachusetts General Hospital, Boston, Massachusetts

Patrick G. O'Malley, M.D., M.P.H., F.A.C.P.
Professor of Medicine, Uniformed Services University, Bethesda, Maryland

Chiadi U. Onyike, M.D., M.H.S.
Assistant Professor of Psychiatry and Behavioral Sciences and Co-Director, FTD & Young-Onset Dementias Clinic, Division of Geriatric Psychiatry and Neuropsychiatry, The Johns Hopkins University and Hospital, Baltimore, Maryland

James A. Owen, Ph.D.
Associate Professor of Psychiatry and of Pharmacology and Toxicology, Queen's University; Director, Psychopharmacology Lab, Providence Care Mental Health Services, Kingston, Ontario, Canada

Olu Oyesanmi, M.D., M.P.H.
Research Analyst, ECRI Institute, Plymouth Meeting, Pennsylvania

Pauline S. Powers, M.D.
Professor of Psychiatry and Behavioral Medicine, Clinical and Translational Science Institute, College of Medicine, University of South Florida, Tampa, Florida

Miguel Ángel Quintanilla, M.D., Ph.D.
Attending Psychiatrist, Hospital Clínico Universitario; and Instructor, Department of Medicine and Psychiatry, Universidad de Zaragoza, Zaragoza, Spain

J. J. Rasimas, M.D., Ph.D.
Associate Professor of Psychiatry, Penn State College of Medicine/Milton S. Hershey Medical Center, Hershey, Pennsylvania; Medical Toxicology Fellow, Penn State College of Medicine, PinnacleHealth Toxicology Center, Harrisburg, Pennsylvania

Keith G. Rasmussen, M.D.
Associate Professor of Psychiatry, Mayo Clinic Department of Psychiatry and Psychology, Rochester, Minnesota

Peter M. Rees, M.D., Ph.D.
Department of Medicine, Burnaby Hospital, Burnaby, British Columbia, Canada

Gary Rodin, M.D., F.R.C.P.C.
Professor, Department of Psychiatry, University of Toronto; Head, Department of Psychosocial Oncology and Palliative Care, Princess Margaret Hospital, University Health Network, Toronto, Ontario, Canada

Donald L. Rosenstein, M.D.
Professor and Director, Comprehensive Cancer Support Program, Department of Psychiatry, University of North Carolina at Chapel Hill, Chapel Hill, North Carolina

Deborah Rosenthal-Asher, M.A.
Doctoral Candidate, Ferkauf Graduate School of Psychology, Albert Einstein College of Medicine, Yeshiva University, Brooklyn, New York

Carlos A. Santana, M.D.
Associate Professor of Psychiatry and Behavioral Medicine, Director of Outpatient Services, Director of Psychiatry Research Division, College of Medicine, University of South Florida, Tampa, Florida

Pedro Saz, M.D., Ph.D.
Professor, Department of Medicine and Psychiatry, Universidad de Zaragoza, Zaragoza, Spain

Ronald Schouten, M.D., J.D.
Psychiatrist, Massachusetts General Hospital; Associate Professor of Psychiatry, Harvard Medical School, Boston, Massachusetts

Peter A. Shapiro, M.D.
Professor of Clinical Psychiatry, Columbia University; Director, Fellowship Training Program in Psychosomatic Medicine; and Associate Director, Consultation-Liaison Psychiatry Service, New York Presbyterian Hospital-Columbia University Medical Center, New York, New York

Michael C. Sharpe, M.A., M.D., F.R.C.P., F.R.C.Psych.
Professor of Psychological Medicine, Psychological Medicine Research, University of Edinburgh, Royal Edinburgh Hospital, Edinburgh United Kingdom

Felicia A. Smith, M.D.
Director, Acute Psychiatry Service, Massachusetts General Hospital, Boston, Massachusetts

Jorge Luis Sotelo, M.D.
Assistant Professor of Clinical Psychiatry, Division of Consultation Psychiatry/Psychosomatic Medicine; Co-Director, Psychiatry Clerkship for Medical Students, Department of Psychiatry and Behavioral Sciences, University of Miami Miller School of Medicine, Miami, Florida

Theodore A. Stern, M.D.
Chief, Psychiatric Consultation Service, Massachusetts General Hospital; Professor of Psychiatry, Harvard Medical School, Boston, Massachusetts

Donna E. Stewart, M.D, F.R.C.P.C.
University Professor and Chair of Women's Health, University of Toronto, University Health Network Women's Health Program, Toronto, Ontario, Canada

Jon Stone, M.B.Ch.B., Ph.D., F.R.C.P.
Consultant Neuropsychiatrist and Part-Time Senior Lecturer, Department of Clinical Neurosciences, Western General Hospital, University of Edinburgh, Edinburgh, United Kingdom

Nada Logan Stotland, M.D., M.P.H.
Professor of Psychiatry and Obstetrics/Gynecology, Rush Medical College, Chicago, Illinois

Margaret Stuber, M.D.
Jane and Marc Nathanson Professor, Psychiatry and Biobehavioral Sciences, David Geffen School of Medicine at UCLA, Los Angeles, California

Glenn J. Treisman, M.D., Ph.D.
Professor, Department of Psychiatry and Behavioral Sciences, Johns Hopkins University School of Medicine, Baltimore, Maryland

Paula T. Trzepacz, M.D.
Senior Medical Fellow, Neurosciences, Lilly Research Laboratories, Eli Lilly & Co., Indianapolis, Indiana; Clinical Professor of Psychiatry, Indiana University School of Medicine, Indianapolis, Indiana; Clinical Professor of Psychiatry, University of Mississippi Medical School, Jackson, Mississippi; Adjunct Professor of Psychiatry, Tufts University School of Medicine, Boston, Massachusetts

Simone N. Vigod, M.D., F.R.C.P.C.
Assistant Professor, Department of Psychiatry, University of Toronto, Women's College Hospital, Toronto, Ontario, Canada

Crystal C. Watkins, M.D., Ph.D.
Clinical Fellow, Mood Disorders and Neuroimaging, Department of Psychiatry and Behavioral Sciences, Johns Hopkins University School of Medicine, Baltimore, Maryland

Michael Weaver, M.D., F.A.S.A.M.
Associate Professor of Internal Medicine and Psychiatry and Medical Director, Substance Abuse Consult Service, Virginia Commonwealth University School of Medicine, Richmond, Virginia

Thomas N. Wise, M.D.
Chairman, Department of Psychiatry, Inova Health System, Falls Church, Virginia; Associate Chair and Professor, Department of Psychiatry, George Washington University School of Medicine, Washington, D.C.; Professor of Psychiatry, Johns Hopkins University School of Medicine, Baltimore, Maryland; Professor of Psychiatry, Virginia Commonwealth University School of Medicine, Inova Campus, Falls Church, Virginia

Lawson Wulsin, M.D.
Professor of Psychiatry and Family Medicine, Department of Psychiatry, University of Cincinnati, Cincinnati, Ohio

Adam Zeman, M.A., D.M., F.R.C.P.
Consultant Neurologist and Part-Time Senior Lecturer, Department of Clinical Neurosciences, Western General Hospital, University of Edinburgh, Edinburgh, United Kingdom

Disclosure of Interests

The following contributors to this book have indicated a financial interest in or other affiliation with a commercial supporter, a manufacturer of a commercial product, a provider of a commercial service, a nongovernmental organization, and/or a government agency, as listed below:

Andrew A. Angelino, M.D. *Grant Support:* Ryan White Care Act; *Honoraria:* Boehringer-Ingelheim.

Oliver Freudenreich, M.D. *Grant Support:* Cephalon; *Speakers Bureau/Honoraria:* Primedin; Reed Medical Education.

Paul L. Kimmel, M.D. *Stock:* 50 shares, Merck.

Elisabeth J. Shakin Kunkel, M.D. *Speakers Bureau:* IntraMed/Forest, Pfizer, Wyeth.

Philip R. Muskin, M.D. *Speakers Bureau:* AstraZeneca, Bristol-Myers Squibb, Eli Lilly, Forest, Jazz, Takeda, Wyeth.

James A. Owen, Ph.D. *Grant Support:* Lundbeck; *Speakers Bureau/Advisory Board:* Lundbeck.

Michael C. Sharpe, M.A., M.D., F.R.C.P., F.R.C.Psych. *Consultant:* AEGON Insurance (interpretation of medical reports).

Theodore A. Stern, M.D. *Speakers Bureau/Honoraria:* Forest, Reed/Elsevier; *Consultant/Honoraria:* Eli Lilly, Janssen; *Editor/Royalties:* McGraw-Hill, Mosby/Elsevier; *Editor/Salary:* Academy of Psychosomatic Medicine.

Donna E. Stewart, M.D, F.R.C.P.C. *Advisory Board:* Boehringer-Ingelheim, Eli Lilly, Wyeth.

Glenn J. Treisman, M.D., Ph.D. *Speakers Bureau/Honoraria:* Abbott, Boehringer-Ingelheim.

Paula T. Trzepacz, M.D. *Full-Time Salaried Employee and Shareholder:* Eli Lilly & Company.

The following contributors stated that they had no competing interests during the year preceding manuscript submission:

Susan E. Abbey, M.D., F.R.C.P.C.; Yesne Alici, M.D.; David J. Axelrod, M.D., J.D.; Rosemary Basson, M.D.; Madeleine Becker, M.D., M.A.; Charles H. Bombardier, Ph.D.; John Michael Bostwick, M.D.; William Breitbart, M.D.; Rebecca W. Brendel, M.D., J.D.; Brenda Bursch, Ph.D.; Alan J. Carson, M.B.Ch.B., M.Phil., M.D., F.R.C.Psych.; Harvey Max Chochinov, M.D., Ph.D., F.R.S.C.; Michael R. Clark, M.D., M.P.H., M.B.A.; Kathy L. Coffman, M.D.; Lewis M. Cohen, M.D.; Catherine C. Crone, M.D.; Daniel Cukor, Ph.D.; Niccolo D. Della Penna, M.D.; Michael J. Devlin, M.D.; Mary Amanda Dew, Ph.D.; Chris Dickens, M.B.B.S., Ph.D.; Andrea F. DiMartini, M.D.; Christopher R. Dobbelstein, M.D.; Ilyse Dobrow DiMarco, Ph.D.; Steven A. Epstein, M.D.; Jesse R. Fann, M.D., M.P.H.; Charles V. Ford, M.D.; Andrew Francis, Ph.D., M.D.; Gregory L. Fricchione, M.D.; Ann Goebel-Fabbri, Ph.D.; Mark S. Groves, M.D.; Madhulika A. Gupta, M.D., F.R.C.P.C.; Elspeth Guthrie, M.B., Ch.B., M.R.C.Psych., M.Sc., M.D.; Daniel Hicks, M.D.; Michael R. Irwin, M.D.; Joel P. Jahraus, M.D.; Richard Kennedy, M.D., Ph.D.; Lois E. Krahn, M.D.; Maeve Leonard, M.B., M.R.C.Psych.; James L. Levenson, M.D.; Madeline Li, M.D., Ph.D., F.R.C.P.C.; Antonio Lobo, M.D., Ph.D.; Constantine G. Lyketsos, M.D., M.H.S.; Dimitri D. Markov, M.D.; Elaine Martin, M.D.; Mary Jane Massie, M.D.; David J. Meagher, M.D., M.R.C.Psych., M.Sc.; Franklin G. Miller, Ph.D.; Kimberley Miller, M.D., F.R.C.P.C.; Gail Musen, Ph.D.; Shamim H. Nejad, M.D.; Patrick G. O'Malley, M.D., M.P.H., F.A.C.P.; Chiadi U. Onyike, M.D., M.H.S.; Olu Oyesanmi, M.D., M.P.H.; Pauline S. Powers, M.D.; Miguel Ángel Quintanilla, M.D., Ph.D.; J. J. Rasimas, M.D., Ph.D.; Keith G. Rasmussen, M.D.; Peter M. Rees, M.D., Ph.D.; Gary Rodin, M.D., F.R.C.P.C.; Donald L. Rosenstein, M.D.; Deborah Rosenthal-Asher, M.A.; Carlos A. Santana, M.D.; Pedro Saz, M.D., Ph.D.; Ronald Schouten, M.D., J.D.; Peter A. Shapiro, M.D.; Michael C. Sharpe, M.A., M.D., F.R.C.P., F.R.C.Psych.; Felicia A. Smith, M.D.; Jorge Luis Sotelo, M.D.; Jon Stone, M.B.Ch.B., Ph.D., F.R.C.P.; Nada Logan Stotland, M.D., M.P.H.; Margaret Stuber, M.D.; Simone N. Vigod, M.D., F.R.C.P.C.; Crystal C. Watkins, M.D., Ph.D.; Michael Weaver, M.D., F.A.S.A.M.; Thomas N. Wise, M.D.; Lawson Wulsin, M.D.; Adam Zeman, M.A., D.M., F.R.C.P.

Foreword

Thomas N. Wise, M.D.

THIS SECOND EDITION of *The American Psychiatric Publishing Textbook of Psychosomatic Medicine* demonstrates the evolution of the medical textbook as well as the field of Psychosomatic Medicine. Both have long and circuitous developmental pathways. Among the first recorded medical texts were classic Egyptian papyri that outlined empirical observations from ancient physicians on burn care, wound management, gastrointestinal ailments, and congestive heart failure (Trevisanato 2006). The Hippocratic and Galenic traditions also carefully described diseases as well as invoked religious etiological explanations but incorporated the role of emotions into the genesis of physical disorders (Schwab 1985). Heinroth is said to have coined the term *psychosomatic* in 1818 (Steinberg 2007), although he emphasized the quasi-religious mechanism of disorders of the "soul" (Steinberg 2004).

The initial "modern" textbooks of psychiatry tended to ignore psychiatric issues interfacing with medical disorders. This was most likely a result of Psychiatry's isolation in the asylum setting. Griesinger's 1867 textbook was one of the first to view Psychiatry as a legitimate field of medicine with a strong organic substrate. Griesinger discussed delirium and dementia but gave only passing reference to hysteria. He felt that hypochondriasis was often due to "moral causes" but noted that such sufferers "often read medical books." Cheyne's (1733/1991) *The English Malady* is a monograph upon what would now be considered severe health anxiety and the proposed diagnosis for DSM-V, complex somatic symptom disorder.

With the rise of sophisticated bacteriology and molecular biology, the role of psychiatric disorders was relegated to the "art" of medicine rather than the "science" of the profession (Brown 1989). In the introduction to the fourteenth edition of Osler's venerable *Principles and Practice of Medicine,* the editor, Dr. Henry Christian, defined psychosomatic medicine as "that part of medicine, which is concerned with an appraisal of both the emotional and the physical mechanisms involved in the disease processes of the individual patient with particular emphasis on the influence that these two factors exert on each other and on the individual as a whole" (Christian 1942, p. 1). This concept is similar to the first of the three basic definitions of psychosomatic medicine discussed by Lipowski (1984): 1) a research approach looking at biological, psychological, and cultural variables; 2) a "holistic" view of patients; and 3) a subspecialized type of psychiatry, commonly called consultation-liaison. Christian followed his own definition by sadly stating that "psychiatry…will need to be correlated with the demonstrable systemic changes and effects of disease before we can make much advance in psychosomatic medicine" (Christian 1942, p. 2). Contemporary medical and psychiatric science has reached such a stage in the development of our field.

Under the able direction of Dr. Levenson, a collection of outstanding authors have compiled the current knowledge of our field, which is now a formal subspecialty of Psychiatry. A thousand or more in the United States have qualified for this designation via the examination rigorously administered by the American Board of Psychiatry and Neurology. Pessimism about our field being marginalized was premature, as was the belief that the name *Psychosomatic Medicine* would not be accepted (Friedman 1988; Steinberg 2004). This volume demonstrates both the breadth and the knowledge base of our field. As a research approach, the database is increasing, both in the mechanisms of interaction between mind and body and in the clinical importance of recognizing the role of psychiatric issues in medical disorders and medical care. Such data complement the unique skills of psychosomatic specialists who seek to systematically understand how each patient's life story affects his or her life trajectory in the face of illness (Engel 1990; Viederman and Perry 1980).

With advances in such information, textbooks are essential and require regular updating. Kraepelin's textbook had nine editions, while Osler's original text went through twenty-four (Hippius and Muller 2008). *Psychosomatic Medicine* is a term that is now clearly recognized within Psychiatry as a body of research and a clinical subspecialty (Fava and Sonino 2010). I am sure that this second iteration is the first of many more as Psychosomatic Medicine continues to accrue knowledge in its quest to alleviate the suffering of patients. As Osler (1921) noted, "Medicine arose out of the primal sympathy of man with man; out of the desire to help those in sorrow, need and sickness" (pp. 6–7). This Textbook clearly offers great help with that task.

References

Brown TM: Cartesian dualism and psychosomatics. Psychosomatics 30:322–331, 1989

Cheyne G: The English Malady (1733). Tavistock Classics in the History of Psychiatry. Edited by Porter R). London, Routledge, 1991

Christian H (ed): Introduction, in The Principles and Practice of Medicine, 24th Edition. New York, Appleton-Century, 1942, pp 1–2

Engel GL: On looking inward and being scientific. A tribute to Arthur H. Schmale, MD. Psychother Psychosom 54:63–69, 1990

Fava GA, Sonino N: Psychosomatic medicine: a name to keep. Psychother Psychosom 79:1–3, 2010

Friedman SB: The concept of "marginality" applied to psychosomatic medicine. Psychosom Med 50:447–453, 1988

Griesinger W: Mental Pathology and Therapeutics, 2nd Edition. 1867. London, New Sydenham Society, 1867

Hippius H, Muller N: The work of Emil Kraepelin and his research group in Munchen. Eur Arch Psychiatry Clin Neurosci 258 (suppl 2):3–11, 2008

Lipowski ZJ: What does the word "psychosomatic" really mean? A historical and semantic inquiry. Psychosom Med 46:153–171, 1984

Osler W: The Evolution of Modern Medicine. New Haven, CT, Yale University, 1921, pp 6–7

Schwab JJ: Psychosomatic medicine: its past and present. Psychosomatics 26:583–589, 592, 1985

Steinberg H: [The birth of the word "psychosomatic" in medical literature by Johann Christian August Heinroth]. Fortschr Neurol Psychiatr 75:413–417, 2007

Steinberg H: The sin in the aetiological concept of Johann Christian August Heinroth (1773–1843). Part 1: Between theology and psychiatry. Heinroth's concepts of "whose being," "freedom," "reason" and "disturbance of the soul." History of Psychiatry 15(59 Pt 3):329–344, 2004

Trevisanato SI: Six medical papyri describe the effects of Santorini's volcanic ash, and provide Egyptian parallels to the so-called biblical plagues. Medical Hypotheses 67:187–190, 2006

Viederman M, Perry SW III: Use of a psychodynamic life narrative in the treatment of depression in the physically ill. Gen Hosp Psychiatry 2:177–185, 1980

Preface

James L. Levenson, M.D.

WHAT IS PSYCHOSOMATIC Medicine? In the past, Psychosomatic Medicine has had ambiguous connotations, alternatively "psychogenic" or "holistic," but it is the latter meaning that has characterized its emergence as a contemporary scientific and clinical discipline (Lipowski 1984). In this book, Psychosomatic Medicine refers to a specialized area of psychiatry whose practitioners have particular expertise in the diagnosis and treatment of psychiatric disorders and difficulties in complex medically ill patients (Gitlin et al. 2004). We treat and study three general groups of patients: 1) those with comorbid psychiatric and general medical illnesses complicating each other's management, 2) those with somatoform and functional disorders, and 3) those with psychiatric disorders that are the direct consequence of a primary medical condition or its treatment. Psychosomatic Medicine practitioners work as hospital-based consultation-liaison psychiatrists (Kornfeld 1996), on medical-psychiatric inpatient units (Kathol and Stoudemire 2002), and in settings in which mental health services are integrated into primary care (Unutzer et al. 2002). Thus, the field's name reflects the fact that it exists at the interface of psychiatry and medicine.

Historical Background

Psychosomatic Medicine is the newest psychiatric subspecialty formally approved by the American Board of Medical Specialties (ABMS). There have been many other names for this specialized field, including consultation-liaison psychiatry, medical-surgical psychiatry, psychological medicine, and psychiatric care of the complex medically ill. In 2001, the Academy of Psychosomatic Medicine applied to the American Board of Psychiatry and Neurology (ABPN) for the recognition of Psychosomatic Medicine as a subspecialty field of psychiatry, choosing to return to the name for the field embedded in our history, our journals, and our national organizations. Subsequent formal approval was received from the American Psychiatric Association, the ABPN, the Residency Review Committee (RRC) of the Accreditation Council for Graduate Medical Education (ACGME), and the ABMS. In the 4 years that have elapsed since the first certifying examination in 2005, 1,078 psychiatrists have been certified in Psychosomatic Medicine in the United States.

Psychosomatic Medicine has a rich history. The term *psychosomatic* was introduced by Johann Heinroth in 1818, and Felix Deutsch introduced the term *psychosomatic medicine* around 1922 (Lipsitt 2001). Psychoanalysts and psychophysiologists pioneered the study of mind-body interactions from very different vantage points, each contributing to the growth of Psychosomatic Medicine as a clinical and scholarly field. The modern history of the field (see Table 1) perhaps starts with the Rockefeller Foundation's funding of psychosomatic medicine units in several U.S. teaching hospitals in 1935. The National Institute of Mental Health made it a priority to foster the growth of consultation-liaison psychiatry through training grants (circa 1975) and a research development program (circa 1985).

Psychosomatic Medicine is a scholarly discipline with classic influential texts (Table 2), many devoted journals (Table 3), and both national (Table 4) and international (Table 5) professional/scientific societies. The Academy of Psychosomatic Medicine (APM) is the only U.S. national organization primarily dedicated to Psychosomatic Medicine as a psychiatric subspecialty. The American Psychosomatic Society (APS), an older cousin, is primarily devoted to psychosomatic research, and its members come from many disciplines (Wise 1995). While consultation-liaison psychiatry and psychosomatic medicine first flourished in the United States, exciting work now comes from around the world. APM's counterpart in Europe is the European Association of Consultation-Liaison Psychiatry and Psychosomatics (EACLPP) (Wise and Lobo 2001), and similar to APS is the European Conference on Psychosomatic Research (ECPR). There are now associations or special interest groups for

Table 1. Key dates in the modern history of psychosomatic medicine

1935	Rockefeller Foundation opens first Consultation-Liaison (C/L)–Psychosomatic Units at Massachusetts General, Duke, and Colorado
1936	American Psychosomatic Society founded
1939	First issue of *Psychosomatic Medicine*
1953	First issue of *Psychosomatics*
1954	Academy of Psychosomatic Medicine (APM) founded
1975	National Institute of Mental Health (NIMH) Training Grants for C/L Psychiatry
1985	NIMH Research Development Program for C/L Psychiatry
1991	APM-recognized fellowships number 55
2001	Subspecialty application for Psychosomatic Medicine
2003	Approval as subspecialty by American Board of Medical Specialties

Table 2. Selected classic texts in psychosomatic medicine

1935	*Emotions and Body Change* (Dunbar)
1943	*Psychosomatic Medicine* (Weiss and English)
1950	*Psychosomatic Medicine* (Alexander)
1968	*Handbook of Psychiatric Consultation* (Schwab)
1978	*Organic Psychiatry* (Lishman)
1978	*Massachusetts General Hospital Handbook of General Hospital Psychiatry* (Hackett and Cassem)
1993	*Psychiatric Care of the Medical Patient* (Stoudemire and Fogel)

Table 3. Selected journals in psychosomatic medicine

Journal name	Date of initial publication
Psychosomatic Medicine	1939
Psychosomatics	1953
Psychotherapy and Psychosomatics	1953
Psychophysiology	1954
Journal of Psychosomatic Research	1956
Advances in Psychosomatic Medicine	1960
International Journal of Psychiatry in Medicine	1970
General Hospital Psychiatry	1979
Journal of Psychosomatic Obstetrics and Gynecology	1982
Journal of Psychosocial Oncology	1983
Stress Medicine	1985
Psycho-Oncology	1986

Table 4. National organizations

Academy of Psychosomatic Medicine
Association for Medicine and Psychiatry
American Psychosomatic Society
American Association for General Hospital Psychiatry
Society for Liaison Psychiatry
Association for Academic Psychiatry—Consultation-Liaison Section
American Neuropsychiatric Association
American Psychosocial Oncology Society
North American Society for Psychosomatic Obstetrics and Gynecology

Table 5. International organizations

European Association for Consultation-Liaison Psychiatry and Psychosomatics
International Organization for Consultation-Liaison Psychiatry
World Psychiatric Association—Section of General Hospital Psychiatry
International College of Psychosomatic Medicine
International Neuropsychiatric Association
International Psycho-Oncology Society

psychosomatic medicine and consultation-liaison psychiatry in many countries, including Argentina, Brazil, Germany, Italy, the Netherlands, Portugal, Spain, and the United Kingdom. The international nature of the field is reflected in this textbook's Editorial Board and the contributors to this text, who include psychiatrists from Austria, Brazil, Canada, Germany, Hong Kong, Ireland, the Netherlands, Spain, the United Kingdom, and the United States. The first edition of this book has been translated into Chinese and Spanish.

Second Edition of the Textbook

There are 97 contributors to the second edition of this textbook, 38 of them new authors. Twenty-three of the contributors are from countries other than the United States, including Canada, Ireland, Spain, and the United Kingdom. Of this textbook's 41 chapters, 2 are new, bringing topics not covered in the first edition. An additional 9 chapters are newly authored. The remaining 30 chapters have all been extensively revised. In sum, about 40% of the content of this edition is new. All 41 chapters have been reviewed by at least one member of the Editorial Board, and most have been reviewed by an expert in the relevant medical specialty or allied health profession. The distinguished Editorial Board includes noted authorities in psychosomatic medicine and consultation-liaison psychiatry from 17 leading academic centers, representing Austria, Brazil, Canada, Germany, Hong Kong, the Netherlands, Spain, the United Kingdom, and the United States.

This book is organized into four sections. Chapters 1–4 cover general principles in evaluation and management, legal and ethical issues, and psychological reactions to illness. Chapters 5–17 are devoted to psychiatric symptoms and disorders in the medically ill. Chapters 18–37 address issues within each of the medical specialties and subspecialties. The final 4 chapters review psychiatric treatment in the medically ill, including psychopharmacology, psychotherapy, electroconvulsive therapy, and palliative care.

This book has attempted to capture the diversity of our field, whose practitioners do not place equal emphasis on the syllables of "bio-psycho-social." There is not unanimity among us on some questions, and diverse opinions will be found in this book. Psychosomatic Medicine has evolved, since its start, from a field based on clinical experience, conjecture, and theorizing into a discipline grounded in empirical research that is growing and spreading its findings into many areas of medical care.

Acknowledgments

I owe an enormous debt of gratitude to the many people who made this book possible. First, to the contributors, who were patient under repeated onslaughts of red track-changes from me. An assertive Editorial Board pushed us all toward the highest standards.

I am particularly grateful to Richard Shaw at Stanford University and my colleagues at Virginia Commonwealth University who generously gave their time to critique chapters in their respective disciplines, including Ericka Breden, Christian Barrett, Christopher Kogut, Susan Kornstein, Julia Nunley, Mary Ellen Olbrisch, and Brandon Wills.

Tina Coltri-Marshall provided invaluable service, going beyond the call of duty to keep everyone organized and on schedule. Editor-in-Chief Bob Hales as well as John McDuffie and Bob Pursell at American Psychiatric Publishing, Inc. (APPI) gave expert advice and encouragement from start to finish, and I am grateful to all of the APPI staff, including Ellie Abedi, Judy Castagna, Bessie Jones, Greg Kuny, Rebecca Richters, and Susan Westrate.

Finally, this book would not have been possible without enthusiastic support from my chair, Joel Silverman; the help of my assistant, Pam Copeland; and the patience and tolerance of my wife, Janet Distelman.

References

Gitlin DF, Levenson JL, Lyketsos CG: Psychosomatic medicine: a new psychiatric subspecialty. Acad Psychiatry 28:4–11, 2004

Kathol RG, Stoudemire A: Strategic integration of inpatient and outpatient medical-psychiatry services, in The American Psychiatric Publishing Textbook of Consultation-Liaison Psychiatry. Edited by Wise MG, Rundell JR. Washington, DC, American Psychiatric Publishing, 2002, pp 871–888

Kornfeld DS: Consultation-liaison psychiatry and the practice of medicine. The Thomas P. Hackett Award lecture given at the 42nd annual meeting of the Academy of Psychosomatic Medicine, 1995. Psychosomatics 37:236–248, 1996

Lipowski ZJ: What does the word "psychosomatic" really mean? A historical and semantic inquiry. Psychosom Med. 46:153–171, 1984

Lipsitt DR: Consultation-liaison psychiatry and psychosomatic medicine: the company they keep. Psychosom Med 63:896–909, 2001

Unutzer J, Katon W, Callahan CM, et al: Collaborative care management of late-life depression in the primary care setting: a randomized controlled trial. JAMA 288:2836–2845, 2002

Wise TN: A tale of two societies. Psychosom Med 57:303–309, 1995

Wise TN, Lobo A: The European Association of Consultation-Liaison Psychiatry and Psychosomatics: a welcome new addition to the global practice of C-L psychiatry. Psychosomatics 42:201–203, 2001

PART I

General Principles in Evaluation and Management

CHAPTER 1

Psychiatric Assessment and Consultation

Felicia A. Smith, M.D.
James L. Levenson, M.D.
Theodore A. Stern, M.D.

PSYCHOSOMATIC MEDICINE IS rooted in the practice of consultation-liaison psychiatry, having expanded from its beginnings on a handful of general medical wards in the 1930s to specialized medical units throughout various parts of the health care delivery system. Practitioners in this psychiatric subspecialty assist with the care of a variety of patients, especially those with complex conditions such as cancer, organ failure, HIV infection, dementia, delirium, agitation, psychosis, substance abuse or withdrawal, somatoform disorders, personality disorders, and mood and anxiety disorders, as well as suicidal ideation, treatment nonadherence, and aggression and other behavioral problems (Gitlin et al. 2004; Hackett et al. 2004). In addition, ethical and legal considerations are often critical elements of the psychiatric consultation. In the medical setting, prompt recognition and evaluation of psychiatric problems are essential because psychiatric comorbidity commonly exacerbates the course of medical illness, causes significant distress in the patient, prolongs hospital length of stay, and increases costs of care.

In this introductory chapter, we present a detailed approach to psychiatric assessment and consultation in medical settings. Successful psychiatric consultants must be flexible when evaluating affective, behavioral, and cognitive disturbances in the medically ill. In the final section of the chapter, we briefly outline the benefits of psychiatric consultation for patients as well as for the greater hospital and medical communities.

Psychiatric Consultation in the General Hospital

Psychiatrists who work in medical settings are charged with providing expert consultation to medical and surgical patients. In many respects, the psychiatric care of such patients is no different from the treatment of patients in a psychiatric clinic or in a private office. However, the constraints of the modern hospital environment demand a high degree of adaptability. Comfort, quiet, and privacy are scarce commodities in medical and surgical units, and the consultant's bedside manner is important in compensating for this. Interruptions by medical or nursing staff, visitors, and roommates erode the privacy that the psychiatrist usually expects. Patients who are sick, preoccupied with their physical condition, and in pain are ill-disposed to engage in the exploratory interviews that often typify psychiatric evaluations conducted in other settings. Monitoring devices replace the plants, pictures, and other accoutrements of a typical office. Nightstands and tray tables are littered with medical paraphernalia commingled with personal effects.

The consultant must be adept at gathering the requisite diagnostic information related to a patient's condition and must be able to tolerate the sights, sounds, and smells of the sickroom. Additional visits for more history are often inevitable. In the end, the diagnosis will likely fall into

TABLE 1–1. Categories of psychiatric differential diagnoses in the general hospital

- Psychiatric presentations of medical conditions
- Psychiatric complications of medical conditions or treatments
- Psychological reactions to medical conditions or treatments
- Medical presentations of psychiatric conditions
- Medical complications of psychiatric conditions or treatments
- Comorbid medical and psychiatric conditions

Source. Adapted from Lipowski 1967.

one (or more) of the categories outlined in Lipowski's (1967) timeless classification (Table 1–1).

Although the consultant is summoned by the patient's physician, in most cases the visit is unannounced and is not requested by the patient, from whom cooperation is expected. Explicitly acknowledging this reality is often sufficient to gain the patient's cooperation. Cooperation is enhanced if the psychiatrist sits down and operates at eye level with the patient. By offering to help the patient get comfortable (e.g., by adjusting the head of the bed, bringing the patient a drink or a blanket, or adjusting the television) before and after the encounter, the consultant can increase the chances of being welcomed then and for follow-up evaluations.

When psychiatrists are consulted for unexplained physical symptoms or for pain management, it is useful to empathize with the distress that the patient is experiencing. This avoids conveying any judgment on the etiology of the pain except that their suffering is real. After introductions, if the patient is in pain, the consultant's first questions should address this issue. Failing to do so conveys a lack of appreciation for the patient's distress and may be taken by the patient as disbelief in his or her symptoms. Starting with empathic questions about the patient's suffering establishes rapport and also guides the psychiatrist in setting the proper pace of the interview. Finally, because a psychiatric consultation will cause many patients to fear that their physician thinks they are "crazy," the psychiatrist may first need to address this fear.

Process of the Consultation

Although it is rarely as straightforward as the following primer suggests, the process of psychiatric consultation should, in the end, include all the components explained below and summarized in Table 1–2.

TABLE 1–2. Procedural approach to psychiatric consultation

- Speak directly with the referring clinician.
- Review the current records and pertinent past records.
- Review the patient's medications.
- Gather collateral data.
- Interview and examine the patient.
- Formulate diagnostic and therapeutic strategies.
- Write a note.
- Speak directly with the referring clinician.
- Provide periodic follow-up.

Speak Directly With the Referring Clinician

Requests for psychiatric consultation are notorious for being vague and imprecise (e.g., "rule out depression" or "patient with schizophrenia"). They sometimes signify only that the team recognizes that a problem exists; such problems may range from an untreated psychiatric disorder to the experience of countertransferential feelings. In speaking with a member of the team that has requested the consultation, the consultant employs some of the same techniques that will be used later in examining the patient; that is, he or she listens to the implicit as well as the explicit messages from the other physician (Murray 2004). Is the physician angry with the patient? Is the patient not doing what the team wants him or her to do? Is the fact that the patient is young and dying leading to the team's overidentification with him or her? Is the team frustrated by an elusive diagnosis? All of these situations generate emotions that are difficult to reduce to a few words conveyed in a consultation request; moreover, the feelings often remain out of the team's awareness. This brief interaction may give the consultant invaluable information about how the consultation may be useful to the team and to the patient.

Review the Current Records and Pertinent Past Records

When it is done with the unfailing curiosity of a detective hot on the trail of hidden clues, reading a chart can be an exciting and self-affirming part of the consultation process. Although it does not supplant the consultant's independent history taking or examination, the chart review provides a general orientation to the case. Moreover, the consultant is in a unique position to focus on details that may have been previously overlooked. For example, nurses often document salient neurobehavioral data (e.g., the level of awareness and the presence of confusion or agitation);

physical and occupational therapists estimate functional abilities crucial to the diagnosis of cognitive disorders and to the choice of an appropriate level of care (e.g., nursing home or assisted-living facility); and speech pathologists note alterations in articulation, swallowing, and language, all of which may indicate an organic brain disease. All of them may have written progress notes about adherence to treatment regimens, unusual behavior, interpersonal difficulties, or family issues encountered in their care of the patient. These notes may also provide unique clues to the presence of problems such as domestic violence, factitious illness, or personality disorders. In hospitals or clinics where nurses' notes are kept separate from the physician's progress notes, it is essential for the consultant to review those sections.

Review the Patient's Medications

Construction of a medication list at various times (e.g., when at home, on admission, on transfer within the hospital, and at present) is a good, if not essential, practice. Special attention should be paid to medications with psychoactive effects and to those associated with withdrawal syndromes (both obvious ones like benzodiazepines and opiates, and less obvious ones like antidepressants, anticonvulsants, and beta-blockers). Review of order sheets or computerized order entries is not always sufficient, because—for a variety of reasons—patients may not always receive prescribed medications; therefore, medication administration records should also be reviewed. Such records are particularly important for determining the frequency of administration of medicines ordered on an as-needed basis. For example, an order for lorazepam 1–2 mg every 4–6 hours as needed may result in a patient receiving anywhere from 0 mg to 12 mg in a day, which can be critical in cases of withdrawal or oversedation.

Gather Collateral Data

Histories from hospitalized medically ill patients may be especially spotty and unreliable, if not nonexistent (e.g., with a patient who is somnolent, delirious, or comatose). Data from collateral sources (e.g., family members; friends; current and outpatient health care providers; case managers; and, in some cases, police and probation officers) may be of critical importance. However, psychiatric consultants must guard against prizing any single party's version of historical events over another's; family members and others may lack objectivity, be in denial, be overinvolved, or have a personal agenda to advance. For example, family members tend to minimize early signs of dementia and to overreport depression in patients with dementia. Confidentiality must be valued when obtaining collateral information. Ideally, one obtains the patient's consent first; however, this may not be possible if the patient lacks capacity or if a dire emergency is in progress (see Chapter 2, "Legal Issues," and Chapter 3, "Ethical Issues"). Moreover, in certain situations there may be contraindications to contacting some sources of information (e.g., an employer of a patient with substance abuse or the partner of a woman who is experiencing abuse). Like any astute physician, the psychiatrist collates and synthesizes all available data and weighs each bit of information according to the reliability of its source.

Interview and Examine the Patient

Armed with information gleaned and elicited from other sources, the psychiatric consultant now makes independent observations of the patient and collects information that may be the most reliable of all because it comes from direct observations. For non-English-speaking patients, a translator is often needed. Although using family members may be expedient, their presence often compromises the questions asked and the translations offered because of embarrassment or other factors. It is therefore important to utilize hospital translators or, for less common languages, services via telephone. This can be difficult, but it may be necessary in obtaining a full and accurate history.

The process and content of the psychiatric interview must be adapted to the consultation setting. To establish rapport and to have a therapeutic impact, the psychiatrist should assume an engaging, more spontaneous stance (typically, after explaining the purpose of the visit and inquiring about the patient's physical complaints) and deviate from the principles of anonymity, abstinence, and neutrality that help form the foundation for psychodynamic psychotherapy (see Perry and Viederman 1981). Long silences common in psychoanalytic psychotherapy are rarely appropriate with medical patients, who have not sought out psychiatric assessment and who lack the stamina for long interviews. Deeply exploring traumatic events shortly after they occur may not be ideal; it is often sufficient to acknowledge the patient's past hardships and provide a perspective of what treatment after discharge can offer. Neither a rigidly biological approach (which can impede rapport) nor an exclusively psychoanalytic inquiry should be adopted. It is especially important to elicit patients' beliefs about their illness (what is wrong, what caused it, what treatment can do) so that emotional responses and behaviors can be placed in perspective. Although the psychiatric consultant often works under pressure of time (e.g., conducting the evaluation between medical tests and procedures), an open-ended interview style should be used.

Mental Status Examination

A thorough mental status examination is central to the psychiatric evaluation of the medically ill patient. Because the examination is hierarchical, care must be taken to complete it in a systematic fashion (Hyman and Tesar 1994). The astute consultant will glean invaluable diagnostic clues from a combination of observation and questioning.

Level of consciousness. Level of consciousness depends on normal cerebral arousal by the reticular activating system. A patient whose level of consciousness is impaired will inevitably perform poorly on cognitive testing. The finding of disorientation implies cognitive failure in one or several domains. It is helpful to test orientation near the start of the mental status examination.

Attention. The form of attention most relevant to the clinical mental status examination is the sustained attention that allows one to concentrate on cognitive tasks. Disruption of attention—often by factors that diffusely disturb brain function, such as drugs, infection, or organ failure—is a hallmark of delirium. Sustained attention is best tested with moderately demanding, nonautomatic tasks such as reciting the months backward or, as in the Mini-Mental State Examination (MMSE; Folstein et al. 1975), spelling *world* backward or subtracting 7 serially from 100. Serial subtraction is intended to be a test of attention, not arithmetic ability, so the task should be adjusted to the patient's native ability and educational level (serial 3s from 50, serial 1s from 20). An inattentive patient's performance on other parts of the mental status examination may be affected on any task requiring sustained focus.

Memory. Working memory is tested by asking the patient to register some information (e.g., three words) and to recall that information after an interval of at least 3 minutes during which other testing prevents rehearsal. This task can also be considered a test of recent memory. Semantic memory is tapped by asking general knowledge questions (e.g., "Who is the president?") and by naming and visual recognition tasks. The patient's ability to remember aspects of his or her history serves as an elegant test of episodic memory (as well as of remote memory). Because semantic and episodic memories can be articulated, they constitute declarative memory. In contrast, procedural memory is implicit in learned action (e.g., riding a bicycle) and cannot be described in words. Deficits in procedural memory can be observed in a patient's behavior during the clinical evaluation.

Executive function. Executive function refers to the abilities that allow one to plan, initiate, organize, and monitor thought and behavior. These abilities, which localize broadly to the frontal lobes, are essential for normal social and professional performance but are difficult to test. Frontal lobe disorders often make themselves apparent in social interaction with a patient and are suspected when one observes disinhibition, impulsivity, disorganization, abulia, or amotivation. Tasks that can be used to gain some insight into frontal lobe function include verbal fluency, such as listing as many animals as possible in 1 minute; motor sequencing, such as asking the patient to replicate a sequence of three hand positions; the go/no-go task, which requires the patient to tap the desk once if the examiner taps once, but not to tap if the examiner taps twice; and tests of abstraction, including questions like "What do a tree and a fly have in common?"

Language. Language disorders result from lesions of the dominant hemisphere. In assessing language, one should first note characteristics of the patient's speech (e.g., nonfluency or paraphasic errors) and then assess comprehension. Naming is impaired in both major varieties of aphasia, and anomia can be a clue to mild dysphasia. Reading and writing should also be assessed. Expressive (Broca's or motor) aphasia is characterized by effortful, nonfluent speech with use of phonemic paraphasias (incorrect words that approximate the correct ones in sound), reduced use of function words (e.g., prepositions and articles), and well-preserved comprehension. Receptive (Wernicke's or sensory) aphasia is characterized by fluent speech with both phonemic and semantic paraphasias (incorrect words that approximate the correct ones in meaning) and poor comprehension. The stream of incoherent speech and the lack of insight in patients with Wernicke's aphasia sometimes lead to misdiagnosis of a primary thought disorder and psychiatric referral; the clue to the diagnosis of a language disorder is the severity of the comprehension deficit. Global dysphasia combines features of Broca's and Wernicke's aphasias. Selective impairment of repetition characterizes conduction aphasia. The nondominant hemisphere plays a part in the appreciation and production of the emotional overtones of language.

Praxis. Apraxia refers to an inability to perform skilled actions (e.g., using a screwdriver, brushing one's teeth) despite intact basic motor and sensory abilities. These abilities can be tested by asking a patient to mime such actions or by asking the patient to copy unfamiliar hand positions. Constructional apraxia is usually tested with the Clock Drawing Test. Gait apraxia involves difficulty in initiating and maintaining gait despite intact basic motor function in the legs. Dressing apraxia is difficulty in dressing caused by an inability to coordinate the spatial arrangement of clothes with the body.

Mood and affect. Mood and affect both refer to the patient's emotional state, mood being the patient's perception and affect being the interviewer's perception. The interviewer must interpret both carefully, taking into account the patient's medical illness. Normal but intense expressions of emotion (e.g., grief, fear, or irritation) are common in patients with serious medical illness but may be misperceived by nonpsychiatric physicians as evidence of psychiatric disturbance. Disturbances in mood and affect may also be the result of brain dysfunction or injury. Irritability may be the first sign of many illnesses, ranging from alcohol withdrawal to rabies. Blunted affective expression may be a sign of Parkinson's disease. Intense affective lability (e.g., pathological crying or laughing) with relatively normal mood occurs with some diseases or injuries of the frontal lobes. In addition, depressed or euphoric affect may be a medication side effect.

Perception. Perception in the mental status examination is primarily concerned with hallucinations and illusions. However, before beginning any part of the clinical interview and the mental status examination, the interviewer should establish whether the patient has any impairment in vision or hearing that could interfere with communication. Unrecognized impairments have led to erroneous impressions that patients were demented, delirious, or psychotic. Although hallucinations in any modality may occur in primary psychotic disorders (e.g., schizophrenia or affective psychosis), prominent visual, olfactory, gustatory, or tactile hallucinations suggest a secondary medical etiology. Olfactory and gustatory hallucinations may be manifestations of seizures, and tactile hallucinations are often seen with substance abuse.

Judgment and insight. The traditional question for the assessment of judgment—"What would you do if you found a letter on the sidewalk?"—is much less informative than questions tailored to the problems faced by the patient being evaluated; for example, "If you couldn't stop a nosebleed, what would you do?" "If you run out of medicine and you can't reach your doctor, what would you do?" Similarly, questions to assess insight should focus on the patient's understanding of his or her illness, treatment, and life circumstances.

Further guidance on mental status examination. An outline of the essential elements of a comprehensive mental status examination is presented in Table 1–3. Particular cognitive mental status testing maneuvers are described in more detail in Table 1–4. More detailed consideration of the mental status examination can be found elsewhere (Strub and Black 2000; Trzepacz and Baker 1993).

TABLE 1–3. The mental status examination

Level of consciousness

- Alert, drowsy, somnolent, stuporous, comatose; fluctuations suggest delirium

Appearance and behavior

- Overall appearance, grooming, hygiene
- Cooperation, eye contact, psychomotor agitation or retardation
- Abnormal movements: tics, tremors, chorea, posturing

Attention

- Vigilance, concentration, ability to focus, sensory neglect

Orientation and memory

- Orientation to person, place, time, situation
- Recent, remote, and immediate recall

Language

- Speech: rate, volume, fluency, prosody
- Comprehension and naming ability
- Abnormalities including aphasia, dysarthria, agraphia, alexia, clanging, neologisms, echolalia

Constructional ability

- Clock drawing to assess neglect, executive function, and planning
- Drawing of a cube or intersecting pentagons to assess parietal function

Mood and affect

- Mood: subjective sustained emotion
- Affect: observed emotion—quality, range, appropriateness

Form and content of thought

- Form: linear, circumstantial, tangential, disorganized, blocked
- Content: delusions, paranoia, ideas of reference, suicidal or homicidal ideation

Perception

- Auditory, visual, gustatory, tactile, and olfactory hallucinations

Judgment and insight

- Understanding of illness and consequences of specific treatments offered

Reasoning

- Illogical versus logical; ability to make consistent decisions

Source. Adapted from Hyman and Tesar 1994.

Physical Examination

Although the interview and mental status examination as outlined above are generally thought to be the primary diagnostic tools of the psychiatrist, the importance of the

TABLE 1–4. Detailed assessment of cognitive domains

Cognitive domain	Assessment
Level of consciousness and arousal	Inspect the patient.
Orientation to place and time	Ask direct questions about both of these.
Registration (recent memory)	Have the patient repeat three words immediately.
Recall (working memory)	Have the patient recall the same three words after performing another task for at least 3 minutes.
Remote memory	Ask about the patient's age, date of birth, milestones, or significant life or historical events (e.g., names of presidents, dates of wars).
Attention and concentration	Subtract serial 7s (adapt to the patient's level of education; subtract serial 3s if less educated). Spell *world* backward (this may be difficult for non-English speakers). Test digit span forward and backward. Have the patient recite the months of the year (or the days of the week) in reverse order.
Language	(Adapt the degree of difficulty to the patient's educational level.)
◆ Comprehension	Inspect the patient while he or she answers questions. Ask the patient to point to different objects. Ask yes-or-no questions. Ask the patient to write a phrase (paragraph).
◆ Naming	Show a watch, pen, or less familiar objects, if needed.
◆ Fluency	Assess the patient's speech. Have the patient name as many animals as he or she can in 1 minute.
◆ Articulation	Listen to the patient's speech. Have the patient repeat a phrase.
◆ Reading	Have the patient read a sentence (or a longer paragraph if needed).
Executive function	Determine if the patient requires constant cueing and prompting.
◆ Commands	Have the patient follow a three-step command.
◆ Construction tasks	Have the patient draw interlocked pentagons. Have the patient draw a clock.
◆ Motor programming tasks	Have the patient perform serial hand sequences. Have the patient perform reciprocal programs of raising fingers.
Judgment and reasoning	Listen to the patient's account of his or her history and reason for hospitalization. Assess abstraction (similarities: dog/cat; red/green). Ask about the patient's judgment about simple events or problems: "A construction worker fell to the ground from the seventh floor of the building and broke his two legs; he then ran to the nearby hospital to ask for medical help. Do you have any comment on this?"

physical examination should not be forgotten, especially in the medical setting. Most psychiatrists do not perform physical examinations on their patients. The consultation psychiatrist, however, should be familiar with and comfortable performing neurological examinations and other selected features of the physical examination that may uncover the common comorbidities in psychiatric patients (Granacher 1981; Summers et al. 1981a, 1981b). At an absolute minimum, the consultant should review the physical examinations performed by other physicians. However, the psychiatrist's examination of the patient, especially of central nervous system functions relevant to the differential diagnosis, is often essential. A more complete physical examination is appropriate on medical-psychiatric units or whenever the psychiatrist has assumed responsibility for the care of a patient's medical problems. Even with a sedated or comatose patient, simple observation and a few maneuvers that involve a laying on of hands may potentially yield a bounty of findings. Although it is beyond the scope of this chapter to discuss a comprehensive physical

TABLE 1–5. Selected elements of the physical examination and significance of findings

Elements	Examples of possible diagnoses
General	
General appearance healthier than expected	Somatoform disorder
Fever	Infection or NMS
Blood pressure or pulse abnormalities	Withdrawal, thyroid or cardiovascular disease
Body habitus	Eating disorders, polycystic ovaries, or Cushing's syndrome
Skin	
Diaphoresis	Fever, withdrawal, NMS
Piloerection ("gooseflesh")	Opioid withdrawal
Dry, flushed	Anticholinergic toxicity, heatstroke
Pallor	Anemia
Changes in hair, nails, skin	Malnutrition, thyroid or adrenal disease, polycystic ovaries
Jaundice	Liver disease
Characteristic stigmata	Syphilis, cirrhosis, or self-mutilation
Bruises	Physical abuse, ataxia, traumatic brain injury
Eyes	
Mydriasis	Opiate withdrawal, anticholinergic toxicity
Miosis	Opiate intoxication, cholinergic toxicity
Kayser-Fleischer rings	Wilson's disease
Neurological	
Tremors	Delirium, withdrawal syndromes, parkinsonism, lithium toxicity
Primitive reflexes present (e.g., snout, glabellar, grasp)	Dementia, frontal lobe dysfunction
Hyperactive deep tendon reflexes	Withdrawal, hyperthyroidism
Ophthalmoplegia	Wernicke's encephalopathy, brain stem dysfunction, dystonic reaction
Papilledema	Increased intracranial pressure
Hypertonia, rigidity, catatonia, parkinsonism	EPS, NMS
Abnormal movements	Parkinson's disease, Huntington's disease, EPS
Abnormal gait	Normal-pressure hydrocephalus, Parkinson's disease, Wernicke's encephalopathy
Loss of position and vibratory sense	Vitamin B_{12} deficiency

Note. EPS = extrapyramidal symptoms; NMS = neuroleptic malignant syndrome.

examination, Table 1–5 provides a broad outline of selected findings of the physical examination and their relevance to the psychiatric consultation.

Formulate Diagnostic and Therapeutic Strategies

By the time the consultant arrives on the scene, routine chemical and hematological tests and urinalyses are almost always available and should be reviewed along with any other laboratory, imaging, and electrophysiological tests. The consultant then considers what additional tests are needed to arrive at a diagnosis. Attempts have been made in the past to correlate biological tests, such as the dexamethasone suppression test, with psychiatric illness; despite extensive research, however, no definitive biological tests are available to identify psychiatric disorders. Before ordering a test, the consultant must consider the likelihood that the test will contribute to making a diagnosis.

While there is an extensive list of studies that could be relevant to psychiatric presentations, the most common screening tests in clinical practice are listed in Table 1–6. It was once common practice for the psychiatrist to order routine batteries of tests, especially in cognitively impaired patients, in a stereotypical diagnostic approach to the eval-

TABLE 1–6. Common tests in psychiatric consultation

Complete blood count
Serum chemistry panel
Thyroid-stimulating hormone (thyrotropin) concentration
Vitamin B_{12} (cyanocobalamin) concentration
Folic acid (folate) concentration
Human chorionic gonadotropin (pregnancy) test
Toxicology
Serum
Urine
Serological tests for syphilis
HIV tests
Urinalysis
Electrocardiogram

uation of dementia or delirium. In modern practice, tests should be ordered selectively, with consideration paid to sensitivity, specificity, and cost-effectiveness. Perhaps most importantly, careful thought should be given to whether the results of each test will affect the patient's management. Finally, further studies may be beneficial in certain clinical situations as described throughout this book.

Routine Tests

A complete blood cell count may reveal anemia that contributes to depression or infection that causes psychosis. Leukocytosis is seen with infection and other acute inflammatory conditions, lithium therapy, and neuroleptic malignant syndrome, whereas leukopenia and agranulocytosis may be caused by certain psychotropic medications. A serum chemistry panel may point to diagnoses as varied as liver disease, eating disorders, renal disease, malnutrition, and hypoglycemia—all of which may have psychiatric manifestations (Alpay and Park 2004). Serum and urine toxicological screens are helpful in cases of altered sensorium and obviously whenever substance abuse, intoxication, or overdose is suspected. Because blood tests for syphilis, thyroid disease, and deficiencies of vitamin B_{12} and folic acid (conditions that are curable) are readily available, they warrant a low threshold for their use. In patients with a history of exposures, HIV infection should not be overlooked. Obtaining a pregnancy test is often wise in women of childbearing age to inform diagnostically as well as to guide treatment options. Urinalysis, chest radiography, and electrocardiography are particularly important screening tools in the geriatric population. Although it is not a first-line test, cerebrospinal fluid analysis should be considered in cases of mental status changes associated with fever, leukocytosis, meningismus, or unknown etiology. Increased intracranial pressure should be ruled out before a lumbar puncture is performed, however. More detailed discussion of specific tests is provided in relevant chapters throughout this text.

Neuroimaging

The psychiatric consultant must also be familiar with neuroimaging studies. Neuroimaging may aid in fleshing out the differential diagnosis of neuropsychiatric conditions, although it rarely establishes the diagnosis by itself (Dougherty and Rauch 2004). In most situations, magnetic resonance imaging (MRI) is preferred over computed tomography (CT). MRI provides greater resolution of subcortical structures (e.g., basal ganglia, amygdala, and other limbic structures) of particular interest to psychiatrists. It is also superior for detection of abnormalities of the brain stem and posterior fossa. Furthermore, MRI is better able to distinguish between gray matter and white matter lesions. CT is most useful in cases of suspected acute intracranial hemorrhage (having occurred within the past 72 hours) and when MRI is contraindicated (in patients with metallic implants). Dougherty and Rauch (2004) suggest that the following conditions and situations merit consideration of neuroimaging: new-onset psychosis, new-onset dementia, delirium of unknown cause, prior to an initial course of electroconvulsive therapy, and an acute mental status change with an abnormal neurological examination in a patient with either a history of head trauma or an age of 50 years or older. Regardless of the modality, the consultant should read the radiologist's report, because other physicians tend to dismiss all but acute focal findings and, as a result, misleadingly record the results of the study as normal in the chart. Psychiatrists recognize, however, that even small abnormalities (e.g., periventricular white matter changes) or chronic changes (e.g., cortical atrophy) have diagnostic and therapeutic implications (see Chapter 6, "Dementia," Chapter 8, "Depression," and Chapter 32, "Neurology and Neurosurgery").

Electrophysiological Tests

The electroencephalogram (EEG) is the most widely available test that can assess brain activity. The EEG is most often indicated in patients with paroxysmal or other symptoms suggestive of a seizure disorder, especially complex partial seizures, or pseudoseizures (see Chapter 32, "Neurology and Neurosurgery"). An EEG may also be helpful in distinguishing between neurological and psychiatric etiologies for a mute, uncommunicative patient. An EEG may be helpful in documenting the presence of generalized slowing in a delirious patient, but it rarely indicates a specific etiology of delirium and it is not indicated in every delirious patient. However, when the diagnosis of delirium is uncertain, electroencephalographic evidence of dysrhythmia may prove useful. For example, when the primary treatment team insists that a patient should be transferred to a psychiatric inpatient service because of a mistaken belief that the symptoms of delirium represent schizophrenia or depression, an EEG may provide concrete data to support the correct diagnosis. EEGs may also facilitate the evaluation of rapidly progressive dementia or profound coma; but because findings are neither sensitive nor specific, they are not often helpful in the evaluation of space-occupying lesions, cerebral infarctions, or head injury (Bostwick and Philbrick 2002). Continuous electroencephalographic recordings with video monitoring or ambulatory electroencephalographic monitoring may be necessary in order to document abnormal electrical activity in cases of complex partial seizures or when factitious seizures are suspected. As with neuroimaging reports, the psychiatric consultant must read the electroencephalographic report, because nonpsychiatrists often misinterpret the absence of dramatic focal abnormalities (e.g., spikes) as indicative of normality, even though psychiatrically significant brain dysfunction may be associated with focal or generalized slowing or with sharp waves. Other electrophysiological tests may be helpful in specific situations; for example, sensory evoked potentials to distinguish multiple sclerosis from conversion disorder, or electromyography with nerve conduction velocities to differentiate neuropathy from malingering.

Other Tests

Other diagnostic tools may also prove useful as adjuncts. Neuropsychological testing may be helpful in diagnosis, prognosis, and treatment planning in patients with neuropsychiatric disorders. Psychological testing can help the consultant better understand a patient's emotional functioning and personality style. For example, elevations on the Hypochondriasis and Hysteria scales of the Minnesota Multiphasic Personality Inventory and a normal or minimally elevated result on the Depression scale constitute the so-called conversion V or psychosomatic V pattern, classically regarded as indicative of a significant psychological contribution to the etiology of somatic symptoms but now recognized as confounded by medical illness.

The amobarbital interview has been used as a tool in the diagnosis and treatment of a variety of psychiatric conditions (e.g., conversion disorder, posttraumatic stress disorder, factitious disorder, psychogenic amnesia, neurosis, and catatonia) for the past 70 years (Kavarirajan 1999). The psychiatric literature has been mixed, however, on the utility of the amobarbital interview, and intravenous lorazepam is now generally regarded as a safer alternative. However, the diagnostic validity of amobarbital and lorazepam interviews has not been systematically assessed.

Write a Note

The consultation note should be clear, concise, and free of jargon and should focus on specific diagnostic and therapeutic recommendations. Although an understanding of the patient's psychodynamics may be helpful, the consultant should usually avoid speculations in the chart regarding unconscious motivations. Consultees fundamentally want to know what is going on with the patient and what they should and can do about it; these themes should dominate the note. Mental health professionals are trained to construct full developmental and psychosocial formulations, but these do not belong in a consultation note (although they may inform key elements of the assessment and recommendations). Finger-pointing and criticism of the primary team or other providers should be avoided. The consultant should also avoid rigid insistence on a preferred mode of management if there is an equally suitable alternative (Kontos et al. 2003).

The consultation note should include a condensed version of all the elements of a general psychiatric note with a few additions (Querques et al. 2004). The consultant should begin the note with a summary of the patient's medical and psychiatric history, the reason for the current admission, and the reason for the consultation. Next should be a brief summary of the current medical illness with pertinent findings and hospital course; this summary is meant to demonstrate an appreciation for the current medical issues rather than to repeat what has already been documented in the chart. It is often helpful for the consultant to include a description of the patient's typical patterns of response to stress and illness, if known. Physical and neurological examinations, as well as germane laboratory results or imaging studies, should also be summarized. The consultant should then list the differential diagnosis in order of decreasing likelihood, making clear which is the working diagnosis or diagnoses. If the patient's symptoms are not likely to be due to a psychiatric disorder, this should be explicitly stated. Finally, the consultant should make recommendations or clearly describe plans in order of decreasing importance. Recommendations include ways to further elucidate the diagnosis as well as therapeutic suggestions. It is especially important to anticipate and address problems that may appear at a later time (e.g., offering a medication recommendation for treatment of agitation in a delirious patient who is currently calm). For medication recommendations, brief notation of side effects and their management is useful. The inclusion of a statement indicating that the consultant will provide follow-up will reassure the consulting team, and the consultant should include contact information in the event that they have further questions.

Speak Directly With the Referring Clinician

The consultation ends in the same way that it began—with a conversation with the referring clinician. Personal contact is especially crucial if diagnostic or therapeutic suggestions are time-sensitive. Some information or recommendations may be especially sensitive, whether for reasons of confidentiality or risk management, and are better conveyed verbally than fully documented in the chart. The medical chart is read by a variety of individuals, including the patient at times, and, thus, discretion is warranted.

Provide Periodic Follow-Up

Many consultations cannot be completed in a single visit. Rather, several encounters may be required before the problems identified by both the consultee and the consultant are resolved. Moreover, new issues commonly arise during the course of the consultative process, and a single consultation request often necessitates frequent visits, disciplined follow-up, and easy accessibility. All follow-up visits should be documented in the chart. Finally, it may be appropriate to sign off of a case when the patient is stabilized or when the consultant's opinion and recommendations are being disregarded (Kontos et al. 2003).

Role of Other Providers

Although the emphasis of this chapter is on the psychiatrist as consultant, the value of members of other professions, working together as a team, should not be overlooked. Psychologists play an essential role in performing neuropsychological and psychological testing and providing psychotherapeutic and behavioral interventions. Psychiatric clinical nurse specialists provide services to the nursing staff that parallel those that the psychiatrist provides to the medical team. They are especially helpful in organizing interdisciplinary care conferences and nursing behavioral treatment plans that include behavioral contracts with patients. Case managers facilitate transfers and set up aftercare. Chaplains address the spiritual needs of patients in distress. Finally, communication with primary care physicians remains of utmost importance, since the primary care physician is well positioned to oversee and coordinate ongoing care after discharge.

Consultation and Collaborative Care in the Outpatient Setting

Whereas the majority of this chapter has focused on psychiatric consultation in the inpatient setting, it could be argued that the consultation psychiatrist provides an even greater impact by working collaboratively with primary care physicians in the outpatient domain (Stern et al. 2004). Many studies over the past 30 years have established both the high prevalence of mental disorders in outpatient medical settings and the fact that more people with mental health disorders present to general medical settings than to psychiatrists (Unützer et al. 2006). In their report for the President's New Freedom Commission on Mental Health, Unützer et al. (2006) described a number of common barriers to effective mental health care at the interface with medicine, including the following: incorrect identification of symptoms by patients or reluctance to seek psychiatric care due to stigma; lack of mental health training for primary care providers; lack of time to fully address mental health issues in brief clinical encounters in the primary care setting; and restrictions in insurance coverage for mental health services. The elderly, children and adolescents, ethnic minorities, and uninsured individuals are especially susceptible to having their needs unmet in this regard (Unützer et al. 2006). Given that general medical settings comprise such a significant portion of the mental health care system, what strategies may be used to improve quality and efficacy of care?

Initial studies that focused on the improvement of mental health care in general medical settings stressed diagnosis and screening techniques (Gilbody et al. 2001; Spitzer et al. 1999) (see a detailed description of screening tools for this population later in this chapter). Subsequent inquiries then combined screening with systematic feedback of diagnoses to the primary care providers. These studies revealed that whereas screening and giving feedback to providers often increase the rate of diagnosis of mental disorders, they are not sufficient to improve patient outcomes (Katon and Gonzales 1994; Klinkman and Okkes 1998). Similar results were obtained when researchers looked at the efficacy of employing treatment guidelines for the care of common psychiatric disorders in primary care settings in combination with developing comprehensive training for providers (Hodges et al. 2001; Simon 2002). A simple referral to a psychiatrist is often inadequate for a myriad of reasons, including lack of access to mental health practitioners (especially for underserved populations), lack of patient follow-through (e.g., the patient never makes it to the appointment), and inability to pay for mental health services. Although adequate screening, use of practice guidelines, provider training, and referral to specialists are all important components of improving mental health care in general medical settings, research has shown that these alone are inadequate (Unützer et al. 2006). The development of collaborative care models represents a potential solution to this problem.

Collaborative care refers to the joining together of mental health care providers with primary care physicians and their teams to deliver specialized care within the outpatient primary care setting. Consultation psychiatrists are uniquely positioned for this role, given the focus of psychosomatic medicine at the interface of medicine and psychiatry. While specific models of collaborative care vary, effective programs generally share certain key components. The first is systematic care management (often by a trained nurse, social worker, or psychologist). The care manager helps identify patients in need, coordinates an initial treatment plan, educates patients, provides follow-up, monitors progress, and helps change the treatment course as needed. These tasks may be performed in person (e.g., in the primary care clinic) or by telephone (Worth and Stern 2003). The next essential piece is consultation and appropriate sharing of information between the primary care provider, the care manager, and the consulting psychiatrist (Unützer et al. 2006). This does not necessarily mean that the psychiatric specialist provides a consultation for every patient; in fact, research has shown that the most efficient and cost-effective measures often involve a stepwise approach in which progressively more intensive interventions are applied until a successful outcome is achieved (Katon et al. 2005, 2008; Richards et al. 2007; Unützer et al. 2001; Von Korff and Tiemens 2000). Thus, stepped care for a patient with depression might involve an initial intervention of prescription of an antidepressant by the primary care provider along with care management either by phone or in person, as detailed above. If the patient remains symptomatic, the next step would be referral for brief psychotherapy or other behavioral interventions and/or a switch to another medication. While much of this process takes place under the supervision of a consulting psychiatrist, referral to mental health specialists is generally reserved for treatment nonresponders. For example, in the IMPACT (Improving Mood—Promoting Access to Collaborative Treatment) randomized trial for depressed elderly patients in primary care, consulting psychiatrists saw only about 10% of patients but served as key members of the collaborative team by providing consultation and education to care managers and primary care providers (Hunkeler et al. 2006; Unützer et al. 2002). Collaborative care models have been shown to improve outcomes and enhance patient function and quality of life as well as to be cost-effective (Schoenbaum et al. 2001, 2004; Simon et al. 2001). Finally, ethnic minorities seem to benefit in particular from collaborative care models (Miranda et al. 2003; Wells et al. 2004).

Screening

As mentioned in the previous section, the use of screening tools may be helpful in specific situations. For example, even though a comprehensive assessment of cognitive function is not required for every patient, even a slim suspicion of the possibility of a cognitive deficit should prompt performance of cognitive screening. Although individualized mental status examinations performed as part of a psychiatrist's clinical interview are much preferred to standardized tests, screening tests may be particularly useful in case finding (e.g., in primary care settings as part of a collaborative care approach) and in research domains. The same has been proposed for a variety of other psychiatric disorders, including depression, anxiety, and substance abuse. An important note in this regard, however, is that screening and case finding are unlikely to be helpful without a systematic approach to treatment (see the discussion of collaborative care above). This is evidenced by a recent meta-analysis, which showed that when used alone, screening questionnaires for depression did not have an impact on the actual detection and management of depression by clinicians in non–mental health settings (Gilbody et al. 2008). Such findings underscore the importance of collaboration between psychosomatic medicine specialists and general medical teams (in both the outpatient and inpatient settings), with screening tools as just one aspect of this collaboration. Selected instruments are described below; others are discussed in the relevant chapters in this book.

Tests such as the MMSE or the Mini-Cog (Borson et al. 2000) are helpful adjuncts in the hands of nonpsychiatrists to quickly identify potential cognitive disorders. The MMSE is a 19-question test that provides an overview of a patient's cognitive function at a moment in time; it includes assessment of orientation, attention, and memory. It is of limited use without modification, however, in patients who are deaf or blind, who are intubated, or who do not speak English. The MMSE is also particularly insensitive in measuring cognitive decline in very intelligent patients, who may appear less impaired than they really are. The Mini-Cog, on the other hand, combines a portion of the MMSE (3-minute recall) with the Clock Drawing Test, as described by Critchley in 1953 (Scanlan and Borson 2001). In screening for dementia, the MMSE and the Mini-Cog have been shown to have similar sensitivity (76%–79%) and specificity (88%–89%) (Borson et al. 2003). However, the Mini-Cog is significantly shorter and enables screening temporoparietal and frontal cortical areas via the Clock Drawing Test, areas that are not fully assessed by the MMSE.

In addition, these tests may be supplemented with others—including Luria maneuvers and cognitive estimations (e.g., How many slices are there in an average loaf of white bread? How long is the human spinal cord?)—that further assess the functioning of frontal-subcortical networks. A formal neuropsychological battery may be useful if these bedside tests produce abnormal results. In a patient with an altered level of awareness or attention, formal cognitive tests should be deferred until the sensorium clears, because clouding of consciousness will produce uninterpretable results.

Other screening instruments may also help to identify patients in medical settings who could benefit from a comprehensive psychiatric interview. The Patient Health Questionnaire (PHQ), an abbreviated form of the Primary Care Evaluation of Mental Disorders (PRIME-MD), is a three-page questionnaire that can be entirely self-administered by the patient (Spitzer et al. 1999). In addition to the assessment of mood, anxiety, eating, alcohol use, and somatization disorders, the PHQ screens for posttraumatic stress disorder and common psychosocial stressors and also elicits a pregnancy history. The PHQ is valid and reliable and has improved the diagnosis of psychiatric conditions in primary care and other ambulatory medical settings (Spitzer et al. 1999); it may also have a role at the bedside. Subsets of the PHQ's items have been validated for specific screening purposes. For example, the nine-item PHQ-9, a self-administered depression-specific questionnaire that can be completed by the patient in roughly 2 minutes (Gilbody et al. 2007a; Kroenke et al. 2001), has been shown to perform as well (in a range of countries, populations, and clinical settings) as longer clinician-administered instruments that screen for depression in medical settings (Gilbody et al. 2007b); it can also be used to monitor the severity of depression. The PHQ-2 for depression, which includes just the items for mood and anhedonia, is sensitive and specific for both major depressive disorder and other depressive disorders, performing almost as well as the PHQ-9 (Löwe et al. 2005).

The PHQ-15 assesses 15 somatic symptoms and is useful as an index of somatization (Kroenke et al. 2009). The Generalized Anxiety Disorder 7-item (GAD-7) scale is a valid and efficient tool for screening for generalized anxiety disorder and assessing its severity (Spitzer et al. 2006).

The Clinical Outcomes in Routine Evaluation—Outcome Measure (CORE-OM; Barkham et al. 2001) is a 34-item instrument that measures a range of mental health problems as well as functional capacity and risk of harm to self or others that has been validated for assessment of depression in the primary care setting (Gilbody et al. 2007a).

The General Health Questionnaire (GHQ) is another instrument originally developed in the 1970s to screen for psychiatric disorders in medical outpatients (Goldberg and Blackwell 1970). The original 60-item version has been replaced with well-validated 28- and 12-item versions. The GHQ has been translated into numerous languages worldwide and is cross-culturally validated (Tait et al. 2003). Because of its emphasis on identifying new symptoms, the GHQ is most useful for assessing state rather than trait conditions (Tait et al. 2003).

The CAGE questionnaire is a well-known screening device developed by Ewing (1984) to identify alcohol abuse. Two or more positive responses on the four-question screen correlate with an 89% chance of alcohol abuse (Mayfield et al. 1974) (see Chapter 17, "Substance-Related Disorders"). Other screening tests are described in the chapters covering specific syndromes (e.g., depression, anxiety, delirium).

Practice Guidelines

Groups from several countries have developed psychosomatic medicine practice guidelines that detail professional standards for psychiatric consultation in nonpsychiatric settings, referencing the appropriate knowledge base as well as delineating integrated clinical approaches, effective methods, and ways to enhance adherence to recommendations made by the consulting psychiatrist (Bronheim et al. 1998; Leentjens et al. 2009; Royal Colleges of Physicians and Psychiatrists 1995). Although a complete review of these guidelines is beyond the scope of this chapter, they may serve as excellent additions to the information provided here. Especially helpful are practice guidelines informing evaluation of specific disorders (e.g., delirium [Leentjens and Diefenbacher 2006]) or specific tasks (e.g., psychosocial evaluation of living unrelated organ donors [Dew et al. 2007]).

Benefits of Psychiatric Services

The benefits of psychiatric services in health care delivery are significant. An extensive body of evidence has demonstrated a link between comorbid psychopathology and increased length of hospital stay and, consequently, increased inpatient costs. Levenson et al. (1990) described a longer median length of hospital stay (a 40% increase) and hospital costs that were 35% higher in medical inpatients with depression, anxiety, cognitive dysfunction, or high levels of pain (independent of severity of medical illness). Cognitively impaired geriatric patients in one sample were shown to have an increased length of stay compared with those without cognitive impairment (Fulop et al. 1998), whereas depressed elderly patients in another sample had more hospitalizations and longer hospital stays (Koenig and Kuchibhatla 1998). Although some have suggested that psychiatric consultation might decrease lengths of stay and inpatient costs (Levitan and Kornfeld 1981; Strain et al. 1991), that is not where its primary value lies. Patients benefit from the reductions in mental suffering and improvements in psychological well-being that result from more accurate diagnosis and more appropriate treatment. The adverse effects of psychopathology on specific medical disorders, and the benefits of treating it, are reviewed in remaining chapters of this textbook. Providers of health care profit from the added diagnostic and therapeutic expertise of the psychiatric consultant as well as from a better understanding of health behaviors. This has been best demonstrated in ambulatory collaborative care models, as discussed earlier in this chapter. The hospital milieu also benefits from having readily available medically knowledgeable psychiatrists, whose assistance improves the care of the complex patients described in the rest of this textbook, contributing to better risk management and a safer and more pleasant work environment.

Conclusion

Psychiatric assessment and consultation can be crucial to seriously ill medical patients. The psychosomatic medicine psychiatrist is an expert in the diagnosis and care of psychopathology in the medically ill. Psychiatric consultation affords a unique ability to offer a panoramic view of the patient, the illness, and the relationship between the two. The psychiatric consultant will be called on to help diagnose, understand, and manage a wide array of conditions; when effective, the consultant addresses the needs of both the patient and the medical–surgical team. In this manner, psychiatric consultation is essential to the provision of comprehensive care in the medical setting.

References

Alpay M, Park L: Laboratory tests and diagnostic procedures, in Massachusetts General Hospital Psychiatry Update and Board Preparation, 2nd Edition. Edited by Stern TA, Herman JB. New York, McGraw-Hill, 2004, pp 251–265

Barkham M, Margison F, Leach C, et al: Service profiling and outcomes benchmarking using the CORE-OM: towards practice-based evidence in the psychological therapies. J Consult Clin Psychol 69:184–196, 2001

Borson S, Scanlan J, Brush M, et al: The Mini-Cog: a cognitive "vital signs" measure for dementia screening in multi-lingual elderly. Int J Geriatr Psychiatry 15:1021–1027, 2000

Borson S, Scanlan JM, Chen P, et al: The Mini-Cog as a screen for dementia: validation in a population-based sample. J Am Geriatr Soc 51:1451–1454, 2003

Bostwick JM, Philbrick KL: The use of electroencephalography in psychiatry of the medically ill. Psychiatr Clin North Am 25:17–25, 2002

Bronheim HE, Fulop G, Kunkel EJ, et al: The Academy of Psychosomatic Medicine practice guidelines for psychiatric consultation in the general medical setting. Psychosomatics 39:S8–S30, 1998

Critchley M: The Parietal Lobes. New York, Hafner, 1953

Dew MA, Jacobs CL, Jowsey SG, et al: Guidelines for the psychosocial evaluation of living unrelated kidney donors in the United States. Am J Transplant 7:1047–1054, 2007

Dougherty DD, Rauch SL: Neuroimaging in psychiatry, in Massachusetts General Hospital Psychiatry Update and Board Preparation, 2nd Edition. Edited by Stern TA, Herman JB. New York, McGraw-Hill, 2004, pp 227–232

Ewing JA: Detecting alcoholism. The CAGE questionnaire. JAMA 252:1905–1907, 1984

Folstein MF, Folstein SE, McHugh PR: "Mini-Mental State": a practical method for grading the cognitive state of patients for the clinician. J Psychiatr Res 12:189–198, 1975

Fulop G, Strain JJ, Fahs MC, et al: A prospective study of the impact of psychiatric comorbidity on length of hospital stays of elderly medical surgical inpatients. Psychosomatics 39:273–280, 1998

Gilbody SM, House AO, Sheldon TA: Routinely administered questionnaires for depression and anxiety: systematic review. BMJ 322:406–409, 2001

Gilbody SM, Richards D, Barkham M: Diagnosing depression in primary care using self-completed instruments: UK validation of PHQ-9 and Core-OM. Br J Gen Pract 57:650–652, 2007a

Gilbody SM, Richards D, Brealey S, et al: Screening for depression in medical settings with the patient health questionnaire (PHQ): a diagnostic meta-analysis. J Gen Intern Med 22:1596–1602, 2007b

Gilbody SM, Sheldon TA, House AO: Screening and case-finding instruments for depression: a meta-analysis. CMAJ 178:997–1003, 2008

Gitlin DF, Levenson JL, Lyketsos CG: Psychosomatic medicine: a new psychiatric subspecialty. Acad Psychiatry 28:4–11, 2004

Goldberg DP, Blackwell B: Psychiatric illness in general practice: a detailed study using a new method of case identification. BMJ 1:439–443, 1970

Granacher RP: The neurologic examination in geriatric psychiatry. Psychosomatics 22:485–499, 1981

Hackett TP, Cassem NH, Stern TA, et al: Beginnings: psychosomatic medicine and consultation psychiatry in the general hospital, in Massachusetts General Hospital Handbook of General Hospital Psychiatry, 5th Edition. Edited by Stern TA, Fricchione GL, Cassem NH, et al. Philadelphia, PA, CV Mosby, 2004, pp 1–7

Hodges B, Inch C, Silver I: Improving the psychiatric knowledge, skills, and attitudes of primary care physicians, 1950–2000: a review. Am J Psychiatry 158:1579–1586, 2001

Hyman SE, Tesar GE: The emergency psychiatric evaluation, including the mental status examination, in Manual of Psychiatric Emergencies, 3rd Edition. Edited by Hyman SE, Tesar GE. Boston, MA, Little, Brown, 1994, pp 3–11

Hunkeler EM, Katon W, Tang L, et al: Long term outcomes from the IMPACT randomized trial for depressed elderly patients in primary care. BMJ 332:259–263, 2006

Katon WJ, Gonzales J: A review of randomized trials of psychiatric consultation-liaison studies in primary care. Psychosomatics 35:268–278, 1994

Katon WJ, Schoenbaum M, Fan MY, et al: Cost-effectiveness of improving primary care treatment of late-life depression. Arch Gen Psychiatry 62:1313–1320, 2005

Katon WJ, Russo JE, Von Korff M, et al: Long-term effects on medical costs of improving depression outcomes in patients with depression and diabetes. Diabetes Care 31:1155–1159, 2008

Kavarirajan H: The amobarbital interview revisited: a review of the literature since 1966. Harv Rev Psychiatry 3:153–165, 1999

Klinkman MS, Okkes I: Mental health problems in primary care: a research agenda. J Fam Practice 47:379–384, 1998

Koenig HG, Kuchibhatla M: Use of health services by hospitalized medically ill depressed elderly patients. Am J Psychiatry 155:871–877, 1998

Kontos N, Freudenreich O, Querques J, et al: The consultation psychiatrist as effective physician. Gen Hosp Psychiatry 25:20–23, 2003

Kroenke K, Spitzer RI, Williams JB: The PHQ-9 validity of a brief depression severity measure. J Gen Intern Med 16:606–613, 2001

Kroenke K, Spitzer RL, Williams JB: The PHQ-15: validity of a new measure for evaluating the severity of somatic symptoms. Psychosom Med 64:258–266, 2009

Leentjens AF, Diefenbacher A: A survey of delirium guidelines in Europe. J Psychosom Res 61:123–128, 2006

Leentjens AFG, Boenink AD, Sno HN, et al: The guideline "consultation psychiatry" of the Netherlands Psychiatric Association. J Psychosom Res 66:531–535, 2009

Levenson JL, Hamer RM, Rossiter LF: Relation of psychopathology in general medical inpatients to use and cost of services. Am J Psychiatry 147:1498–1503, 1990

Levitan SJ, Kornfeld DS: Clinical and cost benefits of liaison psychiatry. Am J Psychiatry 138:790–793, 1981

Lipowski ZJ: Review of consultation psychiatry and psychosomatic medicine, II: clinical aspects. Psychosom Med 29:201–224, 1967

Löwe B, Kroenke K, Gräfe K: Detecting and monitoring depression with a two-item questionnaire (PHQ-2). J Psychosom Res 58:163–171, 2005

Mayfield D, McLeod G, Hall P: The CAGE questionnaire: validation of a new alcoholism screening instrument. Am J Psychiatry 131:1121–1124, 1974

Miranda J, Duan N, Sherbourne C, et al: Improving care for minorities: can quality improvement interventions improve care and outcome for depressed minorities? Results of a randomized, controlled trial. Health Services Research 38:613–630, 2003

Murray GB: Limbic music, in Massachusetts General Hospital Handbook of General Hospital Psychiatry, 5th Edition. Edited by Stern TA, Fricchione GF, Cassem NH, et al. Philadelphia, PA, CV Mosby, 2004, pp 21–28

Perry S, Viederman M: Adaptation of residents to consultation-liaison psychiatry, I: working with the physically ill. Gen Hosp Psychiatry 3:141–147, 1981

Querques J, Stern TA, Cassem NH: Psychiatric consultation to medical and surgical patients, in Massachusetts General Hospital Psychiatry Update and Board Preparation, 2nd Edition. Edited by Stern TA, Herman JB. New York, McGraw-Hill, 2004, pp 507–510

Richards DA, Lovell K, Gilbody S, et al: Collaborative care for depression in UK primary care: a randomized controlled trial. Psychological Med 38:279–287, 2007

Royal Colleges of Physicians and Psychiatrists: The psychological care of medical patients: recognition of need and service provision. A joint working party report. London, Royal College of General Practitioners, 1995

Scanlan JM, Borson S: The Mini-Cog: receiver operation characteristics with expert and naive raters. Int J Geriatr Psychiatry 16:216–222, 2001

Schoenbaum M, Unützer J, Sherbourne C, et al: Cost-effectiveness of practice-initiated quality improvement for depression: results of a randomized controlled trial. JAMA 286:1325–1330, 2001

Schoenbaum M, Miranda J, Sherbourne C, et al: Cost-effectiveness of interventions for depressed Latinos. J Ment Health Policy Econ 7:69–76, 2004

Simon GE: Evidence review: efficacy and effectiveness of antidepressant treatment in primary care. Gen Hosp Psychiatry 24:213–224, 2002

Simon GE, Katon WJ, VonKorff M, et al: Cost-effectiveness of a collaborative care program for primary care patients with persistent depression. Am J Psychiatry 158:1638–1644, 2001

Spitzer RL, Kroenke K, Williams JB: Validation and utility of a self-report version of PRIME-MD: the PHQ Primary Care Study. Primary Care Evaluation of Mental Disorders. Patient Health Questionnaire. JAMA 282:1737–1744, 1999

Spitzer RL, Kroenke K, Williams JB, et al: A brief measure for assessing generalized anxiety disorder: the GAD-7. Arch Intern Med 166:1092–1097, 2006

Stern TA, Herman JB, Slavin PL (eds): Massachusetts General Hospital Guide to Primary Care Psychiatry, 2nd Edition. New York, McGraw-Hill, 2004

Strain JJ, Lyons JS, Hammer JS, et al: Cost offset from a psychiatric consultation-liaison intervention with elderly hip fracture patients. Am J Psychiatry 148:1044–1049, 1991

Strub RL, Black FW: Mental Status Examination in Neurology, 4th Edition. Philadelphia, PA, FA Davis, 2000

Summers WK, Munoz RA, Read MR: The psychiatric physical examination, part I: methodology. J Clin Psychiatry 42:95–98, 1981a

Summers WK, Munoz RA, Read MR, et al: The psychiatric physical examination, part II: findings in 75 unselected psychiatric patients. J Clin Psychiatry 42:99–102, 1981b

Tait RJ, French DJ, Hulse GK: Validity and psychometric properties of the General Health Questionnaire–12 in young Australian adolescents. Aust N Z J Psychiatry 37:374–381, 2003

Trzepacz PT, Baker RW: The Psychiatric Mental Status Examination. New York, Oxford University Press, 1993

Unützer J, Katon W, Williams JW Jr, et al: Improving primary care for depression in late life: the design of a multicenter randomized trial. Medical Care 39:785–799, 2001

Unützer J, Katon W, Callahan CM, et al: Collaborative care management of late-life depression in the primary care setting. A randomized controlled trial. JAMA 288:2836–2845, 2002

Unützer J, Schoenbaum M, Druss BG, et al: Transforming mental health care at the interface with general medicine: report for the President's Commission. Psychiatr Serv 57:37–47, 2006

Von Korff M, Tiemens B: Individualized stepped care of chronic illness. West J Med 172:133–137, 2000

Wells K, Sherbourne C, Schoenbaum M, et al: Five-year impact of quality improvement for depression: results of a group-level randomized controlled trial. Arch Gen Psychiatry 61:378–386, 2004

Worth JL, Stern TA: Benefits of an outpatient Psychiatric Tele-Consultation Unit (PTCU): results of a one-year pilot. Prim Care Companion J Clin Psychiatry 5:80–84, 2003

CHAPTER 2

Legal Issues

Rebecca W. Brendel, M.D., J.D.
Ronald Schouten, M.D., J.D.
James L. Levenson, M.D.

MEDICAL PRACTICE OCCURS in a legal and regulatory context. Concerns often emerge at the intersection of law and medicine, and the field of psychosomatic medicine is no exception. In fact, for a number of reasons, legal questions may arise frequently for the consultation-liaison psychiatrist, and even more often than in many other areas of medicine. One reason is the sensitive nature of communications made by patients to psychiatrists and the historical protections afforded to psychiatric and psychotherapy records that may raise concerns about laws related to confidentiality in the course of a psychiatric evaluation. A second is that medical and surgical practitioners may rely on the psychiatric colleagues' training and expertise in understanding disorders of behavior and cognition for assistance in determining patients' ability to make medical decisions, give informed consent for treatment, or refuse recommended treatment. Third, the complex balancing of individual interests against public policy considerations may lead to questions in the treatment of a particular patient in a number of contexts, including duties to third parties, mandated reporting, and malpractice liability.

For most practitioners, legal concerns are likely background considerations that remain largely unfocused and absent from conscious awareness in daily practice. However, when legal issues arise, they often occur in the context of particularly challenging clinical issues and, if not properly understood and considered, may lead to confusion, departure from sound clinical judgment, and even bad outcomes (Schouten and Brendel 2009). It is therefore critical for clinicians to be aware of relevant legal principles and regulations pertaining to the provision of medical care in jurisdictions relevant to their practice. However, it is also critical for clinicians to appreciate that the best way of minimizing legal complications and providing care to patients is through attention to thorough and sound clinical judgment and care (Brendel and Schouten 2007; Schouten and Brendel 2004, 2009).

This chapter covers a series of legal issues and principles frequently encountered in the practice of psychosomatic medicine, including privacy and confidentiality, capacity and competency, informed consent for treatment and treatment refusal, substitute decision making and guardianship, and malpractice. The information in this chapter should serve as a resource for the general hospital psychiatrist's practice and also as a guide to avoid unnecessary legal entanglements due to misconceptions, overreliance on the law rather than exercise of clinical judgment, and/or failure to be aware of or seek counsel of appropriate legal resources and advice in the course of consultative practice. In addition, this chapter describes principles that are broadly applicable to most United States jurisdictions. That being said, many of these principles reflect practices in other nation's jurisdictions, and variations also occur between U.S. states. Therefore, while this chapter provides an overview, it does not serve as a substitute for practitioners' awareness of legal requirements and resources in the jurisdictions in which they practice.

Confidentiality

The principle of doctor–patient confidentiality was codified in the Hippocratic oath as early as 430 B.C.: "Whatever I see or hear, professionally or privately, which ought not to be divulged, I will keep secret and tell no one" (Lloyd 1983). Since that time, confidentiality has remained a central facet of the doctor–patient relationship on the rationale that it promotes the open and honest exchange of information in the interest of treatment and patient welfare (American Psychiatric Association 1978, 2001; Appelbaum 2002; Brendel and Brendel 2005). Doctor–patient confidentiality is a professional, legal, and ethical requirement. Signs in hospital hallways and elevators reminding staff to respect patient confidentiality serve as just one reminder and symbol of the responsibility of health care providers to their patients. However, the notion of total confidentiality in medicine is, in practice, arcane. Even before the recent expansion of health information systems and electronic medical records over the last decade in particular, medical information was not strictly confidential between doctor and patient in the setting of hospital treatment. For example, even more than 15 years ago, one observer detailed the large number of individuals with access to a patient's medical chart (Siegler 1982). Now, as medical charts have become increasingly electronic, questions about ownership, access, and commoditization are emerging at a rapid pace and will likely further challenge notions of confidentiality as time goes on (Hall and Schulman 2009). In addition, increasing attention has started to focus on the scope of confidentiality after a patient's death (Robinson and O'Neill 2007).

Over time, the principle of strict or absolute confidentiality between one physician and one patient has eroded beyond the sharing of medical information with hospital personnel as described by Siegler (1982). The considerations of a complex society have increasingly led to an erosion of confidentiality as it was understood in the era of Hippocrates and subsequent centuries. Courts and legislatures have created limitations to doctor–patient confidentiality in circumstances where confidentiality is determined to be at odds with public safety or to be more harmful than beneficial for the patient. More recently, federal law has recognized efficiency and effectiveness of the health care system as a principle to be balanced with traditional management and safeguarding of protected health information under the Health Insurance Portability and Accountability Act of 1996 (HIPAA 1996, P.L. 104-191) (Brendel and Bryan 2004).

Public Safety and Welfare Exceptions to Confidentiality

Physicians often express concern that reporting information to government authorities, social service agencies, or other third parties may expose them to potential liability. While protecting patient information and confidentiality is the default rule, there are several situations in which physicians have an affirmative duty to disclose information to authorities. One such example is child and elder abuse and neglect reporting. Every jurisdiction in the United States mandates that physicians report suspected child and elder abuse and neglect (Brendel 2005; Kazim and Brendel 2004; Milosavljevic and Brendel 2008).

Thirty-five years ago, federal law set a minimum standard for what actions or inactions constitute child abuse or neglect, respectively (Child Abuse Prevention and Treatment Act 2003). However, individual states have interpreted the federal definition in different ways, leading to variations in the definition of child abuse among U.S. jurisdictions. As a general rule of thumb, state definitions generally incorporate the concepts of "harm or substantial risk of harm" or "serious threat or serious harm" to a person younger than 18 years who is not emancipated (Milosavljevic and Brendel 2008). Approximately half of states have some form of emancipation law that may exempt an emancipated or mature minor under the chronological age of 18 years from being subject to a child abuse or neglect report. Physicians should be aware of the specific prevailing standards in the jurisdictions in which they practice regarding the definitions and requirements for reporting. In general, liability attaches to a physician for failure to comply with a mandatory child abuse reporting statute rather than for breaching confidentiality by making a report to child protection authorities (this applies even when a report is ultimately unsubstantiated, provided that the report was made in good faith) (Milosavljevic and Brendel 2008).

Beginning in the 1960s, legislation emerged out of the child protection model to protect vulnerable adults, and by the mid-1970s, federal law was passed to establish adult protective services (Milosavljevic and Brendel 2008). Now, every U.S. jurisdiction identifies physicians as mandated reporters of suspected elder abuse and neglect (Milosavljevic and Brendel 2008). Akin to the jurisdictional variations in definitions of child abuse and neglect, the definition of elder abuse and neglect varies from state to state. That being said, most states use a standard incorporating five common elements: infliction of pain or injury, infliction of emotional or psychological harm, sexual assault, material or financial exploitation, and neglect (Kazim and Brendel 2004). Elder abuse standards may also include self-neglect in recognition of the frequency of waning self-care abilities that accompany age-related physical and cognitive decline (Abrams et al. 2002). Unlike reports of suspected child abuse, elder protection laws may recognize the ability of a competent elder to refuse investigation or intervention by protective services agencies.

The psychosomatic medicine practitioner should be aware of the risk factors and manifestations of elder abuse and neglect, especially since they may be more likely to encounter elders at risk due to their presentation with dementia and other mental status changes, as well as when hospitalized for medical consequences of neglect or abuse. As a whole, physicians may be inadequately trained to recognize elder mistreatment, at least in part due to the fact that the manifestations of abuse and neglect may be subtle and may be masked by illness or debility (Alpert et al. 1998; Melton 2002). Simply put, elderly victims of abuse and/or neglect may appear nothing more than frail or sick to the untrained clinician (Kahan and Paris 2003). The psychosomatic medicine physician is in a critically important role to detect elder mistreatment and to intervene to protect vulnerable geriatric patients due to the fact that hospitals and other health care settings may be the only source of help for these individuals. Therefore, practitioners should familiarize themselves with the reporting standards in the jurisdictions in which they practice. As with child abuse reporting, in regard to elder abuse and neglect reporting, physicians are more likely to face legal liability for *failure* to report than for good-faith reporting of suspected abuse and/or neglect, even when reports are "screened out" or found to be unsubstantiated following investigation by elder protective services.

Duties to Third Parties and the Duty to Protect

Since the landmark California Supreme Court Decision in *Tarasoff v. Board of Regents* in 1976, the concept of a duty to protect third parties from physical harm from patients has emerged as a well-known exception to doctor–patient confidentiality (Schouten and Brendel 2004). In this court decision, California's highest court engaged in an analysis of the complex balance between individual patient privacy and the public interest in preventing harm to hold that psychotherapists have a duty to act to protect third parties when the therapist knows or should know that the patient poses a risk of harm to a third party or parties (*Tarasoff v. Board of Regents* 1976). In the more than three decades since this landmark decision, clinicians and lawmakers alike have debated the relative priority of patient confidentiality and public safety in defining the parameters of the duty, for which situations clinicians will face professional and/or legal responsibility, and even whether the duty to warn or protect would apply in different jurisdictions.

Unlike mandated reporting of abuse and neglect, the duty to protect is not recognized in all jurisdictions (Almason 1997; Ginsberg 2004). It is therefore critical for practitioners to familiarize themselves with the law regarding the duty to protect in the jurisdiction(s) in which they practice. In general, many states have enacted statutory laws characterizing the scope of the duty to protect, and others have narrowed the scope of or eliminated the duty (Appelbaum et al. 1989; Kachigian and Felthous 2004). State laws regarding the duty to protect generally limit the situations in which the physician's duty to protect is triggered.

Statutory methods by which the psychiatrist's duty to protect and potential liability may be circumscribed include requiring a specific threat to an identified or identifiable victim, a clinician's knowledge of the patient's having a past history of violence, and/or a reasonable basis to anticipate violence prior to invocation of the duty to protect. In addition to defining and/or limiting the circumstances in which the duty to protect arises, state laws may also specify what measures mental health clinicians may or must take in order to satisfactorily comply with their duty to protect. These measures often include notifying the police or another law enforcement agency, hospitalizing the patient, or warning the potential victim. The Massachusetts statute is one that both limits the scope of the duty and defines measures by which the duty to protect can be discharged (Duty to warn patient's potential victims; cause of action [Mass. Gen. Laws Ch. 123, § 36B, 2005]).

One critical aspect of the duty to protect about which the psychosomatic medicine psychiatrist should be aware is that this duty often applies to psychiatrists and other mental health clinicians, but not to nonpsychiatric physicians and clinicians (Brendel and Cohen 2007; Brendel and Schouten 2007). In the setting of providing consultation to medical and surgical services, psychiatrists may be subject to duties to warn and/or protect that do not apply to the physician of record or the primary treatment team and which may create competing and conflicting obligations for the consultant and the consultee. For example, Massachusetts law requires all physicians to keep HIV-related information confidential unless the patient gives written informed consent for release of that information, but also has a statutory duty to protect that applies to psychiatrists and other mental health professionals (HLTV-III test; confidentiality; informed consent [Mass. Gen. Laws Ch. 11 § 70F, 2005]). In the case of an HIV-positive individual who is putting an unknowing sexual partner at risk, nonpsychiatric physicians are bound to confidentiality under the HIV confidentiality statute whereas psychiatrists have competing obligations under the duty to protect and HIV confidentiality laws (Brendel and Cohen 2007).

The complex tension between doctor–patient confidentiality and protecting patient privacy on one side and public protection and welfare on the other, as highlighted in the above example, is not a new one. In fact, the *Tarasoff* court relied on the precedent of mandated reporting of communicable diseases to public health authorities in its reasoning supporting the duty to protect third parties (*Tarasoff v. Board of Regents* 1976). Infectious disease reporting remains a well-established exception to doctor–patient confidentiality, and individual states, as well as the federal government, have enacted laws about which contagious diseases must be reported—to state public health officials, the Centers for Disease Control and Prevention, or both. Examples of reportable communicable diseases include HIV, varicella, viral hepatitis, severe acute respiratory syndrome, influenza, and syphilis (see, e.g., Averhoff et al. 2006). Reporting requirements vary from jurisdiction to jurisdiction, both in terms of what conditions are reportable and regarding the type and amount of information that must be reported. For example, in the case of HIV, different states vary in what information must accompany a report of a positive test result, including whether the report is anonymized or de-identified and whether partner/spousal notification occurs (Brendel and Cohen 2008; New York State Department of Health 2000, 2003). Physicians should also be aware that both before and following *Tarasoff*, doctors have faced civil liability for failure to disclose a patient's infection status that led to the infection of other individuals, highlighting how critically important it is for physicians to be aware of reporting requirements in the jurisdictions in which they practice (Bradshaw 1993; Gostin and Webber 1998; Liang 2002).

But while clinicians should be aware of the legal and regulatory requirements and constraints applicable to their practice, it is also critical to remember to think and act like clinicians. Simply put, clinicians should resist the tendency to think legally when difficult issues arise and instead act clinically in the setting of an understanding of the law or consultation with appropriate risk management or legal resources (Schouten and Brendel 2009). From the clinical perspective, the starting point for considering the responsibilities to breach confidentiality is the paradigm of doctor–patient confidentiality. The default rule is to protect patient confidentiality and privacy, and breaches for any reason must be carefully weighed and understood. Alternatives to releasing private information (e.g., hospitalization of a patient who has made threats) should be considered before a clinician breaches confidentiality (Beck 1998). In addition, even when a clinician is required to share patient information, only the minimum amount of information necessary to achieve the legal, regulatory, or clinical purpose should be disclosed.

Finally, circumstances may arise in which the consultation psychiatrist is asked to evaluate a patient whose legal status may draw into question the confidentiality of the interview. Examples of these situations include individuals in immigration, police, or correctional custody. In these situations, it is important for the psychiatrist to take steps to maximize the privacy of the interview and also to make the patient aware of the potential limitations on confidentiality inherent in the evaluation given the patient's custodial status. Furthermore, the psychiatrist should follow standard clinical practice regarding communication with law enforcement officials. Specifically, the clinician should consider all information gathered in the course of the interview as covered by doctor–patient confidentiality and limit contact with law enforcement to providing the minimum necessary to meet any mandated reporting obligations and to ensure the patient's safety. Where clinical sign-out is required to ensure the patient's safety, the psychiatrist should work to identify appropriate clinical personnel within the legal system to provide this pass-off and avoid communicating clinical information through nonclinical personnel (Schouten and Brendel 2009). Finally, where law enforcement officials seek to interview patients, clinicians should continue to maintain their therapeutic fiduciary stance relative to the patient and consider principles of patient autonomy, noninterference with medical care, protection of privacy, and maintenance of professional boundaries in making decisions about the appropriateness of these interviews (Jones et al. 2006).

Health Insurance Portability and Accountability Act

The paradigm of doctor–patient confidentiality often conjures up images of records in locked file cabinets and strict confidentiality for all patient information, especially in the field of psychiatry. As discussed above, however, over time, exceptions to the strict rule of doctor–patient confidentiality as codified by Hippocrates have emerged, recognizing that public safety and welfare considerations at times prevail over the safeguarding of private patient information by physicians. With Congress's passage of the HIPAA in 1996 and subsequent adoption of the regulations promulgated to implement HIPAA, the circumstances in which medical information could be released without the patient's explicit written informed consent was substantially broadened—not just for public safety but also for the purposes of payment and health care operations. Perhaps the most common misconception about HIPAA is that it makes it harder, rather than easier, to release a patient's medical information. As will be further elucidated, rather than promoting privacy, HIPAA has had the opposite effect, expanding the situations in which patient consent is *not* required for release of patient health information. If there is a take-home message about HIPAA, it is simple: the "P" in HIPAA is for portability, not privacy (Brendel and Bryan 2004). The effect of HIPAA has been to increase the circumstances in which patient information can be released without the specific informed consent of the patient (Brendel and Bryan 2004; Brendel 2005; Feld 2005).

With the passage of HIPAA, psychiatrists in particular were concerned about what effect it would have on the protection for often-sensitive psychiatric records, protections that until the passage of HIPAA were regulated by state law. HIPAA, a federal law, applies to health care providers performing "certain electronic transactions," and because these functions (e.g., electronic billing, eligibility determinations, claims processing) are performed by hospitals, most if not all psychosomatic medicine psychiatrists are covered by the provisions of HIPAA. HIPAA does not cover all information, but instead governs the management of "protected health information," which includes not only specific medical information about a mental or physical condition but also patient identifiers such as name or social security number, payment information, and records of treatment or services rendered (HIPAA Privacy Rule 2001).

The provisions of HIPAA most relevant to psychosomatic medicine clinicians relate to disclosure of medical information, patient access to information, and a category of records established by and defined by HIPAA known as "psychotherapy notes." When lawmakers passed HIPAA, they specifically aimed to improve the "efficiency and effectiveness" of the health care system (HIPAA 1996). In defining the parameters of what information should be considered protected health information under HIPAA, lawmakers engaged in a balancing between the important principles of confidentiality and privacy and the efficient functioning of an increasingly complex health care system, the functioning of which required regular sharing of information between multiple entities. HIPAA's implementation promoted efficiency by allowing the release of protected health information for treatment, payment, and health care operations purposes without specific informed consent from the patient. This move drew criticism from patient and privacy advocates who believed that the abolition of the consent requirement for release of records would become just the first step in a slippery slope of furthering administrative and operational concerns at the expense of doctor–patient confidentiality—a centuries-old ethical and legal cornerstone of medical treatment (Feld 2005; Friedrich 2001; Gordon 2002).

HIPAA is not a carte blanche for release of medical information. Federal regulations do limit disclosure of protected health information under HIPAA in several ways. First, under HIPAA, covered entities (such as hospitals) are required to inform patients of their practices under HIPAA in the form of privacy notices. In addition, patients may request a record of some disclosures of their protected health information. Finally, HIPAA is preempted by federal and state laws that provide greater protection than HIPAA does to protected health information, including records that are considered especially sensitive. For example, under federal law, records from alcohol and substance abuse treatment programs are considered especially sensitive and written informed consent is specially required for their release. Additionally, state laws vary from jurisdiction to jurisdiction but may require specific written informed consent for release of HIV testing and treatment records as well as records related to domestic violence and sexual assault (Brendel 2005; Brendel and Bryan 2004).

For the psychosomatic medicine psychiatrist pre-HIPAA, distinctions between the handling of medical and psychiatric records often caused confusion. Specifically, psychiatric records were often maintained separately from the general medical record and, even when contained within the medical record, they were subject to limitations on release. For example, at our institution, pre-HIPAA, psychiatric consultation notes contained within the hospital record were redacted before records were released to patients. Post-HIPAA, all psychiatry entries into the medical chart are considered part of the general medical record. The implications of HIPAA's inclusion of psychiatric records in the general medical chart are several. First, under HIPAA, the records may be released for treatment, payment, and health care operations purposes without specific consent. Second, HIPAA grants patients broad rights of access to their medical records. The practical effect of this broad right of access means that a patient's access to psychiatric records and psychiatric entries in the medical record may be denied only if a licensed professional makes a determination that release of the records to the patient would harm, endanger the life, or compromise the physical safety of the patient or another person (Brendel and Bryan 2004). It is especially important for psychosomatic medicine clinicians to be aware that patients have the right to access their records and will be allowed to do so—highlighting the need for careful documentation around sensitive issues, use of nonjudgmental terms and avoidance of jargon, and thoughtful formulation, as if the patient were looking over the clinician's shoulder.

Post-HIPAA, confusion frequently arises among psychiatrists regarding psychotherapy notes. It is critical for practitioners to be aware that while HIPAA affords extra protection for psychotherapy notes in recognition of the sensitive nature of psychiatric treatment, HIPAA's definition of psychotherapy notes is extremely narrow and does not preclude the patient, or others, from accessing the notes (Maio 2003). Very few notes of psychotherapy sessions, inpatient or outpatient, would qualify as psychotherapy notes under HIPAA, which specifically defines psychotherapy notes as a clinician's notes that document or analyze the contents of conversations in private counseling sessions and are kept separate from the rest of the patient's record. In addition, certain information that is more appropriately kept in a medical chart is not subject to the psychotherapy note protection of HIPAA, including medications information, results of tests, diagnosis, prognosis, progress, and treatment plans and goals (Appelbaum 2002; Brendel and Bryan 2004). Notes that qualify under the psychotherapy notes provision of HIPAA may not be released without specific authorization from the patient. In addition, patients do not have the right to access psychotherapy notes, but there is no prohibition on allowing patients to access their psychotherapy notes. Notwithstanding HIPAA, psychotherapy notes are treated as part of the medical record for legal purposes should the record be subpoenaed for litigation (Schouten and Brendel 2004).

Overall, as discussed above, HIPAA has had the effect of facilitating the release of medical information, in large part by departing from the consent requirement each time a patient's protected health information is released for treatment, payment, or health care operations purposes. In addition, HIPAA recognizes that consent is not required to release information in emergency, mandated reporting, and public safety and monitoring situations (Appelbaum 2002; Schouten and Brendel 2004). Clinicians should also be familiar with two additional points about HIPAA. First, HIPAA sets a floor regarding the minimum requirements for the protection of health information and states may enact laws that are more protective of patient privacy and more permissive of patient access. Second, even though HIPAA permits disclosure of protected health information without specific informed consent in many circumstances, clinicians should still use clinical judgment every time a disclosure is made and limit the information released to the minimum necessary amount to achieve the purpose of the disclosure.

Treatment Consent and Refusal

The psychosomatic medicine psychiatrist is often consulted to assess a patient's ability to understand proposed medical and surgical interventions, especially in settings in which the patient is refusing treatment that the treating clinician has determined to be medically necessary and to have a favorable risk-benefit ratio for the patient. The psychiatrist's threshold clinical determination of a patient's ability to make a decision is a capacity assessment. Capacity refers to an individual's ability to perform a task, such as making a medical decision. Competency is the legal analog of capacity and is presumed for all adults. Hence, clinicians make judgments of capacity and incapacity and judges make determinations of competency and incompetency (Appelbaum and Roth 1981; Brendel and Schouten 2007; Schouten and Brendel 2004; Schouten and Edersheim 2008).

Capacity or incapacity may be global or specific. An example of a globally incapacitated person is an individual in a coma. More commonly, psychiatrists are asked to evaluate task-specific capacity, such as the capacity to leave the hospital against medical advice, a frequently encountered capacity determination in the general hospital. Different tasks and decisions require different abilities and levels of understanding, and therefore the first step in any evaluation of capacity is to ask the question "Capacity for what?" In order to assess the degree to which the patient understands the information relevant to a decision, the psychiatrist must first have an understanding of the type of decision and circumstances the patient is facing (see also Chapter 3, "Ethical Issues").

Capacity Assessment

A patient's decisional capacity depends on an understanding of the underlying illness, proposed interventions, prognosis, and consequences of treatment and nontreatment. The most established method of capacity determination for medical decision making is a practical four-pronged analysis developed by Appelbaum and Grisso (Appelbaum 2007; Appelbaum and Grisso 1988). Under this model, the four factors for consideration in determining decisional capacity are preference, factual understanding, appreciation of the facts presented (i.e., how they relate to the specific individual), and rational manipulation of information. All four elements must be met in order for the individual to demonstrate decisional capacity. In practice, a patient's decisional capacity is rarely questioned when the patient is in agreement with the proposed medical interventions.

In assessing the preference element of capacity, the central facet is the patient's ability to communicate a consistent preference over time. A patient who is unable to demonstrate a stable preference regarding a decision—whether it be due to inability or unwillingness—lacks decisional capacity (though this is not meant to preclude patients' changing their mind). The second element of the four-part capacity evaluation is an assessment of the individual's factual understanding of his or her condition and the proposed treatment. It may be assessed through inquiry about the nature of the patient's illness or condition, the treatment options, the recommended treatment, the prognosis with and without treatment, and the risks and benefits of treatment. If the patient does not demonstrate a factual understanding, it is critical for the evaluator to assess why and also if the patient is capable of gaining a factual understanding. For example, a patient may not have a factual understanding of the relevant information because the primary treaters did not provide the information to the patient. A patient who has never been educated about his or her condition and recommended treatment cannot be expected to know the relevant information. On the other hand, if efforts have been made to inform the patient of the relevant information and the patient is unable to retain the relevant information, the patient may not be capable of acquiring the requisite information in order to meet the second prong of the capacity evaluation.

The third element in capacity assessment is a determination of whether the patient appreciates the significance of the information presented to him- or herself. Appreciation goes beyond a recitation of the facts and requires a broad perspective of the implications of the medical decision. Factors that may be explored in assessing appreciation include asking the patient about the consequences to him- or herself both of accepting and of refusing the proposed intervention and the consequences of one decision or another on the individual's future.

The fourth, and final, element of the standard capacity assessment for medical decision making requires the patient to demonstrate that his or her decision-making process is a rational one. The focus of inquiry and assessment is not on the final decision the patient makes, but rather on the process that the individual uses to arrive at that decision, taking into account the individual's past preferences and decisions. An often-used example to illustrate the importance of viewing the individual medical decision in the context of the patient's life, beliefs, and previous choices is that of a Jehovah's Witness who is faced with making a decision about whether to accept or refuse a lifesaving blood transfusion. In this case, the individual's decision to refuse the transfusion and face certain death might seem irrational on the surface, but in the context of this individual's faith-based life decisions and belief that accepting the transfusion would be contrary to religious doctrine would normally meet the rationality requirement. Assessing the rationality of the patient's decision-making process is the key element in determining whether seriously mentally ill patients have sufficient capacity for specific medical decisions. For example a chronic schizophrenic patient who refuses cancer chemotherapy because he does not think the side effects worth the limited benefits may well have sufficient capacity to do so even if he is delusional about other areas of his life. However, if the reason he is refusing is that he thinks the doctors are trying to control his mind through the infusion, he would most likely lack capacity. The question of whether mental illness has distorted a patient's thinking sufficiently to preclude capacity can arise in nonpsychotic disorders like major depression as well and can be particularly difficult when the patient has refused lifesaving treatment (Sullivan and Youngner 1994).

Informed Consent

Decisional capacity is a threshold requirement for the ability to give informed consent or refusal for treatment. In other words, a patient who is unable to make consistent and/or meaningful decisions cannot authorize, or for that matter refuse, proposed medical interventions. The process by which a patient agrees to permit a physician or other treater to do something to or for him or her is informed consent. Informed consent is required before any medical intervention because, in civil law, any unauthorized touching is a battery, including medical intervention. In the treatment context, a patient must therefore give informed consent before any intervention can begin and informed refusal if a treatment intervention is not authorized. Informed consent is an extension of broad principles of individual autonomy and has been a solid cornerstone of medical treatment since the 1960s (Dalla-Vorgia et al. 2001; Mohr 2000).

In hospital settings, informed consent may be equated with having a signed consent form on file. Clinicians should be aware that informed consent is not just signing a form but rather a process characterized by exchange of information, communication, and an active decision by the patient to accept or refuse the treatment. Through this active process, the legal standard of informed consent can be met. Specifically, in addition to decisional capacity, the legal standard for informed consent requires that it must be knowing (or intelligent) and voluntary (Appelbaum et al. 1987; *Salgo v. Leland Stanford Jr. University Board of Trustees* 1957; *Schloendorff v. Society of New York Hospital* 1914). The knowing/intelligent standard varies from jurisdiction to jurisdiction, with two general approaches (Schouten and Edersheim 2008). The first approach to the knowing standard is the reasonable professional standard and considers the information that is required to be presented to the patient in order for informed consent to be what a reasonable practitioner would tell a patient in similar circumstances. A small majority of states use this clinician-centered standard. The second is a patient-centered approach to the knowing requirement, is followed by a substantial minority of states, and defines the information required to meet the knowing standard as the information that an average or reasonable patient would use in coming to a decision. Some states go even further in employing the patient-centered approach and require an inquiry into what information the particular patient would find material or relevant in making a particular decision. This individual patient inquiry is often referred to as the materiality standard (Iheukwumere 2002). Two states use a hybrid approach incorporating both physician and patient focused inquiries in determining the amount of information that must be presented to the patient in order for informed consent to occur (King and Moulton 2006).

As a practical guide to sound clinical practice and risk management, the more information presented to the patient and the more extensive the communication about that information between the doctor and the patient, the better. That being said, there are six broad categories of information that, if presented to the patient, are generally accepted as meeting the standard of how much information needs to be presented, regardless of the particular jurisdictional standard (King and Moulton 2006):

1. The diagnosis and the nature of the condition being treated
2. The reasonably expected benefits from the proposed treatment
3. The nature and likelihood of the risks involved
4. The inability to precisely predict results of the treatment
5. The potential irreversibility of the treatment
6. The expected risks, benefits, and results of alternative, or no, treatment

There are limits to how much information physicians are required to share in the course of the informed consent process. Overall, the ideal of informed consent is a process incorporating a clear and frank discussion and exchange of information between doctor and patient (King and Moulton 2006). The necessity has been recognized of striking a balance among patients' right to know, fairness to physicians, and public policy considerations of avoiding unreasonable burdens on clinicians (*Precourt v. Frederick* 1985).

The second core element of informed consent is voluntariness. The patient must give consent freely and unencumbered by external coercive forces. A decision made under circumstances that limit the patient's ability to exercise a choice is not voluntary and does not meet the standard for informed consent (Faden and Beauchamp 1986; Keeton et al. 1984). Notwithstanding, distinguishing between voluntary and coerced choices requires a complex and nuanced inquiry (Roberts 2002). For example, patients may be under pressure from family members to make certain treatment decisions, and, in these situations, patients are generally determined to have acted voluntarily from both ethical and legal perspectives (although exceptions do exist) (Grisso and Appelbaum 1998; Mallary et al. 1986). However, individuals who are totally dependent on others for their care are generally (notwithstanding some debate on the issue) deemed unable to give voluntary consent to treatment or research because of the inherent inequality between the patient and the institution. Examples of individuals in this category include nursing home residents and prisoners (Gold 1974; Moser et al. 2004; National Commission for the Protection of Human Subjects of Biomedical and Behavioral Research 1976, 1978).

There are certain narrow and circumscribed situations in which informed consent is not required for the initiation of treatment, but these situations are the exception and not the rule (Meisel 1979; Schouten and Brendel 2004; Sprung and Winick 1989). The most common and well-known exception to the informed consent requirement is the emergency exception. For the purposes of exemption from the informed consent requirement, an emergency is a situation in which failure to treat would result in serious and potentially irreversible deterioration of the patient's condition. Invocation of the emergency exception is permissible only until the patient is stabilized, at which time informed consent must be obtained. In addition, the presence of an emergency is not enough to authorize treatment if the physician has knowledge that the patient would have refused the emergency treatment if he or she were able to express his or her wishes. The patient's prior expressed wishes cannot be overridden by an emergency (*Shine v. Vega* 1999).

Two additional narrow exceptions to informed consent are waiver and therapeutic privilege (Meisel 1979; Schouten and Brendel 2004; Sprung and Winick 1989). A competent patient may defer to the clinician or another party, thereby waiving his or her informed consent. In these situations, clinicians should carefully assess and thoroughly document the patient's capacity (Appelbaum et al. 1987). Therapeutic privilege applies when the consent process itself would worsen or contribute to a deterioration in the patient's condition (*Canterbury v. Spence* 1972; Dickerson 1995). In these circumstances, the physician may obtain consent for an intervention from an alternate decision maker. Therapeutic privilege does not apply, however, simply because there is a situation in which providing information to the patient could make the patient less likely to accept the proposed treatment. Over time, the justification for withholding information from a competent patient has narrowed so much that therapeutic privilege is rarely invoked (Bostick et al. 2006). In sum, the default rule is to obtain informed consent for all interventions and to view therapeutic privilege and waiver as two extremely narrow exceptions that should be used in only well-defined and cautiously characterized situations.

Advance Directives and Substitute Decision Making

When a patient lacks capacity to make medical decisions, an alternate decision maker must be identified to authorize medical intervention or to refuse treatment on behalf of the patient. This other person is referred to as a substitute or surrogate decision maker. The surrogate decision maker is charged with making decisions for the patient, and most often for making decisions according to what the patient would have wanted were he or she competent. This standard is known as the substituted judgment standard. In the case of minors and in some limited circumstances where substituted judgment cannot be applied, the substitute decision maker may be charged with making decisions in the patient's best interest (Schouten and Edersheim 2008).

Substitute decision makers may be either informally or formally appointed. Informal appointment occurs without judicial intervention. An advance directive is one common way of appointing a substitute decision maker. An advance directive is a document prepared and executed by an individual at a time when he or she is competent that either gives instructions to guide decisions or appoints a substitute decision maker should the individual become incapacitated at some time in the future. Two types of advance directives are the health care proxy and the durable power of attorney for health care. Both are characterized by a "springing clause," that is, once crafted, they remain inactive until such time as the patient, or principal, is incapacitated. At the time of incapacity and for the duration of the incapacity, the advance directive "springs" into effect. Should the patient regain capacity at a future time, the advance directive would again become inactive.

Since the passage of the federal Patient Self-Determination Act of 1990, hospitals have been legally required to inquire as to whether patients have an advance directive at the time the patient is admitted to the hospital and additionally required to provide information about advance directives. This law also required the provision of education about advance directives to health care personnel and community members about advance directives (Patient Self-Determination Act final revisions [60 C.F.R. 123, 1995]). Notwithstanding passage of this law, it is estimated that the majority of Americans still do not have advance directives (Brendel and Schouten 2007). In the absence of an advance directive, one of several pathways is generally followed. One legally recognized pathway available in some states is the use of a surrogate decision-making statute. In the absence of an advance directive, these laws give priorities to potential surrogate decision makers based on their relationship to the patient. For example, the Illinois law prioritizes the patient's guardian (if any) and then moves on to the patient's spouse, adult child, and then parent as the order in which a surrogate decision maker should be appointed. At the bottom of the list are more distant blood relatives, followed by close friends and the guardian of the estate (Health Care Surrogate Act 2005).

In the absence of an advance directive and of a state surrogate decision-making law, clinicians often defer decisions to family members at the bedside, especially in situations in which there is little or no disagreement about the course of care, about the patient's wishes, and between family members and when the proposed treatment is well established and low risk (Brendel and Cohen 2008; Schouten and Edersheim 2008). In situations where there is less clarity about interventions, proposed interventions are more intrusive, and/or there is disagreement between potential surrogate decision makers, the second type of substitute decision maker, or formal substitute decision maker, is more likely to be appointed. Formal surrogate decision makers are court appointed and are most commonly guardians.

Appointment of guardians is governed by state law. Increasingly, states have adopted guardianship laws and standards that derive from model legislation known as the Uniform Probate Code (UPC). Unlike a clinical finding of incapacity triggering the use of an informal advance directive, guardianship is a legal process that may include appointment of an attorney to represent the patient's values and interests, obtaining of independent medical opinions, and a formal court hearing. In addition, the standard for guardianship requires more than a finding of decisional incapacity. For example, UPC-derived state laws generally require three elements for imposition of a guardian: a clinically diagnosed condition, decision-making inability, and functional impairment. In order to obtain a treatment guardian for a patient, courts may look to neurocognitive assessment and functional testing to determine the need for and scope of the guardianship (Massachusetts Probate and Family Court 2009; Massachusetts UPC 2009). Finally, a guardian may be required, even when the treating clinicians do not believe that an intervention is intrusive. One example of a situation like this is the use of antipsychotic medications in Massachusetts (*Rogers v. Commissioner of Department of Mental Health* 1983).

Treatment Refusal and Involuntary Treatment

Consultation psychiatrists frequently become involved when medical inpatients refuse or are uncooperative with particular interventions, or decline treatment altogether. The legal criteria for involuntary medical treatment are based on capacity criteria and, where applicable, surrogate decision making, as discussed above. In other words, authorization for involuntary medical treatment is based on capacity criteria, and authorization for involuntary medical treatment depends on demonstrating that the patient does not have sufficient capacity to refuse treatment; it does not require that the patient's medical condition be life- or limb-threatening.

In contrast, the legal processes and criteria for temporary psychiatric detention and civil commitment do not as closely follow a decisional capacity–based approach (Byatt et al. 2006). Rather, while laws vary by state, the criteria for involuntary psychiatric detention in general require that the patient have a mental illness and pose a danger to self or to others due to mental illness or be unable to substantially perform self-care or maintain safety due to mental illness. In addition, many jurisdictions follow a bifurcated approach to detention and treatment, meaning that if a patient refuses psychiatric treatment following a psychiatric admission, treatment may proceed only after specific judicial authorization, emergently to prevent imminent harm, and/or with a second psychiatric opinion, depending on the jurisdiction. Some medically ill patients with psychiatric illness may require separate and parallel processes for authorization of medical treatment and for psychiatric admission and/or treatment.

Restraints

The psychiatric-legal issues surrounding the use of physical restraints are complex (Tardiff 1984). As for involuntary medical and psychiatric treatment, the paradigms for use of restraints for medical purposes and for psychiatric purposes are different. In the United States, the Joint Commission (formerly known as the Joint Commission for the Accreditation of Healthcare Organizations [JCAHO]) and the Center for Medicare and Medicaid Services have issued some guidance regarding the use of physical restraints in medical settings. In general, however, the use of restraints is frequent in medical and surgical hospital settings and is generally allowable to prevent interference with medical care. It is therefore commonplace to encounter physical restraint in inpatient medical settings, especially intensive care units (Glezer and Brendel, in press).

Consultation psychiatrists can assist nonpsychiatric colleagues and nurses in determining the risks and benefits of using restraints in general hospital settings. For example, physical restraints may be required in confused, medically unstable patients if chemical restraint is ineffective or contraindicated. If restraints are not used in some patients with delirium or dementia, they may pull out intravenous or arterial lines, endotracheal tubes, or other vital treatment interventions, and this risk often cannot be safely eliminated with sedation alone. Psychiatrists in medical settings can help explore the various options for managing the patient and address the discomfort staff may have in using restraints. It is important to bear in mind that there are clinical and legal risks inherent in using restraints as well as in failing to employ restraints for patient treatment and safety. As a general guideline, the decision about whether to use physical restraints in medical settings should ultimately be determined by what is required to provide necessary medical treatment, and the physician and other clinical staff should document their reasoning for the decision to use physical restraints in the medical record.

In contrast to the use of physical restraints in medical settings, the use of physical restraints on psychiatric units is more limited, and many psychiatric units and facilities have adopted no-restraint policies. Generally, the use of physical restraints in psychiatric settings is legally appropriate only when a patient presents an imminent risk of harm to self or others and a less restrictive alternative is not available.

Discharges Against Medical Advice

Discharges against medical advice (AMA) account for approximately 1% of discharges for general medical patients. AMA discharges commonly occur when patients are experiencing conflict in the doctor-patient relationship, are too anxious about their medical condition or treatment to engage in the treatment, have personal or work pressures to leave the hospital, or have an addictive disorder that has not been adequately diagnosed or treated in the hospital (e.g., nicotine withdrawal or cocaine craving) (Alfandre 2009). Decisions about AMA discharges generally follow the decisional capacity-based model of medical treatment refusal. Specifically, since medical patients are admitted voluntarily to a general hospital, an AMA discharge is akin to a withdrawal of the original consent to hospitalization. Therefore, one role of the consulting psychiatrist is to perform a capacity assessment to determine whether the patient has the requisite capacity to decide to leave the hospital AMA. In addition, the psychiatrist can explore why the patient wants to leave the hospital and, when possible and appropriate, help effect a solution leading to willingness of the patient to remain in the hospital. In other words, the psychiatrist can play a key role in depolarizing a standoff between the patient and the care team.

Care providers often believe that an AMA discharge is an automatic protection from liability (Devitt et al. 2000). Too often, hospital personnel are intent on getting a patient to sign an AMA discharge form, but the form is neither necessary nor sufficient to avoid legal liability. Regardless of whether the patient signs an AMA discharge form, a clear assessment of decisional capacity should be performed, and clear and complete documentation should be made in the medical record of the capacity assessment, the recommendations given to the patient regarding the need for and nature of follow-up care, and the possible risks of premature discharge (Gerbasi and Simon 2003). Medical patients who lack decisional capacity may be kept in the hospital against their will in cases of emergency, until either judicial approval or other authorized surrogate consent can be obtained. Unlike holding a patient involuntarily for psychiatric reasons, involuntary medical hospitalization in these limited circumstances generally does not require a finding of dangerousness to self or to others.

When efforts to convince a competent patient to remain in the hospital fail, a power struggle may ensue and members of the health care team often become angry at the patient. Such anger is not clinically constructive and may contribute to legal liability. For example, some physicians believe that they should refuse to give the departing AMA patient any outpatient prescriptions, thinking that would potentially make them liable for the patient's subsequent clinical course. However, if stopping the medication would endanger the patient (e.g., a beta-blocker after an acute myocardial infarction), it may be both ethical and prudent to give the patient a time-limited prescription, even if the patient wishes to leave the hospital. The patient should be told that he is welcome to return to the hospital if he changes his mind or his symptoms get worse, and robust efforts should be made to secure and convince the patient to accept follow-up care.

Emergency Treatment Requirements and EMTALA

The Emergency Medical Treatment and Active Labor Act (EMTALA), a U.S. federal law enacted in 1986, obligates emergency departments of all hospitals that participate in Medicare to examine patients who seek emergency care and to either stabilize them before discharge or admit or transfer them to another willing facility if medically indicated (Quinn et al. 2002). EMTALA has the effect of preventing health care providers from discriminating against patients who need medical care but are unable to pay. Issues with EMTALA may arise when patients who present to emergency rooms with unstable medical and psychiatric illness are uncooperative with treatment. For example, if a dialysis patient who has been banned from a hospital's outpatient dialysis program because of aggressive behavior toward staff and other patients comes to that hospital's emergency room with severe uremia or hyperkalemia, he or she must be provided with emergent dialysis nonetheless.

Conflicts may also occur between hospitals and between physicians when a patient appears too psychiatrically unstable to be treated in a medical facility and too medically unstable to be transferred to a psychiatric facility. The potential penalties for violations of the law are severe, and as such, in these situations, emergency physicians may admit patients to either a medical or psychiatric setting against the advice of psychiatric and medical colleagues out of fear of EMTALA liability. EMTALA applies only to emergency settings and does not apply to discharges from medical or psychiatric inpatient units, as clarified in 2003 EMTALA rules. However, issues regarding the transfer of psychiatric patients were not addressed in the new rules (Saks 2004).

Malpractice

Like all physicians, the consultation psychiatrist must meet the standard of care in treating patients. The responsibility of the consultant, however, is different than that of the treating physician. Specifically, the consultation psychiatrist's duty is to the consultee, or the physician who requests the consult. The consultant must provide competent consultation to the requesting physician (Brendel and Schouten 2007; Schouten and Brendel 2004). Conversely, the responsibility of the treating clinician is directly to the patient. However, consultants should be cautious in maintaining boundaries between the role of consultant and taking on the role of a treating clinician. For example, if the consultant recommends that the consultee (treating physician) prescribe a medication, the consultant's duty is to provide appropriate recommendations and information to the consultee. But, if the consultant directly enters an order for the medication to be given to the patient, the consultant will generally be held to have assumed a direct treatment role and assumed a direct responsibility to the patient. If the consultant does assume a primary treatment role (and there may be good reasons for the consultant to do so), it is important for the consultant to be cognizant that he or she has assumed the responsibility of a treating psychiatrist, including the responsibility to either monitor and follow-up on the patient's progress or arrange for another clinician to do so.

Physicians—and the psychosomatic medicine psychiatrist is no exception—often fear legal liability and malpractice lawsuits. There is good reason to be concerned, given that defending a malpractice lawsuit, regardless of the outcome, is a personally and professionally burdensome endeavor (Schouten et al. 2008). That being said, the best way to avoid malpractice litigation is to exercise sound clinical judgment, engage in judicious clinical practice, and communicate well with consultees and patients (Schouten et al. 2008). At the same time, familiarity with the legal concept of malpractice and a basic understanding of physicians' responsibilities may help the practitioner contextualize malpractice within the context of treatment and health care delivery.

Malpractice is an area of tort law that covers personal injuries resulting from medical interventions (Brendel and Schouten 2007; Schouten and Brendel 2004; Schouten et al. 2008). To establish a claim of malpractice, four elements must be met. First, a duty must be established, either by the existence of a direct doctor–patient relationship or a consultant–consultee relationship. In some cases, even limited or cursory interactions may be considered by the court to have constituted a doctor–patient relationship. Second, a breach of that duty must have occurred (i.e., a violation of the standard of care). Third, this breach must have directly caused harm to a patient that resulted in the fourth element, or damage to the patient. The legal requirement for malpractice is often summarized as the four *Ds*: duty, dereliction of duty, direct causation, and damage. Malpractice does not require that the physician acted intentionally in causing harm to the patient. Rather, malpractice is an unintentional tort, a tort of negligence, which means that deviation from the accepted standard of care caused damage to the patient.

As a final note, studies of malpractice lawsuits have shown that only a small number of cases involving injury to patients due to medical errors actually lead to malpractice claims or litigation and that defendants prevail in the majority of cases that lead to litigation (Localio et al. 1991; Schouten et al. 2008). Notwithstanding, in a study of paid claims, no medical error was found in up to one-third of claims, highlighting the fact that even error-free practice does not insulate against malpractice liability (Schouten et al. 2008; see also Brennan et al. 1996). As a practical matter, physicians can reduce their risk of malpractice liability by recognizing individual and systemic factors contributing to errors, communicating effectively with colleagues and patients, acknowledging error and preserving relationships, maintaining good records, avoiding overlegalization and focusing on good clinical care, and consulting with colleagues (Schouten et al. 2008).

Conclusion

Issues at the interface of clinical practice and the law may arise frequently in the practice of psychosomatic medicine. Areas in which legal and quasilegal principles emerge include confidentiality and exceptions thereto, HIPAA, capacity determinations, informed consent and refusal, and concerns about malpractice liability. The best rule of thumb is for clinicians to be aware of relevant legal and regulatory provisions in the jurisdictions in which they practice but to leave lawyering to lawyers and, instead, act clinically. At the same time, it is important for the psychiatric consultant to be aware of available legal and risk management resources for consultation when legal issues and concerns arise in the course of treating patients. Finally, it is important for the consulting psychiatrist to be cognizant of his or her role in patients' treatment by maintaining an awareness of his or her role vis-à-vis the patients and to maintain clarity between consultative and direct treatment roles.

References

Abrams LC, Lachs M, McAvay G, et al: Predictors of self-neglect in community-dwelling elders. Am J Psychiatry 159:1724–1730, 2002

Alfandre DJ: "I'm going home": discharges against medical advice. Mayo Clin Proc 84:255–260, 2009

Almason AL: Personal liability implications of the duty to warn are hard pills to swallow: from *Tarasoff* to *Hutchinson v Patel* and beyond. J Contemp Health Law Policy 13:471–496, 1997

Alpert EJ, Tonkin AE, Seeherman AM, et al: Family violence curricula in US medical schools. Am J Prev Med 14:273–282, 1998

American Psychiatric Association: Position Statement on Confidentiality. Washington, DC, American Psychiatric Association, 1978

American Psychiatric Association: The Principles of Medical Ethics With Annotations Especially Applicable to Psychiatry. Washington, DC, American Psychiatric Association, 2001

Appelbaum PS: Privacy in psychiatric treatment. Am J Psychiatry 159:1809–1811, 2002

Appelbaum PS: Clinical practice: assessing patients' competence to consent to treatment. N Engl J Med 357:1834–1840, 2007

Appelbaum PS, Grisso T: Assessing patients' capacities to consent to treatment. N Engl J Med 319:1635–1638, 1988

Appelbaum PS, Roth LH: Clinical issues in the assessment of competency. Am J Psychiatry 138:1462–1467, 1981

Appelbaum PS, Lidz CW, Meisel A: Informed Consent: Legal Theory and Clinical Practice. New York, Oxford University Press, 1987

Appelbaum PS, Zonana H, Bonnie R, et al: Statutory approaches to limiting psychiatrists' liability for their patients' violent acts. Am J Psychiatry 146:821–828, 1989

Averhoff F, Zimmerman L, Harpaz R, et al: Varicella surveillance practices—United States, 2004. Centers for Disease Control and Prevention (CDC). MMWR Morb Mortal Wkly Rep 55(41):1126–1129, 2006

Beck JC: Legal and ethical duties of the clinician treating a patient who is liable to be impulsively violent. Behav Sci Law 16:375–389, 1998

Bostick NA, Sade R, McMahon JW, et al: American Medical Association Council on Ethical and Judicial Affairs: Report of the American Medical Association Council on Ethical and Judicial Affairs: withholding information from patients: rethinking the propriety of "therapeutic privilege." J Clin Ethics 17:302–306, 2006

Bradshaw v Daniel, 854 SW2d 865 (Tenn 1993)

Brendel RW: An approach to forensic issues, in The Ten-Minute Guide to Psychiatric Diagnosis and Treatment. Edited by Stern TA. New York, Professional Publishing Group, 2005, pp 399–412

Brendel RW, Brendel DH: Professionalism and the doctor-patient relationship in psychiatry, in The Ten-Minute Guide to Psychiatric Diagnosis and Treatment. Edited by Stern TA. New York, Professional Publishing Group, 2005, pp 1–7

Brendel RW, Bryan E: HIPAA for psychiatrists. Harv Rev Psychiatry 12:177–183, 2004

Brendel RW, Cohen MA: Ethical issues, advance directives, and surrogate decision-making, in Comprehensive Textbook of AIDS Psychiatry. Edited by Cohen MA, Gorman J. New York, Oxford University Press, 2008, pp 577–584

Brendel RW, Schouten R: Legal concerns in psychosomatic medicine. Psychiatr Clin N Am 30:663–676, 2007

Brennan TA, Sox CM, Burstin HR: Relation between negligent adverse events and the outcomes of medical-malpractice litigation. N Engl J Med 335:1963–1967, 1996

Byatt N, Pinals D, Arikan R: Involuntary hospitalization of medical patients who lack decisional capacity: an unresolved issue. Psychosomatics 47:443–448, 2006

Canterbury v Spence, 464 F2d 772 (DC 1972)

Child Abuse Prevention and Treatment Act, PL 92-273; 42 USC § 5101 (2003)

Dalla-Vorgia P, Skiadas P, Garanis-Papadatos T: Is consent in medicine a concept of only modern times? J Med Ethics 27:59–61, 2001

Devitt PJ, Devitt AC, Dewan M: Does identifying a discharge as "against medical advice" confer legal protection? J Fam Pract 49:224–227, 2000

Dickerson DA: A doctor's duty to disclose life expectancy information to terminally ill patients. Clevel State Law Rev 43:319–350, 1995

Duty to warn patient's potential victims; cause of action. Mass Gen Laws Ch 123, § 36B (2005)

Emergency Medical Treatment and Active Labor Act (EMTALA), 42 USC § 1395dd (1986)

Faden RR, Beauchamp TL: A History and Theory of Informed Consent. New York, Oxford University Press, 1986

Feld AD: The Health Insurance Portability and Accountability Act (HIPAA): its broad effect on practice. Am J Gastroenterol 100:1440–1443, 2005

Friedrich MJ: Practitioners and organizations prepare for approaching HIPAA deadlines [medical news and perspectives]. JAMA 286:1563–1565, 2001

Gerbasi JB, Simon RI: Patients' rights and psychiatrists' duties: discharging patients against medical advice. Harv Rev Psychiatry 11:333–343, 2003

Ginsberg B: Tarasoff at thirty: victim's knowledge shrinks the psychotherapist's duty to warn and protect. J Contemp Health Law Policy 21:1–35, 2004

Glezer A, Brendel RW: Beyond emergencies: the use of restraints in medical and psychiatric settings. Harv Rev Psychiatry (in press)

Gold JA: Kaimowitz v Department of Mental Health: involuntary mental patient cannot give informed consent to experimental psychosurgery. Rev Law Soc Change 4:207–227, 1974

Gordon S: Privacy standards for health information: the misnomer of administrative simplification. Delaware Law Review 5:23–56, 2002

Gostin LO, Webber DW: HIV infection and AIDS in the public health and health care systems: the role of law and litigation. JAMA 279:1108–1113, 1998

Grisso T, Appelbaum PS: Assessing Competence to Consent to Treatment: A Guide for Physicians and Other Health Professionals. New York, Oxford University Press, 1998

Hall MA, Schulman KA: Ownership of medical information. JAMA 301:1282–1284, 2009

Health Care Surrogate Act, 755 Ill Comp Stat 40 (2005)

Health Insurance Portability and Accountability Act of 1996 (HIPAA), PL 104-191

HIPAA Privacy Rule, 45 CFR 164.512 (2001)

HLTV-III test; confidentiality; informed consent. Mass Gen Laws Ch 11 § 70F (2005)

Iheukwumere EO: Doctor: are you experienced? The relevance of disclosure of physician experience to a valid informed consent. J Contemp Health Law Policy 18:373–419, 2002

Jones PM, Appelbaum PS, Siegel DM: Law enforcement interviews of hospital patients: a conundrum for clinicians. JAMA 295:822–825, 2006

Kachigian C, Felthous AR: Court responses to Tarasoff statutes. J Am Acad Psychiatry Law 32:263–273, 2004

Kahan FS, Paris BE: Why elder abuse continues to elude the health care system. Mt Sinai J Med 70:62–68, 2003

Kazim A, Brendel RW: Abuse and neglect, in Massachusetts General Hospital Psychiatry Update and Board Preparation, 2nd Edition. Edited by Stern TA, Herman JB. New York, McGraw-Hill, 2004, pp 539–544

Keeton WP, Dobbs DB, Keeton RE, et al: Prosser and Keeton on the Law of Torts, 5th Edition. St Paul, MN, West Publishing, 1984

King JS, Moulton BW: Rethinking informed consent: the case for shared medical decision-making. Am J Law Med 32:429–493, 2006

Liang BA: Medical information, confidentiality, and privacy. Hematol Oncol Clin North Am 16:1433–1447, 2002

Lloyd GER (ed): Hippocrates: The oath, in Hippocratic Writings. Translated by Chadwick J, Mann WN. London, Penguin Books, 1983, p 67

Localio AR, Lawthers AG, Brennan TA, et al: Relation between malpractice claims and adverse events due to negligence. Results of the Harvard Medical Practice Study III. N Engl J Med 325:245–251, 1991

Maio JE: HIPAA and the special status of psychotherapy notes. Lippincotts Case Manag 8:24–29, 2003

Mallary SD, Gert B, Culver CM: Family coercion and valid consent. Theor Med 7:123–126, 1986

Massachusetts Probate and Family Court, MPC 902 (Instructions to Clinicians for Completing the Medical Certificate for Guardianship or Conservatorship), 2009. Available at: http://www.mass.gov/courts/courtsandjudges/courts/probateandfamilycourt/upc/mpc902-instructions-to-clinicians.pdf. Accessed October 1, 2009.

Massachusetts Uniform Probate Code, Article V (Protection of Persons Under Disability and Their Property), 2009

Meisel A: The "exceptions" to the informed consent doctrine: striking a balance between competing values in medical decision making. Wis L Rev 1979:413–488, 1979

Melton GB: Chronic neglect of family violence: more than a decade of reports to guide US policy. Child Abuse Negl 26:569–586, 2002

Milosavljevic N, Brendel RW: Abuse and neglect, in Comprehensive Clinical Psychiatry. Edited by Stern TA, Rosenbaum JF, Fava M, et al. Philadelphia, PA, Mosby/Elsevier, 2008, pp 1133–1142

Mohr JC: American medical malpractice litigation in historical perspective. JAMA 283:1731–1737, 2000

Moser DJ, Arndt S, Kanz JE, et al: Coercion and informed consent in research involving prisoners. Compr Psychiatry 45:1–9, 2004

National Commission for the Protection of Human Subjects of Biomedical and Behavioral Research: Report and Recommendations: Research Involving Prisoners. Washington, DC, U.S. Government Printing Office, 1976

National Commission for the Protection of Human Subjects of Biomedical and Behavioral Research: Research Involving Those Institutionalized as Mentally Infirm: Report and Recommendations. Washington, DC, U.S. Government Printing Office, 1978

New York State Department of Health: HIV reporting and partner notification questions and answers. 2000. Available at: http://www.health.state.ny.us. Accessed March 26, 2006.

New York State Department of Health AIDS Institute: Identification and ambulatory care of HIV-exposed and -infected adolescents, Appendix B: summary, HIV reporting and partner notification. 2003. Available at: http://www.hivguidelines.org. Accessed April 16, 2006.

Patient Self-Determination Act of 1990, 42 USC 1395 cc(a); final rule: 60 CFR 123 at 33294 (1995)

Precourt v Frederick, 481 NE2d 1144 (Mass 1985)

Quinn DK, Geppert CM, Maggiore WA: The Emergency Medical Treatment and Active Labor Act of 1985 and the practice of psychiatry. Psychiatr Serv 53:1301–1307, 2002

Roberts LW: Informed consent and the capacity for voluntarism. Am J Psychiatry 159:705–712, 2002

Robinson DJ, O'Neill D: Access to health care records after death: balancing confidentiality with appropriate disclosure. JAMA 297:634–636, 2007

Rogers v Commissioner of Department of Mental Health, 458 NE2d 308 (Mass 1983)

Saks SJ: Call 911: psychiatry and the new Emergency Medical Treatment and Active Labor Act (EMTALA) regulations. J Psychiatry Law 32:483–512, 2004

Salgo v Leland Stanford Jr. University Board of Trustees, 154 Cal App 2d 560, 317 P2d 170 (1957)

Schloendorff v Society of New York Hospital, 105 NE 92 (NY 1914)

Schouten R, Brendel RW: Legal aspects of consultation, in The Massachusetts General Hospital Handbook of General Hospital Psychiatry, 5th Edition. Edited by Stern TA, Fricchione GL, Cassem EH, et al. Philadelphia, PA, CV Mosby, 2004, pp 349–364

Schouten R, Brendel RW: Common pitfalls in giving medical-legal advice to trainees and supervisees. Harv Rev Psychiatry 17:291–294, 2009

Schouten R, Edersheim JG: Informed consent, competency, treatment refusal, and civil commitment, in Massachusetts General Hospital Comprehensive Clinical Psychiatry. Edited by Stern TA, Rosenbaum JF, Fava M, et al. Philadelphia, PA, Mosby/Elsevier, 2008, pp 1143–1154

Schouten R, Brendel RW, Edersheim JG: Malpractice and boundary violations, in Massachusetts General Hospital Comprehensive Clinical Psychiatry. Edited by Stern TA, Rosenbaum JF, Fava M, et al. Philadelphia, PA, Mosby/Elsevier, 2008, pp 1165–1175

Shine v Vega, 429 Mass 456, 709 NE2d 58 (Mass 1999)

Siegler M: Sounding Boards. Confidentiality in medicine—a decrepit concept. N Engl J Med 307:1518–1521, 1982

Sprung CL, Winick BJ: Informed consent in theory and practice: legal and medical perspectives on the informed consent doctrine and a proposed reconceptualization. Crit Care Med 17:1346–1354, 1989

Sullivan MD, Youngner SJ: Depression, competence, and the right to refuse lifesaving medical treatment. Am J Psychiatry 151:971–978, 1994

Tarasoff v Board of Regents of the University of California, 17 Cal3d 425 (1976)

Tardiff K (ed): The Psychiatric Uses of Seclusion and Restraint. Washington, DC, American Psychiatric Press, 1984

CHAPTER 3

Ethical Issues

Donald L. Rosenstein, M.D.

Franklin G. Miller, Ph.D.

ETHICAL ISSUES ARE CENTRAL to both the practice of psychosomatic medicine and the professional identity of its practitioners. Psychiatrists who work in medical and surgical settings routinely perform clinical evaluations and make treatment recommendations with deep moral significance. For example, psychiatrists render opinions about whether medically ill patients can make decisions about their own care, whether they pose a danger to themselves or others, or whether they are appropriate candidates to either donate or receive an organ. These clinical assessments bear directly on patients' autonomy and the course of their medical treatment. Similarly, psychiatrists who provide end-of-life care frequently confront the possibility that medical interventions provided to their patients delay death rather than prolong life. The fact that no clear lines of demarcation exist between these types of clinical considerations and their ethical ramifications makes the practice of clinical ethics in psychosomatic medicine both compelling and challenging. All consulting psychiatrists should be adept at identifying ethical issues related to the practice of psychosomatic medicine and be familiar with laws, ethical rules, principles, and standards that provide guidance in solving moral problems in patient care.

Historically, practitioners of psychosomatic medicine and consultation-liaison psychiatry have been active and influential participants in the ethical life of hospitals, hospice settings, and nursing homes. Many serve as members or chairs of ethics committees, institutional review boards (IRBs), and ethics consultation services (Bourgeois et al. 2006). Even for clinical or research psychiatrists who do not participate in these formal ethics activities, the practice of psychosomatic medicine requires a familiarity with the principles of biomedical ethics.

The routine care of medically ill patients usually requires neither psychiatric consultation nor explicit ethical deliberation. However, when difficulties arise in the provision of clinical care, ethical and psychiatric concerns are often packaged together in partially formulated and emotionally charged requests for help (Lederberg 1997). In some cases, a psychiatric disorder may be inaccurately perceived as an ethical problem. For example, a patient's missed dialysis appointments might be interpreted as refusal of treatment when the patient's absences are actually a result of panic attacks. In this case, proper psychiatric evaluation and clinical intervention may obviate misplaced ethical concerns. Conversely, a legitimate ethical dilemma (i.e., an impasse in the clinical care of a patient because of conflicting moral values) can prompt a misguided request for a psychiatric evaluation (e.g., disagreement between family members and the medical team about the value of continued aggressive medical interventions for a severely ill and clearly incompetent patient). This second example requires careful moral deliberation among the relevant stakeholders rather than a specialist's assessment of the patient's decision-making capacity (DMC). Such cases often require a legal opinion and/or the help of an ethics consultant or committee. Nonetheless, the successful resolution of the ethical issues may not be possible un-

The opinions expressed are the views of the authors and do not necessarily reflect the policy of the National Institutes of Health, the Public Health Service, or the U.S. Department of Health and Human Services.

til the presence of psychopathology in the patient, or a systems problem involving the health care team, has been identified and addressed by the psychiatric consultant.

Psychiatrists and ethicists are frequently consulted on the same challenging cases at the same urgent moment. Just as the psychiatrist has been trained to enter carefully into a complex and dynamic health care system, gather information, and formulate the proper questions in the proper sequence, so too must the ethicist. Either consultant may call for a multidisciplinary team meeting to facilitate the critical decision makers talking with one another in the same room rather than through notes in the patient's chart.

Although many of the core skills needed for effective psychiatric intervention are also required for the resolution of ethical dilemmas that arise in the care of medically ill patients, important distinctions exist between the tasks and methods of these two consultative activities. Psychiatric consultation follows the medical model of providing expert advice on diagnosis and therapy. Physicians who request psychiatric consultations are seeking specific answers to specific questions. They want to be told precisely how to manage a certain aspect of their patient's care. Health care professionals often desire the same type of direction from an ethics consultant. However, within the bioethics community, the traditional medical model is one of the least favored approaches to ethics consultation. Instead, most ethics committees and consultation services work to facilitate discussion and conflict resolution between the stakeholders in the case. The purpose of this process-oriented approach is to identify the range of ethically permissible options rather than to provide a single "right answer" or stipulate a specific course of action. The consulting psychiatrist should be able to identify relevant ethical issues that fall outside the scope of the psychiatric question and encourage wider moral deliberation. Similarly, the ethics consultant who can identify unaddressed clinical concerns (e.g., is the patient depressed, anxious, or confused?) can help resolve an apparent ethical problem by bringing the prior clinical questions to the attention of the medical team or psychiatrist.

The purpose of this chapter is to provide a framework for integrating ethical considerations into the practice of psychosomatic medicine. The chapter is organized into two sections. The first section provides an overview of the discipline of ethics and the rules governing the behavior of physicians. The second section includes a case vignette to illustrate the complex interplay among several key clinical and ethical issues encountered in psychosomatic medicine and the process of moral deliberation. The case narrative is interrupted at critical junctures to facilitate a discussion of specific ethical issues as they might unfold in actual practice (e.g., DMC and treatment refusal; involuntary medication; withdrawal of care). The primary focus of the case is on ethical issues related to the provision of clinical care, but we also discuss the relevant differences between the ethics of clinical medicine and the ethics of clinical research.

We do not cover all ethical issues in psychosomatic medicine. Relevant legal considerations are discussed in Chapter 2 ("Legal Issues"). Specific ethical topics covered elsewhere in this book include physician-assisted suicide in Chapter 9 ("Suicidality"), terminal weaning in Chapter 19 ("Lung Disease"), dialysis decisions in Chapter 21 ("Renal Disease"), transplant candidate and donor issues in Chapter 31 ("Organ Transplantation"), sterilization in Chapter 33 ("Obstetrics and Gynecology"), placebos in Chapter 36 ("Pain"), and palliative care in Chapter 41 ("Palliative Care"). Readers are referred to other sources for ethics topics not covered, including confidentiality (Kimball and Silverman 1978), truth telling (Horikawa et al. 1999, 2000), and the scope of the psychiatric consultant's role in medical settings (Agich 1985).

Overview of the Discipline of Ethics

The discipline of ethics consists of systematic investigation and analysis of moral issues, including judgments concerning deliberation and conduct in specific situations, the identification and application of appropriate moral rules or principles, methods of justifying actions and practices, and the development of moral character. In the field of medical ethics, the focus of inquiry is often morally problematic cases involving complex interactions between health care professionals and patients (or research subjects) in which competing moral considerations are relevant. Ethical inquiry aimed at resolving a problem in patient care, or clinical research, proceeds in accordance with a series of connected steps (Fins et al. 1997). First, the factual contours of the case should be investigated, including the pertinent medical facts, the patient's needs and preferences, legal considerations, institutional contexts, and attitudes and actions of involved professionals. Second, the moral considerations relevant to the case are identified and assessed. This calls for discerning the bearing of specific moral rules and principles on the case and their relative weight in determining what to do when such moral considerations conflict. Third, a decision is made on a plan of action to resolve the moral problem. Finally, the plan is implemented, and its results are evaluated. Typically, all these stages of ethical inquiry take place within a process of discussion among the individuals with a stake in the outcome of the case, which may also include ethics consultation with an ethicist or ethics committee in especially difficult situations.

The most general moral considerations guiding ethical inquiry in medical contexts are the principles of biomedical ethics. The leading conception identifies four such principles (Beauchamp and Childress 2009).

1. *Respect for patient autonomy* requires that professionals recognize the right of competent adult individuals to make their own decisions about health care or research participation. This includes the obligation to obtain informed consent and the right of competent patients to refuse recommended diagnostic interventions or therapy or to decline an invitation to enroll in research.
2. In the therapeutic context, *beneficence* directs professionals to promote the health and well-being of particular patients by offering and providing competent medical care; in research, it directs investigators to produce valuable knowledge with the aim of improving medical care for future patients.
3. *Nonmaleficence* enjoins professionals to avoid harming patients or research subjects. Taken together, beneficence and nonmaleficence underlie the obligation of clinicians to assess the risk-benefit ratios of patient care and research interventions.
4. The principle of *justice* requires that medical care and research are performed in a way that is fair and equitable.

Complex moral problems in medicine are rarely resolved by simple application of one of these principles. The specific relevance and weight of principles and subsidiary moral considerations are assessed in the deliberative process of ethical inquiry. An extensive and instructive account of the meaning and application of these principles is presented in *Principles of Biomedical Ethics* by Beauchamp and Childress (2009).

Ethical considerations relevant to the ethical practice of medicine and research are incorporated into various medical oaths (e.g., Hippocratic oath) and codes (e.g., Nuremberg Code, American Medical Association's Code of Medical Ethics; American Medical Association 2001), declarations (Helsinki; World Medical Association 2008) and reports, guidelines, policies, and laws regarding the behavior of physicians. Some of these documents conflict with one another, and some are even internally inconsistent with respect to permissible activities (Miller and Shorr 2002). Indeed, many physicians find their own beliefs at odds with existing laws and policies concerning specific medical practices (e.g., abortion, physician-assisted suicide, use of medical marijuana).

No code of ethics is specific to the practice of psychosomatic medicine. The most relevant professional documents are the American Medical Association's Code of Medical Ethics and the American Psychiatric Association's annotation of this code (American Psychiatric Association 2001). The American Psychiatric Association's annotation goes into substantial detail regarding specific behaviors (e.g., sexual boundary violations, breaches of confidentiality, fee splitting, abandonment of patients) and is directly relevant to all psychiatric practice, including subspecialties. However, certain aspects of the practice of psychosomatic medicine pose ethical challenges that are not specifically addressed by these codes. The following case illustrates several of these difficult issues and suggests a clinically oriented approach to their resolution.

Case Vignette

Mrs. F, a 61-year-old divorced woman, was hospitalized for treatment of advanced breast cancer. She was first diagnosed with breast cancer in her mid-50s and appeared to be free of disease for 5 years after her initial diagnosis. Approximately 6 months ago, she presented with evidence of metastatic disease and received a second course of chemotherapy.

On the day before admission, she went to see her oncologist because of extreme low back pain. Diagnostic imaging identified multiple lesions in her lumbar spine consistent with progressive metastatic breast cancer. Her physician recommended hospitalization for pain management and another course of standard chemotherapy to be followed by radiation therapy. Mrs. F has a history of chronic anxiety and depression and takes paroxetine 20 mg/day and "a couple" of alprazolam "once in a while for nerves."

The morning after her admission, Mrs. F appeared very anxious and short-tempered but was willing to begin chemotherapy. She received intravenous (IV) lorazepam and oral prochlorperazine as part of her chemotherapy regimen. On the third day after admission, her nurse attempted to insert a new IV catheter for the continued administration of chemotherapy. The patient reacted with irritability and pulled her arm away from the nurse. Repeated attempts by the nurse to persuade Mrs. F to allow the IV line to be restarted resulted in an escalation of her anger, and she demanded to be "left alone." She also refused to take any of her oral medications. Psychiatric consultation was requested to determine whether the patient was "competent to refuse treatment."

Informed Consent and Decision-Making Capacity

A patient's refusal of care is a common trigger for psychiatric consultation and raises the related issues of informed consent and the right of competent patients to refuse recommended diagnostic interventions or therapy. Several key points are relevant in the analysis of the case at this point. First, the treatment of a patient without consent can be considered battery (in general, consent makes permissible what would otherwise be a violation of rights). Second, informed consent is meant to serve the values of patient autonomy and well-being by providing the information that patients need to choose for themselves whether to undergo a course of treatment. Third, a necessary condition for informed consent is DMC.

Consultation requests concerning a patient's ability to make his or her own medical decisions pose two questions. The first requires a *clinical judgment:* does this patient have a medical, neurological, or psychiatric disorder that compromises his or her ability to understand, appreciate, and reason with respect to a decision regarding a recommended diagnostic or therapeutic procedure? The second question requires a *moral judgment:* based on this clinical assessment and other relevant factors, should this person be allowed to authorize or refuse medical care? Competent adults are entitled to refuse medical care or demand the withdrawal of lifesaving treatments if they so desire. Consequently, the assessment of Mrs. F's DMC is a critical next task in her care. Furthermore, because impaired DMC often can be improved, it is important to address the clinical question prior to the ethical one.

The domains of legal competence, the capacity to make autonomous decisions, and the ability to provide informed consent are closely related but distinct from one another (Berg and Appelbaum 2001; Faden et al. 1986; Miller and Wertheimer 2010). In our society, we presume that adults are legally competent to make their own decisions. A judgment that someone is incompetent is made by judicial ruling and is typically based on the ability to make specific decisions at a given point in time (e.g., choices concerning medical care, management of finances, designation of a substitute decision maker, execution of a will). Standards for determining competence vary by jurisdiction but are based in large part on clinical assessments of an individual's cognitive state and DMC. From a legal perspective, a person is either competent to make decisions for himself or herself or incompetent to do so, in which case someone else makes decisions on his or her behalf (see also discussion of DMC in Chapter 2, "Legal Issues").

In contrast to the dichotomous nature of competency determinations, DMC varies along a continuum from being unable to make any meaningful decisions to possessing full capacity for complex decision making. In the medical setting, patients commonly manifest diminished DMC in some domains but retain the ability to make decisions in other domains. For example, a patient may have impaired DMC such that he or she does not understand the procedures, risks, and benefits of a complicated medical intervention, but he or she still may be quite capable of designating a spouse or another loved one to make medical decisions for him or her. Furthermore, the nature of comorbid medical and psychiatric illnesses and their treatments is such that DMC often changes over time. Patients with secondary mania, traumatic brain injury, and delirium characteristically manifest fluctuating DMC. Despite the greater prevalence in hospital settings of delirium or comorbid delirium and dementia (Trzepacz et al. 1998), as compared with uncomplicated dementia, the vast majority of published literature on clinical and ethical aspects of impaired DMC has focused on individuals with either stable or progressive cognitive impairment.

The assessment of DMC is particularly challenging in the setting of physical or behavioral communication barriers. Clinical decisions also must be made about patients who are either unable to speak (e.g., due to mechanical ventilation) or unwilling to be interviewed (e.g., due to a personality disorder). The use of written notes or communication boards (often of limited utility because of the patient's fatigue or weakness) and behavioral indicators may allow only tentative conclusions about the patient's DMC. These cases require patience, frequent reassessment, and clinical creativity. Because medically ill patients rarely undergo formal competency evaluations and judicial proceedings, the clinical assessment of DMC carries an extra burden in health care settings to ensure that medical decisions are made by patients with intact DMC or appropriate substitute decision makers for those patients not able to make informed and rational decisions.

Few human activities are as complex and individually determined as how we make decisions. Basic components of DMC include intellectual ability, memory, attention, concentration, conceptual organization, and aspects of "executive function" such as the ability to plan, solve problems, and make probability determinations. Most of the psychiatric literature on DMC has focused on these cognitive functions and used psychometric approaches to the study of subjects with neuropsychiatric illnesses such as dementia, psychosis, major depression, and bipolar disorder (Chen et al. 2002). In contrast, the contributions of mood, motivation, and other influences on risk assessment and decision making have received less attention but have clear implications for the process and quality of informed consent for both clinical procedures and research participation. The extent to which these factors, and less easily quantified concepts such as faith, intuition, trust, or ambivalence, affect the decision-making process is not known. Although much work remains to be done to better understand determinants of decision making, it is clear that focusing exclusively on measures of cognitive impairment is shortsighted.

Medically ill patients are at risk for impaired DMC for multiple reasons. The most common causes for concern are related to the patient's underlying medical problems (e.g., respiratory compromise, hepatic failure, cerebrovascular event, severe pain) or their treatment (e.g., excessive narcotics, high-dose glucocorticoid or cytokine therapy) rather than to a primary psychiatric disorder. In Mrs. F's case, several potential medical causes may account for her treatment-refusing behavior (e.g., delirium due to benzodiazepine withdrawal or selective serotonin reuptake inhibitor withdrawal, inadequate pain control, depression, akathisia). A judgment that Mrs. F is or is not able to refuse treatment would be premature without a careful clinical evaluation of her mental state.

A frequently observed phenomenon on medical and surgical wards is the differential threshold for concern about DMC depending on the degree to which the patient is adherent to medical care. Patients who refuse a diagnostic or therapeutic procedure are often suspected of having impaired DMC and referred for evaluation by psychiatry or neurology. In contrast, decisionally impaired patients who are passive and agreeable with requests from their nurses and physicians rarely engender these same concerns. The diagnosis of delirium, particularly the hypoactive subtype, is often missed in hospital settings (see Chapter 5, "Delirium") and can be very distressing to patients, family members, and health care professionals (Breitbart et al. 2002a). One of several reasons to diagnose and aggressively treat delirium (with or without agitation) is that it may restore DMC and thus allow patients to make important medical decisions for themselves (Bostwick and Masterson 1998).

With respect to determining the adequacy of DMC, it is worth noting that clinicians and ethicists have argued for the legitimate use of a "sliding scale" for assessing competence depending on the consequences for the patient of consent or refusal of treatment (Buchanan and Brock 1990). For example, if Mrs. F urgently needed a lifesaving blood transfusion (low risk and high probability of saving her life), then only a very low threshold of competence would be needed for valid consent. However, in the case as described, Mrs. F is being recommended for a course of chemotherapy for widely metastatic breast cancer, presumably with systemic toxicity and a relatively small prospect of prolonging her survival. Given that risk-benefit scenario, one would want her to show a more sophisticated understanding and appreciation of her circumstances before acting on her decision.

Case Vignette *(continued)*

Dr. M, a psychiatrist specializing in psychosomatic medicine, visited Mrs. F for a psychiatric examination. She observed that Mrs. F was an older woman who appeared tired and poorly groomed. Her temperature was 38.4°C, and her pulse and blood pressure measurements were slightly elevated. When asked if she understood the purpose of the psychiatric evaluation, Mrs. F replied, "I have nothing to say to you or anyone else. I just want to be left alone." Mrs. F was irritable and uncooperative with the interview and after a few minutes of complaining about her nursing care insisted that the psychiatrist leave her room. The nursing report indicated that the patient had been increasingly irritable over the past few days and was briefly disoriented the previous evening.

Suspecting that Mrs. F was experiencing delirium, possibly as a result of benzodiazepine withdrawal, Dr. M recommended treatment with a standing order of lorazepam. Dr. M also considered the possibility that paroxetine withdrawal was contributing to the patient's anxiety and agitation. In addition to restarting the paroxetine, orders were written for a multivitamin, folate, thiamine, and a workup for other metabolic, infectious, or structural causes of delirium (including blood tests, a lumbar puncture, and a magnetic resonance image). However, before completion of this workup, the patient struck a nurse and was placed in a harness and wrist restraints.

Physical Restraint and Involuntary Medical Treatment

Physical restraint of patients should be used only when no less restrictive method is available to protect them and staff from harm. The Centers for Medicare and Medicaid Services (U.S. Department of Health and Human Services 2006) and the Joint Commission (2009) require that hospitals have policies on physical restraint and seclusion. Most physicians and nurses are comfortable deciding whether and when a patient's behavior warrants physical restraint. In cases of extreme agitation and violence, nuanced mental status examinations are unnecessary. However, when the underlying neuropsychiatric disorder is not well characterized, the consulting psychiatrist can provide critical information about the justification for restraint and steps to improve the patient's condition. The medical team is looking for an expert opinion as to the patient's degree of self-control and dangerousness. Is there an imminent risk of harm to the patient or staff, and how can that risk be reduced? If the patient is competent and not dangerous, then forcible restraint violates his or her dignity, privacy, and autonomy. On the other hand, if an incompetent and dangerous patient is not restrained, the rights of staff and other patients, and the patient's safety, have been compromised.

It appears that Mrs. F temporarily lost DMC and that the principal concern at this juncture was her safety and that of her caregivers. Occasionally, health care providers question whether it is ethically and legally permissible to physically restrain patients under these circumstances (see Chapter 2, "Legal Issues"). There should be no confusion in this regard: standard of care and legal precedent for acutely agitated and confused patients are to immediately ensure their safety, even if it requires physical restraint. Compassionate care requires that the patient be treated with dignity and respect under such circumstances and that restraint should be continued only for as long as necessary. The critical distinction to be made at this juncture is between competent, informed refusal of care that warrants respect and refusal behavior due to compromised DMC.

A comprehensive workup for delirium often involves invasive diagnostic procedures and may necessitate the use of force to overcome the patient's resistance. Under what circumstances is it permissible to hold a confused patient down for blood tests (e.g., electrolytes, serum drug levels, or blood cultures), a bladder catheterization, or a lumbar puncture? The clinical presentations that prompt such diagnostic interventions range from true medical emergencies to subacute and self-limiting syndromes. This problem has no simple solution. Such decisions require clinical judgments about the necessity of each diagnostic test, its associated risks, and the degree to which the patient's condition is deemed to threaten life or risk permanent serious injury. For minimally invasive testing judged to be of urgent and critical importance, physicians have an obligation to act in the best medical interests of their patients, even if this entails the use of force. At the other end of the spectrum, a relatively high-risk, low-yield diagnostic test in a stable but incompetent patient is substantially more difficult to justify.

Case Vignette *(continued)*

Mrs. F was divorced 15 years ago and since then has lived alone in the same town as her ex-husband. She has one adult son from a first marriage but had not seen him for many years. Attempts to reach the patient's son were unsuccessful, but her ex-husband came to the hospital to visit her. Mrs. F's ex-husband reported that when they were married, they had filled out an advance directive form that made him the holder of a durable power of attorney for her health care decisions. He did not know where that document was or whether it was still considered valid since their divorce.

Durable Power of Attorney and Advance Directives for Health Care

At this point in Mrs. F's hospitalization, the health care team should attempt to identify the most appropriate substitute decision maker for Mrs. F. Involving a spouse, close relative, or friend in medical decision making for incompetent patients shows respect for them. As with competency standards, laws regarding substitute decision makers vary by jurisdiction. The Patient Self-Determination Act of 1991 (Omnibus Budget Reconciliation Act of 1990) was intended to inform patients of their right to direct their own medical care should they become incompetent or otherwise lose the ability to communicate their preferences. These rights include designating a holder of a durable power of attorney for health care decisions. The completion of a living will, or an advance directive for health care, allows patients to specify in writing the medical care they wish to receive under different medical circumstances (e.g., brain death, persistent vegetative state). Although specific laws and customs vary substantially from country to country, some mechanism for surrogate decision making in the medical setting exists in most developed countries (Lautrette et al. 2008).

Clinicians and caregivers often make false assumptions about the legal status of family members and significant others when it comes to surrogate decision making. Parents of disabled adults (e.g., patients with mental retardation, autism, psychotic disorders) may erroneously conclude that they automatically remain the patient's legal guardian even after their child's eighteenth birthday. In most of these cases, the parents are the logical and most appropriate choices as legal guardians or surrogate decision makers. However, not all parents of incompetent adult patients have the best interests of their children in mind. Similarly, when an unmarried, incompetent patient has more than one adult child, differences of opinion among the children about what is best for that sick or dying parent are common. Consequently, clinicians should clarify the legal status of their patients' substitute decision makers whenever possible to avoid compromised medical care and its legal ramifications.

Research on the use of advance directives and the behavior of substitute decision makers suggests two important conclusions. First, most individuals are reluctant to put in writing the kind of medical care they would like to receive if they were to become gravely ill and incompetent. Several studies found that only 15%–20% of patients fill out an advance directive for health care or research when given an opportunity to do so (Gross 1998; The SUPPORT Principal Investigators 1995; Wendler et al. 2002). Second, regardless of the expressed wishes of patients, substitute decision makers tend to make decisions according to what they would want to happen to themselves or, alternatively, what they consider to be in the best interests of the patient rather than using a substituted judgment standard (i.e., what the patient would have wanted) when making decisions for someone else (Li et al. 2007; Shalowitz et al. 2006).

Case Vignette *(continued)*

The health care team requested a consultation from the hospital's legal department regarding the most appropriate substitute decision maker for Mrs. F. While attempts were made to contact the patient's son, the clinician in charge of Mrs. F's care obtained permission from the patient's ex-husband to continue the physical restraints and complete the diagnostic testing. The medical workup suggested delirium secondary to benzodiazepine withdrawal and a urinary tract infection. Mrs. F was given IV antibiotics, lorazepam, and a low dose of haloperidol to treat her confusion, conceptual disorganization, and agitation.

Two days after treatment with antibiotics, lorazepam, paroxetine, and haloperidol, Mrs. F had a markedly improved sensorium. She was considerably less irritable and was able to complete a detailed psychiatric interview. She was relieved to be able to "think clearly again" and over the course of several sessions developed a trusting relationship with Dr. M. However, as her delirium resolved, she expressed a deepening sadness and sense of hopelessness about her medical condition. She expressed skepticism about the value of more chemotherapy and radiation therapy and reported that what was most important to her at this point was to avoid a painful and lonely death.

Depression in the Medically Ill

In Mrs. F's case, the aggressive treatment of her delirium had the value of restoring her DMC but left her painfully aware of her progressive cancer and feeling depressed as a consequence. The clinicians caring for her again faced a complex clinical problem that raises ethical issues. Mrs. F was contemplating stopping chemotherapy but was manifesting symptoms of depression. Was her depression influencing her decision making, and, if so, what is the proper response from her health care providers? As discussed earlier, clinical considerations should be explored first and in the service of an ethically desirable outcome for Mrs. F.

It is important to recognize that major depression in the medically ill usually does not render the patient incompetent. To be sure, the presence of depression may well influence the patient's ability to tolerate uncomfortable symptoms, maintain hope, or assess a treatment's risk-benefit ratio but not necessarily render him or her unable to make medical decisions for himself or herself (Elliott 1997). Untreated depression has been linked to poor adherence with medical care, increased pain and disability (see also Chapter 8, "Depression"), and a greater likelihood of considering euthanasia and physician-assisted suicide (see also Chapter 9, "Suicidality," and Chapter 41, "Palliative Care"). Depression produces more subtle distortions of decision making than does delirium or psychosis, but refusal of even lifesaving treatment by a depressed patient cannot be assumed to constitute suicidality or lack of competence (Katz et al. 1995; Sullivan and Youngner 1994). Consequently, although a depressed patient should be strongly encouraged to accept treatment for depression, the decision to override a refusal of medical treatment should be based on whether the patient lacks DMC.

Case Vignette *(continued)*

Although Mrs. F was moderately depressed, she declined the recommended adjustment of her antidepressant because she had "lived with depression for years, and another dose or another antidepressant would not change anything for me." She was unwilling to proceed with chemotherapy but did agree to try radiation therapy for palliative treatment of her bone pain. After 4 weeks of radiation therapy, she complained of new chest pain, and it was discovered that she had new bony metastatic lesions in her ribs.

At this point, she asked her oncologist to discharge her to home or hospice. Her oncologist responded that Mrs. F could go home but recommended that she consider enrolling in a Phase I clinical trial of a "very promising" new chemotherapeutic agent. Mrs. F's ex-husband also encouraged her to enroll in the clinical trial and to "keep fighting as long as possible."

Differentiating the Ethics of Clinical Research From the Ethics of Medical Care

In some respects, the option of enrolling in a clinical trial is a logical consideration following the failure of standard medical treatment. However, this decision point in Mrs. F's clinical course warrants a thoughtful exploration of the differences between the practice of medicine and the conduct of clinical research. Clinical medicine aims to provide optimal medical care for particular patients. The risks of diagnostic tests and treatments are justified by the prospect of compensatory medical benefits for the patient. By contrast, clinical research is devoted to answering scientific questions to produce generalizable knowledge. Physician-investigators conduct clinical trials to evaluate experimental treatments in *groups* of patient-subjects, with the ultimate goal of benefiting future patients by improving medical care. The contrast between the group focus of research trials and the individual focus of medical care should not be overstated. Physicians are obligated to practice medicine in the context of a professional standard of care rather than by idiosyncratic judgments about what is best for individual patients. Nonetheless, they are expected to make competent treatment recommendations tailored to the characteristics of their individual patients.

Many patients receive therapeutic benefits from participating in clinical trials, which may even surpass the benefits from standard medical care (Braunholtz et al. 2001). However, clinical trials, especially randomized trials, differ fundamentally from patient care in purpose, characteristic methods, and the justification of risks. Interventions evaluated in these trials are allocated by chance. Double-blind conditions and often placebo controls are used. For scientific reasons, protocols governing clinical trials typically restrict flexibility in dosing of study drugs and use of concomitant medications. Trials often include drug washouts before randomization to establish a drug-free baseline to assess treatment efficacy. Research interventions, such as blood draws, imaging procedures, and biopsies, are often administered to measure trial outcomes. These strictly research interventions pose risks to participants that are not compensated by medical benefits to them but are justified by the potential value of the knowledge to be gained from the trial. Although these differences between research trials and medical care have been frequently noted (Appelbaum et al. 1987; Beecher 1970; Levine 1986; Miller et al. 1998), their ethical significance has not been sufficiently appreciated. Accordingly, clinical trials continue to be conceived from a therapeutic perspective oriented around the physician-patient relationship (Miller and Rosenstein 2003).

Clinical research has changed dramatically in recent years. Two decades ago, most clinical trials were conducted in academic medical centers. Today, they are more likely to be conducted in private practice settings under the direction of clinicians rather than full-time investigators. Increasingly, psychiatrists are being consulted on patients who are either enrolled in or considering a clinical trial. Practitioners of psychosomatic medicine can make several contributions in this context. They may be asked to render an opinion about the psychiatric "appropriateness" of a patient for a clinical trial. Their patients may ask for advice about enrolling in a study. There may be an opportunity to modify the existing study or design a new one that addresses psychiatric aspects of the medical illness or its treatment.

In each of these activities, the consulting psychiatrist is well served by an understanding of the critical aspects of clinical research and how they differ from those related to standard medical care (Emanuel et al. 2000; Miller and Rosenstein 2003). For example, many patients and physicians do not appreciate that the primary purpose of a Phase I trial (what was offered to Mrs. F) is to assess the tolerability and toxicity of a drug rather than to obtain preliminary data on the effectiveness of the drug (Phase II).

Another aspect of research ethics possibly relevant to Mrs. F's case is the issue of research involving subjects considered "mentally disabled" (Rosenstein and Miller 2008). The regulations governing federally funded human subjects research were written more than 20 years ago and mandated additional safeguards for research subjects considered "vulnerable to coercion or undue influence" (U.S. Department of Health and Human Services 1991). Included in this category of vulnerable subjects are the "mentally disabled." These regulations, known as the Common Rule, were clearly intended to prevent the exploitation of individuals for the sake of scientific progress. Unfortunately, the Common Rule does not include a definition of mental disability or of what would constitute the degree of mood, cognitive, or behavioral impairment that would render someone vulnerable in this respect. In practice, a psychiatric consultation often serves as an important additional safeguard by virtue of eliciting an expert opinion about a prospective research subject's DMC and ability to provide informed consent.

The nature of the research protocol, rather than the disorder being studied, also may place research subjects at risk for impaired DMC. Oncology trials in which subjects receive interleukin-2 or interferon-alpha, cytokines associated with central nervous system toxicity, provide examples of protocols that place otherwise competent subjects at risk for losing DMC. In these cases, the concern is less about adequate informed consent on the "front end" of the study than it is about subjects losing their ability to provide adequate consent for continuing participation. For such studies, IRBs can require subjects to appoint a holder of a durable power of attorney as a condition of enrollment. This approach has the advantages of highlighting an important risk of the study (i.e., loss of DMC) and ensuring appropriate initial and ongoing research authorization.

Research Ethics in Psychosomatic Medicine

Guidance on ethical issues raised specifically by research in psychosomatic medicine is needed. For example, obtaining proper authorization for research with individuals who lack DMC is relevant to both research on delirium and research on other conditions in which delirium might develop as a complicating factor. In the case of delirium research, current publication standards for informed consent are variable. Investigators have described research authorization from subjects who provided prospective informed consent (Breitbart et al. 1996). Other articles state that informed consent was obtained from the "subjects or their surrogates" (often without detailing the circumstances of surrogate consent) (Bogardus et al. 2003; Cole et al. 2002; Inouye et al. 1999; Laurila et al. 2002). It also has been argued that prospective IRB review and informed consent are not necessary for studies that involve very little "deviation from (standard) clinical practice" (Breitbart et al. 2002a, 2002b; Lawlor et al. 2000). We contend that this view confuses research with medical care and is inconsistent with the principle of respect for persons and federal regulations for human subjects research (45 CFR 46) (Davis and Walsh 2001). Some reports of delirium research are silent on the issue of IRB review (Lawlor et al. 2000). Finally, we have suggested that published reports of medical and psychiatric research address ethical issues in a more comprehensive fashion (i.e., providing more detail than the standard sentence that the study was approved by a local IRB and that informed consent was obtained from subjects) (Miller et al. 1999; Tanaka 1999).

Case Vignette *(continued)*

After considering the pros and cons of enrolling in the Phase I clinical trial, Mrs. F decided to "face facts and let this thing run its course." She told her oncologist that she was ready to go home but that she was very afraid the cancer would spread to more of her bones. When she told her oncologist that she would rather end her life than suffer through a painful death, her oncologist responded that he would not do anything to "bring on" Mrs. F's death and reconsulted Dr. M because of this request for "physician-assisted suicide."

On psychiatric examination, Mrs. F was judged to be moderately depressed but able to make decisions for herself. She confided that she had cared for her first husband during a "prolonged, excruciating, and undignified" death. She had accepted the inevitability of her death but wished to avoid the kind of experience her first husband had endured. Dr. M then facilitated a discussion between the oncologist and Mrs. F about available options. Mrs. F decided to stop eating and drinking and was discharged to hospice with assurances that she would be kept comfortable while awaiting death. Mrs. F died from terminal dehydration 12 days after her transfer to hospice.

When Patients Express a Wish to Die

Few clinical scenarios generate requests for psychiatric consultation more predictably than when a patient expresses a wish to die. The range of possible meanings underlying this communication is immense, and a comprehensive discussion is beyond the scope of this chapter (see also Chapter 2, "Legal Issues," Chapter 9, "Suicidality," and Chapter 41, "Palliative Care"). Is the patient expressing a passive wish to die, planning to commit suicide, rejecting life-sustaining treatments (withdrawal of care), eliciting help in ending his or her life (physician-assisted suicide), or asking to be killed (euthanasia)? Under any circumstances, an expression of suicidal ideation or a request for help with an intentionally arranged death is a complex message that warrants careful clinical assessment.

Muskin (1998) observed that physicians respond to requests to die by focusing predominantly on determinations of the patient's DMC. He argued persuasively that too often clinicians pay inadequate attention to the underlying meaning and importance of these requests. Although competent subjects have the right to refuse life-sustaining treatments (and in Oregon and Washington in the United States, as well as in Belgium, Luxembourg, and Switzerland, request physician-assisted suicide), a compassionate and comprehensive evaluation by the consulting psychiatrist can help frame both the clinical questions and the ethically permissible medical options.

Just as the clinical issues raised by requests to die are frequently reduced to questions of DMC, the ethical analysis of physician-assisted suicide is often characterized as a simple matter of autonomy versus nonmaleficence. Miller and Brody (1995) articulated an important distinction in the debate on physician-assisted suicide. In considering whether physician-assisted suicide was morally justifiable, they explored whether the practice of physician-assisted suicide as a last resort could be compatible with the professional integrity of physicians.

Ultimately, Mrs. F made an informed and deliberate request for a comfortable and dignified death. Her choice of terminal dehydration was a legal option that did not compromise the professional integrity of her caregivers (Ganzini et al. 2003; Miller and Meier 1998).

Medical care at the end of life often identifies important differences in personal and cultural values held by patients, family members, and health care providers. Psychiatrists may be involved in cases in which a member of the health care team has a moral objection to an ongoing or a proposed treatment plan. When a physician's personal conscience is at odds with a reasonable and legal treatment request from a patient or family member, there should be a mechanism for the transfer of care to another physician. However, it is critical in such cases that the patient not be abandoned in any way before the transfer of care.

Ethics Training in Psychosomatic Medicine

Training in ethics is considered a key component of the educational programs in psychosomatic medicine/consultation-liaison psychiatry fellowships. Recognizing the importance of the interface between psychosomatic medicine and clinical ethics, a task force of the Academy of Psychosomatic Medicine published an annotated bibliography for ethics training (Preisman et al. 1999). Guidelines on ethics, clinical decision making, and professionalism (Roberts and Hoop 2007; Wright and Roberts 2009) and curricula for teaching research ethics in psychiatry (Beresin et al. 2003; Rosenstein et al. 2001) are helpful resources for both students and teachers of psychosomatic medicine. Similarly, a recent analysis of privacy and confidentiality concerns associated with the implementation of the Health Information Portability and Accountability Act is particularly relevant for the practice of psychosomatic medicine (Mermelstein and Wallack 2008). Ethics education should be oriented to developing basic competence in identifying ethical issues in the practice of psychosomatic medicine and in deliberation aimed at satisfactory resolution of moral problems in patient care or research.

Conclusion

The relation between psychosomatic medicine and bioethics is rich and unique for historical, conceptual, and practical reasons. The ethical issues considered in this chapter are often discussed in purely theoretical terms. We have illustrated some of the ways in which clinical considerations can color the expression and resolution of these issues as they are encountered at the bedside. All too often, optimal patient care is hampered by the presence of psychiatric symptoms in the patient or systems problems among the health care team or family members. Practitioners of psychosomatic medicine are ideally positioned to facilitate the resolution of both clinical problems and ethical dilemmas as they arise in an increasingly complex health care environment.

References

Agich GJ: Roles and responsibilities: theoretical issues in the definition of consultation liaison psychiatry. J Med Philos 10:105–126, 1985

American Medical Association: Principles of Medical Ethics, in Code of Medical Ethics. June 2001. Available at: http://www.ama-assn.org/ama/pub/physician-resources/medical-ethics/code-medical-ethics.shtml. Accessed May 5, 2010.

American Psychiatric Association: The Principles of Medical Ethics: With Annotations Especially Applicable to Psychiatry, 2001 Edition. Washington, DC, American Psychiatric Association, 2001. Available at: http://www.psych.org/MainMenu/PsychiatricPractice/Ethics/ResourcesStandards.aspx. Accessed May 5, 2010.

Appelbaum PS, Lidz CW, Meisel JD: Fulfilling the underlying purpose of informed consent, in Informed Consent: Legal Theory and Clinical Practice. New York, Oxford University Press, 1987, pp 237–260

Beauchamp TL, Childress JF: Principles of Biomedical Ethics, 6th Edition. New York, Oxford University Press, 2009

Beecher HK: Research and the Individual: Human Studies. Boston, MA, Little, Brown, 1970

Beresin EV, Baldessarini RJ, Alpert J, et al: Teaching ethics of psychopharmacology research in psychiatric residency training programs. Psychopharmacology (Berl) 171:105–111, 2003

Berg JW, Appelbaum PS: Informed Consent: Legal Theory and Clinical Practice, 2nd Edition. New York, Oxford University Press, 2001

Bogardus ST Jr, Desai MM, Williams CS, et al: The effects of a targeted multicomponent delirium intervention on postdischarge outcomes for hospitalized older adults. Am J Med 114:383–390, 2003

Bostwick JM, Masterson BJ: Psychopharmacological treatment of delirium to restore mental capacity. Psychosomatics 39:112–117, 1998

Bourgeois JA, Cohen MA, Geppert CMA: The role of psychosomatic-medicine psychiatrists in bioethics: a survey study of members of the Academy of Psychosomatic Medicine. Psychosomatics 47:520–526, 2006

Braunholtz DA, Edwards SJL, Lilford RJ: Are randomized clinical trials good for us (in the short term)? Evidence for a "trial effect." J Clin Epidemiol 54:217–224, 2001

Breitbart W, Marotta R, Platt MM, et al: A double-blind trial of haloperidol, chlorpromazine, and lorazepam in the treatment of delirium in hospitalized AIDS patients. Am J Psychiatry 153:231–237, 1996

Breitbart W, Gibson C, Tremblay A: The delirium experience: delirium recall and delirium-related distress in hospitalized patients with cancer, their spouses/caregivers, and their nurses. Psychosomatics 43:183–194, 2002a

Breitbart W, Tremblay A, Gibson C: An open trial of olanzapine for the treatment of delirium in hospitalized cancer patients. Psychosomatics 43:175–182, 2002b

Buchanan AE, Brock DW: Deciding for Others. Cambridge, UK, Cambridge University Press, 1990, pp 51–59

Chen DT, Miller FG, Rosenstein DL: Enrolling decisionally impaired adults in clinical research. Med Care 40:V20–V29, 2002

Cole MG, McCusker J, Bellavance F, et al: Systematic detection and multidisciplinary care of delirium in older medical inpatients: a randomized trial. Can Med Assoc J 167:753–759, 2002

Davis MP, Walsh D: Methadone for relief of cancer pain: a review of pharmacokinetics, pharmacodynamics, drug interactions and protocols of administration. Support Care Cancer 9:73–83, 2001

Elliott C: Caring about risks: are severely depressed patients competent to consent to research? Arch Gen Psychiatry 54:113–116, 1997

Emanuel EJ, Wendler D, Grady C: What makes clinical research ethical? JAMA 283:2701–2711, 2000

Faden RR, Beauchamp TL, King NMP: A History and Theory of Informed Consent. New York, Oxford University Press, 1986

Fins JJ, Bacchetta MD, Miller FG: Clinical pragmatism: a method of moral problem solving. Kennedy Inst Ethics J 7:129–145, 1997

Ganzini L, Goy ER, Miller LL, et al: Nurses' experiences with hospice patients who refuse food and fluids to hasten death. N Engl J Med 349:359–365, 2003

Gross MD: What do patients express as their preferences in advance directives? Arch Intern Med 158:363–365, 1998

Horikawa N, Yamazaki T, Sagawa M, et al: The disclosure of information to cancer patients and its relationship to their mental state in a consultation-liaison psychiatry setting in Japan. Gen Hosp Psychiatry 21:368–373, 1999

Horikawa N, Yamazaki T, Sagawa M, et al: Changes in disclosure of information to cancer patients in a general hospital in Japan. Gen Hosp Psychiatry 22:37–42, 2000

Inouye SK, Bogardus ST Jr, Charpentier PA, et al: A multicomponent intervention to prevent delirium in hospitalized older patients. N Engl J Med 340:669–676, 1999

Joint Commission: Provision of care, treatment, and services, in Revised 2009 Accreditation Requirements as of March 26, 2009: Hospital Accreditation Program, Oakbrook Terrace, IL, Joint Commission Resources, 2009, pp 14–19

Katz M, Abbey S, Rydall A, et al: Psychiatric consultation for competency to refuse medical treatment: a retrospective study of patient characteristics and outcome. Psychosomatics 36:33–41, 1995

Kimball CP, Silverman AJ: The issue of confidentiality in the consultation-liaison process. Bibl Psychiatr 159:82–92, 1978

Laurila JV, Pitkala KH, Strandberg TE, et al: Confusion assessment method in the diagnostics of delirium among aged hospital patients: would it serve better in screening than as a diagnostic instrument? Int J Geriatr Psychiatry 17:1112–1119, 2002

Lautrette A, Peigne V, Watts J, et al: Surrogate decision makers for incompetent ICU patients: a European perspective. Curr Opin Crit Care 14:714–719, 2008

Lawlor PG, Gagnon B, Mancini IL, et al: Occurrence, causes, and outcome of delirium in patients with advanced cancer: a prospective study. Arch Intern Med 160:786–794, 2000

Lederberg MS: Making a situational diagnosis: psychiatrists at the interface of psychiatry and ethics in the consultation-liaison setting. Psychosomatics 38:327–338, 1997

Levine RJ: Ethics and Regulation of Clinical Research. Baltimore, MD, Urban & Schwarzenberg, 1986

Li LL, Cheong KY, Yaw LK, et al: The accuracy of surrogate decisions in intensive care scenarios. Anaesth Intensive Care 35:46–51, 2007

Mermelstein HT, Wallack JJ: Confidentiality in the age of HIPAA: a challenge for psychosomatic medicine. Psychosomatics 49:97–103, 2008

Miller FG, Brody H: Professional integrity and physician-assisted death. Hastings Cent Rep 25:8–17, 1995

Miller FG, Meier DE: Voluntary death: a comparison of terminal dehydration and physician-assisted suicide. Ann Intern Med 128:559–562, 1998

Miller FG, Rosenstein DL: The therapeutic orientation to clinical trials. N Engl J Med 348:1383–1386, 2003

Miller FG, Shorr AF: Unnecessary use of placebo controls: the case of asthma clinical trials. Arch Intern Med 162:1673–1677, 2002

Miller FG, Wertheimer A: The Ethics of Consent: Theory and Practice. New York, Oxford University Press, 2010

Miller FG, Rosenstein DL, DeRenzo EG: Professional integrity in clinical research. JAMA 280:1449–1454, 1998

Miller FG, Pickar D, Rosenstein DL: Addressing ethical issues in the psychiatric research literature [letter to the editor]. Arch Gen Psychiatry 56:763–764, 1999

Muskin PR: The request to die: role for a psychodynamic perspective on physician-assisted suicide. JAMA 279:323–328, 1998

Omnibus Budget Reconciliation Act of 1990, PL 101-508, §§4206, 4751, 42USC, scattered sections (November 5, 1990)

Preisman RC, Steinberg MD, Rummans TA, et al: An annotated bibliography for ethics training in consultation-liaison psychiatry. Psychosomatics 40:369–379, 1999

Roberts LW, Hoop JG: Professionalism and Ethics: A Question and Answer Self-Study Guide for Mental Health Professionals. Washington, DC, American Psychiatric Publishing, 2007

Rosenstein DL, Miller FG: Research involving those at risk for impaired decisionmaking capacity, in The Oxford Textbook of Clinical Research Ethics. Edited by Emanuel EJ, Grady C, Crouch RA, et al. New York, Oxford University Press, 2008, pp 437–445

Rosenstein DL, Miller FG, Rubinow DR: A curriculum for teaching psychiatric research bioethics. Biol Psychiatry 50:802–808, 2001

Shalowitz DI, Garrett-Mayer E, Wendler D: The accuracy of surrogate decision makers: a systematic review. Arch Intern Med 166:493–497, 2006

Sullivan MD, Youngner SJ: Depression, competence, and the right to refuse lifesaving medical treatment. Am J Psychiatry 151:971–978, 1994

Tanaka E: Gender-related differences in pharmacokinetics and their clinical significance. J Clin Pharm Ther 24:339–346, 1999

The SUPPORT Principal Investigators: A controlled trial to improve care for seriously ill hospitalized patients: the Study to Understand Prognoses and Preferences for Outcomes and Risks of Treatments (SUPPORT). JAMA 274:1591–1598, 1995

Trzepacz PT, Mulsant BH, Dew MA, et al: Is delirium different when it occurs in dementia? A study using the Delirium Rating Scale. J Neuropsychiatry Clin Neurosci 10:199–204, 1998

U.S. Department of Health and Human Services: Code of Federal Regulations, Title 42 (Public Health), Part 482 (Conditions of Participation for Hospitals), Section 13 (Patients' Rights), Standard e (Restraint for acute medical and surgical care). 71 FR 71426, Dec. 8, 2006. Available at: http://www.cms.gov/CFCsAndCoPs/downloads/finalpatientrightsrule.pdf. Accessed May 5, 2010.

U.S. Department of Health and Human Services: Code of Federal Regulations, Title 45 (Public Welfare), Part 46 (Protection of Human Subjects). 56 FR 28012, 28022, June 18, 1991. Available at: http://www.hhs.gov/ohrp/humansubjects/guidance/45cfr46.htm. Accessed May 5, 2010.

Wendler D, Martinez RA, Fairclough D, et al: Views of potential subjects toward proposed regulations for clinical research with adults unable to consent. Am J Psychiatry 159:585–591, 2002

Wright MT, Roberts LW: A basic decision-making approach to common ethical issues in consultation-liaison psychiatry. Psychiatr Clin North Am 32:315–328, 2009

World Medical Association: WMA Declaration of Helsinki—Ethical Principles for Medical Research Involving Human Subjects. Adopted by the 18th WMA General Assembly, Helsinki, Finland, June 1964, and amended by the 59th WMA General Assembly, Seoul, South Korea, October 2008. Available at: http://www.wma.net/en/30publications/10policies/b3/index.html. Accessed May 5, 2010.

CHAPTER 4

Psychological Responses to Illness

Mark S. Groves, M.D.

Philip R. Muskin, M.D.

A CENTRAL TASK OF THE psychiatrist working with the medically ill is to understand patients' subjective experiences of illness to design therapeutic interventions that modulate the patients' behavioral or emotional responses, decrease their distress, and improve their medical outcomes. In outpatient practice or in the general hospital, physicians witness tremendous diversity of emotional and behavioral responses to illness. Some individuals seem able to face devastating illnesses for which no cure is currently available with courage and a sense of humor (Cousins 1983; Druss 1995; Druss and Douglas 1988). Others, facing easily treatable illnesses, have difficulty overcoming intense emotions such as anger, fear, or hopelessness. Clinical experience and research indicate that illness variables such as severity, chronicity, or organ system involvement cannot predict an individual's response to any given medical illness (Lipowski 1975; Lloyd 1977; Sensky 1997; Westbrook and Viney 1982). Rather, it is in the realm of the individual's subjective experience of an illness that one can begin to understand his or her emotional and behavioral responses (Lipowski 1970; Lloyd 1977).

During the past few decades, there has been considerable work in the fields of health psychology and psychiatry attempting to explain the interindividual differences in responses to the stresses of illness (see, e.g., Druss 1995; Geringer and Stern 1986; Kahana and Bibring 1964; Lazarus 1999; Perry and Viederman 1981; Peterson 1974; Strain and Grossman 1975; Verwoerdt 1972). In this chapter, we provide a general overview of the stresses that accompany medical illness and hospitalization and review some of the psychological, emotional, and behavioral responses that these stresses frequently elicit.

The concepts of stress, personality types, coping strategies, and defense mechanisms can be integrated into a framework that illustrates the complexity of an individual's behavioral or emotional responses to illness (Figure 4–1). This framework, adapted from the work of Lazarus and Folkman (Lazarus 1999; Lazarus and Folkman 1984), attempts to integrate the psychodynamic concepts of character style and intrapsychic defenses with other psychological concepts such as stress and coping. The importance of individual subjectivity is emphasized in this model through the placement of coping styles, defense mechanisms, personality types, and the appraised meaning of illness as central mediators of the behavioral and emotional responses to the stresses of medical illness.

In this chapter, we do not focus solely on maladaptive responses to illness or psychopathology. A coping strategy or defense mechanism may be relatively maladaptive or ineffective in one context but adaptive and effective in another (Penley et al. 2002). For example, the maladaptive use of denial by a patient just diagnosed with early breast cancer might lead to a long delay in seeking treatment (Zervas et al. 1993). In contrast, the adaptive use of denial by a man diagnosed with untreatable metastatic pancreatic cancer might enable him to maximize his quality of life in the months before his death (Druss 1995).

Psychiatrists do not see most people who become ill, nor will most patients' responses to their illnesses concern their physicians (Patterson et al. 1993; Perry and Vieder-

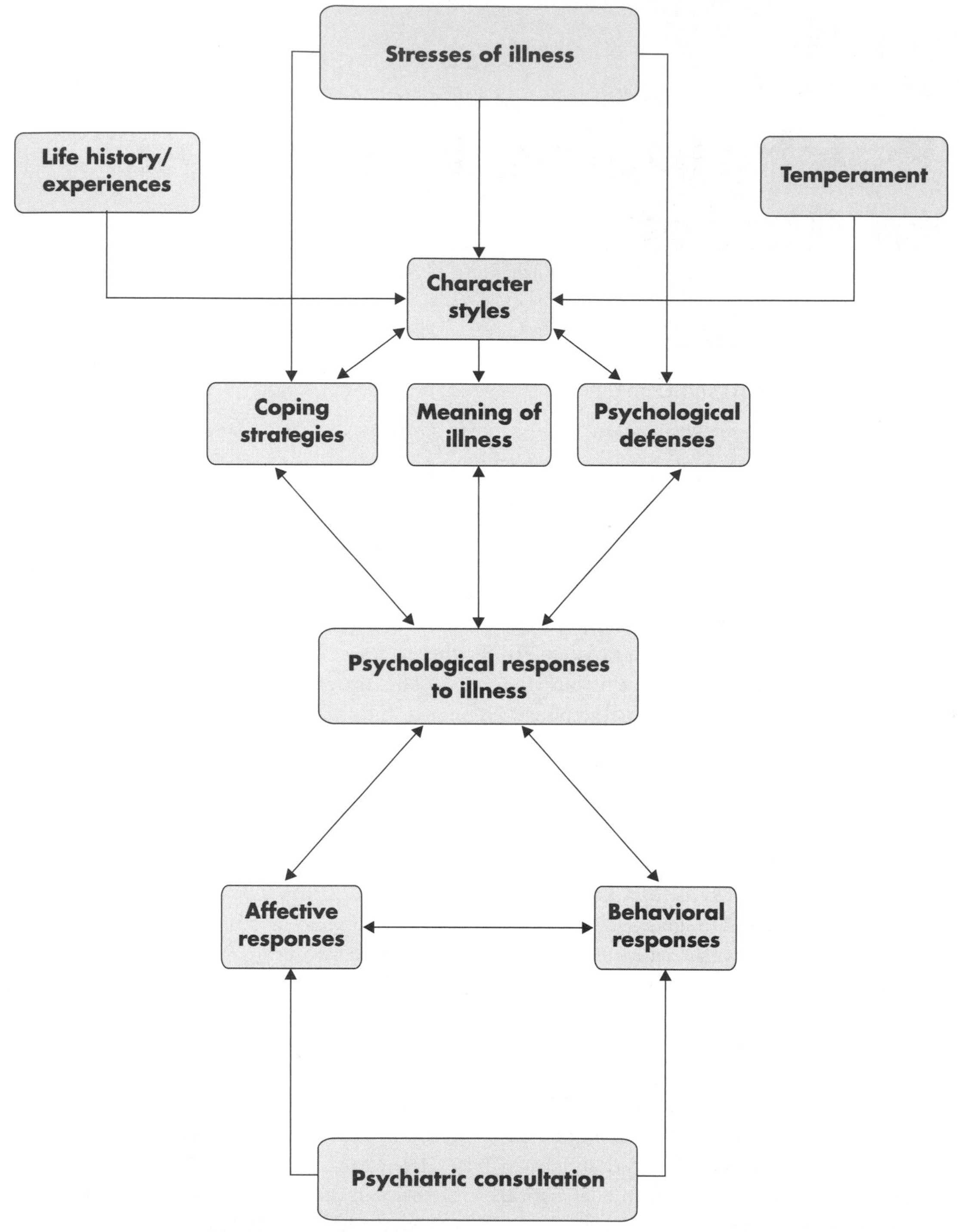

FIGURE 4–1. Framework illustrating the complexity of an individual's behavioral or emotional responses to illness.
Source. Adapted from Lazarus 1999; Lazarus and Folkman 1984.

man 1981). That does not mean, of course, that there is no psychological response to the illness. An overt display of emotion may or may not be appropriate for a patient's racial and cultural background. In addition, patients may feel discouraged from expressing their thoughts and feelings about their illness to family members or physicians. The determination that a psychological response to illness is problematic must be based on the effect the response has on the patient, the patient's adherence to therapeutic plans, and the patient's social functioning.

There is no one correct way to characterize psychological responses to illness. Psychodynamic formulations, coping styles, and personality types offer different perspectives that may or may not be useful in understanding the response of a particular patient. Therefore, in this chapter we provide an overview of the following topics without subscribing exclusively to any single theoretical framework: 1) the stresses of medical illness and hospitalization; 2) the influences of personality types, attachment styles, coping styles, and defense mechanisms on patients' subjective experiences of illness; 3) denial; 4) emotional responses to illness; and 5) behavioral responses to illness.

Stresses of Medical Illness and Hospitalization

The stresses of medical illness and hospitalization are both very significant and numerous (Strain and Grossman 1975). In their frequently cited study from 1967, Holmes and Rahe surveyed many individuals from various countries, asking them to rate the effect of various events on their lives. These ratings generated a ranked list of life events based on relative effect (Lazarus 1999). In this list of stressors, "personal injury or illness" ranked sixth (after death of spouse, divorce, marital separation, death of close family member, and jail term). Some of the stresses accompanying illness are nearly universal, whereas others vary by illness and are more specific (Druss 1995). In this section, we discuss some of the most common stresses experienced by patients in medical settings.

Apart from medical illness, the hospital environment itself can be stressful (Gazzola and Muskin 2003; Kornfeld 1972). To many, the hospital is a frightening place associated with painful personal or family memories. Hospitalization separates patients from their usual environments and social supports; it is by its very nature isolating. The inpatient is asked to wear a hospital gown, which results in deindividualization, loss of control, and loss of privacy (Gazzola and Muskin 2003). The machines, intravenous lines, blood withdrawals, interactions with strangers, and neighboring ill patients all contribute to the stress of hospitalization regardless of the patient's specific illness. In addition, the hospital demands that the patient be largely dependent on others for the most basic tasks—a change that in itself can be very stressful for many individuals (Kornfeld 1972; Muskin 1995; Perry and Viederman 1981). Perry and Viederman (1981) described three successive (although at times overlapping) tasks that patients facing medical illness must go through: 1) acknowledgment to themselves and others that they are ill; 2) regressive dependency on others for care; and 3) resumption of normal functioning after recovery. Perry and Viederman (1981) proposed that all three tasks bring their own stresses and must be confronted for the patient to cope successfully with the illness and the hospitalization.

On a nearly universal level, medical illness results in narcissistic injury—that is, it demands that patients reexamine their views of themselves (Strain and Grossman 1975). Although most people would not overtly claim that they are invulnerable to serious medical illness, they may hold such a belief subconsciously. Unconscious fantasies of invulnerability may be unknown until the person is injured or becomes ill. The development of a medical illness shatters any such conscious or unconscious beliefs. The sick patient may feel "defective," "weak," or less desirable to others.

One determinant of the effect of an illness is whether it is acute or chronic (Verwoerdt 1972). Although an acute, non-life-threatening illness gives the individual little time to adapt, its effects are short term. Chronic illnesses, however, require the individual to change his or her self-view more permanently. The challenges of chronic illness are ongoing and become a part of daily life for the individual. A change in identity or body image is disorienting and often anxiety producing; the patient's previously held self-concept is disturbed, shaken up, or shattered.

Separation from family or friends in the hospital or at home when one is ill produces isolation, disconnection, and stress (Heiskell and Pasnau 1991; Strain and Grossman 1975). This can precipitate conscious or unconscious fears of abandonment. The stress of separation and fear of abandonment are not only experienced by children. Newly diagnosed with AIDS, a 30-year-old Latina mother of three may fear rejection by her community and abandonment by her parents. Or, after many years of chemotherapy for metastatic thyroid cancer, a 55-year-old bank executive may elect to undergo another course of chemotherapy despite the low likelihood of success rather than seek hospice care because the latter would signify giving up. Although not desirous of more treatment, the patient might fear that his oncologist who had worked with him for a decade would abandon him.

The lack of privacy in the hospital environment or clinic places additional stresses on the patient (Kornfeld 1972). Bodily exposure evokes discomfort. Given only a thin gown to wear, patients may be subjected to repeated examinations by doctors, nurses, and medical students. Exposure of the most private aspects of life can occur (Perry and Viederman 1981). A woman presenting with symptoms of a sexually transmitted disease must give a detailed account of her sexual history, and a young patient brought in with acute chest pain and hypertension is asked about use of cocaine, an illegal drug. For the vulnerable individual, such experiences of exposure can evoke feelings of shame and thus require the clinician to be tactful and empathic to put the patient at ease and maintain a therapeutic alliance.

Beyond simple exposure, the medical environment often involves experiences of bodily invasion that are very stressful for the patient (Gazzola and Muskin 2003). From the more invasive experiences of a colonoscopy, the placement of a nasogastric tube, or tracheal intubation to ostensibly more benign procedures such as a fine-needle biopsy of a breast lump or a rectal examination, the fear and discomfort of such interventions are often not fully recognized by the physician for whom such procedures have become routine. Individuals certainly vary in their fears; for example, the victim of repeated physical or sexual abuse might be especially fearful of such experiences and require the doctor to use greater care and psychological preparation than usual.

Pain should not be overlooked as a profound stressor that should be dealt with aggressively (Heiskell and Pasnau 1991). Even the most highly adapted patient with effective coping skills and strong social support can be taxed to the limit by extreme pain. Psychiatrists are frequently asked to evaluate patients for depression and hopelessness. On discovering inadequately treated pain, the consultant can facilitate increased pain control, sometimes leading to full remission of hopelessness and depression without any additional intervention. Like pain, sleep disturbances are extremely common in the medically ill, with significant psychological effects. A patient's outlook, emotional expression, and ability to cope may shift dramatically when insomnia is remedied.

When illness leads to disability—whether due to pain, physical limitations, or psychological effects—the disability is an additional stressor that can have a profound effect on the patient's regular activities of daily life (Westbrook and Viney 1982). What was previously routine and required no conscious planning can become tremendously challenging, both psychologically and practically. For example, on the acute rehabilitation unit, patients are assisted in their efforts to learn to walk again. What was previously automatic has become incredibly difficult and requires new techniques, assistive devices, and the help of others. Disabilities frequently preclude the possibility of an immediate return to work. For many this is a significant loss because it removes the natural opportunities to feel productive, which had provided a sense of accomplishment. For many people, feelings of accomplishment, productivity, and usefulness are important for their self-image. Thus, self-esteem is damaged when they lose this important source of gratification.

Although only a small proportion of medical illnesses signify the imminent or near approach of death and force affected individuals to confront their mortality directly, even minor illnesses can evoke a sense of the fragility and impermanence of life (Perry and Viederman 1981). Psychiatrists for the medically ill are often called to consult on patients who are experiencing anxiety or conflicts facing death (or patients whose illnesses evoke these difficulties in caregivers). Patients may refuse to give do-not-resuscitate orders despite clear evidence that resuscitation would be futile because they equate do-not-resuscitate orders with suicide, which is morally unacceptable to them (Sullivan and Youngner 1993). Facing mortality—whether in the near future or later—can force a person to reflect deeply on life and can shatter previously held dreams of the future. This can stir up regrets and evoke numerous emotions, as described in the work of Elisabeth Kubler-Ross (1969). The various emotions evoked by medical illness are discussed later in this chapter.

Attachment Styles, Personality Types, Coping Styles, and Defense Mechanisms

There is great individual variation in responses to an environmental stressor such as receiving a diagnosis of cancer (Heim et al. 1993). Models of human behavior that involve only environmental stress and reflexive behavioral responses cannot account for this variation in responses and are therefore considered to have limited utility and explanatory power. Richard Lazarus (1999) has reviewed the historical transition in health psychology and other disciplines from the traditional stimulus → response model to the more contemporary stimulus → organism → response model, which emphasizes the importance of understanding individuals' *subjective* experiences. Only through understanding individuals' subjective experiences can the interindividual differences in reactions to a stressor be accounted for.

Although the stressors of a situation and the behavioral responses of the patient may be readily identified by the medical team, the subjective experiences of the patient by their very nature are more elusive and require inquiry. Psychiatrists are often asked to evaluate patients with problematic behavioral or emotional reactions to the hospital setting or to their illnesses. Medical doctors usually can identify the stressors involved—for example, the need for emergent amputation in a 55-year-old diabetic patient with a gangrenous toe. The stated reason for consultation often also identifies the behavioral or emotional responses judged to be problematic, such as displaying anger and threatening to sign out against medical advice. Consulting psychiatrists seek to understand patients' subjective experiences of illness to explain their emotional and behavioral responses and to design interventions to help patients (and their caregivers).

Research investigating subjective variables that influence an individual's response to a given stressor generally has focused on four main areas: attachment styles, personality types, coping styles, and defense mechanisms. These areas are addressed separately in this section.

Attachment Styles

Attachment theory is another fruitful way of examining patients' interactions with the health care setting and their physicians. John Bowlby (1969) developed a theory that emphasized the effect of early interactions with primary caregivers on an individual's internal relationship schemas. Attachment theory has recently been applied to psychosomatic medicine.

Four predominant attachment styles have been described in the literature (a secure style and three insecure styles: preoccupied, dismissing, and fearful; Bartholomew and Horowitz 1991). Several instruments have been developed to assess individuals' predominant styles, such as the Relationship Questionnaire (Griffin and Bartholomew 1994) and the Adult Attachment Interview (Main 1991). Each attachment style implies a view of self and other formed from early life experiences with caregivers; these internal relationship models are stable and enduring over time; thus, they would logically affect patients' experiences, behaviors, and expectations in the doctor–patient relationship. The individual with a secure attachment style is hypothesized to have experienced consistently responsive caregiving in early life and therefore has a positive expectation of others and comfort in depending on others for care. Inconsistently responsive caregiving is proposed as the environmental antecedent to a preoccupied attachment style, characterized by increased effort on the part of the individual to elicit caregiving and a positive expectation of others, with a negative view of self. These individuals may be particularly vulnerable to consciously or unconsciously exaggerated illness behavior or high medical use (Ciechanowski et al. 2002b).

The dismissing attachment style is thought to derive from early experiences with consistently unresponsive caregivers. As an adaptation to such an environment, these individuals come to dismiss their need for others, value being "self-reliant" to an extreme, and have difficulty trusting others. They develop a positive view of themselves as independent and self-reliant and have a negative expectation of others. Individuals with dismissing attachment styles would therefore be averse to reaching out to others or disclosing their emotional experiences. They avoid engaging in psychotherapy but once engaged benefit from the experience (Fonagy et al. 1996).

Hostile, rejecting, or abusive caregiving early in life is thought to originate the fearful attachment style, characterized by negative views of self and others and a desire for support but fear of rejection and difficulty trusting others. These individuals often alternate between help-seeking and help-rejecting behaviors and frequently demand care but are often nonadherent and miss appointments. Individuals may show characteristics of more than one attachment style, but identification of the predominant style can be useful.

Ciechanowski and colleagues' research studies of patients in a specialty diabetes clinic with various attachment styles serve as excellent examples of the richness of the application of this theory to the health care setting and patient–physician interactions. They found that dismissing and fearful attachment styles are associated with worse diabetes self-care, lower adherence to hypoglycemic agents, and higher blood glucose levels. They describe the difficulty such patients have in trusting and depending on others, which affects their interactions with physicians in our fragmented health care system (Ciechanowski and Katon 2006; Ciechanowski et al. 2001). They proposed that awareness of a patient's predominant attachment style can inform understanding of patient–physician dynamics. Skilled clinicians can use this understanding to alter their approach to patients to facilitate patient engagement and treatment adherence.

Other studies have found that attachment style is an important factor associated with 1) frequency of follow-up in a pain management specialty clinic (Ciechanowski et al. 2003); 2) symptom reporting in primary care, health care costs, and utilization (Ciechanowski et al. 2002b); 3) symptom perception or somatization (Ciechanowski et al. 2002b); and 4) medically unexplained symptoms among hepatitis C patients (Ciechanowski et al. 2002a). Reviews, such as Hunter and Maunder (2001) and Thompson and Ciechanowski (2003), provide a more detailed introduction to this rich area of research, particularly applicable to psychosomatic medicine research and clinical practice.

Personality Types

It is important to distinguish between the concepts of personality type or character style and personality disorder. As noted at the outset, we do not focus on psychopathology in this chapter. Personality types may be understood as existing on a continuum with respective personality disorders (Oldham and Skodol 2000). In addition, most patients do not fit exclusively into one type but may show characteristics of several personality types. Although the most accurate and complete understanding of personality may be achieved through a dimensional model, the characterization of discrete personality types is useful in highlighting differences and providing vivid prototypical examples. Much of the literature on personality types consists of contributions from psychodynamic psychiatry. Although this rich literature continues to be tremendously useful for psychiatrists working in the medical setting, it is unfortunately often ignored because of the current emphasis on biological and descriptive psychiatry. In recognition of Kahana and Bibring's (1964) classic and still relevant paper, "Personality Types in Medical Management," we have organized our discussion around the seven personality types they described (altering their terms to fit with more commonly used modern descriptions): 1) dependent, 2) obsessional, 3) histrionic, 4) masochistic, 5) paranoid, 6) narcissistic, and 7) schizoid. Kahana and Bibring's paper is so valuable because of the rich descriptions of these various personality types and the manner in which each type determines the individuals' subjective experiences of the meaning of illness.

Under conditions of stress, an individual's characteristic means of adapting to situations are heightened (Heiskell and Pasnau 1991; Kiely 1972). When confronted with the stress of a medical illness requiring hospitalization, the mildly obsessional patient might appear overly rigid or controlling. Similarly, a moderately dependent individual may appear "clingy" or excessively needy amid the acute stresses of hospitalization. Patients with extreme forms of these personality types can frustrate caregivers, often evoking intense negative emotions. It is important to recognize these countertransference responses because they can be diagnostically useful tools. The negative emotions that patients with these extreme personality types evoke in the physicians and nurses may result in responses from the caregivers that aggravate the situation (Muskin and Epstein 2009).

In another classic paper, "Taking Care of the Hateful Patient," Groves (1978) characterized four types of patients who most challenge physicians: dependent clingers, entitled demanders, manipulative help-rejecters, and self-destructive deniers. Groves also described the typical countertransference responses to each type and provided helpful tips on the management of these challenging patients. In this subsection, we integrate Groves's astute observations and descriptions of these four types with the seven personality types described by Kahana and Bibring.

Table 4-1 summarizes each of the seven personality types described in detail in the following subsections—their characteristics, the meaning of illness to each type, frequent countertransference responses evoked among caregivers, and tips on management—drawing on the contributions of Geringer and Stern (1986), Groves (1978), Kahana and Bibring (1964), Muskin and Haase (2001), and others.

Dependent

The dependent patient is needy and demanding, is seemingly unable to independently solve problems or self-soothe, and continually asks for help from others. Patients with a dependent personality may initially evoke positive feelings from their physicians and are more likely to adhere to treatment recommendations (Bornstein 1994). The physician may enjoy feeling needed or powerful, much as a parent might feel toward a child. The dependent patient, however, can feel "sticky" or seem to have insatiable needs (Miller 2001), making it difficult for the caregiver to leave the room or end an interview. Such patients typically have limited frustration tolerance. Historically described as "oral" personalities, the extreme of this personality type corresponds to a DSM-IV-TR diagnosis of dependent personality disorder and sometimes borderline personality disorder (American Psychiatric Association 2000; Geringer and Stern 1986).

For the patient with a dependent personality, illness evokes an increased desire for care from others. Illness stimulates the patient's fear of abandonment (Perry and Viederman 1981). The person may feel that no one cares about him or her or may frantically cling to caregivers. Extremes of this personality style fit Groves's (1978) description of dependent clingers. These patients evoke aversion in their caregivers. The caregiver becomes overwhelmed by the patient's neediness, may feel manipulated, and may wish to avoid the patient, thus confirming the patient's fear of abandonment (Groves 1978). Tips on managing patients with this personality style, whether in a mild form or at the extreme, include appropriate reassurance that they will be taken care of, setting firm limits regarding what needs will be met, and setting a specific schedule of visits (e.g., 20 minutes three times a week) to establish clear expectations regarding the doctor's time and availability (Miller 2001; Perry and Viederman 1981). For the overdemanding patient, it can be helpful to convey tactfully that behaviors such as incessantly ringing the call bell may have an opposite effect than what is intended and can lead caregivers to avoid the patient (Perry and Viederman 1981).

Obsessional

Individuals with an obsessional personality style are meticulous and orderly and like to feel in control. They place a strong emphasis on rationality, can be self-righteous at times, and are concerned with issues of right and wrong. These patients may be emotionally reserved and focus on details, sometimes to such an extent as to miss the broader picture. Ritual and regularity of schedule are important to them (Miller 2001). They are easily frustrated by the unpredictability of the hospital environment. Patients at the

TABLE 4–1. Personality types

Type	Characteristics	Meaning of illness	Countertransference responses	Tips on management
Dependent	Needy, demanding, clingy Unable to reassure self Seeks reassurance from others	Threat of abandonment	Positive: doctor feels powerful and needed Negative: doctor feels overwhelmed and annoyed; may try to avoid patient	Reassure within limits Schedule visits Mobilize other supports Reward efforts toward independence Avoid tendency to withdraw from patient
Obsessional	Meticulous, orderly Likes to feel in control Very concerned with right/wrong	Loss of control over body/emotions/impulses	May admire When extreme: anger—a "battle of wills"	Try to set routine Give patient choices to increase sense of control Provide detailed information and "homework" Foster collaborative approach/avoid "battle of wills"
Histrionic	Entertaining Melodramatic Seductive, flirtatious	Loss of love or loss of attractiveness	Anxiety, impatience, off-putting Erotic; finds patient attractive	Strike a balance between warmth and formality Maintain clear boundaries Encourage patient to discuss fears Do not confront head-on
Masochistic	"Perpetual victim" Self-sacrificing martyr	Ego-syntonic Conscious or unconscious punishment	Anger, hate, frustration Helplessness, self-doubt	Avoid excessive encouragement Share patient's pessimism Deemphasize connection between symptoms and frequent visits Suggest that patient consider treatment as another burden to endure, or emphasize treatment's positive effect on loved ones
Paranoid	Guarded, distrustful Quick to blame or counterattack Sensitive to slights	Proof that world is against patient Medical care is invasive and exploitative	Anger, feeling attacked or accused May become defensive	Avoid defensive stance Acknowledge patient's feelings without disputing them Maintain interpersonal distance; avoid excessive warmth Do not confront irrational fears
Narcissistic	Arrogant, devaluing Vain, demanding	Threat to self-concept of perfection and invulnerability Shame evoking	Anger, desire to counterattack Activation of feelings of inferiority, or enjoyment of feeling of status of working with an important patient	Resist the desire to challenge patient's entitlement Reframe entitlement to foster treatment adherence Take a humble stance, provide opportunities for patient to show off, offer consultations if appropriate
Schizoid	Aloof, remote Socially awkward Inhibited	Fear of intrusion	Little connection to patient Difficult to engage	Respect patient's privacy Prevent patient from completely withdrawing Maintain gentle, quiet interest in patient Encourage routine and regularity

Source. Derived in large part from Geringer and Stern 1986; Kahana and Bibring 1964; Perry and Viederman 1981.

extreme end of the spectrum with this personality style might meet DSM-IV-TR criteria for obsessive-compulsive personality disorder.

Patients with an obsessional personality style will generally want a lot of information from their physicians regarding their medications, diagnoses, tests, and so forth. The physician may be pleased by the patient's desire to learn about his or her illness and its treatments. Under extreme stress, however, the patient may become increasingly rigid and inflexible, and at times the obsessional patient's only way to feel a sense of control is by refusing treatment or procedures (Kahana and Bibring 1964). A defiant refusal of procedures frequently leads to psychiatric consultation. For example, the obsessional patient who is frustrated by the unpredictability of his hospital care and is angry after hours of fasting for an endoscopy that is subsequently canceled may refuse to allow a phlebotomist to draw his blood the following morning or refuse the second attempt to send him to the endoscopy suite. Conflicts between the extremes of compliance and defiance are common for these individuals.

Illness is experienced by the obsessional patient as a loss of control over the body, and it evokes a fear of loss of control over emotions or impulses (Heiskell and Pasnau 1991; Kahana and Bibring 1964; Miller 2001). When an inflexible or obstinate patient with this personality style confronts the physician, the physician may be tempted to engage in a battle of wills or try to exert greater control over the patient's treatment. Such a response, however, becomes counterproductive and often provokes the patient to resist even harder as in a tug-of-war. Instead, it may be helpful to offer detailed explanations of the procedures and tests and the reasons they are necessary. This emphasizes a collaborative approach, encouraging patients to participate actively in their care. Wherever possible, it is helpful to give patients choices and input into their care. This makes the patient a partner, not an opponent (Gazzola and Muskin 2003). Giving patients information, assigning them "homework," and providing opportunities for their input on decisions, when appropriate, will enable them to feel more in control of their care and will decrease anxiety and interpersonal friction (Muskin and Haase 2001).

Histrionic

Patients with a histrionic personality style can be entertaining, engaging, and at times seductive. This can be charming at times, or it can be uncomfortable or embarrassing for physicians (Miller 2001). Histrionic patients crave attention, approval, and admiration and tend to avoid anxiety-provoking situations through the use of denial. Illness in the patient with a histrionic personality style is experienced as a threat to the patient's masculinity or femininity (Geringer and Stern 1986). Illness activates such patients' fear of loss of love or attractiveness (Kahana and Bibring 1964; Strain and Grossman 1975).

The physician treating the histrionic patient should try to strike a balance between warmth and formality. Maintaining clear boundaries is essential, but an overly formal style will activate the patient's fear of loss of attractiveness or lovability (Heiskell and Pasnau 1991; Miller 2001). Encouraging the patient to discuss his or her fears will help bring to consciousness the anxiety that the patient is attempting to avoid. It is important, however, not to push patients too hard—a supportive and patient stance that gently encourages patients to voice fears when ready will be most helpful. "Confronting denial" head-on usually is counterproductive, as discussed in greater detail later in this chapter.

Masochistic

Patients with a masochistic personality style seem to be perpetual victims and readily recount their woes, experiencing themselves as self-sacrificing martyrs. One typically finds that such patients had miserable, abusive childhoods in which the experiences of physical illness paradoxically may have been bright spots, the only times they may have felt truly loved or cared for by parents or others (Heiskell and Pasnau 1991). The experience of illness, in part, provides reassurance to these patients that they will be able to maintain the attention and care of their physicians. Kahana and Bibring (1964) concretize this wish in the unspoken statement "You have to love me because I suffer so terribly." The patient may feel that the illness (consciously or unconsciously) is punishment for real or fantasized wrongdoings. Other patients may hold an unconscious wish to defeat their physicians (Douglas and Druss 1987; Heiskell and Pasnau 1991). The masochistic personality style can be particularly resistant to change.

Patients with the masochistic personality style may present with somatoform or factitious disorders. When the masochistic patient has no response (or a negative response) to treatment, or the physician's attempts to offer reassurance have no effect, the physician may become extremely frustrated. Encouragement and reassurance may actually have a paradoxical effect, provoking the patient to feel more pessimistic and leading to a worsening of symptoms. Those with an extreme version of this personality style have been described as "help-rejecters" (Groves 1978). They evoke feelings of irritation, depression, self-doubt, and hopelessness in their caregivers, who themselves may believe that such patients engineer their own misfortunes. The idea that someone could obtain psychological benefit from suffering is a concept that is difficult to understand, especially for physicians and other health care professionals.

Managing the patient with a masochistic personality should involve regularly scheduled follow-up visits irrespective of symptoms. It is important to deemphasize the connection between severity of symptoms and frequency of physician contact (Perry and Viederman 1981). Rather than encourage and reassure these patients, it is useful to acknowledge the patients' suffering and to "share their pessimism" (Groves 1978). It is sometimes of benefit for the physician to express to the patient an understanding that the illness and medical treatments are yet another burden for the patient to endure (Gazzola and Muskin 2003). It can also be helpful to emphasize the treatment's potential positive effect on others dear to the patient. This may reframe the treatment as another opportunity for the patient to suffer for the benefit of others (Heiskell and Pasnau 1991).

Paranoid

The paranoid patient is not generally a favorite of the physician. This patient maintains a guarded, distrustful stance; is quick to blame; and readily feels attacked (Heiskell and Pasnau 1991). Patients with a paranoid style do not forgive easily and may maintain lists of grievances. When these patients feel slighted, they tend to counterattack. It may not take much to provoke them because they are extremely sensitive to anything experienced as a slight. When ill, patients with a paranoid personality style may blame others, and they may conceive of the illness as proof that the world is against them. They are prone to feeling hurt, invaded, or exploited by seemingly innocuous medical procedures (Miller 2001). Stress increases such patients' tendency to be suspicious, guarded, or controlling. This results in a request for psychiatric consultation because these patients evoke feelings of anger in their caregivers. They refuse procedures or tests, threaten to sign out against medical advice, and accuse the staff of doing things against them.

The physician assigned the task of treating a patient with this personality style often feels accused. If the physician is not aware of this, it can lead to defensive countertransference (Kahana and Bibring 1964). This may appear as a temptation to argue with the patient or as an attempt to prove the patient wrong. Taking a defensive stance will be counterproductive and can in essence prove the paranoid patient right; a defensive response will only increase the patient's paranoia. A more helpful approach is to acknowledge the patient's feelings without dispute or agreement, explaining in detail the justification for the treatments. Irrational fears often should not be confronted head-on or challenged; the patient will judge caregivers more on their actions and predominant emotional stance than on their words. Avoiding excessive warmth is helpful, as is maintaining sufficient interpersonal distance (Heiskell and Pasnau 1991). A calm, firm, direct stance is preferable to an angry, defensive stance or an intrusive, overly warm stance.

Narcissistic

Patients with a narcissistic personality style are typically easily recognized. Arrogant, devaluing, vain, and demanding, these patients can often be identified by one's immediate reaction. The narcissistic patient frequently begins the interview inquiring about the physician's title and rank. The patient may refuse to be examined by medical students, residents, or junior faculty members. These patients will devalue those believed to be inferior to them and will idealize the few people perceived to be highest in status. At the extreme, some patients will meet the criteria for narcissistic personality disorder. The patient's self-experience is frequently not validated by actual status in the world.

Narcissistic patients will experience an illness as a threat to their self-concept of perfection and invulnerability (Heiskell and Pasnau 1991; Kahana and Bibring 1964). Under such a threat, the patient's characteristic defense of grandiosity will be heightened. The physician or caregiver who is angered by the patient's devaluations and entitlement will be strongly tempted to put the patient in his or her place (Miller 2001). The psychiatric consultant who is called to assist in the management of a narcissistic patient may hear angry staff members say, "Who does he think he is? He's no better than anyone else!" and hear them put down the patient. Groves (1978) described patients at the extreme of this style as "entitled demanders," noting the intense feelings of anger and the desire to counterattack that these patients can evoke in their caregivers. The narcissistic patient can activate the physician's own feelings of inferiority, adding to the desire to avoid or attack the patient. The "power" of narcissistic VIP patients can be very seductive to physicians, who may be tempted to cater to the unreasonable demands with the fantasy of some special status.

Managing patients with a narcissistic personality can be challenging. Resisting the desire to challenge the patient's entitlement is crucial in forming a therapeutic alliance. According to Groves (1978), "Entitlement is the patient's religion and should not be blasphemed." Although it is counterintuitive, the physician should not reflexively support the patient's entitlement but should reframe it in such a way as to foster the patient's adherence to the treatment regimen and working with the team. Frequent use of phrases such as "You deserve the best" can be very helpful (Muskin and Haase 2001). Taking a humble stance can be effective: "Understandably, Mr. Jones, you want the best care and certainly deserve no less—unfortunately, although we strive to provide you with the best care possible, we aren't perfect. We ask your indulgence to work with us so that we can give you the care that you deserve." Such statements can at times have a dramatic effect if delivered genuinely. Judicious use of "narcissistic strokes"—that is, providing opportunities for the patient to brag or show off—can assist in building rapport. Appropriate acknowledgment of mistakes made by the team and offering consultation by specialists can also assist in the management of these challenging patients. If the patient feels recognized as someone unique and special, he or she will feel reassured and will have less need to make demands (Heiskell and Pasnau 1991). The psychiatric consultant can assist members of the team not to take the patient's devaluations personally but instead to understand them as the patient's frantic efforts to maintain self-esteem. If the caregivers can avoid feeling personally attacked, they will find it easier to work with these patients and will be less likely to engage in a counterattack.

Schizoid

Patients with a schizoid personality are seen as aloof, remote, and socially awkward or inhibited; they frequently avoid obtaining medical care until it is absolutely necessary (Kahana and Bibring 1964; Miller 2001). The physician charged with the care of the schizoid patient will find it difficult to build rapport or engage the patient in treatment.

At one end of the spectrum of this personality style are schizoid and avoidant personality disorders (Geringer and Stern 1986). These two personality disorders are distinguished in part by the apparent interest in social contact. The patient with schizoid personality disorder seems uninterested in social contact, whereas the patient with avoidant personality disorder desires social contact but avoids it out of fear of rejection. In the consultation setting, similar management tips apply to either of these two personality disorders and to patients who fall within this spectrum. In general, illness and hospitalization evoke a fear of intrusion and intense anxiety (Geringer and Stern 1986; Heiskell and Pasnau 1991). The physician should respect the patient's need for privacy but should prevent the patient from withdrawing completely (Gazzola and Muskin 2003). Maintaining a quiet, gentle interest in the patient and encouraging a regular, expectable routine can reassure the patient that he or she is safe and will not be intruded on (Miller 2001). Typically, such patients have a fragile sense of self and therefore warrant gentle care but care at a distance.

Summary of Personality Types

These seven prototypical personality styles cannot claim to capture every patient, and many patients fit into multiple categories. Understanding the common features of each style can aid the consulting psychiatrist. Knowing how each personality style experiences illness will inform interactions with such patients. Close monitoring of one's countertransference can also assist in identifying the patient's predominant personality style (e.g., feeling inferior with narcissistic patients or feeling attacked by paranoid patients). Knowledge of these personality types can assist the psychiatric consultant in educating the medical team about the proper management of these challenging patients and in assisting them not to react in counterproductive ways. At times, through understanding of the patient's personality style, the consulting psychiatrist is able to achieve rapid and remarkable therapeutic effects by choosing an appropriate intervention. Such effective interventions are impressive to nonpsychiatric physicians and staff members and confirm the utility of psychodynamic understanding in the psychiatric care of the medically ill.

Coping Styles

In the previous subsection, we illustrated how taking into account personality types can explain some of the interindividual variation in response to the stressors of illness. How individuals cope is another rich area of investigation (Jensen et al. 1991; Lazarus 1999; Penley et al. 2002), and problems in coping with illness have been shown to be a frequent reason for psychiatric consultation (Strain et al. 1993). Health psychologists have developed the concepts of appraisal (the assignment of meaning or value to a particular thing or event) and coping (Lazarus and Folkman 1984). An extensive body of literature developed over the past few decades has examined these processes among patients in health care settings. This psychological literature is often underrecognized by the psychiatric and medical communities but is extremely useful and can complement psychodynamic perspectives.

Coping can be defined as "thoughts and behaviors that the person uses to manage or alter the problem that is causing distress (problem-focused coping) and regulate the emotional response to the problem (emotion-focused coping)" (Folkman et al. 1993, pp. 409–410). A comprehensive review of the literature on the many defined coping strategies in medical illness is beyond the scope of this chapter. The reader is referred to the excellent reviews by Lazarus (1999) and Penley et al. (2002). Some important empirical generalizations that have emerged from decades of research on coping are discussed in this section (Lazarus 1999).

Use of Multiple Coping Styles in Stressful Situations

Folkman and colleagues (1986) identified eight categories of coping styles in a factor analysis of the Ways of Coping Questionnaire–Revised: 1) confrontative coping (hostile or aggressive efforts to alter a situation), 2) distancing (attempts to detach oneself mentally from a situation), 3) self-controlling (attempts to regulate one's feelings or actions), 4) seeking social support (efforts to seek emotional support or information from others), 5) accepting responsibility (acknowledgment of a personal role in the problem), 6) using escape-avoidance (cognitive or behavioral efforts to escape or avoid the problem or situation), 7) planful problem solving (deliberate and carefully thought-out efforts to alter the situation), and 8) conducting positive reappraisal (efforts to reframe the situation in a positive light) (Penley et al. 2002). Research has shown that patients use multiple coping strategies in any given situation (Lazarus 1999). Individuals often prefer or habitually use certain strategies over others, but generally multiple strategies are used for a complex stressful situation such as a medical illness or hospitalization. People use some trial and error in the selection of coping style (Lazarus 1999).

Coping as a Trait and a Process

Preferred coping styles are commonly tied to personality variables; sometimes they can be viewed as traits as well as processes (Heim et al. 1997; Lazarus 1999). Therefore, it is useful to ask patients how they previously dealt with very stressful situations. This can provide useful information for the physician because patients are likely to use strategies in the present that are similar to those they used in the past, whether they were effective or not.

Research on women with breast cancer at various stages of illness has found that coping strategies may change as the nature of the stressor changes (Heim et al. 1993, 1997). For example, on initial detection of breast cancer, a woman may seek social support from her friends and spouse to cope with the uncertainties of her situation. Later, after lumpectomy and staging, she might shift her primary coping strategy to planful problem solving—a plan to follow up regularly for chemotherapy and to adhere fully to her oncologist's prescription of tamoxifen.

Problem-Focused Coping Versus Emotion-Focused Coping

One way to organize various coping styles is whether they are problem focused or emotion focused. Research has shown that patients will tend to choose problem-focused coping strategies when they appraise the situation as being changeable or within their control (Folkman et al. 1993; Schussler 1992). In conditions considered out of their control, patients may choose emotion-focused coping styles (Folkman et al. 1993; Schussler 1992). In the medical setting, consulting psychiatrists can help change the patient's appraisal of the situation and encourage the patient to choose more adaptive coping styles. For example, if a patient newly diagnosed with diabetes mellitus misperceives high blood glucose as being unchangeable or out of his control, he might choose an emotion-focused coping strategy such as avoidance or denial. In educating this patient about how treatable hyperglycemia can be, the physician could encourage the patient to change his coping strategy to a problem-focused strategy such as making dietary changes or increasing exercise.

Variations in Usefulness of Coping Strategies Over Time

Coping is a powerful mediator of how a patient responds emotionally to a given stressor (Folkman and Lazarus 1988; Lipowski 1970). Coping strategies also have been reported to have different effects on health outcomes—some positive, others negative (see Penley et al. 2002 for a meta-analysis on this research). Although some coping strategies may be considered more effective than others, they vary in usefulness depending on the situation. A strategy that is initially effective in dealing with a stressor may no longer be effective when the nature of the stressor changes (Penley et al. 2002). The discussion of maladaptive versus adaptive denial under "Denial" later in this chapter illustrates this point.

Relation Between Coping Styles and the Meaning of Illness

Lipowski (1970) described eight "illness concepts": 1) illness as challenge, 2) illness as enemy, 3) illness as punishment, 4) illness as weakness, 5) illness as relief, 6) illness as strategy, 7) illness as irreparable loss or damage, and 8) illness as value. Lipowski proposed that a patient's choice of coping strategy is partially dependent on the underlying illness concept. In a study of 205 patients with chronic physical illness, the descriptors "illness as challenge" and "illness as value" were found to be related to "adaptive coping and mental well-being." Conversely, "illness as enemy," "illness as punishment," and "illness as relief" were associated with psychological symptoms and maladaptive coping (Schussler 1992).

Defense Mechanisms

Anna Freud (1948), in *The Ego and the Mechanisms of Defense,* first described the psychoanalytic term *defense mechanism* in the literature. Defense mechanisms are automatic psychological processes by which the mind confronts a psychological threat (e.g., the fear of death or deformity) or conflict between a wish and the demands of reality or the dictates of conscience. This psychoanalytic concept has a rich history that is beyond the scope of this chapter. Although there is some overlap of the concept of coping with that of defenses, the psychological concept of coping is more behavioral; it involves action (e.g., seeking social support, or productive problem solving) and is generally a conscious experience. Defenses are usually conceptualized as intrapsychic processes that are largely out of the individual's awareness. In *The Wisdom of the Ego,* George Vaillant (1993) emphasized the usefulness of the concept of defenses:

> Our lives are at times intolerable. At times we cannot bear reality. At such times our minds play tricks on us. Our minds distort inner and outer reality so that an observer might accuse us of denial, self-deception, even dishonesty. But such mental defenses creatively rearrange the sources of our conflict so that they become manageable and we may survive. (p. 1)

He further noted that

> [a] clearly understood nomenclature of defenses not only enables us to understand adaptation to stress; it also offers us a means of uncoding, of translating if you will, much of what seems irrational in human behavior. (p. 28)

A basic understanding of the concept of defense and various defense mechanisms can provide the psychiatrist in the medical setting with another lens through which to examine a patient and to predict or explain the patient's emotional or behavioral responses to medical illness.

Vaillant (1993) identified several aspects of defenses:

1. *Defenses are generally outside of awareness of the individual or unconscious.* They enable the mind to "play tricks on" the individual to lessen distress or conflict.
2. *Defenses by nature distort inner and outer reality.* As is emphasized below, the degree of this distortion varies among defense mechanisms, as does the focus of the distortion: some defenses distort a warded-off internal drive or desire, whereas others distort the external reality or interpersonal situation.
3. *Defenses can appear strange or overt to the observer while going unnoticed by the subject.* The psychiatrist must decide whether directing the patient's awareness to his or her use of certain defenses is indicated.
4. *Defenses are creative.* The mind creates a new perception distinct from reality.
5. *Defenses involve psychological conflict.* Through them the mind attempts to manage the often conflicting demands of inner wishes, conscience, other people, and reality.
6. *Defenses are adaptive and are not all pathological.* Some defenses are more adaptive than others, and the use of defenses is an inherent property of the mind.

Vaillant (1993) proposed a hierarchy of defense mechanisms ranked in four levels of adaptivity: psychotic, immature (or borderline), neurotic, and mature. This hierarchy is based on the degree to which each defense distorts reality and how effectively it enables the expression of wishes or needs without untoward external consequences. Patients often use many different defense mechanisms in different situations or under varying levels of stress. When a patient inflexibly and consistently uses lower-level defenses, this is often consistent with a personality disorder. Table 4–2 lists major defense mechanisms grouped into four levels.

The *psychotic defenses* are characterized by the extreme degree to which they distort external reality. Patients in psychotic states usually employ these defenses; psychotherapy is generally ineffective in altering them, and antipsychotic medication may be indicated.

The *immature defenses* are characteristic of patients with personality disorders, especially the Cluster B personality disorders such as borderline personality disorder. Vaillant (1993) emphasized how many of these defenses are irritating to others and get under other people's skin. "Those afflicted with immature defenses often transmit their shame, impulses and anxiety to those around them" (p. 58).

In contrast to the immature defenses, the *neurotic defenses* do not typically irritate others and are more privately experienced—they are less interpersonal and often involve mental inhibitions. They distort reality less than do immature or psychotic defenses and may go unnoticed by the observer. With appropriate tact and timing, neurotic defenses can be effectively interpreted in exploratory psychotherapy when it is considered appropriate by the treating psychiatrist. "Over the short haul, neurotic defenses make the user suffer; immature defenses make the observer suffer" (Vaillant 1993, p. 66).

The *mature defenses* "integrate sources of conflict...and thus require no interpretation" (Vaillant 1993, p. 67). The use of mature defenses such as humor or altruism in the confrontation of a stressor such as medical illness often earns admiration from others and can be inspirational. Such mature defenses are not interpreted by the psychiatrist but are praised. These defenses maximize expression of drives or wishes without negative consequences or distortion of reality.

Denial

Denial is an important and complex concept and a common reason that physicians request psychiatric consultation. Weisman and Hackett (1961) defined *denial* as "the conscious or unconscious repudiation of part or all of the total available meanings of an event to allay fear, anxiety, or other unpleasant affects" (p. 232). It is to be distinguished from a lack of awareness due to a cognitive deficit such as anosognosia or from the limited insight of a patient with chronic

TABLE 4–2. Defense mechanisms

Mature defenses	
Suppression	Consciously putting a disturbing experience out of mind
Altruism	Vicarious but instinctively gratifying service to others
Humor	Overt expression of normally unacceptable feelings without unpleasant effect
Sublimation	Attenuated expression of drives in alternative fields without adverse consequences
Anticipation	Realistic planning for inevitable discomfort
Neurotic defenses	
Repression	Involuntary forgetting of a painful feeling or experience
Control	Manipulation of external events to avoid unconscious anxiety
Displacement	Transfer of an experienced feeling from one person to another or to something else
Reaction formation	Expression of unacceptable impulses as directly opposite attitudes and behaviors
Intellectualization	Replacing of feelings with facts/details
Rationalization	Inventing a convincing, but usually false, reason why one is not bothered
Isolation of affect	Separating a painful idea or event from feelings associated with it
Undoing	Ritualistic "removal" of an offensive act, sometimes by atoning for it
Immature defenses	
Splitting	Experiencing oneself and others as all good or all bad
Idealization	Seeing oneself or others as all-powerful, ideal, or godlike
Devaluation	Depreciating others
Projection	Attributing unacceptable impulses or ideas to others
Projective identification	Causing others to experience one's unacceptable feelings; one then fears or tries to control the unacceptable behavior in the other person
Acting-out	Direct expression of an unconscious wish or impulse to avoid being conscious of the affect, and thoughts that accompany it
Passive aggression	Expressing anger indirectly and passively
Intermediate denial	Refusal to acknowledge painful realities
Psychotic defenses	
Psychotic denial	Obliteration of external reality
Delusional projection	Externalization of inner conflicts and giving them tangible reality—minimal reality testing
Schizoid fantasy	Withdrawal from conflict into social isolation and fantasizing

Source. Carlat 1999; Muskin and Haase 2001; Vaillant 1993.

schizophrenia. Psychiatrists are often called to see a patient "in denial" about a newly diagnosed illness and may be asked to assess the patient's capacity to consent to or refuse certain treatments. As discussed in this section, denial can be *adaptive,* protecting the patient from being emotionally overwhelmed by an illness, or *maladaptive,* preventing or delaying diagnosis, treatment, and lifestyle changes.

Denial seems to be a very personal response that is prone to a double standard: we are often capable of—even comfortable with—ignoring our own denial but consider other people's denial abnormal. A smoker may minimize his risk of lung cancer, noting that only a small percentage of smokers get the disease, yet simultaneously criticize his son's obesity as a risk factor for diabetes. Physicians urge their patients to adopt healthy lifestyles yet may routinely overwork and get too little sleep (see Gaba and Howard 2002).

Psychiatrists are most likely to be called on when the patient's denial makes the physician uncomfortable, but health care providers sometimes use the term *denial* loosely and inaccurately (Goldbeck 1997; Havik and Maeland 1988; Jacobsen and Lowery 1992). A physician's statement that a patient is "in denial" may refer to various situations: 1) the patient rejects the diagnosis, 2) the patient minimizes symptoms of the illness or does not seem to appreciate its implications, 3) the patient avoids or delays medical treatment, or 4) the patient appears to have no emotional reaction to the diagnosis or illness (Goldbeck 1997). The first task of the psychiatric consultant is to determine specifically what the referring physician means by "denial."

The severity of denial varies by the nature of what is denied, by the predominant defense mechanisms at work (e.g., suppression, repression, psychotic denial), and by the degree of accessibility to consciousness (Goldbeck 1997). Patients who use the mature defense of *suppression* in confronting an illness are not truly in denial. Rather, they have chosen to put aside their fears about illness and treatment until a later time. Their fears are not deeply unconscious but are easily accessible if patients choose to access them. These patients typically accept treatment, face their illnesses with courage, and do not let their emotions overtake them. Such "denial" is considered adaptive (Druss and Douglas 1988). Many authors have proposed that some denial is perhaps necessary for very effective coping with an overwhelming illness (see discussions in Druss 1995; Ness and Ende 1994; Schussler 1992; Wool 1988).

In contrast to suppression, the patient using *repression* as a defense is generally unaware of the internal experience (e.g., fear, thought, wish) being warded off. Repressed thoughts or feelings are not easily accessible to consciousness. Such a patient may feel very anxious without understanding why. For example, a 39-year-old man whose father died of a myocardial infarction at age 41 may become increasingly anxious as his 40th birthday approaches without being aware of the connection.

When it is more severe and pervasive, denial can result in patients flatly denying they are ill and not seeking medical care. If they are already in care, they decline treatment or are nonadherent. Repeated attempts by the medical team to educate them about their illness have no effect. Extreme denial may be severe enough to distort the perception of reality, sometimes described as *psychotic denial*. Most patients with pervasive denial of illness are not psychotic in the usual sense of the word and should be distinguished from those who are. The latter usually have a psychotic illness such as schizophrenia and may pay no attention to signs or symptoms of illness or may incorporate them into somatic delusions. Psychotic patients who deny illness usually do not conceal its signs; others often readily recognize they are ill. In contrast, nonpsychotic patients with pervasive denial often conceal signs of their illness from themselves and others. For example, a nonpsychotic woman with pervasive denial of a growing breast mass avoided medical care and undressing in front of others and kept a bandage over what she regarded as a bruise. Although pregnancy is not a medical illness, a dramatic example of pervasive (sometimes psychotic) denial is the denial of pregnancy (see Chapter 33, "Obstetrics and Gynecology").

Strauss et al. (1990) proposed a new DSM diagnosis—maladaptive denial of physical illness—to describe patients whose denial of illness is maladaptive. How does one determine whether denial is adaptive or maladaptive? For the woman with a growing breast tumor, denial is clearly maladaptive because it has prevented her from receiving potentially lifesaving treatment. In other situations, denial may be quite adaptive. In determining the adaptivity of a patient's denial, it is important to answer the following questions (Goldbeck 1997):

- Does the patient's denial impair or prevent the patient from receiving necessary treatment or lead to actions that endanger the patient's health? If so, then the denial is deemed maladaptive. In cases in which no effective treatment is available, the denial might be judged as adaptive to the extent that it decreases distress and improves quality of life, or it may be maladaptive if it prevents critical life planning (e.g., a single parent with little support and a terminal illness who has made no plans for his or her young children).
- Which component of denial—denial of the facts of illness, denial of the implications of the illness, or denial of the emotional reaction to illness—does the patient show? The latter two components of denial are not as maladaptive as the first component and may be adaptive in some situations. Denying the full implications of a disease, such as inevitable death, might be adaptive because it facilitates hope and improved quality of life. Likewise, denial of certain emotional reactions to the illness such as fear or hopelessness might enable a patient to stay motivated through a completed course of treatment.
- Is the denial a temporary means of "buying time," to accept gradually a diagnosis so that the immediate effect is not so overwhelming, or has the denial been so protracted that it has prevented adaptive action? Many patients are unable to accept a diagnosis immediately, and denial may be a way for them to adjust at their own pace to their emotional distress in a period of gradual acceptance. In many situations, this would be considered adaptive.

Even when denial is adaptive for the patient, it may bother physicians or other caregivers. The following case vignette illustrates this point.

Case Vignette

A psychiatric consultation was requested for a 24-year-old man who was quadriplegic after a gunshot wound to the spine. The physician was insistent that the patient's denial be "broken through" because the patient was convinced that he would walk again. The patient had a thorough understanding of his condition and maintained that his hard work and faith would restore his physical abilities. The physician was concerned that the patient might commit suicide when he realized that there was no chance of recovery of function. Instead of forcing the patient to face the prognosis, the consultant recommended that the physician offer the patient training in the skills necessary to maintain himself in his current state because recovery, in whatever form it took, would take a considerable amount of time. The patient continued to cooperate with physical therapy, learned how to use a motorized wheelchair, and discussed the plans for his living arrangements. The physician felt comfortable with this approach because it was "realistic."

All too often, physicians misjudge patients as being in denial. This tends to occur with three types of patients: 1) patients without an overt emotional reaction to an illness or a diagnosis, 2) patients whose reactions differ from those expected by their caregivers, and 3) patients who have been inadequately informed about their illness. The absence of an overt reaction to medical illness is a style of psychological response. Although it is not evident to an observer, individuals may actually be aware of their emotions and thoughts about their illness. Some physicians have a tendency to misjudge patients as being in denial who do not express an expected emotional response or who seek alternative treatments instead of those recommended by the physician (Cousins 1982). An obsessional middle-aged accountant in the coronary care unit, for example, may be acutely aware of his condition and may be quite concerned about it, yet he may not express any of the fears or anxiety that his caregivers would expect, appearing calm and hopeful. This patient is not denying his illness but may be considered to be doing so by caregivers because he "looks too relaxed and in too good a mood."

One must ensure that patients are fully informed about their illness and treatment before assessing patients as being in denial. Gattelari et al. (1999) found that a portion of patients judged by their caregivers to be using denial were in reality relatively uninformed about the details of their illness or its prognosis. On the contrary, some patients who say that they have not been informed have in fact been repeatedly educated by their health care professionals and really are in denial.

Studies of the effect of denial on medical outcomes have found both beneficial and adverse effects. The literature has several methodological limitations, including sometimes failing to clearly define how denial was measured, treating denial as an all-or-nothing phenomenon, and using a lack of observable negative affect as a primary indicator of denial (problematic for the reasons discussed earlier). The use of different measures of denial and distinct patient populations makes comparisons across studies very difficult (Goldbeck 1997).

Some studies have reported positive effects of denial of physical illness on outcome. Hackett and Cassem (1974) found that "major deniers" in coronary care units after myocardial infarction had a better outcome than did "minor deniers." Levenson et al. (1989) found that among patients with unstable angina, "high deniers" had fewer episodes of angina and more favorable outcomes than did "low deniers." Other studies suggest that denial is useful for specific clinical situations such as elective surgery (Cohen and Lazarus 1973) and wound healing (Marucha et al. 1998). Denial was associated with better survival rates in a small study of patients awaiting heart transplantation (Young et al. 1991).

Other research studies have found a mixed or negative effect of denial on medical outcome. "Major deniers" have shorter stays in the intensive care unit but are more likely to be noncompliant after discharge (Levine et al. 1987). Greater denial was associated with a worse medical outcome but decreased mood symptoms and sleep problems in patients with end-stage renal disease (Fricchione et al. 1992). Denial may be counterproductive in asthma patients (Staudenmeyer et al. 1979). Croog et al. (1971) noted lower treatment adherence among deniers in their large sample of myocardial infarct patients. In a study of women scheduled for breast biopsy, those with a history of habitual use of denial were observed to have been more likely to delay medical evaluation (Greer 1974).

When denial is present and is assessed as maladaptive, interventions usually should be directed toward the underlying emotions provoking the denial (e.g., fear). Direct confrontation of denial generally should be avoided because it is counterproductive (Ness and Ende 1994; Perry and Viederman 1981). For example, a 17-year-old adolescent who is newly diagnosed with diabetes mellitus may not want to accept this diagnosis and the need for changes in his lifestyle because of his painful memories of seeing other family members suffer through complications of diabetes. The physician may be tempted to frighten the patient into compliance with a statement such as, "If you don't change your diet, measure your blood sugar, and take insulin regularly, you will wind up with complications just like your mother's." Such statements are usually counterproductive because they increase anxiety, which is driving the patient's use of denial in the first place. Instead, a gentle, empathic, and nonjudgmental stance is more effective (Ness and Ende 1994). Diminishing the intensity of negative affects such as anxiety through psychopharmacological or psychotherapeutic interventions also can be helpful because these affects may be driving the patient's need for denial.

In addition, the consulting psychiatrist should consider whether a patient's maladaptive denial is fostered by particular interpersonal relationships, such as those with family members, friends, a religious community, physicians, or other caregivers (Goldbeck 1997). In such cases, interventions aimed solely at the individual patient's denial without addressing the reinforcing interpersonal relationships are likely to be unsuccessful.

Emotional Responses to Medical Illness

Psychiatrists in the medical setting are frequently called on to help a patient manage emotional responses to illness and hospitalization (e.g., anger, fear, grief, shame). Usually the patient's emotional response is identified in the consultation request. For example, "Please come see this 25-year-old man just diagnosed with testicular cancer who is angry and refusing treatment." The young man's internist cannot understand why this patient would refuse the very course of therapy needed to treat (and possibly cure) his testicular cancer. With an understanding of the patient's subjective experience of his illness, his predominant coping styles, and his prominent defense mechanisms, the consulting psychiatrist can help the patient and the internist to understand the patient's anger, facilitating an alliance within which treatment is more likely to be accepted.

Because every patient is unique, empathic listening to a patient's story of his or her illness will identify the predominant emotional response, which is a potential clue to the subjective meaning of illness for that patient (Lazarus 1999). Core relational themes for the most common emotions (Lazarus 1999) can serve as hypotheses about the meaning of the illness for the patient (Table 4–3). An illness can evoke multiple emotional responses simultaneously or sequentially. The illness may have multiple meanings, and the meanings may change over the course of the illness. The predominant emotional response should not be the sole focus of the psychiatrist's attention (although it may demand the most attention). For example, the 25-year-old man just diagnosed with testicular cancer is markedly angry and refuses treatment. One can hypothesize that it might be because he feels frightened, weakened, or emasculated or that he fears castration. In viewing the physician as the bearer of bad news, the patient is not only angry about receiving a cancer diagnosis but also angry with his physician. Accepting and attempting to understand the patient's anger aids the psychiatrist in giving this man permission to express his feelings while tactfully helping him to see that he can do so without forgoing his own treatment. The patient's refusal of treatment also may be determined by fear of what the treatment will involve. The psychiatrist might also work with the oncologist and his response to the patient's anger. Education by the physicians about the treatment options and the high likelihood of cure could dramatically shift the patient's emotional and behavioral responses and evoke relief and hope. Assisting the patient in naming his emotional responses and understanding *why* they are present can help the patient feel understood. This can facilitate the acceptance of an individualized treatment plan that appropriately involves medication, psychotherapy, psychoeducation, or other interventions.

TABLE 4–3. Core relational themes underlying affective responses

Anger	A demeaning offense against me and mine
Anxiety	Facing uncertain, existential threat
Fright	An immediate, concrete, and overwhelming danger
Guilt	Having transgressed a moral imperative
Shame	Failing to live up to an ego ideal
Sadness	Having experienced an irrevocable loss
Happiness	Making reasonable progress toward the realization of a goal
Envy	Wanting what someone else has
Relief	A distressing goal-incongruent condition that has changed for the better or gone away
Hope	Fearing the worst but yearning for better

Source. Reprinted from *Emotion and Adaptation* by Richard S. Lazarus, copyright © 1991 by Oxford University Press, Inc. Used by permission of Oxford University Press, Inc.

Anger

Anger is a common emotional response to medical illness and may be the most difficult emotional response for physicians to confront. This is particularly true when the anger is directed toward them or is expressed as treatment refusal. Patients with paranoid, narcissistic, borderline, or antisocial personality styles or disorders are particularly likely to express anger in the face of medical illness (Muskin and Haase 2001). Common reflexive reactions include counterattacking or distancing oneself from the patient. The psychiatrist who is skilled in psychosomatic medicine will convey appropriate empathy along with necessary limit setting for the angry patient. Many maneuvers are possible, such as a tactful redirection of the patient's anger toward more productive targets (e.g., away from refusal of treatment and toward planning with the oncologist to attack the illness through potentially curative chemotherapy). Helping the team respond appropriately to the patient is just as important. Viewing expressed anger as natural and diffusing the intensity of affect can help to reestablish collaborative relationships with the patient.

Anxiety and Fear

Some degree of anxiety is likely to be experienced universally by patients in the medical setting (Lloyd 1977). The degree of anxiety varies tremendously by individual and by situation. Patients with premorbid anxiety disorders are more likely to experience severe anxiety when confronted with medical illness. The patient with a dependent personality style may experience acute anxiety on hospitalization when faced with separation from his or her support system. The obsessional patient is likely to become anxious if the treatment plan or diagnosis remains unclear. The intrusiveness of the medical setting may evoke anxiety in the schizoid patient.

Psychotherapies, education about the illness and treatments, and judicious use of medication can greatly diminish the patient's anxiety (Perry and Viederman 1981). Although fear (usually involving a specific threat or danger) and anxiety (the feeling of nervousness or apprehension experienced on facing uncertain threats) are distinct emotions, their management is similar. It is important to elicit what the patient fears specifically—pain, death, abandonment, disfigurement, dependence, disability, and so forth. Blanket reassurance is usually ineffective and may actually be detrimental because the patient may perceive it as not empathic, superficial, false, or patronizing. Empathy and reassurance tailored to the patient's specific fears can offer significant relief (Perry and Viederman 1981).

Sadness

Situations in which people experience a loss evoke sadness (Lloyd 1977). Medical illness can lead to multiple types of loss: loss of physical function or social role, loss of ability to work, loss of the pursuit of a goal or dream, or loss of a part of one's body. Internal losses of organs or organ functions can be as significant as external losses such as amputation of a limb. Patients with untreated mood disorders may be more likely to develop clinically significant depression in the face of medical illness. Sadness may be the primary manifestation of an adjustment disorder, which is common in medically ill patients (Strain et al. 1998). Drawing an analogy to the process of mourning is often appropriate and helps to normalize the patient's sadness (Fitzpatrick 1999). A fact not well appreciated in medical settings is that mourning a loss takes time. It is important for the physician to convey a sense of appropriate hope. Describing true examples of other patients' positive outcomes in similar situations can often be helpful. Even when the patient's sadness represents a normal grieflike reaction, physicians are often tempted to prescribe antidepressant medication, desiring to make the patient feel better. In such cases, the psychosomatic medicine specialist can redirect the treatment plan to interventions that are more likely to be helpful, such as psychotherapy, pastoral care, and—often most important—more time speaking with the primary treating physician.

Guilt

Some patients experience illness as a punishment for real or imagined sins. Clarifying that illness is not the patient's fault—and thereby confronting the guilt—is a helpful technique. Patients also may experience guilt related to earlier or current illness-promoting behaviors such as smoking cigarettes, nonadherence to medication regimens, or risky sexual practices. Education of family members can be critical if they blame the patient inappropriately for the illness. If the patient is religious, counseling from a hospital chaplain or the appropriate clergy member should be considered.

Shame

Illness is universally experienced as narcissistic injury to some degree. Narcissistic patients are more susceptible to experiencing shame in the face of medical illness. Patients who view their illness as a result of earlier behaviors—such as contracting HIV through impulsive sexual liaisons or developing lung cancer after a long history of smoking—may experience shame in the medical setting. It is important for physicians to take a nonjudgmental stance and avoid blaming patients for their illnesses. Critical, disapproving responses are counterproductive, heighten patients' shame, and frequently lead to treatment avoidance. For example, the noncompliant diabetic patient who is repeatedly admitted to the hospital for diabetic ketoacidosis frustrates her doctors and nurses. They are often tempted to scold the patient, thinking that this is necessary to avoid colluding with her acting-out and failure to take her disease seriously. Such responses are typically humiliating for the patient, are ineffective in motivating behavior change, and often worsen the vicious cycle of noncompliance.

Behavioral Responses to Illness

Patients' behavioral responses to illness vary tremendously within a spectrum ranging from maladaptive to adaptive. Adaptive responses may simply warrant encouragement or praise. Psychiatrists in the medical setting are often asked to see patients whose behavioral responses to illness or hospitalization are maladaptive and are interfering with their treatment. In understanding the patient's subjective experience, personality style, defense mechanisms, and coping strategies, one can design therapeutic interventions to help change the patient's responses to more adaptive behaviors. This section highlights a few of the common behavioral responses to illness.

Adaptive Responses

Support Seeking

Facing a new medical illness or hospitalization can be highly taxing for even the most well-adapted individual. Patients who are fortunate enough to have well-developed social support networks can benefit greatly from support from friends and family. Patients with conflicts about dependency might have more difficulty with this task, and psychotherapy can normalize this need and assist patients in reaching out to others. Referral to patient support groups also can be helpful for many patients; they can learn from the experiences of others facing the same illness and can feel less alone or alienated from other people. Information about self-help organizations can be obtained from various sources on the Internet, such as Dr. John Grohol's "Psych Central" Web site (http://psychcentral.com) and the "Self-Help Group Sourcebook Online" of the American Self-Help Group Clearinghouse (http://mentalhelp.net/selfhelp).

Altruism

Altruistic behavior such as volunteering to raise money for breast cancer, becoming a transplant advocate who meets with preoperative patients and shares experiences with them, or participating in an AIDS walkathon can represent a highly adaptive response to illness. One of the common stresses of illness is the effect on an individual's self-esteem and sense of productivity. Through helping others, patients feel a sense of purpose and gratification that can help improve their mood. Generally, the consulting psychiatrist needs only to support and encourage such behaviors. For many patients with severe illnesses, voluntary participation in research can have the same effect. Particularly for those with terminal illness, participation in research can provide a sense of purpose and hope by contributing to the potential for new treatment options in the future.

Epiphany Regarding Life Priorities

Although no one would generally claim that a medical illness is beneficial for the affected individual, it often helps patients regain perspective on what is most important to them in life. Normal daily hassles of living may no longer seem as stressful, and some patients facing a serious illness experience an epiphany and dramatically change their lives for the better. Patient narratives of the life-affirming effects of illness and stories of personal growth abound in literature (Druss 1995). At times, the consultation psychiatrist can witness and support a patient through a personal transformation. A 47-year-old male executive recently diagnosed with a myocardial infarction may dramatically change his diet, embark on a new exercise regimen, and reconfigure his role at work to reduce emotional stress. Similarly, a woman newly diagnosed with HIV who commits herself to taking her medications regularly, seeks treatment for substance use, and rejoins her church also exemplifies this phenomenon.

There are wonderful opportunities for effective psychotherapy in the medically ill. Patients are under tremendous stress when faced with serious medical illness, and the usual distractions of their daily lives no longer dominate their thoughts. Sometimes a therapeutic alliance can form and work can progress more rapidly than is typical in other settings (Muskin 1990). The regression imposed on patients by the medical illness may set the stage for psychological gains that would take much longer in typical outpatient psychotherapy.

Becoming an Expert in One's Illness

For the obsessional patient in particular, learning as much as possible about the illness can be adaptive and can give the individual a greater sense of control. Although the information itself may not be positive, patients often find that reality can seem more manageable than their imagined fears. However, this response to illness is not appealing to all patients. Some will prefer to put their trust in their physicians and prefer not to know everything. The psychiatrist, armed with an understanding of the patient's personality style, characteristic coping styles, and defense mechanisms, will be able to know whether increased information and knowledge might reduce the patient's distress and augment a sense of control.

Maladaptive Responses: Nonadherence to Treatment Regimens

Treatment nonadherence is more common than most physicians recognize. Estimates suggest that up to 50% of patients fail to adhere to their prescribed medication regimens (Sackett and Haynes 1976). Patients typically overestimate their own adherence to the treatment, and physicians are often unaware of their patients' lack of adherence (Levenson 1998). Physicians working in all medical settings witness the negative effects of nonadherence, and psychiatrists are called frequently to see problem patients who are repetitively noncompliant. For such cases, the consulting psychiatrist is often cast in the role of disciplinarian, detective, or magician; medical colleagues may expect the psychiatrist's interventions to bring rapid change to the patient's adherence patterns. Although it is possible in some cases, this scenario is typically unrealistic. It is possible to undertake interventions that improve patient adherence when the underlying factors accounting for nonadherence are correctly identified and addressed.

Patients do not fully adhere to treatment regimens for numerous reasons. Psychiatric disorders and psychological motivations are not the only factors that may be involved. Other factors, such as cost, side effects, and treatment complexity, may play a role. It is important to determine the degree of a patient's nonadherence and its context. Is the patient occasionally or consistently nonadherent? Is the nonadherence specific to a certain medication or type of recommendation (e.g., dieting), or is it more generalized across different treatments and different physicians? Identifying the context of nonadherence can provide clues to the underlying factors involved when the patient cannot directly give the reasons for nonadherence. In this section, we identify some of the most common reasons for treatment nonadherence and offer 11 general principles for management of this common clinical problem.

Psychologically Motivated Factors for Nonadherence

Perry and Viederman (1981) outlined several distinct psychological reasons that patients do not adhere to treatment recommendations. One reason they discuss is nonadherence to defend against humiliation (Perry and Viederman 1981). Rather than accept the stigma of his illness, a patient with HIV might stop his medications, which remind him daily of his illness. Active empathic work to counteract the illness concepts that cause shame can diminish this motivation for treatment nonadherence.

Another psychological motivation for nonadherence is to counteract a feeling of helplessness (Perry and Viederman 1981). An adolescent with newly diagnosed diabetes mellitus who is struggling with a developmentally appropriate desire to gain autonomy may believe that the only way to feel autonomous and in control is to rebel against her parents and caregivers by not taking insulin. Such nonadherence also may be motivated by the wish to be healthy like her peers.

Anger toward the treating physician or toward the illness or diagnosis itself may be another psychological motivator for treatment nonadherence, whether the anger is appropriate to the situation or is a product of character pathology. Various degrees of denial also may be involved. Specific interventions for clinical situations in which anger and denial are primary motivators for nonadherence were discussed earlier in this chapter in the section "Denial" and in the subsection "Anger" under "Emotional Responses to Medical Illness."

Patients' trust in the physicians recommending their treatment is an important determinant of their likelihood of complying with the treatment regimen. Physicians must earn their patients' trust through building rapport and direct, honest communication. Patients with psychotic disorders or significant character pathology might have particular difficulty placing trust in their caregivers. Mistrust and paranoia may play a role in these patients' noncompliance with treatment regimens.

Comorbid Psychiatric Disorders and Nonadherence

Comorbid psychiatric disorders also may lead to treatment nonadherence. Mood disorders are particularly common. Depressed patients may not have the motivation, concentration, or energy required to comply fully with treatment recommendations. They might even stop treatment as an indirect means of attempting suicide. Manic patients may believe that they no longer need treatment, may abuse substances, or may become disorganized or psychotic. Psychotic disorders, anxiety disorders, substance use disorders, and cognitive disorders are other psychiatric conditions that often play a role in treatment nonadherence. Therefore, a thorough psychiatric history and comprehensive review of symptoms are essential parts of the evaluation of the noncompliant patient.

Other Factors in Nonadherence

Nonadherence may be due to reality factors rather than psychological motivations. Cost of treatment, side effects (whether feared or experienced), and complicated or inconvenient medication dosing schedules are treatment-specific factors that should be considered. Other practical barriers, such as difficulties with transportation, inflexible and lengthy work schedules, or child care responsibilities, may preclude consistent keeping of appointments (Levenson 1998).

A lack of information about the illness or its treatment should always be ruled out as a factor in nonadherence. Patients should understand their illness, their treatment options, and the reasons that treatment is necessary. Patient education should always be provided in the patient's primary language to ensure full understanding. To assess patient understanding, physicians should ask patients to repeat and to explain in their own words what they have been told about their illness. If possible, family members should be involved in the education. Written materials or visual materials may be helpful tools in patient education.

Incongruities between the health beliefs of patients and their physicians can also account for nonadherence and should be identified (Gaw 2001). Physicians of all disciplines must make an effort to understand their patients' cultural and religious backgrounds, paying particular attention to patients' beliefs and values about health and illness. Physicians should attempt to elicit their patients' explanatory models about diseases and the effects of treatments. When possible, attempts can be made to explain treatment plans within patients' explanatory models for illness and treatment. Conversely, at the least, mutual acknowledgment and acceptance of the differences between the explanatory models of the physician and the patient may facilitate treatment adherence and build doctor–patient rapport. When they feel that their caregivers accept and understand their cultural, health, or religious beliefs, patients will be more likely to volunteer information about their use of alternative or herbal treatments.

Interventions to Increase Treatment Adherence

The following general principles may assist the physician in facilitating greater patient adherence to treatment regimens (Becker and Maiman 1980; Chen 1991; Gaw 2001; Levenson 1998):

- Ask patients directly about their adherence, maintaining a nonjudgmental stance. Design a collaborative plan to increase adherence. Normalizing statements and questions—such as "Many patients find it difficult to take their medications on a regular basis. Have you had this experience?"—are more effective in eliciting information about treatment adherence than questions such as "You've been taking your medication regularly, right?"
- Ensure that patients are fully informed about their illness and treatments.
- Rule out cognitive deficits (e.g., mental retardation or dementia) because they may play a role in nonadherence.
- Uncover any underlying psychological motivating factors for nonadherence, and address them specifically.
- Diagnose and treat any comorbid psychiatric disorders.
- Minimize treatment-related factors for nonadherence, such as side effects and cost and complexity of treatment regimens, when possible.
- Identify, acknowledge, and contend with any cultural reasons for nonadherence.
- Avoid shaming, scolding, or frightening the patient. Scolding patients or scaring them with statements such as "If you don't take your medications, you could have a heart attack and die!" is almost always counterproductive (Heiskell and Pasnau 1991). Such statements may shame patients or inflate their fears and can increase the likelihood that they will not return for treatment.
- Use positive reinforcement as a motivator when possible because it is generally more effective than negative reinforcement at facilitating behavior change.
- Involve family members in facilitating patient treatment adherence when they are "on board" with the treatment plan.
- Attend to doctor–patient rapport, and build an effective treatment alliance.

Maladaptive Responses: Signing Out Against Medical Advice

A common reason for urgent psychiatric consultation in the medical hospital is a patient threatening to sign out against medical advice. Of all hospital discharges in the United States, 0.8%–2% are against medical advice (Hwang et al. 2003; Jeremiah et al. 1995; Weingart et al. 1998). Often the psychiatrist is asked to assess the decisional capacity of a patient who wants to sign out against medical advice. Legal aspects of this important assessment are discussed in Chapter 2, "Legal Issues." The patient's threat to sign out is usually not truly motivated by a primary desire to leave but more often reflects another agenda, intense affect, or interpersonal friction with physicians or nursing staff. In some cases, it is a means of expressing anger or frustration toward caregivers (Albert and Kornfeld 1973).

The motivations for signing out against medical advice vary significantly and are similar to those motivating treatment nonadherence. Among the more common motivations are 1) anger with caregivers or dissatisfaction with the treatment received (whether legitimate or partly due to character pathology); 2) overwhelming fear or anxiety; 3) substance craving or withdrawal (sometimes due to the medical team's inadequate use of prophylactic medications such as benzodiazepines or nicotine patches); 4) delirium or dementia; 5) psychosis or paranoia; 6) desire to leave the hospital to attend to outside responsibilities (e.g., child care, work, court dates, or a pet at home alone); and 7) impatience with discharge planning or feeling well enough to leave. In a classic study of patients threatening to sign out against medical advice, the most common underlying motivations were overwhelming fear, anger, and psychosis or confusion (Albert and Kornfeld 1973). In most cases, there had been a progressive increase in the patient's distress that had not been recognized or addressed adequately for days before the threat to sign out (Albert and Kornfeld 1973).

Among interventions, *empathic listening* to the patient's frustrations is critical, in that it provides an opportunity for the patient to ventilate frustrations and to feel understood. Empathic listening will often have a dramatic de-escalating effect and will enable the team to re-engage the patient in treatment. The psychiatrist can also intervene in assisting the team to achieve a better understanding of the patient's behavior and to diminish the patient's feelings of anger and frustration. Other guidelines for intervention are the following:

- Understand the threat as a communication—Does the patient really want to leave, or is he or she expressing frustration, anger, anxiety, or another affect?
- If the patient is justifiably angry, apologize on behalf of the system or hospital.

- Avoid scare tactics or direct confrontation of denial because these techniques are generally counterproductive.
- Design interventions with an understanding of the patient's personality type.
- Diagnose and treat any comorbid psychiatric disorders.
- Involve social supports (if they are allied with the treatment plan).
- Ensure that the patient is adequately informed about the illness and its need for treatment.
- Assess the patient's capacity to sign out, if indicated (discussed further in Chapter 2, "Legal Issues").
- When patients still sign out against medical advice, encourage them to return for treatment if they change their mind.

Conclusion

How does one integrate these various theoretical concepts into the consultation process? How do the psychological responses to illness guide the consultant to use his or her time efficiently, understand the situation, and make useful suggestions? We are aware of no magic formula, but we believe that experienced consultants use their knowledge of human behavior and concepts such as attachment styles, personality types, coping styles, and defense mechanisms to understand their patients and to intervene. Opportunities abound in the medical setting for psychiatric interventions, which can dramatically modify patients' psychological responses to illness. The key to these interventions lies in the development of an understanding of the patient's subjective experience of illness. A curious inquiry into the internal experience of a patient facing medical illness and the appropriate conveyance of empathy is a rewarding experience. We hope the framework, concepts, and guidelines presented in this chapter will prove useful in assisting psychiatrists who have chosen to work with patients in medical settings.

References

Albert HD, Kornfeld DS: The threat to sign out against medical advice. Ann Intern Med 79:888–891, 1973

American Psychiatric Association: Diagnostic and Statistical Manual of Mental Disorders, 4th Edition, Text Revision. Washington, DC, American Psychiatric Association, 2000

Bartholomew K, Horowitz LM: Attachment styles among young adults: a test of a four-category model. J Pers Soc Psychol 61:226–244, 1991

Becker MH, Maiman LA: Strategies for enhancing patient compliance. J Community Health 6:113–135, 1980

Bornstein RF: Adaptive and maladaptive aspects of dependency: an integrative review. Am J Orthopsychiatry 64:622–634, 1994

Bowlby J Attachment and Loss, Vol 1: Attachment. New York, Basic Books, 1969

Carlat DJ: The Psychiatric Interview: A Practical Guide. Philadelphia, PA, Lippincott Williams & Wilkins, 1999

Chen A: Noncompliance in community psychiatry: a review of clinical interventions. Hosp Community Psychiatry 42:282–286, 1991

Ciechanowski P, Katon WJ: The interpersonal experience of health care through the eyes of patients with diabetes. Soc Sci Med 63:3067–3079, 2006

Ciechanowski PS, Katon WJ, Russo JE, et al: The patient-provider relationship: attachment theory and adherence to treatment in diabetes. Am J Psychiatry 158:29–35, 2001

Ciechanowski PS, Katon WJ, Russo JE, et al: Association of attachment style to lifetime medically unexplained symptoms in patients with hepatitis C. Psychosomatics 43:206–212, 2002a

Ciechanowski PS, Walker EA, Katon WJ, et al: Attachment theory: a model for health care utilization and somatization. Psychosom Med 64:660–667, 2002b

Ciechanowski P, Sullivan M, Jensen M, et al: The relationship of attachment style to depression, catastrophizing and health care utilization in patients with chronic pain. Pain 104:627–637, 2003

Cohen F, Lazarus RS: Active coping processes, coping dispositions, and recovery from surgery. Psychosom Med 35:375–398, 1973

Cousins N: Denial: are sharper definitions needed? JAMA 248:210–212, 1982

Cousins N: The Healing Heart. New York, WW Norton, 1983

Croog SH, Shapiro DS, Levine S: Denial among male heart patients: an empirical study. Psychosom Med 33:385–397, 1971

Douglas CJ, Druss RG: Denial of illness: a reappraisal. Gen Hosp Psychiatry 9:53–57, 1987

Druss RG: The Psychology of Illness: In Sickness and in Health. Washington, DC, American Psychiatric Press, 1995

Druss RG, Douglas C: Adaptive responses to illness and disability. Gen Hosp Psychiatry 10:163–168, 1988

Fitzpatrick MC: The psychologic assessment and psychosocial recovery of the patient with an amputation. Clin Orthop 361:98–107, 1999

Folkman S, Lazarus R: The relationship between coping and emotion: implications for theory and research. Soc Sci Med 26:309–317, 1988

Folkman S, Lazarus R, Dunkel-Schetter C, et al: The dynamics of a stressful encounter: cognitive appraisal, coping and encounter outcomes. J Pers Soc Psychol 50:992–1003, 1986

Folkman S, Chesney M, Pollack L, et al: Stress, control, coping and depressive mood in human immunodeficiency virus-positive and -negative gay men in San Francisco. J Nerv Ment Dis 181:409–416, 1993

Fonagy P, Leigh T, Steele M, et al: The relationship of attachment status, psychiatric classification, and response to psychotherapy. J Consult Clin Psychol 64:22–31, 1996

Freud A: The Ego and the Mechanisms of Defense. London, Hogarth Press, 1948

Fricchione GL, Howanitz E, Jandorf L, et al: Psychological adjustment to end-stage renal disease and the implications of denial. Psychosomatics 33:85–91, 1992

Gaba DM, Howard SK: Fatigue among clinicians and the safety of patients. N Engl J Med 347:1249–1255, 2002

Gattelari M, Butow PN, Tattersall HN, et al: Misunderstanding in cancer patients: why shoot the messenger? Ann Oncol 10:39–46, 1999

Gaw AC: Concise Guide to Cross-Cultural Psychiatry. Washington, DC, American Psychiatric Publishing, 2001

Gazzola L, Muskin PR: The impact of stress and the objectives of psychosocial interventions, in Psychosocial Treatment for Medical Conditions: Principles and Techniques. Edited by Schein LA, Bernard HS, Spitz HI, et al. New York, Brunner-Routledge, 2003, pp 373–406

Geringer ES, Stern T: Coping with medical illness: the impact of personality types. Psychosomatics 27:251–261, 1986

Goldbeck R: Denial in physical illness. J Psychosom Res 43:575–593, 1997

Greer S: Delay in the treatment of breast cancer. Proc R Soc Med 6:470–473, 1974

Groves JE: Taking care of the hateful patient. N Engl J Med 298:883–888, 1978

Griffin D, Bartholomew K: Models of the self and other: fundamental dimensions underlying measures of adult attachment. J Pers Soc Psychol 67:430–445, 1994

Hackett TP, Cassem NH: Development of a quantitative rating scale to assess denial. J Psychosom Res 18:93–100, 1974

Havik OE, Maeland J: Verbal denial and outcome in myocardial infarction patients. J Psychosom Res 32:145–157, 1988

Heim E, Augustiny KF, Schaffner L, et al: Coping with breast cancer over time and situation. J Psychosom Res 37:523–542, 1993

Heim E, Valach L, Schaffner L: Coping and psychological adaptation: longitudinal effects over time and stage in breast cancer. Psychosom Med 59:408–418, 1997

Heiskell LE, Pasnau RO: Psychological reaction to hospitalization and illness in the emergency department. Emerg Med Clin North Am 9:207–218, 1991

Holmes TH, Rahe RH: The social readjustment rating scale. J Psychosom Res 11:213–218, 1967

Hunter JJ, Maunder RG: Using attachment theory to understand illness behavior. Gen Hosp Psychiatry 23:177–182, 2001

Hwang SW, Li J, Gupta R, et al: What happens to patients who leave hospital against medical advice? CMAJ 168:417–420, 2003

Jacobsen BS, Lowery BJ: Further analysis of the psychometric properties of the Levine Denial of Illness Scale. Psychosom Med 54:372–381, 1992

Jensen MP, Turner JA, Romano KM, et al: Coping with chronic pain: a critical review of the literature. Pain 47:249–283, 1991

Jeremiah J, O'Sullivan P, Stein MD: Who leaves against medical advice? J Gen Intern Med 10:403–405, 1995

Kahana RJ, Bibring G: Personality types in medical management, in Psychiatry and Medical Practice in a General Hospital. Edited by Zinberg NE. New York, International Universities Press, 1964, pp 108–123

Kiely WF: Coping with severe illness. Adv Psychosom Med 8:105–118, 1972

Kornfeld DS: The hospital environment: its impact on the patient. Adv Psychosom Med 8:252–270, 1972

Kubler-Ross E: On Death and Dying. New York, Macmillan, 1969

Lazarus RS: Stress and Emotion: A New Synthesis. New York, Springer, 1999

Lazarus RS, Folkman S: Stress, Appraisal and Coping. New York, Springer, 1984

Levenson JL: Psychiatric aspects of medical practice, in Clinical Psychiatry for Medical Students, 3rd Edition. Edited by Stoudemire A. Philadelphia, PA, Lippincott-Raven, 1998, pp 727–763

Levenson JL, Mishra A, Hamer RM, et al: Denial and medical outcome in unstable angina. Psychosom Med 51:27–35, 1989

Levine J, Warrenberg S, Kerns R, et al: The role of denial in recovery from coronary heart disease. Psychosom Med 49:109–117, 1987

Lipowski ZJ: Physical illness, the individual and the coping process. Psychiatry Med 1:91–102, 1970

Lipowski ZJ: Psychiatry of somatic diseases: epidemiology, pathogenesis, classification. Compr Psychiatry 16:105–124, 1975

Lloyd G: Psychological reactions to physical illness. Br J Hosp Med 18:352–358, 1977

Main M: Metacognitive knowledge, metacognitive monitoring, and singular (coherent) vs. multiple (incoherent) model of attachment: findings, and directions for future research, in Attachment Across the Life Cycle. Edited by Parkes C, Stevenson-Hinde K, Marris P. London, England, Routledge, 1991, pp 127–160

Marucha PT, Kiecolt-Glaser JK, Favagehi M: Mucosal wound healing is impaired by examination stress. Psychosom Med 60:362–365, 1998

Miller MC: Personality disorders. Med Clin North Am 85:819–837, 2001

Muskin PR: The combined use of psychotherapy and pharmacotherapy in the medical setting. Psychiatr Clin North Am 13:341–353, 1990

Muskin PR: The medical hospital, in Psychodynamic Concepts in General Psychiatry. Edited by Schwartz HJ, Bleiberg E, Weissman SH. Washington, DC, American Psychiatric Press, 1995, pp 69–88

Muskin PR, Epstein LA: Clinical guide to countertransference. Current Psychiatry 8(4):25–32, 2009

Muskin PR, Haase EK: Difficult patients and patients with personality disorders, in Textbook of Primary Care Medicine, 3rd Edition (Noble J, Editor in Chief). St. Louis, MO, Mosby, 2001, pp 458–464

Ness DE, Ende J: Denial in the medical interview. JAMA 272:1777–1781, 1994

Oldham JM, Skodol AE: Charting the future of Axis II. J Personal Disord 14:17–29, 2000

Patterson DR, Everett JJ, Bombardier CH, et al: Psychological effects of severe burn injuries. Psychol Bull 113:362–378, 1993

Penley JA, Tomaka J, Wiebe JS: The association of coping to physical and psychological health outcomes: a meta-analytic review. J Behav Med 25:551–603, 2002

Perry S, Viederman M: Management of emotional reactions to acute medical illness. Med Clin North Am 65:3–14, 1981

Peterson BH: Psychological reactions to acute physical illness in adults. Med J Aust 1:311–316, 1974

Sackett DL, Haynes RB (eds): Compliance With Therapeutic Regimens. Baltimore, MD, Johns Hopkins University Press, 1976

Schussler G: Coping strategies and individual meanings of illness. Soc Sci Med 34:427–432, 1992

Sensky T: Causal attributions in physical illness. J Psychosom Res 43:565–573, 1997

Staudenmeyer H, Kinsman RS, Dirks JF, et al: Medical outcome in asthmatic patients: effects of airways hyperactivity and symptom-focused anxiety. Psychosom Med 41:109–118, 1979

Strain JJ, Grossman S: Psychological reactions to medical illness and hospitalization, in Psychological Care of the Medically Ill: A Primer in Liaison Psychiatry. New York, Appleton-Century-Crofts, 1975, pp 23–36

Strain J, Hammer JS, Huertas D, et al: The problem of coping as a reason for psychiatric consultation. Gen Hosp Psychiatry 15:1–8, 1993

Strain JJ, Smith GC, Hammer JS, et al: Adjustment disorder: a multisite study of its utilization and interventions in the consultation-liaison psychiatry setting. Gen Hosp Psychiatry 20:139–149, 1998

Strauss DH, Spitzer R, Muskin PR: Maladaptive denial of physical illness: a proposal for DSM-IV. Am J Psychiatry 147:1168–1172, 1990

Sullivan MD, Youngner SJ: Depression, competence and the right to refuse lifesaving medical treatment. Am J Psychiatry 151:971–978, 1993

Thompson D, Ciechanowski PS: Attaching a new understanding to the patient-physician relationship in family practice. J Am Board Fam Pract 16:219–226, 2003

Vaillant GE: The Wisdom of the Ego. Cambridge, MA, Harvard University Press, 1993

Verwoerdt A: Psychopathological responses to the stress of physical illness. Adv Psychosom Med 8:119–141, 1972

Weingart SN, Davis RB, Phillips RS: Patients discharged against medical advice from a general medicine service. J Gen Intern Med 13:568–571, 1998

Weisman AD, Hackett TP: Predilection to death: death and dying as a psychiatric problem. Psychosom Med 23:232–256, 1961

Westbrook M, Viney LL: Psychological reactions to the onset of chronic illness. Soc Sci Med 16:899–905, 1982

Wool MS: Understanding denial in cancer patients. Adv Psychosom Med 18:37–53, 1988

Young LD, Schweiger J, Beitzinger J, et al: Denial in heart transplant candidates. Psychother Psychosom 55:141–144, 1991

Zervas IM, Augustine A, Fricchione GL: Patient delay in cancer: a view from the crisis model. Gen Hosp Psychiatry 15:9–13, 1993

PART II

Symptoms and Disorders

CHAPTER

5

Delirium

Paula T. Trzepacz, M.D.

David J. Meagher, M.D., M.R.C.Psych., M.Sc.

Maeve Leonard, M.B., M.R.C.Psych.

DELIRIUM IS AN ACUTE neuropsychiatric disorder that occurs commonly among patients in all health care settings, especially among the elderly and those with preexisting brain lesions or cognitive impairment. It is a disorder of impaired consciousness with inattention, information processing deficits and sleep-wake cycle disruption. Delirium is characterized by generalized impairment of cognition, with inattention as its cardinal feature, but also involves a range of noncognitive symptoms affecting motor behavior, sleep-wake cycle, thinking, language, perception, and affect. It characteristically has an acute onset (hours to days) and a fluctuating course (waxing and waning symptom severity over a 24-hour period), often worsening at night. It may be preceded by a prodromal phase of 2–3 days of malaise, restlessness, poor concentration, anxiety, irritability, sleep and thought disturbances, and nightmares. Delirium has been called *acute organic brain syndrome* and *acute brain failure* because of its breadth of cognitive and behavioral symptoms. Because delirium alters consciousness, it causes broader impairment than do most other psychiatric disorders. Table 5–1 highlights delirium's characteristic features.

Normal consciousness is not easy to define. "At its least, normal human consciousness consists of a serially time-ordered, organized, restricted, reflective awareness of self and the environment. Moreover, consciousness is an experience of graded complexity and quantity" (Schiff and Plum 2000, p. 438). Consciousness is graded in levels, although it can be abruptly lost during coma, general anesthesia, or deep sleep. Consciousness involves intact attentiveness, awareness of both internal states and the external environment, and intact wakefulness—which enable thinking, working memory, intention, perception, cognition, and affect in higher cortical and limbic regions. Consciousness is accompanied by a desynchronized electroencephalogram (EEG) with fast-wave activity.

Delirium is an alteration of consciousness graded along a continuum between normal at one end and stupor and coma at the other end. Delirium must be distinguished from other brain states in which consciousness is lost or even more grossly impaired. Coma and stupor entail loss of consciousness and complete failure of arousal, without an intact sleep-wake cycle. Precise delineation between severe hypoactive delirium and stupor can be difficult. Vegetative states include arousal and intact sleep-wake cycles, but with complete absence of awareness of self or environment due to a disconnection between higher cortical regions and the brain stem/diencephalic areas. Minimally conscious state (MCS) is characterized by partial preservation of consciousness and an intact sleep-wake cycle, but intention is absent, and there is inconsistent ability to follow commands, visually track, verbalize (intelligibly), or gesture (Giacino et al. 2002). MCS can progress to delirium in patients who recover (see Figure 5–1).

Emergence from coma usually involves a period of delirium before normal consciousness is achieved. A prospective study of medical intensive care unit (ICU) patients found that 89% of survivors of stupor or coma progressed to delirium (McNicoll et al. 2003), whereas the small number who progressed directly to normal consciousness without delirium tended to have had drug-induced comatose states (Ely et al. 2004a).

TABLE 5–1. Signs and symptoms of delirium

Diffuse cognitive deficits
Inattention
Disorientation (time, place, person)
Impaired memory (short- and long-term; verbal and visual)
Visuoconstructional impairment
Executive dysfunction
Temporal course
Acute or abrupt onset
Fluctuating severity of symptoms over 24-hour period
Usually reversible
Subclinical syndrome may precede and/or follow
Psychosis
Perceptual disturbances (especially visual), including illusions, hallucinations, metamorphoses
Delusions (usually paranoid and poorly formed)
Thought disorder (tangentiality, circumstantiality, loose associations)
Sleep–wake disturbance
Fragmented throughout 24-hour period
Reversal of normal cycle
Sleeplessness
Motor behavior
Hyperactive
Hypoactive
Mixed
Language impairment
Word-finding difficulty/dysnomia/paraphasia
Comprehension deficits
Altered semantic content
Severe forms can mimic expressive or receptive aphasia
Altered or labile affect
Any mood can occur, usually incongruent to context
Anger or increased irritability common
Hypoactive delirium often mislabeled as depression
Lability (rapid shifts) common
Unrelated to mood preceding delirium

English teacher and marathon runner Jon Stableford experienced delirium after emerging from coma due to sepsis, acute respiratory distress syndrome (ARDS), and heart and renal failure (Stableford 2009): "I learned that the perspective provided by my family can be transient, that hellish fears can still lurk in the lonely hours between visits. My first week of consciousness seemed disjointed and chaotic. I felt like I was sitting in front of a TV set while an invisible stranger clicked the remote control nonstop through the channels—it was all imagery and tone, without any sense."

Delirium is often a brief, transient state when a patient emerges from general anesthesia, an overdose of medication, concussion following a mild traumatic brain injury (TBI), or seizure. Football players who sustain a head injury during a game are removed to the sidelines until the disorienting effects of concussion resolve sufficiently, although repeated injuries increase the severity of subsequent brain effects (Collins et al. 2002).

Most deliria are considered reversible, but in the elderly, cognitive impairment and previously undiagnosed dementia may be found at longer-term follow-up after recovery from delirium. Delirium occurring in patients with serious medical illness frequently remits completely, as illustrated in studies finding that 67%–85% of deliria in hospitalized patients with cancer resolved completely with treatment (Breitbart et al. 2002; Ljubisavljevic and Kelly 2003). Leonard et al. (2008) found that even in terminally ill palliative care patients, delirium was reversible in about 27%.

Delirium is considered a syndrome and not a unitary disorder because a wide variety of underlying etiologies can cause it. Identification of these etiologies, often multiple or occurring serially over time, is a key part of clinical management. Despite these varied etiologies and physiology, delirium symptoms are characteristic and thus may represent dysfunction of a final common neural pathway that includes perturbations of the various brain regions responsible for the abnormal cognition, thinking, sleep, and behaviors (see section "Neuropathogenesis" later in this chapter).

Recent work conceptualizes three core domains of delirium: cognitive, circadian, and higher-level thinking. The *cognitive* domain is comprised primarily of inattention along with other cognitive impairments, the *circadian* domain of sleep–wake cycle disturbance and possibly motor activity abnormalities, and the *higher-level thinking* domain of a combination of semantic language, thought process, and executive function impairments based on research findings that these are the most frequent, consistent, and differentiating symptoms (J.G. Franco et al. 2009; Meagher et al. 2007; Trzepacz et al. 2001c). Furthermore, these deficits in these three domains corresponded to independently diagnosed delirium in post-TBI acute recovery patients, predicting delirium with 97% accuracy (Kean et al., in press).

Unlike most other neuropsychiatric disorders (except Lewy body dementia and subdural hematoma), delirium symptoms typically fluctuate in intensity over any 24-hour period. Symptom fluctuation is measurable (Gagnon et al. 2004a, 2004b) and is an important indicator of delirium emphasized in DSM-IV and DSM-IV-TR (American Psy-

Disorders of Consciousness
Coma
Vegetative state
Minimally conscious state
Delirium
Normal
Complete failure of arousal; unconscious; no sleep–wake cycle
Aroused; complete absence of awareness of self or environment; has sleep–wake cycle
Aroused; partial preservation of consciousness; inconsistently follows commands, visually tracks, and verbalizes or gestures unintelligibly; without intention; has sleep–wake cycle
Aroused with attention deficits; disrupted sleep–wake cycle; impaired higher-level information processing, semantic expression, and comprehension; has intention

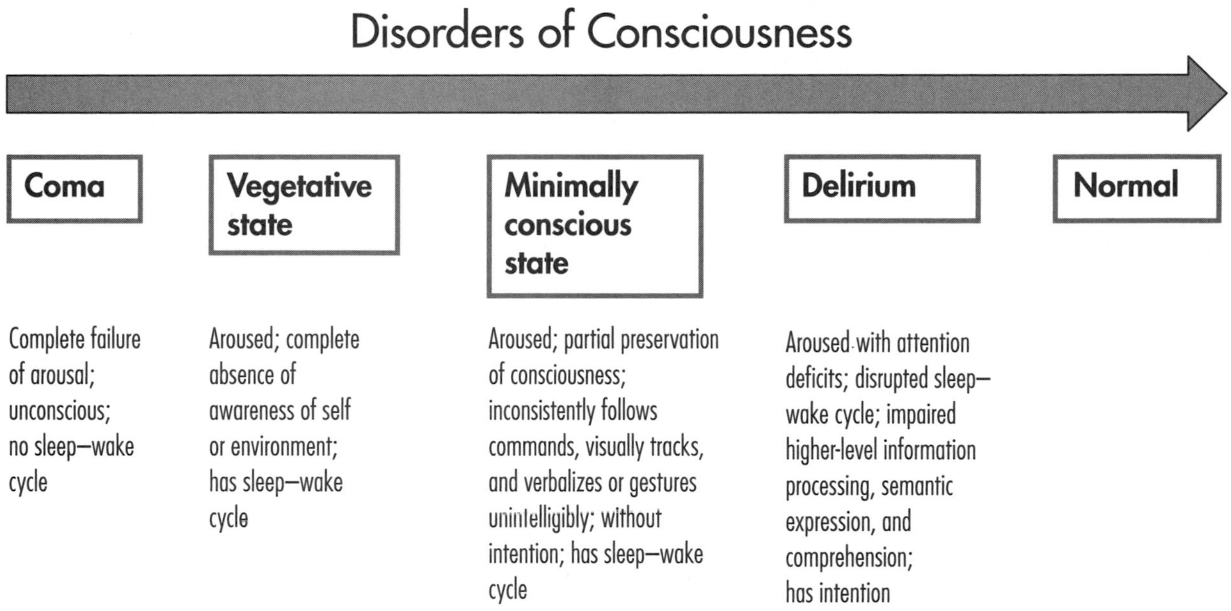

FIGURE 5–1. Disorders of consciousness.

chiatric Association 1994, 2000). This fluctuation is also a key differentiating feature from dementia. During this characteristic waxing and waning of symptoms, relative lucid or quiescent periods often occur, frustrating accurate diagnosis and complicating research severity ratings. In milder cases, such periods involve a significant diminution of delirium symptoms or even a seeming resolution. The underlying reason for this fluctuation in symptom severity is poorly understood—it may relate to shifts in levels of neurotransmitters such as acetylcholine, which supports consciousness; thalamic sensorimotor gating; or fragmentation of the sleep-wake cycle, including daytime rapid eye movement (REM) sleep.

Although not nearly as well studied, the symptom profile of delirium in children appears to be similar to that in adults (Prugh et al. 1980; Turkel et al. 2003, 2006). In the only study of delirium phenomenology in children and adolescents in which a standardized instrument was used, Turkel et al. (2003) retrospectively described 84 consecutively evaluated delirium patients (ages 6 months–19 years) and found scores comparable to those in adults, with the only difference being fewer delusions and hallucinations in younger children. Turkel et al. (2006) also compared delirium symptoms across the life cycle and, despite differences in methodologies, considered them qualitatively to be largely similar. Prugh et al. (1980) noted the importance of educating nursing staff about the difference between visual hallucinations and imaginary friends. Documentation of delirium symptoms in preverbal children or noncommunicative adults is difficult. In these patients, more reliance on inference and observation of changed or unusual behaviors—for example, inferring hallucinations or recording sleep-wake cycle changes—is needed.

Delirium symptoms in adults across the age range are comparable, although the co-occurrence of another cognitive disorder is particularly likely in the elderly as compared with younger adults, usually related to dementia. How the presence of a comorbid dementia alters the phenomenological presentation of delirium in the elderly is not well studied, but existing data suggest that delirium overshadows the dementia symptoms (see section "Differential Diagnosis" later in this chapter). Likewise, diagnosing delirium in mentally retarded patients can be challenging.

One of the challenges for both clinicians and delirium researchers is the myriad of terms applied to the delirious state. Historically, acute global cognitive disturbances have been labeled according to the setting in which they occurred or the apparent etiology for the confusional state, resulting in the many names (see Table 5–2) that exist in practice and the literature. Little evidence supports these as separate entities, and, as such, *delirium* has been adopted as the accepted umbrella term to denote acute disturbances of global cognitive function as defined in both DSM-IV and ICD-10 (World Health Organization 1992) classification systems. Even though the term *delirium* has been used since classical Greek medical writings, different terms unfortunately continue to be used by nonpsychiatric physicians (e.g., *ICU psychosis, hepatic encephalopathy, toxic psychosis, posttraumatic confusion*). These terms inappropriately suggest the existence of independent psychiatric disorders for each etiology rather than recognize delirium as a unitary syndrome. Terms such as *acute brain failure* and

TABLE 5–2. Terms used to denote delirium

Acute brain failure	Cerebral insufficiency	Organic brain syndrome
Acute brain syndrome	Confusional state	Posttraumatic confusion
Acute brain syndrome with psychosis	Dysergastic reaction	Reversible cerebral dysfunction
Acute dementia	Encephalopathy	Reversible cognitive dysfunction
Acute organic psychosis	Exogenous psychosis	Reversible dementia
Acute organic reaction	Infective-exhaustive psychosis	Reversible toxic psychosis
Acute organic syndrome	Intensive care unit (ICU) psychosis	Toxic confusion state
Acute reversible psychosis	Metabolic encephalopathy	Toxic encephalopathy
Acute secondary psychosis	Oneiric state	

acute organic brain syndrome highlight the global nature and acute onset of cerebral cortical deficits in patients with delirium, but they lack specificity in regard to other cognitive mental disorders. The term *delirium* subsumes these many other terms, and its consistent use will enhance medical communication, diagnosis, and research.

Little work has been done with the use of daily delirium ratings to better understand the temporal course of this syndrome. In a study of 432 medical inpatients 65 years or older, Rudberg et al. (1997) found that 15% had delirium, and 69% of those had delirium for only a single day. Mean delirium scores on day 1 were significantly higher (i.e., worse) in those whose delirium occurred for multiple days compared with those whose delirium lasted for 1 day, suggesting a relation between severity and duration in delirium episodes. Systematically monitoring adult bone marrow transplant patients, Fann et al. (2005) found delirium to be more severe in episodes that lasted 3 days or longer. Delirium is common after TBI and can be particularly persistent. The severity of delirium at 1 month post-TBI predicts occupational dysfunction at 1 year (Nakase-Richardson et al. 2007).

Delirium continues to be underrecognized and underdiagnosed. It is commonly misdiagnosed as depression by nonpsychiatric physicians and nurses (Nicholas and Lindsey 1995). Misdiagnosis of delirium is more likely when delirium is hypoactive in presentation and when patients are referred from surgical or intensive care settings (Armstrong et al. 1997). Van Zyl and Davidson (2003) reviewed charts of 31 delirious patients who were referred for psychiatric consultation and found that delirium or a synonym was noted in 55% of the structured discharge summaries and in none of the unstructured summaries, for an overall rate of 16%. Missed cases were denoted as dementia (25%), a functional psychiatric disorder (25%), or no diagnosis noted (50%) (Johnson et al. 1992).

Nondetection of delirium was associated with poorer outcome, including increased mortality, in a study in emergency department patients (Kakuma et al. 2003). In contrast, explicit recognition of delirium was associated with better outcomes in the form of shorter inpatient stays and lower mortality (Rockwood et al. 1994). Detection can be improved to some extent by providing formal educational programs, for example, to house staff (Rockwood et al. 1994). Personal attitudes are important among nursing staff, who often play a key role in identifying and reporting symptoms because the symptoms fluctuate, especially at night (McCarthy 2003). Detection is a challenge in ICU settings, where the sickest patients are at the highest risk for delirium. Ely et al. (2004b) distributed a survey to 912 physicians, nurses, respiratory therapists, and pharmacists attending international critical care meetings and found that 72% thought that ventilated patients experienced delirium, 92% considered delirium a very serious problem, and 78% acknowledged that it was underdiagnosed. Yet only 40% routinely screened for delirium and 16% used a specific tool for assessment. Rincon et al. (2001) reported that critical care unit staff underdiagnosed delirium (and other psychiatric disorders), and used psychotropic medications without any clear documentation of targeted diagnoses.

ICU populations have delirium prevalence rates ranging from 40% to 87% (Ely et al. 2001c). Delirium in the ICU is understudied and neglected in part because it is "expected" to happen during severe illness, and medical resources are preferentially dedicated to managing the more concrete "life-threatening" problems.

With pressure to reduce acute hospital length of stay, elderly patients are discharged, often to nursing homes, before delirium resolves. Kiely et al. (2003) studied 2,158 patients from seven Boston, Massachusetts, area skilled nursing facilities and found that 16% had a full-blown delirium. In general, such facilities are even less well equipped and staffed to diagnose and manage delirium than are acute care hospitals.

Consequences of Delirium

Delirium can have a profound effect on a patient's morbidity and mortality as well as on his or her caregivers and loved ones. Delirious patients have difficulty comprehending and communicating effectively, consenting to procedures, complying with medical management (e.g., removing intravenous lines, tubes, or catheters), benefiting from many therapies, and maintaining expected levels of self-hygiene and eating. They also are at risk for inadvertent self-harm because of confusion about the environment or in response to hallucinations or paranoid delusions. Delirium-recovered patients were uncomfortable discussing their delirium episodes—even to the extent of denial—because they feared that it meant that they were "senile" or "mad" (Schofield 1997). Breitbart et al. (2002) prospectively interviewed and rated 101 cancer patients with a resolved delirium episode, their spouses, and their nurses (see Figure 5–2). About half (43%) of the patients recalled their episode, with recall dependent on delirium severity (100% of patients with mild delirium vs. 16% of patients with severe delirium recalled the episode). Mean distress levels were high for patients and nurses but were highest for spouses. However, among patients with delirium who did not recall the episode, the mean distress level was half that of those who did recall. The experience of the delirium was frightening and stressful for all involved, but for somewhat different reasons—for patients, the presence of delusions; for nurses, the presence of perceptual disturbances or overall severe delirium; and for spouses, the low ability to function was predictive of distress level. Spouses perceived the delirium as indicating a high risk for death and loss of the loved one, contributing to anticipatory bereavement.

Medical complications, including decubitus ulcers, feeding problems, and urinary incontinence, are common in patients with delirium (Gustafson et al. 1988). Effects on hospital length of stay, "persistence" of cognitive impairment, increased rate of institutionalization, and reduced ambulation and activities of daily living (ADL) level have been reported as consequences in elderly patients with delirium.

The Academy of Psychosomatic Medicine (APM) Task Force on Mental Disorders in General Medical Practice

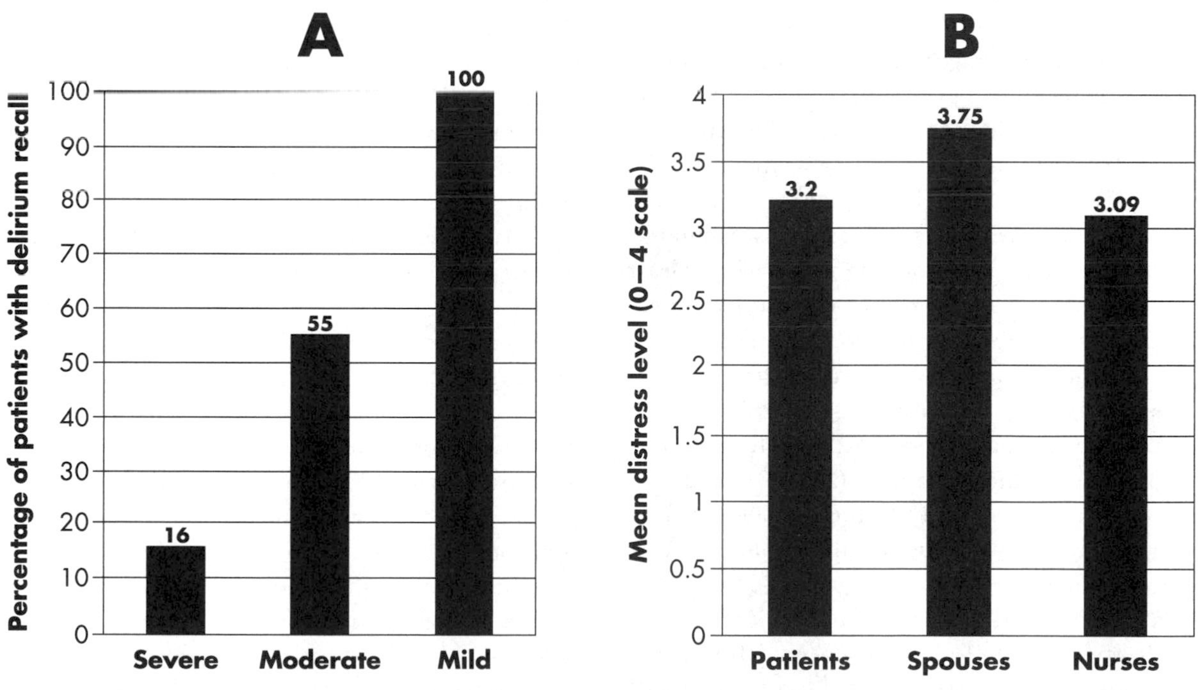

FIGURE 5–2. Relationship of delirium severity to patient recall of the episode, and comparison of delirium-related distress levels, in cancer patients with a resolved delirium episode and their families and caregivers.

(A) Percentage of patients who recalled their episode, by delirium severity. (B) Mean distress levels of patients, spouses or caregivers, and nurses (rated on a 0–4 rating scale).

Source. Reprinted from Breitbart W, Gibson C, Tremblay A: "The Delirium Experience: Delirium Recall and Delirium-Related Distress in Hospitalized Patients With Cancer, Their Spouses/Caregivers, and Their Nurses." *Psychosomatics* 43:183–194, 2002. Copyright 2002, American Psychiatric Publishing, Inc. Used with permission.

(Saravay and Strain 1994) reviewed studies finding that comorbid delirium increased hospital length of stay 100% in general medical patients (R.I. Thomas et al. 1988), 114% in elderly patients (Schor et al. 1992), 67% in stroke patients (Cushman 1988), 300% in critical care patients (Kishi et al. 1995), 27% in cardiac surgery patients, and 200%–250% in hip surgery patients (Berggren et al. 1987). The APM task force noted that delirium contributed to increased length of stay via medical and behavioral mechanisms, including the following: decreased motivation to participate in treatment and rehabilitation, medication refusal, disruptive behavior, incontinence and urinary tract infection, falls and fractures, and decubiti.

Significantly increased length of stay associated with delirium has been reported in many studies in the 1980s and 1990s, and a meta-analysis of eight studies (Cole and Primeau 1993) supported statistically significant differences in length of stay between delirium and control groups. Ely et al. (2004a) found that delirium duration was associated with length of stay in both the medical ICU and the hospital ($P<0.001$) and was the strongest predictor of length of stay even after adjustment for illness severity, age, gender, and days of opioid and narcotic use. McCusker et al. (2003a) studied elderly medical inpatients and found significantly longer length of stay for those with incident, but not prevalent, delirium.

K. Franco et al. (2001) identified the increased costs associated with delirium in a prospective study of 500 elective surgery patients older than 50 years. Delirium occurred in 11.4% of the patients during postoperative days 1–4, and these patients had higher professional, consultation, technical, and routine nursing care costs. Milbrandt et al. (2004) compared costs associated with having at least one delirium episode in 183 mechanically ventilated medical ICU patients and nondelirious control subjects after controlling for age, comorbidity of illness, degree of organ dysfunction, nosocomial infection, and hospital mortality. Median ICU costs per patient were $22,346 for delirious and $13,332 for nondelirious patients ($P<0.001$), and total hospital costs were $41,836 and $27,106 ($P=0.002$), respectively; more severe delirium cases resulted in higher costs than did milder ones.

Decreased independent living status and increased institutionalization during follow-up after a delirium episode were found in many studies of elderly individuals (Cole and Primeau 1993; George et al. 1997; Inouye et al. 1998). Reduction in ambulation and/or ADL level at follow-up is also commonly reported (Francis and Kapoor 1992; Gustafson et al. 1988; Inouye et al. 1998; Minagawa et al. 1996; Murray et al. 1993). Delirium also has an effect in nursing home settings, where incident cases are associated with poor 6-month outcome, including behavioral decline, initiation of physical restraints, greater risk of hospitalization, and increased mortality (Murphy 1999). Even subsyndromal delirium is reported to increase index admission length of stay and postdischarge dysfunction and mortality after adjustment for age, sex, marital status, previous living arrangement, comorbidity, dementia status, and clinical and physiological severity of illness (Cole et al. 2003b).

In nursing home patients, better cognitive function at baseline was associated with better outcome from delirium (Murphy 1999), supporting the notion that impaired brain reserve is an important predelirium factor that needs to be taken into account in any longitudinal outcome assessments. Longitudinal cognitive assessments of postcardiotomy patients who had normal preoperative Mini-Mental State Examination (MMSE) findings compared elderly with middle-aged and younger adults and found that delirium was not a predictor of persistent cognitive impairment at 3-month follow-up, even though it was associated with deficits at the time of discharge from the hospital, and only the elderly group had worse cognitive function at 3 months, whereas the other two groups were similar to the elderly nondelirious control subjects (Monk et al. 2008).

Epidemiology

Delirium can occur at any age, although it is particularly understudied in children and adolescents. Most epidemiological studies have focused on the elderly, who are at higher risk to develop delirium than are younger adults. This is likely because of age-related changes in the brain, including decreased cholinergic functioning, often referred to as *reduced brain reserve.* The frequent occurrence of central nervous system disorders (e.g., stroke, hypertensive and atherosclerotic vessel changes, tumor, dementias) in the elderly further increases their vulnerability to delirium). Improving our understanding and treatment of delirium is thus a considerable health care challenge, especially in countries whose population is aging at a dramatic rate.

Most studies of delirium incidence and prevalence report general hospital populations consisting of either referral samples or consecutive admissions to a given service. Specific patient populations, such as elderly patients who require emergent hip surgery, liver transplant candidates, and hospitalized TBI patients, may be responsible for disparate rates reported in studies. In addition, not all studies use sensitive and specific diagnostic and measurement techniques, risking overestimates or underestimates of the true occurrence of delirium.

Diagnosis is an issue for epidemiological studies. Substantial differences in rates can occur—for example, when DSM-III (American Psychiatric Association 1980), DSM-III-R (American Psychiatric Association 1987), DSM-IV, and ICD-10 criteria were used, only 25% of the patients with delirium received accurate diagnoses by all four systems (Laurila et al. 2003). Lesser diagnostic emphasis on disorganized thinking in the DSM-IV criteria accounted for that system's greater sensitivity and inclusivity (but lower specificity) in comparison with the other systems, whereas ICD-10 criteria were the least inclusive (Cole et al. 2003a). Laurila et al. (2004) concluded that DSM-IV criteria are most inclusive, whereas ICD-10 criteria are overly restrictive. The Confusion Assessment Method may underestimate or overestimate occurrence of delirium when used alone (see section "Diagnosis and Assessment" later in this chapter).

Fann (2000) reviewed prospective studies of delirium in hospitalized patients to report an incidence from 3% to 42%, and prevalence from 5% to 44%. A review of prospective cohort and cross-sectional studies of general medical inpatient settings found prevalence of delirium at admission from 10% to 31%, incidence of new delirium per admission from 3% to 29% and occurrence rate per admission between 11% and 42% (Siddiqi et al. 2006). Table 5-3 describes prospective incidence and prevalence studies of delirium in which DSM diagnostic criteria or rating scales were used. These studies were done in medical, surgical, palliative care, institutional care, intensive care, and community settings, and most focused on geriatric patients.

Prevalence rates for delirium in studies that have been conducted in community-based settings have found highly variable frequencies of delirium (<0.05%–44%) but have involved considerably different methodologies from exclusion of patients with known dementia (Andrew et al. 2006) to the use of the Organic Brain Syndrome scale in settings as diverse as nursing homes along with an emergency hospital (Sandberg et al. 1998). When admitted to a hospital, 10%–15% of elderly patients have delirium, and another 10%–40% receive diagnoses of delirium during the hospitalization. A clinical rule of thumb seems to be that, on average, approximately one-fifth of general hospital patients have delirium sometime during hospitalization. Terminally ill cancer patients have a very high incidence of delirium, with rates from 28% to 42% on admission to a palliative care unit and up to 88% before death (Lawlor et al. 2000a). Also, up to 50% of adults undergoing stem cell transplantation have delirium in the postoperative month (Beglinger et al. 2006; Fann et al. 2002).

In a prospective cohort study of older medical ICU patients, McNicoll et al. (2003) found delirium in 31% on admission and an overall prevalence, and delirium incidences of 62% during the ICU stay and 70% during the entire hospitalization. In addition, 30% had evidence of prior dementia, and these patients were 40% more likely to become delirious, even after controlling for comorbidity, baseline functional status, severity of illness, and invasive procedures. In a prospective study of 275 consecutive mechanically ventilated medical ICU patients that used daily ratings over 5,353 patient days, 51 (18.5%) were comatose; of the remaining 224 patients, 183 (82%) had a delirium at some point during the hospitalization, with a median duration of 2.1 days (Ely et al. 2004b). Delirious patients had numerically higher admission mean comorbidity and critical illness severity scores compared with those who never became delirious, but mean ages were comparable.

Frail elderly individuals living in nursing facilities studied for 3 months during and after an acute medical hospitalization had a high incidence of delirium of 55% at 1 month and 25% at 3 months, which persisted until death or hospitalization in 72% (Kelly et al. 2001).

Thus, irrespective of the diversity of incidence and prevalence rates reported among studies, delirium is very common in medical and institutional settings where its rates generally exceed those for any other serious psychiatric disorder.

Risk Factors

Delirium is particularly common during hospitalization when a confluence of both predisposing (moderating) and precipitating (mediating) factors is present. Several patient, illness, pharmacological, and environmental factors have been identified as being relevant risk factors for delirium. Although some factors are more relevant in certain settings, age, preexisting cognitive impairment, severe comorbid illness, and medication exposure are particularly strong predictors of delirium risk across a range of populations (Inouye et al. 1999). Dementia in older persons is a common risk factor. Korevaar et al. (2005) found the most important independent risk factors in elderly medical inpatients for having a prevalent delirium were premorbid cognitive impairment, functional impairment, and an elevated urea nitrogen level. Terminal illness is a risk factor for delirium (Lawlor et al. 2000a). In stem cell transplant patients, pretransplant risk factors included lower cognition on the Trail Making Test B; higher serum levels of urea nitrogen, magnesium, or alkaline phosphatase; and lower physical functioning (Fann et al. 2002).

Stress-vulnerability models for the occurrence of delirium have been long recognized. Henry and Mann (1965) described "delirium readiness." More recent models of causation involve cumulative interactions between predisposing factors and precipitating insults (Inouye and Charpentier 1996; O'Keeffe and Lavan 1996). Baseline risk is a more potent predictor of delirium likelihood—if baseline vulnerability is low, patients are very resistant to the development of delirium despite exposure to significant precipitating factors, whereas if baseline vulnerability is high, delirium is

TABLE 5–3. Prospective studies of delirium incidence and prevalence

Study	*N*	Sample	Delirium ascertainment	Design	Findings
Erkinjuntti et al. 1986	2,000	Medical inpatients, age ≥55 years	SPMSQ, DSM-III criteria on interview and chart review	Prospective	Prevalence 15%
Cameron et al. 1987	133	Medical inpatients, ages 32–97 years	DSM-III criteria on interview	Prospective	Prevalence 14%, incidence 3%
Gustafson et al. 1988	111	Femoral neck fracture patients, age ≥65 years	OBS Scale, DSM-III criteria on interview	Prospective	Prevalence 33%, incidence 42%
Rockwood 1989	80	Medical inpatients, age ≥65 years	DSM-III criteria on interview	Prospective	Prevalence 16%, incidence 11%
Francis et al. 1990	229	Medical inpatients, age ≥70 years	DSM-III-R criteria on interview and chart review	Prospective	Prevalence 16%, incidence 7%
Johnson et al. 1990	235	Medical inpatients, age ≥70 years	DSM-III criteria on interview	Prospective	Prevalence 16%, incidence 5%
Folstein et al. 1991	810	Community sample	DSM-III criteria on interview	Cross-sectional	Prevalence 0.4% (1.1%, age ≥55)
Williams-Russo et al. 1992	51	Bilateral knee replacement surgery patients receiving postoperative fentanyl	DSM-III-R criteria on interview and chart review	Prospective	Incidence 41%
Jitapunkul et al. 1992	184	Medical inpatients, age ≥60 years	DSM-III-R criteria on chart review	Prospective	Prevalence 22%
Snyder et al. 1992	42	Acquired immunodeficiency syndrome inpatients	DSM-III-R criteria on interview	Prospective	Prevalence 17%
Schor et al. 1992	325	Medical and surgical inpatients, age ≥65 years	DSI	Prospective	Prevalence 11%, incidence 31%
Leung et al. 1992	569	Male medical inpatients, ages 12–99 years	DSM-III criteria on interview	Prospective	Prevalence 9.5%
Kolbeinsson and Jonsson 1993	331	Medical inpatients, age ≥70 years	MSQ, MMSE, and DSM-III-R criteria on interview	Prospective	Prevalence 14%
Rockwood 1993	168	Geriatric medical inpatients, mean age = 79 years	DRS, DSM-III-R criteria on interview	Prospective	Prevalence 18%, incidence 7%
Marcantonio et al. 1994a	1,341	Noncardiac surgery patients, age ≥50 years	CAM, medical records, nursing intensity index	Prospective	Incidence 9%

TABLE 5–3. Prospective studies of delirium incidence and prevalence *(continued)*

Study	*N*	Sample	Delirium ascertainment	Design	Findings
Pompei et al. 1994	432	Medical and surgical inpatients, age ≥65 years	Digit Span, Vigilance "A" Test, CAC, CAM, DSM-III-R criteria on interview	Prospective	Prevalence 5%, incidence 10%
Pompei et al. 1994	323	Medical and surgical inpatients, age ≥70 years	CAM	Prospective	Prevalence 15%, incidence 12%
Kishi et al. 1995	238	Critical care medical unit patients	DSM-III-R criteria on clinical evaluation	Prospective	Incidence 16%
Fisher and Flowerdew 1995	80	Elective orthopedic surgery inpatients, age ≥60 years	CAM	Prospective	Incidence 18%
Inouye and Charpentier 1996	196	Medical inpatients, age ≥70 years	CAM	Prospective	Incidence 18%
	312	Medical inpatients, age ≥70 years	CAM	Prospective	Incidence 15%
Minagawa et al. 1996	93	Terminally ill cancer patients admitted to palliative care unit	MMSE and DSM-III-R criteria on interview	Prospective	Prevalence 28%
Rudberg et al. 1997	432	Medical-surgical patients	DSM-III-R and DRS daily ratings	Prospective	Incidence 15%
Sandberg et al. 1998	717	Institutional care patients, age ≥75 years	OBS Scale	Cross-sectional	Prevalence 44%
Gagnon et al. 2000	89	Hospitalized terminal cancer patients	CAM, CRS	Prospective longitudinal	Incidence 33%, prevalence on admission 20%
Lawlor et al. 2000a	104	Hospitalized advanced cancer patients	DSM-IV, MDAS	Prospective	Incidence 45%, prevalence on admission 42%
Caraceni et al. 2000	393	Multicenter palliative care cancer patients	CAM	Prospective	Prevalence 28%
van der Mast et al. 1999	296	Elective cardiac surgery patients, ages 26–83 years	DSM-III-R criteria on interview and chart review	Prospective	Incidence 14%
Fann et al. 2002	90	Hospitalized hematopoietic stem cell transplant patients	DRS, MDAS	Prospective	Incidence 50%, cumulative incidence 73%
Ely et al. 2004a	275	Consecutive mechanically ventilated medical ICU patients	DSM-IV and CAM-ICU	Prospective	Incidence 82%

TABLE 5–3. Prospective studies of delirium incidence and prevalence *(continued)*

Study	*N*	Sample	Delirium ascertainment	Design	Findings
McNicoll et al. 2003	118	Elderly medical ICU patients	CAM-ICU	Prospective	Incidence on admission 31%, incidence and prevalence combined 62%
Kiely et al. 2003	2,158	Skilled nursing facility elderly patients in Boston area	CAM	Prospective	Prevalence 16%
Spiller and Keen 2006	100	Acute admissions to a palliative care unit	CAM, MDAS	Prospective	Incidence 29% (86% hypoactive)
	109	8 specialist palliative care units	CAM, MDAS	Point prevalence survey	Point prevalence 29.4% (78% hypoactive)
Kalisvaart et al. 2006	603	Elderly hip surgery patients	CAM, DSM-IV	Prospective cohort study	Incidence 12.3%
Furlaneto and Garcez-Leme 2006	103	Elderly hip surgery patients	CAM	Prospective	Incidence 12.6%; prevalence 16.5%
Andrew et al. 2006	1,658	Community dwellers	DSM-III-R	Prospective	Prevalence <0.05%
	1,672	Residents of long-term institutions	DSM-III-R	Prospective	Prevalence <0.05%
Beglinger et al. 2006	30	Adult patients undergoing hematopoietic stem cell transplantation	DRS, MDAS	Prospective	Incidence 43%
Iseli et al. 2007	104	General medical unit	CAM	Prospective	Prevalence 18%; incidence 2%
Bo et al. 2009	121	Acute geriatric ward	CAM	Prospective	Incidence 6.6%
	131	Acute general medical ward	CAM	Prospective	Incidence 15.2%
Nakase-Thompson et al. 2004	171	Acute brain injury rehabilitation unit	DSM-IV, DRS	Prospective	Incident 66%

Note. CAC = Critical Assessment of Confusion; CAM = Confusion Assessment Method; CRS = Confusion Rating Scale; DRS = Delirium Rating Scale; DSI = Delirium Symptom Interview; ICU = intensive care unit; MDAS = Memorial Delirium Assessment Scale; MMSE = Mini-Mental State Examination; MSQ = Mental Status Questionnaire; OBS = Organic Brain Syndrome; SPMSQ = Short Portable Mental Status Questionnaire.

likely even in response to minor precipitants (Inouye and Charpentier 1996). Tsutsui et al. (1996), for example, found that in patients older than 80 years, delirium occurred in 52% after emergency surgery and 20% after elective procedures, whereas no cases of delirium were noted in patients younger than 50 years undergoing either elective or emergency procedures. Kalisvaart et al. (2006) reported that delirium was four times more common in urgent than elective hip surgery patients, with cognitive impairment and age other important risk factors. In addition to the elderly, children are considered at higher risk for delirium, possibly related to ongoing brain development.

Up to two-thirds of the cases of delirium occur superimposed on preexisting cognitive impairment (Wahlund and Bjorlin 1999) which has been reported to increase risk ninefold, making it the strongest risk factor for prevalent delirium (Korevaar et al. 2005). The absence of dementia can be considered an important predictor of recovery (Cole et al. 2007). Delirium is 2.0–3.5 times more common in patients with dementia compared with control subjects without dementia (Erkinjuntti et al. 1986; Jitapunkul et al. 1992). Delirium risk appears to be greater in Alzheimer's disease of late onset and dementia of vascular origin as compared with other dementias, with this increased risk perhaps reflecting the relatively widespread neuronal disturbance associated with these conditions (Robertsson et al. 1998). Voyer et al. (2006) described an association between prior cognitive impairment, low functional autonomy, and benzodiazepine and narcotic use with increased delirium severity in older institutionalized patients admitted to an acute care hospital.

O'Keeffe and Lavan (1996) stratified patients into four levels of delirium risk based on the presence of three factors (chronic cognitive impairment, severe illness, elevated serum urea) and found that the risk of delirium increased as these factors accumulated. Similarly, Inouye and Charpentier (1996) developed a predictive model that included four predisposing factors (cognitive impairment, severe illness, visual impairment, dehydration) and five precipitating factors (more than three medications added, catheterization, use of restraints, malnutrition, and any iatrogenic event). These factors predicted a 17-fold variation in the relative risk of developing delirium. Uremia increases the permeability of the blood–brain barrier, allowing many larger molecules, such as drugs, to enter the brain when they ordinarily would not.

Although the value of reducing risk factors appears self-evident, many may simply be markers of general morbidity; therefore, studies showing preventive effect are important (see subsection "Prevention Strategies" later in this chapter). Some risk factors are potentially modifiable and thus are targets for prevention, although cumulative microstructural effects of aging are not reversible. Thiamine deficiency is an underappreciated cause of and risk factor for delirium in pediatric intensive care and oncology patients (Seear et al. 1992) and nonalcoholic elderly patients (O'Keeffe et al. 1994).

Medication exposure is probably the most readily modifiable risk factor for delirium, implicated as a cause in 20%–40% of cases. Polypharmacy and drug intoxication and withdrawal may be the most common causes of delirium (Hales et al. 1988; Trzepacz et al. 1985). Benzodiazepines, opioids, and drugs with anticholinergic activity have a particular association with delirium (T.M. Brown 2000; Marcantonio et al. 1994b). Many drugs (and their metabolites) can unexpectedly contribute to delirium as a result of unrecognized anticholinergic effects. Ten of the 25 most commonly prescribed drugs for the elderly had sufficient in vitro anticholinergic activity identified by radioreceptor assay to cause memory and attention impairment in nondelirious elderly subjects (Tune et al. 1992). Therefore, drug exposure must be minimized, especially when facing high-risk periods such as the perioperative phase. Although opioids are associated with delirium, Morrison et al. (2003) found in a prospective study of older patients undergoing hip surgery that delirium was nine times more likely in those patients deemed to have undertreated pain.

The temporal relation between exposure to risk factors and development of delirium requires further study. Postoperative delirium (excluding emergence from anesthesia) appears most frequently at day 3. A large multicenter study found age, duration of anesthesia, lower education, second operation, postoperative infection, and respiratory complications to be predictors of postoperative cognitive impairment (Moller et al. 1998).

Low serum albumin is an important risk factor at any age and may signify poor nutrition, chronic disease, or liver or renal insufficiency. Hypoalbuminemia results in a greater bioavailability of many drugs that are transported in the bloodstream by albumin, which is associated with an increased risk of side effects, including delirium (Dickson 1991; Trzepacz and Francis 1990). This increased biological drug activity occurs within the therapeutic range and may not be recognized because increased levels of free drug are not separately reported in most assays. Serum albumin was identified by discriminant analysis, along with Trail Making Test B and EEG dominant posterior rhythm, as sensitively distinguishing delirious from nondelirious liver transplant candidates (Trzepacz et al. 1988b).

Nicotine withdrawal has been implicated as a potential risk factor in the development of delirium, especially in heavy smokers unable to continue their habit during hospital admission. Klein et al. (2002) reported a single case of delirium in such a patient who responded quickly to a transdermal nicotine patch.

The study of genetic factors relevant to delirium has lagged behind other neuropsychiatric conditions and the bulk of work to date has explored candidate genes that regulate factors relevant to alcohol metabolism in alcohol withdrawal delirium. Among these, studies of dopamine receptor genes have produced varied results, with the positive studies (Sander et al. 1997; Wernicke et al. 2002; Wodarz et al. 2003) matched by equivalent negative studies (Kohnke et al. 2005, 2006a; Limosin et al. 2004). Positive associations have been reported for alcohol withdrawal delirium incidence for polymorphisms in genes coding for glutamate receptor (Preuss et al. 2006), tyrosine hydroxylase (Sander et al. 1998), brain-derived neurotrophic factor (BDNF) (Matsushita et al. 2004), and NAD(P)H-quinone oxidoreductase-2 (Okubo et al. 2003), while negative findings have been found in relation to monoamine oxidase A (MAO-A) (Kohnke et al. 2006b), catechol-*O*-methyltransferase (COMT) (Tihonen et al. 1999), neuropeptide Y (Kohnke et al. 2002), and cholecystokinin (Okubo et al. 2000). Two studies of cannabinoid receptors have produced conflicting findings (Preuss et al. 2003; Schmidt et al. 2002).

Genetic factors may increase risk for delirium from medical causes. Some studies have found that the apolipoprotein E (APOE) ε4 allele is associated with an increased risk of delirium in ICU patients (Ely et al. 2007) and poorer prognosis (longer episode duration or nonrecovery) (Adamis et al. 2007b; Ely et al. 2007). Dopaminergic gene polymorphisms may also play a role (Van Munster et al. 2009). While genetic risk factors are a promising avenue for further research, the results to date are inconclusive because of insufficiently powered studies and other methodological issues (Adamis et al. 2009).

Delirium and Mortality

Delirium appears to be associated with high morbidity and mortality both short- and long-term, especially in the elderly. Reported mortality rates during the index hospitalization for a delirium episode have ranged from 4% to 65% (Cameron et al. 1987; Gustafson et al. 1988). Methodological inconsistencies and shortcomings affect the interpretation of many studies of mortality risk associated with delirium. Some earlier studies do not compare patients who have delirium with control groups. Many studies include patients with comorbid dementia, and many earlier studies do not control for severity of medical comorbidity (admittedly difficult to measure). In addition, many early studies do not address the effects of advanced age as a separate risk factor, and specific delirium rating instruments were rarely used. The effect on reducing mortality risk by treatment for the delirium itself, a potential confound, is also not reported in most studies. Attention to whether the sample is incident or prevalent, identification of referral biases, and indication of whether follow-up mortality rates are cumulative to include the original sample are also important issues that vary across study designs. Not all studies have reported a higher mortality rate after delirium (Adamis et al. 2007a; Francis and Kapoor 1992; Inouye et al. 1998).

More recent prospective studies in medically hospitalized patients have found that delirium significantly increases mortality risk, even after controlling for multiple potential confounding factors such as medical comorbidity, demographics, dementia status, and ADL (Curyto et al. 2001; Ely et al. 2004a; Inouye et al. 1998; Leslie et al. 2005; McCusker et al. 2002). Other studies have shown a similar increase in mortality associated with delirium in nursing facilities (Kelly et al. 2001; Marcantonio et al. 2005). Mortality risk may be increased even years later (Curyto et al. 2001). The number of days of delirium is a significant predictor of later mortality (Gonzalez et al. 2009; Pisani et al. 2009). Delirium that is persistent is especially likely to predict poorer prognosis (Cole et al. 2009) and increased mortality (Kiely et al. 2009). Dementia plus delirium appears to carry a higher mortality risk than either diagnosis alone (Bellelli et al. 2007). Longer duration of delirium increases long-term mortality in the elderly, whether measured as number of delirium days in the ICU after controlling for moderating factors (Pisani et al. 2009) or as number of delirium hours in the medically ill (Gonzalez et al. 2009).

Longer-term follow-up of emergency department elderly who were sent home found that delirium increased mortality even after adjustment for age, sex, functional level, cognitive status, comorbidity, and number of medications (Kakuma et al. 2003). However, those with delirium undetected by the emergency department staff had the highest mortality whereas those with detected delirium had comparable long-term mortality to the nondelirious. The latter suggests that detection and intervention may be important determinants in mortality rates, although, in contrast, studies of systematic intervention in delirious patients have failed to show a reduction in mortality or subsequent institutionalization (Cole et al. 1994, 2002; Pitkala 2006).

It is not known whether increased mortality is attributable to the effects of underlying etiologies of delirium; to indirect effects on the body related to perturbations of neuronal, endocrine, and immunological function during delirium; or to damaging effects on the brain from neurochemical abnormalities associated with delirium (i.e., similar to glutamate surges after stroke). Additionally, patients with delirium cannot fully cooperate with their medical care or participate in rehabilitative programs during hospitalization. Their behaviors can directly reduce the effectiveness of procedures meant to treat their medical problems (e.g., removing tubes and intravenous lines, climbing out of bed), which adds to morbidity and possibly to further physiological injury and mortality.

So-called subsyndromal delirium may also be associated with adverse outcomes including increased mortality (Cole et al. 2003b; Levkoff et al. 1992; Marcantonio et al. 2002, 2005), reduced independent living status (Marcantonio et al. 2002), and increased need for postdischarge institutional care (Bourdel-Marchasson et al. 2004). Cole et al. (2003b) prospectively observed that the more delirium symptoms present, especially on admission, the worse the prognosis as evidenced by longer inpatient stays, poorer cognitive and functional status as well as greater subsequent mortality at 12-month follow-up.

Thus, although the mechanism is not understood, the presence of delirium does indeed appear to be an adverse prognostic sign that is associated with an increased risk for mortality, extending well beyond the index hospitalization, even after controlling for other known risk factors like age, medical problems and low function at baseline. To what extent aggressive treatment of both the delirium and its comorbid medical problems would reduce morbidity and mortality is not well studied. There is increasing interest in measuring biological markers of inflammation and other disturbed pathophysiology that may ultimately assist in disentangling the reason for the association between delirium and mortality risk.

Delirium Reversibility and Long-Term Cognitive Impairment in the Elderly

The traditional concept of delirium is of a disorder that is usually reversible, and this attribute has been one of the key characteristics used to distinguish delirium from dementia. In Bedford's (1957) landmark study of delirium, approximately 5% of the patients were still "confused" at 6-month follow-up. Epidemiological reports indicate that a subset of delirium symptoms can persist for months in approximately one-quarter of elderly delirium cases (Marcantonio et al. 2005; McCusker et al. 2003b; Siddiqi et al. 2006). A significant percentage of patients develop enduring cognitive deficits, so-called long-term cognitive impairment (LTCI). A range of studies have documented the occurrence of longer-term cognitive deficits after an index episode of delirium (see Jackson et al. 2004 and MacLullich et al. 2009 for detailed reviews), but it is methodologically challenging to determine causality and distinguish among the many potential causes of LTCI including moderating and mediating factors rather than the delirium itself (see Figure 5–3).

It remains unclear to what extent persistent cognitive difficulties represent ongoing or recurrent delirium symptoms or reflect the development of neuropsychological impairments that differ in character from acute delirium. Zaubler et al. (2009) found that the pattern of neuropsychological impairment at 3 months was unrelated to delirium. Furthermore, Jones et al. (2006) found cognitive impairments in nondelirious ICU patients that persisted following discharge. Both of these findings strengthen the causality argument toward the medical morbidity and not the delirium.

Preexisting cognitive impairment predicts both the risk for delirium and its severity (J.G. Franco et al., in press; Voyer et al. 2007), as well as predicting specific cognitive symptoms of delirium (Voyer et al. 2006). Delirium severity is associated with degree of prior cognitive impairment in the elderly, as well as with baseline low functional autonomy level (i.e., instrumental activities of daily living [IADL]) (Voyer et al. 2007). Ongoing or recurrent delirium symptoms occur in older patients discharged home or to nursing homes before the index delirium episode has resolved (Levkoff et al. 1992, 1994; Rockwood 1993). More recent neuropsychological and longitudinal reports highlight the importance of preexisting moderating factors.

Importantly, both the delirium and LTCI may be caused by another condition, such as an underlying medical illness, brain injury (e.g., hypoxic, traumatic), or a preexisting undiagnosed dementia (Koponen et al. 1994). In such cases, delirium is a marker for risk of future cognitive deterioration. Zaubler et al. (2009) found that greater intraoperative regional oxygen desaturation in frontal lobes as measured by cerebral oximetry predicted a fivefold risk of postoperative delirium, which supports hypoxia as a possible common denominator for both delirium and LTCI, independently.

However, there is the possibility that delirium itself, once precipitated, might be neurotoxic in vulnerable patients, which is an intriguing notion, as it would mean that delirium is an important potentially modifiable risk factor for dementia—the inverse of the current understanding of dementia as a risk factor for delirium. This conclusion is suggested by Fong et al. (2009), who found that the rate of cognitive decline in patients with Alzheimer's disease who had developed delirium was accelerated threefold compared with the rate of decline in those who had not experienced delirium.

Many studies have related persisting cognitive difficulties to "diminished brain reserve" associated with preexisting dementia that has progressed over time (Camus et al. 2000; Koponen et al. 1994; Rahkonen et al. 2000; Rockwood et al. 1999). Thus, persistent deficits may instead reflect an underlying disorder and not the delirium. Comorbid dementia may go unrecognized at the time of the

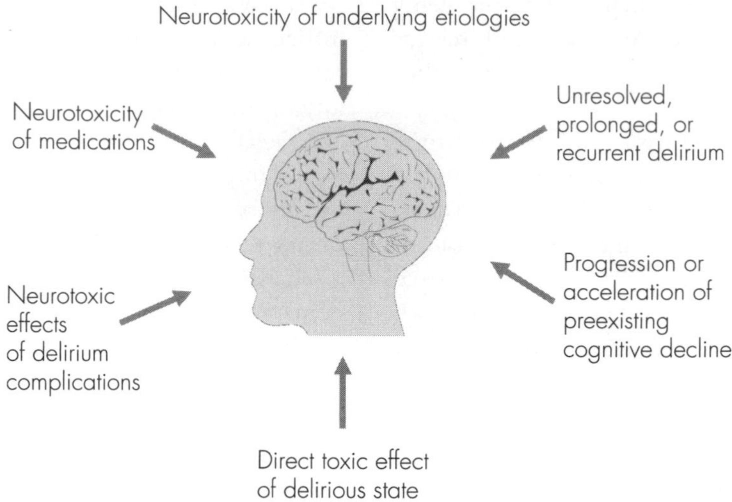

FIGURE 5–3. "Persistent cognitive deficits" following delirium episode: possible mechanisms.

Source. Reprinted from Trzepacz PT, Meagher DJ: "Neuropsychiatric Aspects of Delirium," in *The American Psychiatric Publishing Textbook of Neuropsychiatry and Behavioral Neurosciences,* 5th Edition. Edited by Yudofsky SC, Hales RE. Washington, DC, American Psychiatric Publishing, 2008, pp. 445–517. Copyright 2008, American Psychiatric Publishing, Inc. Used with permission.

delirium index episode in part because it is challenging to adequately assess for preexisting dementia retrospectively. More focal neuropsychological deficits also increase risk for delirium. Several investigators have found that preexisting executive dysfunction and/or attentional difficulties, even in the absence of dementia, predicted delirium (L.J. Brown et al. 2009; I.R. Katz et al. 2001; Lowery et al. 2007; Osse et al. 2008; Rudolph et al. 2006; Smith et al. 2009). Thus, undetected preexisting cognitive deficits may both predict delirium and become manifest as LTCI.

Very interesting are studies that suggest there may be subtypes of delirium with differing vulnerability to poor prognosis. Among elderly delirium survivors there are no significant differences in cognition, function, or institutional status between delirium-recovered and nondelirious groups at 6 and 12 months, after adjustment for multiple moderating and mediating factors (Cole et al. 2008). Following major noncardiac surgery in cognitively normal patients, those with delirium were more likely than age-matched control subjects to have cognitive deficits at discharge but not at 3-month follow-up, when cognitive impairment was instead predicted by baseline IADL (Monk et al. 2008). Furthermore, among the three age groups (young: 18–39 years; middle-aged: 40–59 years; and elderly: 60-plus years), only the elderly group had worse cognitive function than nondelirious control subjects at 3 months.

Although the likelihood of developing both delirium and LTCI is increased in patients with preexisiting cognitive deficits, a number of prospective studies have demonstrated that LTCI may occur in patients who appear cognitively intact prior to experiencing delirium (Benoit et al. 2005; Bickel et al. 2008; Duppils and Wikblad 2004; Fann et al. 2002; Gruber-Baldini et al. 2003; Kat et al. 2008; Lundstrom et al. 2003). However, these studies did not employ the most sensitive assessment methods (usually the MMSE), making it difficult to be sure patients did not have preexisting cognitive deficits.

In summary, whether delirium itself causes irreversible damage remains controversial because of the difficulties disentangling the effects of acute medical burden and preexisting brain damage particularly in those with advanced age. Studies to date have many methodological issues that include a predominance of elderly subjects who are prone to cognitive disorders, inclusion of relatively small sample sizes, use of insensitive screens like the MMSE in lieu of neuropsychological testing, lack of delirium severity measures, inadequate control for baseline cognitive impairment, and other confounders (e.g., severity of illness, exposure to medications), variable length of follow-up, and need to better account for delirium subtype, etiology, severity, and duration, all of which have implications for outcome. These studies do increase awareness that a delirium episode, especially in an older person, is a harbinger of physiological damage in the body and brain that may result from an otherwise unrecognized process which is possibly hastened by the medical or surgical event associated with a delirium episode. Whether the brain sustains enduring damage from the delirium is not discernible at this time, although evidence that delirium is a marker and risk factor for LTCI appears convincing.

Clinical Features

Phenomenology

The classic descriptive study of 106 "dysergastic reaction" (i.e., delirium) patients by Wolff and Curran (1935) is still consistent with current conceptions of delirium phenomenology as a complex neuropsychiatric syndrome that includes a wide range of cognitive and noncognitive disturbances that are of relatively acute onset and fluctuate over the course of an episode. Inconsistent and unclear definitions of symptoms and underuse of standardized symptom assessment tools have hampered subsequent efforts to describe delirium phenomenology or to compare symptom incidences across studies and etiological populations. Moreover, the temporal course of its phenomenological complexity can only be captured by longitudinal studies which are almost entirely lacking. A recent longitudinal study of delirium symptoms in TBI patients using cognitive tests and the sleep-wake cycle item on the Delirium Rating Scale–Revised–98 (DRS-R-98; Trzepacz et al. 2001c) over five ratings found a highly individualized pattern for recovery of each symptom (Abell et al. 2009).

Despite across-study inconsistencies for symptom frequencies, certain symptoms occur more often than others, consistent with the proposal that delirium has core symptoms irrespective of etiology (Trzepacz 1999b, 2000). Multiple etiologies for delirium may "funnel" into a final common neural pathway (Trzepacz 1999b, 2000), so that the phenomenological expression becomes similar despite a breadth of different physiologies. Some symptoms represent core elements of the syndrome (e.g., inattention, sleep-wake cycle disturbances, motor activity changes) while other features are more variable in presentation (e.g., psychosis, affective changes) reflecting the influence of particular etiological underpinnings, comorbidities, exposure to medical treatments for delirium, or individual patient vulnerabilities. Candidates for core symptoms include attention deficits, memory impairment, disorientation, sleep-wake cycle disturbance, thought process abnormalities, motor alterations, and language disturbances, whereas associated or noncore symptoms would include perceptual disturbances (illusions, hallucinations), delusions, and affective changes (Trzepacz 1999b) (see Table 5–4). Relationships between symptoms have received limited study, except through factor analyses of cross-sectional data (J.G. Franco et al. 2009; N. Gupta et al. 2008). These studies indicate some striking similarities regarding which symptoms clustered together typically with 2–3 factor solutions with a composite cognitive and one or more neurobehavioral factors.

Historically, the term *clouding of consciousness* has been used to describe the characteristic cognitive impairment of delirium with diminished capacity to engage with and grasp the external environment. However, a disturbance of consciousness is a better descriptor of delirium as a disorder than as a symptom of it. A disproportionate disturbance of attention has been emphasized as the principal cognitive disruption of delirium, and is the cardinal symptom required for diagnosis of delirium according to current classification systems. However, although inattention correlates highly with other elements of cognitive disturbance (Meagher et al. 2007), it does not account for the breadth of delirium symptoms.

Attention is impaired in all of its aspects such that delirious patients have difficulty in their ability to mobilize, shift, and sustain attention, reflected in apparent distractibility and poor environmental awareness during interview as well as with formal testing (Lipowski 1990). Inattention is a consistent feature, crucial to diagnosis, but also highly prevalent in patients who have subsyndromal or mild delirium (Marquis et al. 2007).

TABLE 5–4. Frequency of phenomenological manifestations in delirium using the Delirium Rating Scale–Revised–98

Core features	Noncore features
Attentional deficits (97%–100%)	Perceptual disturbances (50%–63%)
Disorientation (76%–96%)	Delusions (21%–31%)
Short-term memory deficits (88%–92%)	Affective changes (43%–86%)
Long-term memory deficits (89%–96%)	
Sleep-wake cycle disturbances (92%–97%)	
Thought process abnormalities (54%–79%)	
Visuospatial impairment (87%–96%)	
Motor alterations (24%–94%)	
Language disturbances (57%–67%)	

Source. From N. Gupta et al. 2008.

Patients with delirium also exhibit more generalized cognitive disturbance typically impacting upon short- and long-term memory, orientation, comprehension, vigilance, visuospatial ability, and executive function. Crystallized intelligence is unaffected, however (L.J. Brown et al. 2009). Memory impairment occurs often in delirium, affecting both short- and long-term memory, with particular disruption of recent memory due to diminished capacity to incorporate new experience. Patients are often amnestic for some or all of their delirium episodes (Breitbart et al. 2002). Trzepacz et al. (2001b) found a high correlation between short- and long-term memory items in delirious patients, with attention correlating with short-term memory but not with long-term memory. This is consistent with normally needing to pay attention before information can enter short-term (working) memory, and then selected data from working memory are stored in long-term memory.

Disorientation to time, place, and identity of others is a common feature that is often used as a screen for disturbed cognition in clinical settings but is fraught with potential for inaccuracy in detection due to its fluctuating nature. Visuospatial disturbances impair patients' ability to function in hospital environments. The constructional apraxia measured by performance on the Clock Drawing Test is sensitive to cognitive impairment in general but lacks specificity for delirium (Adamis et al. 2005).

Disorganized thinking is also a prominent feature that was previously emphasized in diagnosis (DSM-III-R) and that ranges from tangentiality and circumstantiality to loose associations. In one study, 21% of the patients with delirium exhibited tangentiality or circumstantiality, while 58% had loose associations (Trzepacz et al. 2001b).

Speech and language disturbances in delirium include abnormal semantic content, dysnomia, paraphasias, impaired comprehension, dysgraphia, and word-finding difficulties. In extreme cases, language resembles a fluent dysphasia. Incoherent speech or speech disturbance is reported commonly. Various forms of dysgraphia (spelling errors, angled and jagged writing, and disturbances of constructional praxis) have been advocated for delirium detection (Baranowski and Patten 2000) but overall writing disturbances appear to be nonspecific in nature (Patten and Lamarre 1989).

Disturbances of the sleep-wake cycle are reported in over 90% of patients with delirium, and the severity and type of disturbances range from napping and nocturnal insomnia to much more severe disturbances (including fragmentation, cycle reversal) which differ considerably from the milder sleep disturbances common in nondelirious hospitalized elderly. The prominence of sleep-wake cycle disturbances has prompted some to advocate delirium as a disorder of sleep and/or circadian rhythms (Matsushima et al. 1997). The extent to which sleep-wake cycle disturbance confounds the hyperactive-hypoactive subtyping of delirium is not known.

Disturbances of motor behavior are almost invariable in delirium (Camus et al. 2000; A.K. Gupta et al. 2005; Meagher et al. 2008c) and include three patterns: hyperactive, hypoactive, and mixed presentations that shift between hyper- and hypoactivity. Often, motor disturbances are characterized as psychomotor behaviors (including hyperalertness, wandering, and uncooperativeness, or hypersomnolence, disinterest, and unawareness) that encompass nonmotor symptoms that may or may not have any specificity for delirium. The relevance of these patterns to clinical subtyping of delirium is discussed below.

Psychotic features such as perceptual disturbances (e.g., hallucinations and delusions) are less frequent than core symptoms (Eriksson et al. 2002; Webster and Holroyd 2000). A retrospective study of 227 patients with delirium found that 26% had delusions, 27% had visual hallucinations, 12% had auditory hallucinations, and 3% had tactile hallucinations (Webster and Holroyd 2000), while O'Keeffe et al. (2005) found that 70% of elderly dementia-free patients with delirium had delusions, misperceptions, or both during delirium. Psychosis is more common in hyperactive presentations but also occurs in hypoactive patients (Breitbart et al. 2002; Meagher et al. 2000). The type of perceptual disturbance and delusion distinguishes delirium from functional psychoses such as schizophrenia (Cutting 1987). Clinically, the occurrence of visual (as well as tactile, olfactory, and gustatory) hallucinations heightens the likelihood of delirium, although primary psychiatric disorders occasionally present with visual misperceptions. Visual hallucinations range from patterns or shapes to complex and vivid animations (Trzepacz 1994). Persecutory delusions that are poorly formed (not systematized) are the most common type in delirium, although other types occur (e.g., somatic or grandiose). Delusional content involves misidentifications, themes of imminent danger, or of bizarre happenings in the immediate environment (Cutting 1987).

Affective lability is typical of delirium and can take many forms (e.g., anxious, apathetic, angry, dysphoric); it reflects a loss of control of emotional expression. In a study of psychiatric consultation referrals for suspected mood disorder who actually had delirium, 24% experienced suicidal thoughts, 52% had frequent thoughts of death, and 32% felt there was no point in taking medications (Farrell and Ganzini 1995). These findings highlight the importance of careful monitoring of mental state in delirious patients. Recent work has highlighted the frequency of more sustained disturbances of mood that complicate differentiation from hypomania in agitated cases and depression in hypoactive presentations (Leonard et al. 2009).

Motor Subtypes

It is not known whether there are meaningful subtypes of delirium based on clinical profiles. The most common proposed subtype has been defined according to alterations in motor activity. Altered motor activity in physically unwell patients with cognitive disturbance has been recognized for over two millennia, with the terms *lethargicus* and *phrenitis* used by the ancient Greeks to denote profiles of decreased and increased activity, respectively. Lipowski (1990) championed the use of "hyperactive" and "hypoactive" as labels for delirium subtypes, before adding a third "mixed" category to account for the observation that many patients experience elements of both within short time frames.

Subsequent work using a range of methodologies applied to a range of populations and treatment settings indicates that subtypes defined by motor presentation have similar neuropsychological and EEG profiles while differing in relationship to a variety of important clinical parameters, including frequency of presence of nonmotor symptoms, etiology, pathophysiology, detection rates, treatment experience, duration of episode, and outcome (Meagher 2009).

One of the most important implications of the different motor presentations of delirium is their impact upon accurate detection. The highly visible and often compelling behavioral disturbances of hyperactive patients tend to attract the attention of clinical staff, but in patients with hypoactive delirium, the frequent absence of overt distress or disturbance causes them to more likely be missed (Inouye et al. 2001) or misdiagnosed as depression.

Symptom fluctuation and acuity of onset are especially evident in hyperactive and mixed cases. Delusions, hallucinations, mood lability, speech incoherence, and sleep disturbances may be somewhat more frequent in hyperactive patients (Meagher and Trzepacz 2000; Ross et al. 1991) but are present in many patients with hypoactive presentations (Breitbart et al. 2002). Studies suggest that delirium occurring in the context of metabolic disorders or organ failure is more frequently hypoactive in presentation while that due to substance intoxication or withdrawal is more typically hyperactive (A. K. Gupta et al. 2005; Meagher et al. 1998; Morita et al. 2001; Ross et al. 1991).

The motor subtypes of delirium occur at differing frequencies in different populations. Hypoactive subtype is reported at higher frequency in palliative care and ICU populations, while psychiatric consultations are more likely to be requested for patients with relatively more hyperactivity. ICU patients have high rates of the mixed subtype. Detailed longitudinal study of delirium symptoms is necessary before any definitive conclusion can be reached regarding the stability of motor subtypes. Mixed cases may reflect different impacts over time of multiple etiological effects on motor behavior or may be a hybrid state; some evidence suggests that mixed types occur in more severe delirium (Meagher 2009).

Few treatment studies in delirium have attempted to assess response for different motor subtypes, and they are small and do not paint a clear or consistent picture (Boettger et al. 2007a, 2007b; Liu et al. 2004; Platt et al. 1994, 2002). Overall, the relationship between motor subtype and treatment remains uncertain, but existing studies do suggest that hypoactive patients may also benefit when given antipsychotic treatment.

A range of studies have linked psychomotor profile and motor subtypes to outcome of delirium The balance of the evidence suggests that hypoactivity is associated with a relatively poorer prognosis, but such differences may reflect differences in underlying causes, recognition rates, and/or treatment practices. Meagher et al. (1996), for example, found that psychotropic medication and supportive environmental ward strategies were more frequently used in the management of patients with hyperactive subtype.

An important methodological issue is that clinical checklist methods of motor subtyping do not focus solely on motor activity but instead include various "psychomotor" symptoms (verbal, affective, sleep, psychotic) that have a questionable phenomenological relationship to motor activity levels (Meagher and Trzepacz 2000). Therefore, Meagher et al. (2008c) studied motor and psychomotor symptoms in a study of delirious patients and nondelirious control patients and on the basis of these analyses developed a new pure motor disturbance clinical subtyping method, the Delirium Motor Subtype Scale (DMSS). DMSS items differentiated delirious subjects from control subjects (Meagher et al. 2008b; see Table 5–5). This scale is recommended for clinical use to replace nonvalidated psychomotor schema that include many nonmotor items. Unlike traditional psychomotor checklists, this scale has been demonstrated to have concurrent validity with objectively measured motor activity recorded via electronic actigraphy (Godfrey et al. 2009; Leonard et al. 2007b; Meagher et al. 2008a). Figure 5–4 depicts the percentage of time spent per hour in dynamic activity for patients with hyperactive, hypoactive, and mixed motor delirium, highlighting the differences among these subtypes (Godfrey et al. 2010).

Diagnosis and Assessment

Diagnosis

The diagnosis of delirium is made according to diagnostic systems where the cardinal symptom is inattention or clouded/impaired level of consciousness or both. Inatten-

TABLE 5–5. Delirium Motor Subtype Scale (DMSS)

A. HYPERACTIVE SUBTYPE if definite evidence in the previous 24 hours (and this should be a deviation from predelirium baseline) of at least two of the following:

(1) Increased quantity of motor activity: Is there evidence of excessive level of activity (e.g., pacing, fidgeting, general overactivity)?

(2) Loss of control of activity: Is the patient unable to maintain levels of activity that are appropriate for the circumstances (e.g., remain still when required)?

(3) Restlessness: Does the patient complain of restlessness or appear agitated?

(4) Wandering: Is the patient wandering (i.e., moving around without clear direction or purpose)?

B. HYPOACTIVE SUBTYPE if definite evidence in the previous 24 hours (and this should be a deviation from predelirium baseline) of two or more of the following:

(1)* Decreased amount of activity: Does the patient engage in less activity than is usual or appropriate for the circumstances (e.g., sits still with few spontaneous movements)?

(2)* Decreased speed of actions: Is the patient slow in initiation and performance of movements (e.g., walking)?

(3) Reduced awareness of surroundings: Does the patient show a relative absence of emotional reactivity to the environment (i.e., show a passive attitude to his or her surroundings)?

(4) Decreased amount of speech: Does the patient have a reduced quantity of speech in relation to the environment (e.g., answers are unforthcoming or restricted to a minimum)?

(5) Decreased speed of speech: Does the patient speak more slowly than usual (e.g., long pauses and slowing of actual verbal output)?

(6) Listlessness: Is the patient less reactive to his/her environment (e.g., responses to activity in surroundings are slow or reduced in amount)?

(7) Reduced alertness/withdrawal: Does the patient appear detached or lacking in awareness of his or her surroundings or their significance?

*At least one of either decreased amount of activity or speed of actions must be present.

C. MIXED MOTOR SUBTYPE if evidence of both hyperactive and hypoactive subtype in the previous 24 hours.

D. NO MOTOR SUBTYPE if evidence of neither hyperactive nor hypoactive subtype in the previous 24 hours.

Source. Adapted from Meagher et al. 2008b.

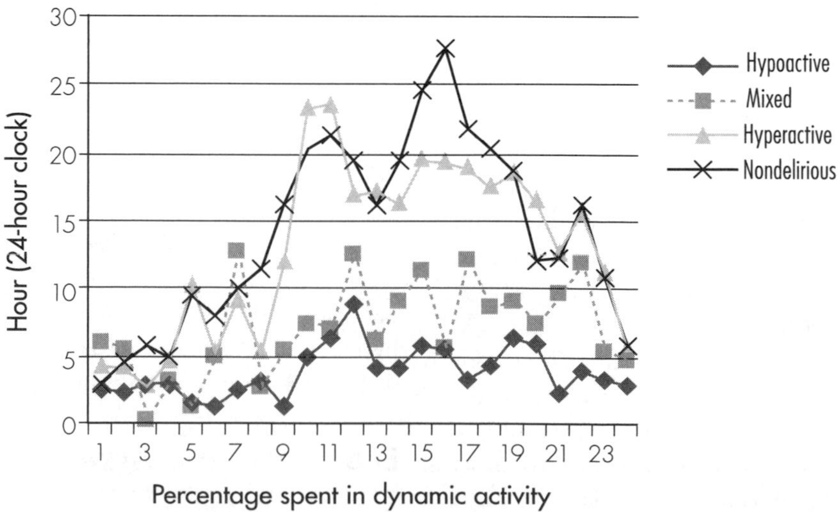

FIGURE 5–4. Percentage of time spent in dynamic activity per hour (24-hour clock; midnight=0) among patients with hyperactive, hypoactive, and mixed motor subtypes of delirium compared with nondelirious control subjects.

Source. Reprinted from Godfrey A, Leonard M, Donnelly S, et al.: "Validating a New Clinical Subtyping Scheme for Delirium With Electronic Motion Analysis." *Psychiatry Research* 178:186–190, 2010. Copyright 2010, Elsevier. Used with permission.

tion is also a consistent feature during the course of a delirious episode, supporting its usefulness as a reliable marker of delirium (Fann et al. 2002; Leonard et al. 2007a). Temporal course is a key indicator—delirium is typically of acute onset and symptom severity fluctuates over the course of the day. In addition, the presence of a potential etiological cause of delirium is also diagnostically valuable.

The demonstration of generalized cognitive disturbance allows distinction from disorders with more discrete neuropsychological disruptions (e.g., amnestic syndromes, mood disorders, attention deficit disorder). Where patients are known or suspected of having prior cognitive impairment, it is essential that a deterioration from baseline is used to identify symptoms that reflect delirium.

In clinical practice, making a diagnosis of delirium usually requires gathering information from multiple sources. A patient's mental status can be assessed by observation, interview, and formal cognitive testing. Further information regarding the course of any deficits is gleaned from the observer's knowledge of the patient, clinical notes, nursing staff, family, and other caregivers. Accurate assessment of attention combines clinical observation with specific cognitive tests, such as digit span, serial sevens test, or recitation of the months of the year in reverse order.

For many centuries the concept of delirium has included altered consciousness with generalized disturbance of higher cortical function. Historically, clouding of consciousness has been emphasized, but this is a concept that lacks precision and encompasses a combination of diminished attention, poor awareness, comprehension and grasp, altered wakefulness levels, and other cognitive disruptions. It does, however, capture delirium as essentially a disorder of impaired consciousness.

Specific diagnostic criteria for delirium first appeared in DSM-III, prior to which delirium was encapsulated in DSM I and DSM II under the general category of acute brain syndrome, characterized by five key symptoms—impairments of orientation, memory, all intellectual functions, and judgment, as well as lability and shallowness of affect. Other disturbances, such as hallucinations and delusions, were considered secondary to the disturbance of the sensorium. Note that inattention was not cardinal. DSM-II (American Psychiatric Association 1968) described two acute organic brain syndromes, psychotic and nonpsychotic types.

DSM-III, DSM-III-R, and DSM-IV included efforts to further clarify the major criterion describing altered states of consciousness, considered as either a disturbance of consciousness or inattention. DSM-III-R is the most inclusive of the breadth of delirium symptoms and tends to be preferred by researchers. DSM-IV requires fewer symptoms and therefore tends to overdiagnose cases. All DSM versions required that symptoms not be better accounted for by a dementia.

DSM-IV (American Psychiatric Association 1994) and its text revision, DSM-IV-TR (American Psychiatric Association 2000), have five categories of delirium; the criteria are the same for each category except the one for etiology. The categories are 1) delirium due to a general medical condition, 2) substance intoxication delirium, 3) substance withdrawal delirium, 4) delirium due to multiple etiologies, and 5) delirium not otherwise specified. This notation of etiology in DSM-IV is reminiscent of that used in DSM-I (American Psychiatric Association 1952).

The ICD-10 (World Health Organization 1992) research diagnostic criteria for delirium are similar to the DSM-IV criteria. However, ICD-10 mandates that disturbances of *both* memory and orientation be evident. Specifically, a disproportionate disturbance of immediate recall and recent memory with relatively intact remote memory is required. Disturbances of memory are notoriously difficult to attribute to delirium in populations with comorbid dementia. In such cases it is helpful to demonstrate that disturbances in memory represent a clear deterioration from a recent baseline or focus inattention. The pattern mandated in ICD-10 is not always evident in delirium research, and orientation is prone to great fluctuation during the course of an episode (Leonard et al. 2007a). This impacts considerably upon detection especially where lucidity is equated with absence of disorientation. The ICD-10 criteria for delirium also require the presence of many features which are highly variable in their frequency (e.g., affective changes, perceptual disturbances). A number of studies have shown that the ICD-10 criteria lack sensitivity, excluding many patients who would be classified as delirious by DSM systems and whose clinical profiles and prognoses are very similar to delirium as diagnosed by these other systems (Cole et al. 2003a; Laurila et al. 2004).

Some studies have suggested that the presence of some features of delirium, although insufficient to meet DSM or ICD criteria, may indicate a subsyndromal condition that is not recognized in DSM. Although delirium is usually characterized by an acute onset replete with many symptoms, it may be preceded by a subclinical delirium with more insidious changes in sleep pattern or cognition (Harrell and Othmer 1987) and background slowing on the EEG (Matsushima et al. 1997). J.G. Franco et al. (2009) found that subsyndromal delirium was comparable to full delirium for sleep-wake cycle and perceptual disturbances, affective lability, short-term memory deficits, motor disturbances, and acute onset but was intermediate in severity between normal controls and full delirium for inattention, delusions, language and thought process abnormalities, disorientation, and long-term memory and visuospatial impairments.

Cognitive Assessment

Because delirium is primarily a cognitive disorder, bedside assessment of cognition is critical to proper diagnosis. All cognitive domains—orientation, attention, short- and long-term memory, visuoconstructional ability, and executive function—are affected in delirium. Use of bedside screening tests (see also Chapter 1, "Psychiatric Assessment and Consultation") such as the MMSE (Folstein et al. 1975) is important clinically to document the presence of a cognitive disorder, but it lacks specificity for delirium (Trzepacz et al. 1988a). The MMSE is too easy for many people (ceiling effect) and has a limited breadth of items, particularly for prefrontal executive and right-hemisphere functions. Despite these shortcomings, some work (O'Keeffe et al. 2005) suggests that serial assessment with the MMSE can identify delirium in older medical patients, with a decrease of 2 or more points on the MMSE sensitive to delirium occurrence. There is evidence that some items are more indicative of delirium (e.g., orientation to current year and date, backwards spelling, copying of a pentagon) (Fayers et al. 2005), whereas others are more consistent with Alzheimer's dementia (e.g., orientation to time, recall of three objects) (Solfrizzi et al. 2001). Lowery et al. (2008) found that a combination of the MMSE with tests of attention and reaction time allowed for a high discrimination of delirium in postoperative patients without dementia. Overall, the MMSE is a useful means of identifying cognitively impaired patients, but the differentiation of delirium and dementia requires additional assessment methods.

The Cognitive Test for Delirium (CTD; Hart et al. 1996) is a bedside test designed specifically for patients with delirium who are often unable to speak or write in a medical setting (e.g., on a ventilator). Unlike the MMSE, the CTD has many nonverbal (nondominant hemisphere) items and abstraction questions. The CTD correlates highly with the MMSE (r=0.82) in patients with delirium and was performable in 42% of the ICU patients in whom the MMSE was not. It has two equivalent forms that correlated highly (r=0.90) in patients with dementia, which makes it better suited for repeated measurements. Cognitive impairment on the CTD correlates highly with scores for the cognitive subscale of the DRS-R-98 (Meagher et al. 2007). However, it correlates less well with symptom rating scales for delirium that also include noncognitive symptoms—for example, the Medical College of Virginia (MCV) Nurses Rating Scale for Delirium (r=–0.02) (Hart et al. 1996) and the DRS-R-98 (r=–0.62) (Trzepacz et al. 2001c). An abbreviated version of the CTD with just two of its nine items (visual attention span and recognition memory for pictures) retained good reliability and discriminant validity (Hart et al. 1997). Kennedy et al. (2003) found that a CTD cutoff score of less than 21 (rather than 19) was more suited to identification of delirium in recovering acute TBI patients. Greater severity on the inattention item of the CTD was found to be predictive of shorter survival time in delirious palliative care patients with cancer diagnoses (Leonard et al. 2008).

The Clock Drawing Test (CDT) assesses constructional praxis, visuospatial ability, executive function, and verbal and semantic memory. While it is a useful screen for cognitive impairment in medically ill patients, it lacks specificity for either presence or severity of delirium (Adamis et al. 2005) and does not discriminate between delirium and dementia (Manos 1997).

More discrete tests focusing on simple and complex attention (e.g., digit or spatial span, Trail Making Test B) can be useful in identifying and monitoring progress in delirious patients (Fann et al. 2002; Meagher and Leonard 2008; O'Keeffe and Gosney 1997; Trzepacz et al. 1988a). Overall, the use of systematic formal testing that focuses on delirium-relevant aspects of cognition (such as attention) can assist in more accurate detection of delirium.

Delirium Assessment Instruments

Delirium assessment tools can serve a variety of functions from clarifying diagnosis to studying the relationship between phenomenology and other clinical variables, including treatment response. A wide range of instruments have been described, but few have been subjected to robust investigation of psychometric properties or applicability across health care settings. Key considerations in choice of instrument include purpose of use (screening vs. diagnosis vs. severity measure vs. phenomenological profiling), ease of use (including time to administer, need for training, and knowledge of assessor—nurse vs. physician), characteristics of the population under study, and evidence to support validity and reliability in different settings and/or population. None are intended to substitute for adequate clinical experience. Furthermore, proper training on administration of these instruments increases their accuracy. There are a variety of delirium tools used but many are not described here due to infrequent use, inadequate validation, or exclusion of some key delirium symptoms (e.g., inattention, sleep-wake disturbance). Several are recommended (Kean and Ryan 2008; Timmers et al. 2005) that can be used together or separately, depending on the purpose. For example, a screening tool can be used for case detection, followed by application of DSM criteria, and then a more thorough rating for symptom severity.

The Confusion Assessment Method (CAM) is the most widely used screening tool for diagnosis of delirium across health care settings (Inouye et al. 1990) and has been translated into many languages. The CAM is based on DSM-III-

R criteria and has two forms: 1) a full scale with 11 items rated as present or absent and 2) the more commonly used algorithm that requires the presence of 3 of 4 key symptoms for a diagnosis of delirium. It has been adapted for use in intensive care settings (Ely et al. 2001a, 2001b), emergency departments (Monette et al. 2001), palliative care (Ryan et al. 2009), and even a telephone interview version (Fisher and Flowerdew 1995).

In general, the CAM has acceptable sensitivity and specificity when used by trained physicians, but it is much less useful when in nonexpert hands (Kean and Ryan 2008). Its sensitivity is much lower when used by nurses (Rolfson et al. 1999). Although the CAM can have utility as a screening tool, it is not adequate for diagnosis (Laurila et al. 2002) and has not been subjected to blind validation against patients with dementia or other psychiatric disorders, which limits its applicability.

Cole et al. (2003a) assessed the sensitivity and specificity of the full CAM in patients with DSM-III-R–diagnosed delirium, dementia, or comorbid delirium and dementia. With a cutoff of 6 of 11 items present, the authors found 95% sensitivity and 83% specificity in delirium-only patients and 98% sensitivity and 76% specificity in comorbid patients; however, use of fewer items (e.g., a minimum cutoff of 3 symptoms) greatly reduced the specificities to 60% for delirium and 47% for comorbid delirium and dementia.

An extension of the CAM is the CAM-ICU (Ely et al. 2001a, 2001b), aimed for use by nurses for severely medically ill patients in the ICU. The CAM-ICU uses specific adjunctive tests and standardized administration to enhance reliability and validity; 95% validity and 0.92–0.96 interrater reliability have been reported, compared with expert psychiatric diagnosis of delirium with DSM-IV criteria, in two different validation studies of 150 patients (Ely et al. 2001a, 2001b). Routine application of the CAM-ICU may permit earlier detection leading to haloperidol use for shorter time periods (Van den Boogaard et al. 2009).

The Delirium Rating Scale (DRS; Trzepacz et al. 1988a) is a 10-item scale assessing a breadth of delirium features and can function both for diagnosis and to assess symptom severity because of its hierarchical nature and anchored item choice descriptions (Trzepacz 1999a; van der Mast 1994). It has been translated into Italian, French, Spanish, Korean, Japanese, Mandarin Chinese, Dutch, Swedish, German, Portuguese, and a language of India. It is generally used by those who have some psychiatric training. The DRS has high interrater reliability and validity, even when compared with other psychiatric diagnoses, and distinguishes delirium from dementia. Factor analysis finds a two- or three-factor structure (Trzepacz 1999a; Trzepacz and Dew 1995). However, it does not function as well for frequent repeated measurements and has been modified by some researchers to a seven- or eight-item subscale. It is useful in children and adolescents (Turkel et al. 2003) and in hypoactive patients who border on stupor.

The DRS-R-98 is a substantially revised version of the DRS that addresses its shortcomings (Trzepacz et al. 2001c). It allows for repeated measurements and includes separate or new items for language, thought process, motor agitation, motor retardation, and five cognitive domains. It is intended for administration by clinicians with appropriate training in psychiatry, delirium, and use of the scale. An administration guide is available (obtainable from Dr. Trzepacz). Factor analysis (J.G. Franco et al. 2009) described two factors—cognition and psychosis/agitation. Inattention, thought process abnormalities, and sleep-wake disturbance loaded onto both factors, consistent with their being core domains of delirium.

The DRS-R-98 Total scale has 16 items, with 3 diagnostic items separable from 13 severity items that form a severity scale that also was validated. Severity is rated for a broad range of symptoms. The total scale is used for initial evaluation of delirium to allow discrimination from other disorders. The DRS-R-98 total score distinguished ($P<0.001$) delirium from dementia, schizophrenia, depression, and other medical illnesses during blind ratings, with sensitivities ranging from 91% to 100% and specificities from 85% to 100%, depending on the cutoff score chosen. The DRS-R-98 has high internal consistency (Cronbach $\alpha=0.90$), correlates well with the DRS ($r=0.83$) and CTD ($r=-0.62$), and has high interrater reliability (intraclass correlation coefficient [ICC]=0.99). Japanese, Korean, Greek, Portuguese, Danish, Dutch, German, Spanish (Colombia and Spain), Lithuanian, Norwegian, Italian, Thai, Hebrew, Turkish, and Chinese (traditional and modern) versions are available. In addition, Japanese, Korean, Dutch, traditional Chinese, Portuguese, and Spanish (Spain and Colombia) versions have been validated (de Negreiros et al. 2008; de Rooij et al. 2006; Fonseca et al. 2005; J.G. Franco et al. 2007; Huang et al. 2009; Kato et al., in press; Lim et al. 2006; Trzepacz et al. 2001a), and Turkish, Thai, Hebrew, Italian, and Greek validations are under way. Revalidations confirm the high sensitivity, specificity, and reliability of the DRS-R-98.

The Memorial Delirium Assessment Scale (MDAS) is a 10-item severity rating scale intended for repeated ratings within a 24-hour period (Breitbart et al. 1997). It takes approximately 10 minutes to complete and is intended for physician use. It was originally developed to assess delirium severity in patients with cancer or AIDS, but subsequent work has included elderly patients in general hospital (Marcantonio et al. 2002) and ICU (Shyamsundar et al. 2009) settings. The MDAS does not include items for temporal onset or fluctuation of symptoms, which are needed to diagnose delirium and help distinguish it from dementia. The MDAS correlated highly with the DRS (r=0.88) and MMSE (r=–0.91). Japanese and Italian versions have been validated (Grassi et al. 2001; Matsuoka et al. 2001). Sensitivity, specificity, and concordance with other delirium measures have varied from excellent to moderate (Kazmierski et al. 2008; Shyamsundar et al. 2009). Factor analyses have shown a two-factor structure for the MDAS (Lawlor et al. 2000b; Shyamsundar et al. 2009). The motor activity items of the MDAS as well as the DRS-R-98 have been used widely to define motor subtypes of delirium (Meagher 2009).

Electroencephalography

In the 1940s, Engel and Romano (1944, 1959; Romano and Engel 1944) wrote a series of classic papers that described the relation of delirium, as measured by cognitive impairment, to EEG generalized slowing. In their seminal work, they showed an association between abnormal electrical activity of the brain and symptoms of delirium, the reversibility of both of these conditions, the ubiquity of EEG changes across different underlying disease states, and the improvement in EEG background rhythm that paralleled clinical improvement. In most cases, EEGs are not needed to make a clinical diagnosis of delirium; instead, they are used when seizures are suspected or differential diagnosis is difficult, as in schizophrenic patients with medical illness. Most often, a careful assessment of behaviors, cognition, and history is sufficient to diagnose delirium. Nonetheless, EEG is the only technological method to assist in delirium diagnosis.

EEG characteristics in delirium include slowing or dropout of the dominant posterior rhythm, diffuse theta or delta waves (i.e., slowing), poor organization of the background rhythm, and loss of reactivity of EEG to eye opening and closing (Jacobson and Jerrier 2000). Similarly, quantitative EEG in delirium shows slowing of power bands' mean frequency, especially in posterior regions (see Figure 5–5).

In burn patients, Andreasen et al. (1977) showed that the time course of EEG slowing could precede or lag behind overt clinical symptoms of delirium, although sensitive delirium symptom ratings were not used. EEG dominant posterior rhythm, along with serum albumin and Trail Making Test B, distinguished delirious from nondelirious cirrhosis patients in another study (Trzepacz et al. 1988b). Although generalized slowing is the typical EEG pattern for both hypoactive and hyperactive presentations of delirium and for most etiologies, delirium tremens is characterized by low-voltage fast activity (Kennard et al. 1945) that is superimposed on slow waves. Intoxication with sedative-hypnotics is associated with fast beta waves. Although diffuse slowing is the most common presentation, false-negative results occur when a person's characteristic dominant posterior rhythm does not slow sufficiently to drop from the alpha to the theta range, thereby being read as normal despite the presence of abnormal slowing for that individual. (Generally, a change of more than 1 cycle per second [cps] from an individual's baseline is considered abnormal.) Jacobson and Jerrier (2000) warned that it can be difficult to distinguish delirium from drowsiness and light sleep unless the technologist includes standard alerting procedures during the EEG. Comparison with prior baseline EEGs is often helpful to document that slowing has in fact occurred. Less commonly, an EEG may detect focal causes of confusion, such as ictal and subictal states, including toxic ictal psychosis, nonconvulsive status, and complex partial status epilepticus (Drake and Coffey 1983; Trzepacz 1994) or a previously unsuspected focal lesion (Jacobson and Jerrier 2000) (see Table 5–6). A toxic ictal state may occur after tricyclic antidepressant (TCA) overdose, in which the seizure threshold is lowered and anticholinergicity contributes to delirium. New-onset complex partial seizures, usually related to ischemic damage (Sundaram and Dostrow 1995), are an underrecognized cause of delirium in the elderly, especially when prolonged confusion occurs during status.

Quantitative EEG (qEEG) has shown promise in delirium assessment. Power spectra reveal decreased alpha and increased theta and delta bands that may help to distinguish delirium from dementia (Jacobson and Jerrier 2000; Jacobson et al. 1993a, 1993b). C. Thomas et al. (2008) found that a prolonged activation procedure combined with spectral analysis for alpha/delta density ratios during qEEG discriminated patients with delirium from patients with comorbid delirium-dementia and cognitively normal frail medically ill elderly subjects.

Evoked potentials also may be abnormal in delirium. Metabolic causes of delirium precipitate abnormalities in visual, auditory, and somatosensory evoked potentials (Kullmann et al. 1995; Trzepacz 1994), whereas somatosensory evoked potentials are abnormal in patients whose delirium is due to TBI. In general, normalization of evoked potentials parallels clinical improvement; however, evoked potentials are not clinically used for assessment of delirium.

EEGs and evoked potentials in children with delirium show patterns similar to those in adults, with diffuse slowing on EEG and increased latencies of evoked potentials (J.A. Katz et al. 1988; Prugh et al. 1980; Ruijs et al. 1993, 1994). The degree of slowing on EEGs and evoked potentials performed serially over time in children and adolescents correlates with the severity of delirium and with recovery from delirium (Foley et al. 1981; Montgomery et al. 1991; Onofrj et al. 1991).

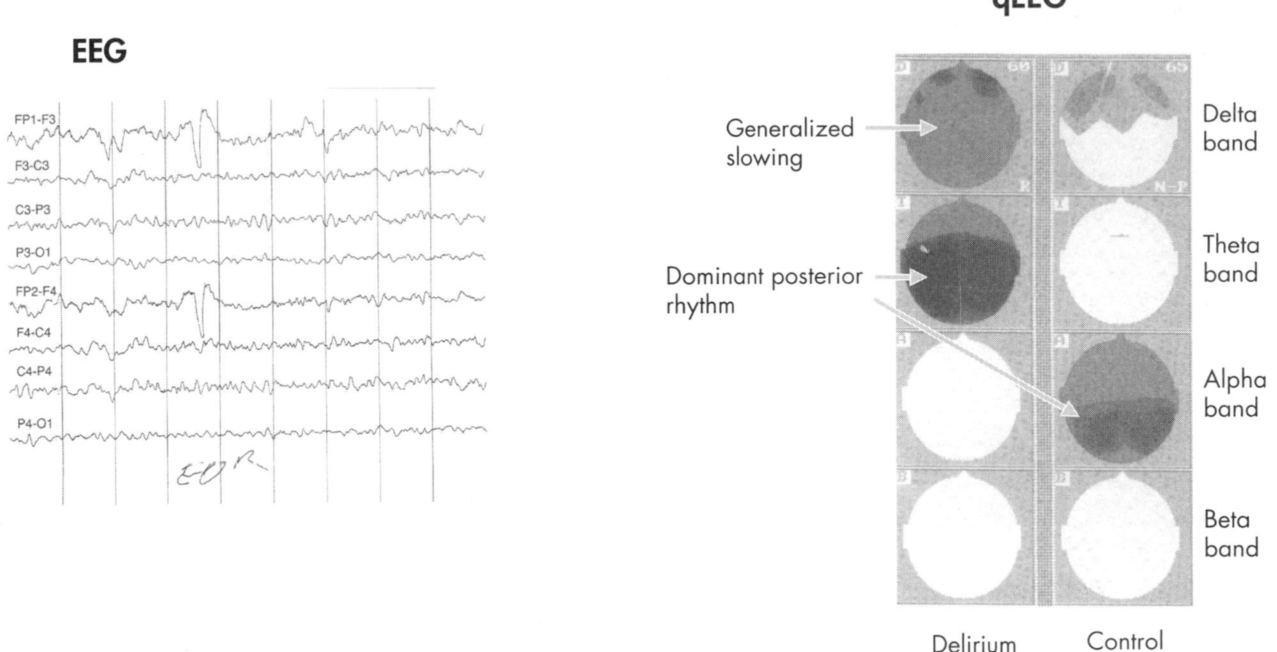

FIGURE 5–5. Typical electroencephalogram (EEG) and quantitative EEG (qEEG) findings in delirium.

Examples of bipolar lead EEG and qEEG in delirium showing diffuse slowing, especially of the dominant posterior rhythm. On qEEG, higher power is shown in darker shading, according to each of the four frequency bands.

Source. Reprinted from Jacobson SA, Jerrier S: "EEG in Delirium." *Seminars in Clinical Neuropsychiatry* 5:86–93, 2000. Copyright 2000, W.B. Saunders Co. Used with permission.

Etiology

Delirium has a wide variety of etiologies, which may occur alone or in combination (see Table 5–7). Single etiology delirium is the exception (Meagher et al. 2007), with most cases involving the contribution of multiple factors, often sequentially, making regular rigorous reassessment of causation essential in its management (Meagher and Leonard 2008). Etiological factors include primary cerebral disorders, systemic disturbances that affect cerebral function, drug and toxin exposure (including intoxication and withdrawal), and a range of factors that can contribute to delirium but have an uncertain etiological role by themselves (including psychological and environmental factors). To be considered causal, an etiology should be a recognized possible cause of delirium and be temporally related in onset and course to delirium presentation; also, the delirium should not be better accounted for by other factors.

Multiple etiologies are common, with between two and six possible causes typically identified, especially in the elderly and those with terminal illness (Breitbart et al. 1996; Francis et al. 1990; Meagher et al. 1996; O'Keeffe and Lavan 1996; Trzepacz et al. 1985). A single etiology is identified in fewer than 50% of cases (Camus et al. 2000; O'Keeffe and Lavan 1999; Olofsson et al. 1996). In frail elderly, Laurila et al. (2008) identified a mean of 3 etiologies per delirious patient, in addition to a mean of 5.2 predisposing factors. The most common etiologies were infectious, metabolic abnormalities, adverse drug effects, and cardiovascular events. Drug classes most commonly associated with delirium in the elderly are benzodiazepines, opioids, and anticholinergics. Delirium in cancer patients can be due to the direct effect of the primary tumor or the indirect effects of metastases, metabolic problems (organ failure or electrolyte disturbance), chemotherapy, central nervous system (CNS) radiation and other treatments, infections, vascular complications, nutritional deficits, and paraneoplastic syndromes. Sagawa et al. (2009) found the most frequent causes of delirium in cancer inpatients were opioids (29%), inflammation (27%), and dehydration and/or sodium level abnormalities (15%), with two or more causes identified in more than 40% of cases. No association between etiology and either reversibility or motor subtype was found. This multifactorial nature has been underemphasized in research—etiological attribution typically is based on clinical impressions that are not standardized (e.g., the most likely cause identified by referring physician) or that are oversimplified by documenting a single etiology for each case. That

TABLE 5–6. Electroencephalographic patterns in patients with delirium

Electroencephalographic finding	Comment	Causes
Diffuse slowing	Most typical delirium pattern	Many causes, including anticholinergicity, posttraumatic brain injury, hepatic encephalopathy, hypoxia
Low-voltage fast activity	Typical of delirium tremens	Alcohol withdrawal; benzodiazepine intoxication
Spikes/polyspikes, frontocentral	Toxic ictal pattern (nonconvulsive)	Hypnosedative drug withdrawal; tricyclic and phenothiazine intoxication
Left/bilateral slowing or delta bursts; frontal intermittent rhythmic delta	Acute confusional migraine	Usually in adolescents
Epileptiform activity, frontotemporal or generalized	Status with prolonged confusional states	Nonconvulsive status and complex partial status epilepticus

delirium due to a single etiology is the exception rather than the rule highlights the importance of considering the possibility of further etiological inputs even when a cause has been identified.

Some causes are more frequently encountered in particular populations. Delirium in children and adolescents involves the same categories of etiologies as in adults, although frequencies of specific causes differ. Delirium related to illicit drugs is more common in younger populations, whereas delirium due to prescribed drugs and polypharmacy is more common in older populations. Cerebral hypoxia is common at age extremes—chronic obstructive airway disease, myocardial infarction, and stroke are common in older patients, whereas hypoxia due to foreign-body inhalation, drowning, and asthma are more frequent in younger patients. Poisonings are also more common in children than in adults, whereas young adults have the highest rates of head trauma.

There are probably a relatively small number of pathophysiological mechanisms utilized by many different etiologies and precipitants to cause the brain disturbance that results in delirium. Major pathophysiological perturbations hypothesized have been reviewed by Maldonado (2008) and include oxygen deprivation, inflammatory, neurotransmitter imbalance, neuronal aging, physiological stress, and cellular signaling. These are often complementary and concurrent; they are both systemic and CNS disturbances or both. For example, proinflammatory cytokines can be produced in the periphery and enter the brain through the ventricular system, and the brain can also produce its own cytokines by glia. Medication adverse effects or toxicities can perturb neurotransmitter systems, leading to imbalance in key brain regions responsible for maintaining consciousness and attention.

Once delirium is diagnosed, a careful and thorough, but prioritized, search for causes must be conducted. Ameliorations of specific underlying causes are important in resolving delirium; however, this should not preclude treatment of the delirium itself, which can reduce symptoms even before underlying medical causes are rectified (Breitbart et al. 1996).

Neuropathogenesis

Delirium is a syndrome which means its symptoms are stereotyped while resulting from numerous different causes. This suggests that different pathophysiological or pharmacological perturbations affecting the brain ultimately culminate into common dysfunction of certain neural circuits (as well as neurotransmitters) which leads to a common clinical expression. This is termed a "final common neural pathway" and refers to a neural network of certain regions and circuits that supports consciousness and higher level thinking and produces characteristic symptom profile when dysfunction occurs (Trzepacz 1999b, 2000). The involvement of certain specific regions and pathways is largely based on interpretation of structural and functional neuroimaging data (Fong et al. 2006; Trzepacz 2000; Trzepacz et al. 2002a). Prefrontal, posterior parietal, and fusiform cortices and basal ganglia are implicated, especially on the right side, plus thalamus especially anterior and medial nuclei. The thalamus is poised at the intersection of the reticular activating system and circuitry to the cerebral cortex. It is reciprocally connected to the cerebral cortex and supports the desynchronized fast-wave EEG of wakeful conscious states. Its intralaminar nucleus, which is highly cholinergic, is involved in sensorimotor gating and supports cerebral cortical activation along with the medial reticular activating system and is important in subserving consciousness (Perry et al. 1999). Dysfunction in both cortical and subcortical regions in delirium has been supported by studies of regional cerebral blood flow,

TABLE 5–7. Selected etiologies of delirium

Central nervous system (CNS)	Metabolic and endocrine disturbance
Meningitis, encephalitis	Hypo- or hyperglycemia
CNS HIV infection	Severe electrolyte disturbance
Stroke	Acidosis or alkalosis
Subarachnoid hemorrhage	Hypoxia
Cerebral edema	Hypercarbia
Seizures	Uremia
Hypertensive encephalopathy	Severe endocrinopathy
Eclampsia	Hepatic failure
CNS vasculitis	Refeeding syndrome (see Chapter 14, "Eating Disorders")
CNS tumor	Other metabolic disorders (e.g., porphyria, carcinoid syndrome)
CNS paraneoplastic syndrome	
	Systemic conditions
Drug intoxication	Sepsis, bacteremia
Alcohol and other drugs of abuse	Minor infection in dementia (e.g., urinary tract infection)
Sedative-hypnotics	Acute graft rejection
Opioids, especially meperidine	Acute graft-versus-host disease
Anticholinergics	Shock
Antihistamines	Postoperative state
Corticosteroids	Disseminated intravascular coagulation and other hypercoagulable states
Drug withdrawal	**Trauma**
Alcohol	Traumatic brain injury
Sedative-hypnotics	Subdural hematoma
	Fat emboli
Hyperthermia	
Heatstroke, neuroleptic malignant syndrome, malignant hyperthermia, serotonin syndrome	

single photon emission computed tomography, positron emission tomography, EEG, and evoked potentials (Trzepacz 1994; Yokota et al. 2003).

The best-established neurotransmitter alteration accounting for many cases of delirium is reduced cholinergic activity (Trzepacz 1996a, 2000). There are numerous lines of evidence to support this and a role for acetylcholine in the classic symptoms of delirium. Furthermore, desynchronized waking EEG patterns and consciousness require muscarinic activity. The cholinergic system has widespread efferents and is involved in cortical activation, induction of REM sleep, EEG fast-wave activity, motor components of behavior, attentional processes, learning and memory, mood, and sensory gating.

Many medications and/or their metabolites have anticholinergic activity and have been reported to cause delirium. Some act postsynaptically; others act presynaptically; and still others, such as normeperidine, have anticholinergic metabolites (Coffman and Dilsaver 1988). Tune et al. (1992) measured the anticholinergic activity of many medications in "atropine equivalents." They identified medications usually not recognized as being anticholinergic (e.g., digoxin, nifedipine, cimetidine, codeine). Delirium induced by anticholinergic drugs is associated with generalized EEG slowing and is reversed by treatment with physostigmine or neuroleptics (Itil and Fink 1966; Stern 1983). Numerous studies find relationships between delirium and higher serum anticholinergic assay levels, and there is a high correlation between cerebrospinal fluid (CSF) and serum anticholinergicity (Plaschke et al. 2007). Serum levels of anticholinergic activity are elevated in patients with postoperative delirium and correlate with severity of cognitive impairment (Tune et al. 1981), improving with resolution of the delirium (Mach et al. 1995). Post–electroconvulsive therapy (ECT) delirium is also associated with higher serum anticholinergic activity (Mondimore et al. 1983).

Both metabolic and structural etiologies of delirium involve anticholinergic effects. Hypoxia and hypoglycemia reduce acetylcholine by affecting the oxidative metabolism of glucose and the production of acetyl coenzyme A, the rate-limiting step for acetylcholine synthesis and thiamine deficiency via being a necessary cofactor for synthesis (Gibson et al. 1975; Trzepacz 1994). Oxidative metabolic stress occurring acutely due to low glucose, hypoxia or reduced perfusion will result in lower choline and adenosine-5′-triphosphate (ATP), required for acetylcholine production. Furthermore, free-radical damage in mitochondria over the years may explain an increased risk of delirium with aging, in addition to alterations in the efficiency of cholinergic neurotransmission. High levels of intraoperative oxygen desaturation, as measured by frontal lobe cerebral oximetry, are associated with postoperative delirium (Zaubler et al. 2009). Clinical indices of oxidative stress (low hemoglobin, low hematocrit, and low oxygen saturation) were associated with ICU delirium, whereas Acute Physiology and Chronic Health Evaluation II (APACHE II) scores were not (Seaman et al. 2006). Parietal cortex levels of choline are reduced in chronic hepatic encephalopathy (Kreis et al. 1991).

Alzheimer's and vascular dementias impair cholinergic neurons and are associated with increased risk for delirium. Dementia with Lewy bodies is associated with significant loss of cholinergic nucleus basalis neurons, and with its fluctuating symptom severity, confusion, hallucinations (especially visual), delusions, and EEG slowing mimics delirium. Its delirium symptoms respond to donepezil (Kaufer et al. 1998). Age-associated changes in cholinergic function also increase delirium propensity. Stroke and TBI are associated with decreased cholinergic activity (Yamamoto et al. 1988) and have enhanced vulnerability to antimuscarinic drugs (Dixon et al. 1994). The low cholinergic state seems to correlate temporally with delirium following the acute event. Thus, there is broad support for an anticholinergic mechanism for many seemingly diverse causes of delirium.

Increased dopamine also may play a major role and its effects are often opposite of that of acetylcholine (Trzepacz 2000). Dopamine has the same effect on the EEG as do anticholinergic drugs. Dopamine release increases during hypoxia (Broderick and Gibson 1989) so this would be expected to exacerbate effects of low acetylcholine. Delirium due to dopamine excess includes intoxication with dopamine agonists (Ames et al. 1992), ECT, alcohol withdrawal (Sander et al. 1997), opiate intoxication, and cocaine toxicity (Wetli et al. 1996). The efficacy of antidopaminergic agents, particularly neuroleptics, in treating delirium, including that arising from anticholinergic causes (Itil and Fink 1966; Platt et al. 1994), also suggests a neuropathogenic role for dopamine. Blockade of D_2 receptors increases acetylcholine release, as does stimulation of D_1 receptors (Ikarashi et al. 1997). Drugs that antagonize D_2 receptors or that agonize/allosterically modulate M_1 and M_4 receptors reverse sensorimotor gating disturbances in rats (Jones et al. 2005), consistent with findings for therapeutics that improve delirium and affect these systems (see section "Treatment" later in this chapter).

The underlying pathophysiology for motor subtypes may be related to neurotransmitter activity. The distribution of dopamine D_3 and D_4 receptor subtypes in the nucleus accumbens can produce hyper- or hypoactivty in rodents, suggesting that an individual's response to excess dopamine in delirium may relate to these receptors. Van der Cammen et al. (2006) reported that hyperactive delirious patients had higher homovanillic acid (HVA) levels than hypoactive patients, consistent with more dopamine turnover.

Both increased and decreased gamma-aminobutyric acid (GABA) levels have been implicated in causing delirium. Increased GABAergic activity is one of several putative mechanisms implicated in hepatic encephalopathy (Mousseau and Butterworth 1994). GABA activity is reduced during delirium following withdrawal from ethanol and sedative-hypnotic drugs. Decreased GABA activity is also implicated in the delirium caused by penicillins, cephalosporins, and quinolones (Akaike et al. 1991; Mathers 1987). Both low and excessive levels of serotonin are also associated with delirium (van der Mast and Fekkes 2000). Serotonin syndrome (see Chapter 38, "Psychopharmacology") is the obvious example of the latter, but serotonergic activity may be increased in patients with hepatic encephalopathy (Mousseau and Butterworth 1994; van der Mast and Fekkes 2000) and sepsis (Mizock et al. 1990). Histamine may play a role in delirium through its effects on arousal and hypothalamic regulation of sleep–wake circadian rhythms. Both H_1 and H_2 antagonists can cause delirium, although both also have anticholinergic properties (Picotte-Prillmayer et al. 1995; Tejera et al. 1994). Glutamate release is increased during hypoxia, and glutamatergic receptors may be activated by quinolone antibiotics (P.D. Williams and Helton 1991). Glutamate surges accompany acute brain damage from stroke or trauma and may mediate neuronal damage that causes preferential basal forebrain and thalamic cholinergic neuron damage that can lead to delirium (Robbins et al. 1997; Weiss et al. 1994).

Whereas some etiologies of delirium alter neurotransmission directly or via general metabolism, others may antagonize or interfere with specific receptors and neurotransmitter precursors. Altered ratios of plasma amino acids during severe illness, surgery, and trauma may affect brain synthesis of neurotransmitters including tryptophan and tyrosine (Pandharipande et al. 2009; Trzepacz and van der Mast 2002; van der Mast and Fekkes 2000). In addition to changes in major neurotransmitter systems, neurotoxic metabolites, such as quinolinic acid from tryptophan metabolism (Basile et al. 1995), and false transmitters, such as octopamine in patients with liver failure, have been implicated in the pathogenesis of delirium. Because glia help to regulate neurotransmitter amounts in the synapse, glial dysfunction also may be involved and may implicate glutamate, which is regulated by astroglia. Increased blood-brain barrier permeability—as occurs in uremia, allowing a host of offending proteins to enter the brain—is another possible mechanism contributing to delirium. Cytokines are increased during stress, rapid growth, inflammation, tumor, trauma, and infection (Hopkins and Rothwell 1995; Rothwell and Hopkins 1995; Stefano et al. 1994). Raised levels of cytokines—whether occurring as part of the body's response to inflammation or infection or from treatment with interferons or interleukins—can cause delirium. The mechanism by which cytokines cause delirium may be through neurotoxicity (Lipton and Gendelman 1995), through effects on a variety of neurotransmitters (Rothwell and Hopkins 1995; Stefano et al. 1994), by altering blood-brain barrier permeability, or through effects on glial function. Proinflammatory cytokines interleukin-6 (IL-6) and interleukin-8 (IL-8) as well as C reactive protein (CRP) and BDNF have been associated with delirium (Adamis et al. 2007b; de Rooij et al. 2007; Pfister et al. 2008; Van Munster et al. 2008).

Differential Diagnosis

Delirium is frequently detected late or not at all in clinical practice. Between one-third and two-thirds of cases are misdiagnosed or completely missed across a range of care settings and by a variety of specialists, including psychiatrists and neurologists (Johnson et al. 1992; Kishi et al. 2007; Meagher and Leonard 2008). The failure to recognize the symptoms or diagnosis of delirium results in poorer outcomes (Kakuma et al. 2003; Rockwood et al. 1994). Poor detection rates are in part explained by delirium's fluctuating nature and complex phenomenology which confer considerable clinical variability and a broad differential diagnosis.

Delirium detection is also hampered by the prevailing stereotype (as in delirium tremens) of an agitated psychotic patient which in fact occurs in approximately one-third of presentations (Meagher 2009), since most patients with delirium have either mixed or hypoactive symptom profiles (Meagher and Trzepacz 2000). The hypoactive presentation is less appreciated because the quiet, untroublesome patient is often presumed to have intact cognition and is more easily overlooked in time-pressured modern health care environments. Nursing staff play a key role in delirium recognition because of their consistency of contact with patient and family but can easily overlook delirium due to limited skills in assessing cognition (Inouye et al. 2001) or a tendency to attribute delirium symptoms to fatigue, anxiety, depression, or patient eccentricities (Irving et al. 2006). Detection can be improved by maintaining a high level of suspicion for delirium, improving awareness of its varied presentations, and routinely assessing cognitive function using a systematic approach supplemented by one of the currently available screening instruments for delirium (Rockwood et al. 1994), such as the CAM or CAM-ICU (Ryan et al. 2009).

Delirium has a wide differential diagnosis. It can be mistaken for dementia, depression, psychosis, anxiety, somatoform disorders, and, particularly in children, behavioral disturbance (see Table 5-8). Accurate diagnosis requires close attention to symptom profile and temporal onset and is further supplemented by a variety of tests (e.g., cognitive, laboratory, EEG). Given that delirium can be the presenting feature of serious medical illness, any patient experiencing a sudden deterioration in cognitive function should be examined for possible delirium.

The most difficult differential diagnosis for delirium is dementia—the other cause of generalized cognitive impairment. Particularly challenging can be diagnosing dementia with Lewy bodies because it may mimic delirium with fluctuation of symptom severity, visual hallucinations, attentional impairment, alteration of consciousness, and delusions (Robinson 2002). Despite this substantial overlap, delirium and dementia can be reliably distinguished by a combination of careful history taking for symptom onset, examination of the patient, and selected clinical tests. Abrupt onset and fluctuating course are highly characteristic of delirium. In addition, level of consciousness and attention are markedly disturbed in delirium but remain relatively intact in uncomplicated dementia. Dementia patients often have nocturnal disturbances of sleep, whereas delirium is characterized by varying degrees of disruption of the sleep-wake circadian cycle, including fragmentation, napping, and sleeplessness. Overall, the presentation of delirium does not seem to be greatly altered by the presence of dementia, with delirium symptoms dominating

TABLE 5–8. Differential diagnosis of delirium

	Delirium	Dementia	Depression	Schizophrenia
Onset	Acute/subacute	Insidious[a]	Variable	Variable
Course	Fluctuating	Often progressive	Diurnal variation	Variable
Reversibility	High[b]	Low	Usually but can be recurrent	No, but has exacerbations
Identifiable medical etiology	Usually; often multifactorial	Neuropathological	Occasionally	Neuropathological
Level of consciousness	Impaired	Clear until late stages	Unimpaired	Unimpaired (perplexity in acute stage)
Attention/memory	Inattention, poor registration and immediate recall, impaired working memory and long-term retrieval	Poor short-term memory; intact attention until later stages (except Lewy body type); confabulation	Poor attention, forgetfulness, ("pseudodementia")	Poor attention; memory intact
Hallucinations	Visual most common; can be auditory, tactile, gustatory, olfactory	Can be visual or auditory	Auditory most common	Auditory most common
Delusions	Fleeting, fragmented, and usually persecutory	Paranoid, often fixed	Complex and mood congruent	Frequent, complex, systematized, and often paranoid
Sleep disturbances	Fragmentation of sleep-wake cycle	Nocturnal insomnia	Initial/middle insomnia, early-morning awakening, hypersomnia	No characteristic pattern
Language	Impaired semantic (fluent aphasia); dysnomia and dysfluencies	Depends on stage and frontal vs. posterior type	Unimpaired	Unimpaired except for neologisms
Thought process	Tangential, circumstantial, and loose associations	Impaired in later stages; distinguish from aphasia, agnosia, apraxia	Unimpaired	Loose associations

[a]Except for large strokes.
[b]Can be chronic (paraneoplastic syndrome, central nervous system adverse events of medications, severe brain damage).

the clinical picture when they co-occur (Cole et al. 2003a; Trzepacz et al. 1998; Voyer et al. 2006).

A range of tools can facilitate differentiation of delirium and dementia. The DRS (Trzepacz and Dew 1995), DRS-R-98, and CTD (Hart et al. 1996) have been shown to distinguish delirium from dementia during validation studies. Although abnormalities of the EEG are common to both delirium and dementia, diffuse slowing occurs more frequently in (81% vs. 33%)—and favors a diagnosis of—delirium. EEG slowing occurs later in the course of most degenerative dementias, although slowing occurs sooner with viral and prion dementias. Percentage theta activity on quantitative EEG may aid differentiation of delirium from dementia (Jacobson and Jerrier 2000). Visual attention and visual perception tasks may also distinguish delirium from dementia.

Several studies have addressed the issue of which symptoms may discriminate between patients with delirium and patients with dementia, or patients with both disorders, with varying results (Liptzin et al. 1993; O'Keeffe 1994; Trzepacz and Dew 1995; Trzepacz et al. 1998, 2002b). Overall, their results suggest that when delirium and dementia are comorbid, delirium phenomenology overshadows that of the dementia, but when the two are assessed as individual conditions, several discriminating symptoms are seen. Temporal onset, degree of inattention, and fluctuating course favor delirium. These research findings are consistent with the clinical rule of thumb that "it is delirium until proven otherwise."

The early behavioral changes of delirium may be mistaken for adjustment reactions to adverse events, particularly in patients who have experienced major trauma or who have cancer. Hypoactive delirium is frequently mistaken for depression (Nicholas and Lindsey 1995; Spiller and Keen 2006). Some symptoms of major depression occur in delirium (e.g., psychomotor slowing, sleep disturbances, irritability). It has been estimated that 7% of patients with delirium attempt self-harm during an episode. However, in major depression, symptom onset tends to be less acute, and mood disturbances typically dominate the clinical picture, with any cognitive impairment more reflective of poor effort. Dehydration or malnutrition can precipitate delirium in severely depressed patients who are unable to maintain food or fluid intake. The distinction of delirium from depression is particularly important because, in addition to delayed treatment, some antidepressants have anticholinergic activity (paroxetine and TCAs) that can aggravate delirium. The overactive, disinhibited presentation of some patients with delirium can closely resemble agitated depression or mania, particularly delirious (Bell's) mania and agitated ("lethal") catatonia, which typically include cognitive impairment.

Abnormalities of thought and perception can occur in both delirium and schizophrenia but are more fluctuant and fragmentary in delirium. Delusions in delirium are rarely as fixed or complex as in schizophrenia, and first-rank symptoms are uncommon (Cutting 1987). Unlike schizophrenia, hallucinations in delirium tend to be visual rather than auditory. Consciousness, attention, and memory are generally less impaired in schizophrenia, with the exception of the pseudodelirious picture that can occur as a result of marked perplexity in the acute stage of illness. Careful examination, coupled with EEG and/or an instrument such as the DRS-R-98, generally distinguishes delirium from these functional disorders.

Treatment

Delirium is an example par excellence of a disorder requiring a multifaceted biopsychosocial approach to assessment and treatment. After the diagnosis of delirium is made, the process of identifying and reversing suspected etiologies begins. Rapid treatment is important because of the high morbidity and mortality associated with delirium. Treatments include medication, environmental manipulation, and patient and family psychosocial support (American Psychiatric Association 1999). However, no drug has a U.S. Food and Drug Administration (FDA) indication for the treatment of delirium, and double-blind, placebo-controlled studies of efficacy and safety of drugs in treating delirium are very limited (American Psychiatric Association 1999).

Psychiatric consultation facilitates identification of predisposing and precipitating factors for delirium. Medication exposure, visual and hearing impairments, sleep deprivation, uncontrolled pain, dehydration, malnutrition, catheterization, and use of restraints are all factors that can be modified, but uncertainty remains as to the precise value of multicomponent interventions that attempt to reduce the incidence and severity of delirium through modification of recognized risk factors (Bogardus et al. 2003; Cole et al. 1998; Inouye et al. 1999) or systematic detection and multidisciplinary care of identified cases (Cole et al. 2002). The effect of such interventions depends on degree of implementation, with evidence that higher adherence leads to lower delirium rates (Inouye et al. 2003). A range of preoperative psychological interventions aimed at patient education and anxiety reduction may have preventive value, but these require more study before they warrant implementation into routine clinical practice.

The principles of management of delirium include ensuring the safety of the patient and his or her immediate surroundings (includes sitters), achieving optimal levels of environmental stimulation, and minimizing the effects of any sensory impediments. The complications of delirium can be minimized by careful attention to the potential for falls and avoidance of prolonged hypostasis. Using orienting techniques (e.g., calendars, night-lights, reorientation by staff) and familiarizing the patient with the environment (e.g., with photographs of family members) are sometimes comforting, although it is important to remember that environmental manipulations alone do not reverse delirium (American Psychiatric Association 1999; Anderson 1995). It also has been suggested that diurnal cues from natural lighting reduce sensory deprivation and incidence of delirium (Wilson 1972), although sensory deprivation alone is insufficient to cause delirium (Francis 1993). Unfortunately, implementation of these environmental interventions occurs primarily in response to agitation rather than the core disturbances of delirium (Meagher et al. 1996).

Supportive interaction with relatives and caregivers is fundamental to good management of delirium. Relatives can play an integral role in efforts to support and reorient patients with delirium, but ill-informed, critical, or anxious caregivers can add to the burden of a delirious patient. A nontherapeutic triangle can emerge whereby health care providers respond to the distress of relatives by medicating patients, which complicates ongoing cognitive assessment. Clarification of the cause and meaning of symptoms combined with recognition of treatment goals can allow better management of what is a distressing experience for both patient and loved ones (Breitbart et al. 2002; Meagher 2001).

Prevention Strategies

Nonpharmacological and pharmacological interventions are available to prevent delirium. Preoperative patient education or preparation was helpful in reducing delirium symptom rates in early studies (Chatham 1978; Owens and Hutelmyer 1982; M.A. Williams et al. 1985), although caregiver education and environmental or risk factor interventions have had mixed results, with two not finding any significant effect on delirium rate (Nagley 1986; Wanich et al. 1992). In contrast, Inouye et al. (1999) studied the effect on delirium of preventive measures that minimized six of the risk factors identified in their previous work with hospitalized elderly patients. They used standardized protocols in a prospective study of 852 elderly inpatients to address cognitive impairment, sleep deprivation, immobility, visual impairment, hearing impairment, and dehydration, which resulted in significant reductions in the number (62 vs. 90) and duration (105 vs. 161 days) of delirium episodes relative to control subjects. Effects of adherence on delirium risk were subsequently reported for 422 elderly patients during implementation of this standardized protocol (Inouye et al. 2003). Adherence ranged from 10% for the sleep protocol to 86% for orientation. Higher levels of adherence by staff resulted in lower delirium rates, up to a maximum of an 89% reduction, even after controlling for confounding variables. At 6-month follow-up of 705 survivors from this intervention study of six risk factors, no differences were found between groups for any of the 10 outcome measures, except for less frequent incontinence in the intervention group (Bogardus et al. 2003), suggesting that the intervention's effect was essentially during the index hospitalization without any longer-lasting benefits. However, in a subset of high-risk patients at baseline, the intervention group had significantly better self-rated health and functional status at follow-up. A recent pediatric surgery report found reduced delirium in a randomized controlled trial of family-centered preparation for surgery (Kain et al. 2007).

Milisen et al. (2001) compared delirium rates in two cohorts of elderly hip surgery patients (N=60 in each)—before and after implementing an intervention consisting of nurse education, cognitive screening, consultation by a nurse or physician geriatric/delirium specialist, and a scheduled pain protocol. They found no effect on delirium incidence but a shorter duration of delirium (median 1 vs. 4 days) and lower delirium severity in the intervention group. Marcantonio et al. (2001) used a different study design and randomly assigned 62 elderly hip fracture patients to either a perioperative geriatric consultation or usual care. On the basis of daily ratings, they found a lower delirium rate (32% vs. 50%) and fewer cases of severe delirium (12% vs. 29%) in the consultation group. Length of stay was not affected, and the effect of consultation was greatest in those patients without preexisting dementia or poor ADL performance.

The cholinergic deficiency hypothesis of delirium suggests that enhancing acetylcholine should reduce delirium incidence or severity. Perioperative piracetam use during anesthesia was reviewed across eight studies, mostly from the 1970s, and was believed to have a positive effect on reducing postoperative delirium symptoms (Gallinat et al. 1999). Citicholine 1.2 mg/day was assessed for delirium prevention in a randomized, placebo-controlled trial of 81 dementia-free hip surgery patients, given 1 day before and each of the 4 days after surgery, but there was no significant difference in delirium incidence between groups (Diaz et al. 2001). More recently, there have been randomized prophylaxis trials using cholinesterase inhibitors. A lack of significant effect on delirium incidence was reported in studies using donepezil (Liptzin et al. 2005; Sampson et al. 2006) and rivastigmine (Gamberini et al. 2009) for acute prophylaxis. In contrast, chronic prophylaxis with rivastigmine in older stroke patients significantly reduced the number of delirium episodes over a 2-year follow-up period when compared with cardioaspirin (Moretti et al. 2004).

Kalisvaart et al. (2005) studied 408 elderly hip surgery patients in a double-blind, randomized comparison of one to two doses of 0.5-mg dose haloperidol or placebo given up to 3 days before and/or 3 days after hip surgery. They found significant differences for shorter delirium duration, lower DRS-R-98 scores, and shorter lengths of stay in the active treatment group, although the study was underpowered to detect an incidence difference. Delirium incidence was significantly reduced in a randomized, double-blind, placebo-controlled prophylaxis trial in elderly joint replacement surgery patients treated perioperatively with low-dose rapidly dissolving olanzapine 5 mg (14.3% vs. 40.2%) (Larsen et al. 2007). Similarly, risperidone 1 mg immediately after surgery significantly reduced delirium incidence in elective cardiac surgery patients as compared with placebo (11.1% vs. 31.7%) (Prakanrattana and Prapaitrakool 2007).

Maldonado et al. (2009) reported significantly reduced delirium incidence (3%) as measured by the DRS when a novel alpha$_2$-adrenergic receptor agonist, dexmedetomidine, was used for postoperative sedation, as compared with propofol (50%) or fentanyl/midazolam (50%), in cardiac valve surgery patients in a randomized open-label trial. In contrast, Pandharipande et al. (2007) did not find a difference in delirium incidence as measured by the CAM-ICU in dexmedetomidine (79%) as compared with. lorazepam (82%) in ventilated ICU patients in a randomized multisite trial, although there was a trend toward more delirium-free days. Improved pain control after hepatectomy surgery in elderly patients who used patient-controlled epidural anesthesia with bupivacaine and fentanyl (n = 14), compared with continuous epidural mepivacaine (n = 16), was associated with lower incidences of moderate and severe delirium (36% vs. 75% and 14% vs. 50%, respectively), and antipsychotic drug use also was lower in the former group (Tokita et al. 2001).

Pharmacological Treatment

Current delirium pharmacotherapies have evolved from their use in the treatment of mainstream psychiatric disorders; hence, psychiatrists are well acquainted with the practicalities of their use. Pharmacological treatment with a neuroleptic agent (D$_2$ antagonist) is the clinical standard for delirium treatment, usually either haloperidol or an atypical antipsychotic. Itil and Fink (1966) found that chlorpromazine reversed experimentally induced anticholinergic delirium and reversed EEG abnormalities. There are over 33 prospective trials studying more than 3,300 patients in neuroleptic treatment of delirium (Bourne et al. 2008), and although only a minority are blinded, randomized, and controlled, the evidence base finds neuroleptic agents to be useful and well tolerated. Nonetheless, there is a need for large randomized multisite trials (Seitz et al. 2007; Trzepacz et al. 2008).

Haloperidol is the conventional neuroleptic most often chosen for the treatment of delirium. It can be administered orally, intramuscularly, or intravenously (American Psychiatric Association 1999; Sanders and Stern 1993; Tesar et al. 1985), although the intravenous route has not been approved by the FDA. Intravenously administered haloperidol is twice as potent as that taken orally (Gelfand et al. 1992). Bolus intravenous doses usually range from 0.5 to 20 mg, although larger doses are sometimes given. In severe, refractory cases, continuous intravenous infusions of 15–25 mg/hour (up to 1,000 mg/day) can be given. Platt et al. (1994) reported that both hypoactive and hyperactive subtypes responded to treatment with haloperidol or chlorpromazine, and they noted improvement within hours of treatment, even before the underlying medical causes were addressed. In delirious patients receiving palliative care, haloperidol can be given subcutaneously (Fonzo-Christe et al. 2005).

Cases of prolonged QTc interval and torsade de pointes (multifocal ventricular tachycardia) have been increasingly recognized and attributed to intravenously administered haloperidol, even in young patients, and therefore patients need to be monitored (Hatta et al. 2001; Kriwisky et al. 1990; Metzger and Friedman 1993; O'Brien et al. 1999; Perrault et al. 2000; Wilt et al. 1993). Risk factors include female sex, heart disease, hypokalemia, higher doses of the offending agent, concomitant use of a QT-prolonging drug, and a history of long QT syndrome (Justo et al. 2005). The American Psychiatric Association (1999) "Practice Guideline for the Treatment of Patients With Delirium" advised that QTc prolongation greater than 450 msec or to greater than 25% over a previous electrocardiogram may warrant telemetry, cardiac consultation, dose reduction, or discontinuation. They also recommend monitoring use of other drugs that can prolong the QTc interval, as well as serum magnesium and potassium, in critically ill patients with delirium whose QTc is 450 msec or greater.

There have been five randomized controlled comparator efficacy trials, all of which found improvement for active agents and, when studied, superiority to placebo or lorazepam (Breitbart et al. 1996; Han et al. 2004; Hua et al. 2006; Kim et al. 2005; Lee et al. 2005). More than two-thirds of delirious patients in these studies experienced rapid clinical improvement, typically after 2–6 days of treatment (Bourne et al. 2008). One of the placebo-controlled studies, a randomized three-arm trial in elderly delirious patients assessed longitudinally with the DRS, reported comparable response rates in the haloperidol (87.5%) and olanzapine (82%) groups that were significantly greater than those in the placebo group (31%) (Hua et al. 2006). In contrast, a three-arm double-blind, randomized, controlled multisite trial of ziprasidone versus haloperidol versus placebo in mechanically ventilated ICU patients found no difference between groups for delirium-free days or mortality, but unfortunately delirium severity was not measured. There may have been confounding, as all three groups also received concomitant open-label haloperidol as needed (Girard et al. 2010). In a double-blind randomized trial in delirious ICU patients, patients treated with quetiapine required less as-needed haloperidol to control agitation, had a shorter duration and faster resolution of delirium, and were discharged to home or rehabilitation at a higher rate compared with those receiving placebo (Devlin et al. 2010).

The atypical antipsychotics olanzapine (5–20 mg), risperidone (1.5–4 mg), and quetiapine (25–750 mg) have been studied in case series, open-label case-control convenience samples, open-label prospective trials using standardized measures, and blinded trials (Bourne et al. 2008; Meagher and Leonard 2008). An open-label trial of the atypical agent perospirone suggested its efficacy (Takeuchi et al. 2007).

Clinical experience with neuroleptics in pediatric delirium supports their beneficial effects, but no controlled studies have been done. A retrospective report of 30 children (ages 8 months–18 years; mean age=7 years) with burn injuries supported the use of haloperidol for agitation, disorientation, hallucinations, delusions, and insomnia (R.L. Brown et al. 1996). The mean haloperidol dose was 0.47 mg/kg, administered intravenously, orally, and intramuscularly. Haloperidol was not efficacious in 17% of the patients (4 of 5 of these failures were via the oral route). Extrapyramidal symptoms (EPS) were not observed, and one episode of hypotension occurred with the intravenous route. In ICU pediatric delirium, 37 were treated with either haloperidol or risperidone (Schieveld et al. 2007) and two of the haloperidol children had acute torticollis as an EPS adverse event. Intravenous haloperidol single doses of 0.15–0.25 mg resulted in prompt resolution of delirium in two young children (28 and 42 months old) (Schieveld and Leentjens 2005).

Antipsychotic agents carry black-box FDA warnings for increased mortality when used in agitated elderly patients with dementia. Whether the risks are applicable to short-term use in delirium is not known. However, a retrospective analysis of haloperidol and risperidone use in 111 of 326 delirium cases found no statistical increased risk of mortality between the exposed (20.7%) and unexposed (17.2%) groups; instead, increased mortality was associated with medical comorbidity and acute physiology scores (Elie et al. 2009).

Other classes of drugs are indicated in particular situations. Benzodiazepines are generally reserved for delirium due to ethanol or sedative-hypnotic withdrawal; lorazepam or clonazepam (the latter for alprazolam withdrawal) is often used. Intravenous lorazepam is sometimes combined with intravenous haloperidol in critically ill patients to lessen EPS and increase sedation. However, benzodiazepine use should be limited because they can be deliriogenic. With the use of standardized assessment methods and a double-blind, randomized, controlled design, Breitbart et al. (1996) found that delirium in patients with AIDS significantly improved with haloperidol or chlorpromazine but worsened with lorazepam. Even at low doses, lorazepam has been reported to be an independent risk factor for causing delirium in ICU patients (Pandharipande et al. 2006). Anticholinergic poisoning-induced delirium and/or agitation was controlled and reversed with physostigmine (87% and 96%, respectively), whereas benzodiazepines controlled agitation in only 24% and were ineffective in treating delirium (Burns et al. 2000). Patients who received physostigmine had a lower incidence of complications (7% vs. 46%) and a shorter time to recovery (median=12 vs. 24 hours). Lorazepam has a significant aggravating effect on delirium in medical ICU patients, but this effect was not found for propofol, morphine, and fentanyl (Ely et al. 2004a; Pandharipande et al. 2006) (see Figure 5–6).

The cholinergic deficiency hypothesis of delirium suggests that treatment with a cholinergic enhancer drug could be therapeutic. Physostigmine reverses anticholinergic delirium (Stern 1983), but its side effects (seizures) and short half-life make it unsuitable for routine clinical treatment of delirium. Three case reports found that donepezil improved delirium postoperatively, in dementia with Lewy bodies, and in alcohol dementia (Burke et al. 1999; Kaufer et al. 1998; Wengel et al. 1998, 1999). Physostigmine administered in the emergency department to patients suspected of having muscarinic toxicity resulted in reversal of delirium in 22 of 39, including several patients in whom the cause could not be determined (Schneir et al. 2003); only 1 patient in 39 had an adverse event (brief seizure). Rivastigmine added to antipsychotics in delirium nonresponders resulted in recovery in 71%, suggesting that a combination of acetylcholine enhancement and D_2 receptor blockade may be beneficial (Dautzenberg et al. 2004).

A single 8-mg intravenous dose of ondansetron, a serotonin$_3$ receptor antagonist, was reported to reduce agitation in 35 postcardiotomy delirium patients (Bayindir et al. 2000). Supplementary oxygen reduced delirium in a

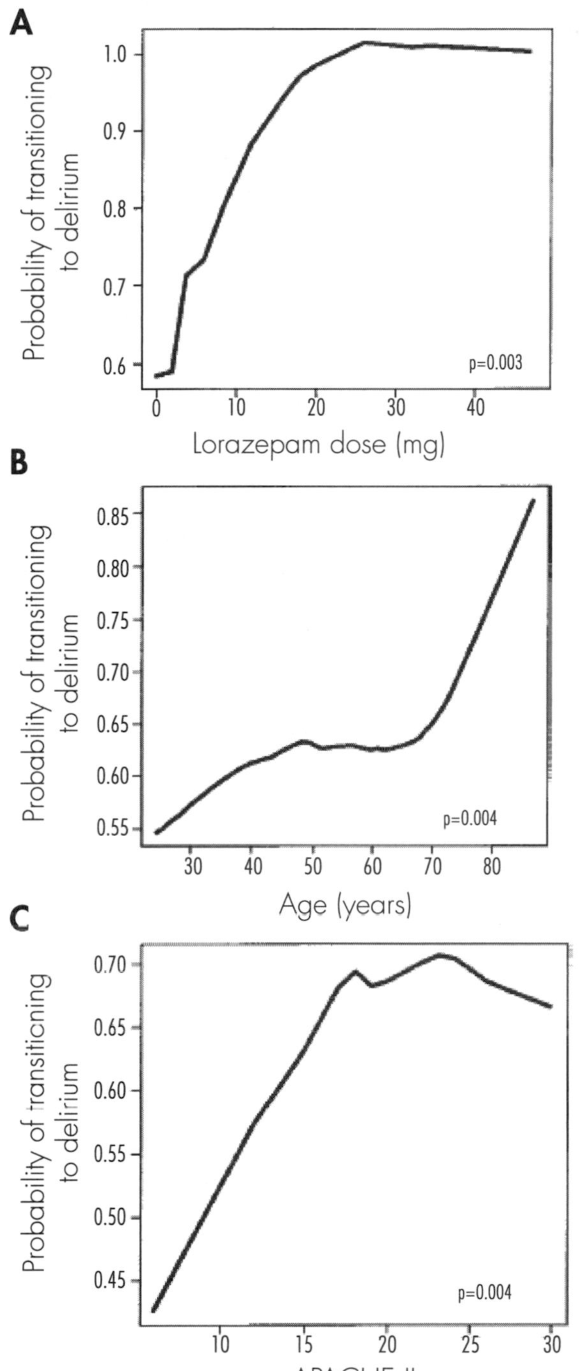

FIGURE 5–6. Probability of transitioning to delirium as a function of sedative lorazepam dosage, patient age, and severity of illness (*left*).

(A) *Lorazepam dosage*—The probability of transitioning to delirium increased with increases in lorazepam dosage administered within the previous 24 hours. This incremental risk was large at low doses and plateaued at around 20 mg/day. **(B)** *Age (years)*—The probability of transitioning to delirium increased dramatically for each year of life after age 65 years. **(C)** *Severity of illness*—The probability of transitioning to delirium increased dramatically for each additional point in the Acute Physiology and Chronic Health Evaluation II (APACHE II) severity-of-illness score until reaching a plateau at an APACHE II score of 18.

Source. Reprinted from Pandharipande PP, Shintani A, Peterson J, et al.: "Lorazepam Is an Independent Risk Factor for Transitioning to Delirium in Intensive Care Unit Patients." *Anesthesiology* 104:21–26, 2006. Copyright 2006, Wolters Kluwer Health, Inc. (Lippincott Williams & Wilkins). Used with permission.

small cohort of postoperative delirium cases who had lower mean arterial oxygen saturation than nondelirious on the night prior to delirium onset (Aakerlund and Rosenberg 1994). Psychostimulants can worsen delirium and are generally not recommended when depressed mood is present (Rosenberg et al. 1991).

Mianserin, a serotonergic tetracyclic antidepressant, has been used in Japan for delirium in elderly medical and postsurgical patients, administered either orally or as a suppository. Several open-label studies found reductions in the DRS scores similar to those seen with haloperidol (Nakamura et al. 1995, 1997a, 1997b; Uchiyama et al. 1996), attributed to enabling improved sleep-wake cycle.

Conclusion

Clearly, further delirium treatment research is needed—especially randomized, placebo-controlled, adequately powered clinical trials addressing both efficacy and safety. However, mounting evidence from prospective trials is supportive of current clinical practice and in a consistent fashion with neurotransmitter hypotheses for delirium.

References

Aakerlund LP, Rosenberg J: Postoperative delirium: treatment with supplementary oxygen. Br J Anesthesia 72:286–290, 1994

Abell M, Kean J, Malec J: Further investigation of resolution of the acute confusion (delirium) of the acute period following traumatic brain injury. Poster presentation at American Congress on Rehabilitation Medicine annual meeting, Denver, CO, October 2009

Adamis D, Morrison C, Treloar A, et al: The performance of the clock Drawing Test in elderly medical inpatients: does it have utility in the identification of delirium. J Geriatr Psychiatry Neurol 18:129–133, 2005

Adamis D, Treloar A, Darwiche F-Z, et al: Associations of delirium with in-hospital and in 6-months mortality in elderly medical inpatients. Age Ageing 36:644–649, 2007a

Adamis D, Treloar A, Martin FC, et al: APOE and cytokines as biological markers for recovery of prevalent delirium in elderly medical inpatients. Int J Geriatr Psychiatry 22:688–694, 2007b

Adamis D, Van Munster BC, Macdonald AJ: The genetics of deliria. Int Rev Psychiatry 21:20–29, 2009

Akaike N, Shirasaki T, Yakushiji T: Quinolone and fenbufen interact with GABA-A receptors in dissociated hippocampal cells of rats. J Neurophysiol 66:497–504, 1991

American Psychiatric Association: Diagnostic and Statistical Manual: Mental Disorders. Washington, DC, American Psychiatric Association, 1952

American Psychiatric Association: Diagnostic and Statistical Manual of Mental Disorders, 2nd Edition. Washington, DC, American Psychiatric Association, 1968

American Psychiatric Association: Diagnostic and Statistical Manual of Mental Disorders, 3rd Edition. Washington, DC, American Psychiatric Association, 1980

American Psychiatric Association: Diagnostic and Statistical Manual of Mental Disorders, 3rd Edition, Revised. Washington, DC, American Psychiatric Association, 1987

American Psychiatric Association: Diagnostic and Statistical Manual of Mental Disorders, 4th Edition. Washington, DC, American Psychiatric Association, 1994

American Psychiatric Association: Practice guideline for the treatment of patients with delirium. Am J Psychiatry 156 (suppl):1–20, 1999

American Psychiatric Association: Diagnostic and Statistical Manual of Mental Disorders, 4th Edition, Text Revision. Washington, DC, American Psychiatric Association, 2000

Ames D, Wirshing WC, Szuba MP: Organic mental disorders associated with bupropion in three patients. J Clin Psychiatry 53:53–55, 1992

Andreasen NJC, Hartford CE, Knott JR, et al: EEG changes associated with burn delirium. Dis Nerv Syst 38:27–31, 1977

Andrew M, Freter S, Rockwood K: Prevalence and outcomes of delirium in community and non-acute care settings in people without dementia: a report from the Canadian Study of Health and Ageing. BMC Med 4:15, 2006

Armstrong SC, Cozza KL, Watanabe KS: The misdiagnosis of delirium. Psychosomatics 38:433–439, 1997

Baranowski SL, Patten SB: The predictive value of dysgraphia and constructional apraxia for delirium in psychiatric inpatients. Can J Psychiatry 45:75–78, 2000

Basile AS, Saito K, Li Y, et al: The relationship between plasma and brain quinolinic acid levels and the severity of hepatic encephalopathy in animal models of fulminant hepatic failure. J Neurochem 64:2607–2614, 1995

Bayindir O, Akpinar B, Can E, et al: The use of the 5-HT3-receptor antagonist ondansetron for the treatment of postcardiotomy delirium. J Cardiothorac Vasc Anesth 14:288–292, 2000

Bedford PD: General medical aspects of confusional states in elderly people. BMJ 2:185–188, 1957

Beglinger LJ, Duff K, Van Der Heiden S, et al: Incidence of delirium and associated mortality in haematopoietic stem cell transplantation patients. Biol Blood Marrow Transplant 12:928–935, 2006

Bellelli G, Frisoni GB, Turco R, et al: Delirium superimposed on dementia predicts 12-month survival in elderly patients discharged from a postacute rehabilitation facility. J Gerontol A Biol Sci Med Sci 62:1306–1309, 2007

Benoit AG, Campbell MI, Tanner JR, et al: Risk factors and prevalence of perioperative cognitive dysfunction in abdominal aneurysm patients. J Vasc Surg 42:884–890, 2005

Berggren D, Gustafson Y, Eriksson B, et al: Postoperative confusion following anesthesia in elderly patients treated for femoral neck fractures. Anesth Analg 66:497–504, 1987

Bickel H, Gradinger R, Kochs E, et al: High risk of cognitive and functional decline after postoperative delirium. A three-year prospective study. Dement Geriatr Cogn Disord 26:26–31, 2008

Bo M, Martini B, Ruatta C, et al: Geriatric ward hospitalization reduced incidence delirium among older medical inpatients. Am J Geriatr Psychiatry 17:760–768, 2009

Boettger S, Alici-Evcimen Y, Breitbart W, et al: An open label trial of aripiprazole in the treatment of delirium. Presentation at the Academy of Psychosomatic Medicine 54th annual meeting, Amelia Island, FL, November 2007a

Boettger S, Alici-Evcimen Y, Breitbart W, et al: Risperidone in the treatment of hypoactive and hyperactive delirium. Presentation at the Academy of Psychosomatic Medicine 54th annual meeting, Amelia Island, FL, November 2007b

Bogardus ST, Desai MM, Williams CS, et al: The effects of a targeted multicomponent delirium intervention on postdischarge outcomes for hospitalized older adults. Am J Med 114:383–390, 2003

Bourdel-Marchasson I, Vincent S, Germain C, et al: Delirium symptoms and low dietary intake in older inpatients are independent predictors of institutionalization: a 1-year prospective population-based study. J Gerontol A Biol Sci Med Sci 59:350–354, 2004

Bourne RS, Tahir TA, Borthwick M, et al: Drug treatment of delirium: past, present and future. J Psychosom Res 65:273–282, 2008

Breitbart W, Marotta R, Platt MM, et al: A double-blind trial of haloperidol, chlorpromazine, and lorazepam in the treatment of delirium in hospitalized AIDS patients. Am J Psychiatry 153:231–237, 1996

Breitbart W, Rosenfeld B, Roth A, et al: The Memorial Delirium Assessment Scale. J Pain Symptom Manage 13:128–137, 1997

Breitbart W, Gibson C, Tremblay A: The delirium experience: delirium recall and delirium-related distress in hospitalized patients with cancer, their spouses/caregivers, and their nurses. Psychosomatics 43:183–194, 2002

Broderick PA, Gibson GE: Dopamine and serotonin in rat striatum during in vivo hypoxic-hypoxia. Metab Brain Dis 4:143–153, 1989

Brown LJ, McGrory S, McLaren L, et al: Cognitive visual perceptual deficits in patients with delirium. J Neurol Neurosurg Psychiatry 80:594–599, 2009

Brown RL, Henke A, Greenhalgh DG, et al: The use of haloperidol in the agitated, critically ill pediatric patient with burns. J Burn Care Rehabil 17:34–38, 1996

Brown TM: Drug-induced delirium. Semin Clin Neuropsychiatry 5:113–125, 2000

Burke WJ, Roccaforte WH, Wengel SP: Treating visual hallucinations with donepezil. Am J Psychiatry 156:1117–1118, 1999

Burns MJ, Linden CH, Graudins A, et al: A comparison of physostigmine and benzodiazepines for the treatment of anticholinergic poisoning. Ann Emerg Med 35:374–381, 2000

Cameron DJ, Thomas RI, Mulvihill M, et al: Delirium: a test of DSM-III criteria on medical inpatients. J Am Geriatr Soc 35:1007–1010, 1987

Camus V, Gonthier R, Dubos G, et al: Etiologic and outcome profiles in hypoactive and hyperactive subtypes of delirium. J Geriatr Psychiatry Neurol 13:38–42, 2000

Caraceni A, Nanni O, Maltoni M, et al: Impact of delirium on the short term prognosis of advanced cancer patients. Cancer 89:1145–1149, 2000

Chatham MA: The effect of family involvement on patients' manifestations of postcardiotomy psychosis. Heart Lung 7:995–999, 1978

Coffman JA, Dilsaver SC: Cholinergic mechanisms in delirium. Am J Psychiatry 145:382–383, 1988

Cole MG, Primeau FJ: Prognosis of delirium in elderly hospital patients. Can Med Assoc J 149:41–46, 1993

Cole MG, Primeau FJ, Bailey RF, et al: Systematic intervention for elderly inpatients with delirium: a randomized trial. Can Med Assoc J 151:965–970, 1994

Cole M, Primeau F, Elie L: Delirium: prevention, treatment, and outcome studies. J Geriatr Psychiatry Neurol 28:551–556, 1998

Cole M, McCusker J, Bellavance F, et al: Systematic detection and multidisciplinary care of delirium in older medical inpatients: a randomized trial. Can Med Assoc J 167:753–759, 2002

Cole MG, Dendukuri N, McCusker J, et al: An empirical study of different diagnostic criteria for delirium among elderly medical inpatients. J Neuropsychiatry Clin Neurosci 15:200–207, 2003a

Cole M, McCusker J, Dendukuri N, et al: The prognostic significance of subsyndromal delirium in elderly medical inpatients. J Am Geriatr Soc 51:754–760, 2003b

Cole M, McCusker J, Ciampi A, et al: An exploratory study of diagnostic criteria for delirium in older medical inpatients. J Neuropsychiatry Clin Neurosci 19:151–156, 2007

Cole MG, You Y, McCusker J, et al: The 6 and 12 month outcomes of older medical inpatients who recover from delirium. Int J Geriatr Psychiatry 23:301–307, 2008

Cole MG, Ciampi A, Belzile E, et al: Persistent delirium in older hospital patients: a systematic review of frequency and prognosis. Age Ageing 38:19–26, 2009

Collins MW, Lovell MR, Iverson GL, et al: Cumulative effects of concussion in high school athletes. Neurosurgery 51:1175–1181, 2002

Curyto KJ, Johnson J, TenHave T, et al: Survival of hospitalized elderly patients with delirium: a prospective study. Am J Geriatr Psychiatry 9:141–147, 2001

Cushman LA: Secondary neuropsychiatric implications of stroke: implications for acute care. Arch Phys Med Rehabil 69:877–879, 1988

Cutting J: The phenomenology of acute organic psychosis: comparison with acute schizophrenia. Br J Psychiatry 151:324–332, 1987

Dautzenberg PL, Mulder LJ, Olde Rikkert MG, et al: Adding rivastigmine to antipsychotics in the treatment of delirium. Age Ageing 33:516–521, 2004

de Negreiros DP, da Silva Meleiro AM, Furlanetto LM, et al: Portuguese version of the Delirium Rating Scale-Revised-98: reliability and validity. Int J Geriatr Psychiatry 23:472–477, 2008

de Rooij SE, van Munster BC, Korevaar JC, et al: Delirium subtype identification and the validation of the Delirium Rating Scale-Revised 98 (Dutch version) in hospitalized elderly patients. Int J Geriatr Psychiatry 27:1–7, 2006

de Rooij SE, van Munster BC, Korevaar JC, et al: Cytokines and acute phase response in delirium. J Psychosomatic Res 62:521–525, 2007

Devlin JW, Roberts RJ, Fong JJ, et al: Efficacy and safety of quetiapine in critically ill patients with delirium: a prospective multicenter randomized double-blind placebo-controlled trial. Crit Care Med 38:419–427, 2010

Diaz V, Rodriguez J, Barrientos P, et al: Use of procholinergics in the prevention of postoperative delirium in hip fracture surgery in the elderly. A randomized controlled trial. Rev Neurol 33:716–719, 2001

Dickson LR: Hypoalbuminemia in delirium. Psychosomatics 32:317–323, 1991

Dixon CE, Hamm RJ, Taft WC, et al: Increased anticholinergic sensitivity following closed skull impact and controlled cortical impact traumatic brain injury in the rat. J Neurotrauma 11:275–287, 1994

Drake ME, Coffey CE: Complex partial status epilepticus simulating psychogenic unresponsiveness. Am J Psychiatry 140:800–801, 1983

Duppils GS, Wikblad K: Cognitive function and health-related quality of life after delirium in connection with hip surgery. A six-month follow-up. Orthop Nurs 23:195–203, 2004

Elie M, Boss K, Cole MG, et al: A retrospective exploratory secondary analysis of the association between antipsychotic use and mortality in elderly patients with delirium. Int Psychogeriatrics 21:588–592, 2009

Ely EW, Inouye SK, Bernard GR, et al: Delirium in mechanically ventilated patients: validity and reliability of the Confusion Assessment Method for the Intensive Care Unit (CAM-ICU). JAMA 286:2703–2710, 2001a

Ely EW, Margolin R, Francis J, et al: Evaluation of delirium in critically ill patients: validation of the Confusion Assessment Method for the Intensive Care Unit (CAM-ICU). Crit Care Med 29:1370–1379, 2001b

Ely EW, Siegel MD, Inouye SK: Delirium in the intensive care unit: an under-recognized syndrome of organ dysfunction. Semin Respir Crit Care Med 22:115–126, 2001c

Ely EW, Shintani A, Truman B, et al: Delirium as a predictor of mortality in mechanically ventilated patients in the intensive care unit. JAMA 291:1753–1762, 2004a

Ely EW, Stephens RK, Jackson JC, et al: Current opinions regarding the importance, diagnosis, and management of delirium in the intensive care unit: a survey of 912 healthcare professionals. Crit Care Med 32:106–112, 2004b

Ely EW, Girard TD, Shintani AK, et al: Apolipoprotein E4 polymorphism as a genetic predisposition to delirium in critically ill patients. Crit Care Med 35:112–117, 2007

Engel GL, Romano J: Delirium, II: reversibility of electroencephalogram with experimental procedures. Arch Neurol Psychiatry 51:378–392, 1944

Engel GL, Romano J: Delirium, a syndrome of cerebral insufficiency. J Chronic Dis 9:260–277, 1959

Eriksson M, Samuelsson E, Gustafson Y, et al: Delirium after coronary bypass surgery evaluated by the organic brain syndrome protocol. Scand Cardiovasc J 36:250–255, 2002

Erkinjuntti T, Wikstrom J, Parlo J, et al: Dementia among medical inpatients: evaluation of 2000 consecutive admissions. Arch Intern Med 146:1923–1926, 1986

Fann JR: The epidemiology of delirium: a review of studies and methodological issues. Semin Clin Neuropsychiatry 5:86–92, 2000

Fann JR, Roth-Roemer S, Burington BE, et al: Delirium in patients undergoing hematopoietic stem cell transplantation. Cancer 95:1971–1981, 2002

Fann JR, Alfano CM, Burington BE, et al: Clinical presentation of delirium in patients undergoing hematopoietic stem cell transplantation. Cancer 103:810–820, 2005

Farrell KR, Ganzini L: Misdiagnosing delirium as depression in medically ill elderly patients. Arch Intern Med 155:2459–2464, 1995

Fayers PM, Hjermstad MJ, Ranhoff AH, et al: Which Mini-Mental State Exam items can be used to screen for delirium and cognitive impairment? J Pain Symp Manage 30:41–50, 2005

Fisher BW, Flowerdew G: A simple model for predicting postoperative delirium in older patients undergoing elective orthopedic surgery. J Am Geriatr Soc 43:175–178, 1995

Foley CM, Polinsky MS, Gruskin AB, et al: Encephalopathy in infants and children with chronic renal disease. Arch Neurol 38:656–658, 1981

Folstein MF, Folstein SE, McHugh PR: "Mini-Mental State": a practical method for grading the cognitive state of patients for the clinician. J Psychiatr Res 12:189–198, 1975

Folstein MF, Bassett SS, Romanoski AJ, et al: The epidemiology of delirium in the community: the Eastern Baltimore Mental Health Survey. Int Psychogeriatr 3:169–176, 1991

Fong TG, Bogardus ST Jr, Daftary A, et al: Cerebral perfusion changes in older delirious patients using 99mTc HMPAO SPECT. J Gerontol A Biol Sci Med Sci 61:1294–1299, 2006

Fong TG, Jones RN, Marcantono ER, et al: Delirium accelerates cognitive decline in Alzheimer disease. Neurology 72:1570–1575, 2009

Fonseca F, Bulbena A, Navarrete R, et al: Spanish version of the Delirium Rating Scale-Revised-98: reliability and validity. J Psychosom Res 59:147–151, 2005

Fonzo-Christe C, Vukasovic C, Wasilewski-Rasca AF, et al: Subcutaneous administration of drugs in the elderly: survey of practice and systematic literature review. Palliat Med 19:208–219, 2005

Francis J: Sensory and environmental factors in delirium. Paper presented at Delirium: Current Advancements in Diagnosis, Treatment and Research, Geriatric Research, Education, and Clinical Center (GRECC), Veterans Administration Medical Center, Minneapolis, MN, September 13–14, 1993

Francis J, Kapoor WN: Prognosis after hospital discharge of older medical patients with delirium. J Am Geriatr Soc 40:601–606, 1992

Francis J, Martin D, Kapoor WN: A prospective study of delirium in hospitalized elderly. JAMA 263:1097–1101, 1990

Franco JG, Mejía MA, Ochoa SB, et al: Escala revisada-98 para valoracion del delirium (DRS-R-98): Adaptacion Columbiana de la version Espanola. Actas Espanolas De Psiquitria 35:170–175, 2007

Franco JG, Trzepacz PT, Mejía MA, et al: Factor analysis of the Colombian translation of the Delirium Rating Scale-Revised-98. Psychosomatics 50:255–262, 2009

Franco JG, Valencia C, Bernal C, Ocampo MV, Trzepacz PT, de Pablo J, Mejia MA: Relationship between cognitive status at admission and incident delirium in older medical inpatients. J Neuropsychiatry Clin Neurosci (in press)

Franco K, Litaker D, Locala J, et al: The cost of delirium in the surgical patient. Psychosomatics 42:68–73, 2001

Furlaneto ME, Garcez-Leme LE: Delirium in elderly individuals with hip fracture: causes, incidence, prevalence, and risk factors. Clinics (Sao Paulo) 61(1):35–40, 2006

Gagnon P, Allard P, Masse B, et al: Delirium in terminal cancer: a prospective study using daily screening, early diagnosis, and continuous monitoring. J Pain Symptom Manage 19:412–426, 2000

Gagnon P, Allard P, Gagnon B, et al: Delirium incidence and associated factors in terminally ill cancer patients. Psychosomatics 45:153, 2004a

Gagnon P, Gandreau JD, Harel F, et al: Delirium incidence and associated factors in hospitalized cancer patients. Psychosomatics 45:154, 2004b

Gallinat J, Möller H-J, Hegerl U: Piracetam in anesthesia for prevention of postoperative delirium [in German]. Anesthesiol Intensivmed Notfallmed Schmerzther 34:520–527, 1999

Gamberini M, Bolliger D, Lurati Buse GA, et al: Rivastigmine for the prevention of postoperative delirium in elderly patients undergoing elective cardiac surgery—a randomized controlled trial. Crit Care Med 37:1762–1768, 2009

Gelfand SB, Indelicato J, Benjamin J: Using intravenous haloperidol to control delirium (abstract). Hosp Community Psychiatry 43:215, 1992

George J, Bleasdale S, Singleton SJ: Causes and prognosis of delirium in elderly patients admitted to a district general hospital. Age Ageing 26:423–427, 1997

Giacino JT, Ashwal S, Childs N, et al: The minimally conscious state: definition and diagnostic criteria. Neurology 58:349–353, 2002

Gibson GE, Jope R, Blass JP: Decreased synthesis of acetylcholine accompanying impaired oxidation of pyruvate in rat brain slices. Biochem J 26:17–23, 1975

Girard T, Pandharipande PP, Carson S, et al: Feasibility, efficacy and safety of antipsychotics for intensive care unit delirium: the MIND randomized placebo-controlled trial. Crit Care Med 38:428–437, 2010

Godfrey A, Conway R, Leonard M, et al: A classification system for delirium subtyping with the use of a commercial mobility monitor. Gait Posture 30:245–252, 2009

Godfrey A, Leonard M, Donnelly S, et al: Validating a new clinical subtyping scheme for delirium with electronic motion analysis. Psychiatry Res 178:186–190, 2010

Gonzalez M, Martinez G, Calderon J, et al: Impact of delirium on short-term mortality in elderly inpatients: a prospective cohort study. Psychosomatics 50:234–238, 2009

Grassi L, Caraceni A, Beltrami E, et al: Assessing delirium in cancer patients: the Italian versions of the Delirium Rating Scale and the Memorial Delirium Assessment Scale. J Pain Symptom Manage 21:59–68, 2001

Gruber-Baldini AL, Zimmerman S, Morrison RS, et al: Cognitive impairment in hip fracture patients: timing of detection and longitudinal follow-up. J Am Geriatr Soc 51:1227–1236, 2003

Gupta AK, Saravay SM, Trzepacz PT, et al: Delirium motor subtypes. Psychosomatics 46:158, 2005

Gupta N, de Jonghe J, Schieveld J, et al: Delirium phenomenology: what can we learn from the symptoms of delirium? J Psychosom Res 65:215–222, 2008

Gustafson Y, Berggren D, Brahnstrom B, et al: Acute confusional states in elderly patients treated for femoral neck fracture. J Am Geriatr Soc 36:525–530, 1988

Hales RE, Polly S, Orman D: An evaluation of patients who received an organic mental disorder diagnosis on a psychiatric consultation-liaison service. Gen Hosp Psychiatry 11:88–94, 1988

Han CS, Kim YK: A double-blind trial of risperidone and haloperidol for the treatment of delirium. Psychosomatics 45:297–301, 2004

Harrell R, Othmer E: Postcardiotomy confusion and sleep loss. J Clin Psychiatry 48:445–446, 1987

Hart RP, Levenson JL, Sessler CN, et al: Validation of a cognitive test for delirium in medical ICU patients. Psychosomatics 37:533–546, 1996

Hart RP, Best AM, Sessler CN, et al: Abbreviated Cognitive Test for Delirium. J Psychosom Res 43:417–423, 1997

Hatta K, Takahashi T, Nakamura H, et al: The association between intravenous haloperidol and prolonged QT interval. J Clin Psychopharmacol 21:257–261, 2001

Henry WD, Mann AM: Diagnosis and treatment of delirium. Can Med Assoc J 93:1156–1166, 1965

Hopkins SJ, Rothwell NJ: Cytokines and the nervous system, I: expression and recognition. Trends Neurosci 18:83–88, 1995

Hua H, Wei D, Hui Y, et al: Olanzapine and haloperidol for senile delirium: a randomized controlled observation. Chinese Journal of Clinical Rehabilitation 10:188–190, 2006

Huang M-C, Lee C-H, Lai Y-C, et al: Chinese version of the Delirium Rating Scale-Revised-98: reliability and validity. Compr Psychiatry 50:81–85, 2009

Ikarashi Y, Takahashi A, Ishimaru H, et al: Regulation of dopamine D1 and D2 receptors on striatal acetylcholine release in rats. Brain Res Bull 43:107–115, 1997

Inouye SK, Charpentier PA: Precipitating factors for delirium in hospitalized elderly patients: predictive model and interrelationships with baseline vulnerability. JAMA 275:852–857, 1996

Inouye SK, van Dyke CH, Alessi CA, et al: Clarifying confusion: the Confusion Assessment Method. Ann Intern Med 113: 941–948, 1990

Inouye SK, Rushing JT, Foreman MD, et al: Does delirium contribute to poor hospital outcome? J Gen Intern Med 13:234–242, 1998

Inouye SK, Bogardus ST, Charpentier PA, et al: A multicomponent intervention to prevent delirium in hospitalized older patients. N Engl J Med 340:669–676, 1999

Inouye SK, Foreman MD, Mion LC, et al: Nurses' recognition of delirium and its symptoms: comparison of nurse and researcher ratings. Arch Intern Med 161:2467–2473, 2001

Inouye SK, Bogardus ST Jr, Williams CS, et al: The role of adherence on the effectiveness of non-pharmacologic interventions: evidence from the Delirium Prevention Trial. Arch Intern Med 163:958–964, 2003

Irving K, Fick D, Foreman M: Delirium: a new appraisal of an old problem. International Journal of Older People Nursing 1(2):106–112, 2006

Iseli R, Brand C, Telford M, et al: Delirium in elderly general medical inpatients: a prospective study. Intern Med J 37:806–811, 2007

Itil T, Fink M: Anticholinergic drug-induced delirium: experimental modification, quantitative EEG, and behavioral correlations. J Nerv Ment Dis 143:492–507, 1966

Jackson JC, Gordon SM, Hart RP, et al: The association between delirium and cognitive decline: a review of the empirical literature. Neuropsychol Rev 14:87–98, 2004

Jacobson SA, Jerrier S: EEG in delirium. Semin Clin Neuropsychiatry 5:86–93, 2000

Jacobson SA, Leuchter AF, Walter DO: Conventional and quantitative EEG diagnosis of delirium among the elderly. J Neurol Neurosurg Psychiatry 56:153–158, 1993a

Jacobson SA, Leuchter AF, Walter DO, et al: Serial quantitative EEG among elderly subjects with delirium. Biol Psychiatry 34:135–140, 1993b

Jitapunkul S, Pillay I, Ebrahim S: Delirium in newly admitted elderly patients: a prospective study. Q J Med 83:307–314, 1992

Johnson JC, Gottlieb GL, Sullivan E, et al: Using DSM-III criteria to diagnose delirium in elderly general medical patients. J Gerontol 45:M113–M119, 1990

Johnson JC, Kerse NM, Gottlieb G, et al: Prospective versus retrospective methods of identifying patients with delirium. J Am Geriatr Soc 40:316–319, 1992

Jones CK, Eberle EL, Shaw DB, et al: Pharmacologic interactions between the muscarinic cholinergic and dopaminergic systems in the modulation of prepulse inhibition in rats. J Pharmacol Exp Ther 312:1055–1063, 2005

Jones C, Griffiths RD, Slater T, et al: Significant cognitive dysfunction in non-delirious patients identified during and persisting following critical illness. Intensive Care Med 32:923–926, 2006

Justo D, Prokhorov V, Heller K, et al: Torsade de pointes induced by psychotropic drugs and the prevalence of its risk factors. Acta Psychiatr Scand 111:171–176, 2005

Kain ZN, Caldwell-Andrews AA, Mayes LC, et al: Family centered preparation for surgery improves perioperative outcomes in children: a randomized controlled trial. Anesthesiology 106:65–74, 2007

Kakuma R, du Fort GG, Arsenault L, et al: Delirium in older emergency department patients discharged home: effect on survival. J Am Geriatr Soc 51:443–450, 2003

Kalisvaart K, de Jonghe JFM, Bogards MJ, et al: Haloperidol prophylaxis for elderly hip surgery patients at risk for delirium: a randomized placebo-controlled study. J Am Geriatr Soc 53:1658–1666, 2005

Kalisvaart K, Vreeswiik R, de Jonghe J, et al: Risk factors and prediction of postoperative delirium in elderly hip surgery patients: implementation and validation of a medical risk factor model. J Am Geriatr Soc 54:817–822, 2006

Kat MG, Vreeswijk R, de Jonghe JF, et al: Long-term cognitive outcome of delirium in elderly hip surgery patients: a prospective matched controlled study over two and a half years. Dement Geriatr Cogn Disord 26:1–8, 2008

Kato M, Kishi Y, Okuyama T, et al: Japanese version of the Delirium Rating Scale–Revised-98 (DRS-R98-J): reliability and validity. Psychosomatics (in press)

Katz IR, Curyto KJ, TenHave T, et al: Validating the diagnosis of delirium and evaluating its association with deterioration over a one year period. Am J Geriatr Psychiatry 9:248–259, 2001

Katz JA, Mahoney DH, Fernbach DJ: Human leukocyte alpha-interferon induced transient neurotoxicity in children. Invest New Drugs 6:115–120, 1988

Kaufer DI, Catt KE, Lopez OL, et al: Dementia with Lewy bodies: response of delirium-like features to donepezil. Neurology 51:1512–1513, 1998

Kazmierski J, Kowman M, Banach M, et al: Clinical utility and use of DSM-IV and ICD-10 criteria and the MDAS in establishing a diagnosis of delirium after cardiac surgery. Psychosomatics 49:73–76, 2008

Kean J, Ryan K: Delirium detection in clinical practice: critique of current tools and suggestions for future development. J Psychosomatic Res 65:255–259, 2008

Kean J, Trzepacz PT, Murray LL, Abell M, Trexler L: The accuracy and validity of a new provisional diagnostic tool for delirium in acquired brain injury. Brain Inj (in press)

Kelly KG, Zisselman M, Cutillo-Schmitter T, et al: Severity and course of delirium in medically hospitalized nursing facility residents. Am J Geriatr Psychiatry 9:72–77, 2001

Kennard MA, Bueding E, Wortis WB: Some biochemical and electroencephalographic changes in delirium tremens. Q J Stud Alcohol 6:4–14, 1945

Kennedy RE, Nakase-Thompson R, Nick TG, et al: Use of the Cognitive Test for Delirium in patients with traumatic brain injury. Psychosomatics 44:283–289, 2003

Kiely DK, Bergmann MA, Murphy KM, et al: Delirium among newly admitted postacute facility patients: prevalence, symptoms, and severity. J Gerontol A Biol Sci Med Sci 58:M441–M445, 2003

Kiely DK, Marcantonio ER, Inouye SK, et al: Persistent delirium predicts greater mortality. J Am Geriatr Soc 57:55–61, 2009

Kim JY, Jung IK, Han C, et al: Antipsychotics and dopamine transporter gene polymorphisms in delirium patients. Psychiatry Clin Neurosci 59:183–188, 2005

Kishi Y, Iwasaki Y, Takezawa K, et al: Delirium in critical care unit patients admitted through an emergency room. Gen Hosp Psychiatry 17:371–379, 1995

Kishi Y, Kato M, Okuyama T, et al: Delirium: patient characteristics that predict a missed diagnosis at psychiatric consultation. Gen Hospital Psychiatry 29:442–445, 2007

Klein M, Payaslian S, Gomez J, et al: Acute confusional syndrome due to acute nicotine withdrawal. Medicina (B Aires) 62:335–336, 2002

Kohnke MD, Schick S, Lutz U, et al: Severity of alcohol withdrawal symptoms and the T1128C polymorphism of the neuropeptide Y gene. J Neural Transm 109:1423–1429, 2002

Kohnke MD, Batra A, Kolb W, et al: Association of the dopamine transporter gene with alcoholism. Alcohol Alcohol 40:339–342, 2005

Kohnke MD, Kolb W, Kohnke AM, et al: DBH*444G/A polymorphism of the dopamine-beta-hydroxylase gene is associated with alcoholism but not with severe alcohol withdrawal symptoms. J Neural Transm 113:869–876, 2006a

Kohnke MD, Lutz U, Kolb W, et al: Allele distribution of a monoamine oxidase A gene promoter polymorphism in German alcoholics and in subgroups with severe forms of alcohol withdrawal and its influence on plasma homovanillic acid. Psychiatr Genet 16:237–238, 2006b

Kolbeinsson H, Jonsson A: Delirium and dementia in acute medical admissions of elderly patients in Iceland. Acta Psychiatr Scand 87:123–127, 1993

Koponen H, Sirvio J, Lepola U, et al: A long-term follow-up study of cerebrospinal fluid acetylcholinesterase in delirium. Eur Arch Psychiatry Clin Neurosci 243:347–351, 1994

Korevaar JC, van Munster BC, de Rooij S: Risk factors for delirium in acutely admitted elderly patients: a prospective cohort study. BMC Geriatrics 5:6, 2005

Kreis R, Farrow N, Ross BN: Localized NMR spectroscopy in patients with chronic hepatic encephalopathy: analysis of changes in cerebral glutamine, choline, and inositols. NMR Biomed 4:109–116, 1991

Kriwisky M, Perry GY, Tarchitsky D, et al: Haloperidol-induced torsades de pointes. Chest 98:482–484, 1990

Kullmann F, Hollerbach S, Holstege A, et al: Subclinical hepatic encephalopathy: the diagnostic value of evoked potentials. J Hepatol 22:101–110, 1995

Larsen K, Kelly S, Stern T: A double-blind, randomized, placebo-controlled study of perioperative administration of olanzapine to prevent postoperative delirium in joint replacement patients. Presentation at the Academy of Psychosomatic Medicine 54th annual meeting, Amelia Island, FL, November 2007

Laurila JV, Pitkala KH, Strandberg TE, et al: Confusion assessment method in the diagnostics of delirium among aged hospital patients: would it serve better in screening than as a diagnostic instrument? Int J Geriatr Psychiatry 17:1112–1119, 2002

Laurila JV, Pitkala KH, Strandberg TE, et al: The impact of different diagnostic criteria on prevalence rates for delirium. Dement Geriatr Cogn Disord 16:156–162, 2003

Laurila JV, Pitkala KH, Strandberg TE, et al: Impact of different diagnostic criteria on prognosis of delirium: a prospective study. Dement Geriatr Cogn Disord 18:240–244, 2004

Laurila JV, Laakkonen M-L, Laurila J, et al: Predisposing and precipitating factors for delirium in a frail geriatric population. J Psychosom Res 65:249–254, 2008

Lawlor PG, Gagnon B, Mancini IL, et al: Occurrence, causes and outcome of delirium in patients with advanced cancer. Arch Intern Med 160:786–794, 2000a

Lawlor PG, Nekolaichuk C, Gagnon B, et al: Clinical utility, factor analysis and further validation of the Memorial Delirium Assessment Scale in patients with advanced cancer: assessing delirium in advanced cancer. Cancer 88:2859–2867, 2000b

Lee KU, Won WY, Lee HK, et al: Amisulpride versus quetiapine for the treatment of delirium: a randomized, open prospective study. Int Clin Psychopharmacol 20:311–314, 2005

Leonard M, Donnelly S, Conroy M, et al: A longitudinal study of phenomenological profile in delirium. Presentation at the European Delirium Association 2nd annual meeting, Limerick, Ireland, November 2007a

Leonard M, Godfrey A, Silberhorn M, et al: Motion analysis in delirium: a novel method of clarifying motoric subtypes. Neurocase 13:272–277, 2007b

Leonard M, Raju B, Conroy M, et al: Reversibility of delirium in terminally ill patients and predictors of mortality. Palliat Med 22:848–854, 2008

Leonard M, Spiller J, Keen J, et al: Symptoms of depression and delirium assessed serially in palliative care inpatients. Psychosomatics 50:506–514, 2009

Leslie DL, Zhang Y, Holford TR, et al: Premature death associated with delirium at 1-year follow up. Arch Intern Med 165:1657–1662, 2005

Leung CM, Chan KK, Cheng KK: Psychiatric morbidity in a general medical ward: Hong Kong's experience. Gen Hosp Psychiatry 14:196–200, 1992

Levkoff SE, Evans DA, Liptzin B, et al: Delirium: the occurrence and persistence of symptoms among elderly hospitalized patients. Arch Intern Med 152:334–340, 1992

Levkoff SE, Liptzin B, Evans D, et al: Progression and resolution of delirium in elderly patients hospitalized for acute care. Am J Geriatr Psychiatry 2:230–238, 1994

Lim K-O, Kim S-Y, Lee Y-H, et al: A validation study of the Korean version of Delirium Rating Scale-Revised-98 (K-DRS-98). J Korean Neuropsychiatr Assoc 45:518–526, 2006

Limosin F, Loze J-Y, Boni C, et al: The A9 allele of the dopamine transporter gene increases the risk of visual hallucinations during alcohol withdrawal in alcohol-dependent women. Neurosci Lett 362:91–94, 2004

Lipowski ZJ: Delirium: Acute Confusional States. New York, Oxford University Press, 1990

Lipton SA, Gendelman HE: Seminars in medicine of the Beth Israel Hospital, Boston. Dementia associated with the acquired immunodeficiency syndrome. N Engl J Med 332:934–940, 1995

Liptzin B, Levkoff SE, Gottlieb GL, et al: Delirium. J Neuropsychiatry Clin Neurosci 5:154–160, 1993

Liptzin B, Laki A, Garb JL, et al: Donepezil in the prevention and treatment of post-surgical delirium. Am J Geriatr Psychiatry 13:1100–1106, 2005

Liu CY, Juang YY, Liang HY, et al: Efficacy of risperidone in treating the hyperactive symptoms of delirium. Int Clin Psychopharmacol 19:165–168, 2004

Ljubisavljevic V, Kelly B: Risk factors for development of delirium among oncology patients. Gen Hosp Psychiatry 25:345–352, 2003

Lowery DP, Wesnes K, Ballard C: Subtle attentional deficits in the absence of dementia are associated with an increased risk of post-operative delirium. Dement Geriatr Cogn Disord 23:390–394, 2007

Lowery DP, Wesnes K, Brewster N, et al: Quantifying the association between computerised measures of attention and confusion assessment method defined delirium: a prospective study of older orthopaedic surgical patients, free of dementia. Int J Geriatr Psychiatry 23:1253–1260, 2008

Lundstrom M, Edlund A, Bucht G, et al: Dementia after delirium in patients with femoral neck fractures. J Am Geriatr Soc 51:1002–1006, 2003

Mach J, Dysken M, Kuskowski M, et al: Serum anticholinergic activity in hospitalized older persons with delirium: a preliminary study. J Am Geriatr Soc 43:491–495, 1995

MacLullich AM, Beaglehole A, Hall RJ, et al: Delirium and long-term cognitive impairment. Int Rev Psychiatry 21:30–42, 2009

Maldonado JR: Pathoetiological model of delirium: a comprehensive understanding of the neurobiology of delirium and an evidence based approach to prevention and treatment. Crit Care Clin 24:789–856, 2008

Maldonado JR, Wysong A, van der Starre PJA, et al: Dexmedetomidine and reduction of postoperative delirium after cardiac surgery. Psychosomatics 50:206–217, 2009

Manos PJ: The utility of the ten-point clock test as a screen for cognitive impairment in general hospital patients. Gen Hosp Psychiatry 19:439–444, 1997

Marcantonio ER, Goldman L, Mangione CM, et al: A clinical prediction rule for delirium after elective noncardiac surgery. JAMA 271:134–139, 1994a

Marcantonio ER, Juarez G, Goldman L, et al: The relationship of postoperative delirium with psychoactive medications. JAMA 272:1518–1522, 1994b

Marcantonio ER, Flacker JM, Wright J, et al: Reducing delirium after hip fracture: a randomized trial. J Am Geriatr Soc 49:516–522, 2001

Marcantonio ER, Simon SE, Orav EJ, et al: Outcomes of elders admitted to post-acute care facilities with delirium, subsyndromal delirium, or no delirium. J Am Geriatr Soc 50:S168, 2002

Marcantonio ER, Kiely DR, Simon DE, et al: Outcomes of older people admitted to postacute facilities with delirium. J Am Geriatr Soc 53:963–969, 2005

Marquis F, Ouimet S, Riker R, et al: Individual delirium symptoms: do they matter? Crit Care Med 35:2533–2537, 2007

Mathers DA: The GABA-A receptor: new insights from single channel recording. Synapse 1:96–101, 1987

Matsuoka Y, Miyake Y, Arakaki H, et al: Clinical utility and validation of the Japanese version of the Memorial Delirium Assessment Scale in a psychogeriatric inpatient setting. Gen Hosp Psychiatry 23:36–40, 2001

Matsushima E, Nakajima K, Moriya H, et al: A psychophysiological study of the development of delirium in coronary care units. Biol Psychiatry 41:1211–1217, 1997

Matsushita S, Kimura M, Miyakawa T, et al: Association study of brain-derived neurotrophic factor gene polymorphism and alcoholism. Alcohol Clin Exp Res 28:1609–1612, 2004

McCarthy MC: Detecting acute confusion in older adults: comparing clinical reasoning of nurses working in acute, long-term, and community health care environments. Res Nurs Health 26:203–212, 2003

McCusker J, Cole M, Abrahamowicz M, et al: Delirium predicts 12-month mortality. Arch Intern Med 162:457–463, 2002

McCusker J, Cole MG, Dendukuri N, et al: Does delirium increase hospital stay? J Am Geriatr Soc 51:1539–1546, 2003a

McCusker J, Cole MG, Dendukuri N, et al: The course of delirium in older medical inpatients: a prospective study. J Gen Intern Med 18:696–704, 2003b

McNicoll L, Pisani MA, Zhang Y, et al: Delirium in the intensive care unit: occurrence and clinical course in older patients. J Am Geriatr Soc 51:591–598, 2003

Meagher DJ: Delirium: the role of psychiatry. Advances in Psychiatric Treatments 7:433–443, 2001

Meagher D: Motor subtypes of delirium: past, present and future. Int Rev Psychiatry 21:59–73, 2009

Meagher DJ, Leonard M: Advances in Psychiatric Treatment 14:292–301, 2008

Meagher DJ, Trzepacz PT: Motoric subtypes of delirium. Semin Clin Neuropsychiatry 5:76–86, 2000

Meagher DJ, O'Hanlon D, O'Mahony E, et al: Use of environmental strategies and psychotropic medication in the management of delirium. Br J Psychiatry 168:512–515, 1996

Meagher DJ, O'Hanlon D, O'Mahony E, et al: Relationship between etiology and phenomenologic profile in delirium. J Geriatr Psychiatry Neurol 11:146–149, 1998

Meagher DJ, O'Hanlon D, O'Mahony E, et al: Relationship between symptoms and motor subtype of delirium. J Neuropsychiatry Clin Neurosci 12:51–56, 2000

Meagher DJ, Moran M, Raju B, et al: Phenomenology of delirium. Assessment of 100 adult cases using standardized measures. Br J Psychiatry 190:135–141, 2007

Meagher D, Leonard M, Donnelly S, et al: Testing the predictive ability of a new motor-based subtyping scheme for delirium (NR5-050), in 2008 New Research Program and Abstracts, American Psychiatric Association 161st Annual Meeting, Washington, DC, May 3–8, 2008. Washington, DC, American Psychiatric Association, 2008a, p 235

Meagher DJ, Moran M, Raju B, et al: A new data-based motor subtype schema for delirium. J Neuropsychiatry Clin Neurosci 20:185–193, 2008b

Meagher DJ, Moran M, Raju B, et al: Motor symptoms in 100 patients with delirium versus control subjects: comparison of subtyping methods. Psychosomatics 49:300–308, 2008c

Metzger E, Friedman R: Prolongation of the corrected QT and torsades de pointes cardiac arrhythmia associated with intravenous haloperidol in the medically ill. J Clin Psychopharmacol 13:128–132, 1993

Milbrandt EB, Deppen S, Harrison PL, et al: Costs associated with delirium in mechanically ventilated patients. Crit Care Med 32:955–962, 2004

Milisen K, Foreman MD, Abraham IL, et al: A nurse-led interdisciplinary intervention program for delirium in elderly hip fracture patients. J Am Geriatr Soc 49:523–532, 2001

Minagawa H, Uchitomi Y, Yamawaki S, et al: Psychiatric morbidity in terminally ill cancer patients: a prospective study. Cancer 78:1131–1137, 1996

Mizock BA, Sabelli HC, Dubin A, et al: Septic encephalopathy: evidence for altered phenylalanine metabolism and comparison with hepatic encephalopathy. Arch Intern Med 150:443–449, 1990

Moller JT, Cluitmans P, Rasmussen LS, et al: Long-term postoperative cognitive dysfunction in the elderly ISPOCD1 study. ISPOCD investigators. International Study of Post-Operative Cognitive Dysfunction. Lancet 351:857–861, 1998 [published erratum appears in Lancet 351:1742, 1998]

Mondimore FM, Damlouji N, Folstein MF, et al: Post-ECT confusional states associated with elevated serum anticholinergic levels. Am J Psychiatry 140:930–931, 1983

Monette J, Galbaud du Fort G, Fung SH, et al: Evaluation of the Confusion Assessment Method (CAM) as a screening tool for delirium in the emergency room. Gen Hosp Psychiatry 23:20–25, 2001

Monk TG, Weldon BC, Garvan CW, et al: Predictors of cognitive dysfunction after major noncardiac surgery. Anesthesiology 108:18–30, 2008

Montgomery EA, Fenton GW, McClelland RJ, et al: Psychobiology of minor head injury. Psychosom Med 21:375–384, 1991

Moretti R, Torre P, Antonello RM, et al: Cholinesterase inhibition as a possible therapy for delirium in vascular dementia: a controlled, open 24-month study of 246 patients. Am J Alzheimers Dis Other Demen 19:333–339, 2004

Morita T, Tei Y, Tsunoda J, et al: Underlying pathologies and their associations with clinical features in terminal delirium of cancer patients. J Pain Symptom Manage 22:997–1006, 2001

Morrison RS, Magaziner J, Gilbert M, et al: Relationship between pain and opioid analgesics on the development of delirium following hip fracture. J Gerontol A Biol Sci Med Sci 58:76–81, 2003

Mousseau DD, Butterworth RF: Current theories on the pathogenesis of hepatic encephalopathy. Proc Soc Exp Biol Med 206:329–344, 1994

Murphy KM: The baseline predictors and 6-month outcomes of incident delirium in nursing home residents: a study using the minimum data set. Psychosomatics 40:164–165, 1999

Murray AM, Levkoff SE, Wetle TT, et al: Acute delirium and functional decline in the hospitalized elderly patient. J Gerontol 48:M181–M186, 1993

Nagley SJ: Predicting and preventing confusion in your patients. J Gerontol Nurs 12:27–31, 1986

Nakamura J, Uchimura N, Yamada S, et al: The effect of mianserin hydrochloride on delirium. Hum Psychopharmacol 10:289–297, 1995

Nakamura J, Uchimura N, Yamada S, et al: Does plasma free 3-methoxy-4-hydroxyphenyl(ethylene)glycol increase the delirious state? A comparison of the effects of mianserin and haloperidol on delirium. Int Clin Psychopharmacol 12:147–152, 1997a

Nakamura J, Uchimura N, Yamada S, et al: Mianserin suppositories in the treatment of post-operative delirium. Hum Psychopharmacol 12:595–599, 1997b

Nakase-Richardson R, Yablon AS, Sherer M: Prospective comparison of acute confusion severity with duration of post-traumatic amnesia in predicting employment outcome after traumatic brain injury. J Neurol Neurosurg Psychiatry 78:872–876, 2007

Nakase-Thompson R, Sherer M, Yablon SA, et al: Acute confusion following traumatic brain injury. Brain Injury 18:131–142, 2004

Nicholas LM, Lindsey BA: Delirium presenting with symptoms of depression. Psychosomatics 36:471–479, 1995

O'Brien JM, Rockwood RP, Suh KI: Haloperidol-induced torsades de pointes. Ann Pharmacother 33:1046–1050, 1999

O'Keeffe ST: Rating the severity of delirium: the Delirium Assessment Scale. Int J Geriatr Psychiatry 9:551–556, 1994

O'Keeffe ST, Gosney MA: Assessing attentiveness in older hospitalized patients: global assessment vs. test of attention. J Am Geriatr Soc 45:470–473, 1997

O'Keeffe ST, Lavan JN: Predicting delirium in elderly patients: development and validation of a risk-stratification model. Age Ageing 25:317–321, 1996

O'Keeffe ST, Lavan JN: Clinical significance of delirium subtypes in older people. Age Ageing 28:115–119, 1999

O'Keeffe ST, Tormey WP, Glasgow R, et al: Thiamine deficiency in hospitalized elderly patients. Gerontology 40:18–24, 1994

O'Keeffe ST, Mulkerrin EC, Nayeem K, et al: Use of serial Mini-Mental State Examinations to diagnose and monitor delirium in elderly hospital patients. J Am Geriatr Soc 53:867–870, 2005

Okubo T, Harada S, Higuchi S, et al: Genetic polymorphism of the CCK gene in patients with alcohol withdrawal symptoms. Alcohol Clin Exp Res 24 (4 suppl):2S–4S, 2000

Okubo T, Harada S, Higuchi S, et al: Association analyses between polymorphisms of the phase II detoxification enzymes (GSTM1, NQO1, NQO2) and alcohol withdrawal symptoms. Alcohol Clin Exp Res 27 (8 suppl):68S–71S, 2003

Olofsson SM, Weitzner MA, Valentine AD, et al: A retrospective study of the psychiatric management and outcome of delirium in the cancer patient. Support Care Cancer 4:351–357, 1996

Onofrj M, Curatola L, Malatesta G, et al: Reduction of P3 latency during outcome from post-traumatic amnesia. Acta Neurol Scand 83:273–279, 1991

Osse RJ, Tulen JHM, van der Mast RC, et al: Preoperative cognitive functioning is associated with delirium in elderly patients undergoing cardiac surgery. Third International Scientific Congress on Delirium, Helsinki, Finland, October 2008

Owens JF, Hutelmyer CM: The effect of postoperative intervention on delirium in cardiac surgical patients. Nurs Res 31:60–62, 1982

Pandharipande PP, Shintani A, Peterson J, et al: Lorazepam is an independent risk factor for transitioning to delirium in intensive care unit patients. Anesthesiology 104:21–26, 2006

Pandharipande PP, Pun BT, Herr DL, et al: Effect of sedation with dexmedetomidine vs. lorazepam on acute brain dysfunction in mechanically ventilated patients: the MENDS randomized controlled trial. JAMA 298:2644–2653, 2007

Pandharipande PP, Morandi A, Adams JR, et al: Plasma tryptophan and tyrosine levels are independent risk factors for delirium in critically ill patients. Intensive Care Med 35:1886–1892, 2009

Patten SB, Lamarre CJ: Dysgraphia (letter). Can J Psychiatry 34:746, 1989

Perrault LP, Denault AY, Carrier M, et al: Torsades de pointes secondary to intravenous haloperidol after coronary artery bypass graft surgery. Can J Anaesth 47:251–254, 2000

Perry E, Walker M, Grace J, et al: Acetylcholine in mind: a neurotransmitter correlate of consciousness? Trends Neurosci 22:273–280, 1999

Pfister D, Siegemund M, Dell-Kuster S, et al: Cerebral perfusion in sepsis-associated delirium. Crit Care 12:R63, 2008

Picotte-Prillmayer D, DiMaggio JR, Baile WF: H2 blocker delirium. Psychosomatics 36:74–77, 1995

Pisani MA, Kong SY, Kasl SV, et al: Days of delirium are associated with 1-year mortality in an older intensive care population. Am J Respir Crit Care Med 180:1092–1097, 2009

Pitkala KH, Laurila JV, Strandberg TE, et al: Multicomponent Geriatric Intervention for elderly inpatients with delirium: a randomized controlled trial. J Gerontol A Biol Sci Med Sci 61:176–181, 2006

Plaschke K, Thomas C, Engelhardt R, et al: Significant correlation between plasma and CSF anticholinergic activity in presurgical patients. Neurosci Lett 417:16–20, 2007

Platt MM, Breitbart W, Smith M, et al: Efficacy of neuroleptics for hypoactive delirium. J Neuropsychiatry Clin Neurosci 6:66–67, 1994

Pompei P, Foreman M, Rudberg MA, et al: Delirium in hospitalized older persons: outcomes and predictors. J Am Geriatr Soc 42:809–815, 1994

Prakanrattana U, Prapaitrakool S: Efficacy of risperidone for prevention of postoperative delirium in cardiac surgery. Anaesth Intensive Care 35:714–719, 2007

Preuss UW, Koller G, Zill P, et al: Alcoholism-related phenotypes and genetic variants of the CB1 receptor. Eur Arch Psychiatry Clin Neurosci 253:275–280, 2003

Preuss UW, Zill P, Koller G, et al: Ionotropic glutamate receptor gene GRIK3 SER310ALA functional polymorphism is related to delirium tremens in alcoholics. Pharmacogenomics J 6:34–41, 2006

Prugh DG, Wagonfeld S, Metcalf D, et al: A clinical study of delirium in children and adolescents. Psychosom Med 42:177–195, 1980

Rahkonen T, Luukkainen-Markkula R, Paanila S, et al: Delirium episode as a sign of undetected dementia among community dwelling elderly subjects: a 2 year follow up study. J Neurol Neurosurg Psychiatry 69:519–521, 2000

Rincon HG, Granados M, Unutzer J, et al: Prevalence, detection and treatment of anxiety, depression and delirium in the adult critical care unit. Psychosomatics 42:391–396, 2001

Robbins TW, McAlonan G, Muir JL, et al: Cognitive enhancers in theory and practice: studies of the cholinergic hypothesis of cognitive deficits in Alzheimer's disease. Behav Brain Res 83:15–23, 1997

Robertsson B, Blennow K, Gottfries CG, et al: Delirium in dementia. Int J Geriatr Psychiatry 13:49–56, 1998

Robinson MJ: Probable Lewy body dementia presenting as delirium. Psychosomatics 43:84–86, 2002

Rockwood K: Acute confusion in elderly medical patients. J Am Geriatr Soc 37:150–154, 1989

Rockwood K: The occurrence and duration of symptoms in elderly patients with delirium. J Gerontol 48:M162–M166, 1993

Rockwood K, Cosway S, Stolee P, et al: Increasing the recognition of delirium in elderly patients. J Am Geriatr Soc 42:252–256, 1994

Rockwood K, Cosway S, Carver D, et al: The risk of dementia and death after delirium. Age Ageing 28:551–556, 1999

Rolfson DB, McElhaney JE, Jhangri GS, et al: Validity of the Confusion Assessment Method in detecting post-operative delirium in the elderly. Int Psychogeriatr 11:431–438, 1999

Romano J, Engel GL: Delirium, I: electroencephalographic data. Archives of Neurology and Psychiatry 51:356–377, 1944

Rosenberg PB, Ahmed I, Hurwitz S: Methylphenidate in depressed medically ill patients. J Clin Psychiatry 52:263–267, 1991

Ross CA, Peyser CE, Shapiro I, et al: Delirium: phenomenologic and etiologic subtypes. Int Psychogeriatr 3:135–147, 1991

Rothwell NJ, Hopkins SJ: Cytokines and the nervous system, II: actions and mechanisms of action. Trends Neurosci 18:130–136, 1995

Rudberg MA, Pompei P, Foreman MD, et al: The natural history of delirium in older hospitalized patients: a syndrome of heterogeneity. Age Ageing 26:169–174, 1997

Rudolph JL, Jones RN, Grande LJ, et al: Impaired executive function is associated with delirium after coronary artery bypass graft surgery. J Am Geriatr Soc 54:937–941, 2006

Ruijs MB, Keyser A, Gabreels FJ, et al: Somatosensory evoked potentials and cognitive sequelae in children with closed head injury. Neuropediatrics 24:307–312, 1993

Ruijs MB, Gabreels FJ, Thijssen HM: The utility of electroencephalography and cerebral CT in children with mild and moderately severe closed head injuries. Neuropediatrics 25:73–77, 1994

Ryan K, Leonard M, Guerin S, et al: Validation of the confusion assessment method in the palliative care setting. Palliat Med 23:40–45, 2009

Sagawa R, Akechi T, Okuyama T, et al: Etiologies of delirium and their relationship to reversibility and motor subtype in cancer patients. Jpn J Oncol 39:175–183, 2009

Sampson EL, Raven PR, Ndhlovu PN, et al: A randomized, double-blind, placebo-controlled trial of donepezil hydrochloride (Aricept) for reducing the incidence of postoperative delirium after elective total hip replacement. Int J Geriatr Psychiatry 22:343–349, 2006

Sandberg O, Gustafson Y, Brannstrom B, et al: Prevalence of dementia, delirium and psychiatric symptoms in various care settings for the elderly. Scand J Soc Med 26:56–62, 1998

Sander T, Harms H, Podschus J, et al: Alleleic association of a dopamine transporter gene polymorphism in alcohol dependence with withdrawal seizures or delirium. Biol Psychiatry 41:299–304, 1997

Sander T, Harms H, Rommelspacher H, et al: Possible allelic association of a tyrosine hydroxylase polymorphism with vulnerability to alcohol-withdrawal delirium. Psychiatr Genet 8:13–17, 1998

Sanders KM, Stern TA: Management of delirium associated with use of the intra-aortic balloon pump. Am J Crit Care 2:371–377, 1993

Saravay SM, Strain JJ: Academy of Psychosomatic Medicine Task Force on Funding Implications of Consultation/Liaison Psychiatry Outcome Studies: Special series introduction: a review of outcome studies. Psychosomatics 35:227–232, 1994

Schieveld JN, Leentjens AF: Delirium in severely ill children in the pediatric intensive care unit (PICU). J Am Acad Child Adolesc Psychiatry 44:392–394, 2005

Schieveld JN, Leroy PL, van Os J, et al: Pediatric delirium in critical illness: phenomenology, clinical correlates and treatment response in 40 cases in the pediatric intensive care unit. Intensive Care Med 33:1033–1040, 2007

Schiff ND, Plum F: The role of arousal and gating systems in the neurology of impaired consciousness. J Clin Neurophysiol 17:438–452, 2000

Schmidt LG, Samochowiec J, Finckh U, et al: Association of a CB1 cannabinoid receptor gene (CNR1) polymorphism with severe alcohol dependence. Drug Alcohol Depend 65:221–224, 2002

Schneir AB, Offerman SR, Ly BT, et al: Complications of diagnostic physostigmine administration to emergency department patients. Ann Emerg Med 42:14–19, 2003

Schofield I: A small exploratory study of the reaction of older people to an episode of delirium. J Adv Nurs 25:942–952, 1997

Schor JD, Levkoff SE, Lipsitz LA, et al: Risk factors for delirium in hospitalized elderly. JAMA 267:827–831, 1992

Seaman JS, Schillerstrom J, Carroll D, et al: Impaired oxidative metabolism precipitates delirium: a study of 101 ICU patients. Psychosomatics 47:56–61, 2006

Seear M, Lockitch G, Jacobson B, et al: Thiamine, riboflavin and pyridoxine deficiency in a population of critically ill children. J Pediatr 121:533–538, 1992

Seitz DP, Gill SS, van Zyl L: Antipsychotics in the treatment of delirium: a systematic review. J Clin Psychiatry 68:11–21, 2007

Shyamsundar G, Raghuthaman G, Rajkumar AP, et al: Validation of memorial delirium assessment scale. J Crit Care 24:530–534, 2009

Siddiqi N, House AO, Holmes J D: Occurrence and outcome of delirium in medical in-patients: a systematic literature review. Age Ageing 35:350–364, 2006

Smith PJ, Attix DK, Weldon BC, et al: Executive function and depression as independent risk factors for postoperative delirium. Anesthesiology 110:781, 2009

Snyder S, Reyner A, Schmeidler J, et al: Prevalence of mental disorders in newly admitted medical inpatients with AIDS. Psychosomatics 33:166–170, 1992

Solfrizzi V, Torres F, Capursi C, et al: Analysis of individual items of MMSE in discrimination between normal and demented subjects. Arch Gerontol Geriatr 7 (suppl):357–362, 2001

Spiller J, Keen J: Hypoactive delirium: assessing the extent of the problem in inpatient specialist palliative care. Palliat Med 20:17–23, 2006

Stableford JA: The longest run. Dartmouth Medicine, Winter 2009; online at dartmed.dartmouth.edu

Stefano GB, Bilfinger TV, Fricchione GL: The immune-neurolink and the macrophage: post-cardiotomy delirium, HIV-associated dementia and psychiatry. Prog Neurobiol 42:475–488, 1994

Stern TA: Continuous infusion of physostigmine in anticholinergic delirium: a case report. J Clin Psychiatry 44:463–464, 1983

Sundaram M, Dostrow V: Epilepsy in the elderly. Neurologist 1:232–239, 1995

Takeuchi T, Furuta K, Hirasawa T, et al: Perospirone in the treatment of patients with delirium. Psychiatry Clin Neurosci 61:67–70, 2007

Tejera CA, Saravay SM, Goldman E, et al: Diphenhydramine-induced delirium in elderly hospitalized patients with mild dementia. Psychosomatics 35:399–402, 1994

Tesar GE, Murray GB, Cassem NH: Use of high-dose intravenous haloperidol in the treatment of agitated cardiac patients. J Clin Psychopharmacol 5:344–347, 1985

Thomas C, Hestermann U, Walther S, et al: Prolonged activation EEG differentiates dementia with and without delirium in frail elderly. J Neurol Neurosurg Psychiatry 79:119–125, 2008

Thomas RI, Cameron DJ, Fahs MC: A prospective study of delirium and prolonged hospital stay. Arch Gen Psychiatry 45:937–946, 1988

Tihonen J, Hallikainen T, Lachman H, et al: Association between the functional variant of the catechol-O-methyltransferase (COMT) gene and type 1 alcoholism. Mol Psychiatry 4:286–289, 1999

Timmers JFM, Kalisvaart KJ, Schuurmans M, et al: A review of assessment scales for delirium, in Primary Prevention of Delirium in the Elderly. Edited by Kalisvaart K. Amsterdam, The Netherlands, Academisch Proefschrift, University of Amsterdam, 2005, pp 21–39

Tokita K, Tanaka H, Kawamoto M, et al: Patient-controlled epidural analgesia with bupivacaine and fentanyl. Masui 50:742–746, 2001

Trzepacz PT: Neuropathogenesis of delirium: a need to focus our research. Psychosomatics 35:374–391, 1994

Trzepacz PT: Anticholinergic model for delirium. Semin Clin Neuropsychiatry 1:294–303, 1996a

Trzepacz PT: Delirium: advances in diagnosis, assessment, and treatment. Psychiatr Clin North Am 19:429–448, 1996b

Trzepacz PT: The Delirium Rating Scale: its use in consultation/liaison research. Psychosomatics 40:193–204, 1999a

Trzepacz PT: Update on the neuropathogenesis of delirium. Dement Geriatr Cogn Disord 10:330–334, 1999b

Trzepacz PT: Is there a final common neural pathway in delirium? Focus on acetylcholine and dopamine. Semin Clin Neuropsychiatry 5:132–148, 2000

Trzepacz PT, Dew MA: Further analyses of the Delirium Rating Scale. Gen Hosp Psychiatry 17:75–79, 1995

Trzepacz PT, Francis J: Low serum albumin and risk of delirium (letter). Am J Psychiatry 147:675, 1990

Trzepacz PT, van der Mast R: Neuropathophysiology of delirium, in Delirium in Old Age. Edited by Lindesay J, Rockwood K, MacDonald A. Oxford, UK, Oxford University Press, 2002, pp 51–78

Trzepacz PT, Teague GB, Lipowski ZJ: Delirium and other organic mental disorders in a general hospital. Gen Hosp Psychiatry 7:101–106, 1985

Trzepacz PT, Baker RW, Greenhouse J: A symptom rating scale for delirium. Psychiatry Res 23:89–97, 1988a

Trzepacz PT, Brenner R, Coffman G, et al: Delirium in liver transplantation candidates: discriminant analysis of multiple test variables. Biol Psychiatry 24:3–14, 1988b

Trzepacz PT, Mulsant BH, Dew MA, et al: Is delirium different when it occurs in dementia? A study using the Delirium Rating Scale. J Neuropsychiatry Clin Neurosci 10:199–204, 1998

Trzepacz PT, Kishi Y, Hosaka T, et al: Delirium Rating Scale—Revised-98 (DRS-R-98), Japanese version. Seishin Igaku (Clinical Psychiatry) 43:1365–1371, 2001a

Trzepacz PT, Mittal D, Torres R, et al: Delirium phenomenology using the Delirium Rating Scale-Revised-98 (DRS-R-98). J Neuropsychiatry Clin Neurosci 13:154, 2001b

Trzepacz PT, Mittal D, Torres R, et al: Validation of the Delirium Rating Scale-Revised-98: comparison with the Delirium Rating Scale and the Cognitive Test for Delirium. J Neuropsychiatry Clin Neurosci 13:229–242, 2001c [published erratum appears in J Neuropsychiatry Clin Neurosci 13:433, 2001]

Trzepacz PT, Meagher DJ, Wise M: Neuropsychiatric aspects of delirium, in The American Psychiatric Publishing Textbook of Neuropsychiatry and Clinical Neurosciences, 4th Edition. Edited by Yudofsky SC, Hales RE. Washington, DC, American Psychiatric Publishing, 2002a, pp 525–564

Trzepacz PT, Mittal D, Torres R, et al: Delirium vs. dementia symptoms: Delirium Rating Scale-Revised-98 (DRS-R-98) and Cognitive Test for Delirium (CTD) item comparisons. Psychosomatics 43:156–157, 2002b

Trzepacz PT, Bourne R, Zhang S: Designing clinical trials for the treatment of delirium. J Psychosomatic Research 65:299–307, 2008

Tsutsui S, Kitamura M, Higachi H, et al: Development of postoperative delirium in relation to a room change in the general surgical unit. Surg Today 26:292–294, 1996

Tune LE, Dainloth NF, Holland A, et al: Association of postoperative delirium with raised serum levels of anticholinergic drugs. Lancet 2(8248):651–653, 1981

Tune L, Carr S, Hoag E, et al: Anticholinergic effects of drugs commonly prescribed for the elderly: potential means for assessing risk of delirium. Am J Psychiatry 149:1393–1394, 1992

Turkel SB, Braslow K, Tavare CJ, et al: The Delirium Rating Scale in children and adolescents. Psychosomatics 44:126–129, 2003

Turkel SB, Trzepacz PT, Tavare J: Comparing symptoms of delirium in adults and children. Psychosomatics 47:320, 2006

Uchiyama M, Tanaka K, Isse K, et al: Efficacy of mianserin on symptoms of delirium in the aged: an open trial study. Prog Neuropsychopharmacol Biol Psychiatry 20:651–656, 1996

Van den Boogaard M, Pickkers P, van der Hoeven H, et al: Implementation of a delirium assessment tool in the ICU can influence haloperidol use. Crit Care 13(4):R131, 2009

van der Cammen TJ, Tiemeier H, Engelhart MJ, et al: Abnormal neurotransmitter metabolite levels in Alzheimer patients with a delirium. Int J Geriatr Psychiatry 21:838–843, 2006

van der Mast RC: Detecting and measuring the severity of delirium with the Symptom Rating Scale for Delirium, in Delirium After Cardiac Surgery. Thesis, Erasmus University Rotterdam, Amsterdam, Benecke Consultants, 1994, pp 78–89

van der Mast RC, Fekkes D: Serotonin and amino acids: partners in delirium pathophysiology? Semin Clin Neuropsychiatry 5:125–131, 2000

van der Mast RC, van den Broek WW, Fekkes D, et al: Incidence of and preoperative predictors for delirium after cardiac surgery. J Psychosom Res 46:479–483, 1999

Van Munster BC, Korevaar JC, Zwinderman AH, et al: Time-course of cytokines during delirium in elderly patients with hip fractures. J Am Geriatr Soc 56:1704–1709, 2008

Van Munster BC, Yazdanpanah M, Tanck MW, et al: Genetic polymorphisms in the DRD2, DRD3, and SLC6A3 gene in elderly patients with delirium. Am J Med Genet 153B:38–45, 2009

van Zyl LT, Davidson PR: Delirium in hospital: an underreported event at discharge. Can J Psychiatry 48:555–560, 2003

Voyer P, McCusker J, Cole MG, et al: Influence of prior cognitive impairment on the severity of delirium symptoms among older patients. J Neurosci Nurs 38:90–101, 2006

Voyer P, McCusker J, Cole MG, et al: Factors associated with delirium severity among older patients. J Clin Nurs 16:819–831, 2007

Wahlund L, Bjorlin GA: Delirium in clinical practice: experiences from a specialized delirium ward. Dement Geriatr Cogn Disord 10:389–392, 1999

Wanich CK, Sullivan-Marx EM, Gottlieb GL, et al: Functional status outcomes of a nursing intervention in hospitalized elderly. Image J Nurs Sch 24:201–207, 1992

Webster R, Holroyd S: Prevalence of psychotic symptoms in delirium. Psychosomatics 41:519–522, 2000

Weiss JH, Yin H-Z, Choir DW: Basal forebrain cholinergic neurons are selectively vulnerable to AMPA/kainate receptor-mediated neurotoxicity. Neuroscience 60:659–664, 1994

Wengel SP, Roccaforte WH, Burke WJ: Donepezil improves symptoms of delirium in dementia: implications for future research. J Geriatr Psychiatry Neurol 11:159–161, 1998

Wengel SP, Burke WJ, Roccaforte WH: Donepezil for postoperative delirium associated with Alzheimer's disease. J Am Geriatr Soc 47:379–380, 1999

Wernicke C, Smolka M, Gallinat J, et al: Evidence for the importance of the human dopamine transporter gene for withdrawal symptomatology of alcoholics in a German population. Neurosci Lett 333:45–48, 2002

Wetli CV, Mash D, Karch SB: Cocaine-associated agitated delirium and the neuroleptic malignant syndrome. Am J Emerg Med 14:425–428, 1996

Williams MA, Campbell EB, Raynor WJ, et al: Reducing acute confusional states in elderly patients with hip fractures. Res Nurs Health 8:329–337, 1985

Williams PD, Helton DR: The proconvulsive activity of quinolone antibiotics in an animal model. Toxicol Lett 58:23–28, 1991

Williams-Russo P, Urquhart BL, Sharrock NE, et al: Post-operative delirium: predictors and prognosis in elderly orthopedic patients. J Am Geriatr Soc 40:759–767, 1992

Wilson LM: Intensive care delirium: the effect of outside deprivation in a windowless unit. Arch Intern Med 130:225–226, 1972

Wilt JL, Minnema AM, Johnson RF, et al: Torsades de pointes associated with the use of intravenous haloperidol. Ann Intern Med 119:391–394, 1993

Wodarz N, Bobbe G, Eichhammer P, et al: The candidate gene approach in alcoholism: are there gender-specific differences? Arch Womens Ment Health 6:225–230, 2003

Wolff HG, Curran D: Nature of delirium and allied states: the dysergastic reaction. Archives of Neurology and Psychiatry 33:1175–1215, 1935

World Health Organization: International Statistical Classification of Diseases and Related Health Problems, 10th Revision. Geneva, World Health Organization, 1992

Yamamoto T, Lyeth BG, Dixon CE, et al: Changes in regional brain acetylcholine content in rats following unilateral and bilateral brainstem lesions. J Neurotrauma 5:69–79, 1988

Yokota H, Ogawa S, Kurokawa A, et al: Regional cerebral blood flow in delirium patients. Psychiatry Clin Neurosci 57: 337–339, 2003

Zaubler T, Slater J, Bustamo R, et al: Intraoperative cerebral oxygen desaturation: a significant risk factor for postoperative delirium in cardiac surgery patients. Oral presentation at the annual meeting of the Academy of Psychosomatic Medicine, Las Vegas, NV, November 2009

CHAPTER

6

Dementia

Antonio Lobo, M.D., Ph.D.

Pedro Saz, M.D., Ph.D.

Miguel Ángel Quintanilla, M.D., Ph.D.

CONCERN IS INCREASING about the worldwide epidemic (Ferri et al. 2005) and consequences of dementia. The high prevalence of dementing conditions in medical settings, often undiagnosed, and the association of dementia with longer hospital stays and greater use of health resources have direct implications for psychosomatic medicine and consultation-liaison psychiatry (Table 6–1). The psychiatric consultant is an invaluable collaborator with other health care professionals in the identification, evaluation, treatment, management, discharge planning, placement, and rehabilitation of the patient with dementia. In this chapter, we focus on the general clinical approach to dementia and its common causes. Some of these and other causes of dementia are also discussed elsewhere in this book: those disorders that are particularly likely to present with other neurological symptoms in Chapter 32, "Neurology and Neurosurgery"; HIV infection in Chapter 28, "HIV/AIDS"; other infections in Chapter 27, "Infectious Diseases"; alcohol and other substance use in Chapter 17, "Substance-Related Disorders"; toxic/metabolic conditions in Chapter 22, "Endocrine and Metabolic Disorders," and Chapter 37, "Medical Toxicology"; rheumatological/inflammatory conditions in Chapter 25, "Rheumatology"; traumatic brain injury in Chapter 35, "Physical Medicine and Rehabilitation"; and paraneoplastic syndromes in Chapter 23, "Oncology."

Concept of Dementia and Clinical Approach

Dementia is defined as a syndrome of global deterioration of intellectual function occurring in clear consciousness and caused by brain disease. It is a paradigm of the disease model in psychiatry (McHugh and Slavney 1998). The notion of deterioration emphasizes the acquired nature of the impairment in dementia, to distinguish it from mental retardation, and the requirement of clear consciousness underlines the difference from delirium, if dementia is the only diagnosis. The impairment of memory is the most frequent and important sign or symptom, but deterioration in at least two other cognitive domains is required in our operational definition (Table 6–2). Also, the deterioration must be severe enough to adversely affect activities of daily living (ADLs). Social or occupational activities are also impaired.

Deterioration in personality and noncognitive psychopathological symptoms are almost universal in dementia (Lyketsos et al. 2002; Steinberg et al. 2008) and are most important for psychiatrists. Although there is general agreement that only the cognitive psychopathology should be included in the diagnostic criteria, we have argued for the inclusion of noncognitive, psychopathological symptoms, particularly negative symptoms in view of their frequency

We gratefully acknowledge research grants from the Fondo de Investigación Sanitaria, Ministry of Health, Spain (PI 042722); Centro de Investigación Biomédica en Red de Salud Mental (CIBERSAM), Ministry of Science and Innovation, Spain. We also wish to thank Olga Ibáñez for her administrative help.

TABLE 6–1. Relevance of dementia in psychosomatic medicine and consultation-liaison psychiatry

General relevance

- Worldwide epidemic (Ferri et al. 2005)
- High prevalence: 9.6% in the U.S. elderly community (Breitner et al. 1999); 74% in nursing homes (Macdonald et al. 2002)
- High incidence: 2.8 per 1,000 person-years in 65- to 69- year age group; increases to 56.1 per 1,000 person-years in the older-than-90-year age group (Kukull et al. 2002)
- Dramatic increase in the projected dementia rates is expected in the next decades (Organization for Economic Cooperation and Development 2002)
- Burden of the disease:
  Patient-related
  Caregiver-related (Colvez et al. 2002)
  DAT leads to earlier institutionalization (Patterson et al. 1999)
  DAT patients occupy two-thirds of nursing home beds (Macdonald et al. 2002)
  Gross annual cost of caring for people with dementia living in the United States (National Institute on Aging 2003): $100 billion
- Mortality rate at least twice that of individuals without dementia (Dewey and Saz 2001)

Specific relevance to psychosomatic medicine and consultation-liaison psychiatry

- High prevalence in general hospital patients (Erkinjuntti et al. 1986)
- High prevalence in specific medical conditions
- One-third of elderly referrals to consultation-liaison psychiatrists go undiagnosed (Huyse et al. 1996)
- Almost all patients have noncognitive neuropsychiatric symptoms (Lyketsos et al. 2002; Saz et al. 2009)
- Most patients with early dementia go undiagnosed, both in the general population (Lobo et al. 1997) and in primary care (Boise et al. 2004)
- Patients with dementia have longer hospital stays, which are associated with higher costs and greater use of health resources after discharge (Lyketsos et al. 2000)

Note. DAT=dementia of the Alzheimer's type.

and relative specificity (Saz et al. 2009). Persistence of the syndrome is important for the diagnosis, and some international committees require that symptoms be present for at least 6 months (World Health Organization 1992). However, exceptions to this norm occur and are important in settings such as the general hospital. Progression of the syndrome is the norm in most cases of dementia but is not included in the concept because some cases of dementia are stable and potentially reversible.

Recent research has identified a construct known as *mild cognitive impairment,* a possible transitional state between the cognitive changes of normal aging and dementia (Petersen 2004). Mild cognitive impairment is defined as an entity of subjective memory difficulties, accompanied by cognitive difficulties documented by neuropsychological tests in individuals who are otherwise functioning well and do not meet the clinical criteria for dementia. Several studies have shown that persons without dementia who have cognitive impairment have a higher chance of progressing to dementia, the annual conversion rate being 10%–15%. However, mild cognitive impairment is a heterogeneous concept (Wahlund et al. 2003), and most cases do not progress to dementia, even after a follow-up period of 10 years (Mitchell 2009).

TABLE 6–2. The dementia syndrome

A. Global deterioration of intellectual function
   Memory
   At least two other cognitive functions

B. Clear consciousness

C. Impairment of personal activities of daily living and social or occupational activities due to the decline in intellectual function

D. Deterioration in emotional control, motivation, or personality frequent but not necessary for diagnosis

E. Duration of at least 6 months (important exceptions, such as in the general hospital)

Epidemiology, Etiology, and Risk Factors

Dementia has been etiologically associated with numerous heterogeneous conditions, as listed in Table 6–3. The adjusted prevalence estimate was 9.6% for all dementias in the U.S. population after age 65 and 6.5% for dementia of the Alzheimer's type (DAT) (Breitner et al. 1999). Similar rates have been reported in Europe (A. Lobo et al. 2000). It has been estimated that the number of patients with DAT will continue to increase in the United States (L.E. Hebert et al. 2001), but most of the dementia epidemic will occur in the developing world (Ferri et al. 2005).

Incidence estimates of dementia show that DAT rates rise from 2.8 per 1,000 person-years (age group: 65–69 years) to 56.1 per 1,000 person-years (age group: older than 90 years) (Kukull et al. 2002). These data are consistent with those in comparable studies in countries outside the United States (Fratiglioni et al. 2000). In all these population studies, both the prevalence and the incidence rates of elderly patients with dementia, and DAT in particular, increase dramatically with age, approximately doubling every 5 years.

DAT and vascular dementia have been reported to be the most frequent types of dementia in population studies (Fratiglioni et al. 2000; Van der Flier and Scheltens 2005). However, research suggests that a clinical diagnosis of dementia made during life may fail to reflect the pathogenic complexity of this condition in very elderly persons because most cases at autopsy have significant mixtures of dementia-related lesions, including DAT and vascular-type lesions (Neuropathology Group, Medical Research Council Cognitive Function and Aging Study 2001; White et al. 2005). Both dementia with Lewy bodies (DLB) and frontotemporal dementia (FTD) in cases of earlier onset may prove to be considerably more common than previously recognized (Campbell et al. 2001).

Dementia is also commonly found in general hospitals. A large-scale study documented that 9.1% of the patients age 55 years and older admitted to a teaching hospital medical service had dementia, but the prevalence was 31.2% in patients age 85 years and older (Erkinjuntti et al. 1986). Dementia is also common in elderly patients with alcoholism (60%–70%) (Kasahara et al. 1996), Parkinson's disease (Aarsland et al. 2001), HIV disease (American Academy of Neurology AIDS Task Force 1991), and traumatic brain injury (TBI; Kraus and Sorenson 1994).

The prevalence of mild cognitive impairment ranges between 3% and 19% in population studies in individuals age 65 years or older (Gauthier et al. 2006). It may account for more than one-third of the patients referred to memory clinics (Wahlund et al. 2003).

Epidemiological studies also have suggested that noncognitive, psychopathological symptoms, sometimes called behavioral and psychological symptoms of dementia, predict a poorer outcome (Shin et al. 2005). They also may be early markers of the disease (E. Teng et al. 2007). Lyketsos et al. (2002) found in their population-based study that the most frequent disturbances among individuals with dementia were apathy (36%), depression (32%), and agitation or aggression (30%). The reported prevalence of depressive syndromes in dementia has ranged widely, from 10% to 54%, across recruitment sites (A. Lobo et al. 1995; Zubenko et al. 2003). The prevalence of depression varies according to diagnostic criteria used and was 44% when National Institute of Mental Health criteria were used (R. Teng et al. 2008). Depression in elderly patients with dementia may have different symptoms from depression in elderly patients without dementia and frequently has negative consequences for both patients and caregivers (Lyketsos and Lee 2004). Psychotic symptoms are also frequent in DAT and are associated with rapid cognitive deterioration (Ropacki and Jeste 2005).

In the first population-based estimate among those with mild cognitive impairment, 29% of the individuals were considered to have clinically significant neuropsychiatric symptoms during the previous month (Lyketsos et al. 2002). The behavior changes observed in mild cognitive impairment are similar to those of DAT and may help identify the subgroup of mild cognitive impairment patients with prodromal dementia (Apostolova and Cummings 2008).

Table 6–4 summarizes the results of recent, sophisticated analytic epidemiological research, including case-control studies in incident cases. Confirmed risk factors for DAT are scarce and limited to age, unalterable genetic factors (the apolipoprotein E epsilon4 [*APOE* ε4] genotype), and mild cognitive impairment. Mild cognitive impairment may have important clinical but also preventive implications (Modrego et al. 2005).

Other probable risk factors and protective factors in DAT are also listed in Table 6–4 (Ravaglia et al. 2005; Van der Flier and Scheltens 2005; Verghese et al. 2003). Recent meta-analytic studies have found evidence to support an association between depression and dementia from both case-control studies and prospective studies (Jorm 2001). Depression has to be seriously considered as a probable risk factor for dementia. The attributable risk of DAT related to cardiovascular risk factors is still debated (Posner et al. 2002), but research has suggested that cerebrovascular disease plays an important role in determining the presence of dementia and specifically DAT (Ivan et al. 2004; Launer 2002). Hypertension may be particularly relevant in this respect because it is very common in the commu-

TABLE 6–3. Disorders and conditions that may produce dementia syndromes

Degenerative disorders
- **Cortical**
  - Alzheimer's disease
  - Frontotemporal dementia
  - Dementia with Lewy bodies
- **Subcortical**
  - Parkinson's disease
  - Huntington's disease
  - Basal ganglia calcification
    - Wilson's disease
    - Striatonigral degeneration
    - Thalamic dementia
  - Progressive supranuclear palsy
  - Spinocerebellar degeneration
- **Others**
  - Demyelinating disorders
    - Multiple sclerosis
    - Others
  - Amyotrophic lateral sclerosis
  - Hallervorden-Spatz disease
  - Lafora myoclonus epilepsy

Vascular dementias
- Multi-infarct dementia
- Multiple large-vessel occlusions
- Strategic infarct dementia
- Lacunar state
- Binswanger's disease
- Chronic ischemia

Hydrocephalic dementias
- Communicating, normal pressure
- Noncommunicating

CNS infection–associated dementias
- HIV-associated dementia
- Creutzfeldt-Jakob disease
- Neurosyphilis
- Chronic meningitis
- Viral encephalitis
- Progressive multifocal leukoencephalopathy
- Fungal meningitis (cryptococcal)

Metabolic disorders
- **Anoxia**
  - Cardiac disease
  - Pulmonary failure
  - Anemia
  - Others
- **Chronic renal failure**
  - Uremic encephalopathy
  - Dialysis dementia
- **Hepatic failure**
  - Portosystemic encephalopathy
  - Acquired hepatocerebral degeneration
- **Endocrinopathies**
  - Thyroid disturbances
  - Cushing's syndrome
  - Parathyroid disturbances
  - Recurrent hypo- or hyperglycemia
- **Porphyria**
- **Vitamin deficiency states**
  - Thiamine (B_1)
  - Cyanocobalamin (B_{12})
  - Folate
  - Niacin
- **Other chronic metabolic abnormalities**
  - Hypo- or hypernatremia
  - Hematological conditions

Toxic conditions
- **Alcohol related**
- **Drugs**
  - Polydrug abuse
  - Psychotropic agents and anticonvulsants
  - Solvents and other inhalants
  - Anticholinergic compounds
  - Antineoplastic therapies
  - Corticosteroids, NSAIDs
  - Antihypertensive and cardiac medications
- **Metals**
  - Lead, mercury, arsenic, nickel, others
- **Industrial agents and pollutants**
  - Carbon monoxide
  - Organophosphate insecticides
  - Organochlorine pesticides
  - Perchloroethylene, toluene
  - Trichloroethane, trichloroethylene
  - Hydrocarbon inhalants
  - Others

Neoplastic dementias
- Meningioma
- Glioblastoma
- Metastases
- Paraneoplastic syndromes
  - Limbic encephalopathy
  - Others
- Others

Traumatic conditions
- Posttraumatic
- Subdural hematoma
- Dementia pugilistica

Chronic inflammatory conditions
- Systemic lupus erythematosus
- Other collagen-vascular disorders

Psychiatric disorders
- Depression
- Others

Note. CNS = central nervous system; NSAIDs = nonsteroidal anti-inflammatory drugs.

nity and may be preventable. However, hypotension also has been suggested as a risk factor (Qui et al. 2003). Until now, insufficient evidence has been found to support some factors hypothesized as increasing the risk for DAT, such as high aluminum levels and hyperhomocysteinemia, or others thought to be protective, such as low cholesterol levels, estrogen therapy, or antioxidants in the diet (Larrieu et al. 2004; Podewils et al. 2005). However, recent studies have suggested social isolation and loneliness as risk factors for DAT (R.S. Wilson et al. 2007) and the potential

TABLE 6–4. Risk factors and protective factors in dementias

Risk factors for dementia of the Alzheimer's type	
Older age	++
Female sex	+
Low education	+
First-degree relative with Alzheimer's	+
Down syndrome	+
Head trauma	+
Apolipoprotein ε4 allele	++
High aluminum levels	+/–
Cigarette smoking	+
Hypertension	+
Hyperhomocysteinemia	+/–
Depression	+
Mild cognitive impairment	++
Social isolation	+
Risk factors for vascular dementia	
Age >60 years	+
Male sex	+
Previous stroke	++
Stroke risk factors	
Hypertension	++
Heart disease/atrial fibrillation	+
Cigarette smoking	++
Diabetes mellitus	++
Excessive alcohol consumption (3 drinks/day)	+
Hyperlipidemia	+
Hyperhomocysteinemia, low serum folate levels	+
Previous mental decline	+/–
Protective factors for dementia of the Alzheimer's type	
Apolipoprotein ε2 allele[a]	++
Low cholesterol levels[a]	+/–
Statin drugs[a]	+/–
Antihypertensive drug treatment[a]	+
Moderate alcohol consumption	+/–
Other	
Hormone replacement therapy (estrogens)	+/–
Aspirin	–
Nonsteroidal anti-inflammatory drugs	+/–
Dietary factors (vitamin E, antioxidants, Mediterranean diet)	+/–
Lifestyle (active life, leisure activities, social support and network)	+/–

Note. ++ = confirmed; + = probable; +/– = controversial; – = negative.
[a]Protective factors also for vascular dementia.

protective effects of physical activity (Buchman et al. 2008; Taaffe et al. 2008) or the Mediterranean diet (Scarmeas et al. 2009). Although the preventive potential of moderate alcohol consumption has stirred considerable interest (Peters et al. 2008), it remains a controversial issue (E. Lobo, C. Dufouil, G. Marcos, B. Quetglas, P. Saz, E. Guallar, and A. Lobo, "Evidence Against and Association Between Alcohol Intake and Cognition in the Elderly: The ZARADEMP Project" [manuscript in review], May 2010).

Risk and protective factors for vascular dementia are also listed in Table 6–4. The risk factors include hyperhomocysteinemia and low serum folate levels, which are potentially reversible and can be identified early.

Genetics

Genetic knowledge about dementing conditions, most relevant if related to pathophysiology, may be summarized as follows. Huntington's disease is inherited as an autosomal dominant trait with complete penetrance, the mutation responsible being in an elongated and unstable trinucleotide (CAG) repeat on the short arm of chromosome 4 (Haskins and Harrison 2000). In DAT, particularly with early onset, several well-documented cases suggest that the disorder is transmitted in families through an autosomal dominant gene, although such transmission is rare. Possible genetic loci for familial DAT have been documented in chromosomes 21 (the amyloid precursor protein [APP] gene), 14 (the presenilin-1 gene), and 1 (the presenilin-2 gene). Furthermore, the *APOE* ε4 gene coded in chromosome 19 has been associated with an increased risk of developing DAT and might advance its age at onset by several years. A gene carried on chromosome 17 is thought to be related to familial multiple system tauopathy, an early-onset dementia similar to DAT.

Wilson's disease is an autosomal recessively inherited defect in the copper-carrying serum protein ceruloplasmin, resulting in the destructive deposition of copper in the basal nuclei, the defective gene being localized on chromosome 13 (Loudianos and Gitlin 2000). Recent advances in the genetics of other dementias include the identification of *tau* gene mutations on chromosome 17 in some familial cases of FTD (H.J. Rosen et al. 2000) and the identification of genetic loci in other disorders that produce dementia, such as Pick's disease; Gerstmann-Straussler-Scheinker syndrome, an autosomal dominant, familial type of prion dementia; cerebral autosomal dominant arteriopathy with subcortical infarcts and leukoencephalopathy; some forms of cerebral amyloid angiopathy; alcoholism; major depression; and some forms of Parkinson's disease (Lev and Melamed 2001).

Important changes in the classification of dementia might soon occur following dramatic advances in the genetics of dementia. Tau aggregates and alpha-synucleinopathy aggregates observed in neurodegenerative disorders have generated the concepts of tauopathies and alpha-synucleinopathies, respectively, to differentiate them from the amyloidopathies such as DAT. Most cases of FTD now tend to be classified as tauopathies, related to mutations in the *tau* gene (Buee et al. 2000), with a large clinical spectrum including Pick's disease, progressive supranuclear palsy (PSP), corticobasal degeneration, and multisystem atrophy (Lebert et al. 2002). Alpha-synucleinopathies include DLB and Parkinson's disease (Ferrer et al. 2002; Litvan 1999), but the findings of both types of pathological aggregates in several diseases have led to some disagreement in classifications (Iseki et al. 2003; Litvan 1999).

General Clinical Features

The Dementia Syndrome

The clinical picture may differ widely according to the type and severity of dementia, and the characteristics are important in the differential diagnosis. In most cases of degenerative processes—in particular, DAT, some types of vascular dementia, and dementias due to endocrinopathies, brain tumors, metabolic disorders, and abuse of medications—the onset of symptoms is gradual, and the signs of the dementia syndrome are subtle and may at first be ignored by both the patient and his or her relatives. In contrast, the onset may be abrupt after severe cerebral infarcts, head trauma, cardiac arrest with cerebral hypoxia, and encephalitis.

The full dementia syndrome progresses through severity levels in degenerative processes and is very characteristic in DAT (Table 6–5). The earliest manifestations, such as impairment of memory, may be very subtle. Individuals with dementia also show impairment in thinking and their capacity for reasoning, but the earliest difficulties can be mistakenly disregarded or explained away as the expression of fatigue, distraction, or discouragement. The deficits may become apparent in the face of more complex problems or when specifically tested, but patients often attempt to compensate for defects by using strategies to avoid showing failures in intellectual performance. Similarly, language is impoverished if carefully observed, and praxic difficulties for complex tasks may be documented, but special examinations may be necessary. A general loss of efficiency in all aspects of thinking as well as disturbances in the executive functions necessary to maintain goal-directed behavior, including planning, organizing, and sequencing, may be apparent, and the patient has difficulties in his or her usual occupation and with ADLs, such as using the telephone, managing small amounts of money, cooking, or taking responsibility for medications.

The dementia syndrome in degenerative disorders such as DAT relentlessly progresses to severe deterioration (see Table 6–5). Eventually, the patient may retain only the earliest learned information; he or she is totally disoriented, with extreme impoverishment of thought, and communication with the patient is impossible. Apraxia and agnosia are severe. The patient is incontinent of urine and feces and is entirely dependent on caregivers. He or she may be totally disconnected from his or her environment, with respect to both input and output. The most severe neurological signs, including primitive reflexes, motor system rigidity, and flexion contractures, are then present, and the patient is confined to bed. The patient may experience a final stage of decortication, but death, from pneumonia or some other infection, commonly occurs before this stage.

Changes in personality and behavior are frequent, and the patient may seem to be less concerned than he or she had been about issues of daily life or about the effects of his or her behavior on others. Catastrophic reactions, with agitation or extreme emotion, also may be observed as a reaction to the subjective awareness of the patient's inability to cope with a problem.

Noncognitive, psychopathological symptoms are often quite disturbing for patients and caregivers (Shin et al. 2005) and may be quite persistent unless treated. The modern classification of these symptoms distinguishes delirium, affective syndrome, psychotic syndrome, drive disturbances (sleep and eating), and specific problem behaviors (usually in late stages). Major depressive episodes are frequent in DAT and other types of dementia (Zubenko et al. 2003) and often have serious adverse consequences for patients and their caregivers. Paranoid ideas are frequent, often representing "logical" conclusions based on misinterpretations, misperceptions, or memory deficits. They may not be persistent, but complex and well-systematized delusions, as well as hallucinations, are also reported (for all modalities). Late-evening agitation (the sundowning phenomenon) may be quite disturbing and has been associated with circadian rhythms in DAT (Volicer et al. 2001).

The course of the syndrome is also variable according to type of dementia and has implications for the differential diagnosis. An incrementally worsening or stepwise course is common in vascular dementia, whereas the deficits may be stable in some types of dementia, such as in dementia related to head trauma. Furthermore, the regression of symptoms is a possibility, once treatment is initiated, in dementias caused by potentially reversible disorders, such as normal-pressure hydrocephalus (NPH); metabolic and toxic conditions; or dementias related to

TABLE 6–5. Clinical findings in patients with dementia of the Alzheimer's type, by severity level

Mild (MMSE score = 18–23; duration of disease = 1–3 years)

- Impaired registration and recent memory (early sign); remote recall mildly impaired
- Defective temporal orientation
- Mild impairment of thinking; bewilderment in the face of complexity
- Impoverishment of language; naming problems
- Mild apraxia for complex tasks
- Agnosia not evident unless tested
- Difficulties in planning, sequencing, and executing instrumental activities of daily living
- Frequent personality changes: irritability, less apparent concern about issues of daily life and effects of their behavior on others
- Depression in approximately 20% of patients; mild apathy; loss of initiative; lack of energy
- Frequent misinterpretations; psychotic phenomena rare
- Urinary incontinence in fewer than 10%
- Other neurological signs and primitive reflexes rare

Moderate (MMSE score = 12–17; duration of disease = 2–8 years)

- Recent memory and remote recall more severely impaired
- Severe temporal disorientation, moderate spatial disorientation
- Obvious impairment of thinking; catastrophic reactions if pressured
- Fluent aphasia, anomia, paraphasic errors, empty quality of language, perseveration
- Praxic difficulties to manage dressing, feeding, manipulations
- Agnosia evident: failure to identify objects, including familiar faces
- Difficulties in planning, sequencing, and executing extend to basic activities of daily living
- Evident personality changes: marked irritability; marked lack of concern about issues of daily life and effects of their behavior on others
- Dysphoric mood, depression less frequent; apathy; loss of initiative
- Frequent psychotic phenomena (delusions, illusions, hallucinations)
- Restlessness, pacing, wandering occasionally, agitation, sporadic aggressiveness
- Urinary incontinence frequent; fecal incontinence rare
- Gait disorder and frequent primitive reflexes

Severe (MMSE score <12; duration of disease = 7–12 years)

- Memory: only earliest learned information retained
- Total disorientation
- Severe impairment of thinking; indifference in the face of failures
- Extreme impoverishment of language; communication impossible
- Complete incapacity to manage dressing, feeding, simple manipulations
- Severe agnosia: does not identify close relatives
- Total dependence for even basic activities of daily living
- Total disconnection from environment
- Affective indifference; severe apathy; loss of initiative
- Double incontinence (urinary and fecal)
- Motor system rigidity and flexion contractures of all limbs; final stage of decortication

Note. MMSE = Mini-Mental State Examination.

the use of medications, to subdural hematoma, or to brain tumors. In fact, studies have found that only 4%–23% of the patients referred to memory clinics had potentially reversible conditions (Hejl et al. 2002), and actual reversal of dementia through treatment is rare (Ovsiew 2003).

Clinicopathological Correlations

Some clinical characteristics suggest the involvement of specific brain areas and should help in clinical recognition of entities with different implications, as well as in understanding the underlying pathology of cognitive and noncognitive phenomena (McHugh and Folstein 1979). *Cortical dementia* is the conceptual term for those dementias in which the predominance of dysfunction is in the cortex, even if coexisting pathology exists in subcortical regions (Cummings and Benson 1984). Together with amnesia, not helped by cues to remember, the most characteristic signs are aphasia, apraxia, and agnosia, which are often designated the four *A*'s (Table 6–6).

Subcortical dementia describes the predominant involvement of the white and deep gray matter structures, such as basal ganglia, thalamus, and their frontal lobe projections. McHugh and Folstein (1975) were among the first to emphasize that parts of the brain other than the cortex have a role in cognitive activity and described the distinctive combination of three features in what they called the "subcortical dementia syndrome": a slowly progressive dilapidation of all cognitive powers; prominent psychic apathy and inertia that may worsen to akinetic mutism; and the absence of aphasia, alexia, or agnosia (see Table 6–6). The same authors also emphasized the early appearance in subcortical dementia of prominent noncognitive symptoms, particularly depression and other affective disturbances considered to be a direct consequence of the cerebral pathology. Rabins et al. (1999) have designated some specific features of subcortical dementia as the four *D*'s:

- Dysmnesia—memory impairment; patients may benefit from cues to remember
- Dysexecutive—related to troubles with decision making
- Delay—related to slowed thinking and moving
- Depletion—reduced complexity of thought

When both cortical and subcortical regions are involved, the clinical characteristics include aspects of cortical dementia, such as aphasia and apraxia, and the apathetic state characteristic of lesions in the subcortical areas.

Clinical Types and Pathophysiology of Dementia

Cortical Dementias

Alzheimer's Disease

Most cases of Alzheimer's disease start after age 65, but an earlier onset is not infrequent. The characteristic general dementia syndrome has been described and includes the cortical signs (see Tables 6–5 and 6–6). The insidious onset and slowly worsening, relentless course are most characteristic and crucial in the diagnostic process. Other char-

TABLE 6–6. Clinical characteristics of cortical and subcortical dementia syndromes

	Cortical	Subcortical
Aphasia	Early	No
Agnosia	Late	No
Apraxia	Rather early	Rare
Alexia	Rather late	No
Apathy, inertia	Rare or late	Very marked, early
Loss of initiative	Frequent, late	Marked
Psychomotor retardation	Rare or late	Very marked, early
Amnesia	Recall and recognition not aided by cues to remember	Recognition better preserved, may be aided by cues to remember
Gait	Normal until late	Abnormal, early
Extrapyramidal signs	Rare or late	Very marked, early
Pathological reflexes (grasp, snout, suck, etc.)	Late	Rare
Affective syndromes	Less frequent	Frequent, severe

acteristic clinical signs and symptoms include 1) a "hippocampal type" of memory difficulty, which is not reliably aided by cues on memory testing and has a high number of intrusions and false recognitions; 2) language difficulties, including a fluent aphasia with anomia, paraphasic errors, and a tendency of the patient to perseverate; 3) the capability of the patient in many cases to continue to recognize objects and to use them appropriately when he or she can no longer name them accurately; and 4) agnosia for faces, including family faces in late stages of the disease. Gait disorder in the middle stages is also common, as well as frontal signs such as grasping and sucking reflexes, along with a change in muscular tone.

The neuropathology of this condition is its defining characteristic (Folstein and McHugh 1983); its extent and severity correlate with the type and severity of the cognitive signs and symptoms. Cortical atrophy occurs, with widened sulci and ventricular enlargement. The most severe changes occur in the medial temporal lobe, including the hippocampus. Areas of association cortex in the parietotemporal lobes, and to a lesser degree the frontal lobes, are also involved. Characteristic microscopic findings are neuronal loss; synaptic loss, particularly in the cortex; senile plaques, with a core of amyloid peptide; neurofibrillary tangles, containing abnormally phosphorylated tau proteins; granulovacuolar degeneration of the neurons; and amyloid angiopathy. The location and abundance of microscopic findings determine the postmortem histological diagnosis of Alzheimer's disease (Cummings et al. 1998). The cause of DAT is not well known. Heredity is important in its causation, and genes implicated have been discussed earlier in this chapter. However, it is likely that DAT is heterogeneous. It is suspected that the primary process may occur many years before clinical symptoms are apparent. This process would initiate a cascade of events leading to neuronal cell death, and this would eventually result in characteristic signs and symptoms.

The amyloid hypothesis gives an important pathogenic role to the APP. The abnormal breakdown of this protein present in neuronal membranes would lead to deposition of the amyloid peptide to form the senile plaques. This is considered to be a central phenomenon in the pathogenesis of DAT. Hope is now placed in studies to disentangle the way in which APP is converted to beta-amyloid because this may lead to specific preventive treatments.

Several studies have supported the cholinergic deficit hypothesis in DAT, including specific degeneration of cholinergic neurons in the nucleus basalis of Meynert; decreases in acetylcholine and choline acetyltransferase concentrations in the brain; and observations about the role of cholinergic agonists and antagonists. Other hypotheses are suggested by the decrease in norepinephrine activity and, more recently, by reports of decreased levels of many neurotransmitters, including serotonin and the neuroactive peptides somatostatin and corticotropin. Evidence also indicates that the excitatory activity of L-glutamate plays a role in the pathogenesis of DAT. However, some research suggests that vascular factors may play an important role in determining the presence and severity of the clinical symptoms of DAT (Launer 2002).

Dementia With Lewy Bodies

DLB is a condition of uncertain nosological status, with cortical signs suggesting DAT alongside the classic, extrapyramidal features of Parkinson's disease (McKeith et al. 1996). However, the typical neuropathological findings of DAT are much less common in this condition. The distinctive feature is the presence of Lewy bodies, intracellular inclusion bodies in the cortex, particularly in limbic areas, whereas in Parkinson's disease they are typically found in subcortical regions. Most authors now include both DLB and Parkinson's disease among the alpha-synucleinopathies on the basis of recent pathological findings (Boeve 2006). Mean age at disease onset varies between 60 and 80 years. Psychotic syndromes and confusional states are common and may be the presenting symptomatology. Other characteristics include relative preponderance of visuospatial and frontal lobe signs and clear day-to-day fluctuations in symptoms and cognitive performance. Parkinsonian features, together with fluctuation in cognitive performance, hallucinations, and delusions, are core features of the diagnosis (McKeith et al. 2005). Patients who have DLB have frequent falls and/or transient, unexplained episodes of loss of consciousness. They have a characteristic vulnerability to neuroleptics, which frequently exacerbate extrapyramidal dysfunction. Such reactions may be severe and may include acute episodes of rigidity, instability, and falls. DLB patients may have a dramatic decline in the late stage of the disease, death coming after a few months of very severe neurological and psychiatric symptoms.

Frontotemporal Dementia

FTD syndromes, often accompanied by cortical signs, are also the result of neurodegenerative diseases. The most characteristic features that distinguish FTD from DAT are personality changes and neuropsychiatric symptoms, which may be quite marked and precede the cognitive decline by several years. The psychiatric symptoms in FTD include marked irritability; poor judgment; defective control of impulses, including violent impulses in some cases; disinhibition; and a general disregard for the conventional rules of social conduct. Restlessness and hyperorality also have been reported. Social withdrawal or overt depression may be the first symptom in some patients. Executive dysfunction is a frequent early sign of the disease. Language disorder may be the initial manifestation when the temporal lobes are the main site of pathology. Onset of FTD is usually earlier than in DAT, in the fifth decade of life, and the average duration is 10 years. In clinical samples, it may be the second most common type of dementia, after DAT.

Neuronal loss and gliosis in the frontotemporal areas define this type of neurodegenerative dementia. Several types of FTD have been described, the differences being related to predominant location of lesions and the corresponding signs and symptoms. They include the frontal lobe subtype, the thalamostriatal subtype, the motor neuron subtype, and the amnestic subtype. Pick's disease, characterized by the presence of distinctive intraneuronal Pick bodies and ballooned Pick cells on microscopic examination, may be diagnosed in up to 25% of cases. This disease and the remaining types of FTDs tend now to be classified as tauopathies, with a large clinical spectrum including Pick's disease, PSP, corticobasal degeneration, and multisystem atrophy (Lebert et al. 2002). PSP is often classified among the subcortical dementias because of the predominance of subcortical signs. Primary progressive aphasia is an atypical dementia typified by insidious and progressive impairments in language, with relative preservation of memory and other cortical functions. Although the disorder was once thought to be rare, it is now recognized as being not uncommon (Mesulam 2003).

Subcortical Dementias

Huntington's Disease

Huntington's disease has the three main characteristics of the subcortical dementia syndrome (Folstein and McHugh 1983), together with the classic choreoathetoid movement disorder and a positive family history. Huntington's disease usually has its onset in the third or fourth decade, although juvenile forms occasionally occur. The psychopathology, both cognitive and noncognitive, may appear before the movement abnormalities. The initial pattern of subcortical dementia evolves into the global impairment seen in mixed dementias. Very severe cognitive loss and profound self-neglect, resembling an akinetic mute state, may be seen in the last stage of the disease. Several authors also have reported prominent symptoms that may be difficult to differentiate from primary mood disorder, particularly depression. However, demoralization and depressive reactions are also frequent, and the risk of suicide is increased (Huntington 1872). Suspiciousness and misinterpretations are quite common, but delusions and hallucinations with paranoid and catatonic features also have been described.

The neuropathology in Huntington's disease includes atrophy of the caudate nucleus and loss of gamma-aminobutyric acid (GABA) interneurons (Lishman 1998).

Parkinson's Disease

A typical subcortical, progressive dementia syndrome may occur in patients with Parkinson's disease, and recent studies suggest that it may eventually affect most patients (Aarsland et al. 2003). However, contrary to Huntington's disease, it tends to occur late in the course of the illness, after the motor symptoms have advanced significantly. Classic parkinsonian signs in a patient with dementia point to the diagnosis. Apathy is particularly prominent and may advance to an akinetic mute state. Individual parkinsonian patients endure a wide variety of psychopathological symptoms, including frequent emotional reactions to the disease, but a depressive disorder identical to that seen in affective illness and responsive to the usual treatments is found in approximately one-third of patients (Miyasaki et al. 2006).

Nigral pathology alone is probably not sufficient for the development of dementia in Parkinson's disease and requires the spread of pathology to other subcortical nuclei, the limbic system, and the cerebral cortex. The main degenerative pathology seems to be Lewy body type, principally made of alpha-synuclein (Duyckaerts et al. 2003). Losses of cholinergic, dopaminergic, and noradrenergic innervation have been suggested to be the underlying neurochemical deficits.

Wilson's Disease

Subcortical dementia with characteristic extrapyramidal signs also may be seen in Wilson's disease. This combination of symptoms, together with onset during adolescence or early adulthood, should suggest the diagnosis. Cognitive deficits are usually mild, and psychosis is infrequent. However, depressive syndromes, irritability, disinhibition, personality changes, and poor impulse control are common, with the severity paralleling the severity of the neurological signs (Shanmugiah et al. 2008). The psychopathological features result from destructive deposition of copper in the basal nuclei (Starosta-Rubinstein 1995) because of an inherited defect in the copper-carrying serum protein ceruloplasmin.

Normal-Pressure Hydrocephalus

NPH can present as a very characteristic neuropsychiatric syndrome, a triad of clinical symptoms combining motoric and psychopathological features (Folstein and McHugh 1983; McHugh 1966): 1) an early gait disturbance, resembling the stiff steps of spastic paraparesis; 2) subcortical dementia with particularly severe apathetic features; and

3) urinary incontinence that may not appear until late in the course. An insidious onset with cognitive difficulties is common, but the illness may eventually progress to a state resembling akinetic mutism if untreated. Studies monitoring cerebrospinal fluid pressure have shown waves of increased pressure that are exaggerated in NPH patients. The resulting mechanical pressure on the subcortex tissue surrounding lateral and third ventricles may lead in chronic hydrocephalus to exhaustion of the normal elasticity of brain tissue and eventually to tissue destruction.

Mixed Dementia and Dementia in Disseminated Brain Diseases

Vascular Dementia

Vascular dementia is defined as the dementia resulting from ischemic, ischemic-hypoxic, or hemorrhagic brain lesions due to cerebrovascular or cardiovascular pathology. Clinical findings in vascular dementia are heterogeneous and depend to a great extent on the speed, total volume, and localization of the lesions (Knopman 2006). Typically, the onset is in the 70s, and the dementia syndrome is the result of small or large brain infarcts, which lead to cognitive deterioration when they have enough cumulative effects on critical areas of the brain. However, cognitive impairment and dementia also can be seen in chronic ischemia without frank infarction. Acute onset usually develops after stroke, either from thrombosis, from an embolism, or rarely from a single massive hemorrhage. Onset and course of dementia are often more gradual in so-called multi-infarct dementia, as a consequence of many minor ischemic episodes, which produce an accumulation of lacunae in the cerebral parenchyma.

Cortical dementia occurs when the infarcts affect primarily the cortex, with focal neurological signs being the norm. Subcortical dementia is typically seen in patients with a history of hypertension and foci of ischemic destruction in the deep white matter of the cerebral hemispheres. A variant of vascular dementia results from extensive subcortical degeneration and white matter loss, known as *leukoaraiosis,* as a result of chronic vascular insufficiency. In such cases, extensive, diffuse demyelination of white matter can be seen in periventricular regions, and recent neuroimaging techniques have shown that the condition is more frequent than previously suspected. Mixed cortical and subcortical syndromes are also common in vascular dementia, with neuroimaging findings or autopsy findings suggesting the presence of lesions in both cerebral areas. Mild cognitive impairment of the vascular type also has been described, with an outcome worse than in nonvascular mild cognitive impairment (Frisoni et al. 2002).

The course of vascular dementia has classically been described as stepwise and patchy, but advances in brain imaging techniques have shown that patients with vascular dementia may have clinical courses as gradual and smooth as in patients with DAT. Noncognitive symptoms are common. Poststroke depression, independent of the disability caused by the disease, is frequent. Emotional lability, with transient depressive mood, weeping, or explosive laughter, is also a classic finding in these patients. Personality is usually relatively preserved, but in a proportion of patients, personality changes may be evident, with apathy or disinhibition or the accentuation of previous traits such as egocentricity, paranoid attitude, or irritability.

In more than two-thirds of vascular dementia patients, the pathological correlate is the lacunar state, characterized by multiple lacunar infarctions in subcortical structures such as the basal ganglia and thalamus. The term *vascular cognitive impairment* has been proposed to broaden the current definitions of vascular dementia to recognize the important part cerebrovascular disease plays in several cognitive disorders, including DAT and other degenerative dementias (O'Brien et al. 2003). It is now estimated that the prevalence of mixed cases of vascular dementia and DAT has been underestimated (Langa et al. 2004); that pure vascular dementia is rare; and that, in addition to simple coexistence, vascular dementia and DAT may share common pathogenetic mechanisms (Jellinger 2002).

Prion Dementias

Prion dementias are uncommon diseases that are now considered to be caused by an abnormal form of a normal cerebral protein named *prion protein.* This protein is encoded by a gene on chromosome 20. Because the diseases are transmissible by transferring the altered prion proteins, they act like infectious agents. Nevertheless, neither immunological response nor viruses have been detected in the process.

Creutzfeldt-Jakob disease is one such dementia and is considered to be a sporadic nonfamilial form. It has an extremely rapid course. Cognitive deterioration is progressive, widespread, very severe, and accompanied by pyramidal and extrapyramidal signs, early characteristic myoclonic jerks, muscle rigidity, and ataxia. The average onset is in the 50s, and death usually occurs in 6–12 months (Will et al. 1996). Pathological findings are widespread in both the cortex and the subcortical structures. Spongiform change in neurons is characteristic, and neuronal loss and astrocytic proliferation occur. The clinical diagnosis is based on the rapid progression of dementia, with myoclonic jerks and a characteristic electroencephalogram (EEG) pattern with bursts of generalized, triphasic complexes in most cases (Bourgeois et al. 2008). Brain imaging may be normal. A specific protein, the "14-3-3 protein" has been reported in the cerebrospinal fluid in a proportion of patients (Waldemar et al. 2007).

A new form of Creutzfeldt-Jakob disease has been detected in Europe. It may begin earlier, before age 40 years, and signs, symptoms, and progression of the disease are similar to those in the original form. It is believed to be the human form of bovine spongiform encephalopathy. An autosomal-dominant familial type, known as Gerstmann-Straussler-Scheinker syndrome, also has been described. This genetic form has similar clinical and pathological features but is less malignant, and death usually occurs after several years.

Infection-Associated Dementias

HIV-associated dementia, formerly called *AIDS dementia complex,* is now the most common dementia caused by an infectious disease (see also Chapter 27, "Infectious Diseases," and Chapter 28, "HIV/AIDS"). Cognitive deterioration is frequently observed in infection with HIV-1 and may be severe enough to fulfill criteria for dementia (World Health Organization 1990). Cognitive dysfunction may be the earliest or the only clinical manifestation of AIDS. At least two types of AIDS-associated dementia have been described. In one of them, the heterogeneity of psychopathological manifestations and the occurrence of both cortical and subcortical features suggest disseminated brain pathology. This is most likely the result of opportunistic infections common in advanced stages of HIV. The other type is a subcortical dementia, with prominent psychomotor retardation. It is considered to be caused directly by HIV, through activation of neurotoxic elements in the immune system.

Noncognitive psychopathology—in particular, depressive syndromes associated with cognitive dysfunction—is also common in patients infected with HIV-1. The incidence of dementia in patients with HIV has declined after the development of antiretroviral therapy, with early treatment. Furthermore, the prior prognosis with typical survival of a few months has now been improved considerably (Bourgeois et al. 2008).

Neurosyphilis may evolve into different types of dementia if left untreated. The most severe form is general paresis, which becomes evident 15–20 years after the original infection. The dementia may be easily recognized in the advanced state and is accompanied by characteristic signs, such as pupillary abnormalities, dysarthria, tremor of the tongue, and hypotonia. However, the onset is commonly insidious, and the diagnosis may be suggested when the initial memory difficulties are accompanied by indifference, facial quivering, tremor, and, sometimes, myoclonus. Intellectual deterioration is progressive and severe, with cortical deficits and often signs suggesting frontal lobe involvement, including disinhibited behavior. Psychotic phenomena, such as grandiose or hypochondriacal delusions, are common.

Chronic meningitis, caused by chronic bacterial, parasitic, or fungal infections, can eventually cause progressive dementia, with fluctuations in arousal and cognitive performance, apathy and lethargy, disorientation, and cranial nerve abnormalities.

Immunosuppressed or debilitated chronically ill patients are at special risk. Herpes simplex encephalitis may cause major neurological and cognitive sequelae. Because herpes encephalitis has a predilection for the temporal lobes, amnestic and aphasic syndromes are common, but dementia also can be seen. Other cortical signs reflect damage to other cortical areas.

Progressive multifocal leukoencephalopathy (PML) is a rare complication of a common subacute viral disorder, most commonly seen in immunosuppressed patients. Clinical signs and symptoms are quite heterogeneous, and the dementia may include both cortical and subcortical signs and symptoms, reflecting widespread lesions in the central nervous system. PML is usually progressive, with motor dysfunction and blindness sometimes developing; death commonly follows in a few months.

Metabolic and Toxic Dementias

Metabolic and toxic dementias (see also Chapter 22, "Endocrine and Metabolic Disorders," and Chapter 37, "Medical Toxicology") form a heterogeneous group of diseases (see Table 6-3) of special interest to the consultant psychiatrist because they are relatively frequent in medical settings and are potentially reversible. Dementia in these conditions has predominantly subcortical features but may have mixed characteristics. Psychomotor slowing may be severe in cases of hypothyroidism. Memory deficits are often accompanied by problems in executive function, with impaired attention and concentration also common. Whether the metabolic and toxic encephalopathies are best conceptualized as reversible dementias or as chronic deliria is unclear, and perhaps the distinction is primarily semantic, particularly in cases of hepatic, renal, and cardiopulmonary failure. Progression of the dementia is usually quite insidious, in relation to the chronicity of the metabolic or toxic condition, and the course tends to be disease specific.

The neuropathology in these conditions is not well known. Hippocampal neurons are probably most vulnerable to anoxic injury but are also vulnerable to severe hypercholesterolemia and to repeated or severe episodes of hypoglycemia, such as may occur in type 1 diabetes mellitus.

Hypothyroidism can produce subcortical damage through a mechanism of relative cerebral hypoxia. Vitamin B_{12} deficiency, as seen in pernicious anemia, has been associated with disseminated degeneration in areas of cortical white matter, the optic tracts, and the cerebellar peduncles. In pellagra, lack of nicotinic acid and probably other vitamin B deficiencies may lead to neuronal destruction.

Alcoholic dementia, one possible complication of chronic alcoholism, is more frequent after age 50 years and is likely multifactorial in etiology. The pathophysiology of this condition is not well known, but thiamine and other vitamin B deficiencies and multiple TBIs have been found in these patients. Pathological findings at autopsy suggest that this condition is probably underdiagnosed. The cognitive deficits are more global here than in pure amnestic syndrome (e.g., Korsakoff's psychosis), and unlike those patients, alcoholic patients with dementia may complain of decreased efficiency of memory and intellectual functioning. Neuropathological changes include cortical atrophy and nerve fiber disintegration with dissolution of myelin sheaths. Dementing syndromes are also seen in distinct brain diseases related to chronic alcoholism, such as Marchiafava-Bignami disease, with degeneration of the corpus callosum and anterior commissure, or in acquired hepatocerebral degeneration.

Dementing syndromes also may occur in chronic intoxication with medications, which can be either prescribed or abused by patients. The onset is insidious, and the course is progressive; physicians should be alert to the possibility of this reversible dementia. Benzodiazepines, including those with high potency and a short half-life, are known to cause anterograde amnesia and impairment of memory consolidation and subsequent memory retrieval. Elderly patients are more vulnerable to developing the dementia syndrome. Syndromes of cognitive deterioration have been reported in cocaine users and also in heavy users of cannabis.

Neoplastic-Associated Dementias

Neoplastic disease may affect any part of the brain and produce essentially any kind of neuropsychiatric symptoms, depending on tumor location and extent, as well as rapidity of tumor growth and propensity to cause increased intracranial pressure (see also Chapter 23, "Oncology," and Chapter 32, "Neurology and Neurosurgery"). Dementia is one such syndrome, and certain symptom clusters that occur with regularity may suggest the general location of lesions.

Initial symptoms of depression and some cognitive loss, with apathy, negativism, and akinesia, suggest the possibility of frontal lobe tumors such as meningioma or some forms of glioblastoma; a low performance on executive function tests further supports a frontal lobe site. Temporal lobe tumors are prone to produce seizures, and the psychiatric symptomatology may be complex and include features such as sexual disturbances, irritability, aggressiveness, and hallucinations. Tumors in the parietal region often cause characteristic language disorders when the location is in the dominant hemisphere. In the nondominant hemisphere, they tend to produce signs such as unilateral neglect or apraxia. Tumors around the third ventricle, such as craniopharyngiomas and colloid cysts, may obstruct the flow of spinal fluid and cause hydrocephalic, subcortical dementia.

Paraneoplastic limbic encephalitis is a nonmetastatic complication of small cell lung carcinoma (and less commonly several other cancers) and may manifest with dramatic, sudden onset of memory loss. A full dementia syndrome may eventually develop (Foster and Caplan 2009). Mood disturbance, behavior change, and sometimes psychotic symptoms are also common. Pathological findings include neuronal loss, astrocytosis, lymphocytic perivascular infiltration, and glial nodules. The psychiatric symptoms may antedate the diagnosis of malignancy by several years. Early medical intervention might considerably improve the outcome of treatment in some cases (Dalmau et al. 2008).

Dementia Following Traumatic Brain Injury

A variety of cognitive difficulties are very frequent after TBI (see also Chapter 35, "Physical Medicine and Rehabilitation"). Symptoms vary depending on the site of the lesion. Cognitive deficits become permanent in more than half of the patients if they do not recover memory and orientation within 2 weeks after injury. Common difficulties include dysmnesia, organic personality disorder, dysphasia, attentional disturbances, and impairments suggestive of frontal lobe damage, particularly executive dysfunction. Dementia also occurs in a minority of cases and may be accompanied by seizures and neurological deficits, as well as secondary psychiatric syndromes, including depression, mania, and psychosis. Dementia in boxers (dementia pugilistica) commonly starts with signs of ataxia, dysarthria, and parkinsonian-like extrapyramidal signs before the global cognitive deficits are appreciated. Dementia due to subdural hematoma is notable because it is potentially reversible. Focal neurological signs, personality changes, and lethargy or agitation may be the presenting symptoms. The history of brain trauma may not be confirmed in a considerable proportion of cases (Bourgeois et al. 2008). In cases of dementia following TBI, diffuse axonal injury, with anatomical disruption and axonal tearing, has been described, and contusional foci in cortical areas and intracerebral hemorrhage also have been reported.

Depression

The relation between dementia and depression is complex. *Pseudodementia,* a term no longer used, referred in the past to depressed patients who perform poorly on cognitive tasks because of lack of interest and motivation. However, it is clear that the dementia syndrome of depression (DSD) is not "pseudo" because it is debilitating and often the harbinger of degenerative diseases (Sáez-Fonseca et al. 2007). DSD may occur during episodes of severe mood disorder (Folstein and McHugh 1978). DSD is probably associated with potentially reversible neurotransmitter dysfunction. It is more frequent in elderly patients with a history of depression, and the presenting depressive syndrome often includes severe psychomotor retardation and other melancholic symptoms, as well as psychotic features such as delusions. Cortical signs such as language disturbances are uncommon, and in DSD, in contrast to DAT, prompting and organization of material tend to improve memory performance (O'Brien et al. 2001). DSD may be potentially reversible and tends to disappear with successful treatment of depression. However, cognitive monitoring and follow-up are recommended because a persistent dementia syndrome may develop in a significant proportion of cases (Chen et al. 2008). Depressive symptoms in the elderly and a history of late-onset depression have been associated with the severity of subcortical white matter lesions, suggesting an etiological role for vascular disease (de Groot et al. 2000). The dissection of apathy and depression in cognitively impaired patients is often difficult, but it is relevant for treatment. Furthermore, apathy and depression may have a differential role in the development of dementia (Vicini Chilovi et al. 2009).

Diagnosis and Differential Diagnosis

Early detection of dementia can play an important role in both the social and the health care dimensions of the disease (Organization for Economic Cooperation and Development 2002). A brief interview can detect the dementia syndrome with reasonable accuracy (Boustani et al. 2003) and can be taught to nonpsychiatrists. However, a systematic search for dementia should follow general screening principles and should be linked ideally to a system prepared to care for all identified patients (J.M.G. Wilson and Junger 1968). Dementia should be suspected in patients at risk referred to psychiatrists, particularly elderly medical patients with delirium or unexpected behavioral disturbances and patients referred by primary care physicians because of subjective complaints or observations by relatives about memory problems or loss of intellectual efficiency. In both cases, the clinical approach to diagnosis follows a classic sequence: first, to identify characteristic signs and symptoms of cognitive impairment; second, to document whether the signs and symptoms cluster in the defined syndrome and to complete a differential diagnosis by discarding false-positive cases; and finally, to search for the etiological type of dementia. A search for associated medical conditions, neuropsychiatric symptoms, and special social needs completes the evaluation process.

Clinical History

A clinical history corroborated through reliable caregivers and a systematic mental status examination are the foundation of the diagnostic process (Rabins et al. 2007). In taking the history, it is important to search for specific evidence of deterioration in memory and other cognitive functions summarized in the general dementia syndrome (see Table 6–5). Specific, convincing examples should be required as support for the diagnosis of dementia. Furthermore, the consultant must assess the presence, extent, and consequences of the cognitive problems in occupational activities and ADLs (see Figure 6–1). An outside informant is crucial for obtaining data about decline in cognitive function measured against premorbid abilities. The Informant Questionnaire on Cognitive Decline in the Elderly (IQCODE; Jorm and Jacomb 1989)—and in particular the short form (Jorm 1994)—is suggested as a useful, simple questionnaire that has good reliability and validity. The onset and pattern of progression of the cognitive difficulties also should be carefully documented. Insidious diseases such as DAT can easily go undetected for years before becoming apparent. Finally, it is also important to determine whether changes in personality and behavior have accompanied the cognitive difficulties and whether psychopathological signs and symptoms, including apathy and loss of initiative, are present.

Mental Status Examination

A systematic, basic bedside or office mental status examination is a minimum requirement in each case of suspected dementia. The cognitive assessment is relatively easy to complete and should include all relevant domains. Table 1–4 ("Detailed assessment of cognitive domains") in Chapter 1, "Psychiatric Assessment and Consultation," summarizes the cognitive areas to cover in the assessment. In-depth examination of recent memory should be emphasized. Other important areas to explore are remote memory and fund of knowledge; attention; language and verbal fluency; visuospatial skills; and abstraction. Figure 6–2 shows the performance on some construction tasks by patients with dementia. It is strongly recommended that the clinician be familiar with a standard assessment method,

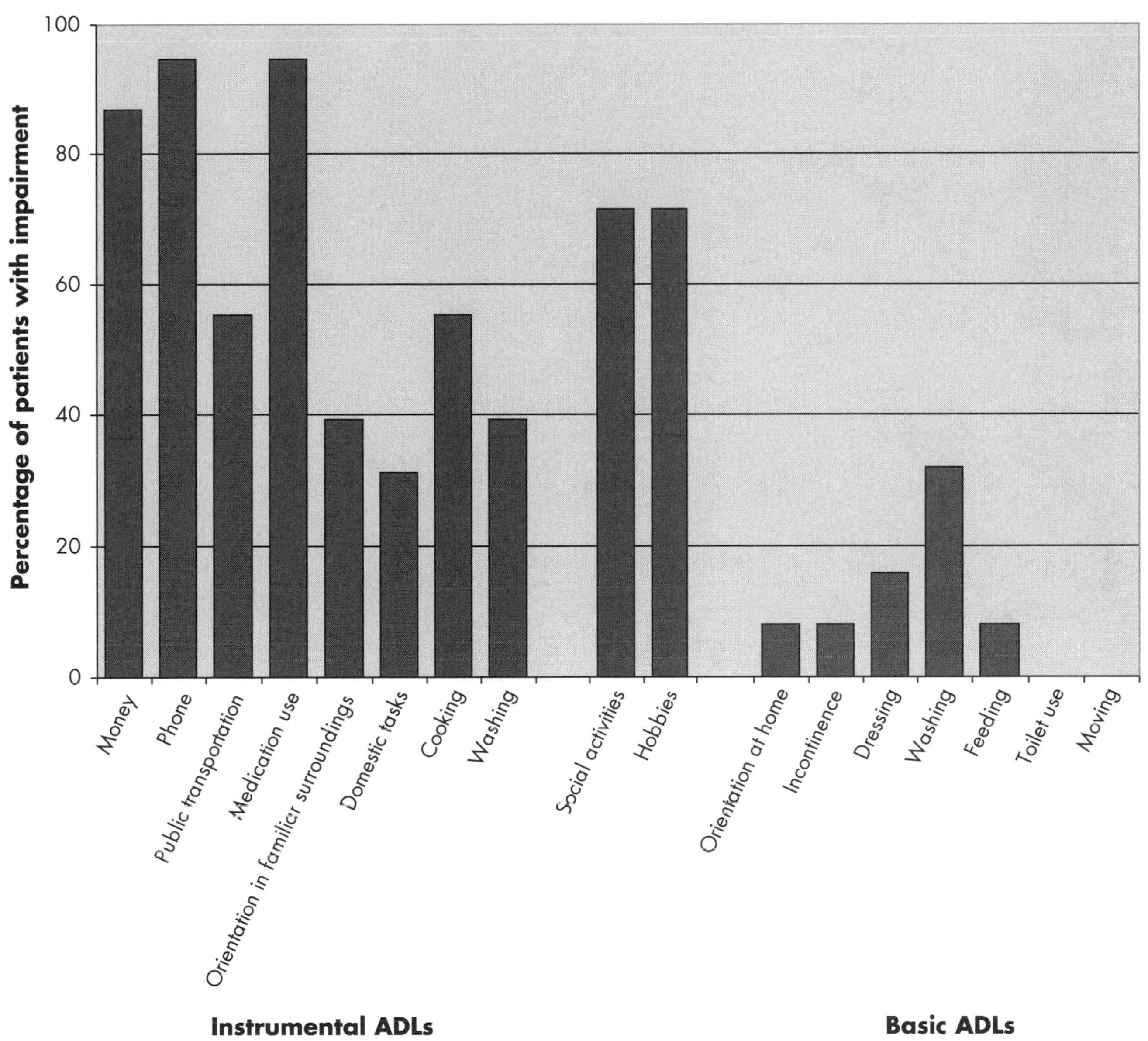

FIGURE 6–1. Impairment in instrumental[a] and basic[b] activities of daily living (ADLs) in patients with dementia of the Alzheimer's type of mild severity (Mini-Mental State Examination score > 18) at time of diagnosis.

Note. Patients were new referrals to a memory clinic in a psychosomatics/consultation-liaison psychiatry service.

[a]Instrumental items in modified Lawton and Brody Scale.

[b]Basic items in Katz Index.

Source. Adapted from A. Lobo and Saz 2004.

ideally one supported by efficiency data. Although no standardized instrument is a substitute for sound clinical assessment, some are quite helpful, provided their limitations are kept in mind.

The Mini-Mental State Examination (MMSE) is one such instrument for screening purposes (sensitivity≥87%; positive predictive value≥79% in clinical populations) (Folstein et al. 1975, 2001) and is widely considered to be the standard measure in most clinical and research studies (Gray and Cummings 2002). It fares very well in different cultures, if the standardization has been adequate (A. Lobo et al. 1999). Data on the efficiency of individual items in the MMSE, remarkable in items such as temporal orientation, may help the consultant in interpreting the results of the test (Table 6–7). A recent meta-analysis supports the accuracy of this brief scale in the detection of dementia (Mitchell 2009) The limits of the MMSE relate to both floor and ceiling effects, and population norms have to be considered

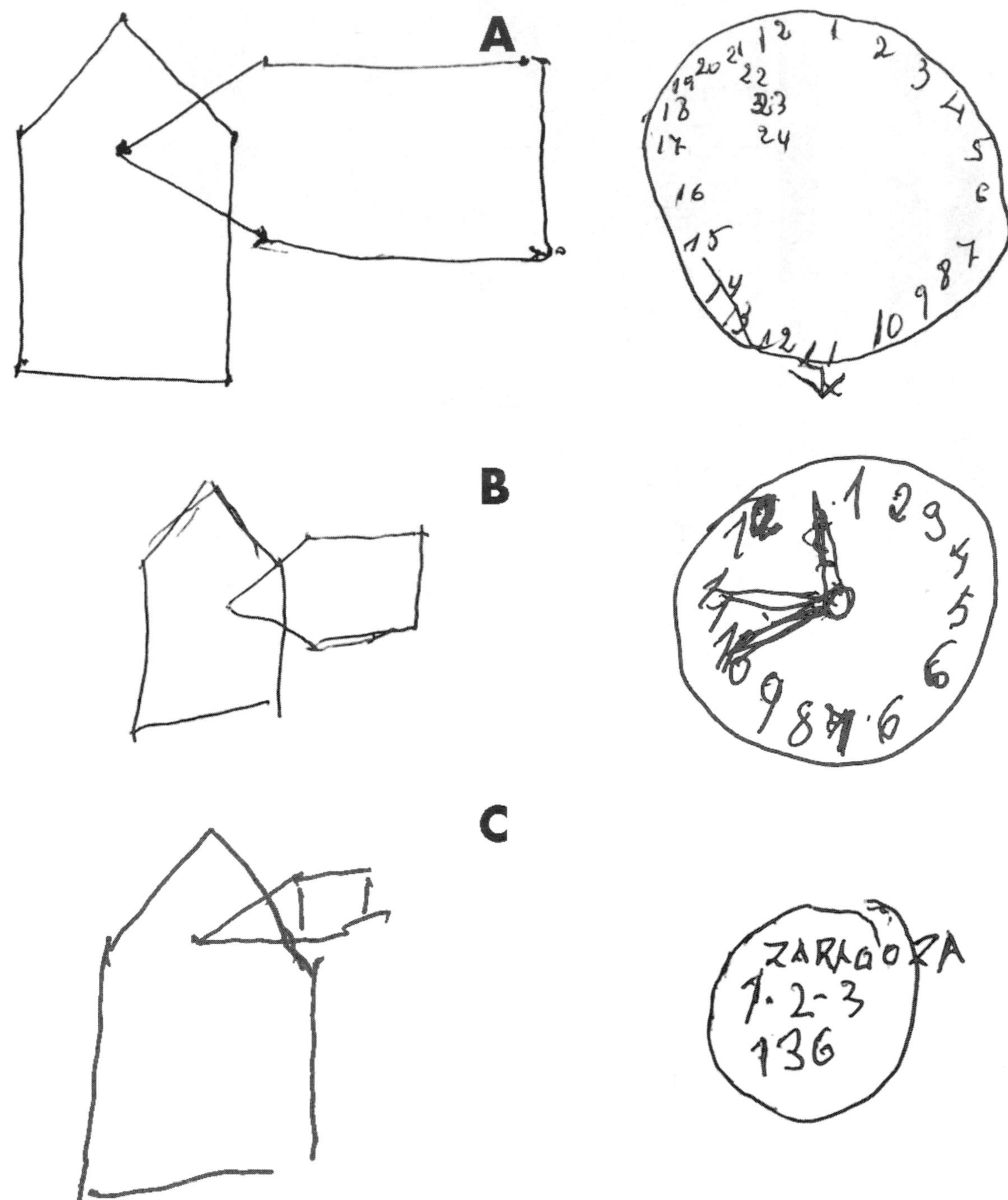

FIGURE 6–2. Performance in construction tasks (commands to draw interlocked pentagons and a clock) by patients with increasing levels of dementia severity.

Impairment in performance appears earlier in clock drawing than in pentagon construction and increases with severity level of dementia. Clock A (Mini-Mental State Examination [MMSE] score = 18) shows executive deficits in planning and organization; construction deficits to place the numbers; probable perseveration (24 hours); and deficits in judgment to correct errors and to place the hands indicating the time (11:10). Pentagon A shows nominal construction deficit. Clock B (MMSE score = 15) shows subtle construction deficits (mild deviation of numbers, but spacing is correct); executive deficits in planning and judgment to indicate the time; and unsuccessful executive attempts to correct errors (in placing number 6; in placing the hands). Pentagon B shows mild construction deficit. Clock C (MMSE score = 14) shows deficits both in remembering and in understanding the command and probable "stimulus dependence syndrome" (the pen in the patient's hand acts as a stimulus and writes inappropriately inside the circle). Pentagon C shows construction and visuomotor coordination deficits.

TABLE 6–7. Validity of individual items of MMSE (administered by lay interviewers)[a]

MMSE items	Cutoff score	Sensitivity (%)	Specificity (%)	PPV (%)[b]	NPV (%)[b]	Misclassifications (%)	AUC
Temporal orientation	3/4	81.3	91.5	93.9	96.3	10.1	0.914
Spatial orientation	4/5	70.8	86.4	45.3	92.5	17.4	0.805
Immediate memory	2/3	14.6	97.7	53.8	86.1	15.2	0.565
Calculation	3/4	78.0	71.4	31.4	95.1	27.6	0.794
Delayed memory	1/2	91.7	49.6	25.4	96.9	43.7	0.774
Nomination	1/2	12.2	98.8	66.7	85.3	15.6	0.555
Articulation	0/1	12.8	94.9	31.6	85.5	17.9	0.540
Verbal commands	2/3	41.7	79.5	27.8	87.8	26.5	0.618
Written commands	0/1	29.0	95.1	45.0	90.8	12.8	0.620
Writing	0/1	60.0	58.6	17.1	91.1	41.2	0.595
Pentagon drawing	0/1	91.9	54.4	24.6	97.6	40.4	0.730

Note. AUC=area under receiver operating characteristics curve; MMSE=Mini-Mental State Examination; NPV=negative predictive value; PPV=positive predictive value.
[a]Gold standard=dementia (diagnosis by psychiatrist, DSM-III-R criteria [American Psychiatric Association 1987], 2-month interval); Lobo et al. (1999).
[b]Predictive values for a prevalence of dementia of 5.5%.

in adjusting the usual cutoff point (23 of 24) (Crum et al. 1993; A. Lobo et al. 1999) to avoid false-positive cases in individuals with limited educational background or, conversely, false-negative cases in highly educated, intelligent patients. The Modified Mini-Mental State (3MS; E.L. Teng and Chui 1987), with minor changes introduced to circumvent these difficulties, works well in clinical practice (McDowell et al. 1997). Executive functions, which are not well covered in the MMSE, may be easily assessed at bedside with the Frontal Assessment Battery (FAB; Dubois et al. 2000). Standardized assessment scales also may be recommended for cases of severe dementia (Rabins and Steele 1996), for noncognitive symptoms in individuals with dementia (Cummings et al. 1994), and specifically for depression (Alexopoulos et al. 1988).

Neurological Examination

The neurological examination is also an integral part of, and informs, the diagnosis and differential diagnosis. The examination should be standard but may be focused on the assessment of neurological signs described in the clinical section, including specific gait difficulties, praxias, and pathological reflexes. Other testing should be included if warranted by clinical information.

Differential Diagnosis

Differential diagnosis starts by ruling out false-positive cases of dementia—namely, previous mental retardation; amnestic syndromes (such as in Korsakoff's psychosis), without the global deficits required for the diagnosis of dementia; cognitive difficulties due to general physical frailty, particularly in elderly patients; and age-related memory impairment (or benign senescent forgetfulness), characterized by a minor degree of memory problems observed as a normal part of aging and not significantly interfering with a person's social or occupational behavior. Pseudodementia syndromes may be the result of motivational or emotional factors interfering with performance. They include acute psychotic episodes, conversion disorder, factitious disorder, and malingering, suggested by reports of relatives, examination, or evidence of primary and/or secondary gains. Schizophrenia may present special diagnostic difficulties, both because of the emotional and psychotic features and because of the cognitive deficits (Zakzanis et al. 2003a). The cardinal symptoms of schizophrenia and longitudinal history should help clarify the diagnosis. The central cognitive functions and ADLs that deteriorate in dementia usually are preserved in schizophrenia.

Ganser's syndrome, or the syndrome of "approximate answers," requires special consideration. This syndrome is characterized by the voluntary production of severe cognitive symptoms (Dwyer and Reid 2004; Lishman 1998). Key features include approximate answers to simple questions (i.e., incorrect answers that imply the person knows the correct answers—e.g., "How many legs does a table have?" "*Three.*" "How much is 2+2?" "*Five.*"). The cause of this rare syndrome remains uncertain. It was previously classified as a factitious disorder, but current classification systems categorize it as a dissociative disorder, the symptoms of which are judged as psychogenic in origin (Wirtz et al. 2008).

Ganser's syndrome is frequently associated with brain injury but may occur in patients with a variety of psychiatric disorders. The differential diagnosis may be very difficult. Objective psychological tests may be useful to document the factitious nature of the cognitive symptoms. The fact that the symptoms are often worse when the patients believe they are being watched also helps in the recognition of this syndrome. A major predisposing factor is the existence of a previous severe personality disorder.

Depressive disorders in elderly patients also should be considered because these patients may have memory difficulties, slowed thinking, and lack of spontaneity, which suggest dementia (see discussion of DSD earlier in this chapter in the "Depression" subsection).

Delirium makes it very difficult to determine whether concurrent dementia is present, and delirium without fluctuating level of consciousness may be very difficult to distinguish from dementia. The diagnosis of delirium is suggested when global cognitive disturbance (including immediate and recent memory) is accompanied by rapid onset, fluctuating level of consciousness, impairment of attention, incoherence of thought, visual illusions or hallucinations or other perceptual disturbances, and disturbances of the sleep-wake cycle, all in the presence of a severe medical condition. Definitive diagnosis often must be postponed until the follow-up after recovery from acute medical illness. A "double" diagnosis of delirium superimposed on dementia is very common in general hospital patients; A. Lobo and Saz (2004) found that a postdischarge diagnosis of dementia is confirmed in approximately half the cases of uncertain diagnosis.

Mild cognitive impairment, as described in the "Concept of Dementia and Clinical Approach" section, merits special consideration because of its high prevalence and the high rate of progression to dementia. Clinical judgment is required for the diagnosis, but neuropsychological assessment is helpful. The screening instruments and rating scales presented in this chapter may be used for this purpose. Scores of 2 or 3 on the Global Deterioration Scale (GDS; Reisberg et al. 1982) or a score of 0.5 on the Clinical Dementia Rating Scale (CDR; Hughes et al. 1982) has been considered to correspond to mild cognitive impairment. Neuroimaging findings helpful in the diagnosis are described in the following sections.

Once false-positive cases are ruled out and a dementia syndrome is confirmed, the consultant determines whether the syndrome has characteristics of cortical, subcortical, or mixed type (see Table 6-6), as described in the previous sections. The onset and progression of the cognitive difficulties, the other psychopathological features, and whether another medical condition is present will give further clues as to the type of dementia. For diagnostic purposes, clinical differences between types of dementia have been emphasized in the "Clinical Types and Pathophysiology of Dementia" section. The search for potentially reversible types of dementia due to medical conditions or toxic effects (see Table 6-3) has long been emphasized and remains an important step in the diagnostic process. Such conditions are more frequent in general hospital patients, although the identification of truly reversible causes has become less common than in the past, and true reversibility has been questioned (Weytingh et al. 1995).

Workup recommendations for the diagnosis of dementia are available (Knopman et al. 2001; Small et al. 1997), although standard workup is applicable to every patient. Table 6-8 lists a screening battery of tests that are

TABLE 6-8. Laboratory tests and other diagnostic procedures in the assessment of dementia

Screening battery[a]

- Complete blood cell count with differential cell type count
- Erythrocyte sedimentation rate
- Blood glucose
- Blood urea nitrogen
- Electrolytes, calcium, magnesium
- Thyrotropin
- Vitamin B_{12} and folate levels
- Urinalysis
- Fluorescent treponemal antibody absorption[b]
- Liver and renal function tests

Neuroimaging

- Computed tomography (CT) head scan
- Magnetic resonance imaging (MRI) head scan[c]
- Single photon emission computed tomography[b,c]

Other tests and procedures[a]

- Blood tests
  - Arterial blood gases
  - Blood and urine screens for alcohol, drugs, and heavy metals
  - Serum HIV test[b,c]
  - Homocysteine level
  - Antinuclear antibody, C3, C4, anti-double-stranded DNA, anticardiolipin antibody
- Other
  - Chest X ray
  - Electrocardiogram
  - Disease-specific tests (e.g., serum copper and ceruloplasmin for Wilson's disease)
  - Lumbar puncture[c] (usually after CT or MRI)

[a]Tests may be selected on the basis of patient age.
[b]May require special consent and counseling.
[c]Tests selected on the basis of specific symptoms (history and physical examination) or patient populations.

commonly used to identify conditions associated with dementia, such as infectious, metabolic, and neoplastic diseases and substance-induced dementia. The specific tests used should be determined by various factors, including the patient's age, medical comorbidities, history, and physical examination. Neuroimaging is often obtained, and neuropsychological testing may be very useful in some cases (Table 6–9). Lumbar puncture should be considered for patients with early onset or atypical clinical features, as well as for patients with positive syphilis serology or suspected hydrocephalus, central nervous system infection, vasculitis, immunosuppression, or metastatic cancer.

The DSM-IV-TR (American Psychiatric Association 2000) diagnostic criteria for dementia overlap with the

TABLE 6–9. Neuroimaging findings in dementia syndromes

Syndrome and findings	Neuroimaging modalities
Dementias treatable by surgical procedures	
Normal-pressure hydrocephalus, brain tumors, subdural hematoma	CT, MRI
Dementia of the Alzheimer's type	
Enlarged ventricles	CT, MRI
General atrophy	CT, MRI
Medial temporal lobe or hippocampus atrophy (early markers)	CT, MRI (combined with SPECT)
Temporoparietal (and sometimes frontal) hypoperfusion	SPECT
Temporoparietal (and sometimes frontal) hypometabolism; relative sparing of visual and sensorimotor cortex	PET
Absence of signs of vascular dementia	CT, MRI
Vascular dementia	
Leukoaraiosis in white matter (very frequent)	CT
Areas of infarct (very characteristic, only half the cases)	CT
Hyperintensities in white matter (more sensitive)	MRI
Frontotemporal dementia	
Frontal (and temporal) atrophy	CT, MRI
Frontal (and temporal) hypoperfusion	SPECT
Normal-pressure hydrocephalus	
Very enlarged ventricles	CT, MRI
Huntington's disease	
Atrophy of caudate nucleus	CT, MRI
Alcoholic dementia	
Enlarged ventricles and atrophy	CT, MRI
HIV dementia	
Atrophy	CT, MRI
Demyelination of subcortical white matter	MRI
Hypermetabolism of thalamus and basal ganglia	PET
Depression	
Frontal hypometabolism, asymmetric (reversible)	PET
Mild cognitive impairment	
Hippocampal and entorhinal volume reduction	MRI, CT
Hypoperfusion or hypometabolism	SPECT, PET

Note. Structural imaging: CT = computed tomography; MRI = magnetic resonance imaging. Functional imaging: PET = positron emission tomography; SPECT = single photon emission computed tomography.

ICD-10 criteria (World Health Organization 1992), and the latter also have been adapted for use in general hospital patients (Malt et al. 1996). It is accepted that a definitive diagnosis of Alzheimer's disease requires histological evidence in the brain at autopsy (McKhann et al. 1984). However, a careful clinical diagnosis coincides with the pathological diagnosis in most cases (Rabins et al. 2007). This diagnosis must be based on the presence of a cortical type of dementia syndrome, an insidious onset with slow deterioration (although plateaus may occur in the progression), and characteristic psychopathological and neurological signs and symptoms (see Table 6–5). The diagnosis is further supported by neuroimaging findings (see Table 6–9); the absence of clinical evidence; or findings from special investigations, which suggest that the mental state may be due to vascular dementia (Table 6–10) or another systemic disease that can induce a dementia syndrome.

Genetic testing for DAT is promising and relies on the fact that two general groups of genes are associated with this disease. Presenilin-1 is a fairly accurate predictor of early-onset Alzheimer's disease, but genetic testing for mutations in presenilin has proven to be ineffective as a screening tool because of its low sensitivity (Kurz et al. 2002). The *APOE* genotype is statistically associated with late-onset Alzheimer's disease, but current genetic testing for the *APOE* ε4 allele cannot be recommended for screening because of its low efficiency (Patterson et al. 2008).

The clinical characteristics supporting a diagnosis of vascular dementia are summarized in Table 6–10, and Table 6–9 includes the characteristic and differential neuroimaging findings. More stringent diagnostic criteria are also available (Roman et al. 1993) and are widely considered important for research purposes. A diagnosis of a mixed DAT and vascular type of dementia or a double diagnosis is usually made when clinical and imaging characteristics of both coexist. This may happen, for example, when cerebrovascular episodes are superimposed on a clinical picture and history suggesting Alzheimer's disease. The presence of cerebrovascular lesions in patients with DAT has been confirmed by recent evidence, including postmortem findings (Kalaria 2000).

TABLE 6–10. Clinical characteristics suggesting vascular dementia

Mixed type of dementia syndrome
Uneven cognitive deterioration
Relative preservation of insight and judgment
Abrupt onset, stepwise course
Emotional incontinence and lability
History of strokes
History of cardiovascular risk factors
Focal neurological signs and symptoms

Neuroimaging and Electroencephalography

Neuroimaging has revolutionized the ability of clinicians to diagnose dementia. It is a useful adjunct to clinical diagnosis and is considered to be mandatory in some stringent diagnostic systems (McKhann et al. 1984; Roman et al. 1993). However, it may be unnecessary in cases of advanced symptoms and long history of the disease. Computed tomography (CT) and magnetic resonance imaging (MRI) are very useful in ruling out reversible conditions such as NPH, subdural hematoma, and brain tumors. Therefore, these imaging modalities should be routinely considered in patients with history or findings suggesting those conditions, specifically when such patients have cognitive impairment with rapid onset or recent head trauma; focal neurological signs or abnormalities in gait; severe headache, papilledema, or visual field defect; early appearance of incontinence; or history of stroke or seizures without known risk factors.

In DAT, both CT and MRI are helpful diagnostic tools (see Table 6–9). However, the findings are not totally specific (in particular, for general atrophy), which may be found in elderly patients without dementia. Images of enlarged ventricles are considered to be better discriminators. Early markers of the disease may be the CT—and particularly the MRI—views of the medial temporal lobe and hippocampus (Chetelat and Baron 2003). Single photon emission computed tomography (SPECT) may be particularly useful in early cases of FTD to detect changes in blood flow. Positron emission tomography (PET) is also a promising technique (see Table 6–9), although not all hospitals have adequate facilities. The utility of both functional techniques has been supported by meta-analytic reviews (Zakzanis et al. 2003b). However, the costs of tests, and whether the results will make a difference in management of the patient, should be considered before routine recommendation in clinical practice. In vascular dementia, neuroimaging can provide strong support for the diagnosis, especially the MRI finding of hyperintensities in the white matter, and some authors suggest that the diagnosis is excluded in the absence of vascular lesions (Roman 2002). However, some hyperintensities are also found in DAT and other degenerative dementias, as well as in control subjects (Pantoni and Garcia 1995).

The EEG has limited utility in the differential diagnosis of dementia because abnormalities are frequent but relatively nonspecific. Slow-wave activity characteristic of delirium does not appear until late in the course of DAT. The EEG is very useful in diagnosing Creutzfeldt-Jakob disease (triphasic, periodic burst patterns) (Waldemar et al. 2007) and in patients with some metabolic dementias, such as hepatic encephalopathy (triphasic waves), although in neither case is the finding pathognomonic.

Neuropsychological Testing

Neuropsychological testing is valuable as an adjunct to the clinical examination but is no substitute for sound clinical judgment. Any battery of tests for the evaluation of dementia should assess a wide range of cognitive abilities, with special emphasis on memory. The age, education, and culture of the population must be considered in standardizing the instruments and interpreting the results. Neuropsychological testing may be particularly useful to differentiate dementia from age-related cognitive impairment and to provide both quantitative and qualitative information that helps differentiate subtypes of dementia (Chertkow et al. 2008). Batteries commonly used include measures of memory, intellect, language, and visuospatial function. Some are exhaustive, with the administration taking several hours—a feature that limits their utility. A rather short battery has been standardized by the Consortium to Establish a Registry for Alzheimer's Disease (Welsh et al. 1992) and has been used in different countries.

Dementia Rating Scales

Aside from the MMSE, screening and assessment instruments for dementia include classic scales, such as the Blessed Mental Status Examination (Blessed et al. 1968). Instruments for specific purposes have been designed; one such instrument, the Alzheimer's Disease Assessment Scale (ADAS; W.G. Rosen et al. 1984), is considered to have improved sensitivity for DAT. The use of these instruments does not replace a careful mental status examination. Educational and cultural factors must be taken into account in interpreting the results of cognitive assessment with any of these instruments. Primary care physicians and nurse practitioners can be trained in their use. Global staging instruments, such as the CDR (Hughes et al. 1982), have come into wide use. A variety of assessments are also available for documenting functional deficits, such as the classic instruments of Lawton and Brody (1969), the Katz Index (Katz et al. 1970), or the Functional Assessment Staging (FAST) procedure, which can be used in conjunction with the GDS staging system (Reisberg et al. 1993).

Clinical Course, Prognosis, and Outcome

The course and prognosis of dementia are generally disease specific but may be influenced by a variety of factors. Timely surgical treatment, before irreversible brain damage occurs, may have spectacular results in subdural hematoma or brain tumors, depending on type and location. Classical studies suggested the improvement of severe apathy in NPH by surgical shunting, although cognitive improvement was not as evident. However, a systematic review concluded that no evidence indicates whether placement of a shunt is effective (Esmonde and Cooke 2002). One would expect that dementia associated with medications or metabolic conditions should be reversible, but this is not always the case in practice (Weytingh et al. 1995).

Medical comorbidity may be present in two-thirds of DAT patients and is strongly associated with greater impairment in cognition and in self-care (Doraiswamy et al. 2002). Optimal management of medical illnesses may offer potential to improve cognition in Alzheimer's disease. Dementias associated with infections have disease-specific prognoses. Untreated HIV dementia generally progresses quickly (over months) to severe global dementia, mutism, and death. However, with careful antiretroviral treatment, patients may survive for years. Adequate treatment with dopamine agonists and other standard treatments significantly improves the prognosis of dementia in Parkinson's disease. Early treatment with thiamine is vital in alcoholic patients with cognitive dysfunction (Blansjaar and van Dijk 1992).

Important events or changes in a patient's routine may precipitate episodes of behavioral disturbance. Medical illness (most often urinary tract infection or pneumonia) or the use of benzodiazepines or alcohol also may precipitate episodes of delirium. Patients with good premorbid adjustment and greater intelligence and education are in general more able to compensate for intellectual deficits and disability. Support from family and caregivers may determine to an important extent the presence or absence of affective and other psychological symptoms, as well as the course of dementia.

Studies suggest that median survival after the onset of DAT is much shorter than has previously been estimated and is strongly associated with age. In the study by Brookmeyer et al. (2002), median survival ranged from 8.3 years for persons who received the diagnosis at age 65 years to 3.4 years for persons who received the diagnosis at age 90 years. No important differences in mean survival have been found between DAT and vascular dementia (Wolfson et al. 2001).

The relative risk of death for DAT is two to three times higher than in persons without DAT, particularly in older women (Dewey and Saz 2001; Dodge et al. 2003). The mean annual rate of progression of cognitive impairment is approximately 2–4 points when degree of impairment is assessed with the MMSE (Ballard et al. 2001). Most researchers have found faster rates of decline in early-onset DAT (Stern et al. 1997). A more recent review (Sarazin et al. 2002) suggested that an increased rate of deterioration was associated with the following factors: low baseline cognitive status, presence of Lewy bodies, language deficits, lower scores on nonverbal neuropsychological tests, extrapyramidal signs, and myoclonus. The relation between *APOE* ε4 and the course of DAT is still debated (Galasko et al. 2000), but the presence of psychotic symptoms at baseline is strongly and independently predictive of a more rapid decline (Paulsen et al. 2000). However, some reports consider that cognitive decline in such cases might be related to neuroleptic treatment (McShane et al. 1997). Neuropsychiatric symptoms tend to fluctuate in the course of dementia in most patients, but depression, agitation, and aggression may show greater persistence as compared with delusions and hallucinations (Devanand et al. 1997).

Functional impairment in DAT is highly correlated with the severity of cognitive impairment (Mohs et al. 2000). Instrumental ADLs demand higher cognitive functions than do the basic ADLs, and, as expected, the former are impaired earlier. Nursing home placement has consistently been related not only to severity of dementia but also to severity of both functional impairment and neuropsychiatric symptoms (Luppa et al. 2008). Strong evidence suggests that caring for patients with dementia has a negative effect on caregivers, often more negative than when caring for a person with physical disabilities (Morris et al. 1988); the ability of caregivers to tolerate neuropsychiatric symptoms reduces the probability of nursing home placement (Luppa et al. 2008).

Considerably less evidence is available regarding the course of other degenerative diseases, but clinical experience and some reports suggest that disease progression is similar to that in DAT. Duration of DLB ranges from 1.8 to 9.5 years (Walker et al. 2000), and early-onset cases might have a more rapid decline. Visual hallucinations tend to be persistent in DLB (Ballard et al. 2001), but psychosis does not appear to predict accelerated decline (Mohs et al. 2000). The increased survival reported in studies might be related to a decrease in the prescription of neuroleptics in patients with DLB (McShane et al. 1997), in view of the greater awareness of their negative side effects, which include rapid cognitive decline.

A faster rate of deterioration in executive functions, but not of other cognitive functions, has been reported in patients with FTD when compared with DAT (Galasko et al. 2000). Loss of autonomy appears early in the course of FTD and is frequently accompanied by behavior changes. In the late stages of subcortical dementias, such as Huntington's disease, apathy may be quite severe and cause profound self-neglect; the patient's condition may resemble the akinetic mute state. Duration of disease varies from 5–10 years in PSP to 10–15 years in Huntington's disease. Survival in Parkinson's disease might be 12–14 years, provided the treatment is adequate, and patients with Wilson's disease may have a normal survival time if their symptoms are adequately treated with penicillamine before irreversible liver and brain damage occurs. The course of vascular dementia is typically stepwise but varies significantly depending on the type of vascular problem. Prognosis is poor, and patients usually die as a result of new cardiovascular events or strokes, but considerable individual variation is seen.

Treatment

General Principles

The general principles for treatment of dementia are summarized in Table 6–11. Extensive clinical guides on how to provide care for patients with dementia are available (Rabins et al. 2006, 2007). Patients with dementia very often have a broad range of medical problems, neuropsychiatric symptoms, and social needs accompanying their cognitive deterioration. Therefore, they usually need a multimodal plan, which should be adapted to the individual and to the specific stage of the disease. Specific recommendations are discussed in the following sections.

Adequate medical care is crucial in all dementias because both cognitive function and behavior may be adversely influenced by medical problems. Specific and frequent problems that must be addressed include the management of pain, urinary tract infections, and decubitus ulcers. Tube feeding to improve survival in hospitalized patients with advanced dementia is controversial, if not contraindicated, because it lacks demonstrated benefits (Meier et al. 2001). Treatment in nonreversible dementia aims at controlling the underlying condition as much as possible and slowing the progression of symptoms. The treatment of cognitive loss with new pharmacological agents has become a major focus, and the identification and treatment of neuropsychiatric symptoms are especially relevant for psychiatrists. General measures include mandatory restrictions on driving. Both patients and families should be informed that dementia increases the risk for accidents, even in the early stages, and patients certainly should not be driving when dementia reaches a moderately severe stage. Psychological and social support and treatment always should be considered for patients. Psychiatrists also should be alert to the potential needs of caregivers. Long-term treatment must be considered in most dementias, and psychiatrists should participate in public health, including public awareness campaigns that

TABLE 6–11. General principles for treatment of dementia and bases for consultation-liaison programs

Use a multimodal treatment plan and individualize it for each patient.

Adjust treatment to stage of disease.

Provide adequate care of emergencies.

Evaluate for suicidal potential, self-harm (e.g., falling or wandering), or accidents (e.g., fires).

Treat agitation and potential for violence.

Initiate early treatment of potentially reversible medical or surgical conditions etiologically related to dementia (e.g., hypothyroidism, subdural hematoma).

See patient on regular basis.

Schedule frequent visits when starting therapy; see for routine follow-up every 4–6 months thereafter (more frequent visits may be required in special circumstances).

Ensure adequate medical care.

Maintain the patient's physical health: nutritious diet, proper exercise.

Identify and treat comorbid medical conditions: cardiopulmonary dysfunction, pain, urinary tract infections, decubitus ulcers, visual and auditory problems, etc.

Care for iatrogenic events, pressure sores, aspiration pneumonia, fecal impaction.

Exert stringent control of unnecessary drugs taken for other medical disorders.

Try to control underlying disease and slow progression in nonreversible dementias.

Prevent and treat vascular problems (in both vascular dementia and dementia of the Alzheimer's type): hypertension, hyperlipidemia, obesity, cardiac disease, diabetes, alcohol dependence, smoking cessation, etc.

Treat cognitive loss: pharmacological, other measures.

Use other general measures.

Use general health measures: recreational and activity therapies, etc.

Restrict driving and use of other dangerous equipment.

Identify neuropsychiatric symptoms; provide vigorous treatment if needed.

Provide psychological support and treatment for patient.

Provide orientation aids (calendars, clocks, television).

Assess activities of daily living and provide assistance as needed.

Use special techniques: stimulation-oriented, reminiscence therapy, cognitive or reality therapy.

Provide social treatment.

Educate family caregivers.

Give advice with arrangements for wills, power of attorney, and general estate matters.

Suggest support groups, community organizations.

Provide support for caregivers and treatment if needed (e.g., for depression).

Arrange long-term treatment and coordinate with care organizations.

Memory clinics

Community resources, geriatric day hospitals

Multidisciplinary rehabilitation in an outpatient setting

Support groups, Alzheimer's Association

Respite care

Long-term facility (including nursing homes, hospice) necessary if caregivers not available

Vigilance regarding neglect or abuse

Incorporate health care strategies.

Public awareness campaigns; campaigns for early detection and treatment of dementia stress the importance of early detection and treatment of dementia (Organization for Economic Cooperation and Development 2002).

Pharmacological Treatment

General guidelines for psychotropic medication use in frail elderly patients are applicable (Spar and La Rue 2002). Specific suggestions for dementia patients are summarized in Table 6–12. Systematic evidence to support the effectiveness of particular psychotropic drugs in dementia patients is limited. Therefore, choice of drug class may be based on clinical evidence, and choice of agent is often based on the side-effect profile and on the characteristics of a given patient. Noncognitive, psychopathological, and behavioral manifestations in patients with dementia may be early targets for psychiatric intervention.

Treatment of Psychosis and Agitation

Some evidence indicates that antipsychotics are effective in controlling agitation, aggressiveness, wandering, and psychotic symptoms in individuals with dementia (Olin and Schneider 2002), mostly in studies of no longer than 12 weeks. The data suggest that improvement is greater for psychosis than for other symptoms. Antipsychotics are often administered in the evening so that maximum levels occur at sleep time. Most antipsychotics have long half-lives, so once-a-day doses may be sufficient. Oral administration is preferred, except in cases of emergency or when the patient is unable to take the medication by mouth. Initial treatment with low doses of a high-potency agent, such as haloperidol (0.5–2.0 mg/day; maximum dosage 5 mg/day), may be recommended, and evidence indicates that it is effective in reducing aggressiveness in agitated dementia (Lonergan et al. 2002). However, the atypical antipsychotics cause fewer extrapyramidal effects, and their use in dementia has been supported by randomized controlled trials (Ballard and Waite 2006; Daiello 2007; L.S. Schneider et al. 2006). Specific antipsychotics and doses recommended are risperidone (0.25–1 mg/day), olanzapine (1.25–5.0 mg/day), quetiapine (12.5–50 mg/day), or aripiprazole (5 mg/day). An increase in mortality associated with the use of atypical antipsychotics has been reported (Ballard and Waite 2006), and a black-box warning has been issued (U.S. Food and Drug Administration 2005). However, similar risks have been suggested for typical antipsychotics (Wang et al. 2005) (see Chapter 38, "Psychopharmacology"). In patients with Parkinson's disease or DLB, atypical antipsychotics with limited extrapyramidal effects may be recommended (Rabins et al. 2007). Another option is clozapine (initial dose 12.5 mg/day; maximum dose 75–100 mg/day).

TABLE 6–12. Suggested guidelines for psychotropic medication use

Consider that agitation and/or behavioral disturbances may be due to

A medical condition, pain, other psychiatric condition, or sleep loss, which would resolve with treatment of the primary condition.

Hunger, constipation, stressful atmosphere, change in living conditions, or interpersonal difficulties.

Use strategies to minimize the total amount of medication required.

Instruct caregivers to appropriately administer sedatives when warranted.

Mild symptoms or limited risk often may resolve with support, reassurance, and distraction.

Remember that dementia patients are often physically frail and have decreased renal clearance and slowed hepatic metabolism.

Be specific in selecting target symptoms.

Use low initial doses, one-quarter to one-third of the usual initial dose; dose increments should be smaller and between-dose intervals longer. Seek lowest effective dose.

Avoid polypharmacy.

Keep especially alert to

Medical conditions and drug interactions.

Frequent and worrying side effects: orthostatic hypotension and central nervous system sedation (may worsen cognition and cause falls); susceptibility to extrapyramidal side effects.

Idiosyncratic drug effects: mental confusion; restlessness; increased sedation; and vulnerability to anticholinergic effects of psychotropic medication.

In cases of extrapyramidal effects, reduce the dose or change to another drug rather than use anticholinergic drugs.

Reassess risks and benefits of psychotropic treatment on an ongoing basis.

The use of cholinesterase inhibitors—namely, donepezil, rivastigmine, and galantamine—is considered to be an appropriate pharmacological strategy for the management of psychotic symptoms and agitation in patients with dementia. Substantial clinical experience is available (Cummings et al. 2006), although the evidence of their efficacy is still limited, in part because of methodological considerations (Rodda et al. 2009). Similarly, some evidence supports the use of memantine in such cases (Wilcock et al. 2008).

There is less empirical support for, but considerable clinical experience with, the use of other medications in cases of agitated behavior, particularly in milder cases or cases unresponsive to neuroleptics. These medications include trazodone (50–400 mg/day; higher doses have been reported by some clinicians) (Rojas-Fernández et al. 2003), buspirone (15–50 mg/day) (Salzman 2001), carbamazepine (400–1,200 mg/day; maximum blood levels: 8–12 ng/mL) (Olin et al. 2001a), and gabapentin (400–1,200 mg/day) (L.J. Miller 2001). These medications may be particularly useful in cases of DLB because the likelihood of severe adverse side effects with the use of neuroleptics is quite high (McKeith et al. 1992). Anticonvulsants require close monitoring because of potential toxic effects. Several other agents have been proposed for the treatment of agitation in patients with dementia, including benzodiazepines and beta-blockers, but evidence of efficacy is very limited, and potential side effects preclude routine recommendation.

Treatment of Depression

Both well-designed studies (Lyketsos et al. 2003) and reviews of randomized controlled trials (Olin and Schneider 2002) suggest that antidepressants may be effective for treating depressive syndromes in patients with dementia. However, because antidepressants do have side effects, clinicians should prescribe with due caution (Bains et al. 2002). The newer antidepressants, particularly the selective serotonin reuptake inhibitors (SSRIs), are widely considered to be first-line treatment and should be preferred because of their favorable side-effect profile (Giron et al. 2001). SSRIs used in dementia include fluoxetine (initial dosage 5–10 mg/day, increase at several-week intervals to 40–60 mg/day); paroxetine (same dosages, increase every 1–2 weeks because of shorter half-life); sertraline (initial dosage 25 mg/day, increase at 1- to 2-week intervals to 150–200 mg/day); and citalopram (initial dosage 10 mg/day, increase at weekly intervals to a maximum dosage of 40 mg/day). Escitalopram (10–20 mg/day) is promising (Lepola et al. 2003). Aside from well-known gastrointestinal symptoms, some potential SSRI side effects, such as agitation, akathisia and other extrapyramidal symptoms, dizziness, and weight loss, require monitoring in dementia patients. Venlafaxine (initial dosage 18.75–37.50 mg twice a day, increase at weekly intervals to 350–375 mg/day) is also recommended, particularly in apathetic patients because of stimulating effects, but it may elevate blood pressure at higher doses. Bupropion (initial dosage 37.5 mg/day, increase slowly to a maximum of 300 mg/day) and mirtazapine (initial dosage 7.5 mg at bedtime, increase slowly to a maximum of 45–60 mg at bedtime) have similarly been recommended. Trazodone (initial dosage 25–50 mg/day, increase at weekly intervals to 300–400 mg/day) is often recommended when sedation and improved sleep are desired. Trazodone's main risks in elderly patients with dementia are orthostatic hypotension and excessive sedation. In depressed patients with FTD, both SSRIs (Swartz et al. 1997) and trazodone (Lebert et al. 1999) have shown some benefit.

Classic cyclic antidepressants usually are not considered first-line treatment because they have more adverse effects such as orthostatic hypotension, delays in cardiac conduction, anticholinergic effects, impaired cognition, and delirium. However, some clinicians prefer these drugs, particularly in treating severe depressive syndromes. In such cases, because of a more favorable side-effect profile, the recommended drugs are nortriptyline, particularly when sedation is needed (initial dosage 10–25 mg/day, increase at weekly intervals to 100–150 mg/day; blood levels should not exceed 100–150 ng/mL), and desipramine (initial dosage 25–50 mg/day, increase at weekly intervals to 200 mg/day; blood levels should not exceed 150–200 ng/mL).

Evidence is limited on the beneficial effects of other drugs recommended in the treatment of depression-associated symptoms in dementia patients, such as buspirone for the treatment of agitation and anxiety associated with depression.

Psychostimulants, such as D-amphetamine and methylphenidate, are sometimes useful in patients with medical illness and depression, but few data are available regarding their use in DSD. Potential side effects of restlessness, agitation, sleep disturbances, and appetite suppression are uncommon at low doses. Apathy in depressed dementia patients also has been treated with bromocriptine and amantadine, but potential side effects include psychosis, confusion, dyskinesias, and anticholinergic effects, including delirium. Bupropion and psychostimulants also have been used to treat apathy (Herrmann et al. 2008). Clinical experience suggests that electroconvulsive therapy (ECT) may be useful in treating severe depression associated with dementia that does not respond to drugs, but the data are limited. In such cases, ECT should be given twice rather than thrice weekly, and less memory loss has been documented with unilateral than with bilateral placement of electrodes (American Psychiatric Association 2001; Rabins et al. 2007) (see also Chapter 40, "Electroconvulsive Therapy").

Treatment of Insomnia and Anxiety

Sleep disturbances, which are frequent in patients with dementia, should be primarily managed by careful attention to sleep hygiene. When the disturbances occur in patients with other neuropsychiatric symptoms requiring psychotropic treatment, a drug with sedating properties, given at bedtime, probably should be selected. Otherwise, trazodone (50–100 mg, once at bedtime) is often prescribed. Clinical experience suggests that low-dose antipsychotics (haloperidol 0.5–1.0 mg or the atypical antipsychotics) can be helpful. Zolpidem (5–10 mg at bedtime) and zopiclone (5–10 mg at bedtime) are good alternatives for short-term use. Clonazepam (0.5 mg/day, with increases in dosage up to 2 mg/day) is recommended by some clinicians in patients with frequent awakening or nocturnal wandering. However, all hypnotics have the potential risk of causing nocturnal confusion, daytime sedation, tolerance, rebound insomnia, worsening cognition, disinhibition, and delirium. Triazolam is not recommended because of its association with amnesia. Many patients use diphenhydramine because it is available in a variety of nonprescription preparations and therefore is erroneously believed to be safe. It is not a good choice because of its anticholinergic properties, which may exacerbate confusion and also counteract the effects of cholinesterase inhibitors.

The use of benzodiazepines for anxiety in patients with dementia is controversial because of the side-effect profile described, which also includes ataxia and falls, respiratory depression, and agitation among the most disturbing effects in dementia patients. Low dosages of relatively short-acting drugs, such as lorazepam (0.5–1.0 mg every 4–6 hours) or oxazepam (7.5–15.0 mg four times per day), are preferred when using benzodiazepines and may be beneficial for brief periods. Antidepressants should be considered for long-term treatment, but empirical evidence is very limited regarding their use for anxiety in dementia patients.

Treatment of Cognitive Deficits

Pharmacological treatment of DAT also should aim at restoring cognitive function and associated functional losses (Farlow and Boustani 2009). Currently, the main drugs approved act by inhibiting acetylcholinesterase and thus providing cholinergic augmentation. They may improve cognitive and behavioral symptoms, as well as functional ADLs, although the degree of benefit achieved is limited or symptomatic (see Cochrane reviews in Table 6–13; Birks and Harvey 2006) with little proven effect on the ultimate outcome. Tacrine, which was approved for treating DAT in 1993, has since been replaced by a group of drugs with fewer adverse effects, which include donepezil, rivastigmine, and galantamine (Mayeux and Sano 1999).

Donepezil used to be the most widely prescribed cholinesterase inhibitor, probably because it was the first one to appear (Organization for Economic Cooperation and Development 2002). More adverse effects with rivastigmine and galantamine had been encountered by clinicians, but they were minimized by careful dose titration. Furthermore, the new transdermal patch for rivastigmine (dosage 4.6–9.5 mg released per 24 hours once a day) and extended-release capsules of galantamine (8–24 mg) now available make all three drugs equally easy to use. Cost-effectiveness analysis of cholinesterase inhibitors supports their use (Loveman et al. 2006), but medical guidelines in many countries recommend that cholinergic augmentation therapy be used only in patients with mild to moderate forms of DAT (MMSE score >10 or 12 points or an equivalent score on the ADAS—cognitive subscale; Gillen et al. 2001). However, the U.S. Food and Drug Administration (FDA) has recently approved donepezil for treatment of severe cases of DAT (Rabins et al. 2007). Positive results also have been documented in moderate to severe cases of DAT with memantine (Reisberg et al. 2003) (see Table 6–13). It blocks the effects of glutamate in stimulating the *N*-methyl-D-aspartate receptor. A Cochrane review concluded that the evidence to date shows that in moderate to severe DAT, memantine improves measures of cognition and functional decline but does not effect clinically discernible change or improve global measures of dementia (Areosa Sastre et al. 2004). Some evidence indicates that the combined administration of cholinesterase inhibitors and memantine may be more effective than either one of the drugs alone (Fillit et al. 2006; Grossberg et al. 2006).

Cholinesterase inhibitors show some promise in the treatment of other dementias, such as DLB (McKeith et al. 2000) and Parkinson's disease (Maidment et al. 2006). Rivastigmine has been approved by the FDA for Parkinson's disease (Rabins et al. 2007).

An antioxidant, vitamin E (200–2,000 IU/day), was in the past recommended for DAT patients to prevent further decline. However, a systematic review found limited evidence to support its use (Isaac et al. 2008), and doubts have been raised about the safety of such doses (E.R. Miller et al. 2005) for treatment of DAT.

Positive results with a wide variety of agents to treat DAT have been reported, and systematic reviews support the benefits of nimodipine (90 mg/day), a calcium channel blocker (López-Arrieta and Birks 2000); nicergoline, an ergot derivative (Fioravanti and Flicker 2001); and selegiline, a monoamine oxidase–B inhibitor (Birks and Flicker 2003). Selegiline (5–10 mg/day) may delay cognitive deterioration and may be worth considering in patients who are intolerant of, or unresponsive to, cholinesterase inhibitors. At this dosage, it requires no dietary limitations as with other

TABLE 6–13. Drug treatments for cognitive and functional losses in dementia of the Alzheimer's type (DAT): Cochrane System Reviews

Drug	Effectiveness[a]	Cognitive[a]	Behavioral[a]	ADL[a]	Indications in DAT	Dosage	Mechanism of action	Side effects
Donepezil[b]	++	++	++	++	Mild or moderate	5–10 mg once daily	AChE inhibitor	Nausea, vomiting, diarrhea
Rivastigmine[c]	++	++	++	++	Mild or moderate	1.5–6 mg twice a day	AChE, BChE inhibitor	Nausea, vomiting, diarrhea
Galantamine[d]	++	++	++	++	Mild or moderate	4–12 mg twice a day	AChE inhibitor	Nausea, vomiting, diarrhea
Memantine[e]	+	++	+	+	Moderate or severe	10–20 mg twice a day	NMDA antagonist	Agitation, urinary incontinence

Note. AChE = acetylcholinesterase; ADL = activity of daily living; BChE = butyrylcholinesterase; NMDA = *N*-methyl-D-aspartate.

[a]++ = evidence considerable; + = some evidence, limited number of controlled trials.

[b]Birks 2006; Birks and Harvey 2006.

[c]Birks et al. 2009.

[d]Birks and Harvey 2006; Olin and Schneider 2002.

[e]Areosa Sastre and Sherriff 2004; McShane et al. 2006.

monoamine oxidase inhibitors, but a major side effect is orthostatic hypotension.

Beneficial effects have been claimed, but not proven, with several agents, including statin therapy to lower serum cholesterol (Scott and Laake 2001); dehydroepiandrosterone (Huppert and Van Niekerk 2001); estrogen replacement therapy in postmenopausal women (Hogervorst et al. 2002); and ginkgo biloba, an extract of the leaves of the maidenhair tree (Birks et al. 2002; DeKosky et al. 2008). No evidence has been found for the use of Hydergine, an ergoloid mesylate, in DAT (Olin et al. 2001b). Preventive treatment with antihypertensive drugs is also controversial (Feigin et al. 2005; McGuinness et al. 2006), although the results of a large international trial with candesartan in mild hypertension are promising (Lithell et al. 2003). In view of recent findings related to vascular factors influencing the cognitive symptoms of DAT, multicomponent vascular care programs combining pharmacological and nonpharmacological interventions have been designed, but results to date have been negative (Richard et al. 2009).

Finally, systematic reviews do not support the use of indomethacin, a nonsteroidal anti-inflammatory drug (Tabet and Feldman 2002); piracetam, a nootropic agent with effects on increasing oxygen and glucose utilization and probable platelet antiaggregation properties (Flicker and Grimley Evans 2001); lecithin, a major dietary source of choline (Higgins and Flicker 2003); omega-3 polyunsaturated fatty acid (Lim et al. 2006); D-cycloserine, an antibiotic that enhances glutamate function (Laake and Oeksengaard 2002); nicotine (López-Arrieta et al. 2001); and folic acid (Malouf and Grimley Evans 2008) or vitamin B_{12} (Malouf and Areosa Sastre 2003).

Future drugs may strategically aim to retard or prevent amyloid deposition and neuronal degeneration and to stimulate neuroprotection (Cutler and Sramek 2001). The development of experimental vaccines directed against the formation and accumulation of amyloid plaques has shown promise. Strategies include the development of drugs focused on reduction of amyloid beta (Aβ) production; promotion of the Aβ degrading catabolic pathway; immunotherapy for Aβ; and inhibition of Aβ aggregation (Hamaguchi et al. 2006).

Drug treatment of mild cognitive impairment is controversial because evidence supporting pharmacological strategies remains limited. Efficacy of nicergoline (Fioravanti and Flicker 2001) and the dopamine receptor agonist piribedil (Nagaraja and Jayashree 2001) has been reported, and results of a meta-analysis support the use of acetyl-L-carnitine (Montgomery et al. 2003). Several long-term clinical trials are still ongoing (antioxidants, nootropics, anticholinesterases). Prevention and disease-modifying strategies raise ethical questions because interventions are focused on nondiseased elderly at risk, which means that long-term safety should be given disproportionate emphasis compared with efficacy. At present, treatment strategies for DAT could be extrapolated to mild cognitive impairment (Jelic and Winblad 2003). We recommend follow-up and monitoring of individuals with mild cognitive impairment, especially when neuroimaging suggests a high probability of conversion to DAT (see subsection "Neuroimaging and Electroencephalography" earlier in this chapter).

Vascular dementia has no standard treatment (Erkinjuntti 2002), but recently, symptomatic cholinergic treatment has shown promise in both DAT with vascular dementia and vascular dementia alone. However, evidence on the efficacy and safety of the drugs is limited (Craig and Birks 2006; Kavirajan and Schneider 2007). Individual patients might be helped with these drugs, but no general recommendations can be issued. Similarly, limited evidence supports the use of memantine (Kavirajan and Schneider 2007; McShane et al. 2006; Rabins et al. 2007), nicergoline (Fioravanti and Flicker 2001), and nimodipine (López-Arrieta and Birks 2000). Evidence is also limited on the primary prevention and secondary prevention of vascular dementia (Roman 2002), but treating associated medical conditions and reducing known cardiovascular and cerebrovascular risk factors seem logical steps. Daily aspirin therapy to inhibit platelet aggregation has been recommended but remains controversial (R. Hebert et al. 2000) and is not supported by the results of a systematic review (Williams et al. 2000). The preventive effects of early treatment of even mild hypertension are also promising for vascular dementia (Lithell et al. 2003), but no convincing evidence has been found so far relating diabetic treatment to the prevention or management of cognitive impairment in type 2 diabetes (Areosa Sastre and Grimley Evans 2002). More studies are needed of the effectiveness and efficacy of prevention and treatment of mild cognitive impairment of vascular origin. In the meantime, good clinical sense recommends symptomatic treatment and control of other treatable risk factors—namely, cardiac disease, hyperlipidemia, obesity, hyperhomocysteinemia, hyperfibrinogenemia, and other conditions that can cause brain hypoperfusion, such as obstructive sleep apnea and orthostatic hypotension (Frisoni et al. 2002). Psychiatrists can play a prominent role in treating and preventing smoking and alcohol dependence. Genetic counseling may be considered in diseases of genetic basis, such as cerebral autosomal dominant arteriopathy with subcortical infarcts and leukoencephalopathy.

Psychological Treatment

Two main goals may be identified in the psychological treatment of dementia: providing support and modifying behavior. Few psychological treatments have been subjected to systematic evaluation, but some research, including single-case studies, along with clinical experience, supports their effectiveness. The supportive techniques are based on the recognition that deterioration of cognitive function and sense of identity has significant psychological meaning for patients with dementia and may be associated with high levels of distress. There is some overlap with cognitive-behavioral techniques because the support is often accompanied by educational measures in which the nature and course of their illness are clearly explained. Psychiatrists also can assist patients and teach other staff to find ways to maximize functioning in preserved areas and to compensate for the defective functions. This includes simple maneuvers, such as taking notes for memory problems or making schedules to help structure activities into a daily routine. In this way, patients with dementia may have a predictable schedule and avoid undue distress, including catastrophic reactions when confronted with unfamiliar activities or environments.

Behavioral treatments are often focused on specific cognitive deficits, and different strategies have been devised. Reality orientation operates through the presentation of orientation-related information (e.g., time-, place-, and person-related), which is thought to provide the person with a greater understanding of his or her surroundings. A systematic review found evidence that reality orientation has benefits for both cognition and behavior in dementia (Spector et al. 2000a). Cognitive stimulation therapy has been reported to have benefits for cognition and may be more cost-effective than treatment as usual (Knapp et al. 2006). Observational studies give some support to other strategies, such as recreational activity, art therapy, dance therapy, and pet therapy. Reminiscence therapy tries to stimulate the patient to talk about the past. Beneficial effects on the patient's mood and/or behavior have been reported with this technique, but the evidence in systematic reviews is limited (Chung et al. 2002; Spector et al. 2000b). Similarly, evidence is insufficient on the effectiveness of other techniques, such as validation therapy (Neal and Briggs 2000).

Family Support and Social Care

The fate of dementia patients is determined to a large extent by their social framework (Organization for Economic Cooperation and Development 2002). Psychiatrists and other providers should pay attention to the family and social structures, community supports, and the potential need for residential treatment. Strong evidence suggests that informal (i.e., family) caregivers very frequently have psychiatric morbidity and possibly also medical morbidity related to the burden of caring for patients with dementia (J. Schneider et al. 1999). Empathic interventions may help them understand the complex mixture of feelings associated with caring for a loved one with a dementing illness. The effectiveness of techniques aimed at improving management of patients with dementia and coping strategies has been reported (Selwood et al. 2007). Referral to support groups is often indicated, and associations of families of patients with dementia exist in many countries and often provide critical support. Education, counseling, and support for family caregivers of DAT patients have been shown to improve the outcomes for both caregivers and patients (Olin and Schneider 2002) and to decrease the likelihood of placing a spouse in a nursing home (Cohen and Pushkar 1999). A book that has been very helpful for family and other caregivers is *The 36-Hour Day* (Mace and Rabins 2006).

Care Provision

Mental health facilities that specialize in treating dementia are varied. Psychiatrists should participate in supporting access to quality care, but no consensus currently exists about what constitutes quality care and how to assess care provision (Innes 2002). Social service referrals are very helpful to inform the family about available resources. Special care units for patients with dementia may offer models of optimal care, but no empirical evidence indicates that this type of unit achieves better outcomes than do traditional facilities.

The most common facility to care for patients with dementia is the memory clinic (Colvez et al. 2002). Such clinics gain value when attached to a psychosomatic medicine/consultation-liaison service, particularly when liaison is developed with primary care (A. Lobo and Saz 2004). Community resources include home health services, day care, or nursing homes. Shortage of nursing home beds is reported in most countries, so residential care remains important and in demand (Organization for Economic Cooperation and Development 2002). Geriatric day hospitals provide multidisciplinary rehabilitation in an outpatient setting. A review of studies documented a significant difference in favor of day hospital attendance when compared with no comprehensive elderly care (Forster et al. 2000). However, the general move toward an increased emphasis on community care is also dependent on the availability of informal caregivers. Respite services are considered very important for informal caregivers, although their effectiveness remains inconclusive.

Long-term care of patients with dementia presents special problems. Delirium, a frequent complication in institutionalized elderly patients with dementia, is discussed in Chapter 5, "Delirium." Another common complication is wandering. DAT patients may, at times, put themselves at risk, creating difficult challenges for caregivers and institutional staff. Traditional interventions to prevent wandering include restraint, drugs, and locked doors. Because cognitively impaired patients may respond to environmental stimuli in different ways, new techniques that might reduce wandering include the design of visual and other selective barriers, such as mirrors and grids or stripes of tape. However, a systematic review has found no evidence that these techniques are effective (Price et al. 2000).

Overuse of medication in long-term institutionalized patients can lead to worsening of the dementia and to harmful side effects. Available alternatives, such as the search for medical, psychiatric, or environmental factors that may be causing agitation or behavior problems, are discussed in a previous section of this chapter ("Epidemiology, Etiology, and Risk Factors") and should be pursued. However, if a patient's behavior is dangerous, psychotropic medications should be used, and additional measures may be needed if no response occurs. Use of physical restraints should be limited to patients with imminent risk of physical harm to themselves or others and only until more definitive treatment is provided or after other measures have been exhausted (or pose greater risk to the patient). Good clinical practice and legal regulations in some countries require careful consideration and documentation of the indications and available alternatives, monitoring of the response, and reassessment of the need for treatment. Structured educational programs for staff may decrease both the abuse of tranquilizers and the use of physical restraints in the institutionalized elderly.

References

Aarsland D, Andersen K, Larsen JP, et al: Risk of dementia in Parkinson's disease: a community-based, prospective study. Neurology 56:730–736, 2001

Aarsland D, Andersen K, Larsen JP, et al: Prevalence and characteristics of dementia in Parkinson disease: an 8-year prospective study. Arch Neurol 60:387–392, 2003

Alexopoulos G, Abrams R, Young R, et al: Cornell scale for depression in dementia. Biol Psychiatry 23:271–284, 1988

American Academy of Neurology AIDS Task Force: Nomenclature and research case definitions for neurologic manifestations of human immunodeficiency virus-type 1 (HIV-1) infection. Neurology 41:778–785, 1991

American Psychiatric Association: Diagnostic and Statistical Manual of Mental Disorders, 3rd Edition, Revised. Washington, DC, American Psychiatric Association, 1987

American Psychiatric Association: Diagnostic and Statistical Manual of Mental Disorders, 4th Edition, Text Revision. Washington, DC, American Psychiatric Association, 2000

American Psychiatric Association: The Practice of Electroconvulsive Therapy: Recommendations for Treatment, Training and Privileging, 2nd Edition. A Task Force Report of the American Psychiatric Association. Washington, DC, American Psychiatric Press, 2001

Apostolova LG, Cummings JL: Neuropsychiatric manifestations in mild cognitive impairment: a systematic review of the literature. Dement Geriatr Cogn Disord 25:115–126, 2008

Areosa Sastre A, Grimley Evans J: Effect of the treatment of Type II diabetes mellitus on the development of cognitive impairment and dementia. Cochrane Database Syst Rev (4):CD003804, 2002

Areosa Sastre A, McShane R, Sherriff F: Memantine for dementia. Cochrane Database Syst Rev (4):CD003154, 2004

Bains J, Birks JS, Dening TR: The efficacy of antidepressants in the treatment of depression in dementia. Cochrane Database Syst Rev (4):CD003944, 2002

Ballard C, Waite J: The effectiveness of atypical antipsychotics for the treatment of aggression and psychosis in Alzheimer's disease. Cochrane Database Syst Rev (1):CD003476, 2006

Ballard CG, O'Brien JT, Morris CM, et al: The progression of cognitive impairment in dementia with Lewy bodies, vascular dementia and AD. Int Psychogeriatr 16:499–503, 2001

Birks J: Cholinesterase inhibitors for Alzheimer's disease. Cochrane Database Syst Rev (1):CD005593, 2006

Birks J, Flicker L: Selegiline for Alzheimer's disease. Cochrane Database Syst Rev (1):CD000442, 2003

Birks J, Harvey RJ: Donepezil for dementia due to Alzheimer's disease. Cochrane Database Syst Rev (1):CD001190, 2006

Birks J, Grimley Evans J, Van Dongen M: Ginkgo biloba for cognitive impairment and dementia. Cochrane Database Syst Rev (4):CD003120, 2002

Birks J, Grimley Evans J, Iakovidou V, et al: Rivastigmine for Alzheimer's disease. Cochrane Database Syst Rev (2):CD001191, 2009

Blansjaar BA, van Dijk JG: Korsakoff minus Wernicke syndrome. Alcohol 27:435–437, 1992

Blessed G, Tomlinson BE, Roth M: The association between quantitative measures of dementia and of senile change in the cerebral grey matter of elderly subjects. Br J Psychiatry 114:797–811, 1968

Boeve BF: A review of non-Alzheimer dementias. J Clin Psychiatry 67:1985–2001, 2006

Boise L, Neal M, Kaye J: Dementia assessment in primary care: results from a study in three managed care systems. J Gerontol Biol Sci Med Sci 59:M621–M626, 2004

Bourgeois JA, Seaman JS, Servis M: Delirium, dementia and amnestic and other cognitive disorders, in The American Psychiatric Publishing Textbook of Psychiatry, 5th Edition. Edited by Hales RE, Yudofsky SC, Gabbard GO. Washington, DC, American Psychiatric Publishing, 2008, pp 303–363

Boustani M, Peterson B, Hanson L, et al: Screening for dementia in primary care: a summary of the evidence for the U.S. Preventive Services Task Force. Ann Intern Med 138:927–937, 2003

Breitner JC, Wyse BW, Anthony JC, et al: APOE-epsilon4 count predicts age when prevalence of AD increases, then declines: the Cache County Study. Neurology 53:321–331, 1999

Brookmeyer R, Corrada MM, Curriero FC, et al: Survival following a diagnosis of Alzheimer disease. Arch Neurol 59:1764–1767, 2002

Buchman AS, Wilson RS, Bennett DA: Total daily activity is associated with cognition in older persons. Am J Geriatr Psychiatry 16:697–701, 2008

Buee L, Bussiere T, Buee-Scherrer V, et al: Tau protein isoforms, phosphorylation and role in neurodegenerative disorders. Brain Res Rev 33:95–130, 2000

Campbell S, Stephens S, Ballard C: Dementia with Lewy bodies: clinical features and treatment. Drugs Aging 18:397–407, 2001

Chen R, Hu Z, Wei L, et al: Severity of depression and risk for subsequent dementia: cohort studies in China and the UK. Br J Psychiatry 193:373–377, 2008

Chertkow H, Massoud F, Nasreddine Z, et al: Diagnosis and treatment of dementia, 3: mild cognitive impairment and cognitive impairment without dementia. CMAJ 178:1273–1285, 2008

Chetelat G, Baron JC: Early diagnosis of Alzheimer's disease: contribution of structural neuroimaging. Neuroimage 18:525–541, 2003

Chung JCC, Lai CKY, Chung PMB, et al: Snoezelen for dementia. Cochrane Database Syst Rev (4):CD003152, 2002

Cohen CA, Pushkar D: Lessons learned from a longitudinal study of dementia care. Am J Geriatr Psychiatry 7:139–146, 1999

Colvez A, Joel ME, Ponton-Sanchez A, et al: Health status and work burden of Alzheimer patients' informal caregivers: comparisons of five different care programs in the European Union. Health Policy 60:219–233, 2002

Craig D, Birks J: Galantamine for vascular cognitive impairment. Cochrane Database Syst Rev (1):CD004746, 2006

Crum RM, Anthony JC, Basset SS, et al: Population based norms for the Mini-Mental State Examination by age and educational level. JAMA 269:2386–2391, 1993

Cummings JL, Benson DF: Subcortical dementia: review of an emerging concept. Arch Neurol 41:874–879, 1984

Cummings JL, Mega M, Gray KF, et al: The Neuropsychiatric Inventory: comprehensive assessment of psychopathology in dementia. Neurology 44:2308–2314, 1994

Cummings JL, Vinters HV, Cole GM, et al: Alzheimer's disease: etiologies, pathophysiology, cognitive reserve, and treatment opportunities. Neurology 51:S2–S17, 1998

Cummings JL, McRae T, Zhang R; Donepezil-Sertraline Study Group: Effects of donepezil on neuropsychiatric symptoms in patients with dementia and severe behavioral disorders. Am J Geriatr Psychiatry 14:605–612, 2006

Cutler NR, Sramek JJ: Review of the next generation of Alzheimer's disease therapeutics: challenges for drug development. Prog Neuropsychopharmacol Biol Psychiatry 25:27–57, 2001

Daiello LA: Atypical antipsychotics for the treatment of dementia-related behaviors: an update. Med Health R I 90:191–194, 2007

Dalmau J, Gleichman AJ, Hughes EG, et al: Anti-NMDA-receptor encephalitis: case series and analysis of the effects of antibodies. Lancet Neurol 7:1091–1098, 2008

de Groot JC, de Leeuw FE, Oudkerk M, et al: Cerebral white matter lesions and depressive symptoms in elderly adults. Arch Gen Psychiatry 57:1071–1076, 2000

DeKosky ST, Williamson JD, Fitzpatrick AL: Ginkgo biloba for prevention of dementia: a randomized controlled trial. JAMA 300:2253–2262, 2008

Devanand DP, Jacobs DM, Tang MX, et al: The course of psychopathologic features in mild to moderate Alzheimer's disease. Arch Gen Psychiatry 54:257–263, 1997

Dewey ME, Saz P: Dementia, cognitive impairment and mortality in persons aged 65 and over living in the community: a systematic review of literature. Int J Geriatr Psychiatry 16:751–761, 2001

Dodge HH, Shen C, Pandav R, et al: Functional transitions and active life expectancy associated with Alzheimer disease. Arch Neurol 60:253–259, 2003

Doraiswamy PM, Leon J, Cummings JL, et al: Prevalence and impact of medical comorbidity in Alzheimer's disease. J Gerontol A Biol Sci Med Sci 57:M173–M177, 2002

Dubois B, Slachevsky A, Litvan I, et al: The FAB: a Frontal Assessment Battery at bedside. Neurology 55:1621–1626, 2000

Duyckaerts C, Verny M, Hauw JJ: Recent neuropathology of parkinsonian syndromes [in French]. Rev Neurol (Paris) 159 (5 pt 2):3S11–3S18, 2003

Dwyer J, Reid S: Ganser's syndrome. Lancet 364:471–473, 2004

Erkinjuntti T: Diagnosis and management of vascular cognitive impairment and dementia. J Neural Transm Suppl 63:91–109, 2002

Erkinjuntti T, Wikstrom J, Palo J, et al: Dementia among medical inpatients: evaluation of 2000 consecutive admissions. Arch Intern Med 146:1923–1926, 1986

Esmonde T, Cooke S: Shunting for normal pressure hydrocephalus (NPH). Cochrane Database Syst Rev (3):CD003157, 2002

Farlow MR, Boustani M: Pharmacological treatment of Alzheimer disease and mild cognitive impairment, in The American Psychiatric Publishing Textbook of Alzheimer Disease and Other Dementias. Edited by Weiner MF, Lipton AM. Washington, DC, American Psychiatric Publishing, 2009, pp 317–331

Feigin V, Ratnasabapathy Y, Anderson C: Does blood pressure lowering treatment prevent dementia or cognitive decline in patients with cardiovascular and cerebrovascular disease? J Neurol Sci 229–230:151–155, 2005

Ferrer I, Barrachina M, Puig B: Glycogen synthase kinase-3 (GSK-3) is associated with neuronal and glial hyper-phosphorylated tau deposits in Alzheimer's disease, Pick's disease, progressive supranuclear palsy and corticobasal degeneration. Acta Neuropathol 104:583–591, 2002

Ferri CP, Prince M, Brayne C, et al: Global prevalence of dementia: a Delphi consensus study. Lancet 366:2112–2117, 2005

Fillit HM, Doody RS, Binaso K, et al: Recommendations for best practices in the treatment of Alzheimer's disease in managed care. Am J Geriatr Pharmacother 4 (suppl):S9–S24, 2006

Fioravanti M, Flicker L: Efficacy of nicergoline in dementia and other age associated forms of cognitive impairment. Cochrane Database Syst Rev (4):CD003159, 2001

Flicker L, Grimley Evans J: Piracetam for dementia or cognitive impairment. Cochrane Database Syst Rev (2):CD001011, 2001

Folstein MF, McHugh PR: Dementia syndrome of depression, in Alzheimer's Disease: Senile Dementia and Related Disorders, Aging, Vol 7. Edited by Katzman R, Terry RD, Bick KL. New York, Raven, 1978, pp 87–93

Folstein MF, McHugh PR: The neuropsychiatry of some specific brain disorders, in Handbook of Psychiatry 2, Mental Disorders and Somatic Illness. Edited by Lader MH. London, Cambridge University Press, 1983, pp 107–118

Folstein MF, Folstein SE, McHugh PR: Mini-Mental State: a practical method for grading the cognitive state of patients for the clinician. J Psychiatr Res 12:189–198, 1975

Folstein MF, Folstein SE, McHugh PR, et al: MMSE: Mini-Mental State Examination: User's Guide. Odessa, FL, PAR Psychological Assessment Resources, 2001

Forster A, Young J, Langhorne P, for the Day Hospital Group: Medical day hospital care for the elderly versus alternative forms of care. Cochrane Database Syst Rev (2):CD001730, 2000

Foster AR, Caplan JP: Paraneoplastic limbic encephalitis. Psychosomatics 50:108–113, 2009

Fratiglioni L, Launer LJ, Andersen K, et al: Incidence of dementia and major subtypes in Europe: a collaborative study of population-based cohorts. Neurology 54 (suppl 5):10–15, 2000

Frisoni GB, Galluzzi S, Bresciani L, et al: Mild cognitive impairment with subcortical vascular features: clinical characteristics and outcome. J Neurol 249:1423–1432, 2002

Galasko DR, Gould RL, Abramson IS, et al: Measuring cognitive change in a cohort of patients with Alzheimer's disease. Stat Med 19:1421–1432, 2000

Gauthier S, Reisberg B, Zaudig M, et al: Mild cognitive impairment. International Psychogeriatric Association Expert Conference on mild cognitive impairment. Lancet 367:1262–1270, 2006

Gillen TE, Gregg KM, Yuan H, et al: Clinical trials in Alzheimer's disease: calculating Alzheimer's Disease Assessment Scale—cognitive subsection with the data from the Consortium to Establish a Registry for Alzheimer's Disease. Psychopharmacol Bull 35:83–96, 2001

Giron MS, Forsell Y, Bernsten C, et al: Psychotropic drug use in elderly people with and without dementia. Int J Geriatr Psychiatry 16:900–906, 2001

Gray KF, Cummings JL: Dementia, in The American Psychiatric Publishing Textbook of Consultation-Liaison Psychiatry: Psychiatry in the Medically Ill, 2nd Edition. Edited by Wise MG, Rundell JR. Washington, DC, American Psychiatric Publishing, 2002, pp 273–306

Grossberg GT, Edwards KR, Zhao Q: Rationale for combination therapy with galantamine and memantine in Alzheimer's disease. J Clin Pharmacol 46 (suppl):17S–26S, 2006

Hamaguchi T, Ono K, Yamada M: Anti-amyloidogenic therapies: strategies for prevention and treatment of Alzheimer's disease. Cell Mol Life Sci 63:1538–1552, 2006

Haskins BA, Harrison MB: Huntington's disease. Curr Treat Options Neurol 2:243–262, 2000

Hebert LE, Beckett LA, Scherr PA, et al: Annual incidence of Alzheimer disease in the United States projected to the years 2000 through 2050. Alzheimer Dis Assoc Disord 15:169–173, 2001

Hebert R, Lindsay J, Verreault R, et al: Vascular dementia: incidence and risk factors in the Canadian study of health and aging. Stroke 31:1487–1493, 2000

Hejl A, Hogh P, Waldemar G: Potentially reversible conditions in 1000 consecutive memory clinic patients. J Neurol Neurosurg Psychiatry 73:390–394, 2002

Herrmann N, Rothenburg LS, Black SE, et al: Methylphenidate for the treatment of apathy in Alzheimer disease: prediction of response using dextroamphetamine challenge. J Clin Psychopharmacol 28:296–301, 2008

Higgins JP, Flicker L: Lecithin for dementia and cognitive impairment. Cochrane Database Syst Rev (3):CD001015, 2003

Hogervorst E, Yaffe K, Richards M, et al: Hormone replacement therapy to maintain cognitive function in women with dementia. Cochrane Database Syst Rev (3):CD003799, 2002

Hughes CP, Berg L, Danziger WL, et al: A new clinical scale for the staging of dementia. Br J Psychiatry 140:566–572, 1982

Huntington G: On chorea. Med Surg Rep 26:317–332, 1872

Huppert FA, Van Niekerk JK: Dehydroepiandrosterone (DHEA) supplementation for cognitive function. Cochrane Database Syst Rev (2):CD000304, 2001

Huyse FJ, Herzog T, Malt UF, et al: The European Consultation-Liaison Workgroup (ECLW) Collaborative Study, I: general outline. Gen Hosp Psychiatry 18:44–55, 1996

Innes A: The social and political context of formal dementia care provision. Ageing Soc 22:483–499, 2002

Isaac MG, Quinn R, Tabet N: Vitamin E for Alzheimer's disease and mild cognitive impairment. Cochrane Database Syst Rev (3):CD002854, 2008

Iseki E, Togo T, Suzuki K, et al: Dementia with Lewy bodies from the perspective of tauopathy. Acta Neuropathol (Berl) 105:265–270, 2003

Ivan CS, Seshadri S, Beiser A, et al: Dementia after stroke: the Framingham Study. Stroke 35:1264–1268, 2004

Jelic V, Winblad B: Treatment of mild cognitive impairment: rationale, present and future strategies. Acta Neurol Scand Suppl 179:83–93, 2003

Jellinger KA: Alzheimer disease and cerebrovascular pathology: an update. J Neural Transm 109:813–836, 2002

Jorm AF: A short form of the Informant Questionnaire on Cognitive Decline in the Elderly (IQCODE): development and cross-validation. Psychol Med 24:145–153, 1994

Jorm AF: History of depression as a risk factor for dementia: an updated review. Aust N Z J Psychiatry 35:776–781, 2001

Jorm AF, Jacomb PA: The Informant Questionnaire on Cognitive Decline in the Elderly (IQCODE): socio-demographic correlates, reliability, validity and some norms. Psychol Med 19:1015–1022, 1989

Kalaria RN: The role of cerebral ischemia in Alzheimer's disease. Neurobiol Aging 21:321–330, 2000

Kasahara H, Karasawa A, Ariyasu T, et al: Alcohol dementia and alcohol delirium in aged alcoholics. Psychiatry Clin Neurosci 50:115–123, 1996

Katz S, Downs TD, Cash HR, et al: Progress in development of the index of ADL. Gerontologist 10:20–30, 1970

Kavirajan H, Schneider LS: Efficacy and adverse effects of cholinesterase inhibitors and memantine in vascular dementia: a meta-analysis of randomised controlled trials. Lancet Neurol 6:782–792, 2007

Knapp M, Thorgrimsen L, Patel A, et al: Cognitive stimulation therapy for people with dementia: cost-effectiveness analysis. Br J Psychiatry 188:574–580, 2006

Knopman DS: Dementia and cerebrovascular disease. Mayo Clin Proc 81:223–230, 2006

Knopman DS, DeKosky ST, Cummings JL, et al: Practice parameter: diagnosis of dementia (an evidence-based review)—report of the Quality Standards Subcommittee of the American Academy of Neurology. Neurology 56:1143–1153, 2001

Kraus JF, Sorenson SB: Epidemiology, in Neuropsychiatry of Traumatic Brain Injury. Edited by Silver JM, Yudofsky SC, Hales RE. Washington, DC, American Psychiatric Press, 1994, pp 3–41

Kukull WA, Higdon R, Bowen JD, et al: Dementia and Alzheimer disease incidence: a prospective cohort study. Arch Neurol 59:1737–1746, 2002

Kurz A, Riemenschneider M, Drzezga A, et al: The role of biological markers in the early and differential diagnosis of Alzheimer's disease. J Neural Transm Suppl 62:127–133, 2002

Laake K, Oeksengaard AR: D-Cycloserine for Alzheimer's disease. Cochrane Database Syst Rev (2):CD003153, 2002

Langa KM, Foster NL, Larson EB: Mixed dementia: emerging concepts and therapeutic implications. JAMA 292:2901–2908, 2004

Larrieu S, Letenneur L, Helmer C, et al: Nutritional factors and risk of incident dementia in the PAQUID longitudinal cohort. J Nutr Health Aging 8:150–154, 2004

Launer LJ: Demonstrating the case that AD is a vascular disease: epidemiologic evidence. Ageing Res Rev 1:61–77, 2002

Lawton MP, Brody E: Assessment of older people: self-maintaining and instrumental activities of daily living. Gerontologist 9:179–186, 1969

Lebert F, Souliez L, Pasquier F, et al: Trazodone in the treatment of behavior in frontotemporal dementia. Hum Psychopharmacol Clin Exp 14:279–281, 1999

Lebert F, Delacourte A, Pasquier F: Treatment of frontotemporal dementia, in Alzheimer's Disease and Related Disorders Annual 2002. Edited by Gauthier S, Cummings JL. London, Taylor & Francis, 2002, pp 171–182

Lepola UM, Loft H, Reines EH: Escitalopram (10–20 mg/day) is effective and well tolerated in a placebo-controlled study in depression in primary care. Int Clin Psychopharmacol 18:211–217, 2003

Lev N, Melamed E: Heredity in Parkinson's disease: new findings. Isr Med Assoc J 3:435–438, 2001

Lim WS, Gammack JK, Van Niekerk J, et al: Omega 3 fatty acid for the prevention of dementia. Cochrane Database Syst Rev (1):CD005379, 2006

Lishman WA: Organic Psychiatry: The Psychological Consequences of Cerebral Disorder, 3rd Edition. London, Blackwell Science, 1998

Lithell H, Hansson L, Skoog I, et al: The Study on Cognition and Prognosis in the Elderly (SCOPE): principal results of a randomized double-blind intervention trial. J Hypertens 21:875–886, 2003

Litvan I: Recent advances in atypical parkinsonian disorders. Curr Opin Neurol 12:441–446, 1999

Lobo A, Saz P: Clínica de la memoria y unidad de demencias: un programa de enlace con atención primaria [A memory clinic and dementia unit: a liaison program with primary care]. Cuadernos de Medicina Psicosomática 69/70:115–123, 2004

Lobo A, Saz P, Marcos G, et al: The prevalence of dementia and depression in the elderly community in a Southern European population: the Zaragoza study. Arch Gen Psychiatry 52:497–506, 1995

Lobo A, Saz P, Marcos G, et al: The Zaragoza Study: Dementia and Depression in the Elderly Community. Barcelona, Spain, Editorial Masson Salvat S.A., 1997

Lobo A, Saz P, Marcos G, et al: Revalidation and standardization of the cognition mini-exam (first Spanish version of the Mini-Mental Status Examination) in the general geriatric population. Med Clin (Barc) 112:767–774, 1999

Lobo A, Launer LJ, Fratiglioni L, et al: Prevalence of dementia and major subtypes in Europe: a collaborative study of population-based cohorts. Neurology 54 (suppl 5):4–9, 2000

Lonergan E, Luxenberg J, Colford J: Haloperidol for agitation in dementia. Cochrane Database Syst Rev (2):CD002852, 2002

López-Arrieta JM, Birks J: Nimodipine for primary degenerative, mixed and vascular dementia. Cochrane Database Syst Rev (2):CD000147, 2000

López-Arrieta JM, Rodríguez JL, Sanz F: Efficacy and safety of nicotine on Alzheimer's disease patients. Cochrane Database Syst Rev (2)CD001749, 2001

Loudianos G, Gitlin JD: Wilson's disease. Semin Liver Dis 2:353–364, 2000

Loveman E, Green C, Kirby J, et al: The clinical and cost-effectiveness of donepezil, rivastigmine, galantamine and memantine for Alzheimer's disease. Health Technol Assess 10:1–160, 2006

Luppa M, Luck T, Brähler E, et al: Prediction of institutionalisation in dementia: a systematic review. Dement Geriatr Cogn Disord 26:65–78, 2008

Lyketsos CG, Lee HB: Diagnosis and treatment of depression in Alzheimer's disease: a practical update for the clinician. Dement Geriatr Cogn Disord 17:55–64, 2004

Lyketsos CG, Sheppard JM, Rabins PV: Dementia in elderly persons in a general hospital. Am J Psychiatry 157:704–707, 2000

Lyketsos CG, Lopez O, Jones B, et al: Prevalence of neuropsychiatric symptoms in dementia and mild cognitive impairment: results from the Cardiovascular Health Study. JAMA 288:1475–1483, 2002

Lyketsos CG, DelCampo L, Steinberg M, et al: Treating depression in Alzheimer disease: efficacy and safety of sertraline therapy, and the benefits of depression reduction: the DIADS. Arch Gen Psychiatry 60:737–746, 2003

Macdonald AJ, Carpenter GI, Box O, et al: Dementia and use of psychotropic medication in non-"Elderly Mentally Infirm" nursing homes in South East England. Age Ageing 31:58–64, 2002

Mace NL, Rabins PV: The 36-Hour Day, 4th Edition: A Family Guide to Caring for People With Alzheimer Disease, Other Dementias, and Memory Loss in Later Life. Baltimore, MD, Johns Hopkins University Press, 2006

Maidment I, Fox C, Boustani M: Cholinesterase inhibitors for Parkinson's disease dementia. Cochrane Database Syst Rev (1):CD004747, 2006

Malouf R, Areosa Sastre A: Vitamin B12 for cognition. Cochrane Database Syst Rev (3):CD004326, 2003

Malouf R, Grimley Evans J: Folic acid with or without vitamin B12 for the prevention and treatment of healthy elderly and demented people. Cochrane Database Syst Rev (4):CD004514, 2008

Malt UF, Huyse FJ, Herzog T, et al: The ECLW Collaborative Study, III: training and reliability of ICD-10 psychiatric diagnoses in the general hospital setting—an investigation of 220 consultants from 14 European countries. J Psychosom Res 41:451–463, 1996

Mayeux R, Sano M: Treatment of Alzheimer's disease. N Engl J Med 341:1670–1679, 1999

McDowell I, Kristjansson B, Hill GB, et al: Community screening for dementia: the Mini Mental State Exam (MMSE) and Modified Mini-Mental State Exam (3MS) compared. J Clin Epidemiol 50:377–383, 1997

McGuinness B, Todd S, Passmore P, et al: The effects of blood pressure lowering on development of cognitive impairment and dementia in patients without apparent prior cerebrovascular disease. Cochrane Database Syst Rev (2):CD004034, 2006

McHugh PR: Hydrocephalic dementia. Bull N Y Acad Med 42:907–917, 1966

McHugh PR, Folstein MF: Psychiatric syndromes of Huntington's chorea: a clinical and phenomenologic study, in Psychiatric Aspects of Neurologic Disease. Edited by Benson DF, Blumer D. New York, Grune & Stratton, 1975, pp 267–285

McHugh PR, Folstein MF: Psychopathology of dementia: implications for neuropathology, in Congenital and Acquired Cognitive Disorders. Edited by Katzman R. New York, Raven, 1979, pp 17–30

McHugh PR, Slavney PR: The Perspectives of Psychiatry. Baltimore, MD, Johns Hopkins University Press, 1998

McKeith I, Fairburn A, Perry R, et al: Neuroleptic sensitivity in patients with senile dementia of Lewy body type. BMJ 305:673–678, 1992

McKeith IG, Galasko D, Kosaka K, et al: Consensus guidelines for the clinical and pathologic diagnosis of dementia with Lewy bodies (DLB): report of the Consortium on DLB International Workshop. Neurology 47:1113–1124, 1996

McKeith I, Del Ser T, Spano P, et al: Efficacy of rivastigmine in dementia with Lewy bodies: a randomised, double-blind, placebo-controlled international study. Lancet 356:2031–2036, 2000

McKeith IG, Dickson DW, Lowe J, et al: Diagnosis and management of dementia with Lewy bodies: third report of the DLB Consortium. Neurology 65:1863–1872, 2005

McKhann G, Drachman D, Folstein M, et al: Clinical diagnosis of Alzheimer's disease: report of the NINCDS-ADRDA Work Group under the auspices of Department of Health and Human Services Task Force on Alzheimer's Disease. Neurology 34:939–944, 1984

McShane R, Gedling D, Reasing M, et al: A prospective study of psychotic symptoms in dementia sufferers: psychosis in dementia. Int Psychogeriatr 9:57–64, 1997

McShane R, Areosa Sastre A, Minakaran N: Memantine for dementia. Cochrane Database Syst Rev (2):CD003154, 2006

Meier DE, Ahronheim JC, Morris J, et al: High short-term mortality in hospitalized patients with advanced dementia: lack of benefit of tube feeding. Arch Intern Med 161:594–599, 2001

Mesulam MM: Primary progressive aphasia—a language-based dementia. N Engl J Med 349:1535–1542, 2003

Miller ER III, Pastor-Barriuso R, Dalal D, et al: Meta-analysis: high-dosage vitamin E supplementation may increase all-cause mortality. Ann Intern Med 142:37–46, 2005

Miller LJ: Gabapentin for treatment of behavioral and psychological symptoms of dementia. Ann Pharmacother 35:427–431, 2001

Mitchell AJ: A meta-analysis of the accuracy of the mini-mental state examination in the detection of dementia and mild cognitive impairment. J Psychiatr Res 43:411–431, 2009

Miyasaki JM, Shannon K, Voon V, et al: Practice Parameter: evaluation and treatment of depression, psychosis, and dementia in Parkinson disease (an evidence-based review): report of the Quality Standards Subcommittee of the American Academy of Neurology. Neurology 66:996–1002, 2006

Modrego PJ, Fayed N, Pina MA: Conversion from mild cognitive impairment to probable Alzheimer's disease predicted by brain magnetic resonance spectroscopy. Am J Psychiatry 162:667–675, 2005

Mohs RC, Schmeidler J, Aryan M: Longitudinal studies of cognitive, functional and behavioral change in patients with Alzheimer's disease. Stat Med 19:1401–1409, 2000

Montgomery SA, Thal LJ, Amrein R: Meta-analysis of double blind randomized controlled clinical trials of acetyl-l-carnitine versus placebo in the treatment of mild cognitive impairment and mild Alzheimer's disease. Int Clin Psychopharmacol 18:61–71, 2003

Morris RG, Morris LW, Britton PG: Factors affecting the emotional wellbeing of the caregivers of dementia sufferers. Br J Psychiatry 153:147–156, 1988

Nagaraja D, Jayashree S: Randomized study of the dopamine receptor agonist piribedil in the treatment of mild cognitive impairment. Am J Psychiatry 158:1517–1519, 2001

National Institute on Aging: Alzheimer's Disease: Unraveling the Mystery. Bethesda, MD, National Institutes of Health, 2003

Neal M, Briggs M: Validation therapy for dementia. Cochrane Database Syst Rev (2):CD001394, 2000

Neuropathology Group, Medical Research Council Cognitive Function and Aging Study: Pathological correlates of late-onset dementia in a multicentre, community-based population in England and Wales. Neuropathology Group of the

Medical Research Council Cognitive Function and Ageing Study (MRC CFAS). Lancet 357:169–175, 2001
O'Brien J, Thomas A, Ballard C, et al: Cognitive impairment in depression is not associated with neuropathologic evidence of increased vascular or Alzheimer-type pathology. Biol Psychiatry 49:130–136, 2001
O'Brien JT, Erkinjuntti T, Reisberg B, et al: Vascular cognitive impairment. Lancet Neurol 2:89–98, 2003
Olin J, Schneider L: Galantamine for Alzheimer's disease. Cochrane Database Syst Rev (3):CD001747, 2002
Olin JT, Fox LS, Pawluczyk S, et al: A pilot randomized trial of carbamazepine for behavioural symptoms in treatment-resistant outpatients with Alzheimer disease. Am J Geriatr Psychiatry 9:400–405, 2001a
Olin J, Schneider L, Novit A, et al: Hydergine for dementia. Cochrane Database Syst Rev (2):CD000359, 2001b
Organization for Economic Cooperation and Development (OECD): Case Study on Dementia Care. OECD Report. Paris, France, Organization for Economic Cooperation and Development, 2002
Ovsiew F: Seeking reversibility and treatability in dementia. Semin Clin Neuropsychiatry 8:3–11, 2003
Pantoni L, Garcia JH: The significance of cerebral white matter abnormalities 100 years after Binswanger's report: a review. Stroke 26:1293–1301, 1995
Patterson CJ, Gauthier S, Bergman H, et al: The recognition, assessment and management of dementing disorders: conclusions from the Canadian Consensus Conference on Dementia. CMAJ 160 (12 suppl):S1–S15, 1999
Patterson C, Feightner, Garcia A, et al: Diagnosis and treatment of dementia, 1: risk assessment and primary prevention of Alzheimer disease. CMAJ 178:548–556, 2008
Paulsen JS, Salmon DP, Thal LJ: Incidence of and risk factors for hallucinations and delusions in patients with probable AD. Neurology 54:1965–1971, 2000
Peters R, Peters J, Warner J, et al: Alcohol, dementia and cognitive decline in the elderly: a systematic review. Age Ageing 37:505–512, 2008
Petersen RC: Mild cognitive impairment as a diagnostic entity. J Intern Med 256:183–194, 2004
Plum AF: Dementia: an approaching epidemic. Nature 279:372–373, 1979
Podewils LJ, Guallar E, Kuller LH, et al: Physical activity, APOE genotype and dementia risk: findings from the Cardiovascular Health Cognition Study. Am J Epidemiol 161:639–651, 2005
Posner HB, Tang MX, Luchsinger J, et al: The relationship of hypertension in the elderly to AD, vascular dementia, and cognitive function. Neurology 58:1175–1181, 2002
Price JD, Hermans DG, Grimley Evans J: Subjective barriers to prevent wandering of cognitively impaired people. Cochrane Database Syst Rev (4):CD001932, 2000
Qui C, von Strauss E, Fastbom J, et al: Low blood pressure and risk of dementia in the Kungsholmen Project: a 6-year follow-up study. Arch Neurol 60:223–228, 2003
Rabins P, Steele C: A scale to measure impairment in severe dementia and similar conditions. Am J Geriatr Psychiatry 4:247–251, 1996
Rabins PV, Lyketsos CG, Steele C: Practical Dementia Care. New York, Oxford University Press, 1999
Rabins P, Lyketsos C, Steele C: Practical Dementia Care, 2nd Edition. New York, Oxford University Press, 2006
Rabins PV, Blacker D, Rovner BW, et al: American Psychiatric Association practice guideline for the treatment of patients with Alzheimer's disease and other dementias. Second edition. Am J Psychiatry 164 (12 suppl):5–56, 2007
Ravaglia G, Forti P, Maioli F, et al: Homocysteine and folate as risk factors for dementia and Alzheimer disease. Am J Clin Nutr 82:636–643, 2005
Reisberg B, Ferris SH, de Leon MJ, et al: The Global Deterioration Scale for assessment of primary degenerative dementia. Am J Psychiatry 139:1136–1139, 1982
Reisberg B, Sclan SG, Franssen E, et al: Clinical stages of normal aging and Alzheimer's disease: the GDS staging system. Neurosci Res Commun 13 (suppl 1):551–554, 1993
Reisberg B, Doody R, Stoffler A, et al: Memantine in moderate-to-severe Alzheimer's disease. N Engl J Med 348:1333–1341, 2003
Richard E, Kuiper R, Dijkgraaf MG, et al: Vascular care in patients with Alzheimer's disease with cerebrovascular lesions—a randomized clinical trial. J Am Geriatr Soc 57:797–805, 2009
Rodda J, Morgan S, Walker Z: Are cholinesterase inhibitors effective in the management of the behavioral and psychological symptoms of dementia in Alzheimer's disease? A systematic review of randomized, placebo-controlled trials of donepezil, rivastigmine and galantamine. Int Psychogeriatr 19:1–12, 2009
Rojas-Fernández CH, Eng M, Allie ND: Pharmacologic management by clinical pharmacists of behavioral and psychological symptoms of dementia in nursing home residents: results from a pilot study. Pharmacotherapy 23:217–221, 2003
Roman GC: Vascular dementia revisited: diagnosis, pathogenesis, treatment, and prevention. Med Clin North Am 86:477–499, 2002
Roman GC, Tatemichi TK, Erkinjuntti T, et al: Vascular dementia: diagnostic criteria for research studies: report on the NINDS-AIREN International Workshop. Neurology 43:250–260, 1993
Ropacki SA, Jeste DV: Epidemiology of and risk factors for psychosis of Alzheimer's disease: a review of 55 studies published from 1990 to 2003. Am J Psychiatry 162:2022–2030, 2005
Rosen HJ, Lengenfelder J, Miller B: Frontotemporal dementia. Neurol Clin 18:979–992, 2000
Rosen WG, Mohs RC, Davis KL: A new rating scale for Alzheimer's disease. Am J Psychiatry 141:1356–1364, 1984
Sáez-Fonseca JA, Lee L, Walker Z: Long-term outcome of depressive pseudodementia in the elderly. J Affect Disord 101:123–129, 2007
Salzman C: Treatment of the agitation of late-life psychosis and Alzheimer's disease. Eur Psychiatry 16 (suppl 1):25S–28S, 2001

Sarazin M, Horne N, Dubois B: Natural history of Alzheimer's disease and other dementing illnesses, in Alzheimer's Disease and Related Disorders Annual. Edited by Gauthier S, Cummings JL. London, Taylor & Francis, 2002, pp 183–197

Saz P, López-Antón R, Dewey M, et al: Prevalence and implications of psychopathological non-cognitive symptoms in dementia. Acta Psychiatr Scand 119:107–116, 2009

Scarmeas N, Stern Y, Mayeux R, et al: Mediterranean diet and mild cognitive impairment. Arch Neurol 66:216–225, 2009

Schneider J, Murray J, Banerjee S, et al: EUROCARE: a cross-national study of co-resident spouse carers for people with Alzheimer's disease, I: factors associated with carer burden. Int J Geriatr Psychiatry 14:651–661, 1999

Schneider LS, Dagerman K, Insel PS: Efficacy and adverse effects of atypical antipsychotics for dementia: meta-analysis of randomized, placebo-controlled trials. Am J Geriatr Psychiatry 14:191–210, 2006

Scott HD, Laake K: Statins for the prevention of Alzheimer's disease. Cochrane Database Syst Rev (4):CD003160, 2001

Selwood A, Johnston K, Katona C, et al: Systematic review of the effect of psychological interventions on family caregivers of people with dementia. J Affect Disord 101:75–89, 2007

Shanmugiah A, Sinha S, Taly AB, et al. Psychiatric manifestations in Wilson's disease: a cross-sectional analysis. J Neuropsychiatry Clin Neurosci 20:81–85, 2008

Shin IS, Carter M, Masterman D, et al: Neuropsychiatric symptoms and quality of life in Alzheimer disease. Am J Geriatr Psychiatry 13:469–474, 2005

Small GW, Rabins PV, Barry PP: Diagnosis and treatment of Alzheimer disease and related disorders: consensus statement of the American Association for Geriatric Psychiatry, the Alzheimer Association, and the American Geriatrics Society. JAMA 278:1363–1371, 1997

Spar JE, La Rue A: Concise Guide to Geriatric Psychiatry, 3rd Edition. Washington, DC, American Psychiatric Publishing, 2002

Spector A, Orrell M, Davies S, et al: Reality orientation for dementia. Cochrane Database Syst Rev (2):CD001119, 2000a

Spector A, Orrell M, Davies S, et al: Reminiscence therapy for dementia. Cochrane Database Syst Rev (2):CD001120, 2000b

Starosta-Rubinstein S: Treatment of Wilson's disease, in Treatment of Movement Disorders. Edited by Kurlan R. Philadelphia, PA, JB Lippincott, 1995, pp 663–664

Steinberg M, Shao H, Zandi P, et al: Point and 5-year period prevalence of neuropsychiatric symptoms in dementia: the Cache County Study. Int J Geriatr Psychiatry 23:170–177, 2008

Stern Y, Tang MX, Albert MS, et al: Predicting time to nursing home care and death in individuals with Alzheimer disease. JAMA 277:806–812, 1997

Swartz JR, Miller BL, Lesser IM, et al: Frontotemporal dementia: treatment response to serotonin selective reuptake inhibitors. J Clin Psychiatry 58:212–216, 1997

Taaffe DR, Irie F, Masaki KH, et al: Physical activity, physical function, and incident dementia in elderly men: the Honolulu-Asia Aging Study. J Gerontol A Biol Sci Med Sci 63:529–535, 2008

Tabet N, Feldman H: Indomethacin for the treatment of Alzheimer's disease patients. Cochrane Database Syst Rev (2): CD003673, 2002

Teng EL, Chui HC: The Modified Mini-Mental State (3MS) Examination. J Clin Psychiatry 48:314–318, 1987

Teng E, Lu PH, Cummings JL: Neuropsychiatric symptoms are associated with progression from mild cognitive impairment to Alzheimer's disease. Dement Geriatr Cogn Disord 24:253–259, 2007

Teng R, Ringman JM, Ross LK, et al: Diagnosing depression in Alzheimer disease with the National Institute of Mental Health provisional criteria. Am J Geriatr Psychiatry 16:469–477, 2008

U.S. Food and Drug Administration: FDA Public Health Advisory: Death With Antipsychotics in Elderly Patients With Behavioral Disturbances, April 11, 2005. Available at: http://www.fda.gov/Drugs/DrugSafety/PublicHealthAdvisories/ucm053171.htm. Accessed May 2010.

Van der Flier WM, Scheltens P: Epidemiology and risk factors of dementia. J Neurol Neurosurg Psychiatry 76:v2–v7, 2005

Verghese J, Lipton RB, Katz MJ, et al: Leisure activities and the risk of dementia in the elderly. N Engl J Med 348:2508–2516, 2003

Vicini Chilovi B, Conti M, Zanetti M, et al: Differential impact of apathy and depression in the development of dementia in mild cognitive impairment patients. Dement Geriatr Cogn Disord 27:390–398, 2009

Volicer L, Harper DG, Manning BC, et al: Sundowning and circadian rhythms in Alzheimer's disease. Am J Psychiatry 158:704–711, 2001

Wahlund LO, Pihlstrand E, Jonhagen ME: Mild cognitive impairment: experience from a memory clinic. Acta Neurol Scand Suppl 179:21–24, 2003

Waldemar G, Dubois B, Emre M, et al: Recommendations for the diagnosis and management of Alzheimer's disease and other disorders associated with dementia: EFNS guideline. Eur J Neurol 14:e1–26, 2007

Walker Z, Allen R, Shergill S, et al: Three years survival in patients with a clinical diagnosis of dementia with Lewy bodies. Int J Geriatr Psychiatry 15:267–273, 2000

Wang PS, Schneeweiss S, Avorn J, et al: Risk of death in elderly users of conventional vs atypical antipsychotic medications. N Engl J Med 353:2335–2341, 2005

Welsh KA, Butters B, Hughes JP, et al: Detection and staging of dementia of Alzheimer's disease: use of the neuropsychological measures developed for the Consortium to Establish a Registry for Alzheimer's Disease. Arch Neurol 49:448–452, 1992

Weytingh MD, Bossuyt PM, van Crevel H: Reversible dementia: more than 10% or less than 1%? A quantitative review. J Neurol 242:466–471, 1995

White L, Small BJ, Petrovich H, et al: Recent clinical-pathologic research on the causes of dementia in late life: update from the Honolulu-Asia Aging Study. J Geriatr Psychiatry Neurol 18:224–227, 2005

Wilcock GK, Ballard CG, Cooper JA, et al: Memantine for agitation/aggression and psychosis in moderately severe to severe

Alzheimer's disease: a pooled analysis of 3 studies. J Clin Psychiatry 69:341–348, 2008

Will RG, Ironside JW, Zeidler M, et al: A new variant of Creutzfeldt-Jacob disease in the UK. Lancet 347:921–925, 1996

Williams PS, Spector A, Orrell M, et al: Aspirin for vascular dementia. Cochrane Database Syst Rev (2):CD001296, 2000

Wilson JMG, Junger G: The Principles and Practice of Screening for Disease (Public Health Papers No 34). Geneva, Switzerland, World Health Organization, 1968

Wilson RS, Scherr PA, Schneider JA, et al: Relation of cognitive activity to risk of developing Alzheimer disease. Neurology 69:1911–1920, 2007

Wirtz G, Baas U, Hofer H, et al: Psychopathology of Ganser's syndrome: literature review and case report. Nervenarzt 79:543–557, 2008

Wolfson C, Wolfson DB, Asgharian M, et al: A reevaluation of the duration of survival after the onset of dementia. N Engl J Med 344:1111–1116, 2001

World Health Organization: Report of the Second Consultation on the Neuropsychiatric Aspects of HIV-1 Infection, Global Programme on AIDS, Geneva, Annex 3 (Ref No WHO/GPA/MNH 90.1). Geneva, Switzerland, World Health Organization, 1990

World Health Organization: The ICD-10 Classification of Mental and Behavioural Disorders: Clinical Descriptions and Diagnostic Guidelines. Geneva, Switzerland, World Health Organization, 1992

Zakzanis KK, Andrikopoulos J, Young DA, et al: Neuropsychological differentiation of late-onset schizophrenia and dementia of the Alzheimer's type. Appl Neuropsychol 10:105–114, 2003a

Zakzanis KK, Graham SJ, Campbell Z: A meta-analysis of structural and functional brain imaging in dementia of the Alzheimer's type: a neuroimaging profile. Neuropsychol Rev 13:1–18, 2003b

Zubenko GS, Zubenko WN, McPherson S, et al: A collaborative study of the emergence and clinical features of the major depressive syndrome of Alzheimer's disease. Am J Psychiatry 160:857–866, 2003

CHAPTER 7

Aggression and Violence

Chiadi U. Onyike, M.D., M.H.S.
Constantine G. Lyketsos, M.D., M.H.S.

AGGRESSION IS UBIQUITOUS in human societies. As an adaptive behavior, it serves the expression of drives and feelings that are intimately connected with survival needs. Aggression is a complex socialized behavior associated with motivations such as self-preservation (which includes protection of offspring), retaliation, material advantage, and power. Thus, in some circumstances, aggression represents the expression of appetitive drives, and in others, it represents defensive behaviors. In an "everyday" perspective, aggressive behaviors range from assertiveness to coercion (including the use of force) and from hostile attitudes and verbal abuse to threats, belligerence, and violence.

Generally psychiatry is concerned with forms of aggression that can be attributed to medical or psychological disorders. Within this narrower context, aggression still encompasses a broad range of behaviors. In this chapter, we cover those aggressive behaviors that are associated with psychiatric, neurological, and general medical conditions. The focus is on fear-inducing and violent behavior: hostility, verbal abuse, and physically aggressive behaviors that threaten or inflict harm on an individual or an object. Definitions of aggression, violence, and related terms used in this chapter are presented in Table 7-1. Although most aggression involves intent to harm, the definition used in this chapter does not require such intent because clinically important aggressive behavior can occur in the absence of demonstrable intent, especially in patients with cognitive impairments, delirium, dementia, or mental retardation. Not included here are behaviors that may be characterized as *agitation,* such as yelling, screaming, and other nonthreatening verbal outbursts; oppositional and resistive behaviors; intrusiveness; and restlessness, pacing, and other hyperkinetic behaviors. We also do not address community violence (e.g., riots, war, terrorism) or criminality.

Psychiatrists primarily encounter aggression and violence when patients present for treatment in acute states. Aggression may manifest as a complication of delusional psychoses, dementia, agitated delirium, intoxication, conduct disorder in children or personality disorders (particularly antisocial, borderline, paranoid, and narcissistic types) in adults, and even adjustment disorder. Aggression also may complicate nonpsychiatric illnesses because it can develop when patients feel disregarded, dissatisfied, frustrated, confused, frightened, thwarted, disenfranchised, and angered by perceived unfairness or mistreatment, or as a "primary" symptom of the illness. Aggression can manifest in both males and females and in individuals of any age (except early infancy) and is seen in all patient care settings—outpatient clinics, inpatient units, rehabilitation programs, residential and custodial care facilities, nursing homes, and emergency departments. Aggressive behavior can result in involuntary confinement (in hospitals and jails), disruption of clinical and custodial care environments, longer hospital stays, and physical injury to patients, their caregivers (family and aides), and their health care providers. Family members, home health aides, and health professionals who are repeatedly exposed to aggression often experience demoralization, which leads to diminished quality of care for patients.

In this chapter, we focus on aggression and violence in the medically ill, beginning with the epidemiology of aggressive and violent behaviors in diverse clinical settings, including risk factors and the causes and precipitants of aggression; we use the epidemiological causal model of

TABLE 7–1. Terms used in this chapter

Aggression	Hostile, threatening, and violent behaviors directed at another person or objects, often with no (or trivial) provocation
Violence	Overt physical aggression directed at another person or object
Domestic violence	A continuum of behaviors directed against an intimate partner, ranging from verbal abuse, to threats and intimidation, to sexual assault and violence
Agitation	A state of pathologically intense emotional arousal and motor restlessness
Disinhibition	A behavioral state in which the individual's capacity for preemptive evaluation and restraint of behavioral responses is decreased or lost
Impulsivity	A behavioral state characterized by a proneness to act without thought or self-restraint; a habitual tendency toward "hair trigger" actions
Irritability	A state of abnormally low tolerance in which the individual is easily provoked to anger and hostility

host, agent, and *environment.* We also discuss elder abuse and intimate partner violence, which are not necessarily manifestations of illness but are important causes and correlates of psychiatric and medical morbidity. (Because our focus is on adults, we do not address child abuse in this chapter.) We then review evaluation, case formulation, and differential diagnosis of aggression. We conclude with a review of the management of aggressive behavior in the general hospital setting, including the emergency department. The content of this chapter is based on empirical evidence, existing care standards, and clinical experience.

Epidemiology

Violence is common among individuals with psychiatric disorders. A 1990 community-based study found that 55.5% of the respondents who reported violent behavior in the previous year had a psychiatric diagnosis, compared with 19.6% of the nonviolent respondents (Swanson et al. 1990). In that study, 8.9%–21.1% of the men and 3.3%–21.7% of the women who had a psychiatric diagnosis reported violent behavior, in contrast to 2.7% of the men and 1.1% of the women who did not have such diagnosis. The association was lowest for anxiety disorders and highest for substance use disorders, major affective disorders, and schizophrenia. More recent data indicate that violence is not the inevitable outcome of mental illness. For example, analyses of longitudinal data on mental disorders and violence collected during the National Epidemiologic Survey on Alcohol and Related Conditions (NESARC) indicated that mental illness alone did not predict future violent behavior (Elbogen and Johnson 2009). Future violence (measured by self-report) was instead associated with various clinical factors (substance abuse and perceived threats), demographic factors (age, sex, and income), historical factors (past violence, juvenile detention, physical abuse, and parental arrests), and social factors (recent divorce, unemployment, history of victimization). These findings indicate that violence among individuals with mental illness is not merely a phenomenon of the illness; rather, the causal relationships are "complex, indirect and embedded in a web" of pertinent personal and contextual factors (Elbogen and Johnson 2009). Other research has found that individuals with severe mental illness attending crisis and inpatient services, and sometimes clinics, are more frequently the *victims* of violence rather than the perpetrators (Choe et al. 2008; Mericle and Havassy 2008).

Whereas most mental illness does not result in violent behavior, subgroups with high potential for aggressive and violent behavior have been described. Violent behavior has been observed in specific clinical conditions, particularly schizophrenia (and other primary psychoses), substance abuse, and personality disorders (antisocial, borderline, paranoid, and narcissistic) (Biancosino et al. 2009; de Barros and de Pádua Serafim 2008; Elbogen and Johnson 2009; Eronen et al. 1998; Fazel et al. 2009; Pulay et al. 2009). Violent behavior has also been observed in primary dementia (Kalunian et al. 1990; Lyketsos 2000) and cognitive disorder resulting from head trauma (Hesdorffer et al. 2009; Rao et al. 2009). Violence is also associated with specific states, such as confusion, intoxication (with alcohol or other substances), akathisia, fearfulness, agitation, paranoid delusions, and command hallucinations (McNiel et al. 2000; Swanson et al. 2006). While the presence of delusions does not necessarily indicate a higher risk for violent behavior (Appelbaum et al. 2000; Colasanti et al. 2008), psychotic illness concurrent with substance use appears to increase synergistically the risk of violent behavior (Elbogen and Johnson 2009).

Although men are generally more aggressive than women, the gender gap in the frequency and severity of aggressive behavior narrows among individuals with major mental illness and may disappear among psychiatric inpatients and patients recently evaluated in the emergency department (Lam et al. 2000; Newhill et al. 1995), although this is not a consistent observation. There is evidence that a gender gap may exist for serious violence, such as assault, but not for lesser forms of aggression, such as threats (Hiday et al. 1998). Other psychosocial correlates of aggression include childhood conduct disorders (Hodgins et al. 2008; Swanson et al. 2008), onset of psychiatric illness at a younger age, previous violence, longer duration of hospitalization (Amore et al. 2008; Bobes et al. 2009; Elbogen and Johnson 2009), and treatment nonadherence and resistance, particularly among patients with psychotic illness (Ehmann et al. 2001; Swartz et al. 1998). Social and functional maladjustment can accentuate background risk for aggression and violence, particularly in patients with psychotic illness (Swanson et al. 1998). Ecological factors such as overcrowding, sensory overload, provocation by other patients, high staff anxiety, poor training, rigid rules, and insensitive staff attitudes and communication styles can predispose psychiatric inpatients to anger and violence (Flannery 2005; Hamrin et al. 2009).

All health care professionals, regardless of training and specialty, may encounter aggressive or violent patients. Aggression has been observed in all ambulatory, hospital, and custodial (or residential) settings, with the frequency generally varying according to the specific population (e.g., diagnostic mix, acuity levels) and the characteristics of the setting (e.g., crowding, staffing levels). Within settings, the frequency of violence may vary by the illness, its acuity and severity, or the mode of presentation of the patient. Aggression is especially common in emergency care settings, where there is typically a confluence of risk factors (e.g., high acuity, high emotions, crowding, overextended staff) to promote its development. Emergency medical services (EMS) personnel, the first responders for community emergencies, must stabilize and transport patients to the emergency department and are therefore at high risk for exposure to violence. It has been estimated that 8.5% of EMS encounters involve aggression (Grange and Corbett 2002); about half of these encounters involve violence. Patients were responsible for 90% of the incidents, and relatives and other bystanders for the remainder. Encounters that involved males, police presence, street gangs, suspected psychiatric disorder, and abuse of alcohol or other substances carried high risk for aggression incidents. Up to 95% of EMS personnel have had to restrain a patient, and more than 60% have been assaulted (with 25% reporting injury from the assault) (Corbett et al. 1998). Other studies have reported similar or higher prevalence estimates of assault and injury (Mock et al. 1998; Pozzi 1998). In the past, the risk to EMS workers exposed to aggression was compounded by limited formal training on how to manage aggressive patients and lack of counseling in the aftermath of an assault. Since 1998, these training needs have been met with comprehensive training curricula developed by the U.S. Department of Transportation.

Aggression in the emergency department (ED) may manifest as threats, belligerent confrontations, assault, and stalking and is especially common in large EDs (i.e., those with volumes of 60,000 or more cases annually) (Behnam et al. 2010). Surveys of such large EDs have shown that staff are threatened by patients every day, that use of restraints is frequently necessary, and that nearly 50% of these facilities have one or more staff members assaulted each month (resulting in injury in 25% of cases) (Blanchard and Curtis 1999). For many patients, the agitation, aggressiveness, or violent behavior may be the reason that they have been brought to the ED, whereas for other patients who were not agitated or aggressive on arrival, threatening and violent behavior may develop as a result of their acute condition or other factors. Furthermore, some patients have guns, knives, or other weapons in their possession when they arrive (Kansagra et al. 2008), which signals a general predisposition to violence. Although health professionals (especially nurses) are the typical victims of patient aggression, sometimes a visitor or another patient is assaulted. In still other cases, a family member or other visitor, not the patient, is the perpetrator of an aggressive act. More recent information, based on retrospective data, indicates that assailants are more likely to be male patients, repeat offenders, residents of deprived communities, and intoxicated (James et al. 2006). Other contributing factors include involuntary transport to the ED; negative perceptions of hospital staff; inadequately trained and/or overextended staff; crowding, noise, discomfort, and long waits; and inadequate security.

Aggression is common beyond the ED, in a variety of inpatient settings. Of the estimated 20% of general hospital staff assaulted by patients, up to 90% of incidents may occur in inpatient units (Whittington et al. 1996). In hospitalized patients, aggressive acts may occur as features or complications of confusion associated with the patients' primary conditions (e.g., thyroid storm, head injuries, hypoxia, encephalitis) or administered treatments (e.g., benzodiazepines or corticosteroids) or may result from co-occurring mental illness. On surgical units, aggression may result from confusion during the immediate postoperative period, undiagnosed alcohol withdrawal, or inadequately controlled postoperative pain. Aggression in the general hospital may also evolve from patients' dissatisfaction with care or frustration from unfulfilled wants and expectations or during patient and staff conflicts.

In a recently reported survey of intensive care units (ICUs) in England and Wales, nurses were subjected to verbal hostility by patients in 87% of the ICUs and by patients' relatives in 74% (Lynch et al. 2003). Nurses were assaulted by patients in 77% of the ICUs, and by patients' relatives in 17%; rates of hostility and assault directed at physicians were lower. Illness severity was associated with aggression committed by patients, whereas emotional distress, alcohol abuse, and sociopathic traits were associated with aggression committed by relatives. A similar pattern of aggressive behaviors may be seen on general medical and surgical wards, although the frequency of aggressive behaviors (particularly those committed by relatives) is likely to be lower.

Substance abuse and sociopathic traits among inpatients may contribute more to aggressive behaviors in hospital wards (as compared with aggression in ICUs). Individuals are more likely to show negative affects and personality traits during times of high stress, including serious medical illness; thus, patients with personality styles high in impulsivity, distrust, and aggressiveness (particularly antisocial or borderline personality disorders) may be more likely to commit violent acts during hospitalization. Substance abusers experiencing withdrawal symptoms or intense cravings are frequent perpetrators of in-hospital aggression. Nicotine dependence can also be a factor; smoking is no longer allowed in hospitals, and although nicotine withdrawal and craving are unlikely to directly cause violence, they can provoke or inflame conflict between patients and staff.

Aggression has serious consequences for patients and for those who care for them. These include disruption of the care environment, longer duration of hospitalization, higher treatment costs (Greenfield et al. 1989), and stigmatization of the mentally ill and their caregivers. Patients may sustain injuries, for example, from punching walls or glass, handling dangerous objects, falling, fighting with another patient, or resisting restraint. In addition, inpatients who are prone to impulsive aggressive acts tend to be at higher risk for flight (Bowers et al. 2000) and impulsive suicidal acts (Giegling et al. 2009).

Although all health care personnel are at risk for injury, nurses and clinical assistants are by far the most likely to be injured by violent patients (Hillbrand et al. 1996; Salerno et al. 2009; Whittington et al. 1996). Patient aggression results in demoralization, physical and psychological disability, absenteeism (as a result of sick days and disability), and job departures among nurses (Gerberich et al. 2004; Nachreiner et al. 2007), as well as higher administrative costs and litigation exposure for the care facility. Violence from patients can cause staff to adopt negative attitudes toward their work and their patients, resulting in impaired job performance, poor patient-staff relationships, and patient dissatisfaction with care; the myriad negative effects on the treatment environment and the overall quality of patient care can lead to a vicious cycle in which a deteriorating environment promotes yet more violence (Arnetz and Arnetz 2001).

Mechanisms of Aggression

Aggression and violence can be categorized as impulsive or premeditated. *Impulsive* aggression is spontaneous behavior that is typically reactive, emotion laden, and sometimes explosive, whereas *instrumental* (or *premeditated*) aggression is purposeful, controlled behavior that may be predatory (committed for material or strategic advantage) or pathological (a deliberate response to misperceptions, hallucinations, or delusions). Generally, patients manifest predominantly impulsive or predominantly instrumental aggressive behaviors. Instrumental aggression is typically pathological, but patients with antisocial or borderline personality disorders frequently manifest predatory behavior. Impulsive aggression may be associated with cognitive deficits, psychotic states, and high emotional sensitivity and is usually accompanied by autonomic arousal (Nelson and Trainor 2007; Siever 2008). Instrumental aggression, on the other hand, may be associated with low sensitivity and low autonomic arousal, such as in conduct disorder and antisocial personality disorder (Nelson and Trainor 2007). Impulsive aggression is not necessarily unintentional; rather, it occurs on a *continuum of intention,* depending on the coalescence of individual susceptibility and context, ranging from entirely unintentional reflexive behaviors (e.g., ill-directed shoving and swinging in a patient with postictal confusion) to resistive behaviors (e.g., thrashing, spitting, and biting during placement of lines or tubes in an agitated patient with delirium) to spur-of-the-moment intentional behaviors (e.g., a patient with borderline personality disorder throwing a telephone at the nurse who is scolding her).

From a pathogenetic perspective, aggression is a heterogeneous behavior associated with background genetic, familial, and social determinants. These include unfavorable prenatal, perinatal, and rearing experiences (such as childhood experience of neglect or abuse); genetic determinants; poor education; and negative cultural and peer influences (Volavka 1999). These factors, and others acquired, such as Axis I conditions, brain injury syndromes, and personality disorders, can be viewed as coalescing in the individual to yield a *host* with a baseline propensity for aggression that interacts with specific provocations (*agents*) and occurs in environments or *circumstances* to produce aggressive behaviors. Examples of *agents* include threats by others, misperceptions, conflicts, or physical discomfort. *Circumstances* are contexts, such as intense (or distant) interpersonal relationships, personal losses, or hospitalization for serious illness, that are captured in a narrative that reveals a vulnerable patient's maladaptive interactions with his or her environment. This framework describes the setting and sequence of events leading to an episode of aggressive behavior, while simultaneously placing these events in the context of the specific circumstances and the individual's psychological assets and liabilities.

The *host–agent–context* framework allows for enhanced understanding of any patient and his or her observed aggressive behavior. In some cases, an aggressive episode is the latest in a pattern of recurring impulsive, predatory, or pathological acts, which may (or may not) be associated with identifiable triggers, in an individual with cognitive or emotional vulnerabilities. In other cases, the act may be an easily discerned complication of the patient's primary condition or a not-so-surprising reaction to distressing circumstances.

Consider the following illustrations:

- Aggression and violence in inpatient settings appear to be relatively frequent in the first 48 hours after admission in acutely psychotic patients and in substance users (Barlow et al. 2000; Sheridan et al. 1990). In contrast, a rapid reduction in the risk of aggression in patients with schizophrenia within a few days after admission also has been reported (Binder and McNiel 1990). Both of these observations are reconciled by realizing that agitation and acute psychosis often lead to more intensive treatment efforts.
- Substance users may become aggressive soon after admission as a result of the irritability that accompanies a withdrawal syndrome. When treatment for the withdrawal syndrome is prescribed preemptively, the risk for aggression is minimized.
- Three types of aggressive behavior have been described in schizophrenia (Hodgins 2008): 1) in the first type, antisocial behaviors that develop in childhood or early adolescence, well before the onset of schizophrenia, persist as psychopathic traits; 2) the largest group develop impulsive aggression at the onset of schizophrenia, and this remains a persistent feature of their illness; 3) in a small group, aggression is not observed for years after illness onset, until serious violence manifests as a complication of acute psychosis. Studies suggest that these types show differences in their neuropsychological profiles and brain morphology (Naudts and Hodgins 2006).
- Patient and staff conflicts—especially those that involve enforcement of rules, denying of requests (e.g., discharge, change in medications, off-unit smoking breaks), and involuntary admission or transfer—can precipitate aggressive acts and violence (Sheridan et al. 1990).

Psychosomatic medicine specialists often encounter recurrent impulsive aggression, which occurs as an inexplicable event or a "hair trigger" response to relatively unimportant stimuli. This form of aggression is usually related to dysfunction of the brain areas involved in the modulation (or suppression) of primitive impulses and drives. It often arises as a consequence of physical illness or injury that directly or indirectly affects these brain areas. It is also true that in the general hospital setting, many episodes of impulsive aggression are not related to physical illness or injury per se but rather arise in an individual in whom impulsivity is a dominant (or prominent) behavioral *trait*—for example, individuals with personality disorders.

The role of the prefrontal cortex in maintaining self-control and prosocial behavior has been recognized for more than a century and a half, ever since the classic case of Phineas Gage (Harlow 1848, 1868), who underwent a dramatic personality change (manifesting as a coarse manner, jocularity, impulsivity, and aggressive outbursts) after sustaining orbitofrontal cortical injury from a projectile. Patients who suffer frontotemporal dementia, a neurodegenerative condition characterized by focal degeneration of the frontal and temporal cortices, frequently manifest a similar phenotype. Acquired antisocial behavior and aggressive behavior has also been observed in adults who suffered injuries of the prefrontal cortex in childhood (Siever 2008). Abnormalities in working memory, abstract thinking, moral reasoning, affective regulation, and behavioral inhibition have been noted in impulsively aggressive patients with antisocial personality disorder or frontal lobe injuries, and in children and adolescents with attention-deficit/hyperactivity disorder (ADHD) or conduct disorder (Brower and Price 2001; Coccaro and Siever 2002; Davidson et al. 2000). Brain imaging studies of impulsively aggressive patients and violent offenders have shown reduced activation in the frontal cortex (Nelson and Trainor 2007). These imaging studies have also shown hyperactivity in the limbic system (particularly the amygdala and cingulate cortex), suggesting that hypervigilance and heightened emotional responsiveness may underlie vulnerability to impulsive aggression, along with low thresholds for activation of fear, anger, and aggressive responses (Siever 2008). In other words, impulsive aggression may arise from a low threshold in the amygdala for activation of negative affects (fear, anger, and aggressive responses) or a failure of the orbitofrontal cortex to suppress negative affects prompted by cues in the environment.

There is considerable interest in the molecular underpinnings of aggressive behavior. Like other complex social behaviors, aggression involves neural circuits that are modulated by a variety of neurotransmitter signals. The principal neurotransmitters identified with the modulation of aggressive behavior are dopamine, norepinephrine, 5-hydroxytryptamine (5-HT; serotonin), acetylcholine, gamma-aminobutyric acid (GABA), and neuropeptides such as opioid peptides, substance P, cholecystokinin, and vasopressin. It is now well established that low levels of 5-HT are correlated with impulsiveness and aggressiveness (Nelson and Trainor 2007; Siever 2008). Lower cerebrospinal fluid (CSF) levels of the 5-HT metabolite 5-hydroxyindoleacetic acid (5-HIAA) have been found in aggressive psychiatric patients, impulsive violent men (including violent offenders), disruptive and aggressive male children and adolescents and victims of violent suicides (Coccaro and Siever 2002). In animal studies, interventions that increase 5-HT activity by any of a variety of mechanisms (e.g., administration of 5-HT precursors and agonists, inhibition of 5-HT reuptake inhibition) reduce impulsive and aggressive behavior, whereas the opposite behavioral effects can be achieved by lowering 5-HT transmission. Furthermore, pharmacological challenge studies show blunted prolactin response to 5-HT agonist challenge (with buspirone or fenfluramine) in aggressive, antisocial, and suicidal individuals, suggesting deficient 5-HT transmission in these individuals (Siever 2008). Thus, it has been proposed that modulatory control of aggressive behavior by the prefrontal cortex is facilitated by 5-HT, and that disruption of 5-HT neurotransmission may lead to loss of inhibitory control of aggressive behavior.

Dopaminergic neurons, which contribute to a variety of motivated behaviors, may be required for the expression of aggressive behavior, although their precise role in modulating aggression remains unclear (Nelson and Trainor 2007). This requirement is reflected in the effectiveness of D_2-receptor antagonism in ameliorating aggressive behaviors (particularly in patients who are experiencing psychosis), although changes in alertness, autonomic arousal, and locomotor activity may partly explain the effects of these antagonists.

Another catecholamine, norepinephrine, has been linked to irritable aggression, although this is not a consistent observation. High levels of norepinephrine, which characterize states of hyperarousal, appear to facilitate aggression, although antagonists do not reliably reduce aggressive behavior in humans. It has been suggested that patients with blunted noradrenergic responsiveness manifest instrumental aggression, whereas impulsive aggression is associated with low 5-HT activity in association with normal or increased noradrenergic activity (Siever 2008).

Roles for other neurotransmitters are more speculative. Glutaminergic–GABAergic balance may play a role in the modulation of aggression. It is noted that benzodiazepines, barbiturates, and other modulators of the $GABA_A$ receptor reduce aggression at high doses, although lower doses may produce a disinhibited state and facilitate aggression. Provocation of violent reactions by benzodiazepines is rare. Abnormalities in acetylcholine transmission have been associated with irritability and aggression. Opioid signaling appears to inhibit aggression, as do high levels of vasopressin and oxytocin, neurotransmitters that appear to be biological facilitators of affiliation behaviors (Miczek et al. 2007; Siever 2008). The notion is that affiliation-promoting effects of vasopressin and oxytocin may reduce proneness to mistrust and hostility, thereby minimizing negative attribution bias and threat perceptions in ambiguous or stressful environments.

Evaluation of Aggression

An episode of belligerence and violence in the general hospital setting typically progresses from a specific clinical state—the *setting*—to a *sequence* of events that culminates in the *outcome*—aggressive behavior (see Figure 7–1). Several factors influence the expression of aggression in the clinic or hospital: aggression may occur if the patient has specific symptoms, mental states, adverse effects of medicines, dissatisfaction with care, or conflicts with staff. However, aggression can be prevented, its intensity reduced, or its consequences avoided or minimized by prompt intervention. The clinical progression of aggressive behavior in the general hospital is depicted in Figure 7–1. The choice of intervention depends on the specific situation as well as the case formulation and the specific diagnosis the patient has received.

Elucidation of the *setting–sequence–outcome* progression involves describing the specific aggressive behavior, the sequence of events preceding it, and the symptoms and factors that may be influencing its expression. This approach has been referred to as a "define and decode" strategy (Lyketsos 2000). The effects of the patient's behavior also should be noted by inquiring about injury to the patient or others, damage to property, disruption of the milieu, and so on. Precipitants such as staff–patient conflicts, end of visiting hours, or recent administration of a medication should be carefully sought, and the history also should clarify the setting in which the behavior has occurred and the temporal relation of the aggressive behavior to any co-occurring symptoms. It is also helpful to know whether the patient is febrile, confused, in pain, craving cigarettes, cognitively impaired or disabled, anxious or fearful, hallucinating or delusional, or if he or she has epilepsy (especially a recent seizure). All prescribed medicines (e.g., insulin, benzodiazepines, anticholinergics, antipsychotics) should

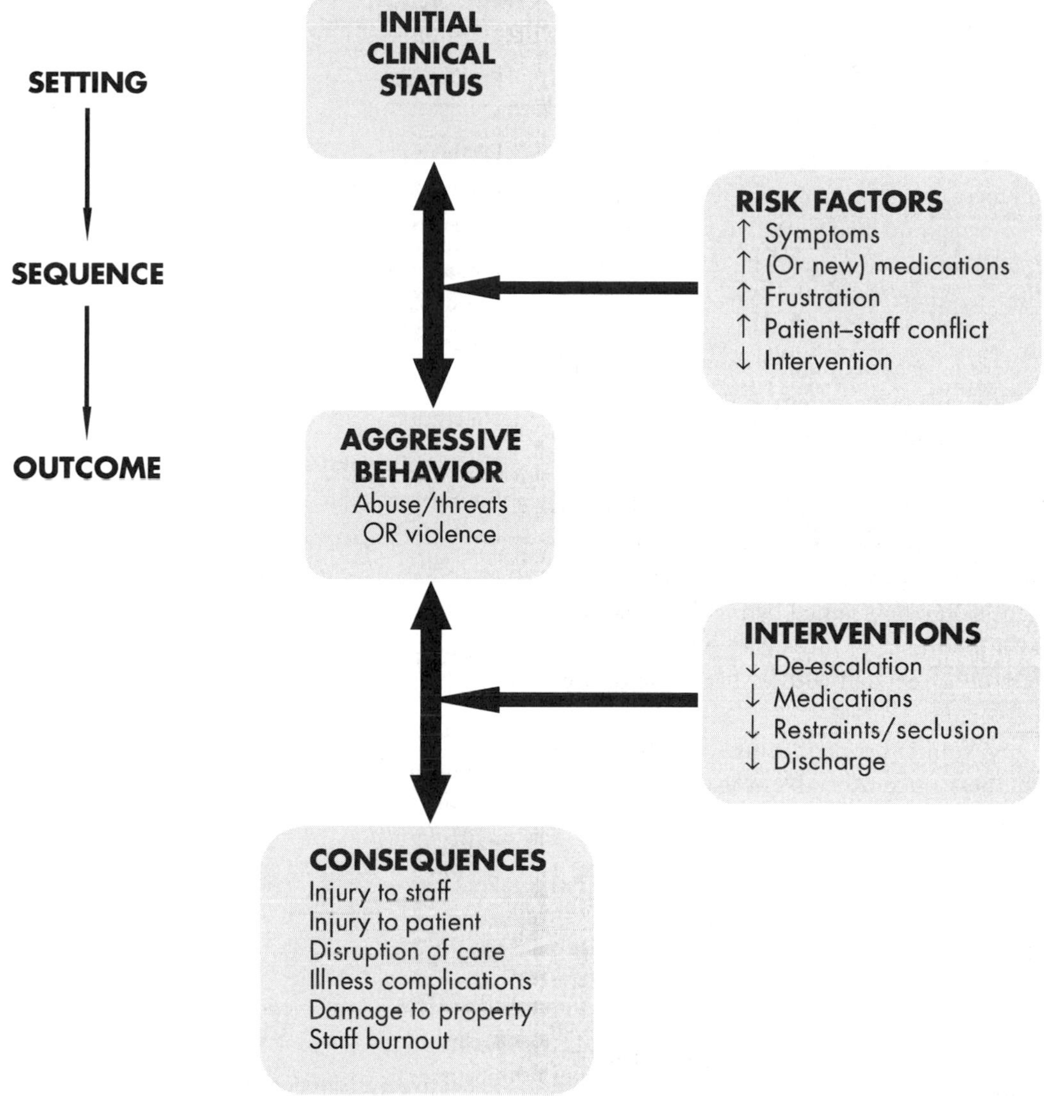

FIGURE 7–1. Clinical progression of aggressive behavior in the general hospital.

be noted. The psychiatrist should systematically search for symptoms such as acute confusion, restlessness, akathisia, or agitation, which require urgent intervention.

In addition to collecting a careful history of the aggressive episode, the evaluation requires describing concurrent illnesses; the patient's personal, social, and family history (including current psychosocial functioning); any substance abuse; and the patient's personality and psychiatric status. General medical, neurological, cognitive, and mental status examinations are focused on describing systems that have been implicated in the history but also should include important "inspections," such as the checking of vital signs, airway and cardiovascular status, exclusion of injuries, repeated assessment of alertness, assessment of dangerousness (inquiring about violent or suicidal ideas), and assessment of reality testing.

In the general hospital setting, laboratory data are often essential for accurate differential diagnosis. Blood tests can help to identify infection, anemia, electrolyte disturbances, or biochemical abnormalities that may explain delirium. Likewise, toxicology screens and serum drug concentrations may help to identify acute intoxications and chronic substance use. Urinalysis, microbiological cultures (of blood and urine), and chest X ray may be helpful in certain circumstances (e.g., in immunosuppressed patients or patients with dementia). If seizures are a possibility, an electroencephalogram (EEG) should be performed. When obtundation, evidence of recent head trauma, or another reason to suspect an acute intracranial event is present, brain imaging (computed tomography [CT] or magnetic resonance imaging [MRI]) should be obtained. In most circumstances, a brain CT is adequate. A high index of suspicion for intracranial hemorrhage (e.g., subdural hematoma) is appropriate because those who are violent toward others are at higher risk for being victims of violence themselves.

The integration of the clinical data leads to a case formulation and differential diagnosis, as well as a summary narrative that depicts the *setting–sequence–outcome* chain of the aggressive episode (and also articulates the contributions of *host, agent,* and *circumstance*). The formulation addresses the following questions:

- Does the patient have a mental illness, personality vulnerability, cognitive impairment, delirium, or other condition that predisposes him or her to aggressive behavior?
- Is the aggression linked to specific aspects of illness such as psychomotor agitation, disinhibition, command hallucinations, aphasia, or acute pain?
- Can the aggression be explained by medications causing confusion, akathisia, or intoxication?
- Is the aggression associated with a specific activity or with interpersonal conflicts?
- How is the environment contributing to the behavior?
- Is the environment uncomfortable, noisy, overcrowded, or frightening?

It is also important for psychiatrists to remember that many impulsively aggressive patients have a relatively high risk for suicidal behavior. Several psychiatric disorders manifesting aggressive and violent behavior, particularly alcohol dependence and personality disorders, are associated with suicidal behavior. Thus, the evaluation of aggression also must include an assessment of the risk for self-injury and suicide.

TABLE 7–2. Differential diagnosis of aggressive and violent behavior

Psychoses
Mania
Depression
Schizophrenia
Delusional disorder
Personality disorders
Antisocial
Borderline
Paranoid
Narcissistic
Other behavior disorders
Intermittent explosive disorder
Episodic dyscontrol
Hypothalamic-limbic rage
Conduct disorder
Substance use disorders
Alcohol
Phencyclidine
Stimulants
Cocaine
Epilepsy
Preictal
Ictal
Postictal
Interictal
Delirium
Executive dysfunction syndromes
Dementia
Developmental disorders
Mental retardation
XYY genotype

Disorders Associated With Aggressive Behavior

Many disorders can manifest with aggression and violence in the general hospital (Table 7–2). Thus, the psychiatrist's task will include a consideration of these disorders in the differential diagnosis of violent behavior in patients.

Psychoses and Chronic Serious Mental Illness

As noted earlier in this chapter, several major mental disorders can produce violent behavior. Irritable patients with mania, depression, schizophrenia, or other major psychoses may commit impulsive violent acts. This risk for impulsive violence is greatest during acute presentations and is particularly high when patients have been brought to treatment against their will. Clinicians should therefore maintain high levels of vigilance when evaluating the irritable psychotic patient, especially when the patient is seen in the ED or soon after being involuntarily hospitalized.

Deliberate premeditated violence also can arise from psychotic disorders—usually as a response to delusional beliefs—but generally the content of psychotic patients' delusions is focused on familiar individuals (people in the patients' daily life), public figures, or imaginary persecutors rather than on the health professionals caring for them. It also should be noted that many patients with chronic mental illness have maladaptive coping responses to stress or conflict and thus may react with violence during interpersonal conflicts. Therefore, a crucial aspect of the psychiatrist's role is to educate nonpsychiatric physicians, nurses, and others caring for these patients. When patients with major mental illness are admitted to nonpsychiatric settings, the psychiatrist's role as consultant should include educating the medical team about the illness (its current status and treatment) and the fact that most such patients can communicate their concerns and symptoms, will cooperate with care, and are nonviolent (even when psychotic). Treatment recommendations should include ways of approaching the patient (e.g., approaching the patient from within his or her visual field and calling out a greeting so that he or she is not startled), ensuring that the patient's current psychotropic regimen is prescribed, and pointing out any known habits or preferences that can be accommodated (e.g., arranging for regular smoking breaks, preferred meals, or a favorite television show). The patient's physicians and nurses should be educated about early signs of agitation, such as pacing, restlessness, staring, and refusal of medications, and contingency plans for managing these symptoms or states should be specified—what behavioral approaches (such as positive reinforcement and pacification) and tranquilization strategies should be used and how the psychiatrist can be contacted when his or her expertise is urgently needed.

Personality Disorders

Violence associated with personality disorders is usually embedded in the individual's behavioral repertoire. Personality disorders that frequently manifest violent behavior are shown in Table 7–2; of these, antisocial personality is the most likely to be associated with habitual aggression. Antisocial individuals usually are thrill seeking, have low frustration tolerance, and have high rates of substance abuse, criminal behavior, and violence. They often present to the ED with injuries resulting from violence (such as stab and gunshot wounds) and with a variety of medical complications of substance abuse (including severe intoxications, wound infections, head injuries, and hepatitis); they often require admission to the medical or surgical ward for treatment of these conditions. Antisocial patients who are intoxicated can become very dangerous because of their mood instability, lowered frustration tolerance, and behavioral disinhibition. While in the hospital, they may become aggressive when their demands—for pain medication, more food, cigarettes, and so on—are not met. In making these demands, they may verbally threaten, intimidate staff with boasts and gestures, or become violent.

Many antisocial patients are repeatedly hospitalized for treatment of problems arising from their lifestyle, especially the medical complications of addictions and risk-taking behaviors. This often arouses resentment and animosity from physicians and nurses, who may believe that their efforts to care for the patient are unwanted and futile. Health care professionals may be provoked into angry verbal (and, rarely, physical) retaliation. Such patients have earned notoriety from their behavior during earlier hospitalizations, which may put them at risk for punitive interventions such as suboptimal care, inadequate pain treatment, and premature discharge. Staff may understandably prefer to focus care on patients who are seen as cooperative, appreciative, and "innocent victims" of disease. This puts the aggressive antisocial patient at higher risk for missed diagnoses and medical errors. Thus, psychiatrists involved in caring for such patients need to know their reputation on the unit and the feelings of the physicians and nurses caring for them. This information is valuable for formulating a plan of care that ensures adequate evaluation and treatment for the patient and appropriate safeguards for the staff. One of the psychiatrist's responsibilities with such patients is to help physicians, nurses, and other staff appropriately handle their anger and frustration, avoiding both overreaction (e.g., yelling at patients, inappropriate precipitous discharge) and underreaction (e.g., failing to set limits, failing to discharge when indicated). Antisocial patients are not immune to other conditions that may explain aggression, including delirium, substance withdrawal, and psychosis. Therefore, psychiatrists should pursue a systematic psychiatric and general medical assessment whenever antisocial patients are encountered in nonpsychiatric settings.

Borderline personality disorder is characterized by intense emotionality, intense relationships, rejection sensitivity, manipulative behaviors, impulsiveness, recklessness, low self-regard, irritability, aggressiveness, and a tendency to extreme reactions. Most patients with borderline personality disorder are women. Their violent acts usually are impulsive and typically occur during interpersonal conflict. They also have a high potential for self-injury and suicidal acts and thus are often seen in the ED. Borderline patients can be very difficult to manage because they may demand specific conditions or individuals before submitting to an interview or examination. They are capable of angrily refusing care or of violent temper tantrums. Thus, a major challenge in their care is maintaining limits on behavior and managing the intense negative countertransference feelings that they may stir up. In caring for them, psychiatrists must maintain an empathic stance and assist the staff in doing so, often despite deliberate provocation.

Individuals with borderline personality seen in the ED should be screened for depression, substance abuse, and domestic violence because these conditions are highly comorbid. On medical units, borderline patients can become disruptive when their expectations are not met. Psychiatrists should educate their physicians and nurses about the need to define behavior limits, meet expectations agreed on with the patient, and maintain a consistent approach to the patient's care. This is best accomplished in an interdisciplinary care conference, with the psychiatrist assisting the staff in constructing a written treatment contract to be negotiated with, and signed by, the patient.

Other personality disorders are less frequently associated with violent behavior, although narcissistic individuals may threaten or act (e.g., slap a nurse) in retaliation for perceived slights or to satiate their sense of entitlement, and individuals with paranoid personality disorder may become aggressive in response to perceived mistreatment.

Intermittent Explosive Disorder, Episodic Dyscontrol Syndrome, and Hypothalamic–Limbic Rage Syndrome

Intermittent explosive disorder, episodic dyscontrol syndrome, and hypothalamic–limbic rage syndrome describe disturbances that are characterized by explosive episodes of aggression and violence. *Intermittent explosive disorder,* as defined by DSM-IV (American Psychiatric Association 1994) and its text revision, DSM-IV-TR (American Psychiatric Association 2000), refers to a disturbance characterized by recurrent episodes of explosive anger not explained by psychosis or some other mental disorder. *Episodic dyscontrol* is a similar construct, denoting recurring episodes of uncontrollable rage. It has been used as a label for males who have a history of conduct disorder, unstable employment, poverty, intimate partner violence and other sexual assaults, criminal behavior, and substance abuse (typically alcohol) (Cummings and Mega 2003). Neurological signs such as short attention span, poor coordination, and mild gait abnormalities have been found in some cases; temporal lobe EEG abnormalities also are sometimes seen. Whereas intermittent explosive disorder denotes a relatively narrow clinical spectrum of explosive aggression, episodic dyscontrol refers to episodic, impulsive violence in a broad, ill-defined group of mostly antisocial individuals. Because episodic dyscontrol syndrome overlaps widely with several psychiatric categories (including intermittent explosive disorder, ADHD, conduct disorder, and antisocial personality disorder), it lacks face validity and is of limited clinical usefulness.

Although rare, rage attacks in association with neoplastic and surgical lesions of the hypothalamus and amygdala have been described (Demaree and Harrison 1996; Tonkonogy and Geller 1992). These attacks, which have been repeatedly reproduced in experimental animals with lesion models and neurophysiological methods, have been termed *hypothalamic rage attacks* or *hypothalamic–limbic rage syndrome.* This disorder is characterized by provoked and unprovoked episodes of uncontrollable rage and may represent an acquired form of intermittent explosive disorder. In addition to rage attacks, patients may have symptoms such as hyperphagia, polydipsia, excessive weight gain, or obesity; clinical findings suggesting thyroid, adrenal, or pituitary disease; a history of recently diagnosed pituitary, midbrain, or temporal lobe tumor; or recent brain surgery. Treatment involves correction of the underlying condition (including surgical resection of tumors) and behavioral and pharmacological approaches targeted at aggression. It should be noted, too, that hypothalamic lesions might be accompanied by "atypical" rage attacks with anxious and social features that suggest multifactorial origins (Savard et al. 2003).

Substance Use Disorders

Alcohol is the psychoactive substance most often associated with violence. Alcohol-related violence may result from a severely intoxicated state that produces gross impairment of self-restraint and judgment and/or a blackout. Pathological intoxication, which occurs in vulnerable individuals following the ingestion of only modest amounts of alcohol, may be associated with disorganized behavior, emotional lability, and violent outbursts. In severe cases, pathological intoxication may be accompanied by a delirium with hyperarousal, hallucinations, delusions, and terror, followed by amnesia for the event after recovery. Alcohol withdrawal also can be accompanied by irritability and low frustration tolerance, which predispose to directed aggression, or by seizures that are followed by aggression during a postictal state. Patients who develop delirium tremens may show poorly coordinated, resistive, or preemptive violence in response to hyperarousal, hallucinations, and terror.

Intoxication with other substances also can result in violence. Cocaine and amphetamine abuse is common and can produce impulsive, disinhibited intoxicated states during which violence may occur. Patients undergoing opioid, sedative, or cocaine withdrawal may experience anxious tension and irritability, during which interpersonal conflict or frustration may result in violent behavior. Although phencyclidine is not commonly abused, phencyclidine intoxication can manifest with severe impulsively directed violence. Even less common is violence that occurs in individuals who have taken Ecstasy, lysergic acid diethylamide (LSD), or other hallucinogens; as an apparent consequence of severe perceptual disturbances; and in patients who abuse anticholinergic agents, in whom delirium may be accompanied by aggressive behavior.

Epilepsy

In evaluating episodes of aggression in patients with epilepsy (see also Chapter 32, "Neurology and Neurosurgery"), psychosomatic medicine psychiatrists must carefully consider whether the aggression is directly related to a seizure, a feature of mental state changes associated with seizures, or a complication of other conditions that increase the risk of aggressive behavior. In addition, psychiatrists must be aware that certain seizures can be misinterpreted as intentional violent behavior. Violent behavior may be observed during complex partial seizures but never during grand mal seizures.

Ictal violence is rare, and most cases are characterized by spontaneous, undirected, stereotyped aggressive behaviors. Typical characteristics are as follows: 1) the seizure episode occurs suddenly, without provocation, and is of very short duration (usually a few minutes); 2) automatisms and other stereotypic phenomena of the patient's habitual seizures accompany the aggressive act, and the act is associated with these phenomena from one seizure to the next; 3) the patient's consciousness is impaired; 4) the aggressive behavior is poorly directed and involves few skills; and 5) purpose and interpersonal interaction are absent (Marsh and Krauss 2000). In practice, it can be difficult to determine whether a violent behavior should be attributed to a seizure event. This determination requires the integration of findings from interview, clinical history, and video EEG monitoring to make the diagnosis. Abnormal nonseizure EEG phenomena (such as sharp waves) are nonspecific findings and should not be used as evidence that violence is ictal. Widely applicable criteria for attributing a specific violent act to an epileptic seizure have been developed (Treiman 1986) and are presented in Table 7–3.

Although uncommon, a prodromal state of affective instability preceding a seizure episode by several hours or days may be associated with directed aggression (Marsh and Krauss 2000). The affective symptoms may be specific to the preictal state or an exacerbation of interictal phenomena; these states and their aggressive features usually resolve after the seizure.

Violent behavior in epilepsy is most frequent during postictal confusional states. These states are usually brief but can vary widely in duration because they are influenced by the type and severity of the preceding seizures. Abnormal moods, paranoia, hallucinations, and delirium may occur and result in violence by heightening aggressive propensities or causing misinterpretations of stimuli in the immediate environment. In general, episodes of postictal violence are longer in duration than episodes of ictal violence, are associated with amnesia for the event, and are out of character for the individual. In some males, stereotypic episodes of severe postictal aggression can occur after clusters of seizures (Gerard et al. 1998). Postictal delirium can be detected clinically by assessing the patient's level of consciousness and awareness and performing an EEG—which shows diffuse slowing (and no ictal activity). Typically, the delirium is brief, and a gradual return to normal consciousness follows, but prolonged or repetitive seizures can extend the duration. Violence occurring during postictal delirium is usually relatively undirected; resistive violence is fairly frequent, usually occurring when attempts are made to help or restrain a patient after the seizure.

TABLE 7–3. Criteria for determining whether a violent act resulted from an epileptic seizure

1. Diagnosis of epilepsy established by an expert neurologist[a]
2. Epileptic automatisms documented by clinical history and closed-circuit-television electroencephalogram
3. Aggression during epileptic automatisms documented on closed-circuit-television electroencephalogram
4. The violent behavior is characteristic of the patient's habitual seizures
5. Clinical judgment by the neurologist that the behavior was part of a seizure

[a]A neurologist with special competence in epilepsy.
Source. Adapted from Treiman 1986.

Many episodes of postictal violence are motivated by a postictal psychosis. The psychosis may emerge from postictal confusion or a lucid state and tends to follow a psychosis-free interval of several hours to a few days after a seizure (or cluster of complex partial seizures) (Marsh and Krauss 2000). Postictal psychosis usually manifests as grandiose affective psychoses (mania or depression with mood-congruent psychotic phenomena) or with thought disorder, hallucinations, and paranoid ideational psychoses reminiscent of schizophrenia. Although usually transient (of no longer than several hours' duration), these states may last up to several weeks. Postictal psychosis has a tendency to recur and may become chronic. Violence in the context of postictal psychosis may be motivated by paranoid delusions and hallucinations, in which case it manifests as well-directed violence. In fact, violence is more likely to occur in individuals with postictal psychosis, compared with those with interictal psychosis or postictal confusion (Kanemoto et al. 1999). Most episodes of postictal psychosis resolve spontaneously or following treatment with low doses of an antipsychotic, and improved control of the epilepsy then becomes the focus of treatment. However, some patients require chronic maintenance treatment with antipsychotics (see also Chapter 10, "Psychosis, Mania, and Catatonia," and Chapter 32, "Neurology and Neurosurgery").

Most violent behaviors in patients with epilepsy have no particular association with ictal or postictal states. For example, studies that report higher prevalence rates of epilepsy in prisoners than in nonprisoners rarely identify connections between criminal acts and specific seizure episodes, and prevalence rates for epilepsy are not higher in violent criminals than in nonviolent criminals (Treiman 1986). Thus, the increased risk for violence in prisoners who have epilepsy can be attributed to other factors such as cognitive dysfunction and adverse social circumstances. The assessment of violence in patients with epilepsy should therefore also elicit a contextualized description (*setting–sequence–outcome*) of the act and other biological and psychosocial factors that may mediate the expression of aggression. These forms of aggression are well directed and are associated with stressors and triggers. They typically occur around other people and are purposeful, nonstereotyped, and highly coordinated. The aggression is "explained" by the situation at hand, is associated with the buildup of negative emotions concerning some circumstance, and may be of relatively prolonged duration.

Brain injury and cognitive impairment are important risk factors for interictal aggressive behavior. In addition, interictal psychiatric phenomena, such as depression, hallucinations, and delusions, and sociopathic personality traits, such as impulsivity, remorselessness, self-absorption, and superficiality, also predispose patients with epilepsy to aggressive behavior. Furthermore, violence can be learned behavior in patients whose educational and social disadvantages are a correlate or result of their epilepsy.

Delirium

States of heightened arousal often accompany the confusion and fluctuating alertness of delirium and may predispose patients to violent behavior. The presence of hallucinations and delusions also increases the potential for violence in patients with delirium, as it does in patients with epilepsy. The presence of delirium in an aggressive patient should prompt a thorough search for an underlying cause. When ambiguity exists about the presence of delirium, the diagnosis can be established by noting day-to-day variability in scores on the Mini-Mental State Examination (or other short cognitive battery) in a relatively short period (several hours) or by slowed cerebral activity on the EEG. A more detailed discussion of delirium is presented in Chapter 5, "Delirium."

Executive Dysfunction Syndromes

Executive dysfunction syndromes, more commonly called *frontal lobe syndromes,* are manifestations of brain injury characterized by varying combinations of inattention, impulsivity, disinhibition, emotional dysregulation, absence of insight, impairment of judgment, and diminished initiative (Lyketsos et al. 2004). These frontal-subcortical syndromes result from a range of etiologies, including trauma, infection, neoplasm, stroke, and neurodegenerative disease. Explosive violence is often a feature, particularly in patients in whom impulsivity, disinhibition, or affective dysregulation predominates. In many individuals with habitual impulsive violence, formal neuropsychological testing indicates deficits in executive cognition (see section "Mechanisms of Aggression" earlier in this chapter); these individuals may be viewed as having occult executive dysfunction syndromes. Further discussion of these syndromes is presented in Chapter 32, "Neurology and Neurosurgery."

Dementia

Aggression is common in patients with dementia, with the risk increasing with dementia severity, concurrent medical illness, crowding, noise, poor quality of interpersonal relationships, and sleep disorder (Lyketsos 2000). The presence of motor restlessness, depression, hallucinations, misinterpretations, paranoia, or delusions in patients with dementia also should alert the clinician to the risk for aggressive behavior. Type of dementia appears to have limited influence on the likelihood of aggression, even though patients with vascular dementia and Huntington's disease may be less cognitively impaired than their counterparts with other forms of dementia.

In elders with dementia, aggression generally manifests as relatively simple behaviors such as throwing objects, pushing, shoving, kicking, pinching, biting, and scratching; destruction of property is uncommon (Cohen-Mansfield and Billig 1986). Impulsive, intrusive, aggressive sexual behaviors may be manifest, and intimacy-seeking sexual behaviors may also be complicated by reactive aggression when the patient is thwarted (de Medeiros et al. 2008). It is unusual for elderly persons with dementia to have well-coordinated and goal-directed physical aggression, but such violence does occur and can be serious, especially when committed by younger patients with dementia.

Aggression in patients with dementia often occurs during routine care activities, such as bathing, morning grooming, and toileting. In these situations, the aggression may result from adversarial interactions with caregivers or from unsophisticated caregiving. Thus, it is important for the physician evaluating violence in the patient with dementia to be cognizant of the circumstances of the act and to search carefully for environmental or caregiver factors that may be triggers for aggression. Careful identification of such "external" factors facilitates their removal or modification (see also Chapter 6, "Dementia").

Developmental Disorders

Violent behavior also occurs in patients with neurodevelopmental syndromes such as mental retardation. Few patients with mental retardation are habitually or impulsively aggressive. However, because many patients with mental retardation also have severe communication or language deficiencies, they may be prone to temper tantrums and violence when frustrated or in discomfort (e.g., from pain). They are also at increased risk for psychiatric symptoms, such as irritability, impulsivity, disinhibition, and low frustration tolerance, and affective and psychotic conditions, which may occasionally contribute to aggressive behavior.

Domestic Aggression Presenting in Medical Settings

Elder Abuse

Elder mistreatment, in the form of abuse or neglect, may provoke aggression by the mistreated elder. Mistreatment begets aggression, but aggressive elders also are more likely to be mistreated by caregivers, whether at home or in an institutional setting. Psychiatrists must be alert to this possibility and screen for mistreatment if an elder presents with an unusual pattern of agitated behavior—for example, if the elder is only aggressive with a particular caregiver or in a particular setting (e.g., while being bathed or dressed) or if he or she presents with physical signs of mistreatment, such as shin bruises or unexplained persistent skin tears. For a comprehensive discussion of elder mistreatment and how to screen for and manage it, the reader is referred to a review published by the National Academies of Sciences (2003).

Intimate Partner Violence

As understanding of violence during intimate relationships has grown, early terms like *wife abuse* that focused on the battery of married women have become obsolete. It is now widely recognized that violence can occur in marital, cohabitation, and dating relationships; in heterosexual and homosexual relationships; and during separation and divorce. *Intimate partner abuse* refers to emotional, psychological, physical, and/or sexual coercion within an intimate relationship, and *intimate partner violence* (IPV) denotes battery of an intimate partner (McHugh and Frieze 2006).

The majority of victims of IPV are women; it has been estimated that 25% of all women and 14% of all men have suffered a lifetime episode (Breiding et al. 2008). It is estimated that 10%–20% of women have received IPV from more than one partner (Thompson et al. 2006), and the frequency is especially high for younger women, single mothers, those who are poorly educated, and those who suffered abuse in their childhood. IPV is a widespread, cross-cultural problem, with high rates worldwide (Garcia-Moreno et al. 2006). Cultural attitudes may contribute to IPV (Uthman et al. 2009a, 2009b), but individual characteristics such as low education, poverty, abuse of alcohol and other substances, and certain psychological attributes appear to be more important. Alcohol abuse is common among both perpetrators and victims of severe IPV (McKinney et al. 2010), with a stronger association in clinical than in nonclinical samples (Foran and O'Leary 2009). Perpetrators also tend to have high rates of exposure to IPV during their childhood (Ernst et al. 2009). Perpetrators of impulsive IPV have been found to have more frequent and severe psychopathology than is the case with perpetrators of premeditated IPV (Stanford et al. 2008).

IPV results in high utilization of health care services (Bonomi et al. 2009a), particularly for mental health. These patients are seen frequently in a variety of ambulatory care settings, in the general hospital, and in psychiatry wards. Victims of IPV experience adverse health outcomes besides injury (and death), such as cigarette smoking, asthma, musculoskeletal disease, complications of pregnancy and childbirth, sexually transmitted diseases (including HIV/AIDS), substance abuse, somatoform and conversion disorders, family and social problems, anxiety, and depression (Bonomi et al. 2009b). Exposed children sustain emotional injury living in an environment of domestic aggression and may themselves be victims of accidental or intentional violence. Many of these children will later in life show a wide range of psychopathology and are prone to becoming abusive men and abused women themselves.

Victims of IPV are frequent visitors to clinics and EDs, and although some are too afraid to discuss their experiences with a physician, many are willing. Unfortunately, most cases remain undetected. Several factors account for this, including inadequate training in the detection and management of IPV, physicians' feelings of discomfort and powerlessness, and pressures on physicians to spend less time with patients. A patient's reluctance may derive from negative past experiences, pessimism, low self-confidence, fear of retaliation, or their emotional and/or financial dependence.

Vigilant clinicians can recognize patterns suggestive of IPV, such as repeat visits for vague or minor complaints or chronic pain (especially pelvic), evasive and anxious behavior, inability to recall events leading to the presenting problem, inadequate or baffling explanations for injuries, domineering and obstructionist behavior in a partner, unexplained nonadherence to medication regimens and treatment plans, and findings of child or elder abuse (Eisenstat and Bancroft 1999). In addition, certain physical findings should raise the possibility of battery: injuries to the head, neck, or mouth; multiple injuries; bruises in various stages of healing; defensive injuries of the forearms; dental trauma; and genital injuries. It is prudent to screen for IPV in patients with somatoform, anxiety, and substance abuse disorders and in those with suicidal ideation or attempts.

Routine screening of all women is widely recommended by advocacy organizations and professional associations but has lately become controversial. Many formal screening tools have been developed, but their psychometric properties have not been fully characterized and their effectiveness remains uncertain (Rabin et al. 2009). Victims of IPV may prefer self-completed questionnaires to face-to-face questioning (MacMillan et al. 2006). Computer-based screening approaches can improve rates of screening in the ED (Trautman et al. 2007) but are not likely to be widely implemented. A simpler screening strategy is to incorporate probe questions into the clinical interview. However, two considerations limit the utility of routine screening for IPV: 1) the uncertain reliability of current tools and methods for detecting (or ruling out) IPV (Wathen et al. 2006) and 2) a dearth of data showing that screening reduces violence. The results of a recent large controlled trial indicated that a screening program did not lead to improved outcomes (MacMillan et al. 2009); however, further study is needed, given that sample attrition in the study reached 43%. Also, it is likely that screening must be coupled with structured, individualized psychosocial and mental health interventions to be effective.

In Table 7–4, we provide some sample questions that may be used to initiate the screening process. Incorporating screening questions into the routine interview process can minimize physician and patient discomfort.

When abuse or IPV is identified, descriptions of current, recent, and past battery, including dates and circumstances, should be elicited and carefully documented. Legal intervention may rely on this documentation so the findings should be described in precise language, quoting the specific words spoken by the patient when possible. A complete history and thorough examination should be performed, all injuries should be carefully described (body maps are very useful for this purpose), and photographs should be taken if the patient consents. Strict confidentiality of the disclosure is needed to protect the patient from retaliation; this may require restricted access or sequestration of the disclosure records. On completion of the medical evaluation, a social work evaluation and referral to services such as the National Domestic Violence Hotline (1-800-799-SAFE) and local advocacy organizations should follow. It is usually best to respect the patient's wishes regarding when to report the violence to legal authorities and when to flee the situation. However, in some states, the physician is required by law to make a report. In the United States, mandatory reporting is the norm whenever evidence of child abuse is found (see also Chapter 2, "Legal Issues").

TABLE 7–4. Helpful questions for intimate partner abuse screening by clinicians

1. Do you and your partner argue a lot? Does it ever get physical? Has either one of you ever hit the other? Has either one of you ever injured the other?
2. Do you ever feel unsafe at home?
3. Has anyone ever hit you or tried to injure you in any way?
4. Has anyone ever threatened you or tried to control you?
5. Have you ever felt afraid of your partner?
6. Is there anything particularly stressful going on now? How are things at home?
7. I see patients in my practice who are being hurt or threatened by someone they love. Is this happening to you? Has this ever happened to you?

Source. Question 1 from J.L. Levenson (personal communication, October 2003); Questions 2–5 from Eisenstat and Bancroft 1999; Questions 6–7 from Gerbert et al. 2000.

Management of Aggressive Behavior

Education and Relationship Building

Ideally, health care providers and staff have been educated about the management of aggression in the general hospital. This is one component of the psychiatrist's liaison role, performed through seminars, bedside teaching, care conferences, and continuing education. Important content includes recognition of the early signs of incipient aggression (e.g., restlessness, staring, pacing) and behavioral interventions, including verbal de-escalation techniques (nonthreatening approaches such as speaking calmly, using gentle eye contact, adopting a problem-solving stance, and knowing when to disengage), and guidance on when and how to use a "show of force," pharmacological tranquilization, and physical restraint. This teaching serves to broaden the skill set of the medical team members and to increase their confidence in their ability to manage these patients, which can result in fewer aggressive incidents, reduced likelihood of patient or staff injury during episodes, more effective treatment of the underlying conditions, and more productive collaboration in patient care.

Safety of the Environment

The safety of the environment should be ensured before any aggressive patient is evaluated. The psychiatrist should check that actual weapons, such as guns and knives, and potential weapons, such as scissors, belts, and ropes, have been removed. In the ED, this is often accomplished by routinely using hand searches and metal detectors and by keeping any discovered items safely locked away. On inpatient units, monitoring and controlling what the patient can keep, conducting periodic room searches, and providing plastic utensils for meals are common interventions. A safe environment also should allow for the examiner's easy escape, as well as observation and easy entry by other health care personnel. The psychiatrist should use what information is available to anticipate what precautions and emergency interventions may be needed before starting the evaluation and should make sure that the medical team is ready to intervene in the event that the patient becomes severely agitated or violent.

Psychiatric Evaluation

Effective management of the aggressive patient requires a comprehensive psychiatric evaluation, ultimately leading to the identification of potentially modifiable factors at which interventions are targeted. In many instances, formulation of the case results in the diagnosis of a psychiatric disorder, and specific treatment is instituted with the expectation that remission of the disorder will lead to resolution of the aggression (e.g., an antipsychotic for acute psychosis in a patient with schizophrenia). However, in many patients with aggression, the psychiatric diagnosis only partially explains the behavior and does not indicate what the appropriate treatment strategy should be. This situation is often observed in patients with personality disorder, brain injury, or dementia but is frequently also true for patients with major mental disorders such as schizophrenia. In most such situations, careful characterization of the patient's background and careful description and decoding of the aggressive behavior will inform the approach to treatment.

Positive Therapeutic Alliance

The first step in the management of the aggressive patient is to develop a positive therapeutic alliance (Beauford et al. 1997). In all cases, and particularly in patients who are chronically aggressive or have recurrent violent episodes, it is crucial to actively seek the patient's collaboration in the treatment process. A positive therapeutic alliance facilitates the patient's compliance with behavioral expectations and with prescribed treatments and makes it easier to mediate patient-staff conflicts and de-escalate aggressive episodes. Also, a positive alliance facilitates the development of a psychotherapeutic relationship that may enable the psychiatrist to eventually reduce the patient's propensity to violent responses when anticipated precipitants occur in the future (O'Connor 2003).

Behavioral Approaches

Verbal de-escalation techniques (shown in Table 7-5) are often effective for controlling and terminating mild to moderate aggression (threats and belligerence) and are used frequently in the ED and acute psychiatric inpatient unit. These techniques can be used in general medical settings by those who have been taught how to use them. Although verbal de-escalation should be conceptualized as a semistructured intervention (see Table 7-5), in practice, it is often deployed as an instinctive, commonsense reaction to the patient's behavior rather than as a systematic intervention. The basic goal of de-escalation is to manage a patient's anger and hostility by conveying empathy and understanding, personalizing the clinician, helping the patient to articulate grievances and frustrations, and actively involving the patient in problem solving and treatment planning (Stevenson 1991). Verbal de-escalation techniques are most useful in situations that involve patient-staff conflict, but they also can be used to manage pathological aggression and to set the stage for pharmacological interventions.

More sophisticated behavioral approaches have been successfully applied to the management of chronic aggression, particularly in patients with dementia and brain in-

TABLE 7-5. Verbal de-escalation techniques

Communication

Nonverbal

- Maintain a safe distance
- Maintain a neutral posture
- Do not stare; eye contact should convey sincerity
- Do not touch the patient
- Stay at the same height as the patient
- Avoid sudden movements

Verbal

- Speak in a calm, clear tone
- Personalize yourself
- Avoid confrontation; offer to solve the problem

Tactics

Debunking

- Acknowledge the patient's grievance
- Acknowledge the patient's frustration
- Shift focus to discussion of how to solve the problem

Aligning goals

- Emphasize common ground
- Focus on the big picture
- Find ways to make small concessions

Monitoring

- Be acutely aware of progress
- Know when to disengage
- Do not insist on having the last word

jury. These approaches include behavioral analysis, operant conditioning, differential reinforcement strategies, validation, manipulation of ambient light and/or sound, activity programs, and environmental modification (Lyketsos 2000). Evidence for the use of these approaches derives primarily from uncontrolled studies.

Seclusion and Restraint

It is not unusual for de-escalation and other behavioral techniques to fail to calm the patient who is very agitated, particularly in the ED and other acute care settings. Also, in some settings, de-escalation techniques may be impractical because the patient is unable to communicate meaningfully (as a result of confusion, cognitive impairment, or communication disorders), is known to be explosive, is too severely agitated to cooperate, or is already engaging in violent behavior. In such cases, the use of physical restraint, which may involve *manual restraint* (wherein the patient is restrained by several health care workers) and *mechanical restraint* (wherein an appliance is used to restrain the patient), may be needed to terminate dangerous behavior. Sometimes, physical restraint is needed to administer tranquilizers or to protect other medical interventions (e.g., to keep the patient from pulling out intravenous lines, chest tubes, urinary catheters, or other vital lines or tubes). For a brief period immediately after the application of physical restraints (or the administration of tranquilizers), it is prudent to observe the patient in isolation (in his or her own room or a designated safe room) to ensure that the violent episode, its consequences, and identifiable triggers have been successfully managed. Because improper use of restraints can result in injury to the patient or to health care workers, such use should be directed and implemented only by experienced personnel. Training courses in the use of manual and physical restraints are widely supported, and many jurisdictions have developed certification programs.

During the past decade, the use of seclusion and physical restraints has come under intense criticism. As a result, governmental and judicial regulation of restraint use has steadily increased (see also Chapter 2, "Legal Issues"). In response to these trends, the Academy of Psychosomatic Medicine issued guidelines (Bronheim et al. 1998, p. S20) that state the following:

> Constant observation and restraints should be implemented for the shortest possible time with the least restrictive, though effective, means available; these interventions must not be made solely for the convenience of medical staff. Assessment and treatment of underlying psychiatric conditions that contribute to the patient's need for these measures should be expeditiously undertaken.

These guidelines are consistent with those developed by other medical associations, with regulatory standards, and with the general opinion of the courts. In general, the standards for the clinical use of restraints are as follows: 1) restraints should be used only when necessary to protect the patient or others from harm; 2) restraints should not be used solely to coerce the patient to accept treatments or remain in the treatment setting; and 3) when restraints are being used, the patient should be closely monitored and his or her condition frequently reassessed. The clinical and regulatory issues involved in the use of restraints are complex; thus, it is often necessary for psychiatrists to help other medical colleagues explore the various options for managing an aggressive patient and to address any staff discomfort with the use of restraints, while keeping in mind the clinical and legal risks involved in using or forgoing restraints.

Pharmacological Approaches

Data indicating that neurotransmitter systems modulate aggression have stimulated the development of pharmacological approaches for the clinical management of aggression. This pharmacotherapy for aggression is based more on contemporary intuitions of the neurotransmitter effects of medications and how these effects modulate the expression of aggressive behavior and less on evidence from controlled trials. Medications are indicated for impulsive and pathological forms of aggression. In general, treatment of clinically relevant aggression falls into two broad categories: 1) treatment of *syndromic* aggression separate from the diagnostic context and 2) focused treatment of conditions that manifest *symptomatic* aggression, such as schizophrenia, delusional disorders, major depressive disorders, and delirium. The discussion that follows focuses mainly on the treatment of syndromic aggression; treatments for specific conditions are covered in detail in other chapters of this text.

Pharmacological agents are indicated for both acute and chronic aggression. In the treatment of acute aggression, the goal is typically rapid tranquilization (which refers to the use of medications to achieve a rapid termination of agitated or aggressive behavior). A survey of U.S. psychiatrists who specialize in emergency psychiatry found that benzodiazepines (particularly lorazepam) were the preferred agents for treating acute aggression (Allen et al. 2001) because they are relatively free of adverse effects that are typically associated with antipsychotics, such as the acute dystonias, akathisia, and parkinsonism. Antipsychotics, especially haloperidol, also were considered first-line agents, particularly for acute aggression associated with psychosis. The survey predates the introduction of parenteral formulations of ziprasidone and olanzapine, which are now used in many centers. A controlled trial found the combination of lorazepam and haloperidol to be superior to lorazepam or haloperidol alone for the treatment of acute agitation in patients with psychosis (Battaglia et al. 1997), suggesting that the combination also may be more effective for acute aggression. Newer antipsychotics—for example, the atypical antipsychotics risperidone and olanzapine—are also being increasingly used for the management of acute agitation and aggression (Allen et al. 2001). For rapid tranquilization, drugs that can be given parenterally are advantageous. Lorazepam (intramuscular, intravenous) and haloperidol (intramuscular, intravenous) are typically used for this purpose. Intramuscular formulations of three atypical antipsychotics—ziprasidone, olanzapine, and aripiprazole—are also available.

A wider range of pharmacological agents is used for the treatment of chronic aggression (see Table 7-6). Of these agents, antipsychotics are the most widely used. The relative dearth of evidence from placebo-controlled trials and the phenotypic and neurobiological heterogeneity of aggression may explain the diversity of agents used to treat chronic aggression. It is noteworthy that placebo-controlled trials of treatments for agitation and aggression in elderly patients have yielded placebo responses as high as 60% in some studies, underscoring the importance of rigorous methodology in the evaluation of treatments (Lyketsos 2000). However, despite the limited availability of data from controlled trials, considerable empirical support exists for the use of several psychotropic classes in treating aggression.

Antipsychotics are the preferred agents for treating agitation and aggression in the general medical setting, especially when these phenomena arise in a patient with delirium. Antipsychotics are also used to treat aggression in psychotic patients and to tranquilize patients with severe aggression (regardless of cause). Tranquilization may terminate an episode of aggression, but sometimes it does not reduce the frequency or severity of future episodes of impulsive aggression.

In clinical trials of typical antipsychotics for the treatment of impulsive aggression in patients with personality disorders, results have been mixed; however, the atypical agents (which selectively block 5-HT_2 receptors—an action associated with reduced aggression in animals) may be more effective in treating chronic impulsive aggression (Coccaro and Siever 2002). In a randomized comparative study, clozapine was the most efficacious agent in reducing hostile aggression (independent of its effectiveness in relieving psychosis); olanzapine, risperidone, and haloperidol were equal in effectiveness (Citrome et al. 2001). Although these results would seem to recommend clozapine as a first choice for treating aggression in psychotic patients, in practice, the drug is typically reserved for severe or treatment-resistant cases because of its adverse-effect profile.

TABLE 7–6. Medications used in the treatment of chronic aggression

Antidepressants
Selective serotonin reuptake inhibitors
Tricyclic antidepressants
Serotonin-norepinephrine reuptake inhibitors
Trazodone
Mirtazapine
Antipsychotics
Haloperidol
Fluphenazine
Loxapine
Risperidone
Paliperidone
Aripiprazole
Ziprasidone
Olanzapine
Clozapine
Quetiapine
Anticonvulsants
Divalproex sodium
Carbamazepine
Oxcarbazepine
Phenytoin
Others
Lithium
Buspirone
Propranolol, nadolol
Amantadine
Progesterone
Leuprolide
Prazosin

Antipsychotics are also used to treat aggression in patients with brain diseases. In multicenter trials in patients with dementia, risperidone and olanzapine were found useful in reducing aggression (Ballard and Waite 2006; Lyketsos 2000), but results from the CATIE-AD (Clinical Antipsychotic Trials in Intervention Effectiveness—Alzheimer's Disease) study indicated that their effects are modest and are offset by adverse effects (Schneider et al. 2006). As with other antipsychotics, both risperidone and olanzapine are associated with cerebrovascular events, extrapyramidal symptoms, and increased mortality in dementia. Clinicians must balance their modest efficacy and associated risks against the risks of untreated aggression in patients with dementia (Salzman et al. 2008). It is prudent to reserve their use for those dementia patients whose aggression poses significant risk or causes marked distress. In cases of aggression in dementia successfully treated with an antipsychotic, planned withdrawal of the drug after 3 months is recommended (Ballard et al. 2008; Onyike 2008). There is a growing consensus among specialists that behavioral interventions should be the first line of treatment for aggression in dementia, with pharmacological interventions reserved for behavioral emergencies and refractory cases. Recent evidence indicates that memantine, a treatment for dementia, can reduce aggression and psychosis (Wilcock et al. 2008). It seems reasonable to consider memantine as the first pharmacological intervention when a patient with dementia becomes aggressive. It is uncertain whether cholinesterase inhibitors reduce agitation, aggression, and violence in dementia (Rodda et al. 2009).

Data showing that experimental and pharmacological modulation of serotonin neurotransmission can reduce levels of aggression in nonhuman primates and smaller animals (Walsh and Dinan 2001), and other results showing low CSF levels of serotonin metabolites in impulsively aggressive patients, violent offenders, and suicide attempters (discussed earlier, in the section "Mechanisms of Aggression"), constitute compelling reasons to treat impulsive aggression with selective serotonin reuptake inhibitors (SSRIs), lithium, buspirone, and other drugs that may enhance central serotonin levels. In addition, SSRIs, lithium, and buspirone have been effective, in small placebo-controlled trials, in reducing impulsive nonviolent aggression in patients with personality disorders, autism, and depressive disorders (Coccaro and Siever 2002), although this is not consistently observed (e.g., Lee et al. 2008).

Anticonvulsants may be effective in reducing impulsive aggression. A recent Cochrane Library review of placebo-controlled clinical trials (Huband et al. 2010) showed that valproate/divalproex, carbamazepine, oxcarbazepine, and phenytoin reduce recurrent impulsive aggression in a broad spectrum of patients, including male psychiatric outpatients and prisoners, adults with personality disorders, and (valproate only) children and adolescents with conduct disorder. It has not been demonstrated that anticonvulsants reduce aggression in children and adolescents with pervasive developmental disorders. Another review of controlled trials, using less stringent inclusion criteria, concluded that topiramate and lamotrigine may reduce impulsive aggression in adults with personality disorders (Stanford et al. 2009). With respect to dementia, a recent controlled trial found that valproate was ineffective and poorly tolerated (Herrmann et al. 2007). In blinded, placebo-controlled trials, carbamazepine reduced aggression in nursing home patients with dementia (Tariot et al. 1998). Oxcarbazepine did not reduce aggression in dementia in another trial (Sommer et al. 2009). Gabapentin is prescribed frequently for impulsive aggression, although no empirical evidence supports this practice. Small trials suggest that topiramate might reduce aggression in individuals with borderline personality disorder (Nickel and Loew 2008; Nickel et al. 2004, 2005). Levetiracetam did not reduce aggression in a recent trial (Mattes 2008), and there is evidence that it causes impulsivity and aggression when used in epilepsy treatment (Helmstaedter et al. 2008).

Because overactivity in the noradrenergic system has been implicated in the expression of aggression, noradrenergic blockade has emerged as another therapeutic strategy. The typically used agents are propranolol and nadolol, both beta-adrenergic blockers. Clinical trials have found them to be effective in patients with traumatic brain injury, dementia, and psychosis (Allan et al. 1996; Ratey et al. 1992; Shankle et al. 1995; Sorgi et al. 1986). Beta-blockers may cause hypotension and bradycardia and therefore should be used with caution. In fact, low-dose treatment may be effective for certain patients; one study found that low-dose propranolol (10–80 mg/day) reduced aggression in patients with dementia (Shankle et al. 1995).

Table 7–6 provides a summary of other medications that may be helpful for treating aggression. Progesterone and leuprolide are used for some patients with aggressive sexual behavior. In routine practice, psychiatrists often use combinations of medications from different classes because the response to single-agent therapy is usually modest.

Conclusion

Aggression is a major clinical and public health problem. In clinical settings, it represents a difficult, disruptive, and dangerous problem for psychiatrists, nonpsychiatric physicians, nurses, and other health care workers. Fortunately, strategies exist to manage this problem. A careful description of the aggressive episode, in the context of a comprehensive psychiatric examination, informs clinical management. Out of the clinical examination comes an appreciation of the fundamental nature of the problem (for instance, whether the aggression is impulsive or premeditated), the factors that have produced and/or sustained it, and the approaches to treatment.

The treatment of aggression requires awareness that psychiatric diagnosis alone is often not enough to inform the treatment and, therefore, an individualized approach is required. For most patients, aggression is managed empirically with a combination of approaches, behavioral, environmental and pharmacological. In the general hospital, the management of aggressive patients involves active collaboration among psychiatrists, nonpsychiatric physicians, nurses, and other health care workers. This collaboration works best when the ground has been prepared beforehand through the liaison efforts of the psychiatrist and will maximize the effectiveness of interventions while minimizing the risk of injury to patients and medical staff.

Finally, it is also important to keep in mind that many aggressive patients, particularly those with impulsive aggression, are also at risk for suicidal behavior and require a careful suicide risk assessment and appropriate interventions. Recent research has yielded much insight into the neurobiology of aggression and violence, but more work is needed to develop predictive methods and more effective preventive and treatment modalities.

References

Allan ER, Alpert M, Sison CE, et al: Adjunctive nadolol in the treatment of acutely aggressive schizophrenic patients. J Clin Psychiatry 57:455–459, 1996

Allen MH, Currier GW, Hughes DH, et al: The Expert Consensus Guideline Series: treatment of behavioral emergencies. Postgrad Med (Spec No):1–88; quiz 89–90, 2001

American Psychiatric Association: Diagnostic and Statistical Manual of Mental Disorders, 4th Edition. Washington, DC, American Psychiatric Association, 1994

American Psychiatric Association: Diagnostic and Statistical Manual of Mental Disorders, 4th Edition, Text Revision. Washington, DC, American Psychiatric Association, 2000

Amore M, Menchetti M, Tonti C, et al: Predictors of violent behavior among acute psychiatric patients: clinical study. Psychiatry Clin Neurosci 62:247–255, 2008

Appelbaum PS, Robbins PC, Monahan J: Violence and delusions: data from the MacArthur Violence Risk Assessment Study. Am J Psychiatry 157:566–572, 2000

Arnetz JE, Arnetz BB: Violence towards health care staff and possible effects on the quality of patient care. Soc Sci Med 52:417–427, 2001

Ballard C, Waite J: The effectiveness of atypical antipsychotics for the treatment of aggression and psychosis in Alzheimer's disease. Cochrane Database Syst Rev (1):CD003476, 2006

Ballard C, Lana MM, Theodoulou M, et al: A randomised, blinded, placebo-controlled trial in dementia patients continuing or stopping neuroleptics (the DART-AD trial). PLoS Med 5:e76, 2008

Barlow K, Grenyer B, Ilkiw-Lavalle O: Prevalence and precipitants of aggression in psychiatric inpatient units. Aust N Z J Psychiatry 34:967–974, 2000

Battaglia J, Moss S, Rush J, et al: Haloperidol, lorazepam, or both for psychotic agitation? A multicenter, prospective, double-blind, emergency department study. Am J Emerg Med 15:335–340, 1997

Beauford JE, McNiel DE, Binder RL: Utility of the initial therapeutic alliance in evaluating psychiatric patients' risk of violence. Am J Psychiatry 154:1272–1276, 1997

Behnam M, Tillotson RD, Davis SM, et al: Violence in the emergency department: a national survey of emergency medicine residents and attending physicians. J Emerg Med 2010 Feb 2 [Epub ahead of print]

Biancosino B, Delmonte S, Grassi L, et al: Violent behavior in acute psychiatric inpatient facilities: a national survey in Italy. J Nerv Ment Dis 197:772–782, 2009

Binder RL, McNiel DE: The relationship of gender to violent behavior in acutely disturbed psychiatric patients. J Clin Psychiatry 51:110–114, 1990

Blanchard JC, Curtis KM: Violence in the emergency department. Emerg Med Clin North Am 17:717–731, 1999

Bobes J, Fillat O, Arango C: Violence among schizophrenia outpatients compliant with medication: prevalence and associated factors. Acta Psychiatr Scand 119:218–225, 2009

Bonomi AE, Anderson ML, Rivara FP, et al: Health care utilization and costs associated with physical and nonphysical-only intimate partner violence. Health Serv Res 44:1052–1067, 2009a

Bonomi AE, Anderson ML, Reid RJ, et al: Medical and psychosocial diagnoses in women with a history of intimate partner violence. Arch Intern Med 169:1692–1697, 2009b

Bowers L, Jarrett M, Clark N, et al: Determinants of absconding by patients on acute psychiatric wards. J Adv Nurs 32:644–649, 2000

Breiding MJ, Black MC, Ryan GW: Prevalence and risk factors of intimate partner violence in eighteen US states/territories, 2005. Am J Prev Med 34:112–118, 2008

Bronheim HE, Fulop G, Kunkel EJ, et al: The Academy of Psychosomatic Medicine practice guidelines for psychiatric consultation in the general medical setting. The Academy of Psychosomatic Medicine. Psychosomatics 39:S8–S30, 1998

Brower MC, Price BH: Neuropsychiatry of frontal lobe dysfunction in violent and criminal behaviour: a critical review. J Neurol Neurosurg Psychiatry 71:720–726, 2001

Choe JY, Teplin LA, Abram KM: Perpetration of violence, violent victimization, and severe mental illness: balancing public health concerns. Psychiatr Serv 59:153–164, 2008

Citrome L, Volavka J, Czobor P, et al: Effects of clozapine, olanzapine, risperidone, and haloperidol on hostility among patients with schizophrenia. Psychiatr Serv 52:1510–1514, 2001

Coccaro EF, Siever LJ: Pathophysiology and treatment of aggression, in Neuropsychopharmacology: The Fifth Generation of Progress. Edited by Davis KL, Charney D, Coyle JT, et al. Philadelphia, PA, Lippincott, Williams & Wilkins, 2002, pp 1709–1723

Cohen-Mansfield J, Billig N: Agitated behaviors in the elderly, I: a conceptual review. J Am Geriatr Soc 34:711–721, 1986

Colasanti A, Natoli A, Moliterno D, et al: Psychiatric diagnosis and aggression before acute hospitalisation. Eur Psychiatry 23:441–448, 2008

Corbett SW, Grange JT, Thomas TL: Exposure of prehospital care providers to violence. Prehosp Emerg Care 2:127–131, 1998

Cummings JL, Mega MS: Violence and aggression, in Neuropsychiatry and Behavioral Neuroscience. New York, Oxford University Press, 2003, pp 360–370

Davidson RJ, Putnam KM, Larson CL: Dysfunction in the neural circuitry of emotion regulation—a possible prelude to violence. Science 289:591–594, 2000

de Barros DM, de Pádua Serafim A: Association between personality disorder and violent behavior pattern. Forensic Sci Int 179:19–22, 2008

de Medeiros K, Rosenberg PB, Baker AS, et al: Improper sexual behaviors in elders with dementia living in residential care. Dement Geriatr Cogn Disord 26:370–377, 2008

Demaree HA, Harrison DW: Case study: topographical brain mapping in hostility following mild closed head injury. Int J Neurosci 87:97–101, 1996

Ehmann TS, Smith GN, Yamamoto A, et al: Violence in treatment resistant psychotic inpatients. J Nerv Ment Dis 189: 716–721, 2001

Eisenstat SA, Bancroft L: Domestic violence. N Engl J Med 341:886–892, 1999

Elbogen EB, Johnson SC: The intricate link between violence and mental disorder: results from the National Epidemiologic Survey on Alcohol and Related Conditions. Arch Gen Psychiatry 66:152–161, 2009

Ernst AA, Weiss SJ, Hall J, et al: Adult intimate partner violence perpetrators are significantly more likely to have witnessed intimate partner violence as a child than nonperpetrators. Am J Emerg Med 27:641–650, 2009

Eronen M, Angermeyer MC, Schulze B, et al: The psychiatric epidemiology of violent behaviour. Soc Psychiatry Psychiatr Epidemiol 33 (suppl 1):S13–S23, 1998

Fazel S, Grann M, Carlström E, et al: Risk factors for violent crime in schizophrenia: a national cohort study of 13,806 patients. J Clin Psychiatry 70:362–369, 2009

Flannery RB Jr: Precipitants to psychiatric patient assaults on staff: review of empirical findings, 1990–2003, and risk management implications. Psychiatr Q 76:317–326, 2005

Foran HM, O'Leary KD: Alcohol and intimate partner violence: a meta-analytic review. Clin Psychol Rev 28:1222–1234, 2009

Garcia-Moreno C, Jansen HA, Ellsberg M, et al: Prevalence of intimate partner violence: findings from the WHO Multi-Country Study on Women's Health and Domestic Violence. Lancet 368:1260–1269, 2006

Gerard ME, Spitz MC, Towbin JA, et al: Subacute postictal aggression. Neurology 50:384–388, 1998

Gerberich SG, Church TR, McGovern PM, et al: An epidemiological study of the magnitude and consequences of work related violence: the Minnesota Nurses' Study. Occup Environ Med 61:495–503, 2004

Gerbert B, Moe J, Caspers N, et al: Simplifying physicians' response to domestic violence. West J Med 172:329–331, 2000

Giegling I, Olgiati P, Hartmann AM, et al: Personality and attempted suicide. Analysis of anger, aggression and impulsivity. J Psychiatr Res 43:1262–1271, 2009

Grange JT, Corbett SW: Violence against emergency medical services personnel. Prehosp Emerg Care 6:186–190, 2002

Greenfield TK, McNiel DE, Binder RL: Violent behavior and length of psychiatric hospitalization. Hosp Community Psychiatry 40:809–814, 1989

Hamrin V, Iennaco J, Olsen D: A review of ecological factors affecting inpatient psychiatric unit violence: implications for relational and unit cultural improvements. Issues Ment Health Nurs 30:214–226, 2009

Harlow JM: Passage of an iron rod through the head. Boston Med Surg J 39:389–393, 1848

Harlow JM: Recovery from the passage of an iron rod through the head. Publications of the Massachusetts Medical Society 2:327–347, 1868

Helmstaedter C, Fritz NE, Kockelmann E, et al: Positive and negative psychotropic effects of levetiracetam. Epilepsy Behav 13:535–541, 2008

Herrmann N, Lanctôt KL, Rothenburg LS, et al: A placebo-controlled trial of valproate for agitation and aggression in Alzheimer's disease. Dement Geriatr Cogn Disord 23:116–119, 2007

Hesdorffer DC, Rauch SL, Tamminga CA: Long-term psychiatric outcomes following traumatic brain injury: a review of the literature. J Head Trauma Rehabil 24:452–459, 2009

Hiday VA, Swartz MS, Swanson JW, et al: Male-female differences in the setting and construction of violence among people with severe mental illness. Soc Psychiatry Psychiatr Epidemiol 33 (suppl 1): S68–S74, 1998

Hillbrand M, Foster HG, Spitz RT: Characteristics and cost of staff injuries in a forensic hospital. Psychiatr Serv 47:1123–1125, 1996

Hodgins S: Violent behaviour among people with schizophrenia: a framework for investigations of causes, and effective treatment, and prevention. Philos Trans R Soc Lond B Biol Sci 363:2505–2518, 2008

Hodgins S, Cree A, Alderton J, et al: From conduct disorder to severe mental illness: associations with aggressive behaviour, crime and victimization. Psychol Med 38:975–987, 2008

Huband N, Ferriter M, Nathan R, et al: Antiepileptics for aggression and associated impulsivity. Cochrane Database Syst Rev (2):CD003499, 2010

James A, Madeley R, Dove A: Violence and aggression in the emergency department. Emerg Med J 23:431–434, 2006

Kalunian DA, Binder RL, McNiel DR: Violence by geriatric patients who need psychiatric hospitalization. J Clin Psychiatry 51:340–343, 1990

Kanemoto K, Kawasaki J, Mori E: Violence and epilepsy: a close relation between violence and postictal psychosis. Epilepsia 40:107–109, 1999

Kansagra SM, Rao SR, Sullivan AF, et al: A survey of workplace violence across 65 U.S. emergency departments. Acad Emerg Med 15:1268–1274, 2008

Lam JN, McNiel DE, Binder RL: The relationship between patients' gender and violence leading to staff injuries. Psychiatr Serv 51:1167–1170, 2000

Lee R, Kavoussi RJ, Coccaro EF: Placebo-controlled, randomized trial of fluoxetine in the treatment of aggression in male intimate partner abusers. Int Clin Psychopharmacol 23:337–341, 2008

Lyketsos CG: Aggression, in The American Psychiatric Press Textbook of Geriatric Neuropsychiatry. Edited by Coffey E, Cummings JL. Washington, DC, American Psychiatric Press, 2000, pp 477–488

Lyketsos CG, Rosenblatt A, Rabins P: The forgotten frontal lobe syndrome or "executive dysfunction syndrome." Psychosomatics 45:247–255, 2004

Lynch J, Appelboam R, McQuillan PJ: Survey of abuse and violence by patients and relatives towards intensive care staff. Anaesthesia 58:893–899, 2003

MacMillan HL, Wathen CN, Jamieson E, et al: Approaches to screening for intimate partner violence in health care settings: a randomized trial. JAMA 296:530–536, 2006

MacMillan HL, Wathen CN, Jamieson E, et al: Screening for intimate partner violence in health care settings: a randomized trial. JAMA 302:493–501, 2009

Marsh L, Krauss GL: Aggression and violence in patients with epilepsy. Epilepsy Behav 1:160–168, 2000

Mattes JA: Levetiracetam in patients with impulsive aggression: a double-blind, placebo controlled trial. J Clin Psychiatry 69:310–315, 2008

McHugh MC, Frieze IH: Intimate partner violence: new directions. Ann N Y Acad Sci 1087:121–141, 2006

McKinney CM, Caetano R, Rodriguez LA, et al: Does alcohol involvement increase the severity of intimate partner violence? Alcohol Clin Exp Res 34:655–658, 2010

McNiel DE, Eisner JP, Binder RL: The relationship between command hallucinations and violence. Psychiatr Serv 51:1288–1292, 2000

Mericle AA, Havassy BE: Characteristics of recent violence among entrants to acute mental health and substance abuse services. Soc Psychiatry Psychiatr Epidemiol 43:392–402, 2008

Miczek KA, de Almeida RM, Kravitz EA, et al: Neurobiology of escalated aggression and violence. J Neurosci 27:11803–11806, 2007

Mock EF, Wrenn KD, Wright SW, et al: Prospective field study of violence in emergency medical services calls. Ann Emerg Med 32:33–36, 1998

Nachreiner NM, Gerberich SG, Ryan AD, et al: Minnesota Nurses' Study: perceptions of violence and the work environment. Ind Health 45:672–678, 2007

National Academies of Sciences: Elder Mistreatment: Abuse, Neglect, and Exploitation in an Aging America. Panel to Review Risk and Prevalence of Elder Abuse and Neglect. Washington, DC, National Academies Press, 2003

Naudts K, Hodgins S: Neurobiological correlates of violent behavior among persons with schizophrenia. Schizophr Bull 32:562–572, 2006

Nelson RJ, Trainor BC: Neural mechanisms of aggression. Nat Rev Neurosci 8:536–546, 2007

Newhill CE, Mulvey EP, Lidz CW: Characteristics of violence in the community by female patients seen in a psychiatric emergency service. Psychiatr Serv 46:785–789, 1995

Nickel MK, Loew TH: Treatment of aggression with topiramate in male borderline patients, part II: 18-month follow-up. Eur Psychiatry 23:115–117, 2008

Nickel MK, Nickel C, Mitterlehner FO, et al: Topiramate treatment of aggression in female borderline personality disorder patients: a double-blind, placebo-controlled study. J Clin Psychiatry 65:1515–1519, 2004

Nickel MK, Nickel C, Kaplan P, et al: Treatment of aggression with topiramate in male borderline patients: a double-blind, placebo-controlled study. Biol Psychiatry 57:495–499, 2005

O'Connor S: Violent behavior in chronic schizophrenia and inpatient psychiatry. J Am Acad Psychoanal Dyn Psychiatry 31:31–44, 2003

Onyike CU: Neuroleptic discontinuation during dementia care: a recent trial and its implications for practice. Nat Clin Pract Neurol 4:528–529, 2008

Pozzi C: Exposure of prehospital providers to violence and abuse. J Emerg Nurs 24:320–323, 1998

Pulay AJ, Dawson DA, Hasin DS, et al: Violent behavior and DSM-IV psychiatric disorders: results from the National Epidemiologic Survey on Alcohol and Related Conditions. J Clin Psychiatry 69:12–22, 2008

Rabin RF, Jennings JM, Campbell JC, et al: Intimate partner violence screening tools: a systematic review. Am J Prev Med 36:439–445.e4, 2009

Rao V, Rosenberg P, Bertrand M, et al: Aggression after traumatic brain injury: prevalence and correlates. J Neuropsychiatry Clin Neurosci 21:420–429, 2009

Ratey JJ, Sorgi P, O'Driscoll GA, et al: Nadolol to treat aggression and psychiatric symptomatology in chronic psychiatric inpatients: a double-blind, placebo-controlled study. J Clin Psychiatry 53:41–46, 1992

Rodda J, Morgan S, Walker Z: Are cholinesterase inhibitors effective in the management of the behavioral and psychological symptoms of dementia in Alzheimer's disease? A systematic review of randomized, placebo-controlled trials of donepezil, rivastigmine and galantamine. Int Psychogeriatr 21:813–824, 2009

Salerno S, Dimitri L, Talamanca IF: Occupational risk due to violence in a psychiatric ward. J Occup Health 51:349–354, 2009

Salzman C, Jeste DV, Meyer RE, et al: Elderly patients with dementia-related symptoms of severe agitation and aggression: consensus statement on treatment options, clinical trials methodology, and policy. J Clin Psychiatry 69:889–898, 2008

Savard G, Bhanji NH, Dubeau F, et al: Psychiatric aspects of patients with hypothalamic hamartoma and epilepsy. Epileptic Disord 5:229–234, 2003

Schneider LS, Tariot PN, Dagerman KS, et al: Effectiveness of atypical antipsychotic drugs in patients with Alzheimer's disease. N Engl J Med 355:1525–1538, 2006

Shankle WR, Nielson KA, Cotman CW: Low-dose propranolol reduces aggression and agitation resembling that associated with orbitofrontal dysfunction in elderly demented patients. Alzheimer Dis Assoc Disord 9:233–237, 1995

Sheridan M, Henrion R, Robinson L, et al: Precipitants of violence in a psychiatric inpatient setting. Hosp Community Psychiatry 41:776–780, 1990

Siever LJ: Neurobiology of aggression and violence. Am J Psychiatry 165:429–442, 2008

Sommer OH, Aga O, Cvancarova M, et al: Effect of oxcarbazepine in the treatment of agitation and aggression in severe dementia. Dement Geriatr Cogn Disord 27:155–163, 2009

Sorgi PJ, Ratey JJ, Polakoff S: Beta-adrenergic blockers for the control of aggressive behaviors in patients with chronic schizophrenia. Am J Psychiatry 143:775–776, 1986

Stanford MS, Houston RJ, Baldridge RM: Comparison of impulsive and premeditated perpetrators of intimate partner violence. Behav Sci Law 26:709–722, 2008

Stevenson S: Heading off violence with verbal de-escalation. J Psychosoc Nurs Ment Health Serv 29:6–10, 1991

Swanson JW, Holzer CE 3rd, Ganju VK, et al: Violence and psychiatric disorder in the community: evidence from the Epidemiologic Catchment Area surveys. Hosp Community Psychiatry 41:761–770, 1990 [published erratum appears in Hosp Community Psychiatry 42:954–955, 1991]

Swanson J, Swartz M, Estroff S, et al: Psychiatric impairment, social contact, and violent behavior: evidence from a study of outpatient-committed persons with severe mental disorder. Soc Psychiatry Psychiatr Epidemiol 33 (suppl 1):S86–S94, 1998

Stanford MS, Anderson NE, Lake SL, et al: Pharmacologic treatment of impulsive aggression with antiepileptic drugs. Curr Treat Options Neurol 11:383–390, 2009

Swanson JW, Swartz MS, Van Dorn RA, et al: A national study of violent behavior in persons with schizophrenia. Arch Gen Psychiatry 63:490–499, 2006

Swanson JW, Van Dorn RA, Swartz MS, et al: Alternative pathways to violence in persons with schizophrenia: the role of childhood antisocial behavior problems. Law Hum Behav 32:228–240, 2008

Swartz MS, Swanson JW, Hiday VA, et al: Taking the wrong drugs: the role of substance abuse and medication noncompliance in violence among severely mentally ill individuals. Soc Psychiatry Psychiatr Epidemiol 33 (suppl 1):S75–S80, 1998

Tariot PN, Erb R, Podgorski CA, et al: Efficacy and tolerability of carbamazepine for agitation and aggression in dementia. Am J Psychiatry 155:54–61, 1998

Thompson RS, Bonomi AE, Anderson M, et al: Intimate partner violence: prevalence, types, and chronicity in adult women. Am J Prev Med 30:447–457, 2006

Tonkonogy JM, Geller JL: Hypothalamic lesions and intermittent explosive disorder. J Neuropsychiatry Clin Neurosci 4:45–50, 1992

Trautman DE, McCarthy ML, Miller N, et al: Intimate partner violence and emergency department screening: computerized screening versus usual care. Ann Emerg Med 49:526–534, 2007

Treiman DM: Epilepsy and violence: medical and legal issues. Epilepsia 27 (suppl 2):S77–S104, 1986

Uthman OA, Lawoko S, Moradi T: Factors associated with attitudes towards intimate partner violence against women: a comparative analysis of 17 sub-Saharan countries. BMC Int Health Hum Rights 9:14, 2009a

Uthman OA, Moradi T, Lawoko S: The independent contribution of individual-, neighbourhood-, and country-level socioeconomic position on attitudes towards intimate partner violence against women in sub-Saharan Africa: a multilevel model of direct and moderating effects. Soc Sci Med 68:1801–1809, 2009b

Volavka J: The neurobiology of violence: an update. J Neuropsychiatry Clin Neurosci 11:307–314, 1999

Walsh MT, Dinan TG: Selective serotonin reuptake inhibitors and violence: a review of the available evidence. Acta Psychiatr Scand 104:84–91, 2001

Wathen CN, Jamieson E, MacMillan HL, et al: Who is identified by screening for intimate partner violence? McMaster Violence Against Women Research Group. Womens Health Issues 18:423–432, 2008

Whittington R, Shuttleworth S, Hill L: Violence to staff in a general hospital setting. J Adv Nurs 24:326–333, 1996

Wilcock GK, Ballard CG, Cooper JA, et al: Memantine for agitation/aggression and psychosis in moderately severe to severe Alzheimer's disease: a pooled analysis of 3 studies. J Clin Psychiatry 69:341–348, 2008

CHAPTER

8

Depression

Madeline Li, M.D., Ph.D., F.R.C.P.C.

Gary Rodin, M.D., F.R.C.P.C.

MEDICAL AND DEPRESSIVE illnesses are common conditions that frequently coexist in the general population. This association is to be expected both because of coincidence and because the risk of depressive disorders is increased in most medical conditions. This elevated risk is due, in part, to the association of most, or all, serious medical illnesses with a variety of nonspecific risk factors for depression. However, there also has been much speculation about whether specific biological mechanisms may account for the comorbidity of depression with particular medical conditions.

Depression is frequently undiagnosed and untreated in medical and primary care populations, despite its frequency, negative effect on health, and responsiveness to a variety of interventions. This diagnostic and therapeutic neglect may occur for several reasons, including the stigma associated with psychological distress, the difficulty of distinguishing normative from pathological distress, the physical symptom overlap between depression and medical illness, the frequent lack of sufficient training in or comfort of medical caregivers with emotional inquiry, and mistaken beliefs among both medical caregivers and patients about the untreatability of depression that is "understandable." Untreated depression is of concern in medical populations because it is associated with greater somatic symptom burden (Katon et al. 2007) and morbidity and with worse quality of life (Katon 2003) in common medical disorders. Depression is also associated with higher rates of health care utilization, with medical costs up to 50% higher than those attributed to medical illness alone, and with poorer medical treatment compliance, functional capacity, and occupational productivity (Unutzer et al. 2009).

In this chapter we review the prevalence and clinical features of depression in the medically ill; describe screening, diagnostic, and treatment approaches to depressive disorders in medical populations; and consider potential mechanisms to account for the etiology, course, and outcome of depression in specific medical illnesses.

The Continuum of Depression: From Experience to Disorder

The experience of sadness is a normal, expectable response to the multiple adverse effects of a serious medical illness. These effects include changes in bodily appearance and functioning; pain and physical distress; limitations in the capacity to work and to engage in pleasurable activities; a perceived alteration in the anticipated life trajectory; fears of disability and dependency; and alterations in intimate relationships, family life, social relationships, and other activities. Nonpathological sadness and grief lie at the milder end of the continuum of depression in medical populations. In the middle lie adjustment disorders and subthreshold depressions, which are the most prevalent depressive disorders among medically ill patients (Rowe and Rapaport 2006). At the more severe end of the continuum are depressive symptoms that may clearly meet diagnostic

We wish to acknowledge the contributions of the coauthors of an earlier version of this chapter in the first edition (Rodin et al. 2004), which has been an important foundation for the present chapter.

criteria for one of the depressive disorders specified in the *Diagnostic and Statistical Manual of Mental Disorders,* 4th Edition, Text Revision (DSM-IV-TR; American Psychiatric Association 2000). These categorical distinctions have heuristic and communicative value but the boundaries that distinguish them from each other and from nonpathological sadness are somewhat arbitrary and often difficult to determine, particularly in medically ill patients.

The six major categories of depressive disorders specified in DSM-IV-TR are major depressive disorder (MDD), dysthymic disorder, mood disorder due to a [specified] general medical condition, substance-induced mood disorder, adjustment disorder with depressed mood, and depressive disorder not otherwise specified, which includes minor depressive disorder. In this chapter, we emphasize the syndromes of MDD and dysthymic disorder. A categorical diagnosis of MDD is based on the presence of five or more symptoms, which must include a depressed mood or anhedonia for at least 2 weeks, representing a significant change from previous functioning. Neurovegetative symptoms in these criteria include impairment in sleep or appetite, loss of energy, and psychomotor retardation or agitation. Psychological criteria include feelings of worthlessness, hopelessness or excessive guilt, cognitive impairment, and recurrent suicidal ideation (American Psychiatric Association 2000). Dysthymic disorder is characterized by less severe depressive symptoms that have been continuously present for at least 2 years, in contrast to minor depression, in which the symptoms of dysthymic disorder need be present for only 2 weeks. Subthreshold disorders that do not meet criteria for MDD can nevertheless substantially impair quality of life and the capacity to comply with medical treatment. Further research is needed to determine their responsiveness to pharmacological and psychosocial interventions.

To avoid pathologizing the profound but normative distress that may follow the loss of a close relationship, the DSM-IV-TR excludes from the diagnostic criteria for a depressive disorder depressive symptoms that persist for up to 2 months following bereavement. Initial grief reactions and subsequent mourning are common following the onset of a serious or terminal illness and can be regarded as normative and nonpathological but have nevertheless not been excluded from the DSM-IV-TR diagnostic criteria for MDD (Horwitz and Wakefield 2007) (reviewed in detail in Chapter 41, "Palliative Care"). Indeed, it may be argued that the onset, exacerbation, or progression of a serious medical illness may be at least as distressing as the loss of a loved one. The diagnosis of adjustment disorder is based on emotional or behavioral symptoms "in excess of what would be expected" from exposure to an identifiable stressor. However, the operational criteria for this diagnosis, including what constitutes an "excessive" response to the multiple and chronic stressors of medical illness, are not clear. Despite this ambiguity, the heuristic and nonstigmatizing appeal of the category of adjustment disorder cause it to remain one of the most common psychiatric diagnoses in medical patients (Li et al. 2010).

Epidemiology

Depressive disorders are extremely common in the general population, with up to 17% of adults in the United States having had at least one episode of MDD during their lifetime (Kessler et al. 2003), and 2%–4% suffering from a current MDD (Burvill 1995). Medical illness has been consistently shown to be a risk factor for depression. Dysthymic disorder and minor depression are the most common depressive syndromes in medical populations, reported in up to 26% of medical outpatients, a rate several times higher than that in the general population (Rowe and Rapaport 2006). Presumably based on differences in medical disease severity, the prevalence of MDD has been found to increase progressively from community samples (2%–4%), to primary care settings (5%–10%), to medical inpatient settings (6%–14%) (Burvill 1995). Similarly, the risk of a depressive episode in patients in primary care (Barkow et al. 2002) and in the community (Wilhelm et al. 1999) rises with the number of comorbid medical diseases. The reported prevalence of MDD in specific medical conditions, including cancer, diabetes, cardiovascular disease, chronic obstructive pulmonary disease (COPD)/asthma, HIV/AIDS, stroke, epilepsy, multiple sclerosis, Alzheimer's disease, and Parkinson's disease, is listed in Table 8–1.

Etiology

Depressive symptoms and depressive disorders have been found to occur at increased rates in virtually all medical conditions in which they have been studied. There have been claims and hypotheses that specific biological mechanisms cause depression in specific medical conditions, including stroke, Parkinson's disease, type 1 diabetes, and some types of cancer. However, such specificity has not been substantiated in any of these conditions, although each is associated with multiple nonspecific risk factors that may increase the prevalence of depression. In fact, depression in the context of medical illness is a prime example of the biopsychosocial model of disease, with interacting pathophysiological and psychosocial factors contributing to this comorbidity. The final common pathway to depression resulting from the interaction of disease-related, psychological, and social risk and protective factors is shown in Figure 8–1.

TABLE 8–1. Prevalence of major depressive disorder in selected medical illnesses

Medical illness	Prevalence (%)	Reference
Cancer	0–38	Massie 2004
Diabetes	9–26	Musselman et al. 2003
Heart disease	17–27	Rudisch and Nemeroff 2003
COPD/asthma	20–50	Cleland et al. 2007; Van Lieshout et al. 2009
HIV/AIDS	5–20	Cruess et al. 2003
Stroke	14–19	Robinson 2003
Epilepsy	20–55	Kanner 2003
Multiple sclerosis	40–60	Wallin et al. 2006
Alzheimer's disease	30–50	Lee and Lyketsos 2003
Parkinson's disease	4–75	McDonald et al. 2003

Note. COPD=chronic obstructive pulmonary disease.

Potential biological contributors to depression in medical illness include the physical effects of illness and treatment, medications, neurological involvement, genetic vulnerability, and systemic inflammation. In this regard, greater pain and treatment intensity (Kaasa et al. 1993), more advanced disease (Manne et al. 2001), and proximity to death (Butler et al. 2003) have all been shown to increase the risk of depression. Individuals with a genetic vulnerability to depression are also more likely to develop it in the context of medical illness (Levinson 2006) and common genetic vulnerabilities may account for the frequent comorbidity of depression and Alzheimer's disease (Kim et al. 2002), Parkinson's disease (Mossner et al. 2001), and coronary artery disease (Su et al. 2009). Immune-activated systemic inflammation (Dantzer et al. 2008), manifest as cytokine-induced sickness behavior, is a recently proposed common pathophysiological mechanism that may underlie depression in a wide range of medical disorders including cancer (Raison and Miller 2003), cardiovascular disease (Parissis et al. 2007), diabetes (Musselman et al. 2003), Alzheimer's disease (Leonard 2007), stroke (Arbelaez et al. 2007), multiple sclerosis (Wallin et al. 2006), asthma (Van Lieshout et al. 2009), and infectious diseases such as HIV/AIDS (Leserman 2003).

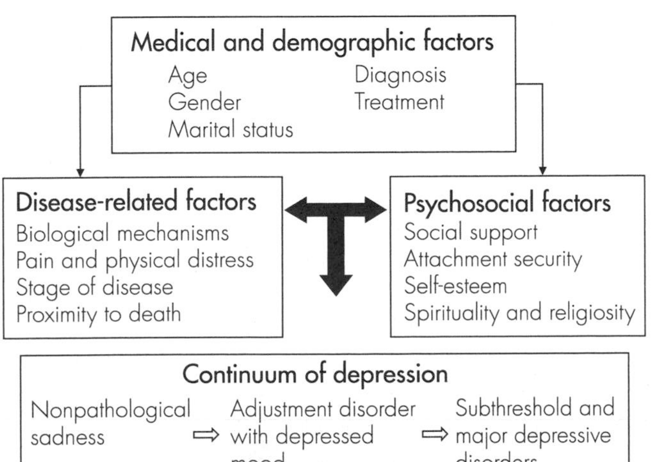

FIGURE 8–1. Pathways to depression.

Psychosocial factors that affect the likelihood of a comorbid depressive disorder in medical illness include the stigma and personal meaning associated with the medical condition, illness-related disability (Talbot et al. 1999), maladaptive coping styles (Wallin et al. 2006), low self-esteem, impaired spiritual well-being (Rodin et al. 2007b), and capacity to express affect (Classen et al. 2008). Low social support (Lewis 2001), including poor communication with medical caregivers (Gurevich et al. 2004), also increases the likelihood of a comorbid depressive disorder. More recent evidence suggests that expectations of support and the capacity for flexible use of social support, captured in the construct of attachment security, may provide protection from the emergence of depressive symptoms in medically ill patients (Rodin et al. 2007b).

Age is inversely related to the severity of depressive symptoms (Cleland et al. 2007; Gottlieb et al. 2004). Postulated explanations for age-related differences in depression severity include greater disruption of the life trajectory and lesser stigma associated with emotional distress in younger patients, a diminishing tendency with more advanced age to experience or communicate distress, and growth in attachment security and spiritual well-being over the life span (Lo et al. 2010). Finally, although depression in the general population has been strongly associated with female gender (Lucht et al. 2003), this gender difference has not been found consistently in depression in medical populations (Cleland et al. 2007; Rodin et al. 2007b; Miller et al. 2010). It may be that the overriding common stressors related to the medical illness obliterate gender-related differences that would otherwise emerge.

Clinical Features and Diagnosis

The diagnosis of depressive disorders in medical populations is fraught with difficulty for a variety of reasons, including the following:

1. Many physical symptoms of medical illness (e.g., fatigue, anorexia, weight loss, insomnia, psychomotor retardation, diminished concentration) resemble those of depression. In addition, a variety of emotional disturbances, such as "emotionalism," pathological crying, apathy, or fatigue, in poststroke patients (Bogousslavsky 2003) or in those with multiple sclerosis (Chwastiak and Ehde 2007), can be mistaken for depression. It may also be difficult to distinguish depression from the apathy associated with hypoactive delirium or dementia, or from the akinesia and masked facies that are the hallmark of Parkinson's disease.
2. Thoughts of death and the desire for death in patients with advanced medical disease have been associated with depression and demoralization in the terminally ill (Breitbart et al. 2000). However, they may also reflect adaptive death acceptance or an attempt at cognitive mastery, rather than depression (Nissim et al. 2009).
3. Physical suffering and disability, in the absence of comorbid depression, may diminish the capacity to experience pleasure in many formerly enjoyable activities. Presence of a depressed mood or withdrawal from social or physical activities that is disproportionate to physical disability increases the likelihood that the loss of pleasure is secondary to depression.
4. In medical populations, depressive symptoms may manifest in atypical or masked forms, including the amplification of somatic symptoms (Katon et al. 2007) and noncompliance with or refusal of medical treatment (DiMatteo et al. 2000). These phenomena may contribute to both the underdiagnosis and the overdiagnosis of MDD in medical populations.
5. The categories of MDD, mood disorder due to a general medical condition, and substance-induced mood disorder may overlap in the context of medical illness. The latter two diagnoses imply that the etiology of the depression is a direct physiological consequence of the specified general medical condition or substance. However, no medical illness or substance has been shown to have a linear causal relationship to depression.

Various approaches have been proposed to diminish the confounding effect of medical symptoms in the diagnosis of MDD. DSM-IV-TR suggests a combined "exclusive" and "etiological" approach, which specifies exclusion of symptoms that are judged by the clinician to be etiologically related to a general medical condition or that are not more frequent in depressed than nondepressed patients with such conditions (Bukberg et al. 1984). This approach is intended to avoid attributing symptoms of physical illness to a depressive syndrome, although the wording in DSM-IV-TR leaves unclear whether the exclusion applies only to the physiological consequences of the medical condition or also extends to psychological reactions to the condition (Koenig et al. 1997). In practice, the exclusive approach is usually applied only to the somatic symptoms of depression, although this does not take into account that depressed medical patients report significantly more physical symptoms than matched nondepressed medical patients (Simon and Von Korff 2006). In any case, the criteria for determining which symptoms are due to a medical illness and which are due to other factors unrelated to the medical illness are unclear.

Another approach to the diagnosis of MDD in the medically ill is "substitutive" (Endicott 1984). In this approach, symptoms that are more likely to be affective in origin—such as irritability, tearfulness, social withdrawal, and feeling punished—are substituted for symptoms that are most likely to be confounded with the effects of medical illness, such as loss of energy, weight loss, and impaired concentration. This substitution eliminates the need to distinguish symptoms of medical illness from those of depression but may underestimate depression prevalence by excluding some somatic symptoms that are core manifestations of more severe forms of depression. Furthermore, the criteria to determine which symptoms should be substituted are not clearly established, and this approach has not been widely adopted.

Evaluating the rates of depression in hospitalized elderly medical patients according to six different diagnostic schemes, Koenig et al. (1997) found no overall advantage of one diagnostic scheme over others. The exclusive/etiological approach identified the most severe persistent depressions, but an inclusive approach was the most sensitive and reliable. In cases in which the diagnosis remains unclear, a trial of treatment may be the most practical means of resolving the question.

Health Outcomes

The World Health Organization (WHO) projects that by the year 2020, depression will be the second leading cause of disability, surpassed only by heart disease (Michaud et al. 2001). Although the impact of depression has often been underestimated, the WHO World Health Survey (Moussavi et al. 2007) found that depression reduces overall health significantly more than do chronic diseases such as angina, arthritis, asthma, or diabetes and that the comorbid state of depression and medical illness worsens health more than any combination of chronic diseases without depression. Comorbid depression is also associated with a significant economic burden, including an almost twofold higher rate of health care utilization and workplace disability (Stein et al. 2006), longer inpatient lengths of stay (Saravay et al. 1996), and at least a twofold increase in emergency room visits (Himelhoch et al. 2004). Comorbid depression is also associated with a threefold risk of noncompliance with medical treatment, thereby contributing to increased morbidity and mortality (DiMatteo et al. 2000). Such noncompliance may include not taking treatments that are prescribed, not following diet or lifestyle recommendations, and not attending medical appointments.

The finding that the comorbidity of depression and medical illness is associated with worse medical outcomes and higher mortality rates has been replicated in a variety of medical conditions. It has been associated with more rapid progression of HIV disease (Leserman 2003) and with increased mortality with cardiovascular disease (van Melle et al. 2004) and in cancer (Onitilo et al. 2006). This increased mortality rate, which persists even after controlling for such factors as smoking, disease severity, and alcohol consumption (Schulz et al. 2000), may be due to several different factors. Biological mechanisms in depression may increase mortality rates in the medically ill via effects on the autonomic nervous system and on related cardiac outcomes. The association of suicide with depression may also increase mortality rates in medical populations, a finding that has been demonstrated in medical conditions, such as cancer (Steel et al. 2007), multiple sclerosis (Stenager et al. 1996), and Huntington's chorea (Almqvist et al. 1999). Depression may be associated with other health risk behaviors—such as cigarette smoking, overeating, physical inactivity, obesity, and excess alcohol consumption—that increase the prevalence of associated medical illness and affect its course adversely.

Screening for and Detection of Depression

Obstacles to Diagnosis in Medical Settings

Depression and other forms of distress are often underdiagnosed and undertreated in medical settings (Fallowfield et al. 2001). In fact, a recent study in the United Kingdom suggests that less than one-half of cases of depression are correctly diagnosed by general practitioners (Mitchell et al. 2009). This is of concern because missing the diagnosis of MDD, or even of a minor depressive disorder, may forgo the opportunity to improve quality of life, decrease the risk of suicide, shorten hospital stay, and improve treatment compliance in the medically ill. There are many explanations for the low rate of detection of clinical depression in medical settings. The structure of medical care, with medical visits often lasting less than 15 minutes, with multiple other clinical concerns that may need to be addressed during each visit, and with the frequent lack of privacy in clinic and hospital settings, may inhibit disclosure or elaboration of symptoms. Furthermore, some clinicians avoid emotional inquiry because they fear that they lack sufficient time or skill to manage emotional reactions. Some patients are reluctant to disclose depressive symptoms because of perceived stigma or anticipated lack of interest of their medical caregivers. However, most patients welcome the opportunity to discuss psychosocial issues that are raised by their health care providers (Rodin et al. 2009). In some cases, both patients and clinicians may have difficulty differentiating the somatic symptoms of depression from those of medical disease. They may also both dismiss clinically significant depression as an "understandable" reaction to the multiple stresses of medical illness, mistakenly assuming that treatment for such reactions is unnecessary or ineffective.

Paradoxically, time-pressured medical clinic visits that preclude adequate assessment of mood can also lead to the overdiagnosis of depression. This may occur due to the misattribution of the symptoms of physical illness to depression and to the employment of low diagnostic thresholds of depression, with a readiness to prescribe antidepressant medications and/or to refer for specialized psychiatric assessment (Boland et al. 1996) because of inadequate resources or training to explore or manage psychological distress (Aragones et al. 2006). The more appropriate utilization of limited specialized psychiatric resources may be facilitated by the use of validated depression screening tools in medical settings.

Screening for Depression: General Considerations

Screening for depression may be particularly helpful in medical settings where routine assessment of mood might otherwise not occur. The ideal screening instrument would be easy to administer and score, acceptable to patients, and, most importantly, accurate. However, the utility of screening for depression depends not only on the measure used but also on whether its results are routinely communicated to medical caregivers and whether such communication leads to timely and effective intervention. Failure to ensure that such a response loop is implemented may account for the failure of distress screening to result in better management of depression or improved outcomes (Palmer and Coyne 2003).

Screening Instruments Commonly Used in Medical Populations

There is no true gold standard for the diagnosis of depression, particularly in the context of medical illness, but clinical interviews have traditionally been used to confirm diagnoses and to establish prevalence rates. Such interviews may be unstructured—with an inclusive or substitutive approach to counting symptoms—or more structured, utilizing diagnostic instruments such as the Structured Clinical Interview for DSM Disorders (SCID; First et al. 1997), the Composite International Diagnostic Interview (CIDI; World Health Organization 1997), the Mini-International Neuropsychiatric Interview (Sheehan et al. 1998), the Present State Examination (PSE; Hall et al. 1999), or the Primary Care Evaluation of Mental Disorders (PRIME-MD; Spitzer et al. 1999).

Depression rating scales can be used to measure depression severity or symptom change over time, but the diagnosis of depression requires a second-stage clinical diagnostic interview with those who score above the cutoff. Numerous psychometric measures have been developed to measure depressive symptoms, with criterion validity and optimal cutoff scores usually established with some form of clinical interview. The cutoff scores selected determine the sensitivity and specificity of the measure, and, therefore, the proportion of false-negative and false-positive cases. Higher cutoffs that avoid false positives may be preferable for research purposes and for determining resource allocation for more severe cases. Lower thresholds may be preferable in well-resourced treatment settings in which a premium is placed on avoiding false negatives and on detecting subthreshold disorders. Table 8–2 lists validation studies of rating scales commonly used to assess and screen for depression in medical populations, including the Center for Epidemiologic Studies Depression Scale (CES-D; Radloff 1977), the Hospital Anxiety and Depression Scale (HADS; Zigmond and Snaith 1983), the Beck Depression Inventory–II (BDI-II; Beck et al. 1996), and the Patient Health Questionnaire–depression module (PHQ-9; Kroenke et al. 2001). A brief discussion of each of these instruments follows.

The CES-D Scale is a 20-item self-report measure of depressive symptoms, in which only 4 of the 20 items are somatic. Originally designed as a measure of depressive distress in nonpsychiatric community samples, the CES-D has also been extensively used in medically ill samples with evidence of good psychometric properties. A cutoff score of 17 was originally recommended to identify clinically significant depression (Radloff 1977), but the low positive predictive value (PPV) of the CES-D suggests that it might be a better measure of general distress than of depression. The reported sensitivity and specificity of various cutoff scores in a variety of medical populations are shown in Table 8–2.

The HADS is a 14-item self-report scale specifically designed for use in the medically ill, with separate 7-item subscales for anxiety and depression. The depression subscale emphasizes anhedonia and does not include somatic items. The HADS is highly acceptable to patients and has been extensively used in the medically ill (Herrmann 1997). It has good concurrent and discriminant validity and acceptable sensitivity to change (Flint and Rifat 1996), but it has not been extensively validated as a screening instrument. There have been conflicting reports regarding its accuracy (Herrmann 1997), and some empirical studies (Chaturvedi et al. 1996; Razavi et al. 1990) have found that the total score (HADS-T) more accurately predicts the presence of MDD or minor depression than does the depressive subscale (HADS-D). The most widely recommended cutoff scores are 8 on the HADS-D (Berard et al. 1998) and 16 on the HADS-T (Chaturvedi et al. 1996).

The BDI-II is the most widely accepted measure of depressive distress. Originally developed as a measure of symptom severity in psychiatric patients, this 21-item self-report scale has been used in numerous studies of depression in the medically ill. Concerns have been raised about its validity in patients with medical illness (because of its preponderance of somatic items) and about the acceptability to patients of its forced-choice format and complex response alternatives (Koenig et al. 1992). However, several studies evaluating the accuracy of the BDI-II as a screening instrument in medically ill samples found it to be an accurate self-report measure of depressive symptoms (Berard et al. 1998; Craven et al. 1987). The cutoff most commonly recommended in the medically ill is 15–16 (Berard et al. 1998).

The PHQ-9 is the nine-item depression module of the PHQ, which is a self-administered version of the PRIME-MD, a freely available diagnostic instrument for common

TABLE 8–2. Validation of depression rating scales in medical illness

Measure	Practical issues/ references	Psychometric properties				
		Validation measure	Cutoff	Sensitivity (%)	Specificity (%)	PPV (%)
CES-D (20 items; self-report)	**Time: 5 minutes Cost: noncopyrighted Translations: multiple**					
Cancer	Hopko et al. 2008	SCID	17	100	79	92
Diabetes	Hermanns et al. 2006	CIDI	23	79	89	54
Heart disease	Koenig 1998	Psychiatric interview	16	73	84	NR
HIV/AIDS	Myer et al. 2008	MINI	NR	79	61	24
Stroke	Shinar et al. 1986	PSE	16	100	73	NR
Epilepsy	J.E. Jones et al. 2005	MINI, SCID	14	96	79	42
Multiple sclerosis	Pandya et al. 2005	Psychiatric interview	16	NR	NR	74
HADS (14 items; self-report)	**Time: 5 minutes Cost: copyrighted Translations: multiple**					
Cancer	Walker et al. 2007	SCID	15	87	85	35
Diabetes	McHale et al. 2008	CIDI	11	64	64	43
Heart disease	Stafford et al. 2007	MINI	8	39	94	72
Stroke	Tang et al. 2004	SCID	4 (HADS-D)	86	78	55
Epilepsy	Phabphal et al. 2007	NR	11	86	91	NR
Parkinson's disease	Mondolo et al. 2006	Ham-D	11	100	95	71
BDI-II (21 items; self-report)	**Time: 10–15 minutes Cost: copyrighted Translations: multiple**					
Cancer	Hopko et al. 2008	SCID	22	92	100	100
Stroke	Aben et al. 2002	SCID	18	80	61	22
Epilepsy	J.E. Jones et al. 2005	MINI, SCID	11	96	78	42
PHQ-9 (9 items; self-report)	**Time: 5 minutes Cost: noncopyrighted Translations: multiple**					
Diabetes	Lamers et al. 2008	MINI	6	96	81	NR
Heart disease	Stafford et al. 2007	MINI	5	82	81	62
HIV/AIDS	Justice et al. 2004	CIDI	10	63	77	42
Stroke	L.S. Williams et al. 2005	SCID	10	91	89	91

Note. All numbers rounded to nearest %. NR=not reported; PPV=positive predictive value; CES-D=Center for Epidemiologic Studies Depression Scale; SCID=Structured Clinical Interview for DSM Disorders (First et al. 1997); CIDI=Composite International Diagnostic Interview (World Health Organization 1977); MINI=Mini-International Neuropsychiatric Interview (Sheehan et al. 1998); PSE=Present State Exam (Hall et al. 1999); HADS=Hospital Anxiety and Depression Scale; HADS-D=Hospital Anxiety and Depression Scale–depressive subscale; Ham-D=Hamilton Rating Scale for Depression (Hamilton 1960); BDI-II=Beck Depression Inventory–II; PHQ-9=Patient Health Questionnaire–depression module.

mental disorders specifically designed for use in primary care settings. The PHQ has been studied in thousands of primary care and medical specialty outpatients in the United States, Europe, and China. Its depression subscale, the PHQ-9, measures each of the nine DSM-IV-TR criteria for a major depressive episode with scores ranging from 0 (not at all) to 3 (nearly every day). When assessed against an independent structured interview performed by mental health professionals, a PHQ-9 cutoff score of 10 or greater had a sensitivity of 88% and a specificity of 88% for the diagnosis of MDD. PHQ-9 scores of 5, 10, 15, and 20 represented mild, moderate, moderately severe, and severe depression, respectively (Spitzer et al. 1999). A recent meta-analysis reported a summary sensitivity of 77% and specificity of 94% with a PPV of 59% in unselected primary care populations and a PPV of 85%–90% in populations at increased risk for depression (Wittkampf et al. 2007).

Single-Item and Very Brief Screening Scales

There has been great interest in single-item screening tests for depression, although recent pooled analyses of such tools in cancer (Mitchell 2007) and in primary care (Mitchell and Coyne 2007) revealed PPVs of only 34% and 38%, respectively. The most widely known single-item scale is the Distress Thermometer, a 0- to 10-point visual analogue scale measuring level of distress in the past week (A.J. Roth et al. 1998). Recommended for distress screening by the National Comprehensive Cancer Network, the Distress Thermometer was found to have 79% sensitivity and 83% specificity but only a 41% PPV for detecting depression in cancer patients (Grassi et al. 2006). Single-item questions such as "Are you depressed?" (Chochinov et al. 1997) demonstrated a sensitivity of 55% and specificity of 74% in detecting MDD in patients on a palliative care ward (Lloyd-Williams et al. 2003) and a sensitivity of 42% and specificity of 86% in cancer patients undergoing radiotherapy (Kawase et al. 2006). The question "Do you often feel sad or depressed?" had a sensitivity of 86%, a specificity of 78%, and a PPV of 82% for depression in stroke patients (Watkins et al. 2001). Pomeroy et al. (2001) demonstrated in elderly medical patients that both the 1-item Mental Health Index (Berwick et al. 1991) and the 4-item Geriatric Depression Scale (Yesavage et al. 1982) were as effective as the 30- or 15-item Geriatric Depression Scales.

Kroenke et al. (2001) evaluated the two-item version of the PHQ (PHQ-2), which was derived from the PHQ-9 module for depression. The PHQ-2 includes the first two items of the PHQ-9: Over the last 2 weeks, how often have you been bothered by 1) little interest or pleasure in doing things and 2) feeling down, depressed, or hopeless? In a sample of 1,619 medical outpatients, the PHQ-2 demonstrated 87% sensitivity and 78% specificity for MDD and 79% sensitivity and 86% specificity for any depressive disorder, validated against the SCID (Lowe et al. 2005). These same two questions were able to identify 99% of cases diagnosed by SCID interview in patients with multiple sclerosis (Mohr et al. 2007).

The lower sensitivity and specificity of single-item or ultrabrief self-report measures of depression may limit their utility, although measures such as the PHQ-2, which focus on the core features of a depressed mood and/or anhedonia, may be most useful. However, the most common shortcoming in the detection of depression is not in the nature of the instrument used or in the questions posed in the clinical setting but rather in the failure to screen for depression using *any* method.

Depression in Specific Medical Conditions

The association of depressive disorders with specific medical diseases is of concern because of their impact on the treatment, course, and outcome of these conditions. There has been particular concern that depression in coronary artery disease (CAD) is associated with increased mortality (see also Chapter 18, "Heart Disease"). There has also been attention to the comorbidity of depression with diabetes mellitus and HIV disease because of its effect on treatment adherence. The occurrence of depression in neurological and other medical conditions has been of interest because of diagnostic complexities related to the clinical features of these conditions. We do not attempt here to review depression in all medical conditions; the reader is referred to the chapters on specific medical conditions in this textbook for more information. In the following subsections we selectively focus on representative medical disorders that have been more extensively investigated in relation to depression.

Coronary Artery Disease

MDD (May et al. 2009; Surtees et al. 2008), and even less severe symptoms of depression (Wulsin 2004), have been associated with a significantly increased relative risk for cardiac complications in patients with coronary artery disease. There has also been speculation that a specific symptom cluster within the MDD profile may account for the association between depression and coronary events. For example, the cluster of vital exhaustion, which includes excessive fatigue, low energy, feelings of demoralization, and irritability, has been observed to predict recurrent coronary events, including myocardial infarction, following percutaneous transluminal coronary angioplasty (Mendes de Leon et al. 1996). However, it remains to be established whether other depressive symptoms, such as anhedonia, psychomotor retardation, and diminished attention and concentration are also associated with CAD disease severity or with prolonged disability in CAD patients.

Depressive symptoms may increase cardiac risk through their impact on the motivation to initiate and sustain heart-healthy lifestyle changes, such as smoking cessation, modification of diet, and exercise programs. CAD patients who are depressed may also have a greater sympathetic and neuroendocrine response to stress, as well as decreased heart rate variability and baroreflex sensitivity, and higher resting heart rate (Huffman et al. 2006; Parissis et al. 2007). These sympathoexcitatory states lower the threshold for hypertension and progression of the atherosclerotic process and for clinically significant cardiac events. Such autonomic effects may partly account for the frequent association between depression and increased mortality (van Melle et al. 2004), although Huffman et al. (2006) suggested that recent improvements in cardiac outcomes may account for the failure to confirm this association in more recent studies.

The American College of Cardiology regards depression as a secondary risk factor for CAD, because of its independent association with CAD; it does not meet their criteria for a Category I risk factor, which would require evidence that a decrease in symptoms of depression leads to a decrease in morbidity or mortality among patients with CAD (Pearson and Fuster 1996). Selective serotonin reuptake inhibitors (SSRIs) have beneficial pleiotropic effects, such as reduction of platelet activity (Serebruany et al. 2003), and improvement in heart rate variability (Yeragani et al. 2002), and have demonstrated effectiveness in treating MDD in CAD (Lesperance et al. 2007). However, randomized trials of antidepressant treatment, such as the Sertraline AntiDepressant Heart Attack Randomized Trial (SADHART; Glassman et al. 2002), and the Myocardial INfarction and Depression—Intervention Trial (MIND-IT; van den Brink et al. 2002) failed to demonstrate a reduction in risk for cardiac events. Similarly, no beneficial effects on cardiac outcomes were found in studies of psychotherapeutic interventions such as the Montreal Heart Attack Readjustment Trial (MHART; Frasure-Smith 1995) and the Enhancing Recovery in Coronary Heart Disease Patients (ENRICHD; Berkman et al. 2003) trials. More recently, a study of enhanced depression treatment in patients with acute coronary syndrome demonstrated a reduction in major adverse cardiac events in intervention patients compared with usual-care patients (Davidson et al. 2010). Unique aspects of this study were a flexible treatment model in which patients could choose problem-solving therapy and/or antidepressants and selection for persistent (>3 months) depression. A better understanding of the temporal and mechanistic relationships between depression and CAD will be crucial for the design of future trials in order to clarify potential medical effects of antidepressant treatment (Dickens et al. 2007). (See also Chapter 18, "Heart Disease.")

Cancer

Prevalence rates for MDD in cancer have varied widely in the literature depending on the conceptualization of depression and on the diagnostic scheme employed, with reported rates ranging from 0% to 38% (Massie 2004). These prevalence rates also vary with disease severity, with consistently higher rates found in patients with more advanced disease, in hospitalized samples, and in patients with lower performance status. There has long been the speculation that pancreatic cancer has a specific association with depression and that depression often precedes the cancer diagnosis. More recently, however, it has been suggested that this association may have been overestimated and that depressive symptoms in this context are closely linked to pain and other physical symptoms (Makrilia et al. 2009). Certain chemotherapeutic agents used to treat cancer, including the cytokines (e.g., interleukin-2, interferon-alpha), corticosteroids (e.g., prednisone, dexamethasone), and *Vinca* alkaloids (e.g., vincristine, vinblastine), are also associated with higher rates of depression (Capuron et al. 2001).

Depression in cancer is associated with many adverse health outcomes. Several studies have suggested that it is an independent predictor of mortality (Lazure et al. 2009; Lloyd-Williams et al. 2009), although others have failed to find such an association (Akechi et al. 2009; Phillips et al. 2008). Other reported adverse sequelae include decreased compliance with medical treatment, increased length of hospital stays, impaired quality of life, and reduced capacity to cope with pain and other physical symptoms (Pelletier et al. 2002; Pirl and Roth 1999). The emergence of MDD has also been associated with significantly higher rates of treatment discontinuation in patients with malignant melanoma receiving interferon-alpha (Musselman et al. 2001) and with a heightened desire for hastened death in hospitalized cancer patients (J.M. Jones et al. 2003) and outpatients with metastatic cancer (Rodin et al. 2007c).

Evidence that treatment of depression in cancer improves medical outcomes is limited. In a randomized controlled trial of a 6-month course of fluoxetine versus placebo in early-stage breast cancer patients undergoing adjuvant therapy, Navari et al. (2008) reported that fluoxetine reduced depressive symptoms, improved quality of life, and increased the percentage of patients who successfully completed adjuvant treatment. Studies have yet to be published on recurrence or survival rates associated with treatment of MDD. Although the question of whether psychotherapy can improve survival in cancer has been a hotly debated one (Coyne et al. 2009; Kraemer et al. 2009), the preponderance of the evidence demonstrates that the psychosocial interventions that are effective in reducing depressive symptoms do not confer a survival benefit in cancer (Kissane 2009). (See also Chapter 23, "Oncology.")

Type 1 Diabetes

Type 1 diabetes mellitus is a chronic medical condition associated with considerable treatment demands, including multiple daily tests of serum glucose levels and injections of insulin, and adherence to a restrictive diet. Individuals with diabetes must also live with the risk of multiple medical complications, including blindness, renal failure, amputations, neuropathy, and cardiovascular disease. The burden of this disease and its frequent medical comorbidity would be expected to increase the risk for depression although it also has been suggested that the metabolic impairment in type 1 diabetes mellitus may contribute to mood disturbances via neurobiological mechanisms (Musselman et al. 2003).

Depression in individuals with diabetes mellitus is an important risk factor because it is associated with poorer adherence to the diabetic dietary and medication regimen and with poorer quality of life (Van Tilburg et al. 2001). Poor glycemic control has been associated with MDD in some studies (Lustman et al. 2000a), although this finding has not been consistently reported (A.M. Jacobson et al. 1990). However, depression has been associated with an increased risk of diabetes-related medical complications, including sexual dysfunction, retinopathy, nephropathy, heart disease, and stroke (de Groot et al. 2001), and with increased mortality (Milano and Singer 2007). Because of the reciprocal relationship between depression and metabolic control, attention to both mood disturbances and measures to enhance diabetes management is necessary to prevent or delay the progression of such complications (see also Chapter 22, "Endocrine and Metabolic Disorders").

Neurological Disease

The relation between neurological disorders and depression has been of particular interest both because of the frequent comorbidity of these conditions and because understanding the interface between depression and disorders of the central nervous system (CNS) may help to clarify the neuroanatomic pathways involved in depression. Sheline (2003) noted that the sites of damage in neurological disorders associated with late life depression, including the frontal cortex, hippocampus, thalamus, amygdala, and basal ganglia, overlap with those implicated in early onset recurrent MDD. In particular, the limbic-cortical-striatal-pallidal-thalamic tract, which is intimately involved in emotional regulation, has been associated with structural brain abnormalities, particularly volume loss, in computed tomography (CT) and magnetic resonance imaging (MRI) studies of patients with primary unipolar depression. Mechanisms that have been postulated to account for this volume loss in early onset recurrent depression include chronic stress-induced hypercortisolemic neurotoxicity, inhibition of neurogenesis, decreased brain-derived growth factor, and loss of neuroplasticity (Benedetti et al. 2006). However, no specific neurobiological lesions or disorders have yet been shown to be associated with elevated rates of depression, after controlling for the effects of disability and disease severity.

Parkinson's Disease

Depressive symptoms are common in patients with Parkinson's disease; indeed, melancholia was included in the original description of the condition by James Parkinson in 1817. Such depression may be caused by the psychosocial stress of this progressive incurable and disabling disorder and its implications for the future of the affected individual. However, neurobiological factors also may play an etiological role. For example, neurodegeneration of subcortical nuclei and disturbances in the circuit connecting the basal ganglia to the thalamus and frontal cortex have been shown to correlate with clinical symptoms of depression in patients with Parkinson's disease (McDonald et al. 2003). It also has been postulated that degeneration of dopamine-, serotonin-, and norepinephrine-containing neurons in the ventral tegmental area and in the substantia nigra, which project to mesocortical, mesolimbic, and striatal areas, may contribute to depression in these patients (McDonald et al. 2003).

The assessment of depression in patients with Parkinson's disease is particularly challenging. It may be difficult to differentiate depressive symptoms, such as psychomotor retardation, affective restriction, fatigue, and disturbances in sleep and concentration, from the core features of Parkinson's disease. Furthermore, the akinesia and restricted facial expression that are characteristic of Parkinson's disease, as well as the apathy and cognitive impairment that may accompany comorbid dementia, may all be mistaken for symptoms of depression. However, evidence indicates that screening instruments, such as the BDI-II, are still useful for assessment of depression in Parkinson's disease, despite the overlap of somatic items with symptoms of Parkinson's (Leentjens et al. 2000). Depressive disorders in patients with Parkinson's disease have been associated with increased impairment of fine motor performance, decrements in cognitive function, and reduced perceived quality of life (McDonald et al. 2003). In fact, in a randomized multisite treatment study, depressive symptoms were the single most important determinant of patient quality-of-life ratings, exceeding the effects of both disease severity and medication (Global Parkinson's Disease Survey Steering Committee 2002).

Stroke

Strokes are the third leading cause of mortality and the most common serious neurological disorder, accounting for 50% of all acute hospitalizations for neurological disease (Robinson 2003). Depression adversely affects functional rehabilitation and cognitive functioning in the poststroke period (Tharwani et al. 2007) and may be associated with a heightened risk of mortality after 1 year (House et al. 2001) and 10 years (Morris et al. 1993), even after controlling for medical and other background variables.

It has been suggested that early poststroke depression is associated with lesions in the left anterior and left basal ganglia regions (Robinson 2003) and that chronic poststroke depression is associated with lesions in the subcortical white matter, thalamus, basal ganglia, and brain stem (Bogousslavsky 2003). However, meta analysis has failed to show any association between poststroke depression and left anterior or left hemisphere lesions (Carson et al. 2000). More recently nonlocalized central nervous system inflammation, resulting in platelet and adrenocortical hyperreactivity, have been proposed to explain the association between depression and stroke (Arbelaez et al. 2007).

Tricyclic antidepressants (TCAs) such as nortriptyline and SSRIs such as citalopram are effective in treating poststroke depression (Robinson et al. 2000) and some evidence suggests that this may also result in a reduction in associated cognitive impairment (Kimura et al. 2000). The evidence has been mixed on whether prophylactic treatment with SSRIs can prevent the emergence of depression or other morbidity in stroke patients. Six months of prophylactic treatment with the SSRI sertraline was not found to prevent this complication (Almeida et al. 2006), and two of three randomized controlled antidepressant trials (Narushima et al. 2002; Rasmussen et al. 2003) found that cardiovascular morbidity and mortality may be reduced in stroke patients who receive antidepressant medication, particularly SSRIs.

Dementing Disorders

Depression is one of the most common neuropsychiatric, noncognitive symptoms of Alzheimer's dementia (Lee and Lyketsos 2003). The prevalence of MDD ranges from 20% to 32% in Alzheimer's dementia (Lyketsos et al. 2002; Migliorelli et al. 1995) with minor depression reported to occur in an additional 25% (Migliorelli et al. 1995). However, symptoms of Alzheimer's dementia, such as emotional lability, may be easily mistaken for depression, and other symptoms, such as apathy, may arise additively from both conditions. In that regard, apathy was found in 27% of patients with Alzheimer's dementia alone and in 56% of those with comorbid MDD (Lyketsos et al. 2001). The diagnosis of depression is often difficult to make, however, in cognitively impaired patients because of the associated impairments in communication and insight (Lee and Lyketsos 2003).

In some circumstances, depressive symptoms have been associated with an increased risk for the development of mild cognitive impairment (Barnes et al. 2006). In particular, both late-onset depression and depression associated with reversible cognitive impairment (i.e., pseudodementia) have been shown to be highly correlated with the eventual diagnosis of Alzheimer's dementia (Alexopoulos et al. 1993). It has been postulated that noradrenergic neuronal loss in the locus coeruleus and serotonergic cell loss in the dorsal raphe nucleus in Alzheimer's dementia may contribute to these high rates of reported antecedent depression (Forstl et al. 1992). However, the findings regarding the treatment of depression in Alzheimer's dementia have been equivocal. Some studies have found antidepressants to be efficacious in the treatment of depression in this population, whereas others have reported minimal treatment effects (Lee and Lyketsos 2003). Further research is needed, given that depression in Alzheimer's dementia is associated with more adverse outcomes, such as earlier nursing home placement, diminished activities of daily living, more rapid cognitive decline, and increased mortality (Kopetz et al. 2000; Lyketsos et al. 1997).

Epilepsy

Depression is the most common psychiatric condition found in patients with epilepsy, with prevalence rates linked to the adequacy of seizure control. MDD has been found in 20%–55% of those with poorly controlled seizures but in only 3%–9% of those whose seizures are well controlled (Kanner 2003). The relation between depression and epilepsy appears to be bidirectional. Depression may be caused by a seizure disorder, particularly with complex partial seizures (Kanner 2003). Conversely, monoamine depletion, which may occur with depression, may contribute to seizure activity (Jobe et al. 1999). The interictal period is a time of increased risk for depression with temporal lobe epilepsy (Quiske et al. 2000), and abnormalities in 5-hydroxytryptamine (5-HT; serotonin) receptor binding have been identified outside of the epileptogenic zone (Savic et al. 2004). A history of depression was found to be 17 times more common in patients with complex partial seizures than in control subjects (Forsgren and Nystrom 1990). Although antidepressants may lower the seizure threshold, this risk is small and more common with TCAs than with SSRIs or venlafaxine (Kanner 2003). Bupropion, maprotiline, and amoxapine are the antidepressants most likely to trigger seizures and should be avoided in this population (Pisani et al. 2002).

Other Neurological Disorders

The lifetime risk for depression in patients with multiple sclerosis ranges from 40% to 60% (Beal et al. 2007; Wallin et al. 2006). Some evidence indicates that depressed patients with multiple sclerosis are more likely than comparable nondepressed patients to have white matter demyelinating plaques involving the arcuate fasciculus (Pujol et al. 1997). Interferon-beta-1b, used to treat multiple sclerosis, is associated with depression in up to 40% of patients with that condition (Mohr et al. 1996). Increased expression of the inflammatory cytokine interferon-gamma is related to depression severity in multiple sclerosis patients, with levels decreasing following psychotherapy or pharmacotherapy (Mohr et al. 2001). Huntington's disease, an autosomal dominant disorder affecting the basal ganglia and characterized by involuntary movements and cognitive impairment, has been associated with MDD in up to 32% and with bipolar disorder in 9% of patients (Folstein et al. 1983). These and other neurological disorders are discussed more fully in Chapters 6 ("Dementia") and 32 ("Neurology and Neurosurgery").

Depression Caused by Medications

A broad range of prescription medications have been purported to be etiologically linked to depression (Sadock et al. 2007). These include many which are standard of care in the treatment of medical illnesses (e.g., L-dopa in Parkinson's disease, calcium channel blockers in hypertension, analgesics and nonsteroidal anti-inflammatory drugs [NSAIDs] in arthritis, phenobarbital in epilepsy). The association of these medications with depression has largely been based on case reports, with relatively few empirical studies, and those conducted have been hampered by methodological and conceptual problems. Some reports in the literature have been uncritical, either misinterpreting drug-induced symptoms as indicative of depression (e.g., weakness, sedation, bradykinesia, fatigue, anorexia, insomnia) or misattributing preexisting depression to the drug. Consequently, controversy surrounds both the claims that specific drugs cause depression (e.g., beta-blockers) and the attempts to quantify the magnitude of risk (e.g., isotretinoin). In their review of the literature on drug-induced depression, Patten and Barbui (2004) concluded that no medications directly cause the typical MDD syndrome, although some may cause substance-induced alterations in mood. Valid evidence linking the drug to atypical depressive syndromes was found only for corticosteroids, interferon-alpha, interleukin-2, gonadotropin-releasing hormone agonists, mefloquine, progestin-releasing implanted contraceptives, and propranolol. Most of these drugs and their psychiatric side effects are discussed in other chapters of this textbook.

Treatment

Several recent studies have reported that both pharmacological and psychotherapeutic interventions are effective for the treatment of depression associated with medical disorders such as type 1 diabetes mellitus (Musselman et al. 2003), CAD (Lesperance et al. 2007), chronic obstructive pulmonary disease (I. Wilson 2006), cancer (Rodin et al. 2007a), HIV infection and AIDS (Olatunji et al. 2006), renal disease (Tossani et al. 2005), stroke (Chen et al. 2006), multiple sclerosis (Wallin et al. 2006), Alzheimer's disease (Thompson et al. 2007), and Parkinson's disease (Lagopoulos et al. 2005). However, despite the evidence for the effectiveness of treatment for depression in medical populations, it has been estimated that more than 60% of primary care patients with depression do not receive adequate care for this condition (Kessler 2003).

Psychopharmacological Management of Depression

SSRIs, heterocyclic antidepressants and TCAs, novel antidepressants, and psychostimulants have been evaluated in the treatment of depression comorbid with medical illness. All antidepressants are discussed more fully in Chapter 38 ("Psychopharmacology"); we summarize some key points here.

Selective Serotonin Reuptake Inhibitors

SSRIs are generally regarded as first-line pharmacological treatment in the management of depression in the medically ill because of their tolerability and relative safety. Randomized controlled trials have shown various SSRIs to be effective and safe in patients with cardiac disease (Glassman et al. 2002), stroke (Wiart et al. 2000), cancer (Pezzella et al. 2001), HIV infection (Rabkin et al. 1999), Alzheimer's disease (Lyketsos et al. 2000), multiple sclerosis (Mohr et al. 2001), and diabetes (Lustman et al. 2000b). SSRIs have been regarded generally as safer and less toxic than TCAs, although significant side effects still may occur with these medications, particularly in the medically ill (Richard et al. 1999). All SSRIs can cause nausea, headache, sexual dysfunction, and tremor. Other frequent side effects include nervousness, insomnia, sedation, diarrhea, constipation, and dry mouth. Rare but potentially serious side effects of

SSRIs include the syndrome of inappropriate antidiuretic hormone secretion and platelet dysfunction leading to bleeding (van Walraven et al. 2001). Some reports indicate that SSRIs may worsen motor symptoms in some patients with Parkinson's disease (Richard et al. 1999).

Drug interactions or hepatic disease may affect SSRI metabolism and excretion and alter antidepressant pharmacokinetics (Hiemke and Hartter 2000). A reduced initial dose with slow titration of the shorter-half-life SSRIs is recommended for patients with hepatic disease because the metabolism of SSRIs is decreased by significant hepatic disease (Joffe et al. 1998). Fluvoxamine should be avoided because of its propensity for drug interactions. Paroxetine is a strong inhibitor of cytochrome P450 (CYP) 2D6, which has been found to decrease levels of the active metabolite of tamoxifen frequently used in breast cancer (Jin et al. 2005). Sertraline and citalopram appear to present the lowest risk for drug interactions. Drug interactions are reviewed in detail in Chapter 38 ("Psychopharmacology") as well as in the chapters in Part III (Specialties and Subspecialties) of this volume.

Novel Antidepressants

Novel antidepressants include venlafaxine, duloxetine, bupropion, mirtazapine, nefazodone, and moclobemide (not available in the United States). Venlafaxine, duloxetine, bupropion, and mirtazapine, in particular, have become increasingly popular as alternatives to SSRIs in the medically ill, although there is little empirical evidence supporting their specific advantages in this population. Moclobemide was shown to be efficacious in reducing depressive symptoms in patients with Alzheimer's disease (M. Roth et al. 1996). A number of open trials point to the effectiveness of other novel antidepressants in patients with stroke (venlafaxine) (Dahmen et al. 1999), cancer (mirtazapine) (Theobald et al. 2002), and HIV infection (nefazodone) (Elliott et al. 1999). It has been suggested that greater depression remission rates may be achieved with the serotonin–norepinephrine reuptake inhibitors (SNRIs) venlafaxine and duloxetine, than with SSRIs (Smith et al. 2002), although this view is controversial. Similar to the SSRIs, venlafaxine is effective for hot flashes in breast cancer (Loprinzi et al. 2000) and both venlafaxine and duloxetine are effective for the treatment of neuropathic pain (Jann and Slade 2007). The main adverse effects of SNRIs are nausea and hypertension, particularly with high doses of venlafaxine, and elevation of serum transaminases and bilirubin with duloxetine. These side effects may limit their use in patients with hepatic or renal insufficiency.

Mirtazapine increases norepinephrine and serotonin concentrations through blockade of inhibitory receptors but does not appear to cause the nausea, insomnia, anxiety, or sexual dysfunction associated with the SSRIs (de Boer 1996). As a result of its serotonin$_3$ receptor–blocking antiemetic effects, mirtazapine may be useful in treating medically ill patients who are experiencing nausea. It may also rapidly improve insomnia and anorexia, which are common in depressed medically ill patients. The most problematic side effects of mirtazapine are sedation and weight gain, although the latter effect may be desirable in some cachectic patients. Mirtazapine has minimal drug interactions (de Boer 1996).

Bupropion is a norepinephrine and dopamine modulator that has not been associated with sedation, weight gain, sexual dysfunction, or cardiotoxicity (Golden et al. 1998). It may be particularly useful in treating patients with prominent neurovegetative symptoms, such as fatigue (Raison et al. 2005). Side effects can include agitation, insomnia, and (at higher dosages) seizures. Because of the latter concern, single doses greater than 150 mg and daily dosages greater than 300 mg should be avoided in patients with brain tumors or a history of seizures (Golden et al. 1998).

Tricyclic Antidepressants

TCAs have been shown to be efficacious in poststroke depression, cancer, HIV infection, Parkinson's disease, Alzheimer's disease, multiple sclerosis, diabetes, and renal failure (Gill and Dansky 2003). They have also proven to be effective as analgesics in the treatment of chronic pain syndromes, including pain related to cancer (reviewed in Magni et al. 1987). Because of their analgesic and sedating effects, TCAs may be particularly useful in depressed patients with significant pain and/or insomnia.

TCAs are variably noradrenergic and/or serotonergic. Their side effects are related to their central and peripheral anticholinergic effects, their central antihistaminic properties, and their effects on cardiac conduction and on the peripheral autonomic nervous system. TCAs should be avoided in patients with cardiac disease in whom they may cause hypotension and arrhythmias (Glassman et al. 1993). TCAs should also be used with caution in patients with diabetes because of their anticholinergic, orthostatic, and other adverse cardiovascular effects (Carney 1998). Anticholinergic side effects of TCAs may also exacerbate cognitive impairment and cause delirium in patients with CNS disorders, especially dementia (Reynolds 1992). TCAs that are more anticholinergic are generally not recommended for the treatment of depression in immunocompromised patients, such as those with HIV or AIDS, because these medications promote candidiasis or thrush infections (Rabkin et al. 1994). TCAs also may not be suitable for patients who are at increased risk for bone fractures or who have skeletal weakness, because the side effect of orthostatic hypotension increases the likelihood of falls (Shuster et al. 1992). TCAs have been associated with seizures, but usually at high plasma levels such as may occur with an overdose (Preskorn and Fast 1992).

Up to one-third of medical patients are unable to tolerate TCAs because of side effects (Benton et al. 2007), and these drugs can be lethal in overdose. For insomnia or pain, doses of TCAs lower than those required for an antidepressant effect may be effective. Among the TCAs, the secondary amines, such as nortriptyline and desipramine, are better tolerated by the medically ill. In addition, nortriptyline has reliable serum levels and a defined therapeutic window that may guide clinical management, particularly in patients with liver disease or malabsorption (Potter et al. 1998).

Psychostimulants

Methylphenidate has been reported to alleviate depressive symptoms in a range of medical conditions, including stroke (Grade et al. 1998), HIV disease (Fernandez et al. 1995), and cancer (Grade et al. 1998), although its efficacy for this purpose has not yet been adequately demonstrated in randomized controlled trials. Psychostimulants are generally well tolerated and at relatively low doses can serve as adjuvant analgesics (Bruera et al. 1987). They may elevate mood rapidly, increase appetite, diminish fatigue, improve attention and concentration, and reduce sedation caused by opiates or other drugs (Orr and Taylor 2007). Many consider psychostimulants to be the antidepressants of choice in the palliative care setting because of their rapid onset of action (K. Wilson et al. 2000). Side effects are typically mild and dose-related and include agitation, nausea, and insomnia. Rarely, psychotic symptoms or tachycardia and hypertension may occur (Masand et al. 1991). Methylphenidate is typically given in divided doses (2.5–10.0 mg) in the morning and afternoon. Modafinil, a newer stimulant not associated with tolerance or dependence, is increasing in use as evidence of its effectiveness is accumulating (Ballon and Feifel 2006).

Electroconvulsive Therapy

Electroconvulsive therapy (ECT) is sometimes used in the medically ill as an alternative to antidepressants in the treatment of severe or refractory depression (Beale et al. 1997). It has been shown to be an effective treatment of depression in Parkinson's disease and also may improve the symptoms of the Parkinson's disease itself (Poewe and Seppi 2001). It has also been shown to improve poststroke depression and depression associated with multiple sclerosis, endocrine disorders, and renal failure (Krystal and Coffey 1997). ECT has been associated with improvements in cognition and mood in patients with dementia (Rao and Lyketsos 2000) and is considered safe for epilepsy patients with severe or refractory depression (Lambert and Robertson 1999). It should be considered early in the course of psychotic depression and for depression associated with severe suicidal ideation or failure to maintain adequate nutritional status. ECT and its risks are reviewed in detail in Chapter 40 ("Electroconvulsive Therapy").

Psychotherapeutic Treatment

The relationship with the primary medical caregiver may be the most important psychotherapeutic tool to prevent or treat depression for many patients with a serious medical illness. In addition, specific psychological therapies may alleviate or prevent depression, without the risk of physical side effects or drug interactions, and may help to modify health behaviors that adversely affect disease outcomes. The indication to refer to a mental health professional for psychotherapy will depend on the severity of the depression and on the skill, interest, and availability of primary care practitioners. The specific psychotherapeutic intervention selected should also take into account the available support network and the patient's capacity to learn new coping strategies and/or to engage in a process that may involve introspection and the expression of feelings. Unique features of psychotherapy in the medically ill are the importance of collaborative relationships between the therapist and the medical caregivers, the likelihood of frequent disruptions in treatment due to complications of the disease, and the need for flexible treatment goals that accommodate shifts in the patient's physical well-being and capacity to participate. In more advanced disease, issues related to hope, existential well-being, and advance care planning may be prominent (Rodin et al. 2009; Vamos 2006).

Specific psychotherapeutic approaches that may alleviate depression in medical populations include cognitive-behavioral therapy (CBT), interpersonal therapy, and supportive-expressive therapy delivered on an individual or a group basis. Peer support, self-help, and cognitive behavioral groups (e.g., psychoeducation, guided imagery/relaxation) also may protect patients from depression by diminishing stigma and feelings of isolation and by promoting self-efficacy and a sense of mastery. A recent Cochrane review of psychotherapy for depression among incurable cancer patients concluded that psychotherapy is effective in decreasing depressive symptoms, although no studies were identified that focused on patients with MDD (Akechi et al. 2008).

There is limited evidence that psychological interventions either reduce or prevent the emergence of depressive symptoms in patients with cancer (C.M. Jacobson et al. 2008), cardiovascular disease (Rivelli and Jiang 2007), diabetes (Musselman et al. 2003), HIV/AIDS (Olatunji et al. 2006), and multiple sclerosis (Wallin et al. 2006). Evidence for the effectiveness of psychological therapies in stroke, heart failure or dialysis is also lacking. A randomized trial of CBT for poststroke depression found no evidence of benefit (Lincoln and Flannaghan 2003), and Cochrane reviews failed to identify any randomized controlled trials of psychological interventions for depression in either heart failure (Lane et al. 2005) or dialysis patients (Rabindranath et al. 2005).

The vast majority of research on psychosocial interventions for depression in medical illness has been conducted in cancer settings. Numerous systematic reviews and meta-analyses of psychosocial interventions in cancer have found treatment effects for depressive symptoms in 22%–83% of randomized controlled trials (Jacobsen 2006; Newell et al. 2002; S. Williams and Dale 2006), and two systematic reviews of psychosocial interventions for categorical diagnoses of MDD demonstrated a treatment effect in 50% of randomized controlled trials (Rodin et al. 2007a; S. Williams and Dale 2006). Based on a meta-analysis of 20 trials, Sheard and Maguire (1999) concluded that psychological interventions have no clinical effect in preventing depression in cancer. However, Kissane et al. (2007) published the first randomized controlled trial demonstrating that supportive-expressive group therapy was effective in preventing the emergence of MDD in women with metastatic breast cancer.

In other medical illnesses, Barrett et al. (2001) found that paroxetine and a problem-solving approach to support active coping strategies were equally effective for the treatment of minor depression or dysthymic disorder in a primary care sample but were no more effective than watchful waiting for the treatment of minor depression. Teri et al. (1997) found that patients with Alzheimer's disease and depressive symptoms showed significant improvement in depressive symptoms following a behavioral intervention for patient–caregiver dyads focused on either pleasant events or caregiver problem solving. Lustman et al. (1998) showed in patients with type 2 diabetes that an intervention that included CBT and diabetes education produced a depression remission rate three times higher than that in a control condition and was associated with a significant improvement in glycosylated hemoglobin 6 months after the end of treatment.

There is growing evidence in medical and nonmedical populations that combined psychotherapy and pharmacotherapy may be more effective than either modality alone. A multicomponent randomized controlled trial in patients with a recent myocardial infarction examined the effects of treatment with CBT plus group therapy when feasible, supplemented with SSRIs in patients who had elevated and/or persistent depressive symptoms. Results revealed improvement in the treatment group that was significantly greater than that in the usual-care group (Berkman et al. 2003). Kelly et al. (1993) found that both cognitive-behavioral and support group brief therapies equally reduced depressive symptoms in depressed HIV-infected individuals, while Markowitz et al. (1998) found that depressed HIV-positive patients had greater improvement in depressive symptoms with interpersonal therapy or supportive psychotherapy plus imipramine than did subjects who received supportive therapy or CBT alone.

These studies of psychotherapeutic interventions to treat depression in a variety of medical populations indicate some degree of effectiveness, which is often improved when combined with antidepressant medication. Numerous other nonspecific psychotherapeutic and educational interventions also may be effective in reducing depressive symptoms and in protecting individuals from their emergence. The full range of psychosocial interventions designed to improve adjustment in medical populations is discussed at more length in Chapter 39 ("Psychotherapy") and in other chapters of this textbook.

Conclusion

Clinical depression, particularly MDD and dysthymic disorder, is common in the medically ill and is associated with impaired quality of life, decreased compliance with medical treatment, and increased medical morbidity and mortality. The elevated prevalence of depression in the medically ill is most often the result of multiple nonspecific risk factors, although there is continued speculation that specific biological mechanisms operate in certain medical conditions. The diagnosis of depressive disorders in medical patients is complicated by the frequent overlap between symptoms of depression and those of medical illness. This overlap may contribute to underdiagnosis, when symptoms of depression are assumed to be features of the medical condition, or to overdiagnosis, when symptoms of a medical illness are attributed to a depressed mood. However, the neglect of simple inquiry about the symptoms of depression may be the most common reason that the diagnosis of depression is overlooked in a medical population. Screening tests may be useful for drawing the attention of clinicians to these symptoms and identifying patients in medical clinics who are most likely to have depressive disorders.

Psychopharmacological and psychotherapeutic approaches are both effective in the treatment of depressive disorders in the medically ill and are often even more effective when used together. Medical patients may be more sensitive to the side effects of pharmacological treatments, and careful attention must be paid to the dosage, to the potential for drug–drug interactions, and to impairment in hepatic or renal function, which can affect drug metabolism.

References

Aben I, Verhey F, Lousberg R, et al: Validity of the Beck Depression Inventory, Hospital Anxiety and Depression Scale, SCL-90, and Hamilton Depression Rating Scale as screening instruments for depression in stroke patients. Psychosomatics 43:386–393, 2002

Akechi T, Okuyama T, Onishi J, et al: Psychotherapy for depression among incurable cancer patients. Cochrane Database Syst Rev (2):CD005537, 2008

Akechi T, Okamura H, Okuyama T, et al: Psychosocial factors and survival after diagnosis of inoperable non-small-cell lung cancer. Psychooncology 18:23–29, 2009

Alexopoulos GS, Meyers BS, Young RC, et al: The course of geriatric depression with "reversible dementia": a controlled study. Am J Psychiatry 150:1693–1699, 1993

Almeida, OP, Waterreus A, Hankey GJ: Preventing depression after stroke: results from a randomized placebo-controlled trial. J Clin Psychiatry 67:1104–1109, 2006

Almqvist EW, Bloch M, Brinkman R, et al: A worldwide assessment of the frequency of suicide, suicide attempts, or psychiatric hospitalization after predictive testing for Huntington disease. Am J Hum Genet 64:1293–1304, 1999

American Psychiatric Association: Diagnostic and Statistical Manual of Mental Disorders, 4th Edition, Text Revision. Washington, DC, American Psychiatric Association, 2000

Aragones E, Pinol JL, Labad A: The overdiagnosis of depression in non-depressed patients in primary care. Fam Pract 23:363–368, 2006

Arbelaez JJ, Ariyo AA, Crum RM, et al: Depressive symptoms, inflammation, and ischemic stroke in older adults: a prospective analysis in the cardiovascular health study. J Am Geriatr Soc 55:1825–1830, 2007

Ballon JS, Feifel D: A systematic review of modafinil: potential clinical uses and mechanisms of action. J Clin Psychiatry 67:554–566, 2006

Barkow K, Maier W, Ustun TB, et al: Risk factors for new depressive episodes in primary health care: an international prospective 12-month follow-up study. Psychol Med 32:595–607, 2002

Barnes DE, Alexopoulos GS, Lopez OL, et al: Depressive symptoms, vascular disease, and mild cognitive impairment: findings from the Cardiovascular Health Study. Arch Gen Psychiatry 63:273–279, 2006

Barrett JE, Williams JW Jr, Oxman TE, et al: Treatment of dysthymia and minor depression in primary care: a randomized trial in patients aged 18 to 59 years. J Fam Pract 50:405–412, 2001

Beal CC, Stuifbergen AK, Brown A: Depression in multiple sclerosis: a longitudinal analysis. Arch Psychiatr Nurs 21:181–191, 2007

Beale MD, Kellner CH, Parsons PJ: ECT for the treatment of mood disorders in cancer patients. Convuls Ther 13:222–226, 1997

Beck AT, Steer RA, Brown GK: Manual for Beck Depression Inventory-II. San Antonio, TX, Psychological Corporation, 1996

Benedetti F, Bernasconi A, Pontiggia A: Depression and neurological disorders. Curr Opin Psychiatry 19:14–18, 2006

Benton T, Staab J, Evans DL: Medical comorbidity in depressive disorders. Ann Clin Psychiatry 19:289–303, 2007

Berard RM, Boermeester F, Viljoen G: Depressive disorders in an outpatient oncology setting: prevalence, assessment, and management. Psychooncology 7:112–120, 1998

Berkman LF, Blumenthal J, Burg M, et al: Effects of treating depression and low perceived social support on clinical events after myocardial infarction: the Enhancing Recovery in Coronary Heart Disease Patients (ENRICHD) Randomized Trial. JAMA 289:3106–3116, 2003

Berwick DM, Murphy JM, Goldman PA, et al: Performance of a five-item mental health screening test. Med Care 29:169–176, 1991

Bogousslavsky J: William Feinberg lecture 2002: emotions, mood, and behavior after stroke. Stroke 34:1046–1050, 2003

Boland RJ, Diaz S, Lamdan RM, et al: Overdiagnosis of depression in the general hospital. Gen Hosp Psychiatry 18:28–35, 1996

Breitbart W, Rosenfeld B, Pessin H, et al: Depression, hopelessness, and desire for hastened death in terminally ill patients with cancer. JAMA 284:2907–2911, 2000

Bruera E, Chadwick S, Brenneis C, et al: Methylphenidate associated with narcotics for the treatment of cancer pain. Cancer Treat Rep 71:67–70, 1987

Bukberg J, Penman D, Holland JC: Depression in hospitalized cancer patients. Psychosom Med 46:199–212, 1984

Burvill PW: Recent progress in the epidemiology of major depression. Epidemiol Rev 17:21–31, 1995

Butler LD, Koopman C, Cordova MJ, et al: Psychological distress and pain significantly increase before death in metastatic breast cancer patients. Psychosom Med 65:416–426, 2003

Capuron L, Bluthe RM, Dantzer R: Cytokines in clinical psychiatry. Am J Psychiatry 158:1163–1164, 2001

Carney C: Diabetes mellitus and major depressive disorder: an overview of prevalence, complications, and treatment. Depress Anxiety 7:149–157, 1998

Carson AJ, MacHale S, Allen K, et al: Depression after stroke and lesion location: a systematic review. Lancet 356:122–126, 2000

Chaturvedi SK, Shenoy A, Prasad K, et al: Concerns, coping and quality of life in head and neck cancer patients. Support Care Cancer 4:186–190, 1996

Chen Y, Guo JJ, Zhan S, et al: Treatment effects of antidepressants in patients with post-stroke depression: a meta-analysis. Ann Pharmacother 40:2115–2122, 2006

Chochinov HM, Wilson KG, Enns M, et al: "Are you depressed?" Screening for depression in the terminally ill. Am J Psychiatry 154:674–676, 1997

Chwastiak LA, Ehde DM: Psychiatric issues in multiple sclerosis. Psychiatr Clin North Am 30:803–817, 2007

Classen CC, Kraemer HC, Blasey C, et al: Supportive-expressive group therapy for primary breast cancer patients: a randomized prospective multicenter trial. Psychooncology 17:438–447, 2008

Cleland JA, Lee AJ, Hall S: Associations of depression and anxiety with gender, age, health-related quality of life and symptoms in primary care COPD patients. Fam Pract 24:217–223, 2007

Coyne JC, Stefanek M, Thombs BD, et al: Time to let go of the illusion that psychotherapy extends the survival of cancer patients: reply to Kraemer, Kuchler, and Spiegel (2009). Psychol Bull 135:179–182, 2009

Craven JL, Rodin GM, Johnson L, et al: The diagnosis of major depression in renal dialysis patients. Psychosom Med 49:482–492, 1987

Cruess DG, Evans DL, Repetto MJ, et al: Prevalence, diagnosis, and pharmacological treatment of mood disorders in HIV disease. Biol Psychiatry 54:307–316, 2003

Dahmen N, Marx J, Hopf HC, et al: Therapy of early poststroke depression with venlafaxine: safety, tolerability, and efficacy as determined in an open, uncontrolled clinical trial. Stroke 30:691–692, 1999

Dantzer R, O'Connor JC, Freund GG, et al: From inflammation to sickness and depression: when the immune system subjugates the brain. Nat Rev Neurosci 9:46–56, 2008

Davidson KW, Rieckmann N, Clemow L, et al: Enhanced depression care for patients with acute coronary syndrome and persistent depressive symptoms: coronary psychosocial evaluation studies randomized controlled trial. Arch Intern Med 170:600–608, 2010

de Boer T: The pharmacologic profile of mirtazapine. J Clin Psychiatry 57 (suppl 4):19–25, 1996

de Groot M, Anderson R, Freedland KE, et al: Association of depression and diabetes complications: a meta-analysis. Psychosom Med 63:619–630, 2001

Dickens C, McGowan L, Percival C, et al: Depression is a risk factor for mortality after myocardial infarction: fact or artifact? J Am Coll Cardiol 49:1834–1840, 2007

DiMatteo MR, Lepper HS, Croghan TW: Depression is a risk factor for noncompliance with medical treatment: meta-analysis of the effects of anxiety and depression on patient adherence. Arch Intern Med 160:2101–2107, 2000

Elliott AJ, Russo J, Bergam K, et al: Antidepressant efficacy in HIV-seropositive outpatients with major depressive disorder: an open trial of nefazodone. J Clin Psychiatry 60:226–231, 1999

Endicott J: Measurement of depression in patients with cancer. Cancer 53:2243–2249, 1984

Fallowfield L, Ratcliffe D, Jenkins V, et al: Psychiatric morbidity and its recognition by doctors in patients with cancer. Br J Cancer 84:1011–1015, 2001

Fernandez F, Levy JK, Samley HR, et al: Effects of methylphenidate in HIV-related depression: a comparative trial with desipramine. Int J Psychiatry Med 25:53–67, 1995

First M, Gibbon M, Spitzer R, et al: Structured Clinical Interview for DSM-IV Axis II Personality Disorders (SCID-II). Washington, DC, American Psychiatric Press, 1997

Flint A, Rifat S: Validation of the Hospital Anxiety and Depression Scale as a measure of severity of geriatric depression. Int J Geriatr Psychiatry 11:991–994, 1996

Folstein S, Abbott MH, Chase GA, et al: The association of affective disorder with Huntington's disease in a case series and in families. Psychol Med 13:537–542, 1983

Forsgren L, Nystrom L: An incident case-referent study of epileptic seizures in adults. Epilepsy Res 6:66–81, 1990

Forstl H, Burns A, Luthert P, et al: Clinical and neuropathological correlates of depression in Alzheimer's disease. Psychol Med 22:877–884, 1992

Frasure-Smith N: The Montreal Heart Attack Readjustment Trial (MHART). J Cardiopulm Rehabil 15:103–106, 1995

Gill JM, Dansky BS: Use of an electronic medical record to facilitate screening for depression in primary care. Prim Care Companion J Clin Psychiatry 5:125–128, 2003

Glassman AH, Roose SP, Bigger JT Jr: The safety of tricyclic antidepressants in cardiac patients. Risk-benefit reconsidered. JAMA 269:2673–2675, 1993

Glassman AH, O'Connor CM, Califf RM, et al: Sertraline treatment of major depression in patients with acute MI or unstable angina. JAMA 288:701–709, 2002

Global Parkinson's Disease Survey Steering Committee: Factors impacting on quality of life in Parkinson's disease: results from an international survey. Mov Disord 17:60–67, 2002

Golden R, Dawkins K, Nicholas L, et al: Trazodone, nefazodone, bupropion, and mirtazapine, in Textbook of Psychopharmacology, 2nd Edition. Edited by Schatzberg AF, Nemeroff CB. Washington, DC, American Psychiatric Press, 1998, pp 549–588

Gottlieb SS, Khatta M, Friedmann E, et al: The influence of age, gender, and race on the prevalence of depression in heart failure patients. J Am Coll Cardiol 43:1542–1549, 2004

Grade C, Redford B, Chrostowski J, et al: Methylphenidate in early poststroke recovery: a double-blind, placebo-controlled study. Arch Phys Med Rehabil 79:1047–1050, 1998

Grassi L, Sabato S, Rossi E, et al: Depressive and anxiety disorders among cancer patients: screening methods by using the Distress Thermometer compared to the ICD-10. Psychooncology 15:s162, 2006

Gurevich M, Devins GM, Wilson C, et al: Stress response syndromes in women undergoing mammography: a comparison of women with and without a history of breast cancer. Psychosom Med 66:104–112, 2004

Hall A, A'Hern R, Fallowfield L: Are we using appropriate self-report questionnaires for detecting anxiety and depression in women with early breast cancer? Eur J Cancer 35:79–85, 1999

Hamilton M: A rating scale for depression. J Neurol Neurosurg Psychiatry 23:56–62, 1960

Hermanns N, Kulzer B, Krichbaum M, et al: How to screen for depression and emotional problems in patients with diabetes: comparison of screening characteristics of depression questionnaires, measurement of diabetes-specific emotional problems and standard clinical assessment. Diabetologia 49:469–477, 2006

Herrmann C: International experiences with the Hospital Anxiety and Depression Scale—a review of validation data and clinical results. J Psychosom Res 42:17–41, 1997

Hiemke C, Hartter S: Pharmacokinetics of selective serotonin reuptake inhibitors. Pharmacol Ther 85:11–28, 2000

Himelhoch S, Weller WE, Wu AW, et al: Chronic medical illness, depression, and use of acute medical services among Medicare beneficiaries. Med Care 42:512–521, 2004

Hopko DR, Bell JL, Armento ME, et al: The phenomenology and screening of clinical depression in cancer patients. J Psychosoc Oncol 26:31–51, 2008

Horwitz AV, Wakefield JC: The Loss of Sadness: How Psychiatry Transformed Normal Sorrow Into Depressive Disorder. New York, Oxford University Press, 2007

House A, Knapp P, Bamford J, et al: Mortality at 12 and 24 months after stroke may be associated with depressive symptoms at 1 month. Stroke 32:696–701, 2001

Huffman C, Smith FA, Quinn DK, et al: Post-MI psychiatric syndromes: six unanswered questions. Harv Rev Psychiatry 14:305–318, 2006

Jacobsen PB: Lost in translation: the need for clinically relevant research on psychological interventions for distress in cancer patients. Ann Behav Med 32:119–120, 2006

Jacobson AM, Adler AG, Wolfsdorf JI, et al: Psychological characteristics of adults with IDDM. Comparison of patients in poor and good glycemic control. Diabetes Care 13:375–381, 1990

Jacobson CM, Rosenfeld B, Pessin H, et al: Depression and IL-6 blood plasma concentrations in advanced cancer patients. Psychosomatics 49:64–66, 2008

Jann MW, Slade JH: Antidepressant agents for the treatment of chronic pain and depression. Pharmacotherapy 27:1571–1587, 2007

Jin Y, Desta Z, Stearns V, et al: CYP2D6 genotype, antidepressant use, and tamoxifen metabolism during adjuvant breast cancer treatment. J Natl Cancer Inst 97:30–39, 2005

Jobe PC, Dailey JW, Wernicke JF: A noradrenergic and serotonergic hypothesis of the linkage between epilepsy and affective disorders. Crit Rev Neurobiol 13:317–356, 1999

Joffe P, Larsen FS, Pedersen V, et al: Single-dose pharmacokinetics of citalopram in patients with moderate renal insufficiency or hepatic cirrhosis compared with healthy subjects. Eur J Clin Pharmacol 54:237–242, 1998

Jones JE, Hermann BP, Woodard JL, et al: Screening for major depression in epilepsy with common self-report depression inventories. Epilepsia 46:731–735, 2005

Jones JM, Huggins MA, Rydall AC, et al: Symptomatic distress, hopelessness, and the desire for hastened death in hospitalized cancer patients. J Psychosom Res 55:411–418, 2003

Justice AC, McGinnis KA, Atkinson JH, et al: Psychiatric and neurocognitive disorders among HIV-positive and negative veterans in care: veterans aging cohort five-site study. AIDS 18 (suppl 1):S49–S59, 2004

Kaasa S, Malt U, Hagen S, et al: Psychological distress in cancer patients with advanced disease. Radiother Oncol 27:193–197, 1993

Kanner AM: Depression in epilepsy: prevalence, clinical semiology, pathogenic mechanisms, and treatment. Biol Psychiatry 54:388–398, 2003

Katon WJ: Clinical and health services relationships between major depression, depressive symptoms, and general medical illness. Biol Psychiatry 54:216–226, 2003

Katon W, Lin EH, Kroenke K: The association of depression and anxiety with medical symptom burden in patients with chronic medical illness. Gen Hosp Psychiatry 29:147–155, 2007

Kawase E, Karasawa K, Shimotsu S, et al: Evaluation of a one-question interview for depression in a radiation oncology department in Japan. Gen Hosp Psychiatry 28:321–322, 2006

Kelly JA, Murphy DA, Bahr GR, et al: Outcome of cognitive-behavioral and support group brief therapies for depressed, HIV-infected persons. Am J Psychiatry 150:1679–1686, 1993

Kessler R: Depression screening. J Fam Pract 52:466; author reply 467, 2003

Kessler RC, Berglund P, Demler O, et al: The epidemiology of major depressive disorder: results from the National Comorbidity Survey Replication (NCS-R). JAMA 289:3095–3105, 2003

Kim JM, Shin IS, Yoon JS: Apolipoprotein E among Korean Alzheimer's disease patients in community-dwelling and hospitalized elderly samples. Dement Geriatr Cogn Disord 13:119–124, 2002

Kimura M, Robinson RG, Kosier JT: Treatment of cognitive impairment after poststroke depression: a double-blind treatment trial. Stroke 31:1482–1486, 2000

Kissane D: Beyond the psychotherapy and survival debate: the challenge of social disparity, depression and treatment adherence in psychosocial cancer care. Psychooncology 18:1–5, 2009

Kissane DW, Grabsch B, Clarke DM, et al: Supportive-expressive group therapy for women with metastatic breast cancer: survival and psychosocial outcome from a randomized controlled trial. Psychooncology 16:277–286, 2007

Koenig HG: Depression in hospitalized older patients with congestive heart failure. Gen Hosp Psychiatry 20:29–43, 1998

Koenig HG, Cohen HJ, Blazer DG, et al: A brief depression scale for use in the medically ill. Int J Psychiatry Med 22:183–195, 1992

Koenig HG, George LK, Peterson BL, et al: Depression in medically ill hospitalized older adults: prevalence, characteristics, and course of symptoms according to six diagnostic schemes. Am J Psychiatry 154:1376–1383, 1997

Kopetz S, Steele CD, Brandt J, et al: Characteristics and outcomes of dementia residents in an assisted living facility. Int J Geriatr Psychiatry 15:586–593, 2000

Kraemer HC, Kuchler T, Spiegel D: Use and misuse of the consolidated standards of reporting trials (CONSORT) guidelines to assess research findings: comment on Coyne, Stefanek, and Palmer (2007). Psychol Bull 135:173–178; discussion 179–182, 2009

Kroenke K, Spitzer RL, Williams JB: The PHQ-9: validity of a brief depression severity measure. J Gen Intern Med 16:606–613, 2001

Krystal AD, Coffey CE: Neuropsychiatric considerations in the use of electroconvulsive therapy. J Neuropsychiatry Clin Neurosci 9:283–292, 1997

Lagopoulos J, Malhi GS, Ivanovski B, et al: A matter of motion or an emotional matter? Management of depression in Parkinson's disease. Expert Rev Neurother 5:803–810, 2005

Lambert MV, Robertson MM: Depression in epilepsy: etiology, phenomenology, and treatment. Epilepsia 40 (suppl 10):S21–S47, 1999

Lamers F, Jonkers CC, Bosma H, et al: Summed score of the Patient Health Questionnaire-9 was a reliable and valid method for depression screening in chronically ill elderly patients. J Clin Epidemiol 61:679–687, 2008

Lane DA, Chong AY, Lip GY: Psychological interventions for depression in heart failure. Cochrane Database Syst Rev (1):CD003329, 2005

Lazure KE, Lydiatt WM, Denman D, et al: Association between depression and survival or disease recurrence in patients with head and neck cancer enrolled in a depression prevention trial. Head Neck 31:888–892, 2009

Lee HB, Lyketsos CG: Depression in Alzheimer's disease: heterogeneity and related issues. Biol Psychiatry 54:353–362, 2003

Leentjens AF, Verhey FR, Luijckx GJ, et al: The validity of the Beck Depression Inventory as a screening and diagnostic instrument for depression in patients with Parkinson's disease. Mov Disord 15:1221–1224, 2000

Leonard BE: Inflammation, depression and dementia: are they connected? Neurochem Res 32:1749–1756, 2007

Leserman J: HIV disease progression: depression, stress, and possible mechanisms. Biol Psychiatry 54:295–306, 2003

Lesperance F, Frasure-Smith N, Koszycki D, et al: Effects of citalopram and interpersonal psychotherapy on depression in patients with coronary artery disease: the Canadian Cardiac Randomized Evaluation of Antidepressant and Psychotherapy Efficacy (CREATE) trial. JAMA 297:367–379, 2007

Levinson DF: The genetics of depression: a review. Biol Psychiatry 60:84–92, 2006

Lewis L: Mood disorders: diagnosis, treatment, and support from a patient perspective. Psychopharmacol Bull 35:186–196, 2001

Li M, Hales S, Rodin G: Adjustment disorders, in Psycho-Oncology, 2nd Edition. Edited by Holland JC. New York, Oxford University Press, 2010, pp 303–310

Lincoln NB, Flannaghan T: Cognitive behavioral psychotherapy for depression following stroke: a randomized controlled trial. Stroke 34:111–115, 2003

Lloyd-Williams M, Spiller J, Ward J: Which depression screening tools should be used in palliative care? Palliat Med 17:40–43, 2003

Lloyd-Williams M, Shiels C, Taylor F, et al: Depression—an independent predictor of early death in patients with advanced cancer. J Affect Disord 113:127–132, 2009

Lo C, Lin J, Gagliese L, et al: Age and depression in patients with metastatic cancer: the protective effects of attachment security and spiritual well-being. Ageing Soc 30:325–336, 2010

Loprinzi CL, Kugler JW, Sloan JA, et al: Venlafaxine in management of hot flashes in survivors of breast cancer: a randomised controlled trial. Lancet 356:2059–2063, 2000

Lowe B, Kroenke K, Grafe K: Detecting and monitoring depression with a two-item questionnaire (PHQ-2). J Psychosom Res 58:163–171, 2005

Lucht M, Schaub RT, Meyer C, et al: Gender differences in unipolar depression: a general population survey of adults between age 18 to 64 of German nationality. J Affect Disord 77:203–211, 2003

Lustman PJ, Griffith LS, Freedland KE, et al: Cognitive behavior therapy for depression in type 2 diabetes mellitus. A randomized, controlled trial. Ann Intern Med 129:613–621, 1998

Lustman PJ, Anderson RJ, Freedland KE, et al: Depression and poor glycemic control: a meta-analytic review of the literature. Diabetes Care 23:934–942, 2000a

Lustman PJ, Freedland KE, Griffith LS, et al: Fluoxetine for depression in diabetes: a randomized double-blind placebo-controlled trial. Diabetes Care 23:618–623, 2000b

Lyketsos CG, Steele C, Baker L, et al: Major and minor depression in Alzheimer's disease: prevalence and impact. J Neuropsychiatry Clin Neurosci 9:556–561, 1997

Lyketsos CG, Sheppard JM, Steele CD, et al: Randomized, placebo-controlled, double-blind clinical trial of sertraline in the treatment of depression complicating Alzheimer's disease: initial results from the Depression in Alzheimer's Disease study. Am J Psychiatry 157:1686–1689, 2000

Lyketsos CG, Sheppard JM, Steinberg M, et al: Neuropsychiatric disturbance in Alzheimer's disease clusters into three groups: the Cache County study. Int J Geriatr Psychiatry 16:1043–1053, 2001

Lyketsos CG, Lopez O, Jones B, et al: Prevalence of neuropsychiatric symptoms in dementia and mild cognitive impairment: results from the cardiovascular health study. JAMA 288:1475–1483, 2002

Magni G, Conlon P, Arsie D: Tricyclic antidepressants in the treatment of cancer pain: a review. Pharmacopsychiatry 20:160–164, 1987

Makrilia N, Indeck B, Syrigos K, et al: Depression and pancreatic cancer: a poorly understood link. JOP 10:69–76, 2009

Manne S, Glassman M, Du Hamel K: Intrusion, avoidance, and psychological distress among individuals with cancer. Psychosom Med 63:658–667, 2001

Markowitz JC, Kocsis JH, Fishman B, et al: Treatment of depressive symptoms in human immunodeficiency virus–positive patients. Arch Gen Psychiatry 55:452–457, 1998

Masand P, Pickett P, Murray GB: Psychostimulants for secondary depression in medical illness. Psychosomatics 32:203–208, 1991

Massie MJ: Prevalence of depression in patients with cancer. J Natl Cancer Inst Monogr 32:57–71, 2004

May HT, Horne BD, Carlquist JF, et al: Depression after coronary artery disease is associated with heart failure. J Am Coll Cardiol 53:1440–1447, 2009

McDonald WM, Richard IH, DeLong MR: Prevalence, etiology, and treatment of depression in Parkinson's disease. Biol Psychiatry 54:363–375, 2003

McHale M, Hendrikz J, Dann F, et al: Screening for depression in patients with diabetes mellitus. Psychosom Med 70:869–874, 2008

Mendes de Leon CF, Kop WJ, de Swart HB, et al: Psychosocial characteristics and recurrent events after percutaneous transluminal coronary angioplasty. Am J Cardiol 77:252–255, 1996

Michaud CM, Murray CJ, Bloom BR: Burden of disease—implications for future research. JAMA 285:535–539, 2001

Migliorelli R, Teson A, Sabe L, et al: Prevalence and correlates of dysthymia and major depression among patients with Alzheimer's disease. Am J Psychiatry 152:37–44, 1995

Milano AF, Singer RB: Mortality in comorbidity (II)—excess death rates derived from a follow-up study on 10,025 subjects divided into 4 groups with or without depression and diabetes mellitus. J Insur Med 39:160–166, 2007

Miller S, Lo C, Gagliese L, et al: Patterns of depression in cancer patients: an indirect test of gender-specific vulnerabilities to depression. Soc Psychiatry Psychiatr Epidemiol, 2010 Jun 25 [Epub ahead of print]

Mitchell AJ: Pooled results from 38 analyses of the accuracy of distress thermometer and other ultra-short methods of detecting cancer-related mood disorders. J Clin Oncol 25:4670–4681, 2007

Mitchell AJ, Coyne JC: Do ultra-short screening instruments accurately detect depression in primary care? A pooled analysis and meta-analysis of 22 studies. Br J Gen Pract 57:144–151, 2007

Mitchell AJ, Vaze A, Rao S: Clinical diagnosis of depression in primary care: a meta-analysis. Lancet 374:609–619, 2009

Mohr DC, Goodkin DE, Likosky W, et al: Therapeutic expectations of patients with multiple sclerosis upon initiating interferon beta-1b: relationship to adherence to treatment. Mult Scler 2:222–226, 1996

Mohr DC, Goodkin DE, Islar J, et al: Treatment of depression is associated with suppression of nonspecific and antigen-specific T(H)1 responses in multiple sclerosis. Arch Neurol 58:1081–1086, 2001

Mohr DC, Hart SL, Julian L, et al: Screening for depression among patients with multiple sclerosis: two questions may be enough. Mult Scler 13:215–219, 2007

Mondolo F, Jahanshahi M, Grana A, et al: The validity of the hospital anxiety and depression scale and the geriatric depression scale in Parkinson's disease. Behav Neurol 17:109–115, 2006

Morris PL, Robinson RG, Samuels J: Depression, introversion and mortality following stroke. Aust N Z J Psychiatry 27:443–449, 1993

Mossner R, Henneberg A, Schmitt A, et al: Allelic variation of serotonin transporter expression is associated with depression in Parkinson's disease. Mol Psychiatry 6:350–352, 2001

Moussavi S, Chatterji S, Verdes E, et al: Depression, chronic diseases, and decrements in health: results from the World Health Surveys. Lancet 370:851–858 2007

Musselman DL, Lawson DH, Gumnick JF, et al: Paroxetine for the prevention of depression induced by high-dose interferon alfa. N Engl J Med 344:961–966, 2001

Musselman DL, Betan E, Larsen H, et al: Relationship of depression to diabetes types 1 and 2: epidemiology, biology, and treatment. Biol Psychiatry 54:317–329, 2003

Myer L, Smit J, Roux LL, et al: Common mental disorders among HIV-infected individuals in South Africa: prevalence, predictors, and validation of brief psychiatric rating scales. AIDS Patient Care STDS 22:147–158, 2008

Narushima K, Kosier JT, Robinson RG: Preventing poststroke depression: a 12-week double-blind randomized treatment trial and 21-month follow-up. J Nerv Ment Dis 190:296–303, 2002

Navari RM, Brenner MC, Wilson MN: Treatment of depressive symptoms in patients with early stage breast cancer undergoing adjuvant therapy. Breast Cancer Res Treat 112:197–201, 2008

Newell SA, Sanson-Fisher RW, Savolainen NJ: Systematic review of psychological therapies for cancer patients: overview and recommendations for future research. J Natl Cancer Inst 94:558–584, 2002

Nissim R, Gagliese L, Rodin G: The desire for hastened death in individuals with advanced cancer: a longitudinal qualitative study. Soc Sci Med 69:165–171, 2009

Olatunji BO, Mimiaga MJ, O'Cleirigh C, et al: A review of treatment studies of depression in HIV. Top HIV Med 14:112–124, 2006

Onitilo AA, Nietert PJ, Egede LE: Effect of depression on all-cause mortality in adults with cancer and differential effects by cancer site. Gen Hosp Psychiatry 28:396–402, 2006

Orr K, Taylor D: Psychostimulants in the treatment of depression: a review of the evidence. CNS Drugs 21:239–257, 2007

Palmer SC, Coyne JC: Screening for depression in medical care: pitfalls, alternatives, and revised priorities. J Psychosom Res 54:279–287, 2003

Pandya R, Metz L, Patten SB: Predictive value of the CES-D in detecting depression among candidates for disease-modifying multiple sclerosis treatment. Psychosomatics 46:131–134, 2005

Parissis JT, Fountoulaki K, Filippatos G, et al: Depression in coronary artery disease: novel pathophysiologic mechanisms and therapeutic implications. Int J Cardiol 116:153–160, 2007

Patten SB, Barbui C: Drug-induced depression: a systematic review to inform clinical practice. Psychother Psychosom 73:207–215, 2004

Pearson T, Fuster V: 27th Bethesda Conference. Matching the Intensity of Risk Factor Management with the Hazard for Coronary Disease Events. September 14–15, 1995. J Am Coll Cardiol 27:957–1047, 1996

Pelletier G, Verhoef MJ, Khatri N, et al: Quality of life in brain tumor patients: the relative contributions of depression, fatigue, emotional distress, and existential issues. J Neurooncol 57:41–49, 2002

Pezzella G, Moslinger-Gehmayr R, Contu A: Treatment of depression in patients with breast cancer: a comparison between paroxetine and amitriptyline. Breast Cancer Res Treat 70:1–10, 2001

Phabphal K, Sattawatcharawanich S, Sathirapunya P, et al: Anxiety and depression in Thai epileptic patients. J Med Assoc Thai 90:2010–2015, 2007

Phillips KA, Osborne RH, Giles GG, et al: Psychosocial factors and survival of young women with breast cancer: a population-based prospective cohort study. J Clin Oncol 26:4666–4671, 2008

Pirl WF, Roth AJ: Diagnosis and treatment of depression in cancer patients. Oncology (Williston Park) 13:1293–1301; discussion 1301–1302, 1305–1306, 1999

Pisani F, Oteri G, Costa C, et al: Effects of psychotropic drugs on seizure threshold. Drug Saf 25:91–110, 2002

Poewe W, Seppi K: Treatment options for depression and psychosis in Parkinson's disease. J Neurol 248 (suppl 3):III12–III21, 2001

Pomeroy IM, Clark CR, Philp I: The effectiveness of very short scales for depression screening in elderly medical patients. Int J Geriatr Psychiatry 16:321–326, 2001

Potter WZ, Manji HK, Rudorfer MV: Tricyclics and tetracyclics, in The American Psychiatric Press Textbook of Psychopharmacology, 2nd Edition. Edited by Schatzberg AF, Nemeroff CB. Washington, DC, American Psychiatric Press, 1998, pp 199–218

Preskorn SH, Fast GA: Tricyclic antidepressant-induced seizures and plasma drug concentration. J Clin Psychiatry 53:160–162, 1992

Pujol J, Bello J, Deus J, et al: Lesions in the left arcuate fasciculus region and depressive symptoms in multiple sclerosis. Neurology 49:1105–1110, 1997

Quiske A, Helmstaedter C, Lux S, et al: Depression in patients with temporal lobe epilepsy is related to mesial temporal sclerosis. Epilepsy Res 39:121–125, 2000

Rabindranath KS, Daly C, Butler JA, et al: Psychosocial interventions for depression in dialysis patients. Cochrane Database Syst Rev (3):CD004542, 2005

Rabkin JG, Rabkin R, Harrison W, et al: Effect of imipramine on mood and enumerative measures of immune status in depressed patients with HIV illness. Am J Psychiatry 151:516–523, 1994

Rabkin JG, Wagner GJ, Rabkin R: Fluoxetine treatment for depression in patients with HIV and AIDS: a randomized, placebo-controlled trial. Am J Psychiatry 156:101–107, 1999

Radloff L: The CES-D Scale: a self-report depression scale for research in the general population. Appl Psychol Meas 1:385–401, 1977

Raison CL, Miller AH: Depression in cancer: new developments regarding diagnosis and treatment. Biol Psychiatry 54:283–294, 2003

Raison CL, Demetrashvili M, Capuron L, et al: Neuropsychiatric adverse effects of interferon-alpha: recognition and management. CNS Drugs 19:105–123, 2005

Rao V, Lyketsos CG: The benefits and risks of ECT for patients with primary dementia who also suffer from depression. Int J Geriatr Psychiatry 15:729–735, 2000

Rasmussen A, Lunde M, Poulsen DL, et al: A double-blind, placebo-controlled study of sertraline in the prevention of depression in stroke patients. Psychosomatics 44:216–221, 2003

Razavi D, Delvaux N, Farvacques C, et al: Screening for adjustment disorders and major depressive disorders in cancer inpatients. Br J Psychiatry 156:79–83, 1990

Reynolds CF 3rd: Treatment of depression in special populations. J Clin Psychiatry 53 (suppl):45–53, 1992

Richard IH, Maughn A, Kurlan R: Do serotonin reuptake inhibitor antidepressants worsen Parkinson's disease? A retrospective case series. Mov Disord 14:155–157, 1999

Rivelli S, Jiang W: Depression and ischemic heart disease: what have we learned from clinical trials? Curr Opin Cardiol 22:286–291, 2007

Robinson RG: Poststroke depression: prevalence, diagnosis, treatment, and disease progression. Biol Psychiatry 54:376–387, 2003

Robinson RG, Schultz SK, Castillo C, et al: Nortriptyline versus fluoxetine in the treatment of depression and in short-term recovery after stroke: a placebo-controlled, double-blind study. Am J Psychiatry 157:351–359, 2000

Rodin G, Nolan R, Katz M: Depression, in Textbook of Psychosomatic Medicine. Edited by Levenson J. Washington, DC, American Psychiatric Publishing, 2004, pp 193–217

Rodin G, Lloyd N, Katz M, et al: The treatment of depression in cancer patients: a systematic review. Support Care Cancer 15:123–136, 2007a

Rodin G, Walsh A, Zimmermann C, et al: The contribution of attachment security and social support to depressive symptoms in patients with metastatic cancer. Psychooncology 16:1080–1091, 2007b

Rodin G, Zimmermann C, Rydall A, et al: The desire for hastened death in patients with metastatic cancer. J Pain Symptom Manage 33:661–675, 2007c

Rodin G, Mackay JA, Zimmermann C, et al: Clinician-patient communication: a systematic review. Support Care Cancer 17:627–644, 2009

Roth AJ, Kornblith AB, Batel-Copel L, et al: Rapid screening for psychologic distress in men with prostate carcinoma: a pilot study. Cancer 82:1904–1908, 1998

Roth M, Mountjoy CQ, Amrein R: Moclobemide in elderly patients with cognitive decline and depression: an international double-blind, placebo-controlled trial. Br J Psychiatry 168:149–157, 1996

Rowe SK, Rapaport MH: Classification and treatment of subthreshold depression. Curr Opin Psychiatry 19:9–13, 2006

Rudisch B, Nemeroff CB: Epidemiology of comorbid coronary artery disease and depression. Biol Psychiatry 54:227–240, 2003

Sadock B, Kaplan H, Sadock V: Kaplan Sadock's Synopsis of Psychiatry: Behavioral Sciences/Clinical Psychiatry. Philadelphia, PA, Lippincott Williams & Wilkins, 2007

Saravay SM, Pollack S, Steinberg MD, et al: Four-year follow-up of the influence of psychological comorbidity on medical rehospitalization. Am J Psychiatry 153:397–403, 1996

Savic I, Lindstrom P, Gulyas B, et al: Limbic reductions of 5-HT1A receptor binding in human temporal lobe epilepsy. Neurology 62:1343–1351, 2004

Schulz R, Beach SR, Ives DG, et al: Association between depression and mortality in older adults: the Cardiovascular Health Study. Arch Intern Med 160:1761–1768, 2000

Serebruany VL, Glassman AH, Malinin AI, et al: Platelet/endothelial biomarkers in depressed patients treated with the selective serotonin reuptake inhibitor sertraline after acute coronary events: the Sertraline AntiDepressant Heart Attack Randomized Trial (SADHART) Platelet Substudy. Circulation 108:939–944, 2003

Sheard T, Maguire P: The effect of psychological interventions on anxiety and depression in cancer patients: results of two meta-analyses. Br J Cancer 80:1770–1780, 1999

Sheehan DV, Lecrubier Y, Sheehan KH, et al: The Mini-International Neuropsychiatric Interview (M.I.N.I.): the development and validation of a structured diagnostic psychiatric interview for DSM-IV and ICD-10. J Clin Psychiatry 59 (suppl 20):22–33; quiz 34–57, 1998

Sheline YI: Neuroimaging studies of mood disorder effects on the brain. Biol Psychiatry 54:338–352, 2003

Shinar D, Gross CR, Price TR, et al: Screening for depression in stroke patients: the reliability and validity of the Center for Epidemiologic Studies Depression Scale. Stroke 17:241–245, 1986

Shuster JL, Stern TA, Greenberg DB: Pros and cons of fluoxetine for the depressed cancer patient. Oncology (Williston Park) 6:45–50, 55; discussion 55–56, 1992

Simon GE, Von Korff M: Medical comorbidity and validity of DSM-IV depression criteria. Psychol Med 36:27–36, 2006

Smith D, Dempster C, Glanville J, et al: Efficacy and tolerability of venlafaxine compared with selective serotonin reuptake inhibitors and other antidepressants: a meta-analysis. Br J Psychiatry 180:396–404, 2002

Spitzer RL, Kroenke K, Williams JB: Validation and utility of a self-report version of PRIME-MD: the PHQ primary care study. Primary Care Evaluation of Mental Disorders. Patient Health Questionnaire. JAMA 282:1737–1744, 1999

Stafford L, Berk M, Jackson HJ: Validity of the Hospital Anxiety and Depression Scale and Patient Health Questionnaire-9 to screen for depression in patients with coronary artery disease. Gen Hosp Psychiatry 29:417–424, 2007

Steel JL, Geller DA, Gamblin TC, et al: Depression, immunity, and survival in patients with hepatobiliary carcinoma. J Clin Oncol 25:2397–2405, 2007

Stein MB, Cox BJ, Afifi TO, et al: Does comorbid depressive illness magnify the impact of chronic physical illness? A population-based perspective. Psychol Med 36:587–596, 2006

Stenager EN, Koch-Henriksen N, Stenager E: Risk factors for suicide in multiple sclerosis. Psychother Psychosom 65:86–90, 1996

Su S, Miller AH, Snieder H, et al: Common genetic contributions to depressive symptoms and inflammatory markers in middle-aged men: the Twins Heart Study. Psychosom Med 71:152–158, 2009

Surtees PG, Wainwright NW, Luben RN, et al: Depression and ischemic heart disease mortality: evidence from the EPIC-Norfolk United Kingdom prospective cohort study. Am J Psychiatry 165:515–523, 2008

Talbot F, Nouwen A, Gingras J, et al: Relations of diabetes intrusiveness and personal control to symptoms of depression among adults with diabetes. Health Psychol 18:537–542, 1999

Tang WK, Ungvari GS, Chiu HF, et al: Detecting depression in Chinese stroke patients: a pilot study comparing four screening instruments. Int J Psychiatry Med 34:155–163, 2004

Teri L, Logsdon R, Yesavage J: Measuring behavior, mood, and psychiatric symptoms in Alzheimer disease. Alzheimer Dis Assoc Disord 11 (suppl 6):50–59, 1997

Tharwani HM, Yerramsetty P, Mannelli P, et al: Recent advances in poststroke depression. Curr Psychiatry Rep 9:225–231, 2007

Theobald DE, Kirsh KL, Holtsclaw E, et al: An open-label, crossover trial of mirtazapine (15 and 30 mg) in cancer patients with pain and other distressing symptoms. J Pain Symptom Manage 23:442–447, 2002

Thompson S, Herrmann N, Rapoport MJ, et al: Efficacy and safety of antidepressants for treatment of depression in Alzheimer's disease: a meta-analysis. Can J Psychiatry 52:248–255, 2007

Tossani E, Cassano P, Fava M: Depression and renal disease. Semin Dial 18:73–81, 2005

Unutzer J, Schoenbaum M, Katon WJ, et al: Healthcare costs associated with depression in medically Ill fee-for-service Medicare participants. J Am Geriatr Soc 57:506–510, 2009

Vamos M: Psychotherapy in the medically ill: a commentary. Aust N Z J Psychiatry 40:295–309, 2006

van den Brink RH, van Melle JP, Honig A, et al: Treatment of depression after myocardial infarction and the effects on cardiac prognosis and quality of life: rationale and outline of the Myocardial INfarction and Depression-Intervention Trial (MIND-IT). Am Heart J 144:219–225, 2002

Van Lieshout RJ, Bienenstock J, MacQueen GM: A review of candidate pathways underlying the association between asthma and major depressive disorder. Psychosom Med 71:187–195, 2009

van Melle JP, de Jonge P, Spijkerman TA, et al: Prognostic association of depression following myocardial infarction with mortality and cardiovascular events: a meta-analysis. Psychosom Med 66:814–822, 2004

Van Tilburg MA, McCaskill CC, Lane JD, et al: Depressed mood is a factor in glycemic control in type 1 diabetes. Psychosom Med 63:551–555, 2001

van Walraven C, Mamdani MM, Wells PS, et al: Inhibition of serotonin reuptake by antidepressants and upper gastrointestinal bleeding in elderly patients: retrospective cohort study. BMJ 323:655–658, 2001

Walker J, Postma K, McHugh GS, et al: Performance of the Hospital Anxiety and Depression Scale as a screening tool for major depressive disorder in cancer patients. J Psychosom Res 63:83–91, 2007

Wallin MT, Wilken JA, Turner AP, et al: Depression and multiple sclerosis: review of a lethal combination. J Rehabil Res Dev 43:45–62, 2006

Watkins C, Daniels L, Jack C, et al: Accuracy of a single question in screening for depression in a cohort of patients after stroke: comparative study. BMJ 323:1159, 2001

Wiart L, Petit H, Joseph PA, et al: Fluoxetine in early poststroke depression: a double-blind placebo-controlled study. Stroke 31:1829–1832, 2000

Wilhelm K, Parker G, Dewhurst-Savellis J, et al: Psychological predictors of single and recurrent major depressive episodes. J Affect Disord 54:139–147, 1999

Williams LS, Brizendine EJ, Plue L, et al: Performance of the PHQ-9 as a screening tool for depression after stroke. Stroke 36:635–638, 2005

Williams S, Dale J: The effectiveness of treatment for depression/depressive symptoms in adults with cancer: a systematic review. Br J Cancer 94:372–390, 2006

Wilson I: Depression in the patient with COPD. International Journal of COPD 1(1):61–64, 2006

Wilson K, Chochinov HM, de Fay B, et al: Diagnosis and management of depression in palliative care, in Handbook of Psychiatry in Palliative Medicine. Edited by Chochinov HM, Breitbart W. New York, Oxford University Press, 2000, pp 25–40

Wittkampf KA, Naeije L, Schene AH, et al: Diagnostic accuracy of the mood module of the Patient Health Questionnaire: a systematic review. Gen Hosp Psychiatry 29:388–395, 2007

World Health Organization: Composite International Diagnostic Interview, Version 2.1. Geneva, Switzerland, World Health Organization, 1997

Wulsin LR: Is depression a major risk factor for coronary disease? A systematic review of the epidemiologic evidence. Harv Rev Psychiatry 12:79–93, 2004

Yeragani VK, Pesce V, Jayaraman A, et al: Major depression with ischemic heart disease: effects of paroxetine and nortriptyline on long-term heart rate variability measures. Biol Psychiatry 52:418–429, 2002

Yesavage JA, Brink TL, Rose TL, et al: Development and validation of a geriatric depression screening scale: a preliminary report. J Psychiatr Res 17:37–49, 1982

Zigmond AS, Snaith RP: The hospital anxiety and depression scale. Acta Psychiatr Scand 67:361–370, 1983

CHAPTER 9

Suicidality

John Michael Bostwick, M.D.

James L. Levenson, M.D.

ONE OF THE MOST COMMON questions posed to any psychiatrist, including psychosomatic medicine specialists, is whether a patient is suicidal. Suicidal ideation, frequent and ubiquitous in medical settings, challenges the psychiatrist to discern what drives the patient's suicidal statement. Compared with suicidal ideation, completed suicide is rare in psychiatric patients and rarer still in medically ill patients.

Completed suicides are statistically uncommon events. Many risk factors are recognized, but none has a high positive predictive value (Mann 1987). As a low-base-rate phenomenon, screening for suicide risk has a high rate of false-positive results. Demographic risk factors alone will identify many more subjects potentially at risk than imminently in danger of dying (Goldberg 1987).

Despite hundreds of studies over decades that have drawn dozens of epidemiological correlations between suicide and particular descriptors, no effective screening paradigm has been identified. This situation is no different with suicidality in medical illness. Many medical illnesses have been associated with increased suicide attempts; for example, in one study, an elevated odds ratio (OR) for suicide was found in lung disease (OR = 1.8) and peptic ulcer disease (OR = 2.1) (Goodwin et al. 2003). A Canadian study showed elevated ORs for completed suicide in cancer (1.73), prostate disease (1.70), and chronic pulmonary disease (1.86) (Quan et al. 2002). In a Swedish study, visual impairment (OR = 7.00), neurological disorders (OR = 3.8), and malignancy (OR = 3.4) were independently associated with suicide (Waern et al. 2002). In U.S. dialysis patients, the OR for suicide was calculated at 1.84 (Kurella et al. 2005). Nevertheless, these increased rates are still too low to consider the medical diagnosis a predictor of suicide. Moreover, no epidemiological risk factor represents an individual's suicide intent—the essential, highly personal variable in suicide prediction (Davidson 1993). Fortunately, the field of suicidology has shifted from trying to predict individual suicides to a more realistic goal of estimating probabilities of risk for particular subpopulations (Hughes and Kleespies 2001). Such data can then be used to inform the psychiatrist's assessment of an individual patient's suicide threat while also considering the personal meaning of the patient's communication.

A focus on probabilities of risk and general categories of psychiatric symptoms rather than individual diagnoses lends itself well to understanding suicidality in the medically ill. Medical illness by itself is rarely a sole determinant of suicide potential. Comorbid factors drive what is best understood as a multidetermined act (Hughes and Kleespies 2001). Shneidman (1989), the father of American suicidology, conceptualized a cubic model of suicidal states, incorporating *perturbation* (the state of being stirred up or upset), *pain* (psychological pain resulting from frustrated psychological needs), and *press* (genetic and developmental susceptibility to particular events). Moscicki (1995) envisioned two distinct but interactive groups of risk factors, with recent events—"proximal risk factors"—unfolding on a substrate of underlying "distal" conditions. According to both models, the assessment of a medically ill person—as with any suicidal person—demands attention not only to current events but also to what past characterological, temperamental, or experiential features push someone toward suicide.

In Mann's (1998) diathesis-stress model of suicidal behavior, *stresses* resemble Moscicki's proximal factors, and *diatheses* resemble her distal ones (Figure 9-1). Noting that

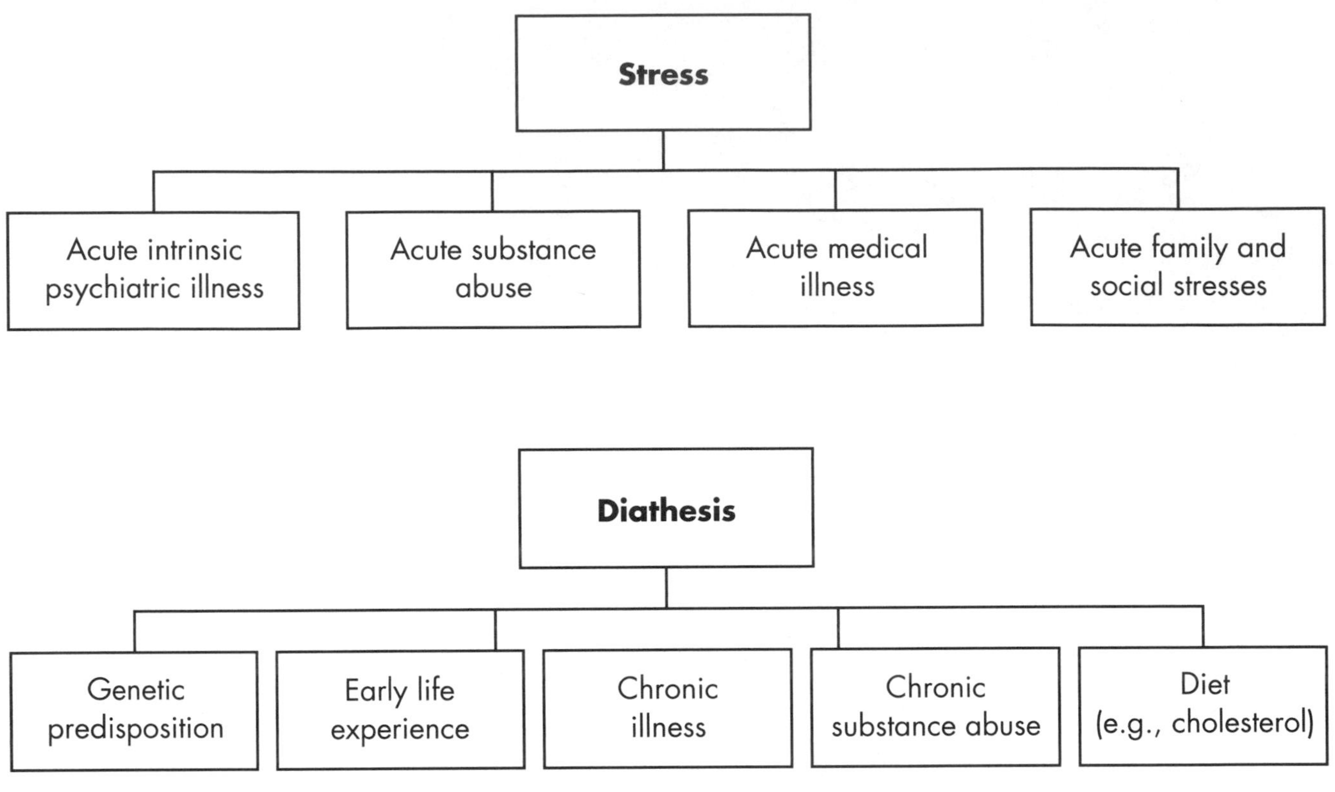

FIGURE 9–1. Diathesis–stress model of suicidal behavior: components of stress and diathesis.
Source. Adapted from Mann JJ: "The Neurobiology of Suicide." *Nature Medicine* 4:25–30, 1998. Copyright 1998. Used with permission.

two groups of patients, each with the same severity of depressive illness, attempt suicide at different rates, Mann proposed suicide diathesis components, including genetic predisposition, early life experience, chronic illness, chronic substance abuse, and certain dietary factors. Extreme stress alone, which Mann defined as acute psychiatric illness, intoxication, medical illness, or family and social stresses, is not typically enough to invoke suicidal behavior. A suicidal individual already has the predisposition, or diathesis, on which the stress is superimposed, resulting in the suicide attempt (Mann 1998).

Mann's subcategories adapt readily to the medically ill. Acute intrinsic psychiatric illness is represented by dementia, depression, delirium, and anxiety in the context of a general medical illness. Acute substance abuse appears in the form of intoxication or withdrawal syndromes. Acute medical illness includes not only the disease itself but also the effects of treatments. Acute family and social stresses could include fears of becoming a burden, financial consequences such as expense of treatment and lost income, and disruption in the family members' lives. These state phenomena occur against the background of trait characteristics, which Mann labels as *diathesis.* Diatheses include genetic predisposition to illness, coping styles and personality characteristics (e.g., pain tolerance), and the long-term effects of chronic physical illness or substance abuse.

The Mann model, though comprehensive, does not inform the psychiatrist whether a particular patient is at immediate risk for suicide. Litman (1989) noted that the 95% prevalence of psychiatric illness among individuals who commit suicide is derived from psychological autopsies and retrospective studies, the scientific equivalent of Monday-morning quarterbacking. At any moment, very few of those who are "at risk" will die by suicide. Identifying the medical patient at high risk is just a first step in evaluation. The search for possible biological markers for suicide has focused on the midbrain dorsal and median raphe nuclei, with their serotonergic inputs to the ventral prefrontal cortex. Responsible for dampening aggressive or impulsive behavior, the ventral prefrontal cortex exerts its inhibitory effects on suicidal behavior less effectively when serotonergic hypofunction occurs (Kamali et al. 2001). A history of child abuse, a familial depression history, substance abuse, head injury, genetic variants, and low cholesterol levels are all associated with both lower serotonergic activity and greater suicide risk (Mann 1998). No practical test based on these psychobiological research advances currently exists. If a test were available, it would likely provide only one more risk factor in a complex biopsychosocial formulation.

Kishi and Kathol (2002) identified four "pragmatic reasons" for suicidality: 1) psychosis, 2) depression, 3) poor impulse control, and 4) philosophical reasons. White et al. (1995) subdivided the suicidal medically ill into three general categories: 1) patients admitted to a medical-surgical bed after a suicide attempt, 2) patients with delirium and resultant agitation and impulsivity, and 3) patients with chronic medical illness causing frustration or hopelessness.

In this chapter, we integrate these two approaches first by reviewing the general epidemiology of suicide and suicide attempts and then by discussing psychodynamic and social factors. The next section concerns the management of the medical and surgical consequences of a suicide attempt and the care of high-risk patients on medical inpatient units. Suicide in the medically ill is reviewed next, exemplified by a focus on cancer, end-stage renal disease, and AIDS. Finally, we address physician-assisted suicide.

Epidemiology

Suicide assessment begins with demographic clues to the patient's relative risk of suicide. Both descriptive and dynamic risk factors are important. In this section, we review descriptive risk factors—comparatively static characteristics of the individual. As the subsequent sections make clear, however, changes in psychiatric status coupled with recent life events are crucial in understanding suicidality in the medically ill.

Completed Suicide

Reported suicide was the eleventh leading cause of death in the United States in 2006, with 33,300 suicides comprising 1.4% of all deaths (McIntosh 2009). The known suicide rate today is nearly identical to what it was in 1900 (Monk 1987), but the epidemiology of suicide has been shifting over the past few decades. Between 1990 and 2001, suicide rates decreased in every age category, with the overall annual rate in the United States declining from 12.4 to 10.8 per 100,000. Over the most recent 5 years for which statistics are available, however, the rate has ticked up in several age groups—as has the overall rate, to 11.1 per 100,000. In 2006, annual suicide rates per 100,000 individuals increased over the life span—from 0.5 in 5- to 14-year-olds and 9.9 in 15- to 24-year-olds to 15.9 in those ages 85 years and older. In 15- to 24-year-olds, suicide ranks behind only accidents and homicide as a leading cause of death (McIntosh 2009). The suicide rate among men is 3.8 times higher than that among women. Nonwhite Americans killed themselves in 2006 at less than half the rate of white Americans (McIntosh 2009).

Over the course of the life cycle, men and women show different patterns of suicide. For men, suicide rates gradually rise during adolescence, increase sharply in early adulthood, and then decrease before starting an upward trajectory in midlife, increasing into the 75- to 84-year age bracket and beyond (Shneidman 1989). Suicide rates for women peak in midlife and then decrease, in contrast to the bimodal peaks for men. Men's suicide methods tend to be more violent and lethal; men are more likely to die by hanging, drowning, and shooting. Women are less likely to die in suicide attempts because they are more likely to choose the less lethal methods of wrist cutting and overdose (Kaplan and Klein 1989; A. Morgan 1989). Traditionally, epidemiological studies have shown that suicide attempters are more likely to be younger, female, and married and to use pills, whereas completers are more likely to be older, male, and single and to use violent means (Fawcett and Shaughnessy 1988). However, anyone at any age may contemplate or execute suicide.

History of a suicide attempt is an important predictor of future suicide risk (Pokorny 1983). One of every 100 suicide attempt survivors will die by suicide within 1 year of the index attempt, a suicide risk approximately 100 times that for the general population (Hawton 1992). Twenty-five percent of chronically self-destructive or suicidal individuals will eventually kill themselves (Litman 1989). Of those who complete suicide, 25%–50% have tried before (Patterson et al. 1983). A Danish study of patients admitted to a psychiatric unit after a suicide attempt reported that 12% successfully completed suicide within the next 5 years, 75% within 6 months of their last admission (Nielsen et al. 1990). Bostwick and Pankratz (2000) found that depressed patients who had suicidal ideation or who had just made a suicide attempt had a lifetime prevalence of suicide of 8.6%. Palmer et al. (2005) determined that three-fourths of suicides in schizophrenic patients occur within 10 years of the first admission or first diagnosis.

It has been repeatedly shown in general population U.S. and European retrospective psychological autopsy studies over the last half-century that psychiatric illness—particularly depression and alcoholism—is associated with the vast majority of completed suicides (Barraclough et al. 1974; Dorpat and Ripley 1960; Robins et al. 1959; Roy 1989). Most patients had not been identified before death as being psychiatrically ill, however, and had not received treatment.

Many suicides are committed by patients with active alcohol and other substance use disorders. In one study, 43% of the suicide attempters were using alcohol at the time of the attempts (Hall et al. 1999). An Australian study of completed suicides by methods other than overdose found that 41% had been drinking alcohol and 20% had been using illicit drugs (Darke et al. 2009). Although alcohol abusers may kill themselves at any age, especially when acute intoxication clouds their judgment and disinhibits them, those with chronic alcoholism tend to commit suicide after their relationships, work performance, and health are all in decay. Murphy and Weitzel (1990) estimated that 3.4% of alcoholic patients kill themselves, a rate that is nearly three times the lifetime risk in the general population (Murphy and Weitzel 1990). Most of the higher suicide rates among men may be accounted for by the higher rates of alcoholism among men (Klerman 1987).

Alcoholic patients often commit suicide in response to crises in their personal lives. One-third of alcoholic individuals who kill themselves have lost a close relationship within the previous 6 weeks, and another one-third anticipate such a loss (Murphy 1992). Alcoholic patients frequently have numerous other suicide risk factors, many resulting from their substance abuse, including comorbid major depression, estrangement from family and social supports, unemployment, and serious medical illness. People who abuse other psychoactive substances also have high suicide rates. For example, opiate-dependent patients kill themselves at 20 times the expected rate (Miles 1977), although inadvertent overdoses may constitute part of this number.

The audience for this chapter constitutes a group at particularly high risk. Physicians kill themselves at much higher rates than the people they treat. In comparison with the general population, male doctors have a relative risk of suicide of up to 3.4; for female doctors, the relative risk has been calculated to be as high as 5.7 (Center et al. 2003). Whereas suicide rates of men and women in the general population are widely disparate, they are nearly equal in male and female physicians (Center et al. 2003). More recent studies have found that the rate in female physicians now exceeds that in males (Lagro-Janssen and Luijks 2008; Petersen and Burnett 2008). Medical students and residents are not immune. Although they begin medical school with the same rates of depression as their nonmedical peers, depression prevalence in medical trainees soon outstrips that in their peers (Rosenthal and Okie 2005). Suicide rates are also higher in trainees than their nonmedical counterparts (Reynolds and Clayton 2009).

Attempted Suicide

An estimated 832,500 suicide attempts occurred in the United States in 2006, 25 times more than completed suicides (McIntosh 2009). Although there are important differences, attempted suicides are not a discrete category from completed ones, particularly in the medically ill. Suicide attempts occur across spectra of lethality of intent and lethality of effect, which may or may not coincide. Some patients deliberately plan death but naively choose a nonlethal method (e.g., benzodiazepine overdose), whereas others only intend gestures but unwittingly select a fatal method (e.g., acetaminophen overdose). At the more severe end of the spectrum, suicide attempters resemble completers. In a New Zealand study, Beautrais (2001) compared individuals who died by suicide with those who made very serious attempts. She found that they shared the same predictors, including current psychiatric disorder, history of suicide attempts, previous psychiatric care and contact, social disadvantage, and exposure to recent stressful life events.

Nonetheless, some characteristics distinguish surviving attempters from those who die. In the study by Hall et al. (1999) of serious suicide attempters, the patients, by and large, did not have long-standing mental illness or carefully considered plans. They did not have command hallucinations and were not particularly ruminative about their suicidal intent. Whereas 80% had symptoms of an anxiety or a depressive disorder, few had chronic symptoms. Patients who overdose are more likely to survive because they have time after the act to reconsider (or be found) and undergo medical treatment, infrequent options after a jump or a gunshot wound. As with completed suicides, demographics change over the life cycle. The ratio of attempts to death in the young is 100–200:1, but by old age, it narrows precipitously to 4:1.

Hackett and Stern (1991) reported that 1%–2% of all patients evaluated in the Massachusetts General Hospital emergency department had overdosed, and 47% of these required admission—one-half to medical-surgical wards and one-half to psychiatric units. Of the patients, 85% had overdosed on benzodiazepines, alcohol, nonnarcotic analgesics, antidepressants, barbiturates, or antihistamines/anticholinergics.

Medical illness is a common factor in suicide attempters admitted to general psychiatry units. In a 1-year sample of admissions to a Danish psychiatry unit, 52% of the individuals had a somatic disease, and 21% took daily analgesic medications for pain. The somatic group was older, and most had neurological or musculoskeletal conditions in conjunction with depression that was more severe than in the nonsomatic group (Stenager et al. 1994). In the study by Hall et al. (1999) of 100 serious suicide attempters, 41% had a chronic, deteriorating medical illness, and 9% had recently received a diagnosis of a life-threatening illness.

Psychodynamic and Social Factors

Litman (1989) described a *presuicidal syndrome,* a change in cognitive set, that characterizes lethal attempts and completed suicides. The presuicidal patient in crisis has constricted choices and perception, a tunnel vision of life as hopeless, physical tension, and emotional perturbation. The tension and distress may be relieved by a fantasy of death. The hopelessness is combined with help rejection and distrust. Often the patient has a long-term disposition toward impulsive action, an all-or-nothing approach to problems, and the characterological attitude "my way or no way."

Klerman (1987) framed the presuicidal crisis in terms of a medical model—as the result of an underlying condition, the patient has lost the capacity for rational thought. The hopelessness and helplessness of severe depression may have reached irrational proportions. Auditory hallucinations may be commanding self-harm. Clouded sensorium, impaired judgment, and the disinhibition and misperceptions of delirium, intoxication, or substance withdrawal all may be causing the patient to act in uncharacteristically self-destructive or dangerous ways.

Gardner and Cowdry (1985) divided suicidal behavior into four categories, each with its own affective state, motivation, and outcome:

1. *True suicidal acts* are characterized by intense melancholia and despair, a wish for release from emotional pain, and the highest risk of completed suicide, given the likelihood of careful planning and a high-risk to low-rescue ratio.
2. *Retributive rage* is characterized by impulsiveness, vengefulness, and a nihilistic, constricted capacity to see other immediate options.
3. *Parasuicidal gesturing*, often repetitive and tinged with strong dependency needs, appears to be a form of communication, designed to extract a response from a significant other.
4. *Self-mutilation* serves the purpose of relieving dysphoria, a form of "indirect self-destructive behaviors" (N. Farberow 2000).

Only the first category includes the *intent* to die, but any of the four can be lethal.

An early study of personality factors and suicide among medically ill patients identified a "dependent-dissatisfied" behavior pattern among the patients who committed suicide (L. Farberow et al. 1966). Many subsequent investigators have added to the picture of the types of personality structure or cognitive styles that lend themselves to suicidal ideation or behavior. Berger (1995) observed that rational-seeming suicides were unusual in his study of the medically ill and that suicides in this population were correlated with maladaptive emotional reactions. Describing the role of hopelessness in the thinking of terminally ill cancer patients who wished for hastened death, Breitbart et al. (2000) found the hopelessness to represent a pessimistic cognitive style rather than an accurate assessment of poor prognosis. That is, patients wished to speed death not because they were mortally ill but because they were chronically pessimistic. A similar finding came from Goodwin and Olfson's (2002) study of suicidal ideation in nearly 2,600 patients with physical illness diagnoses. Perception of poor health was a significant predictor of suicidal ideation, even after controlling for psychiatric disorders, physical conditions, and other factors. While a high score on a commonly used instrument such as the Beck Hopelessness Scale identifies a group at elevated risk, McMillan et al. (2007) caution that poor specificity limits the scale's utility in predicting which individuals in the group will actually kill themselves. Nonetheless, combating hopelessness per se in medically ill patients cannot be a bad thing, even if it doesn't pick out the suicidal among them.

One conclusion to be drawn from these studies is that a tendency of patients and medical providers alike to attribute hopelessness to the disease—the proximal factor—has resulted in a failure to recognize the mental disorder or personality type—the distal condition—that is actually speaking. "There has been a tendency to regard the suicide of a victim of severe medical illness, such as cancer, as a rational alternative to the distress caused by the disease," concluded Suominen et al. (2002) after analyzing a year's worth of suicides in Finland. "On the other hand, most suicide victims with physical illness have suffered from concurrent mental disorder.... Mental disorders may thus have a mediating role between medical disorder and suicide" (p. 412).

Suicide is often a response to a loss, real or imagined. To help assess the meaning of suicidal ideation or behavior, psychiatrists must inquire about recent or anticipated losses and coping strategies that the patient has used with past losses (Davidson 1993). Fantasies of revenge, punishment, reconciliation with a rejecting object, relief from the pain of loss, or reunion with a dead loved one may be evident (Furst and Ostow 1979).

A patient's degree of autonomy and extent of dependency on external sources of emotional support can shed light on the level of psychic resilience (Buie and Maltsberger 1989). A recent loss of a loved one or a parental loss during childhood increases suicide risk. Holidays and anniversaries of important days in the life and death of the deceased person, when the loved one's absence is experienced more intensely, also increase the risk for suicide. In medical settings, what may be lost is a part of one's self. It may be tangible—an organ, a limb, sexual potency—or intangible—a sense of youthfulness, health, or invincibility. Glickman (1980) believed that a suicidal patient cannot be judged safe until he or she has either regained the lost object, accepted its loss, or replaced it with a new object.

A social services intervention is likely to identify remediable contributors to suicidal states, particularly if the medical evaluation has not delved into the patient's social and interpersonal context. In the largest psychological autopsy study conducted to date, which interviewed informants for 100 individuals age 60 years or older who killed themselves, Harwood et al. (2006) found, not unexpectedly, that physical illness—particularly pain and increased physical dependence—contributed to 62 of the suicides. Interpersonal issues, including conflict and health worries about another person, factored in 31, and bereavement—both the recent death of a loved one and long-term social problems resulting from that death—influenced 25. Lesser contributors included impending relocation to a nursing home, financial distress, and occupational or retirement concerns. Once again, separate from whether these contributors to suicidal states are independent suicide predictors, they are stresses that in Mann's model help create the setting for a suicidal crisis.

Psychiatrists must monitor themselves for reactions and countertransference feelings toward suicidal patients. In medical settings, consulting psychiatrists help other health care professionals identify and overcome their countertransference reactions as well. These include the classic reactions of "countertransference hate" (Maltsberger and Buie 1974), in which aversion to the suicidal patient (conscious or unconscious) leads to acting angrily toward the patient or withdrawing to an aloof passivity, both of which increase the risk for suicide. Overidentification with seriously medically ill patients may lead to other countertransference reactions. For example, in response to a hopeless patient, the psychiatrist may become overly pessimistic or too reassuring.

Management in Medical Inpatient Settings

For a patient who survives a recent suicide attempt, the emergency department usually is the first stop for assessment and triage. If the patient is medically cleared, ideally a psychiatrist, but sometimes another mental health professional, evaluates the patient and decides whether psychiatric inpatient or outpatient management is the appropriate disposition. It is important for psychiatrists to form their own judgment about whether patients are truly medically stable enough for transfer out of the medical setting. Countertransference reactions to suicidal states frequently cause nonpsychiatric physicians to minimize the role of medical contributions and prematurely "clear" patients. Once a patient is labeled "psychiatric," tunnel vision in initial evaluators may preclude performance of a comprehensive medical workup. For a patient with self-induced injuries severe enough to require additional medical or surgical care, admission follows, and a psychiatrist is consulted. Patients who are admitted to medical-surgical beds after suicide attempts represent a particularly dangerous subset of suicidal patients. Considering data from all of New Zealand's public hospitals, Conner et al. (2003) showed that individuals hospitalized with self-induced injuries have a relative risk of 105.4 for suicide within the next year and a relative risk of 175.7 for additional self-injury hospitalizations, compared with the New Zealand general population.

Divergent conditions such as delirium, psychosis, personality disorder, and intoxication and withdrawal syndromes have in common the impulsivity that must be anticipated and managed in medical settings. Withdrawal—particularly from alcohol or sedative-hypnotics—epitomizes impulsivity syndromes that can be deadly and must be recognized and aggressively managed with detoxification protocols. In the absence of a suitably equipped psychiatric unit, the psychiatrist will need to arrange medical admission.

In addition to trying to make the environment safe, egress must be controlled. In the general medical hospital, patients should be prevented access to open stairwells, roofs, and balconies, and all windows should be secured (Berger 1995; Bostwick and Rackley 2007). In a classic study of the dangers of hospitalizing impulsive patients in an unsecured environment, Reich and Kelly (1976) described 17 medical inpatients who attempted suicide while on the medical and surgical wards at Peter Bent Brigham Hospital between 1967 and 1973 and survived. They judged 15 of the 17 patients to have mental disorders, but the cardinal characteristics of depression and hopelessness were not present in this sample. "All...were impulsive acts, none of the patients gave warnings, left notes, expressed suicidal thoughts or appeared to be seriously depressed" (Reich and Kelly 1976, p. 300). The investigators considered most of these 17 attempts to be reactions motivated by anger at perceived loss of emotional support, usually from staff. They attributed this underlying impaired impulse control to personality disorders in 8 of the patients, to psychosis in 7, and to delirium in 3.

When a suicidal or an impulsive patient is too medically ill to be cared for on a locked general psychiatry unit, a medical-psychiatry unit—if a hospital has one—is the ideal disposition for such a patient. In the absence of such a specialty unit, medical intensive care units are more likely to provide one-to-one nursing care, although critical care physicians may argue that such observation in the absence of need for critical care is an inappropriate use of their service.

Case Vignette

Ms. C, a 22-year-old woman addicted to crack cocaine, developed severe cardiomyopathy after the birth of her third child. Four months later, no longer able to climb the two flights of stairs to her apartment without becoming short of breath, she was admitted to the hospital with congestive heart failure. A toxicology screen was positive for alcohol and cocaine.

After she arrived on the medical floor, Ms. C curled up in a fetal position and refused to speak to her nurse until she was found lighting a cigarette while receiving oxygen. When the nurse attempted to stop her, Ms. C began cursing and shrieked that if she were not allowed to smoke, she would overdose on digitalis she had hidden in the room.

Ms. C refused to submit to a room search. The psychiatric consultant recommended that security be called so that Ms. C could not leave before he could perform an emergency evaluation. Ms. C had to be placed in leather restraints when she assaulted the officers. After speaking with the psychiatrist, Ms. C agreed to take medication (5 mg of haloperidol and 1 mg of lorazepam). She then consented to a search of her belongings. A bottle of 50 digitalis tablets was found in her suitcase. Because of her threats and impulsivity, the psychiatrist recommended constant observation with sitters.

As Ms. C's case shows, the first task in the medical setting is ensuring the patient's safety (Gutheil and Appelbaum 2000). A safe environment must be created and maintained until the patient is stable enough for psychiatric transfer (Bostwick and Rackley 2007).

Patients who are most intent on suicide, as well as those who are most impulsive and unpredictable, may attempt suicide in the hospital. In order to secure a patient's room, staff must "think like a suicide" (Bostwick and Lineberry 2009)—that is, anything that patients could potentially use to injure themselves must be removed. Luggage and possessions should be searched with a suspicious eye and a morbid imagination. Staff must ferret out sharp objects, lighters, belts, caches of pills—anything that could inflict damage in either an impulsive or a carefully planned way. Special attention should be paid to items that could be used for self-strangulation, including drapery cords, belts, shoelaces, ties, and other items of clothing (Tishler and Reiss 2009). Objects that are being brought into the room must be regarded as potential hazards (e.g., the phlebotomist's needles, the pop-tops from soft drink cans, the custodian's disinfectants, the meal utensils). The rooms of the general medical hospital lack many of the safeguards that are routine on inpatient psychiatric units, such as locked unit entrances, secured windows, and collapsible shower heads, curtain rods, and light fixtures. Normally, in the former, scissors and a variety of paraphernalia that can be "creatively" used for self-harm are easily accessible. The culture on medical inpatient units also differs from that on psychiatric units. On medical units, staff do not usually consider elopement a risk; they assume that patients are fundamentally compliant and that they will press their call buttons when they need help (Kelly et al. 1999).

Early reports focused on jumping as a means of suicide in medically hospitalized patients (N. Farberow and Litman 1970; Glickman 1980; Pollack 1957), a readily available and usually lethal method regardless of whether the patient actually intends to die. In the most recent study, White et al. (1995) identified impulsivity and agitation in many of the 12 patients who jumped from an Australian general hospital during a 12-year period. Five had been noted to be delirious on the day of the jump, 7 were dyspneic, and 10 were in pain. Ten of the 12 had two of these factors, and 1 had all three factors.

Modern hospitals are deliberately built without open stairwells and without windows that open or break easily; however, many older buildings remain in service, indicating the persistent need for corrective precautions. The inpatient suicide rate in a New York hospital dropped fivefold during the first 11 years after the hospital secured the windows and implemented educational programs encouraging staff members to pay closer attention to disruption in the doctor-patient relationship (Pisetsky and Brown 1979; Sanders 1988).

Shah and Ganesvaran (1997) found that one-third of 103 suicides committed by psychiatric inpatients at their hospital involved patients away on pass, and another one-third involved patients away from the hospital without permission. Methods readily available near the hospital include jumping in front of vehicles, leaping from buildings or bridges, and drowning in nearby bodies of water (H. Morgan and Priest 1991). Although these authors studied psychiatric inpatients, the same dangers exist with patients on medical units. Passes are rarely given from contemporary medical units, but elopements are all too common, with resultant ready access to potentially lethal means of suicide.

Constant observation by a one-to-one sitter is indicated for patients judged at high risk for impulsive self-harm. This may require compromising patients' privacy. Patients permitted to use the bathroom unobserved have been known to hang or cut themselves behind the closed door. A moment of privacy granted to the patient out of misplaced civility, or a few minutes of inattention or absence by the sitter, may be all the time a suicidal person needs to execute a suicide plan. All staff guarding suicidal patients should know how to summon security personnel as reinforcements when they perceive that they have lost control of the patient or the situation. In an era of cost cutting, the consultant may feel pressure to limit the use of constant observation. Economizing on sitters could mean the life of a suicidal patient. On the other hand, staff anxiety may lead to overuse, initiating one-to-one sitters for every patient who has expressed any suicidal thoughts. In addition to wasting resources, overuse of sitters may desensitize them to the constant awareness needed for their role. The decision to use constant observation should be made on clinical grounds; constant observation is not just a protective intervention but also one that has therapeutic potential (Cardell and Pitula 1999). However, there are no published data examining whether constant observation reduces the risk of suicide in the hospital (Jaworowski et al. 2008). Prudent risk management supports avoiding under- and overuse of one-to-one sitters.

After the environment is secured, the medical psychiatrist should search for reversible contributors to the impulsive state, including delirium (see Chapter 5, "Delirium"), medical illness or medications that may be contributing to mood (see Chapter 8, "Depression"), anxiety (see Chapter 11, "Anxiety Disorders"), and psychotic disorders (see Chapter 10, "Psychosis, Mania, and Catatonia").

Agitation and active suicide attempts in the hospital often require chemical restraints and, rarely, physical restraints. Antipsychotics should be used in patients with hyperactive delirium or psychosis, and antipsychotics and/or benzodiazepines should be given to other agitated, anxious patients. Physical restraints may be required if other measures prove inadequate. In some cases, emergent electroconvulsive therapy may be necessary (see Chapter 40, "Electroconvulsive Therapy").

Suicide in the Medically Ill

Physical disease is present in a high proportion of people who commit suicide. Several large studies have identified the presence of medical illness in 30%–40% of the patients who committed suicide (Hughes and Kleespies 2001). However, most of these suicides do not occur during medical hospitalization. About 2% of Finnish suicides occurred in medical or surgical inpatients (Suominen et al. 2002). In Montreal, Quebec, about 3% of the suicides were in general hospital inpatients, of which one-third (1%) were medical-surgical patients (Proulx et al. 1997). During a 10-year period in a 3,000-bed Chinese medical hospital, there were 75 self-destructive acts, only 15 of which proved fatal (Hung et al. 2000).

Sanders (1988) reviewed six studies of inpatients at a general hospital who committed suicide. Most had one or more chronic or terminal illnesses or sequelae that were painful, debilitating, or both, including dyspnea, ostomies, or disfiguring surgery. Harris and Barraclough (1994) compiled a list of 63 medical disorders noted in the medical literature as potentially having elevated suicide risk. In their meta-analysis, they concluded that the only disorders that actually elevated suicide risk were HIV and AIDS, Huntington's disease, cancer (particularly head and neck), multiple sclerosis, peptic ulcer disease, end-stage renal disease, spinal cord injuries, and systemic lupus erythematosus. More recent studies confirm or add to a seemingly arbitrary list of medical conditions associated with risk for suicide. In a Canadian study, cancer, prostate disease, and chronic pulmonary disease were associated with suicide ORs of 1.70–1.86 among adults older than 55 years with versus without the diseases (Quan et al. 2002). In the previously cited Chinese study of patients who committed suicide in a general hospital, 40% had cancer, 13% had neurological disease, 13% had cardiovascular disease, and 7% had liver failure (Hung et al. 2000). In the Montreal study, associated diagnoses included cardiovascular disease, abdominal pain, cerebrovascular disease, Parkinson's disease, and rheumatoid arthritis (Proulx et al. 1997). Of 12 patients who jumped from an Australian hospital between 1980 and 1991, 4 had delirium, 4 had terminal cancer, 2 had advanced lung disease, and 1 had irreversible cardiac failure (White et al. 1995). However, these studies were small and did not capture suicides in the medically ill attempted or completed outside the hospital, so they cannot be used to construct a list of "most suicidal" medical disorders.

A study drawing on the U.S. National Comorbidity Survey identified a dozen general medical diagnostic categories with statistically significantly elevated ORs for suicide attempts, most ranging from 1.1 to 3.2, except for AIDS (133.9) and hernia (10.4) (Goodwin et al. 2003). Clinically, however, use of a diagnosis alone in estimating suicide risk is not helpful. Even though the OR in each of the 12 categories achieved statistical significance, substituting a rate only slightly higher than the very low base rate offers little to guide clinical decision making, particularly if this is the only indicator being used to predict suicide.

What does appear useful is evidence that suicides in the medically ill—as in the general population—seem to be related to frequently unrecognized comorbid psychiatric illnesses, including depression, substance-related disorders, delirium, dementia, and personality disorders (Davidson 1993; Kellner et al. 1985). In their study of the role of physical disease in 416 Swedish suicides, Stensman and Sundqvist-Stensman (1988) concluded that although somatic disease was one important factor in the suicidal act, psychiatric conditions such as depression and alcohol abuse had even more significant roles.

Suicidality is also not a static phenomenon over an illness course. For example, there are two time periods during Huntington's disease—1) when the patient has become aware of neurological changes but does not yet have a confirmed diagnosis, and 2) when cognitive and physical symptoms have developed enough to curtail independent living—when suicidal ideation is particularly prominent (Paulsen et al. 2005). A Danish study of suicide risk in epilepsy showed an overall relative risk of 3.17 compared with the general population but found that both illness chronology and the presence of psychiatric comorbidity influenced risk, in some cases synergistically. For the overall group, suicide relative risk in the 6 months after diagnosis was 5.35. Psychiatrically ill patients with epilepsy had an overall relative risk of 13.7, with the relative risk in the first 6 months after epilepsy diagnosis more than double, at 29.2 (Christensen et al. 2007).

The presence of standard risk factors that transcend medical illness may be more predictive of suicidality than particular disease characteristics. In U.S. dialysis patients, advanced age, male sex, Caucasian or Asian race, substance dependence, geographic region of the country, and recent psychiatric hospitalization all reached significance as independent predictors of completed suicide (Kurella et al. 2005). In chronic pain patients, family history of suicide and access to potentially lethal medications, in addition to abdominal pain, were significantly associated with both passive and active suicidal ideation, while severity of pain and depression were not (Smith et al. 2004). Tending to these basic risk factors should not be overlooked, even in the face of devastating physical illness.

Rather than focusing on particular medical diagnoses, it will be more fruitful for the medical psychiatrist to determine whether a suicide-prone psychiatric condition is present in a medically ill patient, whether the patient is at a particularly emotionally difficult time in his or her illness course, and whether secondary effects of the medical illness—pain, physical disfigurement, cognitive dysfunction, and disinhibition—are present that add to the risk. Much can be done to help. In a review of the literature of suicide in chronic pain patients, in whom they estimate that suicide risk is doubled, Tang and Crane (2006) identified specific pain-induced risk factors, including sleep-onset insomnia, hopelessness, catastrophizing, desire for escape, and problem-solving deficits, all of which respond to psychological interventions. Reduction in intensity in any category may de-escalate suicidal urges.

It must be emphasized that no matter how horrific the medical condition, significant suicide risk is not the rule, and when suicidality does emerge, it is frequently linked to specific illness stages or mental states. According to Brown et al. (1986), most terminally ill patients do not develop severe depression, and suicidality is closely associated with the presence of a depressive disorder. In the study of terminally ill cancer patients by Breitbart et al. (2000), only 17% had a high desire for hastened death, for which depression and hopelessness were the strongest predictors. Feeling that one is a burden on others is an important and underestimated factor contributing to suicidality in the terminally ill (Wilson et al. 2005). An important empirical finding in a Canadian study was that the will to live in the terminally ill fluctuates, mostly predicted by depression, anxiety, shortness of breath, and sense of well-being (Chochinov et al. 1999).

Three diagnoses—cancer, end-stage renal disease, and AIDS—are discussed here in detail to illustrate these points further. These comparatively common conditions underscore principles that can be extrapolated to the breadth of diagnoses and situations encountered in medical settings.

Cancer

Recent population studies replicate what has been known for decades: cancer patients have an elevated suicide risk compared with the general population. In a U.S. cohort of nearly 3.6 million individuals diagnosed with cancer between 1973 and 2002, the standardized mortality ratio (SMR) for suicide was 1.9 relative to the general population. Highest risks were found for lung and bronchial (SMR=5.74), stomach (SMR=4.68), oral-pharyngeal (SMR=3.66), and laryngeal cancer (SMR=2.83). As in the general population, older white men were at particularly high risk. The first 5-year period after diagnosis was the time of highest risk, although elevated risk persisted after 15 years (Misono et al. 2008).

In a U.S. sample of 1.3 million cancer patients, Kendal (2007) found that males had 6.2 times the suicide risk of females, a mirroring of general population statistics. Kendal's composite high-risk patient was a widower with metastatic head and neck cancer or myeloma (both painful) with limited social support and limited treatment options. His composite low-risk example was an African American married woman with localized cervical or colorectal cancer. Unlike terminally ill cancer patients, in whom elevated suicide risk is associated with hopelessness, cancer patients in remission had suicide risk factors similar to those established in the general population, including personal or family psychiatric illness and previous history of suicide attempts.

Through the lens of prognosis, a study from Western Australia sharpens the focus on which cancer patients are at increased risk and when (Dormer et al. 2008). With an SMR of 3.39, the poor-prognosis group had nearly four times the suicide risk of the good-prognosis group (SMR=0.86). The first 3 months after diagnosis was the period of highest risk, with particularly marked lethality at this time in the poor-prognosis group confronting the lack of treatment for their conditions. A second period of increased risk occurred at 12–14 months, the likeliest time of recurrence or acknowledgment of treatment failure. A U.K. study found that the relative risk of suicide in cancer patients was greatest in the first year after diagnosis and also greater in individuals diagnosed with cancers with high fatality (Robinson et al. 2009). A study in Taiwan found that almost half of suicides in cancer patients occurred within the first 2 weeks after hospital discharge (Lin et al. 2009).

Consistent with the Australian study, Björkenstam et al. (2005) in Sweden demonstrated a reciprocal relationship between cancer prognosis and suicide risk. The lower the survival rate, the higher the suicide rate, with the highest rates in pancreatic, esophageal, hepatocellular, and pulmonary cancers, conditions known for being painful and having strongly deleterious effects on quality of life. Among medical illnesses, cancer may even have a singular relationship to suicide. In a study using conditional logistic regression in a U.S. sample of 1,408 individuals age 65 years and older, cancer was the only medical diagnosis still associated with suicide in adjusted analyses, with an odds ratio of 2.3 (Miller et al. 2008).

Cancer patients who die by suicide are psychiatrically similar to noncancer patients, particularly when the cancer is in remission. In a case-control study of 60 suicides in individuals with cancer and 60 age- and sex-matched comparison suicides in individuals without a cancer history, Henriksson et al. (1995) found that most of the patients with cancer who committed suicide—as well as the control subjects without cancer—had a diagnosable psychiatric disorder. Terminally ill cancer patients had lower rates of depression and alcohol dependence than did patients in remission (72% vs. 96%), but nearly three-quarters still met criteria for a depressive disorder. As a group, cancer patients had fewer psychotic disorders than did control subjects. Allebeck et al. (1985) observed that the longer the time from diagnosis of cancer, the lower the relative risk for suicide in a Swedish cohort. In the first year after diagnosis, the relative risk was 16.0 for men and 15.4 for women. From 1 to 2 years, the ratio decreased to 6.5 for men and 7.0 for women. By 3–6 years, the ratio was 2.1 for men and 3.2 for women. By 10 years after diagnosis, the rate, at 0.4, was actually less than one-half that in the general population. A study of Japanese cancer patients found the highest risk of suicide soon after patients had been discharged from the hospital, with an elevated relative risk the first 5 years after diagnosis compared with the general population and disappearing thereafter (Tanaka et al. 1999).

The fear of pain, disfigurement, and loss of function that cancer evokes in patients' imaginations can precipitate suicide, especially early in the course if the disease. In a large cohort of Italians with cancer, suicide accounted for only 0.2% of the deaths, but the relative risk during the first 6 months after diagnosis was 27.7 (Crocetti et al. 1998). The high relative risk of suicide just after diagnosis comes at a time of overwhelming fear and cognitive overload. In individual patients, important contributing factors (Filiberti et al. 2001) can include overly pessimistic prognosis, exaggerated impressions of anticipated suffering, a physician unintentionally undermining hope, fear of loss of control, or nihilism about treatment. Patients may fear or experience inadequate pain control, lost dignity, compromised privacy, or guilt at having habits that caused the disease. Surgical treatments may be disfiguring, chemotherapy debilitating, and side effects defeminizing or emasculating. As cancer patients live longer with their disease, most become less frightened and less susceptible to suicide.

End-Stage Renal Disease

More formidable than the suicide risk among cancer patients was the purported increase in relative risk of suicide among patients with end-stage renal disease. Abrams et al. (1971) reported very high rates of suicide and suicidal behavior among 3,478 renal dialysis patients studied at 127 dialysis centers. In their sample, 20 deaths were the result of suicide; 17 suicide attempts were unsuccessful; 22 patients withdrew from the program, knowing that doing so would hasten their deaths; and 117 deaths were attributed to noncompliance with treatment. The authors' calculated suicide rate of 400 times that in the general population has been widely quoted but is misleading. In arriving at a 5% figure for suicidal behavior in dialysis patients, they used an extremely broad definition of suicide that encompassed death caused by a wide range of causes, from willful acts of self-destruction to noncompliance. Contemporary studies place suicide risk in dialysis patients at less than double the risk in the general population (Kurella et al. 2005).

Most of the cases that Abrams et al. (1971) called suicide would never come to the attention of psychiatry today. Although their report has been widely cited, no other subsequent study (there have been nearly 20) has defined suicide so broadly (Bostwick and Pankratz 2000). In extreme cases, noncompliance is better understood as a function of personality-disordered behavior; in less dramatic examples, it can be an understandable human response to a burdensome treatment. Deciding to forgo dialysis is not equivalent to suicide (see also Chapter 21, "Renal Disease"). A U.S. study concluded that "most patients who decide to stop dialysis do not seem to be influenced by major depression or ordinary suicidal ideation" (Cohen et al. 2002, p. 889). Even so, depression may play a significant role in some cases and must therefore be ruled out (Cohen and Germain 2005). Treatment withdrawal, negotiated among the patient, significant others, and the treatment team, has become routine as quality of life during dialysis fades. Using parameters of presence or absence of intent to die and presence or absence of collaboration with physicians and significant others in making the decision to die, a recently published model offers help in separating suicide from life-ending acts such as noncompliance and treatment withdrawal; physician-assisted suicide; and end-of-life decisions regarding palliative care (Bostwick and Cohen 2009). The model proceeds from the premise that lumping multiple acts under the rubric of suicide, as Abrams et al. (1971) did, obscures the complexities of end-of-life decision making and inflames critical conversations best undertaken with rational appreciation for distinctions between these diverse exit strategies from life.

In 1,766 Minnesota dialysis patients followed for 17 years, for example, only 3 killed themselves by frank suicide, representing only 2% of the 155 cases in which dialysis was discontinued (Neu and Kjellstrand 1986). The suicide rate in this sample of dialysis patients was only about 15 times that in the general population, which is a considerable rate but much lower than Abrams and colleagues' figure. Haenel et al. (1980) also found less dramatic suicide rates among European patients undergoing chronic dialysis between 1965 and 1978. In Switzerland, dialysis patients killed themselves at about 10 times the rate in the general population. When patients who refused therapy and died as a result were included in the suicide group, the rate was 25 times higher. They also found no statistically significant difference between suicide rates among patients with functioning cadaveric renal transplants and patients undergoing maintenance dialysis, suggesting that transplantation may not in and of itself be associated with decreased suicide risk. Overall, among dialysis patients pooled from all countries belonging to the European Dialysis and Transplant Association, the suicide rate was 108 per 100,000 per year (Haenel et al. 1980). Whether compared with the general population suicide rate of 4–5 per 100,000 in Mediterranean countries or 20–25 per 100,000 in central European or Scandinavian countries, the figure of 108 per 100,000 represents a higher suicide rate, although not orders of magnitude greater than that in the general population.

After nearly a half-century, during which dialysis has become routine treatment for end-stage renal disease, nephrologists have become more sophisticated at negotiating end-of-life decisions with their patients. Practices judged to be tantamount to suicide in the 1960s and 1970s are now considered the standard of care. A survey of U.S. and Canadian nephrologists found that those who perceived themselves as well prepared to guide end-of-life decisions were more likely to discontinue dialysis in general, to stop dialysis in a patient with permanent and severe dementia, and to recommend time-limited dialysis courses and less likely to refer patients to hospice care (Davison et al. 2006). This last finding may not be a good thing. Compared with patients who withdraw from dialysis but do not use hospice, those who use hospice sustain less than half the patient care costs in the last week of life and have one-third the likelihood of dying in the hospital (Murray et al. 2006).

HIV/AIDS

Although the suicide risk has dropped over the past 30 years as HIV/AIDS has evolved from an almost inevitably terminal illness to a chronic one, HIV/AIDS patients continue to have a higher relative risk of suicide. Early data were primarily based on men who had sex with men in the United States in the 1980s, prior the introduction of antiretroviral agents, when an AIDS diagnosis was a virtual death sentence. Much has changed, both in the demographics and geographic distribution of AIDS and in regard to advances in treatment, availability of mental health services, public education, and reduction in stigma and social hysteria. As rates of completed suicide have dropped, the contributions of comorbid risk factors in populations at highest risk for HIV/AIDS—men who have sex with men, injection drug abusers, and poor minority heterosexual women—have come into focus. These risk factors—substance abuse, psychiatric illness, and intimate partner violence—each contribute an independent elevated suicide risk.

In the first, terror-stricken decade of the AIDS epidemic, Marzuk et al. (1988) found a suicide rate in persons with AIDS 36 times that in an age-matched sample of men without AIDS and 66 times that in the general population in New York City in 1985. A dozen years later (1997), when the same group of investigators reexamined this question based on all suicides in New York City in 1991–1993, they concluding that positive HIV serostatus was associated with (at most) a modest elevation in suicide risk (Marzuk et al. 1997). In California in 1986, the rate was 21 times higher than that in the general population (Kizer et al. 1988). In the largest study to date, Cote et al. (1991) charted a continuous decrease in suicide rates over 3 years among AIDS patients in 45 states and the District of Columbia. From 1987 to 1989, a total of 165 suicides among AIDS patients were reported to the National Center for Health Statistics. Of these, 164 were committed by men. The relative suicide risk calculated for AIDS patients was 10.5 in 1987, 7.4 in 1988, and 6.0 in 1989. The authors attributed the decrease to advances in medical care, diminishing social stigma, and improved psychiatric services, while noting probable underreporting of deaths due to both AIDS and suicide (Cote et al. 1991). Frierson and Lippman (1988) suggested that suicide risk also may be increased among HIV-positive but asymptomatic people who fear the eventual illness, HIV-negative people who are worried about contracting the disease, and people who enter suicide pacts with dying loved ones. In a comparison of 15 HIV-infected active-duty members of the U.S. Air Force who attempted suicide with 15 who did not, Rundell et al. (1992) identified several risk factors equivalent to risk factors for suicide in general, including social isolation, perceived lack of social support, adjustment disorder, personality disorder, alcohol abuse, interpersonal or occupational problems, and history of depression.

More recent studies reflect both the changing demographics of HIV and AIDS and the interplay between HIV-positive status and stable classic risk factors for suicidality. Roy (2003) found that almost half of a cohort of HIV-positive substance-dependent patients had attempted suicide. Significantly more of the patients who attempted suicide were young, female, and had a family history of suicidal behavior. Compared with nonattempters, attempters reported more childhood trauma and more comorbid depression and had higher neuroticism scores. A survey in HIV-infected Americans living in rural areas found that 38% had thoughts of suicide during the past week, associated with greater depression and more stigma-related stress and less coping self-efficacy (Heckman et al. 2002).

In a sample of 611 women, Gielen et al. (2005) compared rates of suicidal thoughts and attempts, anxiety, and depression among four subgroups based on HIV status (HIV-positive and HIV-negative) and experience of intimate partner violence (IPV-positive and IPV-negative). Women who were HIV-negative and IPV-negative were least likely to report ever having had suicidal ideation, suicide attempts, or problems with either anxiety or depression. IPV-positive women were more likely than HIV-positive women to report a history of suicide attempts, depression, and anxiety and equally likely to report suicidal ideation. Women positive for both IPV and HIV outstripped the other three subgroups in all four mental health indicators, being three times more likely to have a history of suicidal ideation, eight times more likely to have a history of suicide attempts, four times more likely to have a history of anxiety, and three times more likely to have a history of depression compared with women who were negative for both HIV and IPV.

In a study of 2,909 HIV-positive individuals, 75% of whom were men, 19% reported having suicidal ideation (albeit without intent in the vast majority) within the previous week (Carrico et al. 2007). Suicidal ideation was not evenly distributed, however, but was more likely to be reported by participants who were nonheterosexual, who were experiencing more severe HIV-related symptoms and medication side effects, who used marijuana regularly, and who had depressive symptoms. Suicidal ideation was less likely in Latinos, individuals with a stable romantic relationship, and those who described themselves as having good coping skills.

In a study integrating elements of the Gielen et al. (2005) and Carrico et al. (2007) studies, Cooperman and Simoni (2005) found that having an AIDS diagnosis, acute psychiatric difficulties, or a physical or sexual abuse history significantly predicted both suicidal ideation and suicide attempts. Unexpectedly, having children and being employed also predicted suicidal ideation and suicide attempts, while possessing a well-developed spirituality was negatively associated with either suicidal ideation or suicide attempts. Alone among the three studies, Cooperman and Simoni (2005) identified specific periods of risk in the illness course. Since first receiving an HIV diagnosis, 26% of their sample had made a suicide attempt, 42% within a month of getting the news, and 27% within a week. Earlier studies have indicated that suicide attempts are more likely at the time that physical symptoms first appear and around the time that full-blown AIDS emerges, although the rate then drops again for those living with AIDS (McKegney and O'Dowd 1992; O'Dowd et al. 1993).

Finally, several studies have underscored the possibility that the contribution of HIV/AIDS status to suicidality is incidental or minimal next to more robust population-specific factors. Two studies, one from Italy (Grassi et al. 2001) and one from Brazil (Malbergier and de Andrade 2001), found that although psychiatric morbidity and suicidal ideation or attempts are common in HIV-positive intravenous drug abusers, they are equally common in those who are HIV-negative. A Swiss study of men having sex with men found a high rate of suicide attempts in both HIV-negative and HIV-positive individuals, with moderately more suicidal ideation in those who were HIV-positive (Cochand and Bovet 1998). Dannenberg et al. (1996) compared 4,147 HIV-positive U.S. military service applicants and 12,437 HIV-negative applicants disqualified from military service because of other medical conditions (matched on age, race, sex, and screening date and location); the relative risk for suicide was similar for each group: 2.08 in the HIV-positive and 1.67 in the HIV-negative applicants. These studies reinforce the point that psychopathology is implicated more potently than any specific medical diagnosis in suicidality.

Prevention and Treatment

The first priority in preventing suicide in the medically ill is the early detection and treatment of the comorbid psychiatric disorders covered throughout this volume. Patient and family education about the medical disease course and its treatment can help prevent excessive fear and pessimism.

Direct questions and frank discussion about suicidal thoughts, ideally part of every primary physician's care for any patient with a serious disease, can reduce suicidal pressures. Nonpsychiatric physicians often fail to recognize medically ill patients at high risk for suicide—for example, misattributing severe vegetative symptoms to medical illness and missing suicidal depression (Copsey Spring et al. 2007). One important role for psychiatrists is to restrain other physicians from automatically prescribing antidepressants for every medically ill patient who expresses a wish to die, particularly without also recommending psychotherapy to address cognitive misconceptions that may be encouraging hopelessness or impulsivity (Mann et al. 2005). Overdiagnosis of depression can lead to inappropriate pharmacotherapy, pathologization of normal feelings, or neglect of relevant personality traits potentially amenable to psychotherapeutic intervention. Soliciting patients' wishes and preferences regarding pain management and end-of-life care early on may reduce the fear of having no control of their dying that lures some patients toward suicide.

Palliative care for the terminally ill is essential in offering relief to those for whom life has become (or is feared) unbearable (see Chapter 41, "Palliative Care"). Psychiatrists can help elicit fears, guilt, impulses, and history that patients may be reluctant to share with their primary physicians. In addition to treating psychiatric symptoms, psychiatrists can monitor for illicit drug use, medication side effects, and emergent neuropsychiatric complications of the underlying medical illness. Psychotherapy can facilitate the exploration and expression of grief and restore a sense of meaning in life (Chochinov 2002; Frierson and Lippman 1988; see also Chapter 39, "Psychotherapy," and Chapter 41, "Palliative Care"). Psychotherapy also may be psychoeducational, reinforcing patients' and family members' accurate knowledge about the disease. Attention to patients' spiritual needs is very important as well; spiritual well-being offers some protection against end-of-life despair (McClain et al. 2003). Finally, for both patients and family, support groups and other community resources may be critical in making the difference between feeling life is worth living and giving up.

Physician-Assisted Suicide

In an editorial in *Medicine,* McHugh (1994) argued that assisted suicides and "naturalistic" ones occurred in different groups of people. Conceptually, physician-assisted suicide follows a rational request from a competent, hopelessly ill patient whose decision is not driven by psychiatric illness. It is legal in very few jurisdictions, where there are practice guidelines and legal safeguards.

In a pair of unanimous 1997 decisions, the U.S. Supreme Court ruled that there is no constitutional right to physician-assisted suicide and that states can prohibit physician conduct in which the primary purpose is to hasten death (Burt 1997). Three states have now legalized physician-assisted death (PAD). Proposals in many other states have been voted down by legislatures or voters. Oregon's Death With Dignity Act was passed in 1994 and enacted in 1997, with the first PAD occurring in 2008. Terminally ill Oregonians can ask their primary care physicians to prescribe lethal doses of medication, but the patients must be able to administer the killing doses themselves. Between 1998 and 2007, only 401 individuals—1 in 900, or 0.11% of Oregon's 365,204 deaths during that time period—elected this option (Oregon Department of Human Services 2008, 2009).

The first PAD in response to Washington State's newly enacted law occurred in May 2009. Montana's PAD law, passed in 2008, has yet to be enacted because of court challenges that are expected to reach the level of the U.S. Supreme Court (O'Reilly 2009).

The safeguards built into the Oregon process closely resemble criteria that have been in place in the Netherlands since 1973, outside the law for nearly three decades, until the Dutch Parliament passed the Termination of Life on Request and Assistance With Suicide Act in 2001 (Cohen-Almagor 2002). To meet the guidelines of the act, the patient must experience his or her situation as intolerable and voluntarily and repeatedly ask the physician for assistance with suicide. The request must be informed, uncoerced, and consistent with the patient's values, and all treatment options must have been exhausted or refused. Finally, the initial physician must seek a second opinion to confirm the diagnosis and prognosis and report the death to the designated municipal authorities (Cohen-Almagor 2002; de Wachter 1989; Singer and Siegler 1990). Quill et al. (1992) suggested an addition to these more legalistic safeguards—that physician-assisted suicide should be carried out only in the context of a meaningful doctor–patient relationship. Three other European countries—Belgium, Luxembourg, and Switzerland—permit variations on PAD (Steinbrook 2008).

The Oregon law is both more conservative and more specific than its Dutch counterpart. It requires supplicants to have the capacity to make their own health care decisions. They must have an illness expected to lead to death within 6 months and must make their requests to the physician in the form of one written and two oral statements separated by 15 days from each other. The primary physician and the consultant giving a second opinion not only must agree on capacity, diagnosis, and terminal prognosis but also have the option of referring the patient for a mental health evaluation if either suspects that depression or another psychiatric disorder is affecting the patient's judgment. Although most patients in Oregon who have received assistance in dying did not have depressive disorders, current practice may have failed to protect some patients whose choice to request a prescription for a lethal drug was influenced by depression (Ganzini et al. 2008). The primary physician is required to inform the patient of all feasible options, such as comfort care, hospice care, and pain management; only then can the patient be given a lethal prescription (Chin et al. 1999). The law specifically forbids active euthanasia, which is distinguished from physician-assisted suicide by the physician actively performing the killing act. Physician-assisted suicide is thus denied to patients who lack motor capacity (e.g., patients with advanced amyotrophic lateral sclerosis) (Rowland 1998). Such individuals may still wish for physician-assisted suicide; Ganzini et al. (2002) reported that one-third of amyotrophic lateral sclerosis patients discussed wanting assisted suicide in the last month of life, particularly those with greater distress at being a burden and those with more insomnia, pain, and other discomfort.

Although he postulated that a request for suicide could be rational, Muskin (1998) advocated a psychodynamic approach to a dialogue between the patient and the physician, a dialogue he believed any such request demands. He saw the query as "an opportunity for patient and physician to more fully understand and know one another" (Muskin 1998, p. 327) and asserted that "every request to die should be subjected to careful scrutiny of its multiple potential meanings" (p. 323). For example, is the patient asking the physician to provide a reason to live? Does the patient harbor revenge fantasies? Is the patient driven by inadequately treated pain or depression, by guilt or hopelessness, or by feelings of already being dead?

In contrast to Muskin's fundamentally intrapsychic approach, Hackett and Stern (1991) outlined diverse interpersonal factors to be considered in evaluating a patient requesting physician-assisted suicide, potentially life-threatening analgesics, or withdrawal of life support. The attending physician and consulting psychiatrist each must take sufficient time to understand the wishes of the patient. What has the patient pictured his or her clinical course to be? What are his or her values? What notions exist about the end of life? Is the patient clinically depressed? Where does the family stand? Do other family members understand the patient's request, and how do they affect it? At what point does the patient specify that the potential for meaning in his or her life has been exhausted? Does the patient fear that he or she will become a financial burden, a caregiving burden, or both? Has any of this been discussed with the family? If the patient considers life devoid of value and meaning for himself or herself, does it have meaning for significant others? Does that affect the patient's thinking? Has the patient made any effort to achieve family consensus so that death can actually be a meaningful shared family experience?

Recent work by Ganzini et al. (2009) contradicts the notion that current physical discomfort or interpersonal issues drive patients' interest in PAD. In this survey of 56 Oregonians who had expressed interest in physician-assisted suicide at end of life, the most important motivations were desire to control the timing and location of death and desire to avoid loss of independence. Worries about future pain, compromised quality of life, and dependence on others for care came next. Least important were limited supports or current physical or mental symptoms. The overall portrait of a typical PAD requester was of a rugged individualist determined to be in charge of his or her destiny, even unto the moment of death.

The psychiatrist's role in physician-assisted suicide is to be available for consultation. In that psychiatrists are almost never primary care providers for terminally ill patients other than dementia patients, who—by definition—lack capacity and are thus not eligible for physician-assisted suicide, Oregon psychiatrists have not been writing lethal prescriptions (Linda Ganzini, personal communication, 2003). Moreover, mental health evaluation is not among the mandatory safeguards in the Oregon law. Despite the fact that numerous investigators have opined that primary care physicians are usually ill-equipped to tease out factors confounding a truly informed decision to take an active role in the timing of one's own death (Billings and Block 1996; Conwell and Caine 1991; Hendin and Klerman 1993), only 12.6% of the 356 patients requesting PAD between 1998 and 2006 were referred for psychiatric evaluation. In 2007, zero of 85 such patients were referred, a trend that continued in 2008, with zero of 60 patients requesting PAD referred (Steinbrook 2008; Linda Ganzini, personal communication, 2009). As Great Britain contemplates instituting a PAD law, Hicks (2006) has expressed concern that requests for PAD can be influenced by coercion, particularly in geriatric patients; can be affected by unconscious and unexamined motives in physicians, caregivers, and patients themselves; and risk being honored inappropriately, given the high rate of depression—often underrecognized by physicians—in terminally ill patients that can influence their decision making.

Block and Billings (1995) outlined five key clinical questions for psychiatrists to explore in clarifying decision-making capacity in terminally ill patients requesting euthanasia or assisted suicide:

1. Does the patient have physical pain that is undertreated or uncontrolled?
2. Does the patient have psychological distress driven by inadequately managed psychiatric symptoms?
3. Does the patient have social disruption resulting from interpersonal relationships strained by fears of burdening others, losing independence, or exacting revenge?
4. Does the patient have spiritual despair in the face of taking the measure of a life nearing its end while coming to terms with personal beliefs about the presence or absence of God?
5. Does the patient have iatrogenic anxiety about the dying process itself and the physician's availability as death encroaches?

Regardless of the status of the law, Block and Billings (1995) argued that requests to hasten death will come, and they explicitly acknowledged in a case example—as others have done in notorious publications ("A Piece of My Mind: It's Over, Debbie" 1988; Quill 1991)—that some physicians participate in extralegal physician-assisted suicide. They enjoin the psychiatrist to perform several functions for a nonpsychiatric colleague wrestling with such a request, including "offering a second opinion on the patient's psychological status, providing a sophisticated evaluation of the patient's decision-making capacity, validating that nothing treatable is being missed, and helping create a setting in which the primary physician and team can formulate a thoughtful decision about how to respond" (Block and Billings 1995, pp. 454–455).

Making time and space for a comprehensive mental health evaluation for the presence of a treatable psychiatric disorder can result in a patient deciding to live longer and withdraw the physician-assisted suicide request (Hendin and Klerman 1993), particularly if "the demoralizing triad" of depression, anxiety, and preoccupation with death is confronted and dispelled. The Oregon experience has shown that intervening in any or all of Block and Billings's five realms can forestall a physician-assisted suicide request actually being carried to completion. Only 1 in 6 requests resulted in the physician issuing a prescription, and only 1 in 10 of those initially requesting physician-assisted suicide ultimately used the medication to hasten death (Ganzini et al. 2001).

Although the U.S. Supreme Court in its 1997 decision specifically denied that physician-assisted suicide was a constitutional right, it endorsed making palliative care more available and acknowledged the legal acceptability of providing pain relief, even if it hastened death (Burt 1997; Quill et al. 1997). Terminal sedation (in which a patient is given narcotics, even to the point of unconsciousness) accompanied by withdrawal or withholding life-prolonging therapies such as ventilatory support (see Chapter 19, "Lung Disease"), antibiotics, food, and water has become normative end-of-life management (see Chapter 41, "Palliative Care").

The distinctions among, and propriety of, physician-assisted suicide, active euthanasia, and passive euthanasia remain controversial and beyond the scope of this chapter, but some clarifications should be noted. At present, all 50 states in the United States continue to outlaw active euthanasia, and since the 1997 Supreme Court ruling, no state is required to permit physician-assisted suicide within its borders. Some have worried that making physician-assisted suicide legal would undermine the availability of appropriate care, partly driven by financial exigencies such as strained health care resources. In the Netherlands, the availability of euthanasia appeared to have stunted the evolution of palliative care (Cohen-Almagor 2002), but in Oregon, the reverse appears to have happened. The availability of physician-assisted suicide has coincided there with a dramatic increase in the use of hospice. In 1994, when voters approved physician-assisted suicide, 22% of Oregonians died in hospice care. By 1999, that figure had risen to 35% without any appreciable increase in the geographic distribution or number of hospice beds in the state (Ganzini et al. 2001). The fear that physician-assisted suicide would become a ubiquitous and convenient way of prematurely disposing of Oregon's dying patients also appears not to have been borne out: In the 11 years for which statistics are available, no more than 1.9% of Oregon deaths resulted from physician-assisted suicide (Oregon Department of Human Services 2008, 2009). Another concern among the public is whether allowing patients to decide to die through refusal of fluids and nutrition will cause undue suffering. The evidence clearly shows that this is not the case (Ganzini et al. 2003).

Psychiatrists will continue to be consulted frequently when patients request withdrawal of treatment or assisted suicide. Evaluation of the patient's capacity for decision making follows the same principles as for other medical decisions (see Chapter 2, "Legal Issues," and Chapter 3, "Ethical Issues"), but psychiatrists should strive to distinguish those who wish to die despite remediable contributors to their despair from those who primarily find the burdens of treatment outweighing the offered benefits. As with any "competency consultation," the psychiatrist should always broaden the scope of examination to a full understanding of the patient and his or her predicament.

Conclusion

Compared with suicidal ideation, completed suicide is rare in psychiatric patients and rarer still in the medically ill. Although identifiable demographic factors are associated with increased suicide risk, these factors by themselves will identify many more persons potentially at risk than imminently in danger of dying. Many medical illnesses have been associated with increased suicide attempts, but medical illness by itself is rarely the sole determinant of suicide potential. The assessment of a suicidal medically ill person—as with any suicidal person—demands attention to the role played by characterological, temperamental, or experiential features in the individual's immediate push toward suicide. Management begins with a search for reversible contributors to impulsivity, such as delirium, psychosis, and intoxication. A priority in preventing suicide in the medically ill is the early detection and treatment of comorbid psychiatric disorders.

One of the most frequent reasons for psychiatric consultation in medical hospitals is for evaluation for transfer of care of patients who have made suicide attempts. Because countertransference issues not infrequently lead nonpsychiatric physicians to prematurely "clear" patients, it is critical for psychiatrists to form their own judgments about whether patients are truly medically stable enough for transfer out of the medical setting. If a suicidal patient must remain on a medical floor, the psychiatric consultant should keep in mind that rooms in the general medical hospital may lack safeguards routinely found on inpatient psychiatric units. Constant observation by a one-on-one sitter is indicated for patients judged to be at high risk.

Suicide is not synonymous with refusal of lifesaving treatment or with requests to hasten death in terminal illness. Psychiatrists are frequently consulted when patients request withdrawal of treatment or assisted suicide; in these situations, the clinician should evaluate the patient's capacity for decision making, the adequacy of pain management, and the role that treatable psychiatric illness may be playing in the request. Psychological distress, social disruption of interpersonal relationships, and spiritual despair must also be explored and addressed. Responding to these issues with concern and comfort may transform a desire for hastened death into a graceful and timely exit from life.

References

Abrams H, Moore G, Westervelt F: Suicidal behavior in chronic dialysis patients. Am J Psychiatry 127:1199–1204, 1971

Allebeck P, Bolund C, Ringback F: Increased suicide rate in cancer patients. J Clin Epidemiol 42:611–616, 1985

A piece of my mind: it's over, Debbie (case report). JAMA 259:272, 1988

Barraclough B, Bunch J, Nelson B, et al: A hundred cases of suicide: clinical aspects. Br J Psychiatry 125:355–373, 1974

Beautrais A: Suicides and serious suicide attempts: two populations or one? Psychol Med 31:837–845, 2001

Berger D: Suicide risk in the general hospital. Psychiatry Clin Neurosci 49:585–589, 1995

Billings JA, Block SD: Slow euthanasia. J Palliat Care 12:21–30, 1996

Björkenstam C, Edberg A, Ayoubi S, et al: Are cancer patients at higher suicide risk than the general population? Scand J Public Health 33:208–214, 2005

Block S, Billings J: Patient requests for euthanasia and assisted suicide in terminal illness: the role of the psychiatrist. Psychosomatics 36:445–457, 1995

Bostwick J, Cohen L: Differentiating suicide from life-ending acts and end-of-life decisions: a model based on chronic kidney disease and dialysis. Psychosomatics 50:1–7, 2009

Bostwick J, Lineberry T: Editorial on "Inpatient suicide: preventing a common sentinal event." Gen Hosp Psychiatry 31:101–102, 2009

Bostwick J, Pankratz V: Affective disorders and suicide risk: a reexamination. Am J Psychiatry 157:1925–1932, 2000

Bostwick J, Rackley S: Completed suicide in medical/surgical patients: who is at risk? Current Psychiatry Reports 9:242–246, 2007

Breitbart W, Rosenfeld B, Pessin H, et al: Depression, hopelessness, and desire for hastened death in terminally ill patients with cancer. JAMA 284:2907–2911, 2000

Brown J, Henteleff P, Barakat S, et al: Is it normal for terminally ill patients to desire death? Am J Psychiatry 143:208–211, 1986

Buie D, Maltsberger J: The psychological vulnerability to suicide, in Suicide: Understanding and Responding. Edited by Jacobs D, Brown H. Madison, CT, International Universities Press, 1989, pp 59–71

Burt R: The Supreme Court speaks—not assisted suicide but a constitutional right to palliative care. N Engl J Med 337:1234–1236, 1997

Cardell R, Pitula CR: Suicidal inpatients' perceptions of therapeutic and nontherapeutic aspects of constant observation. Psychiatr Serv 50:1066–1070, 1999

Carrico AW, Johnson MO, Morin SF, et al.: Correlates of suicidal ideation among HIV-positive persons. AIDS 21:1199–1203, 2007

Center C, Davis M, Detre T, et al: Confronting depression and suicide in physicians: a consensus statement. JAMA 289:3161–3166, 2003

Chin A, Hedberg K, Higginson G, et al: Legalized physician-assisted suicide in Oregon—the first year's experience. N Engl J Med 340:577–583, 1999

Chochinov H: Dignity-conserving care—a new model for palliative care: helping the patient feel valued. JAMA 287:2253–2260, 2002

Chochinov H, Tataryn D, Clinch J, et al: Will to live in the terminally ill. Lancet 354:816–819, 1999

Christensen J, Vestergaard M, Mortensen P, et al.: Epilepsy and risk of suicide: a population-based case-control study. Lancet Neurol 6:693–698, 2007

Cochand P, Bovet P: HIV infection and suicide risk: an epidemiological inquiry among male homosexuals in Switzerland. Soc Psychiatry Psychiatr Epidemiol 33:230–234, 1998

Cohen L, Germain M: The psychiatric landscape of withdrawal. Seminars in Dialysis 18:147–153, 2005

Cohen L, Dobscha S, Hails K, et al: Depression and suicidal ideation in patients who discontinue the life-support treatment of dialysis. Psychosom Med 64:889–896, 2002

Cohen-Almagor R: Dutch perspectives on palliative care in the Netherlands. Issues Law Med 18:111–126, 2002

Conner K, Langley J, Tomaszewski K, et al: Injury hospitalization and risks for subsequent self-injury and suicide: a national study from New Zealand. Am J Public Health 93:1128–1131, 2003

Conwell Y, Caine E: Rational suicide and the right to die. N Engl J Med 324:1100–1103, 1991

Cooperman NA, Simoni JM: Suicidal ideation and attempted suicide among women living with HIV/AIDS. J Behav Med 28:149 156, 2005

Copsey Spring TR, Yanni LM, Levenson JL: A shot in the dark: failing to recognize the link between physical and mental illness. J Gen Intern Med 22:677–680, 2007

Cote T, Biggar R, Dannenberg A: Risk of suicide among persons with AIDS: a national assessment. JAMA 268:2066–2068, 1991

Crocetti E, Arniani S, Acciai S, et al: High suicide mortality soon after diagnosis among cancer patients in central Italy. Br J Cancer 77:1194–1196, 1998

Dannenberg A, McNeail J, Brundage J, et al: Suicide and HIV infection: mortality follow-up of 4147 HIV-seropositive military service applicants. JAMA 276:1743–1746, 1996

Darke S, Duflou J, Torok M: Drugs and violent death: comparative toxicology of homicide and non-substance toxicity suicide victims. Addiction 104:1000–1005, 2009

Davidson L: Suicide and aggression in the medical setting, in Psychiatric Care of the Medical Patient. Edited by Stoudemire A, Fogel B. New York, Oxford University Press, 1993, pp 71–86

Davison SN, Jhangri GS, Holley JL, et al: Nephrologists' reported preparedness for end-of-life decision-making. Clin J Am Soc Nephrol 1:1256–1262, 2006

de Wachter M: Active euthanasia in the Netherlands. JAMA 262:3316–3319, 1989

Dormer NR, McCaul KA, Kristianson LJ: Risk of suicide in cancer patients in Western Australia, 1981–2002. Med J Aust 188:140–143, 2008

Dorpat T, Ripley H: A study of suicide in the Seattle area. Compr Psychiatry 1:349–359, 1960

Farberow L, McKelligott J, Cohen S, et al: Suicide among patients with cardiorespiratory illnesses. JAMA 195:422–428, 1966

Farberow N: Indirect self-destructive behavior, in Comprehensive Textbook of Suicidology. Edited by Maris R, Berman A, Silverman M. New York, Guilford, 2000, pp 427–455

Farberow N, Litman R: Suicide prevention in hospitals, in The Psychology of Suicide. Edited by Shneidman E, Farberow N, Litman R. New York, Science House, 1970, pp 423–458

Fawcett J, Shaughnessy R: The suicidal patient, in Psychiatry: Diagnosis and Therapy. Edited by Flaherty J, Channon R, Davis J. Norwalk, CT, Appleton & Lange, 1988, pp 49–56

Filiberti A, Ripamonti C, Totis A, et al: Characteristics of terminal cancer patients who committed suicide during a home palliative care program. J Pain Symptom Manage 22:544–553, 2001

Frierson R, Lippman S: Suicide and AIDS. Psychosomatics 29:226–231, 1988

Furst S, Ostow M: The psychodynamics of suicide, in Suicide: Theory and Clinical Aspects. Edited by Hankoff L, Einsidler B. Littleton, MA, PSG Publishing, 1979, pp 165–178

Ganzini L, Nelson H, Lee M, et al: Oregon physicians' attitudes about and experiences with end-of-life care since passage of the Oregon Death With Dignity Act. JAMA 285:2363–2369, 2001

Ganzini L, Silveira M, Johnston W: Predictors and correlates of interest in assisted suicide in the final month of life among ALS patients in Oregon and Washington. J Pain Symptom Manage 24:312–317, 2002

Ganzini L, Goy E, Miller L, et al: Nurses' experiences with hospice patients who refuse food and fluids to hasten death. N Engl J Med 349:359–365, 2003

Ganzini L, Goy ER, Dobscha SK: Prevalence of depression and anxiety in patients requesting physicians' aid in dying: cross sectional survey. BMJ 337:a1682, 2008

Ganzini L, Goy E, Dobscha S: Oregonians' reasons for requesting physician aid in dying. Arch Intern Med 169:489–492, 2009

Gardner DL, Cowdry RW: Suicidal and parasuicidal behavior in borderline personality disorder. Psychiatr Clin North Am 8:389–403, 1985

Gielen AC, McDonnell KA, O'Campo PJ, et al: Suicide risk and mental health indicators: do they differ by abuse and HIV status? Womens Health Issues 15:89–95, 2005

Glickman L: Psychiatric Consultation in the General Hospital. New York, Marcel Dekker, 1980

Goldberg R: The assessment of suicide risk in the general hospital. Gen Hosp Psychiatry 9:446–452, 1987

Goodwin R, Olfson M: Self-perception of poor health and suicidal ideation in medical patients. Psychol Med 32:1293–1299, 2002

Goodwin R, Marusic A, Hoven C: Suicide attempts in the United States: the role of physical illness. Soc Sci Med 56:1783–1788, 2003

Grassi L, Mondardini D, Pavanati M, et al: Suicide probability and psychological morbidity secondary to HIV infection: a control study of HIV-seropositive, hepatitis C virus (HCV)-seropositive and HIV/HCV-seronegative injecting drug users. J Affect Disord 64:195–202, 2001

Gutheil T, Appelbaum P: Clinical Handbook of Psychiatry and the Law. Philadelphia, PA, Lippincott Williams & Wilkins, 2000

Hackett T, Stern T: Suicide and other disruptive states, in The Massachusetts General Hospital Handbook of General Hospital Psychiatry. Edited by Cassem N. St. Louis, MO, Mosby-Year Book, 1991, pp 281–307

Harwood D, Hawton K, Hope T, et al: Life problems and physical illness as risk factors for suicide in older people: a descriptive and case-control study. Psychol Med 36:1265–1274, 2006

Haenel T, Brunner F, Battegay R: Renal dialysis and suicide: occurrence in Switzerland and Europe. Compr Psychiatry 21:140–145, 1980

Hall R, Platt D, Hall R: Suicide risk assessment: a review of risk factors for suicide in 100 patients who made severe suicide attempts. Evaluation of suicide risk in a time of managed care. Psychosomatics 40:18–27, 1999

Harris E, Barraclough B: Suicide as an outcome for medical disorders. Medicine 73:281–296, 1994

Hawton K: Suicide and attempted suicide, in Handbook of Affective Disorders. Edited by Paykel E. New York, Guilford, 1992, pp 635–650

Heckman T, Miller J, Kochman A, et al: Thoughts of suicide among HIV-infected rural persons enrolled in a telephone-delivered mental health intervention. Ann Behav Med 24:141–148, 2002

Hendin H, Klerman G: Physician-assisted suicide: the dangers of legalization. Am J Psychiatry 150:143–145, 1993

Henriksson M, Isometsa E, Hietanen P, et al: Mental disorders in cancer suicides. J Affect Disord 36:11–20, 1995

Hicks MHR: Physician-assisted suicide: a review of the literature concerning practical and clinical implications for UK doctors. BMC Family Practice 7:39, 2006

Hughes D, Kleespies P: Suicide in the medically ill. Suicide Life Threat Behav 31 (suppl):48–59, 2001

Hung C, Liu C, Liao M, et al: Self-destructive acts occurring during medical general hospitalization. Gen Hosp Psychiatry 22:115–121, 2000

Jaworowski S, Raveh D, Lobel E, et al: Constant observation in the general hospital: a review. Isr J Psychiatry Relat Sci 45:278–284, 2008

Kamali M, Oquendo M, Mann J: Understanding the neurobiology of suicidal behavior. Depress Anxiety 14:164–176, 2001

Kaplan A, Klein R: Women and suicide, in Suicide: Understanding and Responding. Edited by Jacobs D, Brown H. Madison, CT, International Universities Press, 1989, pp 257–282

Kellner C, Best C, Roberts J, et al: Self-destructive behavior in hospitalized medical and surgical patients. Psychiatr Clin North Am 8:279–289, 1985

Kelly M, Mufson M, Rogers M: Medical settings and suicide, in The Harvard Medical School Guide to Suicide Assessment and Intervention. Edited by Jacobs D. San Francisco, CA, Jossey-Bass, 1999, pp 491–519

Kendal WS: Suicide and cancer: a gender-comparative study. Ann Oncol 18:381–387, 2007

Kishi Y, Kathol RG: Assessment of patients who attempt suicide. Prim Care Companion J Clin Psychiatry 4:132–136, 2002

Kizer K, Green M, Perkins C, et al: AIDS and suicide in California (letter). JAMA 260:1881, 1988

Klerman G: Clinical epidemiology of suicide. J Clin Psychiatry 48:33–38, 1987

Kurella M, Kimmel P, Young B, et al: Suicide in the United States end-stage renal disease program. J Am Soc Nephrol 16:774–781, 2005

Lagro-Janssen AL, Luijks HD: Suicide in female and male physicians [in Dutch]. Ned Tijdschr Geneeskd 152:2177–2181, 2008

Lin HC, Wu CH, Lee HC: Risk factors for suicide following hospital discharge among cancer patients. Psychooncology 18:1038–1044, 2009

Litman R: Suicides: what do they have in mind? in Suicide: Understanding and Responding. Edited by Jacobs D, Brown H. Madison, CT, International Universities Press, 1989, pp 143–154

Malbergier A, de Andrade A: Depressive disorders and suicide attempts in injecting drug use with and without HIV infection. AIDS Care 13:141–150, 2001

Maltsberger J, Buie D: Countertransference hate in the treatment of suicidal patients. Arch Gen Psychiatry 30:625–633, 1974

Mann J: Psychobiological predictors of suicide. J Clin Psychiatry 48:39–43, 1987

Mann J: The neurobiology of suicide. Nat Med 4:25–30, 1998

Mann JJ, Apter A, Bertolote J, et al: Suicide prevention strategies: a systematic review. JAMA 294:2064–2074, 2005

Marzuk PM, Tierney H, Tardiff K, et al: Increased risk of suicide in persons with AIDS. JAMA 259:1333–1337, 1988

Marzuk PM, Tardiff K, Leon A, et al: HIV seroprevalence among suicide victims in New York City, 1991–1993. Am J Psychiatry 154:1720–1725, 1997

McClain C, Rosenfeld B, Breitbart W: Effect of spiritual well-being on end-of-life despair in terminally ill cancer patients. Lancet 361:1603–1607, 2003

McHugh P: Suicide and medical afflictions. Medicine 73:297–298, 1994

McIntosh J: U.S.A. Suicide: Suicide Data, 2006. Washington, DC, American Association of Suicidology, 2009

McKegney FP, O'Dowd MA: Suicidality and HIV status. Am J Psychiatry 149:396–398, 1992

McMillan D, Gilbody S, Beresford E, et al: Can we predict suicide and non-fatal self-harm with the Beck Hopelessness Scale? A meta-analysis. Psychol Med 37:769–778, 2007

Miles C: Conditions predisposing to suicide: a review. J Nerv Ment Dis 164:231–246, 1977

Miller M, Mogun H, Azrael D, et al: Cancer and the risk of suicide in older Americans. J Clin Oncol 26:4720–4724, 2008

Misono S, Weiss NS, Fann JR, et al: Incidence of suicide in persons with cancer. J Clin Oncol 26:4731–4738, 2008

Monk M: Epidemiology of suicide. Epidemiol Rev 9:51–69, 1987

Morgan A: Special issues of assessment and treatment of suicide risk in the elderly, in Suicide: Understanding and Responding. Edited by Jacobs D, Brown H. Madison, CT, International Universities Press, 1989, pp 239–255

Morgan H, Priest P: Suicide and other unexpected deaths among psychiatric inpatients. Br J Psychiatry 158:368–374, 1991

Moscicki E: Epidemiology of suicide. Int Psychogeriatr 7:137–148, 1995

Murphy G: Recognizing the alcoholic risk for suicide. Lifesavers: Newsletter of the American Suicide Foundation 4:3, 1992

Murphy G, Weitzel R: The lifetime risk of suicide in alcoholism. Arch Gen Psychiatry 47:383–392, 1990

Murray AM, Arko C, Chen SC, et al: Use of hospice in the United States dialysis population. Clin J Am Soc Nephrol 1:1248–1255, 2006

Muskin P: The request to die: role for a psychodynamic perspective on physician-assisted suicide. JAMA 279:323–328, 1998

Neu S, Kjellstrand C: Stopping long-term dialysis: an empirical study of withdrawal of life-supporting treatment. N Engl J Med 314:14–20, 1986

Nielsen B, Wang A, Brille-Brahe U: Attempted suicide in Denmark, IV: a five-year follow-up. Acta Psychiatr Scand 81:250–254, 1990

O'Dowd MA, Biderman DJ, McKegney FP: Incidence of suicidality in AIDS and HIV-positive patients attending a psychiatry outpatient program. Psychosomatics 34:33–40, 1993

Oregon Department of Human Services: Death With Dignity Act Annual Reports, Year 11—2008, Table 1: Characteristics and end-of-life care of 401 DWDA patients who died after ingesting a lethal dose of medication, by year, Oregon, 1998–2008. Available at: http://oregon.gov/DHS/ph/pas/docs/yr11-tbl-1.pdf. Accessed September 26, 2009.

Oregon Department of Human Services: Center for Health Statistics—Health Statistics/Data: Death Data. 2009. Available at: http://www.dhs.state.or.us/dhs/ph/chs/data/death/death.shtml. Accessed September 26, 2009.

O'Reilly K: Montana judge rejects stay of physician-assisted suicide ruling. AMNews, posted January 29, 2009 at www.ama-assn.org/amednews/2009/01/26/prsd0129.htm

Palmer B, Pankratz V, Bostwick J: The risk of suicide in schizophrenia: a meta-analysis. Arch Gen Psychiatry 62:247–253, 2005

Patterson W, Dohn H, Bird J, et al: Evaluation of suicidal patients: the SAD PERSONS scale. Psychosomatics 24:348–349, 1983

Paulsen J, Ferneyhough-Hoth K, Nehl K, et al: Critical periods of suicide risk in Huntington's disease. Am J Psychiatry 162:725–731, 2005

Petersen MR, Burnett CA: The suicide mortality of working physicians and dentists. Occup Med (Lond) 58(1):25–29, 2008

Pisetsky J, Brown W: The general hospital patient, in Suicide: Theory and Clinical Aspects. Edited by Hankoff L, Einsidler B. Littleton, MA, PSG Publishing, 1979, pp 279–290

Pokorny A: Prediction of suicide in psychiatric patients: report of a prospective study. Arch Gen Psychiatry 40:249–257, 1983

Pollack S: Suicide in a general hospital, in The Psychology of Suicide. Edited by Shneidman E, Farberow N. New York, McGraw-Hill, 1957, pp 152–176

Proulx F, Lesage A, Grunberg F: One hundred in-patient suicides. Br J Psychiatry 171:247–250, 1997

Quan H, Arboleda-Florez J, Fick G, et al: Association between physical illness and suicide among the elderly. Soc Psychiatry Psychiatr Epidemiol 37:190–197, 2002

Quill T: Death and dignity—a case of individualized decision making. N Engl J Med 324:691–694, 1991

Quill T, Cassel C, Meier D: Care of the hopelessly ill: proposed clinical criteria for physician-assisted suicide. N Engl J Med 327:1380–1384, 1992

Quill T, Lo B, Brock D: Palliative options of last resort: a comparison of voluntarily stopping eating and drinking, terminal sedation, physician-assisted suicide, and voluntary active euthanasia. JAMA 278:2099–2104, 1997

Reich P, Kelly M: Suicide attempts by hospitalized medical and surgical patients. N Engl J Med 294:298–301, 1976

Reynolds C, Clayton P: Out of the silence: confronting depression in medical students and residents. Acad Med 84:159–160, 2009

Robins E, Murphy G, Wilkinson R, et al: Some clinical considerations in the prevention of suicide based on a study of 134 successful suicides. Am J Public Health 49:888–899, 1959

Robinson D, Renshaw C, Okello C, et al: Suicide in cancer patients in South East England from 1996 to 2005: a population-based study. Br J Cancer 101:198–201, 2009

Rosenthal J, Okie S. White coat, mood indigo: depression in medical school. N Engl J Med 353:1085–1088, 2005

Rowland L: Assisted suicide and alternatives in amyotrophic lateral sclerosis. N Engl J Med 339:987–989, 1998

Roy A: Emergency psychiatry: suicide, in Comprehensive Textbook of Psychiatry/V. Edited by Kaplan H, Sadock B. Baltimore, MD, Williams & Wilkins, 1989, pp 1414–1427

Roy A: Characteristics of HIV patients who attempt suicide. Acta Psychiatr Scand 107:41–44, 2003

Rundell J, Kyle K, Brown G, et al: Risk factors for suicide attempts in a human immunodeficiency virus screening program. Psychosomatics 33:24–27, 1992

Sanders R: Suicidal behavior in critical care medicine: conceptual issues and management strategies, in Problems in Critical Care Medicine. Edited by Wise M. Philadelphia, PA, JB Lippincott, 1988, pp 116–133

Shah A, Ganesvaran T: Inpatient suicides in an Australian mental hospital. Aust N Z J Psychiatry 31:291–298, 1997

Shneidman E: Overview: a multidimensional approach to suicide, in Suicide: Understanding and Responding. Edited by Jacobs D, Brown H. Madison, CT, International Universities Press, 1989, pp 1–30

Singer P, Siegler M: Euthanasia—a critique. N Engl J Med 322:1881–1883, 1990

Smith M, Edwards R, Robinson R, et al: Suicidal ideation, plans, and attempts in chronic pain patients: factors associated with increased risk. Pain 111:201–208, 2004

Steinbrook R. Physician-assisted death—from Oregon to Washington State. N Engl J Med 359:2513–2514, 2008

Stenager EN, Stenager E, Jensen K: Attempted suicide, depression, and physical diseases: a 1-year follow-up study. Psychother Psychosom 61:65–73, 1994

Stensman R, Sundqvist-Stensman U: Physical disease and disability among 416 suicide cases in Sweden. Scand J Soc Med 16:149–153, 1988

Suominen K, Isometsa E, Heila H, et al: General hospital suicides—a psychological autopsy study in Finland. Gen Hosp Psychiatry 24:412–416, 2002

Tanaka H, Tsukuma H, Masaoka T, et al: Suicide risk among cancer patients: experience at one medical center in Japan, 1978–1994. Jpn J Cancer Res 90:812–817, 1999

Tang N, Crane C: Suicidality in chronic pain: a review of the prevalence, risk factors, and psychological links. Psychol Med 36:575–586, 2006

Tishler C, Reiss N: Inpatient suicide: preventing a common sentinel event. Gen Hosp Psychiatry 31:103–109, 2009

Waern M, Rubenowitz E, Runeson B, et al: Burden of illness and suicide in elderly people: case-control study. BMJ 324:1355–1358, 2002

White R, Gribble R, Corr M, et al: Jumping from a general hospital. Gen Hosp Psychiatry 17:208–215, 1995

Wilson KG, Curran D, McPherson CJ: A burden to others: a common source of distress for the terminally ill. Cogn Behav Ther 34:115–123, 2005

CHAPTER 10

Psychosis, Mania, and Catatonia

Oliver Freudenreich, M.D.

Shamim H. Nejad, M.D.

Andrew Francis, Ph.D., M.D.

Gregory L. Fricchione, M.D.

PSYCHOSIS, MANIA, AND catatonia can greatly hamper the ability of patients to care for themselves and of medical staff to care for them. We discuss psychosis, mania, and catatonia in three subsections as if they were separate entities, with one of the symptoms dominating (and when the symptom is not the result of delirium or dementia; see Chapter 5, "Delirium," and Chapter 6, "Dementia"); in clinical practice, the distinction cannot always be made: patients with mania can be psychotic, or catatonia may occur in the setting of a manic or psychotic patient. In each of the subsections, we use the "primary/secondary" distinction even though it is not officially sanctioned by our current classification system (i.e., DSM-IV-TR [American Psychiatric Association 2000]). Clinicians, however, base their diagnostic approach on this distinction: are psychiatric symptoms attributable to a primary psychiatric syndrome or are they secondary to medical diseases, substance use, or medication intoxication? In this chapter, we focus on the management principles of medically hospitalized patients who are psychotic, manic, or catatonic and place particular emphasis on the etiologies of secondary psychosis, mania, and catatonia. Psychotic symptoms due to toxic exposures are covered in Chapter 37, "Medical Toxicology."

Psychosis in the Medically Ill

Epidemiology and Risk Factors

The prevalence and etiology of psychosis in the general hospital setting depend on the diagnostic criteria used and on the specifics of the hospital setting and service and its geographic location. In surgical settings, particularly if elderly patients are treated, delirium and dementia are often accompanied by psychosis. When a young patient presents to an inner-city emergency department with psychosis, illicit drug use is likely. In a patient who is evaluated in a first-episode outpatient program, the likelihood that a primary psychotic disorder is present is fairly high. In the seminal Northwick Park study, fewer than 6% of cases referred for a first episode of psychosis were thought to have an "organic" ailment (Johnstone et al. 1987).

Risk factors for the development of psychosis, particularly paranoid symptoms in an elderly patient, include cognitive problems and social isolation (Forsell and Henderson 1998) as well as hearing loss (Thewissen et al. 2005). The prevalence of any psychotic symptom in the general population of dementia-free individuals older than 85 years is about 10% (Ostling and Skoog 2002).

Clinical Features

The hallmarks of psychotic disorder due to a medical condition according to DSM-IV-TR (American Psychiatric Association 2000) are hallucinations and delusions. Hallucinations can occur in any sensory modality, but they lack diagnostic specificity (Carter 1992). If patients retain their insight into the abnormal nature of their hallucinations, the term *pseudohallucinations* is sometimes used (Berrios and Dening 1996). A good example of hallucinations that occur in patients who remain insightful (and as a consequence hesitant to divulge information about the experience unless specifically asked for fear of being labeled as insane) is the Charles Bonnet syndrome (Menon 2005). In this syndrome, generally pleasant, complex visual hallucinations occur in visually impaired individuals who are cognitively intact. Another example of complex visual hallucinations is peduncular hallucinosis, in which vivid, scenic images can emerge after focal damage to the thalamus or mesencephalic structures (Benke 2006; Mocellin et al. 2006). Some hallucinations occur only under very specific conditions. For example, auditory hallucinations heard only when the air conditioner is running are called functional hallucinations. Hypnagogic or hypnopompic hallucinations occur only in the transition to sleep or awakening, respectively.

The second hallmark of psychosis, delusions, can be fleeting and poorly formed or rather elaborate and entrenched. Delusions are often classified by their content and style (as being bizarre or nonbizarre). Some delusional syndromes are best known by their eponyms such as the delusions of infidelity (Othello syndrome) or delusions of nihilism (Cotard's syndrome) (Freudenreich 2007). As with hallucinations, however, the type of delusion lacks diagnostic specificity. For example, although the morbid jealousy in the Othello syndrome is traditionally associated with male alcoholic patients, it can occur as both a primary psychiatric disorder and a manifestation of organic etiology (Yusim et al. 2008). Kurt Schneider described classic psychotic experiences in patients with schizophrenia. His so-called Schneiderian first-rank symptoms include delusional perception; passivity experiences; and thought insertion, withdrawal, or broadcasting. In patients with first-episode psychosis, first-rank symptoms are common; in one representative sample, only 16% of the patients did not experience any first-rank symptoms (Thorup et al. 2007). The presence of a belief in duplicates and replacements is typical for a group of delusions known as *delusional misidentification syndromes* (Weinstein 1994). For example, in the Capgras delusion, a patient believes that a family member or close friend has been replaced by an exact double.

The course and prognosis of secondary psychosis are determined to a large extent by the underlying illness. It can reasonably be expected that a pure drug-induced or medication-induced psychosis resolves once the inciting agent is removed. However, in some cases such as phencyclidine (PCP) psychosis, prolonged psychosis lasting several weeks can result. Some illnesses are treatable but require prolonged treatment with the very medication that caused the psychosis in the first place (e.g., steroids for systemic lupus erythematosus [SLE] or interferon for cancer). Unfortunately, many illnesses in which psychosis emerges are degenerative, progressive, and incurable. The emergence of psychosis in a degenerative disorder greatly complicates its management. For example, in a patient with Alzheimer's disease and psychosis, caregivers are more distressed, and patients are more likely to be transferred to a nursing home (Ballard et al. 2008). A more optimistic picture emerged in the only longitudinal follow-up study that used the DSM diagnosis, psychosis due to a general medical condition (Feinstein and Ron 1998). In this cohort of 44 patients with various neurological conditions who were followed up for an average of 4 years, most required only brief, intermittent treatment with antipsychotics, and none required maintenance treatment with antipsychotics.

Diagnosis and Assessment

Psychotic symptoms in a medically hospitalized patient fall into one of three possibilities:

1. *Primary psychiatric illness*
   - New-onset or an acute exacerbation of psychiatric illness associated with psychosis
2. *Secondary psychosis*
   - Psychosis due to a general medical condition (systemic or brain-based)
   - Substance-induced psychosis
   - Medication-induced psychosis
3. *"Secondary on primary"*
   - A patient with a primary psychotic disorder has psychosis unrelated to his or her primary psychotic disorder

The first step in the evaluation of any new-onset psychosis requires an assessment of the patient's safety and then a careful analysis of the longitudinal history of symptoms and the cross-sectional symptom profile, taking into account the clinical context. A preadmission baseline should be established with the help of collateral sources. For example, new-onset psychosis in an elderly patient is unlikely to result from a primary psychiatric disorder; it is more likely the result of a delirium or another intercurrent event such as a stroke or seizure. A physical examination that identifies abnormal vital signs or focal neurological findings often points toward a secondary cause of psychosis. The possibility of unacknowledged drug abuse (withdrawal or drug use while in the hospital) should always be considered. A chart review should focus on medications administered during the hospitalization.

Determining that psychosis is present if the patient is not cooperating sufficiently during the interview is not always straightforward. A patient might be too suspicious to answer questions. Unless a patient is able to cooperate, cognitive limitations might not be apparent, and a delirium may be overlooked. Patients with a preexisting psychosis pose particular difficulties because psychosis in and of itself might not indicate an "organic" etiology, and exacerbations resulting from intercurrent illnesses that lead to secondary psychosis are missed. Repeat examinations over the course of the day and a comprehensive survey of psychotic phenomena, including Schneiderian first-rank symptoms, hallucinations in all modalities, and misidentification syndromes, may be necessary to make the diagnosis.

Well-established rating scales such as the Brief Psychiatric Rating Scale (BPRS; Overall and Gorham 1988) that were developed for schizophrenia could be used to track secondary psychosis during a hospital stay. However, their clinical utility in this setting is unclear. Routine screening (such as the CAGE questionnaire; Ewing 1984) for substance use problems at the time of hospital admission should be used to identify unrecognized substance use and to avoid withdrawal (including psychosis) during the hospitalization.

Unfortunately, no pathognomonic signs or symptoms differentiate primary from secondary psychosis or allow clinicians to determine the presence of a secondary psychosis on clinical grounds alone. For example, the presence of Schneiderian first-rank symptoms has been reported in a wide variety of "organic" conditions, particularly epilepsy and endocrine disturbances (Marneros 1988). In a chart review of 1,698 patients diagnosed with "organic mental disorder," Schneiderian first-rank symptoms were seen in 7% of the patients (Marneros 1988). Conversely, visual hallucinations, which many clinicians regard as indicative of "organicity," are clearly also part of the symptom spectrum in schizophrenia, bipolar disorder, and psychotic depression (Baethge et al. 2005).

Nevertheless, considering the phenomenology of the reported experience, including the presence or absence of first-rank symptoms, content of delusions, or modality of hallucinations, is still valuable. In a prospective study, Cutting (1987) comprehensively compared the psychopathology of patients with organic psychosis and acute schizophrenia with the Present State Examination (PSE) and found that only 3% of the patients with an organic condition experienced first-rank symptoms and that visual hallucinations were more common in these patients; mistaken identity was a common delusional theme. In an emergency department study that examined differences between substance-induced psychosis and primary psychosis, the presence of visual hallucinations on arrival at the emergency department was one of three key predictors of substance-induced psychosis, as opposed to a primary psychotic disorder (Caton et al. 2005). The other two predictors of substance-induced psychosis were parental substance abuse and dependence on any substance. Patients who experience gustatory or olfactory hallucinations, particularly if they have no associated delusions, might have organic problems, including paroxysmal disorders such as epilepsy or migraines. Delusional misidentification syndromes are possible in those with primary psychiatric disorders but strongly suggest a neurodegenerative process. Josephs (2007) reported that 81% of patients with Capgras' syndrome had a neurodegenerative disorder, mostly Lewy body disease. Even the remaining 19% of the patients with a nondegenerative disorder experienced delusions secondary to methamphetamine abuse or had just had a stroke in addition to primary psychotic disorders.

The extent of the medical evaluation of psychosis in medically ill patients is guided by the clinical picture and likely etiologies. It is important to eliminate causes of a delirium. Therefore, most patients who develop psychosis in the hospital will need a basic laboratory evaluation to assess gross organ dysfunction and infections. The information obtained from a lumbar puncture can be lifesaving. If seizures are considered or if a delirium is high on the list of potential causes, then an electroencephalogram (EEG) is indicated. A normal EEG result makes delirium as a cause of psychosis less likely. Also, a computed tomography (CT) or magnetic resonance imaging (MRI) scan is indicated if brain pathology is suspected. Syphilis and human immunodeficiency virus (HIV) infection are crucial to consider and specifically exclude. If no culprit is found on the basis of history and the initial evaluation, the search needs to be broadened to include less common medical causes of psychosis (such as thyrotoxicosis or Wilson's disease) before making a diagnosis of schizophrenia, which is a diagnosis of exclusion (see Table 10-1 for an initial medical evaluation of secondary psychosis, mania, or catatonia).

However, even if a medical disease, substance, or medication that can be associated with psychosis is discovered, establishing causality is not straightforward. Slater and Beard (1963) discussed this problem of causation in comorbid conditions in a classic essay on the psychosis of epilepsy. They outlined three levels of association: epilepsy and psychosis occurring together by chance; epilepsy precipitating schizophrenia; or epilepsy producing schizo-

TABLE 10–1. Initial medical evaluation for secondary psychosis, mania, and catatonia

Laboratory evaluation
Complete blood count
Electrolytes including calcium and phosphate
Serum urea nitrogen/creatinine
Glucose
Thyrotropin
Liver function tests
Erythrocyte sedimentation rate
Antinuclear antibody
Human immunodeficiency virus test
Fluorescent treponemal antibody absorption (FTA-ABS) test for syphilis (rapid plasma reagin not sufficient)
Vitamin B_{12} and folate
Serum cortisol level
Ceruloplasmin
Urinalysis
Serum toxicology screen
Drug levels of prescribed medications, if indicated
Blood cultures
Urine culture
Brain imaging
Magnetic resonance imaging (generally preferred over computed tomography)
Electroencephalogram
If seizures or delirium are suspected

Note. This list of tests is based on the medical evaluation of a first episode of psychosis and is neither mandatory nor exhaustive. Other tests should be considered if the clinical history and the clinical picture suggest that they might be useful diagnostically (e.g., arterial blood gases, chest X ray, lumbar puncture, genetic testing). Note the overlap with a delirium evaluation.
Other tests such as a serum pregnancy test and an electrocardiogram (to monitor QTc) might need to be added to safely administer treatment.
Source. Based on Freudenreich et al. 2007.

phrenia-like symptoms. Only in the third case would treatment of the underlying illness alone be expected to lead to a concomitant remission of psychosis. In clinical practice, the causality determination is difficult: how much do drugs explain psychosis? Is the old lesion seen on brain scan large enough and located appropriately to "explain" psychosis?

Etiology and Differential Diagnosis

Secondary psychosis can be caused by a multitude of medical conditions, illicit drugs, and toxins, including medications. The diagnostic challenge lies not only in the sheer number of possible conditions that can cause psychosis but also in the possibility that rare diseases (rare because of low absolute incidence or because of low local prevalence) that most clinicians will be unfamiliar with can present with psychosis, either typically (e.g., West African sleeping sickness) or atypically (e.g., adult-onset Niemann-Pick disease type C) (Freudenreich et al. 2009). Table 10–2 provides a comprehensive compilation of disorders that have been associated with psychosis.

Both systemic infections and infections of the brain can cause psychosis in the absence of a frank delirium. The exact pathogens will vary depending on geography, travel history, and immune status and include infective agents leading to tuberculosis, cerebral malaria, toxoplasmosis, and neurocysticercosis. Herpes simplex, neurosyphilis, and HIV are important considerations for any hospitalized patients with unexplained psychosis. In one case series in the antibiotic era, neuropsychiatric symptoms alone were seen in 51% of confirmed cases of neurosyphilis (Timmermans and Carr 2004). (See also Chapter 27, "Infectious Diseases," and Chapter 28, "HIV/AIDS.")

Endocrine diseases can be accompanied by psychotic symptoms. Affective symptoms are most common, but psychosis can also occur. The classic example is thyrotoxicosis (Brownlie et al. 2000). As a special case, in a woman presenting with postpartum psychosis, postpartum thyroiditis must be ruled out (Bokhari et al. 1998). However, psychosis has been reported with a wide variety of endocrine diseases, including hypothyroidism ("myxedema madness"), Addison's disease, Cushing's disease, hyper- and hypoparathyroidism, and hypoglycemia. (See also Chapter 22, "Endocrine and Metabolic Disorders.")

Many neurological conditions can be accompanied by psychosis. Epilepsy and psychosis share a long history, with psychosis potentially occurring ictally, postictally, or interictally (Sachdev 1998; Toone 2000). Temporal lobe epilepsy is most likely to lead to psychosis, but psychosis also can occur with frontal lobe seizures (Lautenschlager and Foerstl 2001). Postictal psychosis typically occurs close in time to a seizure, with psychosis emerging a day or several days after the seizure. Interictal psychosis typically occurs in patients with poorly controlled seizures, after a decade or more of seizures. Dementing illnesses are frequently accompanied by neuropsychiatric symptoms, including psychosis. In Alzheimer's dementia, psychosis emerges in 41% of patients (Ropacki and Jeste 2005). The severity of cognitive impairment is a risk factor for psychosis. Delusions, which are more common than hallucinations, are typically concrete and simple. If seen in the context of cognitive difficulties, delusions are understandable (e.g., delusions of theft in the elderly person who forgot where he put an item, misidentification delusions, or delusions of infidelity) (Klimstra and Mahgoub 2009). In

TABLE 10–2. Selected causes of secondary psychosis

Psychomotor seizures
Head trauma (history of)
Dementias
Alzheimer's disease
Pick's disease
Lewy body disease
Stroke, including CADASIL (cerebral autosomal dominant arteriopathy with subcortical infarcts and leukoencephalopathy)
Space-occupying lesions and structural brain abnormalities
Primary brain tumors
Secondary brain metastases
Brain abscesses and cysts
Tuberous sclerosis
Midline abnormalities (e.g., corpus callosum agenesis, cavum septi pellucidi)
Cerebrovascular malformations (e.g., involving the temporal lobe)
Hydrocephalus
Demyelinating diseases
Multiple sclerosis
Leukodystrophies (metachromatic leukodystrophy, X-linked adrenoleukodystrophy, Marchiafava-Bignami syndrome)
Schilder's disease
Neuropsychiatric disorders
Huntington's disease
Wilson's disease
Parkinson's disease
Friedreich's ataxia
Autoimmune disorders
Systemic lupus erythematosus and other forms of CNS vasculitis
Paraneoplastic syndromes
Infections
Viral encephalitis
Neurosyphilis
HIV infection
CNS-invasive parasitic infections (e.g., cerebral malaria, toxoplasmosis, neurocysticercosis)
Tuberculosis
Sarcoidosis
Cryptococcal meningoencephalitis
Prion diseases (e.g., Creutzfeldt-Jakob disease)
Endocrinopathies
Hypoglycemia
Addison's disease
Cushing's disease
Hyper- and hypothyroidism
Hyper- and hypoparathyroidism
Hypopituitarism
Narcolepsy
Nutritional deficiencies
Magnesium deficiency
Vitamin A deficiency
Niacin deficiency (pellagra)
Thiamine deficiency
Vitamin B_{12} deficiency (pernicious anemia)
Metabolic disorders (partial list)
Amino acid metabolism (Hartnup disease, homocystinuria, phenylketonuria)
Porphyrias (acute intermittent porphyria, porphyria variegata, hereditary coproporphyria)
GM_2 gangliosidosis
Fabry's disease
Niemann-Pick disease type C
Gaucher's disease, adult type
Chromosomal abnormalities
Sex chromosomes (Klinefelter's syndrome, XXX syndrome)
Fragile X syndrome
Velo-cardio-facial syndrome

Note. CNS=central nervous system; HIV= human immunodeficiency virus.
Source. Adapted from Freudenreich et al. 2008.

Lewy body dementia, recurrent and well-formed visual hallucinations are a core feature (McKeith et al. 2005). Rarely, stroke can lead to poststroke psychosis, although the possibility of complicating seizures should be considered (Chemerinski and Robinson 2000). Interestingly, among the demyelinating disorders, rare leukodystrophies are more frequently associated with psychosis than is the prototypical demyelinating disease, multiple sclerosis (Ghaffar and Feinstein 2007). Basal ganglia disorders, including Huntington's disease, are also a cause of psychosis (Rosenblatt and Leroi 2000), although in Parkinson's disease, the effects of treatment with dopamine agonists must be considered.

Numerous legal and illegal drugs can cause psychosis. Some drugs produce psychosis reliably in most people (e.g., PCP). Cannabis rarely leads to anything more than mild, transient paranoia in most people. In susceptible individuals, however, cannabis is considered a risk factor for the emergence of schizophrenia and can trigger a psychotic episode (Moore et al. 2007). Psychosis in alcoholic patients has a large differential diagnosis, including alcohol withdrawal, delirium tremens, alcoholic hallucinosis, Wernicke-Korsakoff syndrome, pellagra, hepatic encephalopathy, Marchiafava-Bignami syndrome, central pontine myelinolysis, and alcohol-associated dementia (Greenberg and Lee 2001). Paranoia and morbid jealousy that can reach delusional conviction (i.e., the Othello syndrome) are well-recognized complications of severe alcoholism (Michael et al. 1995).

Among prescription medications, certain drugs are clearly associated with the potential for inducing psychosis. In reviewing patient charts, particular attention should be paid to drugs with a high potential for medication-induced psychosis, such as high-dose steroids used for autoimmune diseases, L-dopa for the treatment of Parkinson's disease, or interferon for the treatment of chronic hepatitis C. Table 10–3 provides a list of more common offending agents.

TABLE 10–3. Selected medications that can cause psychosis at therapeutic doses

Important offenders

Anticholinergics and antihistaminics

Dopaminergic drugs (e.g., L-dopa, amantadine)

Interferon

Stimulants

Corticosteroids

Others

Cardiovascular drugs: antiarrhythmics, digitalis

Anesthetics

Antimalaria drugs: mefloquine

Antituberculous drugs: D-cycloserine, ethambutol, isoniazid

Antibiotics: ciprofloxacin

Antivirals: human immunodeficiency virus medications (e.g., acyclovir; efavirenz at high plasma levels)

Anticonvulsants (high doses)

Antineoplastics (especially ifosfamide)

Sympathomimetics (including over-the-counter preparations)

Pain medications: opioids (especially meperidine, pentazocine), indomethacin

Miscellaneous: baclofen, disulfiram, cyclosporine, ephedra-containing dietary supplements

Effects of Psychosis on Medical Disorders

The presence of psychosis can greatly jeopardize the cooperation necessary for a successful hospital stay. Psychosis can be disruptive because of ancillary symptom clusters (e.g., fear or agitation) or because of its thought content (e.g., a patient refusing cooperation with surgery because of conspiracy theories). Because patients who are overtly psychotic and agitated may pose a risk to themselves and the ward, staff might be rightly afraid and limit interactions. However, patients also can be quietly psychotic and appear withdrawn (i.e., secondary negative symptoms). Patients who are suspicious, mildly disorganized, or apathetic can get "blamed" for their inability to conform to ward routines or participate in their treatment (Freudenreich and Stern 2003). Lack of insight into the need for psychiatric treatment can require legal involvement, resulting in treatment delays. In any patient who requests discharge against medical advice (AMA), a psychotic process should be ruled out.

Patients with schizophrenia have a reduced life expectancy compared with those in the general population (Brown 1997; Colton and Manderscheid 2006). The reasons for this survival gap include deaths from suicides but also an increased risk for cardiovascular disease (Goff et al. 2005; McEvoy et al. 2005). The reasons for this disparity are complex and not well understood. Added iatrogenic morbidity related to second-generation antipsychotics has possibly increased the mortality gap (Saha et al. 2007). Some factors are the same as in the general population, such as socioeconomic status, unhealthy diet, substance use, or smoking. However, it is also well documented that patients with schizophrenia receive substandard medical care compared with those in the general population (Druss et al. 2001). Unrecognized staff fears, biases, and misconceptions about psychosis therefore almost certainly contribute to the delivery of substandard care in this population (Leucht et al. 2007). Stigma is responsible for the poor care provided to patients who have a psychotic disorder diagnosis, with serious downstream consequences for patients.

Given the already increased medical morbidity and mortality, improving adherence to medical treatment (as opposed to just the psychiatric treatment) is an important long-term management consideration for physicians who care for patients with schizophrenia. In one pharmacy record study of patients with a chronic psychotic disorder, adherence was equally problematic regarding use of antipsychotics and drugs for medical conditions (antihypertensives, antihyperlipidemics, or antidiabetics), with 12-month prescription fill rates ranging from 52% to 64% (Dolder et al. 2003). In another sample of patients with serious mental illnesses and HIV infection, only 40% achieved

90% adherence to prescribed HIV medications (Wagner et al. 2003). The solution to possible nonadherence requires its recognition and a plan to remedy it based on individual patient and organizational factors. Health care systems that integrate medical and psychiatric care offer the best hope for improving medical outcomes for patients with psychotic disorders (Fleischhacker et al. 2008; Goff 2007).

Treatment of Secondary Psychosis

General Principles of Management

Safety for all parties involved, identification of the etiology of psychosis, and treatment of psychosis are the three initial goals in the care of psychotic patients in the hospital. Patients who are psychotic can be quite agitated and restless; they often require a sitter or restraints to prevent injury. Involuntary treatment can be required. During the evaluation, even when the etiology of psychosis seems clear, additional causes should be considered and unnecessary central nervous system (CNS)–active medications discontinued. In the early phase of treatment, frequent reassessment of the clinical situation is required to determine the best course of action and to assess the efficacy and ongoing necessity of interventions. Although benzodiazepines are routinely used as an ancillary treatment to calm patients with primary psychotic disorders, they should be used only judiciously in medical settings because they might paradoxically worsen agitation in medically compromised patients.

Psychiatric consultants can perform important liaison functions (including making judgments about potential dangerousness, helping with an appropriate disposition [e.g., Can the patient be discharged home? Does he need further inpatient psychiatric care? Is the psychiatric facility able to handle medical complexity?]), and coordinating care with the outpatient psychiatrist. Education about psychosis can be provided to patients, family members, and staff.

Discharge planning should take into account dangerousness and iatrogenic morbidity and mortality. Dangerousness to self or others must be considered when the patient has command hallucinations, and dangerousness to other people must be considered if the patient has delusions such as the Othello syndrome or delusional misidentification syndromes (Leong et al. 1994; Silva et al. 1994). Patients should be discharged with a plan that takes into account effects of psychosis on behavior and only when the patient has the ability to follow the treatment plan. In some cases, medication supervision by a family member or a visiting nurse will be required. Discharge planning also should take into account the long-term risks of antipsychotics, particularly the risk for tardive dyskinesia (TD) and metabolic problems such as dyslipidemias and glucose intolerance. In one prospective study of patients older than 45 years who were taking first-generation antipsychotics, about a quarter of the patients developed TD after 1 year of treatment (Jeste et al. 1995). Given the age-related increase in TD risk, the cumulative dose of antipsychotics should be kept to the absolute minimum in all patients but particularly in the elderly. Patients successfully treated with an antipsychotic for delirium or secondary psychosis who do not require long-term antipsychotic maintenance treatment should have a clear plan in place for the discontinuation of the antipsychotic (if this has not been accomplished prior to transfer).

Specific Treatment Considerations for Secondary Psychosis

Often, antipsychotics are needed to treat secondary psychosis. Antipsychotics may be withheld if psychosis is mild and expected to resolve within hours (e.g., substance-induced psychosis). Instead, benzodiazepines such as diazepam (10 mg orally) can be given to alleviate distress. However, in instances when distress from psychosis is severe; when psychosis can be expected to last longer than a few hours; or when psychosis jeopardizes the medical treatment and safety of patients, staff, or visitors, antipsychotics are the treatment of choice for psychosis. Depending on the underlying cause of psychosis, treatment strategies other than antipsychotics are sometimes indicated. For example, in dementia of the Lewy body type, rivastigmine has been shown in a controlled trial to have beneficial behavioral effects, perhaps through reversing a proposed cholinergic deficit (McKeith et al. 2000). If psychosis is the result of alcohol or sedative withdrawal, benzodiazepines are the treatment of choice. Thiamine must be administered when Wernicke's encephalopathy arises and should always be given before glucose in cases of suspected hypoglycemia. Valproate was effective for alcoholic hallucinosis in one controlled treatment trial (Aliyez and Aliyez 2008).

In the ideal situation, the medical team will effectively treat the medical disease responsible for the psychosis, and the psychiatrist will control psychosis until the medical condition is cured. With time, psychosis resolves, and the antipsychotic can be reduced and discontinued. In some instances, control of the medical condition alone, without using antipsychotics, might resolve the psychosis—as, for example, in the case of seizures (Nadkarni et al. 2007), although the best course of action for psychosis in epilepsy is not well established (Farooq and Sherin 2008). If the underlying medical disease (e.g., a degenerative condition) cannot be cured, then a decision must be made as to the duration of antipsychotic treatment. Interestingly, in the earlier-mentioned longitudinal study of patients diagnosed with psychosis due to a general medical condition, no temporal association between the neurological illness and psychosis was seen, and intermittent but not maintenance treatment was sufficient for the treatment of psychosis (Feinstein and Ron 1998).

The choice of an antipsychotic should be determined by the specifics of the situation (including urgency, access, medical comorbidities, and tolerability). In general, second-generation antipsychotics were, until recently, considered preferred for the long-term management of schizophrenia (and, by inference, medical disorders that require long-term management with antipsychotics) because of their better tolerability, particularly with regard to extrapyramidal symptoms (EPS) and TD risk (Correll et al. 2004). Tolerability of antipsychotics is clearly a concern in medically complex patients with secondary psychosis. Patients with HIV infection or AIDS, for example, are very sensitive to first-generation antipsychotics. However, in schizophrenia care, the assumption of better effectiveness (i.e., efficacy and tolerability) of second-generation antipsychotics over first-generation antipsychotics is increasingly being challenged by large randomized trials (Jones et al. 2006; Kahn et al. 2008; Leucht et al. 2009; Lieberman et al. 2005; Sikich et al. 2008), with particular concerns being raised about the development of metabolic syndrome (Stahl et al. 2009). Both first- and second-generation antipsychotics have now been shown to also be associated with sudden cardiac death (Ray et al. 2009).

Antipsychotics might not be effective and safe for all instances of psychosis either. For example, they have been shown to be relatively ineffective for the neurobehavioral problems associated with Alzheimer's disease (Schneider et al. 2006). In a randomized trial, nursing home patients with Alzheimer's disease who took antipsychotics for 1 year were 7% more likely to have died compared with patients who were switched to placebo (Ballard et al. 2009), leaving clinicians with no good options for the treatment of psychosis in demented patients (Jeste et al. 2008). In all patients, but particularly in the elderly, treatments that increase anticholinergic tone (e.g., low-potency first-generation antipsychotics or high-potency antipsychotics requiring ancillary anticholinergics) are to be avoided to reduce the risk of delirium or anticholinergic-associated cognitive problems.

Mania in the Medically Ill

Mania associated with a variety of conditions has been described in the literature. It was not, however, until Krauthammer and Klerman's (1978) classic article on secondary mania that a category was created to separate this condition from "functional" primary bipolar mood disorder.

Epidemiology and Risk Factors

Goodwin and Jamison (2007) reported that the annual risk of having a manic episode is 0.24%–0.77% in the general U.S. population; however, no studies have used formal instruments to report the incidence or prevalence of mania in the medically ill. In a retrospective chart review of 755 patients evaluated by a psychiatry consultation service in a general hospital, Rundell and Wise (1989) found that in a 1-year period, 13 of the 15 (87%) patients diagnosed with mania met criteria for secondary mania. A positive family or personal history of bipolar illness might steer clinicians toward diagnosing primary mania, but such a history could merely indicate an increased susceptibility for secondary mania. Postpartum mania might be considered a special case of secondary mania in which sudden hormonal changes induce a manic episode in a patient with increased (genetic) susceptibility to mood episodes. Vascular disease is a risk factor that seems to predispose some elderly to late-onset mania (Subramaniam et al. 2007).

Clinical Features

The clinical features of secondary mania mimic those of mania in bipolar disorder and often develop in stages, potentially extending from mild hypomania to delirious psychotic mania (Carlson and Goodwin 1973). Early symptoms in secondary mania include mood lability, feeling "high," and disrupted sleep. As in primary mania, grandiosity, racing thoughts, euphoria, irritability, and hostility may appear, and progression to flight of ideas, gross disorganization, and frank psychosis may occur.

The course and prognosis of secondary mania depend in part on the underlying illness. When secondary mania is caused by drugs such as methamphetamine, cocaine, or methylenedioxymethamphetamine, the behavior and mood changes generally resolve once the offending agent is stopped. However, when mania arises via CNS injury, infections, neoplasm, or neurodegenerative processes, symptoms may persist. In addition, medications to treat the underlying illness also may precipitate secondary mania, often presenting treatment dilemmas, because their continued use may be required for ongoing care (e.g., interferon for cancer, steroids for organ transplantation or autoimmune disorders). In these cases, the consultation psychiatrist may play a critical role in controlling the symptoms of secondary mania to ensure that optimal medical treatment can be delivered safely.

Diagnosis and Assessment

Although the symptoms of secondary mania are the same as those seen in primary mania, a DSM-IV-TR diagnosis of secondary mania requires only a prominent and persistently elevated, expansive, or irritable mood. DSM-IV-TR makes no mention of number or duration of symptoms. Because both delirium and mania have similar clinical presentations, their differentiation can be difficult. Both syndromes are abrupt in onset and have accompanying symptoms of inattention, agitation, erratic sleep, and the presence of paranoia and psychosis. The waxing and waning course of delirium, along with decreased arousal and clouding of consciousness, should help differentiate it from secondary mania.

Once new-onset mania is diagnosed, the differentiation between primary mania due to bipolar disorder and secondary mania should be attempted. Secondary mania often develops within a short period (e.g., hours or days) from the physiological insult and may occur throughout the life span. In contrast, episodes due to bipolar disorder typically occur during the first three decades of life (Goodwin and Jamison 2007), and although there has been increasing discussion about late-onset bipolar illness, new-onset primary mania tends to be rare after age 50 (Oostervink et al. 2009). In addition, the diagnosis of secondary mania is more likely when cognitive dysfunction or focal neurological signs are present, no personal history or family history of bipolar disorder exists, or treatment of the mood disorder with standard interventions is ineffective (Arora and Daughton 2007).

As with psychosis, the clinical history, physical examination, and laboratory evaluations are important elements in distinguishing primary and secondary mania (see Table 10–1 for laboratory evaluation). In addition, the neurological examination should particularly focus on the presence of nondominant hemispheric lesions associated with secondary mania, including left-sided hemiparesis, hyperactive deep tendon reflexes, presence of Hoffmann's and Babinski's signs, along with the snout, palmomental, and glabellar reflexes. Attentional deficits, including left-sided neglect, anosognosia, and constructional dyspraxia, also should be assessed. Other regions of the brain that have been associated with manic states include lesions related to the anterior cerebral artery, with associated frontal lobe deficits, and lesions of the basal ganglia, which may manifest with symptoms such as chorea, athetosis, parkinsonism, or hemiballismus.

Although the evaluation of mania is based on a clinical assessment, rating scales can track the severity of symptoms. A well-accepted scale often used in clinical trials is the 11-item Young Mania Rating Scale (YMRS; Young et al. 1978).

Etiology and Differential Diagnosis

Secondary mania has been ascribed to numerous conditions (Table 10–4). Many are reported as cases, linked tem-

TABLE 10–4. Selected causes of secondary mania

Neurological conditions
Tumors (gliomas, meningiomas, thalamic metastasis)
Cerebrovascular lesions (right hemispheric)
Multiple sclerosis
Traumatic brain injury
Complex partial seizures
Viral encephalitis (acute and postinfectious)
Human immunodeficiency virus infection
Cryptococcal meningoencephalitis
Neurosyphilis
Huntington's disease
Parkinson's disease (including treatment with deep brain stimulation)
Frontotemporal dementia
Wilson's disease
Fahr's disease
Klinefelter's syndrome
Kleine-Levin syndrome
Systemic conditions
Cushing's disease
Vitamin B_{12} deficiency
Niacin deficiency
Antiphospholipid antibody syndrome
Hyponatremia
Carcinoid syndrome
Hyperthyroidism
Medications and substances of abuse
Amantadine
Amphetamines
Anabolic steroids
Antidepressants
Baclofen (administration and withdrawal)
Buspirone
Captopril
Cimetidine
Clonidine withdrawal
Cocaine
Corticosteroids/corticosteroid withdrawal
Didanosine
Hallucinogens
Isoniazid
L-Dopa
Methylphenidate
Phencyclidine
Procainamide
Thyroxine
Zidovudine

porally to the development of mania, but some have proven to be more consistently associated with the development of manic syndromes and are discussed in more detail below.

Mania Secondary to Neurological Diseases

Cerebrovascular injury. Poststroke mania occurs in about 1% of strokes (Jorge et al. 1993; Starkstein et al. 1989). Manic syndromes have been reported following cerebrovascular lesions in multiple areas, including following a right middle cerebral artery territory stroke with ischemic lesions involving the medial and basal temporal lobes (Bornke et al. 1998), right thalamic infarcts and hemorrhage (Leibson 2000; Vuilleumier et al. 1998), and isolated strokes of the right caudate nuclei (Mendez et al. 1989). Berthier et al. (1996) reported a case series of nine patients with development of poststroke bipolar illness, with predominant involvement of subcortical structures of the right hemispheres, including the lentiform nucleus, internal capsule, caudate nucleus, thalamus, periventricular white matter, and brain stem. Most cases in the literature attribute the development of vascular-associated mania to right-sided infarcts, but left-sided lesions also have been described (Berthier et al. 1990; Fenn and George 1999).

Traumatic brain injury (TBI). Up to 50% of all patients with TBI may develop posttraumatic depression (Mendez 2000), whereas mania tends to be relatively infrequent. In a study of 66 patients with a head injury, 41% had symptoms of depression, 9% developed mania, and one patient was diagnosed with bipolar disorder within 1 year of the injury (Jorge et al. 1993). Post-TBI manic patients were typically less euphoric and less likely to have depressive episodes, with 85% of patients being irritable and 70% being more aggressive (Jorge et al. 1993; Shukla et al. 1987).

Neurodegenerative processes. Dementing processes also have been associated with the development of mania. Although mania tends to be rare in Alzheimer's disease, it has been reported to occur in greater frequency in patients with frontotemporal dementia (FTD) (Arciniegas 2006; Galvez-Andres et al. 2007; Woolley et al. 2007). Emotional changes (such as depression, mania, irritability, lability, and anger) are common in patients with FTD, as are obsessive symptoms. Neurodegenerative movement disorders also have been associated with mania. Manic episodes have been shown to occur in 2%–12% of patients with Huntington's disease, and often the mood change may precede the appearance of a movement disorder (Folstein 1989; Mendez 1994). Symptoms of mania also have been described in Fahr's disease (idiopathic basal ganglia calcification), Wilson's disease, and postencephalitic Parkinson's disease, along with a case report of mania following treatment of Parkinson's symptoms with subthalamic nucleus stimulation (Krauthammer and Klerman 1978; Raucher-Chene et al. 2008; Rosenblatt and Leroi 2000).

Epilepsy. Although depression is more common in those with epilepsy, mania also may arise. Investigators have reported a frequency of bipolar illness of 3%–22% (Robertson 1992) in depressed patients with epilepsy, and these disorders occasionally can be clinically difficult to distinguish from primary bipolar disorder (Himmelhoch 1984). Mania may follow right temporal lobe epileptiform discharges (Hurwitz et al. 1985) and tends to occur with an increase in seizures or intermittent epileptiform activity (Barczak et al. 1988; Ramchandani and Riggio 1992). Mania associated with epilepsy also may present with compulsive behavior and elements of psychosis (such as thought insertion and hallucinations) (Himmelhoch 1984). In one retrospective review of patients seen by psychiatric consultants, two of four manic epileptic patients had peri-ictal mania and poor seizure control (Lyketsos et al. 1993b). In addition, patients in the immediate postictal state may show intermixed epileptiform activity without clinical signs of seizures (Mendez and Grau 1991). Patients may experience postictal psychosis with features of mania 12–48 hours after a burst of seizures, which may continue for weeks or even months, but this is rare (Chakrabarti et al. 1999; Mendez and Grau 1991).

Mania Secondary to Infectious Diseases

Several infections involving the CNS may produce manic syndromes. Mania may be the first manifestation of neurosyphilis, cryptococcal meningoencephalitis, or viral encephalitides, including herpes simplex encephalitis (Mendez 2000). Mania also may occur as a postencephalitic process following recovery from the acute stage of illness.

In a study conducted in the Department of Veterans Affairs (VA) health care system, 4% of HIV-infected patients were reported by their providers to have mania or bipolar disorder; however, the prevalence of mania directly as a result of HIV is not known (Kilbourne et al. 2001). In some settings, the prevalence of secondary mania might be quite high. In a study of mania in Uganda (a country with a high prevalence of HIV infection), 61 of 141 (43%) patients admitted to a psychiatric ward for mania were judged to have HIV-related secondary mania (Nakimuli-Mpungu et al. 2006). In this cohort, patients with secondary mania had more manic symptoms (including irritability and aggression) and showed more cognitive impairment compared with the patients admitted with primary mania. Almost all patients with secondary mania experienced psychosis (including visual hallucinations in 67% of patients). This recent cohort confirms earlier clinical descriptions of increased irritability and pressured speech with neurocognitive changes in patients with advanced HIV disease who developed mania (Lyketsos et al. 1997). Compared with patients with primary bipolar disorder, patients with secondary mania are less likely to have a personal or family history of mood disorder. Secondary mania is associated with evidence of structural brain changes (as seen on CT or MRI scans) (Boccellari et al. 1988; Kieburtz et al. 1991; Lyketsos et al. 1993a). Certain antiretroviral medications have been implicated in medication-induced mania, including zidovudine (Maxwell et al. 1988; Wright et al. 1989), didanosine (Brouillette et al. 1994), abacavir (Brouilette and Routy 2007), and efavirenz (Shah and Balderson 2003). In addition, both ethambutol and clarithromycin have been reported to be associated with manic symptoms in the setting of treatment for *Mycobacterium avium* complex in individuals with AIDS (Nightingale et al. 1995; Pickles and Spelman 1996).

Mania Secondary to Endocrine Diseases

Several endocrine diseases have been associated with the development of manic states, including Cushing's disease and diseases of the thyroid. Typically, mania has been associated with hyperthyroidism (Clower 1984; C.S. Lee and Hutto 2008; Villani and Weitzel 1979), whereas hypothyroidism has been linked with depression and severe hypothyroidism with psychosis (Clower 1984). However, reports also have noted depression associated with hyperthyroidism (Thomsen et al. 2005) and mania associated with hypothyroidism (Balldin et al. 1987; Levitte 1993; Stowell and Barnhill 2005).

Treatment with corticosteroids is likely the most common cause of secondary mania (Rundell and Wise 1989). In a prospective study by Naber et al. (1996), of 50 patients with ophthalmic conditions being administered high-dose corticosteroids for 8 days, 13 patients (26%) developed symptoms of (mild) mania, and 5 patients (10%) developed depression. Most mood-related symptoms developed early in the course of treatment, typically within 3 days of starting corticosteroids.

Effects of Mania on Medical Disorders

Like patients with psychotic disorders, patients with bipolar disorder have medical comorbidity (Kilbourne et al. 2004) that can complicate treatment of the psychiatric disorder. Because of its unpredictable nature, bipolar illness may cause significant periods in which the patient has little or no contact with providers, especially during a manic episode (Keck et al. 1997). This lack of contact may lead to poor adherence, social instability, and increased medical comorbidity. Manic and hypomanic episodes can increase the risk of infectious diseases (e.g., cervical cancer, hepatitis C, HIV infection) through sexual indiscretions or drug use (el-Serag et al. 2002).

During an inpatient hospitalization, the development of mania may cause refusal of care proposed by medical-surgical teams. If secondary hypomania or mania is not suspected, the medical team may attribute the patient's behavior to personality traits or to being "difficult," often causing a schism between the patient and his or her providers, potentially jeopardizing the necessary medical evaluation and care.

Treatment of Secondary Mania

General Principles of Management

Similar to the management of psychotic patients, ensuring the safety of the patient and staff is of paramount importance and is the initial goal of care for the acutely manic patient. Patients with mania are unpredictable, disinhibited, and easily agitated, especially in an unknown medical environment with an overabundance of stimuli (e.g., ancillary staff, frequent vital sign checks, laboratory blood draws, medical procedures). The psychiatry consultant can assess the patient's medical and neuropsychiatric condition and help to minimize any unnecessary interventions (including medications with CNS effects that may contribute to or exacerbate the patient's symptoms). Once safety has been addressed, the focus should be helping to elucidate the underlying etiology of secondary mania.

Psychopharmacology

Medications used for the treatment of secondary mania are generally the same as those used in primary bipolar illness. The choice of medication is based on the severity of mania, the patient's willingness or ability to receive oral medications, the etiology of the mania, and the patient's comorbid medical illnesses. For example, lithium may be difficult to administer safely in patients with fluid shifts, electrolyte abnormalities, acute or chronic renal dysfunction, or already established thyroid dysfunction. Valproate may be relatively contraindicated in patients with hepatic disease or a history of pancreatitis. Carbamazepine also may pose difficulties in patients with hepatic disease and is associated with potential hematological toxicity (e.g., leukopenia or aplastic anemia), antidiuretic actions, and quinidine-like effects on cardiac conduction. In addition, carbamazepine is a potent inducer of cytochrome P450 3A4, and a review of current active medications is necessary to help prevent drug-drug interactions. Although benzodiazepines may provide rapid symptom reduction, they may also potentiate CNS depression by decreasing respiratory drive, and their use is relatively contraindicated in patients with chronic obstructive pulmonary disease who are at risk for carbon dioxide retention. In addition, paradoxical disinhibition with worsening behavior may occur, especially in patients with a TBI. First- and second-generation antipsychotics are often used for the treatment of secondary mania, particularly in agitated patients. Second-generation antipsychotics are generally preferred for the short-term treatment of secondary mania because of lower propensity to cause EPS. Nevertheless, monitoring for neuroleptic-induced catatonia is still warranted. If long-term use of antipsychotics for the management of secondary mania is contemplated, potential morbidity and mortality risks associated with antipsychotics should be considered (e.g., risk for metabolic syndrome or TD).

Electroconvulsive Therapy

Electroconvulsive therapy (ECT) has been used in the management of acute mania and may be especially helpful to treat mania and marked physical activity that is poorly responsive to pharmacological interventions. Delirious mania, a syndrome of acute onset characterized by excitement, psychosis, and delirium, has been described and treated successfully with ECT and benzodiazepines, with administration of lithium and/or antipsychotics possibly worsening the underlying condition (Fink 1999). If ECT is used, lithium should be avoided because this may prolong the neuromuscular blockade induced before ECT administration (Rudorfer et al. 1987). ECT may present higher risk in some medically ill patients (see Chapter 40, "Electroconvulsive Therapy").

Catatonia in the Medically Ill

Initially described in Kahlbaum's 1874 monograph, catatonia has long been associated with psychiatric, neurological, and medical disorders (Kahlbaum 1973). Modern theorists view catatonia as a syndrome of motor signs in association with disorders of affect, thought, and behavior. Some motor features are classic but infrequent (e.g., echopraxia and waxy flexibility), whereas others are common in psychiatric patients (e.g., agitation and withdrawal) but denoted as catatonic because of their duration and severity. The sometimes subtle presentation of catatonia may go undetected, which could account for the impression of a declining incidence. For example, in one study, clinicians diagnosed catatonia in only 2% of 139 patients, whereas a research team identified it in 18% (van der Heijden et al. 2005).

Epidemiology and Risk Factors

The rate of catatonia in the psychiatric population varies according to study design and diagnostic criteria. In a series of prospective studies of patients hospitalized with acute psychotic episodes, the incidence of catatonia was within the 7%–17% range (Caroff et al. 2004a). When mood disorders were the focus, rates ranged from 13% to 31%. Catatonia secondary to medical illness with a variety of "organic" etiologies accounts for 4%–46% of cases in various series, underscoring the need for a thorough medical evaluation when catatonic signs are present. In pediatric settings, catatonia is sometimes reported in patients with mental retardation and autistic spectrum disorders (Wing and Shah 2006).

Certain conditions may increase the risk of developing neuroleptic malignant syndrome (NMS)—an important iatrogenic form of catatonia (Mann et al. 1994). A history of simple catatonia is a major risk factor for the progression to NMS (White and Robins 1991). Other risk factors include schizophrenia, mood disorders, neurological disorders (e.g., basal ganglia disorders), alcoholism, and substance abuse disorders. Alcohol or sedative-hypnotic withdrawal may increase the risk of NMS as a result of altered thermoregulation and autonomic dysfunction. Agitation, dehydration, and exhaustion also may increase the risk for NMS. Up to one-third of patients who have had NMS will have a subsequent episode when rechallenged with neuroleptics.

Clinical Features

Stupor, mutism, negativism, motoric immobility, catalepsy, posturing, but also excitement are considered the core clinical features of catatonia. These features are the same regardless of whether the condition occurs in the context of a mood, psychotic, or medical state. Catatonia may have rapid or insidious onset and may be associated with high morbidity and mortality. It may be described in a variety of ways by clinicians on medical, surgical, and neurological wards—as a stupor, as a fever of unknown origin, as an acute encephalopathic syndrome, or falsely as "schizophrenic" or "conversion disorder."

The clinician must be cognizant of the fact that diametrically opposed subtypes of catatonia have been described. Catatonic withdrawal, with posturing, rigidity, mutism, and repetitive actions, is the most commonly recognized form, and the term *catatonia* is sometimes used as shorthand for this retarded motor state, occasionally referred to as "Kahlbaum's syndrome" (Fink and Taylor 2009). Patients with severe catatonia will be stuporous and may even present with low Glasgow Coma Scale scores. However, patients also can present with hyperactivity, hyperproductive pressured speech, and restless, agitated behavior accompanied by catatonic features (bizarre stereotypies, mannerisms, grimacings, echo phenomena, perseverations) and an acute confusional state. Catatonic excitement has at times been called "delirious mania" or "Bell's mania" (Bell 1849; Fink 1999).

In 1934, Stauder described a syndrome of "lethal catatonia." It was marked by the acute onset of a manic delirium, high fever, and catatonic stupor and a mortality rate of greater than 50%. Because not all cases are lethal, Philbrick and Rummans (1994) suggested the term *malignant catatonia* to describe critically ill cases marked by autonomic instability or hyperthermia, in contrast to cases of "simple, nonmalignant catatonia."

NMS is a form of malignant catatonia (Caroff et al. 2004b; Fink and Taylor 2003). It is characterized by fever, autonomic dysfunction with tachycardia and elevated blood pressure, rigidity (sometimes "lead pipe" in nature), mutism, and stupor. NMS usually develops over the course of a few days (Caroff 1980; Mann and Caroff 1990). It commonly begins with rigidity and mental status changes followed by signs of a hypermetabolic state. Hyperthermia, which can climb to higher than 42°C, is reported in 98% of the cases. The patient with NMS may be alert, delirious, stuporous, or comatose. Once neuroleptics are stopped and supportive measures are begun, the course is usually self-limited, lasting 2 days to 1 month. Persistent cases are usually secondary to use of depot neuroleptics, and ECT is highly effective in these cases. Although the mortality rate has been reduced through better recognition and management, a 10% risk of death remains.

The prognosis in catatonia reflects the nature and severity of the underlying etiology of the catatonia, which largely accounts for the severity and chronicity of the catatonic state itself (Levenson and Pandurangi 2004). Those with catatonia secondary to a mood disorder often do better than do those with underlying schizophrenia; and those with catatonia secondary to toxic-metabolic disorders often have better prognoses than do those with catatonia secondary to brain lesions. When the catatonia becomes chronic, as it does in certain cases of catatonic schizophrenia, the prognosis is poorer.

Diagnosis and Assessment

The signs and symptoms of the catatonic syndrome based on the Modified Bush-Francis Catatonia Rating Scale (BFCRS) are outlined in Table 10–5 (Bush et al. 1996a).

The BFCRS 23-item rating scale operationally defines each catatonic sign, rates its severity, and provides a standardized schema for clinical examination (see Table 10–6), leading to reliable ratings that are sensitive to change (Bush et al. 1996b).

With the BFCRS, a case is defined by the presence of at least 2 of the first 14 items from this scale. However, the number of signs and symptoms required to make a diagnosis of catatonia is controversial. DSM-IV-TR stipulates the presence of only one catatonic motor sign to make a diagnosis of catatonic disorder due to a general medical condition if evidence confirms a medical etiology. A nosological difficulty with DSM-IV-TR is that this diagnosis is prevented for an episode that occurs "exclusively during the course of a delirium," an issue currently under debate for DSM-V.

A general evaluation to exclude secondary catatonia is provided in Table 10–1. Other entities to consider in the differential diagnosis that are not secondary catatonia but may be mistaken for it include stiff-person syndrome (Lockman and Burns 2007), malignant hyperthermia (Ali et al. 2003), locked-in syndrome (Smith and Delargy 2005), and other hyperkinetic and hypokinetic states (Fink and Taylor 2003). Akinetic Parkinson's disease can produce a catatonia-like state (i.e., mute, immobilized), but it occurs well after the diagnosis of Parkinson's disease. Selective mutism and conversion disorder are psychiatric conditions that can be confused with catatonia.

Diffuse, nonspecific changes on the EEG will be found most often in patients with secondary catatonias. An EEG read as normal would be most consistent with primary catatonia, although psychiatric patients may have abnormal EEG findings. Generalized slowing that is consistent with encephalopathy is found in approximately half of NMS cases. Occasionally, EEG evidence of nonconvulsive status epilepticus is found in catatonic patients (Louis and Pflaster 1995). Neuroimaging, especially MRI of the brain, should be obtained, although a negative result does not rule out an "organic" etiology. Brain imaging is important because strokes, hematomas, and space-occupying lesions can all present with new-onset catatonia, and these conditions may worsen with prolonged benzodiazepine treatment (Carroll and Goforth 2004). Head CT and cerebrospinal fluid studies are normal in 95% of NMS cases. Creatine kinase levels are often elevated in malignant catatonias but also can be high in simple catatonias.

Etiology and Differential Diagnosis

Catatonia erroneously became exclusively associated with schizophrenia through the influence of Kraepelin and Bleuler, and this nosological error continued into DSM, despite long-standing linkage of catatonia to affective disorders and to organic conditions (Abrams and Taylor 1976; Gelenberg 1976; Wilcox and Nasrallah 1986). Some now advocate a separate nosology for catatonia based on the syndromic nature of the diagnosis and its unique treatment with lorazepam and ECT (Taylor and Fink 2003). Clinically, the catatonic syndrome is perhaps best divided into primary (psychiatric) and secondary ("organic") varieties on the basis of etiologies as well as into simple and malignant types on the basis of severity (see Table 10–7).

TABLE 10–5. Catatonic symptoms (based on the Modified Bush-Francis Catatonia Rating Scale)

Catatonia can be diagnosed by the presence of 2 or more of the first 14 signs listed below.

Sign	Description
1. Excitement	Severe hyperactivity and constant motor unrest, which is manifestly purposeless (not to be attributed to akathisia or goal-directed agitation)
2. Immobility/stupor	Severe hypoactivity, immobility, and minimal response to stimuli
3. Mutism	Verbal unresponsiveness or minimal responsiveness
4. Staring	Fixed gaze, little or no visual scanning of environment, and decreased eye blink
5. Posturing/catalepsy	Spontaneous maintenance of posture(s), including everyday ones (e.g., sitting/standing for long periods without reacting)
6. Grimacing	Maintenance of bizarre facial expressions
7. Echolalia/echopraxia	Mimicking of an examiner's speech and/or movements
8. Stereotypy	Perseverative, non-goal-directed, not inherently abnormal motor activity (e.g., playing with fingers, or repetitively touching, patting, or rubbing oneself)
9. Mannerisms	Bizarre, inherently abnormal movements (e.g., hopping or walking on tiptoe, saluting those passing by, or exaggerating caricatures of mundane movements)
10. Verbigeration	Repetition of phrases (like a scratched record)
11. Rigidity	Maintenance of a rigid posture despite efforts to be moved; exclude if cogwheeling or tremor present
12. Negativism	Seemingly motiveless resistance to instructions or attempts to move or examine the patient; patient does the exact opposite of the instruction
13. Waxy flexibility	During repositioning, patient first offers resistance before allowing repositioning (similar to that of a bending candle)
14. Withdrawal	Refusal to eat, drink, do activities of daily living, or make eye contact
15. Impulsivity	Sudden inappropriate behaviors (e.g., running down a hallway, screaming, or taking off clothes) without provocation and without appropriate explanation
16. Automatic obedience	Exaggerated cooperation with the examiner's request or spontaneous continuation of the movement requested
17. *Mitgehen*	Exaggerated arm raising in response to light pressure of finger, despite instructions to the contrary; like an "Anglepoise lamp"
18. *Gegenhalten*	Resistance to passive movement that is proportional to strength of the stimulus; appears automatic rather than willful
19. Ambitendency	Appearance of being "stuck" in indecisive, hesitant movement
20. Grasp reflex	As in the neurological examination
21. Perseveration	Repeatedly returns to the same topic or persistence with movement
22. Combativeness	Aggressive in an undirected manner, with no or only inadequate or inappropriate explanation afterward
23. Fever and autonomic abnormality	Abnormal temperature, blood pressure, pulse, or respiratory rate, and diaphoresis

Note. The full 23-item Bush-Francis Catatonia Rating Scale (BFCRS) measures the severity of 23 signs on a 0–3 continuum for each sign. The first 14 signs combine to form the Bush-Francis Catatonia Screening Instrument (BFCSI). The BFCSI measures only the presence or absence of the first 14 signs, and it is used for case detection. Item definitions on the two scales are the same.
Source. Modified from the BFCRS (Bush et al. 1996a; Fricchione et al. 2004).

TABLE 10–6. Bedside examination for catatonia

This standardized method is used to complete the 23-item Bush-Francis Catatonia Rating Scale (BFCRS) and the 14-item Bush-Francis Catatonia Screening Instrument (BFSCI). Item definitions on the two scales are the same. The BFCSI measures only the presence or absence of the first 14 signs.

Ratings are based on observed behaviors during the examination, with the exception of completing the items for "withdrawal" and "autonomic abnormality," which may be based on directly observed behavior or chart documentation.

Generally, only those items that are clearly present should be rated. If uncertain about the presence of an item, it should be rated as "0."

Procedure

1. Observe the patient while attempting to involve in conversation.
2. The examiner should scratch his or her head in an exaggerated manner.
3. The arm should be examined for cogwheeling. Attempt to reposture, and instruct the patient to "keep your arm loose." Move the arm with alternating lighter and heavier force.
4. Ask the patient to extend his or her arm. Place one finger under his or her hand and state, "Do *not* let me raise your arm," and try to raise the arm slowly.
5. Extend the hand stating, "Do *not* shake my hand."
6. Reach into your pocket and state, "Stick out your tongue. I want to stick a pin in it."
7. Evaluate for grasp reflex.
8. Evaluate the chart for reports from the previous 24 hour period. Check for oral intake, vital signs, and any incidents.
9. Evaluate the patient indirectly, at least for a brief period each day, regarding the following:
    - Activity level
    - Abnormal movements
    - Abnormal speech
    - Echopraxia
    - Rigidity
    - Negativism
    - Waxy flexibility
    - *Gegenhalten*
    - *Mitgehen*
    - Ambitendency
    - Automatic obedience
    - Grasp reflex

Source. Adapted from Bush et al. 1996a; Fricchione et al. 2004.

TABLE 10–7. Clinical classification of catatonia

Based on etiology

Primary catatonia
- Due to mood disorder
- Due to psychotic disorder
- Due to other psychiatric disorder

Secondary catatonias
- Due to neurological condition
- Due to medical condition
- Due to substance toxicity[a]

Based on severity

Simple (nonmalignant) catatonia[b]

Malignant ("lethal"[c]) catatonia

[a]Neuroleptic malignant syndrome is an iatrogenic cause of a secondary malignant catatonia (i.e., antipsychotic-induced malignant catatonia).
[b]Kahlbaum's syndrome is a hypokinetic form of nonmalignant catatonia.
[c]Not all cases of "lethal" catatonia are deadly.
Source. Based on Philbrick and Rummans 1994; Taylor and Fink 2003.

The numerous causes of catatonia are summarized in Table 10–8 (Carroll et al. 1994; Fricchione et al. 2004; Philbrick and Rummans 1994).

When catatonic stupor occurs in the setting of delirium, limbic encephalitis should be considered in the differential diagnosis (Ali et al. 2008). Limbic encephalitis can present acutely or subacutely with confusion, cognitive impairment, seizures, and catatonia. Infectious, autoimmune, paraneoplastic, and idiopathic etiologies of limbic encephalitis should be ruled out (Eker et al. 2008; Foster and Caplan 2009; Tüzün and Dalmau 2007).

Effects of Catatonia on Medical Disorders

Major medical complications that frequently will be manifested in patients with persistent catatonic stupor need close monitoring and management if the patient is to escape morbidity and mortality (Levenson and Pandurangi 2004). Some of this risk stems from the clinical challenge of diagnosing medical conditions in patients who are mute, rigid, and unable to cooperate. But the risk is sometimes compounded by "therapeutic nihilism" when catatonic patients are viewed as hopeless or demented. In addition, those in chronic catatonic states often wind up in long-term care centers such as nursing homes or state facilities without the proper medical resources to adequately address their conditions.

Pulmonary Complications

Aspiration is the most common pulmonary complication of catatonia. It can result in pneumonitis or pneumonia.

TABLE 10–8. Selected causes of catatonia

Primary
Acute psychoses
Conversion disorder
Dissociative disorders
Mood disorders
Obsessive-compulsive disorder
Personality disorders
Schizophrenia
Secondary
Cerebrovascular causes
Arterial aneurysms
Arteriovenous malformations
Arterial and venous thrombosis
Bilateral parietal infarcts
Temporal lobe infarct
Subarachnoid hemorrhage
Subdural hematoma
Third ventricle hemorrhage
Hemorrhagic infarcts
CNS vasculitis (e.g., systemic lupus erythematosus)
Other CNS disorders
Akinetic mutism
Alcoholic degeneration and Wernicke's encephalopathy
Cerebellar degeneration
Cerebral anoxia
Cerebromacular degeneration
Traumatic brain injury
Frontal lobe atrophy
Multiple sclerosis and acute disseminated encephalomyelitis
Hydrocephalus
Lesions of thalamus and globus pallidus
Narcolepsy
Parkinsonism
Postencephalitic states
Seizure disorders[a]
Tuberous sclerosis
Tumors
Angioma
Frontal lobe tumors
Gliomas
Langerhans' carcinoma
Paraneoplastic encephalopathy (e.g., oat cell carcinoma, teratomas)
Periventricular diffuse pinealoma
Toxins
Coal gas
Organic fluorides
Tetraethyl lead poisoning
Infections[a]
Bacterial meningoencephalitis
Bacterial sepsis
Hepatic amoebiasis
HIV/AIDS
Cerebral malaria
Subacute sclerosing panencephalitis
Tertiary syphilis
Typhoid fever
Viral encephalitis (especially herpes)
Metabolic causes[a]
Acute intermittent porphyria
Addison's disease
Cushing's disease
Diabetic ketoacidosis
Hepatic encephalopathy
Hereditary coproporphyria
Homocystinuria
Hyperparathyroidism
Pellagra
Uremia
Drug-associated causes
Antipsychotics[a] (both typical and atypical have been associated)
Antidepressants (tricyclics, monoamine oxidase inhibitors, and others)
Anticonvulsants (e.g., carbamazepine, primidone)
Disulfiram[a]
Efavirenz
Metoclopramide
Dopamine depleters (e.g., tetrabenazine)
Dopamine withdrawal (e.g., abrupt discontinuation of L-dopa)
Hallucinogens (e.g., mescaline, phencyclidine,[a] and lysergic acid diethylamide)
Lithium carbonate
Sedative-hypnotic withdrawal
Corticosteroids[a]
Stimulants (e.g., amphetamines, methylphenidate, and possibly cocaine)

Note. CNS=central nervous system.
[a]Signifies most common medical conditions associated with catatonic disorder from literature review done by Carroll et al. 1994.
Source. Adapted from Fricchione et al. 2004; Philbrick and Rummans 1994.

Risk factors for pneumonia include atelectasis, malnutrition, poor respiratory effort, and institutional settings, which also make nosocomial infections with antibiotic-resistant organisms more likely. Prophylactic antibiotics are not beneficial in patients who are considered at high risk for aspiration. Prophylactic administration of antacids, H_2 blockers, or proton pump inhibitors is also not recommended; although they would neutralize gastric acidity and therefore would be expected to reduce pneumonitis, gastric acidity normally keeps stomach contents sterile. Hence neutralization may promote colonization by pathogenic organisms, making aspiration pneumonia more likely (Levenson and Pandurangi 2004). Respiratory failure may result when respiratory effort is severely inadequate (Boyarsky et al. 1999). Catatonic patients are also more susceptible to pulmonary emboli. Immobility increases the likelihood of venous stasis, which can then promote thrombosis, which can lead to pulmonary embolism (Lachner and Sandson 2003; McCall et al. 1995; Woo 2007). Prophylactic measures such as hydration, physical therapy, support hose, and anticoagulation can be helpful.

Dehydration, Malnutrition, and Gastrointestinal Complications

Catatonia leads to dehydration and malnutrition. Infection, skin breakdown, constipation, and ileus may be sequelae (Kaufmann et al. 2006; Thomas 2001). Persistent catatonia may necessitate the use of enteral feeding, which can result in complications from the feeding tubes.

Oral and Cutaneous Complications

Dental caries, oral infections, and gum disease are common in chronic catatonia. Skin breakdown and decubitus ulcers are very common as a result of immobility and pressure (Thomas 2001).

Genitourinary Tract Complications

Urinary retention, urinary incontinence, and urinary tract and vaginal infections are frequent complications in the persistently catatonic patient.

Neuromuscular Complications

The immobility of catatonia can result in flexion contractures and nerve palsies. Mobilization through physical therapy can help prevent these complications. Muscle breakdown as a result of immobilization may lead to rhabdomyolysis, particularly in malignant catatonias.

Treatment of Catatonia

Catatonia when properly treated typically resolves completely, but an underlying psychosis will often remain. Benzodiazepines and ECT are the most frequently recommended treatments. Bush et al. (1996b) in an open trial with 13 acute catatonic patients reported that 2 mg of intravenous lorazepam reduced catatonia scores on the BFCRS by 60% within 10 minutes. Although no published randomized controlled trials for acute catatonia are available, many case series and prospective open trials over the past 20 years with parenteral or oral benzodiazepines (such as lorazepam) showed a response rate of 60%–80% within hours or days (Rosebush and Mazurek 2004). Given the consistent benefit with low risk in these studies along with extensive clinical experience, a benzodiazepine given parenterally has been advocated as appropriate initial treatment for catatonia (Bush et al. 1996b; Rosebush and Mazurek 2004). Arguments favoring benzodiazepines include familiarity in contemporary psychiatric practice, a favorable therapeutic index, and the availability of flumazenil, a specific antagonist for benzodiazepines. It is of interest that flumazenil reversed the benefit of lorazepam in a case of catatonia (Wetzel et al. 1987). Initial dosages of 2–6 mg/day of lorazepam by any route of administration are recommended, but some patients may require higher doses.

Benzodiazepines are effective for both simple and malignant catatonia attributed to primary psychiatric illness, neuroleptic toxicity, and a variety of other secondary conditions. Treatment response is not predicted by age, sex, or severity of catatonia, but underlying chronic schizophrenia may predict a poorer response (Bush et al. 1996b; J.W.Y. Lee et al. 2000; Rosebush et al. 1990; Ungvari et al. 1999). Because underlying psychiatric disorders are difficult to assess in mute catatonic patients, specific treatment may be delayed until resolution of the catatonic state.

Since the 1930s, ECT has had a well-deserved reputation as the most effective treatment for catatonia. Clinical experience and case series have determined that ECT produces remission of catatonia even when other treatments such as lorazepam have failed. An added benefit of ECT is its effectiveness for the mood or psychotic disorders frequently associated with the catatonic syndrome. A synergism between ECT and lorazepam has been reported in the treatment of catatonia; therefore, embarking on an ECT course does not preclude continued lorazepam use (Petrides et al. 1997). (See also Chapter 40, "Electroconvulsive Therapy.")

One damaging consequence of the nosological error linking catatonia prominently to schizophrenia was the reflexive use of neuroleptic medication in catatonic patients. Many patients likely have been pushed into NMS as a result. The use of antipsychotics for catatonia requires caution because of this risk of changing a simple catatonia into a malignant one. Several reports indicated that both the older high-potency agents, such as haloperidol, and the second-generation antipsychotics failed to improve catatonia, induced or worsened catatonia, or led to progression from catatonia to NMS (Lopez-Canino and Francis 2004; Rosebush and Mazurek 2004; White and Robins 1991). Nevertheless, second-generation antipsychotics may have a role in the treatment of catatonia (Van Den Eede et al. 2005). In one double-blind study, 14 of 68 patients with nonaffective disorder and catatonia who had failed to respond to lorazepam were randomly assigned to receive risperidone plus sham ECT (n=6) or bilateral ECT plus placebo (n=8). After 3 weeks, scores on the BFCRS declined more than 90% with ECT and approximately 50% with risperidone (Girish and Gill 2003).

Unfortunately, ECT may not be available or permitted, and the clinician may be motivated to consider use of second-generation antipsychotics. Use of antipsychotic agents in the treatment of malignant catatonia is contraindicated because of the risk of exacerbation. In this setting, prompt use of ECT is advocated (Mann et al. 2004). In a review of 18 cases of malignant catatonia, 11 of 13 patients who received ECT survived, whereas only 1 of 5 who did not receive ECT lived (Mann et al. 2004). In another series, 16 of 19 patients who had received ECT within 5 days of symptom onset survived, whereas none of the 14 patients who had received ECT after 5 days did (Philbrick and Rummans 1994). Thus, when a patient presents with malignant catatonia of any type, ECT should be used expeditiously (i.e., within 5 days if possible) if a medication trial is unsuccessful.

Conclusion

Secondary psychosis, mania, and catatonia can occur in a wide range of medical diseases and toxic states. Prompt recognition of these neuropsychiatric complications allows for specific syndromal treatments that can lead to a complete resolution of the psychiatric symptoms, even if the underlying illness cannot be cured. If the neuropsychiatric symptoms are not recognized or poorly treated, substantial morbidity or even death can result.

References

Abrams R, Taylor MA: Catatonia: a prospective clinical study. Arch Gen Psychiatry 33:579–581, 1976

Ali SZ, Taguchi A, Rosenberg H: Malignant hyperthermia. Best Pract Res Clin Anaesthesiol 17:519–533, 2003

Ali S, Welch CA, Park LT, et al: Encephalitis and catatonia treated with ECT. Cogn Behav Neurol 21:46–51, 2008

Aliyez ZN, Aliyez NA: Valproate treatment of acute alcohol hallucinosis: a double-blind, placebo-controlled study. Alcohol Alcohol 43:456–459, 2008

American Psychiatric Association: Diagnostic and Statistical Manual of Mental Disorders, 4th Edition, Text Revision. Washington, DC, American Psychiatric Association, 2000

Arciniegas DB: New-onset bipolar disorder in late life: a case of mistaken identity. Am J Psychiatry 163:198–203, 2006

Arora M, Daughton J: Mania in the medically ill. Curr Psychiatry Rep 9:232–235, 2007

Baethge C, Baldessarini RJ, Freudenthal K, et al: Hallucinations in bipolar disorder: characteristics and comparison to unipolar depression and schizophrenia. Bipolar Disord 7:136–145, 2005

Ballard C, Day S, Sharp S, et al: Neuropsychiatric symptoms in dementia: importance and treatment considerations. Int Rev Psychiatry 20:396–404, 2008

Ballard C, Hanney ML, Theodoulou M, et al: The Dementia Antipsychotic Withdrawal Trial (DART-AD): long-term follow-up of a randomised placebo-controlled trial. Lancet Neurol 8:151–157, 2009

Balldin J, Berggren U, Rybo E, et al: Treatment-resistant mania with primary hypothyroidism: a case of recovery after levothyroxine. J Clin Psychiatry 48:490–491, 1987

Barczak P, Edmunds E, Betts T: Hypomania following complex partial seizures: a report of three cases. Br J Psychiatry 152:137–139, 1988

Bell L: On a form of disease resembling some advanced stages of mania and fever. Am J Insanity 6:97–127, 1849

Benke T: Peduncular hallucinosis: a syndrome of impaired reality monitoring. J Neurol 253:1561–1571, 2006

Berrios GE, Dening TR: Pseudohallucinations: a conceptual history. Psychol Med 26:753–763, 1996

Berthier ML, Starkstein SE, Robinson RG, et al: Limbic lesions in a patient with recurrent mania. J Neuropsychiatry Clin Neurosci 2:235–236, 1990

Berthier ML, Kulisevsky J, Gironell A, et al: Poststroke bipolar affective disorder: clinical subtypes, concurrent movement disorders, and anatomical correlates. J Neuropsychiatry Clin Neurosci 8:160–167, 1996

Boccellari A, Dilley JW, Shore MD: Neuropsychiatric aspects of AIDS dementia complex: a report on a clinical series. Neurotoxicology 9:381–389, 1988

Bokhari R, Bhatara VS, Bandettini F, et al: Postpartum psychosis and postpartum thyroiditis. Psychoneuroendocrinology 23:643–650, 1998

Bornke C, Postert T, Przuntek H, et al: Acute mania due to a right hemisphere infarction. Eur J Neurol 5:407–409, 1998

Boyarsky BK, Fuller M, Early T: Malignant catatonia-induced respiratory failure with response to ECT. J ECT 15:232–236, 1999

Brouilette MJ, Routy JP: Abacavir sulfate and mania in HIV. Am J Psychiatry 164:979–980, 2007

Brouillette MJ, Chouinard G, Lalonde R: Didanosine-induced mania in HIV infection. Am J Psychiatry 151:1839–1840, 1994

Brown S: Excess mortality of schizophrenia: a meta-analysis. Br J Psychiatry 171:502–508, 1997

Brownlie BE, Rae AM, Walshe JW, et al: Psychoses associated with thyrotoxicosis—"thyrotoxic psychosis": a report of 18 cases, with statistical analysis of incidence. Eur J Endocrinol 142:438–444, 2000

Bush G, Fink M, Petrides G, et al: Catatonia, I: rating scale and standardized examination. Acta Psychiatr Scand 93:129–136, 1996a

Bush G, Fink M, Petrides G, et al: Catatonia, II: treatment with lorazepam and electroconvulsive therapy. Acta Psychiatr Scand 93:137–143, 1996b

Carlson GA, Goodwin FK: The stages of mania: a longitudinal analysis of the manic episode. Arch Gen Psychiatry 28:221–228, 1973

Caroff S: The neuroleptic malignant syndrome. J Clin Psychiatry 41:79–83, 1980

Caroff SN, Mann SC, Campbell EC, et al: Epidemiology in catatonia: from psychopathology to neurobiology, in Catatonia: From Psychopathology to Neurobiology. Edited by Caroff SN, Mann SC, Francis A, et al. Washington, DC, American Psychiatric Publishing, 2004a, pp 15–31

Caroff SN, Mann SC, Francis A, et al (eds): Catatonia: From Psychopathology to Neurobiology. Washington, DC, American Psychiatric Publishing, 2004b

Carroll BT, Goforth HW: Medical catatonia, in Catatonia: From Psychopathology to Neurobiology. Edited by Caroff SN, Mann SC, Francis A, et al. Washington, DC, American Psychiatric Publishing, 2004, pp 121–127

Carroll BT, Anfinson TJ, Kennedy JC, et al: Catatonic disorder due to general medical conditions. J Neuropsychiatry Clin Neurosci 6:122–133, 1994

Carter JL: Visual, somatosensory, olfactory, and gustatory hallucinations. Psychiatr Clin North Am 15:347–358, 1992

Caton CL, Drake RE, Hasin DS, et al: Differences between early phase primary psychotic disorders with concurrent substance use and substance-induced psychoses. Arch Gen Psychiatry 62:137–145, 2005

Chakrabarti S, Aga VM, Singh R: Postictal mania following primary generalized seizures. Neurol India 47:332–333, 1999

Chemerinski E, Robinson RG: The neuropsychiatry of stroke. Psychosomatics 41:5–14, 2000

Clower CG: Organic affective syndromes associated with thyroid dysfunction. Psychiatr Med 2:177–181, 1984

Colton CW, Manderscheid RW: Congruencies in increased mortality rates, years of potential life lost, and causes of death among public mental health clients in eight states. Prev Chronic Dis 3:A42, 2006

Correll CU, Leucht S, Kane JM: Lower risk for tardive dyskinesia associated with second-generation antipsychotics: a systematic review of 1-year studies. Am J Psychiatry 161:414–425, 2004

Cutting J: The phenomenology of acute organic psychosis: comparison with acute schizophrenia. Br J Psychiatry 151:324–332, 1987

Dolder CR, Lacro JP, Jeste DV: Adherence to antipsychotic and nonpsychiatric medications in middle-aged and older patients with psychotic disorders. Psychosom Med 65:156–162, 2003

Druss BG, Bradford WD, Rosenheck RA, et al: Quality of medical care and excess mortality in older patients with mental disorders. Arch Gen Psychiatry 58:565–572, 2001

Eker A, Saka E, Dalmau J, et al: Testicular teratoma and anti-N-methyl-D-aspartate receptor-associated encephalitis. J Neurol Neurosurg Psychiatry 79:1082–1083, 2008

el-Serag HB, Kunik M, Richardson P, et al: Psychiatric disorders among veterans with hepatitis C infection. Gastroenterology 123:476–482, 2002

Ewing JA: Detecting alcoholism: the CAGE questionnaire. JAMA 252:1905–1907, 1984

Farooq S, Sherin A: Interventions for psychotic symptoms concomitant with epilepsy. Cochrane Database Syst Rev (4):CD006118, 2008

Feinstein A, Ron M: A longitudinal study of psychosis due to a general medical (neurological) condition: establishing predictive and construct validity. J Neuropsychiatry Clin Neurosci 10:448–452, 1998

Fenn D, George K: Post-stroke mania late in life involving the left hemisphere. Aust N Z J Psychiatry 33:598–600, 1999

Fink M: Delirious mania. Bipolar Disord 1:54–60, 1999

Fink M, Taylor MA: Catatonia: A Clinician's Guide to Diagnosis and Treatment. Cambridge, UK, Cambridge University Press, 2003

Fink M, Taylor MA: The catatonia syndrome: forgotten but not gone. Arch Gen Psychiatry 66:1173–1177, 2009

Fleischhacker WW, Cetkovich-Bakmas M, De Hert M, et al: Comorbid somatic illnesses in patients with severe mental disorders: clinical, policy, and research challenges. J Clin Psychiatry 69:514–519, 2008

Folstein S. Huntington's Disease: A Disorder of Families. Baltimore, MD, Johns Hopkins University Press, 1989

Forsell Y, Henderson AS: Epidemiology of paranoid symptoms in an elderly population. Br J Psychiatry 172:429–432, 1998

Foster AR, Caplan JP: Paraneoplastic limbic encephalitis. Psychosomatics 50:108–113, 2009

Freudenreich O: Psychotic Disorders: A Practical Guide. Baltimore, MD, Lippincott Williams & Wilkins, 2007

Freudenreich O, Stern TA: Clinical experience with the management of schizophrenia in the general hospital. Psychosomatics 44:12–23, 2003

Freudenreich O, Holt DJ, Cather C, et al: The evaluation and management of patients with first episode schizophrenia: a selective, clinical review of diagnosis, treatment, and prognosis. Harv Rev Psychiatry 15:189–211, 2007

Freudenreich O, Weiss AP, Goff DC: Psychosis and schizophrenia, in Massachusetts General Hospital Comprehensive Clinical Psychiatry. Edited by Stern TA, Rosenbaum JF, Fava M, et al. Philadelphia, PA, Mosby/Elsevier, 2008, pp 371–389

Freudenreich O, Schulz SC, Goff DC: Initial medical work-up of first-episode psychosis: a conceptual review. Early Intervention in Psychiatry 3:10–18, 2009

Fricchione GL, Huffman JC, Stern TA, et al: Catatonia, neuroleptic malignant syndrome, and serotonin syndrome, in Massachusetts General Hospital Handbook of General Hospital Psychiatry, 5th Edition. Edited by Stern TA, Fricchione GL, Cassem NH, et al. Philadelphia, PA, Mosby/Elsevier, 2004, pp 513–530

Galvez-Andres A, Blasco-Fontecilla H, Gonzalez-Parra S, et al: Secondary bipolar disorder and Diogenes syndrome in frontotemporal dementia: behavioral improvement with quetiapine and sodium valproate. J Clin Psychopharmacol 27:722–723, 2007

Gelenberg AJ: The catatonic syndrome. Lancet 2:1339–1341, 1976

Ghaffar O, Feinstein A: The neuropsychiatry of multiple sclerosis: a review of recent developments. Curr Opin Psychiatry 20:278–285, 2007

Girish K, Gill NS: Electroconvulsive therapy in lorazepam nonresponsive catatonia. Indian J Psychiatry 45:21–25, 2003

Goff DC: Integrating general health care in private community psychiatry practice. J Clin Psychiatry 68 (suppl 4):49–54, 2007

Goff DC, Sullivan LM, McEvoy JP, et al: A comparison of ten-year cardiac risk estimates in schizophrenia patients from the CATIE study and matched controls. Schizophr Res 80:45–53, 2005

Goodwin FK, Jamison KR: Manic-Depressive Illness: Bipolar Disorder and Recurrent Depression, 2nd Edition. New York, Oxford University Press, 2007

Greenberg DM, Lee JW: Psychotic manifestations of alcoholism. Curr Psychiatry Rep 3:314–318, 2001

Himmelhoch J: Major mood disorders related to epileptic changes, in Psychiatric Aspects of Epilepsy. Edited by Blumer D. Washington, DC, American Psychiatric Press, 1984, pp 271–294

Hurwitz TA, Wada JA, Kosaka BD, et al: Cerebral organization of affect suggested by temporal lobe seizures. Neurology 35:1335–1337, 1985

Jeste DV, Caligiuri MP, Paulsen JS, et al: Risk of tardive dyskinesia in older patients: a prospective longitudinal study of 266 outpatients. Arch Gen Psychiatry 52:756–765, 1995

Jeste DV, Blazer D, Casey D, et al: ACNP White Paper: update on use of antipsychotic drugs in elderly persons with dementia. Neuropsychopharmacology 33:957–970, 2008

Johnstone EC, Macmillan JF, Crow TJ: The occurrence of organic disease of possible or probably aetiological significance in a population of 268 cases of first episode schizophrenia. Psychol Med 17:371–379, 1987

Jones PB, Barnes TR, Davies L, et al: Randomized controlled trial of the effect on Quality of Life of second- vs first-generation antipsychotic drugs in schizophrenia: Cost Utility of the Latest Antipsychotic Drugs in Schizophrenia Study (CUtLASS 1). Arch Gen Psychiatry 63:1079–1087, 2006

Jorge RE, Robinson RG, Starkstein SE, et al: Secondary mania following traumatic brain injury. Am J Psychiatry 150:916–921, 1993

Josephs KA: Capgras syndrome and its relationship to neurodegenerative disease. Arch Neurol 64:1762–1766, 2007

Kahlbaum K: Catatonia. Baltimore, MD, Johns Hopkins University Press, 1973

Kahn RS, Fleischhacker WW, Boter H, et al: Effectiveness of antipsychotic drugs in first-episode schizophrenia and schizophreniform disorder: an open randomised clinical trial. Lancet 29:1085–1097, 2008

Kaufmann RM, Schreinzer D, Strnad A, et al: Case report: intestinal atonia as an unusual symptom of malignant catatonia responsive to electroconvulsive therapy. Schizophr Res 84:178–179, 2006

Keck PE Jr, McElroy SL, Strakowski SM, et al: Compliance with maintenance treatment in bipolar disorder. Psychopharmacol Bull 33:87–91, 1997

Kieburtz K, Zettelmaier AE, Ketonen L, et al: Manic syndrome in AIDS. Am J Psychiatry 148:1068–1070, 1991

Kilbourne AM, Justice AC, Rabeneck L, et al: General medical and psychiatric comorbidity among HIV-infected veterans in the post-HAART era. J Clin Epidemiol 54 (suppl 1):S22–S28, 2001

Kilbourne AM, Cornelius JR, Han X, et al: Burden of general medical conditions among individuals with bipolar disorder. Bipolar Disord 6:368–373, 2004

Klimstra S, Mahgoub N: Psychosis of Alzheimer's disease. Psychiatr Ann 39:10–14, 2009

Krauthammer C, Klerman GL: Secondary mania: manic syndromes associated with antecedent physical illness or drugs. Arch Gen Psychiatry 35:1333–1339, 1978

Lachner C, Sandson NB: Medical complications of catatonia: a case of catatonia-induced deep venous thrombosis. Psychosomatics 44:512–514, 2003

Lautenschlager NT, Foerstl H: Organic psychosis: insight into the biology of psychosis. Curr Psychiatr Rep 3:319–325, 2001

Lee CS, Hutto B: Recognizing thyrotoxicosis in a patient with bipolar mania: a case report. Ann Gen Psychiatry 7:3, 2008

Lee JWY, Schwartz DI, Hallmayer J: Catatonia in a psychiatric intensive care facility: incidence and response to benzodiazepines. Ann Clin Psychiatry 12:89–96, 2000

Leibson E: Anosognosia and mania associated with right thalamic haemorrhage. J Neurol Neurosurg Psychiatry 68:107–108, 2000

Leong GB, Silva JA, Garza-Trevino ES, et al: The dangerousness of persons with the Othello syndrome. J Forensic Sci 39:1445–1454, 1994

Leucht S, Burkard T, Henderson J, et al: Physical illness and schizophrenia: a review of the literature. Acta Psychiatr Scand 116:317–333, 2007

Leucht S, Corves C, Arbter D, et al: Second-generation versus first-generation antipsychotic drugs for schizophrenia: a meta-analysis. Lancet 373:31–41, 2009

Levenson JL, Pandurangi AK: Prognosis and complications, in Catatonia: From Psychopathology to Neurobiology. Edited by Caroff SN, Mann SC, Francis A, et al. Washington, DC, American Psychiatric Publishing, 2004, pp 161–172

Levitte SS: Coexistent hypomania and severe hypothyroidism. Psychosomatics 34:96–97, 1993

Lieberman JA, Stroup TS, McEvoy JP, et al: Effectiveness of antipsychotic drugs in patients with chronic schizophrenia. N Engl J Med 353:1209–1223, 2005

Lockman J, Burns TM: Stiff-person syndrome. Curr Treat Options Neurol 9:234–240, 2007

Lopez-Canino A, Francis A: Drug induced catatonia, in Catatonia: From Psychopathology to Neurobiology. Edited by Caroff SN, Mann SC, Francis A, et al. Washington, DC, American Psychiatric Publishing, 2004, pp 129–140

Louis ED, Pflaster NL: Catatonia mimicking nonconvulsive status epilepticus. Epilepsia 36:943–945, 1995

Lyketsos CG, Hanson AL, Fishman M, et al: Manic syndrome early and late in the course of HIV. Am J Psychiatry 150:326–327, 1993a

Lyketsos CG, Stoline AM, Longstreet P, et al: Mania in temporal lobe epilepsy. Neuropsychiatry Neuropsychol Behav Neurol 6:19–25, 1993b

Lyketsos CG, Schwartz J, Fishman M, et al: AIDS mania. J Neuropsychiatry Clin Neurosci 9:277–279, 1997

Mann S, Caroff SN: Lethal catatonia and the neuroleptic malignant syndrome, in Psychiatry: A World Perspective. Edited by Stefanis C, Soldatos C, Rambazilas A. Amsterdam, The Netherlands, Elsevier Science, 1990, pp 287–292

Mann SC, Caroff SN, Keck PE, et al: Neuroleptic Malignant Syndrome and Related Conditions, 2nd Edition. Washington, DC, American Psychiatric Press, 1994

Mann SC, Caroff SN, Fricchione GL, et al: Malignant catatonia, in Catatonia: From Psychopathology to Neurobiology. Edited by Caroff SN, Mann SC, Francis A, et al. Washington, DC, American Psychiatric Publishing, 2004, pp 105–120

Marneros A: Schizophrenic first-rank symptoms in organic mental disorders. Br J Psychiatry 152:625–628, 1988

Maxwell S, Scheftner WA, Kessler HA, et al: Manic syndrome associated with zidovudine treatment. JAMA 259:3406–3407, 1988

McCall WV, Mann SC, Shelp FE, et al: Fatal pulmonary embolism in the catatonic syndrome: two case reports and a literature review. J Clin Psychiatry 56:21–25, 1995

McEvoy JP, Meyer JM, Goff DC, et al: Prevalence of the metabolic syndrome in patients with schizophrenia: baseline results from the Clinical Antipsychotic Trials of Intervention Effectiveness (CATIE) schizophrenia trial and comparison with national estimates from NHANES III. Schizophr Res 80:19–32, 2005

McKeith I, Del Ser T, Spano P, et al: Efficacy of rivastigmine in dementia with Lewy bodies: a randomised, double-blind, placebo-controlled international study. Lancet 356:2031–2036, 2000

McKeith IG, Dickson DW, Lowe J, et al: Diagnosis and management of dementia with Lewy bodies: third report of the DLB consortium. Neurology 65:1863–1872, 2005

Mendez MF: Huntington's disease: update and review of neuropsychiatric aspects. Int J Psychiatry Med 24:189–208, 1994

Mendez MF: Mania in neurologic disorders. Curr Psychiatry Rep 2:440–445, 2000

Mendez MF, Grau R: The postictal psychosis of epilepsy: investigation in two patients. Int J Psychiatry Med 21:85–92, 1991

Mendez MF, Adams NL, Lewandowski KS: Neurobehavioral changes associated with caudate lesions. Neurology 39:349–354, 1989

Menon GJ: Complex visual hallucinations in the visually impaired: a structured history-taking approach. Arch Ophthalmol 123:349–355, 2005

Michael A, Mirza S, Mirza KA, et al: Morbid jealousy in alcoholics. Br J Psychiatry 167:668–672, 1995

Mocellin R, Walterfang M, Velakoulis D: Neuropsychiatry of complex visual hallucinations. Aust N Z J Psychiatry 40:742–751, 2006

Moore TH, Zammit S, Lingford-Hughes A, et al: Cannabis use and risk of psychotic or affective mental health outcomes: a systematic review. Lancet 370:319–328, 2007

Naber D, Sand P, Heigl B: Psychopathological and neuropsychological effects of 8-days' corticosteroid treatment: a prospective study. Psychoneuroendocrinology 21:25–31, 1996

Nadkarni S, Arnedo V, Devinsky O: Psychosis in epilepsy patients. Epilepsia 48 (suppl 9):17–19, 2007

Nakimuli-Mpungu E, Musisi S, Kiwuwa Mpungu S, et al: Primary mania versus HIV-related secondary mania in Uganda. Am J Psychiatry 163:1349–1354, 2006

Nightingale SD, Koster FT, Mertz GJ, et al: Clarithromycin-induced mania in two patients with AIDS. Clin Infect Dis 20:1563–1564, 1995

Oostervink F, Boomsma MM, Nolen WA, et al: Bipolar disorder in the elderly; different effects of age and of age of onset. J Affect Disord 116:176–183, 2009

Ostling S, Skoog I: Psychotic symptoms and paranoid ideation in a nondemented population-based sample of the very old. Arch Gen Psychiatry 59:53–59, 2002

Overall JE, Gorham DR: The Brief Psychiatric Rating Scale (BPRS): recent developments in ascertainment and scaling. Psychopharmacol Bull 24:97–99, 1988

Petrides G, Divadeenam KM, Bush G, et al: Synergism of lorazepam and electroconvulsive therapy in the treatment of catatonia. Biol Psychiatry 42:375–381, 1997

Philbrick K, Rummans T: Malignant catatonia. J Neuropsychiatry Clin Neurosci 6:1–13, 1994

Pickles RW, Spelman DW: Suspected ethambutol-induced mania. Med J Aust 164:445–446, 1996

Ramchandani D, Riggio S: Periictal mania: a case report. Psychosomatics 33:229–231, 1992

Raucher-Chene D, Charrel CL, de Maindreville AD, et al: Manic episode with psychotic symptoms in a patient with Parkinson's disease treated by subthalamic nucleus stimulation: improvement on switching the target. J Neurol Sci 273:116–117, 2008

Ray WA, Chung CP, Murray KT, et al: Atypical antipsychotic drugs and the risk of sudden cardiac death. N Engl J Med 360:225–235, 2009

Robertson MM: Affect and mood in epilepsy: an overview with a focus on depression. Acta Neurol Scand Suppl 140:127–132, 1992

Ropacki SA, Jeste DV: Epidemiology of and risk factors for psychosis of Alzheimer's disease: a review of 55 studies published from 1990 to 2003. Am J Psychiatry 162:2022–2030, 2005

Rosebush P, Mazurek M: Pharmacotherapy, in Catatonia: From Psychopathology to Neurobiology. Edited by Caroff SN, Mann SC, Francis A, et al. Washington, DC, American Psychiatric Publishing, 2004, pp 141–150

Rosebush PI, Hildebrand AM, Furlong BG, et al: Catatonic syndrome in a general psychiatric inpatient population: frequency, clinical presentation, and response to lorazepam. J Clin Psychiatry 51:357–362, 1990

Rosenblatt A, Leroi I: Neuropsychiatry of Huntington's disease and other basal ganglia disorders. Psychosomatics 41:24–30, 2000

Rudorfer MV, Linnoila M, Potter WZ: Combined lithium and electroconvulsive therapy: pharmacokinetic and pharmacodynamic interactions. Convuls Ther 3:40–45, 1987

Rundell JR, Wise MG: Causes of organic mood disorder. J Neuropsychiatry Clin Neurosci 1:398–400, 1989

Sachdev P: Schizophrenia-like psychosis and epilepsy: the status of the association. Am J Psychiatry 155:325–336, 1998

Saha S, Chant D, McGrath J: A systematic review of mortality in schizophrenia: is the differential mortality gap worsening over time? Arch Gen Psychiatry 64:1123–1131, 2007

Schneider LS, Tariot PN, Dagerman KS, et al: Effectiveness of atypical antipsychotic drugs in patients with Alzheimer's disease. N Engl J Med 355:1525–1538, 2006

Shah MD, Balderson K: A manic episode associated with efavirenz therapy for HIV infection. AIDS 17:1713–1714, 2003

Shukla S, Cook BL, Mukherjee S, et al: Mania following head trauma. Am J Psychiatry 144:93–96, 1987

Sikich L, Frazier JA, McClellan J, et al: Double-blind comparison of first- and second-generation antipsychotics in early onset schizophrenia and schizo-affective disorder: findings from the treatment of early onset schizophrenia spectrum disorders (TEOSS) study. Am J Psychiatry 165:1420–1431, 2008

Silva JA, Leong GB, Weinstock R, et al: Delusional misidentification syndromes and dangerousness. Psychopathology 27:215–219, 1994

Slater E, Beard AW: The schizophrenia-like psychoses of epilepsy, V: discussion and conclusions. Br J Psychiatry 109:143–150, 1963

Smith E, Delargy M: Locked-in syndrome. BMJ 330:406–409, 2005

Stahl SM, Mignon L, Meyer JM: Which comes first: atypical antipsychotic treatment or cardiometabolic risk? Acta Psychiatr Scand 119:171–179, 2009

Starkstein SE, Berthier ML, Lylyk PL, et al: Emotional behavior after a Wada test in a patient with secondary mania. J Neuropsychiatry Clin Neurosci 1:408–412, 1989

Stauder K: Die tödliche Katatonie. Arch Psychiatrie Nervenkr 102:614–634, 1934

Stowell CP, Barnhill JW: Acute mania in the setting of severe hypothyroidism. Psychosomatics 46:259–261, 2005

Subramaniam H, Dennis MS, Byrne EJ: The role of vascular risk factors in late onset bipolar disorder. Int J Geriatr Psychiatry 22:733–737, 2007

Taylor MA, Fink M: Catatonia in psychiatric classification: a home of its own. Am J Psychiatry 160:1233–1241, 2003

Thewissen V, Myin-Germeys I, Bentall R, et al: Hearing impairment and psychosis revisited. Schizophr Res 76:99–103, 2005

Thomas DR: Prevention and treatment of pressure ulcers: what works? what doesn't? Cleve Clin J Med 68:704–707, 710–714, 717–722, 2001

Thomsen AF, Kvist TK, Andersen PK, et al: Increased risk of affective disorder following hospitalisation with hyperthyroidism—a register-based study. Eur J Endocrinol 152:535–543, 2005

Thorup A, Peterson T, Jeppesen L, et al: Frequency and predictive values of first rank symptoms at baseline among 362 young adult patients with first-episode schizophrenia: results from the Danish OPUS study. Schizophr Res 97:60–67, 2007

Timmermans M, Carr J: Neurosyphilis in the modern era. J Neurol Neurosurg Psychiatry 75:1727–1730, 2004

Toone BK: The psychoses of epilepsy. J Neurol Neurosurg Psychiatry 69:1–3, 2000

Tüzün E, Dalmau J: Limbic encephalitis and variants: classification, diagnosis and treatment. Neurologist 13:261–271, 2007

Ungvari GS, Chiu HF, Chow LY, et al: Lorazepam for chronic catatonia: a randomized double-blind, placebo-controlled cross-over study. Psychopharmacology 142:393–398, 1999

Van Den Eede F, Van Hecke J, Van Dalfsen A, et al: The use of atypical antipsychotics in the treatment of catatonia. Eur Psychiatry 20:422–429, 2005

van der Heijden FM, Tuinier S, Arts NJ, et al: Catatonia: disappeared or under-diagnosed? Psychopathology 38:3–8, 2005

Villani S, Weitzel WD: Secondary mania. Arch Gen Psychiatry 36:1031, 1979

Vuilleumier P, Ghika-Schmid F, Bogousslavsky J, et al: Persistent recurrence of hypomania and prosopoaffective agnosia in a patient with right thalamic infarct. Neuropsychiatry Neuropsychol Behav Neurol 11:40–44, 1998

Wagner GJ, Kanouse DE, Koegel P, et al: Adherence to HIV antiretrovirals among persons with serious mental illness. AIDS Patient Care STDS 17:179–186, 2003

Weinstein EA: The classification of delusional misidentification syndromes. Psychopathology 27:130–135, 1994

Wetzel H, Heuser I, Benkert O: Stupor and affective state: alleviation of psychomotor disturbances by lorazepam and recurrence of symptoms after Ro 15-1788. J Nerv Ment Dis 175:240–242, 1987

White DA, Robins AH: Catatonia: harbinger of the neuroleptic malignant syndrome. Br J Psychiatry 158:419–421, 1991

Wilcox JA, Nasrallah HA: Organic factors in catatonia. Br J Psychiatry 149:782–784, 1986

Wing L, Shah A: A systematic examination of catatonia-like clinical pictures in autism spectrum disorders. Int Rev Neurobiol 72:21–39, 2006

Woo BK: Basal ganglia calcification and pulmonary embolism in catatonia. J Neuropsychiatry Clin Neurosci 19:472–473, 2007

Woolley JD, Wilson MR, Hung E, et al: Frontotemporal dementia and mania. Am J Psychiatry 164:1811–1816, 2007

Wright JM, Sachdev PS, Perkins RJ, et al: Zidovudine-related mania. Med J Aust 150:339–341, 1989

Young RC, Biggs JT, Ziegler VE, et al: A rating scale for mania: reliability, validity and sensitivity. Br J Psychiatry 133:429–435, 1978

Yusim A, Anbarasan D, Bernstein C, et al: Normal pressure hydrocephalus presenting as Othello syndrome: case presentation and review of the literature. Am J Psychiatry 165:1119–1125, 2008

CHAPTER 11

Anxiety Disorders

Steven A. Epstein, M.D.

Daniel Hicks, M.D.

ANXIETY IS AN EXTREMELY common problem in primary care and specialty medical settings. Because the 1-year prevalence rate of any anxiety disorder in the general population is approximately 18% (Kessler et al. 2005), many medically ill patients will have concurrent anxiety unrelated to the experience of medical illness. The profound physical and psychological stressors of medical illness often precipitate anxiety, particularly in individuals with preexisting vulnerability. Therefore, when evaluating a medically ill patient, the psychosomatic medicine psychiatrist should always determine whether anxiety symptoms are present. Although the presence of anxiety may reflect a mood disorder or other psychiatric disorder, formal assessment for the presence of an anxiety disorder should be considered in all patients. Unfortunately, medical professionals often neglect to screen for these highly treatable disorders. Even when they recognize anxiety, some practitioners minimize its significance by considering it to be a "normal" response to the uncertainty and adversity associated with having a disease.

Once the psychiatrist has determined that a patient has anxiety, the more complex task of ascertaining etiology must be undertaken. Although it is advisable to use a biopsychosocial approach to formulation, surprisingly few data are available regarding medical and pharmacological causes of anxiety. Nonetheless, the psychiatrist must carefully assess their potential etiological roles. Finally, it is important to consider medical comorbidity when designing pharmacological and psychotherapeutic treatment plans. In this chapter, we discuss each of these topics. For detailed reviews of anxiety among individuals with specific medical comorbidities, the reader is referred to the corresponding chapters in this text.

General Features and Diagnostic Considerations

Anxiety may reflect the presence of an anxiety disorder but also may be a symptom of another psychiatric disorder such as depression. In the medical setting, it is also important to remember that anxiety may be a symptom of delirium, dementia, or a somatoform disorder such as hypochondriasis. Anxiety also may be the result of a medical disorder (e.g., hyperthyroidism) or a medication side effect. Furthermore, some symptoms and signs of medical disorders (e.g., tachycardia, dyspnea, and diaphoresis) may be mistaken for anxiety.

An interview during which DSM-IV-TR (American Psychiatric Association 2000) criteria are used is the gold standard for diagnosis of an anxiety disorder. In primary care settings, it is often useful to ask brief screening questions to determine whether a full diagnostic assessment is necessary. A 7-item anxiety screen, the Generalized Anxiety Disorder (GAD)-7 scale, has been reported to be an effective screen for GAD, panic, posttraumatic stress disorder (PTSD), and social phobia (Kroenke et al. 2007). The Hospital Anxiety and Depression Scale (HADS), a 14-item scale, also has been shown to be a valid screening instrument for both anxiety and depression (Bjelland et al. 2002).

Many patients with anxiety do not present to mental health providers. Of all anxiety disorder visits in the National Ambulatory Medical Care Survey in 1998, 48% were to primary care physicians (Harman et al. 2002). Among a sample of 3,000 adult primary care patients, 11% were diagnosed with an anxiety disorder (Spitzer et al. 1999). Individuals with chronic medical conditions such as arthritis, heart disease, gastrointestinal disease, and hypertension are more likely to have anxiety disorders (Sareen et al. 2006). Unfortunately, many individuals treated in primary care settings do not receive appropriate care for anxiety (Roy-Byrne et al. 1999; Young et al. 2001). Some physicians lack the skill or time to treat anxiety. In addition, some primary care patients are reluctant to consider either psychosocial or pharmacological treatment for their conditions (Hazlett-Stevens et al. 2002).

Anxiety disorders have clearly been shown to impair functioning and well-being among individuals with chronic medical conditions (Kessler et al. 2003; Sherbourne et al. 1996). Anxiety may be a risk factor for the development of medical illness and may physiologically exacerbate some conditions (e.g., angina, arrhythmias, movement disorders, labile hypertension, and irritable bowel syndrome). Some evidence indicates that phobic anxiety is a risk factor for fatal coronary artery disease (Albert et al. 2005; Kawachi et al. 1994), but some studies have shown no relation between anxiety and mortality (e.g., Herrmann et al. 2000; Lane et al. 2001). Anxiety also may lead to increased risk of developing hypertension (Jonas et al. 1997) and cardiovascular morbidity (Smoller et al. 2007). In a recent analysis of National Comorbidity Survey data, lifetime PTSD was associated with a higher prevalence of hypertension (Kibler et al. 2009). For an excellent recent review of anxiety disorders and their relation to medical illnesses, see Roy-Byrne et al. (2008).

Although depression is more clearly a predictor of poor adherence to medical treatment (DiMatteo et al. 2000), excessive anxiety might reduce adherence to medical treatment in some individuals (Martín-Santos et al. 2008). Anxiety may lead some individuals to refuse diagnostic procedures or surgery and even to sign out of the hospital against medical advice.

TABLE 11–1. DSM-IV-TR criteria for panic attack

Note: A panic attack is not a codable disorder. Code the specific diagnosis in which the panic attack occurs (e.g., 300.21 panic disorder with agoraphobia).

A discrete period of intense fear or discomfort, in which four (or more) of the following symptoms developed abruptly and reached a peak within 10 minutes:

(1) palpitations, pounding heart, or accelerated heart rate
(2) sweating
(3) trembling or shaking
(4) sensations of shortness of breath or smothering
(5) feeling of choking
(6) chest pain or discomfort
(7) nausea or abdominal distress
(8) feeling dizzy, unsteady, lightheaded, or faint
(9) derealization (feelings of unreality) or depersonalization (being detached from oneself)
(10) fear of losing control or going crazy
(11) fear of dying
(12) paresthesias (numbness or tingling sensations)
(13) chills or hot flushes

Source. American Psychiatric Association 2000.

Specific Anxiety Disorders

Panic Disorder

Primary care patients with panic attacks (see Table 11–1 for diagnostic criteria) are high utilizers of medical care (Roy-Byrne et al. 1999). In particular, many patients who present with chest pain are found to have panic disorder. For example, in one study, panic disorder was found in approximately 25% of 441 patients presenting to an emergency department with chest pain (Fleet et al. 1996). Researchers estimate that at least one-third of individuals with chest pain and normal coronary arteries have panic disorder (e.g., Bringager et al. 2008; Fleet et al. 1998; Maddock et al. 1998). These rates contrast with 12-month prevalence rates of 2.7% found in the National Comorbidity Survey Replication (Kessler et al. 2005). A meta-analysis identified five variables that correlate with higher rates of panic disorder among individuals seeking treatment for chest pain in emergency departments or cardiology clinics: 1) absence of coronary artery disease; 2) atypical quality of chest pain; 3) female gender; 4) younger age; and 5) high level of self-reported anxiety (Huffman and Pollack 2003).

Patients with benign palpitations have high rates of panic disorder (Barsky et al. 1994; Ehlers et al. 2000). One explanation for such high rates is that individuals with panic disorder may have heightened cardiac sensitivity to symptoms such as chest pain and palpitations (Barsky 2001; Mayou 1998). Panic symptoms also may be linked to physiological changes in peripheral organ systems. Panic attacks may be difficult to distinguish symptomatically from paroxysmal atrial tachycardia; both occur frequently in young, otherwise healthy women, and they are frequently comorbid. Before palpitations are attributed to anxiety, it is important for patients to undergo cardiac evaluation (e.g., ambulatory electrocardiographic monitoring) to rule out arrhythmias. There have been many reports of comorbidity of panic disorder and mitral valve prolapse, but data are not sufficiently strong to support a clear association (Filho et al. 2008). (See also Chapter 18, "Heart Disease.")

Panic disorder also leads patients to present to other medical specialists. For example, patients who present for evaluation of dizziness have elevated rates of this disorder (N.M. Simon et al. 1998; Wiltink et al. 2009; Yardley et al. 2001). Panic disorder also has significant comorbidity with irritable bowel syndrome (Kumano et al. 2004; Sugaya et al. 2008). In patients with irritable bowel syndrome, anxiety may be due to locus coeruleus activation by afferent signals from the bowel. Thus, with irritable bowel syndrome and other medical disorders such as asthma, anxiety symptoms may be due to central nervous system responses to afferent information from the viscera (Zaubler and Katon 1998). Finally, many patients with negative evaluations for pheochromocytoma are found to have anxiety disorders, including panic disorder (Eisenhofer et al. 2008).

Collaborative care interventions can improve outcomes for primary care patients with panic disorder. In one model, collaborative care consisted of patient education, treatment with paroxetine, two visits with an on-site consulting psychiatrist, and follow-up telephone calls. Patients who received this intervention, compared with those receiving usual primary care, had significant reductions in anxiety (Katon et al. 2002; Roy-Byrne et al. 2005).

(For further discussion of panic disorder in cardiac patients, see Chapter 18, "Heart Disease.")

Posttraumatic Stress Disorder

The National Comorbidity Survey estimated the 12-month prevalence of DSM-IV-TR PTSD in the general population to be 3.5% (Kessler et al. 2005). Prevalence in medical settings appears to be higher. For example, in one primary care sample, the current prevalence of PTSD was approximately 12% (M.B. Stein et al. 2000). Trauma victims and individuals with PTSD are frequent users of health care (Seng et al. 2006). PTSD also has been linked to adverse medical outcomes. For example, in a study of Vietnam veterans, PTSD was associated prospectively with heart disease mortality (Boscarino 2006). In a large study of former prisoners of war from World War II, risk of cardiovascular disease was associated with PTSD (Kang et al. 2006).

It is not surprising that PTSD symptoms are common among individuals who experience acute physical traumas. For example, burn victims have been reported to have PTSD at rates ranging from 20% to 45% (Difede et al. 2002; McKibben et al. 2008; Yu and Dimsdale 1999). In one study, 30%–40% of survivors of a motor vehicle crash or an assault reported PTSD symptoms for months after the trauma. Higher symptom levels were associated with female gender, stimulant intoxication, and greater prior trauma (Zatzick et al. 2002). PTSD also has been reported among individuals with automatic implantable cardioverter defibrillators (Hamner et al. 1999). In one recent study of patients with an implanted cardioverter defibrillator, high levels of PTSD symptoms were associated with increased mortality over an average of 5 years of follow-up (Ladwig et al. 2008).

Intensive care unit experiences can result in PTSD symptoms. In one study, recall of "delusional memories" (paranoia, hallucinations, or nightmares presumably due to delirium) from an intensive care unit hospitalization was shown to be associated with the development of PTSD symptoms (C. Jones et al. 2001). PTSD symptoms may occur after many other medical conditions or treatments, including myocardial infarction (Gander and von Kanel 2006) and the diagnosis of HIV infection. For reviews, see the articles by Tedstone and Tarrier (2003) and Davydow et al. (2008).

Acute stress disorder also may occur after life-threatening illnesses or injuries. In one study, 19% of 83 hospitalized adult burn patients developed acute stress disorder within 2 weeks of injury. The presence of acute stress disorder strongly predicted the presence of PTSD at least 6 months later (Difede et al. 2002; McKibben et al. 2008). Similarly, the degree of fright experienced at the time of myocardial infarction was associated with PTSD symptoms 3 months later (Bennett et al. 2001).

Life-threatening illness such as cancer is a stressor that can precipitate PTSD (Kangas et al. 2002; Smith et al. 1999). However, this trauma is different from more usual PTSD stressors such as rape in two principal ways: 1) the threat arises from one's own body; and 2) once the patient has been treated, the ongoing stressor is often not the memory of past events but the fear of recurrence (Green et al. 1997). Some researchers have speculated that the trauma associated with the diagnosis and treatment of serious medical illness might be sufficient to cause PTSD even in the absence of a catastrophic event. The rate of current PTSD in cancer survivors is approximately 3%–5%, but many more patients experience some symptoms of PTSD (Alter et al. 1996; Andrykowski and Cordova 1998; Green et al. 1998). The likelihood of developing PTSD symptoms after cancer treatment has been shown to be increased among individuals with past trauma, prior psychiatric diagnoses, lower levels of social support, and recent life stressors (Green et al. 2000; Jacobsen et al. 2002). As is the case with other medical illnesses, severity of cancer is not a strong predictor of the development of PTSD.

Other Anxiety Disorders

There are relatively few studies regarding the characteristics and significance of other anxiety disorders in medical settings. Although the 12-month prevalence rate of GAD in community samples is approximately 3% (Kessler et al. 2005), an international study found the 1-month prevalence rate in primary care to be 7.9%. In that study, GAD was usually comorbid with other psychiatric conditions

(Maier et al. 2000). GAD also may lead to excess health care use (G.N. Jones et al. 2001). GAD symptoms such as fatigue, muscle tension, and insomnia often lead the patient to present initially to a primary care physician. As is the case with depression, it is important for physicians to consider GAD in the differential diagnosis for such patients. A simple screening question can be extremely useful in helping the physician to determine whether GAD may be present; for example, "In the past 4 weeks, how often have you been bothered by feeling nervous, anxious, on edge, or worrying a lot about different things?" (Spitzer et al. 1999).

Although specific phobias are quite common, they rarely come to the attention of medical professionals. Exceptions include blood-injection-injury phobias and claustrophobia. Blood-injection-injury phobias may lead to fainting during medical procedures or to avoidance of injections and blood tests. In the Baltimore Epidemiologic Catchment Area study, approximately 3% of the sample was found to have one of these phobias. Of that sample of 60 individuals, 23% reported fear of blood; 47%, fear of injections; and 78%, fear of dentists. Although this condition may have serious implications for an affected individual, little is known about its public health significance (Bienvenu and Eaton 1998). Syncope or presyncope in individuals with health care phobias may be due to an underlying predisposition toward neurally mediated syncope (Accurso et al. 2001). Claustrophobia comes to medical attention most commonly when individuals need a magnetic resonance imaging (MRI) procedure. The procedure commonly causes anxiety that is severe enough to require sedation (e.g., with a short-acting benzodiazepine such as midazolam or lorazepam). Behavioral techniques such as relaxation exercises also may be helpful.

Compulsive skin picking or scratching may be a manifestation of obsessive-compulsive disorder (OCD). In a recent study of 60 individuals with skin picking, 15% were found to have OCD (Odlaug and Grant 2008). Among 31 individuals with psychogenic excoriation seen in a dermatology clinic, 45% had OCD (Calikusu et al. 2003). However, in another study of 34 patients with psychogenic excoriation, OCD was not a common disorder (Arnold et al. 1998). (For further discussion, see Chapter 29, "Dermatology.")

Causes of Anxiety in the Medically Ill

In evaluating an anxious patient who is also medically ill, it is essential for the psychiatrist to consider the full range of potential causes of anxiety. In addition to the possibility of a preexisting primary anxiety disorder, three categories of causes of anxiety should be considered for every patient. First, is the patient having a psychological reaction to the experience of medical illness? Second, is the patient's anxiety directly due to the biological effects of a substance? Third, is the patient's anxiety directly due to the biological effects of a medical illness? As is the case for many medically ill patients, the etiology of anxiety is often multifactorial and may vary with the course of illness.

Anxiety as a Psychological Reaction to the Experience of Illness

The importance of one's health added to the often unavoidable uncertainty associated with medical illness leads many medically ill patients to feel anxious. Particularly for individuals with a predisposition to anxiety, the psychosocial stress of illness may be sufficient to induce an anxiety disorder. Just as when evaluating a depressed patient, psychiatrists should never make assumptions regarding the cause of anxiety in an individual patient. For example, it is easy to assume that the patient who is awaiting cardiac surgery is afraid of dying, when in fact the patient might actually be more concerned about potential disability. When approaching the anxious patient, the psychiatrist should consider all potential psychological causes of anxiety. The following discussion reviews the major causes among medically ill populations. For seminal reviews of this topic, the reader is referred to the work of Strain and Grossman (1975) and Kahana and Bibring (1964) (see also Chapter 4, "Psychological Responses to Illness").

Uncertainty Regarding Medical Diagnosis

Some individuals worry excessively that they might have a serious illness. Routine evaluations may cause anxiety, especially in those with a personal or family history of illness. For example, an individual with a family history of breast cancer might become quite anxious in the period preceding routine mammography. Anxiety also may occur during the period between initial evaluation and receipt of the definitive result—for example, after the physician tells the patient, "It's probably nothing, but let's perform a brain MRI just to be sure." Prolonged uncertainty regarding diagnosis is even more anxiety-provoking, such as when the patient is told, "Your PSA [prostate-specific antigen] is slightly elevated, but at this point we should simply wait and reevaluate your level in a few months." Although physicians are acutely aware that there is significant uncertainty inherent in medical diagnoses, patients are generally not reassured by this fact.

Uncertainty Regarding Medical Prognosis

For most medical illnesses and medical procedures, prognosis is uncertain. Many patients will experience ongoing fears of recurrence, especially when they have illnesses that frequently do recur (e.g., arrhythmias, cancer, and multiple sclerosis). Similarly, many fear that their treatments will fail, even if they are initially successful. Examples include fear of rejection of a transplanted organ and development of graft-versus-host disease. Physicians often realize that the potential for a poor prognosis—for example, in cases of relatively advanced cancer—often leads to anxiety. However, it is important to keep in mind that patients who have favorable prognoses often experience anxiety. For example, a 95% cure rate is reassuring to many patients, but some will have difficulty coping with the prospect of a 5% recurrence rate. Complicating the problem is the fact that prognoses may be inaccurate when they are derived from aggregate data, which may have been based on treatments that are now outmoded. For patients who learn about their prognoses through personal medical searches, physicians may be able to provide reassurance by reminding the anxious patients of this information: "You are not a statistic; those data were published before the newest treatments became available."

Anxiety About One's Body

Many individuals experience anxiety about the future effects of illness on their bodies (see Strain and Grossman 1975). Patients may fear that they will lose body parts (e.g., due to amputation). Ongoing fears of amputation are particularly problematic for some patient populations (e.g., those with diabetes mellitus and peripheral vascular disease). Others may fear that they will lose functional capacities or that they will become overly dependent on others. For example, individuals with diabetes mellitus may fear eventual blindness, patients with chronic obstructive pulmonary disease may fear "being hooked to a breathing machine," and men with prostate cancer may fear impotence. Others are afraid of the experience of pain. For example, individuals with metastatic cancer are often afraid that they will have unremitting, severe pain. Knowledge of these fears can help the physician to provide appropriate reassurances (e.g., that pain will be aggressively treated).

Fear of Death

All individuals, regardless of their physical health, fear death at some time in their lives. The experience of physical illness often heightens that fear because everyone either has faced life-threatening illness or has known someone who has died from a physical illness. Physicians must be comfortable assessing fears of death in both patients and their families. This assessment must include an exploration of specific reasons for fear of death (e.g., a patient may fear death from childbirth because that occurred many years earlier to a close relative). Exploration of the reasons for an irrationally high estimate of risk of death may lead to straightforward reassurance. Assessment of death anxiety also should include the opportunity for individuals to discuss existential thoughts about dying (e.g., reflections about the meaning of one's life [Adelbratt and Strang 2000]). When interviewing the patient with a fear of dying, the physician should assess for particular dying-related fears (e.g., a patient may actually be at peace with dying but may be afraid that her family will not be able to survive without her). In that case, involvement of the family may lead to reassurance and a more peaceful dying process (see also Chapter 41, "Palliative Care").

Anxiety About the Effect of Illness on Identity and Livelihood

Even if illness alone is not sufficient to cause anxiety, patients may be concerned about the potential effect of illness on their ability to work, to perform essential household functions, or to maintain income. Uncertainties about medical reimbursements may make insured individuals justifiably concerned. The uninsured are often so anxious about how they would pay for medical procedures that they avoid medical visits altogether. Patients may be anxious that the costs of medical treatment might cause financial burdens for their families, and they may decline treatment for this reason. In these situations, meetings with family members and health care financial counselors may help to assuage unjustifiable fears that treatments will cause more harm than good.

Anxiety About Strangers and Being Alone in the Hospital

Individuals with medical illnesses become anxious even when their own personal physician performs a medical procedure. Thus, it is not unusual for an acutely ill patient to become intensely anxious when asked to trust his or her life to the new physician he or she has just met in the emergency department or the intensive care unit. Patients who are so anxious that they refuse a medical procedure may be labeled as noncompliant when, in fact, fear is the underlying explanation. As noted by Muskin (1995), acceptance of the involvement of unfamiliar clinicians may be particularly difficult for individuals with preexisting problems with trust (e.g., those with paranoia or borderline personality disorder). Similarly, it is often difficult for some patients to tolerate being alone in the hospital. Because many individuals regress while hospitalized, it is not surprising that patients with dependency needs might become unduly anxious when left alone in an unfamiliar environment.

Anxiety About Negative Reactions From Physicians

Many individuals with medical illness worry about their physician's opinion of them. Excessive concern may lead to reluctance to seek health care. Persons who feel guilty for not following their physician's recommendations might cancel appointments for fear of being scolded (e.g., for failure to lose weight, stop smoking, or check blood sugar levels more reliably). Similarly, some individuals' anxiety might lead them to deny or fail to disclose important information (e.g., regarding sexual risk factors or level of alcohol intake). Anxiety may be particularly prominent among patients who have caused or aggravated their own illness. It is important for the physician to be vigilant for clues that a patient might have excessive anxiety. Awareness of negative countertransference is essential; it is appropriate to provide consistent, firm reminders of the need for proper medical care, but harsh criticism is unwarranted and may contribute to poor adherence.

Substance-Induced Anxiety

In evaluating the anxious medical patient, it is important to consider whether medications or medication withdrawal might be contributory. Because they can be obtained without prescriptions, caffeine and over-the-counter sympathomimetics are common causes of anxiety in the general population. Caffeine is widely used and commonly causes anxiety. It may be present in significant quantities in coffee, tea, caffeinated soda, caffeinated water, and coffee ice cream, as well as in over-the-counter preparations for alertness (e.g., NoDoz), weight loss, and headache (e.g., Excedrin). Even at low doses, caffeine may induce anxiety in susceptible individuals (Childs et al. 2008). In individuals with anxiety disorders, reduction of caffeine intake often reduces anxiety symptoms. Over-the-counter sympathomimetics used as decongestants (e.g., pseudoephedrine) frequently cause anxiety, and tachyphylaxis develops rapidly. Some individuals may use large quantities in the form of nasal spray. Similarly, the widely used herbal preparation ephedra also may cause anxiety.

The most important medication classes that are associated with anxiety are summarized in Table 11-2, which includes examples of specific medications in each class. Where appropriate, notes have been added for further clarification. General references in this area are *The Medical Letter on Drugs and Therapeutics* ("Drugs That May Cause Psychiatric Symptoms" 2008) and the *Physicians' Desk Reference* (2009).

Anxiety Secondary to General Medical Conditions

Many medical problems have been reported to cause anxiety, but data are limited to case reports for many associations. Nonetheless, it is important for the psychosomatic medicine physician to consider medical causes of anxiety when evaluating an anxious patient. It is particularly important to evaluate medical causes when the history is not typical for a primary anxiety disorder (e.g., lack of personal or family history, lack of psychosocial stressors) and when the onset of anxiety is at a later age. In addition, it is important to evaluate medical causes when the anxiety is accompanied by disproportionate physical symptoms (e.g., marked dyspnea, tachycardia, or tremor) or atypical physical symptoms (e.g., syncope, confusion, or focal neurological symptoms).

It is important for the clinician to keep in mind the distinction between anxiety that is physiologically secondary to a general medical condition and anxiety that is comorbid with, or a psychological reaction to, a general medical condition. (For example, hyperthyroidism appears to biologically cause anxiety, whereas diabetes mellitus usually does not.) The DSM-IV-TR diagnosis of anxiety due to a general medical condition refers to the former, not the latter. This difference has not been clearly articulated in some reviews in this area, and it can also be confusing for patients. One source of confusion results from the assumption of causality when there is an epidemiological association between anxiety and a specific medical condition. For example, anxiety disorders are common among individuals with migraine (Torelli and D'Amico 2004), but the onset of anxiety disorders generally precedes that of migraine (Merikangas and Stevens 1997).

Components of the medical evaluation of the anxious patient should be determined by the patient's specific medical symptoms. For example, it may be necessary to obtain electroencephalograms and a neurological consultation for a patient with seizurelike episodes. The general evaluation of all anxious patients should include the following elements (Colon and Popkin 2002):

- History and physical examination, including neurological examination
- Evaluation of the potential role of medications and substances (see Table 11-2)
- Screening diagnostic studies (e.g., routine blood chemistries, complete blood cell count, calcium concentration, thyroid hormone levels, electrocardiogram)

In the following subsections, we discuss common medical conditions that are associated with anxiety for which data are strongly supportive of a causal relation.

Thyroid Disease

Anxiety symptoms commonly occur among individuals with thyroid disease. Patients with subclinical and clinical hyperthyroidism have been shown to have elevated anxiety levels (Gulseren et al. 2006; Sait Gönen et al. 2004) (see also Chapter 22, "Endocrine and Metabolic Disorders"). Hyperthyroidism may be difficult to distinguish from a primary

TABLE 11–2. Substances that may cause anxiety

Class	Example(s)	Notes
Androgens	Methyltestosterone, nandrolone	Most problems occur when abused.
Angiotensin-converting enzyme inhibitors	Captopril, lisinopril	They are often stimulating.
Anticholinergics	Atropine, benztropine, dicyclomine, hyoscyamine	
Anticataplexy agent	Sodium oxybate	
Antidepressants	Bupropion, serotonin reuptake inhibitors, tricyclics	
Antiemetics	Droperidol, prochlorperazine, promethazine	Anxiety may actually be akathisia.
Antiepileptics	Pregabalin, zonisamide	
Antimalarial agents	Mefloquine	
Antimycobacterial agents	Isoniazid	
Antineoplastic agents	Ifosfamide, vinblastine	
Antipsychotics	Haloperidol, thiothixene	Anxiety may actually be akathisia.
Antiviral agents	Acyclovir, efavirenz, ganciclovir, valganciclovir	
Beta-adrenergic agonists	Albuterol, metaproterenol	
Cannabinoids	Dronabinol	
Class I antiarrhythmics	Lidocaine, procainamide, quinidine	
Corticosteroids	Methylprednisolone, prednisone	
Dopaminergic agents	Amantadine, carbidopa-levodopa	
Estrogens	Conjugated estrogens, ethinyl estradiol, levonorgestrel implant	They may cause panic attacks and depression.
Gonadotropin-releasing hormone active agents	Leuprolide	
Histamine H_2 receptor antagonists	Cimetidine, famotidine, nizatidine	
Interferons	Interferon-alpha, interferon-beta	
Methylxanthines	Caffeine, theophylline	
Sympathomimetics	Ephedrine, epinephrine, phenylephrine nasal, pseudoephedrine	
Nonsteroidal anti-inflammatory drugs	Indomethacin, naproxen, salicylates	
Opiates	Meperidine	Anxiety may be a symptom of delirium.
Opioid antagonists	Naltrexone	Observe patient for opiate withdrawal.
Progestins	Medroxyprogesterone acetate, norethindrone	
Prokinetic agents	Metoclopramide	Anxiety may be due to akathisia.
Psychostimulants	Dextroamphetamine, methylphenidate	
Sedative-hypnotics	Alcohol, barbiturates, benzodiazepines	Anxiety occurs with drug withdrawal.

anxiety disorder. Signs that may be suggestive of thyrotoxicosis include persistent tachycardia, palms that are warm and dry (not cold and clammy), and fatigue accompanied by the desire to be active (Colon and Popkin 2002). However, data differentiating the two are not definitive in this regard (see Iacovides et al. 2000), and much of the research in this area is not current. Some individuals with hyperthyroidism also may have cognitive impairment. Improvement in anxiety usually parallels successful treatment of the hyperthyroidism. Therefore, specific antianxiety treatment may not be necessary. Nonetheless, antianxiety treatment should be considered during normalization of thyroid hormone levels, particularly for individuals with moderate to severe symptoms. Beta-blockers, which are used routinely for acute treatment of hyperthyroidism, will relieve peripheral manifestations of anxiety.

Because thyroid dysfunction is so common among individuals with anxiety, a screening thyroid stimulating hormone (TSH) assay should be considered for patients with new-onset anxiety disorders and treatment-resistant anxiety, particularly when the anxiety is generalized and accompanied by prominent physical symptoms. If the TSH level is abnormal, further evaluation of the thyroid axis is recommended (e.g., free thyroxine index or free thyroxine measurement).

There are several putative mechanisms for the association between abnormalities of the thyroid axis and mood or anxiety symptoms. A blunted TSH response to thyrotropin-releasing hormone stimulation had been reported to occur in some depressed patients, but little recent research is available, and the test does not have clinical utility. The adrenergic overreactivity that accompanies hyperthyroidism provides a ready explanation for its association with anxiety. Finally, thyroid hormones interact with brain neurotransmitters (e.g., the serotonergic and noradrenergic systems; Altshuler et al. 2001). Nonetheless, the association between the thyroid axis and anxiety is not well understood.

Anxiety also has been reported to be a symptom of hypothyroidism (Hall and Hall 1999; Sait Gönen et al. 2004). Its association may be better explained by the association between depression and hypothyroidism, in which anxiety is conceptualized as a symptom of depression as opposed to a direct biological result of a hypothyroid state.

Pulmonary Disease

Patients with pulmonary disease often experience symptoms of anxiety. Rates of anxiety disorders among individuals with asthma and chronic obstructive pulmonary disease are higher than among the general population (e.g., Goodwin and Pine 2002; Goodwin et al. 2003; Hasler et al. 2005; Rockhill et al. 2007). The psychological stress and uncertainty of living with asthma certainly make important contributions to this association. In addition, it is essential to consider physiological factors intrinsic to asthma. For example, both hypercapnia and hyperventilation may lead to symptoms of a panic attack; in one model, hypercapnia may lead to increased locus coeruleus activity, which could cause panic and hyperventilation (Zaubler and Katon 1998). Furthermore, carbon dioxide inhalation has been shown to precipitate panic attacks among individuals with panic disorder. Asthma also may be associated with panic attacks through a process of classical conditioning. In this paradigm, because a severe asthma attack is so terrifying, a future sensation of mild dyspnea might precipitate a full-blown panic episode (Carr 1998). In addition, anxiety may worsen asthma, thereby contributing to a vicious circle in which pulmonary and anxiety symptoms exacerbate each other (Carr 1998; Deshmukh et al. 2008). Several asthma medications may cause anxiety (see Table 11–2). Pulmonary emboli also may lead to symptoms of anxiety (Tapson 2007); this diagnosis is more easily missed when the emboli are small (see also Chapter 19, "Lung Disease").

Parkinson's Disease

Anxiety is often seen in individuals with Parkinson's disease (Richard 2005; Walsh and Bennett 2001). Most studies of the prevalence of anxiety disorders among patients with Parkinson's disease involve small samples, but they indicate that these disorders are much more common among Parkinson's disease patients than in the general population (Richard 2005). Anxiety often appears after the manifestations of symptoms of Parkinson's disease. For example, some individuals may develop social anxiety disorder symptoms because they are embarrassed about manifestations of the Parkinson's disease (e.g., tremor) (American Psychiatric Association 2000). Anxiety also may be due to the uncertainty associated with Parkinson's disease, with respect to both day-to-day functioning and long-term prognosis. Anxiety in some patients may be worse during "off" periods compared with "on" periods, but in others, anxiety symptoms do not correlate with motor fluctuations (Richard 2005; Richard et al. 2004). Depression and anxiety symptoms often coexist among individuals with Parkinson's disease (Richard 2005).

The neurobiology of anxiety in Parkinson's disease has not been clearly delineated, but limited evidence supports the roles of neurotransmitter abnormalities, particularly in central noradrenergic systems (Richard 2005). The dopaminergic neural circuits implicated in Parkinson's disease have intimate connections with systems involved with anxiety (e.g., serotonin). Anxiety also may be due to medications used to treat Parkinson's disease, such as L-dopa (see Table 11–2). Deep brain stimulation of the subthalamic nucleus was shown to reduce anxiety in one recent study (Witt et al. 2008).

Poststroke Anxiety

Although poststroke depression has been more widely described, many individuals also have anxiety after a stroke (Angelelli et al. 2004; De Wit et al. 2008). It may appear alone or comorbid with depression (Barker-Collo 2007; Kimura et al. 2003; Wise and Rundell 1999). When they appear after a stroke, anxiety symptoms have been shown to persist in many individuals. For example, in one large study, 40% of the patients with initial anxiety remained anxious at 6 months (De Wit et al. 2008). Stroke also has been reported to result in PTSD (Bruggimann et al. 2006). Limited literature has found anxiety to be associated with right-hemisphere lesions, whereas depression and mixed depression and anxiety are more commonly associated with left-hemisphere lesions (Aström 1996; Castillo et al. 1993).

Seizures

Anxiety symptoms may be caused by seizures. For example, complex partial seizures may be accompanied by symptoms of panic disorder, including fear, depersonalization, derealization, dizziness, and paresthesias (Kim et al. 2007; S.A. Thompson et al. 2000). One group used ambulatory electroencephalographic monitoring with sphenoidal electrodes to study patients with atypical panic attacks (i.e., panic attacks with concomitant neurological symptoms such as change in level of consciousness, aphasia, and focal paresthesias). Focal paroxysmal electroencephalographic changes were found in 5 of 11 patients who had panic attacks during monitoring (Weilburg et al. 1995).

For further discussion of neurophysiological and neuroanatomical aspects of anxiety disorders, the reader is referred to Chapter 32, "Neurology and Neurosurgery," and D.J. Stein and Hugo (2002).

Other Conditions

In addition to the disorders discussed earlier, anxiety has reportedly been caused by many other medical conditions. For example, anxiety may be associated with hypocalcemia and hypomagnesemia. Relatively rare conditions for which there are only limited data supporting a causal relation include carcinoid syndrome, hyperparathyroidism, and pheochromocytoma (Colon and Popkin 2002). In the absence of other findings suggestive of one of these rare disorders, it is not advisable to screen for them (e.g., serotonin metabolites to rule out carcinoid, parathyroid hormone levels to rule out hyperparathyroidism, or catecholamine metabolites to rule out pheochromocytoma).

Treatment of Anxiety in the Medically Ill

Treatment of anxiety disorders has been shown to be safe and effective. Treatment of anxiety associated with medical illness can also improve physical symptoms, decrease disability, lower high rates of frequent medical use, and improve quality of life (Roy-Byrne et al. 2008). Most people with anxiety disorders seek care from their primary care physicians, complaining of the physical symptoms of anxiety such as pain, insomnia, or gastrointestinal symptoms, and often not recognizing the underlying emotional disorder. In a study of three academic primary care outpatient clinics (M.B. Stein et al. 2004), fewer than one-third of identified patients with anxiety disorders received adequate treatment with psychotherapy or medication. Collaboration between psychiatrists and primary care providers is important to ensure effective treatment. Several current models of collaborative care and stepped care interventions in primary care treatment of anxiety and depression show cost-effective outcomes and improved patient satisfaction (Katon et al. 2002; G.E. Simon et al. 2004; Veer-Tazelaar et al. 2009).

Psychotherapy

An overemphasis on psychopharmacology in the care of medically ill patients sometimes results in overlooking the value of psychotherapy. The first step in treatment is to spend time listening to and talking with the patient. Just as in psychotherapy with any patient, empathic listening is a powerful tool to relieve distress. With medically ill patients, the goal is to help patients understand and discuss their emotional reactions to their illness so that they can then manage these feelings by using their own coping mechanisms. Psychotherapeutic approaches include supportive, cognitive-behavioral, and psychodynamic therapies.

Supportive Therapy

Supportive therapy involves listening and providing reassurance, sympathy, education about the medical process and the underlying illness, advice, and suggestions. The process includes listening for fears and misperceptions about illness or its treatment and giving patients appropriate information so that they can be as prepared as possible (House and Stark 2002). Effective communication, using language the patient and family can understand, can lead to a great decrease in anxiety. It is also helpful to give patients as much choice in their treatment decisions as possible so that they feel they have some control over the course of their treatment.

Reassurance is an important skill that all physicians use in treating patients. In some highly anxious patients, however, simple reassurance can actually cause increased anxiety and lead to a cycle of maladaptive behavior. For example, if a patient who has been told that a procedure is simple or painless subsequently experiences pain or untoward results, the resulting anxiety can lead to more reassurance-seeking behavior, mistrust, and decreased cooperation. Many anxious patients tend to interpret bodily symptoms as evidence of serious disease, and as a result, they may seek multiple consultations for reassurance. Understanding the patient's beliefs, concerns, and perceptions can be helpful in challenging misperceptions, educating the patient about his or her illness, and devising a realistic plan to monitor symptoms. Having a realistic plan to help patients differentiate minor symptoms from those that may need medical attention will reduce anxiety and decrease the excessive need for reassurance (Stark and House 2000). It is also important that the physician not assume that a patient's anxiety is due to fear of dying. When reassurance is directed at the wrong fear, it may accentuate anxiety and lead patients to believe that their physician does not understand them.

The consultant can serve as a liaison between the patient and the health care team. For example, the psychiatrist might help the primary physician understand the importance of clarifying the risks and benefits of treatment and of informing the anxious patient when delays in scheduling arise. It also may be helpful for the treatment team to consult directly with the psychiatrist about how to care for the anxious patient. Facilitating communication among the patient and members of the treatment team can help avoid misperceptions or mistrust that will only serve to heighten anxiety.

Another important aspect of supportive therapy is the involvement of the patient's support system of family, friends, and spiritual/religious community. Some patients may need assistance in expanding their support network (e.g., to reach out to friends with whom they may have lost contact). Some family members may need supportive psychotherapy to reduce their anxieties about the patient's medical condition. Hospital staff such as nurses and chaplains can be instrumental in reducing patient's fears.

Patients confronting life-threatening or terminal illnesses such as cancer may experience death anxiety (Yalom 1980). Open discussions with patients about death help to reduce anxiety and distress (Spiegel et al. 1981), and psychological interventions alone can help patients manage their death anxiety (Payne and Massie 2000). Maintaining hope is an important aspect of minimizing anxiety, although goals can change from full recovery to having more time to accomplish specific short-term goals. Helping patients find meaning and value in their lives, despite their illness and suffering, helps to relieve emotional distress (Frankl 1987). For example, anxiety can be reduced when patients see that they are still important to their families or that they still have unfinished business to address. Dignity-oriented therapy has extended this approach to the care of terminally ill patients (G.N. Thompson and Chochinov 2008). The hospice movement has been instrumental in helping provide relief for many patients (Byock 1997). Despite recent improvements in physician education, some caregivers need more training to be able to overcome their own death anxiety so that they can provide comfort to end-of-life patients (Adelbratt and Strang 2000) (see Chapter 41, "Palliative Care").

Supportive group interventions have been shown to be effective in reducing anxiety and distress in medically ill patients, and support groups for HIV, cancer, cardiac, and other medical illnesses have proliferated in recent years (Wallis 2004). They can be quite helpful in providing emotional support, improving coping skills, and providing information about health promotion and wellness (Sherman et al. 2007).

Cognitive-Behavioral Therapy

Cognitive-behavioral therapy has been proven to be as effective as medication in treating many anxiety disorders, including GAD, PTSD, and panic disorder ("Generalized anxiety disorder: toxic worry" 2003; Stanley et al. 2009). Cognitive techniques are used to uncover and correct misinterpretations and irrational thoughts that lead to increased anxiety and distress. Behavioral techniques, such as systematic desensitization, can be used to help overcome fears that can interfere with effective treatment, such as claustrophobia during MRI (Goldberg and Posner 2000). A brief course of cognitive-behavioral therapy can have long-lasting effects, but occasional "booster" sessions may be needed.

A variety of therapies that involve teaching self-awareness and self-regulation of body functions have been found effective in reducing anxiety and physical symptoms in medically ill patients. These include muscle relaxation techniques (such as Jacobson's progressive muscle relaxation), autogenic training (such as biofeedback, which uses technology to control internal processes), and relaxation techniques (such as meditation, breathing exercises, and self-hypnosis). Stress management interventions may improve quality of life (e.g., by decreasing anxiety in the course of medical treatments; Antoni et al. 2006). Relaxation techniques may help to wean patients from the ventilator as well as to reduce dyspnea and anxiety in patients with chronic obstructive pulmonary disease (Smoller et al. 1999). A review of studies that have examined efficacy of meditation and relaxation techniques indicates that they are safe and may have some benefit in reducing anxiety in medically ill patients (Arias et al. 2006).

Psychodynamic Therapy

For patients who are not too ill and who have sufficient emotional resilience, brief dynamic psychotherapy can be useful in uncovering the conscious and unconscious meaning of the illness to the patient. Understanding patients' developmental history, interpersonal dynamics, and defense mechanisms can help the psychiatrist to assist them in finding healthier ways to cope with medical illness (Viederman 2000). What coping strategies have helped in the past? When did the individual feel most fulfilled in his or her life? How can those memories and skills be used now, even in the presence of significant medical illness? Psychotherapy can uncover areas leading to increased distress, such as real or imagined guilt, unhealthy coping strategies such as avoidance and denial, and recognition of past conflicted relationships that may be repeated in the current doctor–patient relationship. An understanding of the patient's underlying dynamics can help identify and resolve conflicts with the treatment team that may be interfering with recovery. An understanding of psychodynamic principles can also help psychiatrists in working with the primary treatment team that is caring for the anxious patient.

Countertransference reactions can cause problems for providers of anxious patients. For example, physicians may overidentify with their patients, leading to frustration because of lack of progress or poor prognosis. As a result, they may then overcompensate by offering excessive reassurance, or they may minimize or overlook symptoms in an unconscious attempt to reduce their own anxiety. Caregivers also may become withdrawn and distant, providing care mechanically with little empathy or awareness of the emotional needs of the patient. Psychiatrists can play a role in helping the health care team to be cognizant of these defenses so that they do not interfere with the provision of optimal patient care. (See Chapter 39, "Psychotherapy," for further discussion of psychotherapy for the medically ill.)

Pharmacotherapy

Psychotherapeutic techniques are often not sufficient to manage anxiety in the medically ill. An increasingly broad range of psychopharmacological agents can be used safely with this population. (For further details, see Chapter 38, "Psychopharmacology," as well as specific discussions in Chapters 18–37 of Part III, "Specialties and Subspecialties.")

Benzodiazepines and Hypnotics

For acute anxiety symptoms, the most immediately effective and frequently used agents are the benzodiazepines (Table 11–3). Diazepam and chlordiazepoxide were among the first of these to be used. They also have established efficacy for other conditions—diazepam as an anticonvulsant and muscle relaxant and chlordiazepoxide for alcohol detoxification. Newer benzodiazepines have better safety profiles and shorter half-lives, so they tend to be used more frequently.

Alprazolam works rapidly and is eliminated quickly, but as a result there may be rebound anxiety and withdrawal symptoms. Because lorazepam can be given orally, intravenously, or intramuscularly and does not have an active metabolite, it is often a preferred medication in hospitalized patients. Lorazepam can be given in an intravenous bolus or drip, but as doses increase to provide sedation and treat delirium tremens, respiratory status must be watched closely. Lorazepam and oxazepam are metabolized through conjugation, and temazepam is metabolized almost exclusively through conjugation (Trevor and Way 2007). As a result, those benzodiazepines may be less problematic in patients with liver disease than are the other benzodiazepines, which are oxidatively metabolized (Crone et al. 2006). Midazolam, a benzodiazepine with a very short half-life that can only be given intravenously or intramuscularly, is used for short-term procedures such as bone marrow biopsies, endoscopies, and MRI scans in claustrophobic patients. For patients who need long-term benzodiazepines, it is often helpful to change to a medication with a longer half-life, such as clonazepam.

All benzodiazepines can cause excessive sedation. They may also cause motor and cognitive disturbances, especially in older persons and individuals with impaired brain functioning (e.g., due to dementia, head injury, or mental retardation). Therefore, they should be used with caution, if at all, in these patients. Anxiety in delirious patients is usually better treated with antipsychotics than with benzodiazepines (Breitbart et al. 1996). Benzodiazepines can cause respiratory suppression, so they should be used cautiously in persons with pulmonary disease who retain carbon dioxide, or in patients with sleep apnea. Because of potential teratogenicity, benzodiazepines should be avoided in the first trimester of pregnancy. They should also be avoided at the very end of pregnancy because there are reports of sedation and withdrawal symptoms in the fetus (McGee and Pies 2002). All benzodiazepines can lead to tolerance and dependence, so they should be avoided or used judiciously (i.e., for detoxification) in persons with a substance abuse history. However, compared with barbiturates and earlier sedative-hypnotics such as meprobamate, they are much safer in overdose and have fewer side effects. In persons who are conscientious and do not have a history of chemical dependence, benzodiazepines often can be used safely for years without causing problems or tolerance. As an individual

TABLE 11–3. Selected benzodiazepines used for anxiety in the medically ill

Medication	Route of administration	Dosage	Elimination half-life (hours)	Comments
Alprazolam	Oral	0.25–1.0 mg tid	9–20	Rapid onset. Interdose withdrawal a problem, but new extended-release form is available.
Chlordiazepoxide	Oral, intramuscular	5–25 mg qid	28–100 (including metabolites)	Useful for alcohol withdrawal.
Clonazepam	Oral	0.25–1 mg bid–tid	19–60	Also used for absence seizures, periodic leg movements, and neuropathic pain.
Diazepam	Oral, intravenous	2–10 mg qid	30–200 (including metabolites)	Also used as an anticonvulsant and muscle relaxant.
Lorazepam	Oral, intramuscular, intravenous	0.5–2.0 mg up to qid	8–24	Intravenous availability is an advantage. Metabolized by conjugation. Also approved for chemotherapy-related nausea and vomiting.
Midazolam	Intramuscular, intravenous	Intramuscular: 5 mg single dose Intravenous: 0.02–0.10 mg/kg/h	1–20 (including metabolites)	Used for preoperative sedation and intravenous induction.
Oxazepam	Oral	10–30 mg qid	3–25	Metabolized by conjugation. May also be useful for alcohol withdrawal.

Note. bid=twice a day; qid=four times a day; tid=three times a day.
Source. Adapted from Bezchlibnyk-Butler and Jeffries 2006; Physicians' Desk Reference 2009.

ages, use should be reevaluated. Similarly, long-term benzodiazepine use may need to be reduced or discontinued among patients who develop specific medical conditions (e.g., end-stage liver disease, dementia, chronic obstructive pulmonary disease, and cerebellar dysfunction).

Hypnotics are commonly used in medically ill patients who are kept awake by their anxiety. Newer agents such as zolpidem, zaleplon, and eszopiclone are nonbenzodiazepines that act on the benzodiazepine receptor. They are preferred for short-term use because they have very short half-lives and generally cause less daytime sedation, impaired coordination, and cognitive disturbance than do the benzodiazepines. Ramelteon is a melatonin receptor agonist that is thought to act on the suprachiasmatic nucleus to help with sleep induction (Roth and Culpepper 2008). Generally all of the hypnotics are best used for short intervals to decrease the chance of side effects, to maintain effectiveness (i.e., prevent tolerance), and to prevent dependence (National Institutes of Health 2005).

Antidepressants

The pharmacological treatment of choice for GAD, panic disorder, PTSD, OCD, and social anxiety disorder is a medication that can increase serotonin, such as the selective serotonin reuptake inhibitors (SSRIs): fluoxetine, sertraline, paroxetine, citalopram, escitalopram, and fluvoxamine. All antidepressants now have a black-box warning to monitor for increased suicidality, especially in children through young adults. These medications have few side effects and therefore are generally quite safe for the medically ill; they do not result in cardiac conduction problems, orthostatic hypotension, or physical dependence. Because antidepressants may take 2–6 weeks to relieve anxiety, the patient may need initial treatment with benzodiazepines. Once the patient has been stabilized on the antidepressant medication, the benzodiazepines usually can be gradually withdrawn without recurrence of anxiety. The antidepressant should be used for at least 3–6 months before stopping it, and it should be tapered to avoid discontinuation symptoms.

Antidepressants can be used safely on a long-term basis if anxiety returns.

One of the main side effects of the SSRIs is a relatively high incidence of sexual dysfunction in both men and women. This side effect may be particularly problematic for persons with medical problems already associated with sexual dysfunction, such as diabetes or vascular disease (see Chapter 16, "Sexual Dysfunction"). In addition, psychiatrists must be concerned about the potential for drug interactions—for example, with fluoxetine and paroxetine (cytochrome P450 2D6 inhibitors) and fluvoxamine (a cytochrome P450 3A4 inhibitor; see Chapter 38, "Psychopharmacology"). Serotonin reuptake inhibitors may cause initial gastrointestinal distress and nausea, so they are generally given with food. It is important to reassure the patient with gastrointestinal disease that these side effects are almost always transient. SSRIs are also associated with the syndrome of inappropriate secretion of antidiuretic hormone, especially in older patients. Caution is advised when using serotonin medications with the antibiotic linezolid because of the potential for hypertensive crisis and serotonin syndrome, although they are thought to occur rarely (Sola et al. 2006). SSRIs may help decrease frequency of migraine headaches, but they can also exacerbate headaches. Caution is advised in using triptans with SSRIs because of the potential for serotonin syndrome. It has been reported that SSRIs can exacerbate parkinsonism in individuals with Parkinson's disease; however, this appears to be an uncommon side effect (Dell'Agnello et al. 2001; Hedenmalm et al. 2006). Because all SSRIs are equally efficacious, medication choice is often based on side-effect profile. For example, the more sedating SSRIs (e.g., fluvoxamine and paroxetine) may be advantageous for the highly anxious patient with insomnia, whereas fluoxetine may be more stimulating. For medically ill patients taking multiple medications, agents with the fewest drug interactions are preferred: sertraline, citalopram, and escitalopram.

Serotonin-norepinephrine reuptake inhibitors (SNRIs), including venlafaxine, duloxetine, and desvenlafaxine, also may be useful for anxiety (Katzman 2009). Venlafaxine and duloxetine have been approved for treatment of some anxiety disorders and, based on their mechanism of action, are probably effective agents for treating all anxiety disorders. Blood pressure should be monitored when these drugs are being initiated and with each dosage increase. If diastolic blood pressure increases, the dosage should be reduced or the drug stopped. These medications also can cause sexual dysfunction and should be given with food to decrease gastrointestinal side effects.

Mirtazapine—an alpha-adrenergic receptor antagonist and an antagonist at serotonin 5-HT_{2A}, 5-HT_{2C}, and 5-HT_3 receptors—may be helpful in reducing anxiety. Its use in medically ill patients has increased recently for two reasons: 1) it has few drug interactions, and 2) the side effects of sedation and increased appetite may be helpful in patients who have insomnia and anorexia with weight loss (Cankurtaran et al. 2008). Trazodone is a weak antidepressant; it is most commonly used as a hypnotic because of its sedative properties and lack of tolerance or dependence. In some cases, it has been used for anxiety and agitation in patients, mainly because of its sedative properties.

Tricyclic antidepressants and monoamine oxidase inhibitors are well established as effective treatments for anxiety disorders and for depression. Tricyclics can be efficacious for the treatment of anxiety in the medically ill (e.g., in patients with chronic pain or diarrhea-predominant irritable bowel syndrome). The main reasons these medications are currently not used frequently as first-line treatment are their numerous side effects and their toxicity in overdose. Tricyclics often cause dry mouth, weight gain, constipation, sedation, orthostatic hypotension, urinary retention, and falls, especially in elderly patients. In addition, because of their quinidine-like effects, they can cause heart block and arrhythmias. Because the margin of safety between efficacy and toxicity is relatively small, overdose can be dangerous and even fatal. Persons with liver and kidney disease may develop toxicity as a result of impaired metabolism and excretion. Monoamine oxidase inhibitors can cause dizziness, orthostatic hypotension, and weight gain. These side effects, as well as the potential for serious hypertensive crises, limit their usefulness in medically ill patients. Selegiline recently has been introduced as a transdermal patch, which offers the advantage of fewer food restrictions than with oral monoamine oxidase inhibitors at the lower dose. However, the risks of hypertensive crisis with many medications remain, so it probably will not be used widely in medically ill persons.

Antipsychotics

Antipsychotic medications are not approved for the treatment of anxiety, although limited data support their efficacy (Gao et al. 2006). Psychosomatic medicine psychiatrists often find them to be efficacious and safe to use in selected medical populations. Long-term use may lead to adverse side effects such as metabolic syndrome. Because antipsychotics do not cause confusion or respiratory compromise, they may be preferable to benzodiazepines for the more severe anxiety associated with agitation or delirium or in patients with respiratory compromise. For example, antipsychotics may be helpful in assisting the anxious patient who is being weaned from a ventilator (Rosenthal et al. 2007). The antipsychotic agent used most often in medically ill patients is haloperidol, which can be given orally, intramuscularly, or intravenously. In acutely agitated patients who may be violent or psychotic, 5–10 mg of haloperidol is often given orally or intramuscularly, usually in conjunction with a benzodiazepine such as lorazepam, and sometimes with benztropine to prevent a dystonic reaction. For mild agitation, 0.5–2.0 mg might be given, but much higher doses can be used. If a high-potency typical antipsychotic such as haloperidol is used in treating anxiety, it is important to monitor for akathisia because it can be mistaken for worsening anxiety.

Newer atypical antipsychotics such as olanzapine, risperidone, quetiapine, ziprasidone, and aripiprazole are also used selectively in the management of anxiety, especially in lower doses. Ziprasidone, olanzapine, and aripiprazole are now available in intramuscular formulation. The intramuscular formulations may be helpful in those with severe anxiety or agitation, especially if they are unable to take oral medications. Olanzapine, risperidone, and aripiprazole are available as orally disintegrating tablets, which may be useful for patients who cannot swallow pills. Current data suggest that ziprasidone and aripiprazole may have less propensity to cause weight gain and metabolic syndrome than do the other atypical antipsychotics.

Buspirone

Buspirone is a partial serotonin agonist that may be effective in the treatment of anxiety (Lee et al. 2005). It may be useful in treating anxiety in medically ill patients because it has few drug interactions and does not cause respiratory depression. It can be used safely in substance abusers because it does not cause dependence, and its metabolism is not greatly affected by liver disease (Stahl 2004). The main drawbacks with buspirone are that it may take 2–4 weeks to become effective, and its benefits seem modest. Because of its short half-life, it needs to be given two to three times a day. Some patients complain of dizziness and excessive sedation when first beginning the medication, but it is usually well tolerated.

Beta-Blockers

Beta-adrenergic blockers produce anxiolytic effects by blocking autonomic hyperarousal (elevated pulse, elevated blood pressure, sweating, tremors) associated with anxiety responses. They work best for specific anxiety-producing situations, such as performance anxiety and public speaking, and are less efficacious for panic disorder and social phobias. All beta-blockers are contraindicated in persons with asthma or chronic obstructive lung disease, and they can worsen peripheral vascular disease (Barnes 2005). Patients with type 1 diabetes should not be prescribed nonselective beta-blockers; those medications block the sympathetic nervous system response to hypoglycemia, resulting in lack of awareness of symptoms (Kaplan 2007). The reported association between beta-blockers and depression has not been supported by data from clinical trials (Ko et al. 2002).

Antihistamines

Sedating histamine H_1 receptor blockers are sometimes used to treat anxiety and insomnia. Hydroxyzine has been shown to be as effective and safe as benzodiazepines in treating anxiety (Llorca et al. 2002) in a general study population. Diphenhydramine, which is often used to treat insomnia, is available in over-the-counter preparations. Because these medications are not addicting, many physicians consider them to be benign. However, they can cause dizziness, excessive sedation, incoordination, and confusion, especially when used with alcohol or other central nervous system depressants. Elderly patients and those with brain disease or injury are more sensitive to these medications and may become delirious even with low doses. Despite these risks, these medications are still an option when benzodiazepines must be avoided because of concerns about dependence or respiratory depression.

Anticonvulsants

Anticonvulsants are primarily prescribed by psychiatrists for patients with bipolar disorder who cannot tolerate or do not respond to lithium, but they can also be helpful for some individuals with anxiety (Mula et al. 2007). Divalproex sodium may be helpful in calming agitated, anxious patients, especially those with brain injury, mental retardation, or dementia. Newer anticonvulsants such as lamotrigine and pregabalin have shown some promise in treating mood and anxiety symptoms and may prove to have some role in treating anxiety in medically ill patients.

Conclusion

The experience of medical illness often leads to clinically significant anxiety symptoms. Although many individuals with medical illnesses have anxiety disorders, these disorders are often underrecognized and undertreated. Both psychotherapy and pharmacotherapy can significantly ameliorate anxiety symptoms, even among patients with severe medical problems. Thus, careful assessment and treatment of anxiety disorders are important components of the psychiatric care of the medically ill.

References

Accurso V, Winnicki M, Shamsuzzaman AS, et al: Predisposition to vasovagal syncope in subjects with blood/injury phobia. Circulation 104:903–907, 2001

Adelbratt S, Strang P: Death anxiety in brain tumour patients and their spouses. Palliat Med 14:499–507, 2000

Albert CM, Chae CU, Rexrode KM, et al: Phobic anxiety and risk of coronary heart disease and sudden cardiac death among women. Circulation 111:480–487, 2005

Alter CL, Pelcovitz D, Axelrod A, et al: Identification of PTSD in cancer survivors. Psychosomatics 37:137–143, 1996

Altshuler LL, Bauer M, Frye MA, et al: Does thyroid supplementation accelerate tricyclic antidepressant response? A review and meta-analysis of the literature. Am J Psychiatry 158:1617–1622, 2001

American Psychiatric Association: Diagnostic and Statistical Manual of Mental Disorders, 4th Edition, Text Revision. Washington, DC, American Psychiatric Association, 2000

Andrykowski MA, Cordova MJ: Factors associated with PTSD symptoms following treatment for breast cancer: test of the Andersen model. J Trauma Stress 11:189–203, 1998

Angelelli P, Paolucci S, Bivona U, et al: Development of neuropsychiatric symptoms in poststroke patients: a cross-sectional study. Acta Psychiatr Scand 110:55–63, 2004

Antoni MH, Wimberly SR, Lechner SC, et al: Reduction of cancer-specific thought intrusions and anxiety symptoms with a stress management intervention among women undergoing treatment for breast cancer. Am J Psychiatry 163:1791–1797, 2006

Arias AJ, Steinberg K, Banga A, et al: Systematic review of the efficacy of meditation techniques as treatments for medical illness. J Altern Complement Med 12:817–832, 2006

Arnold LM, McElroy SL, Mutasim DF, et al: Characteristics of 34 adults with psychogenic excoriation. J Clin Psychiatry 59:509–514, 1998

Aström M: Generalized anxiety disorder in stroke patients: a 3-year longitudinal study. Stroke 27:270–275, 1996

Barker-Collo SL: Depression and anxiety 3 months post stroke: prevalence and correlates. Arch Clin Neuropsychol 22:519–531, 2007

Barnes PJ: Airway pharmacology, in Textbook of Respiratory Medicine, 4th Edition. Edited by Mason RJ, Murray JF, Broaddus VC, et al. Philadelphia, PA, WB Saunders, 2005, pp 235–248

Barsky AJ: Palpitations, arrhythmias, and awareness of cardiac activity. Ann Intern Med 134:832–837, 2001

Barsky AJ, Cleary PD, Coeytaux RR, et al: Psychiatric disorders in medical outpatients complaining of palpitations. J Gen Intern Med 9:306–313, 1994

Bennett P, Conway M, Clatworthy J, et al: Predicting posttraumatic symptoms in cardiac patients. Heart Lung 30:458–465, 2001

Bezchlibnyk-Butler KZ, Jeffries JJ: Benzodiazepines, in Clinical Handbook of Psychotropic Drugs, 16th Edition. Seattle, WA, Hogrefe & Huber, 2006, pp 134–147

Bienvenu OJ, Eaton WW: The epidemiology of blood-injection-injury phobia. Psychol Med 28:1129–1136, 1998

Bjelland I, Dahl AA, Haug TT, et al: The validity of the Hospital Anxiety and Depression Scale: an updated literature review. J Psychosom Res 52:69–77, 2002

Boscarino JA: Posttraumatic stress disorder and mortality among U.S. Army veterans 30 years after military service. Ann Epidemiol 16:248–256, 2006

Breitbart W, Marotta R, Platt M, et al: A double-blind trial of haloperidol, chlorpromazine, and lorazepam in the treatment of delirium in hospitalized AIDS patients. Am J Psychiatry 153:231–237, 1996

Bringager CB, Friis S, Arnesen H, et al: Nine-year follow-up of panic disorder in chest pain patients: clinical course and predictors of outcome. Gen Hosp Psychiatry 30:138–146, 2008

Bruggimann L, Annoni JM, Staub F, et al: Chronic posttraumatic stress symptoms after nonsevere stroke. Neurology 66:513–516, 2006

Byock I: Dying Well: The Prospect for Growth at the End of Life. New York, Riverhead Books, 1997

Calikusu C, Yücel B, Polat A, et al: The relation of psychogenic excoriation with psychiatric disorders: a comparative study. Compr Psychiatry 44:256–261, 2003

Cankurtaran ES, Ozalp E, Soygur H, et al: Mirtazapine improves sleep and lowers anxiety and depression in cancer patients: superiority over imipramine. Support Care Cancer 16:1291–1298, 2008

Carr RE: Panic disorder and asthma: causes, effects and research implications. J Psychosom Res 44:43–52, 1998

Castillo CS, Starkstein SE, Fedoroff JP, et al: Generalized anxiety disorder after stroke. J Nerv Ment Dis 181:100–106, 1993

Childs E, Hohoff C, Deckert J, et al: Association between ADORA2A and DRD2 polymorphisms and caffeine-induced anxiety. Neuropsychopharmacology 33:2791–2800, 2008

Colon EA, Popkin MK: Anxiety and panic, in The American Psychiatric Publishing Textbook of Consultation-Liaison Psychiatry, 2nd Edition. Edited by Wise MG, Rundell JR. Washington, DC, American Psychiatric Publishing, 2002, pp 393–415

Crone CC, Gabriel GM, DiMartini A: An overview of psychiatric issues in liver disease for the consultation-liaison psychiatrist. Psychosomatics 47:188–205, 2006

Davydow DS, Gifford JM, Desai SV, et al: Posttraumatic stress disorder in general intensive care unit survivors: a systematic review. Gen Hosp Psychiatry 30:421–434, 2008

Dell'Agnello G, Ceravolo R, Nuti A, et al: SSRIs do not worsen Parkinson's disease: evidence from an open-label, prospective study. Clin Neuropharmacol 24:221–227, 2001

Deshmukh VM, Toelle BG, Usherwood T, et al: The association of comorbid anxiety and depression with asthma-related quality of life and symptom perception in adults. Respirology 13:695–702, 2008

De Wit L, Putman K, Baert I, et al: Anxiety and depression in the first six months after stroke: a longitudinal multicentre study. Disabil Rehabil 30:1858–1866, 2008

Difede J, Ptacek JT, Roberts J, et al: Acute stress disorder after burn injury: a predictor of posttraumatic stress disorder? Psychosom Med 64:826–834, 2002

DiMatteo MR, Lepper HS, Croghan TW: Depression is a risk factor for noncompliance with medical treatment: meta-analysis of the effects of anxiety and depression on patient adherence. Arch Intern Med 160:2101–2107, 2000

Drugs that may cause psychiatric symptoms. Med Lett Drugs Ther 50:100–103, 2008

Ehlers A, Mayou RA, Sprigings DC, et al: Psychological and perceptual factors associated with arrhythmias and benign palpitations. Psychosom Med 62:693–702, 2000

Eisenhofer G, Sharabi Y, Pacak K: Unexplained symptomatic paroxysmal hypertension in pseudopheochromocytoma: a stress response disorder? Ann N Y Acad Sci 1148:469–478, 2008

Filho AS, Maciel BC, Martin-Santos R, et al: Does the association between mitral valve prolapse and panic disorder really exist? Prim Care Companion J Clin Psychiatry 10:38–47, 2008

Fleet RP, Dupuis G, Marchand A, et al: Panic disorder in emergency department chest pain patients: prevalence, comorbidity, suicidal ideation, and physician recognition. Am J Med 101:371–380, 1996

Fleet RP, Dupuis G, Marchand A, et al: Panic disorder in coronary artery disease patients with noncardiac chest pain. J Psychosom Res 44:81–90, 1998

Frankl V: Man's Search for Meaning. London, Hoddard-Stoughton, 1987

Gander ML, von Känel R: Myocardial infarction and post-traumatic stress disorder: frequency, outcome, and atherosclerotic mechanisms. Eur J Cardiovasc Prev Rehabil 13:165–172, 2006

Gao K, Muzina D, Gajwani P, et al: Efficacy of typical and atypical antipsychotics for primary and comorbid anxiety symptoms or disorders: a review. J Clin Psychiatry 67:1327–1340, 2006

Generalized anxiety disorder: toxic worry. Harv Ment Health Lett 19:1–5, 2003

Goldberg R, Posner D: Anxiety in the medically ill, in Psychiatric Care of the Medical Patient, 2nd Edition. Edited by Stoudemire A, Fogel BS, Greenberg DB. New York, Oxford University Press, 2000, pp 165–180

Goodwin RD, Pine DS: Respiratory disease and panic attacks among adults in the United States. Chest 122:645–650, 2002

Goodwin RD, Jacobi F, Thefeld W: Mental disorders and asthma in the community. Arch Gen Psychiatry 60:1125–1130, 2003

Green BL, Epstein SA, Krupnick JL, et al: Trauma and medical illness: assessing trauma-related disorders in medical settings, in Assessing Psychological Trauma and PTSD. Edited by Wilson JP, Keane TM. New York, Guilford, 1997, pp 160–191

Green BL, Rowland JH, Krupnick JL, et al: Prevalence of posttraumatic stress disorder in women with breast cancer. Psychosomatics 39:102–111, 1998

Green BL, Krupnick JL, Rowland JH, et al: Trauma history as a predictor of psychologic symptoms in women with breast cancer. J Clin Oncol 18:1084–1093, 2000

Gulseren S, Gulseren L, Hekimsoy Z, et al: Depression, anxiety, health-related quality of life, and disability in patients with overt and subclinical thyroid dysfunction. Arch Med Res 37:133–139, 2006

Hall RC, Hall RC: Anxiety and endocrine disease. Semin Clin Neuropsychiatry 4:72–83, 1999

Hamner M, Hunt N, Gee J, et al: PTSD and automatic implantable cardioverter defibrillators. Psychosomatics 40:82–85, 1999

Harman JS, Rollman BL, Hanusa BH, et al: Physician office visits of adults for anxiety disorders in the United States, 1985–1998. J Gen Intern Med 17:165–172, 2002

Hasler G, Gergen PJ, Kleinbaum DG, et al: Asthma and panic in young adults: a 20-year prospective community study. Am J Respir Crit Care Med 171:1224–1230, 2005

Hazlett-Stevens H, Craske MG, Roy-Byrne PP, et al: Predictors of willingness to consider medication and psychosocial treatment for panic disorder in primary care patients. Gen Hosp Psychiatry 24:316–321, 2002

Hedenmalm K, Guzey C, Dahl ML, et al: Risk factors for extrapyramidal symptoms during treatment with selective serotonin reuptake inhibitors, including cytochrome P-450 enzyme, and serotonin and dopamine transporter and receptor polymorphisms. J Clin Psychopharmacol 26:192–197, 2006

Herrmann C, Brand-Driehorst S, Buss U, et al: Effects of anxiety and depression on 5-year mortality in 5,057 patients referred for exercise testing. J Psychosom Res 48:455–462, 2000

House A, Stark D: Anxiety in medical patients. BMJ 325:207–209, 2002

Huffman JC, Pollack MH: Predicting panic disorder among patients with chest pain: an analysis of the literature. Psychosomatics 44:222–236, 2003

Iacovides A, Fountoulakis K, Grammaticos P, et al: Difference in symptom profile between generalized anxiety disorder and anxiety secondary to hyperthyroidism. Int J Psychiatry Med 30:71–81, 2000

Jacobsen PB, Sadler IJ, Booth-Jones M, et al: Predictors of posttraumatic stress disorder symptomatology following bone marrow transplantation for cancer. J Consult Clin Psychol 70:235–240, 2002

Jonas BS, Franks P, Ingram DD: Are symptoms of anxiety and depression risk factors for hypertension? Longitudinal evidence from the National Health and Nutrition Examination Survey I Epidemiologic Follow-Up Study. Arch Fam Med 6:43–49, 1997

Jones C, Griffiths RD, Humphris G, et al: Memory, delusions, and the development of acute posttraumatic stress disorder-related symptoms after intensive care. Crit Care Med 29:573–580, 2001

Jones GN, Ames SC, Jeffries SK, et al: Utilization of medical services and quality of life among low-income patients with generalized anxiety disorder attending primary care clinics. Int J Psychiatry Med 31:183–198, 2001

Kahana RJ, Bibring GL: Personality types in medical management, in Psychiatry and Medical Practice in a General Hospital. Edited by Zinberg N. New York, International Universities Press, 1964, pp 108–123

Kang HK, Bullman TA, Taylor JW: Risk of selected cardiovascular diseases and posttraumatic stress disorder among former World War II prisoners of war. Ann Epidemiol 16:381–386, 2006

Kangas M, Henry JL, Bryant RA: Posttraumatic stress disorder following cancer: a conceptual and empirical review. Clin Psychol Rev 22:499–524, 2002

Kaplan N: Systemic hypertension: therapy, in Braunwald's Heart Disease: A Textbook of Cardiovascular Medicine, 8th Edition. Edited by Libby P, Bonow RO, Mann DL, et al. Philadelphia, PA, WB Saunders, 2007, pp 1049–1068

Katon WJ, Roy-Byrne P, Russo J, et al: Cost-effectiveness and cost offset of a collaborative care intervention for primary care patients with panic disorder. Arch Gen Psychiatry 59:1098–1104, 2002

Katzman MA: Current considerations in the treatment of generalized anxiety disorder. CNS Drugs 23:103–120, 2009

Kawachi I, Colditz GA, Ascherio A, et al: Prospective study of phobic anxiety and risk of coronary heart disease in men. Circulation 89:1992–1997, 1994

Kessler RC, Ormel J, Demler O, et al: Comorbid mental disorders account for the role impairment of commonly occurring physical disorders: results from the National Comorbidity Survey. J Occup Environ Med 45:1257–1266, 2003

Kessler RC, Chiu WT, Demler O, et al: Prevalence, severity, and comorbidity of 12-month DSM-IV disorders in the National Comorbidity Survey Replication. Arch Gen Psychiatry 62:617–627, 2005

Kibler JL, Joshi K, Ma M: Hypertension in relation to posttraumatic stress disorder and depression in the US National Comorbidity Survey. Behav Med 34:125–132, 2009

Kim HF, Yudofsky SC, Hales RE, et al: Neuropsychiatric aspects of seizure disorders, in The American Psychiatric Publishing Textbook of Neuropsychiatry and Behavioral Neurosciences. Edited by Yudofsky SC, Hales RE. Washington, DC, American Psychiatric Publishing, 2007, pp 649–676

Kimura M, Tateno A, Robinson RG: Treatment of poststroke generalized anxiety disorder comorbid with poststroke depression: merged analysis of nortriptyline trials. Am J Geriatr Psychiatry 11:320–327, 2003

Ko DT, Hebert PR, Coffey CS, et al: Beta-blocker therapy and symptoms of depression, fatigue, and sexual dysfunction. JAMA 288:351–357, 2002

Kroenke K, Spitzer RL, Williams JB, et al: Anxiety disorders in primary care: prevalence, impairment, comorbidity, and detection. Ann Intern Med 146:317–325, 2007

Kumano H, Kaiya H, Yoshiuchi K, et al: Comorbidity of irritable bowel syndrome, panic disorder, and agoraphobia in a Japanese representative sample. Am J Gastroenterol 99:370–376, 2004

Ladwig KH, Baumert J, Marten-Mittag B, et al: Posttraumatic stress symptoms and predicted mortality in patients with implantable cardioverter-defibrillators: results from the prospective living with an implanted cardioverter-defibrillator study. Arch Gen Psychiatry 65:1324–1330, 2008

Lane D, Carroll D, Ring C, et al: Mortality and quality of life 12 months after myocardial infarction: effects of depression and anxiety. Psychosom Med 63:221–230, 2001

Lee ST, Park JH, Kim M: Efficacy of the 5-HT1A agonist, buspirone hydrochloride, in migraineurs with anxiety: a randomized, prospective, parallel group, double-blind, placebo-controlled study. Headache 45:1004–1011, 2005

Llorca PM, Spadone C, Sol O, et al: Efficacy and safety of hydroxyzine in the treatment of generalized anxiety disorder: a 3-month double-blind study. J Clin Psychiatry 63:1020–1027, 2002

Maddock RJ, Carter CS, Tavano-Hall L, et al: Hypocapnia associated with cardiac stress scintigraphy in chest pain patients with panic disorder. Psychosom Med 60:52–55, 1998

Maier W, Gansicke M, Freyberger HJ, et al: Generalized anxiety disorder (ICD-10) in primary care from a cross-cultural perspective: a valid diagnostic entity? Acta Psychiatr Scand 101:29–36, 2000

Martín-Santos R, Díez-Quevedo C, Castellví P, et al: De novo depression and anxiety disorders and influence on adherence during peginterferon-alpha-2a and ribavirin treatment in patients with hepatitis C. Aliment Pharmacol Ther 27:257–265, 2008

Mayou R: Chest pain, palpitations and panic. J Psychosom Res 44:53–70, 1998

McGee M, Pies R: Benzodiazepines in primary practice: risks and benefits. Resid Staff Physician 48:42–49, 2002

McKibben JB, Bresnick MG, Wiechman Askay SA, et al: Acute stress disorder and posttraumatic stress disorder: a prospective study of prevalence, course, and predictors in a sample with major burn injuries. J Burn Care Res 29:22–35, 2008

Merikangas KR, Stevens DE: Comorbidity of migraine and psychiatric disorders. Neurol Clin 15:115–123, 1997

Mula M, Pini S, Cassano GB: The role of anticonvulsant drugs in anxiety disorders: a critical review of the evidence. J Clin Psychopharmacol 27:263–272, 2007

Muskin PR: The medical hospital, in Psychodynamic Concepts in General Psychiatry. Edited by Schwartz HJ. Washington, DC, American Psychiatric Press, 1995, pp 69–88

National Institutes of Health: NIH State-of-the-Science Conference Statement on manifestations and management of chronic insomnia in adults. NIH Consens State Sci Statements 22(2):1–30, 2005

Odlaug BL, Grant JE: Clinical characteristics and medical complications of pathologic skin picking. Gen Hosp Psychiatry 30:61–66, 2008

Payne D, Massie MJ: Anxiety in palliative care, in Handbook of Psychiatry in Palliative Medicine. Edited by Chochinov HM, Breitbart W. New York, Oxford University Press, 2000, pp 63–74

Physicians' Desk Reference, 63rd Edition. Montvale, NJ, Thomson Reuters, 2009

Richard IH: Anxiety disorders in Parkinson's disease. Adv Neurol 96:42–55, 2005

Richard IH, Frank S, McDermott MP, et al: The ups and downs of Parkinson disease: a prospective study of mood and anxiety fluctuations. Cogn Behav Neurol 17:201–207, 2004

Rockhill CM, Russo JE, McCauley E, et al: Agreement between parents and children regarding anxiety and depression diagnoses in children with asthma. J Nerv Ment Dis 195:897–904, 2007

Rosenthal LJ, Kim V, Kim DR: Weaning from prolonged mechanical ventilation using an antipsychotic agent in a patient with acute stress disorder. Crit Care Med 35:2417–2419, 2007

Roth T, Culpepper L: Insomnia management in primary care. Clinical Symposia 58(1):23–25, 2008

Roy-Byrne PP, Stein MB, Russo J, et al: Panic disorder in the primary care setting: comorbidity, disability, service utilization, and treatment. J Clin Psychiatry 60:492–499, 1999

Roy-Byrne P, Stein MB, Russo J, et al: Medical illness and response to treatment in primary care panic disorder. Gen Hosp Psychiatry 27:237–243, 2005

Roy-Byrne PP, Davidson KW, Kessler RC, et al: Anxiety disorders and comorbid medical illness. Gen Hosp Psychiatry 30:208–225, 2008

Sait Gönen M, Kisakol G, Savas Cilli A, et al: Assessment of anxiety in subclinical thyroid disorders. Endocr J 51:311–315, 2004

Sareen J, Jacobi F, Cox BJ, et al: Disability and poor quality of life associated with comorbid anxiety disorders and physical conditions. Arch Intern Med 166:2109–2116, 2006

Seng JS, Clark MK, McCarthy AM, et al: PTSD and physical comorbidity among women receiving Medicaid: results from service-use data. J Trauma Stress 19:45–56, 2006

Sherbourne CD, Wells KB, Meredith LS, et al: Comorbid anxiety disorder and the functioning and well-being of chronically ill patients of general medical providers. Arch Gen Psychiatry 53:889–895, 1996

Sherman AC, Pennington J, Latif U, et al: Patient preferences regarding cancer group psychotherapy interventions. Psychosomatics 48:426–432, 2007

Simon GE, Ludman EJ, Tutty S, et al: Telephone psychotherapy and telephone care management for primary care patients starting antidepressant treatment. JAMA 292:935–942, 2004

Simon NM, Pollack MH, Tuby KS, et al: Dizziness and panic disorder: a review of the association between vestibular dysfunction and anxiety. Ann Clin Psychiatry 10:75–78, 1998

Smith MY, Redd WH, Peyser C, et al: Post-traumatic stress disorder in cancer: a review. Psychooncology 8:521–537, 1999

Smoller JW, Simon NM, Pollack MH, et al: Anxiety in patients with pulmonary disease: comorbidity and treatment. Semin Clin Neuropsychiatry 4:84–97, 1999

Smoller JW, Pollack MH, Wassertheil-Smoller S, et al: Panic attacks and risk of incident cardiovascular events among postmenopausal women in the Women's Health Initiative observational study. Arch Gen Psychiatry 64:1153–1160, 2007

Sola CL, Bostwick JM, Hart DA, et al: Anticipating potential linezolid-SSRI interaction in the general hospital setting: an MAOI in disguise. Mayo Clin Proc 81:330–334, 2006

Spiegel D, Bloom J, Yalom I: Group support for patients with metastatic cancer. Arch Gen Psychiatry 38:527–533, 1981

Spitzer RL, Kroenke K, Williams JB: Validation and utility of a self-report version of PRIME-MD: the PHQ primary care study. Primary Care Evaluation of Mental Disorders. Patient Health Questionnaire. JAMA 282:1737–1744, 1999

Stahl SM: Essential Psychopharmacology. New York, Cambridge University Press, 2004

Stanley MA, Wilson NL, Novy DM, et al: Cognitive behavior therapy for generalized anxiety disorder among older adults in primary care: a randomized clinical trial. JAMA 301:1460–1467, 2009

Stark D, House A: Anxiety in cancer patients. Br J Cancer 83:1261–1267, 2000

Stein DJ, Hugo FJ: Neuropsychiatric aspects of anxiety disorders, in The American Psychiatric Publishing Textbook of Neuropsychiatry and Clinical Neurosciences, 4th Edition. Edited by Yudofsky SC, Hales RE. Washington, DC, American Psychiatric Publishing, 2002, pp 1049–1068

Stein MB, McQuaid JR, Pedrelli P, et al: Posttraumatic stress disorder in the primary care medical setting. Gen Hosp Psychiatry 22:261–269, 2000

Stein MB, Sherbourne CD, Creske MG, et al: Quality care for primary care patients with anxiety disorders. Am J Psychiatry 161:2230–2237, 2004

Strain JJ, Grossman S: Psychological Care of the Medically Ill. New York, Appleton-Century-Crofts, 1975

Sugaya N, Kaiya H, Kumano H, et al: Relationship between subtypes of irritable bowel syndrome and severity of symptoms associated with panic disorder. Scand J Gastroenterol 43:675–681, 2008

Tapson VF: Pulmonary embolism, in Cecil Textbook of Medicine, 23rd Edition. Edited by Goldman L, Ausiello D. Philadelphia, PA, WB Saunders, 2007, pp 688–695

Tedstone JE, Tarrier N: Posttraumatic stress disorder following medical illness and treatment. Clin Psychol Rev 23:409–448, 2003

Thompson GN, Chochinov HM: Dignity-based approaches in the care of terminally ill patients. Curr Opin Support Palliat Care 2:49–53, 2008

Thompson SA, Duncan JS, Smith SJ: Partial seizures presenting as panic attacks. BMJ 321:1002–1003, 2000

Torelli P, D'Amico D: An updated review of migraine and co-morbid psychiatric disorders. Neurol Sci 25 (suppl 3):S234–S235, 2004

Trevor AJ, Way WL: Sedative-hypnotic drugs, in Basic and Clinical Pharmacology, 10th Edition. Edited by Katzung BG. New York, McGraw-Hill, 2007, pp 347–362

Veer-Tazelaar PJ, Van Marwijk HWJ, van Oppen P, et al: Stepped-care prevention of anxiety and depression in later life. Arch Gen Psychiatry 66:297–302, 2009

Viederman M: The supportive relationship, the psychodynamic narrative, and the dying patient, in Handbook of Psychiatry in Palliative Medicine. Edited by Chochinov HM, Breitbart W. New York, Oxford University Press, 2000, pp 215–222

Wallis JM: Support Groups for People With HIV. Focus, A Guide to AIDS Research and Counseling, March 2004

Walsh K, Bennett G: Parkinson's disease and anxiety. Postgrad Med J 77:89–93, 2001

Weilburg JB, Schacter S, Worth J, et al: EEG abnormalities in patients with atypical panic attacks. J Clin Psychiatry 56:358–362, 1995

Wiltink J, Tschan R, Michal M, et al: Dizziness: anxiety, health care utilization and health behavior—results from a representative German community survey. J Psychosom Res 66:417–424, 2009

Wise MG, Rundell JR: Anxiety and neurological disorders. Semin Clin Neuropsychiatry 4:98–102, 1999

Witt K, Daniels C, Reiff J, et al: Neuropsychological and psychiatric changes after deep brain stimulation for Parkinson's disease: a randomised, multicentre study. Lancet Neurol 7:605–614, 2008

Yalom I: Death and Dying. New York, Basic Books, 1980

Yardley L, Owen N, Nazareth I, et al: Panic disorder with agoraphobia associated with dizziness: characteristic symptoms and psychosocial sequelae. J Nerv Ment Dis 189:321–327, 2001

Young AS, Klap R, Sherbourne CD, et al: The quality of care for depressive and anxiety disorders in the United States. Arch Gen Psychiatry 58:55–61, 2001

Yu B-H, Dimsdale JE: Posttraumatic stress disorder in patients with burn injuries. J Burn Care Rehabil 20:426–433, 1999

Zatzick DF, Kang SM, Muller HG, et al: Predicting posttraumatic distress in hospitalized trauma survivors with acute injuries. Am J Psychiatry 159:941–946, 2002

Zaubler TS, Katon W: Panic disorder in the general medical setting. J Psychosom Res 44:25–42, 1998

CHAPTER

12

Somatization and Somatoform Disorders

Susan E. Abbey, M.D., F.R.C.P.C.
Lawson Wulsin, M.D.
James L. Levenson, M.D.

SOMATIZATION IS A POORLY understood "blind spot" of medicine (Quill 1985). Somatoform disorders remain neglected by psychiatrists and primary care clinicians despite their associated significant functional impairments and economic burden (Bass et al. 2001). Important conceptual and clinical questions exist about the validity and utility of the concepts, particularly in primary care settings, where they appear most commonly, and new paradigms might lead to more effective management (Epstein et al. 1999; Mayou et al. 2003; Sharpe and Carson 2001). Recent proposals for major revisions in the definitions of somatoform disorders are likely to guide these new paradigms (Dimsdale and Creed 2009; Fink et al. 2005; Kroenke et al. 2007; Oken 2007).

Somatization and somatoform disorders challenge consulting psychiatrists, who often wade into emotionally charged clinical situations in which diagnosis is difficult, both the referring physician and the patient are frustrated and angry, and the involvement of a psychiatrist may be stigmatizing. The complex set of emotions that patients with somatoform disorders engender has resulted in the application of disparaging names both to these patients (e.g., "crocks") (Lipsitt 1970) and to the discipline (e.g., "psychoceramic medicine"). The DSM diagnostic terms themselves may offend patients and are often not used (Stone et al. 2002b). The evidence base for diagnosing and treating these patients remains suboptimal, but there is a strong clinical literature that can help psychiatrists to work effectively with these patients, produce substantial improvements in the patients' and their families' well-being, and decrease direct and indirect costs of their illness. The medical training of psychosomatic medicine psychiatrists facilitates management of difficult cases, such as patients who somatize or have a somatoform disorder and have a concurrent general medical condition with overlapping symptoms.

We begin this chapter with a discussion of the process of somatization, followed by a review of the DSM-IV-TR (American Psychiatric Association 2000) somatoform disorders. The sections for each disorder include diagnostic dilemmas to be addressed in DSM-V and key treatment approaches for that disorder. The chapter concludes with principles of management and treatment. Our focus in this chapter is on adults; somatization and somatoform disorders in children are discussed in Chapter 34, "Pediatrics," and in several reviews (Garralda 1999; Silber and Pao 2003). Conversion disorder is also discussed in Chapter 32, "Neurology and Neurosurgery."

Somatization as a Process

Somatization can be conceptualized in a variety of different ways, but fundamentally it appears to be a way of responding to stress. It is a ubiquitous human phenomenon that at times becomes problematic and warrants clinical attention. Somatization is extremely common in medical settings and among the patients referred to psychosomatic medicine psychiatrists. Not all somatizing patients have a somatoform disorder. Many have another Axis I disorder or transiently somatize in the context of significant life stress.

Definitions and Clinically Useful Theoretical Concepts

The area of somatization is complicated by a lack of uniformity in the use of terminology. Theoretical concepts that are clinically useful in management are described below.

Somatization as a Dimension of Distress

Historically, *somatization* was defined by Steckel as a deep-seated neurosis that produced bodily symptoms (Lipowski 1988). In the past 20 years, the term *somatization* has been used to describe the tendency of certain patients to experience and communicate psychological and interpersonal problems in the form of somatic distress and medically unexplained symptoms for which they seek medical help (Katon et al. 1984; Kleinman 1986; Lipowski 1988). Although it has become a widely used term, Sharpe (2002) cautioned that its use should be restricted to cases in which the somatic symptoms are an expression of an identifiable emotional disorder. In essence, somatization is a culturally sanctioned idiom of psychosocial distress (Katon et al. 1984; Kleinman 1986). Kirmayer and Young (1998) noted that depending on circumstances, somatization "can be seen as an index of disease or disorder, an indication of psychopathology, a symbolic condensation of intrapsychic conflict, a culturally coded expression of distress, a medium for expressing social discontent, and a mechanism through which patients attempt to reposition themselves within their local worlds" (p. 420).

Because severity of somatic symptoms, when related to either psychiatric or medical illness, is associated with increasing functional impairment, disability days, and use of health care services (Kroenke et al. 2002), some experts have proposed considering somatization as a dimension in all illnesses and measuring somatic symptom number and severity, regardless of whether the symptom can be medically explained.

Three components of somatization described by Lipowski (1988) can offer targets for intervention: experiential, cognitive, and behavioral (Table 12–1).

Medically Unexplained Symptoms

Somatization is frequently implicated in medically unexplained symptoms (MUS), defined as symptoms that are not attributable to or are out of proportion to identifiable physical disease (Sharpe 2002). Medically unexplained symptoms are discussed in other chapters in this volume, including noncardiac chest pain (see Chapter 18, "Heart Disease"), hyperventilation syndrome (see Chapter 19, "Lung Disease"), irritable bowel and functional upper gastrointestinal tract disorders (see Chapter 20, "Gastrointestinal Disorders"), chronic fatigue syndrome and fibromyalgia (see Chapter 26, "Chronic Fatigue and Fibromyalgia Syndromes"), idiopathic pruritus (see Chapter 29, "Dermatology"), chronic pelvic pain and vulvodynia (see Chapter 33, "Obstetrics and Gynecology"), pain syndromes (see Chapter 36, "Pain"), and multiple chemical sensitivity (see Chapter 37, "Medical Toxicology").

Clinicians and cultures vary widely in how they explain symptoms (i.e., causes) and what they consider a sufficient medical explanation for a symptom. Recent proposals to discard "medically unexplained symptoms" as a diagnostic criterion note the following disadvantages: 1) it is not clear what counts as a medical explanation, 2) it is a negative explanation that can feel dismissive to patients, 3) MUS foster mind–body dualism, 4) the concept is difficult to operationalize into reliable measures, and 5) the evidence for causality is often sketchy (Dimsdale and Creed 2009).

Somatosensory Amplification

Symptoms are the result of bodily sensations and their subsequent cortical interpretation. *Somatosensory amplification* refers to the tendency to experience somatic sensations as intense, noxious, or disturbing (Barsky et al. 1988b). It is composed of three elements: 1) hypervigilance to bodily sensations, 2) predisposition to select out and concentrate on weak or infrequent bodily sensations, and 3) reaction to sensations with cognitions and affect that intensify them and make them more alarming (Duddu et al. 2006; Nakao and Barsky 2007). It has both trait and state components.

Illness Versus Disease

The distinction between illness and disease (Eisenberg 1977) is useful for psychosomatic medicine psychiatrists. *Illness* is the response of the individual and his or her family to symptoms; this contrasts with *disease,* which is defined by physicians and is associated with pathophysiological processes and documentable lesions. Mismatches between illness and disease are common and are at the root of many management problems. Hypertensive patients may not perceive themselves as ill and therefore might not comply with treatment regimens. Patients with somatoform disorders view themselves as very ill despite not having a disease. In somatizing patients with some disease component, their subjective illness experience is assessed to be disproportionate to the degree of disease.

Illness Behavior and Abnormal Illness Behavior

Illness behavior refers to "the manner in which individuals monitor their bodies, define and interpret their symptoms,

TABLE 12–1. Clinical implications of the components of somatization

Component	Potential intervention
Experiential	Techniques to decrease somatic sensations (e.g., biofeedback, pharmacotherapy for concomitant psychiatric disorder)
Cognitive	Reattribution of sensation from sinister to benign cause Distraction techniques
Behavioral	Operant techniques to reduce medication consumption Contract to "save" symptoms for regular visit with primary care physician rather than visiting emergency room

take remedial action, and utilize sources of help as well as the more formal health care system. It also is concerned with how people monitor and respond to symptoms and symptom change over the course of an illness and how this affects behavior, remedial actions taken, and response to treatment" (Mechanic 1986, p. 1). Illness behavior may be regarded as a syndrome, as a symptom, as a dimension, or as an explanation of behavior (Mayou 1989). Illness behavior is affected by a wide variety of social, psychiatric, and cultural factors and can be used "to achieve a variety of social and personal objectives having little to do with biological systems of the pathogenesis of disease" (Mechanic 1986, p. 3).

Abnormal illness behavior is identified by a physician when there is an "inappropriate or maladaptive mode of perceiving, evaluating or acting in relation to one's own health status, which persists despite the fact that a doctor (or other appropriate social agent) has offered an accurate and reasonably lucid explanation of the nature of the illness and the appropriate course of management to be followed, based on a thorough examination of all parameters of functioning, and taking into account the individual's age, educational and sociocultural background" (Pilowsky 1987, p. 89). The behavior may be somatically or psychologically focused and may be either illness affirming or illness denying. The construct has been criticized as dangerous in that it places physicians in the position of defining what is normal and what is abnormal. It has been counterargued that a corresponding physician behavioral pattern of "abnormal treatment behavior" might also be proposed.

Somatization as a Clinical Problem

Somatization becomes clinically significant when it is associated with significant occupational and social dysfunction or with excessive health care use. The relation between acute and persistent forms of somatization is unclear; they may form a continuum or may be discrete conditions. Although individual somatic symptoms are notoriously unstable, clusters of somatic symptoms tend to persist. A literature review concluded that patients with at least three bothersome somatic symptoms typically continue to have multiple somatoform symptoms at 1 year (86%) and at 5 years (67%) (Rief and Rojas 2007). Somatization and somatoform disorders pose a significant economic burden (Bass et al. 2001). In addition to the higher-than-average inpatient, ambulatory, and physician service costs of care of such patients, there are social costs, including decreased occupational productivity. Many patients with somatization also have severe distress, particularly depression and anxiety. In addition, somatizing patients are at increased risk of iatrogenic disease and injury. For example, in pseudoseizures, the most frequent cause of morbidity and death is the misdiagnosis of epilepsy and resulting aggressive treatment with anticonvulsants (Kanner 2003).

Relation Among Psychiatric Disorders, Somatization, and Medically Unexplained Symptoms

Strong interrelations exist among somatization, psychiatric disorders, and health care utilization. Four models (Figure 12–1) have been advanced to explain these interrelationships (Simon 1991). Different models may apply to different patients.

Somatization as Cause and Consequence of Psychiatric Illness

Physical symptoms are an integral part of most psychiatric disorders, at times triggering their onset, at others complicating their course (Lieb et al. 2007). Somatizing patients may focus on their physical symptoms to the exclusion of psychological symptoms. They may then attribute the psychological symptoms to the distress resulting from the physical symptoms (e.g., "Yes, doctor, I am sad, but you would be too if you couldn't sleep or eat and had no energy!"). This "masking" of the psychiatric syndrome is important, because major depressive disorder and anxiety disorders are significantly underrecognized in patients presenting with somatic complaints (Kirmayer et al. 1993). Somatization does not appear to be a defense against acknowledging the presence of a psychiatric disorder (Hotopf et al. 2001). On the contrary, more than half of primary care patients with significant somatization ac-

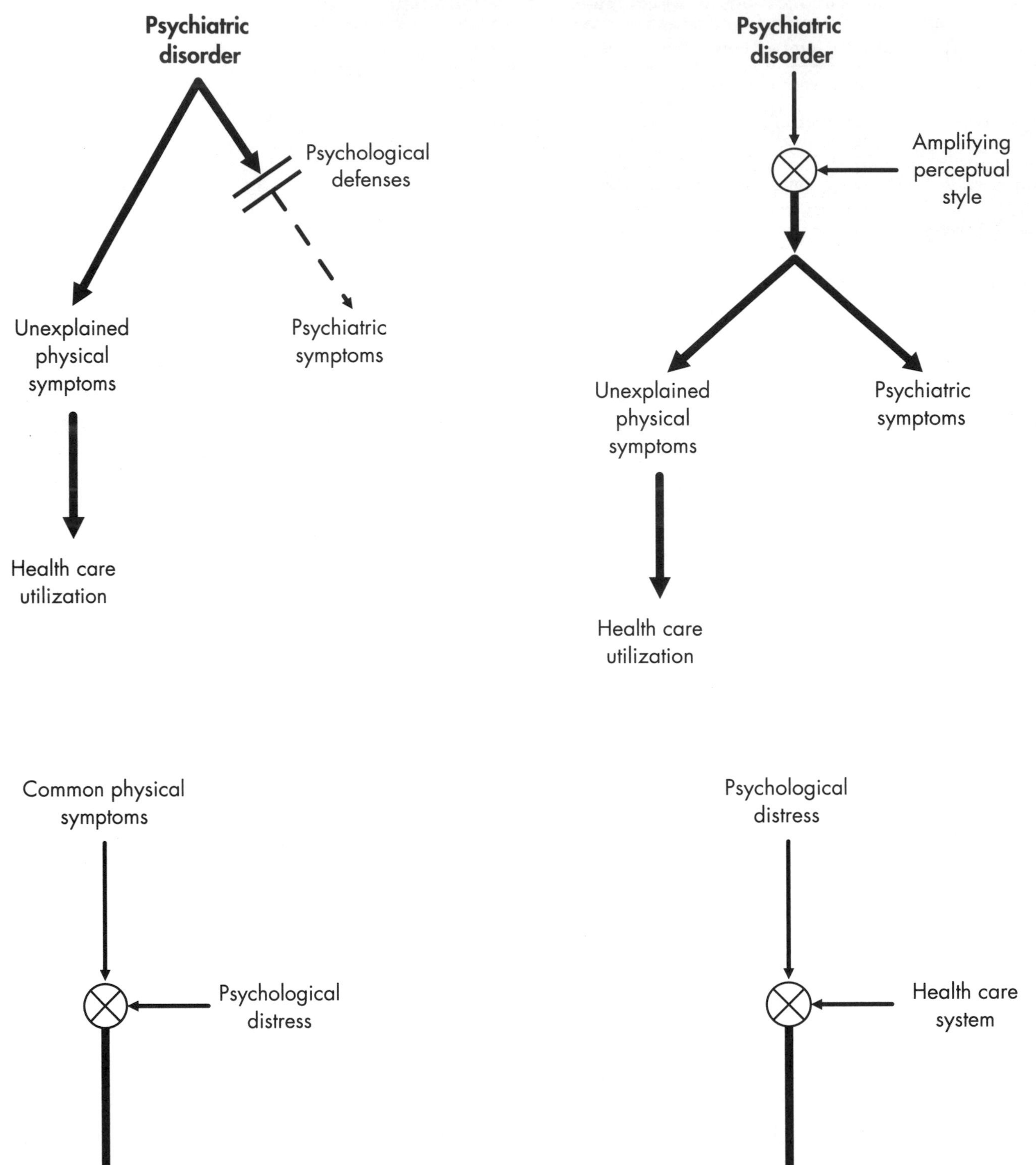

FIGURE 12–1. Four models of the relation between psychiatric symptomatology and psychiatric disorder.

Source. Reprinted from Simon GE: "Somatization and Psychiatric Disorder," in *Current Concepts of Somatization: Research and Clinical Perspectives.* Edited by Kirmayer LJ, Robbins JM. Washington, DC, American Psychiatric Press, 1991, pp. 37–62. Used with permission.

knowledge significant anxiety and/or depression (Lowe et al. 2008). Although depression and anxiety frequently overlap with somatization, they also occur independently (see Figure 12–2). Furthermore, depression and anxiety often amplify the perception and the distress of somatic symptoms in the presence of common chronic illnesses like diabetes, arthritis, and pulmonary disease (Katon et al. 2007). Ironically, the physical symptom burden in depression and anxiety, as measured by the number and severity of physical symptoms, may exceed that in many common chronic illnesses that are relatively asymptomatic or limited to a single bothersome symptom (e.g., hypertension, diabetes, coronary artery disease, arthritis, asthma).

Depression and somatization. Physical symptoms are common in major depressive disorder (Simon et al. 1999; see also Chapter 8, "Depression"). The mechanism by which they are produced is unclear and may be related to 1) psychophysiological concomitants of depression, 2) somatosensory amplification, and 3) a depressive attributional style in which symptoms are perceived as indicating poor health. Primary care patients with depression have higher health care utilization and report more somatic symptoms than do patients without depression (Kroenke 2003). It is estimated that 50% or more of the patients presenting in primary care with major depressive disorder do so with predominantly somatic complaints rather than with cognitive or affective symptoms of depression (Lowe et al. 2008; Simon and Gureje 1999). These somatic presentations of depression have been referred to as *masked depression* or *depressive equivalents.* Somatic symptoms in depression are related to concomitant anxiety, the tendency to amplify somatic distress, and difficulty identifying and communicating emotional distress (Sayar et al. 2003). Comorbidity among depression, somatization, and somatoform disorders is high (G.R. Smith 1992). Consequently, it has been argued that medically unexplained symptoms are a manifestation of an affective-spectrum disorder (Hudson et al. 2003).

Anxiety and somatization. Anxiety disorders (especially panic disorder) are also accompanied by prominent physical symptoms and are frequently mistaken for or associated with somatization in patients presenting in primary care and medical subspecialty settings (Lowe et al. 2008; Sullivan et al. 1993; see also Chapter 11, "Anxiety Disorders"). Somatization and hypochondriacal fears and beliefs are common among patients with panic disorder, particularly those who also have agoraphobia and focus more on seeking an explanation for, than on treatment of, their symptoms (Starcevic et al. 1992). In addition, posttraumatic stress disorder (PTSD) often presents with somatic complaints (Andreski et al. 1998; Moreau and Zisook 2002).

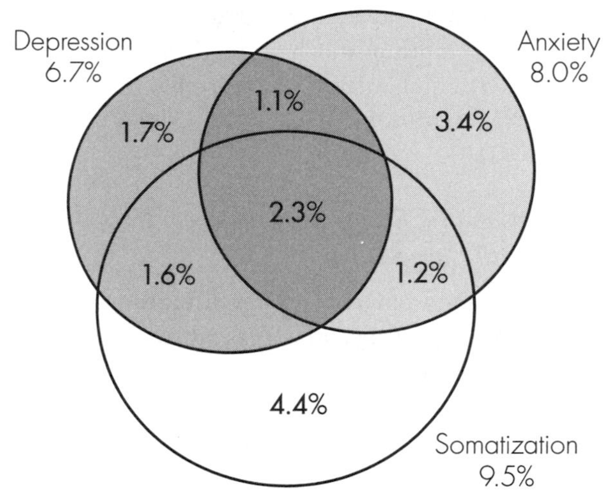

FIGURE 12–2. Overlap of severe depression, severe anxiety, and severe somatization as percentage of total sample (*N* = 2,091).

Source. Reprinted from Lowe B, Spitzer RL, Williams JB, et al.: "Depression, Anxiety and Somatization in Primary Care: Syndrome Overlap and Functional Impairment. *General Hospital Psychiatry* 30(3):191–199, 2008. Copyright 2008, Elsevier/North-Holland. Used with permission.

Other Axis I diagnoses. Substance abuse is associated with somatization (Mehrabian 2001) and is reported in subsets of patients with substance abuse. Finally, somatization is also prevalent in patients with schizophrenia and is associated with emotional distress, medication side effects, and expressed emotion within families. One study found that more than a quarter of patients with schizophrenia had five or more unexplained medical symptoms, both at admission and 12 months later (Ritsner 2003). Psychotic somatic symptoms (somatic delusions, hallucinations, and misperceptions) are common in schizophrenia and in somatic delusional disorders such as delusions of parasitosis (see Chapter 29, "Dermatology").

Somatization as an Amplifying Personal Perceptual Style

An amplifying personal perceptual style may be a stable personality trait or a consequence of abnormal neuropsychological information processing (Barsky et al. 1988a). Some somatizing patients show a lowered threshold for reporting physical symptoms (Barsky et al. 1988b; Pennebaker and Watson 1991).

Somatization as a Tendency to Seek Care for Common Symptoms

This model posits that emotional distress prompts people to seek care for common symptoms for which they would not seek care in the absence of emotional distress. It is supported by research in patients with a variety of medically unexplained symptoms in whom medical help seeking is associated with higher levels of emotional distress rather than physical symptoms (Drossman 1999; McBeth and Silman 2001).

Somatization as a Response to the Incentives of the Health Care System

The health care system tends to reinforce illness behavior and symptom reporting and may produce "iatrogenic somatization" (Henningsen et al. 2007; Simon 1991).

Etiological Factors in Somatization and Somatoform Disorders

Pathophysiological Mechanisms

Understanding and acknowledging the physiological as well as the psychological mechanisms associated with somatization helps both patient and physician to avoid dualistic "mind versus body" thinking—which often devolves into stigmatized notions of "imaginary" versus "real" symptoms—and to develop a therapeutic alliance (Sharpe and Bass 1992). Some of the proposed pathophysiological mechanisms of somatization are summarized in Table 12–2. Occasionally, what appears to be a pattern of somatization is subsequently found to be a medical syndrome or disorder, such as multiple sclerosis, obstructive sleep apnea, or celiac disease; however, rates of misdiagnosis of patients with somatoform disorders have been in the range of 2%–10%—not high, though not negligible (Rief and Rojas 2007; Stone et al. 2005).

TABLE 12–2. Pathophysiological mechanisms of somatization

Physiological mechanisms
Autonomic arousal
Muscle tension
Hyperventilation
Vascular changes
Cerebral information processing
Physiological effects of inactivity
Sleep disturbance
Brain cytokines
Psychological mechanisms
Perceptual factors
Beliefs
Mood
Personality factors
Interpersonal mechanisms
Reinforcing actions of relatives and friends
Health care system
Disability system

Source. Adapted from Mayou 1993; Sharpe and Bass 1992.

Genetic Factors

Somatization and somatization disorder appear to have a genetic component (Guze 1993; Kendler et al. 1995). Adoption studies of Swedish men suggested that the psychiatric processes associated with somatization in men and women may be qualitatively different (Cloninger et al. 1986). There have been no recent studies of genetic factors in somatization disorder, but recent twin studies illustrate complex relationships between genetic factors and the co-occurrence of functional somatic syndromes, anxiety, and depression (Kato et al. 2006, 2009).

Developmental Factors

The cognitive appraisals patients make of somatic symptoms often have some of their roots in early family experiences. Physical symptoms are a major form of interpersonal communication in some families (Stuart and Noyes 1999). Childhood exposure to parental chronic illness or abnormal illness behavior appears to increase the risk of somatization in later life (Bass and Murphy 1995; Craig et al. 1993; Gilleland et al. 2009). Negative parenting styles are associated with somatization in irritable bowel syndrome patients (Lackner et al. 2004). Children with poor awareness of emotional experiences are more likely to experience impairing, unexplained somatic complaints (Gilleland et al. 2009). Anxious attachment behavior arising from early life experiences may also be the basis for persistent care-seeking behavior that frustrates both health care professionals and family members (Noyes et al. 2003; Stuart and Noyes 1999).

Cognitive Theories

Cognitive distortions and preferential memory bias for disorder-congruent information have been demonstrated in patients with somatoform disorders (Brown et al. 1999; Pauli and Alpers 2002). For a recent review, see Escobar et al. 2007 and Woolfolk et al. 2007.

Personality Characteristics

A variety of psychological traits or personality factors have been linked with somatization, although it is unclear whether they primarily influence symptom production and help-seeking behavior or are a consequence of living with chronic symptoms. Introspectiveness (i.e., the tendency to think about oneself) is associated with increased symptom reporting, greater physical and psychological distress, and more medical help seeking (Mechanic 1986). Negative affectivity, a construct based on negative mood, poor self-concept, and pessimism, is also considered an important contributor to somatization (De Gucht et al. 2004) and was found to be a prospective predictor of somatization among victims of acute trauma (Elklit and Christiansen 2009).

Psychodynamic Factors

Bodily symptoms have been interpreted as metaphors through which a patient expresses emotional distress or psychic conflict (McDougall 1989). Self psychologists argue that bodily preoccupation develops in response to a fragmented sense of self and can be best understood as an attempt to restore a sense of integration (Rodin 1984). *Alexithymia* refers to impairment in the ability to verbalize affect and elaborate fantasies that results from deficits in the cognitive processing and regulation of emotions (Taylor 2000). It has been implicated as a mechanism of some forms of somatization. Although repressed anger or aggression was thought by classical psychodynamic theorists to be important, Kellner et al. (1985) found no evidence that anger or hostility plays a specific etiological role in somatization and hypochondriasis.

Sexual and Physical Abuse

Sexual and physical abuse, in both childhood and adulthood, has been linked with somatization, medically unexplained symptoms, and somatoform disorders in numerous studies since the late 1980s. The development of insight into the relation of the abuse to subsequent somatization is helpful for some patients and may decrease subsequent health care use (Walling et al. 1994). The mechanisms by which physical and sexual trauma is associated with somatization are poorly understood. Sexual abuse negatively affects "embodiment" (i.e., the experience of the self in and through the body) (Young 1992). Abuse also causes a tendency to dissociate, and dissociation is associated with a tendency to report increased physical symptoms (Salmon et al. 2003). Higher hypnotic susceptibility, a marker of the capacity to self-evoke dissociative experiences, has been found to partially mediate the relationship between abuse and conversion symptoms in patients with conversion disorder (Roelofs et al. 2002).

Sociocultural Factors

Somatization was originally thought to be more common among non-Western cultures, but recent work suggests that somatization is ubiquitous, although prevalence and specific features vary across cultures (Kirmayer and Young 1998). The World Health Organization Cross-National Study of Mental Disorders in Primary Care found that all sites (14 countries) reported high rates of somatization (Gureje et al. 1997) and correlation of somatic symptoms and emotional distress (Simon et al. 1996). The stigmatization of psychiatric distress may be a powerful factor promoting somatization. "Organic" or physical illnesses are seen as more real and less blameworthy than psychiatric disorders, which are seen as being under voluntary control and are often associated with connotations of malingering and weak moral fiber (Kirmayer and Robbins 1991). Somatization may be the only form of communication permissible for the socially powerless.

Gender

The relation between gender and somatization is complex and poorly understood. Although it has traditionally been believed that women somatize more than men, the literature is problematic (Barsky et al. 2001b). An international study of somatization in primary care found few sex differences (Piccinelli and Simon 1997). A longitudinal study of primary care attendees found that somatizers were more likely to be men (Kirmayer and Robbins 1996), whereas data from the Epidemiologic Catchment Area study found that women report more unexplained symptoms overall (Liu et al. 1997).

Iatrogenesis

The health care insurance and disability systems may foster somatization by providing reinforcement (Ford 1983; Henningsen et al. 2007; Simon 1991). Insurance policies with better coverage and fewer barriers for nonpsychiatric medical care than mental health care also provide incentives to somatize (Ford 1992). Well-intentioned but uninformed actions by physicians may also contribute, through unnecessary diagnostic testing and treatments (and their adverse effects) and reinforcement of the sick role (Page and Wessely 2003).

Assessment and Diagnosis of Somatization

Assessment for somatization or somatoform disorders is often difficult and requires special interviewing skills (Creed and Guthrie 1993; Sharpe et al. 1992).

Building an Alliance With the Patient

Early in the interview, the patient's ambivalence about seeing a psychiatrist must be addressed, as well as what the patient has been told about the consultation process. The specific approach to the examination will vary according to the patient. For very resistant patients, the initial interview is often dominated by gaining sufficient cooperation to allow a more detailed assessment to take place at a later time. The initial phase of the assessment should focus on the history of physical symptoms. Allowing the patient to report a detailed history of his or her physical symptoms provides reassurance that the symptoms are being taken seriously, which aids immeasurably in later phases of the assessment and treatment process. The psychiatrist's use of empathic comments such as "You have had a terrible time" or "The symptoms sound very difficult" help to build an alliance and may lead the patient to volunteer information (Creed and Guthrie 1993). The question "How has this illness or symptom affected your life?" may go a long way toward answering the question "How has your life affected this illness?" Making interpretive or linking statements that bring together the patient's physical and emotional states may encourage the patient to be more forthcoming with regard to emotional distress and may further the sense of engagement (Creed and Guthrie 1993). However, caution must be exercised because premature or maladroit interpretations can be detrimental to the developing trust between patient and physician. For especially skeptical patients, the psychiatrist can emphasize his or her expertise in helping people develop the skills they need to cope with symptoms, regardless of the "cause."

Collaborating With the Referral Source

Collaboration with the referral source is essential for a clear understanding of the reason for referral and of what the patient has been told about it. Psychiatrists can provide guidance about how to explain the psychiatric referral to the patient to make it more acceptable.

Reviewing the Medical Records

Medical records should be reviewed before the consultation to help the psychiatrist devise an approach to the patient. Familiarity with the history fosters an alliance. The type, number, and frequency of the patient's symptoms, as well as comments about the patient's prior attitude toward symptoms and behavior, should be documented (Creed and Guthrie 1993). The importance of a thorough chart review cannot be overestimated, because the psychosomatic medicine psychiatrist may be the first person to thoroughly review the typically thick chart and thus may be in a better position than any other member of the medical team to reach a diagnosis of either a general medical condition or a psychiatric disorder.

Gathering Collateral Information From Family and Friends

Collateral information can be invaluable to the accurate assessment of current and past functional capacity and current and past psychosocial stressors.

Performing a Psychiatric and Mental Status Examination

In addition to routine psychiatric observations, the examination of the patient with somatic symptoms should include observations about abnormal illness behavior, symptom amplification, and the quality of the patient's description of his or her symptoms. It is essential to evaluate the individual's ideas about the meaning, cause, implications, and significance of his or her symptoms and the individual's emotional response to his or her situation (Barsky 1998; Creed and Guthrie 1993; Sharpe et al. 1992). If it is performed after taking a history of the physical complaints (but not before), a mental status examination is usually acceptable to the patient.

Assessing the severity of somatic distress by self-report measures adds clarity and consistency to the assessment process. The 15-item somatic symptom Patient Health Questionnaire (PHQ-15; Kroenke et al. 2002) is perhaps the most useful measure for screening and monitoring somatic symptom severity. It is brief, easy to complete, easy to score, and available through public access. The PHQ-15 assesses the number and severity of symptoms that account for 90% of physical complaints in the outpatient setting (aside from upper respiratory tract symptoms). Patients who reported that three or more somatic symptoms "bothered [me] a lot" during the previous 4 weeks reported significantly more functional impairment, number of sick days, and health care utilization. In a primary care sample of more than 900 men and women in which a cutoff of three or more severe somatic symptoms during the past 4 weeks was used, the PHQ-15 detected somatoform disorders with a sensitivity of 78% and a specificity of 71% (van Ravesteijn et al. 2009). Although not a diagnostic instrument for somatoform disorders, the PHQ-15 is useful as a measure of somatic symptom severity.

Performing a Physical Examination

A physical examination of the patient is a prerequisite for accurate diagnosis and treatment for several reasons. In some cases, elements of the physical examination should be performed by the psychiatrist (see Chapter 1, "Psychiatric Assessment and Consultation"), who may be in the best position to diagnose a general medical condition because "something about the patient (personality, behavior, affect, odd cognition) has effectively distracted the primary physician and other consultants from the diagnosis" (Cassem and Barsky 1991, p. 132). A case vignette follows.

Case Vignette

Ms. P, a 42-year-old woman who had had a renal transplant 2 months earlier, was referred for psychiatric evaluation of "suspected conversion disorder in a patient with history of obsessive-compulsive disorder" after she developed "constant rocking movement that she can voluntarily stop." The psychiatrist found on examination that the patient had an obvious resting rhythmic truncal tremor. The psychiatrist's examination revealed subtle choreiform movements in the patient's tongue and fingers. Noting that metoclopramide had been started at the time of the transplant, the psychiatrist diagnosed a movement disorder, which resolved after drug discontinuation.

The physician who is managing a persistently somatizing patient must also tolerate the patient's perpetual concern about symptoms with some degree of equanimity. A medical education that repeatedly emphasizes the danger of "missed diagnoses" and the current medicolegal climate mean that the physician must be confident that a thorough medical evaluation has been completed.

The physical examination may also help to establish a positive diagnosis of somatization disorder. For example, awareness of physical signs associated with stress (e.g., tender anterior chest wall, tender abdomen, spurious breathing, short breath-holding time) leads to a more confident diagnosis rather than a diagnosis of exclusion, the latter of which always has an implication of doubt associated with it (Sharpe and Bass 1992). A variety of physical signs may be useful, but some are controversial in making a diagnosis of a somatoform disorder (see Fishbain et al. 2003). A somatoform disorder should be diagnosed (as the sole diagnosis) only if the examination also confirms normal functioning of the system being tested (Newman 1993).

Somatoform Disorders

The DSM-IV-TR somatoform disorders are somatization disorder, undifferentiated somatoform disorder, conversion disorder, pain disorder, hypochondriasis, body dysmorphic disorder, and somatoform disorder not otherwise specified (American Psychiatric Association 2000). The feature they have in common is the presence of unexplained physical symptoms that are not intentionally produced. In DSM-IV-TR, it is emphasized that these disorders are grouped together because of the need to exclude medical and substance-induced etiologies (American Psychiatric Association 2000).

Somatoform disorders are more common in ambulatory than in inpatient settings. They have been diagnosed in 3%–4% of psychiatric consultations in general hospitals in Australia (G.C. Smith et al. 2000) and the Netherlands (Thomassen et al. 2003). In the latter study the somatoform diagnoses were conversion disorder, 40%; hypochondriasis, 24%; somatoform pain disorder, 20%; and somatization disorder, 17%. Studies of the general population have reported more variable rates. One study of German adolescents and young adults found a lifetime rate for somatoform disorders of 3%; a further 11% of subjects had subsyndromal conditions (Lieb et al. 2000).

There are a number of difficulties in the clinical application of the somatoform diagnoses as defined in DSM. First, excluding a medical cause for symptoms is problematic, particularly for those with comorbid medical diseases. The focus on exclusion promotes dualistic thinking, but failure to demonstrate a medical cause for symptoms does not necessarily mean the patient has a psychiatric disorder (Kirmayer and Young 1998). Second, the question of intentionality or consciousness in symptom production is a vexing one. Distinguishing somatoform disorders from the factitious disorders and malingering is discussed in Chapter 13 ("Deception Syndromes: Factitious Disorders and Malingering"), but these disorders can overlap. Third, dimensional rather than categorical approaches may be more helpful in describing hypochondriacal preoccupation, medically unexplained symptoms, and help seeking. Fourth, the clinical descriptions of specific disorders are largely derived from tertiary care or psychiatric hospital samples and emphasize chronicity. Diagnostic dilemmas specific to each disorder are described below.

Finally, the separate existence of a discrete category of somatoform disorders reinforces the mind-body dualism of Western medicine and implies a separation of affective, anxiety, dissociative, and somatic symptoms (Kirmayer and Young 1998). In fact, somatic symptoms and somatization cut across DSM-IV-TR diagnostic categories. Although somatization is commonly observed in primary care settings, somatoform disorder diagnoses are relatively rarely used by either primary care clinicians or mental health specialists. It may be that the DSM-IV-TR somatoform disorders are too numerous and are too narrowly defined, separated by distinctions for which there is only limited evidence. Some recent critics have suggested extensive reformulation, reclassification, and even abolition of the somatoform disorders (Fink et al. 2005; Kroenke et al. 2007; Oken 2007).

Somatization Disorder

Definition

Somatization disorder is based on the earlier diagnosis of Briquet's syndrome, which required 25 of 59 physical symptoms, an illness onset before age 30 years, and a pattern of recurrent physical complaints and was shown to have validity, reliability, and internal consistency (Feighner et al. 1972). The long-term stability of the diagnosis was documented by the finding that 80%–90% of patients continued to meet diagnostic criteria at 6- to 8-year follow-up (Guze et al. 1986). DSM-III (American Psychiatric Association 1980) criteria for somatization disorder were a modification of Feighner's criteria, with a total symptom count of 14 symptoms in women and 12 symptoms in men from a total list of 36 physical symptoms. In DSM-III-R (American Psychiatric Association 1987), the criteria were further modified by simplifying the requirement to 13 of 35 physical symptoms and specifically excluding symptoms occurring only during a panic attack. The diagnostic criteria were again simplified in DSM-IV (American Psychiatric Association 1994), and they have been found to be concordant with prior criteria (Yutzy et al. 1995).

Diagnostic Dilemmas

Critics have argued that complexity of the criteria for somatization disorder (i.e., four sets of symptoms across different body sites/functions: four pain, two gastrointestinal, one sexual, and one pseudoneurological) defy memory or reliable application in all but the most rigorous research settings (Creed 2006; Kroenke et al. 2007). Can a simpler definition be devised that captures the more common patterns of somatization and its distress and impaired functioning and thus proves more useful to clinicians? Several less restrictive alternatives have been proposed and are described under "Undifferentiated Somatoform Disorder" later in this chapter.

Epidemiology

The lifetime prevalence of somatization disorder has varied widely across studies, ranging from 0.2% to 2.0% among women and less than 0.2% in men (American Psychiatric Association 2000), reflecting variations in research methodology and study samples. Because patients with somatization disorder actively seek medical help, their prevalence in medical settings is higher than in the general population. Somatization disorder has been diagnosed in 1%–5% of primary care patients (Simon and Gureje 1999). Changes in practice patterns have likely led to fewer somatization disorder patients being admitted to hospitals. Patients with somatization disorder accounted for 0.7% of Dutch psychiatric consultations (Thomassen et al. 2003) and 0.2% of Australian consultations to medical and surgical inpatients (G.C. Smith et al. 2000). Recent work has emphasized the instability of recall of somatic symptoms, with implications for underdiagnosing somatization disorder (Simon and Gureje 1999). By definition, the syndrome must begin before age 30, but most often symptoms begin in the teens, often with menarche, or less commonly in the early 20s. The risk for depression, alcohol abuse, and antisocial personality disorder is increased in the first-degree relatives of individuals with somatization disorder (Golding et al. 1992).

Specific Culture and Gender Factors

There is cultural variability in the presentation of somatization disorder. Symptoms used in DSM-IV-TR are those that have been found to be most diagnostic in the United States (American Psychiatric Association 2000). The disorder is uncommon in American men (Golding et al. 1991), although in an American sample women and men with somatization disorder had similar clinical characteristics, including comorbid psychopathology (Golding et al. 1991). Women with somatization disorder are more likely to have a history of sexual abuse than are women with primary mood disorders (Morrison 1989).

Case Vignette

Ms. L is a 28-year-old woman referred for psychiatric assessment based on 25 primary care visits, 18 emergency room visits, and 2 hospitalizations in the past 12 months for a variety of symptoms, including unexplained headaches, pelvic pain, dysmenorrhea, back pain, nausea, dysphagia, and irregular menses. She has been "sickly" since childhood; is unemployed as a result of her multiple medical problems; and is socially isolated, having had difficulties in interpersonal relationships for many years.

Clinical Features

The classic patient with somatization disorder is a woman who subjectively is "sickly" and who began to experience medically unexplained symptoms in early adolescence. Her condition has shown a waxing and waning course over the years, with a medical history that documents repeated, unexplained physical complaints. Patients with somatization disorder are often difficult historians who provide dramatic and colorful but vague descriptions of their medical history (Cassem and Barsky 1991) and may present as odd or anxious (Rost et al. 1992). There is often more to be learned in a review of their medical records.

Associated features. Patients with somatization disorder have high rates of psychiatric comorbidity. As many as 75% of patients with somatization disorder have comorbid Axis I diagnoses (Katon et al. 1991), of which the most common are major depressive disorder, dysthymia, panic disorder, simple phobia, and substance abuse. Because patients with somatization disorder have a low threshold for endorsing symptoms, in some cases comorbid diagnoses may reflect an amplifying response tendency rather than significant symptomatology. However, many patients do have bona fide comorbid Axis I disorders with significant negative impact on functioning. Personality disorders appear to be especially common in patients with somatization disorder. The most common comorbid Axis II diagnoses in psychiatric settings are Cluster B diagnoses, whereas in primary care settings Cluster C and paranoid personality diagnoses are more frequent (Rost et al. 1992). The association between personality disorder and somatization disorder may result from a common biological substrate or social-environmental factors such as childhood abuse (G.R. Smith 1991). Patients with somatization disorder often have multiple social problems and chaotic lifestyles characterized by poor interpersonal relationships, disruptive or difficult behavior, and substance abuse (Cassem and Barsky 1991) and show significant occupational and social impairment.

Clinical course and prognosis. Somatization disorder is "a chronic but fluctuating disorder that rarely remits completely. A year seldom passes without the individual's seeking some medical attention prompted by unexplained somatic complaints" (American Psychiatric Association 2000, p. 488). Patients may experience iatrogenic disease or injury secondary to unnecessary diagnostic investigations, polypharmacy, and polysurgery. They are particularly at risk for abuse and dependence on drugs prescribed for symptom control (e.g., analgesics, sedative-hypnotics).

Differential Diagnosis

Occult medical diseases affecting multiple organ systems and manifesting with vague or nonspecific symptoms (e.g., systemic lupus erythematosus, sarcoidosis, lymphoma) should be excluded. Patients with these diagnoses, in contrast to somatization disorder, look chronically ill and usually have abnormal physical examinations or laboratory tests. *Panic disorder* may be mistakenly diagnosed as somatization disorder, given a history of many physicians and extensive diagnostic investigations, although symptom patterns differ, with panic disorder patients describing acute symptoms occurring simultaneously, in contrast to the chronic, protean, and fluctuating symptoms of somatization disorder. Chronic physical symptoms may be a part of a *depressive disorder* but occur in the context of the mood disturbance without the long duration and dramatic symptom fluctuations seen in somatization disorder. Some patients with *schizophrenia* or *delusional disorder* develop multiple somatic delusions, distinguished from somatization disorder by their bizarre content. By definition, somatization disorder includes symptoms compatible with other *somatoform disorders,* and diagnostic overlap is common. Somatization disorder differs from *factitious disorder* and *malingering* by the lack of intentional symptom production.

Specific Treatments

The most effective treatments for somatization disorder (discussed in greater detail later in this chapter under "Management of Somatization and Somatoform Disorders") include cognitive-behavioral therapy (CBT), short-term group therapy, and a psychiatric consultation letter to the primary care physician about strategies for managing the somatizing patient.

Undifferentiated Somatoform Disorder

Definition

Undifferentiated somatoform disorder is a residual category for individuals who do not meet the full criteria for somatization disorder or another somatoform disorder. The diagnosis requires one or more physical complaints persisting for more than 6 months that cannot be accounted for by a general medical condition, direct effects of a substance, or another psychiatric disorder.

Epidemiology

No studies of undifferentiated somatoform disorder per se have been conducted, but investigators have studied variously defined subsyndromal somatization syndromes. *Abridged somatization disorder,* defined by a cutoff score of four DSM-III-R somatization symptoms for men and six symptoms for women, identified patients whose characteristics, including increased medical utilization, resembled those of patients meeting the full criteria for somatization disorder (Escobar et al. 1987, 1989). Studies of distressed high utilizers of medical care documented significant increased health care utilization by patients endorsing functional somatic symptoms falling below the DSM-III-R cutoff score of 13 symptoms (Katon et al. 1991). It is estimated that 4%–11% of the population have multiple medically unexplained symptoms that are consistent with a subsyndromal form of somatization disorder (Escobar et al. 1987, 1989).

Other diagnoses have been proposed as being more clinically useful than undifferentiated somatoform disorder. *Multisomatoform disorder* is characterized by three or more medically unexplained, currently bothersome physical symptoms in addition to a greater than 2-year history of somatization (Kroenke et al. 1997). Criteria for multisomatoform disorder were met in 8% of primary care patients, and the diagnosis was associated with worse functional status, and higher health care utilization (Jackson and Kroenke 2008). *Specific somatoform disorder* requires at least one unexplained physical impairment and a substantial impairment in more than one life domain (Rief and Hiller 1998, 1999) and identifies a more impaired group than does the DSM-IV-TR diagnosis of undifferentiated somatoform disorder (Grabe et al. 2003).

Clinical Course, Prognosis, and Differential Diagnosis

It is likely that the course of this heterogeneous disorder is variable, although there has been little systematic study

(American Psychiatric Association 2000). The differential diagnosis is similar to that of somatization disorder.

Specific Treatments

There are no good studies of the effectiveness of specific treatments for undifferentiated somatoform disorder per se. Beneficial effects have been shown in two small randomized controlled trials (RCTs) of antidepressants in multisomatoform disorder (Kroenke et al. 2006; Muller et al. 2008) and one RCT of a care recommendation letter to primary care physicians (Dickinson et al. 2003). There is an ongoing trial of CBT for abridged somatization disorder (Magallon et al. 2008).

Conversion Disorder

Definition

Conversion symptoms have been described since antiquity (Mace 1992). DSM-IV-TR diagnostic criteria for conversion disorder include neurological (voluntary motor or sensory) symptoms or deficits that are associated with psychological factors (American Psychiatric Association 2000). Conversion presentations can be quite dramatic and can include paralysis, pseudoseizures, amnesia, ataxia, or blindness (see Chapter 32, "Neurology and Neurosurgery").

Controversies surrounding the diagnosis of conversion disorder include whether 1) it is a symptom rather than a disorder, because it has not been validated on the basis of longitudinal or family studies (Martin 1992); 2) it is better classified with the dissociative disorders as in ICD-10 (Phillips et al. 2003; Toone 1990); and 3) the determination that the symptom is unconsciously produced can be a valid and reliable judgment. Critics have also questioned what constitutes "relevant psychological conflict," how malingering is excluded, and the extent to which organic disorders can and should be excluded (Halligan et al. 2000).

Diagnostic Dilemmas

Some have argued for moving conversion disorder to the dissociative disorders category, given that the conversion experience, as in pseudoseizures, usually includes features of dissociation. In most cases the clinician can at best only speculate about the psychological factors whose presence is required by criterion B—the patient is often unaware of or unwilling to divulge such factors, and the psychological factors may not emerge for a long time or even at all. Because the psychological factors are not usually measurable, there is little research to support the value of this criterion. The requirement in criterion C that the symptoms not be intentionally produced or feigned is untestable and unfairly suggests that patients with conversion symptoms are more likely to be dishonest. Because neurologists tend to arrive at the diagnosis of conversion disorder in a manner that differs from the methods of the psychiatrist, future diagnostic revisions may attempt to reduce these differences.

Epidemiology

The reported prevalence of conversion disorder has varied and is likely influenced by several factors. Toone's 1990 review noted rates of 0.3% in the general population, 1%–3% in medical outpatients, and 1%–4.5% in hospitalized neurological and medical patients. Settings such as combat, in which substantial secondary gain may be involved, have increased rates of conversion. Studies of associations of conversion disorder with social class and urban versus rural distribution have yielded equivocal findings (Murphy 1990). A large prospective cohort study found that one-third of new referrals to general neurology clinics had symptoms that were poorly explained by identifiable organic disease (Carson et al. 2000).

Onset is typically in adolescence or early adulthood, but cases have been described in children as well as in older adults. An often-quoted early study cautioned that many patients given a conversion disorder diagnosis subsequently received a diagnosis of a neurological or medical condition that explained the symptom (Slater and Glithero 1965). Later studies have found lower (5%–12%) rates of explanatory neurological diagnoses (Crimlisk et al. 1998; Moene et al. 2000), and the most recent systematic review found an overall rate of misdiagnosis of conversion disorder of only 4% (Stone et al. 2005). These more recent findings may be partially explained by increasing caution on the part of clinicians in making a diagnosis of conversion disorder and by modern neuroimaging and electrophysiological tests. The relationship between childhood traumatization, particularly physical and sexual abuse, and the subsequent development of conversion disorder was first described by Freud and is supported by empirical research (e.g., Roelofs et al. 2002), although this association has not been found in all samples (Binzer and Eisemann 1998). Clinically, this association appears especially frequently among patients with pseudoseizures, with trauma reported by 84%, which included sexual abuse by 67%, physical abuse by 67%, and other traumas by 73% in one study (Bowman and Markand 1996).

Specific Culture and Gender Factors

Much higher prevalence rates have been described in developing countries (Murphy 1990) and in isolated rural American settings (Ford 1983). Women outnumber men with the disorder in a ratio varying from 2:1 to 10:1 (Murphy 1990). Men are more likely to present with conversion symptoms related to military service and industrial accidents (Ford 1983).

Case Vignette

Mr. T is a 36-year-old male payroll officer presenting with frequent seizures despite a 10-year history of excellent anticonvulsant control after originally developing seizures following a severe head injury sustained in a motor vehicle accident. There is a strong family history of epilepsy and a history of childhood febrile seizures. Anticonvulsant levels remained therapeutic, and there were no changes in his neurological examination. Detailed history taking revealed markedly increased workplace stress with little chance of changing jobs and a precarious marital relationship. His wife noted that the first seizure occurred on the morning after he had been reprimanded at work.

Clinical Features

Conversion symptoms typically begin abruptly and dramatically. Common conversion symptoms include motor symptoms (e.g., paralysis, disturbances in coordination or balance, localized weakness, akinesia, dyskinesia, aphonia, urinary retention, and dysphagia), sensory symptoms (e.g., blindness, double vision, anesthesia, paresthesias, deafness), and seizures or convulsions that may have voluntary motor or sensory components. Unilateral symptoms may be more likely to occur on the left side of the body, as may be true for other somatoform disorders, although the neurophysiological basis for this finding is unclear (Toone 1990) and not all data support it (Roelofs et al. 2000; Stone et al. 2002a). Some patients with conversion symptoms also have or had the same symptoms from a neurological disease (e.g., conversion pseudoseizures in a patient with epilepsy, as in the case vignette above; Iriarte et al. 2003). In many patients with conversion disorder there is a discrepancy between the presumably frightening symptoms and the patient's bland, even cheerful emotional response *(la belle indifférence),* but this is not a pathognomonic sign and if present does not have prognostic value (Toone 1990). In fact, a review of 11 studies found the frequency of la belle indifférence to be 21% in patients with conversion disorder and 29% in patients with organic disease (Stone et al. 2006). The authors recommended abandoning la belle indifférence as a clinical sign since it failed to discriminate between conversion symptoms and symptoms of organic disease.

Psychological factors are associated with symptom onset or exacerbation. Psychodynamic views of conversion focus on the etiological role of *primary gain,* which refers to "the effectiveness of the conversion symptom in providing a satisfactory symbolic expression for the repressed wishes" (Engel 1970, p. 660). For example, a conflict about aggression might be symbolically expressed through a paralyzed arm. *Secondary gain* refers to the potential tangible benefits accruing from the sick role, which may include alterations in the behavior of significant others that are deemed positive by the patient (e.g., increased attentiveness) and permission to withdraw from disliked responsibilities. Secondary gain is believed to occur, but not to be consciously sought, in patients with conversion disorder. This contrasts with malingering, in which symptoms are produced intentionally and are motivated by external incentives, or factitious disorders, in which symptoms are produced intentionally from the unconscious motivation of assuming the sick role. Caution must be exercised in making judgments about secondary gain because it is intrinsic to the sick role and may be found in patients with any medical or psychiatric illness.

Associated features. Although there has been little systematic study of comorbid Axis I diagnoses, conversion disorder frequently co-occurs with PTSD and other somatoform, dissociative, and mood disorders. The literature on associated personality features suggests that "hysterical personality may be seen, but only in a minority of conversion cases; other forms of personality disorder of immature, dependent type are more usual" (Toone 1990, p. 229). Protracted conversion reactions may be associated with secondary physical changes (e.g., disuse atrophy).

Clinical course and prognosis. The course of conversion disorder is difficult to predict. Individual episodes of conversion are usually of short duration with sudden onset and resolution, although recurrence of symptoms over time is common (American Psychiatric Association 2000; Murphy 1990). In some cases, conversion symptoms may last years. Factors reported to predispose to conversion disorder are antecedent physical disorders in the individual or a close contact, which provides a model for the symptoms occurring, and severe social stressors, including bereavement, rape, incest, warfare, and other forms of psychosocial trauma (Toone 1990). The prognosis depends on a number of factors, including acuity of onset, presence of major stressors, duration of symptoms before treatment, symptom pattern, personality, and sociocultural context within which the illness developed. Most patients show a rapid response to treatment, but some do not. Patients with pseudoseizures, tremor, and amnesia are particularly likely to have a poor outcome (Toone 1990). In the Scottish Neurological Symptom Study (Sharpe et al. 2010), two-thirds of the patients reported poor outcome (symptom worsening) at 1 year, with the best predictors of poor outcome being patients' illness beliefs (expectation of nonrecovery) and receipt of financial benefits.

Differential Diagnosis

The differential diagnosis of conversion disorder includes *neurological conditions* that present with evanescent signs and symptoms (e.g., multiple sclerosis, complex partial seizures, myasthenia gravis). *Pain disorder* is diagnosed in DSM-IV-TR if pain is the only conversion symptom. Conversion symptoms may occur in *other psychiatric disorders* (e.g., pseudoseizures as a manifestation of panic disorder or PTSD [Bowman and Coons 2000]) or during *bereavement.* Psychogenic amnesia, fugue, or stupor may represent conversion or *dissociative disorders,* although this appears to be an arbitrary semantic distinction. As with other somatoform disorders, symptoms are generated unconsciously, whereas they are intentional in *factitious disorder* and *malingering,* although in practice the distinction may be blurry.

Specific Treatments

The most effective treatments for conversion disorder (discussed in detail later in this chapter under "Management of Somatization and Somatoform Disorders") include supportive therapy, physical therapy, and hypnosis. Clinical trials of pharmacotherapy for conversion disorder have reported inconclusive results (Kroenke 2007).

Pain Disorder

Pain disorder in DSM-IV-TR is the latest incarnation of somatoform pain disorder (DSM-III-R) and psychogenic pain disorder (DSM-III) (see Chapter 36, "Pain").

Hypochondriasis

Definition

Hypochondriasis is characterized by persistent fears of having a disease or the belief that one has a serious disease based on the misinterpretation of one or more bodily symptoms that persist despite medical reassurance (American Psychiatric Association 2000). The validity of the construct in medical outpatients has been documented (Barsky et al. 1986b; Noyes et al. 1993). Secondary hypochondriasis (i.e., hypochondriasis developing in the context of another Axis I psychiatric disorder, a major life stress, or a medical disorder) has been described (Barsky et al. 1992), although it is not recognized in DSM-IV-TR.

Diagnostic Dilemmas

The obsessional preoccupation and phobic distress of hypochondriasis have led some to propose reclassifying it as an anxiety disorder, perhaps under the less stigmatizing name of "health anxiety" (Olatunji et al. 2009). Although hypochondrias includes some features of obsessive-compulsive disorder (OCD), only 10% of patients with hypochondriasis also have OCD.

Epidemiology

No large-scale epidemiological studies of hypochondriasis have been conducted. Prevalence rates for primary and secondary forms of hypochondriasis of 3%–13% have been reported for study samples from medical and psychiatric settings (Kellner 1986) and 4%–6% of general medical outpatients (Barsky 2001). The prevalence in the general population is thought to be 1%–5% (American Psychiatric Association 2000), but the diagnosis has not been included in large psychiatric epidemiological studies. The disorder can begin at any age, but onset is most commonly in early adulthood (American Psychiatric Association 2000).

Specific Culture and Gender Factors

The reported data on ethnic and cultural differences are equivocal (Barsky et al. 1986a; Kellner 1986), and these factors may be most important when an individual's concerns are reinforced by a traditional or alternative healer who disagrees with the medical reassurance provided (American Psychiatric Association 2000). Gender has received little attention, but there does not seem to be a female predominance (Creed and Barsky 2004).

Case Vignette

Mr. J, a 44-year-old sales manager, was referred for assessment of anxiety by an infectious disease doctor who felt that the patient did not have chronic fatigue syndrome. Mr. J was reluctant to speak with a psychiatrist but was grateful to have someone listen in detail to his various medical concerns. On the second assessment interview, he confided that he was convinced that he had multiple sclerosis or amyotrophic lateral sclerosis and that he repeatedly measured the muscle mass in his legs, tested for changes in strength, and watched for "muscle twitches." His preoccupation with his health had negatively affected his work, because he spent much of the day searching the Internet for information, and he reported feeling distant from his wife and children as he "prepared to go downhill and die."

Clinical Features

The core feature of hypochondriasis is fear of disease or a conviction that one has or is at risk for a disease despite normal physical examination results and investigations and physician reassurance. Bodily preoccupation (i.e., increased observation of and vigilance toward bodily sensations) is common. The preoccupation may be with a particular bodily function or experience (e.g., heartbeat); a trivial abnormal physical state that is taken as evidence of disease (e.g., cough); a vague physical sensation; or a particular organ (e.g., heart) or diagnosis (e.g., cancer). Patients with hypochondriasis believe that good health is a relatively symptom-free state, and compared with control patients, they are more likely to consider symptoms to be indicative of disease (Barsky et al. 1993). They also have an exaggerated appraisal of their risk of developing disease (Barsky et al. 2001a).The concern about the feared illness "often becomes a central feature of the individual's self-image, a topic of social discourse, and a response to life stresses" (American Psychiatric Association 2000, p. 504).

Associated features. Patients with hypochondriasis have a high rate of psychiatric comorbidity, with the most common comorbid diagnoses being generalized anxiety disorder, dysthymia, major depressive disorder, somatization disorder, and panic disorder (Barsky et al. 1992). Personality disorders as assessed by questionnaire were three times more likely to be diagnosed in hypochondriacal patients compared with a control group (Barsky et al. 1992). High medical utilization is common, and the potential exists for iatrogenic damage from repeated investigations. Involvement with complementary health care practices is common. Interpersonal relationships typically deteriorate because of the preoccupation with disease. Occupational functioning is often compromised, with increased time taken off from work and decreased performance when the individual is at work because of the preoccupation with disease.

Clinical course and prognosis. The clinical course and prognosis of hypochondriasis are poorly understood. There appear to be multiple pathways to the diagnosis. Primary hypochondriasis appears to be a chronic condition, and therefore some have argued that it might be better classified as a personality style or trait (Barsky and Klerman 1983; Fallon and Feinstein 2001; Mayou et al. 2003; Tyrer et al. 1990). In DSM-IV-TR the course is described as "usually chronic, with waxing and waning symptoms, but complete recovery sometimes occurs" (American Psychiatric Association 2000, p. 506). Positive prognostic features include an acute onset, brief duration, mild symptoms, absence of secondary gain, presence of a comorbid general medical condition, and absence of psychiatric comorbidity (American Psychiatric Association 2000). Secondary hypochondriasis may develop in the context of either current or past serious illness in the patient or family, bereavement, and psychosocial stressors or during the course of another Axis I disorder, principally a mood or anxiety disorder characterized by prominent somatic symptoms. Some forms of secondary hypochondriasis remit with resolution or treatment of the underlying condition (e.g., major life stressors, mood or anxiety disorders). A prospective study found that hypochondriacal patients had a considerable decline in symptoms and improvement in role functioning over 4–5 years, but two-thirds still met diagnostic criteria (Barsky et al. 1998). A large international primary care study reported that at 1-year follow-up, of those with hypochondriasis at baseline, 18% still had it, and an additional 16% continued to report hypochondriacal worries. Forty-five percent of those with hypochondriasis at follow-up also met criteria for DSM-IV anxiety or depressive disorders (Simon et al. 2001).

Differential Diagnosis

The differential diagnosis of hypochondriasis includes *general medical conditions,* particularly the early stages of a variety of rheumatological, immunological, endocrine, and neurological diseases in which the patient may notice symptoms that may not be associated with signs detectable on physical examination or with abnormal laboratory investigation. Of course, hypochondriasis may coexist with medical pathology (Barsky et al. 1986a). Transient hypochondriacal preoccupations related to medical illness do not constitute hypochondriasis (American Psychiatric Association 2000). Hypochondriacal concerns may accompany *other psychiatric diagnoses* characterized by prominent somatic symptoms (e.g., *major depressive disorder, dysthymia, panic disorder, generalized anxiety disorder, obsessive-compulsive disorder*). *Psychotic disorders* are characterized by the fixed quality of the patient's delusional belief, in contrast to the hypochondriacal patient, who is convinced of the veracity of his or her concerns but is able to consider the possibility that the feared disease is not present. In clinical practice sorting out delusional from nondelusional hypochondriasis is sometimes difficult.

Specific Treatments

The most effective treatments for hypochondriasis (discussed in detail later in this chapter under "Management of Somatization and Somatoform Disorders") include CBT, exposure and response prevention, and systematic desensitization (Thomson and Page 2007). There is also evidence for the efficacy of selective serotonin reuptake inhibitors (SSRIs) (Fallon et al. 2008; Greeven et al. 2007).

Body Dysmorphic Disorder

Definition

The hallmark of body dysmorphic disorder (BDD) is the preoccupation with an imagined defect in appearance (if a slight physical anomaly is present, the individual's concern with it is judged to be markedly excessive) that is accompanied by significant distress or impairment in social or occupational functioning (American Psychiatric Association 2000). Although BDD is classified in DSM-IV-TR as a somatoform disorder, it is increasingly seen as an obsessive-compulsive spectrum disorder (Chosak et al. 2008; Phillips and Stout 2006).

Diagnostic Dilemmas

Future revisions of DSM may reclassify BDD as a subtype of OCD, although there are some differences between the disorders (Chosak et al. 2008).

Epidemiology

The prevalence of BDD is greater than many clinicians recognize (Phillips 1998). BDD has been reported to occur in about 5% of patients seeking cosmetic surgery in the United Kingdom (Veale et al. 2003), 5% of female Turkish college students (Cansever et al. 2003), and 9% of Turkish patients presenting for acne treatment (Uzun et al. 2003). See also Chapter 29, "Dermatology." The prevalence of BDD in Dutch psychiatric outpatients who were referred for depressive, anxiety, or somatoform disorders was 0.8% (Vinkers et al. 2008). Otto et al. (2001) estimated a point prevalence of 0.7% in a community sample of women ages 36–44 years in Boston, Massachusetts. Structured interviewing is more likely to identify cases (Zimmerman and Mattia 1998), supporting the claim that it is an underrecognized disorder. Onset is typically in adolescence (Phillips 1998), although the disorder may begin in childhood (Albertini and Phillips 1999). Many years may pass before diagnosis because of the individual's reluctance to reveal symptoms (American Psychiatric Association 2000).

Specific Culture and Gender Factors

Cultural variation in BDD has received relatively little attention, although it is clear that concerns about physical appearance vary across cultures and likely color the presentation in different cultures. A comparative study of American and German college students concluded that body image concerns and preoccupation were significantly greater in American than in German students, although the prevalence of probable BDD was not (Bohne et al. 2002). The sex distribution of BDD varies across case series (Phillips 1998). Men and women describe differential preoccupations in line with cultural norms: women are more likely to be preoccupied with their hips and weight, and men with body build, genitals, and thinning hair (Phillips and Diaz 1997).

Case Vignette

Ms. Y is a 32-year-old woman who was referred to a psychiatrist for "support" by a plastic surgeon whom she had consulted regarding revisions of a rhinoplasty ("still not right") and breast augmentation ("I don't look balanced"). The breast augmentation had been complicated by infection, and there was an objective imbalance and excessive scarring, but her nose appeared aesthetically pleasing. She believed that plastic surgery would make her more attractive, thus "allowing" her to leave her married abusive boyfriend and find a new partner. Collateral information from her mother revealed long-standing bodily preoccupation dating from early adolescence, difficulties in relationships with men, and poor occupational functioning and underemployment.

Clinical Features

Most patients with BDD have concerns about more than one body part (Phillips 1998). The intensity of the preoccupation with the bodily "defect" has been described as "torturing" and "tormenting," dominating the patients' lives and severely limiting social and occupational functioning. Many patients engage in compulsive "checking" behaviors, such as observing themselves in the mirror or measuring the body part of concern. Medical intervention, including surgery, is sought by many patients—75% in one study, with 66% receiving treatment (Phillips et al. 2001b). Delusional BDD—classified as delusional disorder, somatic type—may reflect a difference in insight rather than a distinct syndrome (Phillips et al. 1994).

Associated features. BDD has substantial comorbidity. Major depressive disorder is the most common comorbid disorder, with a current comorbidity rate of about 60% and a lifetime rate of more than 80% (Phillips and Diaz 1997). Other disorders with lifetime rates of more than 30% include social phobia, substance use disorders, and OCD. Some case series have lower rates of comorbidity (Veale et al. 1996). Social phobia usually begins before the onset of BDD, whereas depression and substance use disorders typically develop after the onset of BDD (Gunstad and Phillips 2003). Personality disorder is common (Phillips 2001), with the most common diagnosis being avoidant personality disorder (Veale et al. 1996). Psychosocial dysfunction is often profound, with social withdrawal and occupational functioning below capacity (Phillips 1998) as well as suicidal behavior (Phillips et al. 1993). BDD can profoundly reduce quality of life; BDD subjects' scores in all mental health domains of the Medical Outcomes Study 36-Item Short-Form Health Survey (SF-36) were worse than norms for patients with depression, diabetes, or a recent myocardial infarction (Phillips 2000).

Clinical course and prognosis. Case series suggest that BDD is usually chronic, with few symptom-free intervals. The one prospective study found that psychosocial functioning remained stably poor over 1–3 years follow-up (Phillips et al. 2008). The intensity of the symptoms may vary over time (American Psychiatric Association 2000). Patients with BDD often seek and obtain inappropriate medical and surgical treatment (Phillips et al. 2001b). Cosmetic surgeons have recognized the importance of identifying BDD, because it occurs in 7%–15% of those seeking surgery, and operating on BDD patients may worsen the BDD, placing the surgeon at risk of litigation and physical harm (Sarwer et al. 2003).

Differential Diagnosis

A diagnosis of BDD is not made when another Axis I disorder (e.g., mood disorder, schizophrenia, anorexia nervosa) better accounts for the behavior. Distinguishing between BDD and delusional disorder, somatic type, can be difficult (Phillips 2001; Phillips et al. 1993), as can sorting out "normal body dissatisfaction" (Murphy 1990), because concerns about appearance are common and are reinforced by unrealistic media ideals.

Specific Treatments

The most effective treatments for BDD (discussed in detail later in this chapter under "Management of Somatization and Somatoform Disorders") include CBT, SSRIs, and clomipramine (Ipser et al. 2009).

Management of Somatization and Somatoform Disorders

The key to clinical management of chronic somatization and somatoform disorders is to adopt caring rather than curing as a goal. Management is a much more realistic goal than cure in these patients (Bass and Benjamin 1993; Creed and Guthrie 1993; Epstein et al. 1999; Sharpe et al. 1992; G.C. Smith et al. 2000). Management must be tailored to the individual's somatic symptoms, thoughts and beliefs, behavior, and emotional state (Epstein et al. 1999). Three potential management approaches to the patient with somatization disorder have been described:

1. A *reattribution approach* emphasizes helping the patient to link his or her physical symptoms with psychological or stressful factors in his or her life. This is accomplished via a three-step process that links psychosocial stressors (e.g., marital strife) through physiological mechanisms (e.g., increased muscle tension) to physical symptoms (e.g., headache) (Goldberg et al. 1989).
2. A *psychotherapeutic approach* concentrates on developing a close and trusting relationship with the patient (Guthrie et al. 1991).
3. A *directive approach* treats the patient as though he or she has a physical problem, and interventions are framed in a medical model (Benjamin 1989).

The three management approaches vary in their suitability for different patients. The reattribution approach is particularly useful in primary care settings, in medical-surgical inpatient settings with patients who have a fair degree of insight, and in psychiatric settings with patients who have less lengthy histories of somatization. The reattribution technique can be easily taught to primary care practitioners (Goldberg et al. 1989). The psychotherapeutic approach is most suitable for patients with persistent somatization who are willing to explore the effect of psychosocial factors on their symptoms. The directive approach is most useful for hostile patients who deny the importance of psychological or social factors in their symptoms.

A systematic review of 34 RCTs of treatments for somatoform disorders, almost all published in 1995–2007, concluded that CBT is the best-established treatment for a variety of somatoform disorders (Kroenke 2007). CBT was effective in 11 of 13 studies, and antidepressants were effective in 4 of 5 studies. For the treatment of somatization disorder, 3 of 4 studies found that a psychiatric consultation letter to the primary care physician about strategies for managing the somatizing patient was effective in improving patient functional status, though none found this intervention to reduce patient psychological distress.

Principles of Management

The fundamental principles of management are similar for patients with somatization and with somatoform disorders.

Providing a Positive Explanation of Symptoms

In order to engage in treatment, patients require a sense that their primary physician is taking them seriously, appreciates the magnitude of their distress, and has a rationale for the proposed management plan. Most somatizing patients hold explanatory models of their symptoms that are in conflict with their physician's model (Salmon et al. 1999). The clinical challenge is therefore to provide explanations that empower patients with tangible mechanisms, exculpation, and encouragement of self-management rather than explanations that reject or collude with the patient's model (Salmon et al. 1999). Reassurance is helpful to many patients (Page and Wessely 2003), but it must be carefully dosed and targeted. Facile or excessive reassurance may exacerbate disease fears or cause patients to redouble efforts to prove they are sick and may undermine the doctor–patient relationship (Warwick 1992). It is important to emphasize to patients that the psychiatrist is not dismissing their symptoms as being "all in their head" but rather sees the symptoms as being "real" and "in their body" and wants to explore all opportunities for symptom control. The use of metaphors and analogies is often helpful. The metaphor of a radio has been reported to be particularly useful (N.H. Cassem, personal communication,

July 1985). The radio channel playing is the symptom that is of concern, and given that it cannot be changed by medical or surgical interventions, the patient must gain greater control over the volume control knob (i.e., factors that exacerbate or relieve symptoms) or the sensitivity of the antenna (i.e., factors that amplify symptoms). Physiological mechanisms underlying symptoms may be usefully explained (see Table 12-2) (Sharpe and Bass 1992). Understanding the personal meaning of the symptoms to the patient and tailoring one's explanations and reassurance in light of this meaning may improve the doctor–patient relationship (Epstein et al. 1999; Priel et al. 1991).

Ensuring Regular Follow-Up

Regular follow-up is the key to effective management; it results in decreased health care utilization overall and is less stressful for both patients and physicians than symptom-driven visits. The best choice for most patients is management by their primary care practitioner in consultation with a psychiatrist. However, the psychiatrist may provide primary follow-up if significant comorbid Axis I or Axis II pathology is present or if the primary care physician cannot manage the symptoms.

Treating Mood or Anxiety Disorders

Mood or anxiety disorders have significant morbidity in their own right and interfere with participation in rehabilitation and psychotherapy. Their physiological concomitants may fuel the somatization process or heighten somatic amplification.

Minimizing Polypharmacy

Polypharmacy may produce iatrogenic complications. Unnecessary medications, especially those that are potentially addictive, should be tapered and withdrawn using a staged approach over time with small, realistically achievable steps.

Providing Specific Therapy When Indicated

A variety of specific therapies have been recommended for the somatoform disorders and are discussed below. For example, physiotherapy or massage may be helpful in diminishing musculoskeletal pain for patients with somatoform disorders.

Changing Social Dynamics That Reinforce Symptoms

Many patients' lives come to revolve around their symptoms and their use of the health care system. Regularly scheduled follow-up means that the patient no longer has to present a symptom as a "ticket of admission" to the physician's office. Important members of the patient's social support system may be persuaded to consistently reward non-illness-related behaviors. Social skills building, life skills training, assertiveness training, and physical reactivation programs may be indicated. Group therapy may be useful because it provides social support, increases interpersonal skills, and provides a nonthreatening environment in which to learn to experience and express emotions and desires more directly.

Resolving Difficulties in the Doctor–Patient Relationship

Somatizing patients often have difficult relationships with their caregivers because of attention seeking, demands, and anger. These difficulties have multiple determinants, including problematic early attachment (Stuart and Noyes 1999), differences in expectations and beliefs about the meaning and management of symptoms, and prior frustrating experiences with the health care system (Page and Wessely 2003). Consequently, addressing shortcomings in doctor–patient interactions can be helpful (Page and Wessely 2003).

Recognizing and Controlling Negative Reactions or Countertransference

Somatizing patients can evoke powerful emotional responses in physicians, which may result in less than optimal clinical care (Hahn et al. 1994; Sharpe et al. 1994). The range of emotions experienced by physicians may include guilt for failing to help the patient, fear that the patient will make a complaint, and anger at the patient's entitlement. The physician may be dismissive of the patient or, alternatively, may collude with the patient in excessive investigations to exclude physical disease in "a suspension of professional judgment" (Bass and Murphy 1990). Excessive investigation might result from a conscious attempt to avoid a "painful, embarrassing and time-consuming confrontation" (Bass and Murphy 1990) or may represent an unconscious solution to the conflicts and emotions that the patient evokes in the physician. The treating physician should seek to identify something about the patient that is either likable or interesting that will help to sustain his or her involvement—in the most difficult patients, it may simply be a sense of amazement at the degree of somatization. A physician caring for these patients must also set clear limits as to his or her availability. If all else fails, the physician should transfer the care of the patient to a colleague, either temporarily or permanently.

Because many patients with somatoform disorders refuse mental health treatment, the psychiatrist's role is often that of a consultant developing a management plan that integrates multiple treatment modalities and different health care disciplines. Several reviews have discussed psychosocial treatments for unexplained physical symptoms (Looper and Kirmayer 2002; Woolfolk et al. 2007). Cost-effective integrated programs have shown decreased health care utilization (Hiller et al. 2003). Treatment interventions can be tailored to the relevant underlying mechanisms in specific patients, as illustrated in Figure 12-3 (Looper and Kirmayer 2002).

Therapeutic Interventions

Approach to the Patient

Specific management strategies have been described for patients with conversion disorder that also apply to patients with other somatoform disorders. These include 1) explaining to the patient that his or her conversion (or somatic) symptoms are not caused by a serious disease, 2) refraining from confronting the patient, and 3) providing some form of "face-saving" mechanism for symptom resolution such as physical therapy or the suggestion that the patient will improve over a specified period. Eisendrath (1989) observed that "when dealing with behavior with prominent unconscious motivation such as conversion reactions...the therapist provides no benefit by revealing understanding of the psychological processes too early in the treatment" (p. 386). Although many clinicians feel uncomfortable about the risks inherent in "legitimizing" the illness, this approach seems justified based on considerable anecdotal experience of good outcome with treatment and prolonged disability without it. The consulting psychiatrist often must help the referring physician and other health care professionals manage their emotional responses to these patients, whom they may view as deceiving them. The choice of words in talking to patients is very important: terms such as *stress-related seizures* or *functional seizures* are much more acceptable, while remaining truthful, than *pseudoseizures* or *psychogenic seizures,* which may be seen as offensive or pejorative (Stone et al. 2003).

There has been little study of the treatment preferences of patients. Walker et al. (1999) studied 23 volunteers with a diagnosis of hypochondriasis and found that CBT was rated as more acceptable than medications and was perceived as more likely to be effective in the short and long term. CBT was the first choice of 74% of participants, in contrast to medication in 4% and equal preference in 22%. Of note, 48% reported they would accept only CBT. Stone et al. (2004) reported that the majority of neurology clinic patients, and not just those with medically unexplained symptoms, have largely negative beliefs about antidepressants.

Cognitive Therapy

In Kroenke's (2007) systematic review of the efficacy of treatments for somatoform disorders, cognitive therapy proved effective in 11 of 13 RCTs. These trials spanned the range of somatoform disorders and drew from samples that included psychiatric outpatients, medical outpatients, and community respondents. Cognitive therapy has been shown to be beneficial for somatization disorder, hypochondriasis, BDD, and medically unexplained symptoms.

The use of cognitive therapy is predicated on cognitive models such as the one shown in Figure 12-4 for hypochondriasis. The cognitive model directs attention to factors that maintain preoccupation with worries about health, including attentional factors, avoidant behaviors, beliefs, and misinterpretation of symptoms, signs, and medical communications (Salkovskis 1989). Cognitive therapy has been helpful in decreasing health care visits and physical complaints in patients with multiple unexplained physical symptoms (Sumathipala et al. 2008). In a 15-month follow-up of a 10-week RCT of CBT, primary care patients with somatization disorder showed improvements in functioning, fewer somatic symptoms, and a decrease in health care costs (Allen et al. 2006). A controlled treatment study using both individual and group CBT demonstrated cost-effectiveness and decreased health care utilization in a mixed group of patients with somatoform disorders (Hiller et al. 2003).

Cognitive therapy programs for hypochondriasis have been described in considerable detail (Salkovskis 1989) and are based on a model of hypochondriasis as a disorder of perception and cognition in which somatic sensations are perceived as abnormally intense and are attributed to serious medical disease. Barsky et al. (1988a) described a 6-week group program for patients with hypochondriasis. At 12-month follow-up, a randomized usual-care control trial of a 6-session individual CBT intervention demonstrated significant, persistent reductions in hypochondriacal beliefs and attitudes; in health-related anxiety; and in impairment in social role functioning and activities of daily living, but no improvement in hypochondriacal somatic symptoms (Barsky and Ahern 2004). Cognitive therapy achieved a somewhat higher rate of response than paroxetine (45% vs. 30%) in a comparative RCT in psychiatric outpatients with hypochondriasis, and response rates for both treatments were significantly greater than the response rate for placebo (14%) (Greeven et al. 2007). Four of the five studies of CBT in patients with medically unexplained symptoms reported a positive response rate (Kroenke 2007), and two of three studies of CBT in BDD patients reported significant reduction in symptom severity (Ipser et al. 2009).

Pharmacotherapy

The evidence base for pharmacological treatment of somatoform disorders is limited to studies of small heteroge-

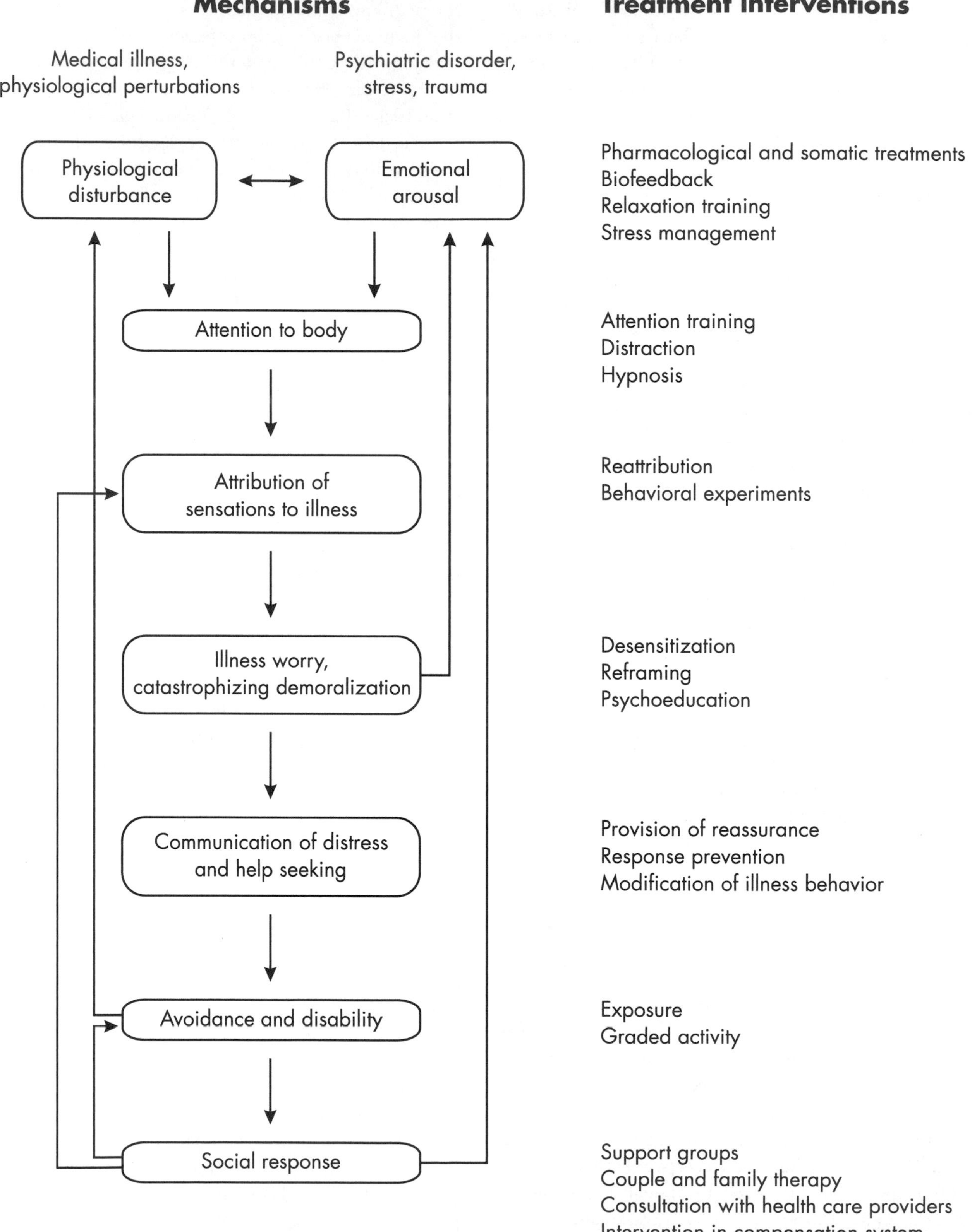

FIGURE 12–3. Matching mechanisms and interventions in the management of somatoform disorders.

Source. Reprinted from Looper KJ, Kirmayer LJ: "Behavioral Medicine Approaches to Somatoform Disorders." *Journal of Consulting and Clinical Psychology* 70:810–827, 2002, p. 812. Copyright 2002, the American Psychological Association. Used with permission.

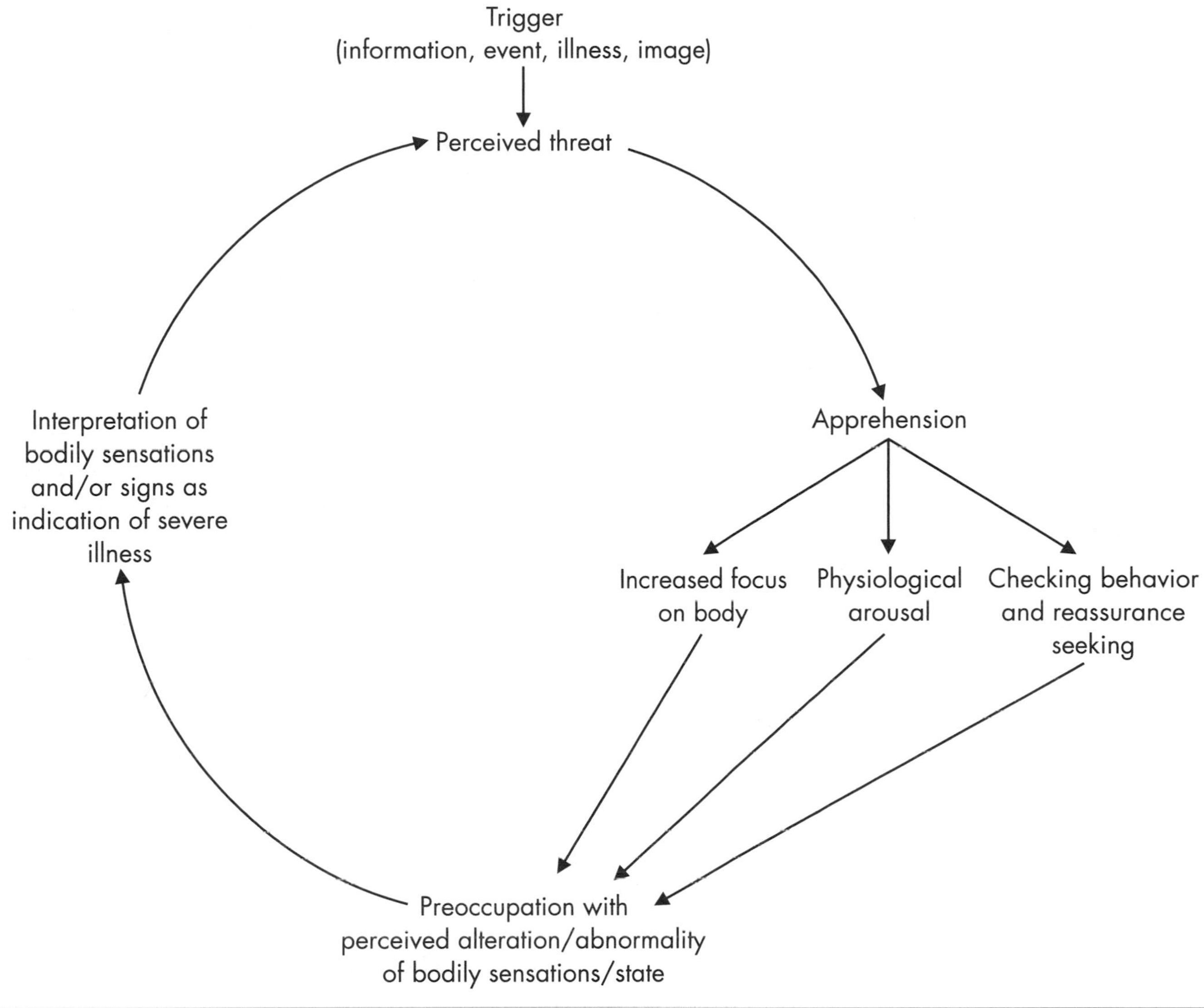

FIGURE 12–4. A cognitive model for hypochondriasis.

Source. Reprinted from Salkovskis PM: "Somatic Problems," in *Cognitive Behaviour Therapy for Psychiatric Problems.* Edited by Hawton K, Salkovskis PM, Kirk J, et al. New York, Oxford University Press, 1989, pp. 235–276. Copyright 1989, Oxford University Press (www.oup.com). Used with permission.

neous samples, chart reviews, open-label trials, and a small number of RCTs. There is great interest in the potential role of antidepressants in ameliorating somatic symptoms associated with depression, as well as functional somatic symptoms in nondepressed patients (Stahl 2003). Norepinephrine and serotonin have important functions in mediating physical symptoms, and therefore their modulation with antidepressants may bring about changes in somatic experiences (Stahl 2003). An open-label trial of fluoxetine found moderate improvement in 61% of 29 patients with a variety of somatoform disorders (Noyes et al. 1998). In a European placebo-controlled trial, opipramol (a histamine H_1, serotonin 5-HT_2, and dopamine D_2 blocker) demonstrated efficacy in a diverse group of somatoform patients with high rates of depressive and anxiety comorbidity (Volz et al. 2000).

Pharmacotherapy has shown limited evidence of effectiveness in somatization disorder except for treatment of comorbid mood and anxiety disorders. Drugs that have been studied for hypochondriasis include high-dose fluoxetine (average dosage 51 mg/day), which improved the response rate to 63% versus 33% for placebo in one RCT (Fallon et al. 2008), and paroxetine, which proved better than placebo in another RCT (Greeven et al. 2007). Secondary hypochondriasis in patients with depression has been treated with amitriptyline (Kellner et al. 1986). A number of studies of BDD have reported success with SSRIs in about two-thirds of patients treated (Phillips 1998; Phillips et al. 2001a, 2008). In one RCT, fluoxetine proved effective in reducing BDD beliefs and behaviors (Phillips et al. 2002). It has also been reported that augmentation strategies and changing antidepressants may be helpful in BDD patients who are nonresponsive to SSRIs (Phillips et al. 2001a). High relapse rates in BDD were reported with discontinuation of pharmacotherapy (Phillips et al. 2001a). Clomipramine (a potent serotonin reuptake inhibitor) was more effective than desipramine (a norepinephrine reuptake inhibitor) in treating BDD in a 16-week double-blind crossover trial (Hollander et al. 1999). The SSRIs appear to be effective even among patients with a delusional variant of BDD (Hollander et al. 1999; Phillips et al. 2001a). The time to response is longer than with major depression for at least one-third of patients.

Physical Reactivation and Physical Therapy

Physical reactivation via a gradually escalating program of exercise (e.g., walking, swimming) often improves the quality of life in patients with a variety of somatoform disorders. It may be difficult to engage patients in exercise, but once they become more active, they often find it pleasurable and report feelings of accomplishment, reduced stress, and greater confidence in their body. Physical reactivation should start at a level just below what the patient can do on his or her worst day, and the patient should then strive for consistency with activity at least 5 days a week. Physical therapy is invaluable for patients who have conversion disorder and may be the only treatment required to restore physical function in some cases (Delargy et al. 1986; Dvonch et al. 1991). In a recent report of 34 consecutive referrals for inpatient rehabilitation treatment of conversion disorder patients with motor paralysis, 9 had complete recovery, 10 had partial recovery, and 15 remained unchanged (Heruti et al. 2002).

Relaxation Therapies, Meditation, and Hypnotherapy

Various forms of relaxation therapies, biofeedback, meditation, and hypnotherapy have been used with somatoform disorder patients. Relaxation therapies modulate somatic sensations and may be used as part of a more comprehensive group treatment program for hypochondriasis (Barsky et al. 1988a). These therapies may be used either as a primary form of treatment based on a psychophysiological model or as an adjuvant to other forms of treatment. Hypnosis has been used diagnostically and therapeutically in patients with conversion disorder (see review by Van Dyck and Hoogduin 1989), and it showed sustained benefits for 6 months in an RCT (Moene et al. 2003). Hypnotherapy may be combined with intravenous sedation (Toone 1990) and eclectic behavioral treatment programs (Moene et al. 2003). Although abreaction or catharsis under hypnosis or sedation has had dramatic anecdotal effects in some individuals in whom the conversion was precipitated by extreme trauma, such interventions are not helpful for most patients (Toone 1990).

Behavioral Treatment

Learning theory models have been proposed for the treatment of several somatoform disorders. Hypochondriasis has been treated with exposure and response prevention individually tailored to the patient's specific problem behaviors (Visser and Bouman 1992, 2001; Warwick and Marks 1988). Prevention of reassurance seeking was a key component of treatment because it is conceptualized as an anxiety-reducing ritual that is reinforced by the reassurance received (Warwick 1992). This program, which required a median of seven treatment sessions and 11 therapist hours, was associated with improvement that was maintained in half of the patients at follow-up (mean duration, 5 years; range, 1–8 years). Exposure therapy may decrease hypochondriacal fears and beliefs in agoraphobic patients (Fava et al. 1988). Exposure plus response prevention for hypochondriasis was found to be as effective as cognitive therapy, and both treatments demonstrated results that were superior to a wait-list control group (Visser and Bouman 2001). Behavioral stress management is helpful in treating hypochondriasis (Clark et al. 1998). In some patients, BDD has been successfully treated with behavioral techniques such as desensitization, live and fantasy exposure, and assertiveness training (Marks and Mishan 1988).

Suggestion and Reassurance

The use of suggestion or reassurance requires clinical acumen in framing the intervention and ensuring that one does not give an explanation that is heard as "It's all in your head." Explanations should empower patients, reframe the symptoms, and emphasize the possibility of improvement over time, particularly with active involvement from the patient. For example, the psychiatrist may tell the patient, "The sudden weakness in your legs really laid you up. The good news is that you don't have multiple sclerosis, a stroke, a tumor, or anything else like that. This sort of weakness typically disappears as mysteriously as it initially appears, but our experience is that you can speed up your recovery through physical therapy."

Dynamic Psychotherapy

Psychotherapy has a role in the management of some somatoform disorders. In general, psychoeducational and supportive techniques predominate, although insight-oriented therapy may be indicated in some patients. Explanatory therapy for hypochondriasis has been described

(Kellner 1986) and showed an impact superior to the waiting-list control condition (Fava et al. 2000). Explanatory therapy has been described as "providing accurate information, teaching the principles of selective perception (attention to one part of the body makes the patient more aware of sensations in that part of the body than in other parts), reassurance, clarification and repetition" (Fava et al. 2000). Unlike CBT, explanatory therapy is simpler, uses fewer therapeutic components, does not introduce specific behavioral techniques, and is not based on a specific theoretical framework (Fava et al. 2000). Insight-oriented psychotherapy for somatizing patients has been advocated (McDougall 1989; Rodin 1984), but there is no empirical evidence supporting it, and it will appeal to only a minority of patients.

Group Psychotherapy

Group therapy may be particularly useful in the management of somatoform disorders. When social and affiliative needs are gratified via the group, patients' need to somatize to establish or maintain relationships may be reduced (Ford 1984). Confrontation by fellow group members about secondary gain is usually better tolerated than that by an individual therapist or primary physician. Anger at physicians and family and dependence needs may be better tolerated in the group setting, which tends to diffuse intense affects. Group therapy also may be useful in increasing interpersonal skills and in enhancing more direct forms of communication regarding thoughts, feelings, and desires (Ford 1984). Helplessness has been identified as a central psychotherapeutic issue that can be effectively addressed in group therapy for patients with somatoform disorder (Levine et al. 1993). Various forms of group therapy have been reported for patients with somatoform disorder (see review by Levine et al. 1993). Short-term group therapy appears to be effective in primary care patients with somatization disorder (Kashner et al. 1995).

Marital and Family Therapy

Most families will benefit from information and psychoeducational approaches. More intensive forms of therapy are required when patients have significant marital or family pathology and when somatic symptoms are an important form of social communication within the family. It is important to identify the family's attitude and response because they may have a conscious or unconscious interest in maintaining a symptom in a patient.

References

Albertini RS, Phillips KA: Thirty-three cases of body dysmorphic disorder in children and adolescents. J Am Acad Child Adolesc Psychiatry 38:453–459, 1999

Allen LA, Woolfolk RL, Escobar JI, et al: Cognitive-behavioral therapy for somatization disorder: a randomized controlled trial. Arch Intern Med 166:1512–1518, 2006

American Psychiatric Association: Diagnostic and Statistical Manual of Mental Disorders, 3rd Edition. Washington, DC, American Psychiatric Association, 1980

American Psychiatric Association: Diagnostic and Statistical Manual of Mental Disorders, 3rd Edition, Revised. Washington, DC, American Psychiatric Association, 1987

American Psychiatric Association: Diagnostic and Statistical Manual of Mental Disorders, 4th Edition. Washington, DC, American Psychiatric Association, 1994

American Psychiatric Association: Diagnostic and Statistical Manual of Mental Disorders, 4th Edition, Text Revision. Washington, DC, American Psychiatric Association, 2000

Andreski P, Chilcoat H, Breslau N: Post-traumatic stress disorder and somatization symptoms: a prospective study. Psychiatry Res 79:131–138, 1998

Barsky AJ: A comprehensive approach to the chronically somatizing patient. J Psychosom Res 45:301–306, 1998

Barsky AJ: The patient with hypochondriasis. N Engl J Med 345:1395–1399, 2001

Barsky AJ, Ahern DK: Cognitive behavior therapy for hypochondriasis: a randomized controlled trial. JAMA 291:1464–1470, 2004

Barsky AJ, Klerman GL: Overview: hypochondriasis, bodily complaints, and somatic styles. Am J Psychiatry 140:273–283, 1983

Barsky AJ, Wyshak G, Klerman GL: Hypochondriasis: an evaluation of the DSM-III criteria in medical outpatients. Arch Gen Psychiatry 43:493–500, 1986a

Barsky AJ, Wyshak G, Klerman GL: Medical and psychiatric determinants of outpatient medical utilization. Med Care 24:548–560, 1986b

Barsky AJ, Geringer E, Wood CA: A cognitive-educational treatment for hypochondriasis. Gen Hosp Psychiatry 10:322–327, 1988a

Barsky AJ, Goodson JD, Lane RS, et al: The amplification of somatic symptoms. Psychosom Med 50:510–519, 1988b

Barsky AJ, Wyshak G, Klerman GL: Psychiatric co-morbidity in DSM-III-R hypochondriasis. Arch Gen Psychiatry 49:101–108, 1992

Barsky AJ, Coeytaux RR, Sarnie MK, et al: Hypochondriacal patients' beliefs about good health. Am J Psychiatry 150:1085–1089, 1993

Barsky AJ, Fama JM, Bailey ED, et al: A prospective 4- to 5-year study of DSM-III-R hypochondriasis. Arch Gen Psychiatry 55:737–744, 1998

Barsky AJ, Ahern DK, Bailey ED, et al: Hypochondriacal patients' appraisal of health and physical risks. Am J Psychiatry 158:783–787, 2001a

Barsky AJ, Peekna HM, Borus JF: Somatic symptom reporting in women and men. J Gen Intern Med 16:266–275, 2001b

Bass C, Benjamin S: The management of chronic somatisation. Br J Psychiatry 162:472–480, 1993

Bass C, Murphy M: The chronic somatizer and the Government White Paper. J R Soc Med 83:203–205, 1990

Bass C, Murphy M: Somatoform and personality disorders: syndromal comorbidity and overlapping developmental pathways. J Psychosom Res 39:403–427, 1995

Bass C, Peveler R, House A: Somatoform disorders: severe psychiatric illnesses neglected by psychiatrists. Br J Psychiatry 179:11–14, 2001

Benjamin S: Psychological treatment of chronic pain: a selective review. J Psychosom Res 33:121–131, 1989

Binzer M, Eisemann M: Childhood experiences and personality traits in patients with motor conversion symptoms. Acta Psychiatr Scand 98:288–295, 1998

Bohne A, Keuthen NJ, Wilhelm S, et al: Prevalence of symptoms of body dysmorphic disorder and its correlates: a cross-cultural comparison. Psychosomatics 43:486–490, 2002

Bowman ES, Coons PM: The differential diagnosis of epilepsy, pseudoseizures, dissociative identity disorder, and dissociative disorder not otherwise specified. Bull Menninger Clin 64:164–180, 2000

Bowman ES, Markand ON: Psychodynamic and psychiatric diagnoses of pseudoseizure subjects. Am J Psychiatry 153:57–63, 1996

Brown HD, Kosslyn SM, Delamater B, et al: Perceptual and memory biases for health-related information in hypochondriacal individuals. J Psychosom Res 47:67–78, 1999

Cansever A, Uzun O, Donmex E, et al: The prevalence and clinical features of body dysmorphic disorder in college students: a study in a Turkish sample. Compr Psychiatry 44:60–64, 2003

Carson AJ, Ringbauer B, Stone J, et al: Do medically unexplained symptoms matter? A prospective cohort study of 300 new referrals to neurology outpatient clinics. J Neurol Neurosurg Psychiatry 68:207–210, 2000

Cassem NH, Barsky AJ: Functional somatic symptoms and somatoform disorders, in Massachusetts General Hospital Handbook of General Hospital Psychiatry, 3rd Edition. Edited by Cassem NH. St. Louis, MO, Mosby Year Book, 1991, pp 131–157

Chosak A, Marques L, Greenberg JL, et al: Body dysmorphic disorder and obsessive-compulsive disorder: similarities, differences and the classification debate. Expert Rev Neurother 8:1209–1218, 2008

Clark DM, Salkovskis PM, Hackmann A, et al: Two psychological treatments for hypochondriasis: a randomised controlled trial. Br J Psychiatry 173:218–225, 1998

Cloninger CR, Martin RL, Guze SB, et al: A prospective follow-up and family study of somatization in men and women. Am J Psychiatry 143:873–878, 1986

Craig TK, Boardman AP, Mills K, et al: The South London somatisation study, I: longitudinal course and the influence of early life experiences. Br J Psychiatry 163:579–588, 1993

Creed F: Can DSM-V facilitate productive research into the somatoform disorders? J Psychosom Res 60:331–334, 2006

Creed F, Barsky A: A systematic review of the epidemiology of somatisation disorder and hypochondriasis. J Psychosom Res 56:391–408, 2004

Creed F, Guthrie E: Techniques for interviewing the somatising patient. Br J Psychiatry 162:467–471, 1993

Crimlisk HL, Bhatia K, Cope H, et al: Slater revisited: 6-year follow-up study of patients with medically unexplained motor symptoms. BMJ 316:582–586, 1998

De Gucht V, Fischler B, Heiser W: Personality and affect as determinants of medically unexplained symptoms in primary care: a follow-up study. J Psychosom Res 56:279–285, 2004

Delargy MA, Peatfield RC, Burt AA: Successful rehabilitation in conversion paralysis. BMJ 292:1730–1731, 1986

Dickinson WP, Dickinson LM, deGruy FV, et al: A randomized clinical trial of a care recommendation letter intervention for somatization in primary care. Ann Fam Med 1:228–235, 2003

Dimsdale J, Creed F: The proposed diagnosis of somatic symptom disorders in DSM-V to replace somatoform disorders in DSM-IV—a preliminary report. J Psychosom Res 66:473–476, 2009

Drossman DA: Do psychosocial factors define symptom severity and patient status in irritable bowel syndrome? Am J Med 107(5A):41S–50S, 1999

Duddu V, Isaac MK, Chaturvedi SK: Somatization, somatosensory amplification, attribution styles and illness behaviour: a review. Int Rev Psychiatry 18:25–33, 2006

Dvonch VM, Bunch WH, Siegler AH: Conversion reactions in pediatric athletes. J Pediatr Orthop 11:770–772, 1991

Eisenberg L: Disease and illness: distinctions between professional and popular ideas of sickness. Cult Med Psychiatry 1:9–23, 1977

Eisendrath SJ: Factitious physical disorders: treatment without confrontation. Psychosomatics 30:383–387, 1989

Elklit A, Christiansen DM: Predictive factors for somatization in a trauma sample. Clin Pract Epidemiol Ment Health 5:1, 2009

Engel GL: Conversion symptoms, in Signs and Symptoms: Applied Pathologic Physiology and Clinical Interpretation, 5th Edition. Edited by MacBryde CM. Philadelphia, PA, JB Lippincott, 1970, pp 650–668

Epstein RM, Quill TE, McWhinney IR: Somatization reconsidered: incorporating the patient's experience of illness. Arch Intern Med 159:215–222, 1999

Escobar JI, Burnam MA, Karno M, et al: Somatization in the community. Arch Gen Psychiatry 44:713–718, 1987

Escobar JI, Manu P, Matthews D, et al: Medically unexplained physical symptoms, somatization disorder and abridged somatization: studies with the Diagnostic Interview Schedule. Psychiatr Dev 3:235–245, 1989

Escobar JI, Gara MA, Diaz-Martinez AM, et al: Effectiveness of a time-limited cognitive behavior therapy type intervention among primary care patients with medically unexplained symptoms. Ann Fam Med 5:328–335, 2007

Fallon BA, Feinstein S: Hypochondriasis, in Somatoform and Factitious Disorders (Review of Psychiatry Series, Vol 20, No 3; Oldham JM and Riba MB, series eds). Edited by Phillips KA. Washington, DC, American Psychiatric Press, 2001, pp 27–66

Fallon BA, Petkova E, Skritskaya N, et al: A double-masked, placebo-controlled study of fluoxetine for hypochondriasis. J Clin Psychopharmacol 28:638–645, 2008

Fava GA, Kellner R, Zielezny M, et al: Hypochondriacal fears and beliefs in agoraphobia. J Affect Disord 14:239–244, 1988

Fava GA, Silvana G, Rafanelli C, et al: Explanatory therapy in hypochondriasis. J Clin Psychiatry 61:317–322, 2000

Feighner JP, Robins E, Guze SB, et al: Diagnostic criteria for use in psychiatric research. Arch Gen Psychiatry 26:57–63, 1972

Fink P, Rosendal M, Olesen F: Classification of somatization and functional somatic symptoms in primary care. Aust N Z J Psychiatry 39:772–781, 2005

Fishbain DA, Cole B, Cutler RB, et al: A structured evidence-based review on the meaning of nonorganic physical signs: Waddell signs. Pain Med 4:141–181, 2003

Ford CV: The Somatizing Disorders: Illness as a Way of Life. New York, Elsevier, 1983

Ford CV: Somatizing disorders, in Helping Patients and Their Families Cope With Medical Problems. Edited by Roback HB. Washington, DC, Jossey-Bass, 1984, pp 39–59

Ford CV: Illness as a lifestyle: the role of somatization in medical practice. Spine 17:S338–S343, 1992

Garralda ME: Assessment and management of somatisation in childhood and adolescence: a practical perspective. J Child Psychol Psychiatry 40:1159–1167, 1999

Gilleland J, Suveg C, Jacob ML, et al: Understanding the medically unexplained: emotional and familial influences on children's somatic functioning. Child Care Health Dev 35:383–390, 2009

Goldberg D, Gask L, O'Dowd T: The treatment of somatization: teaching techniques of reattribution. J Psychosom Res 33:689–695, 1989

Golding JM, Smith GR Jr, Kashner TM: Does somatization disorder occur in men? Clinical characteristics of women and men with multiple unexplained somatic symptoms. Arch Gen Psychiatry 48:231–235, 1991

Golding JM, Rost K, Kashner TM, et al: Family psychiatric history of patients with somatization disorder. Psychiatr Med 10:33–47, 1992

Grabe HJ, Meyer C, Hapke U, et al: Specific somatoform disorder in the general population. Psychosomatics 44:304–311, 2003

Greeven A, van Balkom AJ, Visser S, et al: Cognitive behavior therapy and paroxetine in the treatment of hypochondriasis: a randomized controlled trial. Am J Psychiatry 164:91–99, 2007

Gunstad J, Phillips KA: Axis I comorbidity in body dysmorphic disorder. Compr Psychiatry 44:270–276, 2003

Gureje O, Simon GE, Ustun TB, et al: Somatization in cross-cultural perspective: a World Health Organization study in primary care. Am J Psychiatry 154:989–995, 1997

Guthrie EA, Creed F, Dawson D, et al: A controlled trial of psychological treatment for the irritable bowel syndrome. Gastroenterology 100:450–457, 1991

Guze SB: Genetics of Briquet's syndrome and somatization disorder. A review of family, adoption, and twin studies. Ann Clin Psychiatry 5:225–230, 1993

Guze SB, Cloninger CR, Martin RL, et al: A follow-up and family study of Briquet's syndrome. Br J Psychiatry 149:17–23, 1986

Hahn SR, Thompson KS, Wills TA, et al: The difficult doctor-patient relationship: somatization, personality and psychopathology. J Clin Epidemiol 47:647–657, 1994

Halligan PW, Bass C, Wade DT: New approaches to conversion hysteria. BMJ 320:1488–1489, 2000

Henningsen P, Zipfel S, Herzog W: Management of functional somatic syndromes. Lancet 369:946–955, 2007

Heruti RJ, Reznik J, Adunski A, et al: Conversion motor paralysis disorder: analysis of 34 consecutive referrals. Spinal Cord 40:335–340, 2002

Hiller W, Fichter MM, Rief W: A controlled treatment study of somatoform disorders including analysis of healthcare utilization and cost-effectiveness. J Psychosom Res 54:369–380, 2003

Hollander E, Allen A, Kwon J, et al: Clomipramine vs desipramine crossover trial in body dysmorphic disorder. Arch Gen Psychiatry 56:1033–1039, 1999

Hotopf M, Wadsworth M, Wessely S: Is "somatisation" a defense against the acknowledgement of psychiatric disorder? J Psychosom Res 50:119–124, 2001

Hudson JL, Mangweth B, Pope HG, et al: Family study of affective spectrum disorder. Arch Gen Psychiatry 60:170–177, 2003

Ipser JC, Sander C, Stein DJ: Pharmacotherapy and psychotherapy for body dysmorphic disorder. Cochrane Database Syst Rev (1):CD005332, 2009

Iriarte J, Parra J, Urrestarazu E, et al: Controversies in the diagnosis and management of psychogenic pseudoseizures. Epilepsy Behav 4:354–359, 2003

Jackson JL, Kroenke K: Prevalence, impact, and prognosis of multisomatoform disorder in primary care: a 5-year follow-up study. Psychosom Med 70:430–434, 2008

Kanner AM: More controversies on the treatment of psychogenic pseudoseizures: an addendum. Epilepsy Behav 4:360–364, 2003

Kashner TM, Rost K, Cohen B, et al: Enhancing the health of somatization disorder patients: effectiveness of short-term group therapy. Psychosomatics 36:462–470, 1995

Kato K, Sullivan PF, Evengård B, et al: Chronic widespread pain and its comorbidities: a population-based study. Arch Intern Med 166:1649–1654, 2006

Kato K, Sullivan PF, Evengard B, et al: A population-based twin study of functional somatic syndromes. Psychol Med 39:497–505, 2009

Katon W, Ries RK, Kleinman A: The prevalence of somatization in primary care. Compr Psychiatry 25:208–215, 1984

Katon W, Lin E, Von Korff M, et al: Somatization: a spectrum of severity. Am J Psychiatry 148:34–40, 1991

Katon W, Lin EH, Kroenke K: The association of depression and anxiety with medical symptom burden in patients with chronic medical illness. Gen Hosp Psychiatry 29:147–155, 2007

Kellner R: Somatization and Hypochondriasis. New York, Praeger, 1986

Kellner R, Slocumb J, Wiggins RG, et al: Hostility, somatic symptoms and hypochondriacal fears and beliefs. J Nerv Ment Dis 173:554–560, 1985

Kellner R, Fava GA, Lisansky J, et al: Hypochondriacal fears and beliefs in DSM-III melancholia: changes with amitriptyline. J Affect Disord 10:21–26, 1986

Kendler KS, Walters EE, Truett KR, et al: A twin-family study of self-report symptoms of panic-phobia and somatization. Behav Genet 25:499–515, 1995

Kirmayer LJ, Robbins JM (eds): Current Concepts of Somatization: Research and Clinical Perspectives. Washington, DC, American Psychiatric Press, 1991

Kirmayer LJ, Robbins JM: Patients who somatize in primary care: a longitudinal study of cognitive and social characteristics. Psychol Med 26:937–951, 1996

Kirmayer LJ, Young A: Culture and somatization: clinical, epidemiological and ethnographic perspectives. Psychosom Med 60:420–430, 1998

Kirmayer LJ, Robbins JM, Dworkind M, et al: Somatization and the recognition of depression and anxiety in primary care. Am J Psychiatry 150:734–741, 1993

Kleinman A: Social Origins of Distress and Disease: Depression, Neurasthenia, and Pain in Modern China. New Haven, CT, Yale University Press, 1986

Kroenke K: Patients presenting with somatic complaints: epidemiology, psychiatric comorbidity and management. Int J Methods Psychiatr Res 12:34–43, 2003

Kroenke K: Efficacy of treatment for somatoform disorders: a review of randomized controlled trials. Psychosom Med 69:881–888, 2007

Kroenke K, Spitzer RL, deGruy FV, et al: Multisomatoform disorder: an alternative to undifferentiated somatoform disorder for the somatizing patient in primary care. Arch Gen Psychiatry 54:352–358, 1997

Kroenke K, Spitzer RL, Williams JB: The PHQ-15: validity of a new measure for evaluating the severity of somatic symptoms. Psychosom Med 64:258–266, 2002

Kroenke K, Messina N 3rd, Benattia I, et al: Venlafaxine extended release in the short-term treatment of depressed and anxious primary care patients with multisomatoform disorder. J Clin Psychiatry 67:72–80, 2006

Kroenke K, Sharpe M, Sykes R: Revising the classification of somatoform disorders: key questions and preliminary recommendations. Psychosomatics 48:277–285, 2007

Lackner JM, Gudleski GD, Blanchard EB: Beyond abuse: the association among parenting style, abdominal pain, and somatization in IBS patients. Behav Res Ther 42:41–56, 2004

Levine JB, Irving KK, Brooks JD, et al: Group therapy and the somatoform patient: an integration. Psychotherapy 30:625–634, 1993

Lieb R, Meinlschmidt G, Araya R: Epidemiology of the association between somatoform disorders and anxiety and depressive disorders: an update. Psychosom Med 69:860–863, 2007

Lieb R, Pfister H, Mastaler M, et al: Somatoform syndromes and disorders in a representative population sample of adolescents and young adults: prevalence, comorbidity and impairments. Acta Psychiatr Scand 101:194–208, 2000

Lipowski ZJ: Somatization: the concept and its clinical application. Am J Psychiatry 145:1358–1368, 1988

Lipsitt DR: Medical and psychological characteristics of "crocks." Psychiatr Med 1:15–25, 1970

Liu G, Clark MR, Eaton WW: Structural factor analyses for medically unexplained somatic symptoms of somatization disorder in the Epidemiologic Catchment Area study. Psychol Med 27:617–626, 1997

Looper KJ, Kirmayer LJ: Behavioral medicine approaches to somatoform disorders. J Consult Clin Psychol 70:810–827, 2002

Lowe B, Spitzer RL, Williams JB, et al: Depression, anxiety and somatization in primary care: syndrome overlap and functional impairment. Gen Hosp Psychiatry 30:191–199, 2008

Mace CJ: Hysterical conversion, I: a history. Br J Psychiatry 161:369–377, 1992

Magallon R, Gili M, Moreno S, et al: Cognitive-behaviour therapy for patients with Abridged Somatization Disorder (SSI 4,6) in primary care: a randomized, controlled study. BMC Psychiatry 8:47, 2008

Marks I, Mishan J: Dysmorphophobic avoidance with disturbed bodily perception: a pilot study of exposure therapy. Br J Psychiatry 152:674–678, 1988

Martin RL: Diagnostic issues for conversion disorder. Hosp Community Psychiatry 43:771–773, 1992

Mayou R: Illness behavior and psychiatry. Gen Hosp Psychiatry 11:307–312, 1989

Mayou R: Somatization. Psychother Psychosom 59:69–83, 1993

Mayou R, Levenson J, Sharpe M: Somatoform disorders in DSM-V. Psychosomatics 44:449–451, 2003

McBeth J, Silman AJ: The role of psychiatric disorders in fibromyalgia. Curr Rheumatol Rep 3:157–164, 2001

McDougall J: Theaters of the Body: A Psychoanalytic Approach to Psychosomatic Illness. New York, WW Norton, 1989

Mechanic D: The concept of illness behaviour: culture, situation and personal predisposition. Psychol Med 16:1–7, 1986

Mehrabian A: General relations among drug use, alcohol use, and major indexes of psychopathology. J Psychol 135:71–86, 2001

Moene FC, Landberg EH, Hoogduin KAL: Organic syndromes diagnosed as conversion disorder: identification and frequency in a study of 85 patients. J Psychosom Res 46:7–12, 2000

Moene FC, Spinhoven P, Hoogduin KA, et al: A randomized controlled clinical trial of a hypnosis-based treatment for patients with conversion disorder, motor type. Int J Clin Exp Hypn 51:29–50, 2003

Moreau C, Zisook S: Rationale for a posttraumatic stress spectrum disorder. Psychiatr Clin North Am 25:775–790, 2002

Morrison J: Childhood sexual histories of women with somatization disorder. Am J Psychiatry 146:239–241, 1989

Muller JE, Wentzel I, Koen L, et al: Escitalopram in the treatment of multisomatoform disorder: a double-blind, placebo-controlled trial. Int Clin Psychopharmacol 23:43–48, 2008

Murphy MR: Classification of the somatoform disorders, in Somatization: Physical Symptoms and Psychological Illness. Edited by Bass C. Boston, MA, Blackwell Scientific, 1990, pp 10–39

Nakao M, Barsky AJ: Clinical application of somatosensory amplification in psychosomatic medicine. Biopsychosoc Med 1:17, 2007

Newman NJ: Neuro-ophthalmology and psychiatry. Gen Hosp Psychiatry 15:102–114, 1993

Noyes R Jr, Kathol RG, Fisher MM, et al: The validity of DSM-III-R hypochondriasis. Arch Gen Psychiatry 50:961–970, 1993

Noyes R Jr, Happel RL, Muller BA, et al: Fluvoxamine for somatoform disorders: an open trial. Gen Hosp Psychiatry 20:339–344, 1998

Noyes R Jr, Stuart SP, Langbehn DR, et al: Test of an interpersonal model of hypochondriasis. Psychosom Med 65:292–300, 2003

Pennebaker JW, Watson D: The psychology of somatic symptoms, in Current Concepts of Somatization: Research and Clinical Perspectives. Edited by Kirmayer LJ, Robbins JM. Washington, DC, American Psychiatric Press, 1991, pp 21–36

Oken D: Evolution of psychosomatic diagnosis in DSM. Psychosom Med 69:830–831, 2007

Olatunji BO, Deacon BJ, Abramowitz JS: Is hypochondriasis an anxiety disorder? Br J Psychiatry 194:481–482, 2009

Otto MW, Wilhelm S, Cohen LS, et al: Prevalence of body dysmorphic disorder in a community sample of women. Am J Psychiatry 158:2061–2063, 2001

Page LA, Wessely S: Medically unexplained symptoms: exacerbating factors in the doctor-patient encounter. J R Soc Med 96:223–227, 2003

Pauli P, Alpers GW: Memory bias in patients with hypochondriasis and somatoform pain disorder. J Psychosom Res 52:45–53, 2002

Phillips KA: Body dysmorphic disorder: clinical aspects and treatment strategies. Bull Menninger Clin 62 (4 suppl A):A33–A48, 1998

Phillips KA: Quality of life for patients with body dysmorphic disorder. J Nerv Ment Dis 188:170–175, 2000

Phillips KA: Body dysmorphic disorder, in Somatoform and Factitious Disorders (Review of Psychiatry Series, Vol 20, No 3; Oldham JM and Riba MB, series eds). Edited by Phillips KA. Washington, DC, American Psychiatric Press, 2001, pp 67–94

Phillips KA, Diaz SF: Gender differences in body dysmorphic disorder. J Nerv Ment Dis 185:570–577, 1997

Phillips KA, Stout RL: Associations in the longitudinal course of body dysmorphic disorder with major depression, obsessive-compulsive disorder, and social phobia. J Psychiatr Res 40:360–369, 2006

Phillips KA, McElroy SL, Keck PE, et al: Body dysmorphic disorder: 30 cases of imagined ugliness. Am J Psychiatry 150:302–308, 1993

Phillips KA, McElroy SL, Keck PE, et al: A comparison of delusional and nondelusional body dysmorphic disorder in 100 cases. Psychopharmacol Bull 30:179–186, 1994

Phillips KA, Albertini RS, Siniscalchi JM: Effectiveness of pharmacotherapy for body dysmorphic disorder: a chart-review study. J Clin Psychiatry 62:721–727, 2001a

Phillips KA, Grant J, Siniscalchi J, et al: Surgical and nonpsychiatric medical treatment of patients with body dysmorphic disorder. Psychosomatics 42:504–510, 2001b

Phillips KA, Albertini RS, Rasmussen SA: A randomized placebo-controlled trial of fluoxetine in body dysmorphic disorder. Arch Gen Psychiatry 59:381–388, 2002

Phillips KA, Price LH, Greenberg BD, et al: Should the DSM diagnostic groupings be changed? in Advancing DSM: Dilemmas in Psychiatric Diagnosis. Edited by Phillips KA, First MB, Pincus HA. Washington, DC, American Psychiatric Association, 2003, pp 57–84

Phillips KA, Quinn G, Stout RL: Functional impairment in body dysmorphic disorder: a prospective, follow-up study. J Psychiatr Res 42:701–707, 2008

Piccinelli M, Simon G: Gender and cross-cultural differences in somatic symptoms associated with emotional distress. An international study in primary care. Psychol Med 27:433–444, 1997

Pilowsky I: Abnormal illness behavior. Psychiatr Med 5:85–91, 1987

Priel B, Rabinowitz B, Pels RJ: A semiotic perspective on chronic pain: implications for the interaction between patient and physician. Br J Med Psychol 64:65–71, 1991

Quill TE: Somatization disorder: one of medicine's blind spots. JAMA 254:3075–3079, 1985

Rief W, Hiller W: Somatization—future perspectives on a common phenomenon. J Psychosom Res 44:529–536, 1998

Rief W, Hiller W: Toward empirically based criteria for classification of somatoform disorders. J Psychosom Res 46:507–518, 1999

Rief W, Rojas G: Stability of somatoform symptoms—implications for classification. Psychosom Med 69:864–869, 2007

Ritsner M: The attribution of somatization in schizophrenia patients: a naturalistic follow-up study. J Clin Psychiatry 64:1370–1378, 2003

Rodin G: Somatization and the self: psychotherapeutic issues. Am J Psychother 38:257–263, 1984

Roelofs K, Naring GW, Moene FC, et al: The question of symptom lateralization in conversion disorder. J Psychosom Res 49:21–25, 2000

Roelofs K, Keijsers GP, Hoogduin KA, et al: Childhood abuse in patients with conversion disorder. Am J Psychiatry 159:1908–1913, 2002

Rost KM, Akins RN, Brown FW, et al: The comorbidity of DSM-III-R personality disorders in somatization disorder. Gen Hosp Psychiatry 14:322–326, 1992

Salkovskis PM: Somatic problems, in Cognitive Behaviour Therapy for Psychiatric Problems. Edited by Hawton K, Salkovskis PM, Kirk J, et al. New York, Oxford University Press, 1989, pp 235–276

Salmon P, Peters S, Stanley I: Patients' perceptions of medical explanations for somatisation disorders: qualitative analysis. BMJ 318:372–376, 1999

Salmon P, Skaife K, Rhodes J: Abuse, dissociation, and somatization in irritable bowel syndrome: towards an explanatory model. J Behav Med 26:1–18, 2003

Sarwer DB, Crerand CE, Didie ER: Body dysmorphic disorder in cosmetic surgery patients. Facial Plast Surg 19:7–17, 2003

Sayar K, Kirmayer LJ, Taillefer SS: Predictors of somatic symptoms in depressive disorder. Gen Hosp Psychiatry 25:108–114, 2003

Sharpe M: Medically unexplained symptoms and syndromes. Clin Med 2:501–504, 2002

Sharpe M, Bass C: Pathophysiological mechanisms in somatization. Int Rev Psychiatry 4:81–97, 1992

Sharpe M, Carson A: "Unexplained" somatic symptoms, functional syndromes, and somatization: do we need a paradigm shift? Ann Intern Med 134:926–930, 2001

Sharpe M, Peveler R, Mayou R: The psychological treatment of patients with functional somatic symptoms: a practical guide. J Psychosom Res 36:515–529, 1992

Sharpe M, Mayou R, Seagroatt V, et al: Why do doctors find some patients difficult to help? Q J Med 87:187–193, 1994

Sharpe M, Stone J, Hibberd C, et al: Neurology out-patients with symptoms unexplained by disease: illness beliefs and financial benefits predict 1-year outcome. Psychol Med 40:689–698, 2010

Silber TJ, Pao M: Somatization disorders in children and adolescents. Pediatr Rev 24:255–264, 2003

Simon GE: Somatization and psychiatric disorders, in Current Concepts of Somatization: Research and Clinical Perspectives. Edited by Kirmayer LJ, Robbins JM. Washington, DC, American Psychiatric Press, 1991, pp 37–62

Simon GE, Gureje O: Stability of somatization disorder and somatization symptoms among primary care patients. Arch Gen Psychiatry 56:90–95, 1999

Simon G, Gater R, Kisely S, et al: Somatic symptoms of distress: an international primary care study. Psychosom Med 58:481–488, 1996

Simon GE, VonKorff M, Piccinelli M, et al: An international study of the relation between somatic symptoms and depression. N Engl J Med 341:1329–1335, 1999

Simon GE, Gureje O, Fullerton C: Course of hypochondriasis in an international primary care study. Gen Hosp Psychiatry 23:51–55, 2001

Slater E, Glithero E: A follow-up of patients diagnosed as suffering from "hysteria." J Psychosom Res 9:9–13, 1965

Smith GC, Clarke DM, Handrinos D, et al: Consultation-liaison psychiatrists' management of somatoform disorders. Psychosomatics 41:481–489, 2000

Smith GR: Somatization Disorder in Medical Settings. Washington, DC, American Psychiatric Press, 1991

Smith GR: The epidemiology and treatment of depression when it coexists with somatoform disorders, somatization, or pain. Gen Hosp Psychiatry 14:265–272, 1992

Stahl SM: Antidepressants and somatic symptoms: therapeutic actions are expanding beyond affective spectrum disorders to functional somatic syndrome. J Clin Psychiatry 64:745–746, 2003

Starcevic V, Kellner R, Uhlenhuth EH, et al: Panic disorder and hypochondriacal fears and beliefs. J Affect Disord 24:73–85, 1992

Stone J, Sharpe M, Carson A, et al: Are functional motor and sensory symptoms really more frequent on the left? A systematic review. J Neurol Neurosurg Psychiatry 73:578–581, 2002a

Stone J, Wojcik W, Durrance D, et al: What should we say to patients with symptoms unexplained by disease? The "number needed to offend." BMJ 325:1449–1450, 2002b

Stone J, Campbell K, Sharma N, et al: What should we call pseudoseizures? The patient's perspective. Seizure 12:568–572, 2003

Stone J, Durrance D, Wojcik W, et al: What do medical outpatients attending a neurology clinic think about antidepressants? J Psychosom Res 56:293–295, 2004

Stone J, Smyth R, Carson A, et al: Systematic review of misdiagnosis of conversion symptoms and "hysteria." BMJ 331:989, 2005

Stone J, Smyth R, Carson A, et al: La belle indifference in conversion symptoms and hysteria: systematic review. Br J Psychiatry 188:204–209, 2006

Stuart S, Noyes R: Attachment and interpersonal communication in somatization. Psychosomatics 40:34–43, 1999

Sullivan M, Clark MR, Katon WJ, et al: Psychiatric and otologic diagnoses in patients complaining of dizziness. Arch Intern Med 153:1479–1484, 1993

Sumathipala A, Siribaddana S, Abeysingha MR, et al: Cognitive-behavioural therapy v. structured care for medically unexplained symptoms: randomised controlled trial. Br J Psychiatry 193:51–59, 2008

Taylor GJ: Recent developments in alexithymia theory and research. Can J Psychiatry 45:134–142, 2000

Thomassen R, van Hemert AM, Huyse FJ, et al: Somatoform disorders in consultation-liaison psychiatry: a comparison with other mental disorders. Gen Hosp Psychiatry 25:8–13, 2003

Thomson AB, Page LA: Psychotherapies for hypochondriasis. Cochrane Database Syst Rev (4):CD006520, 2007

Toone BK: Disorders of hysterical conversion, in Somatization: Physical Symptoms and Psychological Illness. Edited by Bass C. Boston, MA, Blackwell Scientific, 1990, pp 207–234

Tyrer P, Fowler-Dixon R, Ferguson B, et al: A plea for the diagnosis of hypochondriacal personality disorder. J Psychosom Res 34:637–642, 1990

Uzun O, Basoglu C, Akar A, et al: Body dysmorphic disorder in patients with acne. Compr Psychiatry 44:415–419, 2003

Van Dyck R, Hoogduin K: Hypnosis and conversion disorders. Am J Psychother 43:480–493, 1989

van Ravesteijn H, Wittkampf K, Lucassen P, et al: Detecting somatoform disorders in primary care with the PHQ-15. Ann Fam Med 7:232–238, 2009

Veale D, Boocock A, Gournay K, et al: Body dysmorphic disorder. A survey of fifty cases. Br J Psychiatry 169:196–201, 1996

Veale D, De Haro L, Lambrou C: Cosmetic rhinoplasty in body dysmorphic disorder. Br J Plast Surg 56:546–551, 2003

Vinkers DJ, van Rood YR, van der Wee NJ: [Prevalence and comorbidity of body dysmorphic disorder in psychiatric outpatients]. Tijdschr Psychiatr 50:559–565, 2008

Visser S, Bouman TK: Cognitive-behavioural approaches in the treatment of hypochondriasis: six single case cross-over studies. Behav Res Ther 30:301–306, 1992

Visser S, Bouman TK: The treatment of hypochondriasis: exposure plus response prevention vs cognitive therapy. Behav Res Ther 39:423–442, 2001

Volz HP, Moller HJ, Reimann I, et al: Opipramol for the treatment of somatoform disorders results from a placebo-controlled trial. Eur Neuropsychopharmacol 10:211–217, 2000

Walker J, Vincent N, Furer P, et al: Treatment preference in hypochondriasis. J Behav Ther Exp Psychiatry 30:251–258, 1999

Walling MK, O'Hara MW, Reiter RC, et al: Abuse history and chronic pain in women, II: a multivariate analysis of abuse and psychological morbidity. Obstet Gynecol 84:200–206, 1994

Warwick H: Provision of appropriate and effective reassurance. Int Rev Psychiatry 4:76–80, 1992

Warwick HMC, Marks IM: Behavioural treatment of illness phobia and hypochondriasis: a pilot study of 17 cases. Br J Psychiatry 152:239–241, 1988

Woolfolk RL, Allen LA, Tiu JE: New directions in the treatment of somatization. Psychiatr Clin North Am 30:621–644, 2007

Young L: Sexual abuse and the problem of embodiment. Child Abuse Negl 16:89–100, 1992

Yutzy SH, Cloninger CR, Guze SB, et al: DSM-IV field trial: testing a new proposal for somatization disorder. Am J Psychiatry 152:97–101, 1995

Zimmerman M, Mattia JI: Body dysmorphic disorder in psychiatric outpatients: recognition, prevalence, comorbidity, demographic, and clinical correlates. Compr Psychiatry 39:265–270, 1998

CHAPTER

13

Deception Syndromes

Factitious Disorders and Malingering

Charles V. Ford, M.D.

> Disease has been simulated in every age, and by all classes of society. The monarch, the mendicant, the unhappy slave, the proud warrior, the lofty statesman, even the minister of religion as well as the condemned malefactor and boy "creeping like a snail unwillingly to school," have sought to disguise their purposes, or obtain their desires, by feigning mental or bodily infirmities.
>
> Gavin 1838, p. i

THE ABOVE INTRODUCTORY PARAGRAPH to Hector Gavin's 1838 book *On the Feigned and Factitious Diseases of Soldiers and Seamen,* in which he described clinical features of factitious disorders and malingering, indicates the pervasiveness of simulated disease. Also noteworthy is that in the second century A.D., the Roman physician Galen devoted a chapter to simulated disease in one of his medical texts (Adams 1846).

In the current diagnostic classification, that of DSM-IV-TR (American Psychiatric Association 2000), simulated diseases such as somatization disorder are placed within the category of *somatoform disorders.* These disorders are considered to be of unconscious etiology. *Factitious disorders,* considered to be of conscious production but of unconscious motivation, are included among Axis I diagnoses in a separate category. *Malingering,* considered to be of both conscious production and motivation, is assigned a V code. Imprecise criteria (e.g., conscious vs. unconscious motivation) are bound to result in imprecise diagnoses, and in fact illness behavior is frequently motivated by a variety of conscious and unconscious objectives. Furthermore, a person may feign illness to achieve different goals at different times (Eisendrath 1996). Thus, an originally unconsciously motivated symptom may evolve into a consciously driven symptom so that the patient may achieve secondary gains.

Anticipation of the development and publication of new diagnostic criteria and categories of DSM-V (work in progress) has generated debate within the medical community regarding factitious disorders. Some authors (Bass and Halligan 2007; Ford 2005; Turner 2006) have proposed that factitious disease production is a syndrome of misbehavior, while others (Hamilton et al. 2009; Krahn et al. 2008) note its similarities to somatization disorder and advocate maintaining factitious disorder as an Axis I diagnosis. The draft proposed DSM-V criteria for *factitious disorder on self* and *factitious disorder imposed on another* (previously, factitious disorder by proxy) places these disorders within a new category, Somatic Symptom Disorders. The proposed criteria for *factitious disorder on self* require "a pattern of falsification of physical or psychological signs or symptoms associated with identified deception" and state that "this pattern of presentation to others as ill or impaired is evident even in the absence of obvious external rewards." Exclusion criteria are that the behavior is neither due to an acute psychosis or delusional belief system nor better accounted for by another mental disorder. The proposed criteria for *factitious disorder imposed on another* are the same, except that there is the presentation of another person (the victim) to others as ill or impaired (Dimsdale and Creed 2009).

Illness behavior includes a wide continuum of symptoms and motivations. At one extreme are behaviors that might be considered normal in view of their commonality, such as using a complaint of a physical symptom (e.g., a headache) to avoid some undesired social obligation. In this chapter, I focus on the other extreme of consciously initiated illness behavior: factitious disorders and malingering. As noted earlier, the primary difference between these two forms of illness behavior is the perceived role of conscious versus unconscious motivation. Such a distinction is useful for textbook descriptions, but unfortunately in actual clinical situations the determination of motivation becomes a highly subjective process. A complicating factor is the unreliability of information provided by persons who are, by definition, deceptive.

There are two primary forms of factitious behavior. The first is self-induced or simulated disease, known at times by the eponym Munchausen syndrome, and the second is factitious disease induced or simulated in others, also commonly known as Munchausen syndrome by proxy. Although these two forms of factitious illness overlap at certain points, they are discussed separately here to provide clarity on various important clinical and legal issues. Malingering, not a medical diagnosis per se, is discussed separately from the factitious disorders.

Interest in factitious disorders has increased markedly since the publication of Richard Asher's seminal paper in 1951. As of 2010, there are more than 2,500 publications in the medical literature focused on factitious disorders. There have been descriptions of several other syndromes related to factitious disorder, such as factitious allegations of sexual abuse (Feldman et al. 1994; Feldman-Schorrig 1996; Gibbon 1998), the "angel of death" syndrome (Yorker et al. 2006) (in which a nurse creates emergency situations in his or her patients), and even production of disease in one's pets (Munro and Thrusfield 2001). There are increasing reports of the use of the Internet to obtain medical information and even download medical reports to present as one's own (Levenson et al. 2007). Persons also may assume a false identity to enter chat rooms and support groups for chronic diseases (Feldman 2000).

Hardie and Reed (1998) described the overlaps in characteristics of persons who have pseudologia fantastica (Table 13–1), create factitious disorders, and engage in impostorship. They proposed the term *deception syndrome* to describe these syndromes—a concept that would provide more unity than does the current tendency to create increasing numbers of new syndromes and eponyms.

TABLE 13–1. Pseudologia fantastica

A form of pathological lying characterized by
Matrix of fact and fiction
Enduring repetitive quality
Presentation of the storyteller in a grandiose manner and/or as a victim
The syndrome is often associated with
Cognitive dysfunction
Learning disabilities
Factitious disorders
Childhood traumatic experiences

Factitious Disorders

Persons who have factitious disorders intentionally feign, exaggerate, aggravate, or self-induce symptoms or disease. They are conscious of their behaviors, although the underlying motivation may be unconscious. By convention, this diagnosis is also characterized by the surreptitious nature of the behavior. Patients who acknowledge that they have produced their own self-harm (e.g., self-mutilators) are not included in this diagnostic group. Inherent in factitious disorders is a paradox: the patient presents to a physician or other health care provider with the request for medical care but simultaneously conceals the known cause of the problem.

Risk factors for factitious disorder vary according to the subtype of the clinical syndrome. The most common subtype is common factitious disorder (or nonperegrinating factitious disorder), in which the person does not use aliases or travel from hospital to hospital. In this syndrome, female gender, unmarried status, age in the 30s, prior work or experience in the health care professions (e.g., nursing), and Cluster B personality disorders with borderline features are frequently found. For full-blown Munchausen syndrome, in which the patient uses aliases and travels from hospital to hospital (and often from state to state), risk factors include male gender, single marital status, age often in the 40s, and a personality disorder of the Cluster B type with at least some antisocial features. In their review of 93 cases of factitious disorder diagnosed at the Mayo Clinic, Krahn et al. (2003) found that 72% were women, of whom 65.7% had some association with health-related occupations. The mean age for women was 30.7 years, and the mean age for men was 40.0 years.

Few epidemiological data are available for factitious disorders. An Italian community study found a lifetime prevalence of 0.1% (Faravelli et al. 2004). Most investigators believe that factitious disorder is a relatively uncommon but not extremely rare disorder. For example, Sutherland and Rodin (1990) noted that 10 of 1,288 psychiatric consultations at a large teaching hospital in Toronto, Ontario, included a diagnosis of factitious disorder. A similar percentage of 0.6% was reported for a German university hospital psychiatric consultation service (Kapfhammer et al. 1998). These differing methods of determining incidence reflect a very large range. If the number of diagnoses established by psychiatric consultation is used as an estimate, then—with the assumption that no more than 1 in 10 medical inpatients is seen in psychiatric consultation—the incidence would be less than 1 in 10,000 admissions to medical-surgical services. However, many patients with factitious disorder may successfully evade detection and thereby go through the system undiagnosed.

Clinical Features: Phenomenology, Course, and Prognosis

Self-induced factitious disorders fit into two major syndromes. Unfortunately, the terminology in the general medical literature is inconsistent, and the terms *Munchausen syndrome* and *factitious disorder* are often used interchangeably (Fink and Jensen 1989). In this chapter, *Munchausen syndrome* refers specifically to the subtype of factitious disorders originally described by Richard Asher in 1951.

Classic Munchausen syndrome consists of three essential components: the simulation or self-induction of disease, pseudologia fantastica, and travel from hospital to hospital, often using aliases to disguise identity. These patients frequently present in the emergency department with dramatic symptoms such as hemoptysis, acute chest pain suggesting a myocardial infarction, or coma from self-induced hypoglycemia. Munchausen patients may make a career out of illness and hospitalizations; as many as 423 separate hospitalizations for an individual patient have been reported (von Maurer et al. 1973).

The types of symptoms and different diseases that have been simulated defy the imagination (Table 13-2). Essentially every subspecialty journal has published case reports of self-induced illness related to that particular subspecialty. Among the most common presentations have been chest pain, endocrine disorders such as hyperthyroidism or Cushing's syndrome, coagulopathies, infections, and neurological symptoms. The Munchausen patient often presents during evening or weekend hours, presumably in order to be evaluated by less senior or experienced clinicians. The patient is frequently admitted to an inpatient service, where he or she may become the "star patient" in view of the dramatic nature of the symptoms or the rarity of the presumed diagnosis. In addition, the patient may call attention to himself or herself by providing false information such as claiming to be a former professional football player, a recipient of the Medal of Honor, or perhaps the president of a foreign university. Despite such reputed prominence, these patients and their physicians rarely receive telephone calls from concerned family members or friends. The Munchausen patient is usually willing to undergo multiple diagnostic studies. When inconsistencies in history, medical findings, or laboratory examinations create suspicions, caregivers often become more confrontational. At this point, the patient generally responds with irritation, new complaints, disruptive behavior, or threats to file a lawsuit. He or she may request discharge against medical advice or may simply disappear. Embarrassed and angry clinicians on the treatment team may console themselves by preparing a case presentation for grand rounds or perhaps for publication.

Munchausen syndrome is the most dramatic form of factitious behavior, and the eponym certainly has great popularity, but much more frequently seen is what has been termed *common factitious disorder*. In this syndrome, the patient does not use aliases and tends to seek treatment repetitively with the same physician or within the same health system. She may carry a diagnosis—which, on careful reflection, was made with imprecise criteria—such as a bleeding coagulopathy or a collagen disease. In retrospect, when the true diagnosis is discovered, it can be determined that the history, both medical and personal, was inaccurate. These patients are not, however, as inclined to pseudologia fantastica as are patients with full-blown Munchausen syndrome.

Symptoms and signs for patients with common factitious disorder tend to be less dramatic, and their complaints are often more chronic or subjective. Some common symptoms include joint pain, recurrent abscesses, failure to heal following operations, hypoglycemic episodes, simulated renal colic, and blood dyscrasias. Factitious disorder as a cause for these patients' symptoms may not be suspected for months or even years. When the diagnosis is finally established, there may be disbelief among the medical care providers. "Splitting" behavior, in which the patient plays one group of providers against another group, is frequently seen.

Factitious Disorder With Psychological Symptoms

The large majority of published cases of factitious disorder describe physical symptoms alone. When factitious psychological symptoms are recognized, they are generally in association with either authentic or fabricated physical complaints. The reason for this may be that subspecialists in psychosomatic medicine are more likely to encounter patients with factitious psychological symptoms who are hospitalized on medical-surgical wards, or in the emer-

TABLE 13–2. Examples of factitious diseases

Symptom/disease	Method of production	Diagnostic clue
Infections	Injections of saliva or feces	Polymicrobial cultures
Hypoglycemic coma	Self-injection of insulin	Low C-peptide
	Oral hypoglycemic agents	Glyburide in urine
Fever of unexplained etiology[a]	Manipulation of thermometer	Dissociation of fever/pulse
Neurological disease	Anisocoria secondary to anticholinergic eyedrops	Variable reactivity of pupils
Diarrhea	Laxative abuse	Laxative in stool
Pheochromocytoma	Epinephrine in urine	Low blood chromogranin A
Electrolyte imbalance	Diuretics	High urinary potassium
Vomiting	Ipecac	Increased urinary potassium with low chloride
Coagulopathies	Warfarin	Serum assay
Anemia	Self-bloodletting	No bleeding site or iron malabsorption
Pancytopenia	Methotrexate	Serum assay
Proteinuria	Egg white in urine	Large daily variations of urine protein
Purpura	Quinidine	Serum or urinary assay
Hyperthyroidism	Exogenous thyroid	Low serum thyroglobulin
Hematuria	Finger-prick blood to urine	

[a]Now uncommon because of the use of instantaneous electronic thermometers.
Source. Adapted from Wallach 1994.

gency department, than to see such patients on psychiatric units. One study of Spanish psychiatric inpatients found that 8% had factitious symptoms (Catalina et al. 2008). These were interpreted as largely being exaggeration or invention of symptoms to find support, social relationships, and safety in the hospital. Patients with factitious psychological symptoms fabricate a wide range of symptoms. The most commonly reported include depression and suicidal thinking tied to claims of bereavement (Phillips et al. 1983; Snowden et al. 1978). The patient reports that his or her emotional distress is due to the death of someone close such as a parent or child. Distress appears genuine, is often accompanied by tears, and characteristically elicits sympathy from medical personnel. Later, staff members may discover that the mourned person is very much alive, that the circumstances of the death were less dramatic than the patient reported, or that the death was many years in the past. Case reports of factitious psychological symptoms also describe feigned multiple personality disorder, substance dependence, dissociative and conversion reactions, memory loss, and posttraumatic stress disorder. Multiple feigned psychological symptoms may be present in the same patient (Parker 1993). Some authors urge caution in diagnosing factitious disorder with predominantly psychological symptoms, especially factitious psychosis, because some patients with these symptoms eventually manifest clear-cut severe mental illness (Nicholson and Roberts 1994; Rogers et al. 1989).

Ganser's syndrome is closely related to factitious disorder, with predominantly psychological symptoms (Wirtz et al. 2008). This syndrome is characterized by the provision of approximate answers (*Vorbeireden*) to questions (e.g., the examiner asks, "What is the color of snow?" and the patient answers, "Green"). Complaints of amnesia, disorientation, and perceptual disturbance are generally present as well. This syndrome was originally described by the nineteenth-century German psychiatrist Sigbert Ganser (1965) as a form of malingering seen in prisoners, but it also has been described in other settings, including general hospital units (Dalfen and Anthony 2000; Weiner and Braiman 1955). Ganser's syndrome was described in one patient who also had clear-cut factitious physical and psychological symptoms (Parker 1993). The etiology of this syndrome remains in question, and malingering, dissociation, and organic brain disease (Sigal et al. 1992) have been proposed as contributing factors.

When the patient presents with both physical and psychological factitious symptoms and neither predominates, the appropriate diagnosis is factitious disorder with combined physical and psychological symptoms. The aforementioned case reported by Parker (1993) included pseudodementia (Ganser's syndrome), feigned bereavement, factitious rape, pseudoseizures, and simulated renal failure.

The prognosis of patients with factitious symptoms is unclear. Some patients may, at some point in their life, abandon their behavior. Death, probably as a result of the patient's miscalculations of the risk of the behavior, also has been reported (Eisendrath and McNeil 2004; Nichols et al. 1990).

Diagnosis and Assessment

The diagnosis of factitious disorder may be suggested by inconsistent laboratory results, physical findings that do not conform to reported symptoms, failure to respond as predicted to effective treatment for the disorder in question, or, most frequently, the accidental discovery of medical paraphernalia on the patient's person or in the room. For example, a syringe may be found taped onto the inside portion of a toilet lid or a nurse may come into a patient's room unannounced and find the patient digging in a surgical wound with a foreign body. Ultimately, the diagnosis of factitious disorder is made via detective work by health care providers who have a high index of suspicion. A review of past medical records from other institutions may be essential to establish the diagnosis (Krahn et al. 2003). On the surface the patient may appear normal, and a psychiatric interview per se cannot establish the diagnosis unless there is a "confession." The patient, even when confronted with irrefutable evidence of factitious behavior, typically denies that the illness was self-induced.

The differential diagnosis of factitious disorder includes unusual, rare, or as-yet undescribed and unknown diseases; somatoform disorders; and overt malingering.

Etiology

The reasons that a person might engage in factitious illness behavior are to a large extent speculative. Even when seen in long-term treatment, these patients are resistant to articulating their motivations. Furthermore, the essential quality of these persons—the need to deceive—creates a question of validity. Proposed underlying motivations are outlined in Table 13–3.

TABLE 13–3. Proposed motivations for factitious disorder

Need to be the center of attention
Longing to be cared for
Maladaptive reaction to loss or separation
Anger at physicians or displaced onto physicians
Pleasure derived from deceiving others ("duping delight")

The large majority of patients with factitious disorder have an underlying severe personality disorder, usually of the Cluster B type. Factitious behavior can be seen as a form of acting out, similar to other acting-out behaviors seen in Cluster B personality disorders. Axis I comorbidity, including major depression and schizophrenia, has been described but is not common. However, it must be kept in mind that psychiatric symptoms also may be simulated.

Few patients have been extensively studied with regard to developmental history because very few will agree to see a psychotherapist, and even fewer open up honestly. In the very select few who have, a childhood history of parental illness, death, or abandonment, or personal illness or institutionalization, is common (Ford 1973). As a result of these childhood experiences, factitious behavior may be viewed, at least in some circumstances, as a learned coping mechanism.

The possible role of cerebral dysfunction for at least some patients has been proposed. Pankratz and Lezak (1987) reported that approximately one-third of the Munchausen patients in their series had deficits in conceptual organization. Abnormal findings on brain imaging also have been reported (Babe et al. 1992; Fenelon et al. 1991). Brain dysfunction also has been reported in approximately 20%–25% of persons with pseudologia fantastica and/or Munchausen syndrome (Ford 1996; King and Ford 1988).

Management and Treatment

In the past, it was suggested that blacklists should be created, disseminated, and maintained at various hospitals to identify Munchausen patients when they present for care (Mohammed et al. 1985). A variant of this concept for an individual hospital is to mark the old chart in some conspicuous manner to identify the patient when he or she presents to an emergency department. Such blacklists have found disfavor in the United States largely because of legal and ethical concerns and would be considered a violation of regulations under the Health Insurance Portability and Accountability Act of 1996 (P.L. 104-191). However, identification of past factitious illness behavior is facilitated in systems with a common electronic medical record (e.g., U.S. Department of Veterans Affairs). Diagnosis of a factitious disorder by use of an electronic medical record (EMR) search was reported by Van Dinter and Welch (2009). These authors emphasized the importance of attention to legal and ethical issues in reviews of EMRs.

A major question in management is how to deal with a patient once a definitive diagnosis of factitious disorder has been established. No matter how understandable the anger at these deceptive patients might be, the temptation to "let them have it" must be resisted. To act out in an angry way only plays into the patient's pathology by drawing the physician into a dramatized scene. A direct, accusative confrontation is likely to result in anger from the patient and in his or her subsequent departure from the hospital, often against medical advice, or with threats to bring a lawsuit for defamation. It has been suggested that the confrontation be more indirect, in a manner that allows face-saving for the patient or an opportunity for therapy. For example, a patient may be told, "When some patients are very upset, they often do something to themselves to create illness as a way of seeking help. We believe that something such as this must be going on, and we would like to help you focus on the true nature of your problem, which is emotional distress." Unfortunately, such an approach, although logical and humane, does not usually result in the patient's acknowledgment of factitious illness behavior and acceptance of psychological treatment.

When present, comorbid psychiatric disorders such as depression (if not believed to be also factitious) should be appropriately treated; in at least one case in the literature, remission of factitious behavior with antidepressant medication was reported (Earle and Folks 1986). Psychotherapy with the patient who engages in factitious behavior is, at best, extremely difficult. Treatment for these patients should be conceptualized essentially as being for a severe underlying personality disorder manifested by acting-out defenses. M.H. Stone (1977) proposed vigorous persistent confrontation of the behavior, but most clinicians who have had experience with these patients find that such confrontation results in abandonment of treatment or increase in acting-out behaviors. Instead of direct confrontation, the patient may be provided with indirect confrontation or interpretation in ongoing supportive psychotherapy (Eisendrath 2001). This technique is based on the premise that if the patient can maintain a relationship with a physician that is not contingent on development of new physical symptoms, factitious behavior may be reduced. Such a treatment approach must be viewed as primarily symptomatic with no expectation of changes in the basic personality structure that predisposes a person to factitious illness behavior. Experience with this type of treatment indicates that there may be remissions that last a few months but that they are often followed by the patient leaving treatment without warning and reengaging in factitious illness behavior elsewhere. A systematic review of all known published reports of the management and outcome of patients with diagnosed factitious disorder found no evidence for any effective treatment (Eastwood and Bisson 2008). A nonsignificant trend was that patients who had longer treatments had better outcomes.

In the medical care of patients with any somatizing disorder (including factitious illness and malingering), the physician should proceed with invasive diagnostic and treatment procedures only when objective evidence is available. Furthermore, physicians must be cautious when prescribing any potentially dangerous or habituating medication (Ford 1992).

Legal and ethical issues frequently arise in the assessment and treatment of patients with factitious disorder. In the past, the paternalistic model of medicine suggested that the physician was permitted to do essentially anything that would help establish the diagnosis. More recently, particularly in the United States, medical practice has emphasized patients' rights and informed consent. This creates a dilemma. On one hand, a failure to do all that is necessary to establish the diagnosis might be regarded as abdication of medical responsibility and ultimately harmful to the patient. On the other hand, even patients suspected of factitious behavior have rights to personal privacy, including privacy in one's belongings, confidentiality, and informed consent. One approach is to tell the patient that factitious illness behavior is suspected and request permission to rule this out. This has the risk of alienating a patient who does not have factitious illness. It may result in the patient with factitious disorder refusing permission, leaving the hospital, and perpetuating the same behavior at another medical facility.

Physicians may believe that the patient's outrageous behavior of factitious disease production would leave them free from the risk of malpractice suits. This is untrue, and there have been numerous reports of lawsuits initiated by these patients (Eisendrath and McNeil 2004; Janofsky 1994). The reasons for lawsuits may include overt greed, rage at a physician who was previously idealized (borderline behavior), or perhaps the opportunity to change one's highly dramatized role as a patient in a hospital to an equally dramatized role as a plaintiff in a courtroom.

Because patients with factitious disorder do create legal and ethical problems, it is prudent for the psychiatric consultant to suggest that the management plan require careful multidisciplinary collaboration and appropriate consultation with hospital administrators, hospital and personal attorneys, and the hospital ethics committee. It cannot be overemphasized that any decision to deviate from usual medical practice with such patients should not be made by a solitary individual. Such decisions should be carried out, and their rationale noted, with the patient's best interests at heart and should be documented in the chart. When factitious disorder is suspected, chart documentation in a factual, nonspeculative manner is highly recommended.

In view of these patients' self-destructive nature, many physicians, including psychiatrists, may question whether involuntary psychiatric hospitalization is indicated. Thresholds for involuntary commitment vary from state to state and from country to country. In the United States, because factitious disorder represents chronic behavior, which is not immediately suicidal, these patients usually do not meet the criteria for involuntary psychiatric hospitalization. In one case in Oregon, outpatient commitment resulted in lower medical costs and less iatrogenic morbidity for a patient with factitious disorder (McFarland et al. 1983).

Factitious Disorders by Proxy (Factitious Disorder Not Otherwise Specified)

In DSM-IV-TR, the diagnostic code *factitious disorder not otherwise specified* includes a variety of factitious diseases and symptoms described or induced by another person. This particular syndrome is far better known by the eponym Munchausen syndrome by proxy, and most case reports describe parents (particularly mothers) who have induced disease in their children. The appropriateness of the term *Munchausen by proxy* has been debated (Pankratz 2006). Some authors prefer terms such as *illness falsification,* whereas others prefer to describe the behavior simply as "child abuse." The latter removes any implication of motivation (Stirling 2007). There are, however, some reports of adults inducing disease in other adults, particularly when in a caregiver setting; for example, a nurse caring for a bedridden patient (Meadow 1998; Yorker 1996).

Munchausen syndrome by proxy is an invidious behavior that, when it involves children, should be considered a form of child abuse. The syndrome was initially described by Meadow (1977), who coined the term; subsequent to his initial report, there have been numerous reports from around the world, including non-Western cultures (Bappal et al. 2001).

The incidence of Munchausen syndrome by proxy is sufficiently high that children's hospitals see several cases per year. Denny et al. (2001) found the incidence in New Zealand to be 2.0 per 100,000 in children younger than 16 years. McClure et al. (1996) computed the annual incidence in the United Kingdom to be at least 2.8 per 100,000 for children younger than 1 year and 0.5 per 100,000 for those between ages 1 and 16 years.

Clinical Features: Phenomenology, Course, and Prognosis

The typical presentation of Munchausen syndrome by proxy is that of a child admitted to a hospital with symptoms such as seizures, bleeding, diarrhea, or respiratory difficulties (including apnea). The mother, who often has a history of some medical training, characteristically assists the nurses and readily consents to any invasive diagnostic procedures proposed for the child. Discovery of the mother's role in the production of the child's symptoms may occur accidentally, such as by finding her smothering the child with a pillow or introducing a toxic substance into the child's mouth or intravenous tubing. Suspicions also may arise if symptoms or episodes of the illness occur only when the mother is alone with the child, if another child in the family has had unexplained illnesses, or if the child's medical problems do not have a predictable response to appropriate treatment.

Sheridan (2003) reviewed and summarized published data from 451 cases of Munchausen syndrome by proxy. Her findings indicated no gender bias of the child victims, who were usually age 4 years or younger. In most of the situations, the perpetrator actively produced symptoms by smothering or poisoning the child, although some instances involved exaggeration or lying about symptoms. The most frequently noted symptoms of the child victims were, in order, apnea, anorexia, feeding problems, diarrhea, seizures, and cyanosis. The mortality rate for identified children victims was 6.0%, but 25% of known siblings were known to be dead! This implies a much higher mortality rate (than 6.0%) when the diagnosis is unrecognized. Other reports also have emphasized the high mortality rate associated with Munchausen syndrome by proxy (Bools et al. 1993; Rosenberg 1987).

Diagnosis and Assessment

The diagnosis of Munchausen by proxy should be assigned only after a careful consideration of differential diagnoses such as somatization by proxy (Table 13–4) because it is, in essence, an accusation of child abuse. As noted in the previous subsection, the diagnosis may become apparent by fortuitous findings such as the discovery of secret paraphernalia or drugs or the accidental observation of the mother smothering the child. However, when Munchausen syndrome by proxy is suspected but not confirmed, several procedures to confirm the diagnosis have been proposed. These include 1) a review of medical records of other siblings, looking for a pattern of chronic illness or unexplained death; 2) the separation of the child from the parent to determine whether a change occurs in the child's course of illness (e.g., many children suddenly recover when separated from the parent for several days or weeks); and 3) the controversial technique of video surveillance with a hidden camera. Ethical and legal questions may arise as to whether video surveillance involves an invasion of privacy. Such a procedure should be undertaken only after appropriate consultation with hospital legal staff, administration, and child protective services; such surveillance may place the child at risk (Hall et al. 2000; Southall et al. 1997).

Ayoub et al. (2002) stated that perpetrators of factitious disorder by proxy should be diagnosed with factitious disorder not otherwise specified, DSM-IV-TR code

TABLE 13–4. Differential diagnosis of Munchausen syndrome by proxy

Pediatric somatization syndromes
Somatoform disorder by proxy (parent's anxiety projected/displaced onto child)
Infanticide/murder
Psychosis in parent
Child abuse (garden variety)
Factitious behavior initiated by child
Malingering by child (e.g., school rejection)
Unrecognized physical disease

300.19. However, providing a DSM-IV-TR diagnosis to any person who perpetuates factitious behavior is controversial because an official diagnosis might imply mitigation for misbehavior—criminal behavior in the case of Munchausen syndrome by proxy (Ford 2005).

The differential diagnosis of Munchausen syndrome by proxy, of course, always includes the possibility of underlying genuine physical disease and the fact that at times an older child may produce illness in himself or herself (Libow 2000; Peebles et al. 2005) (see Table 13–4). There also may be "blended cases" in which the child or adolescent self-produces symptoms but with the active help of the parent, who may coach the behavior (Libow 2002). At present, most pediatricians and child protection caseworkers are well aware of Munchausen syndrome by proxy, and there is a risk of becoming overly zealous in making the diagnosis. Rand and Feldman (1999) reported 4 cases of misdiagnosed Munchausen syndrome by proxy and identified another 11 cases in their review of more than 200 articles and books.

Etiology

In Munchausen syndrome by proxy, the identified patient is the victim of misbehavior by another. Adults who perpetrate this disorder may superficially seem quite normal, and frequently evaluation of them does not result in a psychiatric diagnosis (Sanders and Bursch 2002). Others may meet criteria for a somatoform disorder or a personality disorder or have previously produced factitious disease in themselves (Bools et al. 1994). Most explanations for perpetrating this behavior revolve around the idea that the perpetrator is motivated by the need to become the center of attention by playing the role of concerned parent in the high drama of life and death in a hospital.

Characteristics of perpetrators as computed by Sheridan (2003) include motherhood (76.5%); some features of personal Munchausen syndrome (29.3%); a psychiatric diagnosis (22.8%), usually depression or personality disorder; and a personal history of abuse (21.0%).

Family dynamics and the individual psychodynamics of the perpetrator are believed to be important, but there has not been any large-scale systematic study (Mercer and Perdue 1993). Griffith (1988) studied some families with Munchausen syndrome by proxy and proposed several commonly observed features that reflect multigenerational dysfunctional families. Mercer and Perdue (1993) suggested that the mother may be both victim and perpetrator, and her behavior is an attempt to gain power and control in a powerless existence.

Management and Treatment

Ethical and Legal Issues

The primary and immediate goal in treatment of Munchausen syndrome by proxy is cessation of the behavior that perpetrates symptoms. Separation between the perpetrator and the victim is usually necessary to accomplish cessation of the behavior. In the most common form of factitious disorder by proxy (parent-perpetrated), it is necessary to place the child into some type of foster care. Visits by the parents during these separations must be carefully monitored. Such placement requires a legal hearing and involvement of the agencies that have responsibility for protecting child welfare. It is amazing to see how a chronically sick child blooms when separated from the perpetrating parent. Permanent separation of parent and child is a major legal and ethical issue; courts are understandably reluctant to act in such a manner without very serious consideration. The key question is whether the parent has been sufficiently rehabilitated to reduce risk to the child, but the nature of the support system (other parent, other family members, availability of caseworkers) is also crucial (Sanders and Bursch 2002).

Therapy for the Perpetrator

The perpetrator, who is usually the mother, should receive psychological treatment. The effectiveness of such intervention is dependent on the perpetrator's open and honest acknowledgment of his or her behavior. Unfortunately, this does not usually occur.

Treatment of the Victim

It is recognized that victims of factitious disorder by proxy experience a high incidence of varied psychiatric disorders (Bools et al. 1993; Bryk and Siegel 1997). To date, no systematic studies of treatment have been done. The specifics of treatment are dependent on the nature of the problem. One role of psychotherapy is to help the victim deal with feelings about an abusive parent.

Hospital Epidemics of Factitious Disorder by Proxy

The term *angel of death syndrome* was first used in newspaper reports (later proven to be inaccurate) in which a Las Vegas, Nevada, nurse was accused of tampering with patients' life-support equipment. The motivation was allegedly to help friends win a betting pool dealing with times of patients' deaths (Kalisch et al. 1980).

Although the case against the Las Vegas nurse was disproved, there have been multiple subsequent reports in which health care providers have been accused of causing epidemics of acute cardiac or pulmonary arrests and unusual patterns of deaths (Yorker et al. 2006). Tragically, many of these epidemics have been shown to be caused by the very persons entrusted with the patients' care. In their detailed review of multiple hospital epidemics, Yorker et al. (2006) concluded that the perpetrators were usually nurses or nurse's aides and that the victims were physically compromised: critically ill, elderly, or very young.

The epidemics tended to cluster on evening and night shifts and also involved numerous—often successful—resuscitations. Yorker et al. (2006) proposed that one motive of the perpetrators is the excitement and exhilaration derived from participating in "codes."

This kind of behavior constitutes serial murder, and prosecution has resulted in several convictions. Epidemiological techniques have been used to identify probable perpetrators, but such evidence is circumstantial and cannot be used alone to establish guilt (Sacks et al. 1988).

Malingering

By definition, individuals with malingering are motivated by specific, recognizable external incentives to produce, exaggerate, or simulate physical or psychological illness (American Psychiatric Association 2000). Incentives may be deferment for military service, avoidance of hazardous work assignments, escape from incarceration (e.g., being judged not guilty by reason of insanity), or procurement of controlled substances. Perhaps the most common incentive is financial gain, such as the receipt of disability payments or the hope of damages to be awarded in a lawsuit. It must be kept in mind that malingering is less a diagnosis than a socially unacceptable behavior with legal ramifications (Szasz 1956). Malingering often must be considered in a differential diagnosis, but much caution must be exercised in making such a "diagnosis" (Drob et al. 2009).

Malingering is most common in settings where there are external and tangible gains accrued by illness. Among these settings are prisons, military service, courtroom settings that involve personal or industrial injury, and the offices of physicians who perform disability evaluations. Frueh et al. (2005) found that of men seeking Veterans Affairs specialty care for combat-related posttraumatic stress disorder, 5% had made false claims of Vietnam military service, and another 32%, while serving in Vietnam, had no documentation of combat exposure. Kay and Morris-Jones (1998) found clear-cut surveillance videotape evidence that at least 20% of the litigants registered in a pain clinic were overtly malingering their symptoms. Financial incentives *do* make a difference in symptoms and disability. In their meta-analysis of 2,353 subjects, Binder and Rohling (1996) found more abnormality and disability in patients with mild closed head injury who had financial incentives than in those who did not have such an incentive. Similarly, Paniak et al. (2002) found that when financial compensation was at issue, patients with mild traumatic brain injury had significantly increased symptoms. In contrast, Mayou (1995) conducted a prospective study in the United Kingdom on the outcome of persons involved in motor vehicle accidents and found that malingering to gain compensation was remarkably uncommon. He suggested that the high rates found in some tertiary care centers represent atypical and selected samples. The legal climate regarding lawsuits varies widely from country to country.

Clinical Features: Phenomenology, Course, and Prognosis

Malingering symptoms fall into four major categories: 1) production or simulation of an illness, 2) exacerbation of a previous illness, 3) exaggeration of symptoms, and 4) falsification of laboratory samples or laboratory reports. Embellishment of previous or concurrent illness is probably the form of malingering most frequently encountered by psychosomatic subspecialists. Bellamy (1997) noted that most exaggerated illnesses in compensation situations are a result of a combination of suggestion, somatization, and rationalization. Symptoms are usually subjective and difficult to quantify and include feigned dizziness, weakness, seizures or spells, and features of posttraumatic stress disorder (Sparr and Pankratz 1983). Patients may intensify their complaints when they are asked directly about their symptoms or when they think they are being observed. When distracted, they become physically more relaxed and at times may be seen to engage in physical activities incompatible with their symptom reports.

The malingered symptom generally disappears when the person either obtains the desired goal or is confronted with irrefutable evidence of malingering. However, it has been noted that some malingered symptoms persist even after these occurrences. It may be that the person maintains symptoms as a face-saving mechanism, or perhaps the symptom has in some way been incorporated as a habit into the individual's lifestyle.

Diagnosis and Assessment

As noted earlier, identification of malingering is more an issue of socially unacceptable behavior, an accusation of a person's external motives, than a psychiatric diagnosis. The clinician should consider malingering when symptom complaints and objective data are incongruent. However, the presence of secondary gains, concurrent litigation, and seeking disability are *not* evidence of malingering per se. Thus, there must be not only verification of an external motivation but also objective evidence to confirm the probability of malingering. For example, a patient who cannot walk independently when seen in the consultation suite might later be seen walking normally on a sidewalk outside the hospital. Insurance companies at times engage private investigators who use video surveillance to obtain objective evidence of malingering. For example, a man who claimed an inability to raise his arms above his shoulder was videotaped climbing a ladder onto his roof and installing a television antenna.

Psychological testing is often helpful in identifying malingering patients. The Minnesota Multiphasic Personality Inventory–2 is a useful test for patients who distort their presentations (Arbisi and Butcher 2004; McCaffrey and Bellamy-Campbell 1989; Wetzler and Marlowe 1990). This test and others have diagnostic value in assessing those who exaggerate physical and psychological symptoms (Cliffe 1992; Rawling 1992; Walters et al. 2008). Screening instruments with face validity such as the Beck Depression Inventory and the Hopkins Symptom Checklist–90 are easily distorted by patients who embellish their symptoms (Lees-Haley 1989a, 1989b), and these instruments have very limited value in the determination of malingering. Forced-choice psychological tests may be valuable in detecting malingering. If a person makes more errors than would be expected by chance, a statistical probability can be determined as to whether the person actually knew the correct answers. A recent review (McDermott and Feldman 2007) describes many of the findings and psychological tests that have been used in attempts to distinguish malingering from genuine illness.

Functional neuroimaging has been used in experimental situations to distinguish patients with feigned weakness from those with motor conversion symptoms (J. Stone et al. 2007) and to detect feigned memory impairment (Browndyke et al. 2008). However, the use of functional magnetic resonance imaging for forensic evaluations is fraught with ethical and legal questions (Moriarty 2008).

No single evaluation technique will unequivocally identify malingerers. This is particularly true when the examiner makes a subjective assessment of a feature such as sincerity of effort (Lechner et al. 1998; Main and Waddell 1998). Rather, patients must be evaluated from a complete physical and psychosocial perspective that includes various other possibilities, such as "pseudomalingering" (Ford 1983). Pseudomalingering arises when the patient uses an external incentive as a rationalization for malingered symptoms, thereby shielding himself or herself from awareness of unconscious determinants (Ford 1983; Schneck 1962). For example, a genuinely psychotic person may believe he or she is feigning psychosis to escape punishment for a crime. By believing that one is feigning the psychosis, the person is defensively shielded from conscious awareness of actual mental illness and thus incorrectly believes that he or she is in control of his or her thought processes. Another form of pseudomalingering may exist when a person consciously exaggerates a symptom because he or she truly believes that there is an underlying problem. An underlying problem may exist, but the examiner who picks up on the malingering may mistakenly attribute the entire problem to malingering.

The differential diagnosis of malingering includes somatoform disorders as well as factitious disorders. These clinical syndromes have indistinct boundaries, and a person may meet criteria for different disorders at different times (Ford 1992; Jonas and Pope 1985; Nadelson 1985). Relevant factors that may play a role in assessment include evidence of past somatization as well as coexistence of anxiety, mood, substance, or personality disorders. Patients with unconsciously determined somatoform disorders (e.g., conversion) are usually consistent in their symptom presentation irrespective of their audience or whether they believe they are being observed.

Etiology

By definition, the etiology of malingering is to obtain external gain as a result of the symptoms. However, malingering does tend to be more common in persons who may have hysteroid features. Because of personality characteristics (e.g., histrionic or sociopathic) or cognitive style, some persons may be more inclined toward simulated illness.

Management and Treatment

Malingering is more a management problem than a therapeutic issue. With this in mind, the primary physician and psychosomatic subspecialist must be circumspect in their approach to the patient. Every note must be written with the thought in mind that it may be read by the patient or even become a courtroom exhibit. Malingering is often listed among diagnostic possibilities but is rarely proved conclusively in medical settings.

The person who is suspected of malingering, as a rule, should not be confronted with a direct accusation. Instead, subtle communication can indicate that the physician is "on to the game" (Kramer et al. 1979). One technique is to mention, almost in passing, that diagnostic tests indicate no "serious" basis for the symptoms. The malingerer may feel freer to discard the symptom if the physician suggests that patients with similar problems usually recover after a certain procedure is performed or a particular length of time has passed. Such suggestions are often followed by perceptible improvement, if not recovery. This technique provides face-saving mechanisms for the patient to discard the symptom. Still, some patients, particularly those seeking drugs, will leave treatment and seek medical care elsewhere. Others, in an effort to prove the existence of their disease, may vastly intensify their symptoms. In doing so, they may create such caricatures of illness that their efforts to malinger become obvious to all.

Conclusion

Requests for psychiatric consultation on patients with suspected factitious disorder or malingering are relatively infrequent. However, when the psychosomatic medicine subspecialist does become involved with one of these cases, a disproportionate amount of time is typically required. Issues of diagnosis, legal and ethical considerations, and the need to provide liaison with the medical staff may make one of these patients the primary focus of one's clinical activities for several days. Nevertheless, they are fascinating patients who demonstrate the extreme end of the continuum of abnormal illness behavior. They are rarely forgotten.

References

Adams F: The Seven Books of Paulus Aegineta, Vol 2. London, England, Sydenham Society, 1846

American Psychiatric Association: Diagnostic and Statistical Manual of Mental Disorders, 4th Edition, Text Revision. Washington, DC, American Psychiatric Association, 2000

Arbisi PA, Butcher JN: Psychometric perspectives on detection of malingering of pain: use of the Minnesota Multiphasic Personality Inventory-2. Clin J Pain 20:383–391, 2004

Asher R: Munchausen's syndrome. Lancet 1:339–341, 1951

Ayoub CC, Alexander R, Beck D, et al: Position paper: definitional issues in Munchausen by proxy. Child Maltreat 7:105–111, 2002

Babe KS Jr, Peterson AM, Loosen PT, et al: The pathogenesis of Munchausen syndrome: a review and case report. Gen Hosp Psychiatry 14:273–276, 1992

Bappal B, George M, Nair R, et al: Factitious hypoglycemia: a tale from the Arab world. Pediatrics 107:180–181, 2001

Bass C, Halligan PM: Illness related deception: social or psychiatric problem? J R Soc Med 100:81–84, 2007

Bellamy R: Compensation neurosis: financial reward for illness as nocebo. Clin Orthop Relat Res 336:94–106, 1997

Binder LM, Rohling ML: Money matters: a meta-analytic review of the effects of financial incentives on recovery after closed-head injury. Am J Psychiatry 153:7–10, 1996

Bools CN, Neale BA, Meadow SR: Follow up of victims of fabricated illness (Munchausen syndrome by proxy). Arch Dis Child 69:625–630, 1993

Bools C, Neale B, Meadow R: Munchausen syndrome by proxy: a study of psychopathology. Child Abuse Negl 18:773–788, 1994

Browndyke JN, Paskavitz J, Sweet LH, et al: Neuroanatomical correlates of malingered memory impairment: event-related fMRI of deception on a recognition memory task. Brain Inj 22:481–489, 2008

Bryk M, Siegel PT: My mother caused my illness: the story of a survivor of Munchausen by proxy syndrome. Pediatrics 100:1–7, 1997

Catalina ML, Gomez Macias V, de Cos A: Prevalence of factitious disorder with psychological symptoms in hospitalized patients. Actas Esp Psiquiatr 36:345–349, 2008

Cliffe MJ: Symptom-validity testing of feigned sensory or memory deficits: a further elaboration for subjects who understand the rationale. Br J Clin Psychol 31:207–209, 1992

Dalfen AK, Anthony F: Head injury, dissociation and the Ganser syndrome. Brain Inj 14:1101–1105, 2000

Denny SJ, Grant CC, Pinnock R: Epidemiology of Munchausen syndrome by proxy in New Zealand. J Paediatr Child Health 37:340–343, 2001

Dimsdale J, Creed F: The proposed diagnosis of somatic symptom disorders in DSM-V to replace somatoform disorders in DSM-IV—a preliminary report. J Psychosom Res 66:473–476, 2009

Drob SL, Meehan KB, Waxman SE: Clinical and conceptual problems in the attribution of malingering in forensic evaluations. J Am Acad Psychiatry Law 37:98–106, 2009

Earle JR Jr, Folks DG: Factitious disorder and coexisting depression: a report of a successful psychiatric consultation and case management. Gen Hosp Psychiatry 8:448–450, 1986

Eastwood S, Bisson JL: Management of factitious disorders: a systematic review. Psychother Psychosom 77:209–218, 2008

Eisendrath SJ: When Munchausen becomes malingering; factitious disorders that penetrate the legal system. Bull Am Acad Psychiatry Law 24:471–481, 1996

Eisendrath SJ: Factitious disorders and malingering, in Treatments of Psychiatric Disorders, 3rd Edition, Vol 2. Edited by Gabbard GO. Washington, DC, American Psychiatric Press, 2001, pp 1825–1842

Eisendrath SJ, McNeil DE: Factitious physical disorders, litigation and mortality. Psychosomatics 45:350–353, 2004

Faravelli C, Abrardi L, Bartolozzi D, et al: The Sesto Fiorentino study: background, methods and preliminary results: lifetime prevalence of psychiatric disorders in an Italian community sample using clinical interviewers. Psychother Psychosom 73:216–225, 2004

Feldman MD: Munchausen by Internet: detecting factitious illness and crisis on the Internet. South Med J 93:669–672, 2000

Feldman MD, Ford CV, Stone T: Deceiving others/deceiving oneself: four cases of factitious rape. South Med J 87:736–738, 1994

Feldman-Schorrig S: Factitious sexual harassment. Bull Am Acad Psychiatry Law 24:387–482, 1996

Fenelon G, Mahieux F, Roullet E, et al: Munchausen's syndrome and abnormalities on magnetic resonance imaging of the brain. BMJ 302:996–997, 1991

Fink P, Jensen J: Clinical characteristics of the Munchausen syndrome: a review and 3 new case histories. Psychother Psychosom 52:164–171, 1989

Ford CV: The Munchausen syndrome: a report of four new cases and a review of psychodynamic considerations. Psychiatr Med 4:31–45, 1973

Ford CV: The Somatizing Disorders: Illness as a Way of Life. New York, Elsevier, 1983

Ford CV: Illness as a lifestyle: the role of somatization in medical practice. Spine 17:S338–S343, 1992

Ford CV: Lies! Lies!! Lies!!! The Psychology of Deceit. Washington, DC, American Psychiatric Press, 1996

Ford CV: Factitious disorders: diagnosis or misbehavior? (commentary), in Somatoform Disorders: WPA Series, Evidence and Experience in Psychiatry. Edited by Maj M, Akiskal HS, Mezzick JE, et al. Chichester, England, Wiley, 2005, pp 354–357

Frueh BC, Elhai JD, Grubaugh AL, et al: Documented combat exposure of US veterans seeking treatment for combat-related post-traumatic stress disorder. Br J Psychiatry 186:467–472, 2005

Ganser SJM: A peculiar hysterical state. Br J Criminol 5:120–126, 1965

Gavin H: On the Feigned and Factitious Diseases of Soldiers and Seamen. Edinburgh, Scotland, University Press, 1838

Gibbon KL: Munchausen's syndrome presenting as an acute sexual assault. Med Sci Law 38:202–205, 1998

Griffith JL: The family systems of Munchausen syndrome by proxy. Fam Process 27:423–437, 1988

Hall DE, Eubanks L, Meyyazhagan LS, et al: Evaluation of covert video surveillance in the diagnosis of Munchausen syndrome by proxy: lessons from 41 cases. Pediatrics 105:1305–1312, 2000

Hamilton JC, Feldman MD, Janata JW: The A, B, C's of factitious disorder: a response to Turner. Medscape J Med 11:27, 2009 (published online)

Hardie TJ, Reed A: Pseudologia fantastica, factitious disorder and impostership: a deception syndrome. Med Sci Law 38:198–201, 1998

Health Insurance Portability and Accountability Act of 1996, Pub. L. No. 104-191

Janofsky JS: The Munchausen syndrome in civil forensic psychiatry. Bull Am Acad Psychiatry Law 22:489–497, 1994

Jonas JM, Pope HG: The dissimulating disorders: a single diagnostic entity? Compr Psychiatry 26:58–62, 1985

Kalisch PA, Kalisch BJ, Livesay E: The "Angel of Death": the anatomy of 1980s major news story about nursing. Nurs Forum 19:212–241, 1980

Kapfhammer HP, Rothenhauster HB, Dietrich E, et al: Artifactual disorders—between deception and self-mutilation: experiences in consultation psychiatry at a university clinic (in German with English abstract). Nervenarzt 69:401–409, 1998

Kay NR, Morris-Jones H: Pain clinic management of medico-legal litigants. Injury 29:305–308, 1998

King BH, Ford CV: Pseudologia fantastica. Acta Psychiatr Scand 77:1–6, 1988

Krahn LE, Li H, O'Connor MK: Patients who strive to be ill: factitious disorder with physical symptoms. Am J Psychiatry 160:1163–1168, 2003

Krahn LE, Bostwick JM, Stonnington CM: Looking toward DSM-V: should factitious disorder become a subtype of somatoform disorder? Psychosomatics 49:277–287, 2008

Kramer KK, La Piana FG, Appleton B: Ocular malingering and hysteria: diagnosis and management. Surv Ophthalmol 24:89–96, 1979

Lechner DE, Bradbury SF, Bradley LA: Detecting sincerity of effort: a summary of methods and approaches. Phys Ther 78:867–888, 1998

Lees-Haley PR: Malingering emotional distress on the SCL-90R: toxic exposure and cancerphobia. Psychol Rep 65:1203–1208, 1989a

Lees-Haley PR: Malingering traumatic mental disorder on the Beck Depression Inventory: cancerphobia and toxic exposure. Psychol Rep 65:623–626, 1989b

Levenson JL, Chafe W, Flanagan P: Factitious ovarian cancer: feigning via resources on the Internet. Psychosomatics 48:71–73, 2007

Libow JA: Child and adolescent illness falsification. Pediatrics 105:336–342, 2000

Libow JA: Beyond collusion: active illness falsification. Child Abuse Negl 26:525–536, 2002

Main CJ, Waddell G: Behavioral responses to examination: a reappraisal of the interpretation of "non-organic" signs. Spine 23:2367–2371, 1998

Mayou R: Medico-legal aspects of road traffic accidents. J Psychosom Res 39:789–798, 1995

McCaffrey RJ, Bellamy-Campbell R: Psychometric detection of fabricated symptoms of combat-related post-traumatic stress disorder: a systematic replication. J Clin Psychol 45:76–79, 1989

McClure RJ, Davis PM, Meadow SR, et al: Epidemiology of Munchausen syndrome by proxy, non-accidental poisoning, and non-accidental suffocation. Arch Dis Child 75:57–61, 1996

McDermott BE, Feldman MD: Malingering in the medical setting. Psychiatr Clin North Am 30:645–662, 2007

McFarland BH, Resnick M, Bloom JD: Ensuring continuity of care for a Munchausen patient through a public guardian. Hosp Community Psychiatry 34:65–67, 1983

Meadow R: Munchausen syndrome by proxy: the hinterland of child abuse. Lancet 2:343–345, 1977

Meadow R: Munchausen syndrome by proxy perpetrated by men. Arch Dis Child 78:210–216, 1998

Mercer SO, Perdue JD: Munchausen syndrome by proxy: social work's role. Soc Work 38:74–81, 1993

Mohammed R, Goy JA, Walpole BG, et al: Munchausen's syndrome: a study of the casualty "black books" of Melbourne. Med J Aust 143:561–563, 1985

Moriarty JC: Flickering admissibility: neuroimaging in the U.S. courts. Behav Sci Law 26:29–49, 2008

Munro HM, Thrusfield MV: "Battered pets": Munchausen syndrome by proxy (factitious illness by proxy). J Small Anim Pract 42:385–389, 2001

Nadelson T: False patients/real patients: a spectrum of disease presentation. Psychother Psychosom 44:175–184, 1985

Nichols GR II, Davis GJ, Corey TS: In the shadow of the Baron: sudden death due to Munchausen syndrome. Am J Emerg Med 8:216–219, 1990

Nicholson SD, Roberts GA: Patients who (need to) tell stories. Br J Hosp Med 51:546–549, 1994

Paniak C, Reynolds S, Toller-Lobe G, et al: A longitudinal study of the relationship between financial compensation and symptoms after treated mild traumatic brain injury. J Clin Exp Neuropsychol 24:187–193, 2002

Pankratz L: Persistent problems with the Munchausen by proxy label. J Am Acad Psychiatry Law 34:90–95, 2006

Pankratz L, Lezak MD: Cerebral dysfunction in the Munchausen syndrome. Hillside J Clin Psychiatry 9:195–206, 1987

Parker PE: A case report of Munchausen syndrome with mixed psychological features. Psychosomatics 34:360–364, 1993

Peebles R, Sabella C, Franco K, et al: Factitious disorder and malingering in adolescent girls: case report and literature review. Clin Pediatr 44:237–243, 2005

Phillips MR, Ward NG, Ries RK: Factitious mourning: painless patienthood. Am J Psychiatry 140:420–425, 1983

Rand DC, Feldman MD: Misdiagnosis of Munchausen syndrome by proxy, a literature review and four new cases. Harv Rev Psychiatry 7:94–101, 1999

Rawling PJ: The Simulation Index: a reliability study. Brain Inj 6:381–383, 1992

Rogers R, Bagby RM, Rector N: Diagnostic legitimacy of factitious disorder with psychological symptoms. Am J Psychiatry 146:1312–1314, 1989

Rosenberg DA: Web of deceit: a literature review of Munchausen syndrome by proxy. Child Abuse Negl 11:547–563, 1987

Sacks JJ, Herndon JL, Lieg SH, et al: A cluster of unexplained deaths in a nursing home in Florida. Am J Public Health 78:806–808, 1988

Sanders MJ, Bursch B: Forensic assessment of illness falsification, Munchausen by proxy and factitious disorder NOS. Child Maltreat 7:112–124, 2002

Schneck JM: Pseudo-malingering. Dis Nerv Syst 23:396–398, 1962

Sheridan MS: The deceit continues: an updated literature review of Munchausen syndrome by proxy. Child Abuse Negl 27:431–451, 2003

Sigal M, Altmark D, Alfici S, et al: Ganser syndrome: a review of 15 cases. Compr Psychiatry 33:134–138, 1992

Snowden J, Solomons R, Druce H: Feigned bereavement: twelve cases. Br J Psychiatry 133:15–19, 1978

Southall DP, Plunkett MC, Banks MW, et al: Covert video recordings of life-threatening child abuse: lessons for child protection. Pediatrics 199:735–760, 1997

Sparr L, Pankratz LD: Factitious posttraumatic stress disorder. Am J Psychiatry 140:1016–1019, 1983

Stirling J Jr, American Academy of Pediatrics Committee on Child Abuse and Neglect: Beyond Munchausen syndrome by proxy: identification and treatment of child abuse in a medical setting. Pediatrics 119:1026–1030, 2007

Stone J, Zeman A, Simonotto E, et al: FMRI in patients with motor conversion symptoms and controls with simulated weakness. Psychosom Med 69:961–969, 2007

Stone MH: Factitious illness: psychological findings and treatment recommendations. Bull Menninger Clin 41:239–254, 1977

Sutherland AJ, Rodin GM: Factitious disorders in a general hospital setting: clinical features and a review of the literature. Psychosomatics 31:392–399, 1990

Szasz TS: Malingering: diagnosis or social condemnation? Analysis of the meaning of diagnosis in the light of some interrelations of social structure, value judgment, and the physician's role. AMA Arch Neurol Psychiatry 76:432–443, 1956

Turner MA: Factitious disorders: reformulating the DSM-IV criteria. Psychosomatics 47:23–32, 2006

Van Dinter TJ Jr, Welch BJ: Diagnosis of Munchausen's syndrome by an electronic health record search. Am J Med 122(10):e3, 2009

von Maurer K, Wasson KR, DeFord JW, et al: Munchausen's syndrome: a thirty year history of peregrination par excellence. South Med J 66:629–632, 1973

Wallach J: Laboratory diagnosis of factitious disorders. Arch Intern Med 154:1690–1696, 1994

Walters GD, Rogers R, Berry DTR, et al: Malingering as a categorical or dimensional construct: the latent structure of feigned psychopathology as measured by the SIRS and MMPI-2. Psychol Assess 20:238–247, 2008

Weiner H, Braiman A: The Ganser syndrome. Am J Psychiatry 111:767–773, 1955

Wetzler S, Marlowe D: "Faking bad" on the MMPI, MMPI-2, and Millon-II. Psychol Rep 67:1117–1118, 1990

Wirtz G, Baas U, Hofer H, et al: [Psychopathology of Ganser's syndrome: literature review and case report] (German). Nervenarzt 79:543–557, 2008

Yorker BC: Hospital epidemics of factitious disorder by proxy, in The Spectrum of Factitious Disorders. Edited by Feldman MD, Eisendrath SJ. Washington, DC, American Psychiatric Press, 1996, pp 157–174

Yorker BC, Kizer KW, Lampe P, et al: Serial murder by healthcare professionals. J Forensic Sci 51:1362–1371, 2006

CHAPTER 14

Eating Disorders

Michael J. Devlin, M.D.
Joel P. Jahraus, M.D.
Ilyse Dobrow DiMarco, Ph.D.

ALTHOUGH FULL-SYNDROME eating disorders are relatively rarely diagnosed in medical settings, eating disorder symptoms—such as uncontrolled eating, excessive dieting, and marked body image distress—occur quite commonly. Two important trends may account, at least in part, for the upsurge in these symptoms: 1) the well-documented increase in the prevalence of overweight and obesity in the United States (Ford and Mokdad 2008); and 2) the marked decrease in percentage of body fat of the culturally defined "ideal woman," as exemplified by Miss America pageant winners (Rubinstein and Caballero 2000). Caught between the reality of an obesity-promoting environment and an increasingly unattainable body image ideal, it is perhaps unsurprising that growing numbers of individuals, particularly women, engage in the desperate attempts to lose weight and the dysregulated eating that characterize the eating disorders.

The mortality and morbidity rates in eating disorders are considerable. Anorexia nervosa is among the most lethal of psychiatric disorders, with mortality rates of approximately 5% per decade of illness in the longest follow-up studies (Papadopoulos et al. 2009). Although the lethality of bulimia nervosa is much less than that of anorexia nervosa, the purging behaviors characteristic of this disorder can lead to significant medical and dental morbidity. Binge eating, to the degree that it contributes to the onset or maintenance of obesity, may contribute to obesity-related morbidity and death (Schelbert 2009). But perhaps the greater costs of eating disorders are the time and energy spent on the pursuit of thinness, often to the exclusion of interpersonal, vocational, and recreational sources of satisfaction; the shame and secrecy that often accompany these illnesses; and the ultimate loss of function when the symptoms remain untreated.

Among the most puzzling of psychiatric illnesses for practitioners who regard eating as a healthy and satisfying part of life, eating disorders are also among the most difficult to treat. Yet, as summarized in this chapter, progress is being made in the conceptualization, characterization, and treatment of eating disorders.

Definitions and Clinical Features

The diagnosis and treatment of disordered eating in the medical setting are among the most poorly studied and most important areas for ongoing clinical research. To fully appreciate the spectrum of eating disorders presenting in primary care and general medical settings, it is useful to apply both a categorical and a dimensional approach. The major eating disorder syndromes, including the DSM-IV-TR (American Psychiatric Association 2000) diagnostic categories for eating disorders, are discussed in the subsections that follow. Paradoxically, the most common eating disorder, eating disorder not otherwise specified (NOS), is also the most poorly defined and studied, and the dimensional approach to assessment may be of particular use in patients with this diagnosis.

Anorexia Nervosa and Bulimia Nervosa

Anorexia Nervosa

Anorexia nervosa is first and foremost a syndrome of voluntary starvation. However, the term *voluntary* must be interpreted with caution. Although it is true that patients with anorexia nervosa in some sense choose to restrict their eating, this choice is greatly influenced by genetic vulnerabilities, cultural forces, and life events. Patients in the late stages of anorexia nervosa will often clearly describe that any sense of free will they once may have had regarding their condition has, to a great degree, vanished.

The phenomenon of unexplained starvation, or "nervous consumption," in an otherwise healthy individual was reported as long ago as the late seventeenth century (Morton 1689). Although the practice of extreme food restriction for reasons generally unrelated to body image occurred before the nineteenth century (Brumberg 1988), it was not until the 1870s that the modern syndrome of anorexia nervosa was recognized nearly simultaneously by Lasègue (1873) and Gull (1874), the latter of whom coined the term *anorexia nervosa.* This modern concept was further refined in the 1960s by psychiatrist Hilde Bruch (1973) and others, who recognized low self-esteem and body image distortion as core features of the disorder.

In keeping with earlier conceptions, the current definition of anorexia nervosa is centered on the behavioral feature of starvation. To be diagnosed with anorexia nervosa, patients must manifest weight loss, or the absence of expected weight gain, leading to a state of significant undernourishment, as reflected by a weight markedly (i.e., at least 15%) lower than expected for gender and height. However, to meet modern (DSM-IV-TR) criteria for anorexia nervosa, an individual must manifest the more recently identified psychological features. The diagnosis requires an overconcern with weight and shape, which may or may not take the form of an actual misperception of body fatness but must reflect an overinvestment in thinness as a central feature of one's self-worth. In addition, amenorrhea is a requirement for postmenarchal women. A non-fat-phobic variant of anorexia nervosa has been described, particularly in non-Western societies; interestingly, it appears to be associated with milder eating pathology (Thomas et al. 2009) and a lower likelihood of progressing to bulimia nervosa in outcome studies (Lee et al. 2003).

Although patients with anorexia nervosa often view their illness as that which makes them unique or special, there is a surprising uniformity in the way they present, and there are a number of associated features that occur quite predictably. In addition to severely restricting their intake of food, many individuals with anorexia nervosa are also compulsive exercisers. Some anorexic patients engage in strict dieting without any binge eating or purging (restricting type), whereas others periodically engage in purging (e.g., vomiting, laxative abuse) or uncontrolled binge eating (binge-eating/purging type). Patients with anorexia nervosa are often rigid and perfectionistic, not only in their adherence to restrictive eating and compulsive exercise practices but also in other areas of life. Interestingly, the narrowing of interests, increasing focus on food, and peculiar food-related rituals (toying with food, consumption of unusual food combinations, possessiveness toward food) were also observed in the Minnesota semistarvation study subjects. These subjects were male World War II conscientious objectors who volunteered to participate in a study of the physiological and psychological effects of starvation, eventually losing 25% of their body weight (Franklin et al. 1948). The fact that these men, who had no prior histories of eating disorders, exhibited behaviors so reminiscent of those seen in anorexia nervosa suggests the degree to which these features of the illness are driven by the physiological effects of starvation.

Bulimia Nervosa

The other major eating disorder currently defined in DSM-IV-TR is bulimia nervosa, popularly known as the binge-purge syndrome. This syndrome, first described as a variant of anorexia nervosa (Russell 1979) and later applied to individuals of normal weight, comprises regular uncontrolled consumption of objectively large amounts of food (binge eating), regular use of unhealthy compensatory methods intended to undo the effects of eating, and preoccupation with weight and/or shape as a central component of self-worth. Eating binges typically consist of more than 2,000 kcal and, contrary to popular belief, are not primarily composed of carbohydrate (Walsh et al. 1989). Compensatory behaviors include purging methods (i.e., elimination of food and fluids from the body by the use of vomiting, laxatives, diuretics, or enemas) and nonpurging methods (such as fasting or excessive exercise) for preventing weight gain. Patients with diabetes mellitus who have bulimia nervosa may attempt to purge by reducing or omitting their insulin dosage to promote glycosuria, thereby eliminating calories from the body. Although most individuals who present for treatment for bulimia nervosa are of normal weight, the diagnosis can also be made in overweight or obese individuals. Under the current diagnostic system, individuals who simultaneously meet criteria for anorexia nervosa and bulimia nervosa are diagnosed as having anorexia nervosa, binge-eating/purging type. In fact, the progression from anorexia nervosa to bulimia nervosa is quite common, occurring in about one-half of patients with restricting anorexia nervosa (Bulik et al. 1997). Normal-weight patients with bulimia nervosa progress to anorexia nervosa somewhat less frequently.

Psychiatric Comorbidity of Anorexia Nervosa and Bulimia Nervosa

Individuals with anorexia nervosa and bulimia nervosa often manifest comorbid symptoms of depression and anxiety. Many studies suggest that, at least in clinical samples, a majority or significant minority of individuals with eating disorders also have a lifetime diagnosis of affective or anxiety disorder (Godart et al. 2007; D.B. Herzog and Eddy 2007; Hudson et al. 2007; Kaye et al. 2004). Among affective disorders, major depressive disorder occurs most frequently, although eating disorders also appear prevalent among patients with bipolar disorders and are associated with obesity and other psychiatric morbidity (Wildes et al. 2008). Among anxiety disorders, obsessive-compulsive disorder (OCD) is particularly prominent (Kaye et al. 2004) and has been of particular interest because eating- and exercise-related practices, particularly in individuals with anorexia nervosa, may include the repetitive, ritualized behaviors characteristic of OCD. According to a recent report, a history of overanxious disorder of childhood is present in nearly 40% of individuals with anorexia nervosa and usually precedes onset of the eating disorder. Individuals with this history reported more severe eating disorder pathology than the noncomorbid group (Raney et al. 2008). Although in some cases anxiety or depressive symptoms may be secondary to disordered eating, it is likely that shared etiological factors largely account for the observed comorbidity (Bulik 2002). In any case, a diagnosis of depression or anxiety disorder, particularly in an individual at risk for an eating disorder (i.e., adolescent and young adult women) should raise the clinician's level of suspicion that an eating disorder may also be present. In addition, the comorbid diagnosis must of course be taken into account in devising the treatment plan. In general, treatment can proceed simultaneously with the emphasis, for individuals with anorexia nervosa, on weight restoration as a precondition for successful treatment of comorbid conditions.

The relationship between eating disorders and substance use disorders is of great theoretical as well as practical interest, because the idea of "food addiction" suggests the possibility of common underlying pathophysiological mechanisms (Del Parigi et al. 2003). It is certainly the case that eating and substance abuse disorders co-occur at a rate significantly higher than that explainable by chance (Holderness et al. 1994), and substance use disorders are particularly associated with bulimic symptomatology (Root et al. 2010). However, in contrast to the data on the overlap between eating, affective, and anxiety disorders, the available data on familial transmission of eating and substance abuse disorders fail to support the existence of common genetic risk factors (von Ranson et al. 2003; Wilson 2002). An exception to this general pattern for eating disorders is binge-eating disorder, for which there is evidence for shared transmission with substance use disorders (Lilenfeld et al. 2008). At a phenomenological level, the experience of patients with eating disorders, and even the terminology patients use (e.g., "compulsive" exercise, "going on a binge"), can often mimic the argot of substance abuse. Of course, the one major difference is that, to the degree that food is considered the abused substance, abstinence is not a therapeutic option. For patients with comorbid eating and substance use disorders, it is recommended that the substance abuse problem be prioritized. For patients in whom substance abuse is not severe, treatment for the two disorders may proceed simultaneously (Wilson 2002). Substance use disorders may significantly affect the outcome of eating disorders. In one large-scale study, severity of alcohol use disorder was a significant predictor of death in anorexia nervosa, with a significant minority of patients apparently developing alcoholism subsequent to the onset of their eating disorder. This finding suggests that patients with eating disorders should be carefully assessed over time for the emergence or worsening of a substance use disorder (Keel et al. 2003).

Published rates of Axis II comorbidity in eating disorder samples have been highly variable. However, it is clear that there is no one personality type that characterizes individuals with anorexia nervosa or bulimia nervosa. Rather, in an examination of individuals with eating disorders across diagnoses, Westen and Harnden-Fischer (2001) reported that three personality clusters emerged: high-functioning/perfectionistic, constricted/overcontrolled, and emotionally dysregulated/undercontrolled. These personality subtypes have also been observed in adolescents with eating disorders (Thompson-Brenner et al. 2008). The assessment of personality dimensions may be important when planning treatment for individuals with eating disorders (Tasca et al. 2009).

Eating Disorders and Obesity

Although obesity is not, in and of itself, an eating disorder (Devlin et al. 2000), obese individuals may have eating disorders such as binge-eating disorder (BED), night-eating syndrome, and sleep-related eating disorders (Howell et al. 2009; Stunkard and Allison 2003). BED (uncontrolled binge eating in the absence of regular compensatory behavior) has been a particular focus of research since it was identified in Appendix B of DSM-IV (American Psychiatric Association 1994) as a criteria set requiring further study. Although the status of BED is uncertain (Devlin et al. 2003), the phenomenon of binge eating among the obese has been clearly identified, and its associated features have been studied (Dingemans et al. 2002). In particular, binge eating in the obese has been found to be associated with higher rates of major medical disorders, greater health dissatisfaction, and a higher lifetime prevalence of depression, panic, phobias, and alcohol dependence (Bulik et al. 2002), and stopping binge eating has a favorable effect on weight loss outcomes (Gorin et al. 2008).

Night-eating syndrome—characterized by a disrupted circadian eating rhythm with excessive consumption at the end of the day—has been much less thoroughly studied, but preliminary studies suggest that it has distinct behavioral/psychological and physiological features. Nocturnal sleep-related eating disorders among the obese represent a similar phenomenon but are characterized by recurrent episodes of eating after arousal from sleep, sometimes with amnesia or consumption of unusual food items, often with associated sleep disorders (Howell et al. 2009). Similar patterns have been noted to occur as a side effect of zolpidem (Najjar 2007) and similar hypnotics. Although the best methods for sequencing or combining treatments for obesity and eating disorders have not yet been fully worked out, approaches for simultaneously treating eating disorders and obesity have been described (Devlin 2001).

Atypical Eating Disorders

A final category of eating disorders in DSM-IV-TR is eating disorder NOS, defined as a clinically significant eating disorder that does not meet diagnostic criteria for any defined eating disorder diagnosis. Examples are 1) regular occurrence of subjective binge episodes (i.e., uncontrolled consumption of amounts of food not deemed large) followed by purging, 2) strict dieting and weight loss without amenorrhea, or 3) continuous uncontrolled snacking throughout the day with no discrete binge episodes. Notably, the phenomenon of purging in the absence of binge eating has recently received consideration as an independent eating disorder called purging disorder (Keel et al. 2005). Preliminary studies have demonstrated that this disorder appears to be distinct from bulimia nervosa in regard to subjective and physiological responses to a test meal (Keel et al. 2007). In addition, patients who have behaviors typical of eating disorders, such as food avoidance or vomiting, but who deny body image concern—attributing their symptoms instead to somatic sensations such as bloating, nausea, intolerable fullness, or extreme discomfort after eating—may be diagnosed as having eating disorder NOS once medical etiologies have been ruled out. Community-based studies have typically found that these atypical eating disorders are more common than anorexia nervosa and bulimia nervosa. Nonetheless, they have received relatively little attention in the literature and are poorly understood at this point. Although much of the literature is based on samples seen in eating disorder clinics that are geared toward treating patients with full-blown anorexia nervosa and bulimia nervosa, individuals seen in the medical setting who are not specifically presenting for treatment of an eating disorder may be particularly likely to manifest eating disorder NOS.

Given this state of affairs, it is perhaps useful to transcend conventional diagnostic categories and consider a transdiagnostic or dimensional approach to the classification (Fairburn et al. 2003) and treatment (Fairburn 2008) of eating disorders. One dimension of the patient's condition is *nutritional,* with the spectrum ranging from undernourished to severely obese. A second dimension is *behavioral,* with behaviors of interest including binge eating, nighttime eating, uncontrolled eating of some other variety, extreme dieting, purging, and so forth. A third dimension is *psychological.* This dimension includes body image distress—perhaps the most unifying feature of individuals with eating disorders, be they emaciated, of normal weight, or obese—and psychiatric comorbidity. In addition to assessing the psychological dimension, it is important to assess the patient's *motivation for change.* In contrast to anorexia nervosa, which is often embraced by patients as a lifestyle choice that they are ambivalent about relinquishing, patients with bulimia nervosa are generally more motivated to break the binge-purge cycle, although they may be less enthusiastic about confronting the dieting and body obsession that underlie the behavior. Obese patients with eating disorders may be highly motivated to lose weight but may have unrealistic expectations of thinness that continually undermine their weight-control attempts. A consideration of the various dimensions of a given patient's eating disorder syndrome and the particular history of the patient (e.g., chronicity, rapidity of change, and functional impairment) may assist the practitioner in the difficult task of applying findings from clinical studies of typical eating disorders to the atypical eating disorders more commonly observed in the medical setting.

Eating Disorders in Children

Eating disorders in children and adolescents represent a particular concern because, if not diagnosed and treated, they may have lifelong psychological and medical consequences (see also Chapter 34, "Pediatrics"). As is the case for adult eating disorders, the classification of child and adolescent eating disturbances is the subject of active debate (Bravender et al. 2007). Disordered eating patterns occurring before puberty include food avoidance emotional disorder, selective eating, pervasive refusal syndrome, food phobias, functional dysphagia, and full-syndrome anorexia nervosa (Lask and Bryant-Waugh 1997; Nicholls and

Bryant-Waugh 2009; Rosen 2003). *Food avoidance emotional disorder* is similar to but less severe than anorexia nervosa and carries a better prognosis. *Selective eating* is diagnosed in children who eat only a small number of foods but whose growth and development are generally normal. *Pervasive refusal syndrome* is a severe disorder in which refusal to eat is accompanied by refusal to function in other spheres (e.g., walking, talking, self-care) and is probably not best viewed as an eating disorder. Similarly, specific *food phobias* are often reflective of more pervasive anxiety disorders, and obsessional fears related to food may be particularly common in boys presenting with childhood anorexia nervosa. Children with *functional dysphagia* avoid food due to a fear of swallowing, choking, or vomiting for which no organic etiology can be identified. Bulimia nervosa is thought to occur quite rarely before puberty. Problems of food refusal, selective eating, phobias, failure to thrive, pica, and rumination in children are discussed in detail in Chapter 34, "Pediatrics." However, it is notable that symptoms such as eating conflicts, struggles with food, and unpleasant meals in early childhood have been found to be associated with the later development of eating disorders (Kotler et al. 2001) and therefore should be followed closely.

As reviewed in a Society for Adolescent Medicine position paper (Rome et al. 2003), dieting among school-age girls is increasingly common, and prevention and screening for eating disorders may avert the progression from pathological dieting to clinically significant eating disorders. Just as for adults, eating disorder symptoms in adolescents carry significant medical and psychiatric comorbidity (Herpertz-Dahlmann 2009). Thus, the identification of a significant eating disorder symptom, even in the absence of a formal diagnosis, should trigger some form of intervention to address the problem rather than a wait-and-see approach, which may allow the problem to become more entrenched. Pathological dieting is in some cases difficult to differentiate from normative dieting, but extreme distress about weight or shape, rapid weight loss, frequent weight or size checking, rigid adherence to dietary or exercise regimens, and use of unhealthy dietary practices are all worrisome signs. From a prevention standpoint, eating disorder NOS should probably be the most commonly diagnosed eating disorder in this group.

Feeding Disorders of Infancy or Early Childhood

Quite distinct from the eating disorders described in the preceding subsections are the feeding disorders seen in infants and children, including pica, rumination disorder, and feeding disorder of infancy or early childhood (Nicholls and Bryant-Waugh 2009). *Pica* refers to the consumption of nonnutritive substances such as hair, dirt, pebbles, or clay, sometimes but not always occurring in individuals with mental retardation, but meriting a separate diagnosis only if it is sufficiently severe to warrant independent clinical attention. Pica may be associated with poisoning (e.g., from lead paint) or mechanical obstruction. *Rumination* refers to the regurgitation, rechewing, and reswallowing of ingested food. Although most commonly seen in infants, rumination may also be seen in older children with mental retardation. Interestingly, a small proportion of adolescent and adult patients with anorexia nervosa and bulimia nervosa report rumination.

Finally, feeding disorder of infancy or early childhood is usually diagnosed in the first year of life but sometimes in children up to 3 years of age, for whom food intake is inadequate to support normal growth and development. As reviewed by Rudolph and Link (2002), the early recognition of feeding problems and diagnostic workup to exclude gastrointestinal, metabolic, sensory, or other general medical etiologies can lead to more appropriate management of affected children and their families.

Epidemiology

A number of researchers have attempted to establish incidence and prevalence rates for anorexia nervosa, bulimia nervosa, and (to a lesser extent) BED, and findings have been well summarized (Keski-Rahkonen et al. 2008). Anorexia nervosa is thought to have a lifetime prevalence of approximately 0.9%–2.2% in women and 0.2%–0.3% in men. Its incidence appears to have increased during the decades of the 1960s and 1970s but to have stabilized thereafter. In the United States, the National Comorbidity Survey Replication yielded a lifetime prevalence of 0.9% in women and 0.3% in men (Hudson et al. 2007). Studies of anorexia in non-Western countries demonstrate that it does occur, but overall at lower rates than in Western societies. However, subgroups in these countries (e.g., the minority mixed and white population in Curaçao) may show incidence rates similar to those in Western developed countries (Hoek et al. 2005).

Bulimia nervosa is somewhat more prevalent than anorexia nervosa, with lifetime prevalence rates of 1.5%–2% in women and 0.5% in men (Keski-Rahkonen et al. 2008). The National Comorbidity Survey Replication yielded lifetime prevalence rates of 1.5% and 0.65% among women and men, respectively (Hudson et al. 2007). Like anorexia nervosa, bulimia nervosa most often affects Western Caucasian adolescents and young adults. Regarding time trends, the most recent evidence suggests that rates of bulimia nervosa peaked in the early 1990s and have begun to decrease in Western developed countries though its clinical prevalence in non-Western countries may be rising (Lee et al. 2010). Some research has suggested that certain segments of the population, such as elite athletes (Smolak et al. 2000) and dancers (Dotti et al. 2002), are at particular risk for developing symptoms of bulimia nervosa or anorexia nervosa.

There have been few studies of the epidemiology of BED. The limited data that have been collected suggest that BED has a lifetime prevalence similar to or slightly higher than that of bulimia nervosa, with the National Comorbidity Survey Replication yielding rates of 3.5% and 2.0% for women and men respectively (Hudson et al. 2007). Roughly 5%–10% of those seeking treatment for obesity have BED. Unlike anorexia nervosa and bulimia nervosa, approximately a quarter of those with BED are male, and most patients with BED present with the illness in their 40s.

In establishing epidemiological data for eating disorders, it is important to consider not only individuals who meet diagnostic criteria for anorexia nervosa, bulimia nervosa, and BED but also the large numbers of individuals who are diagnosed with eating disorder NOS or who do not fulfill all DSM-IV-TR criteria for an eating disorder but nonetheless have serious eating pathology. In terms of eating disorder NOS, Fairburn and Harrison (2003) cited three community-based case series studies that all found eating disorder NOS to be a more common diagnosis than anorexia nervosa or bulimia nervosa. In addition, studies of subsyndromal anorexia nervosa, bulimia nervosa, and BED indicate that these subthreshold diagnoses are strikingly similar to their diagnostic counterparts in terms of distress and functional impairment. Therefore, to make a truly accurate assessment of the degree of eating pathology in the general population, epidemiologists must consider both eating disorder NOS and subthreshold eating disorders in addition to anorexia nervosa, bulimia nervosa, and BED.

Course and Outcome

Studies of the long-term course of anorexia nervosa suggest that there is no one typical outcome. Rather, the illness tends to require long-term treatment, with some patients achieving full recovery, others experiencing a longer course of partially remitted or unremitted illness, and some dying as a direct or indirect result of the illness (Pike 1998), with risk of suicide particularly pronounced (Berkman et al. 2007). Mortality rates are as high as 5% per decade of illness in the longest follow-up studies (Nielsen 2001); of surviving patients, fewer than half recover fully, one-quarter to one-third recover partially, and one-fifth remain chronically ill (Steinhausen 2002, 2009). These figures are cross-nationally consistent (Lee et al. 2003). The outcome of patients treated as adolescents appears to be more favorable (Strober et al. 1997), underscoring the importance of early intervention or, ideally, prevention. Bulimia nervosa generally has a more favorable course than anorexia nervosa. Unlike anorexia nervosa, bulimia nervosa does not appear to be associated with increased mortality risk (Berkman et al. 2007). However, long-term follow-up studies suggest that 10 years after presentation, nearly one-third of patients continue to binge and purge regularly (Keel et al. 1999). The outcome of eating disorder NOS is less well defined. However, it is clear that these atypical eating disorders often represent partial recovery from full-syndrome eating disorders or evolve into fully developed anorexia nervosa and bulimia nervosa (Fairburn and Harrison 2003); careful diagnosis and aggressive treatment are therefore warranted.

Several studies have identified specific historical and medical factors that predict good versus poor outcome in eating disorders (Table 14–1). In addition, treatment-related and posttreatment characteristics may predict response. For anorexia nervosa, a high rate of weight gain during inpatient treatment (Lund et al. 2009), higher post-treatment body mass index (BMI), lower rate of weight loss and lack of excessive exercise during the initial weeks following inpatient discharge (Carter et al. 2004; Kaplan et al. 2009), high motivation to change at discharge (Castro-Fornieles et al. 2007), low residual concern about shape and weight (Carter et al. 2004), higher percentage body fat following weight restoration (Mayer et al. 2007), and higher dietary energy density and diet variety score following weight restoration (Schebendach et al. 2008) are all predictive of good outcome. For bulimia nervosa, early change in treatment (Agras et al. 2000a; Fairburn et al. 2004), post-treatment binge abstinence, less-restricted food intake, low cue reactivity (i.e., urges to binge eat in response to cues) (Bulik et al. 1998), and less preoccupation with and ritualization of eating following treatment (Halmi et al. 2002) are all predictive of good outcome.

Assessment and Diagnosis

Assessment

The assessment of patients with symptoms suggestive of eating disorders presents several challenges. The clinical presentation may be confusing in that it may be difficult to determine whether behaviors such as food restriction or vomiting are driven by psychological or somatic distress, and the medical history is often vague and nonspecific. Moreover, as summarized above under "Psychiatric Comorbidity of Anorexia Nervosa and Bulimia Nervosa," comorbid psychiatric conditions frequently occur and may further complicate the presentation. It is often difficult to

TABLE 14–1. Prognostic factors in eating disorders

Factors predicting negative outcome	Factors predicting favorable outcome
Anorexia nervosa	
History of premorbid development or clinical abnormalities	Early age at onset
Binge eating and/or purging	Hospitalization for an affective disorder before baseline assessment
Long duration of illness	Short interval between symptom onset and beginning of treatment
Low body mass index at hospital admission	Conflict-free child–parent relationships
High serum uric acid level	Histrionic personality traits
High serum creatinine level	
Low serum albumin level	
Obsessive-compulsive personality traits	
Comorbid affective disorder	
Comorbid substance abuse	
Severity of alcohol use disorder during follow-up	
Bulimia nervosa	
Poor pretreatment global functioning	Younger age
Premorbid parental obesity	Shorter duration of symptoms
History of obesity	Less severe symptoms
Low self-esteem	Absence of concurrent disruptive pathology
Comorbid major depression	Strong motivation for treatment
Comorbid anxiety disorder	High self-directedness (TCI)
Comorbid alcohol abuse	
Impulsivity	
Comorbid personality disorders (particularly borderline)	

Note. TCI=Temperament and Character Inventory (Cloninger CR: The Temperament and Character Inventory [TCI]: A Guide to Its Development and Use. St. Louis, MO, Center for Psychobiology of Personality, Washington University, 1994).
Source. Adapted from Bulik et al. 1998; Hebebrand et al. 1997; D.B. Herzog et al. 2000; W. Herzog et al. 1997; Keel et al. 2003; Richards et al. 2000; Steinhausen 2002, 2009.

ascertain whether the comorbid psychiatric illness is causally related to the eating disorder or is more indirectly involved in the manifestation of the eating disorder. As an illustration of the latter, an individual with comorbid social phobia may experience a flare-up of eating disorder symptoms in social situations.

Probably the single most important component of the workup for eating disorders is a thorough history, covering the nutritional, behavioral, psychological, and motivational features discussed above under "Atypical Eating Disorders." The history should include past and recent patterns of eating, abnormal weight control behavior, associated beliefs and attitudes, timing of emergence of issues with eating and weight, lifetime weight course, and attitudes toward body image. Although obesity and extreme emaciation are readily apparent, the behaviors associated with these bodily states are not. Normal-weight patients with eating disorders may appear entirely healthy, and patients with anorexia nervosa may attempt to persuade the clinician that they are "naturally thin." Patients with eating disorders may hide their symptoms for several reasons. Behaviors such as binge eating and purging are often experienced by patients as shameful or disgusting. Patients with anorexia nervosa often feel that they must hide their restrictive dieting and compulsive exercise to avoid being prevented from continuing them. Obese patients with eating disorders may be particularly likely to minimize contact with health care providers because they fear being blamed or because they blame themselves for their obesity. Bearing this in mind, clinicians should employ a nonjudgmental assessment style that recognizes the patient's ambivalence and engages the patient in a medically informed discussion of the nature of the illness and the options for treatment. A useful approach to the assessment of eating disorder symptoms in a primary care setting was described by Kreipe and Yussman (2003).

Of particular importance to psychosomatic medicine specialists is the medical evaluation of patients with eating disorders. When the patient displays behaviors and attitudes characteristic of eating disorders (e.g., a classic binge-purge pattern, an unhealthy and excessive dieting regimen, or a lack of concern about weight loss or abnormal eating behaviors), the workup to establish a diagnosis of an eating disorder need not be exhaustive in ruling out primary organic disorders. No laboratory testing is required to make the diagnosis of an eating disorder unless the historical or physical evidence suggests the possibility of an organic etiology. However, for patients with an atypical presentation or those in whom an eating disorder is essentially a diagnosis of exclusion, the workup should be more extensive and the level of suspicion for an underlying organic etiology or sociocultural explanations should remain high. In patients known to have an eating disorder, physical examination and laboratory testing are key in evaluating any medical complications (see "Medical Complications" later in this chapter) or comorbid medical illnesses and in guiding treatment.

When the medical provider is seeing the patient for the first time, he or she must, in collaboration with the mental health provider, determine the level of care that is needed and the urgency of intervention. As outlined in the American Psychiatric Association (2006) "Practice Guideline for the Treatment of Patients With Eating Disorders," the physical assessment of the patient should include 1) complete physical examination, with attention to evidence of dehydration, acrocyanosis, lanugo, salivary gland enlargement, and scarring on the dorsum of the hands (Russell's sign); 2) vital signs with orthostatic determination of blood pressure and pulse; 3) assessment of physical and sexual growth and development, including height and weight (for pediatric patients a review of the patient's growth chart may be helpful); and 4) dental examination.

Laboratory evaluation should be individualized for the particular patient. In accordance with the American Psychiatric Association (2006) "Practice Guideline for the Treatment of Patients With Eating Disorders," the routine workup should include serum electrolytes, blood urea nitrogen and creatinine, liver enzymes, serum albumin, thyroid function tests, complete blood cell count, and urinalysis. Severely malnourished patients should receive additional blood chemistry assessments—including calcium, magnesium, phosphate, and ferritin levels—and an electrocardiogram, as well as 24-hour urine for creatinine clearance. Patients who are chronically underweight should be assessed for osteopenia and osteoporosis using dual-energy X-ray absorptiometry, and serum estradiol (or testosterone in males) may be assessed. Other tests that are not performed routinely but may be indicated in particular clinical situations include serum amylase, luteinizing hormone (LH) and follicle-stimulating hormone (FSH) levels; computed tomography or magnetic resonance imaging (MRI) of the brain; screening stool for blood, and screening stool or urine for bisacodyl, emodin, aloe-emodin, and rhein in patients with suspected laxative abuse. Although elevated serum amylase concentration is a frequent concomitant of vomiting, this test is not sufficiently sensitive or specific to serve as a useful screening tool for unreported vomiting (Walsh et al. 1990).

Large-scale screening for eating disorders may be a priority in some settings, particularly those in which the prevalence is known to be relatively high, such as high school or university health services. Although a variety of self-report and interview-based assessment tools are frequently used in research settings, one well-established instrument that can be recommended for its brevity and ease of use is the Eating Attitudes Test (EAT-26), originally developed to assess attitudes and behaviors characteristic of anorexia nervosa and also useful in detecting bulimia nervosa (Garner et al. 1982). Another more recently developed screening tool is the SCOFF, a five-item scale that, in initial studies, has good sensitivity and specificity for detecting anorexia nervosa and bulimia nervosa in adults (Morgan et al. 1999). The SCOFF questions are 1) Do you make yourself **S**ick because you feel uncomfortably full? 2) Do you worry you have lost **C**ontrol over how much you eat? 3) Have you recently lost more than **O**ne stone (14 pounds) in a 3-month period? 4) Do you believe yourself to be **F**at when others believe you are too thin? and 5) Would you say **F**ood dominates your life?

Differential Diagnosis

Hyperphagia, hypophagia, and altered eating patterns occur as features of a variety of medical and psychiatric illnesses and do not, in and of themselves, constitute formal eating disorders according to the standard of DSM-IV-TR. Table 14-2 lists some medical and psychiatric illnesses to consider in the differential diagnosis of an eating disorder. Two conditions of particular interest are Prader-Willi syndrome and Kleine-Levin syndrome.

Prader-Willi syndrome (PWS) is a multisystem disorder characterized by neonatal hypotonia, later obesity, hyperphagia, hypogonadotropic hypogonadism, and mental retardation. In contrast to most obese individuals, those with PWS have markedly elevated levels of ghrelin, an enteric hormone that stimulates growth hormone secretion and food intake (Haqq et al. 2003). PWS occurs sporadically, as a result of either microdeletion of chromosome 15p (70%) or maternal disomy of chromosome 15 (30%).

TABLE 14–2. Medical and psychiatric differential diagnosis of eating disorders

System	Diagnosis
Endocrine	Diabetes mellitus, hyperthyroidism, Addison's disease, Sheehan's syndrome (postpartum pituitary necrosis), panhypopituitarism
Gastrointestinal	Malabsorption, pancreatitis, cystic fibrosis, inflammatory bowel disease, peptic ulcer disease, superior mesenteric artery syndrome, Zenker's diverticulum, dysmotility disorders, gastric adenocarcinoma
Neurological	Psychomotor or limbic seizures, degenerative neurological conditions (Pick's disease, Alzheimer's disease, Huntington's disease, Parkinson's disease), hypothalamic or diencephalic tumor
Other medical	Malignancies (especially lymphoma and gastrointestinal cancers), collagen vascular disorders, chronic infections (especially tuberculosis, human immunodeficiency virus, fungal disease), parasitic infections, chronic renal failure, drug-induced appetite/weight change (e.g., corticosteroids, novel antipsychotics)
Psychiatric	Body dysmorphic disorder, melancholic major depression, atypical depression, obsessive-compulsive disorder, substance use disorder, dementia, factitious disorder, somatization disorder, psychotic disorder

Care of individuals with PWS can be challenging, primarily due to hyperphagia, food seeking and obesity, and conduct disorder, particularly manifested as tantrums or oppositional behavior (Couper 1999).

Kleine-Levin syndrome is a rare self-limited disorder of unknown origin that usually affects adolescent males and is characterized by episodic hypersomnia, increased appetite, and behavioral and psychiatric disturbances. Individuals typically function normally between episodes (Papacostas and Hadjivasilis 2000).

The presence of body image disturbance or intentional weight manipulation is usually quite useful in differentiating true eating disorders from other eating-related disorders. In the absence of these features, the diagnosis of an eating disorder should be regarded as provisional, and medical disorders such as those listed in Table 14–2 should be thoroughly considered in the differential diagnosis.

Risk Factors and Etiology

As research on the etiology of eating disorders has progressed, it has become clear that the onset of an eating disorder results from a confluence of factors: sociocultural, biological, and genetic. Most of what is currently known about the etiology of eating disorders focuses on anorexia nervosa and bulimia nervosa. Risk factors for BED may overlap with—but are not the same as—those for anorexia nervosa and bulimia nervosa and are considered briefly below under "Etiology of Binge-Eating Disorder."

Culture

Although eating disorders were once thought to affect mainly upper-class, Western women from majority cultures, they are increasingly prevalent among individuals from lower socioeconomic sectors and minority ethnic groups, both in the United States and in other countries (Gard and Freeman 1996; Striegel-Moore 1997). Despite the limitations of existing research in this area, a few facts have been reasonably well established. Across cultures, female gender is a robust risk factor for eating disorders, and the period of greatest risk of onset is during adolescence. Media exposure to the idealization of thinness appears to confer increased risk at least in the short term (Striegel-Moore and Bulik 2007). As Polivy and Herman (2002) explain, the "idealization of thinness" in cultures of abundance may trigger for some an intense focus on their body shape and weight. This intense focus, in turn, may precipitate the development of eating disorder pathology. Thus, a culture of abundance (and the thin ideal that comes with that culture) may be a necessary, but not sufficient, precursor to the development of eating disorders.

Some have suggested that the process of cultural change may be associated with increased vulnerability to eating disorders, especially as developing cultures embrace the modern Western body ideal of thinness. Such change may occur across time within a given society or on an individual level (Lee et al. 2010; M.N. Miller and Pumariega 2001). Cross-cultural differences in the presentation and meaning of eating disorders contribute to challenges in classifying eating disorders, and suggest the need for a more flexible or dimensional classification system that reflects cross-cultural differences (Becker 2007).

Family and Individual Environment

Along with cultural pressures toward thinness, familial and peer pressures to uphold the thin ideal have been cited as potential contributors to eating disorder pathology (Branch and Eurman 1980; Levine et al. 1994; Shisslak et al. 1998; Stice 1998; Wertheim et al. 1997). Furthermore, it has been argued that certain types of familial environments—namely, those in which parents are overly critical, hostile, and coercive and are overly enmeshed in their children's lives (e.g., Haworth-Hoeppner 2000; Minuchin et al. 1978)—may more readily breed eating disorder behaviors. However, none of these assertions concerning the role of peers and family in the development of eating disorders have been proven conclusively, and therefore further study encompassing a wide range of adversities is necessary (Stice 2002). Risk factor research is only now reaching a level of sophistication that will allow the identification of particular risk factors that interact with specific genetic vulnerabilities to increase a given individual's risk for developing a particular form of disordered eating (Mazzeo and Bulik 2009).

Certain environmental risk factors have received particular attention and have both heuristic value and important implications for the treatment of affected individuals. A predisposition to eating disorders has been noted among individuals who participate in certain activities that promote thinness, such as ballet dancing, modeling, and some sports that emphasize weight and body shape (Kann et al. 2000). A history of sexual abuse or trauma appears to be a nonspecific risk factor for developing eating problems and is particularly associated with bulimic disorders. Trauma is associated with greater comorbidity in eating disorders, including posttraumatic stress disorder (Brewerton 2007; Kendler et al. 2000).

Genetics

Although the research discussed above under "Culture" implicates culture as an important risk factor for the development of eating disorders, it is clear that individual vulnerabilities play a substantial role. Specifically, such traits as perfectionism, impulsivity, negative affect, and low self-esteem have all been cited as potential risk factors (Fairburn et al. 1999; Polivy and Herman 2002; Stice 2002) and may account for the fact that only a minority of young women in a high-risk cultural environment actually develop clinical eating disorders. In addition, a vulnerability to obesity appears to increase risk for bulimia nervosa and BED (Fairburn et al. 1997, 1998), possibly by promoting dieting. Many such trait vulnerabilities may be largely genetically determined, and the genetics of eating disorders is a rapidly developing area of interest (Bulik et al. 2007; Monteloene and Maj 2008; Steiger and Bruce 2007; Treasure 2007).

Results of some genetic epidemiological studies have suggested that anorexia nervosa, bulimia nervosa, and atypical eating disorders aggregate in families, and it appears that at least some of the risk factors are common to both anorexia nervosa and bulimia nervosa. In other words, relatives of persons with an eating disorder are significantly more likely than members of the general population to develop either the same or an alternative eating disorder. Twin studies have also suggested that genetic factors contribute substantially to the development of eating disorders (Bulik et al. 2000). In light of the evidence supporting the importance of genetic risk factors for eating disorders, the challenge of identifying meaningful intermediate phenotypes, subphenotypes, and associated biological endophenotypes that interact with environmental factors to promote the onset and maintenance of eating disorders looms large. For anorexia nervosa, obsessive-compulsive traits and perfectionism, weak set shifting, and bias toward detail may be intermediate phenotypes that confer risk. The "emotional phenotype" with abnormalities in reward and fear-anxiety systems may additionally confer risk or influence the particular symptom picture (Treasure 2007). For bulimia nervosa, relevant subphenotypes may include psychologically intact/perfectionistic, overregulated/compulsive, and dysregulated/impulsive personality traits (Steiger and Bruce 2007). At the level of genotype, the 5-hydroxytryptamine (5-HT; serotonin) 2A receptor (*5HT2A*) and brain-derived neurotrophic factor (*BDNF*) genes are promising candidates for association with the restricting subtype of anorexia nervosa (Monteleone and Maj 2008). A predisposition to obesity, particularly in its interaction with cultural values promoting thinness, may secondarily increase risk for bulimia nervosa and binge-eating disorder; genotypes of interest in this regard include variants of the melanocortin-4 receptor (*MC4R*) and fat mass and obesity-associated (*FTO*) genes (Hebebrand and Hinney 2009).

Neurotransmitters, Neuropeptides, and Neuroanatomy

A great deal of research has focused on abnormalities in the functioning of neurotransmitters, particularly serotonin, in the development and maintenance of eating pathology (Kaye 2008). A confluence of evidence suggests that serotonergic activity is increased in women who have recovered from anorexia nervosa and bulimia nervosa but is decreased in underweight individuals with anorexia nervosa and actively symptomatic women with bulimia nervosa. These findings are consistent with the idea that at baseline these patients are characterized by perfectionism and behavioral overcontrol but that when symptomatic, they may be more impulsive and undercontrolled (Kaye 2002). More recently, dopaminergic systems have been investigated in eating disorders, particularly with regard to their role in affect regulation and reward systems (Kaye 2008; Davis and Carter 2009).

Additionally, researchers have been interested in the role of appetite- and weight-regulating peptides, including those that stimulate appetite (such as neuropeptide Y, peptide YY, and galanin) and those that reduce appetite (such as leptin and corticotropin-releasing hormone). Most, but not all, of the reported abnormalities normalize after recovery, suggesting that they may reflect the operation of physiological mechanisms triggered by malnutrition or weight loss. However, increased cerebrospinal fluid concentrations of peptide YY in women who have recovered from bulimia nervosa and reduced cerebrospinal fluid concentrations of galanin in women with anorexia nervosa who have had long-term weight restoration may represent trait abnormalities rather than transient states resulting from eating disorder symptoms. The role of these peptides in the etiology of eating disorders requires further study (Kaye 2002). Other neuropeptide systems that could play a role in eating disorders include melanocortin and cannabinoid systems (Kaye 2008).

One relatively new avenue of research into the biological underpinnings of eating disorders is brain imaging, recently reviewed by Van den Eynde and Treasure (2009). Computed tomographic and MRI studies have consistently detected ventricular enlargement and diffuse atrophy in underweight patients with anorexia nervosa. Most reported abnormalities appear to reverse with weight restoration, suggesting that they represent secondary effects of malnutrition, although there is some evidence that gray matter volume reduction persists even after weight regain. While it is unlikely to be etiological, this persistent abnormality may reflect the effect of long-term malnutrition on the brain and may be related to the high rate of relapse in recovered anorexia nervosa patients.

Functional imaging studies have not yet provided a consistent picture of the relationship between abnormal functioning in particular brain regions and eating disorder symptoms, but provocative findings are beginning to emerge. There is evidence for both global and regional (frontal and parietal cortices) decreased metabolic activity, particularly in underweight patients with anorexia nervosa. Brain activation, as gauged by regional blood flow, in response to food-related cues has been reported in several studies to differ between patients with eating disorders and unaffected individuals, although a consistent pattern of difference has yet to be established. This is an area of active research, and we are approaching the point at which neuroimaging studies, taken together with neurobiological and genetic findings, may allow for an integrative pathophysiological understanding of the onset and maintenance of eating disorders.

Etiology of Binge-Eating Disorder

It should be noted that risk factors for BED may differ in degree and kind from those for anorexia nervosa and bulimia nervosa. A case-control community study found that risk factors for the development of BED were less numerous and weaker than those for anorexia nervosa and bulimia nervosa. Specific risk factors for BED include parental depression, vulnerability to obesity, and repeated exposure to negative comments about shape, weight, and eating (Fairburn et al. 1998). Genetic and environmental factors appear to interact in determining whether an individual progresses toward bulimia nervosa or BED. Genetic risk factors for binge eating and bulimia nervosa may be similar, whereas nonshared environment may be important in influencing the risk for bulimia nervosa once binge eating is initiated (Wade et al. 2000). In regard to obesity, most findings suggest that risk for binge eating is partially or largely independent of risk for obesity (Bulik et al. 2003; Hudson et al. 2006), although binge eating may contribute to the full expression of obese potential.

Medical Complications

The pathological processes associated with eating disorders are multisystemic in nature and result from the altered eating and compensatory behaviors that characterize these disorders. Medical morbidity in eating disorders results from severe restriction with extensive weight loss; self-induced vomiting; use of laxatives, diuretics, or appetite suppressants; or binge eating with excessive weight gain. These symptoms and the resultant pathological processes may occur singly, as in patients with restricting anorexia nervosa or normal-weight bulimia nervosa, or may co-occur, as in patients with anorexia nervosa purging subtype or eating disorder NOS. It is important to note that individuals with normal or above-normal body weight who lose an excessive amount of weight may manifest similar changes in medical status as those who start at normal or low body weight and lose even more. Eating disorder symptoms and their effects on medical status are summarized in Table 14–3. Medical morbidity related to obesity has been extensively reviewed elsewhere (Guh et al. 2009) and is beyond the scope of this chapter.

System-Focused Review of Medical Complications

Metabolic/Endocrine Effects

The primary pathophysiological response to starvation is reduced energy expenditure which likely occurs in two phases. Phase 1 involves a physiological adaptation with a decrease in the metabolic rate as a means of increasing metabolic efficiency. Phase 2 occurs after 2–3 weeks of undernutrition and reflects the actual loss of tissue (Winter et al. 2005). This reduction in energy expenditure has been clearly demonstrated in anorexia nervosa. Underlying the reduced metabolic rate is a change in thyroid hormone

TABLE 14–3. Eating disorder symptoms and medical effects

Symptom	Medical effect
Restrictive eating	Cognitive impairment, fatigue, cold intolerance, constipation, dizziness, hypoglycemia, acrocyanosis, orthostatic pulse and blood pressure, edema, amenorrhea
Vomiting	Dehydration, metabolic alkalosis, hypokalemia, arrhythmias, esophagitis/gastritis, esophageal tears, dental caries, parotid/submandibular gland hypertrophy, gastroesophageal reflux disease, pharyngitis
Binge eating/overeating (with increasing weight)	Obesity, dyslipidemia, hypertension, type 2 diabetes, coronary artery disease, stroke, gallbladder disease, osteoarthritis, sleep apnea, respiratory disorders
Laxative abuse	Cathartic colon, dehydration, hypokalemia, metabolic acidosis or mild metabolic alkalosis
Diuretic abuse	Dehydration, electrolyte imbalance (hypokalemia and hypomagnesemia)
Appetite-suppressant abuse	Hypertension, tremor, arrhythmias
Ipecac abuse	Generalized myopathy, cardiomyopathy
Compulsive exercise	Bradycardia, overuse syndrome, stress fractures
Water loading	Hyponatremia, headache, nausea, dizziness, seizure

synthesis characterized by normal thyroid-stimulating hormone level, low or normal thyroxine (T_4) concentration, low or normal levels of triiodothyronine (T_3), and elevated concentration of reverse T_3—a pattern known as the euthyroid sick syndrome. It is important to remember that this is a physiological adaptation; therefore, in most cases, thyroid hormone supplementation is not warranted (Lawson and Klibanski 2008). The concept of bulimia nervosa and BED as states of intermittent starvation is controversial, and the data on energy expenditure in these conditions are inconsistent (de Zwaan et al. 2002). The typical endocrine features of starvation (increased cortisol and growth hormone levels; decreased estrogen, LH, and FSH levels in women; decreased testosterone level in men) are also seen in anorexia nervosa and resolve with weight restoration (Devlin and Walsh 1988). Cortisol excess is associated with comorbid mood disorders, neurocognitive deficits, hippocampal atrophy, amenorrhea, myopathy, and bone loss. At least in the case of bone loss, there is evidence that the level of hypercortisolemia seen in adolescent girls with anorexia nervosa is sufficient to contribute (Misra et al. 2004). The change in growth hormone represents a nutritionally mediated, acquired resistance to this hormone that is also linked to low insulin-like growth factor-1 (IGF-1) levels and lower IGF-1 bioactivity. Acute starvation blocks IGF-1 production by the liver; thus, growth hormone excess is attributed in part to lack of IGF-1–mediated negative feedback due to low IGF-1 levels. The potential consequences of growth hormone resistance include muscle atrophy, growth failure, and bone loss (Lawson and Klibanski 2008).

Starvation is also associated with a reduction in noradrenergic activity in the central and peripheral nervous systems of patients with eating disorders. This reduction can lead to hypotension, bradycardia, hypothermia, and depression (Pirke 1996). It is not uncommon for body temperature to drop to 95°F (35°C) or even lower with continued weight loss, and marked bradycardia is common in underweight patients and in those who exercise extensively. Altered autonomic control of heart rate and blood pressure appears to return to normal with refeeding and resolution of eating disorder–related symptoms (Rechlin et al. 1998).

Another metabolic concomitant of starvation is hypoglycemia which is often seen in underweight patients with anorexia nervosa (Bhanji and Mattingly 1988) and sometimes in normal-weight patients with bulimia nervosa (Devlin et al. 1990). Symptomatic hypoglycemia is uncommon, but there are case reports of coma and death attributed to severe hypoglycemia in anorexia nervosa.

Renal Failure, Loss of Fluids, and Electrolyte Imbalance

Eating disorder–related behaviors such as vomiting, laxative or diuretic use, fluid restriction, or water loading may result in substantial fluctuations in fluid status and lead to life-threatening states such as severe dehydration with hypotension, acid–base disturbances, and electrolyte imbalances. Fluid loss, particularly from vomiting, often leads to metabolic alkalosis. Patients who abuse laxatives often develop metabolic acidosis. The most common electrolyte imbalance is hypokalemia, which, if chronic and persistent, can lead to nephropathy and chronic renal failure requiring dialysis, as well as to nephrogenic diabetes insipidus, metabolic alkalosis, renal hypochloremia, rhabdomyolysis, and intestinal ileus. Hypokalemia is a significant side effect of laxative and thiazide diuretic abuse. In one study, the creatinine clearance was found to be most reduced by chronic laxative abuse when compared with chronic vomiting or restricting (Takakura et al. 2006). Cardiac arrhythmias secondary to hypokalemia can be life-threatening; patients with arrhythmias must be given supplemental potassium as soon as possible to correct the imbalance. An electrocardiogram should be obtained and the patient should be placed on cardiac monitoring with intravenous potassium replacement if there are significant electrocardiographic abnormalities. Otherwise, oral potassium replacement is usually safe and effective if retention of the medication after ingestion can be assured. Hypomagnesemia may also be present, especially during refeeding (Birmingham et al. 2004), and may interfere with potassium normalization if it is not corrected as well. Hypocalcemia is uncommon, but when present, it (like hypomagnesemia) may be associated with prolongation of the QTc interval (see "Cardiovascular Effects" subsection below).

Serum phosphate levels also must be monitored because they are frequently low in patients with eating disorders, particularly those with low body weight. Although total body phosphate can be depleted through malnutrition, refeeding can also cause a drop to dangerous levels, and oral phosphate replacement is typically needed. During the first week of refeeding in inpatients, electrolyte including calcium, magnesium, and phosphate levels should be obtained at baseline and then monitored at least every other day for the remainder of the week. Thereafter, they can be monitored less frequently if they remain stable (Mehler and Andersen 1999). Hyponatremia can result from purging behaviors or from water loading. Significant hyponatremia is associated with increased seizure risk and therefore requires prompt detection, treatment, and close monitoring. Free water intake may need to be restricted until the sodium imbalance is corrected. Patients with normal kidney function will typically correct their fluid imbalance via spontaneous diuresis.

Plasma volume depletion and hypovolemic hyponatremia are common in the most severely malnourished patients with anorexia nervosa. Because of malnutrition, common indices of hemoconcentration may be within the normal range. In addition, hemoconcentration, when present, may mask anemia (Caregaro et al. 2005). Blood urea nitrogen is an unreliable indicator of hydration because it may be both reduced by inadequate protein intake and elevated by dehydration or increased protein catabolism.

Fluid losses caused by vomiting or abuse of diuretics, laxatives, or caffeine stimulate the renin-angiotensin system. Particularly in laxative abusers, this stimulation results in an increase in aldosterone concentration and subsequent fluid retention that may persist for weeks, leading to significant weight gain and even frank edema that is difficult for patients to tolerate. Maintenance of proper fluid status over time will correct the fluid retention, and diuresis will eventually ensue. Erratic release of vasopressin from the posterior pituitary may result in symptoms of diabetes insipidus, including excessive urination and hypernatremia (Gold et al. 1983).

Approximately 20% of all patients with anorexia nervosa develop some form of peripheral edema during refeeding. In anorexia nervosa, as refeeding progresses, insulin levels increase. Insulin promotes sodium reabsorption through changes in tubular transport of the nephron, leading to fluid retention, weight gain, and localized—or, more rarely, generalized—edema. Refeeding edema usually resolves spontaneously but must be closely monitored (Ehrlich et al. 2006).

Central Nervous System Effects

Both structural and functional changes in the brain are seen in adults and adolescents with anorexia nervosa. Studies have shown evidence of ventricular and cortical sulcal enlargement as well as functional impairment in attention and concentration, visual associative learning, visuospatial abilities, problem solving, and attentional-perceptual motor functions. Other impairments include psychomotor slowing, poor planning, and lack of insight. Some reversal of these changes has been demonstrated with weight restoration (Chowdhury and Lask 2001; Ehrlich et al. 2008; Kerem and Katzman 2003).

From a symptomatic perspective, headaches are common in patients with eating disorders, and the incidence of migraines in patients with anorexia and bulimia is very high (75%) in comparison with that in the general population (12.5%) (Ostuzzi et al. 2008). The biochemical profiles, particularly in relation to tyrosine metabolism, suggest that migraine may constitute a risk factor for development of eating disorders in young females (D'Andrea et al. 2008).

Cardiovascular Effects

Individuals with very low body weight lose significant cardiac muscle over time. The left ventricle is particularly affected, with hypotrophy characterized by myocardial degeneration (Ulger et al. 2006). Tissue doppler imaging has shown evidence of left ventricular dysfunction (Galetta et al. 2005). Undernourished individuals may also develop clinically silent pericardial effusions (McCallum et al. 2006) as well as conduction abnormalities with arrhythmias or a prolonged QTc interval. The latter has been shown to be a marker for risk of sudden death and therefore requires close monitoring. Prolongation of the QTc interval is often associated with hypokalemia, hypocalcemia, or hypomagnesemia but may also be caused or exacerbated by medication (Lesinskiene et al. 2008). QT dispersion is an index of variation in ventricular repolarization, which may increase susceptibility to ventricular arrhythmias. One study showed significantly increased measures of QT dispersion in subjects with chronic anorexia nervosa compared with age-matched controls, although the QT interval did not differ between the two groups (Krantz et al. 2005). Another study found decreased levels of heart rate variability in women with anorexia nervosa. This finding is significant in that low heart rate variability may predict sudden death in patients with cardiac disorders (Melanson et al. 2004). The most common cardiovascular abnormality in anorexia is sinus bradycardia secondary to vagal hyperactivity. Mitral valve prolapse has also been noted, although its clinical significance is not fully understood; it occurs more commonly in patients with anorexia nervosa and is perhaps secondary to physical remodeling of the heart with starvation (Cooke and Chambers 1995). The cardiovascular system is particularly vulnerable to substances used by patients with eating disorders for weight loss, including ipecac, diuretics, and appetite suppressants. The effects of these substances are noted in Table 14–3. Long-term use of ipecac is particularly dangerous, because it can be associated with the development of cardiomyopathy.

Gastrointestinal Effects

Gastrointestinal complications of eating disorders vary according to the specific eating disorder symptoms the patient manifests. Restrictive eating with marked weight loss leads to a slowing of gastrointestinal motility, resulting in gastroparesis and constipation. Impaired gastrointestinal motility may also result from ongoing abuse of laxatives, often in escalating amounts due to the development of tolerance. This condition, known as *cathartic colon,* can be associated with hemorrhoids and rectal prolapse from chronic straining. Delayed gastric emptying is also problematic for individuals with both the binge/purging and the restricting subtype of anorexia; it may serve to perpetuate disordered eating behaviors due to the prolonged sensation of fullness commonly reported by these patients. In one study that followed treatment of anorexic patients over a 20-week period of refeeding, gastric emptying times normalized in the restricting subgroup but not in the binge/purging subgroup. This suggests that long-term nutritional rehabilitation may improve both dyspeptic symptoms and gastric emptying, particularly for patients with the restricting subtype of anorexia nervosa (Benini et al. 2004). Elevation of hepatic transaminases is common in underweight patients with anorexia nervosa. Autophagy has been proposed as a cause for major hepatocyte dysfunction in anorexia nervosa with severe malnourishment even without cell death. Autophagy is a well-known survival strategy under stress conditions (Rautou et al. 2008). Steatosis is also encountered with refeeding and necessitates a reduction in the daily caloric amount and serial testing of transaminases until levels normalize. Nevertheless, continued refeeding is essential to normalization of liver function, which typically occurs quite rapidly (Narayanan et al. 2010).

Vomiting may cause complications related to acid reflux such as enlargement of salivary glands, dental caries, esophagitis, and gastritis. Gastrointestinal dysmotility, when present, is often related to hypokalemia. Forced vomiting may result in hematemesis, which may be secondary to a pharyngeal scratch from induction of vomiting but may also be secondary to gastritis, esophagitis, or (less frequently) gastric or esophageal tears. Binge eating in bulimia or anorexia can cause acute gastric dilatation, as can rapid refeeding in anorexia nervosa. This requires decompression with a nasogastric tube and fluid and electrolyte replacement. There are also case reports of acute and chronic pancreatitis in anorexia nervosa and bulimia.

Genitourinary Effects

In women with anorexia nervosa, amenorrhea is due to hypothalamic amenorrhea syndrome, in which pulsatile secretion of gonadotropin-releasing hormone (GnRH) is diminished. This reduced secretion in turn causes lower levels of LH and FSH along with low blood levels of estradiol, estrone, progesterone, and testosterone, leading to a physiological return to the prepubertal state. Although weight loss is a common precipitant of amenorrhea, a minority of patients develop amenorrhea before the onset of weight loss, indicating that other factors such as caloric restriction, excessive exercise, or psychogenic stress may also be important contributors (Morgan 1999). Menstrual cycling typically resumes with weight restoration at approximately 90% of standard body weight, although resumption may be delayed up to 6 months after that weight is achieved. Additionally, a substantial number of individuals (up to 26% in one study) require an above-average BMI to reestablish normal menstruation (Kaplan and Noble 2007; Vyver et al. 2008). Except in cases in which ovulation is induced, pregnancy is rare in women with active anorexia nervosa. However, in a study of 140 women with anorexia nervosa, 50 had conceived at 10-year follow-up, 20% of whom appeared to have done so while actively anorectic (Brinch et al. 1988).

About half of women with bulimia nervosa become amenorrheic or oligomenorrheic despite having no apparent change in percentage body fat. As in anorexia nervosa, this condition is commonly associated with impaired follicular maturation due to reduced LH concentrations and pulse frequency. Women with abnormal menstrual cycles in bulimia nervosa appear to be underweight in relationship to their own lifetime high body weight but not to average or expected body weight for their age and height (Devlin et al. 1989; Morgan 1999). A recent study that excluded underweight participants found that high school girls who reported vomiting for weight control once per week or more often were more than three times as likely to experience irregular menses as girls who did not report such vomiting (Austin et al. 2008). Another study examined the relationship between bulimic symptoms and fluctuations in ovarian hormones in bulimic women with intact menstrual cycles (Edler et al. 2006). The researchers found that decreases in estradiol and increases in progesterone were associated with marked increases in binge eating. Despite the profound effects of eating disorders on reproductive function, outcome studies suggest that with full recovery, fertility may not be compromised (Crow et al. 2002; Mitchell-Gieleghem et al. 2002).

Musculoskeletal Effects

Severe protein-energy malnutrition gives rise to a metabolic myopathy with significant loss of muscle mass and function. Cases of rhabdomyolysis have been reported in anorexia nervosa. However, muscle is very responsive to refeeding. One study found that muscle performance improved long before the nutritional compromise was entirely corrected, with some improvement noted as early as the eighth day of refeeding (Rigaud et al. 1997).

Osteopenia and osteoporosis are relatively unique among complications of eating disorders in that they appear not to be readily reversible with weight recovery. These conditions are chronic rather than acute effects of malnutrition, because clinically significant bone loss does not usually begin until 12 months after onset of illness. Thereafter, bone loss progresses at an average annual rate of 2.5% in young women with active anorexia nervosa (K.K. Miller et al. 2006). In their study of adolescent women with anorexia nervosa, Castro et al. (2000) found that the following factors were related to development of osteopenia: more than 12 months since onset of the disorder, more than 6 months of amenorrhea, BMI less than 15 kg/m^2, calcium intake less than 600 mg/day, and less than 3 hours/week of physical activity. It is estimated that osteoporosis occurs in more than half of adolescent and young adult females who struggle with eating disorders, and patients with anorexia nervosa have a fracture rate seven times higher than that in healthy women (Kaplan and Noble 2007). These conditions can result in painful fractures, disfiguring kyphosis, and loss of height. The pathophysiology of bone loss in anorexia nervosa is complex (Golden 2003; Mehler 2003; Rosenblum and Forman 2002). Whereas estrogen deficiency has been thought to mediate bone loss in anorexia nervosa, there are other factors integral to this process as well. IGF-1, a nutritionally dependent bone trophic hormone that stimulates osteoblasts to increase bone formation, is decreased in anorexic females, possibly due to decreased dehydroepiandrosterone (DHEA) in adolescent and young women with anorexia nervosa. More recently, receptor activator of nuclear factor kB ligand (RANKL) and osteoprotegerin (OPG) have been identified as important regulators of bone turnover. Serum OPG levels may be increased by a compensatory mechanism for malnutrition and estrogen deficiency that induces an increase in bone resorption (Ohwada et al. 2007). Depression has also been associated with osteoporosis in adults, and one study suggested that comorbid depression is associated with increased risk of osteoporosis in girls with anorexia nervosa (Konstantynowicz et al. 2005). Osteopenia and osteoporosis occur in men with anorexia nervosa as well, perhaps due to a relative lack of testosterone, which is a major substrate for estrogen production (Andersen et al. 2000).

The treatment of low bone density in anorexia nervosa requires—first and foremost—refeeding. Weight restoration is found to be effective in increasing bone mass, although not to pre-illness levels (Mehler and MacKenzie 2009). Resumption of menses is critical to this process as well. In women with anorexia nervosa whose menstrual cycles recover, spine bone mass density significantly increases independently of weight gain (Lawson and Klibanski 2008). Moderate weight-bearing exercise has been shown to be protective, although strenuous activity is detrimental. The uncertain status of pharmacological treatment for osteoporosis in these individuals has been well reviewed (Golden 2003; Mehler 2003). Growth hormone has direct and indirect (via IGF-1) anabolic effects on bone. Growth hormone resistance and low IGF-1 is characteristic of anorexia nervosa. Recombinant human IGF-1 is the only medical therapy shown thus far to improve bone mass density in women with anorexia nervosa, but it is not currently approved for this indication (Lawson and Klibanski 2008). The benefit of supplemental calcium is not clear; however, the current standard practice in the treatment of anorexia nervosa is to give daily calcium (1,300–1,500 mg/day) and vitamin D (400 IU/day). There is no evidence that estrogen replacement therapy either reverses or prevents bone loss in anorexia nervosa. It may even be contraindicated, given that hormone-induced withdrawal bleeding may be misinterpreted by patients as evidence of the return of normal menstrual function, thereby offering spurious assurance that they are at a healthy body weight despite ongoing malnutrition and emaciation (Kaplan and Noble

2007). Research examining the efficacy of oral bisphosphonates in anorexia nervosa has been promising, but use of drugs in this class is not currently recommended due to a lack of long-term safety studies (Jayasinghe et al. 2008). They are contraindicated in women who may become pregnant. There is no evidence supporting the use of calcitonin in anorexia nervosa.

Integumentary Effects

The cutaneous signs of eating disorders result from malnutrition and self-induced vomiting. Findings related to malnutrition include dry, scaly skin; lanugo hair; carotenodermia; brittle nails; and hair loss. Those related to self-induced vomiting include calluses on the dorsum of the hands from constant abrasion against the front teeth with induction of vomiting (Russell's sign), and purpura and petechiae from recurrent Valsalva maneuvers to induce vomiting. Purpura and petechiae can also be seen as a result of thrombocytopenia secondary to malnutrition (Mitchell and Crow 2006). See also Chapter 29, "Dermatology."

Other Effects

Bone marrow suppression with leukopenia, anemia, and thrombocytopenia is common in states of starvation, but these abnormalities reach clinically significant levels only in the most severe cases. Particularly in regard to leukopenia, IGF-1 deficiency may play a role (Polli et al. 2008). Pulmonary complications of eating disorders are rare but include pneumomediastinum and aspiration pneumonitis from forced vomiting, and chronic starvation may promote emphysema-like lung changes (Coxson et al. 2004). Dyspnea in long-standing malnourished states is often secondary to respiratory muscle weakness, which does not always show prompt recovery with refeeding and improved nutrition (Birmingham and Tan 2003).

Eating Disorders and Pregnancy

Eating disorders affect women during the period of reproductive functioning. Several studies have shown that one-third to one-half of women attending infertility clinics have full or subsyndromal eating disorders (Kaplan and Noble 2007). However, pregnant women with eating disorders rarely disclose their eating disorder to their clinician. Poor maternal or fetal weight gain should serve as red flags regarding the possibility of a hidden eating disorder. The diagnosis of an eating disorder has clinical significance, and the timely identification of an eating disorder may enable the clinician to more effectively manage the patient and optimize outcome (Micali et al. 2007).

Although the majority of women with eating disorders have normal pregnancies resulting in healthy babies, and eating disorder symptoms may improve during pregnancy, rates of caesarean section and of postpartum depression are elevated in women with eating disorders (Franko et al. 2001). Low prepregnancy weight and low weight gain during pregnancy are associated with low infant birth weight and a higher incidence of congenital malformations. Other maternal complications include an increase in bulimic symptoms during pregnancy as well as restrictive eating. Both low and high maternal weight gain may occur, miscarriage is more common, and hypertension is reported more often among bulimic women (Morgan et al. 2006). Considerations for hospital admission include degree of weight loss, hypokalemia and other electrolyte abnormalities, and electrocardiographic changes, as well as fetal growth and physiological profile. Birth complications seen with both anorexia nervosa and bulimia nervosa include stillbirth, low birth weight, low Apgar scores, and cleft lip and palate (Mitchell-Gieleghem et al. 2002).

Breast-feeding problems in women with eating disorders have been noted. These include complaints of insufficient lactation or of allergies or negative reactions to breast milk in the infant, resulting in early transition to bottle feeding. For women whose eating disorder treatment includes medication, the risks and benefits of breast-feeding should be carefully reviewed. Child-rearing practices may also be affected by the presence of an unresolved eating disorder in the mother. In a small proportion of cases, inadequate feeding of children has been reported with a secondary effect on the child's growth (Fairburn and Harrison 2003; Mitchell-Gieleghem et al. 2002).

A recent study examined the relationship between obstetric complications and temperament in eating disorder subjects. The findings suggest that neonatal dysmaturity and elevated harm avoidance may have a mediating role in vulnerability to and maintenance of an eating disorder (Favaro et al. 2008).

Eating Disorders and Diabetes Mellitus

Some evidence suggests that there is an increase in disordered eating in chronic medical conditions for which dietary restraint is part of the treatment plan (see also Chapter 22, "Endocrine and Metabolic Disorders"). This is particularly true of type 1 diabetes mellitus. Several studies have examined personality, temperament, and character in type 1 diabetic patients with eating disorders. Weight preoccupation was associated with the presence of an eating disorder, and borderline personality characteristics were related to withholding insulin (Mitchell and Crow 2006). The presence of a comorbid eating disorder has been associated with markedly worse outcome. A study of mortality of individuals with type 1 diabetes and anorexia nervosa reported crude mortality rates of 2.5% for type 1 diabetes, 6.5% for anorexia nervosa, and 34.8% for concurrent cases (Nielsen et al. 2002). Individuals with anorexia nervosa and bulimia nervosa may withhold their daily insulin to prevent uptake of glucose and, in effect, purge. However, they may also manifest other symptoms such as restricting, laxative use, vomiting, use of appetite suppressants, and compulsive exercise. Blood glucose level is typically elevated, and there is an increased risk of ketoacidosis and other complications (Rodin 2002). Mean glycosylated hemoglobin has been found to be higher in subjects with diabetes mellitus who have an eating disorder (9.4%) compared with those without an eating disorder (8.6%) (Affenito and Adams 2001). Of all the problematic behavioral factors related to eating disorders, the duration of severe insulin omission is the factor most closely associated with retinopathy and nephropathy in type 1 diabetic females with eating disorders (Takii et al. 2008). The multidisciplinary team treatment of these individuals should include close endocrinological supervision. There is an ongoing need for frequent insulin changes with progression of the meal plan and activity level, or with symptom fluctuation.

Treatment

Given the contributions of cultural, familial, environmental, and genetic factors to the development of eating disorders, it is not difficult to appreciate why a biopsychosocial approach to understanding eating disorders and a multidisciplinary approach to treatment are seen as the foundation of current practice. This approach includes, at a minimum, team members to provide psychotherapy and medication management, medical monitoring and treatment, dietary management, and social service needs. The intensity of treatment and of the setting in which treatment is delivered may vary from self-help or support groups for the least symptomatic patients to weekly outpatient treatment, intensive outpatient treatment, day hospital treatment, or inpatient treatment for the most severely compromised (Kaplan et al. 2001). Patients with anorexia nervosa who are significantly underweight often require inpatient treatment, at least in the initial phase of weight restoration. Those with bulimia nervosa and BED can most often be treated as outpatients, although medical or psychiatric instability or failure of outpatient treatment options may indicate hospitalization. The treatment guidelines published by the American Psychiatric Association (2006) and by Great Britain's National Institute for Clinical Excellence (2004) provide a useful set of standards for determining the appropriate initial level of care. In addition, the American Dietetic Association (2006) has published a position paper on nutrition intervention in the treatment of eating disorders.

Nutritional Approaches

Nutritional rehabilitation is a fundamental and often extremely challenging component of treatment. Body weight may range from extremely low in patients with anorexia nervosa to high or markedly unstable in patients with bulimia nervosa and BED. Dietary history at intake may reveal various abnormalities, including avoidance of particular foods, overconsumption of low-calorie foods such as artificial sweeteners, uncontrolled binge eating, or food rituals. The latter are common and include preferences for unusually seasoned foods or combinations of foods, prolonged mealtimes, and eating alone. Strikingly, even in patients who eat very little themselves, food obsessions and a tendency to work around food are common (Rock and Curran-Celentano 1996).

Weight restoration is of primary importance for the individual with low body weight, whereas weight stabilization may be needed in individuals with normal or above-normal body weight. For obese patients, weight loss may be a goal, but this is usually best deferred until treatment for the eating disorder is well under way. An inpatient program should be considered for the most seriously nutritionally compromised patients, including those whose weight is less than 75% of ideal body weight or for those, especially children and adolescents, whose weight loss may not be as severe but who are losing weight at a rapid rate. Structured behavioral inpatient programs typically utilize multidisciplinary treatment teams in an effort to help patients meet set nutritional goals (Attia and Walsh 2009). The initial plan calls for establishment of a healthy weight target and a plan to restore weight safely and effectively while addressing body image and related concerns. A target weight for discharge from inpatient treatment is typically set at a range greater than or equal to approximately 90% of average for age and height. It is important that patients understand that this is a *minimum acceptable* rather than a recommended weight range.

Body composition is characterized by an extremely low percentage of body fat in emaciated patients with anorexia nervosa that increases rapidly with refeeding. Measurement of skinfold thickness provides a reliable estimate of body fat in these patients (Probst et al. 2001). Studies of body composition during the process of refeeding in patients with anorexia nervosa reveal that most of the nonfluid weight regained is represented by fat, accounting for 32%–77% of total weight gained (Rock and Curran-Celentano 1996), whereas muscle mass appears to lag behind (Polito et al. 1998). The initial distribution of weight regain is often disproportionately centripetal (Grinspoon et al. 2001), with redistribution occurring in the months following achievement of target weight.

Patients with anorexia nervosa may be unwilling or unable to accept food, at least initially. According to the American Psychiatric Association (2006) Practice Guideline, intake levels should usually start at 30–40 kcal/kg/day (approximately 1,000–1,600 kcal/day) and should be advanced progressively to yield a rate of weight gain of 2–3 lb/week for inpatients and 0.5–1 lb/week for outpatients. Patients may require levels of energy intake as high as 70–100 kcal/kg/day or more to accomplish this rate of weight gain, and nutritional supplements are often used in patients with high caloric requirements for weight regain. Although the oral feeding route is preferred, nasogastric feeding is utilized in the initial stage of treatment in some treatment centers. In particular, some clinicians support progressive nocturnal nasogastric supplemental feeding for individuals with low body weight as a means of minimizing somatic and psychological distress during initial weight regain and of speeding weight restoration (Robb et al. 2002; Zuercher et al. 2003). As weight gain progresses, regular meal portion sizes are gradually increased until nasogastric supplements are no longer required. If nasogastric feeding is necessary, it is recommended that normal eating behaviors (i.e., consuming foods orally during the daytime) be reinstated as soon as is feasible (Attia and Walsh 2009). Parenteral nutrition may be utilized in extreme circumstances; however, parenteral feedings are usually not given because of the associated risks of infection and increased risk of refeeding syndrome (described below in this subsection). Although weight regain is rarely steady, a particularly erratic weight-gain pattern or inability to gain weight despite increasing caloric intake may reflect covert disposal of food, exercise, purging, or water loading to make weight, and more stringent monitoring may be in order.

Physical activity during weight restoration should be adapted to the food intake and energy expenditure of the patient, taking into account the patient's history of excessive exercise. Adherence to the refeeding protocol is often linked with greater freedom to participate in activities and other rewards. Increases in physical activity must be balanced with medical stability, weight restoration, and control of eating disorder symptoms, including excessive activity. Strict limitations are required for individuals who struggle with compulsive exercise, and more intensive monitoring may be needed for those found to be exercising covertly. In most programs, activity is progressively advanced to include regimens of stretching, strengthening, and aerobic activity when appropriate (Rosenblum and Forman 2002).

Careful medical monitoring is essential throughout the refeeding period and typically includes monitoring of vital signs, renal function, food and fluid intake and output, and routine electrolytes plus magnesium, calcium, and phosphate. In addition, patients should be observed for edema and rapid weight regain. If present, these may suggest fluid overload or congestive heart failure. Gastrointestinal symptoms of constipation, bloating, and abdominal pain should also be monitored. Cardiac monitoring may be indicated for severely malnourished individuals (below 70% of ideal body weight), especially children and adolescents and those individuals with severe electrolyte disturbances, arrhythmias, or prolonged QTc interval (Al-Khatib et al. 2003; American Dietetic Association 2006; Sylvester and Forman 2008; Yager and Andersen 2005).

Cholesterol levels in anorexia nervosa are usually normal or high despite low cholesterol intake. These levels do not result from the de novo synthesis of cholesterol. Rather, abnormal thyroid hormone status, low serum estrogen levels, hypercortisolism, and impaired clearance of cholesterol explain or contribute to hypercholesterolemia in this setting. Weight restoration is typically accompanied by reduction in cholesterol level and apolipoprotein B (Feillet et al. 2000), and no effort should be made to further reduce dietary fat or cholesterol (Rock and Curran-Celentano 1996). Other laboratory abnormalities that characterize starvation and early recovery such as low white blood cell count or elevated liver transaminases typically normalize with weight recovery.

One of the most serious complications of weight restoration is the refeeding syndrome, characterized by marked fluid and electrolyte abnormalities, including low serum phosphate levels. The combination of depletion of total body phosphate stores during catabolic starvation and increased cellular influx of phosphate during anabolic refeeding leads to severe extracellular hypophosphatemia. This well-recognized complication of refeeding, particularly in individuals who have very low body weight, can lead to cardiac arrhythmias, delirium, and even sudden death (Solomon and Kirby 1990). Other potential symptoms of the refeeding syndrome include abnormal sodium and fluid balance; alterations in the metabolism of glucose, protein, and fat; thiamine deficiency; hypokalemia; and hypomagnesemia (Mehanna et al. 2008). This syndrome has most often been noted in refeeding with total parenteral nutrition but can occur with oral and nasogastric refeeding regimens as well (American Psychiatric Association 2006).

In a recent review of studies of the refeeding syndrome, Mehanna et al. (2008) recommend adhering to the National Institute for Clinical Excellence (2004) guidelines for prevention of the refeeding syndrome. Per the guidelines, individuals who have "eaten little or nothing for more than 5 days" should initially be given no more than 50% of their required energy intake. Energy intake should be increased slowly, depending on each individual's needs. Individuals who are very malnourished (BMI ≤14 kg/m^2; or have had little food intake for 2+ weeks) should be fed no more than 0.021 MJ/kg/24 hours and should be monitored for any cardiac problems. Vitamin supplements (i.e., potassium, phosphate, calcium, magnesium) should be given before and during the first 10 days of refeeding, unless blood levels are high. There is no need to address electrolyte and fluid imbalances prior to refeeding; they will be corrected during the feeding process. Mehanna et al. (2008) note that there is no consensus in the field about the best method for repletion of electrolytes during feeding.

As refeeding progresses, specific laboratory markers can be used to assess improvement or deterioration in nutritional status and in effect measure the transition from protein catabolism to anabolism. A number of different parameters have been used, including serum albumin, prealbumin, retinol-binding protein, transferrin, and C reactive protein. Serum prealbumin has a short half-life and responds rapidly to low energy intake even in the presence of adequate protein intake, making it an excellent marker of nutritional response to refeeding in severely malnourished individuals. Serum prealbumin levels of 20–40 mg/dL are considered normal, levels in the range of 10–15 mg/dL indicate mild malnutrition, levels of 5–10 mg/dL indicate moderate malnutrition, and levels of less than 5 mg/dL suggest severe depletion (Mears 1996). Caregaro et al. (2001) have studied the use of IGF-1 as a biochemical marker of malnutrition and a sensitive index of nutritional repletion in patients with eating disorders.

For patients with binge eating and/or purging, nutritional rehabilitation is geared toward the establishment of a regular eating pattern, moderation of dietary restraint, and elimination of unhealthy dieting practices. Inpatients with bulimia nervosa may require constant observation after meals to keep them from vomiting and to help them learn to tolerate the sensation of fullness following a meal. For obese patients with bulimia nervosa, weight loss may be medically indicated after resolution of the eating disorder. It is an important principle of treatment that cessation of binge eating/purging and simultaneous weight loss are incompatible goals (Rock and Curran-Celentano 1996). In contrast, for obese patients with BED, some have proposed treatments that concurrently target both obesity and binge eating (Devlin 2001).

Psychopharmacological Approaches

A number of studies have evaluated the efficacy of medications in the treatment of eating disorders, and findings are thoroughly summarized in recent reviews (Crow et al. 2009; Reas and Grilo 2008; Shapiro et al. 2007). An important related area, the psychopharmacological management of obesity associated with mental disorders, is beyond the scope of this chapter but has been reviewed (Malhotra and McElroy 2002).

The most widely studied class of drugs for eating disorders is antidepressants, including tricyclic antidepressants (TCAs), monoamine oxidase inhibitors (MAOIs), and selective serotonin reuptake inhibitors (SSRIs). For patients with bulimia nervosa, antidepressants are significantly more effective than placebo in reducing binge-eating and purging behaviors. Furthermore, it appears that all antidepressants work equally effectively; however, SSRIs yield fewer side effects than MAOIs and TCAs, and fluoxetine is the only medication approved by the U.S. Food and Drug Administration for the treatment of bulimia nervosa. However, longer-term studies of antidepressant treatment with bulimia nervosa suggest that these medications alone are not sufficient to facilitate long-term remission (Romano et al. 2002; Walsh et al. 1991). In BED, SSRIs have been found to significantly reduce binge frequency relative to placebo in the short term (Reas and Grilo 2008). For patients with anorexia nervosa, antidepressant treatment has, for the most part, not been found to be effective (Crow et al. 2009).

Although they are less well studied than antidepressants, other classes of drugs have been reported to be useful in the treatment of BED and bulimia nervosa. Anticonvulsants (carbamazepine, phenytoin, valproate) and other psychotropic medications (lithium, naltrexone, methylphenidate) have been reported to be effective in reducing binge eating in bulimia nervosa or BED, but their routine use has not been clearly established. Topiramate has been found to curb binge-eating episodes in patients with BED and bulimia nervosa and also to cause weight loss in obese patients, a potentially useful side effect that has not been observed with other medications used for these disorders (Arbaizar et al. 2008). Studies have found sibutramine to be significantly more effective than placebo in reducing binge frequency and decreasing weight in obese patients with BED (Appolinario et al. 2003; Milano et al. 2005; Wilfley et al. 2008). In their review of medication for BED, Reas and Grilo (2008) suggested that antiobesity medications (i.e., sibutramine) and antiepileptic medications (i.e., topiramate) may be more clinically useful than SSRIs, as they have been shown to enhance weight loss in trials of cognitive-behavioral therapy and behavioral weight loss treatments for BED and are associated with greater reductions in binge frequency than are SSRIs. Finally, Grilo et al. (2005a) examined orlistat, a lipase inhibitor, as an adjunct to guided self-help cognitive-behavioral therapy for BED. Results indicated that those taking orlistat experienced significantly greater remission from binge eating at posttreatment than did those taking placebo; this difference did not persist at follow-up. However, at follow-up, those taking orlistat had experienced significantly, although quite modestly greater weight loss than did those taking placebo. This relatively minimal benefit, along with the gastrointestinal effects of orlistat somewhat limit clinical enthusiasm for its use in this setting.

In general, patients with anorexia nervosa have not responded favorably to pharmacotherapy (Crow et al. 2009). However, recent evidence suggests that the antipsychotic medication olanzapine may be a useful tool in the treatment of anorexia nervosa, both for its ability to target the delusions, anxiety, and obsessions that often characterize those with anorexia nervosa and its documented side effect of weight gain (Bissada et al. 2008; Dunican and Del-Dotto 2007), though the knowledge of the latter effect may heighten fat concern and cause many anorectic patients to decline it. In addition, some earlier studies found fluoxetine to be a useful tool for relapse prevention in weight-restored patients with prior anorexia nervosa (Kaye et al. 1991, 2001); a more recent study however failed to replicate these findings (Walsh et al. 2006). It has recently been suggested that D-cycloserine, an antibiotic, may help facilitate fear extinction in exposure therapy for anorexia nervosa (Steinglass et al. 2007). However, this has yet to be evaluated in a randomized controlled trial.

Psychotherapeutic Approaches

Mental health professionals employ a wide variety of therapeutic techniques in their efforts to treat the symptoms of anorexia nervosa, bulimia nervosa, and BED. However, only a few of these psychotherapies, such as cognitive-behavioral therapy (CBT) and interpersonal therapy, have been systematically studied in randomized controlled trials, and not all forms of psychotherapy have been studied across eating disorder diagnoses.

CBT, the most widely studied method of psychotherapy for eating disorders, targets the two broad areas of eating disorder symptoms: 1) cognitive and attitudinal disturbances, such as low self-esteem and overemphasis on and distortion of weight and shape; and 2) behavioral aspects of eating and weight regulation, such as purging and food intake restriction. The goals of CBT are to challenge rigid rules about eating and weight that patients with eating disorders have imposed on themselves and to help these patients develop healthier behaviors and cognitions. CBT for bulimia nervosa was first put into manualized format in the early 1990s (Fairburn et al. 1993b) and has subsequently been modified for patients with anorexia nervosa and BED (Garner et al. 1997; Marcus 1997). CBT has been administered in an individual format, in a group setting, and via a self-help manual. Most recently, Fairburn, one of the authors of the original CBT manual (Fairburn et al. 1993b) developed a "transdiagnostic" treatment protocol to be used with all forms of eating disorder pathology. This protocol allows a clinician to flexibly tailor CBT interventions to the specific eating disorder pathology with which a given patient presents (Fairburn 2008).

Most studies of CBT have examined patients with bulimia nervosa. In general, it has been shown that CBT is more effective than minimal treatment, supportive psychotherapy, and purely behavioral interventions in reducing both the behavioral and the cognitive disturbances of patients with bulimia nervosa. Studies assessing the effectiveness of CBT alone, medication alone, and their combination in the treatment of bulimia nervosa have shown that CBT alone is more effective than medication alone and leads to more successful long-term maintenance of change. Antidepressants have not been conclusively shown to confer significant additional benefits to CBT treatment for bulimia nervosa. They are thought to be most useful for targeting comorbid symptoms of depression and anxiety (Walsh et al. 1997; Wilson et al. 2007). Studies of CBT in patients with BED have shown that CBT is significantly more effective than no treatment (American Psychiatric Association 2006) or treatment with antidepressants alone (Grilo et al. 2005b). While an early study indicated that CBT was no more efficacious than a behavioral weight loss program (Agras et al. 1994), more recent findings have suggested that CBT may be superior to behavioral weight loss treatment in terms of binge remission (Grilo and Masheb 2005; Munsch et al. 2007; Wilson et al. 2010). Further, adding an individual CBT component to a group behavioral weight loss treatment enhances reduction in binge frequency and abstinence (Devlin et al. 2005, 2007). Great Britain's National Institute for Clinical Excellence (2004) assigned an "A" grade to CBT for bulimia nervosa and BED, indicating that there is solid empirical evidence to support the efficacy of these treatments. Studies of CBT for anorexia nervosa have been too small in scope and methodologically unsound to yield firm conclusions about the use of CBT in this population.

As mentioned, Fairburn (2008) recently developed a "transdiagnostic" CBT treatment, which can be flexibly tailored to a patient's specific eating pathology. This treatment can be implemented in two forms—a "focused" form, which resembles traditional CBT for eating disorders, as well as a "broad form," in which one or more broad maintaining mechanisms of the eating disorder (mood intolerance, clinical perfectionism, core low self-esteem, and interpersonal problems) are addressed. Treatment length varies according to an individual's specific eating pathology and the treatment modules that are selected. In the first randomized controlled trial of this treatment (Fairburn et al. 2009), individuals across eating disorder diagnoses exhibited significant improvement in eating disorder pathology relative to a wait-list control. Further, both forms of CBT ("focused" and "broad") were equally effective, prompting the authors to suggest that the "broad" form is indicated only when there is significant comorbid psychopathology that could be addressed by one of the "broad" treatment modules.

Several additional nonpharmacological forms of treatment for eating disorders deserve mention. Interpersonal therapy was originally developed as a treatment for depression (Klerman et al. 1984) and was subsequently adapted for use with bulimia nervosa and BED (Fairburn 1997; Wilfley et al. 1993). Interpersonal therapy focuses on a person's interpersonal relationships rather than on the specific behavioral or attitudinal disturbances of the eating disorder. Studies comparing CBT and interpersonal therapy for bulimia nervosa have shown that although CBT appears to exert its effects more quickly, the two treatments both lead to significant long-term symptom change (Agras et al. 2000b; Fairburn et al. 1993a). In patients with BED, CBT and interpersonal therapy appear to be equally effective (Wilfley et al. 2002).

It has been suggested that the behavioral therapy technique of exposure and response prevention (EX/RP) might be effective for individuals with anorexia and bulimia nervosa (e.g., Leitenberg et al. 1988; Steinglass et al. 2007). In patients with anorexia nervosa, EX/RP entails exposing individuals to feared foods and asking them to eat them, thereby challenging their typical response (i.e., to avoid the food). Patients with bulimia nervosa are exposed to binge foods and are then asked to refrain from vomiting after eating these foods. Data on the efficacy of this approach for bulimia nervosa is mixed (American Psychiatric Association 2006), and data on EX/RP for anorexia nervosa is lacking. Some research has supported the efficacy of dialectical behavior therapy (DBT) for bulimia nervosa (Safer et al. 2001) and BED (Telch et al. 2001). These studies must be replicated before firm conclusions can be drawn.

As mentioned above, one alternative to CBT treatment for BED is behavioral weight loss treatment, which focuses on improving the patient's diet and exercise regimen and restricting his or her caloric intake. In general, it appears that behavioral weight loss is effective in the short term in reducing episodes of binge eating and yielding modest weight loss; however, as discussed above, CBT may be more effective for decreasing binge frequency (Latner and Wilson 2008). Furthermore, few studies have examined the long-term effects of behavioral programs, a key issue in obesity treatment. Some patients who have BED associated with obesity may also pursue weight-loss surgery, the most common procedure being the Roux-en-Y gastric bypass (see Chapter 30, "Surgery"). For these patients, the long-term prognostic significance of an eating disorder is uncertain and merits further study.

There have been few systematic studies of treatment for anorexia nervosa. Patients with anorexia nervosa can be treated either on an inpatient or an outpatient basis. Often treatment is sequenced, starting out with inpatient therapy or partial hospitalization followed by outpatient therapy aimed at relapse prevention. Inpatient therapy usually involves some combination of individual therapy, family therapy, nutritional counseling, and occupational/recreational therapy, typically with behavioral incentives in place for encouraging weight gain. Outpatient therapies used for anorexia nervosa have been eclectic, ranging from nutritional counseling to supportive psychotherapy to CBT. Recently, researchers have begun to empirically evaluate some forms of outpatient treatment for anorexia nervosa. For example, a group from the Maudsley Hospital in London developed a manualized outpatient family therapy for adolescents with anorexia nervosa that seeks to empower parents to refeed their child at home (Lock et al. 2001). Results from a number of studies suggest that the Maudsley method is extremely effective for long-term weight restoration in adolescents with an early onset of anorexia nervosa and a short duration of illness (Eisler et al. 2007; Le Grange et al. 2005; Russell et al. 1987). Recent evidence suggests that the Maudsley method might also be effective for adolescents with bulimia nervosa (Le Grange et al. 2007).

Involuntary Treatment

A critical issue concerning treatment for eating disorders, particularly anorexia nervosa, is the question of involuntary hospitalization for critically ill patients. Patients with anorexia nervosa often experience their illness as an important component of their identity, and they are therefore quite reluctant to undertake treatment. Many patients are hospitalized against their will by loved ones or health care providers with serious concerns about their medical stability. Some countries (e.g., the United Kingdom) have established clear guidelines outlining the conditions under which compulsory treatment for anorexia nervosa is indicated. However, the United States has no such guidelines, and American clinicians treating patients with anorexia nervosa must therefore consult more general standards for involuntary treatment. (See Thiels [2008] and Thiels and Curtice [2009] for comprehensive reviews of involuntary treatment for anorexia nervosa.)

The question of whether involuntary treatment for anorexia nervosa is ethical is a controversial one (Beumont and Carney 2004; Russell 2001; Thiels 2008; Thiels and Curtice 2009). Supporters of involuntary treatment claim that extremely low-weight patients with anorexia nervosa are incapable of making treatment decisions for themselves, due to both the cognitive effects of semistarvation and their distorted thinking surrounding food and body image. Detractors of involuntary treatment cite a host of concerns. Some believe that conceptualizing anorexia nervosa as an illness meriting compulsory treatment overemphasizes its medical aspects and ignores the many pertinent emotional and social factors that may contribute to the illness. Others argue that prospective patients are generally neither psychotic nor grossly impaired in cognitive function and therefore do not lack capacity to make treatment decisions. An additional concern is that patients who are forced into treatment will not be willing to continue treatment once their dire medical situation is resolved and that clinicians who take action to commit their patients against their wishes will destroy the therapeutic relationship (Russell 2001). The American Psychiatric Association (2006) practice guidelines state the following regarding involuntary treatment: "There is general agreement that children and adolescents who are severely malnourished and in grave medical danger should be re-fed, involuntarily if necessary, but that every effort should be made to gain their cooperation as cognitive function improves" (p. 44). In a recent study of involuntary hospitalization of adults and adolescents with eating disorders, Guarda et al. (2007) found that of the 46 patients who initially denied needing admission to the hospital, 20 patients changed their minds after 2 weeks in the hospital and agreed that hospitalization was indicated. This led the authors to speculate that engagement in treatment changed patients' perceptions of their need for help.

Four studies, only one of which took place in the United States, compared the outcomes of patients who had been hospitalized involuntarily with those of voluntary patients (Ayton et al. 2008; Griffiths et al. 1997; Ramsay et al. 1999; Watson et al. 2000). Results of all studies indicated that, in the short term, voluntary and involuntary patients made equally strong progress in terms of weight gain, although in some cases involuntary patients required a longer hospital stay to achieve their target weights. Based on the examination of a national mortality register roughly 5 years after hospitalization, Ramsay et al. (1999) reported higher mortality rates in involuntary patients. Ayton et al. (2008) followed their adolescent patients for 1 year posthospitalization and found nonsignificant trends indicating that a larger proportion of involuntary patients had a good outcome and a lower proportion of these patients required rehospitalization. In interpreting studies of involuntary versus voluntary treatment, it is important to note that randomized designs are not feasible; thus, the possibility that observed outcomes might be influenced by unidentified differences in patient characteristics or treatment cannot be dismissed. Further study of both the ethical basis and the practical utility of involuntary treatment is needed.

Conclusion

Disordered eating is an important component of the clinical presentation of a variety of patients with weights ranging from emaciated to severely obese. In some cases, disordered eating is of sufficient severity to warrant an eating disorder diagnosis in its own right, whereas in other cases, eating disorder symptoms may complicate the clinical picture of patients with other medical or psychiatric illness. Although the most common eating disorder diagnosis is eating disorder NOS, it is also the most inadequately studied. However, knowledge of the assessment, differential diagnosis, medical complications, and treatment of the classic eating disorders will aid the psychiatric practitioner in developing a treatment approach for patients with a wide range of eating disorder symptoms and in contributing to the multidisciplinary treatment of severely ill patients who are medically compromised by their eating disorder.

References

Affenito SG, Adams CH: Are eating disorders more prevalent in females with type 1 diabetes mellitus when the impact of insulin omission is considered? Nutr Rev 59:179–182, 2001

Agras WS, Telch CF, Arnow B, et al: Weight loss, cognitive-behavioral, and desipramine treatments in binge eating disorder. An additive design. Behav Ther 25:209–224, 1994

Agras WS, Crow SJ, Halmi KA, et al: Outcome predictors for the cognitive behavior treatment of bulimia nervosa: data from a multisite study. Am J Psychiatry 157:1302–1308, 2000a

Agras WS, Walsh BT, Fairburn CG, et al: A multicenter comparison of cognitive-behavioral therapy and interpersonal psychotherapy for bulimia nervosa. Arch Gen Psychiatry 57:459–466, 2000b

Al-Khatib SM, LaPointe NM, Kramer JM, et al: What clinicians should know about the QT interval. JAMA 289:2120–2127, 2003

American Dietetic Association: Position of the American Dietetic Association: Nutrition intervention in the treatment of anorexia nervosa, bulimia nervosa, and other eating disorders. J Am Diet Assoc 106:2073–2082, 2006

American Psychiatric Association: Diagnostic and Statistical Manual of Mental Disorders, 4th Edition. Washington, DC, American Psychiatric Association, 1994

American Psychiatric Association: Diagnostic and Statistical Manual of Mental Disorders, 4th Edition, Text Revision. Washington, DC, American Psychiatric Association, 2000

American Psychiatric Association: Practice guideline for the treatment of patients with eating disorders (revision). Am J Psychiatry 163 (suppl):1–54, 2006

Andersen AE, Watson T, Schlechte J: Osteoporosis and osteopenia in men with eating disorders (letter). Lancet 355:1967–1968, 2000

Appolinario JC, Bacaltchuk J, Sichieri R, et al: A randomized, double-blind, placebo-controlled study of sibutramine in the treatment of binge-eating disorder. Arch Gen Psychiatry 60:1109–1116, 2003

Arbaizar B, Gómez-Acebo I, Llorca J: Efficacy of topiramate in bulimia nervosa and binge-eating disorder: a systematic review. Gen Hosp Psychiatry 30:471–475, 2008

Attia E, Walsh BT: Behavioral management for anorexia nervosa. N Engl J Med 360:500–506, 2009

Austin SB, Ziyadeh NJ, Vohra S, et al: Irregular menses linked to vomiting in a nonclinical sample: findings from the national eating disorders screening program in high schools. J Adolesc Health 42:450–457, 2008

Ayton A, Keen C, Lask B: Pros and cons of using the Mental Health Act for severe eating disorders in adolescents. Eur Eat Disord Rev 17:14–23, 2008

Becker AE: Culture and eating disorders classification. Int J Eat Disord 40:S111–S116, 2007

Benini L, Todesco T, Grave RD, et al: Gastric emptying in patients with restricting and binge/purging subtypes of anorexia nervosa. Am J Gastroenterol 99:1448–1454, 2004

Berkman ND, Lohr KN, Bulik CM: Outcomes of eating disorders: a systematic review of the literature. Int J Eat Disord 40:293–309, 2007

Beumont P, Carney T: Can psychiatric terminology be translated into legal regulation? The anorexia nervosa example. Aust N Z J Psychiatry 38:819–829, 2004

Bhanji S, Mattingly D: Medical Aspects of Anorexia Nervosa. Boston, MA, Wright, 1988

Birmingham CL, Tan AO: Respiratory muscle weakness and anorexia nervosa. Int J Eat Disord 33:230–233, 2003

Birmingham CL, Puddicombe D, Hlynsky J: Hypomagnesemia during refeeding in anorexia nervosa. Eat Weight Disord 9:236–237, 2004

Bissada H, Tasca GA, Barber AM, et al: Olanzapine in the treatment of low body weight and obsessive thinking in women with anorexia nervosa: a randomized, double-blind, placebo-controlled trial. Am J Psychiatry 165:1281–1288, 2008

Branch CHH, Eurman LJ: Social attitudes toward patients with anorexia nervosa. Am J Psychiatry 137:631–632, 1980

Bravender T, Bryant-Waugh R, Herzog D, et al: Classification of child and adolescent eating disturbances. Workgroup for Classification of Eating Disorders in Children and Adolescents (WCEDCA). Int J Eat Disord 40 (suppl):S117–S122, 2007

Brewerton TD: Eating disorders, trauma, and comorbidity: focus on PTSD. Eat Disord 15:285–304, 2007

Brinch M, Isager T, Tolstrup K: Anorexia nervosa and motherhood: reproduction pattern and mothering behavior of 50 women. Acta Psychiatr Scand 77:98–104, 1988

Bruch H: Eating Disorders: Obesity, Anorexia Nervosa, and the Person Within. New York, Basic Books, 1973

Brumberg JJ: Fasting Girls: The Emergence of Anorexia Nervosa as a Modern Disease. Cambridge, MA, Harvard University Press, 1988

Bulik CM: Anxiety, depression, and eating disorders, in Eating Disorders and Obesity: A Comprehensive Handbook, 2nd Edition. Edited by Fairburn CG, Brownell KD. New York, Guilford, 2002, pp 193–198

Bulik CM, Sullivan PF, Fear J, et al: Predictors of the development of bulimia nervosa in women with anorexia nervosa. J Nerv Ment Dis 185:704–707, 1997

Bulik CM, Sullivan PF, Joyce PR, et al: Predictors of 1-year treatment outcome in bulimia nervosa. Compr Psychiatry 39:206–214, 1998

Bulik CM, Sullivan PF, Wade TD, et al: Twin studies of eating disorders: a review. Int J Eat Disord 27:1–20, 2000

Bulik CM, Sullivan PF, Kendler KS: Medical and psychiatric morbidity in obese women with and without binge eating. Int J Eat Disord 32:72–78, 2002

Bulik CM, Sullivan PF, Kendler KS: Genetic and environmental contributions to obesity and binge eating. Int J Eat Disord 33:293–298, 2003

Bulik CM, Hebebrand J, Keski-Rahkonen A, et al: Genetic epidemiology, endophenotypes, and eating disorder classification. In J Eat Disord 40:S52–S60, 2007

Caregaro L, Favaro A, Santonastaso P, et al: Insulin-like growth factor 1 (IGF-1), a nutritional marker in patients with eating disorders. Clin Nutr 20:251–257, 2001

Caregaro L, Di Pascoli L, Favaro A, et al: Sodium depletion and hemoconcentration: overlooked complications in patients with anorexia nervosa. Nutrition 21:438–445, 2005

Carter JD, Blackmore E, Sutandar-Pinnock K, et al: Relapse in anorexia nervosa: a survival analysis. Psychol Med 34:671–679, 2004

Castro J, Lazaro L, Pons F, et al: Predictors of bone mineral density reduction in adolescents with anorexia nervosa. J Am Acad Child Adolesc Psychiatry 39:1365–1370, 2000

Castro-Fornieles J, Casulà V, Saura B, et al: Predictors of weight maintenance after hospital discharge in adolescent anorexia nervosa. Int J Eat Disord 40:129–135, 2007

Chowdhury U, Lask B: Clinical implications of brain imaging in eating disorders. Psychiatr Clin North Am 24:227–234, 2001

Cooke RA, Chambers JB: Anorexia nervosa and the heart. Br J Hosp Med 54:313–317, 1995

Couper R: Prader-Willi syndrome. J Paediatr Child Health 35:331–334, 1999

Coxson HO, Chan IH, Mayo JR, et al: Early emphysema in patients with anorexia nervosa. Am J Respir Crit Care Med 170:748–752, 2004

Crow SJ, Thuras P, Keel PK, et al: Long-term menstrual and reproductive function in patients with bulimia nervosa. Am J Psychiatry 159:1048–1050, 2002

Crow SJ, Mitchell JE, Roerig JD, et al: What potential role is there for medication treatment in anorexia nervosa? Int J Eat Disord 42:1–8, 2009

D'Andrea G, Ostuzzi R, Bolner A, et al: Study of tyrosine metabolism in eating disorders. Possible correlation with migraine. Neurol Sci 29:588–592, 2008

Davis C, Carter JC: Compulsive overeating and an addiction disorder. A review of theory and evidence. Appetite 53:1–8, 2009

Del Parigi A, Chen K, Salbe AD, et al: Are we addicted to food? Obes Res 11:493–495, 2003

Devlin MJ: Binge eating disorder and obesity—a combined treatment approach. Psychiatr Clin North Am 24:325–335, 2001

Devlin MJ, Walsh BT: The neuroendocrinology of anorexia nervosa, in Neuroendocrinology of Mood (Current Topics in Neuroendocrinology, Vol 8). Edited by Ganten D, Pfaff D. New York, Springer-Verlag, 1988, pp 291–307

Devlin MJ, Walsh BT, Katz JL, et al: Hypothalamic-pituitary-gonadal function in anorexia nervosa and bulimia. Psychiatry Res 28:11–24, 1989

Devlin MJ, Walsh BT, Kral JB, et al: Metabolic abnormalities in bulimia nervosa. Arch Gen Psychiatry 47:144–148, 1990

Devlin MJ, Yanovski SZ, Wilson GT: Obesity: what mental health professionals need to know. Am J Psychiatry 157:854–866, 2000

Devlin MJ, Goldfein JA, Dobrow I: What is this thing called BED? current status of binge eating disorder nosology. Int J Eat Disord 34 (suppl):S2–S18, 2003

Devlin MJ, Goldfein JA, Petkova E, et al: Cognitive behavioral therapy and fluoxetine as adjuncts to group behavioral therapy for binge eating disorder. Obes Res 13:1077–1088, 2005

Devlin MJ, Goldfein JA, Petkova E, et al: Cognitive behavioral therapy and fluoxetine for binge eating disorder: two-year follow-up. Obesity 15:1702–1709, 2007

de Zwaan M, Aslam Z, Mitchell JE: Research on energy expenditure in individuals with eating disorders: a review. Int J Eat Disord 31:361–369, 2002

Dingemans AE, Bruna MJ, van Furth EF: Binge eating disorder: a review. Int J Obes 26:299–307, 2002

Dotti A, Fioravanti M, Balotta M, et al: Eating behavior of ballet dancers. Eat Weight Disord 7:60–67, 2002

Dunican KC, DelDotto D: The role of olanzapine in the treatment of anorexia nervosa. Ann Pharmacother 41:111–115, 2007

Edler C, Lipson SF, Keel PK: Ovarian hormones and binge eating in bulimia nervosa. Psychol Med 37:131–141, 2006

Ehrlich S, Querfeld U, Pfeiffer E: Refeeding oedema: an important complication in the treatment of anorexia nervosa. Eur Child Adolesc Psychiatry 15:241–243, 2006

Ehrlich S, Burghardt R, Weiss D, et al: Glial and neuronal damage markers in patients with anorexia nervosa. J Neural Transm 115:921–927, 2008

Eisler I, Simic M, Russell GF, et al: A randomised controlled treatment trial of two forms of family therapy in adolescent anorexia nervosa: a five-year follow-up. J Child Psychol Psychiatry 48:552–560, 2007

Fairburn CG: Interpersonal psychotherapy for bulimia nervosa, in Handbook of Treatment for Eating Disorders, 2nd Edition. Edited by Garner DM, Garfinkel PE. New York, Guilford, 1997, pp 278–294

Fairburn CG: Cognitive Behavior Therapy and Eating Disorders. New York, Guilford, 2008

Fairburn CG, Harrison PJ: Eating disorders. Lancet 361:407–416, 2003

Fairburn CG, Jones R, Peveler RC, et al: Psychotherapy and bulimia nervosa: the longer-term effects of interpersonal psychotherapy, behavior therapy, and cognitive behavior therapy. Arch Gen Psychiatry 50:419–428, 1993a

Fairburn CG, Marcus MD, Wilson GT: Cognitive-behavioral therapy for binge eating and bulimia nervosa: a comprehensive treatment manual, in Binge Eating: Nature, Assessment, and Treatment. Edited by Fairburn CG, Wilson GT. New York, Guilford, 1993b, pp 361–404

Fairburn CG, Welch SL, Doll HA, et al: Risk factors for bulimia nervosa: a community-based case-control study. Arch Gen Psychiatry 54:509–517, 1997

Fairburn CG, Doll HA, Welch SL, et al: Risk factors for binge eating disorder: a community-based, case-control study. Arch Gen Psychiatry 55:425–432, 1998

Fairburn CG, Cooper Z, Doll HA, et al: Risk factors for anorexia nervosa: three integrated case-control comparisons. Arch Gen Psychiatry 56:468–476, 1999

Fairburn CG, Cooper Z, Shafran R: Cognitive behaviour therapy for eating disorders: a "transdiagnostic" theory and treatment. Behav Res Ther 41:509–528, 2003

Fairburn CG, Agras WS, Walsh BT, et al: Prediction of outcome in bulimia nervosa by early change in treatment. Am J Psychiatry 161:2322–2324, 2004

Fairburn CG, Cooper Z, Doll HA, et al: Transdiagnostic cognitive-behavioral therapy for patients with eating disorders: a two-site trial with 60-week follow-up. Am J Psychiatry 166:311–319, 2009

Favaro A, Tenconi E, Santonastaso P: The relationship between obstetric complications and temperament in eating disorders: a mediation hypothesis. Psychosom Med 70:372–377, 2008

Feillet F, Feillet-Coudray C, Bard JM, et al: Plasma cholesterol and endogenous cholesterol synthesis during refeeding in anorexia nervosa. Clin Chim Acta 294:45–56, 2000

Ford ES, Mokdad AH: Epidemiology of obesity in the western hemisphere. J Clin Endocrinol Metab 93:S1–S8, 2008

Franklin JC, Schiele BC, Brozek J, et al: Observations of human behavior in experimental semistarvation and rehabilitation. J Clin Psychol 4:28–45, 1948

Franko DL, Blais MA, Becker AE, et al: Pregnancy complications and neonatal outcomes in women with eating disorders. Am J Psychiatry 158:1461–1466, 2001

Galetta F, Franzoni F, Cupisti A, et al: Early detection of cardiac dysfunction in patients with anorexia nervosa by tissue Doppler imaging. Int J Cardiol 101:33–37, 2005

Gard MCE, Freeman CP: The dismantling of a myth: a review of eating disorders and socioeconomic status. Int J Eat Disord 20:1–12, 1996

Garner DM, Olmsted MP, Bohr Y, et al: The Eating Attitudes Test: psychometric features and clinical correlates. Psychol Med 12:871–878, 1982

Garner DM, Vitousek KM, Pike KM: Cognitive-behavioral therapy for anorexia nervosa, in Handbook of Treatment for Eating Disorders, 2nd Edition. Edited by Garner DM, Garfinkel PE. New York, Guilford, 1997, pp 94–144

Godart NT, Perderau F, Rein Z, et al: Comorbidity studies of eating disorders and mood disorders. Critical review of the literature. J Affect Disord 97:37–49, 2007

Gold PW, Kaye W, Robertson GL, et al: Abnormalities in plasma and cerebrospinal-fluid arginine vasopressin in patients with anorexia nervosa. N Engl J Med 308:1117–1123, 1983

Golden N: Osteopenia and osteoporosis in anorexia nervosa. Adolesc Med 14:97–108, 2003

Gorin AA, Niemeier HM, Hogan P, et al: Binge eating and weight loss outcomes in overweight and obese individuals with type 2 diabetes. Results from the Look AHEAD trial. Arch Gen Psychiatry 65:1447–1455, 2008

Griffiths RA, Beumont PJV, Russell J et al: The use of guardianship legislation for anorexia nervosa: a report of 15 cases. Aust N Z J Psychiatry 31:525–531, 1997

Grilo CM, Masheb RM: A randomized controlled comparison of guided self-help cognitive behavioral therapy and behavioral weight loss for binge eating disorder. Behav Res Ther 43:1509–1525, 2005

Grilo CM, Masheb RM, Salant SL: Cognitive behavioral therapy guided self-help and orlistat for the treatment of binge eating disorder: a randomized, double-blind, placebo-controlled trial. Biol Psychiatry 57:1193–1201, 2005a

Grilo CM, Masheb RM, Wilson GT: Efficacy of cognitive behavioral therapy and fluoxetine for the treatment of binge eating disorder: a randomized double-blind placebo-controlled comparison. Biol Psychiatry 57:301–309, 2005b

Grinspoon S, Thomas L, Miller K, et al: Changes in regional fat redistribution and the effects of estrogen during spontaneous weight gain in women with anorexia nervosa. Am J Clin Nutr 73:865–869, 2001

Guarda AS, Marinilli Pinto A, Coughlin JW, et al: Perceived coercion and change in perceived need for admission in patients hospitalized for eating disorders. Am J Psychiatry 164:108–114, 2007

Guh DP, Bansback N, Amarsi Z, et al: The incidence of co-morbidities related to obesity and overweight: a systematic review and meta-analysis. BMC Public Health 9:88, 2009

Gull WW: Anorexia nervosa (apepsia hysterica, anorexia hysterica). Transactions of the Clinical Society of London 7:22–28, 1874

Halmi KA, Agras WS, Mitchell J, et al: Relapse predictors of patients with bulimia nervosa who achieved abstinence through cognitive behavior therapy. Arch Gen Psychiatry 59:1105–1109, 2002

Haqq AM, Farooqi S, O'Rahilly S, et al: Serum ghrelin levels are inversely correlated with body mass index, age, and insulin concentrations in normal children and are markedly increased in Prader-Willi syndrome. J Clin Endocrinol Metab 88:174–178, 2003

Haworth-Hoeppner S: The critical shapes of body image: the role of culture and family in the production of eating disorders. J Marriage Fam 62:212–227, 2000

Hebebrand J, Hinney A: Environmental and genetic risk factors in obesity. Child Adolesc Psychiatric Clin N Am 18:83–94, 2009

Hebebrand J, Himmelmann GW, Herzog W, et al: Prediction of low body weight at long-term follow-up in acute anorexia nervosa by low body weight at referral. Am J Psychiatry 154:566–569, 1997

Herpertz-Dahlmann: Adolescent eating disorders: definitions, symptomatology, epidemiology and comorbidity. Child Adolesc Psychiatric Clin N Am 18:31–47, 2009

Herzog DB, Eddy KT: Comorbidity in eating disorders, in Annual Review of Eating Disorders Part I—2007. Edited by Wonderlich S, Mitchell JE, de Zwaan M, et al. Oxford, England, Radcliffe Publishing, 2007, pp 35–50

Herzog DB, Greenwood DN, Dorer DJ, et al: Mortality in eating disorders: a descriptive study. Int J Eat Disord 28:20–26, 2000

Herzog W, Deter HC, Fiehn, et al: Medical findings and predictors of long-term physical outcome in anorexia nervosa: a prospective 12-year follow-up study. Psychol Med 27:269–279, 1997

Hoek HW, van Harten PN, Hermans KMS, et al: The incidence of anorexia nervosa on Curaçao. Am J Psychiatry 162:748–752, 2005

Holderness CC, Brooks-Gunn J, Warren MP: Co-morbidity of eating disorders and substance abuse: review of the literature. Int J Eat Disord 16:1–34, 1994

Howell MJ, Schenck CK, Crow SJ: A review of nighttime eating disorders. Sleep Med Rev 13:23–34, 2009

Hudson JI, Lalonde JK, Berry JM, et al: Binge eating disorder as a distinct familial phenotype in obese individuals. Arch Gen Psychiatry 63:313–319, 2006

Hudson JI, Hiripi E, Pope HG Jr, et al: The prevalence and correlates of eating disorder in the National Comorbidity Survey Replication. Biol Psychiatry 61:348–358, 2007

Jayasinghe Y, Grover SR, Zacharin M: Current concepts in bone and reproductive health in adolescents with anorexia nervosa. BJOG 115:304–315, 2008

Kann L, Kinchen SA, Williams BI, et al: Youth risk behavior surveillance—United States, 1999. MMWR CDC Surveill Summ 49(5):1–32, 2000

Kaplan AS, Noble S: Medical complications of eating disorders, in Annual Review of Eating Disorders Part I—2007. Edited by Wonderlich S, Mitchell JE, de Zwaan M, et al. Oxford, England, Radcliffe Publishing, 2007, pp 101–112

Kaplan AS, Olmsted MP, Carter JC, et al: Matching patient variables to treatment intensity—the continuum of care. Psychiatr Clin North Am 24:281–292, 2001

Kaplan AS, Walsh BT, Olmsted M, et al: The slippery slope: prediction of successful weight maintenance in anorexia nervosa. Psychol Med 39:1037–1045, 2009

Kaye WH: Central nervous system neurotransmitter activity in anorexia nervosa and bulimia nervosa, in Eating Disorders and Obesity: A Comprehensive Handbook, 2nd Edition. Edited by Fairburn CG, Brownell KD. New York, Guilford, 2002, pp 272–277

Kaye W: Neurobiology and anorexia and bulimia nervosa. Physiol Behav 94:121–135, 2008

Kaye WH, Weltzin TE, Hsu LK, et al: An open trial of fluoxetine in patients with anorexia nervosa. J Clin Psychiatry 52:464–471, 1991

Kaye WH, Nagata T, Weltzin TE, et al: Double-blind placebo-controlled administration of fluoxetine in restricting- and restricting-purging-type anorexia nervosa. Biol Psychiatry 49:644–652, 2001

Kaye WH, Bulik CM, Thornton L, et al: Comorbidity of anxiety disorders with anorexia and bulimia nervosa. Am J Psychiatry 161:2215–2221, 2004

Keel PK, Mitchell JE, Miller KB, et al: Long-term outcome of bulimia nervosa. Arch Gen Psychiatry 56:63–69, 1999

Keel PK, Dorer DJ, Eddy KT, et al: Predictors of mortality in eating disorders. Arch Gen Psychiatry 60:179–183, 2003

Keel PK, Haedt A, Edler C: Purging disorder: an ominous variant of bulimia nervosa? Int J Eat Disord 38:191–199, 2005

Keel PK, Wolfe BE, Liddle RA, et al: Clinical features and physiological response to a test meal in purging disorder and bulimia nervosa. Arch Gen Psychiatry 64:1058–1066, 2007

Kendler KS, Bulik CM, Silberg J, et al: Childhood sexual abuse and adult psychiatric and substance use disorders in women: an epidemiological and cotwin control analysis. Arch Gen Psychiatry 57:953–959, 2000

Kerem NC, Katzman DK: Brain structure and function in adolescents with anorexia nervosa. Adolesc Med 14:109–118, 2003

Keski-Rahkonen A, Raevuori A, Hoek HW: Epidemiology of eating disorders: an update, in Annual Review of Eating Disorders Part 2—2008. Edited by Wonderlich S, Mitchell JE, de Zwaan M, et al. Oxford, England, Radcliffe Publishing, 2008, pp 58–68

Klerman GL, Weissman MM, Rounsaville BJ, et al: Interpersonal psychotherapy of depression. New York, Basic Books, 1984

Konstantynowicz J, Kadziela-Olech H, Kaczmarski M, et al: Depression in anorexia nervosa: a risk factor for osteoporosis. J Clin Endocrinol Metab 90:5382–5385, 2005

Kotler LA, Cohen P, Davies M, et al: Longitudinal relationships between childhood, adolescent, and adult eating disorders. J Am Acad Child Adolesc Psychiatry 40:1434–1440, 2001

Krantz MJ, Donahoo WT, Melanson EL, et al: QT interval dispersion and resting metabolic rate in chronic anorexia nervosa. Int J Eat Disord 37:166–170, 2005

Kreipe RE, Yussman SE: The role of the primary care practitioner in the treatment of eating disorders. Adolesc Med 14:133–147, 2003

Lasègue C: De l'anorexie hystérique. Archives Générales de Médecine 1:384–403, 1873

Lask B, Bryant-Waugh R: Prepubertal eating disorders, in Handbook of Treatment for Eating Disorders, 2nd Edition. Edited by Garner DM, Garfinkel PE. New York, Guilford, 1997, pp 476–483

Latner JD, Wilson GT: Obesity and binge eating disorder, in Handbook of Obesity, 3rd Edition. Edited by Bray A, Bouchard C. New York, Informa Healthcare, 2008, pp 553–567

Lawson EA, Klibanski A: Endocrine abnormalities in anorexia nervosa. Nat Clin Pract Endocrinol Metab 4:407–414, 2008

Lee S, Chan YYL, Hsu LKG: The intermediate term outcome of Chinese patients with anorexia nervosa in Hong Kong. Am J Psychiatry 160:967–972, 2003

Lee S, Ng KL, Kwok K, et al: The changing profile of eating disorders at a tertiary psychiatric clinic in Hong Kong (1987–2007). Int J Eat Disord 43:307–314, 2010

Le Grange D, Binford R, Loeb KL: Manualized family-based treatment for anorexia nervosa: a case series. J Am Acad Child Adolesc Psychiatry 44:41–46, 2005

Le Grange D, Crosby RD, Rathouz PJ, et al: A randomized controlled comparison of family based treatment and supportive psychotherapy for adolescent bulimia nervosa. Arch Gen Psychiatry 64:1049–1056, 2007

Leitenberg H, Rosen JC, Gross J, et al: Exposure plus response-prevention treatment of bulimia nervosa. J Consult Clin Psychol 56:535–541, 1988

Lesinskiene S, Barkus A, Ranceva N, et al: A meta-analysis of heart rate and QT interval alteration in anorexia nervosa. World J Biol Psychiatry 9:86–91, 2008

Levine MP, Smolak L, Moodey AF, et al: Normative developmental challenges and dieting and eating disturbances in middle school girls. Int J Eat Disord 15:11–20, 1994

Lilenfeld LR, Ringham R, Kalarchian MA, et al: A family history study of binge-eating disorder. Compr Psychiatry 49:247–254, 2008

Lock J, le Grange D, Agras WS, et al: Treatment Manual for Anorexia Nervosa: A Family Based Approach. New York, Guilford, 2001

Lund BC, Hernandez ER, Yates WR, et al: Rate of inpatient weight restoration predicts outcome in anorexia nervosa. Int J Eat Disord 42:301–305, 2009

Malhotra S, McElroy SL: Medical management of obesity associated with mental disorders. J Clin Psychiatry 63 (suppl 4):24–32, 2002

Marcus MD: Adapting treatment for patients with binge-eating disorder, in Handbook of Treatment for Eating Disorders, 2nd Edition. Edited by Garner DM, Garfinkel PE. New York, Guilford, 1997, pp 484–493

Mayer LE, Roberto CA, Glasofer DR, et al: Does percent body fat predict outcome in anorexia nervosa? Am J Psychiatry 164:970–972, 2007

Mazzeo SE, Bulik CM: Environmental and genetic risk factors for eating disorders: what the clinician needs to know. Child Adolesc Psychiatric Clin N Am 18:67–82, 2009

McCallum K, Bermudez O, Ohlemeyer C, et al: How should the clinician evaluate and manage the cardiovascular complications of anorexia nervosa. Eat Disord 14:73–80, 2006

Mears E: Outcomes of continuous process improvement of a nutritional care program incorporating serum prealbumin measurements. Nutrition 12:479–484, 1996

Mehanna JM, Moledina J, Travis J: Refeeding syndrome: what it is and how to treat it. BMJ 336:1495–1498, 2008

Mehler PS: Osteoporosis in anorexia nervosa: prevention and treatment. Int J Eat Disord 33:113–126, 2003

Mehler PS, Andersen AE: Eating Disorders—A Guide to Medical Care and Complications. Baltimore, MD, Johns Hopkins University Press, 1999

Mehler PS, MacKenzie TD: Treatment of osteopenia and osteoporosis in anorexia nervosa: a systematic review of the literature. Int J Eat Disord 42:195–201, 2009

Melanson EL, Donahoo WT, Krantz MJ, et al: Resting and ambulatory heart rate variability in chronic anorexia nervosa. Am J Cardiol 94:1217–1220, 2004

Micali N, Simonoff E, Treasure J: Risk of major adverse perinatal outcomes in women with eating disorders. Br J Psychiatry 190:255–259, 2007

Milano W, Petrella C, Casella A, et al: Use of sibutramine, an inhibitor of the reuptake of serotonin and noradrenaline, in the treatment of binge eating disorder: a placebo-controlled study. Adv Ther 22:25–31, 2005

Miller KK, Lee EE, Lawson EA, et al: Determinants of skeletal loss and recovery in anorexia nervosa. J Clin Endocrinol Metab 91:2931–2937, 2006

Miller MN, Pumariega AJ: Culture and eating disorders: a historical and cross-cultural review. Psychiatry 64:93–110, 2001

Minuchin S, Rosman BL, Baker L: Psychosomatic families: anorexia nervosa in context. Cambridge, MA, Harvard University Press, 1978

Misra M, Miller KK, Almazan C, et al: Alterations in cortisol secretory dynamics in adolescent girls with anorexia nervosa and effects on bone metabolism. J Clin Endocrinol Metab 89:4972–4980, 2004

Mitchell JE, Crow S: Medical complications of anorexia nervosa and bulimia nervosa. Curr Opin Psychiatry 19:438–443, 2006

Mitchell-Gieleghem A, Mittelstaedt ME, Bulik CM: Eating disorders and childbearing: concealment and consequences. Birth 29:182–191, 2002

Monteleone P, Maj M: Genetic susceptibility to eating disorders: associated polymorphisms and pharmacogenetic suggestions. Pharmacogenomics 9:1487–1520, 2008

Morgan JF: Eating disorders and reproduction. Aust NZ J Obstet Gynaecol 39:167–173, 1999

Morgan JF, Reid F, Lacey JH: The SCOFF questionnaire: assessment of a new screening tool for eating disorders. BMJ 319:1467–1468, 1999

Morgan JF, Lacey JH, Chung E: Risk of postnatal depression, miscarriage, and preterm birth in bulimia nervosa: retrospective controlled study. Psychosom Med 68:487–492, 2006

Morton R: Phthisiologia, seu exercitationes de phthisi. London, S. Smith, 1689

Munsch S, Biedert E, Meyer A, et al: A randomized comparison of cognitive behavioral therapy and behavioral weight loss treatment for overweight individuals with binge eating disorder. Int J Eat Disord 40:102–113, 2007

Najjar M: Zolpidem and amnestic sleep related eating disorder. J Clin Sleep Med 3:637–638, 2007

Narayanan V, Gaudiani JL, Harris RH, et al: Liver function test abnormalities in anorexia nervosa—cause or effect. Int J Eat Disord 43:378–381, 2010

National Institute for Clinical Excellence: Eating disorders: core interventions in the treatment and management of anorexia nervosa, bulimia nervosa and related eating disorders. NICE Clinical Guideline No. 9. London: NICE, 2004. Available at: http://www.nice.org.uk. Accessed June 2, 2009.

Nichols D, Bryant-Waugh R: Eating disorders of infancy and childhood: definition, symptomatology, epidemiology, and comorbidity. Child Adolesc Psychiatric Clin N Am 18:17–30, 2009

Nielsen S: Epidemiology and mortality of eating disorders. Psychiatr Clin North Am 24:201–214, 2001

Nielsen S, Emborg C, Molbak AG: Mortality in concurrent type 1 diabetes and anorexia nervosa. Diabetes Care 25:309–312, 2002

Ohwada R, Hotta M, Sato K, et al: The relationship between serum levels of estradiol and osteoprotegerin in patients with anorexia nervosa. Endocr J 54:953–959, 2007

Ostuzzi R, D'Andrea G, Francesconi F, et al: Eating disorders and headache: coincidence or consequence? Neurol Sci 29:583–587, 2008

Papacostas SS, Hadjivasilis V: The Kleine-Levin syndrome. Report of a case and review of the literature. Eur Psychiatry 15:231–235, 2000

Papadopoulos FC, Ekborn A, Brandt L, et al: Excess mortality, causes of death and prognostic factors in anorexia nervosa. Br J Psychiatry 194:10–17, 2009

Pike KM: Long-term course of anorexia nervosa: response, relapse, remission, and recovery. Clin Psychol Rev 18:447–475, 1998

Pirke KM: Central and peripheral noradrenalin regulation in eating disorders. Psychiatry Res 62:43–49, 1996

Polito A, Cuzzolaro M, Raguzzini A, et al: Body composition changes in anorexia nervosa. Eur J Clin Nutr 52:655–662, 1998

Polivy J, Herman CP: Causes of eating disorders. Annu Rev Psychol 53:187–213, 2002

Polli N, Scacchi M, Giraldi FP, et al: Low insulin-like growth factor I and leukopenia in anorexia nervosa. Int J Eat Disord 41:355–359, 2008

Probst M, Goris M, Vandereycken W, et al: Body composition of anorexia nervosa patients assessed by underwater weighing and skinfold-thickness measurements before and after weight gain. Am J Clin Nutr 73:190–197, 2001

Ramsay R, Ward A, Treasure J, et al: Compulsory treatment in anorexia nervosa: short-term benefits and long-term mortality. Br J Psychiatry 175:147–153, 1999

Raney TJ, Thornton LM, Berrettini W, et al: Influence of overanxious disorder of childhood on the expression of anorexia nervosa. Int J Eat Disord 41:326–332, 2008

Rautou PE, Cazals-Hatem D, Moreau R, et al: Acute liver cell damage in patients with anorexia nervosa: a possible role of starvation-induced hepatocyte autophagy. Gastroenterology 135:840–848, 2008

Reas DL, Grilo CM: Review and meta-analysis of pharmacotherapy for binge-eating disorder. Obesity 16:2024–2038, 2008

Rechlin T, Weis M, Ott C, et al: Alterations of autonomic cardiac control in anorexia nervosa. Biol Psychiatry 43:358–363, 1998

Richards PS, Baldwin BM, Frost HA, et al: What works for treating eating disorders? A synthesis of 28 outcome reviews. Eating Disorders: The Journal of Treatment and Prevention 8:189–206, 2000

Rigaud D, Moukaddem M, Cohen B, et al: Refeeding improves muscle performance without normalization of muscle mass and oxygen consumption in anorexia nervosa patients. Am J Clin Nutr 65:1845–1851, 1997

Robb AS, Silber TJ, Orrell-Valente JK, et al: Supplemental nocturnal nasogastric refeeding for better short-term outcome in hospitalized adolescent girls with anorexia nervosa. Am J Psychiatry 159:1347–1353, 2002

Rock CL, Curran-Celentano JC: Nutritional management of eating disorders. Psychiatr Clin North Am 19:701–713, 1996

Rodin GM: Eating disorders in diabetes mellitus, in Eating Disorders and Obesity: A Comprehensive Handbook, 2nd Edition. Edited by Fairburn CG, Brownell KD. New York, Guilford, 2002, pp 286–290

Romano SJ, Halmi KA, Sarkar NP, et al: A placebo-controlled study of fluoxetine in continued treatment of bulimia nervosa after successful acute fluoxetine treatment. Am J Psychiatry 159:96–102, 2002

Rome ES, Ammerman S, Rosen DS, et al: Children and adolescents with eating disorders: the state of the art. Pediatrics 111:e98–e108, 2003

Root TL, Pinheiro AP, Thornton L, et al: Substance use disorders in women with anorexia nervosa. Int J Eat Disord 43:14–21, 2010

Rosen DS: Eating disorders in children and young adolescents: etiology, classification, clinical features, and treatment. Adolesc Med 14:49–59, 2003

Rosenblum J, Forman S: Evidence-based treatment of eating disorders. Curr Opin Pediatr 14:379–383, 2002

Rubinstein S, Caballero B: Is Miss America an undernourished role model? (letter) JAMA 283:1569, 2000

Rudolph CD, Link DT: Feeding disorders in infants and children. Pediatr Clin North Am 49:97–112, 2002

Russell GFM: Bulimia nervosa: an ominous variant of anorexia nervosa. Psychol Med 9:429–448, 1979

Russell GFM: Involuntary treatment in anorexia nervosa. Psychiatr Clin North Am 24:337–349, 2001

Russell GFM, Szmukler GI, Dare C, et al: An evaluation of family therapy in anorexia nervosa and bulimia nervosa. Arch Gen Psychiatry 44:1047–1056, 1987

Safer DL, Telch CF, Agras WS: Dialectical behavior therapy for bulimia nervosa. Am J Psychiatry 158:632–634, 2001

Schebendach JE, Mayer LE, Devlin MJ, et al: Dietary energy density and diet variety as predictors of outcome in anorexia nervosa. Am J Clin Nutr 87:810–816, 2008

Schelbert KB: Comorbidities of obesity. Prim Care 36:271–285, 2009

Shapiro JR, Berkman ND, Brownley KA, et al: Bulimia nervosa treatment: a systematic review of randomized controlled trials. Int J Eat Disord 40:321–336, 2007

Shisslak CM, Crago M, McKnight KM, et al: Potential risk factors associated with weight control behaviors in elementary and middle school girls. J Psychosom Res 44:301–313, 1998

Smolak L, Murnen SK, Ruble AE: Female athletes and eating problems: a meta-analysis. Int J Eat Disord 27:371–380, 2000

Solomon SM, Kirby DF: The refeeding syndrome: a review. JPEN J Parenter Enteral Nutr 14:90–97, 1990

Steiger H, Bruce KR: Phenotypes, endophenotypes, and genotypes in bulimia spectrum eating disorders. Can J Psychiatry 52:220–227, 2007

Steinglass J, Sysko R, Schebendach J, et al: The application of exposure therapy and D-cycloserine to the treatment of anorexia nervosa: a preliminary trial. J Psychiatr Pract 13:238–245, 2007

Steinhausen HC: The outcome of anorexia nervosa in the 20th century. Am J Psychiatry 159:1284–1293, 2002

Steinhausen HC: Outcome of eating disorders. Child Adolesc Psychiatric Clin N Am 18:225–242, 2009

Stice E: Modeling of eating pathology and social reinforcement of the thin-ideal predict onset of bulimic symptoms. Behav Res Ther 36:931–944, 1998

Stice E: Risk and maintenance factors for eating pathology: a meta-analytic review. Psychol Bull 128:825–848, 2002

Striegel-Moore R: Risk factors for eating disorders. Ann N Y Acad Sci 817:98–109, 1997

Striegel-Moore RH, Bulik CM: Risk factors for eating disorders. Am Psychol 62:181–198, 2007

Strober M, Freeman R, Morrell W: The long-term course of severe anorexia nervosa in adolescents: survival analysis of recovery, relapse, and outcome predictors over 10–15 years in a prospective study. Int J Eat Disord 22:339–360, 1997

Stunkard AJ, Allison KC: Two forms of disordered eating in obesity: binge eating and night eating. Int J Obes Relat Metab Disord 27:1–12, 2003

Sylvester CJ, Forman SF: Clinical practice guidelines for treating restrictive eating disorder patients during medical hospitalization. Curr Opin Pediatr 20:390–397, 2008

Takakura S, Nozaki T, Nomura Y, et al: Factors related to renal dysfunction in patients with anorexia nervosa. Eating Weight Disord 11:73–77, 2006

Takii M, Uchigata Y, Tokunaga S, et al: The duration of severe insulin omission is the factor most closely associated with the microvascular complications of type 1 diabetic females with clinical eating disorders. Int J Eat Disord 41:259–264, 2008

Tasca GA, Demidenko N, Krysanski V, et al: Personality dimensions among women with an eating disorder: towards reconceptualizing DSM. Eur Eat Disord Rev 17:281–289, 2009

Telch CF, Agras WS, Linehan MM: Dialectical behavior therapy for binge eating disorder. J Consult Clin Psychol 69:1061–1065, 2001

Thiels C: Forced treatment of patients with anorexia. Curr Opin Psychiatry 21:495–498, 2008

Thiels C, Curtice M Jr: Forced treatment of anorexic patients: part 2. Curr Opin Psychiatry 22:497–500, 2009

Thomas JJ, Vartanian LR, Brownell KD: The relationship between eating disorder not otherwise specified (EDNOS) and officially recognized eating disorders: meta-analysis and implications for DSM. Psychol Bull 135:407–433, 2009

Thompson-Brenner H, Eddy KT, Satir DA, et al: Personality subtypes in adolescents with eating disorders: validation of a classification approach. J Child Psychol Psychiatry 49:170–180, 2008

Treasure JL: Getting beneath the phenotype of anorexia nervosa: the search for viable endophenotypes and genotypes. Can J Psychiatry 52:212–219, 2007

Ulger Z, Gurses D, Ozyurek AR, et al: Follow-up of cardiac abnormalities in female adolescents with anorexia nervosa after refeeding. Acta Cardiol 61:43–49, 2006

Van den Eynde F, Treasure J: Neuroimaging in eating disorders and obesity: implications for research. Child Adolesc Psychiatric Clin N Am 18:95–116, 2009

von Ranson KM, McGue M, Iacono WG: Disordered eating and substance use in an epidemiological sample, II: associations within families. Psychol Addict Behav 17:193–201, 2003

Vyver E, Steinegger C, Katzman D: Eating disorders and menstrual dysfunction in adolescents. Ann N Y Acad Sci 1135:253–264, 2008

Wade TD, Bulik CM, Sullivan FP, et al: The relation between risk factors for binge eating and bulimia nervosa: a population-based female twin study. Health Psychol 19:115–123, 2000

Walsh BT, Kissileff HR, Cassidy SM, et al: Eating behavior of women with bulimia. Arch Gen Psychiatry 46:54–58, 1989

Walsh BT, Wong LM, Pesce MA, et al: Hyperamylasemia in bulimia nervosa. J Clin Psychiatry 51:373–377, 1990

Walsh BT, Hadigan CM, Devlin MJ, et al: Long-term outcome of antidepressant treatment for bulimia nervosa. Am J Psychiatry 148:1206–1212, 1991

Walsh BT, Wilson GT, Loeb KL, et al: Medication and psychotherapy in the treatment of bulimia nervosa. Am J Psychiatry 154:523–531, 1997

Walsh BT, Kaplan AS, Attia E, et al: Fluoxetine after weight restoration in anorexia nervosa: a randomized controlled trial. JAMA 295:2605–2612, 2006

Watson TL, Bowers WA, Andersen AE: Involuntary treatment of eating disorders. Am J Psychiatry 157:1806–1810, 2000

Wertheim EH, Paxton SJ, Schutz HK, et al: Why do adolescent girls watch their weight? An interview study examining sociocultural pressures to be thin. J Psychosom Res 42:345–355, 1997

Westen D, Harnden-Fischer J: Personality profiles in eating disorders: rethinking the distinction between Axis I and Axis II. Am J Psychiatry 158:547–562, 2001

Wildes JE, Marcus MD, Fagiolini A: Prevalence and correlates of eating disorder co-morbidity in patients with bipolar disorder. Psychiatry Res 161:51–58, 2008

Wilfley DE, Agras WS, Telch CF, et al: Group cognitive-behavioral therapy and group interpersonal psychotherapy for the nonpurging bulimic: a controlled comparison. J Consult Clin Psychol 61:296–305, 1993

Wilfley DE, Welch RR, Stein RI, et al: A randomized comparison of group cognitive-behavioral therapy and group interpersonal psychotherapy for the treatment of overweight individuals with binge eating disorder. Arch Gen Psychiatry 59:713–721, 2002

Wilfley DE, Crow SJ, Hudson JI, et al: Efficacy of sibutramine for the treatment of binge eating disorder: a randomized multicenter placebo-controlled double-blind study. Am J Psychiatry 165:51–58, 2008

Wilson GT: Eating disorders and addictive disorders, in Eating Disorders and Obesity: A Comprehensive Handbook, 2nd Edition. Edited by Fairburn CG, Brownell KD. New York, Guilford, 2002, pp 199–203

Wilson GT, Grilo CM, Vitousek KM: Psychological treatment of eating disorders. Am Psychol 62:199–216, 2007

Wilson GT, Wilfley DE, Agras WS, et al: Psychological treatments of binge eating disorder. Arch Gen Psychiatry 67:94–101, 2010

Winter TA, O'Keefe SJ, Callanan M, et al: The effect of severe undernutrition and subsequent refeeding on whole-body metabolism and protein synthesis in human subjects. JPEN J Parenter Enteral Nutr 29:221–228, 2005

Yager J, Andersen AE: Clinical practice: anorexia nervosa. N Engl J Med 353:1481–1488, 2005

Zuercher JN, Cumella EJ, Woods BK, et al: Efficacy of voluntary nasogastric tube feeding in female inpatients with anorexia nervosa. JPEN J Parenter Enteral Nutr 27:268–276, 2003

CHAPTER

15

Sleep Disorders

Lois E. Krahn, M.D.

OBTAINING SUFFICIENT quantity and quality of sleep is important for good health. Chronic partial sleep deprivation, also known as insufficient sleep, is common in our society. The consequences include depressed mood, interpersonal irritability, decreased daytime vigilance, and cognitive impairment (Pilcher and Huffcutt 1996). However, determining the appropriate amount of required sleep is difficult for several reasons. Sleep duration gradually decreases from a starting length of 16 hours per 24-hour day as human beings make the transition from infancy to adulthood. Interindividual differences in the optimal amount of sleep range from 6 to 12 hours with a mean of 7.5 hours for adults. When a primary sleep disorder, such as obstructive sleep apnea, is present, the continuity and depth of sleep may be compromised independently of sleep duration. These complexities preclude a simplistic identification of a precise target of sleep duration for any individual. Nonetheless, there is consensus that chronically inadequate sleep is detrimental.

Physiological Mechanisms of Normal Sleep

Sleep can be subdivided into two major components: rapid eye movement sleep (REM), which is characterized by high levels of cortical activation in the presence of muscle atonia to prevent corresponding movements, and non-rapid eye movement sleep (NREM), which is separated into three distinct stages. The international classification of sleep was updated in 2007 with the most significant change relating to NREM sleep which previously had four distinct phases (Iber et al. 2007). Table 15-1 summarizes the characteristics and percentage of time spent in each sleep stage by healthy middle-aged adults.

Normal sleep progresses from wakefulness to stage N1 NREM sleep. From this stage of twilight sleep, a patient can be easily awakened by environmental stimuli. Stage N2 NREM sleep is deeper, and moderate environmental stimuli, such as a crack of thunder, no longer cause arousal but rather result in a distinctive electrophysiological event, the K complex. Sleep spindles and K complexes are used to identify stage N2 sleep. When the electroencephalographic (EEG) tracing slows until at least 20% of the activity consists of higher-voltage slow waves, the sleep is rated stage N3. Previously subdivided into Stage III and IV sleep, stage N3 is also called *delta wave sleep, deep sleep,* or *slow-wave sleep.* A person awakes from this sleep only when environmental stimuli are marked, such as the prolonged loud noise of an alarm.

As the normal sleep cycle progresses, the EEG activity gradually returns to the most common stage, N2 sleep. Stage N2 sleep evolves into the first REM sleep episode of the night. REM sleep, now called stage R, consists of high-frequency EEG activity, episodic bursts of vertical eye movements, muscle atonia, and penile tumescence. The first REM episode is often brief and typically occurs 70–100 minutes after the person falls asleep. There is marked interindividual variability in arousal threshold in REM sleep (Carskadon and Dement 1994). The sleep cycle repeats four or five times during the night, subsequent REM episodes being of longer duration. In general, slow-wave sleep is more common early in the night, and REM periods become longer toward morning. Because the last REM episode occurs at the very end of the major sleep period, people recall their dreams, and men experience morning erections.

The data in Table 15-1 are useful as normative data because sleep study reports typically describe the percentage of the night spent in each complete stage, and thus subjects with normal sleep patterns can be compared with sub-

TABLE 15–1. Sleep stages in healthy adults

Stage	Percentage	Polysomnographic characteristics	Physiological changes
Stage N1	2–5	Slow eye movements	Easy to arouse
Stage N2	45–55	Spindles, K complexes	More difficult to arouse
Stage N3	13–23	Slow EEG frequency	Difficult to arouse
Stage R	20–25	Rapid eye movements Muscle atonia Increased EEG frequency	Variable arousal threshold Penile engorgement

Note. EEG=electroencephalographic; REM=rapid eye movement.

jects with pathology. In healthy elderly subjects, the relative percentage of time spent in slow-wave sleep decreases, and sleep is generally more fragmented. Figure 15–1 is based on a meta-analysis of distribution of sleep stages over the life span and shows in the absence of pathology a progressive decrease in total sleep time plus stages N3 and R (Ohayon et al. 2004). Patients with disrupted sleep often spend most of the night in stages N1 and N2 and have little slow-wave or REM sleep. The exact roles of slow-wave sleep and REM sleep in a refreshing night's sleep are not well understood, but significant reductions in either state can lead to undesirable results, including daytime sleepiness, depressed mood, and cognitive impairment. In animal studies, prolonged absolute sleep deprivation has resulted in death attributed to sepsis because of suspected underlying compromise of immune function (Bergmann et al. 1996).

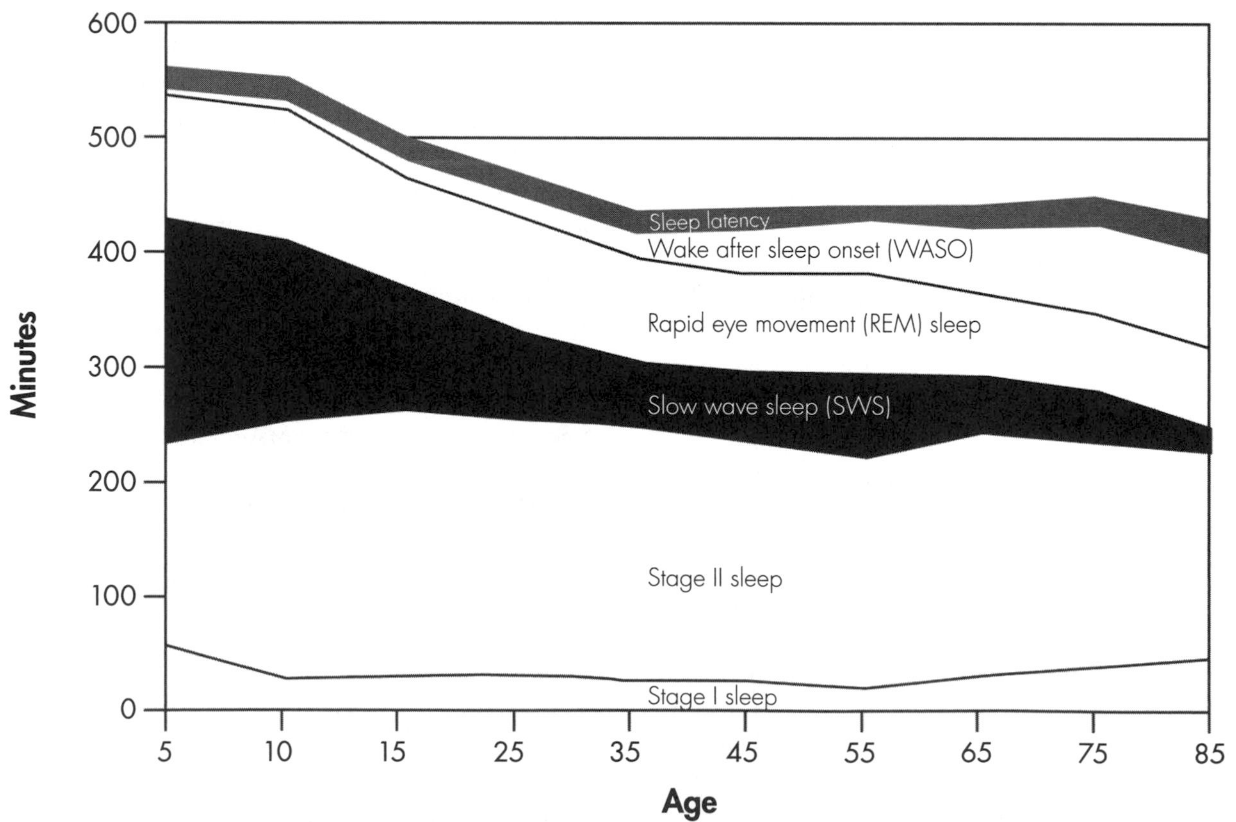

FIGURE 15–1. Changes in sleep architecture throughout the life cycle

Source. Ohayon et al. 2004.

Evaluation of Sleep

Office Evaluation

A detailed diagnostic interview and physical examination remain the foundation of the sleep evaluation. Table 15-2 lists the many issues that must be evaluated in an assessment for a possible sleep disorder. The decision to refer for a specialty evaluation and diagnostic testing is based on the findings at the history and physical examination conducted by the primary care provider or referring physician. Sleep studies are not necessary for some disorders (e.g., restless legs syndrome) and can be avoided if the classic symptoms of the disease are identified in the absence of any other factors. Clinicians need to obtain both thorough medical and psychiatric histories because many illnesses and disorders can alter sleep. As people age, sleep complaints become more common, not because of primary sleep disorders but because of comorbid conditions (Vitiello et al. 2002). Tables 15-3 and 15-4 list disorders that may lead to sleep problems. Treatment should therefore stabilize the underlying disease.

An interview with a bed partner is of great value, if feasible, especially in regard to snoring, respiratory pauses, and unusual behaviors. A screening interview is available to help collect data from family members concerning possible REM sleep behavior disorder and other common conditions (Figure 15-2). The more attentive the bed partner, the more likely it is the clinician will be able to obtain a useful history of what actually happens while the patient sleeps. Presbycusis and sound sleep may limit the ability of a bed partner to provide observations.

Sometimes, even if the patient sleeps alone, a family member can provide useful information if the partner moved out of a shared bedroom because of intolerable snoring or unusual behaviors. Although this interview results in limited specific information about current symptoms, it clearly increases the likelihood that a pathological condition is present.

During the physical examination, the examiner should note the patient's level of alertness (in the waiting room and during the appointment), body mass index, neck circumference, nasopharyngeal abnormalities, protrusion of mandible, thyroid size, pulmonary findings, findings at cardiac auscultation, and cognition. Valuable laboratory tests include measurement of thyroid-stimulating hormone, ferritin, cobalamin, and folate and a complete blood cell count. The findings of these studies are helpful in identifying medical disorders that can enter into the differential diagnosis of several sleep disorders.

Because of the cost and inconvenience of sleep studies, a clear need exists for cost-effective screening tools for determining which patients are good candidates for more definitive diagnostic testing. In children, careful visualization of tonsillar size has been found highly sensitive and specific as a screening test for obstructive sleep apnea (A. Li et al. 2002). In adults, other factors, the most significant of

TABLE 15-2. Essential issues in a sleep diagnostic interview of patients and bed partners

Presenting complaint?	Previous sleep evaluations?
Sleep interruptions—Parenting issues? Caregiver issues?	Work schedule—Rotating shifts? On call?
Preferred sleep time—Early or late bedtime? Sleep position?	Exercise schedule—Late in the evening?
Sleep environment—Bed partner? Comfortable bedding? Bright light? Noisy? Vibrations? Excessive heat/cold? Pets?	Insomnia—Early? Middle? Late? Sleep walking? Somnambulism? Sleep eating?
Nap schedule—Frequent or prolonged?	Motor vehicle accident due to sleepiness?
Excessive daytime somnolence?	Alcohol, street drug, or caffeine use, abuse, or dependence?
Cataplexy? Sleep paralysis? Hallucinogenic experiences?	Snoring? Observed pauses?
Nocturnal movements?	Pain—Chronic? Acute? Medications wear off?
Gastrointestinal reflux—Diagnosed? Partially treated?	Hangover effect? Amnesia?
Erectile problems? Urinary frequency? Enuresis?	Vivid dreams, nightmares?
Depression, mania, or panic attacks?	Herbal preparations?
Prescription drug use, abuse, or dependence?	Childhood sleep history?
Family sleep history?	

TABLE 15–3. Selected causes of insomnia

Primarily medical
Obstructive sleep apnea
Chronic obstructive pulmonary disease
Asthma
Gastroesophageal reflux
Acute pain
Angina
Hypoglycemia
Congestive heart failure (orthopnea, paroxysmal nocturnal dyspnea)
Hyperthyroidism
Chronic pain
Primarily neurological
Central sleep apnea
Dementia
Restless legs syndrome
Fatal familial insomnia
Primarily psychiatric
Medication-induced (xanthines, psychostimulants, etc.)
Psychophysiological insomnia
Anxiety disorders
Altered sleep-wake schedule
Withdrawal-related (alcohol, benzodiazepines, etc.)
Sleep state misperception
Mood disorders (depression, mania)
Primarily environmental
Community noise (traffic, alarms, neighbors, gunshots, etc.)
Altered temperature (too hot, too cold)

which is body mass index, confound clinical prediction models that rely solely on the findings of the nasopharyngeal examination. In one large-scale study with a community-based sample, investigators found that in adults, male sex, older age, higher body mass index, greater neck circumference, snoring, and repeated respiratory pauses were all independent correlates of moderate to severe breathing-related sleep disorder (Young et al. 2002b).

Because many patients minimize excessive daytime sleepiness or slowly adapt to it, they may lose insight into the degree of their excessive daytime sleepiness. History from other sources, such as family members, may be necessary. Daytime symptoms related to excessive sleepiness can be evaluated with the brief and convenient Epworth Sleepiness Scale (Johns 1991) (Table 15–5). Unfortunately, no similar scale or questionnaire has been used widely in clinical practice to screen for nocturnal sleep symptoms and disorders.

TABLE 15–4. Selected causes of excessive daytime sleepiness

Primarily neurological
Idiopathic narcolepsy or hypersomnia
Delirium
Kleine-Levin syndrome
Narcolepsy caused by lesion near the third ventricle
Central sleep apnea
Prader-Willi syndrome
Primarily medical
Obstructive sleep apnea
Gastroesophageal reflux
Primarily psychiatric
Medication-induced disorder (alcohol, hypnotic, sedative, etc.)
Mood disorder
Stimulant withdrawal
Altered sleep-wake schedule

Diagnostic Procedures

Techniques for measuring sleep and body functions during sleep have evolved since the initial description of REM sleep in 1953 (Aserinsky and Kleitman 1953). Currently, most sleep studies are conducted in facilities using sophisticated computerized equipment that is steadily replacing the older paper-and-ink polygraph units. These recording devices typically monitor and store the multiple physiological measurements considered essential for a polysomnographic study (Table 15–6). Trained technologists attend the patient during the study, making adjustments and assisting as needed. Sleep disorders centers designed for the evaluation and treatment of the full spectrum of sleep disorders are free-standing or located in a hospital. Although there is considerable interest in portable systems with which sleep studies can be performed in the patient's home, these systems have not been widely available owing to quality and reimbursement issues. In the United States, Medicare recently approved the use of portable devices that collect no less than three types of physiological data for patients suspected to be at high risk of obstructive sleep apnea. Many patients welcome the availability of portable studies that can be conducted the privacy and comfort of their home. For carefully selected patients where there is a high degree of suspicion about obstructive sleep apnea and the absence of insomnia, the procedure is cost-effective. When the differential diagnosis includes sleep

Mayo Sleep Questionnaire—*Informant*

Do you live with the patient? ☐ Yes ☐ No (If No, END FORM HERE)

Do you sleep in the same room as the patient? ☐ Yes ☐ No

If no, is it because of his/her sleep behaviors (i.e., snores too loud, acts out dreams, etc.)? ☐ Yes ☐ No

Please mark "Yes" if the described event has occurred *at least 3 times.*

1. Have you ever seen the patient appear to "act out his/her dreams" while sleeping? (punched or flailed arms in the air, shouted or screamed)
   - ☐ 0 no
   - ☐ 1 yes
   - If Yes,
     - a. How many months or years has this been going on?
       - ___ year(s)
       - ___ months
     - b. Has the patient ever been injured from these behaviors (bruises, cuts, broken bones?
       - ☐ No
       - ☐ Yes
     - c. Has a bedpartner ever been injured from these behaviors (bruises, blows, pulled hair)?
       - ☐ No
       - ☐ Yes
       - ☐ No bedpartner
     - d. Has the patient told you about dreams of being chased, attacked or that involve defending himself/herself?
       - ☐ No
       - ☐ Yes
       - ☐ Never told you about dreams
     - e. If the patient woke up and told you about a dream, did the details of the dream match the movements made while sleeping?
       - ☐ No
       - ☐ Yes
       - ☐ Never told you about dreams
2. Do the patient's legs repeatedly jerk or twitch during sleep (not just when falling asleep)?
   - ☐ No
   - ☐ Yes
3. Does the patient complain of a restless, nervous, tingly, or creepy-crawly feeling in his/her legs that disrupts his/her ability to fall or stay asleep?
   - ☐ No
   - ☐ Yes
   - If Yes,
     - a. Does the patient tell you that these leg sensations decrease when he/she moves them or walks around?
       - ☐ No
       - ☐ Yes
     - b. When do these sensations seem to be the worst?
       - ☐ before 6 pm
       - ☐ after 6 pm
4. Has the patient ever walked around the bedroom or house while asleep?
   - ☐ No
   - ☐ Yes
5. Has the patient ever snorted or choked him/herself awake?
   - ☐ No
   - ☐ Yes
6. Does the patient ever seem to stop breathing during sleep?
   - ☐ No
   - ☐ Yes
   - If Yes,
     - a. Is the patient currently being treated for this (e.g., CPAP)?
       - ☐ No
       - ☐ Yes
7. Does the patient have leg cramps at night? (e.g., also called a "charlie horse" with intense pain in certain muscles in the leg)?
   - ☐ No
   - ☐ Yes
8. Rate the patient's general level of alertness for the past 3 weeks on a scale from 0 to 10.

0	1	2	3	4	5	6	7	8	9	10
Sleep all day										Fully and normally awake

FIGURE 15–2. Mayo Sleep Questionnaire.

TABLE 15–5. Epworth Sleepiness Scale

Each item is rated 0–3 by the patient.

____ Sitting and reading

____ Sitting inactive in a public place

____ Passenger in a car (>60 minutes)

____ Lying down to rest in the afternoon

____ Sitting and talking

____ Sitting after lunch (without alcohol)

____ Sitting in traffic

Source. Adapted from Johns 1991.

TABLE 15–6. Components of polysomnography

Essentials

Electroencephalography (typically three channels)

Electromyography (surface)—chin and lower extremity

Electro-oculography (two channels)

Electrocardiography

Respiratory effort measurement

Airflow monitoring (nasal pressure or temperature)

Pulse oximetry

Options

Videotaping (conventional or digital) with infrared lighting

Transcutaneous carbon dioxide monitoring

Esophageal pressure monitoring

Esophageal pH monitoring

Additional electromyography (upper extremities, intercostal muscles)

Additional electroencephalography (seizure detection)

disorders other than obstructive sleep apnea or when a patient sleeps poorly increasing the chance that monitors get dislodged, portable studies have not been demonstrated to be appropriate. In these cases the sleep study may need to be repeated in a laboratory setting, in effect increasing the overall cost and inconvenience.

In some tertiary-care hospitals, polysomnographic equipment can be transported to the medical-surgical floor or intensive care unit. In selected cases of a primary sleep disorder coexisting with another process, such as severe chronic obstructive pulmonary disease, identifying and treating the sleep disorder may be necessary before a patient can be stabilized and discharged (Olson 2001). Less research has been conducted on how to screen or test for primary sleep disorders in other settings, such as nursing homes. Sleep diaries, completed by patients or caregivers, can be used but often are inaccurate owing to the poor recall of sleep parameters, lack of adherence to daily documentation, or distorted perception (Mercer et al. 2002).

Use of devices such as wrist actigraphs has been studied in the hospital setting, but these devices are used mostly in ambulatory practices (Krahn et al. 1997). Precise determination of sleep-wake status is impossible with actigraphs because the equipment measures limb acceleration and does not record EEG activity. Accordingly, specific sleep stages cannot be identified. One distinct advantage of actigraphy, however, is that the compact device can be worn 24 hours per day for 1–4 weeks. This longitudinal monitoring also allows identification of irregular sleep-wake patterns while the patient is pursuing routine activities.

Other portable monitoring devices, which do not enable the full complement of measures obtained with polysomnography, have been marketed, but all have limitations. Several models monitor only respiratory function without EEG data. Similarly, overnight pulse oximetry measures only oxygen saturation and heart rate. With this equipment, the clinician does not know heart rhythm, body position, or whether the patient is asleep or awake or in NREM versus REM sleep (Netzer et al. 2001). False-negative results can be obtained from patients with obstructive sleep apnea so severe that they cannot fall asleep. Oxygen saturation looks deceptively normal while patients are lying awake in bed at night. Only after patients fall asleep do they begin to experience significant oxygen desaturation. The setting of the oximeter unit can greatly influence the appearance of the compressed overnight printout and contribute to false-positive and false-negative impressions regarding sleep-related breathing conditions (Davila et al. 2002). The results should specify the time settings. Setting up the equipment to acquire data with briefer time periods—for example, 3 seconds rather than 12 seconds—is preferable in screening for breathing-related sleep disorder.

The multiple sleep latency test is used to identify disorders of excessive daytime sleepiness, including narcolepsy (Krahn et al. 2001a). Patients must first undergo an overnight sleep study for exclusion of other sleep disorders caused by disrupted nocturnal sleep. If the patient has had, at minimum, 6 hours of sleep to preclude sleep deprivation, then a valid multiple sleep latency test can be conducted the next day. Patients are asked to take four or five scheduled naps wearing a simplified set of leads including only EEG, electromyographic, and electro-oculographic leads. The test is used to measure initial sleep latency and initial REM latency, if present, for each nap. Patients are asked to stay awake between naps, to refrain from stimulants such as caffeine and prescribed medications, and to undergo drug screening for occult sedative use. The maintenance of wakefulness test is a similar procedure with slight modifications. Instead of being asked to fall asleep, patients are asked to stay awake during four or five specified daytime sessions (Mitler et al. 1982). The data can be used to document that a patient with a treated sleep disorder such as obstructive sleep apnea or narcolepsy can sustain wakefulness sufficiently to drive or operate equipment requiring sustained vigilance. The result of this test is sometimes used as a marker of successful treatment outcome.

Sleep Disorders

Several disorders with signs and symptoms closely linked with sleep or the 24-hour sleep-wake schedule are generally classified as sleep disorders. Many other disease states—for example, tumor growth and chemotherapy tolerability—vary according to a 24-hour schedule, but are not classified as sleep disorders because circadian rhythmicity is not the defining feature (Mormont and Levi 2003). The clearest example of this distinction would be restless legs syndrome where periodicity and timing set this condition apart from other painful neurological diseases.

Narcolepsy and Other Disorders of Excessive Daytime Sleepiness

Narcolepsy is an excellent example of a disorder with dysfunction of a specific sleep state, in this case REM sleep. Isolated fragments of REM sleep intrude into wakefulness, and the result is the characteristic symptoms that invariably cause excessive daytime sleepiness. Narcolepsy in humans was first described in 1880 by the French neurologist Gelineau. Since that time, this sleep disorder has been observed in several dog breeds as well as in horses and sheep. These naturally occurring animal models have greatly facilitated investigations into the pathophysiological mechanisms of narcolepsy.

Prevalence

Narcolepsy is a more common disorder than many recognize. As a result, the need to identify and treat it offers a valuable opportunity to prevent medical, occupational, and social complications. When patients present with sleepiness, many other conditions, including insufficient sleep and breathing-related sleep disorder, should be suspected before narcolepsy is considered. The average delay between onset of symptoms and diagnosis is 10 years.

In a U.S. community sample, narcolepsy was observed to have prevalence of 0.06% (Silber et al. 2001). All cases of narcolepsy met the diagnostic criteria on the basis of excessive daytime sleepiness and laboratory findings. In 64% of these cases, the patient had cataplexy. Incidence data from the same study confirmed the long-standing impression that narcolepsy is slightly more common in men (1.72 per 100,000) than women (1.05 per 100,000). The disease most commonly starts in the second decade of life and is a chronic condition.

Narcolepsy is no longer believed to be a familial disease, although rare cases of familial clusters have been identified (Overeem et al. 2001). When narcolepsy is familial, the mode of inheritance is neither a simple recessive or dominant one. The debate continues about whether narcolepsy is the result of an autoimmune or neurodegenerative process. The association between 85% of cases of narcolepsy with cataplexy and a specific human leukocyte antigen (HLA) allele (DQB1*0602) is the basis of postulation about an autoimmune mechanism; despite several investigations, no confirmatory evidence had been found as of early 2004 (Black et al. 2001). The possibility of the presence of an extremely selective degenerative process stems from the autopsy finding of gliosis in the hypothalamus of narcolepsy patients (Thannickal et al. 2000).

Clinical Features

Narcolepsy is characterized by chronic excessive daytime sleepiness with episodic sleep attacks. Approximately 65%–75% of patients with narcolepsy have cataplexy, which is a condition in which an emotional trigger, most commonly laughter, provokes abrupt muscle atonia without loss of consciousness. Other associated symptoms of narcolepsy include sleep paralysis (isolated loss of muscle tone associated with REM in normal sleep) and hypnagogic and hypnopompic hallucinations (vivid dreaming occurring at the time of sleep onset and awakening that can be difficult to distinguish from reality). When related to the dissociated components of REM sleep, such as muscle atonia (cataplexy and sleep paralysis) and vivid dreams (hypnagogic and hypnopompic hallucinations), these phenomena can intrude into wakefulness. Disturbed nocturnal sleep has been added as a fifth part of this constellation of symptoms.

Pathophysiological Mechanism

In 2000, patients with narcolepsy were reported to have undetectable levels of a newly identified neuropeptide, hypocretin (also known as orexin), in cerebrospinal fluid. Hypocretin is synthesized by a small number of neurons in the anterior hypothalamus that project widely throughout the central nervous system (CNS). After studies of other sleep and neurological disorders, the absence of this neuropeptide appears to be highly specific (99%) for narcolepsy (Mignot et al. 2002). Hypocretin influences sleep, appetite, and temperature. As of early 2004, the relevance of hypocretin as a neuromodulator in diseases other than narcolepsy was unknown. The genes for the ligands and receptors for hypocretin have been knocked out in mice with the development of excessive sleepiness, cataplexy, and obesity (Smart and Jerman 2002). An autoimmune mechanism has been suspected ever since the association between narcolepsy and a specific HLA allele was recognized 25 years ago. Recent work has demonstrated a strong association between narcolepsy and polymorphisms in the T cell lymphocyte receptors, which may point to a new autoimmune mechanism for neuropsychiatric disease (Hallmayer et al. 2009).

Diagnostic Testing

The most important part of an evaluation for narcolepsy is a careful interview to screen for long-standing excessive daytime sleepiness and spells triggered by emotions. The definitive bedside test for cataplexy is demonstrating the transient absence of deep tendon reflexes during the episode (Krahn et al. 2000). This procedure also aids in differentiating cataplexy from pseudocataplexy (Krahn et al. 2001b). However, cataplexy is difficult to provoke, and the episode is often too brief to allow a physical examination.

In most cases diagnostic testing in a sleep disorders center is necessary to supplement the clinical interview. The diagnosis must be as certain as possible before a lifelong course of treatment is begun. An overnight sleep study is important for ruling out other causes of excessive daytime sleepiness. This study is ideally preceded by wrist actigraphy to confirm adequate sleep in the weeks before testing and to eliminate sleep deprivation as the cause. If polysomnography reveals that the patient has obstructive sleep apnea or another primary sleep disorder, these conditions must be stabilized before reliable daytime testing can be conducted. The multiple sleep latency test quantifies the time to fall asleep during daytime naps and confirms the presence of inappropriate daytime REM sleep. Testing for hypocretin in the cerebrospinal fluid is not yet part of clinical practice.

Complications

Narcolepsy is associated with a poorer quality of life than epilepsy (Broughton and Broughton 1994). Without treatment, patients are at risk of motor vehicle accidents and occupational injuries related to sleepiness. Patients with narcolepsy have a higher-than-expected rate of obstructive sleep apnea, REM sleep behavior disorder, and periodic limb movements (Krahn et al. 2001a). New data indicate that patients with narcolepsy have higher rates of obesity, which potentially may be linked to the hypocretin deficiency. Current pharmacological treatments for sleepiness do not appear to have a significant mitigating effect on weight gain (Schuld et al. 2002).

Treatment

Patient education should emphasize the importance of a consistent sleep–wake schedule, the need for adequate sleep, the value of brief daytime naps, and refraining from driving a car when sleepy. Pharmacological treatment options for narcolepsy include methylphenidate or amphetamines, which target excessive daytime sleepiness (Mitler and Hayduk 2002). Extended-release preparations of methylphenidate and amphetamines have the advantage of continuous drug delivery, which reduces the daytime variability in alertness that may occur with the immediate-release forms, which are taken twice or three times a day. Modafinil is a unique wake-promoting medication that was approved by the U.S. Food and Drug Administration (FDA) in 1999. Modafinil, lacking sympathomimetic activity, is not considered a psychostimulant. The mechanism of action is not well understood (U.S. Modafinil in Narcolepsy Multicenter Study Group 1998). Sodium oxybate (also known as gamma-hydroxybutyrate), approved by the FDA in 2002, is a medication indicated for the treatment of narcolepsy. This novel hypnotic was approved initially for the treatment of cataplexy and subsequently permitted for all narcoleptic symptoms. Recently armodafinil, a longer-acting R-enantiomer, was shown to reduce excessive daytime sleepiness in narcolepsy and to be more suitable than modafinil for administration once a day (Keam and Walker 2007).

An endogenous substance, sodium oxybate, increases slow-wave sleep and also improves sleep continuity (Lammers et al. 1993). Although somewhat counterintuitive, clinical trials in narcolepsy have demonstrated that sodium oxybate decreases excessive daytime sleepiness by increasing nighttime sleep (Black and Houghton 2006). Improving the quality of nocturnal sleep also appears to reduce the severity of cataplexy, sleep paralysis, and hypnagogic hallucinations and improve overall quality of life (Weaver and Cuellar 2006). Because of its expense and the inconvenience of taking a liquid medication twice during the night (upon retiring for bed and again 4 hours later), this medication is reserved for patients whose condition is more refractory to treatment. Taken as prescribed, sodium oxybate is well tolerated. Risks arise from combining it with other sedative agents and taking it in excessive amounts. Tricyclic antidepressants and, to a lesser degree, selective serotonin reuptake inhibitors (SSRIs) historically have been used to treat cataplexy. These agents increase the level of norepinephrine in the brain and thus suppress REM sleep–related symptoms. Sodium oxybate needs to be used with caution. Historically known as gamma-hydroxybutyric acid (GHB), it is sought by drug abusers to increase euphoria and libido. Overdoses with illicit use, leading to coma and respiratory depression, are common because of the difficulty in titrating the dosage. Likely because of the short half-life, fatality with overdose is relatively rare unless GHB is mixed with other substances (Knudsen et al. 2008).

Idiopathic Hypersomnia

Idiopathic hypersomnia is a disorder of unknown etiology characterized by excessive daytime sleepiness in the absence of other specific symptoms. Patients typically have a prolonged duration of nocturnal sleep as well as unrefreshing daytime naps. The prevalence of idiopathic hypersomnia is unknown, but the condition appears to develop at equal rates in both male and female patients. As in narcolepsy, symptoms first appear in adolescence or young adulthood. This condition increases the risk of motor vehicle accidents and occupational or educational problems due to sleepiness. Depression may be another consequence (Bassetti and Aldrich 1997).

The clinical interview should concentrate on the duration of excessive daytime sleepiness, the sleep–wake schedule, and the presence of mood disorders. The presence of a mood disorder complicates the evaluation because both depression and antidepressant medications can alter sleep architecture. Because of the broad differential diagnosis, the evaluation for idiopathic hypersomnia must be in-depth. Ideally the diagnostic testing consists of wrist actigraphy, polysomnography, multiple sleep latency testing, and drug screening. The testing for respiratory arousals must be particularly rigorous, since any degree of upper airway resistance syndrome or subclinical sleep-related breathing disorder can produce persisting excessive daytime sleepiness. The diagnosis of idiopathic hypersomnia is established on the basis of the finding of quantifiable excessive daytime sleepiness on the multiple sleep latency test. Unlike patients with narcolepsy, those with idiopathic hypersomnia have no sleep-onset REM episodes and have normal levels of hypocretin in the cerebrospinal fluid.

There is less consensus on the treatment approach to idiopathic hypersomnia than with other sleep disorders. Patient education regarding adequate sleep is critical. A common strategy is initially to request patients to extend sleep time by at least an hour with the intent to aid patients whose sleepiness may be related to inadequate nocturnal sleep. Long sleepers, who require an hour or more sleep than typical persons to obtain adequate sleep, may be erroneously identified as having idiopathic hypersomnia. Apart from sleep extension, treatment is otherwise similar to that used for narcolepsy. In contrast to narcolepsy, daytime naps are not encouraged because they are not refreshing. If the results at evaluation suggest the presence of a coexisting mood disorder after sleep tests are completed, use of an antidepressant is appropriate and does not cause problems. More stimulating antidepressants are preferred.

Kleine-Levin syndrome, also known as recurrent hypersomnia, is an important part of the differential diagnosis of idiopathic hypersomnia. Patients with recurrent hypersomnia are generally male adolescents who engage in binge eating and have periodic hypersomnia that lasts several weeks (Minvielle 2000). The typical pattern is recurrent episodes, each lasting approximately a week, spanning 8 years, Depressed mood has been reported in 48% of affected patients (Arnulf et al. 2005). In the absence of any randomized controlled trials in Kleine-Levin syndrome, psychostimulants and lithium have been reported to prevent relapses (Oliveira et al. 2009).

Parasomnias

Parasomnias are disorders in which patients have inappropriate intermittent motor behaviors during sleep. REM sleep behavior disorder is arguably of most interest because of the distressing behaviors and the relationship with other neurological conditions. Patients with REM sleep behavior disorder appear to "act out their dreams" by yelling or gesturing during REM sleep. They lack the muscle atonia normally found in REM sleep and move in response to dream imagery. REM sleep behavior disorder appears more common than originally suspected, although the prevalence has not been established. Risk factors for this sleep disorder are male sex (90% of patients described in the literature) and advanced age (most patients have been 50 years or older) (Olson et al. 2000). SSRIs and venlafaxine have been suggested as possible triggers. Patients and their bed partners can be seriously injured by hitting, kicking, rolling, and other more complex behaviors. REM sleep behavior disorder is associated with several neurological disorders, including Parkinson's disease (15%–33% of patients), multiple system atrophy (69%–90%), and dementia with Lewy bodies (50%–80%) (Boeve et al. 2007; Comella et al. 1998). These neurodegenerative disorders share the pathological finding of cerebral intracellular inclusion bodies containing alpha-synuclein.

Polysomnography optimally with extra electromyographic leads and synchronized videotaping can be useful for documenting increased electromyographic tone during REM sleep. Patients can have an inappropriate degree of muscle tone without reports of disruptive or inappropriate behaviors. These patients are not yet considered to have REM sleep behavior disorder, but the disease is expected to evolve. Polysomnography also helps identify complicating disorders, such as obstructive sleep apnea, which is of particular importance if benzodiazepines are used later. Nocturnal seizures should be excluded from the diagnosis. Treatment includes modifying the bedroom to reduce injury to the patient and bed partner. Bed partners often choose to sleep apart. Clonazepam has become the medication of choice because it reduces the muscle movement that occurs during REM sleep, reducing the risk of injury (Schenck and Mahowald 1990), but there are no randomized controlled trials of treatment for REM sleep behavior disorder.

NREM parasomnias, unlike REM sleep behavior disorder, are markedly more common in children and adolescents than in adults. Patients act unusually, walk, or eat when not fully alert. Polysomnography is not always needed because the behaviors are often intermittent and therefore difficult to observe with a single night of monitoring. Sleep deprivation, nocturnal arousals, shifting bedtimes, and consumption of alcohol can precipitate episodes in susceptible individuals. In one study sleep deprivation was used as a trigger of sleepwalking.

Treatment of NREM parasomnias includes modifying the sleeping environment to promote safety, adhering to a consistent sleep schedule, reducing nocturnal awakenings, and, if warranted, using medications such as hypnotics to prevent arousal (Pilon et al. 2008). The relationship between parasomnias and posttraumatic stress disorder remains unclear.

Nocturnal panic disorder is increasingly regarded as a rare disorder. However, panic disorder with attacks occurring both during the day and at night is not rare. Treatment of this condition ideally includes a combination of medications and behavioral measures. When panic or anxiety exists exclusively at night, most typically in NREM sleep, a broad differential diagnosis should be used to screen for breathing-related sleep disorder, nightmares, and medical disorders (e.g., arrhythmia, angina, and gastroesophageal reflux) triggering the anxiety. Confirmed treatment of nocturnal panic disorder relies on medications because behavioral measures are less feasible when an attack develops while the patient sleeps. Hypnosis at bedtime has been tried (Hauri et al. 1989).

Whenever a patient presents with unusual behavior at night, the differential diagnosis must include epilepsy. In particular, seizures arising from a locus in the frontal lobe can result in stereotypical but bizarre events during slow wave sleep (Dyken et al. 2001).

Sleep-Related Breathing Disorder and Snoring

Sleep-related breathing disorder comprises obstructive sleep apnea, central sleep apnea, and obesity hypoventilation syndrome. Obstructive sleep apnea is the most notable of these conditions because of its high prevalence and association with numerous medical conditions if untreated (Walker 2001). Obstructive apnea is defined as cessation of airflow that lasts at least 10 seconds owing to impedance of respiratory effort as the result of airway obstruction. Hypopnea is defined as reduction in airflow resulting in at least a 4% decrease in oxygen saturation. Table 15–7 outlines the diagnostic criteria for obstructive sleep apnea. Apnea and hypopnea both are considered clinically significant markers of disease and as a result are reported together as the apnea–hypopnea index. Since these criteria were published, sleep specialists have recognized that hypopnea with an oxygen desaturation greater than or equal to 4% must be quantified in addition to pure apnea.

TABLE 15–7. American Academy of Sleep Medicine diagnostic criteria for obstructive sleep apnea

Essential signs and symptoms

1. Excessive daytime sleepiness
2. Obstructed breathing during sleep

Essential polysomnographic findings

1. More than five episodes of apnea (>10 seconds) per hour of sleep with evidence of respiratory muscle effort and one of the following:
   a. Apnea causing frequent arousals
   b. Apnea causing oxygen desaturation ≥4%
   c. Bradytachycardia

Source. Adapted from American Academy of Sleep Medicine 2005.

Prevalence

Patients with obstructive sleep apnea are the largest subgroup of patients referred to sleep disorders centers. This disorder, which affects at least 2% of women and 4% of men ages 30–60 years (Young et al. 1993), is strongly associated with obesity. Obstructive sleep apnea is more common without marked obesity in several racial groups, including Asians, in whom craniofacial anatomic features can produce a narrower nasopharyngeal airway (K. Li et al. 2000). Advanced age, male sex, and postmenopausal state are all associated with a higher prevalence of this condition (Young et al. 2002a). In subpopulations of patients with hypertension, heart disease, and adult-onset diabetes mellitus, as many as 30%–40% of patients can have obstructive sleep apnea (Partinen 1995).

Clinical Features

Most patients with obstructive sleep apnea snore. Family members may observe disruptive snoring intermixed with quiet periods and reduced respiration. Although essentially all patients with obstructive sleep apnea snore, the reverse is not the case. Snoring is an extremely common phenomenon in the community, affecting 25% of men and 15% of women. For this reason, screening for obstructive sleep apnea must rely on more than simply a history of snoring. Patients may have restless sleep at times, to the point they are suspected to have a parasomnia such as REM behavior disorder. Excessive sweating and morning headaches can be present. Patients may report choking or being awakened by their snoring. An increased rate of nocturia has been described, possibly because the patient is more aware of bladder fullness when awakened by the breathing disorder (Pressman et al. 1996). Obstructive apnea can lead to respiratory arousals and oxygen desaturation, which can cause transient elevations in blood pressure initially at night (Dart et al. 2003). Hypertension is common, especially in patients with severe obstructive sleep apnea. Initially, blood pressure increases follow each obstructive event, but if apneic or hypopneic episodes are frequent, blood pressure can remain elevated throughout the night and day. Pulmonary hypertension also has been an associated finding, particularly with severe obstructive sleep apnea.

The hemodynamic alterations of obstructive sleep apnea include systemic hypertension, increased right and left ventricular afterload, and increased cardiac output. Earlier reports attributed the association between obstructive sleep apnea and cardiovascular disease to the common risk factors such as age, sex, and obesity. However, newer epidemiological data confirm an independent association between obstructive sleep apnea and these cardiovascular diseases. Possible mechanisms include a combination of intermittent hypoxia and hypercapnia, repeated arousals, sustained increase in sympathetic tone, increased platelet aggregation, reduced baroreflex sensitivity, and elevated plasma fibrinogen and homocysteine levels (Bradley and Floras 2009).

Pathophysiological Mechanism

Patients with obstructive sleep apnea experience intermittent collapse of the upper airway. The most common site of obstruction is the pharynx, a tube unsupported by cartilage or bone that contorts during swallowing and speech. The pharyngeal musculature serves to keep the upper airway open and opposes the subatmospheric pressure in the pharynx itself. The genioglossus muscles also pull forward to keep the upper airway clear of obstruction. This balance is further influenced by anatomic structures (adipose tissue, tongue size, mandible, soft palate, and tonsils) and neuromuscular mechanisms (activity of the pharyngeal muscles affected by sleep state, degree of muscle relaxation, and hypnotic medications) (Rama et al. 2002). The obstructed upper airway leads to cessation or reduction of airflow resulting in a cortical arousal. Snoring or increased effort to ventilate due to narrowing but no actual collapse of the airway is called *upper airway resistance syndrome,* a potentially distressing but subclinical form of obstructive sleep apnea that occurs more often in women than in men (Guilleminault et al. 2001).

Diagnostic Testing

Polysomnographic data generated in a sleep disorders center have been the standard for the diagnosis of breathing-related sleep disorder (Bresnitz et al. 1994). Overnight pulse oximetry has not been demonstrated to be cost-effective, reliable, or sufficiently sensitive but newer multichannel portable monitors are available that are utilized with straightforward cases. Many centers use "split-night" sleep studies. Under these circumstances, patients are monitored while asleep, ideally until they experience both NREM and REM sleep in both the supine and nonsupine positions. Once a diagnosis of breathing-related sleep disorder is established, the technologist introduces nasal continuous positive airway pressure (CPAP). Nasal CPAP is applied through a nasal mask connected to a blower that can be adjusted so that pressurized air is delivered to the upper airway. Having positive pressure keep open the airway is particularly important during expiration, when the airway most commonly collapses in patients with obstructive sleep apnea. The nasal CPAP pressure setting can be carefully titrated in response to airway narrowing during the rest of the sleep study. In the morning, the patient can be asked about comfort and acceptance of this therapy. A split-night study is an opportunity for clinician and patient to compare the untreated versus the newly treated state. The procedure is controversial because of the limited time available for both the diagnostic study and the treatment trial. In most cases, a split-night study eliminates the need for a second night in the laboratory (Strollo et al. 1996).

Complications

The complications of obstructive sleep apnea lead to significant morbidity and mortality. Risk factors for obstructive sleep apnea (see section "Evaluation of Sleep" earlier in this chapter) are male sex, older age, high body mass index, greater neck circumference, snoring, and observed pauses in breathing at night (Young et al. 2002b). Untreated obstructive sleep apnea has been associated with systemic hypertension, right-sided heart failure, cerebrovascular accidents, type 2 diabetes, cognitive impairment and depression (Rakel 2009). The excessive daytime sleepiness that can result from untreated obstructive sleep apnea can put patients at risk of motor vehicle accidents, cognitive problems, and interpersonal difficulties. An association has been described between obstructive sleep apnea and gastroesophageal reflux. Nevertheless, treatment with antireflux medication reduces arousals but not apneic episodes, and intervention for obstructive sleep apnea with nasal CPAP does reduce reflux (Ing et al. 2000).

Treatment

Since the early 1980s, the treatment of obstructive sleep apnea has been revolutionized by the use of nasal CPAP. This treatment involves delivering pressurized air (typically 3–18 cm of water pressure) to sites of upper airway collapse (generally the oropharynx and less commonly the nasopharynx) and forcing the airway open. Apnea and snoring are eliminated, allowing the patient to sleep continuously without being aroused to breathe. Nasal CPAP is generally introduced when the patient is sleeping in the sleep laboratory, where staff can adjust the pressure appropriately and assist with mask fit. Newer technology entails the use of self-titrating devices that modify the pressure setting breath by breath without requiring technologist involvement (Berry et al. 2002). The extent to which these more sophisticated machines may replace nasal CPAP titrations conducted in a sleep laboratory is not clear.

Patients with severe obstructive sleep apnea often report marked improvement, within days, in their mood and energy. This improvement provides positive reinforcement that leads to good compliance with nasal CPAP treatment (Sullivan and Grunstein 1994). Patients with mild to moderate obstructive sleep apnea have more adherence problems, the compliance rate being estimated at 10%–50%. Optimizing compliance with CPAP is a challenge but recent studies show that providing a safe hypnotic medication (zolpidem or eszopiclone) short term may be beneficial presumably by increasing sleep duration (Collen et al. 2009). Certain medications, especially long-acting benzodiazepines and opioids, can exert a similar effect and can depress the reticular activating system to reduce the arousal threshold and prevent arousals that effectively interrupt prolonged episodes of apnea (Dolly and Block 1982). Patients with obstructive sleep apnea who consume alcohol close to bedtime pose a challenge, because alcohol has been observed to increase the collapse of the upper airway. These patients often need higher nasal CPAP settings to prevent apnea. In addition, if the sleep study is done when the patient has not been consuming alcohol often, the selected pressure settings are insufficient on nights when the patient has ingested alcohol (Berry et al. 1991).

Another treatment of obstructive sleep apnea is bilevel positive airway pressure. This therapy represents a modification of CPAP whereby the positive pressure fluctuates depending on whether the airflow is inspiratory or expiratory. Bilevel pressure therapy is considerably more expensive than conventional CPAP and is reserved for patients who cannot tolerate CPAP because of discomfort or emergence of central apnea at necessary pressure settings. Supplemental oxygen alone is inadequate for obstructive sleep apnea because the oxygen cannot pass the obstruction to reach the lungs. Patients with both breathing-related sleep disorder and intrinsic lung disease who have persistent hypoxia despite CPAP can benefit from supplemental oxygen delivered through the nasal CPAP mask.

For patients who have apnea only in the supine position, effective treatment may include preventing them from lying on their backs. Inflatable devices resembling backpacks can serve the same purpose. Few data are available regarding long-term adherence with these interventions. Some patients who refuse CPAP and have severe apnea during REM sleep have been offered a REM-suppressant medication such as a monoamine oxidase inhibitor. No published data are available regarding this practice. Abrupt discontinuation of the pharmacological agent should be avoided because of REM rebound, which can increase the risk of apnea.

Weight loss through diet and exercise is a critical component of the treatment plan for any overweight patient with breathing-related sleep disorder (Flemons 2002). Motivated patients can succeed. Weight loss should be the primary treatment only of patients with mild to moderate disease, particularly if they are not interested in other modalities. Gastric bypass surgery can be especially important for management of medically complicated obesity (see Chapter 30, "Surgery"). In general, a 20-pound weight loss can reduce the required CPAP pressure; however, many patients eventually seem to gain rather than lose weight with the result that CPAP pressure needs to be increased.

Patients with abnormalities of the soft tissue or skeletal structures surrounding the upper airway may consider surgery. Surgical procedures include laser-assisted uvulopalatopharyngoplasty, tonsillectomy, mandibular advancement, and tracheostomy (Littner et al. 2001). Patients must be carefully selected. They must have upper airway obstructions that are resectable, for example, large tonsils, and have no other comorbid conditions, such as a high body mass index that compromises upper airway patency at multiple points. Oral appliances that pull the tongue or mandible forward are also a valuable option (Smith 2007).

Central Sleep Apnea and Obesity Hypoventilation

Central sleep apnea and obesity hypoventilation are two additional breathing-related sleep disorders of interest. Central sleep apnea is more likely to be asymptomatic than is obstructive sleep apnea, given that it is less likely to be associated with sleep disruption. Because the patient's airway is not narrowed and vibrating, snoring is not a typical warning sign. Patients often present with insomnia rather than excessive daytime sleepiness. Patients with central sleep apnea are often older and have associated cardiac or cerebrovascular disease. Central sleep apnea can be differentiated from obstructive sleep apnea by the absence of snoring, this differentiation being confirmed by the presence of polysomnographic features of the apnea (Quaranta et al. 1997). Treatment can include a hypnotic agent to decrease arousals or supplemental oxygen to reduce hypoxia (Guilleminault and Robinson 1998). When central apnea and obstructive sleep apnea coexist, treatment may include CPAP or bilevel positive airway pressure therapy.

In some patients with marked obesity, obstructive sleep apnea with repetitive desaturation is occasionally absent, but patients still have a sleep-related breathing condition. Particularly during REM sleep, when muscle atonia affects all muscles but the diaphragm, patients may be unable to properly ventilate because of the difficulty in expanding their lungs owing to their body mass. In obesity hypoventilation, polysomnography shows persisting oxygen desaturation without the fluctuating cessation of airflow and oxygen desaturation that occur in obstructive sleep apnea. Arterial blood gas panels typically reveal hypercapnia (Kessler et al. 2002). Obese patients commonly have both obesity hypoventilation and obstructive sleep apnea, in which case CPAP is indicated. Other treatment options include weight loss, avoiding any factor that may aggravate hypoventilation (e.g., discontinuing sedatives), CPAP with supplemental oxygen, and bilevel positive airway pressure therapy.

Restless Legs Syndrome and Periodic Limb Movements

Patients with restless legs syndrome describe subjective discomfort of the lower extremities that worsens at night. Patients can have an irresistible need to move their legs in bed or during prolonged periods of sedentary activity, such as airplane flights. This condition was first described by Ekblom in 1945. As a result of these distressing symptoms, patients can experience insomnia or have unrefreshing sleep.

Prevalence

Restless legs syndrome is often unrecognized but is far from rare. For years, all data about this condition were collected in clinical settings and the prevalence in community samples was essentially unknown. A community-based survey showed a prevalence of restless legs syndrome of 3% in respondents ages 18–29 years, 10% in those ages 30–79 years, and 19% in those age 80 years and older. The overall prevalence was 10% with equal rates for male and female respondents. In the study, risk factors for restless legs syndrome were identified as greater age and high body mass index as well as nicotine dependence, diabetes mellitus, and lack of exercise (Phillips et al. 2000). Another survey of community-dwelling adults in five European countries had slightly different findings. The prevalence of restless legs syndrome according to the criteria of the International Classification of Sleep Disorders (Table 15–8) was 5.5% and associated with older age, female sex, musculoskeletal disease, hypertension, use of an SSRI, and engaging in physical activities close to bedtime (Ohayon and Roth 2002).

Restless legs syndrome sometimes occurs in association with anemia and iron deficiency. The condition can develop during the third trimester of pregnancy, likely because of the presence of functional anemia (Allen and Earley 2001a). Case reports have shown that patients with restless legs syndrome who donate blood may have an exacerbation of the condition, which warrants more medication. Patients with restless legs syndrome should carefully consider the condition a risk of donating blood (Silber and Richardson 2003).

Restless legs syndrome is known to be secondary to diabetes, peripheral neuropathy, and uremia; 20%–30% of patients with renal failure experience restless legs syndrome (Winkelmann et al. 1996). Familial occurrence of restless legs syndrome has been described. In several large families, an autosomal dominant mode of inheritance has been observed. In a large French Canadian kindred, restless legs syndrome was mapped to chromosome 12q (Desautels et al. 2001). In familial restless legs syndrome, the disorder can have a childhood onset.

Clinical Features

Periodic limb movement disorder is a condition that frequently overlaps with restless legs syndrome. Approximately 80% of patients with restless legs syndrome have intermittent muscle twitches called periodic limb movements (Montplaisir et al. 1997). These movements are involuntary leg jerks that occur at night. They can cause insomnia and, as a result, excessive daytime sleepiness. Almost all patients with restless legs syndrome have periodic limb movements, but many patients with periodic limb movements have no symptoms (Chaudhuri et al. 2001). The periodic limb

TABLE 15–8. Clinical characteristics of restless legs syndrome

Desire to move the limbs because of subjective discomfort
Motor restlessness
Symptoms worse or exclusively associated with sedentary activities
Symptoms at least partially relieved by activity
Symptoms worse in the evening or during the night

movements can affect a variety of muscles in the legs or arms. Periodic limb movements in the absence of subjective symptoms of restlessness are of uncertain clinical significance (Nicolas et al. 1999).

Periodic limb movements must be differentiated from nocturnal leg cramps, which are extremely painful sustained muscle contractions, particularly involving the gastrocnemius and soleus muscles. Predisposing factors include pregnancy, diabetes mellitus, electrolyte disturbances, and prior vigorous exercise. Nocturnal leg cramps are not periodic and usually occur, at most, several times a night. The differential diagnosis of restless legs syndrome and periodic limb movement disorder includes neuropathic pain, arthritis, restless insomnia, and drug-induced akathisia.

Complications

Patients with restless legs syndrome experience irritability, depressed mood, or cognitive disturbance due to disturbed sleep; headache, especially on awakening; depressed mood; social isolation; and reduced libido (Ulfberg et al. 2001).

Pathophysiological Mechanism

Restless legs syndrome is believed to be a condition associated with decreased dopamine levels. Treatment with dopamine antagonists aggravates the symptoms, and this syndrome occurs with increased frequency in Parkinson's disease. Positron emission tomographic studies of restless legs syndrome have shown decreased dopaminergic functioning in the caudate and putamen regions of the brain (Ruottinen et al. 2000). Treatment with dopaminergic agonists, even low dosages, leads to marked improvement. Restless legs syndrome has been strongly associated with anemia. Deficient iron stores appear to play a role in the pathophysiological mechanism because iron is hypothesized to be a cofactor for tyrosine hydroxylase, the enzyme for the rate-limiting step in the synthesis of dopamine (Earley et al. 2000).

Diagnostic Testing

A rating scale for restless legs syndrome has facilitated diagnosis (Allen and Earley 2001b). Attempts to develop a self-administered screening survey for restless legs syndrome in dialysis populations have been less successful because of low specificity and a high false-positive rate (Cirignotta et al. 2002).

An overnight sleep study is not essential, because the diagnosis of restless legs syndrome can be based on the patient's history. Polysomnography is valuable when a patient may have a coexisting sleep disorder, such as obstructive sleep apnea, or if the patient does not respond to treatment of restless legs syndrome diagnosed on the basis of history alone. Useful laboratory tests include complete blood count to assess for anemia and ferritin, especially when levels are less than 50 μg/L.

Treatment

Treatment of restless legs syndrome is primarily with dopaminergic medications. Direct dopamine receptor agonists, such as pramipexole and ropinirole have become first-line agents (Trenkwalder 2008). These drugs have replaced low-dose, controlled-release carbidopa and levodopa because of a lower incidence of side effects and improved efficacy. There have been encouraging reports about the benefits of gabapentin, although this anticonvulsant lacks an FDA indication for restless legs syndrome (Garcia-Borreguero et al. 2002). Long-acting benzodiazepines, such as clonazepam, and opioids, including codeine and methadone, also have been used. Medications that can lead to physical dependence require careful monitoring for tolerance. As a result, these drugs are not preferred treatment choices. Most clinicians use drug treatment of restless legs syndrome. Nonpharmacological options include physical therapy and exercise consisting of lower body resistance training plus walking on a treadmill (Aukerman et al. 2006). Pneumatic compression devices have recently been demonstrated to improve symptom severity, daytime sleepiness, and quality of life (Lettieri and Eliasson 2009).

Insomnia

As outlined in Table 15–4, insomnia can be caused by a variety of medical, neurological, psychiatric, and environmental conditions. If possible, any factors that cause or exacerbate insomnia, such as gastric regurgitation, should be corrected (Ohayon and Roth 2003). However, many patients have no specific triggers of insomnia, and insomnia is not a symptom of an underlying disorder.

Prevalence

Insomnia is the most common sleep disorder, with 24% of adults reporting that sleep problems affect their daily activities (National Sleep Foundation Web site 2005). The manifestations range from frequent nighttime awakenings (33%) to premature awakenings with inability to return to sleep (23%) and difficulty falling asleep (18%). Women experience even more difficulties, with 67% reporting sleep problems on a weekly basis and 29% using either a prescription or an over-the-counter agent a few nights a week (National Sleep Foundation Web site 2008).

Patients with the classic type of, or psychophysiological (conditioned), insomnia learn to associate sleeplessness with certain circumstances, such as their own bedrooms. These patients become progressively more tense as bedtime approaches. The prevalence of this condition is unknown. Polysomnography is not generally useful in establishing the diagnosis. Sometimes a patient's best sleep in years occurs in the unfamiliar setting of the sleep disorders center (Chesson et al. 2000).

Treatment

Treatment of insomnia includes improvement in sleep hygiene with the techniques listed in Table 15–9; behavioral techniques, such as relaxation strategies including tapes, self-hypnosis, and music; and occasional doses of hypnotic medication (Toney and Ereshefsky 2000).

More medications are now available that were specifically developed as hypnotics. The newer nonbenzodiazepine hypnotics zolpidem and zaleplon have a short half-life that reduces the hangover effect. Patients have been shown to have alertness adequate for driving and other activities that require sustained vigilance (Richardson et al. 2001). Unusual sleep behaviors, including somnambulism and sleep eating, have been reported, especially with zolpidem. The dosage is often supratherapeutic or combined with a cross-tolerant substance such as alcohol. The prevalence of these phenomena is unknown (Tsai et al. 2009). Physical dependence has not been reported with the short-term use approved by the FDA. Ramelteon is a novel hypnotic that acts as a selective melatonin agonist which also has been demonstrated to be well tolerated and free of morning residual effects (Devi and Shankar 2008). Benzodiazepines, although less expensive than some nonbenzodiazepine hypnotics, can cause dependence and alter cognition the morning after use. Several antidepressants with prominent sedative side effects, such as mirtazapine and trazodone, are valuable therapeutic options, especially if the patient has a coexisting mood or anxiety disorder. Mirtazapine has prominent antihistaminergic side effects at doses of 15 mg or less; however, undesirable weight gain can occur (Artigas et al. 2002). Tricyclic antidepressants like low-dose doxepin have a role in carefully selected patients, considering their cardiac and anticholinergic side effects. Antihistamines such as diphenhydramine are generally a poor choice because they quickly lose effectiveness and can exacerbate confusion in the medically ill. Hypnotic medications have an important role in the management of short-term or intermittent insomnia, but most sleep specialists prefer a meaningful trial of nonpharmacological interventions in the care of patients with the chronic form of primary insomnia. The intent is to alter the thoughts and behaviors that lead to the development of poor-quality nocturnal sleep.

More specific behavioral studies have produced basic information about sleep habits that can be helpful to patients who have disturbed sleep. These sleep hygiene factors have been found to have particular efficacy in the care of patients with chronic insomnia. Establishing a regular waking time 7 days a week optimizes biological rhythms. This regimen is particularly helpful for patients who need to keep morning commitments but tend to naturally be "night owls" or have problems falling asleep at the needed bedtime. However, the clock tends to drift rapidly back to the old schedule as soon as there is variability in arising time (Brown et al. 2002). Discipline and consistency are important.

TABLE 15–9. Sleep hygiene

Circadian issues
Avoid daytime naps
Limit time in bed to 8 hours
Get daily exercise, preferably finishing at least 4 hours before bedtime
Keep regular sleep-wake cycle 7 days per week
Avoid bright light in the evening or at night
Seek bright light in the morning
Reduction of sleep disruption
Avoid large quantities of fluids in the evening
Minimize caffeine; a hot drink without caffeine may be beneficial
Avoid alcoholic drinks
Keep the bedroom quiet, dark, and at a comfortable temperature
Develop a relaxing bedtime ritual
Avoid worrying in bed by using tools such as list writing during the day
Manage stress optimally during the day
Do not use the bed and bedroom except for sleep and for sexual activity
Get assistance with pets and children
Avoid large meals soon before bedtime
Pursue medical intervention for problems such as gastroesophageal reflux, pain, and nausea

When regular exercise is an option, exercising in the late afternoon several hours before bedtime may improve sleep. One postulated mechanism is that a decrease in body temperature is associated with sleep, and body temperature decreases approximately 4 hours after exercise (Montgomery and Dennis 2002). Avoiding "clock watching" can help reduce the arousal effects of becoming annoyed when tracking the slow passage of time throughout the night. Most people recall only periods of wakefulness at night, so clock watching can reinforce the perception that no sleep has occurred. Patients should avoid alcohol and stimulants, including nicotine and caffeine, at any time during the day. Patients, particularly patients prone to gastroesophageal reflux, should not sleep on a full stomach. Introducing relaxing routines around bedtime can be helpful to many patients with sleep complaints. Treating gastroesophageal reflux with antacids and histamine$_2$-blocking medication before sleep can be beneficial.

More specific behavioral evaluation may lead to suggestions that a patient learn relaxation techniques or develop stress management strategies (Morin et al. 1999). Psychotherapy can be helpful for sleep-related anxiety. One of the techniques recommended to those who find that they spend inordinate amounts of time worrying when awake at night is called "worry time" or "thinking time." This technique entails the recommendation that patients take 15–30 minutes in the late afternoon or early evening (not near bedtime) during which there is time to devote attention to worries. Patients are expected to use this time to list their concerns and then identify which they may be able to have some control over and which they do not. When patients awaken at night and begin to worry about a "new" problem, this worry is added to the list, to be included in the next day's session. Eventually the energy and time spent worrying at night diminish, and wakefulness is not perpetuated by anxious thought content (Hauri and Esther 1990).

Stimulus control techniques have been used to help patients with psychophysiological, or conditioned, insomnia (Bootzin and Perlis 1992). These patients find they are sleepy near bedtime, but as soon as they enter the sleeping environment, they become aroused and unable to sleep. This conditioned association between sleeplessness and the bedroom may need to be interrupted by instructing patients to avoid "trying to sleep." Patients who find they are hyperaroused while lying in bed should not try to sleep. They are advised instead to get up and go to a different setting and engage in a different activity (e.g., reading a book, watch relaxing television, or listening to music) until they become sleepy again and return to bed. They should repeat this process as often and as long as needed to extinguish the arousal state conditioned to the bedroom. Some patients find that rather than getting out of bed or leaving the bedroom, they can achieve the same results by watching a monotonous videotape in the bedroom with the VCR set to turn off automatically (Pallesen et al. 2003).

For patients with severe persistent insomnia, a sleep restriction management method may be helpful. In this modality, patients are instructed to allow no more hours in bed than they estimated they slept the previous night. Initially this period may be considerably less than 7.5 hours. When they are able to sleep for essentially all the time in bed for several nights, patients are advised to increase their time in bed by half-hour increments until they achieve optimal sleep time and sleep efficiency. Although pharmacological and behavioral treatments are effective for insomnia management over the initial weeks of treatment, results of a randomized controlled trial of these treatments in the care of elderly patients suggested that behavioral treatment was associated with more sustained improvement than was pharmacological therapy (Morin et al. 1999). Research has successfully demonstrated that as little as one to two session may be beneficial (Morin and Espie 2004). The availability of medication may reduce patients' motivation and confidence in behavioral techniques.

Paradoxical Insomnia

Paradoxical insomnia, previously known as sleep state misperception, is a rare type of primary insomnia. Patients with this disorder describe subjective sleep disturbances that are not consistent with objective data. For the criteria for this diagnosis to be met, polysomnography must demonstrate normal duration and quality of sleep (American Academy of Sleep Medicine 2005). As the understanding of sleep increases, specific sleep disorders may eventually be diagnosed in some of these patients. Treatment involves discussing with the patient the discrepancy between subjective and objective data. Behavioral techniques and hypnotic medications have been used successfully in this group of patients.

Medications and Sleep

Any substance that crosses the blood–brain barrier will very likely have an effect on CNS receptors that affect sleep and wakefulness. Essentially all drugs that have been studied have been found to have some effects, and many that have not been formally studied are known by clinicians to influence sleep and wakefulness. The hypothalamus is a key center for sleep regulation in addition to the classically understood brain stem sleep influences. Sleep mechanisms were previously thought to be predominantly due to the interactions of acetylcholine, dopamine, serotonin, and norepinephrine primarily in the brain stem. More recent research findings indicated that the hypothalamic neurotransmitters adenosine, dopamine, gamma-aminobutyric acid (GABA), histamine, and hypocretin also play an important role in the physiological mechanisms of sleep. The newest observations suggest that connections between the thalamus (cortical activation, sleep spindle formation, and EEG synchronization), hypothalamus (sleep–wake switch), suprachiasmatic nucleus (circadian clock), and the brain stem (ascending cortical activation and REM sleep-wake switch) organize circadian, ultradian, and intrinsic sleep function (Saper et al. 2005).

Some CNS substances affect intrinsic sleep parameters, such as sleep latency, awakenings, percentage of various stages of sleep, nocturnal wakefulness, and evidence of sleep interruptions manifested primarily at a sleep EEG study. Many drugs have known effects on primary sleep disorders such as restless legs syndrome, obstructive sleep apnea, and insomnia from many causes. The known effects of drugs on sleep are summarized in Table 15–10.

Few drugs have uniformly beneficial effects on sleep. Rather than assume that these various factors are too complex to be useful in the psychiatric care of a medically ill patient, the consultation psychiatrist can learn the few basic groups of drugs with empirically demonstrated significant effects on sleep (see Table 15–11 for a summary of hypnotic effects). Combining this information with knowledge of the physiological mechanisms of sleep will allow the clinician to logically infer the effects of most other drugs on sleep. The interactions of hypnotics with other medications are reviewed in Chapter 38, "Psychopharmacology."

The following general rules about drugs can assist in the application of sleep knowledge to patient care:

1. Most CNS drugs decrease slow-wave and REM sleep, at least acutely. It is reasonable to learn the relatively short list of drugs known to increase REM sleep and to assume that others will suppress or disrupt normal REM sleep function. The medications that increase REM sleep are reserpine, yohimbine (and other alpha-antagonists), and physostigmine (and other cholinomimetic drugs, perhaps including cholinesterase inhibitors such as donepezil) (Slatkin et al. 2001).
2. Many drugs cause daytime sedation. It is reasonable to learn the short list of drugs that cause increased daytime alertness and perhaps anxiety as well (psychostimulants, modafinil, and caffeine) and to presume that most others will either be neutral or negative toward daytime alertness.
3. Stopping drugs suddenly commonly produces adverse effects. The condition suppressed will likely rebound. Thus, stopping drugs that suppress REM sleep (most CNS agents) will often lead to REM sleep rebound, which can be associated with insomnia, nightmares, and even hallucinations.
4. Stopping drugs that stimulate the CNS (and that have depleted or displaced stimulating neurotransmitters) can lead to temporary depression. This effect is surprisingly uncommon, even in patients who have taken high doses of stimulants for a long time. Depression and decreased alertness are common after stopping stimulants but usually are transient.
5. Many drugs continue their activity on sleep and wakefulness far beyond the intended therapeutic time. Many medications used to promote sleep are associated with some "hangover" experience the next day. The few exceptions are drugs with an ultrashort half-life, such as zaleplon (definitely demonstrated) and perhaps triazolam and zolpidem (less clearly demonstrated) (see Table 15–11).
6. Alternative therapies and herbal preparations may be helpful, but little definitive information is available (although more formal controlled studies are increasingly common). Many of these agents are pharmacologically active in the CNS, and some have interactions with prescribed medications.

Herbal and Alternative Therapies for Sleep Problems

Herbal agents have been used for centuries as traditional remedies for sleep problems. A review of complementary therapies from an Eastern perspective describes in detail an extensive list of Chinese herbal treatments and their potential toxicities (Cheng 2000). Melatonin, 5-hydroxytryptamine, catnip, chamomile, gotu kola, hops, L-tryptophan, lavender, passionflower, skullcap, and valerian are agents that have been used to manage sleep disorders (Cauffield and Forbes 1999). The toxicities of herbal substances most commonly used for sedative or stimulant purposes among consultation-liaison populations are shown in Table 15–12 (Crone and Wise 1998).

Melatonin is a readily available and popular sleep aid. Evaluating clinical trials of melatonin is complicated by the varying bioavailability of oral doses, even in pharmacologically pure preparations, resulting in as much as a 20-fold difference in plasma levels of the agent (Di et al. 1997). Actual doses range markedly, from 0.5 to 10 mg, with lower doses of 1.8–3 mg being more common (Morgenthaler et al. 2007). Some practice guidelines have found support for melatonin's use to promote daytime sleep in night shift workers, to combat jet lag, and to treat sleep phase disorder (advanced or delayed). Research findings for jet lag are somewhat mixed, but on balance, carefully timed administration of melatonin appears to have moderate effectiveness in preventing jet lag (Suhner et al. 2001). The literature on insomnia is replete with contradictory reports concerning the dosage and efficacy of melatonin. There is evidence that a low dose (0.5 mg) of melatonin improves initial sleep quality, for example, in elderly persons with insomnia (Olde Rikkert and Rigaud 2001). Overall adverse effects of melatonin are rare but include autoimmune hepatitis, optic neuropathy, fragmented sleep, psychosis, nys-

TABLE 15–10. Effects of medications on sleep

Substance	TST	A	SL	II	SWS	REM	REML	Insomnia	Vigilance	Sedation	Nightmares, parasomnias
Acetylcholinesterase inhibitors							+	+/–			
Alcohol											
Alcohol, acute	+	–	–		+	–	+	+/–			+
Alcohol, withdrawal	–	+	+		–	+	–	+	+		+
Analgesics											
Opioids, acute	+/–	+	–	–	–	–		+/–		+	+
Opioids, withdrawal	–	+	+			–		+/–			
Antibiotics											
Anticholinergics		–		+		–	+			+/–	+/–
Quinolones						–		+			
Anticonvulsants											
Gabapentin		–			++						
Lamotrigine					–	+					
Phenytoin			–		–	–					
Valproate										+	
Vigabatrin		+			+						
Antidepressants											
Bupropion								+		–	
Duloxetine		+	+		–	–	+				
MAOI, acute	–					–	+				+
Mirtazapine		–	–		+	+	+			–	
Nefazodone	–	–				+/–	+/–	–			
SSRI	+/–	+/–	+/–			–	+	+/–		+/–	
TCAs	+	–	+/–	+		–	–				
TCAs, withdrawal	–	+	+			+	+	+			
Trazodone		–	–		+		+			+	
Venlafaxine		+			–	–	+				

TABLE 15–10. Effects of medications on sleep *(continued)*

Substance	TST	A	SL	II	SWS	REM	REML	Insomnia	Vigilance	Sedation	Nightmares, parasomnias
Antihistamines											
Histamine$_1$ agonists		++									
Histamine$_1$ antagonists		–								+	
Antihypertensives											
ACE inhibitors											+
Alpha$_2$ agonists	+		+	+	+	–	+			+	+
Alpha$_1$ antagonists										+	
Beta-blocker, lipophilic		+				–			–		+
Calcium channel agonist								+			
5-HT$_2$ agonist					+	–					
Methyldopa				–	–						
Reserpine		–				+	–				+
Antineoplastic agents											
Aminoglutethimide							+			+	+
Flutamide								+		+	+
Interferon					+			+			
Procarbazine								+		+	+
Antiparkinsonism agents											
Amantadine								+			
L-Dopa, acute					+			–			
L-Dopa, chronic	–	+			–	–		+			+
Pramipexole										+[a]	
Selegiline	+	–						–			
Antipsychotics											
Acute	+	–	–			–	+			+	
Withdrawal	–	+	+			+					

TABLE 15–10. Effects of medications on sleep *(continued)*

Substance	TST	A	SL	II	SWS	REM	REML	Insomnia	Vigilance	Sedation	Nightmares, parasomnias
Anxiolytics											
Barbiturates and benzodiazepines, acute	+	–	–	–	–	+					
Barbiturates and benzodiazepines, caffeine combination product	–	+	+					+			
Barbiturates and benzodiazepines, withdrawal	–	+	+		+			+			
Buspirone								+			
Other drugs											
Corticosteroids		+						+		+	+
Lithium	+	–		+	+	–	+			+	
Nicotine, acute	–	–	+			–					
Nicotine, withdrawal		+								+	
Stimulants	–	+	+			–	+	+	+		
Tetrahydrocannabinol		+			–						
Yohimbine						+		+			

Note. A=number of arousals; ACE=angiotensin converting enzyme; 5-HT_2=serotonin$_2$ receptor; MAOI=monoamine oxidase inhibitor; REM=percentage of REM sleep; REML=initial REM latency; SL=sleep latency; SSRI=selective serotonin reuptake inhibitor; SWS=percentage of slow-wave sleep; TCA=tricyclic antidepressant; TST=total sleep time; II=percentage of Stage II sleep; +=drug is known to produce an increase in the sleep parameter or phenomenon; –=drug is known to produce a decrease in the sleep parameter or phenomenon; +/–=drug is known to produce variable effects on the sleep parameter or phenomenon; no symbol=there are no reliable data on the effect of this drug on sleep parameters.

[a]At high doses.

Source. Armitage 2000; Dietrich 1997; Nicholson 1994; Nicholson et al. 1994; Novak and Shapiro 1997; Obermeyer and Benca 1996; Parrino and Terzano 1996; Pascoe 1994; Placidi et al. 2000; Winokur et al. 2001.

TABLE 15–11. Effects of hypnotic drugs (including their active metabolites) on sleep

Drug	Half-life (h)	SL	REML	TST	WASO	SWS	REM	Rebound?	Tolerance?	Carryover
Chloral hydrate	4–12	–	–	+	–	?	–	?	Yes	Yes
Flurazepam	40+	–	+	+	–	–	–	Yes	Yes	Yes
Quazepam	25–41	–	+/–	+	–			No	Yes	No
Ramelteon	1–3	–	+/–	+	–	+/–	+/–	No	?	No
Temazepam	10+	–	+	+	–	–	–	Yes	Yes	No
Trazodone (25–50 mg)	4–7	–	+	+	–	?	?	?	?	Yes
Triazolam	1–5	–	+/–	+	–	–	–	Yes	Yes	No
Zaleplon	1	–	?	+	?	?	?	No	?	No
Zolpidem	1–2	–	–	+	–	+/–	+/–	Yes	Yes	Yes

Note. REML = initial rapid eye movement (REM) latency; REM = REM sleep; SL = sleep latency; SWS = slow-wave sleep; TST = total sleep time; WASO = wakefulness after sleep onset; + = increased; – = decreased; +/– = variable effects.

TABLE 15–12. Herbal medications with sleep–wake toxicity

Medication	Toxicity
Herbal medications used as sedatives	
Broom *(Cytisus scoparius)*	Vomiting, uterine contractions, and bradycardia
Kava kava *(Piper methysticum)*	Dermatitis, hallucinations, and shortness of breath
Passionflower *(Passiflora caerulea)*	Seizures, hypotension, and hallucinations
Valerian *(Valeriana officinalis)*	Dystonic reactions and hepatotoxicity
Miscellaneous herbal preparations with excessive stimulation and insomnia as side or toxic effects	
Echinacea *(Echinacea angustifolia* or *E. purpurea)*	Central nervous system stimulation, dermatitis, and anaphylaxis
Ginseng *(Panax ginseng)*	Hypertension, mastalgia, agitation, anxiety, depression, and insomnia
Goldenseal *(Hydrastis canadensis)*	Nausea and vomiting, central nervous system stimulation, paralysis and paresthesia, and respiratory failure
Ma huang *(Ephedra sinica)*	Mania and psychosis, hypertension, and tachycardia
Yohimbine bark *(Pausinystalia yohimbine* or *Corynanthe yohimbe)*	Hallucinations and anxiety, hypertension and tachycardia, and nausea and vomiting

tagmus, seizures, headache, skin eruption, and confusion from overdose (Morera et al. 2001). In general, the risks of melatonin appear to be low (Morgenthaler et al. 2007).

Conclusion

Sleep takes up one-third of a typical day. Obtaining adequate quantity and quality of sleep is optimal for good health and the prevention of complications. We have addressed the major sleep disorders by discussing their clinical features, diagnostic testing, and treatment. Sleep medicine is a vibrant medical specialty with recent scientific advances in understanding of the mechanisms of sleep disorders and their treatment. Interventions can prevent undesirable medical, psychiatric, and social consequences of sleep disorders. Patients can benefit from these discoveries when dysfunctional sleep is recognized and carefully assessed. A growing menu of treatment options is available once the diagnosis of a specific sleep disorder is made.

References

Allen R, Earley C: Restless legs syndrome: a review of clinical and pathophysiologic features. J Clin Neurophysiol 18:128–147, 2001a

Allen R, Earley C: Validation of the Johns Hopkins Restless Legs Severity Scale (JHRLSS). Sleep Med 3:239–242, 2001b

American Academy of Sleep Medicine: International Classification of Sleep Disorders, Second Edition. Westchester, IL, American Academy of Sleep Medicine, 2005

Armitage R: The effects of antidepressants on sleep in patients with depression. Can J Psychiatry 45:803–809, 2000

Arnulf I, Zeitzer JM, File J, et al: Kleine-Levin syndrome: a systematic review of 186 cases in the literature. Brain 128:2763–2776, 2005

Artigas F, Nutt D, Shelton R: Mechanism of action of antidepressants. Psychopharmacol Bull 36 (suppl 2):123–132, 2002

Aserinsky E, Kleitman N: Regularly occurring periods of eye motility, and concomitant phenomena during sleep. Science 118:273–274, 1953

Aukerman MM, Aukerman D, Bayard M, et al: Exercise and restless legs syndrome: a randomized controlled trial. J Am Board Fam Med 19:487–493, 2006

Bassetti C, Aldrich M: Idiopathic hypersomnia: a series of 42 patients. Brain 120:1423–1435, 1997

Bergmann B, Gilliland M, Feng P, et al: Are physiological effects of sleep deprivation in the rat mediated by bacterial invasion? Sleep 19:554–562, 1996

Berry R, Deas M, Light R: Effect of ethanol on the efficacy of nasal continuous positive airway pressure as a treatment for obstructive sleep apnea. Chest 99:339–341, 1991

Berry R, Parish J, Hartse K: The use of auto-titrating continuous positive airway pressure for the treatment of adult obstructive sleep apnea: an American Academy of Sleep Medicine review. Sleep 25:148–173, 2002

Black J, Houghton W: Sodium oxybate improves excessive daytime sleepiness in narcolepsy. Sleep 29:939–946, 2006

Black J, Krahn L, Silber M: A pilot study of serologic markers of autoimmunity in patients with narcolepsy (abstract). Sleep 24 (suppl):A318–A319, 2001

Bootzin R, Perlis M: Nonpharmacologic treatments of insomnia. J Clin Psychiatry 53 (suppl):37–41, 1992

Boeve BF, Silber MH, Saper CB, et al: Pathophysiology of REM sleep behaviour disorder and relevance to neurodegenerative disease. Brain 130(pt 11):2770–2788, 2007

Bradley TD, Floras JS: Obstructive sleep apnoea and its cardiovascular consequences. Lancet 373:82–93, 2009

Bresnitz E, Goldberg R, Kosinski R: Epidemiology of obstructive sleep apnea. Epidemiol Rev 16:210–227, 1994

Broughton W, Broughton R: Psychosocial impact of narcolepsy. Sleep 17 (8 suppl):s45–s49, 1994

Brown FC, Buboltz WC Jr, Soper B: Relationship of sleep hygiene awareness, sleep hygiene practices, and sleep quality in university students. Behav Med 28:33–38, 2002

Carskadon M, Dement W: Normal human sleep: an overview, in Principles and Practice of Sleep Medicine, 2nd Edition. Edited by Kryger M, Roth T, Dement W. Philadelphia, PA, WB Saunders, 1994, pp 16–25

Cauffield J, Forbes H: Dietary supplements used in the treatment of depression, anxiety, and sleep disorders. Lippincotts Prim Care Pract 3:290–304, 1999

Chaudhuri K, Appiah-Kubi L, Trenkwalder C: Restless legs syndrome. J Neurol Neurosurg Psychiatry 71:143–146, 2001

Cheng JT: Review: drug therapy in Chinese traditional medicine. J Clin Pharmacol 40:445–450, 2000

Chesson A Jr, Hartse K, Anderson W, et al: Practice parameters for the evaluation of chronic insomnia: an American Academy of Sleep Medicine report—Standards of Practice Committee of the American Academy of Sleep Medicine. Sleep 23:237–241, 2000

Cirignotta F, Mondini S, Santoro A, et al: Reliability of a questionnaire screening restless legs syndrome in patients on chronic dialysis. Am J Kidney Dis 40:302–306, 2002

Collen J, Lettieri K, Roop S: Clinical and polysomnographic predictors of short-term continuous positive airway compliance. Chest 135:704–709, 2009

Comella CL, Nardine TM, Diedrich NJ, et al: Sleep-related violence, injuries and REM behavior disorder in Parkinson's disease. Neurology 51:526–529, 1998

Crone C, Wise T: Use of herbal medicines among consultation-liaison populations: a review of current information regarding risks, interactions, and efficacy. Psychosomatics 39:3–13, 1998

Dart R, Gregoire J, Gutterman D, et al: The association of hypertension and secondary cardiovascular disease with sleep-disordered breathing. Chest 123:244–260, 2003

Davila D, Richards K, Marshall B, et al: Oximeter performance: the influence of acquisition parameters. Chest 122:1654–1660, 2002

Desautels A, Turecki G, Montplaisir J, et al: Identification of a major susceptibility locus for restless legs syndrome on chromosome 12q. Am J Hum Genet 69:1266–1270, 2001

Devi V, Shankar PK: Ramelteon: a melatonin receptor agonist for the treatment of insomnia. J Postgrad Med 54:45–48, 2008

Di W, Kadva A, Johnston A, et al: Variable bioavailability of oral melatonin (letter). N Engl J Med 336:1028–1029, 1997

Dietrich B: Polysomnography in drug development. J Clin Pharmacol 37 (1 suppl):70S–78S, 1997

Dolly F, Block A: Effect of flurazepam on sleep-disordered breathing and nocturnal oxygen desaturation in asymptomatic subjects. Am J Med 73:239–243, 1982

Dyken M, Yamada T, Lin-Dyken D: Polysomnographic assessment of spells in sleep: nocturnal seizures versus parasomnias. Semin Neurol 21:377–390, 2001

Earley C, Allen R, Beard J, et al: Insight into the pathophysiology of restless legs syndrome. J Neurosci Res 62:623–628, 2000

Ekblom K: Restless legs. Acta Med Scand Suppl 158:1–123, 1945

Flemons W: Obstructive sleep apnea. N Engl J Med 347:498–504, 2002

Garcia-Borreguero D, Larrosa O, de la Llave Y, et al: Treatment of restless legs syndrome with gabapentin: a double-blind, cross-over study. Neurology 59:1573–1579, 2002

Gelineau J: De la narcolepsie. Lancette Francaise 53:626–628, 1880

Guilleminault C, Robinson A: Central sleep apnea. Otolaryngol Clin North Am 31:1049–1065, 1998

Guilleminault C, Do Kim Y, Chowdhuri S, et al: Sleep and daytime sleepiness in upper airway resistance syndrome compared to obstructive sleep apnoea syndrome. Eur Respir J 17:838–847, 2001

Hallmayer J, Faraco J, Lin L, et al: Narcolepsy is strongly associated with the T-cell receptor alpha locus. Nat Genet 41:708–711, 2009

Hauri P, Esther M: Insomnia. Mayo Clinic Proc 65:869–882, 1990

Hauri P, Friedman M, Ravaris C: Sleep in patients with spontaneous panic attacks. Sleep 12:323–337, 1989

Iber C, Ancoli-Israel S, Chesson A, et al: The Academy of Sleep Medicine Manual for the Scoring of Sleep and Associated Events. Westchester, IL, American Academy of Sleep Medicine, 2007

Ing A, Ngu M, Breslin A: Obstructive sleep apnea and gastroesophageal reflux. Am J Med 108 (suppl 4a):120S–125S, 2000

Johns M: A new method for measuring daytime sleepiness: the Epworth Sleepiness Scale. Sleep 14:540–545, 1991

Keam S, Walker MC: Therapies for narcolepsy with or without cataplexy: evidence-based review. Curr Opin Neurol 20:699–703, 2007

Kessler R, Chaouat A, Schinkewitch P, et al: The obesity-hypoventilation syndrome revisited: a prospective study of 34 consecutive cases. Chest 120:369–376, 2002

Knudsen K, Greter J, Verdicchio M: High mortality rates among GHB abusers in Western Sweden. Clin Toxicology 46:187–192, 2008

Krahn L, Lin S, Wisbey J, et al: Assessing sleep in psychiatric inpatients: nurse and patient reports versus wrist actigraphy. Ann Clin Psychiatry 19:203–210, 1997

Krahn L, Boeve B, Olson E, et al: A standardized test for cataplexy. Sleep Med 1:125–130, 2000

Krahn L, Black J, Silber M: Narcolepsy: new understanding of irresistible sleep. Mayo Clinic Proc 76:185–194, 2001a

Krahn L, Hansen M, Shepard J: Pseudocataplexy. Psychosomatics 42:356–358, 2001b

Lammers G, Arends J, Declerck A, et al: Gammahydroxybutyrate and narcolepsy: a double blind placebo-controlled study. Sleep 16:216–220, 1993

Lettieri CJ, Eliasson AH: Pneumatic compression devices are an effective therapy for restless legs syndrome: a prospective, randomized, double-blinded sham-controlled trial. Chest 135:74–80, 2009

Li A, Wong E, Kew J, et al: Use of tonsil size in the evaluation of obstructive sleep apnoea. Arch Dis Child 87:156–159, 2002

Li K, Kushida C, Powell N, et al: Obstructive sleep apnea syndrome: a comparison between Far-East Asian and white men. Laryngoscope 110:1689–1693, 2000

Littner M, Kushida C, Hartse K, et al: Practice parameters for the use of laser-assisted uvulopalatoplasty: an update for 2000. Sleep 24:603–619, 2001

Mercer J, Bootzin R, Lack L: Insomniacs' perception of wake instead of sleep. Sleep 25:564–571, 2002

Mignot E, Lammers GJ, Ripley B, et al: The role of cerebrospinal fluid measurement in the diagnosis of narcolepsy and other hypersomnias. Arch Neurol 59:1553–1562, 2002

Minvielle S: Kleine-Levin syndrome: a neurological disease with psychiatric symptoms. Encephale 26:71–74, 2000

Mitler M, Hayduk R: Benefits and risks of pharmacotherapy for narcolepsy. Drug Saf 25:790–809, 2002

Mitler M, Gujavarty K, Sampson M, et al: Multiple daytime nap approaches to evaluating the sleepy patient. Sleep 5 (suppl 2):S119–S127, 1982

Montgomery P, Dennis J: Physical exercise for sleep problems in adults aged 60+. Cochrane Database Syst Rev (4):CD003404, 2002

Montplaisir J, Boucher S, Poirier G, et al: Clinical, polysomnographic and genetic characteristics of restless legs syndrome: a study of 133 patients with new standard criteria. Mov Disord 12:61–65, 1997

Morera A, Henry M, de La Varga M: Safety in melatonin use [in Spanish]. Actas Esp Psiquiatr 29:334–347, 2001

Morgenthaler T, Lee-Chiong T, Alessi C, et al: Practice parameters for the clinical evaluation and treatment of circadian rhythm sleep disorders. An American Academy of Sleep Medicine Report. Sleep 30:1445–1459, 2007

Morin C, Hauri P, Espie C, et al: Nonpharmacologic treatment of chronic insomnia: an American Academy of Sleep Medicine review. Sleep 22:1134–1156, 1999

Morin C, Espie C: Insomnia: A Clinical Guide to Assessment and Treatment. New York, Springer, 2004

Mormont M, Levi F: Cancer chronotherapy: principles, applications, and perspectives. Cancer 97:155–169, 2003

National Sleep Foundation: Sleep in America poll, 2005. Available at: http://www.sleepfoundation.org.

National Sleep Foundation: Sleep in America poll, 2008. Available at: http://www.sleepfoundation.org.

Netzer N, Eliasson A, Netzer C, et al: Overnight pulse oximetry for sleep-disordered breathing in adults: a review. Chest 120:625-633, 2001

Nicholson A: Hypnotics clinical pharmacology and therapeutics, in Principles and Practice of Sleep Medicine, 2nd Edition. Edited by Kryger M, Roth T, Dement W. Philadelphia, PA, WB Saunders, 1994, pp 355–363

Nicholson A, Bradley C, Pascoe P: Medications: effects on sleep and wakefulness, in Principles and Practice of Sleep Medicine, 2nd Edition. Edited by Kryger M, Roth T, Dement W. Philadelphia, PA, WB Saunders, 1994, pp 364–373

Nicolas A, Michaud M, Lavigne G, et al: The influence of sex, age and sleep/wake state on characteristics of periodic leg movements in restless legs syndrome patients. J Clin Neurophysiol 110:1168–1174, 1999

Novak M, Shapiro C: Drug-induced sleep disturbances: focus on nonpsychotropic medications. Drug Saf 16:133–149, 1997

Obermeyer W, Benca R: Effects of drugs on sleep. Neurol Clin 14:827-840, 1996

Ohayon M, Roth T: Prevalence of restless legs syndrome and periodic movement disorder in the general population. J Psychosom Res 53:547–554, 2002

Ohayon M, Roth T: Place of chronic insomnia in the course of depressive and anxiety disorders. J Psychiatr Res 37:9–15, 2003

Ohayon MM, Carskadon MA, Guilleminault C, et al: Meta-analysis of quantitative sleep parameters from childhood to old age in healthy individuals: developing normative sleep values across the human life span. Sleep 27:1255–1273, 2004

Olde Rikkert MG, Rigaud AS: Melatonin in elderly patients with insomnia: a systematic review. Z Gerontol Geriatr 34:491–497, 2001

Oliveira MM, Conti C, Saconato H, et al: Pharmacological treatment for Kleine-Levin syndrome. Cochrane Database Syst Rev (2):CD006685, 2009

Olson E: Obstructive sleep apnea consultation in hospitalized patients: review of a center's experience. Sleep 24 (abstract suppl):A310, 2001

Olson E, Boeve B, Silber M: Rapid eye movement sleep behavior disorder: demographic, clinical and laboratory findings in 93 cases. Brain 123:331–339, 2000

Overeem S, Mignot E, Gert van Dijk, J, et al: Narcolepsy: clinical features, new pathophysiologic insights, and future perspectives. J Clin Neurophysiol 18:78–105, 2001

Pallesen S, Nordhus I, Kvale G, et al: Behavioral treatment of insomnia in older adults: an open clinical trial comparing two interventions. Behav Res Ther 41:31–48, 2003

Parrino L, Terzano M: Polysomnographic effects of hypnotic drugs: a review. Psychopharmacology 126:1–16, 1996

Partinen M: Epidemiology of obstructive sleep apnea syndrome. Curr Opin Pulm Med 1:482–487, 1995

Pascoe P: Drugs and the sleep-wakefulness continuum. Pharmacol Ther 61:227–236, 1994

Phillips B, Young T, Finn L, et al: Epidemiology of restless legs syndrome in adults. Arch Intern Med 160:2137–2141, 2000

Pilcher J, Huffcutt A: Effects of sleep deprivation on performance: a meta-analysis. Sleep 19:318–326, 1996

Pilon M, Montplaisir J, Zadra A: Precipitating factors of somnambulism: impact of sleep deprivation and forced arousals. Neurology 70:2274–2275, 2008

Placidi F, Scalise A, Marciani M, et al: Effect of antiepileptic drugs on sleep. Clin Neurophysiol 111 (suppl 2):S115–S119, 2000

Pressman M, Figueroa W, Kendrick-Mohamed J, et al: Nocturia: a rarely recognized symptom of sleep apnea and other occult sleep disorders. Arch Intern Med 156:545–550, 1996

Quaranta A, D'Alonzo G, Krachman S: Cheyne-Stokes respiration during sleep in congestive heart failure. Chest 111:467–473, 1997

Rakel R: Clinical and societal consequences of obstructive sleep apnea and excessive daytime sleepiness. Postgrad Med 121:86–95, 2009

Rama A, Tekwani S, Kushida C: Sites of obstruction in obstructive sleep apnea. Chest 122:1139–1147, 2002

Richardson G, Roth T, Hajak G, et al: Consensus for the pharmacological management of insomnia in the new millennium. Int J Clin Pract 55:42–52, 2001

Ruottinen H, Partinen M, Hublin C, et al: An FDOPA positron emission tomography study in patients with periodic limb movement disorder and restless legs syndrome. Neurology 54:502–504, 2000

Saper CB, Cano G, Scammell TE: Homeostatic, circadian, and emotional regulation of sleep. J Comp Neurol 493:92–98, 2005

Schenck C, Mahowald M: Polysomnographic, neurologic, psychiatric, and clinical outcome report on 70 consecutive cases with the REM behavior disorder (RBD): sustained clonazepam efficacy in 89.5% of 57 treated patients. Cleve Clin J Med 57:S10–S24, 1990

Schuld A, Blum W, Pollmacher T: Low CSF hypocretin (orexin) and altered energy metabolism in human narcolepsy. Ann Neurol 51:660–661, 2002

Silber M, Richardson J: Multiple blood donations associated with iron deficiency in patients with restless legs syndrome. Mayo Clin Proc 78:52–56, 2003

Silber M, Krahn L, Olson E, et al: Epidemiology of narcolepsy in Olmsted County, Minnesota: a population-based study. Sleep 24 (abstract suppl):A98, 2001

Slatkin N, Rhiner M, Bolton T: Donepezil in the treatment of opioid-induced sedation: report of six cases. J Pain Symptom Manage 21:425–438, 2001

Smart D, Jerman J: The physiology and pharmacology of the orexins. Pharmacol Ther 94:51–61, 2002

Smith SD: Oral appliances in the treatment of obstructive sleep apnea. Atlas Oral Maxillofac Surg Clin North Am 15:193–211, 2007

Strollo PJ, Sanders M, Costantino J, et al: Split-night studies for the diagnosis and treatment of sleep-disordered breathing. Sleep 19 (10 suppl):S255–S259, 1996

Suhner A, Schlagenhauf P, Johnson R, et al: Comparative study to determine the optimal melatonin dosage form for the alleviation of jet lag. Aviation Space and Environmental Medicine 72:638–646, 2001

Sullivan C, Grunstein R: Continuous positive airway pressure in sleep-disordered breathing, in Principles and Practice of Sleep Medicine, 2nd Edition. Edited by Kryger M, Roth T, Dement W. Philadelphia, PA, WB Saunders, 1994, pp 694–705

Thannickal T, Moore R, Nienhuis R, et al: Reduced number of hypocretin neurons in human narcolepsy. Neuron 27:469–474, 2000

Toney G, Ereshefsky L: Sleep disorders: assisting patients to a good night's sleep. J Am Pharm Assoc (Wash) 40 (5 suppl 1): S46–S47, 2000

Trenkwalder C, Hening W, Montagna P, et al: Treatment of restless legs syndrome: an evidence-based review and implications for clinical practice. Mov Disord 22:2267–2302, 2008

Tsai J, Yang P, Chen C, et al: Zolpidem-induced amnesia and somnambulism: rare occurrence? Eur Neuropsychopharmacol 19:74–76, 2009

Ulfberg J, Nystrom B, Carter N, et al: Prevalence of restless legs syndrome among men aged 18 to 64 years: an association with somatic disease and neuropsychiatric symptoms. Move Disord 16:1159–1163, 2001

U.S. Modafinil in Narcolepsy Multicenter Study Group: Randomized trial of modafinil for the treatment of pathological somnolence in narcolepsy. Ann Neurol 43:88–97, 1998

Vitiello M, Moe K, Prinz P: Sleep complaints cosegregate with illness in older adults: clinical research informed by and informing epidemiological studies of sleep. J Psychosom Res 53:555–559, 2002

Walker R: Long-term health consequences of mild to moderate obstructive sleep apnea. Arch Otolaryngol Head Neck Surg 127:1397–1400, 2001

Weaver T, Cuellar N: A randomized trial evaluating the effectiveness of sodium oxybate therapy on quality of life in narcolepsy. Sleep 29:1189–1194, 2006

Winkelmann J, Chertow G, Lazarus J: Restless legs syndrome in end-stage renal disease. Am J Kidney Dis 28:372–378, 1996

Winokur A, Gary K, Rodner S, et al: Depression, sleep physiology, and antidepressant drugs. Depress Anxiety 14:19–28, 2001

Young T, Palta M, Dempsey J, et al: The occurrence of sleep-disordered breathing among middle-aged adults. N Engl J Med 328:1230–1235, 1993

Young T, Peppard P, Gottlieb D: Epidemiology of obstructive sleep apnea: a population health perspective. Am J Respir Crit Care Med 165:1217–1239, 2002a

Young T, Shahar E, Nieto F, et al: Predictors of sleep-disordered breathing in community dwelling adults: the Sleep Heart Health Study. Arch Intern Med 162:893–900, 2002b

CHAPTER

16

Sexual Dysfunction

Rosemary Basson, M.D.

Peter M. Rees, M.D., Ph.D.

ADVANCES IN SURGICAL and medical treatment have greatly improved survival from a variety of chronic illnesses including many types of cancer. However, frequently, sexual function is negatively affected. Approximately 30% of the general population reports recently acquired sexual difficulties, and about 10% reports long-lasting problems that cause distress, but in some medical conditions, such as end-stage renal disease (ESRD), sexual dysfunction seems almost inevitable: the prevalence of hypoactive sexual desire disorder in men and women may reach 100% (Steele et al. 1996). In contrast, some studies find little increase in sexual dysfunction in women with diabetes compared with control subjects (Basson et al. 2001).

The distress that accompanies sexual dysfunction in the context of illness also varies: a sizable proportion of individuals living with spinal cord injury—regardless of the segmental level of their injury—rate regaining sexual function as either the first or the second priority (Anderson 2004). A recent survey of patients with compensated heart failure in New York Heart Association Classes I–III reported that despite the associated fatigue, some 52% of men and 40% of women still considered sexual activity to be important and felt that their quality of life was reduced by their sexual difficulties (Schwarz et al. 2008). It is important for psychiatrists to routinely address sexual health during their assessments: the attending physician may have avoided this subject entirely. Chronic illness may even increase the need for sexual intimacy (Owen and Tepper 2003). For other persons with chronic illness, for whom sexual activity was never particularly rewarding, being unable to engage may be completely acceptable.

Chronic medical illness can affect sexual function in a variety of ways, both directly and indirectly (Table 16–1). Disease-related interruption of the neurovascular pathways and the hormonal milieu may not be the major determinant of dissatisfaction. For instance, sexual function in both men and women with ESRD is mostly governed by presence or absence of depression (Peng et al. 2005, 2007). Similarly, depression is the major factor influencing sexual function after bone marrow transplantation (Humphreys et al. 2007) and in women with multiple sclerosis (Zivadinov et al. 1999) or diabetes (Bhasin et al. 2007); this knowledge is important to a psychiatrist.

Chronic illness commonly alters a person's sense of self (Anderson et al. 2007a, 2007b). Qualitative studies have shown that new issues in sexuality emerge as people live with a chronic illness (Kralik et al. 2001), including the need to adapt to and accept changes in the body. The realization that part of sexual intimacy involves meeting the needs of others is a further factor. A third factor is the major importance of being able to communicate one's changed sexual needs and meet those of the partner.

Sexual dysfunction can be a harbinger of otherwise asymptomatic systemic disease. Of 32,616 healthy male participants in a U.S. study reporting erectile dysfunction (ED) in 1986, a fourfold higher risk of developing Parkinson's disease was found over the next 16 years of follow-up, suggesting that erectile difficulties can precede the onset of the classic motor features of parkinsonism by a substantial margin (Gao et al. 2007). In a retrospective cohort study of 26,000 men (mean age=40) in good general health, and followed up for an average of just 1 year, a twofold increase in the risk of myocardial infarction was identified among the 13,000 men noted to have ED at baseline (Blumentals et al. 2004).

TABLE 16–1. Factors involved in sexual dysfunction associated with chronic disease

Type	Factor	Examples
Direct	Change in sexual desire from disease	Typically reduced (e.g., from high prolactin level and anemia of chronic renal failure)[a]; may be increased (e.g., from some brain injuries)[b]
	Disruption of genital response from disease	ED from multiple sclerosis,[c] hypertension[d]; orgasmic disorder from multiple sclerosis[e]
	Disruption of genital response from surgery	Radical prostatectomy and ED[f]; radical hysterectomy and reduced genital congestion, reduced lubrication[g]; orgasmic disorder after radical vulvectomy[h]
	Disruption of genital response from radiation	ED from vascular and neurological damage after radiotherapy for prostate cancer[i]; vaginal stenosis and friability from radiation for pelvic cancer[j]
	Dyspareunia and disruption of sexual desire and response from chemotherapy	Ovarian failure after chemotherapy for breast cancer[k]; testicular failure after intensive chemotherapy for hematopoietic transplantation[l]
	Disruption of sexual desire and response from antiandrogen treatment	GnRH therapy for prostate cancer[m]
	Disruption of genital response from estrogen depletion by aromatase inhibitors	Loss of sexual genital sensitivity, and exacerbation of vaginal atrophy from aromatase inhibition following breast cancer[n]
	Disruption of sexual desire and response from pain	Pain from any chronic condition is a potent sexual distraction
	Disruption of sexual desire and response from nonhormonal medications	Narcotics can depress desire through gonadotropin suppression[o]; selective serotonin reuptake inhibitors reduce desire and response[p]
Indirect	Reduction of self-image	Reduced by disfiguring surgeries, stomas, incontinence, altered appearance (e.g., drooling and altered facies of Parkinson's disease; altered skin color and muscle wasting of renal failure)
	Depressed mood	Depression and mood lability commonly accompany chronic illness; depression is a major determinant of sexual function in men and women with renal failure[q] and women with multiple sclerosis[r] or diabetes[s]; strong link between ED and subsequent depression[t]
	Impaired mobility	Reduced ability to caress, hug, and hold a partner; to sexually self-stimulate; to stimulate a partner; to move into positions for intercourse; to pelvically thrust after spinal cord injury, Parkinson's disease, brain injury, or postamputation
	Reduced energy	Fatigue may take its toll on sexuality, especially desire (e.g., from renal failure or chemotherapy)
	Partnership difficulties	Difficulties in finding a partner; lack of privacy from institutionalization; dysfunction in the partner who assumes a caregiver role; fears of inability to satisfy partner; fear of becoming a burden to a partner; lack of independence; relationship discord from stressors of living with medicalized lives (e.g., three times weekly hemodialysis)
	Sense of loss of sexuality from imposed infertility	From surgery removing gonads or uterus, or from chemotherapy or radiotherapy causing gonadal failure
	Fear of sexual activity worsening medical condition	Avoiding sexual intercourse because of fear that a pregnancy would provoke cancer recurrence; fearing that a genital cancer could be contagious; fearing that sexual activity will cause another myocardial infarction

Note. ED=erectile dysfunction; GnRH=gonadotropin-releasing hormone.

[a]Finkelstein et al. 2007; [b]Absher et al. 2000; [c]Rees et al. 2007; [d]Doumas and Douma 2006; [e]Tzortzis et al. 2008; [f]Penson et al. 2005; [g]Bergmark et al. 1999; [h]Likes et al. 2007; [i]Incrocci 2006; [j]Bruner et al. 1993; [k]Kornblith and Ligibel 2003; [l]Syrjala et al. 2008; [m]Basaria et al. 2002; [n]Fallowfield et al. 2004; [o]Hallinan et al. 2008; [p]Clayton et al. 2007; [q]Peng et al. 2005; [r]Zivadinov et al. 1999; [s]Bhasin et al. 2007; [t]Korfage et al. 2009.

Assessment

The details of assessment of sexual dysfunction are shown in Table 16–2. A holistic approach is needed because sexual disorders in illness and in health reflect the interaction of mind and body. For instance, psychological stress alone can induce hypothalamic amenorrhea or male hypogonadotrophic hypogonadism to potentially cause dysfunction from reduced sex hormones. Alternatively, nerve damage from multiple sclerosis or radical pelvic surgery leads to orgasmic dysfunction or ED; these problems undermine sexual self-confidence and mood, thereby compounding the sexual dysfunction. Detailed respectful inquiry is necessary, without assumptions about orientation, but with an acceptance of the range of sexual expression.

The assessment is guided by current models of human sexual response. The traditional model of human sexual response stemming from the research of Masters, Johnson, and Kaplan was of a linear progression from desire to arousal to a plateau of high arousal, culminating in orgasm or ejaculation; a phase of resolution then followed. However, in the past 10 years, empirical and clinical studies have focused on the complexity, variability, flexibility, and more circular nature of human sexual response (see Figure 16–1). In both men and women, the relation between desire and arousal is variable and complex; women are mostly unable to separate the two (Brotto et al. 2009; Janssen et al. 2008). The motivations and incentives for sex are multiple and varied, with a wish to increase emotional intimacy between the partners being important for both men and women (Carpenter et al. 2009; Meston and Buss 2007). Sexual "desire"—as in "lust" or "drive"—is only one of many reasons that people engage in sexual activity. Thus, models have been constructed that reflect the multiple reasons to initiate or agree to sexual activity, the need for sexual stimuli in a context that is conducive to sexual arousal, and a variable order and overlap of the phases of desire and arousal (Bancroft 2008; Basson 2001; Basson and Schultz 2007; Janssen et al. 2000; Meuleman and van Lankveld 2005). The circular nature allows a building of arousal, inviting more intense stimulation, thereby triggering more powerful feelings of both arousal and desire.

Overview of Therapy for Sexual Dysfunction in the Medically Ill

In subsequent sections, we address specific therapies shown to benefit dysfunction precipitated by the particular illness or cancer. However, it is usually necessary first to explain the formulation—that is, the summary of the most important underlying causes of their difficulties—to the patient or couple. Reference to current models of human sexual response can be particularly helpful. Debility, fatigue, and pain frequently lessen any innate or spontaneous desire, so that a sexual encounter beginning prior to sensing arousal or desire becomes the norm. This may be rather different from that before illness, especially for men: the type of sexual stimulation, context of the encounter, and ability to stay focused all may need to be modified, as well as prescribing a needed medical adjunct (e.g., a phosphodiesterase type 5 [PDE-5] inhibitor or local estrogen therapy). In addition, if the interpersonal relationship is troubled, the chances that the couple will move on to enjoy a newly modified type of sexual interaction are slim. This may need to be explained and a necessary resource found. The knowledge that the partner of the less well person also may have developed major sexual dissatisfaction (Schulzer et al. 2003; Wasner et al. 2004) encourages provision of therapy for both partners.

Standard therapies include psychoeducation, cognitive-behavioral therapy (CBT), and sex therapy. The latter usually involves sensate focus therapy, whereby each partner is encouraged to take turns giving or receiving sensual and later sexual touches, caresses, and kisses. Initially, genital areas and breasts are off limits. Past goals and expectations are put aside. Encouragement to stay in the moment is needed. Couples plan 15- to 20-minute sessions two to three times per week for 3–4 weeks. The clinician guides as to when breast and genital areas are included and when ultimately intercourse (if still possible) is also "on the menu."

Mindfulness, although practiced for some 3,500 years, is a new addition to therapy for sexual dysfunction. Early studies show benefit for sexual dysfunction in health and after pelvic cancer (Brotto et al. 2008a, 2008b). Randomized wait-list-controlled studies are in progress. CBT can be very helpful in challenging a distorted self-view or catastrophic thinking from the changes imposed by the illness. In clinical experience, sick persons may view their sexual disability as so unattractive to their partner that they do not deserve care and attention. Some may even stay in a relationship in which they experience emotional, physical, or sexual abuse.

Specific themes in therapy are shown in Table 16–3.

When sexual function deteriorates coincident with beginning a medication, the latter may be able to be changed (see Table 16–4). When this is not possible, the patient is advised that at least part of the problem is the needed medication, and adjustments can be suggested. The context might be made more erotic, more intense sexual stimulation may be provided, and specific goals can be removed (e.g., that intercourse or orgasm must necessarily occur).

TABLE 16–2. Assessment of sexual dysfunction associated with chronic illness

Review medical and psychiatric history.

Review current medical status: consider respiratory, cardiac, mobility, and continence requirements for sexual activity, including intercourse, self-stimulation, and orgasm.

Review current medications.

List the sexual dysfunctions and their duration.

Clarify relationship status and quality.

Review the environment for sexual activity: home/institution/"medicalization" (e.g., hemodialysis machines, respirators, lack of independence in daily living).

Review any chronic pain.

Assess current mood.

Assess consequences of illness on sexual self-image (concerns regarding attractiveness, physical appearance).

Review dysfunctions in detail; ask what the sexual difficulties are:

- For each complaint, clarify if the difficulty is the same with self-stimulation as with partnered sex; for ED, also check erections on waking from sleep.
- Clarify motivations for sexual activity, including desire or drive and desire to satisfy partner; identify reasons for avoiding sexual activity.
- Clarify subjective arousal or excitement and pleasure.
- Clarify genital congestion or erection.
- Review variety and usefulness of sexual stimuli and sexual context.
- Assess couple's sexual communication.
- Inquire about distracting thoughts or negative emotions during sexual intercourse.
- Determine whether wanted orgasms are possible, very delayed, nonintense, or painful.
- Identify ejaculation difficulties: delayed, too early, painful, or absent.
- Determine whether intercourse is possible.
- Assess female dyspareunia: introital, deeper, how constant, exacerbation from partner's ejaculation fluid, postcoital burning, postcoital dysuria.
- Assess male dyspareunia: immediate, delayed, any physical changes.

Clarify sexual response preillness: any dysfunction, how rewarding and how important sexual activity was, any desire discrepancy or paraphilia.

Review effect of medications on desire and response.

Review treatment of sexual dysfunction to date.

Complete a full physical examination, including genital examination; usually necessary because of the medical condition, particularly important for neurological illness and whenever generalized ED, dyspareunia, or pain with arousal occurs.

Perform laboratory investigations—as necessary, especially when needed to monitor anemia, high prolactin level, thyroid replacement, or testosterone levels (in men). Estrogen levels usually are assessed by the history and the genital or pelvic examination.

Complete specialized testing of genital blood flow (e.g., Doppler studies of cavernosal flow for ED; rarely indicated because results do not alter treatment options).

Note. ED=erectile dysfunction.

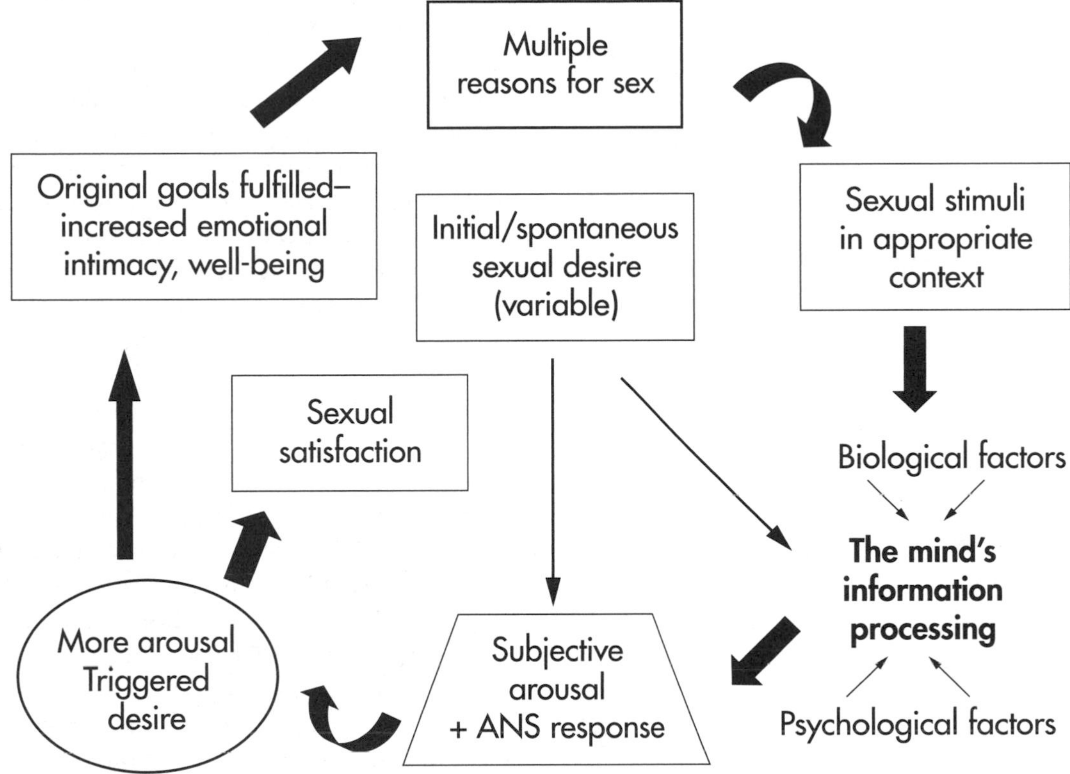

FIGURE 16–1. Sexual response cycle.

A circular sexual response cycle of overlapping phases may be experienced many times during any one sexual encounter. Desire may or may not be present initially; it is triggered by the arousal to sexual stimuli. The sexual and nonsexual outcomes influence future sexual motivation. ANS = autonomic nervous system.

Source. Reprinted with permission from Basson R: "Human Sex Response Cycles." *Journal of Sex and Marital Therapy* 27(1):33–43, 2001. Copyright 2001, Brunner Rutledge. Used with permission.

Sexual Function in Various Medical Conditions

Cardiac Disease

Factors known to strongly influence sexual function in patients with cardiac disease include the ease of treating any associated ED, concomitant depression, and personal or partner's fears that sexual activity is dangerous (Montorsi et al. 2003). Most patients report reduced frequency of sexual activity after myocardial infarction, and 10%–54% do not resume sexual activity at all (Drory et al. 2000). However, it is important to advise patients that risk of further cardiac damage is low and short-lasting. Energy requirements for sexual stimulation, intercourse, and orgasm are estimated to be 3–4 metabolic equivalents (METs)—similar to climbing a flight of stairs. For a 50-year-old patient with a previous myocardial infarction, the risk of a recurrent myocardial infarction during the 2-hour period after sexual intercourse has been calculated to increase from 10 chances to 20 chances in a million per hour (Muller et al. 1996). The patient can be advised that threatening symptoms are unlikely to occur if no cardiac symptoms arise during exercise testing to 6 METs. Prescribing exercise will increase tolerance for sexual activity. Two consensus panels have developed similar guidelines for the resumption of sexual activity in patients with cardiac disease according to degree of cardiovascular risk (Cheitlin et al. 1999; DeBusk et al. 2000) (see Table 16–5). To date, such guidelines have focused on men. Unfortunately, discussion of sexual activity by patients' physicians is often minimal: for instance, in one study, only 24% of cardiac patients were given information on the safety of sex and erection-enhancing medication before receiving a prescription for such medication (Bedell et al. 2002).

Of patients having symptomatic coronary artery disease (CAD), 44%–65% have ED. Erectile difficulty, as mentioned in the introduction, is now considered a warning symptom of CAD. The associated endothelial dysfunction, structural atheromatous change, and loss of cavernosal smooth muscle from ischemia lead to suboptimal venous trapping of blood within the penis subserving erection.

TABLE 16–3. Themes in management of sexual dysfunction in the context of medical disorders

Treat comorbid depression: consider using "sexually neutral" antidepressants, including mirtazapine, bupropion, and possibly agomelatine (an agonist of melatonin receptors MT_1 and MT_2 and an antagonist at serotonin type 2C receptors[a]) in the future.
When current beneficial antidepressants appear to have compounded sexual dysfunction, consider use of PDE-5 inhibitors in men[b,c]; possible benefit from sildenafil for orgasmic dysfunction induced by SSRIs in women.[d]
Address pain relief: suggest planning of sexual encounters at times of better pain control.
Share formulations of sexual dysfunctions with patients (and with partners when possible), referring to the human sexual response model.
Address logistics: privacy, safety from STDs, pregnancy, need of assistance from health care providers, particularly when immobility is a problem.
Encourage openness between the sexual partners: fears of being physically unattractive, that scars are ugly, that the stoma is upsetting to the "well" partner may not be accurate.
Encourage non-goal-oriented sexual activity. Acceptance that sexual activity will not be the same as preillness but need not be less satisfying is a realistic approach.

Note. PDE-5=phosphodiesterase type 5; SSRIs=selective serotonin reuptake inhibitors; STDs=sexually transmitted diseases.
[a]Montgomery 2006; [b]Nurnberg et al. 2007; [c]Segraves et al. 2007; [d]Nurnberg 2008.

Some 60%–90% of patients with heart failure complain of ED (Al-Ameri and Kloner 2009). Although minimally studied, evidence suggests that sexual function does not always recover after cardiac transplantation. Desire may improve, but both preexisting dysfunction and interpersonal difficulties appear to limit attainment of sexual satisfaction posttransplantation (Basile et al. 2001). One of the immunosuppressive drugs given to prevent rejection, sirolimus, can cause primary gonadal failure (Kaczmarek et al. 2004).

The PDE_5 inhibitors such as sildenafil can be used in men with cardiac disease provided there is no risk of hypotension from concomitant prescription of nitrates or nonselective alpha-adrenergic blockers. Inhibitors of cytochrome P450 (CYP) 3A4 (e.g., cimetidine, efavirenz, erythromycin, ketoconazole, itraconazole, ritonavir) can significantly decrease metabolism of PDE-5 inhibitors to cause unwanted accumulation. All three available PDE-5 inhibitors (sildenafil, vardenafil, tadalafil) improve endothelial function (Al-Ameri and Kloner 2009). Sildenafil does not change the time to 1 mm ST segment depression during stress testing in men with chronic stable angina but can prolong the time to angina (Jackson 2002). In contrast, vardenafil may prolong the duration of ST depression in such men. The clinical significance of this is unclear. Vardenafil should not be prescribed to persons with the long QT syndrome, nor should it be prescribed to patients taking quinidine, procainamide, amiodarone, or sotalol because of further increase to the QT interval. The PDE-5 inhibitors should not be used in low-cardiac-output states (e.g., severe aortic stenosis). Intracavernosal injection of prostaglandin E_1 (PGE_1; alprostadil injection) by self or partner can be taught if PDE-5 inhibitors are contraindicated.

More than 50% of patients with CAD are depressed. The mutually reinforcing triad of depression, ischemic heart disease, and ED (Goldstein 2000) should encourage screening for the other two conditions if one is present. To date, studies indicate benefit to sexual function and to depression from sildenafil in men with heart failure (Freitas et al. 2006; Webster et al. 2004). Antidepressant-induced ED can be ameliorated with PDE-5 inhibitors (Nurnberg et al. 2007). Cardiac drugs rarely alter depression, although some (e.g., thiazides, spironolactone, digoxin) may reduce erectile function. Contrary to previous belief, a meta-analysis of 35,000 patients (Ko et al. 2002) suggested that beta-blockers cause only minimal ED—and only if nonselective and higher doses are used (Franzen et al. 2001).

Chronic Obstructive Pulmonary Disease

Studies of sexual dysfunction in patients with chronic obstructive pulmonary disease (COPD) are limited. Of 53 men with mostly moderate or severe COPD, 55% had moderate or severe ED (Köseoglu et al. 2005). Although erectile function, orgasmic function, and general sexual satisfaction decreased with COPD severity, desire did not.

One study showed that about one-third of patients with chronic respiratory failure using noninvasive mechanical ventilation were sexually active (Schönhofer et al. 2001). Sexual activity increased in 12% of the patients after the introduction of noninvasive mechanical ventilation and lessened in 36%. Causes of this decline were not investigated, but progression of the disease rather than the inclusion of noninvasive mechanical ventilation was thought to be responsible. For some patients, noninvasive mechanical ventilation allowed intercourse that had been impossible for several years. These men could not come off the ventilator for intercourse, and the ventilator settings for frequency and tidal volume had to be increased for the patients to reach orgasm.

Limited studies are available on supplementing testosterone for men with COPD. Given the debility associated with COPD alongside the weight loss and loss of lean body mass, testosterone was administered in a randomized,

TABLE 16–4. Frequently noted sexual side effects of commonly used medications

Medication	Sexual side effects	Comments
Antidepressants	SSRIs may cause low desire and delayed orgasm in 30%–50% of women and men[a] and new-onset ED in 22%–41% when patients are asked directly.[a] Trazodone may rarely cause priapism.	PDE-5 inhibitors[b,c] can reverse sexual side effects in men. Limited evidence of reversal of orgasmic delay in women by sildenafil.[d] Limited evidence that bupropion can reverse SSRI-induced dysfunction.[e] Agomelatine, available in Europe, appears sexually neutral.[f]
Antipsychotics	Low desire in 50%–73%,[g] new-onset ED in up to 70% of patients taking traditional antipsychotics when patients are asked directly[g]; retrograde ejaculation[h]	Second-generation antipsychotics, which do not raise prolactin level, may be preferable,[i] but other mechanisms may still cause dysfunction.[j]
Antihypertensives	Low desire: When compared with ACE inhibitors[k] and angiotensin II antagonists,[l] beta-blockers reduce desire in men. Beta-blockers reduce desire in women when compared with angiotensin II antagonists[m]; probably applies to agents with selective and nonselective beta-blockade ED: Increased by centrally acting alpha-blockers; beta-blockers (conflicting data); little evidence from meta-analysis of 35,000 patients[n]; probably only if nonselective and higher dose[o] Priapism: rarely from centrally acting alpha-blockers	Use instead ACE inhibitors, angiotensin receptor antagonists, calcium channel blockers, or peripherally acting alpha-blockers.
Diuretics	ED from thiazides, chlorthalidone, spironolactone[p]	Choose nonthiazide alternatives.
Antiandrogens	Agents such as GnRH agonists, flutamide, cyproterone acetate, and spironolactone in high doses will suppress GnRH, LH, and/or antagonism of androgen receptor, inhibiting sexual desire and response. Finasteride may lower desire, delay ejaculation, and cause ED.	Selective androgen receptor modulators not currently available
Anabolic steroids (chronic use)	Low desire, ED, anejaculation, testicular atrophy	
Narcotics	Low desire in men via suppression of GnRH; limited evidence in women	Testosterone supplementation for men but minimal data
Antiepileptic drugs	May increase SHBG and reduce free testosterone[q]	Studies needed to confirm whether there is less sexual dysfunction from enzyme-neutral AEDs (e.g., oxcarbazepine, lamotrigine, levetiracetam)
Antiparkinsonian drugs	Hedonistic homeostatic dysregulation from early use of dopamine agonists[r] with levodopa Paraphilias from dopamine agonists plus levodopa	Reversible side effects if dopamine agonist is discontinued

Note. ACE=angiotensin-converting enzyme; AED=antiepileptic drug; ED=erectile dysfunction; GnRH=gonadotropin-releasing hormone; LH=luteinizing hormone; PDE-5=phosphodiesterase type 5; SHBG=sex hormone–binding globulin; SSRIs=selective serotonin reuptake inhibitors.
[a]Kennedy et al. 1999; [b]Nurnberg et al. 2007; [c]Segraves et al. 2007; [d]Nurnberg et al. 2008; [e]Clayton et al. 2004; [f]Montejo et al. 2010; [g]MacDonald et al. 2003; [h]Dossenbach et al. 2005; [i]Knegtering et al. 2006; [j]Atmaca et al. 2005; [k]Fogari et al. 1998; [l]Fogari et al. 2002; [m]Fogari et al. 2004; [n]Ko et al. 2002; [o]Franzen et al. 2001; [p]Düsing 2005; [q]Rees et al. 2007; [r]Klos et al. 2005.

TABLE 16–5. Management recommendations based on graded cardiovascular risk assessment

Grade of risk	Cardiovascular disease categories	Management recommendations
Low	Asymptomatic, <3 major risk factors for CAD, excluding age and gender Controlled hypertension Mild, stable angina After successful coronary revascularization Uncomplicated past MI (>6–8 weeks) Mild valve disease LVD/CHF (NYHA Class I)	Primary care management Consider all first-line therapies Reassess at regular intervals (6–12 months)
Intermediate	≥3 major risk factors for CAD, excluding gender Moderate, stable angina Recent MI (>2, <6 weeks) LVD/CHF (NYHA Class II) Noncardiac sequelae of atherosclerotic disease (e.g., CVA, peripheral vascular disease)	Evaluation by a cardiologist prior to initiation of any therapy for erectile dysfunction because of risk of myocardial ischemia during sexual activity and orgasm Specialized cardiovascular testing (e.g., ETT, Echo) Restratification into high risk or low risk based on the results of cardiovascular assessment
High	Unstable or refractory angina Uncontrolled hypertension LVD/CHF (NYHA Class III/IV) Recent MI (<2 weeks), CVA High-risk arrhythmias Hypertrophic obstructive and other cardiomyopathies Moderate or severe valve disease	Priority referral for specialized cardiovascular management Treatment for sexual dysfunction to be deferred until cardiac condition stabilized and dependent on specialist recommendations

Note. CAD=coronary artery disease; CHF=congestive heart failure; CVA=cerebrovascular accident; Echo=echocardiogram; ETT=exercise tolerance test; LVD=left ventricular dysfunction; MI=myocardial infarction; NYHA=New York Heart Association.

double-blind trial and found to increase fat-free mass, decrease fat mass, and improve ED and sexual quality of life (Svartberg et al. 2004).

Rheumatic Disease

Clinical experience confirms that the sexual lives of men and women with rheumatic disease are frequently negatively affected by pain, debility, loss of mobility, comorbid depression, and genital tissue changes in some of the disorders. However, not all studies confirm increased prevalence of sexual dysfunction. When patients with different types of rheumatic disease were studied and long-term couples in which one partner did or did not have rheumatic disease were compared, no differences in sexual satisfaction were found. However, sexual dissatisfaction of both partners was shown to be related to degree of functional impairment (Majerovitz and Revenson 1994).

Impaired mobility can interfere with sexual caressing and specific sexual stimulation of the partner or the self. The movements needed to engage in intercourse may be too painful or impossible. Altered mobility can negatively affect self-image, particularly in adolescents, leading to difficulties forming relationships. It has been shown that when the hip is substantially involved, as in rheumatoid arthritis, hip replacement has a one in two chance of improving sexual function back to previous levels (Yoshino et al. 1984).

Because pain and depression have major negative effects on sexual function, their control is primary when addressing sexual dysfunction in these patients. Particularly in women, pain, age, and depression have been shown to be important modulators of sexual function in the context of rheumatoid arthritis (Abdel-Nasser and Ali 2006). In a recent survey of 552 men (mostly) and women with ankylosing spondylitis, 38% reported that the disease had "quite a bit" or "extreme" negative effects on their sexual relationships (Healey et al. 2009). Depression, greater disease activity, unemployment, and poor self-efficacy were independently associated with a greater impact on sexual function.

Interestingly, the degree of early-morning articular stiffness has been related to both the degree of sexual dissatisfaction in women with rheumatoid arthritis (Gutweniger et al. 1999) and the degree of ED in men with ankylosing spondylitis (Pirildar et al. 2004).

Aside from changes to the joints, other tissue changes may interfere with sexual function. Sjögren's syndrome is associated with vaginal dryness and dyspareunia such that these complaints are at least twice as common as in control subjects (Marchesoni et al. 1995). Moreover, in women with systemic sclerosis, loss of vaginal elasticity is common, as is vaginal dryness and even ulcerations (Bhadauria et al. 1995). ED from associated vasculitis is common in systemic sclerosis, with a prevalence of up to 80% (Tristano 2009). PDE-5 inhibitors are shown to be effective in some but not all studies when the context is systemic sclerosis.

Neurological Disease

Neurological disease can alter sexual motivation, sexual self-image, sexual desire, and ability to communicate sexual needs between partners. Its presence can increase vulnerability to sexual exploitation or coercion. Moreover, neurological disease frequently causes disruption of the sexual response system at brain, spinal cord, and peripheral nerve levels.

For the most part, neurological deficit leads to sexual deficit, but problematic increases can occur, such as hypersexuality from dopaminergic agonists given to treat Parkinson's disease or disinhibited hypersexuality from severe trauma to the prefrontal lobes or bilateral amygdaloid damage in the Klüver-Bucy syndrome.

Ironically, sometimes the imposed neurological deficits can lead to a more rewarding and more intimate sexuality compared with preillness (e.g., after spinal cord injury) (Owen and Tepper 2003).

Brain Injury

Whether from trauma or from stroke, brain injury is frequently associated with sexual problems, the prevalence of which can be difficult to estimate when the patient has extensive bodily injuries other than to the brain or when the patient who has had a stroke has comorbid impairment of genital blood supply because of vascular disease. Depression affecting sexuality is common in both vascular injury and traumatic injury to the brain. Published prevalence levels of depression in the chronic phase following moderate and severe brain injuries are as high as 50% (Kelly et al. 2006). Depression is the most sensitive single predictor of sexual outcome after mechanical injury to the brain (Hibbard et al. 2000).

Damage to the deeply located limbic structures or to their connections is the main cause of organic sexual dysfunction following stroke (Rees et al. 2007). Middle cerebral artery stroke causes injury to multiple limbic and paralimbic areas. Anterior cerebral artery ischemia damages the medial frontal cortex and adjoining cingulate gyrus receiving massive projections from limbic areas. Anterior choroidal artery strokes cause injury to the medial temporal limbic structures.

No clear relation has been found between the focality of brain injury or the duration of coma and the degree of sexual impairment (Sandel et al. 1996). Prevalence figures range from 36% to 54% for more severe head injuries compared with 15% for healthy control subjects (Ponsford 2003). Most studies lack input from the sexual partners, thereby probably lowering the true prevalence of dysfunction, especially when the patient has frontal lobe damage and distorted sense of reality. The most common dysfunctions are ED, premature or delayed ejaculation, and loss of lubrication leading to dyspareunia. At least one-quarter of cases of ejaculatory failure are related to psychotropic medication (Glass and Soni 1999).

Severe head trauma can lead to pituitary injury. This is suspected when a basal skull fracture involves the sphenoid bone that surrounds the pituitary gland or when diffuse cerebral edema compresses the third ventricle with pressure on the hypothalamus and the connecting portal veins alongside the pituitary stalk. Published rates of pituitary hypogonadism after brain injury have shown a wide range of up to 22%, but these studies did not assess sexual symptoms (i.e., the diagnosis was based on only biochemical results). Although brain trauma can induce hyperprolactinemia, which reduces sexual interest and sexual response in both sexes, the most common cause of hyperprolactinemia in the head-injured population is the use of antidepressants (Lieberman et al. 2001) and antipsychotics (Bancroft 2005). Clinicians should screen for pituitary injury at 3 and 12 months following severe brain injury (Ghigo et al. 2005). If the patient has early diabetes insipidus, serious panhypopituitarism may already be present.

The brain trauma also may have led to impaired insight and cognition, causing difficulties in social interaction (Sandel et al. 1996). Many survivors of brain trauma are young men; engaging in the subtleties involved in forming and maintaining a sexual relationship may be particularly challenging.

Parkinson's Disease

Given that Parkinson's disease involves components of the autonomic, limbic, and somatomotor systems, sexual dysfunction rates are high. Further dysfunction from dopamine replacement therapy is possible. Traditionally, dopamine has been thought to play a major role in promoting sexual motivation, sexual arousal, and reward. Recent reviews support the idea that dopamine is important not only for motor function but also for general arousal, thereby explaining most of the effects observed on sexual behavior in parkinsonism (Paredes and Agmo 2004). Prevalence rates of sexual dysfunction in Parkinson's disease vary from 40% to

68% in men and 30% to 88% in women (Meco et al. 2008), including problems with erections and ejaculations (both premature and delayed); difficulties with arousal, lubrication, and orgasm in women; and impaired sexual satisfaction and desire in both sexes. Despite the documented interruption of dopaminergic pathways in Parkinson's disease, it has been found that for men and women, attitudes about their sexuality and Parkinson's disease can be more important to their sexual functioning than are biomedical factors (De Lamater and Sill 2005). Some studies have suggested that healthy female partners of patients with Parkinson's disease are more sexually dissatisfied than are women afflicted with Parkinson's disease (Basson 1996).

Sexual dysfunction is almost invariably present in the parkinsonian variant of multiple system atrophy. The most frequent first symptom of multiple system atrophy in men is ED. Some 50% of women with multiple system atrophy report reduced genital sensitivity compared with only 4% of women with idiopathic Parkinson's disease (Oertel et al. 2003). It is recognized that symptoms of disruption of the autonomic nervous system can occur at any stage of Parkinson's disease or can predate it, so that sexual symptoms do not by themselves indicate the presence of multiple system atrophy.

Some authors have attributed a negative effect on desire and sexual function to L-dopa and dopamine agonists (Bronner et al. 2004). On the contrary, these same agents may increase sexual function and motivation through direct stimulation of the dopamine type 2 (D_2) receptors in the medial preoptic area. Also, prolactin is inhibited and oxytocin is increased at the lumbar sacral spinal cord to potentially facilitate erections. Thus, there is a theoretical reason that dopaminergic therapy allows resumption of sexual activity in some patients but perhaps leads to hypersexuality in others. An open-label, prospective 6-month follow-up study showed that pergolide, 3 mg/day, improved sexual function in young men with Parkinson's disease (Pohanka et al. 2004).

Aberrant sexual behavior has been reported in patients with Parkinson's disease. The term *hedonistic homeostatic dysregulation* has been coined to signify exhibitionism and excessive use of phone-sex lines, prostitution services, and sex shops. Eventually, there can be a vicious cycle of dysregulation of brain reward systems resulting in compulsive use of dopamine agonist medications promoting other behavior disorders such as pathological gambling, obsessive shopping, and aggression (Giovannoni et al. 2000). Hedonistic homeostatic dysregulation may not be rare in milder forms of Parkinson's disease: retrospective case-control studies suggest that a history of mood disorder, alcohol intake, personal traits of novelty seeking, early onset of Parkinson's disease, and early use of dopamine agonists are risk factors for this syndrome (Evans et al. 2005; Pezzella et al. 2005). Of 300 patients with Parkinson's disease taking dopamine agonists, including ropinirole and pramipexole, 25 had sexual compulsions and 28 had comorbid or separate compulsive gambling, of whom 17 met criteria for pathological gambling. These concerns were more common in men than in women (Singh et al. 2007). In several case reports, paraphilias were clearly iatrogenic from use of high-dose dopamine agonists (pergolide, ropinirole, bromocriptine, pramipexole) or use of the monoamine oxidase–B (MAO-B) inhibitor selegiline. It is currently thought that administration of dopamine agonists, especially if combined with L-dopa, may cause these disorders through excessive stimulation of D_2 receptors, particularly the D_3 subclass (Klos et al. 2005). Sexual compulsions can be completely resolved by discontinuing the dopamine agonist despite continuing L-dopa therapy (Klos et al. 2005).

It is interesting that positron emission tomography scans of healthy volunteers experiencing orgasm and ejaculation show strong activation in the dopamine-rich mesodiencephalic and ventral tegmental areas that are also activated during the orgasmlike rush experienced by heroin-addicted persons (Park et al. 2001). The sad irony is that this potential hypersexuality in Parkinson's disease is so diametrically opposed to the disrupted genital function brought about by the neurodegenerative process. The combination of heightened desire with impaired genital function can be enormously problematic for a couple or in a nursing home environment.

Multiple Sclerosis

The prevalence of sexual dysfunction in men and women with multiple sclerosis is high, with the disease eventually affecting 75% of men because of ED predominantly and up to 62% of women because of loss of genital sensation (Rees et al. 2007). Even at diagnosis, when symptoms of MS averaged 2.7 years, sexual dysfunction was present in 35% of women compared with 21% of healthy control subjects (Tzortzis et al. 2008). Fatigue, spasticity, pain, and incontinence all contribute to sexual dysfunction in both men and women. Sexual dysfunction can be a presenting symptom of MS: reduced sensation in the genital area was a presenting symptom in 4 of 63 women with early disease (Tzortzis et al. 2008).

PDE-5 inhibitors are effective for ED. One small study in women showed that these inhibitors improved vaginal lubrication (Dasgupta 2004) but without benefit to the women's overall sexual response. Baclofen, tizanidine, botulinum toxin, and sclerosing agents can lessen spasticity that interferes with sexual activity.

Amyotrophic Lateral Sclerosis

Published data on amyotrophic lateral sclerosis (ALS) are few. Patients with ALS have intact nerve supply to the genitalia because the sensory and autonomic nerve pathways are spared. Consequently, the effect of ALS on sexuality is largely by way of motor incapacity through damaged efferent pathways of brain stem and spinal cord.

Wasner et al. (2004) evaluated sexuality in 62 persons with ALS and found that 62% of the patients and 75% of their partners reported sexual difficulties, compared with 19% and 20%, respectively, before onset of the disease, yet sexual interest and activity remained. Fear of rejection and inhibition by physical limitation were important. The topic of sexuality was rarely discussed with medical personnel. Restricted pulmonary function made penetrative sexual intercourse difficult or impossible: however, five of the six ventilated patients in the study reported having intercourse at least once per month, which is consistent with an unexpectedly high importance of sexuality even in advanced disease.

Spinal Cord and Cauda Equina Injury

Data suggest that some 86% of patients with spinal cord injury retain sexual desire (Anderson et al. 2007a, 2007b), but such injuries are associated with the highest rate of sexual dysfunction from any neurological condition. Depending on the level and completeness of the spinal cord injury, the sexual dysfunction is variable. Very low lesions involving S2, S3, and S4 allow mental excitement to cause a degree of erection and vaginal lubrication and vulval swelling, but reflexive erection of the penis and vulval swelling are lost. The T10–L2 sympathetic outflow from the spinal cord is thought to signal sexual excitement.

In men and women with complete lower motor neuron dysfunction, orgasms are usually lost (Anderson et al. 2007a, 2007b). However, women with complete lesions at any level of the cord still may experience orgasm from cervical vibrostimulation, possibly mediated through an intact neural supply to the cervix traveling separately in the vagus nerve outside of the spinal neuraxis (Komisaruk et al. 2004). Injuries to the medullary cone or to the cauda equina will interrupt the innervation to the genitalia from the autonomic nerves. Trauma to the cauda equina (e.g., from spinal fracture below L1 or severe stenosis of the central canal below L1) can cause complete loss of genital sensation together with loss of voluntary control of the bladder and bowel.

As time progresses postinjury, it is thought that neuroplasticity (Anderson et al. 2007a, 2007b; Duggal et al. 2010) occurs in the ascending pathways of the spinal cord with the result that body areas, including the torso, shoulders, and neck, can be highly sexually arousing when stimulated, even in injuries that have precluded any sensation in the anal or genital areas and any motor function below the lesion level.

PDE-5 inhibitors and intracavernosal PGE_1 are effective to augment reflex and psychogenic erections. Tadalafil has shown benefit in erectile and ejaculatory function at all spinal levels (Giuliano et al. 2007). Similarly, vardenafil has resulted in a significant increase in awareness of orgasm and in ejaculation success (Giuliano et al. 2008). Ejaculation is also facilitated by midodrine combined with penile vibratory stimulation and is more effective than penile vibratory stimulation alone (Soler et al. 2007). Injuries below T10 show less improvement. Sildenafil has been shown to produce a minor increase in vaginal lubrication (Sipski et al. 2000).

Epilepsy

Hyposexuality commonly follows but does not predate the onset of epilepsy and is particularly common in temporal lobe epilepsy (Rees et al. 2007). Epilepsy also can provoke involuntary sexual gestures during a seizure. This occurs when the seizure arises in the mesolimbic temporal structures or the interhemispheric parietal cortex subserving genital sensation. Also, an erotic aura can precede a seizure. Given that automatisms typically occur during the amnestic phase of the seizure, their frequency is probably underreported: video-electroencephalography detected sexual automatisms in 11% of 200 selected patients having medically refractive seizures (Dobesberger et al. 2004). Characteristically, women who have reflex orgasms with their seizures are profoundly hyposexual.

Enzyme-inducing antiepileptic drugs, including phenytoin, barbiturates, and carbamazepine (but not oxcarbazepine), increase the level of sex hormone–binding globulin by an unknown mechanism. Although the total (free plus bound) serum concentration of testosterone is generally unchanged by these anticonvulsants, the increase in sex hormone–binding globulin raises the proportion of bound testosterone and reduces the level of free or bioavailable testosterone. These older antiepileptic drugs impair male sexuality, but data on women are inconclusive. The CYP enzyme-*inhibiting* antiepileptic drug valproic acid may increase serum androgen levels and estradiol level in both men and women. At least in theory, enzyme-*neutral* antiepileptic drugs are less likely to cause sexual side effects. The latter include oxcarbazepine, gabapentin, pregabalin, levetiracetam, and lamotrigine. Some evidence indicates that lamotrigine has the lowest profile of sexual side effects (Devinsky 2005).

Dementia

Patients with dementia may lose the normal inhibitory control of sexual behavior. Inappropriate sexual gestures to caregivers or to other patients when institutionalized, or public self-stimulation, may occur. These difficulties can be compounded by frustration with inability to have sexual release. The typical patient is male, and self-stimulation is ineffective in producing orgasm because of ED. Although such behavior is not usually dangerous, it can cause immense distress to all concerned. It is important to confirm that what appears to be inappropriate or disinhibited sexual behavior is not simply a result of frustration or lack of privacy to be alone to self-stimulate or to be with the intimate partner. Still, in some health care facilities, there is no recognition and acceptance of the sexual needs of the institutionalized patient. Psychiatrists may well be consulted not only to assess the problematic sexual behavior but also to negotiate a necessary environment and willingness of hospital staff to allow their patients sexual expression.

When medical treatment is necessary to prevent harm to the patient or others, antiandrogen therapy is considered. Scientific study is very limited, but spironolactone, medroxyprogesterone acetate (MPA), and gonadotropin-releasing hormone agonists are of some benefit. When spironolactone is prescribed, caution is necessary to avoid hyperkalemia and hypotension. Gonadotropin-releasing hormone agonists will cause a brief increase in testosterone level before it declines, which may produce a temporary increase in sexual behaviors. When decisions concerning the use of pharmacological therapy for limiting sexual behavior of demented patients are made, the inclusion of health care team members, the family, and possibly legal advice is recommended.

Diabetes

Diabetes poses risk for sexual dysfunction in both men and women. In diabetic men, diabetic control and length of disease correlate with the incidence of ED, but generally no such correlations between diabetes and sexual dysfunction are observed in women. However, one recent study indicated that longer duration of diabetes did correlate with sexual dysfunction in women (Abu Ali et al. 2008). Insulin resistance and increased adiposity are associated with low levels of testosterone in men, whereas insulin resistance in women is associated with high testosterone levels (Ding et al. 2006).

Some studies suggest that ED may affect some 75% of men with diabetes; both type 1 and type 2 are mixed in many sampled cohorts. In uncomplicated type 2 diabetes without other risk factors for CAD, ED can signal silent cardiac ischemia (Gazzaruso et al. 2004). Etiology of the ED is multifactorial, including endothelial and smooth muscle dysfunction, autonomic neuropathy, and interpersonal or psychological issues. Men with both diabetes and ED tend to have poor metabolic control, untreated hypertension, peripheral neuropathy, micro- and macroalbuminuria, retinopathy, cardiovascular disease, diuretic treatment, obesity-related testosterone decrease, and psychological vulnerability (Bhasin et al. 2007). Peyronie's disease is an important comorbid disorder in older diabetic men with ED (Bhasin et al. 2007).

PDE-5 inhibitors are the first-line treatment in diabetes; however, these drugs are less effective in some men with diabetes than in others (Bhasin et al. 2007). Calculation of free testosterone concentrations recently has been advocated for patients whose ED is not improved with PDE-5 inhibitors (Traish and Guay 2006).

Ejaculatory problems are common. Retrograde ejaculation consists of propulsion of all or some seminal fluid into the bladder as a result of autonomic nerve damage to the internal urethral sphincter. Sometimes emission happens, but the expulsion phase is completely inhibited so that semen seeps out of the penis, and orgasmic intensity may be less.

Case studies show that ejaculatory dysfunction in diabetes can benefit from treatment with methoxamine, imipramine, or midodrine. When infertility is an issue, sperm can be retrieved by bladder washing after either sexual stimulation or electrostimulation of the prostatic nerve plexus per rectum, prior to intrauterine insemination (Gerig et al. 1997).

A recent review of women's sexual dysfunction in the context of diabetes noted that differentiation between type 1 and type 2 diabetes was often neglected (Bhasin et al. 2007). In addition, most studies did not separate pre- and postmenopausal women, and estrogen status was not controlled. Importantly, sexual dysfunction was linked consistently to comorbid depression. The rates of decreased desire were similar in women with diabetes (17%–85%) and control subjects (16%–90%). However, decreased arousal was high in women with diabetes (76%) compared with control subjects (41%). About twice as common in women with diabetes were reduced lubrication, dyspareunia, orgasmic difficulty, and sexual dissatisfaction in some but not all series. A recent study differentiated the generalized blunting of desire and of all phases of response in women older than 50 years compared with control subjects from the apparently unaffected sexual responses of younger women with diabetes, who showed increased problems only with low desire (Abu Ali et al. 2008).

In another recent study of women enrolled in the long-term Epidemiology of Diabetes, Interventions and Complications (EDIC) study, 35% of participants in a follow-up assessment met criteria for sexual dysfunction (Enzlin et al. 2009). Among these women, low desire was reported by 57%; problems with orgasm, arousal, and lubrication by 38%; and pain by 21%. In a multivariate analysis, only depression and marital status predicted sexual dysfunction.

As in prior research, no association between sexual function and glucose control, duration of diabetes, or hypertension was found in a very recent study of 595 women with type 2 diabetes (Esposito et al. 2010). Moreover, both depression and marital status were again found to be independent predictors of sexual dysfunction. This particular study did show some association between sexual dysfunction and presence of metabolic syndrome and dyslipidemia.

Because of cardiovascular risk, systemic estrogen is generally avoided in diabetes. Topical estrogen can be prescribed via a vaginal ring, tablet, or cream. One small study showed improved genital congestion with sildenafil (Caruso et al. 2006). Screening for treatable comorbid depression is strongly recommended.

Male Hypogonadism

Investigating and treating the primary pathology in secondary hypogonadism is vital. The underlying disease may be life threatening, as in hemochromatosis or a prolactinoma, and the presenting symptoms are typically sexual. Once the underlying disorder leading to secondary hypogonadism is addressed, as well as in cases of primary testicular failure, testosterone replacement usually improves sexual desire and the delayed ejaculation, diminished ejaculate, low sperm count, and variable ED. Transdermal, as opposed to parenteral, preparations are recommended to avoid peaks and troughs in testosterone levels, which tend to cause both erythrocytosis and mood changes. Addressing the vaguer symptoms of late-onset hypogonadism in older men is less straightforward. All levels of the hypothalamic-pituitary-gonadal axis are blunted, and sexual benefit is not seen unless definite clinical symptoms and clear, repeated biochemical deficit are evident (Bhasin et al. 2007). See also Chapter 22, "Endocrine and Metabolic Disorders."

End-Stage Renal Disease

Sexual dysfunction is extremely common in men and women with ESRD. The etiology is complex because of comorbidities, including diabetes, hypertension, CAD, and depression (Peng et al. 2005, 2007). Associated symptoms relevant to sexual activity include pain in bones and joints from osteodystrophy, fatigue, anorexia, nausea, stomatitis, pruritis, and malnutrition. Reported prevalence of ED is as high as 85%, with anemia, endothelial dysfunction, uremia, and autonomic nerve dysfunction all contributing (Basson et al. 2010). PDE-5 inhibitors can be used if no contraindications are identified; the dose is reduced in renal insufficiency but not during dialysis. Transplantation may improve ED, and sildenafil is both effective and safe posttransplant (Basson et al. 2010). Recombinant human erythropoietin therapy is guided by hemoglobin levels and can improve ED in men who are receiving dialysis but not when uremia is present. Low desire is present in up to 100% of men with ESRD; low testosterone, high prolactin, anemia, depression, chronic pain, and psychosexual factors, including altered self-image and medicalization of the bedroom in home hemodialysis, all contribute. Testosterone therapy has been of limited benefit, in part because of the anemia and high prolactin level. Erythropoietin partially corrects low testosterone levels (Basson et al. 2010).

Low sexual desire is present in up to 100% of women with ESRD and those undergoing hemodialysis and is as high as 80% posttransplantation (Basson et al. 2010). Multiple factors are involved, including anemia, negative outcomes to sexual interactions, estrogen deficiency with vaginal atrophy, high prolactin level, depression, chronic pain, and psychosexual and interpersonal issues. In addition, 40% of women with ESRD are totally amenorrheic, and fewer than 10% have regular menstrual periods. Premature menopause is common.

Children with ESRD will face many obstacles when it comes time to form sexual relationships. Their lives have been medicalized, which limits social interaction. Puberty may have been delayed, reducing sexual self-confidence. Their situation is compounded by the negative effects of medical interventions on sexual responsiveness.

Cancer

Advances in the management of malignant disease have allowed more lives to be saved, so now the emphasis is also on the quality of those lives. Negative sexual sequelae are present in most cancer patients, 50% of whom would definitely seek treatment for sexual dysfunction were it available (Huyghe et al. 2009). The most pertinent causes of sexual dysfunction are shown in Tables 16–6 and 16–7.

Nerve Damage

Surgical or tumor-induced damage to the inferior hypogastric plexus and cavernous nerves interrupts genital congestion, leading to ED, decreased lubrication, and reduced pain, together with impoverished genital sensitivity, which delays or prevents orgasm. Enhancement of orgasm is possible (for instance, with a vibrator) because sympathetic fibers to the genital structures take multiple routes. Nerve-sparing techniques in radical hysterectomy are in their infancy, but early studies confirm a conservation of genital congestion in response to erotica (Pieterse et al. 2008). ED

TABLE 16–6. Possible direct effects of malignant disease and its treatment on sexual function

Insult	Dysfunction
Loss of sexual organs: breast, vulva, penis	Reduced desire and response; intercourse possibly precluded
Chemotherapy-induced gonadal failure	Reduced desire and response
Surgical section of pelvic autonomic nerves causing failure of erection, vulval and vaginal congestion	Reduced desire and arousal, ED, dyspareunia
Retroperitoneal lymph node dissection for testicular cancer or lymphoma	Failure of emission
Pelvic radiation damage to tissues, including vagina, to autonomic nerve and vascular supply of penis, vagina, vulva; higher doses causing neurogenic orgasmic disorder	Reduced desire and arousal, ED, dyspareunia or inability to accommodate penis or dildo, orgasmic disorder
Hormonal manipulation depleting testosterone, as in androgen deprivation therapy, and estrogen, as with aromatase inhibitors, bilateral oophorectomy, withdrawal of estrogen therapy	Reduced desire and arousal, ED, orgasmic and ejaculatory disorder, dyspareunia

Note. ED=erectile dysfunction.

TABLE 16–7. Indirect effects of malignant disease on sexual function[a]

Knowledge of potentially terminal disease
Pain and depression
Fear of inability to satisfy partner, especially when vagina is stenosed from radiation or when ED from radical pelvic surgery or radiation is not improved by PDE_5 inhibitors or intracavernosal PGE_1
Fear of transmitting cancer through intercourse
Fear that sexual intercourse was causative of the cancer (e.g., anal or cervical cancer)
Feeling "neutered" from loss of sexual organs
Feeling asexual because no longer fertile after chemotherapy
Perception of premature aging with premature menopause
Feeling unattractive from presence of stoma, ileal conduit, surgical disfigurement

Note. ED=erectile dysfunction; PDE_5=phosphodiesterase type 5; PGE_1=prostaglandin E_1.
[a]All may lower sexual motivation and response.

is still in the range of 53%–86% following attempts at bilateral nerve sparing during radical prostatectomy (Penson et al. 2005). "Penile rehabilitation" with daily or intermittent PDE-5 inhibitors is frequently advocated. However, a recently published randomized controlled trial of vardenafil did not show benefit (Montorsi et al. 2008). Nerve sparing for rectal and colon cancer is also being pursued (Liang et al. 2008; Rees et al. 2007).

Abrupt Loss of Gonadal Hormones

Although studies have confirmed premature ovarian failure from chemotherapy to be a major factor influencing sexual outcome, it has not yet been shown that hormonal changes per se are responsible. A pilot study of women with past breast cancer and complex endocrine status as a result of ongoing antiestrogen therapy used multiple regression analysis to determine what influenced the sexual outcome (Alder et al. 2008). The study found that relationship factors predicted desire, but a history of chemotherapy predicted problematic arousal, lubrication, orgasm, and pain. However, no relation was seen between sexual function and androgen levels, including androgen metabolites. The researchers concluded that the chemotherapy-associated decline in sexual function was mediated by androgen-independent pathways.

Androgen deprivation therapy for prostate cancer may be continuous or intermittent. In the latter group, desire improves when patients are in the "off" phase of therapy (Tunn 2007); ED can be treated with PDE-5 inhibitors.

Preservation of fertility in patients with cancer is now sometimes possible (Jeruss and Woodruff 2009). Whereas sperm banking for men is relatively straightforward, for women, delaying cancer treatment to allow one cycle of hormone stimulation followed by cryopreservation of either a mature oocyte or an embryo may be a very difficult decision. Moreover, in some situations (e.g., after hormone receptor–positive breast cancer), pregnancy may increase the risk of recurrence. It is helpful for psychiatrists to have some understanding of the current and emerging options to preserve fertility for their patients as they prepare for definitive cancer treatment.

Positive Sexual Sequelae in Cancer Survivors

Positive effects on sexuality also can be seen. For example, when therapy for the cancer has been extreme, as in bone marrow transplantation, survivors have described how they treasure life and focus on each moment, including the sexually intimate moments. Sexual "performance" is no longer a goal; indeed, sexual dysfunction may remain some 5 years after marrow transplantation, especially in women (Syrjala et al. 2008), but closeness and sharing erotic touches can be reported as more rewarding than sexual intercourse was before cancer.

Surgeries Resulting in Ostomies

Sexual difficulties associated with stomas range from hesitancy to even begin a relationship to fear that a current partner will now be offended by odor, leakage, or noise from passing flatus. Sexual self-image is vulnerable, particularly in adolescents who already may be feeling unattractive. However, limited study suggests that by young adulthood, marked adaptation may occur such that sexual confidence nevertheless emerges (Erwin-Toth 1999). For older patients, one case-control study suggested that male veterans with stomas had a higher prevalence of ED and less sexual activity than did those requiring major intestinal surgery that did not involve stoma creation (Symms et al. 2008). Of men with stomas, those discontinuing sexual activity adapted less well generally, reporting more isolation and interference with social activities.

Lower Urinary Tract Symptoms in Men and Women

Various urinary symptoms are common and are associated with an increased prevalence of sexual dysfunction in both men and women.

In men, symptoms include urgency, frequency, and nocturia; benign prostatic hyperplasia is often present. ED and lower urinary tract symptoms co-occur and likely share the same etiology. Surgery for benign prostatic hyperplasia precipitates ED in some 10% of cases, and the risk of delayed ejaculation is approximately 20% (Miner et al. 2006).

Pharmacological therapy for lower urinary tract symptoms (traditionally, alpha-adrenergic antagonists and 5-alpha-reductase inhibitors, and more recently, antimuscarinics and PDE-5 inhibitors) may negatively or positively affect sexual function. Combination treatment with alpha-adrenergic receptor antagonists and 5-alpha-reductase inhibitors produces cumulative risks of sexual side effects (Roehrborn et al. 2008). By contrast, treatment of sexual dysfunction with PDE-5 inhibitors can improve lower urinary tract symptoms.

In women, symptoms of lower urinary tract infection include frequency, urgency, nocturia, urinary incontinence, hesitancy, and postvoiding dribbling. When infection is absent, the combination of urinary urgency, frequency, and nocturia, with or without incontinence, constitutes the overactive bladder syndrome. Urinary urgency, frequency, nocturia, pelvic pain, and dyspareunia constitute painful bladder syndrome or interstitial cystitis. Well-designed studies are lacking, and the pathophysiology of sexual dysfunction is unclear. Data are sparse on the effects of medications (oxybutynin, tolterodine, and solifenacin) for lower urinary tract symptoms on women's sexual function. Pelvic floor muscle training is effective for lower urinary tract symptoms and can benefit sexual function (Giuseppe et al. 2007). The effect of urogynecological therapy, including suburethral slings and prolapse surgeries for lower urinary tract symptoms, on women's sexual function is variable.

Simple Hysterectomy for Benign Disease

Prospective studies have now confirmed that most women report improved sexual function after hysterectomy for benign disease, regardless of operative method (Kuppermann et al. 2004; Roovers et al. 2003). The autonomic nerves traveling to the vulva in the cardinal and uterosacral ligaments are spared in a simple hysterectomy because the incisions in those ligaments are near the midline, whereas the autonomic nerves are in the more lateral portions of the ligaments. Probably underlying the postoperative improvement in sexual function is the lessening of dyspareunia and better sexual self-image resulting from the relief of prolapse or chronic menorrhagia.

Bilateral Salpingo-Oophorectomy

Three recent prospective studies have shown that perimenopausal women receiving bilateral salpingo-oophorectomy along with a simple hysterectomy for benign disease did not develop negative sexual effects when followed up over the next 1–3 years (Aziz et al. 2005; Farquhar et al. 2006; Teplin et al. 2007). A recent large national survey of 2,207 American women found an increased prevalence of *distress* about low sexual desire in women with relatively recent bilateral salpingo-oophorectomy but not an increased prevalence of low desire per se (West et al. 2008). The indications for undertaking bilateral salpingo-oophorectomy in this large survey were not given; almost certainly, some would have been for malignant disease.

Conclusion

Neither the debility nor the interruption of sexual response caused by disease or iatrogenesis removes the sexual needs of most persons with chronic illness. When physicians treating the disease or cancer avoid the subject of sexual health, patients may be reluctant to initiate this discussion, an all-too-common situation. By routinely addressing sexual health, psychiatrists are well suited to assess, diagnose, and direct the management of sexual disorders while treating comorbid depression or other psychiatric disorders (Stevenson 2004).

References

Abdel-Nasser AM, Ali E: Determinants of sexual disability and dissatisfaction in female patients with rheumatoid arthritis. Clin Rheumatol 25:822–830, 2006

Absher JR, Vogt BA, Clark DG, et al: Hypersexuality and hemiballism due to subthalamic infarction. Neuropsychiatry Neuropsychol Behav Neurol 13:220–229, 2000

Abu Ali RM, Al Hajeri RM, Khader YS, et al: Sexual dysfunction in Jordanian diabetic women. Diabetes Care 31:1580–1581, 2008

Al-Ameri H, Kloner RA: Erectile dysfunction and heart failure: the role of phosphodiesterase type 5 inhibitors. Int J Impot Res 21:149–157, 2009

Alder J, Zanetti R, Wight E, et al: Sexual dysfunction after premenopausal stage I and II breast cancer: do androgens play a role? J Sex Med 5:1898–1906, 2008

Anderson KD: Targeting recovery: priorities of the spinal cord-injured population. J Neurotrauma 21:1371–1383, 2004

Anderson KD, Borisoff JF, Johnson RD, et al: Long-term effects of spinal cord injury on sexual function in men: implications for neuroplasticity. Spinal Cord 45:338–348, 2007a

Anderson KD, Borisoff JF, Johnson RD, et al: Spinal cord injury influences psychogenic as well as physical components of female sexual ability. Spinal Cord 45:349–359, 2007b

Atmaca M, Kuloglu M, Tezcan E: A new atypical antipsychotic: quetiapine-induced sexual dysfunctions. Int J Impot Res 17:201–203, 2005

Aziz A, Brannstrom M, Bergquist C, et al: Perimenopausal androgen decline after oophorectomy does not influence sexuality or psychological well-being. Fertil Steril 83:1021–1028, 2005

Bancroft J: The endocrinology of sexual arousal. J Endocrinol 186:411–427, 2005

Bancroft J: Sexual arousal and response: the psychosomatic circle, in Human Sexuality and Its Problems, 3rd Edition. Edited by Bancroft JHJ. Edinburgh, UK, Churchill, Livingstone, Elsevier, 2008, pp 96–106

Basaria S, Lieb J 2nd, Tang AM, et al: Long-term effects of androgen deprivation therapy in prostate cancer patients. Clin Endocrinol (Oxf) 56:779–786, 2002

Basile A, Maccherini M, Diciolla F, et al: Sexual disorders after heart transplantation. Transplant Proc 33:1917–1919, 2001

Basson R: Sexuality and Parkinson's disease. Parkinsonism Relat Disord 2:177–185, 1996

Basson R: Human sex-response cycles. J Sex Marital Ther 27:33–43, 2001

Basson R, Schultz WW: Sexual sequelae of general medical disorders. Lancet 369:409–424, 2007

Basson RJ, Rucker BM, Laird PG, et al: Sexuality of women with diabetes. J Sex Reprod Med 1:11–20, 2001

Basson R, Rees P, Wang R, et al: Sexual function in chronic illness. J Sex Med 7(1 Pt 2):374–388, 2010

Bedell S, Graboys T, Duperval M, et al: Sildenafil in the cardiologist's office: patients' attitudes and physicians' practices toward discussions about sexual functioning. Cardiology 97:79–82, 2002

Bergmark K, Avall-Lundqvist E, Dickman PW, et al: Vaginal changes and sexuality in women with a history of cervical cancer. N Engl J Med 340:1383–1389, 1999

Bhadauria S, Moser DK, Clements PJ, et al: Genital tract abnormalities and female sexual function impairment in systemic sclerosis. Am J Obstet Gynecol 172:580–587, 1995

Bhasin S, Enzlin P, Coviello A, et al: Sexual dysfunction in men and women with endocrine disorders. Lancet 369:597–611, 2007

Blumentals WA, Gomez-Caminero A, Joo S, et al: Should erectile dysfunction be considered as a marker for acute myocardial infarction? Results from a retrospective cohort study. Int J Impot Res 16:350–353, 2004

Bronner G, Royter V, Korczyn AD, et al: Sexual dysfunction in Parkinson's disease. J Sex Marital Ther 30:95–105, 2004

Brotto LA, Basson R, Luria M: In mindfulness-based group psychoeducational intervention targeting sexual arousal disorder in women. J Sex Med 5:1646–1659, 2008a

Brotto LA, Heiman J, Goff B, et al: A psychoeducational intervention for sexual dysfunction in women with gynecologic cancer. Arch Sex Behav 37:317–329, 2008b

Brotto LA, Heiman JR, Tolman D: Narratives of desire in mid-age women with and without arousal difficulties. J Sex Res 46:387–398, 2009

Bruner DW, Lanciano R, Keegan M, et al: Vaginal stenosis and sexual dysfunction following intracavitary radiation for the treatment of cervical and endometrial carcinoma. Int J Radiat Oncol Biol Phys 27:825–830, 1993

Carpenter LM, Nathanson CA, Kim YJ: Physical women, emotional men: gender and sexual satisfaction in midlife. Arch Sex Behav 38:87–107, 2009

Caruso S, Rugolo S, Agnello C, et al: Sildenafil improves sexual functioning in premenopausal women with type 1 diabetes who are affected by sexual arousal disorder: a double-blind, crossover, placebo-controlled pilot study. Fertil Steril 85:1496–1501, 2006

Cheitlin MD, Hutter AM Jr, Brindis RG, et al: ACC/AHA expert consensus document. Use of sildenafil (Viagra) in patients with cardiovascular disease. American College of Cardiology/American Heart Association. J Am Coll Cardiol 33:273–282, 1999

Clayton AH, Warnock JK, Kornstein SG, et al: A placebo-controlled trial of bupropion SR as an antidote for selective serotonin reuptake inhibitor–induced sexual dysfunction. J Clin Psychiatry 65:62–67, 2004

Clayton A, Kornstein S, Prakash A, et al: Changes in sexual functioning associated with duloxetine, escitalopram, and placebo in the treatment of patients with major depressive disorder. J Sex Med 4:917–929, 2007

Dasgupta R, Wiseman OJ, Kanabar G, et al: Efficacy of sildenafil in the treatment of female sexual dysfunction due to multiple sclerosis. J Urol 171:1189–1193, 2004

De Lamater JD, Sill M: Sexual desire in later life. J Sex Res 42:138–149, 2005

DeBusk R, Drory Y, Goldstein I, et al: Management of sexual dysfunction in patients with cardiovascular disease: recommendations of the Princeton Consensus Panel. Am J Cardiol 86:175–181, 2000

Devinsky O: Neurologist-induced sexual dysfunction: enzyme-inducing antiepileptic drugs. Neurology 65:980–981, 2005

Ding EL, Song Y, Malik VS, et al: Sex differences of endogenous sex hormones and risks of type 2 diabetes: a systematic review and meta-analysis. JAMA 295:1288–1299, 2006

Dobesberger J, Walser G, Unterberger I, et al: Genital automatisms: a video-EEG study in patients with medically refractory seizures. Epilepsia 45:777–780, 2004

Dossenbach M, Hodge A, Anders M, et al: Prevalence of sexual dysfunction in patients with schizophrenia: international variation and underestimation. Int J Neuropsychopharmacol 8:195–201, 2005

Doumas M, Douma S: Sexual dysfunction in essential hypertension: myth or reality? J Clin Hypertens 8:269–274, 2006

Drory Y, Karvetz S, Weingarten M: Comparison of sexual activity of women and men after first acute myocardial infarction. Am J Cardiol 85:1283–1287, 2000

Duggal N, Rabin D, Bartha R, et al: Brain reorganization in patients with spinal cord compression evaluated using fMRI. Neurology 74:1048–1054, 2010

Düsing R: Sexual dysfunction in male patients with hypertension: influence of antihypertensive drugs. Drugs 65:773–786, 2005

Enzlin P, Rosen R, Wiegel M, et al: Sexual dysfunction in women with type 1 diabetes: long-term findings from the DCCT/EDIC study cohort. Diabetes Care 32:780–785, 2009

Esposito K, Maiorino MI, Bellastella G, et al: Determinants of female sexual dysfunction in type 2 diabetes. Int J Impot Res 22:179–184, 2010

Erwin-Toth P: The effect of ostomy surgery between the ages of 6 and 12 years on psychosocial development during childhood, adolescence, and young adulthood. J Wound Ostomy Continence Nurs 26:77–85, 1999

Evans AH, Lawrence AD, Potts J, et al: Factors influencing susceptibility to compulsive dopaminergic drug use in Parkinson disease. Neurology 65:1570–1574, 2005

Fallowfield L, Cella D, Cuzick J, et al: Quality of life of postmenopausal women in the Arimidex, Tamoxifen, Alone or in Combination (ATAC) Adjuvant Breast Cancer Trial. J Clin Oncol 22:4261–4271, 2004

Farquhar CM, Harvey SA, Yu Y, et al: A prospective study of 3 years of outcomes after hysterectomy with and without oophorectomy. Am J Obstet Gynecol 194:711–717, 2006

Finkelstein FO, Shirani S, Wuerth D, et al: Therapy insight: sexual dysfunction in patients with chronic kidney disease. Nat Clin Pract Nephrol 3:200–207, 2007

Fogari R, Zoppi A, Corradi L, et al: Sexual function in hypertensive males treated with lisinopril or atenolol: a cross-over study. Am J Hypertens 11:1244–1247, 1998

Fogari R, Preti P, Derosa G, et al: Effect of antihypertensive treatment with valsartan or atenolol on sexual activity and plasma testosterone in hypertensive men. Eur J Clin Pharmacol 58:177–180, 2002

Fogari R, Preti P, Zoppi A, et al: Effect of valsartan and atenolol on sexual behavior in hypertensive postmenopausal women. Am J Hypertens 17:77–81, 2004

Franzen D, Metha A, Siefert N, et al: Effects of beta-blockers on sexual performance in men with coronary heart disease: a prospective, randomized and double blinded study. Int J Impot Res 13:348–351, 2001

Freitas D, Athanazio R, Almeida D, et al: Sildenafil improves quality of life in men with heart failure and erectile dysfunction. Int J Impot Res 18:210–212, 2006

Gao X, Chen H, Schwarzschild MA, et al: Erectile function and risk of Parkinson's disease. Am J Epidemiol 166:1446–1450, 2007

Gazzaruso C, Giordanetti S, De Amici E, et al: Relationship between erectile dysfunction and silent myocardial ischemia in apparently uncomplicated type 2 diabetic patients. Circulation 110:22–26, 2004

Gerig NE, Meacham RB, Ohl DA: Use of electroejaculation in the treatment of ejaculatory failure secondary to diabetes mellitus. Urology 49:239–242, 1997

Ghigo E, Masel B, Aimaretti G, et al: Consensus guidelines on screening for hypopituitarism following traumatic brain injury. Brain Inj 19:711–724, 2005

Giovannoni G, O'Sullivan JD, Turner K, et al: Hedonistic homeostatic dysregulation in patients with Parkinson's disease on dopamine replacement therapies. J Neurol Neurosurg Psychiatry 68:423–428, 2000

Giuliano F, Sanchez-Ramos A, Löchner-Ernst D, et al: Efficacy and safety of tadalafil in men with erectile dysfunction following spinal cord injury. Arch Neurol 64:1584–1592, 2007

Giuliano F, Rubio-Aurioles E, Kennelly M, et al: Vardenafil improves ejaculation success rates and self-confidence in men with erectile dysfunction due to spinal cord injury. Spine 33:709–715, 2008

Giuseppe PG, Pace G, Vicentini C: Sexual function in women with urinary incontinence treated by pelvic floor transvaginal electrical stimulation. J Sex Med 4:702–707, 2007

Glass C, Soni B: ABC of sexual health: sexual problems of disabled patients. BMJ 318:518–521, 1999

Goldstein I: The mutually reinforcing triad of depressive symptoms, cardiovascular disease and erectile dysfunction. Am J Cardiol 86(suppl):41F–45F, 2000

Gutweniger S, Kopp M, Mur E, et al: Body image of women with rheumatoid arthritis. Clin Exp Rheumatol 17:413–417, 1999

Hallinan R, Byrne A, Agho K, et al: Erectile dysfunction in men receiving methadone and buprenorphine maintenance treatment. J Sex Med 5:684–692, 2008

Healey EL, Haywood KL, Jordan KP, et al: Ankylosing spondylitis and its impact on sexual relationships. Rheumatology (Oxford) 48:1378–1381, 2009

Hibbard MR, Gordon WA, Flanagan S, et al: Sexual dysfunction after traumatic brain injury. NeuroRehabilitation 15:107–120, 2000

Humphreys CT, Tallman B, Altmaier EM, et al: Sexual functioning in patients undergoing bone marrow transplantation: a longitudinal study. Bone Marrow Transplant 39:491–496, 2007

Huyghe E, Sui D, Odensky E, et al: Needs assessment survey to justify establishing a reproductive health clinic at a comprehensive cancer center. J Sex Med 6:149–163, 2009

Incrocci L: Sexual function after external-beam radiotherapy for prostate cancer: what do we know? Crit Rev Oncol Hematol 57:165–173, 2006

Jackson G: Phosphodiesterase type-5 inhibitors in cardiovascular disease: experimental models and potential clinical applications. Eur Heart J 4:H19–23, 2002

Janssen E, Everaerd W, Spiering M, et al: Automatic processes and the appraisal of sexual stimuli: toward an information processing model of sexual arousal. J Sex Res 37:8–23, 2000

Janssen E, McBride KR, Yarber W, et al: Factors that influence sexual arousal in men: a focus group study. Arch Sex Behav 37:252–265, 2008

Jeruss JS, Woodruff TK: Preservation of fertility in patents with cancer. N Engl J Med 360:902–911, 2009

Kaczmarek I, Groetzner J, Adamidis I, et al: Sirolimus impairs gonadal function in heart transplant recipients. Am J Transplant 4:1084–1088, 2004

Kelly DF, McArthur DL, Levin H, et al: Neurobehavioral and quality of life changes associated with growth hormone insufficiency after complicated mild, moderate, or severe traumatic brain injury. J Neurotrauma 23:928–942, 2006

Kennedy SH, Dickens SC, Eisfeld BS, et al: Sexual dysfunction before antidepressant therapy in major depression. J Affect Disord 56:201–208, 1999

Klos KJ, Bower JH, Josephs KA, et al: Pathological hypersexuality predominantly linked to adjuvant dopamine agonist therapy in Parkinson's disease and multiple system atrophy. Parkinsonism Relat Disord 11:381–386, 2005

Knegtering H, Boks M, Blijd C, et al: A randomized open-label comparison of the impact of olanzapine versus risperidone on sexual functioning. J Sex Marital Ther 32:315–326, 2006

Ko DT, Hebert PR, Coffey CS, et al: Beta-blocker therapy and symptoms of depression, fatigue, and sexual dysfunction. JAMA 288:351–357, 2002

Komisaruk BR, Whipple B, Crawford A, et al: Brain activation during vaginocervical self-stimulation and orgasm in women with complete spinal cord injury: fMRI evidence of mediation by the vagus nerves. Brain Res 1024:77–88, 2004

Korfage IJ, Pluijm S, Roobol M, et al: Erectile dysfunction and mental health in a general population of older men. J Sex Med 6:505–512, 2009

Kornblith AB, Ligibel J: Psychological and sexual functioning of survivors of breast cancer. Semin Oncol 30:799–813, 2003

Köseoglu N, Köseoglu H, Ceylan E, et al: Erectile dysfunction prevalence in sexual function status in patients with chronic obstructive pulmonary disease. J Urol 174:249–252, 2005

Kralik D, Koch T, Telford K: Constructions of sexuality for midlife women living with chronic illness. J Adv Nurs 35:180–187, 2001

Kuppermann M, Varner RE, Summit RL Jr, et al: Effect of hysterectomy vs medical treatment on health related quality of life and sexual functioning: the medicine or surgery (Ms) randomized trial. JAMA 291:1447–1455, 2004

Liang JT, Lai HS, Lee PH, et al: Laparoscopic pelvic autonomic nerve-preserving surgery for sigmoid colon cancer. Ann Surg Oncol 15:1609–1616, 2008

Lieberman SA, Oberoi AL, Gilkison CR, et al: Prevalence of neuroendocrine dysfunction in patients recovering from traumatic brain injury. J Clin Endocrinol Metab 86:2752–2756, 2001

Likes MW, Stegbauer C, Tillmanns T, et al: Pilot study of sexual function and quality of life after excision for vulvar intraepithelial neoplasia. J Reprod Med 52:23–30, 2007

MacDonald S, Halliday J, MacEwan T, et al: Nithsdale Schizophrenia Surveys 24: sexual dysfunction. Case-control study. Br J Psychiatry 182:50–56, 2003

Majerovitz SD, Revenson TA: Sexuality and rheumatic disease: the significance of gender. Arthritis Care Res 7:29–34, 1994

Marchesoni D, Mozzanega B, De Sandre P, et al: Gynaecological aspects of primary Sjögren's syndrome. Eur J Obstet Gynecol Reprod Biol 63:49–53, 1995

Meco G, Rubino A, Caravona N, et al: Sexual dysfunction in Parkinson's disease. Parkinsonism Relat Disord 14:451–456, 2008

Meston CM, Buss DM: Why humans have sex. Arch Sex Behav 36:477–507, 2007

Meuleman EJ, van Lankveld JJ: Hypoactive sexual desire disorder: an underestimated condition in men. BJU Int 95:291–296, 2005

Miner M, Rosenberg M, Perelman M: Treatment of lower urinary tract symptoms in benign prostatic hyperplasia and its impact on sexual function. Clin Ther 28:13–25, 2006

Montejo A, Prieto N, Terleira A, et al: Better sexual acceptability of agomelatine (25 and 50 mg) compared with paroxetine (20 mg) in healthy male volunteers: an 8-week, placebo-controlled study using the PRSEXDQ-SALSEX scale. J Psychopharmacol 24:111–120, 2010

Montgomery SA: Major depressive disorders: clinical efficacy and tolerability of agomelatine, a new melatonergic agonist. Eur Neuropsychopharmacol 16 (suppl 5):S633–S638, 2006

Montorsi F, Briganti A, Salonia A, et al: Erectile dysfunction prevalence, time of onset and association with risk factors in 300 consecutive patients with acute chest pain and angiographically documented coronary artery disease. Eur Urol 44:360–365, 2003

Montorsi F, Brock G, Lee J, et al: Effect of nightly versus on-demand vardenafil on recovery of erectile function in men following bilateral nerve-sparing radical prostatectomy. Eur Urol 54:924–931, 2008

Muller JE, Mittleman MA, Malcolm M, et al: Triggering myocardial infarction by sexual activity. Low absolute risk and prevention by regular physical exertion. Determinants of Myocardial Infarction Onset Study Investigators. JAMA 275:1405–1409, 1996

Nurnberg HG, Fava M, Gelenberg AJ, et al: Open-label sildenafil treatment of partial and non-responders to double-blind treatment in men with antidepressant-associated sexual dysfunction. Int J Impot Res 19:167–175, 2007

Nurnberg HG, Hensley PL, Heiman JR, et al: Sildenafil treatment of women with antidepressant-associated sexual dysfunction. JAMA 300:395–404, 2008

Oertel WH, Wächter T, Quinn NP, et al: Reduced genital sensitivity in female patients with multiple system atrophy of parkinsonian type. Mov Disord 18:430–432, 2003

Owen AF, Tepper MS: Chronic illnesses and disabilities affecting women's sexuality. Female Patient 28:45–50, 2003

Paredes RG, Agmo A: Has dopamine a physiological role in the control of sexual behavior? A critical review of the evidence. Prog Neurobiol 73:179–226, 2004

Park K, Seo JJ, Kang HK, et al: A new potential of blood oxygenation level dependent (BOLD) functional MRI for evaluating cerebral centers of penile erection. Int J Impot Res 17:73–81, 2001

Peng YS, Chiang CK, Kao TW, et al: Sexual dysfunction in female hemodialysis patients: a multicenter study. Kidney Int 68:760–765, 2005

Peng YS, Chiang CK, Hung KY, et al: The association of higher depressive symptoms and sexual dysfunction in male haemodialysis patients. Nephrol Dial Transplant 22:857–861, 2007

Penson DF, McLerran D, Feng Z, et al: 5-Year urinary and sexual outcomes after radical prostatectomy: results from the Prostate Cancer Outcomes Study. J Urol 173:1701–1705, 2005

Pezzella FR, Colosimo C, Vanacore N, et al: Prevalence and clinical features of hedonistic homeostatic dysregulation in Parkinson's disease. Mov Disord 20:77–81, 2005

Pieterse QD, Ter Kuile MM, Deruiter MC, et al: Vaginal blood flow after radical hysterectomy with and without nerve sparing: a preliminary report. Int J Gynecol Cancer 18:576–583, 2008

Pirildar T, Müezzinoglu T, Pirildar S: Sexual function in ankylosing spondylitis: a study of 65 men. J Urol 171:1598–1600, 2004

Pohanka M, Kanovsky P, Bares M, et al: Pergolide mesylate can improve sexual dysfunction in patients with Parkinson's disease: the results of an open, prospective, 6-month follow-up. Eur J Neurol 11:483–488, 2004

Ponsford J: Sexual changes associated with traumatic brain injury. Neuropsychol Rehabil 13:275–289, 2003

Rees PM, Fowler CJ, Maas CP: Sexual function in men and women with neurological disorders. Lancet 369:512–525, 2007

Roehrborn CG, Siami P, Barkin J, et al: The effects of dutasteride, tamsulosin and combination therapy on lower urinary tract symptoms in men with benign prostatic hyperplasia and prostatic enlargement: 2-year results from the CombAT study. J Urol 179:616–621, 2008

Roovers JP, van der Bom JG, van der Vaart CH, et al: Hysterectomy and sexual wellbeing: a prospective observational study of vaginal hysterectomy, subtotal hysterectomy and total abdominal hysterectomy. BMJ 327:774–778, 2003

Sandel ME, Williams KS, Dellapietra L, et al: Sexual functioning following traumatic brain injury. Brain Inj 10:719–728, 1996

Schönhofer B, Von Sydow K, Bucher T, et al: Sexuality in patients with noninvasive mechanical ventilation due to chronic respiratory failure. Am J Respir Crit Care Med 164:1612–1617, 2001

Schulzer M, Mak E, Calne SM: The psychometric properties of the Parkinson's Impact Scale (PIMS) as a measure of quality of life in Parkinson's disease. Parkinsonism Relat Disord 9:291–294, 2003

Schwarz ER, Kapur V, Bionat S, et al: The prevalence and clinical relevance of sexual dysfunction in women and men with chronic heart failure. Int J Impot Res 20:85–91, 2008

Segraves RT, Lee J, Stevenson R, et al: Tadalafil for treatment of erectile dysfunction in men on antidepressants. J Clin Psychopharmacol 27:62–66, 2007

Singh A, Kandimala G, Dewey RB, et al: Risk factors for pathologic gambling and other compulsions among Parkinson's disease patients taking dopamine agonists. J Clin Neurosci 14:1178–1181, 2007

Sipski ML, Rosen RC, Alexander CJ, et al: Sildenafil effects on sexual and cardiovascular responses in women with spinal cord injury. Urology 55:812–815, 2000

Soler JM, Previnaire JG, Plante P, et al: Midodrine improves ejaculation in spinal cord injured men. J Urol 178:2082–2086, 2007

Steele TE, Wuerth D, Finkelstein S, et al: Sexual experience of the chronic peritoneal dialysis patient. J Am Soc Nephrol 8:1165–1168, 1996

Stevenson R: Sexual medicine: why psychiatrists must talk to their patients about sex. Can J Psychiatry 49:673–676, 2004

Svartberg J, Aasebø U, Hjalmarsen A, et al: Testosterone treatment improves body composition and sexual function in men with COPD, in a 6-month randomized controlled trial. Respir Med 98:906–913, 2004

Symms MR, Rawl SM, Grant M, et al: Sexual health and quality of life among male veterans with intestinal ostomies. Clin Nurse Spec 22:30–40, 2008

Syrjala KL, Kurland BF, Abrams JR, et al: Sexual function changes during the 5 years after high-dose treatment and hematopoietic cell transplantation for malignancy, with case-matched controls at 5 years. Blood 111:989–996, 2008

Teplin V, Vittinghoff E, Lin F, et al: Oophorectomy in premenopausal women: health-related quality of life and sexual functioning. Obstet Gynecol 109:347–354, 2007

Traish AM, Guay AT: Are androgens critical for penile erections in humans? Examining the clinical and preclinical evidence. J Sex Med 3:382–407, 2006

Tristano AG: The impact of rheumatic diseases on sexual function. Rheumatol Int 29:853–860, 2009

Tunn U: The current status of intermittent androgen deprivation (IAD) therapy for prostate cancer: putting IAD under the spotlight. BJU Int 99:19–22, 2007

Tzortzis V, Skriapas K, Hadjigeorgiou G, et al: Sexual dysfunction in newly diagnosed multiple sclerosis women. Mult Scler 14:561–563, 2008

Wasner M, Bold U, Vollmer TC, et al: Sexuality in patients with amyotrophic lateral sclerosis and their partners. J Neurol 251:445–448, 2004

Webster LJ, Michelakis ED, Davis T, et al: Use of sildenafil for safe improvement of erectile function and quality of life in men with New York Heart Association classes II and III congestive heart failure: a prospective, placebo-controlled, double-blind crossover trial. Arch Intern Med 164:514–520, 2004

West SL, D'Aloisio AA, Agans RP, et al: Prevalence of low sexual desire and hypoactive sexual desire disorder in a nationally representative sample of US women. Arch Intern Med 168:1441–1449, 2008

Yoshino S, Fujimori J, Morishige T, et al: Bilateral joint replacement of hip and knee joints in patients with rheumatoid arthritis. Arch Orthop Trauma Surg 103:1–4, 1984

Zivadinov R, Zorzon M, Bosco A, et al: Sexual dysfunction in multiple sclerosis: correlation analysis. Mult Scler 5:428–431, 1999

CHAPTER

17

Substance-Related Disorders

Michael Weaver, M.D., F.A.S.A.M.

PSYCHIATRIC CONSULTANTS in hospital settings often encounter patients with alcohol or drug addiction. Patients who are intoxicated are more likely to be injured in traumatic accidents, and there is a significant association between having a substance use disorder (SUD) and injury from physical trauma (Soderstrom et al. 1997). Risk-taking behavior associated with drug use can lead to sexually transmitted diseases and other infections, including those acquired through injection drug use (e.g., cellulitis, endocarditis, HIV, hepatitis C virus [HCV]). Several terms are used to distinguish different patterns of drug use (Table 17-1). Illicit drug abuse is more prevalent in patients who have depression or anxiety disorders or other psychiatric comorbidities (including personality disorders) and in those who use tobacco or abuse alcohol. Patients with a dual diagnosis (i.e., both an SUD and another major psychiatric disorder) may present with complex clinical histories and symptoms that make diagnosis challenging. Intoxication and withdrawal symptoms may be mistaken for other psychiatric or medical symptoms. Hospitalization may be prolonged by delirium due to intoxication or withdrawal.

Assessment

The prevalence rate for alcohol and substance abuse among hospitalized patients is 15%–30% (Katz et al. 2008; Kouimtsidis et al. 2003; McDuff et al. 1997), and this is even higher among trauma or psychiatric inpatients. With rates this high, it is important to be alert for an SUD in inpatients. However, even careful assessment by clinicians looking for an SUD may not identify all current users. A combination of universal questionnaire screening and urine toxicology for those at high risk is more effective than either alone (Christmas et al. 1992). Findings from physical examination and laboratory studies can provide important clues to an SUD (Tables 17-2 and 17-3). Although many of these findings can be caused by other diseases, the differential diagnosis should include SUD, and additional information can help verify this.

A good general health history can elicit risk factors for SUD. Erratic occupational history, relational problems with partners and children, accidents, burns and fractured bones, and charges for driving under the influence may be clues to probe further into possible SUD. A simple screening tool for problems of alcohol use is the CAGE questionnaire, which has been modified for screening for drug use and is known as the CAGE-AID (Adapted to Include Drugs) questionnaire (Brown and Rounds 1995). The more responses that are affirmative, the more likely that the person answering has an SUD warranting further investigation by the clinician (Buchsbaum et al. 1991). The CAGE-AID is especially useful in settings where there is a high likelihood of an SUD, such as emergency departments, sexually transmitted disease clinics, and student health centers.

Asking directly about alcohol and drug use is important and even therapeutic for the patient. Often, the clinician should ask first about socially accepted substances, such as nicotine and caffeine (coffee, tea, soda, and energy drinks). This will establish an initial level of comfort for the patient in addressing questions about use of substances. The clinician should inquire next about alcohol use. Specifically, the clinician should ask about beer, wine, and whiskey because many patients do not consider beer to be "alcohol," which they equate with hard liquor. Then the clinician should ask about misuse of over-the-counter and prescription medications. Finally, the clinician should ask about illicit drugs. By this time, the patient will have a sense that the practitioner is soliciting information in a nonjudgmental fashion for the purpose of helping. The clinician should ask about marijuana first because it is

TABLE 17–1. Definitions

Term	Definition
Use	Sporadic consumption of alcohol or drugs with no adverse consequences of that consumption
Abuse	Frequency of consumption of alcohol or drugs may vary, although some adverse consequences of that use are experienced by the user
Physical dependence	State of adaptation that is manifested by a drug class–specific withdrawal syndrome that can be produced by abrupt cessation or rapid dose reduction of a drug or by administration of an antagonist (American Society of Addiction Medicine 2003)
Psychological dependence	Subjective sense of a need for a specific psychoactive substance, either to experience its positive effects or to avoid negative effects associated with its abstinence (American Society of Addiction Medicine 2003)
Substance use disorder	Incorporates both abuse and dependence (American Psychiatric Association 2000)
Substance-induced disorder	Incorporates effects such as intoxication and withdrawal (American Psychiatric Association 2000)
Addiction	A primary chronic neurobiological disease, with genetic, psychosocial, and environmental factors influencing its development and manifestations; it is characterized by behaviors that include impaired control over drug use, compulsive use, continued use despite harm, and craving (American Society of Addiction Medicine 2003)
Dual diagnosis	Patients with co-occurring psychiatric and addiction diagnoses, which often carry a worse prognosis than either disorder alone (Oscher and Kofoed 1989)

Source. American Psychiatric Association 2000; American Society of Addiction Medicine 2003; Oscher and Kofoed 1989.

considered less problematic by users, its use is prevalent, and it carries less social stigma. Inquiries should then be made about cocaine and heroin use, as well as other illicit substances. The amount of money spent on a daily, weekly, or monthly basis for drugs also may be used to quantify drug use. It is important to ask whether the patient has ever injected drugs in the past or shared needles.

Hospitalized patients frequently will be using more than a single drug. Polysubstance abuse is the norm rather than the exception. Patients with one SUD diagnosis often will have another. Of the patients with an alcohol use disorder (AUD), 13% also have a drug use disorder, and patients with a drug use disorder are highly likely to have an AUD, from 23% of those with sedative dependence to 100% of those with hallucinogen dependence (Stinson et al. 2005). Approximately 22% of adults in the United States use both alcohol and tobacco (Falk et al. 2006).

Recreational drug use is often opportunistic. Users will have a specific drug of choice but will use other drugs when presented with the opportunity or when they do not have access to their drug of choice. Certain drug combinations are more common. Users coadminister drugs to offset unpleasant side effects of one drug by another. Heroin is used with stimulants such as cocaine (this combination is known as a *speedball*) to enhance euphoria and to diminish overstimulation and anxiety (Weaver and Schnoll 1999). Alcohol is used with drugs such as marijuana or stimulants to lessen anxiety during the "high" (euphoria) or to induce sleep during the "crash" (withdrawal). Ethylcocaine (cocaethylene) is a metabolite of cocaine formed by the liver only in the presence of alcohol; this metabolite has a potency equal to cocaine, which allows users to have a longer period of euphoria but also heightens the risk of toxicity (severe hypertension or vasoconstriction leading to myocardial infarction or cerebrovascular accident) from cocaine when it is taken with alcohol (Benowitz 1993; Farooq et al. 2009).

In the United States, many states require hospitals to report pregnant women suspected of heavy alcohol or other drug use to local public health authorities when the women present for delivery. Fifteen states consider substance abuse during pregnancy to be child abuse under civil statutes, and three consider it grounds for civil commitment. Fourteen states require physicians to report suspected substance abuse in pregnant women, and four require drug testing if abuse is suspected (for a specific listing, see Guttmacher Institute 2009). This reporting may cause women to be even more wary of acknowledging that they have a problem (Weaver 2003). Indeed, in 1988, some hospitals in South Carolina started testing pregnant women for drug use without their consent and turning them over for criminal prosecution. The practice was ultimately ended by a ruling of the U.S. Supreme Court that it constituted an unconstitutional search (*Ferguson v. City of Charleston* 2001). Therefore,

TABLE 17–2. Physical examination indications of substance use disorders

Body system	Examination finding	Medical indication	Substance(s)
Eyes	Scleral icterus	Cirrhosis (alcoholic or viral)	Alcohol, any injected drug
	Conjunctival injection		Marijuana
	Pinpoint pupils	Opioid intoxication	Opioids
	Horizontal nystagmus	Acute intoxication	Alcohol
	Vertical nystagmus	Acute phencyclidine intoxication	Hallucinogen
Head and neck	Smell of alcohol on breath	Recent ingestion	Alcohol
	Nasal septal perforation	Snorting drugs	Stimulants
	Poor dentition	Inadequate oral hygiene	Stimulants, opioids
Cardiac	Irregular heart rhythm	Atrial fibrillation ("holiday heart")	Alcohol
	New murmur	Endocarditis from injection drug use	Opioids, stimulants, other injected drugs
	Tachycardia	Intoxication	Stimulants, marijuana
		Acute withdrawal	Alcohol
Abdomen	Enlarged, tender liver	Acute hepatitis (alcoholic or viral)	Alcohol, any injected drug
	Shrunken, hard, or nodular liver	Cirrhosis (alcoholic or viral)	Alcohol, any injected drug
	Caput medusae	Cirrhosis (alcoholic or viral)	Alcohol, any injected drug
	Epigastric tenderness	Pancreatitis, gastritis	Alcohol
	Enlarged colon	Constipation	Opioids
Extremities	Tremulousness, hyperreflexia	Acute withdrawal	Alcohol
	Ataxia	Acute intoxication	Alcohol
		Wernicke's encephalopathy	Alcohol
	Reduced light touch sensation	Peripheral neuropathy	Alcohol
	Reduced strength	Muscle atrophy	Alcohol
Skin	Jaundice	Cirrhosis (alcoholic or viral)	Alcohol, any injected drug
	Spider angiomas	Cirrhosis (alcoholic or viral)	Alcohol, any injected drug
	Track marks, fresh needle marks	Injection drug use	Opioids, stimulants, other injected drugs

it is important to assess pregnant women in a nonjudgmental manner for possible SUD. Some studies have shown that comprehensive treatment programs for addicted pregnant women can be successful (Mondanaro and Reed 1987), but the data are insufficient to support any specific intervention (Lui et al. 2008; Stade et al. 2009; Terplan and Lui 2007). Some women may relapse as they near the end of pregnancy. They may confuse early signs of labor with signs of acute withdrawal, so they may medicate themselves during the early hours of labor and arrive at the hospital in labor with high serum levels of drugs from recent use. This increases the chances of fetal stress and distress.

Some patients are able to use illicit substances while hospitalized. They may bring in drugs and paraphernalia at admission in clothing, or visitors may bring drugs to a patient during the inpatient stay. Occasionally, a patient may obtain drugs from another patient or from hospital personnel. Intoxication may present with altered mental status, unexpected resolution of withdrawal symptoms, or a change in patient behavior. Drug use while in the hospital may be verified by urine drug testing, especially confirmatory testing for specific substances not prescribed. Hospital security personnel may be able to search the room and possibly the patient's belongings. The hospital's risk management department should be notified of any illicit drug use on the premises by a patient. Depending on circumstances, this need not result in a drastic response such as immediate discharge of the patient but may be used as an opportunity for brief intervention to address the seriousness of the patient's addiction.

TABLE 17–3. Laboratory indications of substance use disorders

Laboratory test	Change in result	Medical indication	Substance(s)
Albumin	Reduced	Malnutrition, cirrhosis	Any
Blood alcohol level	Alcohol present	Recent alcohol ingestion	Alcohol
Folate	Reduced	Malnutrition	Alcohol
International normalized ratio, prothrombin time	Increased	Cirrhosis (alcoholic or viral)	Alcohol, any injected drug
Mean corpuscular volume	Increased	Bone marrow suppression, B_{12} deficiency	Alcohol
Thiamine	Reduced	Wernicke-Korsakoff syndrome	Alcohol
Transaminases (alanine aminotransferase, aspartate aminotransferase)	Increased	Acute hepatitis (alcoholic or viral)	Alcohol, any injected drug
Urine drug test	Positive	Recent drug use	Any
White blood cell count	Reduced	Bone marrow suppression, human immunodeficiency virus	Alcohol, any injected drug

Alcohol and Sedatives

In the United States, 90% of men and 70% of women consume alcohol (Johnston et al. 2002) in the form of beer, wine, or liquor. AUDs result in 25,000 deaths per year from accidents and 175,000 deaths annually from heart disease, cancer, and suicide (Schuckit and Tapert 2004).

In addition to alcohol, sedative drugs include benzodiazepines, barbiturates, and other sleeping pills. The newer medications zolpidem, zaleplon, and eszopiclone act on the benzodiazepine subtype 1 receptor (Richardson and Roth 2001) and thus are similar to typical benzodiazepines (e.g., diazepam, alprazolam). Zolpidem and eszopiclone abuse is relatively rare when compared with benzodiazepine abuse, but patients with a history of SUD or psychiatric comorbidity are at higher risk for abuse of these medications (Hajak et al. 2003; Victorri-Vigneau et al. 2007).

Intoxication

The clinical features of acute sedative intoxication (including alcohol) are slurred speech, incoordination, unsteady gait, and impaired attention or memory; severe overdose may lead to stupor or coma. Psychiatric manifestations include inappropriate behavior, labile mood, and impaired judgment. Physical signs include nystagmus and decreased reflexes.

A benzodiazepine antagonist, flumazenil, is available for the treatment of acute benzodiazepine intoxication. Nausea and vomiting are its most common side effects. It may not completely reverse respiratory depression and may provoke withdrawal seizures in patients with benzodiazepine dependence. In a mixed overdose with tricyclic antidepressants, flumazenil can precipitate arrhythmias that had been suppressed by the sedative (Weinbroum et al. 1997). Flumazenil appears safe in patients with stable ischemic heart disease (Croughwell et al. 1990). Flumazenil should be withheld in patients with a history of or current seizures and in patients who have overdosed on drugs that lower the seizure threshold. Flumazenil should not routinely be administered to comatose patients when the identity of ingested drug(s) is not certain. Repeat doses should be administered slowly in patients who are physically dependent on benzodiazepines. Flumazenil is short acting, and sedation may recur after an initial awakening. This can be treated by repeating doses at 20-minute intervals as needed.

Withdrawal

Patients may develop an acute alcohol withdrawal syndrome when chronic alcohol use is interrupted by hospital admission. An identical syndrome occurs in patients chronically taking benzodiazepines or other sedatives if the medication is not continued during inpatient admission. Acute withdrawal is most safely managed in an inpatient setting if the patient has been using high doses of sedatives, has a history of seizures or delirium tremens, or has unstable comorbid medical or psychiatric problems (Saitz 1998). The severity of the withdrawal syndrome is affected by concurrent medical illness. Up to 20% of patients develop delirium tremens if left untreated (Cross and Hennessey 1993). Recognition and effective treatment of alcohol withdrawal are important to prevent excess mortality or prolonged hospitalization resulting from complications.

Even when patients acknowledge heavy drinking, they often underestimate the amount, which may be because of minimization or because alcohol is an amnestic agent, and drinkers quickly lose count of how much they have had to drink. It is simplest to ask all patients admitted to the hospital in a nonjudgmental manner about drinking and to be alert for signs of acute alcohol withdrawal in all patients. Individual variability in the threshold at which a patient may develop withdrawal is significant, and those who drink most days of the week are more likely to develop withdrawal as a result of tolerance. Not all daily drinkers will develop withdrawal, but it is difficult to predict who will and who will not. The best predictor of whether a patient will develop acute withdrawal while hospitalized is a history of acute alcohol withdrawal.

The alcohol withdrawal syndrome has two phases: early withdrawal and late withdrawal (Table 17–4). The signs and symptoms of early withdrawal usually develop within 48 hours of the last drink. This time frame may be prolonged if the patient has taken long-acting sedatives or accelerated in extremely heavy users such that patients may begin to withdraw while still mildly intoxicated. The initial indication of withdrawal is an elevation of vital signs (heart rate, blood pressure, temperature). Tremors develop next: first, a fine tremor of the hands and fasciculation of the tongue, sometimes followed by gross tremors of the extremities. Disorientation and mild hallucinations (often auditory, occasionally visual) may develop as the syndrome progresses, accompanied by diaphoresis. Seizures are an early sign of alcohol withdrawal and may be the presenting symptom. However, a large case-control study found that 16% of first seizures in drinkers occurred outside the conventionally defined withdrawal period, and the timing after the last drink of the other 84% seemed random (Ng et al. 1988).

Late alcohol withdrawal is also known as *delirium tremens* ("the DTs") and consists of worsening autonomic dysregulation that is responsible for much of the morbidity and mortality attributed to alcohol withdrawal. It begins after early withdrawal, usually 72 hours or more after the last drink, and peaks around 5 days (Blondell et al. 2004).

Some patients do not progress from early to late withdrawal, and the symptoms simply subside after a few days with or without treatment, but it is impossible to predict which patients will progress. The signs of late withdrawal consist of worsening diaphoresis; nausea and vomiting (which may result in aspiration pneumonia); delirium with frank hallucinations; and rapid, severe fluctuation in vital signs (Monte Secades et al. 2008). Sudden changes in blood pressure and heart rate may result in complications such as myocardial infarction or a cerebrovascular event, and increased QT variability elevates the risk for serious cardiac arrhythmias (Bar et al. 2007). Hyperthermia is also associated with higher mortality (Khan et al. 2008). Progression to late withdrawal results in significant morbidity and even death (Monte Secades et al. 2008), but adequate treatment of early withdrawal helps prevent progression to late withdrawal.

The revised Clinical Institute Withdrawal Assessment for Alcohol (CIWA-Ar) is commonly used to assess severity of withdrawal (Sullivan et al. 1989). The CIWA-Ar is just as useful for evaluation and treatment of withdrawal in hospitalized patients on general medical wards and emergency departments as it is in chemical dependency units. It also can be used to determine appropriate pharmacotherapy dose for patients in withdrawal who also have other med-

TABLE 17–4. Alcohol withdrawal signs

Sign	Early withdrawal	Late withdrawal (delirium tremens)
Time of onset	<48 hours after last drink	After onset of early withdrawal
Heart rate	80–110 beats/minute	>120 beats/minute
Temperature	<101.5°F	>101.5°F
Blood pressure	Slight increase (especially systolic)	Significant hypotension and hypertension
Respiratory rate	12–20 breaths/minute	>20 breaths/minute
Tremors	Fine tremor of hands and tongue	Gross tremors, all extremities
Consciousness	Agitated	Delirious
Orientation	Mildly disoriented	Completely disoriented
Hallucinations	Mild auditory and/or visual	Visual, auditory, tactile
Seizures	Possible	Unusual

ical illnesses (Weaver et al. 2006). Regular assessment should continue until the withdrawal syndrome has come under control (CIWA-Ar score <6) for at least 24 hours. If no withdrawal signs have manifested after 48 hours, then it is usually safe to discontinue monitoring for withdrawal. Standardized algorithms with frequent assessment for signs of withdrawal also facilitate efficient treatment of postoperative patients at risk for withdrawal (Lansford et al. 2008).

Pharmacotherapy is indicated for management of moderate to severe withdrawal, and any cross-tolerant medication may be used. It is inappropriate to give beverage alcohol to prevent or treat alcohol withdrawal. Use of intravenous alcohol infusion is reserved for poisoning with methanol, isopropanol, or ethylene glycol and should not be given for treatment of acute alcohol withdrawal because of complications such as intoxication with delirium or development of gastritis (Weaver 2007). Both benzodiazepines and barbiturates effectively treat alcohol withdrawal (Mayo-Smith 1997). In the United States, it is most often managed with benzodiazepines, but barbiturates also have been used successfully to treat acute alcohol withdrawal syndrome in general medical inpatients, and phenobarbital has been used most commonly (Weaver et al. 2009). Several alternative non-sedative-hypnotic medications are available for the treatment of acute alcohol withdrawal. Beta-adrenergic blockers (atenolol, propranolol), clonidine, and anticonvulsant agents (carbamazepine, valproate) decrease alcohol withdrawal symptoms and have been used successfully in treatment of mild withdrawal. However, they are not cross-tolerant with alcohol and may result in progression of the withdrawal syndrome. These alternative medications are not appropriate as single agents to treat moderate or severe withdrawal.

In addition to pharmacotherapy for alcohol withdrawal, some patients need intravenous glucose because many individuals with AUD are hypoglycemic as a result of poor diet and hepatic dysfunction. It is essential to administer thiamine and folate (see discussion below), as well as magnesium and phosphate, before or concurrently with glucose.

Severe withdrawal (delirium tremens), manifested by abnormal and fluctuating vital signs with delirium, should be treated aggressively in an intensive care environment with sufficiently large doses of medication to suppress the withdrawal (Weaver 2007). Medications with a rapid onset of action should be used intravenously for immediate effect. Lorazepam and diazepam have a rapid onset of action when given intravenously, although the duration of action is shorter than when given orally. For example, lorazepam, 1–4 mg every 10–30 minutes, should be given until the patient is calm but awake and the heart rate is less than 120 beats/minute (Weaver 2007). A continuous intravenous infusion may be warranted to control withdrawal symptoms, and the infusion rate can be titrated to the desired level of consciousness. After stabilization, the clinician can substitute an equivalent dose of a long-acting sedative-hypnotic that will be tapered.

Nearly 10% of intensive care unit (ICU) admissions are alcohol related (Baldwin et al. 1993), and 5% will develop severe withdrawal, which carries a mortality rate of 15% (Turner et al. 1989). Prevention strategies include screening ICU patients for SUD and assessment for development of acute withdrawal syndromes (De Wit et al. 2008). The key to treating withdrawal syndromes in the ICU is to anticipate when they may occur and treat vigorously to prevent new problems in critically ill patients (Weaver and Schnoll 1996). No specific benzodiazepine is superior to any other for alcohol withdrawal treatment in the ICU, although longer-acting benzodiazepines may allow for a smoother withdrawal course (Ritson and Chick 1986). Severe alcohol withdrawal that is refractory to high-dose benzodiazepines has been treated successfully with the addition of phenobarbital (Gold et al. 2007) or propofol (McCowan and Marik 2000).

Patients who abuse alcohol often have some degree of liver dysfunction when admitted to the hospital, either from acute alcohol-induced hepatitis or from cirrhosis due to long-term consumption. Hepatically metabolized sedatives such as benzodiazepines and barbiturates may worsen hepatic encephalopathy in patients with cirrhosis. These types of medications should be used with caution to avoid adverse outcomes from accumulation of metabolites requiring liver metabolism. Lorazepam and oxazepam are intermediate-acting benzodiazepines that have no active metabolites (hepatic metabolism of these involves only glucuronidation for excretion), unlike other benzodiazepines, which makes them safer in severe liver disease. Despite the long half-life and metabolism by the liver, phenobarbital is still safe to use for patients with liver disease who are not at risk for hepatic encephalopathy because approximately 30% is excreted unchanged in the urine (Hadama et al. 2001) and not metabolized by the liver. This is an advantage over most long-acting benzodiazepines (e.g., chlordiazepoxide and diazepam), which undergo extensive liver metabolism to additional active metabolites (Olkkola and Ahonen 2008).

Effects on Medical Disorders

An individual with AUD reduces his or her life span by 10–15 years. Chronic alcohol use causes many potential medical problems (Table 17–5). Alcohol use disorders are independent risk factors for the development of community-acquired pneumonia (De Roux et al. 2006). Magnesium

TABLE 17–5. Long-term effects of alcohol use

Cardiovascular	**Gastrointestinal**	**Obstetric**
Hypertension	Malnutrition	Sexual dysfunction
Arrhythmias	Gastritis	Intrauterine growth retardation
Cardiomyopathy	Peptic ulcer disease	Fetal alcohol syndrome/fetal alcohol effects
	Gastrointestinal bleeding	
Central nervous system	Acute hepatitis	**Other**
Seizures	Pancreatitis	Bone marrow suppression
Delirium	Fatty liver	Peripheral neuropathy
Dementia	Cirrhosis	Rhabdomyolysis
Cerebral atrophy		
	Malignancy	
Endocrine	Mouth, pharynx, larynx	
Diuresis	Esophagus	
Hyperglycemia	Pancreas	
Male feminization	Liver	

excretion is increased by alcohol intake, so magnesium repletion is important to prevent hypokalemia, which can lead to acute cardiac arrhythmias and muscle weakness (Elisaf et al. 2002). Alcohol dependence is also associated with persistent vascular endothelial damage leading to atherosclerosis with complications such as hypertension and other cardiovascular diseases; this heightened cardiovascular and metabolic risk persists even after 2 years of abstinence (Di Gennaro et al. 2007). Behavior problems may occur in hospitalized patients with AUD, including surgical patients. These may include agitation, sleep disturbances, and verbal abuse (G. Williams et al. 2008). Alcohol also interacts with many different medications in many ways (Table 17–6).

TABLE 17–6. Interactions between alcohol and medications

Medication	Clinical interaction
Warfarin, oral anticoagulants	Acute: increased anticoagulant effect Chronic: decreased anticoagulant effect
Disulfiram Chlorpropamide Griseofulvin Metronidazole Quinacrine	Nausea and vomiting, flushing, palpitations, dyspnea, hypotension, headache, and sympathetic overactivity
Diazepam	Increased sedation (increased absorption)
Antihistamines Benzodiazepines Opioids	Increased sedation
Chloral hydrate Chlorpromazine Cimetidine	Increased intoxication (decreased alcohol metabolism)

Patients with AUD have longer surgical ICU length of stay, higher rates of ICU readmission, and increased risk of death (Delgado-Rodriguez et al. 2003). A history of alcohol use is an important independent risk factor for delirium and other neurocognitive complications in an ICU setting (Dubois et al. 2001). Acute intoxication or withdrawal from illicit substances may result in delirium and can be easily missed by failing to obtain appropriate history of substance abuse from the patient or family members or by failing to use urine or blood toxicology testing on admission. Even patients admitted with minor injuries have higher morbidity with significantly longer hospital length of stay, including ICU stays with days on mechanical ventilation (Bard et al. 2006), when they have AUD. Alcohol abuse results in postoperative complications, especially from development of alcohol withdrawal syndrome (Chang and Steinberg 2001), so patients at risk for alcohol withdrawal should have elective surgical procedures postponed until they have achieved 7–10 days of abstinence (Bard et al. 2006); if this is not feasible, adequate prophylaxis for alcohol withdrawal should be provided.

Alcohol dependence leads to vitamin deficiency states as a result of reduced transport across the intestinal lining, reduced capacity of the liver to store vitamins, and low vitamin content in alcoholic beverages (Thomson 2000).

Vitamin repletion, especially thiamine and folate, is important for all patients with AUD. Wernicke's encephalopathy results from thiamine deficiency and consists of ophthalmoplegia, ataxia, and altered mental status; this may be difficult to differentiate from acute alcohol intoxication. It is a medical emergency requiring immediate treatment with parenteral thiamine (250–500 mg/day for 3–5 days) to prevent development of Korsakoff's syndrome, the irreversible form of thiamine deficiency consisting of chronic loss of working memory accompanied by confabulation (Sechi and Serra 2007). Thiamine must be given before or concurrently with intravenous glucose because giving glucose alone to a thiamine-deficient patient can precipitate Wernicke's encephalopathy due to thalamic neuronal damage (Thomson et al. 2002).

Pharmacological Treatment

Three medications have been approved by the U.S. Food and Drug Administration (FDA) for treatment of alcohol dependence. Disulfiram has been used for 60 years. It does not reduce craving for alcohol but acts as an aversive agent by inhibition of aldehyde dehydrogenase, which prevents metabolism of alcohol to acetaldehyde. When alcohol is ingested, this results in accumulation of acetaldehyde in the blood with unpleasant effects. The drinker experiences nausea and vomiting, flushing, palpitations, dyspnea, hypotension, headache, and sympathetic overactivity. This reaction to alcohol consumption discourages further drinking. However, disulfiram may have serious side effects, including hepatotoxicity, depression, and psychotic reactions (O'Shea 2000). These potential toxicities limit its utility in medically ill patients, including long-term drinkers who may have developed liver damage over time, as well as patients with major depression or psychotic disorders. It is contraindicated in patients with severe cardiac disease or cirrhosis and during pregnancy because of its association with specific birth defects (Jessup and Green 1987). Ingestion of even small amounts of alcohol, such as that in over-the-counter cough medicines or mouthwash, can result in aversive symptoms; oral liquid medications dissolved in alcohol (elixirs) can also trigger the reaction. Alcohol is present in hundreds of oral, parenteral, and topical (including inhalational) prescription and nonprescription drugs (Parker 1982–1983). Metronidazole has been reported to cause a disulfiram-like effect when alcohol is consumed while taking it, but this has been disputed; however, current recommendations are that patients avoid alcohol while taking metronidazole and for at least 48 hours after stopping it (C.S. Williams and Woodcock 2000).

Naltrexone affects alcohol consumption through blockade of opioid receptors because some reinforcing effects of alcohol are mediated through the endogenous opioid system. Naltrexone reduces the pleasurable effects of alcohol, which reduces the risk of relapse, especially among those with a family history of alcoholism and those with strong cravings (Johnson 2008). Naltrexone is available as a daily pill or as a monthly intramuscular depot injection given in a physician's office. The primary side effect is nausea, which occurs somewhat less with the depot version. Naltrexone has been reported to cause transaminase elevation and potential hepatotoxicity, with recommendations to monitor this periodically. Although this has been disputed (Brewer and Wong 2004), an FDA black-box warning now states that naltrexone is contraindicated in severe hepatic disease and may cause hepatotoxicity above the recommended dose. Depot naltrexone provides a lower total exposure to naltrexone and bypasses first-pass hepatic metabolism and thus has potential for improved hepatic safety (Dunbar et al. 2006). Naltrexone should be used with caution in patients with hepatic dysfunction, but this is not an absolute contraindication. Because naltrexone is an opioid blocker, treatment of acute or postoperative pain can be challenging in a patient who is using naltrexone for treatment of AUD. For unexpected severe pain such as trauma, nonopioid analgesics should be considered, including nonsteroidal anti-inflammatory agents, or local anesthesia with a nerve block or epidural catheter can be used (Vickers and Jolly 2006). It also may be feasible to titrate typical opioid analgesics upward to patient comfort under medical observation without causing oversedation or significant respiratory depression.

Acamprosate antagonizes *N*-methyl-D-aspartate glutamate receptors, restoring balance between excitatory and inhibitory neurotransmission that was deregulated by chronic alcohol consumption (De Witte et al. 2005), which reduces negative affect and craving during abstinence (Spanagel and Zeiglgansberger 1997). The primary side effects are diarrhea and nervousness, usually only at high doses. This drug has no contraindication to use with liver damage, but the dose should be reduced in patients with renal impairment (Mason et al. 2002); it is contraindicated in renal failure. Acamprosate has no known drug interactions. Compared with disulfiram and naltrexone, which have multiple drug interactions and potential complications (hepatotoxicity), acamprosate may be a good choice for patients with medical and/or psychiatric comorbidities, especially those taking other medications.

Timely follow-up after hospitalization is essential to monitor effectiveness and adverse effects of medications for abstinence. For patients who are motivated to remain abstinent, one of these medications may be started in the inpatient setting. These medications should be started only if a practitioner is identified to continue them in the outpatient setting.

Opioids

The most commonly used illicit opioid is heroin, with more than 2 million chronic users in the United States (Substance Abuse and Mental Health Services Administration 2006). The all-cause mortality rate of heroin dependence is more than 60 times that expected for nonusers of the same age and sex (Gronbladh et al. 1990). Prescription opioid analgesic abuse is the fastest-growing form of drug abuse in the United States (Cicero et al. 2005) and is predominantly localized in rural, suburban, and small urban areas (Cicero et al. 2007).

Pseudoaddiction is an iatrogenic syndrome of aberrant medication-taking behaviors that occurs when pain is undertreated with opioid analgesics (Weissman and Haddox 1989). This may revert to normal behavior when pain is adequately treated. The best course of action to differentiate addiction from pseudoaddiction is to titrate the dose of medication upward rapidly to control pain quickly (Weaver and Schnoll 2002). Opioid abuse can be differentiated from pseudoaddiction by continuing inappropriate behavior, such as oversedation despite complaints of severe pain and requests for additional opioids despite multiple upward titrations of the opioid dose.

Intoxication

Acute opioid intoxication is characterized by decreased level of consciousness, substantially decreased respiration, miotic pupils, and absent bowel sounds. Prescription opioid analgesics may be abused and can lead to intoxication or overdose. Oral controlled-release oxycodone has been abused by crushing the tablets and then snorting the powder; when taken in this way by people who have no tolerance to the drug, a single 80-mg dose (the highest strength available in a single tablet) can be fatal. Propoxyphene, meperidine, or tramadol can cause seizures in overdose. Meperidine, in particular, can cause an agitated delirium due to accumulation of normeperidine, which is a neuroexcitatory toxic metabolite; this is most prevalent in patients with acute or chronic renal impairment and results in reduced clearance of normeperidine (Adunsky et al. 2002).

Opioid overdose is treated with naloxone. It is given intravenously as an initial dose of 0.4 mg, but if no response is seen in 3–5 minutes, an additional dose of 1–2 mg is given. The duration of action of naloxone is 20–40 minutes, so repeated doses or a continuous infusion may be necessary for patients who have taken long-acting opioids such as methadone. It is advisable to restrain patients prior to administration of naloxone because patients may become agitated and even violent when awakened in acute withdrawal in an unfamiliar setting.

Withdrawal

Opioid withdrawal has very apparent physical symptoms (Table 17–7) and fairly consistent time to onset from the last use (about 8 hours for short-acting opioids such as heroin or oxycodone), which is a prominent factor in repeated administration after development of tolerance. This is in contrast to delirium tremens from alcohol and sedatives, in which minor signs of acute withdrawal often do not progress to severe withdrawal; onset and severity of opioid withdrawal are consistent and predictable for the vast majority of daily users. Opioid withdrawal is treated with substitution of a long-acting opioid (methadone or buprenorphine) for detoxification over several days.

Hospitalization is usually unnecessary for opioid withdrawal alone unless the patient has concurrent medical or psychiatric illness that warrants hospitalization (e.g., unstable angina, brittle diabetes mellitus, suicidality). Methadone is frequently used to treat acute withdrawal from opioids, but current U.S. federal regulations restrict the use of methadone for treatment of opioid dependence. Methadone may be used by a physician for temporary maintenance or detoxification when an opioid-dependent patient is admitted to a hospital for an illness other than opioid addiction. A method of titrating the amount of methadone based on symptoms has been used extensively to titrate methadone for opioid withdrawal, without causing oversedation or severe patient discomfort (Weaver et al. 1999). The severity of 11 symptoms (see Table 17–7) is rated with a score of 0 to 2 points (0 = symptom is absent; 1 = symptom is present; 2 = symptom is severe). The total score for all symptoms is determined; each point is equiv-

TABLE 17–7. Opioid withdrawal signs

Sign	None	Mild	Severe
Nausea/vomiting	0	1	2
Abdominal cramps	0	1	2
Diarrhea	0	1	2
Chills/hot flashes	0	1	2
Myalgias/arthralgias	0	1	2
Piloerection	0	1	2
Restlessness	0	1	2
Twitching/jerks	0	1	2
Lacrimation	0	1	2
Rhinorrhea	0	1	2
Yawning	0	1	2

alent to a requirement of 1 mg of methadone, but no methadone is given for a score of less than 5 points because such a low score indicates only mild withdrawal. The patient should be evaluated and the symptom score reassessed every 6 hours for the first 24 hours. After 24 hours, the total dose of methadone administered is calculated; this dose is approximately equivalent to the dose of opioid the individual was taking. After being stabilized on this dose of methadone for 24 hours, the patient can be tapered off by approximately 10%–20% per day. The duration of action of methadone allows it to be given once daily as a single dose (when treating opioid withdrawal in contrast to pain treatment). Most patients do not experience euphoria with methadone administration. Buprenorphine is also used to treat opioid withdrawal.

Clonidine is not approved by the U.S. FDA for the treatment of opioid withdrawal, although it is commonly used for this purpose. A transdermal clonidine patch is effective for mild withdrawal symptoms and can be left on the skin for 7 days. Typical clonidine protocols use 0.1–0.3 mg of clonidine every 2–4 hours for the first 24 hours, usually 0.8–1.2 mg/day. Subsequently, clonidine is given three to four times a day, with the total daily dose reduced by 0.1 or 0.2 mg on each subsequent day. The total duration for this regimen is 10–14 days. It is important to monitor for hypotension during clonidine therapy and then to taper clonidine gradually to avoid a hypertensive rebound (Gowing et al. 2004). Clonidine should be avoided in hypotensive patients (systolic blood pressure < 100 mm Hg). In addition to orthostatic hypotension, side effects of clonidine include sedation, dry mouth, and constipation; these are more likely at higher doses.

Certain medications may be given for relief of other symptoms of opioid withdrawal: muscle relaxants reduce spasms and twitching; nonsteroidal anti-inflammatory drugs treat aches; antiemetics are used for nausea; an antidiarrheal agent such as bismuth subsalicylate may be useful; and a sleeping medication that has low abuse potential (such as trazodone) will help insomnia.

Opioid withdrawal syndrome during pregnancy can lead to fetal distress and premature labor as a result of increased oxygen consumption by both the mother and the fetus (Cooper et al. 1983). Even minimal symptoms in the mother may indicate fetal distress because the fetus may be more susceptible to withdrawal symptoms than is the mother. Buprenorphine is not recommended for pregnant women yet. Naloxone should not be given to a pregnant woman except as a last resort for severe opioid overdose because withdrawal precipitated by an opioid antagonist can result in spontaneous abortion, premature labor, or stillbirth.

Effects on Medical Disorders

Chronic infection with HCV can lead to cirrhosis and need for liver transplant, and the rate of HCV infection among methadone maintenance (MM) patients is 70% (Weaver et al. 2005). Accurate data about drug and alcohol use among patients with liver disease or liver transplant candidates are difficult to obtain because patients underreport this use because they believe that divulging this information will harm their chances of receiving further care, especially access to a liver transplant (Weinrieb et al. 2000). The standard of care for patients with severe liver disease receiving MM is to continue methadone during evaluation, transplant surgery, and thereafter rather than attempting to taper the patient off methadone (Lucey and Weinrieb 2009). Continuation of MM has superior outcomes in terms of relapse to heroin use when compared with tapering off methadone (Ball and Ross 1991). Therefore, it is inappropriate to require patients who are stable on methadone (or buprenorphine) to discontinue this treatment before any surgical procedure or other intervention.

Individuals admitted to the hospital with opioid dependence may have pain from various sources, including trauma or infection. Acute opioid withdrawal syndrome also may be painful because of myalgias and intestinal cramping. Adequate treatment of pain with opioid analgesics will also ameliorate opioid withdrawal signs. It may be difficult to distinguish pain due to opioid withdrawal from pain due to other causes; the best course of action is to give the patient the benefit of the doubt and provide appropriate amounts of opioid analgesics to treat complaints of pain adequately (Weaver and Schnoll 2002). Sedation and mild reduction in respiratory rate are indicators that the pain and withdrawal are adequately being treated; additional requests for opioids despite these signs may indicate that the patient is seeking higher doses in an attempt to achieve euphoria beyond just relief of pain and withdrawal symptoms. Narcotic bowel syndrome is a form of bowel hyperalgesia that has been proposed but not well studied. Patients have chronic or recurring abdominal pain that is worsened with continued or escalating dosages of opioids (Grunkemeier et al. 2007); improvement in symptoms is observed following gradual tapering off opioids.

Some opioids, including tramadol, meperidine, dextromethorphan, and methadone, are weak serotonin reuptake inhibitors (Gillman 2005). When given—especially at high doses—with monoamine oxidase inhibitors (such as phenelzine, tranylcypromine, selegiline, and even the antibiotic linezolid), this can result in serotonin syndrome (see "Serotonin Syndrome" in Chapter 38, "Psychopharmacology"). Opioids that do not have serotonin activity are morphine, codeine, oxycodone, and buprenorphine;

these would be better choices to use for patients taking other serotonergic medications.

Pharmacological Treatment

Methadone may be used for chronic addiction only by a licensed opioid treatment program. Prescribing methadone for withdrawal or long-term treatment of drug dependence requires a special state and federal license; however, methadone can be prescribed in the United States for treatment of acute or chronic pain by any physician with a Drug Enforcement Administration (DEA) license, similar to laws for other Schedule II medications. If an MM client is hospitalized, such as for a traumatic injury or medical illness, the maintenance dose should be continued throughout hospitalization. The hospital physician should contact the MM program to verify the client's current dose and arrange for dosing to resume after discharge.

Acutely ill or injured hospital patients often experience pain; MM clients experience the same pain despite receiving methadone because methadone reaches steady-state levels in the body and does not provide additional analgesia. Patients receiving MM with acute pain should be treated for pain with opioid or nonopioid medications, as would be appropriate if they were not receiving MM. The patient's usual MM dose should be continued and short-acting opioid analgesics administered additionally. These should be given on a schedule and not ordered as needed. Higher-than-usual opioid analgesic doses may be required because of opioid cross-tolerance (Alford et al. 2006). If the patient cannot take oral medication, methadone can be given by the intramuscular or subcutaneous route. The parenteral dose should be given as one-half to two-thirds of the maintenance dose, divided into two to four equal doses per day. Mixed agonist and antagonist opioid analgesics, such as pentazocine, nalbuphine, and butorphanol, should not be administered because they precipitate acute withdrawal and block the analgesic effects of agonist opioids. Combination products with fixed doses of acetaminophen and an opioid should be avoided for most patients because higher opioid dose requirements may expose patients to potentially hepatotoxic doses of acetaminophen.

Many different medications affect methadone metabolism primarily because it is metabolized by cytochrome P450 3A4. Risperidone, rifampicin, and many antiretrovirals can lower serum methadone levels, resulting in opioid withdrawal symptoms. These interactions usually do not have life-threatening consequences for patients, other than acute discomfort and risk of relapse to opioid abuse (Ferrari et al. 2004). Diazepam, fluoxetine, and erythromycin can elevate methadone serum levels and increase the risk of opioid intoxication. Methadone use can prolong the QTc interval. A dose relation has been observed between methadone and QTc interval (Martell et al. 2005), with most problems occurring at dosages greater than 40 mg/day (Ehret et al. 2006). Torsade de pointes has been reported with very high doses of methadone in outpatient settings, occurring in a few patients who had risk factors for arrhythmias (Krantz et al. 2002). The risk of QTc prolongation is increased when methadone is given intravenously; is used in conjunction with other QTc-prolonging drugs (e.g., antipsychotics, amiodarone, erythromycin) or drugs that inhibit cytochrome P450 3A4; and is administered to patients with hypokalemia, hypocalcemia, hypomagnesemia, or impaired liver function (Ehret et al. 2006).

Buprenorphine, a partial opioid agonist, reduces illicit opioid use with long-term therapy (Kakko et al. 2003). Buprenorphine is taken sublingually. It is available alone or in a combination preparation with naloxone, an opioid antagonist that has poor oral absorption. Buprenorphine has a lower potential for causing respiratory depression than does methadone, and the typical treatment dose (16–32 mg) can be tolerated by opioid-naive users. It does not appear to prolong the QTc interval (Wedam et al. 2007), unlike methadone. Buprenorphine does have the potential to be misused as an injectable agent. It is less restricted than methadone but may be used in the United States only by certified and specially trained physicians who have registered with the Substance Abuse and Mental Health Services Administration. Administration of buprenorphine or buprenorphine/naloxone may precipitate an acute opioid withdrawal syndrome in patients with opioid dependence (Walsh and Eissenberg 2003).

As with MM, patients taking buprenorphine who develop acute pain should be given appropriate pain medications. Short-acting opioid analgesics should be used in higher-than-usual doses, on a set schedule, and mixed agonist–antagonist opioid analgesics should be avoided. Buprenorphine has fewer drug interactions than methadone does, so it is safer when used for patients with medical comorbidities such as HIV who are taking antiretroviral medications. However, buprenorphine may cause elevation of liver transaminase levels in patients with chronic HCV infection (Petry et al. 2000), which has a very high prevalence among patients who have injected opioids and are receiving maintenance treatment, and monitoring of liver enzymes may be necessary. Buprenorphine toxicity has been linked to use of benzodiazepines (Tracqui et al. 1998), so patients who require chronic benzodiazepine therapy for anxiety disorders or who have a history of sedative dependence may not be appropriate candidates for buprenorphine maintenance.

MM is the treatment of choice for opioid-addicted pregnant women (Center for Substance Abuse Treatment 1993; Winklbaur et al. 2008), although other opioids have been used (Minozzi et al. 2008). Illicitly bought heroin is adulterated with other compounds that may be harmful to the fetus, so elimination of heroin use with adequate doses of methadone prevents harm to the fetus from exposure to these other compounds. Pregnant women who are opioid dependent should be referred for prenatal care and to a local MM program, if available. Most programs assign high priority to pregnant women, so the patient may be able to enter treatment sooner than if she were not pregnant. Split dosing of methadone rather than the standard once-a-day dose appears to have fewer neurobehavioral effects on the fetus (Jansson et al. 2009). Women can breast-feed while receiving MM as long as they are not abusing any drugs (McCarthy and Posey 2000) and are not HIV positive. Sublingual buprenorphine is not yet approved for use in pregnancy but has been used successfully for opioid maintenance in pregnant women (Fischer et al. 2000). This medication has been well tolerated by mothers, and the newborns have had a similar incidence of neonatal abstinence syndrome compared with newborns of mothers receiving MM (Jones et al. 2005).

Naltrexone is also used as a medication to assist with maintaining abstinence in patients with opioid addiction. Daily oral dosing or monthly intramuscular injections result in blockade of opioid effects if opioids are used. The intramuscular formulation has been approved by the U.S. FDA for the treatment of alcohol dependence but not for the treatment of opioid dependence. Naltrexone causes immediate withdrawal symptoms if administered prior to detoxification. Patients who discontinue antagonist therapy and resume opioid use should be made aware of the risk of serious overdose. This risk may be a result of loss of tolerance to opioids and a resulting misjudgment of dose at the time of relapse (Strang et al. 2003).

Stimulants

Stimulants are drugs that stimulate the central nervous system (CNS) to produce increased psychomotor activity. Amphetamines, including methamphetamine, and cocaine are the most prevalent abused stimulants, but this class also includes prescription stimulants such as methylphenidate and dextroamphetamine, as well as "designer drugs" such as methylenedioxymethamphetamine (MDMA; Ecstasy). More than 40 million people worldwide have used methamphetamine (United Nations Office on Drugs and Crime 2003).

Caffeine is a mild stimulant found in coffee, tea, soda, and energy drinks. Reports of caffeine intoxication have been rising because of the availability of energy drinks with high caffeine content, and this can mimic symptoms of anxiety disorders. Compelling evidence indicates that caffeine can produce a substance dependence syndrome in some individuals (Reissig et al. 2009). Energy drink consumption is associated with progression to nonmedical use of prescription stimulants, and caffeine increases the reinforcing effects of nicotine and may increase the rate of alcohol-related injuries (Reissig et al. 2009). It is important to ask all patients about consumption of caffeine and use of other drugs.

Khat is a plant with psychostimulant properties that has been long used socially and in religious ritual in some African and Middle Eastern countries and more recently by immigrants from them. Although the psychoactive compounds in khat leaves are much less potent than amphetamines, addiction does occur in a minority of its users. Adverse medical effects are uncommon with low-level use, but high levels may cause hypertension, arrhythmia, insomnia, and anorexia. In addition, khat users appear to be at increased risk for gastrointestinal cancers (Manghi et al. 2009; Pennings et al. 2008).

Intoxication

Stimulant intoxication includes behavior changes such as hypervigilance, psychomotor agitation, grandiosity, and impaired judgment. People should approach acutely intoxicated stimulant users in a subdued manner, avoid speaking in a loud voice or moving quickly, not approach the patient from behind, and avoid touching the patient unless absolutely sure that it is safe to do so (Weaver et al. 1999). Treatment of acute toxicity includes acute stabilization of airway, breathing, and circulation; administration of activated charcoal; seizure control with benzodiazepines; aggressive management of hypertension; and management of hyperthermia.

Many experts advise that beta-blockers should not be considered first-line agents for controlling chest pain or hypertension in patients using cocaine because that would leave alpha-adrenergic stimulation unopposed, but this remains controversial (Dattilo et al. 2008; Page et al. 2007).

Effects on Medical and Psychiatric Disorders

Use of stimulants may result in many health consequences that can bring users into the hospital or complicate existing medical and/or psychiatric conditions (Table 17–8). Known psychiatric disorders may be exacerbated by stimulant use. Schizophrenia is more susceptible to relapse, and panic attacks may increase in intensity and frequency. Chronic use of MDMA can lead to paranoid psychosis that is clinically indistinguishable from that in schizophrenia, but this usually abates after a prolonged period of abstinence (Buchanan and Brown 1988). Several studies suggest that MDMA use can lead to cognitive decline in otherwise healthy young people (Gouzoulis-Mayfrank et al.

TABLE 17–8. Effects of stimulant use

Psychological
Emotional lability
Irritability
Insomnia
Exaggerated startle reactions
Paranoia
Aggressive behavior
Aberrant sexual behavior
Anxiety
Depression
Hallucinations
Psychosis
Delirium

Obstetric
Placenta previa
Premature rupture of membranes
Placental abruption
Spontaneous abortion

Fetal
Intrauterine growth retardation
Fetal hypertension
Congenital malformations

Cardiovascular
Hypertension
Arrhythmias
Cardiomyopathy
Myocardial ischemia/infarction

Central nervous system
Headache
Transient focal neurological deficits
Tremor
Myoclonus
Bradykinesia
Dyskinesia
Cerebral vasculitis
Cerebral edema
Cerebral hemorrhage
Cerebral infarction
Cerebral atrophy
Toxic encephalopathy

Gastrointestinal
Anorexia
Nausea/vomiting
Diarrhea
Intestinal ischemia
Gastroduodenal perforation

Endocrine
Hyperprolactinemia
Elevated thyroxin level

Pulmonary
Chronic productive cough
Asthma exacerbation
Pulmonary edema
Pulmonary hemorrhage
Pneumothorax
Pneumomediastinum
Bronchiolitis obliterans

Head and neck
Dental enamel erosion
Gingival ulceration
Mydriasis
Chronic rhinitis
Nasal septal perforation

Other
Postural abnormalities
Hyperthermia
Rhabdomyolysis
Acute renal failure

2000); this neurotoxicity occurs at typical recreational doses. Patients presenting with these signs should be suspected of stimulant abuse and screened carefully.

Stimulants are used therapeutically for multiple conditions and are prescribed appropriately for attention-deficit disorder, narcolepsy, fatigue in multiple sclerosis, refractory depression, and palliative care. Stimulants potentiate arrhythmias (Wilkerson 1988), and long-term use can lead to cardiomyopathy (Virmani et al. 1988). When prescribed stimulants such as methylphenidate or dextroamphetamine are abused by patients who have valid prescriptions for them, clinicians may see unintended side effects such as elevation in resting heart rate or other cardiovascular complications; these effects may be a clue to the prescriber that unauthorized dosage escalation is occurring. Patients prescribed stimulants who also have cardiovascular disease are at higher risk for complications. Cocaine is the most frequent drug-related cause of emergency department visits (Drug Abuse Warning Network 2003), and chest pain is the most common reason to seek emergency care. Stimulant abuse is a major cause of cerebrovascular and cardiovascular disease in young adults (O'Connor et al. 2005). In numerous case reports, MDMA (Ecstasy) use resulted in rhabdomyolysis, hyperthermia, serotonin syndrome, hyponatremia with cerebral edema, fulminant hepatic failure, and stroke (Hall and Henry 2006). Both prescribed and illicit stimulants interact with other medications, which may result in serious adverse reactions, often cardiovascular in nature (Table 17–9).

Pharmacological Treatment

Abrupt discontinuation of stimulants does not cause gross physiological sequelae, so they are not tapered off or replaced with a cross-tolerant drug during medically supervised withdrawal (Weaver and Schnoll 1999). Most pharmacological agents have not proven significantly better than placebo for long-term management of abstinence for stimulant-dependent patients (Schuckit 1994).

TABLE 17–9. Interactions between stimulants and other drugs

Medication	Clinical interaction
Alcohol Beta-blockers Caffeine Carbamazepine Monoamine oxidase inhibitors Nonsteroidal anti-inflammatory medications	Increased blood pressure, increased heart rate
Anticholinergics Bromocriptine Digoxin Halothane anesthetics	Arrhythmias
Calcium channel blockers Haloperidol	Reduced blood pressure

Nicotine

Around the world, 57% of men and 10% of women smoke tobacco products, primarily cigarettes (Mackay and Eriksen 2002). In the United States, about 21% of the adult population smokes cigarettes (Centers for Disease Control and Prevention 2005). Clinically significant medication interactions with smoking include reduced levels of estradiol, haloperidol, imipramine, pentazocine, propranolol, and theophylline (Smith 2009).

Withdrawal

Symptoms of nicotine withdrawal are similar with all tobacco products, whether cigarettes, chewing tobacco, or snuff. Withdrawal symptoms include irritability, difficulty concentrating, restlessness, anxiety, depression, and increased appetite (Karan et al. 2003). Reaction time and attention are also impaired. Withdrawal symptoms peak around 48 hours after the last use, then gradually diminish over several weeks. Symptoms of dysphoria, anhedonia, and depression may continue for several months after cessation. The withdrawal syndrome from nicotine is similar to that of other stimulants.

Nicotine replacement therapy (NRT) is used in hospitalized smokers to treat acute nicotine withdrawal symptoms and to promote smoking cessation (Rigotti et al. 2008). Recent research supports including NRT in interventions for hospitalized smokers, along with counseling, because pharmacotherapy and counseling may be synergistic. Nicotine replacement products include a patch, gum, lozenge, nasal spray, and inhaler; all provide similar relief from withdrawal symptoms and efficacy for smoking cessation (Hajek et al. 1999). Even patients with hypertension and/or cardiovascular disease benefit from NRT, including those in an inpatient hospital setting (Joseph and Fu 2003). However, NRT is not routinely recommended for smokers with acute coronary syndromes because safety has not been established, and most of these patients have minimal nicotine withdrawal symptoms when they are hospitalized in a tobacco-free environment (Joseph and Fu 2003). Counseling for smoking cessation is appropriate for smokers hospitalized with acute cardiovascular complications. Clinically significant drug interactions of NRT include reduced analgesia from opioids and reduced sedation from benzodiazepines (Kroon 2006).

Pharmacological Treatment

Varenicline is a partial nicotinic receptor agonist (Mihalak et al. 2006) that signals dopamine release and creates reinforcing effects similar to those of nicotine but not to the full extent because of its partial binding of the receptor, and it acts as a physical antagonist by binding to the nicotine receptor and blocking the effects of nicotine. Varenicline is recommended as monotherapy because it blocks the effects of NRT as well as nicotine from tobacco. Varenicline's psychiatric side effects, including depression, agitation, hostility, and suicidality, have prompted an FDA black-box warning. Varenicline is renally excreted, so dose reductions are recommended in patients with renal insufficiency. It is without significant drug interactions. Varenicline's side effects of nausea and vomiting may be problematic in some medically ill patients.

Sustained-release bupropion increases smoking cessation rates by inhibiting dopamine uptake in the mesolimbic dopamine system (reward center) of the brain (Hurt et al. 1997). Bupropion may cause insomnia and may lower the seizure threshold (Dunner et al. 1998), so it is relatively contraindicated in patients with epilepsy or a recent seizure and should be used with caution in patients at risk for seizures (such as those at risk for acute alcohol withdrawal).

Both varenicline and bupropion exert their beneficial effects on smoking cessation over time and are usually started around 10 days prior to quitting smoking, so they may not be appropriate to start in hospitalized patients who are only beginning to consider smoking cessation.

Cannabis

Marijuana is the most frequently abused drug in the United States, with a prevalence of approximately 4% of the adult population that uses regularly. This rate has remained relatively steady since the early 1990s (Compton et al. 2004).

Intoxication

The onset of acute marijuana intoxication is within minutes when smoked, and the effects last for 3–4 hours (American Psychiatric Association 2000). Impairment of concentration and motor performance lasts for 12–24 hours as a result of accumulation of marijuana in adipose tissue, with slow release of tetrahydrocannabinol from fatty tissue stores and enterohepatic recirculation. Thus, a marijuana user may think that he or she is no longer impaired several hours after use when the acute mood-altering effects wear off. However, impairment of cognition, coordination, and judgment lasts much longer than the subjective feeling of being "high." Impairment is intensified by combination with other drugs, especially alcohol. This explains why fatal traffic accidents occur more often among individuals who have positive test results for marijuana use (Laumon et al. 2005).

Acute intoxication with marijuana alone rarely requires medical treatment, although dysphoria may result in distress that causes the user to seek help. First-time users, older persons, users of high-potency marijuana, and those predisposed to psychiatric illness are at higher risk for experiencing unpleasant effects during intoxication. Unpleasant effects of acute intoxication, such as anxiety, paranoia, or palpitations, are managed with supportive treatment. Placing the distraught user in a quiet environment and maintaining gentle contact is often sufficient until the acute effects subside; more severe paranoia or psychosis may require close observation with possible administration of a benzodiazepine or haloperidol for sedation.

Withdrawal

Heavy marijuana use for more than 3 weeks results in a withdrawal syndrome after abrupt cessation (Wiesbeck et al. 1996). Marijuana withdrawal begins within 10 hours of the last dose and consists of irritability, agitation, depression, insomnia, nausea, anorexia, and tremor. Most symptoms peak in 48 hours and last for 5–7 days. Some symptoms, such as unusual dreams and irritability, can persist for weeks (Budney et al. 2004). Marijuana withdrawal is uncomfortable but not life-threatening. Thus, treatment is entirely supportive and nearly always accomplished without the need for adjunctive medications.

Effects on Medical Disorders

Chronic marijuana use results in multiple psychiatric and medical consequences (Table 17–10). Marijuana use results in cognitive deficits that persist for at least hours after acute intoxication. Very heavy use is associated with persistent decrements in neurocognitive performance, even after 28 days of abstinence (Bolla et al. 2002). Marijuana abuse results in measurable health consequences and increases in health care costs (Pacula et al. 2008). A 1999 Institute of Medicine report (Watson et al. 2000) concluded that marijuana has potential therapeutic value for pain relief, control of nausea and vomiting, and appetite stimulation, but smoking it is a poor delivery system. Better alternatives are now available for nausea and vomiting caused by cancer chemotherapy. Data do not support its use for glaucoma. The literature to date suggests the plausibility of an association of marijuana smoking with lung cancer and head and neck cancer, but the data to date have not established it as a risk factor for either cancer (Berthiller et al. 2009; Mehra et al. 2006).

Hallucinogens

Drugs considered hallucinogens are a diverse group of compounds, including lysergic acid diethylamide (LSD), designer drugs, and many others (phencyclidine [PCP; angel dust], ketamine). Hallucinogens produce perceptual distortions and cognitive changes with a clear sensorium, without impairment in level of consciousness or attention (Abraham et al. 1996). Use of LSD dropped off in the 1980s but has increased in the 2000s, with a lifetime prevalence of use of 13% among young adults (Wu et al. 2006).

Intoxication

In general, acute physiological complications of hallucinogen intoxication rarely require medical treatment. However, malignant hyperthermia and seizures may occur with hallucinogen intoxication. Warning signs for hallucinogen hyperthermia are agitation, dry skin, and increased muscle tension. Intoxication with PCP causes a characteristic vertical nystagmus (it can also cause horizontal or rotatory nystagmus), which helps to identify it as the cause when a patient presents with intoxication by an unknown drug (Weaver and Schnoll 2007).

Effects on Medical and Psychiatric Disorders

Hallucinogen use may result in long-term psychiatric consequences, such as anxiety, depression, or psychosis. The risk of a prolonged psychiatric reaction depends on the user's underlying predisposition to develop psychopathology, the amount of prior hallucinogen use, the use of other drugs, and the dose and purity of the hallucinogen taken (Strassman 1984). Patients may present with apathy, hypomania, paranoia, delusions, hallucinations, formal thought disorder, or dissociative states. Treatment of prolonged anxiety, depression, or psychosis is the same as when these conditions are not associated with hallucinogen use.

Hallucinogen use also may result in medical consequences. Up to a third of frequent ketamine users experi-

TABLE 17–10. Effects of marijuana use

System	Acute effects	Chronic effects
Psychiatric	Euphoria Time distortion Anxiety Depression Paranoia Psychosis	Apathy, amotivation Exacerbation of schizophrenia
Cognitive	Impaired reaction time Impaired short-term memory	Verbal memory impairment Impaired attention
Respiratory	Tachypnea	Chronic obstructive pulmonary disease Lung cancer?
Other	Dry mouth Increased appetite Conjunctival injection	

ence severe gastrointestinal cramping known as "k-cramps," but the cause is unknown, and no treatment exists currently (Meutzelfeldt et al. 2008). PCP may cause hypertensive encephalopathy or life-threatening hyperthermia (Weaver and Schnoll 2008).

No pharmacological treatment is available for hallucinogen abuse (Abraham et al. 1996). Treatment settings for hallucinogen abuse focus on behavioral components such as individual and group counseling.

Gamma-Hydroxybutyrate

Gamma-hydroxybutyrate (GHB) is a sedative that is both a precursor and a metabolite of gamma-aminobutyric acid (GABA). It has been used as a sleep aid and for treatment of narcolepsy; it also increases episodic secretion of growth hormone, so some bodybuilders use it to promote muscle growth. After reports of GHB's toxicity resulted in its regulation by the U.S. government, 1,4-butanediol and gamma-butyrolactone, another precursor of GHB and an industrial solvent, began to be marketed as dietary supplements, both of which have similar effects and risk for abuse as GHB (Zvosec et al. 2001).

Intoxication

GHB's effects have been likened to those of alcohol, with mild euphoria, mild numbing, and pleasant disinhibition. GHB is not detectable by routine drug screening. The dose-response curve for GHB is exceedingly steep, so small increases in the amount ingested may lead to significant intensification of effects and onset of CNS depression. Concurrent use of sedatives or alcohol may increase the risk of vomiting, aspiration, or cardiopulmonary depression; use with stimulants may increase the risk of seizure. In cases of acute GHB intoxication, physicians should provide physiological support and maintain a high index of suspicion for intoxication with other drugs. Most patients who overdose on GHB or related compounds recover completely if they receive proper medical attention, but there have been deaths (Zvosec et al. 2001). Management of GHB ingestion in a spontaneously breathing patient (Li et al. 1998) includes oxygen supplementation, intravenous access, and comprehensive physiological and cardiac monitoring. Atropine can be used for persistent symptomatic bradycardia. Patients whose breathing is labored should be managed in the ICU.

Withdrawal

The symptoms of GHB withdrawal include anxiety, tremor, insomnia, and "feelings of doom," which may persist for several weeks after stopping the drug (Galloway et al. 1997). Severe withdrawal involves agitation, delirium, and psychosis (McDaniel and Miotto 2001). The treatment of GHB withdrawal is with benzodiazepines, which may require very high doses (Dyer et al. 2001). Antipsychotics or pentobarbital (Sivilotti et al. 2001) may have some utility in treatment of severe GHB withdrawal.

Inhalant Abuse

Inhalants are volatile substances that produce chemical vapors that can be inhaled for psychoactive effects. Examples of abused inhalants include glue, dry-cleaning fluids (carbon tetrachloride), gasoline, aerosol propellants from whipped cream cans or deodorant sprays, amyl nitrite, butyl nitrite, nitrous oxide ("laughing gas"), and some industrial solvents. Inhalants are second only to marijuana in likelihood of use by adolescents in the United States (Johnston et al. 2003), and about 10% continue to use beyond adolescence for more than 6 years (Neumark et al. 1998).

Many of the inhalants are similar to general anesthetics and sensitize the myocardium to catecholamines; fatal arrhythmias have been reported resulting from inhalant abuse (Shepherd 1989). Antiarrhythmic medications can be given as needed, and supplemental oxygen is administered for hypoxia and to enhance clearance of the inhalant. Chronic inhalant use by industrial workers has caused peripheral neuropathies (Lolin 1989), as well as hepatic, renal, and bone marrow damage (Marjot and McLeod 1989). Cases of methemoglobinemia have been reported secondary to butyl nitrite abuse (Bogart et al. 1986). Chronic complications of abuse usually clear if the patient remains abstinent, but impairment of working memory and executive cognitive function may persist. (See also Chapter 37, "Medical Toxicology.")

Linkage to Addiction Treatment

A psychiatric consultant can address acute issues of intoxication and withdrawal in the inpatient setting. Hospitalization affords an excellent opportunity ("teachable moment") for advising patients to decrease their substance use and for engaging them in treatment (Martins et al. 2007). Brief interventions with trauma patients who have a positive blood alcohol concentration at the time of injury can reduce their future alcohol intake and risk of trauma recidivism (Gentilello et al. 1999). Several inpatient substance abuse consultation services have been described in the literature, but there has been little formal assessment of their efficacy (Fleming et al. 1995; Fuller et al. 1995; McDuff et al. 1997; Murphy et al. 2009).

Acute and long-term treatments are necessary once the diagnosis of SUD is made (McLellan et al. 2000). Recovery from SUD is possible, and those who receive treatment have less disability than do those who do not receive treatment (Hasin et al. 2007). Hospitalized patients identified with SUD should be provided with information linking them to local community addiction treatment resources. In the United States, physicians certified in treatment of addictive disorders can be found through the American Society of Addiction Medicine (www.asam.org) or the American Academy of Addiction Psychiatry (www.aaap.org). At times, it may be more expedient and cost-effective to refer the patient to a nonphysician counselor, which can be found through the Association for Addiction Professionals (www.naadac.org). Nonpharmacological interventions such as stepped care interventions, contingency management (incentive-based interventions), and needle exchange programs are an essential part of treatment programs for substance abuse. However, for the medically ill, they are usually not a primary focus during hospitalization and consequently are beyond the scope of this chapter.

Impaired Health Care Providers

Some health care workers are at increased risk for addiction because of high-stress occupations and access to controlled substances. Rates of SUD among physicians are 10%–12%, approximately equivalent to the prevalence in the general population (DuPont et al. 2009). Anesthesiologists, emergency department physicians, and psychiatrists have higher rates of identified SUD (Berge et al. 2009). Health care practitioners have higher rates of abuse of opioids and benzodiazepines because of familiarity with and availability of these drugs in a health care setting. Impaired physicians usually have a history of substance abuse that began before medical training (McAuliffe et al. 1987). Initial problems usually affect personal relationships, but deterioration in clinical performance is often one of the last signs of an SUD (Table 17–11). Professionals often have the resources to conceal the addiction for a long time and so may have advanced disease by the time they seek treatment. Impaired performance as a result of drug use may have a significant effect on patient care (Baldisseri 2007).

A definitive diagnosis of SUD in a colleague is not required in order to take action by reporting. There are 49 active physician health programs in 48 states and the District of Columbia (DuPont et al. 2009). These programs are an alternative pathway to disciplinary action by state boards of medicine and are not designed to be punitive unless the physician refuses to comply with recommendations. Most European countries lag behind on national or hospital policies to deal with impaired physicians (Magnavita 2006). Basic elements of treatment for impaired physicians are similar to addiction treatment for nonphysicians, including detoxification, psychiatric and medical evaluation, group counseling, and 12-step attendance, but is often more intensive. Physicians have better outcomes than the general population and other impaired health care workers, with abstinence rates of 75% and successful return to work in 95% of those who complete monitoring (Ganley et al. 2005; McLellan et al. 2008).

TABLE 17–11. Signs of physician impairment

Behavioral	Physical	Workplace	Patient care	Other
Mood swings	Fatigue	Disorganized schedule	Missed appointments	Vague letters of reference
Defensiveness	Change in sleep pattern	Missed deadlines	Inaccessible	New jobs in different geographic areas
Impulsiveness	Weight loss or gain	Decreased work performance	Rounds at odd hours	Unexplained time off between jobs
Anxiousness	Pupil dilation	Frequent breaks	Inappropriate behavior	Prescriptions for family members
Personality changes	Conjunctival injection	Frequent lateness	Inappropriate orders	Heavy drinking at hospital functions
Strained communication	Stumbling	Frequent absences	Conflicts with patients	
Social isolation	Tremulousness	Inappropriate behavior with colleagues		
Changes in long-term relationships	Frequent colds and infections	Inaccessible to staff		
	Deterioration in physical fitness	Conflicts with staff and colleagues		
	Deterioration in personal hygiene	Ordering of large quantities of drugs		

Conclusion

The hospital setting is a good place to identify an SUD and initiate a brief intervention. Treating an SUD patient is not a hopeless process, and the long-term treatment of any chronic disorder can be challenging. Addiction treatment is cost-effective (Harwood et al. 2002), and even multiple episodes of treatment are worthwhile. It can be very rewarding for any health care practitioner to assist a patient who was impaired by addiction to return to normal functioning in society.

References

Abraham HD, Aldridge AM, Gogia P: The psychopharmacology of hallucinogens. Neuropsychopharmacology 14:285–298, 1996

Adunsky A, Levi R, Heim M: Meperidine analgesia and delirium in aged hip fracture patients. Arch Gerontol Geriatr 35:253–259, 2002

Alford DP, Compton P, Samet JH: Acute pain management for patients receiving maintenance methadone or buprenorphine therapy. Ann Intern Med 144:127–134, 2006

American Psychiatric Association: Diagnostic and Statistical Manual of Mental Disorders, 4th Edition, Text Revision. Washington, DC, American Psychiatric Association, 2000

American Society of Addiction Medicine: ASAM addiction terminology, in Principles of Addiction Medicine, 3rd Edition. Edited by Graham AW, Shultz TK. Chevy Chase, MD, American Society of Addiction Medicine, 2003, pp 1601–1606

Baldisseri MR: Impaired healthcare professional. Crit Care Med 35 (2 suppl):S106–S116, 2007

Baldwin WA, Rosenfeld BA, Breslow MJ, et al: Substance abuse-related admissions to adult intensive care. Chest 103:21–25, 1993

Ball J, Ross A: The Effectiveness of Methadone Maintenance Treatment. New York, Springer-Verlag, 1991

Bar K-J, Boettger MK, Koschke M, et al: Increased QT interval variability index in acute alcohol withdrawal. Drug Alcohol Depend 9:259–266, 2007

Bard MR, Goettler CE, Toschlog EA, et al: Alcohol withdrawal syndrome: turning minor injuries into a major problem. J Trauma 6:1441–1445, 2006

Benowitz NL: Clinical pharmacology and toxicology of cocaine. Pharmacol Toxicol 72:3–12, 1993

Berge KH, Seppala MD, Schipper AM: Chemical dependency and the physician. Mayo Clin Proc 84:625–631, 2009

Berthiller J, Lee YC, Boffetta P, et al: Marijuana smoking and the risk of head and neck cancer: pooled analysis in the INHANCE consortium. Cancer Epidemiol Biomarkers Prev 18:1544–1551, 2009

Blondell RD, Powell GE, Dodds HN, et al: Admission characteristics of trauma patients in whom delirium develops. Am J Surg 187:332–337, 2004

Bogart L, Bonsignore J, Carvalho A: Massive hemolysis following inhalation of volatile nitrites. Am J Hematol 22:327–329, 1986

Bolla KI, Brown K, Eldreth D, et al: Dose-related neurocognitive effects of marijuana use. Neurology 59:1337–1343, 2002

Brewer C, Wong VS: Naltrexone: report of lack of hepatotoxicity in acute viral hepatitis, with a review of the literature. Addict Biol 9:81–87, 2004

Brown RL, Rounds LA: Conjoint screening questionnaires for alcohol and other drug abuse: criterion validity in a primary care practice. Wis Med J 94:135–140, 1995

Buchanan JF, Brown CR: "Designer drugs": a problem in clinical toxicology. Med Toxicol Adverse Drug Exp 3:1–17, 1988

Buchsbaum DG, Buchanan RG, Centor RM, et al: Screening for alcohol using CAGE scores and likelihood ratios. Ann Intern Med 115:774–777, 1991

Budney AJ, Hughes JR, Moore BA, et al: Review of the validity and significance of cannabis withdrawal syndrome. Am J Psychiatry 161:1967–1977, 2004

Center for Substance Abuse Treatment (CSAT): Treatment Improvement Protocol 2: Pregnant Substance-Abusing Women. Rockville, MD, Center for Substance Abuse Treatment, 1993

Centers for Disease Control and Prevention (CDC): Cigarette smoking among adults—United States, 2004. MMWR Morb Mortal Wkly Rep 54:1121–1124, 2005

Chang PH, Steinberg MB: Alcohol withdrawal. Med Clin North Am 85:1191–1212, 2001

Christmas JT, Knisely JS, Dawson KS, et al: Comparison of questionnaire screening and urine toxicology for detection of pregnancy complicated by substance use. Obstet Gynecol 80:750–754, 1992

Cicero TJ, Inciardi JA, Munoz A: Trends in abuse of Oxycontin and other opioid analgesics in the United States: 2002–2004. J Pain 6:662–672, 2005

Cicero TJ, Dart RC, Inciardi JA, et al: The development of a comprehensive risk-management program for prescription opioid analgesics: researched abuse, diversion and addiction-related surveillance (RADARS). Pain Med 8:157–170, 2007

Compton WM, Grant BF, Colliver JD, et al: Prevalence of marijuana use disorders in the United States: 1991–1992 and 2001–2002. JAMA 291:2114–2121, 2004

Cooper JR, Altman F, Brown BS, et al: Research on the Treatment of Narcotic Addiction—State of the Art (NIDA Treatment Research Monograph Series). Rockville, MD, U.S. Department of Health and Human Services, 1983

Cross GM, Hennessey PT: Principles and practice of detoxification. Prim Care 20:81–93, 1993

Croughwell ND, Reves JG, Will CJ, et al: Safety of rapid administration of flumazenil in patients with ischaemic heart disease. Acta Anaesthesiol Scand Suppl 92:55–58, 1990

Dattilo PB, Hailpern SM, Fearon K, et al: Beta-blockers are associated with reduced risk of myocardial infarction after cocaine use. Ann Emerg Med 51:117–125, 2008

De Roux A, Cavalcanti M, Marcos MA, et al: Impact of alcohol abuse in the etiology and severity of community-acquired pneumonia. Chest 129:1219–1225, 2006

De Wit M, Gennings C, Zilerberg M, et al: Drug withdrawal, cocaine and sedative use disorders increase the need for mechanical ventilation in medical patients. Addiction 103:1500–1508, 2008

De Witte P, Littleton J, Parot P, et al: Neuroprotective and abstinence-promoting effects of acamprosate: elucidating the mechanism of action. CNS Drugs 19:517–537, 2005

Delgado-Rodríguez M, Gómez-Ortega A, Mariscal-Ortiz M, et al: Alcohol drinking as a predictor of intensive care and hospital mortality in general surgery: a prospective study. Addiction 98:611–616, 2003

Di Gennaro C, Biggi A, Barilli AL, et al: Endothelial dysfunction and cardiovascular risk profile in long-term withdrawing alcoholics. J Hypertens 25:367–373, 2007

Drug Abuse Warning Network (DAWN): Emergency department trends from DAWN: final estimates 1995–2002 (DAWN Series D-24, DHHS Publ. No. SMA 03-3780). Rockville, MD, Substance Abuse and Mental Health Services Administration, August 2003

Dubois MJ, Bergeron N, Dumont M, et al: Delirium in an intensive care unit: a study of risk factors. Intensive Care Med 27:1297–1304, 2001

Dunbar JL, Turncliff RZ, Dong Q, et al: Single- and multiple-dose pharmacokinetics of long-acting injectable naltrexone. Alcohol Clin Exp Res 30:480–490, 2006

Dunner DL, Zisook S, Billow AA, et al: A prospective safety surveillance study for bupropion sustained-release in the treatment of depression. J Clin Psychiatry 59:366–373, 1998

DuPont RL, McLellan AT, Carr G, et al: How are addicted physicians treated? A national survey of Physician Health Programs. J Subst Abuse Treat 37:1–7, 2009

Dyer J, Roth B, Hyma BA: Gamma-hydroxybutyrate withdrawal syndrome. Ann Emerg Med 37:147–153, 2001

Ehret GB, Voide C, Gex-Fabry M, et al: Drug-induced long QT syndrome in injection drug users receiving methadone: high frequency in hospitalized patients and risk factors. Arch Intern Med 166:1280–1287, 2006

Elisaf M, Liberopoulos E, Bairaktari E, et al: Hypokalaemia in alcoholic patients. Drug Alcohol Rev 21:73–76, 2002

Falk DE, Yi HY, Hiller-Stermhofel S: An epidemiologic analysis of alcohol and tobacco use and disorders: findings from the National Epidemiologic Survey on Alcohol and Related Conditions. Alcohol Res Health 29:162–171, 2006

Farooq MU, Bhatt A, Patel M: Neurotoxic and cardiotoxic effects of cocaine and ethanol. J Med Toxicol 5:134–138, 2009

Ferguson v City of Charleston, 532 U.S. 67 (2001)

Ferrari A, Coccia CP, Bertolini A, et al: Methadone—metabolism, pharmacokinetics and interactions. Pharmacol Res 50:551–559, 2004

Fischer G, Johnson RE, Eder H, et al: Treatment of opioid-dependent pregnant women with buprenorphine. Addiction 95:239–244, 2000

Fleming MF, Wilk A, Kruger J, et al: Hospital-based alcohol and drug specialty consultation service: does it work? South Med J 88:275–282, 1995

Fuller MG, Diamond DL, Jordan ML, et al: The role of a substance abuse consultation team in a trauma center. J Stud Alcohol 56:267–271, 1995

Galloway GP, Frederick SL, Staggers FE, et al: Gamma-hydroxybutyrate: an emerging drug of abuse that causes physical dependence. Addiction 92:89–96, 1997

Ganley OH, Pendergast WJ, Wilkerson MW, et al: Outcome study of substance impaired physicians and physician assistants under contract with North Carolina Physicians Health Program for the period 1995–2000. J Addict Dis 24:1–12, 2005

Gentilello LM, Rivara FP, Donovan DM, et al: Alcohol interventions in a trauma center as a means of reducing the risk of injury recurrence. Ann Surg 230:473–480, 1999

Gillman PK: Monoamine oxidase inhibitors, opioid analgesics and serotonin toxicity. Br J Anaesth 95:434–441, 2005

Gold JA, Rimal B, Nolan A, et al: A strategy of escalating doses of benzodiazepines and phenobarbital administration reduces the need for mechanical ventilation in delirium tremens. Crit Care Med 35:724–730, 2007

Gouzoulis-Mayfrank E, Daumann J, Tuchtenhagen F, et al: Impaired cognitive performance in drug free users of recreational ecstasy (MDMA). J Neurol Neurosurg Psychiatry 68:719–725, 2000

Gowing L, Farrell M, Ali R, et al: Alpha2 adrenergic agonists for the management of opioid withdrawal. Cochrane Database Syst Rev (4):CD002024, 2004

Gronbladh L, Ohlund LS, Gunne LM: Mortality in heroin addiction: impact of methadone treatment. Acta Psychiatr Scand 82:223–227, 1990

Grunkemeier DM, Cassara JE, Dalton CB, et al: The narcotic bowel syndrome: clinical features, pathophysiology, and management. Clin Gastroenterol Hepatol 5:1126–1139, 2007

Guttmacher Institute: Substance abuse during pregnancy [State Policies in Brief]. August 1, 2009. Available at: http://www.guttmacher.org/statecenter/spibs/spib_SADP.pdf. Accessed August 16, 2009

Hadama A, Ieiri I, Morita T, et al: P-hydroxylation of phenobarbital: relationship to (S) mephenytoin hydroxylation (CYP2C19) polymorphism. Ther Drug Monit 23:115–118, 2001

Hajak G, Muller WE, Wittchen HU, et al: Abuse and dependence potential for the non-benzodiazepine hypnotics zolpidem and zopiclone: a review of case reports and epidemiological data. Addiction 98:1371–1378, 2003

Hajek P, West R, Foulds J, et al: Randomized comparative trial of nicotine polacrilex, a transdermal patch, nasal spray, and an inhaler. Arch Intern Med 159:2033–2038, 1999

Hall AP, Henry JA: Acute toxic effects of 'Ecstasy' (MDMA) and related compounds: overview of pathophysiology and clinical management. Br J Anaesth 96:678–685, 2006

Harwood HJ, Malhotra D, Villarivera C, et al: Cost Effectiveness and Cost Benefit Analysis of Substance Abuse Treatment: A Literature Review. Falls Church, VA, The Lewin Group for the Center for Substance Abuse Treatment, Substance Abuse and Mental Health Services Administration, 2002

Hasin DS, Stinson FS, Ogburn E, et al: Prevalence, correlates, disability, and comorbidity of DSM-IV alcohol abuse and dependence in the United States. Arch Gen Psychiatry 64:830–842, 2007

Hurt RD, Sachs DP, Glover ED, et al: A comparison of sustained-release bupropion and placebo for smoking cessation. N Engl J Med 337:1195–1202, 1997

Jansson LM, Dipietro JA, Velez M, et al: Maternal methadone dosing schedule and fetal neurobehaviour. J Matern Fetal Neonatal Med 22:29–35, 2009

Jessup M, Green JR: Treatment of the pregnant alcohol-dependent woman. J Psychoactive Drugs 19:193–203, 1987

Johnson BA: Update on neuropharmacological treatments for alcoholism: scientific basis and clinical findings. Biochem Pharmacol 75:34–56, 2008

Johnston LD, O'Malley PM, Bachman JG: Monitoring the Future National Survey Results on Drug Use, 1975–2001, Vol 1: Secondary School Students. Rockville, MD, National Institute on Drug Abuse, 2002

Johnston LD, O'Malley PM, Bachman JG: Monitoring the Future National Results on Adolescent Drug Use: Overview of Key Findings. Bethesda, MD, National Institute on Drug Abuse, 2003

Jones HE, Johnson RE, Jasinski DR, et al: Randomized controlled study transitioning opioid-dependent pregnant women from short-acting morphine to buprenorphine or methadone. Drug Alcohol Depend 79:1–10, 2005

Joseph AM, Fu SS: Smoking cessation for patients with cardiovascular disease: what is the best approach? Am J Cardiovasc Drugs 3:339–349, 2003

Kakko J, Svanborg KD, Kreek MJ, et al: 1-Year retention and social function after buprenorphine-assisted relapse prevention treatment for heroin dependence in Sweden: a randomised, placebo-controlled trial. Lancet 361:662–668, 2003

Karan LD, Dani JA, Benowitz N: The pharmacology of nicotine and tobacco, in Principles of Addiction Medicine, 3rd Edition. Edited by Graham AW, Shultz TK. Chevy Chase, MD, American Society of Addiction Medicine, 2003, pp 225–248

Katz A, Goldberg D, Smith J, et al: Tobacco, alcohol, and drug use among hospital patients: concurrent use and willingness to change. J Hosp Med 3:369–375, 2008

Khan A, Levy P, Dehorn S, et al: Predictors of mortality in patients with delirium tremens. Acad Emerg Med 15:788–790, 2008

Kouimtsidis C, Reynolds M, Hunt M, et al: Substance use in the general hospital. Addict Behav 28:483–499, 2003

Krantz MJ, Lewkowiez L, Hays H, et al: Torsade de pointes associated with very-high-dose methadone. Ann Intern Med 137:501–504, 2002

Kroon LA: Drug interactions and smoking: raising awareness for acute and critical care providers. Crit Care Nurs Clin North Am 18:53–62, 2006

Lansford CD, Guerriero CH, Kocan MJ, et al: Improved outcomes in patients with head and neck cancer using a standardized care protocol for postoperative alcohol withdrawal. Arch Otolaryngol Head Neck Surg 134:865–872, 2008

Laumon B, Gadegbeku B, Martin JL, et al: Cannabis intoxication and fatal road crashes in France: population based case-control study. BMJ 331:1371–1376, 2005

Li J, Stokes S, Woeckener A: A tale of novel intoxication: a review of the effects of gamma-hydroxybutyric acid with recommendations for management. Ann Emerg Med 31:729–736, 1998

Lolin Y: Chronic neurological toxicity associated with exposure to volatile substances. Hum Toxicol 8:293–300, 1989

Lucey MR, Weinrieb RM: Alcohol and substance abuse. Semin Liver Dis 29:66–73, 2009

Lui S, Terplan M, Smith EJ: Psychosocial interventions for women enrolled in alcohol treatment during pregnancy. Cochrane Database Syst Rev (3):CD006753, 2008

Mackay J, Eriksen M: The Tobacco Atlas. Geneva, Switzerland, World Health Organization, 2002, pp 24–27

Magnavita N: Management of impaired physicians in Europe. Med Lav 97:762–773, 2006

Manghi RA, Broers B, Khan R, et al: Khat use: lifestyle or addiction? J Psychoactive Drugs 41:1–10, 2009

Marjot R, McLeod AA: Chronic non-neurological toxicity from volatile substance abuse. Hum Toxicol 8:301–306, 1989

Martell BA, Arnsten JH, Krantz MJ, et al: Impact of methadone treatment on cardiac repolarization and conduction in opioid users. Am J Cardiol 95:915–918, 2005

Martins SS, Copersino ML, Soderstrom CA, et al: Sociodemographic characteristics associated with substance use status in a trauma inpatient population. J Addict Dis 26:53–62, 2007

Mason BJ, Goodman AM, Dixon RM, et al: A pharmacokinetic and pharmacodynamic drug interaction study of acamprosate and naltrexone. Neuropsychopharmacology 27:596–606, 2002

Mayo-Smith MF: Pharmacological management of alcohol withdrawal: a meta-analysis and evidence-based practice guideline. JAMA 278:144–151, 1997

McAuliffe WE, Santangelo S, Magnuson E, et al: Risk factors of drug impairment in random samples of physicians and medical students. Int J Addict 22:825–841, 1987

McCarthy JJ, Posey BL: Methadone levels in human milk. J Hum Lact 16:115–120, 2000

McCowan C, Marik P: Refractory delirium tremens treated with propofol: a case series. Crit Care Med 28:1781–1784, 2000

McDaniel CH, Miotto KA: Gamma hydroxybutyrate (GHB) and gamma butyrolactone (GBL) withdrawal: five case studies. J Psychoactive Drugs 33:143–149, 2001

McDuff DR, Solounias BL, Beuger M, et al: A substance abuse consultation service: enhancing the care of hospitalized substance abusers and providing training in addiction psychiatry. Am J Addict 6:256–265, 1997

McLellan AT, Lewis DC, O'Brien CP, et al: Drug dependence, a chronic medical illness: implications for treatment, insurance, and outcomes evaluation. JAMA 284:1689–1695, 2000

McLellan AT, Skipper GS, Campbell M, et al: Five year outcomes in a cohort study of physicians treated for substance use disorders in the United States. BMJ 337:a2038, 2008

Mehra R, Moore BA, Crothers K, et al: The association between marijuana smoking and lung cancer: a systematic review. Arch Intern Med 166:1359–1367, 2006

Meutzelfeldt L, Kamboj SK, Rees H, et al: Journey through the K-hole: phenomenological aspects of ketamine use. Drug Alcohol Depend 95:219–229, 2008

Mihalak KB, Carroll FI, Luetje CW: Varenicline is a partial agonist at alpha4beta2 and a full agonist at alpha7 neuronal nicotinic receptors. Mol Pharmacol 70:801–805, 2006

Minozzi S, Amato L, Vecchi S, et al: Maintenance agonist treatments for opiate dependent pregnant women. Cochrane Database Syst Rev (2):CD006318, 2008

Mondanaro J, Reed B: Current Issues in the Treatment of Chemically Dependent Women (NIDA Research Monograph Series). Rockville, MD, U.S. Department of Health and Human Services, 1987

Monte Secades R, Casariego Vales E, Pértega Díaz S, et al: [Clinical course and features of the alcohol withdrawal syndrome in a general hospital]. Rev Clin Esp 208:506–512, 2008

Murphy MK, Chabon B, Delgado A, et al: Development of a substance abuse consultation and referral service in an academic medical center: challenges, achievements and dissemination. J Clin Psychol Med Settings 16:77–86, 2009

Neumark YD, Delva J, Anthony JC: The epidemiology of adolescent inhalant drug involvement. Arch Pediatr Adolesc Med 152:781–786, 1998

Ng SK, Hauser WA, Brust JC, et al: Alcohol consumption and withdrawal in new-onset seizures. N Engl J Med 319:666–673, 1988

O'Connor AD, Rusyniak DE, Bruno A: Cerebrovascular and cardiovascular complications of alcohol and sympathomimetic drug abuse. Med Clin North Am 89:1343–1358, 2005

O'Shea B: Disulfiram revisited. Hosp Med 61:849–851, 2000

Olkkola KT, Ahonen J: Midazolam and other benzodiazepines. Handb Exp Pharmacol 182:335–360, 2008

Oscher FC, Kofoed LL: Treatment of patients with psychiatric and psychoactive substance use disorders. Hosp Community Psychiatry 40:1025–1030, 1989

Pacula RL, Ringel J, Dobkin C, et al: The incremental inpatient costs associated with marijuana comorbidity. Drug Alcohol Depend 92:248–257, 2008

Page RL 2nd, Utz KJ, Wolfel EE: Should beta-blockers be used in the treatment of cocaine-associated acute coronary syndrome? Ann Pharmacother 41:2008–2013, 2007

Parker WA: Alcohol-containing pharmaceuticals. Am J Drug Alcohol Abuse 9:195–209, 1982–1983

Pennings EJ, Opperhuizen A, van Amsterdam JG: Risk assessment of khat use in the Netherlands: a review based on adverse health effects, prevalence, criminal involvement and public order. Regul Toxicol Pharmacol 52:199–207, 2008

Petry NM, Bickel WK, Piasecki D, et al: Elevated liver enzyme levels in opioid-dependent patients with hepatitis treated with buprenorphine. Am J Addict 9:265–269, 2000

Reissig CJ, Strain EC, Griffiths RR: Caffeinated energy drinks—a growing problem. Drug Alcohol Depend 99:1–10, 2009

Richardson GS, Roth T: Future directions in the management of insomnia. J Clin Psychiatry 62 (suppl 10):39–45, 2001

Rigotti NA, Munafo MR, Stead LF: Smoking cessation interventions for hospitalized smokers: a systematic review. Arch Intern Med 168:1950–1960, 2008

Ritson B, Chick J: Comparison of two benzodiazepines in the treatment of alcohol withdrawal: effects on symptoms and cognitive recovery. Drug Alcohol Depend 18:329–334, 1986

Saitz R: Introduction to alcohol withdrawal. Alcohol Health Res World 22:5–12, 1998

Schuckit MA: The treatment of stimulant dependence. Addiction 89:1559–1563, 1994

Schuckit MA, Tapert S: Alcohol, in The American Psychiatric Publishing Textbook of Substance Abuse Treatment, 3rd Edition. Edited by Galanter M, Kleber HD. Washington, DC, American Psychiatric Publishing, 2004, pp 151–166

Sechi G, Serra A: Wernicke's encephalopathy: new clinical settings and recent advances in diagnosis and management. Lancet Neurol 6:442–455, 2007

Shepherd RT: Mechanism of sudden death associated with volatile substance abuse. Hum Toxicol 8:287–291, 1989

Sivilotti ML, Burns MJ, Aaron CK, et al: Pentobarbital for severe gamma-butyrolactone withdrawal. Ann Emerg Med 38:660–665, 2001

Smith RG: An appraisal of potential drug interactions in cigarette smokers and alcohol drinkers. J Am Podiatr Med Assoc 99:81–88, 2009

Soderstrom CA, Smith GS, Dischinger PC, et al: Psychoactive substance use disorders among seriously injured trauma center patients. JAMA 277:1769–1774, 1997

Spanagel R, Zeiglgansberger W: Anti-craving compounds for ethanol: new pharmacological tools to study addictive processes. Trends Pharmacol Sci 18:54–59, 1997

Stade BC, Bailey C, Dzendoletas D, et al: Psychological and/or educational interventions for reducing alcohol consumption in pregnant women and women planning pregnancy. Cochrane Database Syst Rev (2):CD004228, 2009

Stinson FS, Grant BF, Dawson DA, et al: Comorbidity between DSM-IV alcohol and specific drug use disorders in the United States: results from the national epidemiologic survey on alcohol and related conditions. Drug Alcohol Depend 80:105–116, 2005

Strang J, McCambridge J, Best D, et al: Loss of tolerance and overdose mortality after inpatient opiate detoxification: follow up study. BMJ 326:959–960, 2003

Strassman RJ: Adverse reactions to psychedelic drugs: a review of the literature. J Nerv Ment Dis 172:577–595, 1984

Substance Abuse and Mental Health Services Administration (SAMHSA): Results From the 2005 National Survey on Drug Use and Health: National Findings (Office of Applied Studies, NSDUH Series H-30, DHHS Publ No SMA 06-4194). Rockville, MD, Substance Abuse and Mental Health Services Administration, 2006

Sullivan JT, Sykora K, Schneiderman J, et al: Assessment of alcohol withdrawal: the Revised Clinical Institute Withdrawal Assessment for Alcohol Scale (CIWA-Ar). Br J Addict 84:1353–1357, 1989

Terplan M, Lui S: Psychosocial interventions for pregnant women in outpatient illicit drug treatment programs compared to other interventions. Cochrane Database Syst Rev (4):CD006037, 2007

Thomson AD: Mechanisms of vitamin deficiency in chronic alcohol misusers and the development of Wernicke-Korsakoff syndrome. Alcohol Alcohol 35(suppl):2–7, 2000

Thomson AD, Cook CCH, Touquet R, et al: The Royal College of Physicians report on alcohol: guidelines for managing Wernicke's encephalopathy in the accident and emergency department. Alcohol Alcohol 37(suppl):513–521, 2002

Tracqui A, Kintz P, Ludes B: Buprenorphine-related deaths among drug addicts in France: a report on 20 fatalities. J Anal Toxicol 22:430–434, 1998

Turner RC, Lichstein PR, Peden JG Jr, et al: Alcohol withdrawal syndromes: a review of pathophysiology, clinical presentation, and treatment. J Gen Intern Med 4:432–444, 1989

United Nations Office on Drugs and Crime: Ecstasy and Amphetamines, Global Survey. New York, United Nations Publications, 2003

Vickers AP, Jolly A: Naltrexone and problems in pain management. BMJ 332:132–133, 2006

Victorri-Vigneau C, Dailly E, Veyrac G, et al: Evidence of zolpidem abuse and dependence: results of the French Centre for Evaluation and Information on Pharmacodependence (CEIP) network survey. Br J Clin Pharmacol 64:198–209, 2007

Virmani R, Robinowitz M, Smialek JE, et al: Cardiovascular effects of cocaine: an autopsy study of 40 patients. Am Heart J 115:1068–1076, 1988

Walsh SL, Eissenberg T: The clinical pharmacology of buprenorphine: extrapolating from the laboratory to the clinic. Drug Alcohol Depend 70:S13–S27, 2003

Watson SJ, Benson JA Jr, Joy JE: Marijuana and medicine: assessing the science base: a summary of the 1999 Institute of Medicine report. Arch Gen Psychiatry 57:547–552, 2000

Weaver MF: Perinatal addiction, in Principles of Addiction Medicine, 3rd Edition. Edited by Graham AW, Shultz TK. Chevy Chase, MD, American Society of Addiction Medicine, 2003, pp 1231–1246

Weaver MF: Dealing with the DTs: managing alcohol withdrawal in hospitalized patients. Hospitalist 11:22–25, 2007

Weaver MF, Schnoll SH: Drug overdose and withdrawal syndromes. Curr Opin Crit Care 2:242–247, 1996

Weaver MF, Schnoll SH: Stimulants: amphetamines and cocaine, in Addictions: A Comprehensive Guidebook. Edited by McCrady BS, Epstein EE. New York, Oxford University Press, 1999, pp 105–120

Weaver MF, Schnoll SH: Abuse liability in opioid therapy for pain treatment in patients with an addiction history. Clin J Pain 18:S61–S69, 2002

Weaver MF, Schnoll SH: Phencyclidine and ketamine, in Gabbard's Treatments of Psychiatric Disorders, 4th Edition. Glen O. Gabbard, M.D., Editor in Chief. Washington, DC, American Psychiatric Publishing, 2007, pp 271–280

Weaver MF, Schnoll SH: Hallucinogens and club drugs, in The American Psychiatric Publishing Textbook of Substance

Abuse Treatment, 4th Edition. Edited by Galanter M, Kleber HD. Washington, DC, American Psychiatric Publishing, 2008, pp 191–200

Weaver MF, Jarvis MAE, Schnoll SH: Role of the primary care physician in problems of substance abuse. Arch Intern Med 159:913–924, 1999

Weaver MF, Cropsey KL, Fox S: HCV prevalence in methadone maintenance: self-report versus serum test. Am J Health Behav 29:387–394, 2005

Weaver MF, Hoffman HJ, Johnson R, et al: Alcohol withdrawal pharmacotherapy for inpatients with medical comorbidity. J Addict Dis 25:17–24, 2006

Weaver MF, Jewell C, Tomlinson J: Phenobarbital for alcohol withdrawal. J Addict Nurs 20:1–5, 2009

Wedam EF, Bigelow GE, Johnson RE, et al: QT-interval effects of methadone, levomethadyl, and buprenorphine in a randomized trial. Arch Intern Med 167:2469–2475, 2007

Weinbroum AA, Flaishon R, Sorkine P, et al: A risk-benefit assessment of flumazenil in the management of benzodiazepine overdose. Drug Saf 17:181–196, 1997

Weinrieb RM, Van Horn DH, McLellan AT, et al: Interpreting the significance of drinking by alcohol-dependent liver transplant patients: fostering candor is the key to recovery. Liver Transpl 6:769–776, 2000

Weissman DE, Haddox JD: Opioid pseudoaddiction: an iatrogenic syndrome. Pain 36:363–366, 1989

Wiesbeck GA, Schuckit MA, Kalmijn JA, et al: An evaluation of the history of a marijuana withdrawal syndrome in a large population. Addiction 91:1469–1478, 1996

Wilkerson RD: Cardiovascular toxicity of cocaine. NIDA Res Monogr 88:304–324, 1988

Williams CS, Woodcock KR: Do ethanol and metronidazole interact to produce a disulfiram-like reaction? Ann Pharmacother 34:255–257, 2000

Williams G, Daly M, Proude EM, et al: The influence of alcohol and tobacco use in orthopaedic inpatients on complications of surgery. Drug Alcohol Rev 27:55–64, 2008

Winklbaur B, Kopf N, Ebner N, et al: Treating pregnant women dependent on opioids is not the same as treating pregnancy and opioid dependence: a knowledge synthesis for better treatment for women and neonates. Addiction 103:1429–1440, 2008

Wu LT, Schlenger WE, Galvin DM: Concurrent use of methamphetamine, MDMA, LSD, ketamine, GHB, and flunitrazepam among American youths. Drug Alcohol Depend 84:102–113, 2006

Zvosec DL, Smith SW, McCutcheon JR, et al: Adverse events, including death, associated with the use of 1,4-butanediol. N Engl J Med 344:87–94, 2001

PART III

Specialties and Subspecialties

CHAPTER

18

Heart Disease

Peter A. Shapiro, M.D.

CARDIOVASCULAR DISEASE is the cause of death for one-third of American adults (Lloyd-Jones et al. 2009) and the leading cause of death in the developed world. Although some patients experience sudden fatal illness, many have a disease with chronic course that has a marked impact on their life experience. The interface between psychiatry and cardiovascular disease is complex, including both the effects of psychosocial factors on the heart and vascular system and the effects of cardiovascular disease on the brain, psychological function, and psychopathology. Many psychological states and traits have been identified as contributing to risk for the development or exacerbation of heart disease, especially coronary disease, including anxiety, panic, anger, Type A behavior pattern, depression, stress, Type D personality, and sleep disorders. Treatments for psychiatric disorders may also increase cardiovascular disease risk. Behavioral disorders, some associated with psychiatric illness, such as sedentary lifestyle, overeating, smoking, and alcohol abuse also add to the risk of heart disease, especially coronary disease. Conversely, the experience of heart disease seems to contribute to risk for numerous psychiatric problems, especially depression, anxiety, and cognitive disorders. Not only are the psychological effects of dealing with cardiac illness complicated and profound, but also medications and other treatments for heart diseases often have psychiatric effects. Because heart disease is so common, psychiatrists must expect to deal with the effects of cardiovascular comorbidity in the care of their patients, evaluating the role of medical factors in their mental health and recognizing the potential impact of psychiatric interventions on the cardiovascular system (Birkenaes et al. 2006; Rathore et al. 2008). Unfortunately, patients with serious mental disorders tend to receive insufficient screening and treatment for heart disease (Albert et al. 2009; Kisely et al. 2009; Laursen et al. 2009; Osborn et al. 2006; Rathore et al. 2008), and many patients with heart disease rely on untested complementary and alternative medicine techniques to address emotional stress, depression, and anxiety (Yeh et al. 2006).

Coronary Artery Disease

Aggressive attention to primary prevention measures has reduced the incidence of coronary artery disease (CAD) in the United States over the past 20 years, and early mortality after acute coronary events (Lloyd-Jones et al. 2009). Traditional CAD risk factors include hypertension, smoking, dyslipidemia, diabetes mellitus, male sex, and family history. Increased public awareness about modifiable coronary risk factors and dissemination of effective treatments have resulted in reduction in the prevalence of some of these factors. Nevertheless, the incidence of first acute myocardial infarction (MI) is about 650,000 cases per year in the United States, and of recurrent MI about 350,000 per year (Lloyd-Jones et al. 2009). One-third of patients die within the first hour after the onset of symptoms, before receiving any treatment. Aggressive use of thrombolysis and revascularization procedures, beta-adrenergic blockers, angiotensin-converting enzyme (ACE) inhibitors and angiotensin II receptor blockers, statins, and aspirin and other antiplatelet agents has reduced mortality in those who survive long enough to receive acute care. Estimated 28-day survival after acute MI for patients who survive to hospital admission is over 90%.

Congestive Heart Failure

The prevalence of congestive heart failure (CHF) in the United States is over 2%—a figure essentially unchanged over the past two decades. In individuals older than 65 years, the incidence of heart failure approaches 1% per year. By and large, heart failure is characterized by an inexorable if gradual downhill course. The 5-year mortality of CHF is 50%, generally within 1 year after the onset of advanced symptoms, although rescue therapies such as ventricular assist devices may alter this trajectory. The primary modes of death in heart failure are pump failure and cardiac arrhythmias (Jessup and Brozena 2003). Treatment with beta-adrenergic blockers, ACE inhibitors, angiotensin II receptor blockers, spironolactone, and implantable cardiac defibrillators reduces the risk of death, whereas inotropic agents have largely failed to do so, although they improve functional status in severely ill patients (Cohn 1996; Jessup and Brozena 2003). New treatments in heart failure include the use of biventricular pacing and long-term ventricular assist devices, which hold the promise of improving survival and quality of life (Cazeau et al. 2001; Jessup and Brozena 2003; Rose et al. 2001; Slaughter et al. 2009).

Psychiatric Disorders in Heart Disease

The development of cardiac disease in a previously well individual is associated with a variety of psychological reactions. Perhaps most fundamentally, it is difficult to maintain denial about one's mortality after a cardiac event. Viewing oneself as having heart disease has effects at every level of psychological development: increasing concerns about dependency, autonomy, control, and ability to provide for others; provoking loss of self-esteem and concern about loss of love; and inciting fears about vitality, sexuality, and mortality. The maintenance of denial has been associated with mental well-being (Levenson et al. 1989; Levine et al. 1987) and may manifest as minimizing the severity of the event ("I just had a small attack") or attributing symptoms to a noncardiac source ("gas pains"), but excessive denial can be detrimental to health because of delay in seeking treatment or failure to accept the need to maintain a treatment regimen (Cassem 1985). In contrast, inadequate denial, or exaggeration of the illness, can lead to invalidism or mental disorder in the cardiac patient.

Attention to one's heartbeat, conscious experience of twinges of chest pain or palpitations, and other preoccupations with minor physical symptoms may result in hypochondriacal avoidance of activity and increased visits to the doctor and emergency room. Research with hypochondriacal, somatizing, and panic disorder patients, who make up a large portion of patients presenting to emergency rooms with noncardiac chest pain, has demonstrated the high level of somatic awareness common in such patients (Barsky 1992; Barsky et al. 1994b, 1996).

Depression

Depression in Coronary Artery Disease

Depression appears to be the most common psychiatric disorder in CAD patients (Barth et al. 2004; Glassman and Shapiro 1998; Rugulies 2002; van Melle et al. 2004; Wulsin and Singal 2003). Numerous surveys of patients with established coronary disease, acute MI, and unstable angina consistently indicate a point prevalence of depression in the range of 15%–20% (Barth et al. 2004; Shapiro et al. 1997; van Melle et al. 2004). In a study of 200 patients interviewed after diagnostic coronary angiography confirmed a diagnosis of CAD, 16% met the criteria for major depressive disorder, and 17% met the criteria for minor depression. Most patients with major depression and about half of those with minor depression were found to have major depression at 1-year follow-up (Hance et al. 1996). Studies in post-MI patients in Europe, Canada, and the United States also converge on a point prevalence of depression of about 15% (Barth et al. 2004; Frasure-Smith et al. 1993; Ladwig et al. 1991; Schleifer et al. 1989; van Melle et al. 2004). This figure is remarkable in light of national surveys indicating a lifetime prevalence of depression of approximately 16% in the general population (Kessler et al. 2003). Three studies of patients following coronary artery bypass graft surgery also demonstrate a point prevalence of depression in the range of 20%–30% (Blumenthal et al. 2003; Connerney et al. 2001; Shapiro et al. 1998). Elevated symptom scores on depression rating scales such as the Beck Depression Inventory are even more common and may predict subsequent major depression (Frasure-Smith et al. 1995a, 1995b).

Many studies indicate a widespread failure to diagnose and treat depression in CAD patients (Frasure-Smith et al. 1993; Luutonen et al. 2002). In a Finnish study (Luutonen et al. 2002) of 85 consecutive post-MI patients with 18-month follow-up, the prevalence of Beck Depression Inventory scores of 10 or greater was 21% in the hospital, 30% at 6 months, and 33.9% at 18 months. Only 6 patients received mental health treatment; 2 received benzodiazepines; none received adequate antidepressant therapy. In the Montreal Heart Institute sample, none of 35 patients identified with major depression by research interviews in the post-MI hospital stay received antidepressants (Frasure-Smith et al. 1993). In another study of patients with newly diagnosed CAD, one-sixth of the sample met the criteria for major depression; at 1-year follow-up, only one-sixth of those who were depressed had received treatment (Hance et al. 1996). The availability of good social support reduces the likelihood of persistent depression after an acute coronary event (Frasure-Smith et al. 1995b, 2000). Current guidelines (Davidson et al. 2006; Lichtman et al. 2008) recommend screening for depression in patients with CAD, but the added value of screening is not established (Thombs et al. 2008).

Depression in Congestive Heart Failure

Fewer studies have examined the prevalence of depression in patients with CHF, but as in patients with coronary disease, a point prevalence of major depression around 20% is suggested by available data (Faris et al. 2002; Freedland et al. 2003; Jiang et al. 2001; Rutledge et al. 2006; Westlake et al. 2005). An additional 30%–35% of patients have subsyndromal or mild depression symptoms (Jiang et al. 2001; Westlake et al. 2005). Patients with more severe depression symptoms tend to have worse New York Heart Association (NYHA) functional class and exercise tolerance (Westlake et al. 2005). In the Randomized Evaluation of Mechanical Assistance for the Treatment of Congestive Heart Failure (REMATCH) trial, a study comparing left ventricular assist device (LVAD) implantation with medical therapy for patients with chronic, end-stage CHF, the mean baseline Beck Depression Inventory score was over 16, indicating moderate to severe depression symptoms, and more than two-thirds of patients had a score over 10 (mild depression) (Rose et al. 2001).

Anxiety

Anxiety in Coronary Artery Disease

The prevalence of anxiety disorders in CAD has not been as well studied as that of depression, but anxiety symptoms are clearly elevated in patients with acute coronary disease and in more than 5%–10% of patients with chronic heart disease (Sullivan et al. 2000). A study of more than 800 patients with stable CAD found a prevalence of generalized anxiety disorder of 5.3%, and elevated anxiety symptoms in 41% (Frasure-Smith and Lesperance 2008). Intense subjective distress and fear of dying immediately after an acute coronary event increase the risk for clinically significant anxiety 1 week to several weeks after the event (Whitehead et al. 2005). Some patients with coronary disease have a family history of death of the parent of the same sex as a result of the same illness. This history is often associated with the conscious fantasy that the patient's death at the age at which the parent died is inevitable, leading to considerable vigilance, avoidance, and other anxiety behaviors.

Anxiety in Congestive Heart Failure

Until recently there have been very few studies of the prevalence of anxiety disorders in CHF patients (MacMahon and Lip 2002). In a survey of ambulatory outpatients with dilated cardiomyopathy, anxiety symptoms rated by the Hospital Anxiety and Depression Scale were significantly increased in comparison with population norms, suggesting a substantial prevalence of anxiety disorders, but no diagnostic information was obtained (Steptoe et al. 2000). A 2009 review (Yohannes et al. 2009) identified only 8 studies, all from 2005 to 2009, assessing anxiety in samples of only 50–208 CHF patients. The prevalence of elevated anxiety symptoms was 12%–45%. Only one of the reviewed studies, which included 100 ambulatory CHF patients, reported prevalence of anxiety disorders; 11% had generalized anxiety disorder, and 8% had panic disorder (Haworth et al. 2005). Another recent study reported a 10% prevalence of panic disorder in CHF patients treated in cardiology clinic practice (Muller-Tasch et al. 2008). Predictors of anxiety disorder in CHF patients were previous history of mental illness, diabetes, angina, and NYHA functional class. Both anxiety symptoms (Tsuchihashi-Makaya et al. 2009) and diagnosed anxiety disorders (Cully et al. 2009) have been associated with increased health care utilization in CHF patients.

Panic Disorder and Mitral Valve Prolapse

An association of mitral valve prolapse with panic disorder was proposed in the past on the basis of symptoms associated with prolapse (fluttering or palpitation experiences) in patients with panic disorder and echocardiographic findings of prolapse (R.M. Carney et al. 1990; Gorman et al. 1988). Depending on the echocardiographic criteria employed, 5%–20% or more of patients with panic disorder have mitral valve prolapse (Dager et al. 1986; Liberthson et al. 1986; Margraf et al. 1988). Individuals with mitral valve prolapse may be asymptomatic or may experience occasional palpitations or "fluttering" sensations in the precordium, and it has been proposed that these sensations give rise to catastrophic cognitions that stimulate panic attacks in predisposed individuals (Barlow 1988). The link has been questioned, however, because panic attacks do not occur at higher-than-expected rates in patients with echocardiographic mitral valve prolapse, and because mitral valve prolapse occurs in many other psychiatric disorder populations. Confusion has been created by varying criteria for mitral valve prolapse, small sample sizes, and poorly controlled studies. A 2008 systematic review found the evidence of association inconclusive at best (Filho et al. 2008). A possible link, in at least some cases, comes from genetic studies in panic disorder that have identified a syndrome of joint hyperlaxity, bladder and renal abnormalities, mitral valve prolapse, and panic attacks that is linked to chromosome 13 (Hamilton et al. 2003; Martin-Santos et al. 1998).

Anxiety and Automatic Implantable Cardioverter-Defibrillators

Malignant ventricular arrhythmias account for a substantial fraction of fatal events in patients with ischemic heart disease and CHF. The use of automatic implantable cardioverter-defibrillators (AICDs) reduces mortality (DiMarco 2003; Epstein et al. 2008), but the experience of defibrillation is unpleasant, likened to being "kicked in the chest." Implantable defibrillator discharges are associated with iatrogenic anxiety, particularly in patients who experience repetitive, frequent, or early discharges after device implantation (Heller et al. 1998). Early experience indicated a 50% incidence of psychiatric disorders after AICD implantation (adjustment disorders, major depression, and panic disorder) (Morris et al. 1991), but the incidence of psychopathology has apparently diminished over time (Crow et al. 1998). However, significant anxiety and depression symptoms are still present more than 12 months after implantation in 15%–30% of AICD patients (Magyar-Russell et al. 2009).

Although anxiety symptoms, anxiety disorders, and impaired quality of life are more common in patients who have received shocks (Irvine et al. 2002; Jacq et al. 2009; Schron et al. 2002), the likelihood of developing anxiety is also associated with predisposing personality traits such as social inhibition, negative affectivity, and sensitivity to anxiety (Bostwick and Sola 2007; van den Broek et al. 2008). In one study, individual psychological trait factors such as optimism, past history of depression, trait anxiety, and perceived social support accounted for 25%–40% of the variance in self-reported quality of life of patients 9–18 months following AICD implantation, while the experience of having been shocked accounted for only 1%–7% of the variance (Sears et al. 2005). Anxiety is more common in women than in men (Spindler et al. 2009). Although full-fledged posttraumatic stress disorder (PTSD) appears to occur in fewer than 5% of AICD patients, symptoms of the disorder such as avoidance, hypervigilance, and reexperiencing are common, especially if patients experience multiple sequential shocks while conscious, which they endure with a sense of helplessness. A variety of other reactions to implanted defibrillators have been described, including feelings of invulnerability, dependency, and withdrawal (Fricchione et al. 1989; Morris et al. 1991). Despite the potential for unpleasant experiences, most patients with implanted defibrillators report satisfaction with their experience with the device (Bostwick and Sola 2007).

In patients with atrial fibrillation, a trial of defibrillator-delivered pacing and shock therapy for atrial fibrillation found improvement in quality of life at 6-month follow-up after implantation. In patients in whom the device fired during the follow-up period, there was no decrement in quality of life compared with that of patients who did not experience defibrillator discharges (D.M. Newman et al. 2003).

Anxiety and Supraventricular Tachycardia

Patients with supraventricular tachycardia often experience anxiety, especially with paroxysmal arrhythmias (e.g., paroxysmal supraventricular tachycardia; see the section "Diagnostic Issues" later in this chapter).

Posttraumatic Stress Disorder in Cardiac Disease

PTSD rates ranging from 0% to 38% have been reported for patients with cardiac disease (Spindler and Pedersen 2005; Wiedemar et al. 2008). Proposed risk factors include personality traits such as repressive coping, alexithymia, and neuroticism, history of depression or of previous trauma, younger age, female gender, limited social support, dissociative symptoms and acute stress reactions immediately during index cardiac events, and subjective factors related to the experience of the event. Changes in the diagnostic criteria for PTSD in DSM-IV (American Psychiatric Association 1994) compared with DSM-III (American Psychiatric Association 1980) made it easier to diagnose PTSD in patients who experienced frightening events in the course of illness (Spindler and Pedersen 2005).

Anxiety and Cardiac Surgery

Heart-focused anxiety increases before cardiac surgery but tends to return to normal levels within 1–6 months after surgery. About 20% of patients continue to experience clinically significant heart-focused anxiety 6 months after surgery (Hoyer et al. 2008). A 10-year retrospective study of 440 coronary artery bypass graft (CABG) patients found increased anxiety symptoms before surgery to be associated with increased mortality risk, after adjusting for other known mortality risk factors (Tully et al. 2008).

Delirium and Neurocognitive Dysfunction

In the cardiac surgery intensive care unit (ICU), delirium, like beauty, is very much in the eye of the beholder. After coronary bypass graft surgery and open-heart procedures, it is evident that many patients have altered mental status with an impaired level of consciousness for some days. Whether these patients are identified as experiencing delirium appears to depend on the sensitivity of the observer and on the degree to which the patient's obtundation or agitation interferes with the clinical management of the postoperative state. Even with the use of structured diagnostic criteria (ICD-10, DSM-IV) and various validated rating scales, incidence rates for delirium in post–cardiac surgery patients range from 6% to over 50% (Detroyer et al. 2008; Kazmierski et al. 2008; Koster et al. 2009; Rudolph et al. 2009). Pioneering studies in the 1960s of the psychiatric aspects of heart disease included observations of the psychiatric complications of mitral commissurotomy and mitral and aortic valve replacement (Kornfeld et al. 1965). These studies documented a high prevalence of delirium in early open-heart surgery patients, which led to changes in ICU design and attention to preservation of sleep-wake cycles and appropriate use of narcotic analgesia in open-heart surgery. Studies demonstrating the importance of emboli from valvular structures or intracardiac thrombus, and from the cardiopulmonary bypass circuit, for subsequent cognitive impairment led to alterations of surgical technique and bypass circuit filters (S. Newman 1989; S. Newman et al. 1988; Willner and Rodewald 1991).

Frequency of adverse cerebral effects after CABG was estimated at 6% at hospital discharge in a multicenter study of 2,104 patients, with about half of these events being focal neurological events; other problems included persistent cognitive impairment, diminished level of consciousness, and seizures (Roach et al. 1996). Risk factors included advanced age, history of alcohol abuse, systolic hypertension, pulmonary disease, and aortic arch atherosclerosis. A longitudinal study of 261 patients found that 53% of post-CABG patients demonstrated neurocognitive impairment 1 week after surgery; the prevalence of impairment fell to 24% at 6 months (M.F. Newman et al. 2001). Predictors of delirium after open-heart surgery include older age, cerebrovascular disease, prolonged sedation, metabolic derangement, and narcotic use (Giltay et al. 2006; Kazmierski et al. 2008; Norkiene et al. 2007). Off-pump coronary bypass surgery has been studied as a means of reducing delirium and neuropsychological impairment after surgery (Diegeler et al. 2000). Avoidance of the heart–lung bypass machine reduces the production of inflammatory cytokines and reduces emboli to the brain; these factors appear to correlate with at best modestly improved neuropsychological outcome (Lee et al. 2003; Van Dijk et al. 2002, 2007). Delirium after heart surgery is commonly related to the duration of postoperative sedation with narcotics and benzodiazepines. Substitution of dexmedetomidine for fentanyl, midazolam, or lorazepam sedation reduces the incidence of delirium (Maldonado et al. 2009; Pandharipande et al. 2007).

Psychiatric Side Effects of Cardiac Drugs

A few cardiac medications have psychiatric side effects. These include digoxin, ACE inhibitors, amiodarone, lidocaine, and beta-blockers. Beta-blockers are often blamed for depression, fatigue, and sexual dysfunction; however, it has been demonstrated that fatigue, but not depression, is likely to be exacerbated by beta-blockers (Ko et al. 2002). An exhaustive review is available (Brown and Stoudemire 1998) (Table 18–1).

Psychogenic Cardiac Disability Syndromes

A psychogenic disability syndrome with overvalued ideas or convictions about the severity of one's cardiac illness sometimes occurs after a patient experiences symptoms attributed to heart disease, whether or not actual heart disease exists. In some patients, apparent clinging to symptoms of disease and the resulting disability serve as an unconscious face-saving means to escape otherwise intolerable life stress related to work, troubled intimate rela-

TABLE 18–1. Selected psychiatric side effects of cardiac drugs

Drug/class	Effects
Digoxin	Visual hallucinations (classically, yellow rings around objects), delirium, depression
Beta-blockers	Fatigue, sexual dysfunction
Alpha-blockers	Depression, sexual dysfunction
Lidocaine	Agitation, delirium, psychosis
Carvedilol	Fatigue, insomnia
Methyldopa	Depression, confusion, insomnia
Reserpine	Depression
Clonidine	Depression
ACE inhibitors	Mood elevation or depression (rare)
Pressors (dobutamine, milrinone, dopamine)	Psychiatric effects (rare)
Angiotensin II receptor blockers	Psychiatric effects (rare)
Amiodarone	Mood disorders secondary to thyroid effects
Diuretics	Hypokalemia, hyponatremia resulting in anorexia, weakness, apathy

Note. ACE=angiotensin-converting enzyme.

tionships, or other demands. Remaining in the sick role provides respite from negative affects related to one's previous psychosocial role. Such patients may have a previous history of hard work; denial of dependent needs; and relatively poor capacity for introspection, psychological insight, and verbalization of affects (alexithymia). In other patients, preexisting hypochondriasis, somatization, or panic is directed toward awareness of cardiac symptoms after an initial episode of symptoms. Less commonly, a patient with depression or a chronic psychosis becomes fixated and delusional about cardiac disease. Factitious illness and malingering must also be considered in the differential diagnosis for patients who appear to cling to cardiac disability (Rief et al. 2004).

Sexual Dysfunction

Sexual dysfunction after the onset of heart disease occurs as a consequence of both physical and psychological factors. Physical factors include medications, comorbid medical conditions such as peripheral vascular disease and diabetes mellitus, endothelial dysfunction, and low cardiac output (Kapur et al. 2007). Psychological factors include depression, anxiety, and fear of inducing a heart attack. Coital angina makes up 5% of angina attacks, but it is rare in patients who do not have angina during strenuous physical exertion. The metabolic demand of coitus is about 2–4 metabolic equivalents in men age 33 years, about equal to the demand of walking 2–3 miles/hour. The metabolic demand may be less in older men (DeBusk 2003) (see Chapter 16, "Sexual Dysfunction"). Erectile dysfunction in men with CHF can often be treated with phosphodiesterase type 5 (PDE-5) inhibitors, with appropriate precautions about contraindicated concurrent treatment with nitrates and alpha-adrenergic blockers, which may result in concomitant improvement in mood (Mandras et al. 2007; Webster et al. 2004). Avoidance of intercourse due to fear is associated with greater anxiety and depression in CAD patients, but not with the extent of coronary disease (Kazemi-Saleh et al. 2007).

Effects of Psychological Factors on the Heart and Heart Disease Risk

Depression and Risk of Coronary Heart Disease

Community prospective studies of several different populations demonstrate that a history of depressive disorder or elevated symptoms of depression as evaluated by questionnaire ratings are associated with increased risk for the subsequent development of ischemic heart disease and for coronary disease death. In studies of American, Danish, and Swedish populations, the estimated magnitude of the risk of incident disease associated with depression is 1.5- to 2.0-fold (Anda et al. 1993; Barefoot and Schroll 1996; Barefoot et al. 1996; Herbst et al. 2007; Rugulies 2002; Wulsin and Singal 2003). Meta-analyses have converged on an estimated 1.6-fold increased relative risk of coronary disease for those with a history of depression (Rugulies 2002; Wulsin and Singal 2003). The risk is probably higher in individuals with major depressive disorder (Surtees et al. 2008). Depression also heightens risk of defibrillator shocks for ventricular tachycardia/ventricular fibrillation and of cardiac arrest, independent of other established CAD risk factors (Empana et al. 2006; Whang et al. 2005, 2009). In patients with preexisting CAD, the risk of death for patients with depression is three- to fourfold higher than that for nondepressed coronary patients (R.M. Carney et al. 2003; Barth et al. 2004; Frasure-Smith et al. 1993, 1995a; Ladwig et al. 1991; van Melle et al. 2004). The association cannot be explained by confounding of depression with severity of heart disease (Kronish et al. 2009). Onset of depression after an acute coronary syndrome, severity of depression measured shortly after the acute coronary syndrome, and persistence of depression (with or without active treatment) all increase risk for long-term mortality after acute coronary syndromes (R.M. Carney and Freedland 2009; R.M. Carney et al. 2009; de Jonge et al. 2006, 2007; Dickens et al. 2008; Glassman et al. 2009; Grace et al. 2005; Kaptein et al. 2006; Parker et al. 2008). Although trends in recent years toward decreased mortality and better outcome after MI and more recognition and treatment of post-MI depression may have diminished the effect of depression on prognosis (Spijkerman et al. 2006), recent studies continue to demonstrate the importance of depression as a risk factor after MI (R.M. Carney et al. 2009).

Depression following CABG surgery predicts recurrent cardiac events at 12 months (Connerney et al. 2001), and both moderate and severe depression symptoms before surgery, and even mild depression persisting from baseline to 6-month follow-up after surgery, are predictors of mortality over several years of follow-up, with hazard ratios of more than 2.0 (Blumenthal et al. 2003).

Vital exhaustion, defined as a mental state of unusual fatigue, feelings of dejection or defeat, and increased irritability, has been associated with increased risk of incident coronary disease in European studies, and a psychotherapeutic intervention to reduce exhaustion has been reported to reduce angina complaints, but not recurrent cardiac events, after angioplasty (Appels and Mulder 1989; Appels et al. 2005, 2006). Although the entity has been conceptualized as distinct from depression (e.g., it does not include self-critical thoughts, and hypothalamic-pituitary-adrenal (HPA) axis activity is diminished rather than increased) (Appels et al. 2005), its overlap with depression is substantial, and the independent effect of nondepression components of vital exhaustion on CAD risk is uncertain (McGowan et al. 2004).

In contrast to depression, positive emotional characteristics such as optimism and "emotional vitality" have been associated with reduced incidence of CAD (Davidson et al. 2010a). Investigators have tended to view these positive characteristics as independent of depression, rather than simply an absence of depression (Giltay et al. 2004; Kubzansky and Thurston 2007). Absence of positive emotion, independent of other depression symptoms, was associated with increased death and recurrent MI in a 2-year follow-up of patients after coronary stenting (Denollet et al. 2008; Davidson et al. 2010a).

Depression clearly adversely affects patients' perceptions of their heart disease status and quality of life. Ruo et al. (2003) examined 1,024 patients with stable CAD to evaluate the contributions of depressive symptoms and objective measures of cardiac function to their health status. The patients who had depressive symptoms (20%) were more likely to report coronary disease symptom burden, physical limitations, diminished quality of life, and impaired health. In multivariate analyses, depression symptoms had significant independent association with these health status outcomes. In contrast, exercise capacity, left ventricular ejection fraction, and myocardial ischemia (measured by stress echocardiography) were not related to worse health status. These findings suggest that efforts to improve subjective health and functional status in coronary disease patients should address depression symptoms. A subsequent study (Ruo et al. 2006) in 2,675 postmenopausal women found that new or persistent depression had as powerful an impact on patients' self-ratings of their health as recent acute coronary events, heart failure, and coronary bypass surgery. Somatic symptoms associated with depression have a stronger effect on CAD prognosis than cognitive-affective symptoms (Linke et al. 2009; Martens et al. 2010).

Mechanisms Linking Depression and Coronary Artery Disease

Candidate psychophysiological mechanisms linking depression to adverse coronary disease outcomes include platelet dysfunction, autonomic dysfunction, and abnormalities of inflammation, but there is not yet compelling evidence comprehensively demonstrating that any of these mechanisms account for depression-related effects on heart disease (R.M. Carney et al. 2002; York et al. 2009). Persons with depression have increased platelet reactivity to orthostatic challenge (Musselman et al. 1996) and heightened circulating levels of beta-thromboglobulin and platelet factor 4, two markers of platelet activation (Laghrissi-Thode et al. 1997; Pollock et al. 2000). This implies that depressed patients have increased likelihood of thrombus formation in response to thrombogenic stimuli. Serotonin is stored in platelets, and serotonin release is a crucial intermediate step in platelet aggregation and thrombus formation. Serotonin storage in platelets is dependent on a serotonin transporter protein on the platelet cell membrane. Serotonin reuptake inhibitors may reduce the capacity of platelets to store serotonin, and thereby reduce their capacity to initiate thrombus formation. A large case-control study of first MI patients demonstrated that use of serotonergic antidepressants with high affinity for the serotonin transporter protein reduced the risk of MI in comparison with the risk for those using other antidepressant agents (Sauer et al. 2003).

Several measures of cardiac autonomic control, derived from time series or power spectral analyses of heart rate variability (HRV), are also deranged in depression. These measures indicate elevated sympathetic activation, suppression of vagal tone, and increased propensity to cardiac arrhythmias (R.M. Carney et al. 2001; Stein et al. 2000). Some studies have attributed this association primarily to antidepressant drug use (Licht et al. 2008). Similar changes in heart rate variability have been described as common in CAD patients and predict mortality after MI (Bigger et al. 1992, 1993). However, HRV measures were no different in depressed and nondepressed patients with stable CAD in a large patient cohort in the Heart and Soul Study, raising doubt about the importance of the autonomic derangements seen in depression in explaining subsequent cardiovascular events (Gehi et al. 2005b). Other HRV measures less specifically linked to sympathetic nervous system activation may account for a part of the mortality risk attributable to depression after MI (R.M. Carney et al. 2005).

Inflammation has been widely recognized as another process involved in the development of atherosclerosis and acute coronary events (Libby et al. 2002). Inflammatory cytokines are elevated in coronary disease patients, and the extent of elevation of specific markers such as interleukin-6 (IL-6), tumor necrosis factor-alpha, and C reactive protein (CRP), predicts coronary and cerebrovascular disease events and progression of heart failure (Cesari et al. 2003; Fisman et al. 2006). Depression has been shown to be associated with increased circulating levels of IL-6, CRP, and intercellular adhesion molecule 1 (ICAM-1) (Empana et al. 2005; Liukkonen et al. 2006; G.E. Miller et al. 2002; Vaccarino et al. 2007), but depression adds to risk of CAD incidence and events even after controlling for inflammation (Empana et al. 2005; Vaccarino et al. 2007).

It has also been suggested that antidepressant drugs are the cause of excess cardiovascular events and deaths in patients with depression. There are numerous reports of increased risk of cardiac events and mortality in healthy subjects and coronary disease patients treated with tricyclic antidepressants (TCAs) and/or selective serotonin reuptake inhibitors (SSRIs) (Blanchette et al. 2008; H.W. Cohen et al. 2000; Krantz et al. 2009; Meier et al. 2001; Monster et al. 2004; Rosenberg et al. 2009; Tata et al. 2005; Xiong et al. 2006). None of these studies were randomized trials, however, and they cannot exclude the confounding effect of depression itself on outcomes (O'Connor et al. 2008).

Depression may also exert a negative effect on cardiovascular outcomes through its negative effects on adherence to treatment recommendations. Poor adherence to the medical regimen in CAD patients is associated with increased recurrent cardiac events and mortality (Gehi et al. 2007; J.N. Rasmussen et al. 2007). Demonstrated effects of depression in coronary disease patients include lower rates of smoking cessation, exercise, dietary modification, and adherence to medication regimen (Gehi et al. 2005a; Glassman 1993; Ziegelstein et al. 2000). In fact, differences in adherence behavior between nondepressed and depressed patients with coronary disease may be the most important factor underlying the variance in survival and morbidity associated with depression in coronary disease patients (Hamer et al. 2008; Kronish et al. 2006; Whooley et al. 2008). Improvement in depression symptoms is followed by improved adherence to the medical regimen in heart disease patients (Rieckmann et al. 2006). It remains to be demonstrated in an intervention trial that depression treatment changes any of these candidate mechanisms in a way that accounts for any part of the variance in any cardiovascular outcome.

Intervention Trials

If depression exerts a negative effect on cardiac outcomes in coronary disease, a natural and important question is whether treatment of depression improves coronary disease outcomes. Three large-scale randomized clinical trials have now investigated this question. In the first of these studies, the Sertraline Antidepressant Heart Attack Randomized Trial (SADHART; Glassman et al. 2002), 369 patients with major depression after hospitalization for unstable angina or acute MI were randomized in a double-blind study to receive treatment with sertraline (50–200 mg/day) or placebo. The primary goal of the trial was to assess the safety of sertraline treatment, but a secondary goal was to obtain an estimate of the effect on cardiac outcomes. Although the trial was not powered to adequately test an effect on morbidity or mortality (i.e., only seven deaths occurred during the follow-up period), sertraline was superior in absolute numerical terms to placebo in the rate of recurrent MI, mortality, heart failure, and angina, suggesting that a larger study of treatment effects on mortality would be worthwhile. However, long-term follow-up (mean: 7 years) of the SADHART cohort showed that although more severe depression and failure to improve after short-term treatment were associated with increased mortality, treatment (antidepressant vs. placebo) had no effect on long-term survival (Glassman et al. 2009).

Concurrent with the SADHART, the Enhancing Recovery in Coronary Heart Disease (ENRICHD) trial was directed primarily at addressing the effects of treatment on mortality in post-MI patients (Writing Committee for the ENRICHD Investigators 2003). In ENRICHD, patients with low social support or depression after MI were enrolled in usual care or a cognitive-behavioral therapy (CBT) intervention group. Patients in the intervention group received 6–10 sessions of treatment over 6 months following acute MI. Mortality was assessed at 30-month follow-up. A confounding element of the trial was the use of antidepressants, primarily sertraline, in both arms of the trial in patients with more severe depressive symptoms. The CBT intervention was not effective in reducing mortality, and subgroup analyses did not demonstrate an effect of the intervention even in the depression subgroup. Although the use of sertraline was not randomized, it was notable that all-cause mortality in the sertraline-treated patients was only 7.4%, compared with 15.3% and 10.6% in patients who did not receive drug therapy and patients treated with TCAs, respectively. However, sertraline did not reduce the risk of recurrent nonfatal MI (Taylor et al. 2005).

Suggestive convergent evidence of a possible benefit of SSRI treatment of depression on cardiovascular disease outcomes in cardiovascular disease patients comes from a study of prophylaxis of depression after stroke (A. Rasmussen et al. 2003). In this study, 137 patients with acute ischemic stroke who were not depressed at screening assessment within 4 weeks of the index stroke were randomly assigned to placebo or sertraline treatment for 12 months. The study demonstrated a strong prophylactic effect of sertraline on the incidence of depression, and cardiovascular adverse events during the 12-month follow-up were reduced by two-thirds in the sertraline group compared with the patients receiving placebo.

Myocardial INfarction and Depression—Intervention Trial (MIND-IT), the third major clinical trial, compared a variety of depression interventions against usual care in patients with post-MI depression. A subsample of the MIND-IT patients participated in a randomized, placebo-controlled trial of mirtazapine, but other pharmacotherapy and psychotherapy interventions were also available for intervention group subjects, making this a complicated trial to understand. Although active treatment was modestly more effective than usual care for depression outcome, there was no effect of treatment on cardiac outcomes (Honig et al. 2007; van Melle et al. 2007).

It is notable that in all of these post-MI depression intervention trials, persistence of depression was associated with higher cardiac morbidity and mortality over long-term follow-up (R.M. Carney and Freedland 2009; R.M. Carney et al. 2004; de Jonge et al. 2007; Glassman et al. 2009). Recovery from depression was associated with better long-term cardiac prognosis, but treatment was not. A congruent effect was observed in an observational study of patients following coronary artery bypass surgery, in which patients whose depression improved in the 6 months after surgery had better cardiac prognosis than patients whose depression persisted or worsened (Blumenthal et al. 2003). Conversely, patients with new onset or worsening of depression in the months following myocardial infarction appear to have worse cardiac prognosis (Dickens et al. 2008; Parker et al. 2008).

Depression Effects on CHF Outcome

Depression arising de novo in patients after the diagnosis of coronary disease is associated with 1.5-fold increased risk of subsequent development of CHF, even after adjusting for confounding factors (May et al. 2009). Depression is associated with myocardial fibrosis, a characteristic finding in heart failure (Kop et al. 2010), and also appears to be associated with a two- to threefold increased mortality risk in patients hospitalized with CHF (Albert et al. 2009; Jiang et al. 2001; O'Connor et al. 2008; Sherwood et al. 2007). Depressed CHF patients in the hospital receive lower intensity of invasive interventions and referral to outpatient disease management programs, which may contribute to their risk of death (Albert et al. 2009). Prospective cohort studies in ambulatory CHF patients with 2–6 years of follow-up also demonstrate that depression is associated with substantially increased subsequent mortality and recurrent cardiac events (Faris et al. 2002; Junger et al. 2005; Murberg and Furze 2004; Sherwood et al. 2007).

A multicenter study of 460 outpatients with CHF showed that compared with nondepressed patients, patients with significant depression symptoms had both worse subjective health status at baseline (even after adjustment for objective measures of illness) and more deterioration in health status over short-term follow-up. Depression predicted worsening of heart failure symptoms, physical and social functioning, and quality of life. Depression symptoms were the strongest predictor of decline in health status (Rumsfeld et al. 2003).

Mechanisms like those postulated to underlie the relationship of depression and coronary disease have been proposed to account for the effect of depression on CHF outcomes (Joynt et al. 2004), but little pathophysiological research has been performed specifically in depressed patients with heart failure.

Anxiety and CAD Risk

The relationship of anxiety symptoms and disorders to CAD remains unsettled. Several recent reports demonstrate that anxiety symptoms increase risk of incident CAD (Eaker et al. 2005; Shen et al. 2008), and in middle-aged and older men without heart disease, anxiety is associated with incident MI even after controlling for demographic and metabolic risk factors, smoking, alcohol use, and blood pressure, and for depression, Type A behavior, anger, and treatments for hypertension, diabetes, and dyslipidemia during follow-up (Shen et al. 2008). But lifetime anxiety disorders were not associated with risk of CAD in a large epidemiological survey of older adults (Herbst et al. 2007). Anxiety symptoms and tension also modestly increase risk of incident atrial fibrillation (Eaker et al. 2005).

Large-scale prospective epidemiological studies do demonstrate an association of anxiety with sudden cardiac death. In a study involving 33,999 male, middle-aged health professionals with 2-year follow-up, there were 168 new cases of CAD, including 40 fatal and 128 nonfatal events. Fatal but not nonfatal cardiac events increased with the level of phobic anxiety; the excess risk was limited to cases of sudden cardiac death, with a sixfold increased risk associated with high anxiety (Kawachi et al. 1994a). The second study assessed 2,280 men free of chronic disease at baseline, with 32 years of follow-up. After adjustment for potential confounding variables, men with anxiety scores above the ninety-eighth percentile had a 4.46-fold increased risk of sudden cardiac death and a 1.94-fold increased risk of fatal CAD, but no excess risk for angina or nonfatal MI (Kawachi et al. 1994b). In patients with CAD, phobic anxiety is also associated with increased risk of ventricular arrhythmias, and the co-occurrence of anxiety and depression symptoms elevates this risk further (Watkins et al. 2006).

For patients with preexisting CAD, anxiety increases the risk of future events. In hospitalized acute MI patients, high anxiety symptoms are associated with a more than twofold increased risk of death during the hospitalization (Moser and Dracup 1996). In longer-term follow-up after MI, and in patients with stable CAD, anxiety confers increased risk of recurrent major cardiac events and mortality, independent of depression (Frasure-Smith and Lesperance 2008; Frasure-Smith et al. 1995b; Shibeshi et al. 2007; Strik et al. 2003). Preoperative anxiety symptoms have also been associated with a near-doubling of long-term mortality after CABG surgery, after adjustment for other prognostic factors (Tully et al. 2008).

Panic disorder was associated with increased cardiovascular morbidity (MI and stroke) in a large community sample (Weissman et al. 1990) and an anxiety disorders clinic sample (Coryell 1988; Coryell et al. 1986), but these early studies had significant methodological limitations. Newer studies, however, have supported the finding. A very large prospective epidemiological cohort study found a nearly twofold increased incidence of CAD in panic disorder patients, controlling for tobacco use, comorbid depression, medications, and obesity (Gomez-Caminero et al. 2005), and in the Women's Health Initiative panic attacks were common in healthy postmenopausal women and were associated with risk of subsequent CAD, stroke, and all-cause mortality (Smoller et al. 2007).

Increased CHD incidence also occurs in association with elevated posttraumatic stress symptom severity (Kubzansky et al. 2007). PTSD in patients with established coronary disease is associated with physical symptom burden and impaired quality of life and has a stronger association with self-reported cardiovascular health status than objective measures of cardiac function (B.E. Cohen et al. 2009). Vietnam-era military combat veterans with PTSD have higher rates of heart disease and heart disease mortality than peer veterans without PTSD, and their risk increases in proportion to the severity of their PTSD symptoms (Boscarino 2008).

Anxiety in post-acute coronary syndrome (ACS) patients is associated with reduced adherence to smoking cessation and exercise (Kuhl et al. 2009).

Anger, Type A Behavior, and Hostility

Type A behavior pattern—characterized by anger, impatience, aggravation, and irritability—was linked to incident coronary disease in men in the 1970s. The Western Collaborative Group Study of more than 3,000 middle-aged men demonstrated that Type A behavior was associated with a more than twofold-increased risk of incident MI and of fatal coronary events (Rosenman et al. 1975). One of the few large-scale clinical trials in psychosomatic cardiology, the Recurrent Coronary Prevention Project, examined the effect of group counseling in reducing the impact of Type A behavior pattern on mortality and recurrent infarction. Patients were survivors of an acute MI and were randomly assigned to usual care or Type A behavior modification groups. Follow-up at 4.5 years demonstrated a significant reduction in recurrent infarction in those assigned to Type A counseling (M. Friedman et al. 1986). Subsequent studies of Type A behavior pattern and CAD have been inconclusive or negative, perhaps because of the difficulty in measuring Type A behavior or changes in cardiovascular therapeutics, especially the widespread use of beta-adrenergic blockers in patients with coronary disease (Booth-Kewley and Friedman 1987).

Anger and hostility, considered as "toxic components" within the Type A concept, have also been studied as risk factors for coronary disease but with mixed results in longitudinal observations (Barefoot et al. 1994, 1995). Low hostility is protective against incident coronary disease (Shekelle et al. 1983); a majority of (but not all) studies find that high anger and high hostility are linked to increased cardiovascular risk (Krantz et al. 2006). In women with ischemic symptoms undergoing evaluation for coronary disease, high hostility was equally likely in those with and without angiographic CAD, but a tendency to overtly aggressive angry responding to angry feelings was associated with CAD, and over 3- to 6-year follow-up, high hostility was associated with more CAD events and lower likelihood of event-free survival (Krantz et al. 2006; Olson et al. 2005). In the Normative Aging Study analysis, anger predicted the incidence of a combined endpoint of coronary death, nonfatal MI, and angina, but it did not predict coronary death or nonfatal MI to a statistically significant degree (Kawachi et al. 1996).

Type D Personality

The combination of tendency to experience negative affects and to inhibit expression of negative emotions in social interactions has been coined Type D (for "distressed") personality (Denollet 2005; Pelle et al. 2009). This construct, explored almost exclusively in European studies, has been repeatedly associated with increased coronary disease risk (Denollet et al. 1995, 1996, 2006). Type D personality interacts with anxiety to increase arrhythmia risk (Van den Broek et al. 2009).

Acute Mental Stress

George Engel, who championed the biopsychosocial model in medicine, provided vivid examples from the news media of acute mental stress preceding acute coronary events (Engel 1976), and epidemiological studies of disasters have helped to demonstrate the relationship of acute stress to risk for sudden cardiac death (Dimsdale 2008). Even sports events, such as World Cup soccer matches, can have an epidemiologically significant stress effect on the incidence of coronary events (Wilbert-Lampen et al. 2008). In animal models of sudden cardiac death, ventricular tachycardia and fibrillation can be provoked by classically conditioned emotionally aversive stimuli. Interestingly, this effect depends on the presence of myocardial ischemia and can be disrupted by the use of intracerebral beta-adrenergic blockade (DeSilva 1983, 1993; Lown 1990; Lown et al. 1980; Skinner 1985; Skinner and Reed 1981; Skinner et al. 1975). The Northridge, California, earthquake in 1994 caused a surge in sudden cardiac deaths over the subsequent 2 days in individuals who were not physically endangered by the earthquake but resided in the immediate area (Leor et al. 1996). Other earthquake events have provided serendipitous data demonstrating deleterious effects of sudden massive psychological stress on hemoconcentration and procoagulant activity, incidence of pulmonary embolism, autonomic activity, heart rate and blood pressure, and incidence of MI (Dimsdale 2008; Nakagawa et al. 2009). In the aftermath of the destruction of the World Trade Center in New York in September 2001, patients with implanted defibrillators had increased frequency of ventricular tachycardia and ventricular fibrillation episodes, even if they were geographically distant and at no risk of physical harm from the disaster (Shedd et al. 2004; Steinberg et al. 2004). Acute emotional stress can provoke a variety of supraventricular arrhythmias as well as ventricular tachycardia and fibrillation (Ziegelstein 2007).

Acute stress in the laboratory, provoked by standardized tasks such as mirror drawing, the Stroop color-word test, mental arithmetic, video games, and public speaking, results in elevation in heart rate and blood pressure and alteration in indices of cardiac autonomic regulation, with diminished parasympathetic and elevated sympathetic activation, in both healthy volunteers and patients with CAD (Blumenthal et al. 1995; Manuck and Krantz 1986; Rozanski et al. 1988, 1999; Sheps et al. 2002). In addition, coronary vasospasm and mental stress-induced platelet activation appear to be mechanisms of mental stress-induced ischemia in at least some cases (Reid et al. 2009; Yeung et al. 1991). One-third to one-half of patients with CAD experience ischemia during mental stress testing, and ischemia occurs at lower levels of rate-pressure product elevation during mental stress than during exercise stress. Most patients with mental stress-induced ischemia also have exercise-induced ischemia. Wall motion abnormality appears to be a more sensitive indicator of ischemia than ST segment depression, for unknown reasons (Strike and Steptoe 2003). Mental stress-induced ischemia is usually silent (Blumenthal et al. 1995; Rozanski et al. 1988, 1999). The technique of ecological momentary assessment has been used to demonstrate that emotional arousal, and especially anger during daily events, is associated with similar alterations in hemodynamic and autonomic state, and it has been estimated that acute emotional stress is a trigger for up to 20%–30% of acute coronary events (Muller et al. 1994). In patients with coronary disease, mental stress-induced ischemia, indicated by wall motion abnormalities on radionuclide ventriculography or echocardiography, is associated with more than a doubling in the risk of death, even after adjustment for other prognostic variables (Jiang et al. 1996; Sheps et al. 2002). Mental stress-induced myocardial ischemia in CAD patients is associated with increased QT interval variability, increasing proarrhythmic risk (Hassan et al. 2009). Genetic polymorphisms of the beta-adrenergic receptor substantially affect susceptibility to the development of mental stress-induced myocardial ischemia (Hassan et al. 2008).

Acute stress cardiomyopathy, sometimes referred to as Takotsubo cardiomyopathy or broken heart syndrome, is a rare illness occurring in the setting of sudden emotional stress or surprise. Affected individuals, who are predominantly female, experience abrupt onset of ventricular dysfunction, with characteristic ventricular apical ballooning seen on echocardiography (Tsai et al. 2009), with chest pain and/or hypotension, in the absence of atherosclerosis or CAD. Most patients recover, with improvement in ventricular function over several days to weeks (Bielecka-Dabrowa et al. 2010; Wittstein 2007; Wittstein et al. 2005). An abrupt surge in circulating catecholamines and/or sympathetic nervous system activation is believed to cause the ventricular dysfunction by provoking myocardial hypercontractility, and so-called contraction band necrosis has been reported on myocardial biopsy (Samuels 1993; Wittstein 2007; Wittstein et al. 2005). Takotsubo cardiomyopathy has also been reported as a complication of electroconvulsive therapy (ECT) (Kent et al. 2009; O'Reardon et al. 2008).

Midbrain control of vagal withdrawal and sympathetic nervous system activation during mental stress, and its relationship to cardiac events, can be demonstrated through functional brain imaging (Critchley et al. 2005; Thayer and Lane 2007).

Chronic Mental Stress

The cumulative effect of chronic or recurring emotional stressors on risk of myocardial infarction has been strikingly demonstrated in the INTERHEART study (Rosengren et al. 2004), a 52-country investigation evaluating chronic stress in more than 11,000 MI patients and more than 13,000 matched control subjects. Work stress, family stress, and general stress over the past year were each associated with significantly increased risk of MI (odds ratios > 2). The total number of stressors reported was also correlated with MI risk. Similarly, a prospective cohort study of 972 individuals after a first MI found that chronic job strain was associated with a doubling of risk for recurrent CAD events (Aboa-Eboulé et al. 2007).

Sleep Apnea

Sleep apnea is associated with hypertension and CHF (Bradley and Floras 2003a, 2003b). Two studies of chronic heart failure patients found the prevalence of obstructive sleep apnea to range from 11% to 37%, and the presence of sleep apnea increases the risk of developing heart failure. Obstructive apnea results in hypoxia, elevated intrathoracic pressure, and sympathetic nervous system activation, with increases in heart rate and blood pressure. These physiological derangements may contribute to the development of heart failure, ischemic events, and arrhythmias (Shamsuzzaman et al. 2003). A randomized trial showed that continuous positive airway pressure for 1 month leads to improvement in the number of apnea episodes, systolic blood pressure, heart rate, left ventricular end-systolic dimension, and left ventricular ejection fraction (Kaneko et al. 2003). Central sleep apnea does not severely exacerbate negative intrathoracic pressure, but it does produce periodic sympathetic arousals and increased afterload and myocardial work (Bradley and Floras 2003b) (see also Chapter 15, "Sleep Disorders").

Low Social Support

Although social support is an omnibus term covering a variety of quantitative (i.e., how many relationships?) and qualitative (i.e., what kind of relationships?) aspects of social relationships, a preponderance of studies have shown an association between low support and coronary disease risk and prognosis. The effect of social support is moderated by socioeconomic status, depression, and cultural factors (Lett et al. 2005; H.X. Wang et al. 2006). In two trials, efforts to improve social support for post-MI patients with low social support did not improve cardiac outcomes (Burg et al. 2005; Frasure-Smith et al. 1997).

Excess Cardiovascular Disease–Related Mortality Associated With Other Psychiatric Disorders

Increased cardiovascular mortality risk is also associated with schizophrenia and bipolar disorder (Sowden and Huffman 2009). Adults with bipolar I disorder have increased rates and earlier age at onset of hypertension and CAD compared with the general population, even after controlling for demographic factors, smoking, obesity, substance use, and comorbid anxiety (B.I. Goldstein et al. 2009). The extent to which the pathophysiology of these psychiatric illnesses itself affects cardiovascular risk, as opposed to the effects of lifestyle and associated behaviors (e.g., smoking) and treatments (e.g., antipsychotic drugs, lithium, anticonvulsants), is unknown. These psychiatric disorders also have increased comorbidity with a variety of other medical disorders (C.P. Carney and Jones 2006; C.P. Carney et al. 2006).

Stress Management and Health Education Interventions in CAD Patients

A large meta-analysis of a variety of health-education and stress-reduction interventions in patients with CAD concluded that these interventions reduce the incidence of recurrent MI (29% reduction) and death (34% reduction) at 2- to 10-year follow-up. The mechanism of the effect is unclear; these analyses do not consistently demonstrate a reduction in mental symptoms (i.e., anxiety and depression ratings are not reduced) (Dusseldorp et al. 1999). Psychoeducational programs may include varying components of health education, stress management, and supervised exercise training; and many individual reports fail to give specific details of the interventions. Successful effects on proximal targets such as systolic blood pressure, cholesterol, body weight, smoking behavior, physical exercise, and emotional distress or some combination of these mediate the beneficial effects for mortality. For recurrent MI, protective effects of psychoeducational intervention were associated with beneficial effects on systolic blood pressure, smoking behavior, physical exercise, and emotional distress. Patients who participate in psychoeducational programs are three times more likely to be successful in quitting smoking (Dusseldorp et al. 1999). Longer intervention programs with more hours of intervention and more tailoring of program content to individual needs appear to have greater long-term effect on cardiac outcomes (Linden 2000; Linden et al. 1996). Subsequent meta-analyses have been critical of the quality of individual trials and more guarded in their assessment of the benefits of psychological interventions in CAD patients, suggesting effects ranging from limited to modest benefits for anxiety and depression symptoms only (Rees et al. 2004) to reductions in cardiac and all-cause mortality and nonfatal MI associated with interventions with behavioral components (Welton et al. 2009). Psychosocial interventions including specific efforts to change targeted behaviors are most effective for reducing all-cause mortality and cardiac mortality, while improved psychosocial support has its strongest effect on reducing nonfatal MI. Psychosocial interventions with an educational component (e.g., providing information) are most effective in reducing anxiety, while interventions with a cognitive component (e.g. reframing, changing beliefs about factors leading to heart disease) are most effective for reducing depression symptoms (Welton et al. 2009). In a carefully done randomized trial, both stress management and supervised exercise training in patients with stable CAD were superior to usual care in reducing emotional distress and improving several physiological parameters associated with cardiovascular risk (Blumenthal et al. 2005).

Diagnostic Issues

Most psychiatric diagnoses are reached in a straightforward fashion in patients with heart disease, but confusion may arise because of the overlap of symptoms of heart disease with symptoms of psychiatric disorder and because treatments for heart disease may cause psychiatric side effects. The most frequent problem in psychiatric diagnosis is the attribution of symptoms of depression to the underlying cardiac disease or to a "normal" reaction to the illness, with a resultant underdiagnosis of depression. Generally in practice, however, an inclusive approach is appropriate, counting symptoms such as fatigue and poor sleep toward a diagnosis of depression even if those symptoms might also be attributable to the patient's cardiac condition (Cohen-Cole and Kauffman 1993) (see also Chapter 8, "Depression"). In an analysis of the 222 patients with acute MI included in the landmark Montreal Heart Institute depression mortality study, the investigators considered the specificity of various symptoms from the depression criteria set for a diagnosis of depression. Sleep disturbance and appetite disturbance did not help to distinguish between patients who met criteria for depressive episode and those who did not (i.e., these symptoms were common in both depressed and nondepressed patients), but fatigue and especially sadness and loss of pleasure occurred almost exclusively in patients who met criteria for a major depressive episode (Lesperance et al. 1996). This finding suggests that patients who report somatic symptoms of depression should be evaluated for the presence of the cardinal mood and interest symptoms, and they should be considered depressed if these symptoms are also present. Patients with advanced heart failure often develop appetite loss and cachexia, but in the absence of loss of self-esteem, loss of interest in ordinarily enjoyable events, or depressed mood, these patients should not be diagnosed with a depressive disorder.

Paroxysmal supraventricular tachycardia (PSVT) occurs in young and middle-aged adults and may manifest with symptoms of shortness of breath, chest discomfort, and apprehension. Because these features may overlap with those of generalized anxiety symptoms and panic attacks, there is a significant risk of misdiagnosis. In a retrospective study of 107 patients with PSVT, DSM-IV (American Psychiatric Association 1994) criteria for panic disorder were met in 59 patients (67%); PSVT had been unrecognized after initial medical evaluation in 55% and remained unrecognized for a median of 3.3 years. Prior to the eventual identification of PSVT, nonpsychiatric physicians attributed symptoms to panic, anxiety, or stress in 32 (54%) of the 59 patients (Lessmeier et al. 1997). Of course, some patients may have both PSVT and an anxiety disorder, with symptomatic attacks including elements of each.

Atypical Chest Pain and Palpitations

Typical anginal chest pain in CAD occurs with exertion or after eating; is not exacerbated by palpation of the chest or by inspiration; is described as dull, pressure-like, or burning rather than sharp or stabbing; and is experienced across the precordium rather than in a pinpoint area of the left side of the chest. Many patients present for evaluation of atypical chest pain (Sheps et al. 2004). While atypical features do not rule out a diagnosis of CAD, 40%–70% of patients with no history of documented CAD and few CAD risk factors have panic disorder, somatoform disorders, or depression (Alexander et al. 1994; Fleet et al. 2000). Patients with noncardiac chest pain demonstrate a high prevalence of anxiety disorders (approximately 40%–60%), including panic and social phobia, depression (approximately 5%–25%), and somatoform disorders (2%–15%), and a substantial portion of the remaining patients have subsyndromal symptoms of these disorders (Hocaoglu et al. 2008; Jonsbu et al. 2009; White et al. 2008). More than half of children with noncardiac chest pain have an anxiety disorder, usually panic disorder (Lipsitz et al. 2005). A small randomized trial found a benefit of 8 weeks of paroxetine treatment in noncardiac chest pain patients who did not meet criteria for panic disorder or depression (Doraiswamy et al. 2006).

In the absence of CAD, characteristics of chest pain patients predicting panic disorder include female sex, atypical chest pain quality, younger age, lower education and income, and high self-reported anxiety (Dammen et al. 1999; Huffman and Pollack 2003). Panic disorder is twice as likely in chest pain patients without CAD as in patients with CAD (Dammen et al. 1999; Fleet et al. 2000).

Psychiatric disorders are also common in patients complaining of palpitations. In one study using structured diagnostic interviews and self-report questionnaires for patients undergoing ambulatory electrocardiogram (ECG) monitoring, the lifetime prevalence of any disorder was 45%, and 25% of the patients had a current disorder. The lifetime prevalences of panic disorder and major depression were 27% and 21%, respectively, and 19% had panic disorder at the time of evaluation (Barsky et al. 1994a). Rates of anxiety, depressive, and somatoform disorders were similar in another study 15 years later (Jonsbu et al. 2009). These rates are probably somewhat higher than in the general population, because they derive from tertiary-care clinic settings. Even when a patient with palpitations has a history of panic disorder, clinical examination alone may not be sufficient to exclude significant arrhythmias. Ambulatory electrocardiographic monitoring with loop recording is the most sensitive method for identifying the presence of a specific arrhythmia in patients with palpitations (Thavendiranathan et al. 2009).

Special Issues

Heart Transplantation

Heart transplantation has been the treatment of last resort for patients with severe heart failure, and occasionally for patients with intractable recurrent myocardial ischemia or ventricular arrhythmias, for the past three decades (see also Chapter 31, "Organ Transplantation"). Because of donor scarcity, the number of heart transplants performed annually in the United States has reached a plateau of approximately 2,100 per year. Patients eligible for heart transplantation typically have an expected survival of less than 2 years unless they receive a transplant. With transplantation, expected 5-year survival is now around 67%–73% (Organ Procurement and Transplant Network 2010). Complications can occur, and the care regimen for heart transplant patients is challenging, especially in the first few months after surgery, so transplant programs generally screen patients and exclude from candidacy those with significant relative contraindications.

These facts provide the context for the "normal" psychological experience of patients entering the process (Shapiro 1990). Patients generally fear that they are close to death or will experience a sudden catastrophic deterioration in the future and believe that a transplant is their best hope for survival. Although they may be anxious about the dangers of transplantation, they are even more often anxious about being excluded from candidacy. Consequently, the evaluation period is a time of heightened concern, and patients meeting with a psychiatrist as part of the evaluation process wonder whether they will "pass" this examination. Patients awaiting transplantation often experience depression symptoms, because they perceive themselves as helpless to fundamentally affect their own chances of survival. During the waiting period, depression is often enhanced by a sense of guilt over wishes for the death of a suitable donor. Patients sometimes describe a kind of psychological "ambulance chasing," hearing a siren and wondering whether this might signal the availability of a donor. Before, at the time of evaluation, and up to the time of receiving a transplant, patients may also display variable levels of denial of the seriousness of their illness and ambivalence about undergoing transplant surgery. This minimization or denial of illness can fluctuate and coexist with other emotional responses, including fear, depression, and anxiety. Patients who come to heart transplantation after an acute catastrophic cardiac event, without a prior chronic heart failure syndrome, are especially prone to experience a combination of denial, shock, anger, and fear all at the same time, as they must rapidly assimilate an altered view of their health status, appreciate the associated risks, and appraise the possible risks and benefits of transplantation, before having much opportunity to mourn the loss of their previous health and associated social role. If they are sedated or in a state of altered consciousness because of cardiogenic shock, medication, or metabolic disarray, their capacity to psychologically adjust is further reduced, with more adaptation forced on them after the fact.

Following heart transplant surgery, patients receive multiple immunosuppressive anti-rejection medications, along with vitamins; minerals; antibacterial, antifungal, and antiviral medications; and treatments as needed for hypertension, arrhythmias, fluid retention, or other conditions. Most patients are hospitalized for 10–20 days after surgery, undergoing surveillance for allograft rejection as the immunosuppressive medication doses are adjusted. (These medications are discussed in Chapter 31, "Organ Transplantation.") High doses of intravenous and then oral corticosteroids are the rule in the initial weeks after transplant surgery, and predictably they induce increased appetite, fluid retention, and mood lability. Most patients experience an initial euphoria at awakening from surgery, knowing that they have now been delivered from end-stage heart failure, but the emotional reaction depends in part on the patient's previous expectations in comparison with the state of subjective well-being in the early days after surgery. Positive feelings tend to subside as complications occur and as the patient settles into the work of rehabilitation and adjustment to the new medication regimen. One or more episodes of rejection are not uncommon in the early period after surgery; if transient corticosteroid dose increases are employed to treat rejection episodes, a medication-exacerbated emotional roller coaster may ensue.

Psychiatric complications after heart transplantation are fairly common (see Chapter 31, "Organ Transplantation," for a fuller discussion). In addition to postoperative delirium, steroid-induced mood disorders and depression not attributable to steroids occur in perhaps 20%–40% of patients in the first year after surgery. Many cases occur in the setting of medical complications, but role transitions are often difficult for the recovering patient, and stressors such as increased demand for autonomous function or the need to provide for others in the family, difficulty negotiating return to work, or financial concerns that were previously ignored often stimulate increased emotional distress (Shapiro 1990; Shapiro and Kornfeld 1989). Some heart transplant patients experience transplantation-related posttraumatic stress disorder following particularly frightening or troubling episodes during their care, appear psychologically fixated on these events and subjectively distressed, and are impaired in their daily functioning long after the transplant (Dew et al. 2001).

Left Ventricular Assist Devices

The shortage of available donors of hearts for transplantation and the large number of patients dying of CHF provided impetus even early in the era of heart transplantation for the development of artificial heart technology (D.J.

Goldstein and Oz 2000). In addition to attempting to devise a total artificial heart, researchers have developed and tested a variety of ventricular assist pumps over the past decade. To date, experience with total artificial hearts has been characterized by limited success, although they may be helpful as short-term bridges to heart transplantation (Copeland et al. 2004). Ventricular assist devices, however, have been more successful and are in more widespread use as bridges to heart transplantation or in some cases bridges to recovery after acute myocardial injury (D.J. Goldstein and Oz 2000). Early experience with use of LVADs designed to be used for periods of weeks to months as a bridge to transplantation indicated that significant neuropsychiatric issues were delirium, stroke, cognitive impairment, pain, and depressed mood. Depression seemed especially linked to frustration with ongoing limitations in function as a result of tethering to the device, and cerebrovascular and cognitive problems were associated with a history of even minor or transient cerebrovascular disease symptoms before LVAD surgery (Shapiro et al. 1996). For most patients, quality of life with LVADs was superior to that while they were in severe heart failure (Dew et al. 1998, 1999a, 1999b). Ongoing improvements in device design have reduced the mechanical problems of attachment to an external device to a considerable degree (D.J. Goldstein and Oz 2000).

The success of LVAD use as a bridge to transplantation led to study of permanent ("destination") LVAD treatment for patients with end-stage heart failure who could not receive a heart transplant (Rose et al. 1999). The REMATCH trial, a randomized clinical study providing either optimized medical therapy or LVAD therapy for patients with severe chronic heart failure, demonstrated a substantial survival benefit associated with LVADs, along with improved quality of life outcomes (Rose et al. 2001). Interestingly, somatic dimensions of quality of life were substantially better in LVAD recipients, but mental-emotional components did not differ from those of medically treated heart failure patients (Shapiro et al. 2002). Postoperative delirium was the most important psychiatric problem seen in LVAD patients in this study (Lazar et al. 2004). The success of LVAD treatment in extending survival without worsening quality of life in the REMATCH trial led to approval by the U.S. Food and Drug Administration (FDA) of destination LVAD therapy for nonexperimental use in the United States in 2002. However, quality of life in patients with LVADs is not as good as that in patients who receive heart transplants or who are able to be weaned off of mechanical assist devices (Dew et al. 1999b; Wray et al. 2007).

Ventricular assist device design has evolved over the past decade; pulsatile devices are being superseded by continuous flow systems with better durability and better associated neurocognitive outcomes and quality of life (L.W. Miller et al. 2007; Petrucci et al. 2009; Slaughter et al. 2009). In addition to their use as bridges to transplantation and as destination therapy, ventricular assist devices are also being used for "bridge to recovery," with current trials investigating the adjunctive use of the beta-adrenergic agonist clenbuterol, stem cell therapy, and other means of promoting ventricular remodeling and recovery of ventricular function (Terracciano et al. 2010). While most patients receive ventricular assist devices for chronic heart failure, and therefore have opportunity for education and consideration of their options before implantation, emergency implantation in the setting of acute cardiogenic shock has become more common. Patients in this situation may not have been able to participate in decision making, and have greater difficulty with initial emotional adjustment to living with the assist device.

Hypertension

The relationship of psychological factors to the development of hypertension has been a subject of controversy, with mixed findings in large-scale observational studies. Several cross-sectional studies found no relationship between psychological variables and risk of hypertension (Davies et al. 1999; R. Friedman et al. 2001; Hildrum et al. 2007; Licht et al. 2009). In one study comparing the blood pressure of subjects with current and past history of depression and/or anxiety and healthy control subjects, current and remitted depression were associated with lower likelihood of hypertension and lower mean systolic blood pressure, but use of TCAs, SSRIs, and noradrenergic agents increased the risk of hypertension (Licht et al. 2009). Another study found a significant association of hypertension with co-occurrence of generalized anxiety disorder and major depressive disorder, but not either disorder alone (Carroll et al. 2010).

Large-scale prospective studies with longitudinal follow-up ranging from 11 to 22 years have come to different conclusions. A 15-year prospective study of psychosocial risk factors for hypertension based on a follow-up of more than 3,000 young white and black adults from four metropolitan areas of the United States found that two components of Type A behavior—namely, "time urgency-impatience" and "hostility"—were each associated with almost double the rate of incident hypertension. In contrast, anxiety symptoms, depression symptoms, and "achievement-striving-competitiveness" (another Type A component) did not predict hypertension (Yan et al. 2003). In a Norwegian epidemiological study, high baseline depression and anxiety symptoms were both associated with low systolic blood pressure at 11-year follow-up, and the magnitude and direction of anxiety or depression symptom changes over time were inversely associated with the magnitude of the change in systolic blood pressure. These effects were not accounted for by use of antihypertensive and antidepressant medication (Hildrum et al. 2008). However, 22-year follow-up of a population-based cohort of 3,310 normotensive persons without chronic diseases from the National Health and Nutrition Examination Survey I (NHANES I) Epidemiologic Follow-up Study found that combined symptoms of depression and anxiety ("negative affect") were associated with increased risk for hypertension. The risk for treated hypertension was increased in both men and women and was most pronounced (more than threefold) in black women (Jonas and Lando 2000). A review (Rutledge and Hogan 2002) of 15 prospective studies of psychological traits affecting the development of hypertension, with sample sizes varying from 78 to 4,650 subjects and follow-up for 2.5–21 years, found small but significant effects of anger, anxiety, depression, and other variables, with an overall magnitude of effect suggesting an 8% increase in prospective hypertension risk associated with a high level of one or more of the psychological variables. A smaller number of studies separately reported the effect of psychological factors on hypertension in African Americans and in women. In African Americans, the same psychological predictors appeared to be associated with hypertension. In women, the results were equivocal.

The main psychiatric consequence of hypertension seems to be long-term neurocognitive impairment and increased risk of dementia (Frishman 2002). Treatment that successfully controls blood pressure reduces the risk (Forette et al. 2002; Guo et al. 1999; Launer et al. 1995; Vinyoles et al. 2008). In patients older than 60 years, adherence to antihypertensive therapy is associated with better blood pressure control and better cognitive function (Vinyoles et al. 2008). White-coat hypertension, defined as repeatedly high blood pressure at visits to the doctor's office, with normal ambulatory and self-measured blood pressure, is associated with increased long-term risk of stroke but not of heart disease (Angeli et al. 2005). Behavioral treatments appear to have a modest effect at best on hypertension (Linden and Moseley 2006; Perez et al. 2009), but combined treatments may help in paroxysmal hypertension, especially if paroxysmal episodes of high blood pressure are linked to panic or anxiety (Pickering and Clemow 2008).

Congenital Heart Disease

The prevalence of psychiatric disorders in adult survivors of congenital heart disease has not been extensively studied. The existence of this clinical population depends largely on advances in pediatric cardiac surgery over the past three decades. Lifetime rates of mood and anxiety disorders may be as high as 50% (Kovacs et al. 2009), but some investigators have not found elevated rates of psychiatric symptoms (Cox et al. 2002; Geyer et al. 2006). Sexual dysfunction is common in men who have had surgery for congenital heart disease (Vigl et al. 2009).

Psychological maladjustment is common in children after surgery for congenital heart disease (Latal et al. 2009). Overall IQ scores are typically in the normal range but lower than healthy control subjects, and subtle neuropsychological deficits are common (Forbess et al. 2002; Miatton et al. 2007). For cyanotic conditions, but not for acyanotic lesions, delayed repair appears to exacerbate intellectual impairment (Newburger et al. 1984). Other common psychological problems among children and young adults with congenital heart disease include concerns about exclusion from participation in peer group activities such as sports and gym class, problems with appearance (short stature, cyanosis, drug side effects on appearance), concerns about attractiveness, capacity to develop intimate relationships, exclusion from work, and fears about mortality (Kendall et al. 2001).

Treatment Issues

Psychotherapy

Psychological reactions to the experience of heart disease include feelings of anxiety and sadness as well as concerns about survival and well-being and their effects on social roles, relationships, and the impact on loved ones. Denial is nearly universal as an initial reaction to illness, and it can be helpful in staving off depressed and anxious mood or hurtful because of nonadherence to the treatment program. Conversely, preoccupation with disease can lead to abnormal illness behavior, unnecessary disability, and impaired quality of life. Few systematic studies of psychotherapy have been reported that specifically targeted psychological symptoms or psychiatric disorders in heart patients. As was described previously, a larger number of studies have described stress management or health education effects on cardiac outcomes in cardiac rehabilitation settings; meta-analyses of these studies do show beneficial effects on cardiac outcomes and suggest that reducing emotional distress and changing health-related behaviors may be correlated with better cardiac disease outcomes (Dusseldorp et al. 1999; Linden et al. 1996; Welton et al. 2009).

The ENRICHD trial tested the effects of a CBT intervention versus usual care in patients who had a recent MI and either low social support and/or major depression or minor depression with a history of prior major depression in a randomized trial. Patients in the intervention arm participated in either individual or group therapy sessions; treatment was manualized; and therapist adherence to treatment methods was assessed during the trial. Most patients received 6–10 therapy sessions. The trial demonstrated a modest benefit of the CBT intervention on measures of social support and depression. However, the improvement on these measures seen in the usual-care group was higher than expected, so that the effect of treatment, although statistically significant, was of small magnitude (Writing Committee for the ENRICHD Investigators 2003).

As described previously, the Recurrent Coronary Prevention Project tested the effect of group Type A behavior modification in reducing the impact of Type A behavior pattern on mortality and recurrent infarction in a cohort of post-MI patients (M. Friedman et al. 1986). In retrospect, although the term was not used at the time, this was clearly a cognitive-behavioral psychotherapy intervention. The intervention had a strong beneficial effect on Type A behavior as rated using a videotaped structured interview for the assessment of Type A behavior.

Interpersonal psychotherapy (IPT) of depression focuses on present-day interpersonal problems linked to depressed mood, such as interpersonal disputes, grief after object loss, interpersonal deficits, and social role transitions. One such role transition may occur with the change in social role imposed by development of a chronic or acute medical illness (Klerman et al. 1984). Therefore IPT would seem to be readily applicable to the treatment of patients who experience depression after the onset or exacerbation of heart disease. However, the only published controlled trial of interpersonal therapy for depression in patients with CAD, the CREATE trial (Lesperance et al. 2007), found no added benefit of interpersonal therapy compared with clinical management alone.

An innovative collaborative care model was successful in reducing depression symptoms and improving health-related quality of life in patients with depression following coronary bypass surgery in a recent randomized controlled trial (Rollman et al. 2009). Patients met criteria for at least mild depression through screening with the 9-item Patient Health Questionnaire (PHQ-9). This trial intervention included having a nurse perform telephone monitoring of patient status with education about depression, provision of self-help materials, and encouragement of exercise and treatment adherence. Depending on patient preference and response to initial supportive interventions, referral to a mental health specialist or pharmacotherapy by the patient's primary care physician was coordinated by the psychiatric study nurse, with support by a supervising study psychiatrist. Patients who received pharmacotherapy generally received an SSRI, but treatment was open and could be adjusted according to patient response to try other categories of medication.

Psychopharmacological Treatment

Common adverse cardiac effects of psychiatric drugs are shown in Table 18–2 (see also Chapter 38, "Psychopharmacology").

Antidepressants

Antidepressants must be used in therapeutically effective doses in cardiac patients with depression, and it is counterproductive to use inadequate doses out of fear of side effects or prolongation of metabolism. Unless the patient has severe right heart failure resulting in hepatic congestion, ascites, and jaundice, it is unlikely that metabolism of oral psychotropic medication (except for lithium) will be substantially impaired because of heart disease.

TCAs cause orthostatic hypotension, cardiac conduction delay (bundle branch block or complete atrioventricular nodal block), and, in overdose, ventricular arrhythmias (ventricular premature depolarization, ventricular tachycardia, and ventricular fibrillation). QRS interval prolongation results from interference with phase 1 depolarization (slow Na^+ channel activity) of the action potential across the membrane of the specialized conduction tissue of the ventricle. Prolongation of the QT interval is predominantly caused by prolongation of the QRS interval, and ventricular tachycardia or fibrillation can occur if marked prolongation of the QT interval (over 500 msec) results in the R-on-T phenomenon. Nortriptyline and desipramine tend to cause less orthostatic hypotension than tertiary amine tricyclic drugs and are better tolerated by patients with cardiac disease (Roose and Glassman 1989; Roose et al. 1986, 1987, 1989). Cardiac pacemakers can obviate the risk of heart block associated with TCAs. More commonly problematic, however, is orthostatic hypotension, which can result in syncope and falls.

TCAs have quinidine-like effects on cardiac conduction and are classified as Type 1A antiarrhythmic agents. Drugs of this class have been shown to increase rather than decrease mortality in post-MI patients with premature ventricular contractions (CAST Investigators 1989; CAST II Investigators 1992; Morganroth and Goin 1991), an effect believed to be mediated by episodic myocardial ischemia (Lynch et al. 1987). Consequently, TCAs should generally not be used as first-line agents for treatment of depression in ischemic heart disease patients. This is not to say that they should never be used, however, because their efficacy may offset the risk for selected patients. Consideration should be given to the totality of the clinical situation, including the severity of depression, past treatment responses, concomitant medications, and ECG (Glassman et al. 1993).

SSRIs have little to no cardiac effect in healthy subjects. The most commonly observed effect is slowing of heart rate,

TABLE 18–2. Selected cardiac side effects of psychotropic drugs

Drug/class	Cardiac effects
Lithium	Sinus node dysfunction and arrest
SSRIs	Slowing of heart rate; occasional sinus bradycardia or sinus arrest
TCAs	Orthostatic hypotension; atrioventricular conduction disturbance; Type IA antiarrhythmic effect; proarrhythmia in overdose and in setting of ischemia
MAOIs	Orthostatic hypotension
First-generation antipsychotics	Orthostatic hypotension (especially low-potency drugs); QT interval prolongation; torsade de pointes
Second-generation antipsychotics	Variable; QT interval prolongation; ventricular arrhythmias; metabolic syndrome
Clozapine	Above plus orthostatic hypotension; myocarditis
Carbamazepine	Type IA antiarrhythmic effects; AV block; hyponatremia
Cholinesterase inhibitors	Decreased heart rate

Note. AV=atrioventricular; MAOIs=monoamine oxidase inhibitors; SSRIs=selective serotonin reuptake inhibitors; TCAs=tricyclic antidepressants.

generally by a clinically insignificant 1–2 beats/minute. Occasional cases of sinus bradycardia or sinus arrest, with light-headedness or syncope, have been reported (Roose et al. 1994, 1998a, 1998b). The combination of beta-adrenergic blockade and serotonin reuptake inhibitors may result in additive slowing of heart rate with increased risk of symptoms. In addition, some SSRIs (fluoxetine, paroxetine, fluvoxamine) inhibit metabolism through the cytochrome P450 (CYP) 2D6 pathway responsible for metabolism of many beta-blockers. Therefore, the blood level and effect of beta-adrenergic blockers may be increased.

In patients with preexisting heart disease, the effects of SSRIs on cardiac function have been evaluated in several studies (Sheline et al. 1997). Some studies using fluoxetine and paroxetine in mixed groups of stable patients with ischemic and nonischemic heart disease demonstrate that ejection fraction may actually improve to a small extent in patients with preexisting ventricular dysfunction. The effects on heart rate are similar to those seen in patients who are free of cardiac disease, and no blood pressure, cardiac conduction, or arrhythmia effects have been noted (Roose et al. 1994, 1998a, 1998b). The SADHART study, as described previously, was a double-blind, placebo-controlled, randomized trial examining the effect of sertraline in patients with major depression immediately after an acute coronary syndrome. Sertraline had no effect on heart rate, blood pressure, arrhythmias, ejection fraction, or cardiac conduction, and adverse events were rare. All patients in SADHART began medication within 30 days of the index acute coronary event (Glassman et al. 2002). Sertraline was effective for treatment of depression in those patients with a prior history of depression, but it did not differ from placebo in response rate for those patients with no prior history of depression. Other prognostic factors associated with response to sertraline were onset of depression before the index cardiac event and more severe depression (Glassman et al. 2006).

The CREATE trial (Lesperance et al. 2007) was a 12-week randomized controlled trial utilizing a two-by-two factorial design to compare citalopram (20–40 mg/day) with placebo treatment, while simultaneously comparing clinical management with and without interpersonal psychotherapy, for treatment of depression in 284 patients with stable coronary disease. The effect of citalopram on depression symptoms and remission rate was significant. Compared with subjects in the placebo group, those receiving citalopram had a 3.3-point larger drop in Hamilton Depression Rating Scale scores and a higher likelihood of response (53% vs. 40%) and remission (36% vs. 23%). In a study in CHF patients, treatment of depression with citalopram was not more effective than placebo treatment; a high response rate was observed in both treatment groups (Fraguas et al. 2009).

Mirtazapine treatment (30–45 mg/day) of depression in patients who had had an acute coronary syndrome was evaluated in a randomized placebo-controlled trial as a part of the MIND-IT trial (Honig et al. 2007). This study enrolled 94 patients and employed several measures of depression at 8 and 24 weeks. Findings were mixed, but mirtazapine was superior to placebo on some measures at both follow-up assessments. Mirtazapine was well tolerated by the patients in this trial, with no effects on heart rate, blood pressure or electrocardiographic parameters, and no difference from placebo in the rate of major adverse cardiac events.

A randomized double-blind, placebo-controlled trial of controlled-release paroxetine for depression treatment in 28 patients with chronic heart failure found paroxetine superior to placebo in reducing Beck Depression Inventory symptoms. No blinded observer rating of treatment response was obtained. The paroxetine dose was 12.5–25 mg/day. Paroxetine treatment was generally well tolerated, although one patient in the active treatment arm died of CHF (Gottlieb et al. 2007).

The cardiovascular effects of other antidepressants have been less fully studied, especially in patients with cardiac disease. Bupropion appears to have few cardiovascular effects in small studies but may increase blood pressure occasionally (Roose et al. 1991). The serotonin-norepinephrine reuptake inhibitor venlafaxine behaves as an SSRI at low doses and displays a noradrenergic effect at higher doses. The main cardiovascular effect of this dual action is a tendency to increase blood pressure in a dose-dependent fashion at a dosage of 150 mg/day or higher. There may be a diminution of this hypertensive effect of venlafaxine with its extended-release formulation. The effect on patients with preexisting heart disease or hypertension has not been evaluated. Clinical experience with mirtazapine in patients with hypertension has also demonstrated instances of worsening hypertension, but the frequency of this adverse effect is unknown. Monoamine oxidase inhibitors (MAOIs) cause hypotension and orthostatic hypotension; dietary indiscretions resulting in high circulating levels of tyramine cause hypertensive crises. Consequently, there has been little interest in use of MAOIs in patients with heart disease. Sympathomimetic agents increase blood pressure in patients on MAOIs, though hypertensive crises are actually infrequent. Caution with the use of intravenous pressors (epinephrine, isoproterenol, norepinephrine, dopamine, dobutamine) is required (Krishnan 1995).

Antipsychotics

Antipsychotics are used in cardiac disease patients with comorbid schizophrenia, schizoaffective disorder, bipolar disorder, and other psychotic disorders and in the management of delirium in acute cardiac care settings, such as after cardiac surgery or in ICU management of pulmonary edema, arrhythmias, or acute MI. Although first-generation antipsychotic medications are losing primacy as agents of choice for management of chronic psychosis because of their extrapyramidal side effects, they continue to play a role in management of acute psychotic symptoms in delirium. In part this is because of the availability of parenteral formulations for haloperidol, few cardiovascular effects, and extensive experience with use of intravenous haloperidol in the critically ill (see Chapter 5, "Delirium").

For chronically psychotic patients with heart disease, the choice of antipsychotic is based on side-effect profile. The principal cardiovascular effects of antipsychotic agents are orthostatic hypotension and QT interval prolongation. Orthostatic hypotension secondary to antipsychotic drugs is related to their alpha-adrenergic receptor-blocking effect, seen especially with the low-potency antipsychotic agents such as chlorpromazine and often accompanied by sedative effects. There are few data about the frequency or clinical significance of orthostatic effects of antipsychotic drugs in patients with heart disease. More attention has been paid to the less common but much more dramatic and dangerous side effect of cardiac arrest secondary to ventricular tachyarrhythmias in patients on antipsychotic drugs. The characteristic tachyarrhythmia is torsade de pointes, a polymorphic tachycardia with the appearance of "twisting of the points" of the QRS complex. QT prolongation as a result of antipsychotic agents, unlike that caused by TCAs, appears to be an effect of impaired repolarization of the ventricular conduction tissue at the end of systole, specifically an effect on the so-called potassium rectifier channel. The QT interval normally is less than 450 msec. Because the normal QT interval is dependent on heart rate, evaluation customarily adjusts for heart rate to yield a corrected QT interval (QTc). QTc greater than 500 msec greatly increases the risk of torsade de pointes. Thioridazine is the agent most commonly associated with torsade and sudden cardiac death, and sertindole was withdrawn in the United States because of its QT prolongation effects and the rate of sudden cardiac deaths observed overseas. Intravenous haloperidol is frequently employed in delirious open-heart surgery patients, and although it does have the potential to prolong the QT interval, its use in dosages up to 1,000 mg/24 hours has been reported without complications (Tesar et al. 1985). The one exception appears to be aripiprazole, which has not been reported to cause QTc prolongation even in overdose (Young et al. 2009). Clearly, electrocardiographic monitoring is important in ICU settings, and patients with a QTc interval greater than 450 msec should be closely monitored. A QTc interval over 500 msec is generally considered a contraindication to use of haloperidol and other QT-prolonging agents.

In considering the use of drugs that may prolong the QT interval, risk factors for torsade should be reviewed, including female sex, familial long QT syndrome; family or personal history of sudden cardiac death, syncope, or unexplained seizure; arrhythmias; personal history of hypertension; other medications that prolong the QT interval or that may interfere with metabolism of other QT-prolonging agents; valvular heart disease; and bradycardia. Laboratory values of particular importance are magnesium and potassium levels. Class IA and III antiarrhythmic drugs, dolasetron, droperidol, tacrolimus, levomethadyl acetate, other antipsychotic agents, many antibiotics ("floxacins"), and antifungal agents may increase the risk of torsade de pointes (Al-Khatib et al. 2003; Glassman and Bigger 2001; Moss 2003; Roden 2008).

A large cohort study taking advantage of statewide Medicaid prescription data found that antipsychotic drug use was associated with doubling of sudden cardiac death risk; the increase in the absolute risk of sudden cardiac death associated with antipsychotic drug use was about 0.15%, meaning that one extra death would occur for every 666 persons treated for 1 year with antipsychotic drugs (Ray et al. 2009). It seems clear that this risk would be higher in patients with preexisting cardiac disease maintained on antipsychotic agents. For elderly patients receiving antipsychotic drugs for agitation or behavioral disturbance (e.g., psychotic symptoms in dementia), it is now clear that the risk of death associated with antipsychotic drugs is substantially higher. In the past several years, several studies (Gill et al. 2007; Kales et al. 2007; Liperoti et al. 2005; Rochon et al. 2008; Schneider et al. 2005; Suh and Shaw 2005; P.S. Wang et al. 2005) have drawn attention to the mortality risk associated with antipsychotic drug use in elderly patients with behavioral disturbance, and an FDA black-box warning was applied to all first- and second-generation antipsychotic agents. Studies have been conducted primarily in nursing home populations over short time frames (typically, one to several months) and demonstrate an increased absolute risk of death of about 1.9%, implying a number needed to harm of about 50. Most of these deaths were attributed to either cardiovascular or infectious causes. None of these studies directly address treatment of delirium, but the psychiatrist venturing to treat delirium or acute psychotic symptoms in patients with heart disease must be guided by an appreciation of these risks.

Of course, polymorphic ventricular tachycardia can also occur in the absence of long QT interval. Brugada syndrome is a rare disorder also characterized by history of syncope and risk of sudden death due to polymorphic ventricular tachyarrhythmias. In contrast to the defect in potassium channel–mediated ventricular repolarization underlying antipsychotic-induced prolongation of the QT interval, in Brugada syndrome the conduction abnormality is mediated by a sodium channel, prolonging ventricular depolarization, particularly in the right ventricle. ECG demonstrates an RSR′ pattern and ST segment elevation in the right precordial leads, resembling right bundle branch block. Lithium has been reported to provoke Brugada syndrome, and drugs that interfere with the sodium channel, prolonging the depolarization phase of the action potential, including phenothiazines, tricyclic antidepressants, and carbamazepine, might also increase risk (Laske et al. 2007).

Second-generation antipsychotic agents also increase cardiovascular disease risk indirectly through promotion of the metabolic syndrome (dyslipidemia, obesity, hypertension, and impaired glycemic control). Olanzapine and clozapine may be most likely, and aripiprazole and ziprasidone least likely, to induce metabolic syndrome. In the Clinical Antipsychotic Trials of Intervention Effectiveness (CATIE) study, olanzapine and quetiapine were associated with a slight increase, and risperidone, ziprasidone, and perphenazine with a slight decrease, in the 10-year risk of heart disease (Bobes et al. 2007; Correll et al. 2006, 2009; Daumit et al. 2008; Newcomer et al. 2007).

Myocarditis has been estimated to occur in 0.01%–1.0% of patients treated with clozapine, generally within the first few weeks of treatment (Merrill et al. 2005). Cardiomyopathy has also been reported, with onset up to a few years after starting clozapine, even without prior acute myocarditis (Mackin 2008).

Anxiolytics

Benzodiazepines have no specific cardiac effects. Reduction of anxiety tends to reduce sympathetic nervous system activation and, therefore, to slow heart rate, reduce myocardial work, and reduce myocardial irritability. Before the introduction of beta-blockers to acute coronary care, benzodiazepines were widely used for prophylaxis of infarct extension and arrhythmias in acute coronary syndrome patients, but this practice has largely been abandoned. Lorazepam can be given by intramuscular (or intravenous) injection; for most other benzodiazepines this route should be avoided because of poor absorption. Oxazepam, lorazepam, and temazepam do not undergo Phase I hepatic metabolism and may be easier for patients with heart failure to tolerate. Buspirone has no cardiovascular effects.

Stimulants

Stimulants are often useful for treating of depressed, medically ill patients, particularly those with pronounced apathy, fatigue, or psychomotor slowing. A review (Wilens et al. 2005) of several trials of stimulant treatment of attention-deficit/hyperactivity disorder (ADHD) in adults concluded that treatment increases systolic and diastolic blood pressure by about 5 mm Hg, but the doses that would be employed for ADHD treatment would typically be higher than would be used in cardiac patients. At dosages of 5–30 mg/day, dextroamphetamine and methylphenidate are well tolerated by heart disease patients, including patients with cardiac arrhythmias and angina (Masand and Tesar 1996), and have no effects on heart rate and blood pressure. Clinical response generally occurs within days rather than weeks. The safety of a long-term treatment that raises blood pressure by 5 mm Hg has been questioned (Nissen 2006), and arrhythmia/sudden cardiac death risk associated with stimulants might be increased in children and adolescents (Gould et al. 2009) or if there is unrecognized structural heart disease (Nissen 2006), but a 10-year review of Florida Medicaid data (Winterstein et al. 2007) did not find increased mortality in children treated with stimulants for ADHD, and a recent Cochrane review did not find substantial evidence for cardiovascular harm from stimulant treatment (Candy et al. 2008). In view of the lack of consensus on the cardiovascular risks of stimulants, cardiology consultation may be prudent before prescribing stimulants for patients with heart disease.

Lithium

Lithium occasionally causes sinus node dysfunction and even sinus arrest (Mitchell and Mackenzie 1982). There are no studies of the use of lithium in patients with heart disease. Generally, even in patients with heart disease with reduced cardiac output, lithium can be safely used by adjusting the dosage downward. Because renal function is sometimes impaired in advanced heart failure, lithium dosing requires further reduction. Caution is necessary for patients taking ACE inhibitors, angiotensin II receptor blockers, and diuretics, especially thiazides, and for those on salt restricted diets. In patients with acute CHF exacerbations and acute coronary syndromes, rapid electrolyte and fluid balance shifts can occur; lithium is best avoided during such episodes because of the difficulty managing fluctuations in lithium level as cardiac therapy is adjusted.

Other Mood Stabilizers

Valproic acid and lamotrigine have no cardiovascular effects. Carbamazepine resembles TCAs in having a quinidine-like Type IA antiarrhythmic effect and may cause atrioventricular conduction disturbances.

Cholinesterase Inhibitors and NMDA Receptor Antagonists

The elderly are prone to co-occurrence of dementia and heart disease, and treatments for dementia, including cholinesterase inhibitors (donepezil, rivastigmine, galantamine) and *N*-methyl-D-aspartic acid (NMDA) inhibitors (memantine), may be used in patients with concurrent heart disease. The procholinergic effect of cholinesterase inhibitors may cause vagotonic effects, including bradycardia or heart block. For memantine, hypertension is the only cardiac effect described by the manufacturer on the basis of premarketing controlled trials.

Electroconvulsive Therapy

ECT leads to an initial sympathetic discharge, with tachycardia and hypertension, followed by a parasympathetic reflex response, with instances of bradycardia and arrhythmia. Asystole can occur rarely but can be prevented by premedication with atropine. Excessive sympathetic response may evoke myocardial ischemia; for the elderly or those with known coronary disease, monitoring the ECG is essential, and treatment with intravenous beta-blockers is sometimes required. Takotsubo cardiomyopathy has been reported after ECT; a case of successful reintroduction of ECT after prior Takotsubo cardiomyopathy response to ECT has also been reported (Kent et al. 2009; O'Reardon et al. 2008). Cardiac effects of ECT are discussed further in Chapter 40, "Electroconvulsive Therapy." ECT has been used safely in patients with ischemic heart disease, heart failure, and heart transplants. Acute MI or recent malignant tachyarrhythmias are relatively strong contraindications.

Cardiac–Psychiatric Drug Interactions

A few drug interactions between psychotropic and cardiovascular drugs are worth noting (Table 18–3). Many psychotropic drugs lower blood pressure; their interaction with antihypertensive medications, vasodilators, and diuretics may potentiate hypotension. TCAs and antipsychotic drugs that prolong the QT interval may interact with antiarrhythmic agents such as quinidine, procainamide, moricizine, and amiodarone and result in further QT prolongation or atrioventricular block. Although SSRIs may increase risk of bleeding, most do not appear to have a clinically significant effect on the international normalized ratio (INR) in patients treated with warfarin. The largest INR effects occur with fluoxetine and fluvoxamine (Holbrook et al. 2005; Sansone and Sansone 2009). In patients undergoing CABG, SSRIs do not increase bleeding risk or hospital mortality, even when administered along with warfarin, antiplatelet therapies, and nonsteroidal anti-inflammatory agents (Kim et al. 2009).

Drug Interactions: Cytochrome P450 Issues

CYP 2D6 is responsible for the metabolism of many beta-blockers, carvedilol, and antiarrhythmic agents; this metabolic pathway is inhibited by haloperidol, fluoxetine, and paroxetine, with resulting elevation of blood levels of CYP 2D6 substrates. Conversely, amiodarone is a 2D6 inhibitor and can elevate blood levels of amitriptyline, nortriptyline, clomipramine, codeine, desipramine, fluoxetine, and risperidone. CYP 3A4 is responsible for metabolism of alprazolam, midazolam, triazolam, zolpidem, buspirone, carbamazepine, and haloperidol and of calcium channel blockers, cyclosporine, many statin agents, and tacrolimus.

TABLE 18–3. Selected psychotropic drug interactions with cardiovascular drugs

Psychotropic agent	Cardiovascular agent	Effect
SSRIs	Beta-blockers	Additive bradycardic effects
	Warfarin	Increased bleeding risk, especially with paroxetine and fluoxetine, despite little effect on INR
MAOIs	Epinephrine, dopamine	Hypertension
Lithium	Thiazide diuretics	Increased lithium level
TCAs	Type IA antiarrhythmic agents, amiodarone	Prolonged QT interval, increased AV block
Lithium	ACE inhibitors, angiotensin II receptor blockers	Increased lithium level
Phenothiazines	Beta-blockers	Hypotension

Note. ACE=angiotensin-converting enzyme; AV=atrioventricular; INR=international normalized ratio; MAOIs=monoamine oxidase inhibitors; SSRIs=selective serotonin reuptake inhibitors; TCAs=tricyclic antidepressants.

The 3A4 system is inhibited by amiodarone, diltiazem, verapamil, grapefruit juice, and nefazodone, and to a lesser degree by fluoxetine and sertraline. The combination of nefazodone and haloperidol might increase the risk of ventricular arrhythmias, because increased haloperidol levels may result in greater QT prolongation. Carbamazepine and St. John's wort are inducers of CYP 3A4 activity. An evolving reference listing for CYP interactions is available on the World Wide Web (Flockhart 2009), and these interactions are also reviewed in Chapter 38, "Psychopharmacology."

References

Aboa-Eboulé C, Brisson C, Maunsell E, et al: Job strain and risk of acute recurrent coronary heart disease events. JAMA 298:1652–1660, 2007

Albert NM, Fonarow GC, Abraham WT, et al: Depression and clinical outcomes in heart failure: an OPTIMIZE-HF analysis. Am J Med 122:366–373, 2009

Alexander PJ, Prabhu SG, Krishnamoorthy ES, et al: Mental disorders in patients with noncardiac chest pain. Acta Psychiatr Scand 89:291–293, 1994

Al-Khatib SM, LaPointe NMA, Kramer JM, et al: What clinicians should know about the QT interval. JAMA 289:2120–2127, 2003

American Psychiatric Association: Diagnostic and Statistical Manual of Mental Disorders, 3rd Edition. Washington, DC, American Psychiatric Association, 1980

American Psychiatric Association: Diagnostic and Statistical Manual of Mental Disorders, 4th Edition. Washington, DC, American Psychiatric Association, 1994

Anda R, Williamson D, Jones D, et al: Depressed affect, hopelessness, and the risk of ischemic heart disease in a cohort of US adults. Epidemiology 4:285–294, 1993

Angeli F, Verdecchia P, Gattobigio R, et al: White-coat hypertension in adults. Blood Press Monit 10:301–305, 2005

Appels A, Mulder P: Fatigue and heart disease. The association between "vital exhaustion" and past, present, and future coronary heart disease. J Psychosom Res 3:727–738, 1989

Appels A, Bar F, van der Pol G, et al: Effects of treating exhaustion in angioplasty patients on new coronary events: results of the randomized Exhaustion Intervention Trial (EXIT). Psychosom Med 67:217–223, 2005

Appels A, van Elderen T, Bar F, et al: Effects of a behavioural intervention on quality of life and related variables in angioplasty patients: results of the EXhaustion Intervention Trial. J Psychosom Res 61:1–7, 2006

Barefoot J, Schroll M: Symptoms of depression, acute myocardial infarction, and total mortality in a community sample. Circulation 93:1976–1980, 1996

Barefoot JC, Patterson JC, Haney TL, et al: Hostility in asymptomatic men with angiographically confirmed coronary artery disease. Am J Cardiol 74:439–442, 1994

Barefoot JC, Larsen S, Von der Lieth L, et al: Hostility, incidence of acute myocardial infarction, and mortality in a sample of older Danish men and women. Am J Epidemiol 142:477–484, 1995

Barefoot JC, Helms MJ, Mark DB, et al: Depression and long-term mortality risk in patients with coronary artery disease. Am J Cardiol 78:613–617, 1996

Barlow DH: Anxiety and Its Disorders. New York, Guilford, 1988

Barsky AJ: Palpitations, cardiac awareness, and panic disorder. Am J Med 92 (suppl 1A):31S–34S, 1992

Barsky AJ, Cleary PD, Coeytaux RR, et al: Psychiatric disorders in medical outpatients complaining of palpitations. J Gen Intern Med 9:306–313, 1994a

Barsky AJ, Cleary PD, Sarnie MK, et al: Panic disorder, palpitations, and the awareness of cardiac activity. J Nerv Ment Dis 182:63–71, 1994b

Barsky AJ, Delamater BA, Clancy SA, et al: Somatized psychiatric disorder presenting as palpitations. Arch Intern Med 156:1102–1108, 1996

Barth J, Schumacher M, Herrmann-Lingen C: Depression as a risk factor for mortality in patients with coronary heart disease: a meta-analysis. Psychosom Med 66:802–813, 2004

Bielecka-Dabrowa A, Mikhailidis DP, Hannam S, et al: Takotsubo cardiomyopathy—the current state of knowledge. Int J Cardiol 142:120–125, 2010

Bigger JT, Fleiss JL, Steinman RC, et al: Frequency domain measures of heart period variability and mortality after myocardial infarction. Circulation 85:164–171, 1992

Bigger JT, Fleiss JL, Rolnitzky LM, et al: Frequency domain measures of heart period variability to assess risk late after myocardial infarction. J Am Coll Cardiol 21:729–736, 1993

Birkenaes AB, Sogaard AJ, Engh JA, et al: Sociodemographic characteristics and cardiovascular risk factors in patients with severe mental disorders compared with the general population. J Clin Psychiatry 67:425–433, 2006

Blanchette CM, Simoni-Wastila L, Zuckerman IH, et al: A secondary analysis of a duration response association between selective serotonin reuptake inhibitor use and the risk of acute myocardial infarction in the aging population. Ann Epidemiol 18:316–321, 2008

Blumenthal JA, Jiang W, Waugh RA, et al: Mental stress-induced ischemia in the laboratory and ambulatory ischemia during daily life. Association and hemodynamic features. Circulation 92:2102–2108, 1995

Blumenthal JA, Lett HS, Babyak MA, et al: Depression as a risk factor for mortality after coronary artery bypass surgery. Lancet 362:604–609, 2003

Blumenthal JA, Sherwood A, Babyak MA, et al: Effects of exercise and stress management training on markers of cardiovascular risk in patients with ischemic heart disease: a randomized controlled trial. JAMA 293:1626–1634, 2005

Bobes J, Arango C, Aranda P, et al: Cardiovascular and metabolic risk in outpatients with schizophrenia treated with antipsychotics: results of the CLAMORS Study. Schizophr Res 90:162–173, 2007

Booth-Kewley S, Friedman HS: Psychological predictors of heart disease: a quantitative review. Psychol Bull 101:343–362, 1987

Boscarino JA: A prospective study of PTSD and early-age heart disease mortality among Vietnam veterans: implications for surveillance and prevention. Psychosom Med 70:668–676, 2008

Bostwick JM, Sola CL: An updated review of implantable cardioverter/defibrillators, induced anxiety, and quality of life. Psychiatr Clin North Am 30:677–688, 2007

Bradley TD, Floras JS: Sleep apnea and heart failure, I: obstructive sleep apnea. Circulation 107:1671–1678, 2003a

Bradley TD, Floras JS: Sleep apnea and heart failure, II: central sleep apnea. Circulation 107:1822–1826, 2003b

Brown TM, Stoudemire A: Cardiovascular agents, in Psychiatric Side Effects of Prescription and Over-the-Counter Drugs. Washington, DC, American Psychiatric Press, 1998, pp 209–238

Burg MM, Barefoot J, Berkman L, et al: Low perceived social support and post-myocardial infarction prognosis in the Enhancing Recovery in Coronary Heart Disease clinical trial: the effects of treatment. Psychosom Med 67:879–888, 2005

Candy M, Jones L, Williams R, et al: Psychostimulants for depression. Cochrane Database Syst Rev (2):CD006722, 2008

Carney CP, Jones LE: Medical comorbidity in women and men with bipolar disorders: a population-based controlled study. Psychosom Med 68:684–691, 2006

Carney CP, Jones L, Woolson RF: Medical comorbidity in women and men with schizophrenia: a population-based controlled study. J Gen Intern Med 21:1133–1137, 2006

Carney RM, Freedland KE: Treatment-resistant depression and mortality after acute coronary syndrome. Am J Psychiatry 166:410–417, 2009

Carney RM, Freedland KE, Ludbrook PA, et al: Major depression, panic disorder, and mitral valve prolapse in patients who complain of chest pain. Am J Med 89:757–760, 1990

Carney RM, Blumenthal JA, Stein PK, et al: Depression, heart rate variability, and acute myocardial infarction. Circulation 104:2024–2028, 2001

Carney RM, Freedland KE, Miller GE, et al: Depression as a risk factor for cardiac mortality and morbidity. A review of potential mechanisms. J Psychosom Res 53:897–902, 2002

Carney RM, Blumenthal JA, Catellier D, et al: Depression as a risk factor for mortality after acute myocardial infarction. Am J Cardiol 92:1277–1281, 2003

Carney RM, Blumenthal JA, Freedland KE, et al: Depression and late mortality after myocardial infarction in the Enhancing Recovery in Coronary Heart Disease (ENRICHD) Study. Psychosom Med 66:466–474, 2004

Carney RM, Blumenthal JA, Freedland KE, et al: Low heart rate variability and the effect of depression on post-myocardial infarction mortality. Arch Intern Med 165:1486–1491, 2005

Carney RM, Freedland KE, Steinmeyer B, et al: History of depression and survival after acute myocardial infarction. Psychosom Med 71:253–259, 2009

Carroll D, Phillips AC, Gale CR, et al: Generalized anxiety and major depressive disorders, their comorbidity, and hypertension in middle-aged men. Psychosom Med 72:16–19, 2010

Cassem NH: The person confronting death, in The New Harvard Guide to Psychiatry. Edited by Nicholi AM Jr. Cambridge, MA, Harvard University Press, 1985, pp 728–758

CAST Investigators: Preliminary report: effect of encainide and flecainide on mortality in a randomized trial of arrhythmia suppression after myocardial infarction. N Engl J Med 321:406–412, 1989

CAST II Investigators: Effect of the antiarrhythmic agent moricizine on survival after myocardial infarction. N Engl J Med 327:227–233, 1992

Cazeau S, Leclercq C, Lavergne T, et al: Effects of multisite biventricular pacing in patients with heart failure and intraventricular conduction delay. N Engl J Med 344:873–880, 2001

Cesari M, Penninx BW, Newman AB, et al: Inflammatory markers and onset of cardiovascular events: results from the health ABC study. Circulation 108:2317–2322, 2003

Cohen BE, Marmar CR, Neylan TC, et al: Posttraumatic stress disorder and health-related quality of life in patients with coronary heart disease: findings from the Heart and Soul Study. Arch Gen Psychiatry 66:1214–1220, 2009

Cohen HW, Gibson G, Alderman MH: Excess risk of myocardial infarction in patients treated with antidepressant medications: association with use of tricyclic agents. Am J Med 108:2–8, 2000

Cohen-Cole SA, Kauffman KG: Major depression in physical illness: diagnosis, prevalence, and antidepressant treatment. A ten year review, 1982–1992. Depression 1:181–204, 1993

Cohn JN: The management of chronic heart failure. N Engl J Med 335:490–498, 1996

Connerney I, Shapiro PA, McLaughlin JS, et al: Relation between depression after coronary artery bypass surgery and 12-month outcome: a prospective study. Lancet 358:1766–1771, 2001

Copeland JG, Smith RG, Arabia FA, et al: Cardiac replacement with a total artificial heart as a bridge to transplantation. N Engl J Med 351:859–867, 2004

Correll CU, Frederickson AM, Kane JM: Metabolic syndrome and the risk of coronary heart disease in 367 patients treated with second-generation antipsychotic drug. J Clin Psychiatry 67:575–583, 2006

Correll CU, Manu P, Olshanskiy V, et al: Cardiometabolic risk of second-generation antipsychotic medications during first-time use in children and adolescents. JAMA 302:1765–1773, 2009

Coryell W: Panic disorder and mortality. Psychiatr Clin North Am 2:433–440, 1988

Coryell W, Noyes R, House JD: Mortality among outpatients with anxiety disorders. Am J Psychiatry 143:508–510, 1986

Cox D, Lewis G, Stuart G, et al: A cross-sectional study of the prevalence of psychopathology in adults with congenital heart disease. J Psychosom Res 52:65–68, 2002

Critchley HD, Taggart P, Sutton PM, et al: Mental stress and sudden cardiac death: asymmetric midbrain activity as a linking mechanism. Brain 128:75–85, 2005

Crow SJ, Collins J, Justic M, et al: Psychopathology following cardioverter defibrillator implantation. Psychosomatics 39:305–310, 1998

Cully JA, Johnson M, Moffett ML, et al: Depression and anxiety in ambulatory patients with heart failure. Psychosomatics 50:592–598, 2009

Dager SR, Comess KA, Dunner DL: Differentiation of anxious patients by two-dimensional echocardiographic evaluation of the mitral valve. Am J Psychiatry 143:533–535, 1986

Dammen T, Ekeberg O, Arnesen H, et al: The detection of panic disorder in chest pain patients. Gen Hosp Psychiatry 21:323–332, 1999

Daumit GL, Goff DC, Meyer JM, et al: Antipsychotic effects on estimated 10-year coronary heart disease risk in the CATIE schizophrenia study. Schizophr Res 105:175–187, 2008

Davidson KW, Kupfer DJ, Bigger JT, et al: Assessment and treatment of depression in patients with cardiovascular disease: National Heart, Lung, and Blood Institute Working Group Report. Psychosom Med 68:645–650, 2006

Davidson KW, Mostofsky E, Whang W: Don't worry, be happy: positive affect and reduced 10-year incident coronary heart disease: The Canadian Nova Scotia Health Survey. Eur Heart J 31:1065–1070, 2010a

Davidson KW, Burg MM, Kronish IM, et al: Association of anhedonia with recurrent major adverse cardiac events and mortality 1 year after acute coronary syndrome. Arch Gen Psychiatry 67:480–488, 2010b

Davies SJ, Ghahramani P, Jackson PR, et al: Association of panic disorder and panic attacks with hypertension. Am J Med 107:310–316, 1999

DeBusk RF: Sexual activity in patients with angina. JAMA 290:3129–3132, 2003

de Jonge P, van den Brink RH, Spijkerman TA, et al: Only incident depressive episodes after myocardial infarction are associated with new cardiovascular events. J Am Coll Cardiol 48:2204–2208, 2006

de Jonge P, Honig A, van Melle JP, et al: Nonresponse to treatment for depression following myocardial infarction: association with subsequent cardiac events. The Mind-It Investigators. Am J Psychiatry 164:1371–1378, 2007

Denollet J: DS14: standard assessment of negative affectivity, social inhibition, and type D personality. Psychosom Med 67:89–97, 2005

Denollet J, Sys S, Brutsaert DL: Personality and mortality after myocardial infarction. Psychosom Med 57:582–591, 1995

Denollet J, Sys SU, Stroobant N, et al: Personality as independent predictor of long-term mortality in patients with coronary heart disease. Lancet 347:417–421, 1996

Denollet J, Pedersen SS, Vrints CJ, et al: Usefulness of type D personality in predicting five-year cardiac events above and beyond concurrent symptoms of stress in patients with coronary heart disease. Am J Cardiol 97:970–973, 2006

Denollet J, Pedersen SS, Daemen J, et al: Reduced positive affect (anhedonia) predicts major clinical events following implantation of coronary-artery stents. J Intern Med 263:203–211, 2008

DeSilva RA: Central nervous system risk factors for sudden cardiac death. J S C Med Assoc 79:561–572, 1983

DeSilva RA: Cardiac arrhythmias and sudden cardiac death, in Medical-Psychiatric Practice. Edited by Stoudemire A, Fogel BS. Washington, DC, American Psychiatric Press, 1993, pp 199–236

Detroyer E, Dobbels F, Verfaillie E, et al: Is preoperative anxiety and depression associated with onset of delirium after cardiac surgery in older patients? A prospective cohort study. J Am Geriatr Soc 56:2278–2284, 2008

Dew MA, Kormos RL, Nastala C, et al: Psychiatric and psychosocial issues and intervention among ventricular assist device patients, in Quality of Life and Psychosomatics in Mechanical Circulation and Heart Transplantation. Edited by Albert W, Bittner A, Hetzer R. New York, Springer, 1998, pp 17–27

Dew MA, Kormos RL, Winowich S, et al: Human factors in ventricular assist device recipients and their family caregivers. Paper presented at the American Society for Artificial Internal Organs, San Diego CA, June 1999a

Dew MA, Kormos RL, Winowich S, et al: Quality of life outcomes in left ventricular assist system inpatients and outpatients. ASAIO J 45:218–225, 1999b

Dew M, Kormos R, DiMartini A, et al: Prevalence and risk of depression and anxiety-related disorders during the first three years after heart transplantation. Psychosomatics 42:300–313, 2001

Dickens C, McGowan L, Percival C, et al: New onset depression following myocardial infarction predicts cardiac mortality. Psychosom Med 70:450–455, 2008

Diegeler A, Hirsch R, Schneider F, et al: Neuromonitoring and neurocognitive outcome in off-pump versus conventional coronary bypass operation. Ann Thorac Surg 69:1162–1166, 2000

DiMarco JP: Implantable cardioverter-defibrillators. N Engl J Med 349:1836–1847, 2003

Dimsdale JE: Psychological stress and cardiovascular disease. J Am Coll Cardiol 51:1237–1246, 2008

Doraiswamy PM, Varia I, Hellegers C, et al: A randomized controlled trial of paroxetine for noncardiac chest pain. Psychopharmacol Bull 39:15–24, 2006

Dusseldorp E, Van Elderen T, Maes S, et al: A meta-analysis of psychoeducational programs for coronary heart disease patients. Health Psychol 18:506–519, 1999

Eaker ED, Sullivan LM, Kelly-Hayes M, et al: Tension and anxiety and the prediction of the 10-year incidence of coronary heart disease, atrial fibrillation, and total mortality: the Framingham Offspring Study. Psychosom Med 67:692–696, 2005

Empana JP, Sykes DH, Luc G, et al: Contributions of depressive mood and circulating inflammatory markers to coronary heart disease in healthy European men: the Prospective Epidemiological Study of Myocardial Infarction (PRIME). Circulation 111:2299–2305, 2005

Empana JP, Jouven X, Lemaitre RN, et al: Clinical depression and risk of out-of-hospital cardiac arrest. Arch Intern Med 166:195–200, 2006

Engel GL: Psychologic factors in instantaneous cardiac death. N Engl J Med 294:664–665, 1976

Faris R, Purcell H, Henein MY, et al: Clinical depression is common and significantly associated with reduced survival in patients with non-ischaemic heart failure. Eur J Heart Fail 4:541–551, 2002

Epstein AE, DiMarco JP, Ellenbogen KA, et al: ACC/AHA/HRS 2008 guidelines for device-based therapy of cardiac rhythm abnormalities: a report of the American College of Cardiology/American Heart Association Task Force on Practice Guidelines (Writing Committee to Revise the ACC/AHA/NASPE 2002 Guideline Update for Implantation of Cardiac Pacemakers and Antiarrhythmia Devices) developed in collaboration with the American Association for Thoracic Surgery and Society of Thoracic Surgeons. J Am Coll Cardiol 51:e1–62, 2008

Filho AS, Maciel BC, Martín-Santos R, et al: Does the association between mitral valve prolapse and panic disorder really exist? Prim Care Companion J Clin Psychiatry 10:38–47, 2008

Fisman EZ, Benderly M, Esper RJ, et al: Interleukin-6 and the risk of future cardiovascular events in patients with angina pectoris and/or healed myocardial infarction. Am J Cardiol 98:14–18, 2006

Fleet R, Lavoie K, Beitman PD: Is panic disorder associated with coronary artery disease? J Psychosom Res 48:347–356, 2000

Flockhart DA: Drug Interactions: Cytochrome P450 Drug Interaction Table, Version 5.0. Indianapolis, IN, Indiana University School of Medicine, Division of Clinical Pharmacology, January 2009. Available at: http://www.drug-interactions.com. Accessed January 30, 2010.

Forbess JM, Visconti KJ, Hancock-Friesen C, et al: Neurodevelopmental outcome after congenital heart disease surgery: results from an institutional registry. Circulation 106 (12 suppl 1):I95–I102, 2002

Forette F, Seux ML, Staessen JA, et al: The prevention of dementia with antihypertensive treatment: new evidence from the Systolic Hypertension in Europe (Syst-Eur) study. Arch Intern Med 162:2046–2052, 2002

Fraguas R, da Silva Telles RM, Alves TC, et al: A double-blind, placebo-controlled treatment trial of citalopram for major depressive disorder in older patients with heart failure: the relevance of the placebo effect and psychological symptoms. Contemp Clin Trials 30:205–211, 2009

Frasure-Smith N, Lesperance F: Depression and anxiety as predictors of 2-year cardiac events in patients with stable coronary artery disease. Arch Gen Psychiatry 65:62–71, 2008

Frasure-Smith N, Lesperance F, Talajic M: Depression following myocardial infarction. Impact on 6-month survival. JAMA 270:1819–1825, 1993

Frasure-Smith N, Lesperance F, Talajic M: Depression and 18-month prognosis following myocardial infarction. Circulation 91:999–1005, 1995a

Frasure-Smith N, Lesperance F, Talajic M: The impact of negative emotions on prognosis following myocardial infarction: is it more than depression? Health Psychol 14:388–398, 1995b

Frasure-Smith N, Lesperance F, Prince RH, et al: Randomised trial of home-based psychosocial nursing intervention for patients recovering from myocardial infarction. Lancet 350:473–479, 1997

Frasure-Smith N, Lesperance F, Gravel G, et al: Social support, depression, and mortality during the first year after myocardial infarction. Circulation 101:1919–1924, 2000

Freedland KE, Rich MW, Skala JA, et al: Prevalence of depression in hospitalized patients with congestive heart failure. Psychosom Med 65:119–128, 2003

Fricchione GL, Olson LC, Vlay SC: Psychiatric syndromes in patients with the automatic internal cardioverter defibrillator: anxiety, psychological dependence, abuse, and withdrawal. Am Heart J 117:1411–1414, 1989

Friedman M, Thoresen CE, Gill JJ, et al: Alteration of type A behavior and its effect on cardiac recurrences in post myocardial infarction patients: summary results of the recurrent coronary prevention project. Am Heart J 112:653–665, 1986

Friedman R, Schwartz JE, Schnall PL, et al: Psychological variables in hypertension: relationship to casual or ambulatory blood pressure in men. Psychosom Med 63:19–31, 2001

Frishman WH: Are antihypertensive agents protective against dementia? A review of clinical and preclinical data. Heart Dis 4:380–386, 2002

Gehi A, Haas D, Pipkin S, et al: Depression and medication adherence in outpatients with coronary heart disease: findings from the Heart and Soul Study. Arch Intern Med 165:2508–2513, 2005a

Gehi A, Mangano D, Pipkin S, et al: Depression and heart rate variability in patients with stable coronary heart disease: findings from the Heart and Soul Study. Arch Gen Psychiatry 62:661–666, 2005b

Gehi AK, Ali S, Na B, et al: Self-reported medication adherence and cardiovascular events in patients with stable coronary heart disease: the Heart and Soul Study. Arch Intern Med 167:1798–1803, 2007

Geyer S, Norozi K, Zoege M, et al: Psychological symptoms in patients after surgery for congenital cardiac disease. Cardiol Young 16:540–548, 2006

Gill SS, Bronskill SE, Normand S-LT, et al: Antipsychotic drug use and mortality in older adults with dementia. Ann Intern Med 146:775–786, 2007

Giltay EJ, Geleijnse JM, Zitman FG, et al: Dispositional optimism and all-cause and cardiovascular mortality in a prospective cohort of elderly Dutch men and women. Arch Gen Psychiatry 61:1126–1135, 2004

Giltay EJ, Huijskes RVHP, Kho KH, et al: Psychotic symptoms in patients undergoing coronary artery bypass grafting and heart valve operation. Eur J Cardiothorac Surg 30:140–147, 2006

Glassman AH: Cigarette smoking: implications for psychiatric illness. Am J Psychiatry 150:546–553, 1993

Glassman AH, Bigger JT Jr: Antipsychotic drugs: prolonged QTc interval, torsade de pointes and sudden death. Am J Psychiatry 158:1774–1782, 2001

Glassman AH, Shapiro PA: Depression and the course of coronary artery disease. Am J Psychiatry 155:4–11, 1998

Glassman AH, Roose SP, Bigger JT Jr: The safety of tricyclic antidepressants in cardiac patients. Risk-benefit reconsidered. JAMA 269:2673–2675, 1993

Glassman AH, O'Connor CM, Califf RM, et al: Sertraline treatment of major depression in patients with acute MI or unstable angina. JAMA 288:701–709, 2002

Glassman AH, Bigger JTJ, Gaffney M, et al: Onset of major depression associated with acute coronary syndromes. Relationship of onset, major depressive disorder history, and episode severity to sertraline benefit. Arch Gen Psychiatry 63:283–288, 2006

Glassman AH, Bigger JT Jr, Gaffney M: Psychiatric characteristics associated with long-term mortality among 361 patients having an acute coronary syndrome and major depression: seven-year follow-up of SADHART participants. Arch Gen Psychiatry 66:1022–1029, 2009

Goldstein BI, Fagiolini A, Houck P, et al: Cardiovascular disease and hypertension among adults with bipolar I disorder in the United States. Bipolar Disord 11:657–662, 2009

Goldstein DJ, Oz MC: Cardiac Assist Devices. Armonk, NY, Futura, 2000

Gomez-Caminero A, Blumentals WA, Russo LJ, et al: Does panic disorder increase the risk of coronary heart disease? A cohort study of a national managed care database. Psychosom Med 67:688–691, 2005

Gorman JM, Goetz RR, Fyer M, et al: The mitral valve prolapse-panic disorder connection. Psychosom Med 50:114–122, 1988

Gottlieb SS, Kop WJ, Thomas SA, et al: A double-blind placebo-controlled pilot study of controlled-release paroxetine on depression and quality of life in chronic heart failure. Am Heart J 153:868–873, 2007

Gould MS, Walsh BT, Munfakh JL, et al: Sudden death and use of stimulant medications in youths. Am J Psychiatry 166:992–1001, 2009

Grace SL, Abbey SE, Kapral MK, et al: Effect of depression on five-year mortality after an acute coronary syndrome. Am J Cardiol 96:1179–1185, 2005

Guo Z, Fratiglioni L, Zhu L, et al: Occurrence and progression of dementia in a community population aged 75 years and older: relationship of antihypertensive medication use. Arch Neurol 56:991–996, 1999

Hamer M, Molloy GJ, Stamatakis E: Psychological distress as a risk factor for cardiovascular events: pathophysiological and behavioral mechanisms. J Am Coll Cardiol 52:2156–2162, 2008

Hamilton SP, Fyer AJ, Durner M, et al: Further genetic evidence for a panic disorder syndrome mapping to chromosome 13q. Proc Natl Acad Sci U S A 100:2550–2555, 2003

Hance M, Carney RM, Freedland KE, et al: Depression in patients with coronary heart disease. Gen Hosp Psychiatry 18:61–65, 1996

Hassan M, York KM, Li H, et al: Association of beta1-adrenergic receptor genetic polymorphism with mental stress-induced myocardial ischemia in patients with coronary artery disease. Arch Intern Med 168:763–770, 2008

Hassan M, Mela A, Qin L, et al: The effect of acute psychological stress on QT dispersion in patients with coronary artery disease. Pacing Clin Electrophysiol 32:1178–1183, 2009

Haworth JE, Moniz-Cook E, Clark AL, et al: Prevalence and predictors of anxiety and depression in a sample of chronic heart failure patients with left ventricular systolic dysfunction. Eur J Heart Fail 7:803–808, 2005

Heller SS, Ormont MA, Lidagoster LC, et al: Psychosocial outcome after ICD implantation: a current perspective. Pacing Clin Electrophysiol 21:1207–1215, 1998

Herbst S, Pietrzak RH, Wagner J, et al: Lifetime major depression is associated with coronary heart disease in older adults: results from the National Epidemiologic Survey on Alcohol and Related Conditions. Psychosom Med 69:729–734, 2007

Hildrum B, Mykletun A, Stordal E, et al: Association of low blood pressure with anxiety and depression: the Nord-Trøndelag Health Study. J Epidemiol Community Health 61:53–58, 2007

Hildrum B, Mykletun A, Holmen J, et al: Effect of anxiety and depression on blood pressure: 11-year longitudinal population study. Br J Psychiatry 193:108–113, 2008

Hocaoglu C, Gulec MY, Durmus I: Psychiatric comorbidity in patients with chest pain without a cardiac etiology. Isr J Psychiatry Relat Sci 45:49–54, 2008

Holbrook AM, Pereira JA, Labiris R, et al: Systematic overview of warfarin and its drug and food interactions. Arch Intern Med 165:1095–1106, 2005

Honig A, Kuyper AM, Schene AH, et al: Treatment of post-myocardial infarction depressive disorder: a randomized, placebo-controlled trial with mirtazapine. Psychosom Med 69:606–613, 2007

Hoyer J, Eifert GH, Einsle F, et al: Heart-focused anxiety before and after cardiac surgery. J Psychosom Res 64:291–297, 2008

Huffman JC, Pollack MH: Predicting panic disorder among patients with chest pain: an analysis of the literature. Psychosomatics 44:222–236, 2003

Irvine J, Dorian P, Baker B, et al: Quality of life in the Canadian Implantable Defibrillator Study (CIDS). Am Heart J 144:282–289, 2002

Jacq F, Foulldrin G, Savoure A, et al: A comparison of anxiety, depression and quality of life between device shock and non-shock groups in implantable cardioverter defibrillator recipients. Gen Hosp Psychiatry 31:266–273, 2009

Jessup M, Brozena S: Heart failure. N Engl J Med 348:2007–2018, 2003

Jiang W, Babyak M, Krantz DS, et al: Mental stress-induced myocardial ischemia and cardiac events. JAMA 275:1651–1656, 1996

Jiang W, Alexander J, Christopher E, et al: Relationship of depression to increased risk of mortality and rehospitalization in patients with congestive heart failure. Arch Intern Med 161:1849–1856, 2001

Jonas BS, Lando JF: Negative affect as a prospective risk factor for hypertension. Psychosom Med 62:188–196, 2000

Jonsbu E, Dammen T, Morken G, et al: Cardiac and psychiatric diagnoses among patients referred for chest pain and palpitations. Scand Cardiovasc J 43:256–259, 2009

Joynt KE, Whellan DJ, O'Connor CM: Why is depression bad for the failing heart? A review of the mechanistic relationship between depression and heart failure. J Card Fail 10:258–271, 2004

Junger J, Schellberg D, Muller-Tasch T, et al: Depression increasingly predicts mortality in the course of congestive heart failure. Eur J Heart Fail 7:261–267, 2005

Kales HC, Valenstein M, Kim HM, et al: Mortality risk in patients with dementia treated with antipsychotics versus other psychiatric medications. Am J Psychiatry 164:1568–1576, 2007

Kaneko Y, Floras JS, Usui K, et al: Cardiovascular effects of continuous positive airway pressure in patients with heart failure and obstructive sleep apnea. N Engl J Med 348:1233–1241, 2003

Kaptein KI, de Jonge P, van den Brink RH, et al: Course of depressive symptoms after myocardial infarction and cardiac prognosis: a latent class analysis. Psychosom Med 68:662–668, 2006

Kapur V, Schwarz ER: The relationship between erectile dysfunction and cardiovascular disease, part I: pathophysiology and mechanisms. Rev Cardiovasc Med 8:214–219, 2007

Kawachi I, Colditz GA, Ascherio A, et al: Prospective study of phobic anxiety and risk of coronary heart disease in men. Circulation 89:1992–1997, 1994a

Kawachi I, Sparrow D, Vokonas PS, et al: Symptoms of anxiety and risk of coronary heart disease. The normative aging study. Circulation 90:2225–2229, 1994b

Kawachi I, Sparrow D, Spiro A III, et al: A prospective study of anger and coronary heart disease: the normative aging study. Circulation 94:2090–2095, 1996

Kazemi-Saleh D, Pishgou B, Assari S, et al: Fear of sexual intercourse in patients with coronary artery disease: a pilot study of associated morbidity. J Sex Med 4:1619–1625, 2007

Kazmierski J, Kowman M, Banach M, et al: Clinical utility and use of DSM-IV and ICD-10 criteria and the Memorial Delirium Assessment Scale in establishing a diagnosis of delirium after cardiac surgery. Psychosomatics 49:73–76, 2008

Kendall L, Lewin RJ, Parsons JM, et al: Factors associated with self-perceived state of health in adolescents with congenital cardiac disease attending paediatric cardiologic clinics. Cardiology in the Young 11:431–438, 2001

Kent LK, Weston CA, Heyer EJ, et al: Successful retrial of ECT two months after ECT-induced Takotsubo cardiomyopathy. Am J Psychiatry 166:857–862, 2009

Kessler RC, Berglund P, Demler O, et al: The epidemiology of major depressive disorder: results from the national comorbidity survey replication (NCS-R). JAMA 289:3095–3105, 2003

Kim DH, Daskalakis C, Whellan DJ, et al: Safety of selective serotonin reuptake inhibitor in adults undergoing coronary artery bypass grafting. Am J Cardiol 103:1391–1395, 2009

Kisely S, Campbell LA, Wang Y: Treatment of ischaemic heart disease and stroke in individuals with psychosis under universal healthcare. Br J Psychiatry 195:545–550, 2009

Klerman GL, Weissman MM, Rounsaville BJ, et al: Interpersonal Psychotherapy of Depression. New York, Basic Books, 1984

Ko DT, Hebert PR, Coffey CS, et al: Beta-blocker therapy and symptoms of depression, fatigue, and sexual dysfunction. JAMA 288:351–357, 2002

Kop WJ, Kuhl EA, Barasch E, et al: Association between depressive symptoms and fibrosis markers: the Cardiovascular Health Study. Brain Behav Immun 24:229–235, 2010

Kornfeld DS, Zimberg S, Malm JR: Psychiatric complications of open heart surgery. N Engl J Med 273:287–292, 1965

Koster S, Hensens AG, van der Palen J: The long-term cognitive and functional outcomes of postoperative delirium after cardiac surgery. Ann Thorac Surg 87:1469–1474, 2009

Kovacs AH, Saidi AS, Kuhl EA, et al: Depression and anxiety in adult congenital heart disease: predictors and prevalence. Int J Cardiol 137:158–164, 2009

Krantz DS, Olson MB, Francis JL, et al: Anger, hostility, and cardiac symptoms in women with suspected coronary artery disease: the Women's Ischemia Syndrome Evaluation (WISE) Study. J Womens Health (Larchmt) 15:1214–1223, 2006

Krantz D, Whittaker KS, Francis JL, et al: Psychotropic medication use and risk of adverse cardiovascular events in women with suspected coronary artery disease: outcomes from the Women's Ischemia Syndrome Evaluation (WISE) Study. Heart 95:1901–1906, 2009

Krishnan KRR: Monoamine oxidase inhibitors, in American Psychiatric Press Textbook of Psychopharmacology. Edited by Schatzberg AF, Nemeroff CB. Washington, DC, American Psychiatric Press, 1995, pp 183–193

Kronish IM, Rieckmann N, Halm EA, et al: Persistent depression affects adherence to secondary prevention behaviors after acute coronary syndromes. J Gen Intern Med 21:1178–1183, 2006

Kronish IM, Rieckmann N, Schwartz JE, et al: Is depression after an acute coronary syndrome simply a marker of known prognostic factors for mortality? Psychosom Med 71:697–703, 2009

Kubzansky LD, Thurston RC: Emotional vitality and incident coronary heart disease: benefits of healthy psychological functioning. Arch Gen Psychiatry 64:1393–1401, 2007

Kubzansky LD, Koenen KC, Spiro A 3rd, et al: Prospective study of posttraumatic stress disorder symptoms and coronary heart disease in the Normative Aging Study. Arch Gen Psychiatry 64:109–116, 2007

Kuhl EA, Fauerbach JA, Bush DE, et al: Relation of anxiety and adherence to risk-reducing recommendations following myocardial infarction. Am J Cardiol 103:1629–1634, 2009

Ladwig KH, Kieser M, Konig J, et al: Affective disorders and survival after acute myocardial infarction. Results from the post-infarction late potential study. Eur Heart J 12:959–964, 1991

Laghrissi-Thode F, Wagner WR, Pollack BG, et al: Elevated platelet factor 4 and beta-thromboglobulin plasma levels in depressed patients with ischemic heart disease. Biol Psychiatry 42:290–295, 1997

Laske C, Soekadar SR, Laszlo R, et al: Brugada syndrome in a patient treated with lithium. Am J Psychiatry 164:1440–1441, 2007

Latal B, Helfricht S, Fischer JE, et al: Psychological adjustment and quality of life in children and adolescents following open-heart surgery for congenital heart disease: a systematic review. BMC Pediatr 9:6, 2009

Launer LJ, Masaki K, Petrovitch H, et al: The association between midlife blood pressure levels and late-life cognitive function. The Honolulu-Asia Aging Study. JAMA 274:1846–1851, 1995

Laursen TM, Munk-Olsen T, Agerbo E, et al: Somatic hospital contacts, invasive cardiac procedures, and mortality from heart disease in patients with severe mental disorder. Arch Gen Psychiatry 66:713–720, 2009

Lazar RM, Shapiro PA, Jaski BE, et al: Neurological events during long-term mechanical circulatory support for heart failure: the REMATCH experience. Circulation 109:2423–2427, 2004

Lee JD, Lee SJ, Tsushima WT, et al: Benefits of off-pump bypass on neurologic and clinical morbidity: a prospective randomized trial. Ann Thorac Surg 76:18–25, 2003

Leor WJ, Poole WK, Kloner RA: Sudden cardiac death triggered by an earthquake. N Engl J Med 334:413–419, 1996

Lesperance F, Frasure-Smith N, Talajic M: Major depression before and after myocardial infarction: its nature and consequences. Psychosom Med 58:99–110, 1996

Lesperance F, Frasure-Smith N, Koszycki D, et al: Effects of citalopram and interpersonal psychotherapy on depression in patients with coronary artery disease: the Canadian Cardiac Randomized Evaluation of Antidepressant and Psychotherapy Efficacy (CREATE) trial. JAMA 297:367–379, 2007

Lessmeier TJ, Gamperling D, Johnson-Liddon V, et al: Unrecognized paroxysmal supraventricular tachycardia. Potential for misdiagnosis as panic disorder. Arch Intern Med 157:537–543, 1997

Lett HS, Blumenthal JA, Babyak MA, et al: Social support and coronary heart disease: epidemiologic evidence and implications for treatment. Psychosom Med 67:869–878, 2005

Levenson JL, Mishra A, Bauernfeind RA: Denial and medical outcome in unstable angina. Psychosom Med 51:27–35, 1989

Levine J, Warrenberg S, Kerns R: The role of denial in recovery from coronary heart disease. Psychosom Med 49:109–117, 1987

Libby P, Ridker PM, Maseri A: Inflammation and atherosclerosis. Circulation 105:1135–1143, 2002

Liberthson R, Sheehan DV, King ME, et al: The prevalence of mitral valve prolapse in patients with panic disorders. Am J Psychiatry 143:511–515, 1986

Licht CM, de Geus EJ, Zitman FG, et al: Association between major depressive disorder and heart rate variability in the Netherlands Study of Depression and Anxiety (NESDA). Arch Gen Psychiatry 65:1358–1367, 2008

Licht CM, de Geus EJC, Seldenrijk A, et al: Depression is associated with decreased blood pressure, but antidepressant use increases the risk for hypertension. Hypertension 53:631–638, 2009

Lichtman JH, Bigger JT Jr, Blumenthal JA, et al: Depression and coronary heart disease: recommendations for screening, referral, and treatment. A science advisory from the American Heart Association Prevention Committee of the Council on Cardiovascular Nursing, Council on Clinical Cardiology, Council on Epidemiology and Prevention, and Interdisciplinary Council on Quality of Care and Outcomes Research. Circulation 118:1768–1775, 2008

Linden W: Psychological treatments in cardiac rehabilitation: review of rationales and outcomes. J Psychosom Res 48:443–454, 2000

Linden W, Moseley JV: The efficacy of behavioral treatments for hypertension. Appl Psychophysiol Biofeedback 31:51–63, 2006

Linden W, Stossel C, Maurice J: Psychosocial interventions for patients with coronary artery disease. Arch Intern Med 156:745–752, 1996

Linke SE, Rutledge T, Johnson BD, et al: Depressive symptom dimensions and cardiovascular prognosis among women with suspected myocardial ischemia: a report from the National Heart, Lung, and Blood Institute–sponsored Women's Ischemia Syndrome Evaluation. Arch Gen Psychiatry 66:499–507, 2009

Liperoti R, Gambassi G, Lapane KL, et al: Conventional and atypical antipsychotics and the risk of hospitalization for ventricular arrhythmias or cardiac arrest. Arch Intern Med 165:696–701, 2005

Lipsitz JD, Masia C, Apfel H, et al: Noncardiac chest pain and psychopathology in children and adolescents. J Psychosom Res 59:185–188, 2005

Liukkonen T, Silvennoinen-Kassinen S, Jokelainen J, et al: The association between C-reactive protein levels and depression:

results from the northern Finland 1966 birth cohort study. Biol Psychiatry 60:825–830, 2006

Lloyd-Jones D, Adams R, Carnethon M, et al: Heart disease and stroke statistics—2009 update: a report from the American Heart Association Statistics Committee and Stroke Statistics Subcommittee. Circulation 119(3):e21–e181, 2009

Lown B: Role of higher nervous activity in sudden cardiac death. Jpn Circ J 54:581–602, 1990

Lown B, De Silva RA, Reich P, et al: Psychophysiologic factors in sudden cardiac death. Am J Psychiatry 137:1325–1335, 1980

Luutonen S, Holm H, Salminen JK, et al: Inadequate treatment of depression after myocardial infarction. Acta Psychiatr Scand 106:434–439, 2002

Lynch JJ, Dicarlo LA, Montgomery DG, et al: Effects of flecainide acetate on ventricular tachyarrhythmia and fibrillation in dogs with recent myocardial infarction. Pharmacology 35:181–193, 1987

Mackin P: Cardiac side effects of psychiatric drugs. Hum Psychopharmacol Clin Exp 23:3–14, 2008

MacMahon KMA, Lip GYH: Psychological factors in heart failure: a review of the literature. Arch Intern Med 162:509–516, 2002

Magyar-Russell G, Cai JX, Bavja T, et al: The prevalence of anxiety and depression in patients with implantable cardioverter defibrillators: a systematic review of the literature. Psychosom Med 71:A36–A37, 2009

Maldonado JR, Wysong A, van der Starre PJ, et al: Dexmedetomidine and the reduction of postoperative delirium after cardiac surgery. Psychosomatics 50:206–217, 2009

Mandras SA, Uber PA, Mehra MR: Sexual activity and chronic heart failure. Mayo Clin Proc 82:1203–1210, 2007

Manuck SB, Krantz DS: Psychophysiologic reactivity in coronary heart disease and essential hypertension, in Handbook of Stress, Reactivity, and Cardiovascular Disease. Edited by Matthews KA, Weiss SM, Detre T, et al. New York, Wiley, 1986, pp 11–34

Margraf J, Ehlers A, Roth WT: Mitral valve prolapse and panic disorder: a review of their relationship. Psychosom Med 50:93–113, 1988

Martens EJ, Hoen PW, Mittelhaeuser M, et al: Symptom dimensions of post-myocardial infarction depression, disease severity and cardiac prognosis. Psychol Med 40:807–814, 2010

Martin-Santos R, Bulbena A, Porta M, et al: Association between joint hypermobility syndrome and panic disorder. Am J Psychiatry 155:1578–1583, 1998

Masand PS, Tesar GE: Use of stimulants in the medically ill. Psychiatr Clin North Am 19:515–548, 1996

May HT, Horne BD, Carlquist JF, et al: Depression after coronary artery disease is associated with heart failure. J Am Coll Cardiol 53:1440–1447, 2009

McGowan L, Dickens C, Percival C, et al: The relationship between vital exhaustion, depression and comorbid illnesses in patients following first myocardial infarction. J Psychosom Res 57:183–188, 2004

Miatton M, De Wolf D, Francois K, et al: Neuropsychological performance in school-aged children with surgically corrected congenital heart disease. J Pediatr 151(1):73–78, 78.e1, 2007

Meier CR, Schlienger RG, Jick H: Use of selective serotonin reuptake inhibitors and risk of developing first-time acute myocardial infarction. Br J Clin Pharmacol 52:179–184, 2001

Merrill DB, Dec GW, Goff DC: Adverse cardiac effects associated with clozapine. J Clin Psychopharmacol 25:32–41, 2005

Miller GE, Stetler CA, Carney RM, et al: Clinical depression and inflammatory risk markers for coronary heart disease. Am J Cardiology 90:1279–1283, 2002

Miller LW, Pagani FD, Russell SD, et al: Use of a continuous-flow device in patients awaiting heart transplantation. N Engl J Med 357:885–896, 2007

Mitchell JE, Mackenzie TB: Cardiac effects of lithium therapy in man: a review. J Clin Psychiatry 43:47–51, 1982

Monster TB, Johnsen SP, Olsen ML, et al: Antidepressants and risk of first-time hospitalization for myocardial infarction: a population-based case-control study. Am J Med 117:732–737, 2004

Morganroth J, Goin JE: Quinidine-related mortality in the short-to-medium-term treatment of ventricular arrhythmias. Circulation 84:1977–1983, 1991

Morris PL, Badger J, Chmielewski C, et al: Psychiatric morbidity following implantation of the automatic implantable cardioverter defibrillator. Psychosomatics 32:58–64, 1991

Moser DK, Dracup K: Is anxiety early after myocardial infarction associated with subsequent ischemic and arrhythmic events? Psychosom Med 58:395–401, 1996

Moss AJ: Long QT syndrome. JAMA 289:2041–2044, 2003

Muller JE, Abela GS, Nesto RW, et al: Triggers, acute risk factors and vulnerable plaques: the lexicon of a new frontier. J Am Coll Cardiol 23:809–813, 1994

Muller-Tasch T, Frankenstein L, Holzapfel N, et al: Panic disorder in patients with chronic heart failure. J Psychosom Res 64:299–303, 2008

Murberg TA, Furze G: Depressive symptoms and mortality in patients with congestive heart failure: a six-year follow-up study. Med Sci Monit 10:CR643–CR6438, 2004

Musselman DL, Tomer A, Manatunga AK, et al: Exaggerated platelet reactivity in major depression. Am J Psychiatry 153:1313–1317, 1996

Nakagawa I, Nakamura K, Oyama M, et al: Long-term effects of the Niigata-Chuetsu earthquake in Japan on acute myocardial infarction mortality: an analysis of death certificate data. Heart 95:2009–2013, 2009

Newburger JW, Silbert AR, Buckley LP, et al: Cognitive function and age at repair of transposition of the great arteries in children. N Engl J Med 310:1495–1499, 1984

Newcomer JW, Hennekens CH: Severe mental illness and risk of cardiovascular disease. JAMA 298:1794–1796, 2007

Newman DM, Dorian P, Paquette M, et al: Effect of an implantable cardioverter defibrillator with atrial detection and shock therapies on patient-perceived, health-related quality of life. Am Heart J 145:841–846, 2003

Newman MF, Kirchner JL, Phillips-Bute B, et al: Longitudinal assessment of neurocognitive function after coronary-artery bypass surgery. N Engl J Med 344:395–402, 2001

Newman S: Incidence and nature of neuropsychological morbidity following cardiac surgery. Perfusion 4:93–100, 1989

Newman S, Pugsley W, Klinger L, et al: Neuropsychological consequences of circulatory arrest with hypothermia. J Clin Exp Neuropsychol 11:529–538, 1988

Nissen SE: ADHD drugs and cardiovascular risk. N Engl J Med 354:1445–1448, 2006

Norkiene I, Ringaitiene D, Misiuriene I, et al: Incidence and precipitating factors of delirium after coronary artery bypass grafting. Scand Cardiovasc J 41:180–185, 2007

O'Connor CM, Jiang W, Kuchibhatla M, et al: Antidepressant use, depression, and survival in patients with heart failure. Arch Intern Med 168:2232–2237, 2008

Olson MB, Krantz DS, Kelsey SF, et al: Hostility scores are associated with increased risk of cardiovascular events in women undergoing coronary angiography: a report from the NHLBI-sponsored WISE Study. Psychosom Med 67:546–552, 2005

O'Reardon J, Lott J, Akhtar U, et al: Acute coronary syndrome (Takotsubo cardiomyopathy) following electroconvulsive therapy in the absence of significant coronary artery disease: case report and review of the literature. J ECT 24:277–280, 2008

Organ Procurement and Transplant Network, U.S. Department of Health and Human Services. 2010. Available at: http://optn.transplant.hrsa.gov/latestData/viewDataReports.asp. Accessed May 12, 2010.

Osborn DP, Nazareth I, King MB: Risk for coronary heart disease in people with severe mental illness: cross-sectional comparative study in primary care. Br J Psychiatry 188:271–277, 2006

Pandharipande PP, Pun BT, Herr DL, et al: Effect of sedation with dexmedetomidine vs lorazepam on acute brain dysfunction in mechanically ventilated patients: the MENDS randomized controlled trial. JAMA 298:2644–2653, 2007

Parker GB, Hilton TM, Walsh WF, et al: Timing is everything: the onset of depression and acute coronary syndrome outcome. Biol Psychiatry 64:660–666, 2008

Pelle AJ, Denollet J, Zwisler AD, et al: Overlap and distinctiveness of psychological risk factors in patients with ischemic heart disease and chronic heart failure: are we there yet? J Affect Disord 113:150–156, 2009

Perez MI, Linden W, Perry T, et al: Failure of psychological interventions to lower blood pressure: a randomized controlled trial. Open Med 3:e92–e100, 2009

Petrucci RJ, Wright S, Naka Y, et al KD: Neurocognitive assessments in advanced heart failure patients receiving continuous-flow left ventricular assist devices. J Heart Lung Transplant 28:542–549, 2009

Pickering TG, Clemow L: Paroxysmal hypertension: the role of stress and psychological factors. J Clin Hypertens 10:575–581, 2008

Pollock BG, Laghrissi-Thode F, Wagner WR: Evaluation of platelet activation in depressed patients with ischemic heart disease after paroxetine or nortriptyline treatment. J Clin Psychopharmacol 20:137–140, 2000

Rasmussen A, Lunde M, Poulsen DL, et al: A double-blind, placebo-controlled study of sertraline in the prevention of depression in stroke patients. Psychosomatics 44:216–221, 2003

Rasmussen JN, Chong A, Alter DA: Relationship between adherence to evidence-based pharmacotherapy and long-term mortality after acute myocardial infarction. JAMA 297:177–186, 2007

Rathore SS, Wang Y, Druss BG, et al: Mental disorders, quality of care, and outcomes among older patients hospitalized with heart failure: an analysis of the National Heart Failure Project. Arch Gen Psychiatry 65:1402–1408, 2008

Ray WA, Chung CP, Murray KT, et al: Atypical antipsychotic drugs and the risk of sudden cardiac death. N Engl J Med 360:225–235, 2009

Rees K, Bennett P, West R, et al: Psychological interventions for coronary heart disease. Cochrane Database Syst Rev (2): CD002902, 2004

Reid GJ, Seidelin PH, Kop WJ, et al: Mental-stress-induced platelet activation among patients with coronary artery disease. Psychosom Med 71:438–445, 2009

Rieckmann N, Gerin W, Kronish IM, et al: Course of depressive symptoms and medication adherence after acute coronary syndromes: an electronic medication monitoring study. J Am Coll Cardiol 48:2218–2222, 2006

Rief W, Nanke A, Emmerich J, et al: Causal illness attributions in somatoform disorders: associations with comorbidity and illness behavior. J Psychosom Res 57:367–371, 2004

Roach GW, Kanchuger M, Mangano CM, et al: Adverse cerebral outcomes after coronary bypass surgery. N Engl J Med 335:1857–1863, 1996

Rochon PA, Normand S-L, Gomes T, et al: Antipsychotic therapy and short-term serious events in older adults with dementia. Arch Intern Med 168:1090–1096, 2008

Roden DM: Long QT syndrome. N Engl J Med 358:169–176, 2008

Rollman BL, Belnap BH, LeMenager MS, et al: Telephone-delivered collaborative care for treating post-CABG depression: a randomized controlled trial. JAMA 302:2095–2103, 2009

Roose SP, Glassman AH: Cardiovascular effects of tricyclic antidepressants in depressed patients with and without heart disease. J Clin Psychiatry 50:S1–S18, 1989

Roose SP, Glassman AH, Giardina EGV, et al: Nortriptyline in depressed patients with left ventricular impairment. JAMA 256:3253–3257, 1986

Roose SP, Glassman AH, Giardina EGV, et al: Tricyclic antidepressants in depressed patients with cardiac conduction disease. Arch Gen Psychiatry 44:273–275, 1987

Roose SP, Glassman AH, Dalack GW: Depression, heart disease, and tricyclic antidepressants. J Clin Psychiatry 50:12–16, 1989

Roose SP, Dalack GW, Glassman AH, et al: Cardiovascular effects of bupropion in depressed patients with heart disease. Am J Psychiatry 148:512–516, 1991

Roose SP, Glassman AH, Attia E, et al: Comparative efficacy of selective serotonin reuptake inhibitors and tricyclics in the treatment of melancholia. Am J Psychiatry 151:1735–1739, 1994

Roose SP, Glassman AH, Attia E, et al: Cardiovascular effects of fluoxetine in depressed patients with heart disease. Am J Psychiatry 155:660–665, 1998a

Roose SP, Laghrissi-Thode F, Kennedy JS, et al: Comparison of paroxetine and nortriptyline in depressed patients with ischemic heart disease. JAMA 279:287–291, 1998b

Rose EA, Moskowitz AJ, Packer M, et al: The REMATCH trial: rationale, design, and end points. Ann Thorac Surg 67:723–730, 1999

Rose EA, Gelijns AC, Moskowitz AJ, et al: Long-term mechanical circulatory support for end stage heart failure: the REMATCH trial. N Engl J Med 345:1435–1443, 2001

Rosenberg LB, Whang W, Shimbo D, et al: Exposure to tricyclic antidepressants is associated with an increased risk of incident CHD events in a population-based study. Int J Cardiol 2009 Jul 14. [Epub ahead of print]

Rosengren A, Hawken S, Ôunpuu S, et al: Association of psychosocial risk factors with risk of acute myocardial infarction in 11,119 cases and 13,648 controls from 52 countries (the INTERHEART study): a case-control study. Lancet 364:953–962, 2004

Rosenman RH, Brand RJ, Jenkins CD, et al: Coronary heart disease in the Western Collaborative Group Study. Final follow-up experience of 8½ years. JAMA 233:872–877, 1975

Rozanski A, Bairey CN, Krantz DS, et al: Mental stress and the induction of silent myocardial ischemia in patients with coronary artery disease. N Engl J Med 318:1005–1012, 1988

Rozanski A, Blumenthal JA, Kaplan J: Impact of psychological factors on the pathogenesis of cardiovascular disease and implications for therapy. Circulation 99:2192–2217, 1999

Rudolph JL, Jones RN, Levkoff SE, et al: Derivation and validation of a preoperative prediction rule for delirium after cardiac surgery. Circulation 119:229–236, 2009

Rugulies R: Depression as a predictor for coronary heart disease: a review and meta-analysis. Am J Prev Med 23:51–61, 2002

Rumsfeld JS, Havranek E, Masoudi FA, et al: Depressive symptoms are the strongest predictors of short-term declines in health status in patients with heart failure. J Am Coll Cardiol 42:1811–1817, 2003

Ruo B, Rumsfeld JS, Hlatky MA, et al: Depressive symptoms and health-related quality of life. The Heart and Soul Study. JAMA 290:215–221, 2003

Ruo B, Bertenthal D, Sen S, et al: Self-rated health among women with coronary disease: depression is as important as recent cardiovascular events. Am Heart J 152:921.e1–e7, 2006

Rutledge T, Hogan BE: A quantitative review of prospective evidence linking psychological factors with hypertension development. Psychosom Med 64:758–766, 2002

Rutledge T, Reis VA, Linke SE, et al: Depression in heart failure: a meta-analytic review of prevalence, intervention effects, and associations with clinical outcomes. J Am Coll Cardiol 48:1527–1537, 2006

Samuels M: Neurally induced cardiac damage. Definition of the problem. Neurol Clin 11:273–292, 1993

Sauer WH, Berlin JA, Kimmel SE: Effect of antidepressants and their relative affinity for the serotonin transporter on the risk of myocardial infarction. Circulation 108:32–36, 2003

Sansone RA, Sansone LA: Warfarin and antidepressants: happiness without hemorrhaging. Psychiatry (Edgmont) 6:24–29, 2009

Schleifer SJ, Macari-Hinson MM, Coyle DA, et al: The nature and course of depression following myocardial infarction. Arch Intern Med 149:1785–1789, 1989

Schneider LS, Dagerman KS, Insel P: Risk of death with atypical antipsychotic drug treatment for dementia: meta-analysis of randomized placebo-controlled trials. JAMA 294:1934–1943, 2005

Schron EB, Exner DV, Yao Q, et al: Quality of life in the antiarrhythmics versus implantable defibrillators trial: impact of therapy and influence of adverse symptoms and defibrillator shocks. Circulation 105:589–594, 2002

Sears SF, Lewis TS, Kuhl EA, et al: Predictors of quality of life in patients with implantable cardioverter defibrillators. Psychosomatics 46:451–457, 2005

Shamsuzzaman AS, Gersh BJ, Somers VK: Obstructive sleep apnea: implications for cardiac and vascular disease. JAMA 290:1906–1914, 2003

Shapiro PA: Life after heart transplantation. Prog Cardiovasc Dis 32:405–418, 1990

Shapiro PA, Kornfeld DS: Psychiatric outcome of heart transplantation. Gen Hosp Psychiatry 11:352–357, 1989

Shapiro PA, Levin HR, Oz MC: Left ventricular assist devices: psychosocial burden and implications for heart transplant programs. Gen Hosp Psychiatry 18:30S–35S, 1996

Shapiro PA, Lidagoster L, Glassman AH: Depression and heart disease. Psychiatr Ann 27:347–352, 1997

Shapiro PA, DePena M, Lidagoster L, et al: Depression after coronary artery bypass graft surgery (abstract). Psychosom Med 60:108, 1998

Shapiro PA, Park SJ, Gupta L, et al: Quality of life outcomes in heart failure patients treated with optimal medical management vs. long-term mechanical assist device therapy: results from the REMATCH trial. Circulation 106 (suppl II):606–607, 2002

Shedd OL, Sears SF, Harvill JL, et al: The World Trade Center attack: increased frequency of defibrillator shocks for ventricular arrhythmias in patients living remotely from New York City. J Am Coll Cardiol 44:44:1265–1267, 2004

Shekelle RB, Gale M, Ostfeld AM, et al: Hostility, risk of coronary heart disease, and mortality. Psychosom Med 45:109–114, 1983

Sheline YI, Freedland KE, Carney RM: How safe are serotonin reuptake inhibitors for depression in patients with coronary heart disease? Am J Med 102:54–59, 1997

Shen BJ, Avivi YE, Todaro JF, et al: Anxiety characteristics independently and prospectively predict myocardial infarction in men: the unique contribution of anxiety among psychologic factors. J Am Coll Cardiol 51:113–119, 2008

Sheps DS, McMahon RP, Becker L, et al: Mental stress-induced ischemia and all-cause mortality in patients with coronary artery disease: results from the Psychophysiological Investigations of Myocardial Ischemia study. Circulation 105:1780–1784, 2002

Sheps DS, Creed F, Clouse R: Chest pain in patients with cardiac and noncardiac disease. Psychosom Med 66:861–867, 2004

Sherwood A, Blumenthal JA, Trivedi R, et al: Relationship of depression to death or hospitalization in patients with heart failure. Arch Intern Med 167:367–373, 2007

Shibeshi WA, Young-Xu Y, Blatt CM: Anxiety worsens prognosis in patients with coronary artery disease. J Am Coll Cardiol 49:2021–2027, 2007

Skinner JE: Regulation of cardiac vulnerability by the cerebral defense system. J Am Coll Cardiol 5:88B–94B, 1985

Skinner JE, Reed JC: Blockade of a frontocortical-brain stem pathway prevents ventricular fibrillation of ischemic heart. Am J Physiol 240:H156–H163, 1981

Skinner JE, Lie JT, Entman ML: Modification of ventricular fibrillation latency following coronary artery occlusion in the conscious pig. Circulation 51:656–667, 1975

Slaughter MS, Rogers JG, Milano CA, et al: Advanced heart failure treated with continuous-flow left ventricular assist device. N Engl J Med 361:2241–2251, 2009

Smoller JW, Pollack MH, Wassertheil-Smoller S, et al: Panic attacks and risk of incident cardiovascular events among postmenopausal women in the Women's Health Initiative Observational Study. Arch Gen Psychiatry 64:1153–1160, 2007

Sowden GL, Huffman JC: The impact of mental illness on cardiac outcomes: a review for the cardiologist. Int J Cardiol 132:30–37, 2009

Spijkerman TA, van den Brink RH, May JF, et al: Decreased impact of post-myocardial infarction depression on cardiac prognosis? J Psychosom Res 61:493–499, 2006

Spindler H, Pedersen SS: Posttraumatic stress disorder in the wake of heart disease: prevalence, risk factors, and future research directions. Psychosom Med 67:715–723, 2005

Spindler H, Johansen JB, Andersen K, et al: Gender differences in anxiety and concerns about the cardioverter defibrillator. Pacing Clin Electrophysiol 32:614–621, 2009

Stein PK, Carney RM, Freedland KE, et al: Severe depression is associated with markedly reduced heart rate variability in patients with stable coronary heart disease. J Psychosom Res 48:493–500, 2000

Steinberg JS, Arshad A, Kowalski M, et al: Increased incidence of life-threatening ventricular arrhythmias in implantable defibrillator patients after the World Trade Center attack. J Am Coll Cardiol 44:1261–1264, 2004

Steptoe A, Mohabir A, Mahon NG, et al: Health related quality of life and psychological well-being in patients with dilated cardiomyopathy. Heart 83:645–650, 2000

Strik JJ, Denollet J, Lousberg R, et al: Comparing symptoms of depression and anxiety as predictors of cardiac events and increased health care consumption after myocardial infarction. J Am Coll Cardiol 42:1801–1807, 2003

Strike PC, Steptoe A: Systematic review of mental stress induced myocardial ischemia. Eur Heart J 24:690–703, 2003

Suh GH, Shah A: Effect of antipsychotics on mortality in elderly patients with dementia: a 1-year prospective study in a nursing home. Int Psychogeriatr 17:429–441, 2005

Sullivan MD, LaCroix AZ, Spertus JA, et al: Five-year prospective study of the effects of anxiety and depression in patients with coronary artery disease. Am J Cardiol 86:1135–1138, 2000

Surtees PG, Wainwright NW, Luben RN, et al: Depression and ischemic heart disease mortality: evidence from the EPIC-Norfolk United Kingdom prospective cohort study. Am J Psychiatry 165:515–523, 2008

Tata LJ, West J, Smith C, et al: General population based study of the impact of tricyclic and selective serotonin reuptake inhibitor antidepressants on the risk of acute myocardial infarction. Heart 91:465–471, 2005

Taylor CB, Youngblood ME, Catellier D, et al: Effects of antidepressant medication on morbidity and mortality in depressed patients after myocardial infarction. Arch Gen Psychiatry 62:792–798, 2005

Terracciano CM, Miller LW, Yacoub MH: Contemporary use of ventricular assist devices. Ann Rev Med 61:255–270, 2010

Tesar GE, Murray GB, Cassem NH: Use of high dose intravenous haloperidol in the treatment of agitated cardiac patients. J Clin Psychopharmacol 5:344–347, 1985

Thavendiranathan P, Bagai A, Khoo C, et al: Does this patient with palpitations have a cardiac arrhythmia? JAMA 302:2135–2143, 2009

Thayer JF, Lane RD: The role of vagal function in the risk for cardiovascular disease and mortality. Biol Psychol 74:224–242, 2007

Thombs BD, de Jonge P, Coyne JC, et al: Depression screening and patient outcomes in cardiovascular care: a systematic review. JAMA 300:2161–2171, 2008

Tsai TT, Nallamothu BK, Prasad A, et al: Clinical problem-solving. A change of heart. N Engl J Med 361:1010–1016, 2009

Tsuchihashi-Makaya M, Kato N, Chishaki A, et al: Anxiety and poor social support are independently associated with adverse outcomes in patients with mild heart failure. Circ J 73:280–287, 2009

Tully PJ, Baker RA, Knight JL: Anxiety and depression as risk factors for mortality after coronary artery bypass surgery. J Psychosom Res 64:285–290, 2008

Vaccarino V, Johnson BD, Sheps DS, et al: Depression, Inflammation, and incident cardiovascular disease in women with suspected coronary ischemia: the National Heart, Lung, and Blood Institute–Sponsored WISE Study. J Am Coll Cardiol 50:2044–2050, 2007

Van den Broek KC, Nyklícek I, Van der Voort PH, et al: Shocks, personality, and anxiety in patients with an implantable defibrillator. Pacing Clin Electrophysiol 31:850–857, 2008

van den Broek KC, Nyklicek I, van der Voort PH, et al: Risk of ventricular arrhythmia after implantable defibrillator treatment in anxious type D patients. J Am Coll Cardiol 54:531–537, 2009

Van Dijk D, Jansen EWL, Hijman R, et al: Cognitive outcome after off-pump and on-pump coronary artery bypass graft surgery: a randomized trial. JAMA 287:1405–1412, 2002

van Dijk D, Spoor M, Hijman R, et al: Cognitive and cardiac outcomes 5 years after off-pump vs on-pump coronary artery bypass graft surgery. JAMA 297:701–708, 2007
van Melle JP, de Jonge P, Spijkerman TA, et al: Prognostic association of depression following myocardial infarction with mortality and cardiovascular events: a meta-analysis. Psychosom Med 66:814–822, 2004
van Melle JP, de Jonge P, Honig A, et al: Effects of antidepressant treatment following myocardial infarction. Br J Psychiatry 190:460–466, 2007
Vigl M, Hager A, Bauer U, et al: Sexuality and subjective well-being in male patients with congenital heart disease. Heart 95:1179–1183., 2009
Vinyoles E, De la Figuera M, Gonzalez-Segura D: Cognitive function and blood pressure control in hypertensive patients over 60 years of age: COGNIPRES study. Curr Med Res Opinion 24:3331–3340, 2008
Wang HX, Mittleman MA, Leineweber C, et al: Depressive symptoms, social isolation, and progression of coronary artery atherosclerosis: the Stockholm Female Coronary Angiography Study. Psychother Psychosom 75:96–102, 2006
Wang PS, Schneeweiss S, Avorn J, et al: Risk of death in elderly users of conventional vs. atypical antipsychotic medications. N Engl J Med 353:2335–2341, 2005
Watkins LL, Blumenthal JA, Davidson JRT, et al: Phobic anxiety, depression, and risk of ventricular arrhythmias in patients with coronary heart disease. Psychosom Med 68:651–656, 2006
Webster LJ, Michelakis ED, Davis T, et al: Use of sildenafil for safe improvement of erectile function and quality of life in men with New York Heart Association classes II and III congestive heart failure: a prospective, placebo-controlled, double-blind crossover trial. Arch Intern Med 164:514–520, 2004
Weissman MM, Markowitz JS, Ouellette R, et al: Panic disorder and cardiovascular/cerebrovascular problems: results from a community survey. Am J Psychiatry 147:1504–1508, 1990
Welton NJ, Caldwell DM, Adamopoulos E, et al: Mixed treatment comparison meta-analysis of complex interventions: psychological interventions in coronary heart disease. Am J Epidemiol 169:1158–1165, 2009
Westlake C, Dracup K, Fonarow G, et al: Depression in patients with heart failure. J Card Fail 11:30–35, 2005
Whang W, Albert CM, Sears SF Jr, et al: Depression as a predictor for appropriate shocks among patients with implantable cardioverter-defibrillators: results from the Triggers of Ventricular Arrhythmias (TOVA) study. J Am Coll Cardiol 45:1090–1095, 2005
Whang W, Kubzansky LD, Kawachi I, et al: Depression and Risk of sudden cardiac death and coronary heart disease in women: results from the Nurses' Health Study. J Am Coll Cardiol 53:950–958, 2009
White KS, Raffa SD, Jakle KR, et al: Morbidity of DSM-IV Axis I disorders in patients with noncardiac chest pain: psychiatric morbidity linked with increased pain and health care utilization. J Consult Clin Psychol 76:422–430, 2008
Whitehead DL, Strike P, Perkins-Porras L, et al: Frequency of distress and fear of dying during acute coronary syndromes and consequences for adaptation. Am J Cardiol 96:1512–1516, 2005
Whooley MA, de Jonge P, Vittinghoff E, et al: Depressive symptoms, health behaviors, and risk of cardiovascular events in patients with coronary heart disease. JAMA 300:2379–2388, 2008
Wiedemar L, Schmid JP, Muller J, et al: Prevalence and predictors of posttraumatic stress disorder in patients with acute myocardial infarction. Heart Lung 37:113–121, 2008
Wilbert-Lampen U, Leistner D, Greven S, et al: Cardiovascular events during World Cup soccer. N Engl J Med 358:475–483, 2008
Wilens TE, Hammerness PG, Biederman J, et al: Blood pressure changes associated with medication treatment of adults with attention-deficit/hyperactivity disorder. J Clin Psychiatry 66:253–259, 2005
Willner A, Rodewald G: The Impact of Cardiac Surgery on the Quality of Life: Neurological and Psychological Aspects. New York, Plenum, 1991
Winterstein AG, Gerhard T, Shuster J, et al: Cardiac safety of central nervous system stimulants in children and adolescents with attention-deficit/hyperactivity disorder. Pediatrics 120:e1494–e1501, 2007
Wittstein IS: The broken heart syndrome. Cleve Clin J Med 74 (suppl 1):S17–S22, 2007
Wittstein IS, Thiemann DR, Lima JAC, et al: Neurohumoral features of myocardial stunning due to sudden emotional stress. N Engl J Med 352:539–548, 2005
Wray J, Hallas CN, Banner NR: Quality of life and psychological well-being during and after left ventricular assist device support. Clin Transplant 21:622–627, 2007
Writing Committee for the ENRICHD Investigators: Effects of treating depression and low perceived social support on clinical events after myocardial infarction: the enhancing recovery in coronary heart disease patients (ENRICHD) randomized trial. JAMA 289:3106–3116, 2003
Wulsin LR, Singal BM: Do depressive symptoms increase the risk for the onset of coronary disease? A systematic quantitative review. Psychosom Med 65:201–210, 2003
Xiong GL, Jiang W, Clare R, et al: Prognosis of patients taking selective serotonin reuptake inhibitors before coronary artery bypass grafting. Am J Cardiol 98:42–47, 2006
Yan LL, Liu K, Matthews KA, et al: Psychosocial factors and risk of hypertension: the coronary artery risk development in young adults (CARDIA) study. JAMA 290:2138–2148, 2003
Yeh GY, Davis RB, Phillips RS: Use of complementary therapies in patients with cardiovascular disease. Am J Cardiol 98:673–680, 2006
Yeung AC, Vekshstein VI, Krantz DS, et al: The effect of atherosclerosis on the vasomotor response of coronary arteries to mental stress. N Engl J Med 325:1551–1556, 1991
Yohannes AM, Willgoss TG, Baldwin RC, et al: Depression and anxiety in chronic heart failure and chronic obstructive pulmonary disease: prevalence, relevance, clinical implications

and management principles. Int J Geriatr Psychiatry 2009 Dec 23. [Epub ahead of print]

York KM, Hassan M, Sheps DS: Psychobiology of depression/distress in congestive heart failure. Heart Fail Rev 14:35–50, 2009

Young MC, Shah N, Cantrell FL, et al: Risk assessment of isolated aripiprazole exposures and toxicities: a retrospective study. Clin Toxicol (Phila) 47:580–583, 2009

Ziegelstein RC, Fauerbach JA, Stevens SS, et al: Patients with depression are less likely to follow recommendations to reduce cardiac risk during recovery from a myocardial infarction. Arch Intern Med 160:1818–1823, 2000

Ziegelstein RC: Acute emotional stress and cardiac arrhythmias. JAMA 298:324–329, 2007

CHAPTER 19

Lung Disease

Kathy L. Coffman, M.D.

James L. Levenson, M.D.

IN THIS CHAPTER, we review psychiatric aspects of the major pulmonary disorders, as well as lung transplantation and the use of psychiatric drugs in pulmonary patients.

Common Pulmonary Disorders

Asthma

Asthma is the most common chronic disease in the United States, affecting 5%–7% of the population, or approximately 17 million people (American Lung Association 2000; Barnes and Woolcock 1998). In this chapter, we focus on asthma in adults (see Chapter 34, "Pediatrics," for discussion of asthma in children). Mortality has risen steadily since the early 1980s. Age-adjusted mortality of asthma varies among ethnic groups: Puerto Ricans, 40.9 per million; non-Hispanic blacks, 38.1 per million; Cuban Americans, 15.8 per million; non-Hispanic whites, 14.7 per million; and Mexican Americans, 9.2 per million (National Center for Health Statistics 2000).

Comorbidity With Psychiatric Disorders

Many investigators have assessed psychiatric comorbidity in asthma. Asthma patients have double the rate of anxiety and mood disorders as those without asthma (Rosenkranz and Davidson 2009). Nearly half of asthma patients at tertiary care centers have major depressive disorder (Van Lieshout et al. 2009). A study of 230 outpatients with asthma found that almost half had a positive screen for depressive symptoms (Mancuso et al. 2000). Goodwin et al. (2003a) found that asthma was associated with significantly elevated odds ratios of anxiety disorders, including panic, social phobia, generalized anxiety, and specific phobias. Youths with asthma have almost twice the prevalence of comorbid DSM-IV (American Psychiatric Association 1994) anxiety and depressive disorders compared with control youths (Katon et al. 2007).

Anxiety disorders are more frequent in patients with asthma for several reasons (ten Thoren and Petermann 2000). Anxiety increases risk for asthma, and asthma increases risk for anxiety. Anxiety is increased by asthma attacks, chronic sensations of breathlessness, and anticipation of attacks in response to certain triggers. Respiratory distress causes a wide array of anxiety symptoms (panic attacks, generalized and anticipatory anxiety, phobic avoidance), and audible wheezing aggravates social anxiety. Prospective epidemiological studies indicate that the primary risk factor for development of panic disorder in young adulthood is history of asthma as a child (Goodwin et al. 2003b). An additional reason for frequent anxiety is that many of the drugs used to treat asthma have anxiety as a potential side effect.

Asthma sometimes may be mistakenly diagnosed as an anxiety disorder, especially panic disorder, and some anxiety disorders (panic, social anxiety) may be mislabeled as asthma. This differentiation can be difficult because shortness of breath, palpitations, sweating, chest pain, lightheadedness, fear of losing control, and even fear of dying can represent either asthma or panic anxiety. When the diagnosis is unclear, a negative methacholine inhalation challenge test indicates no airway hyperresponsiveness and, therefore, a diagnosis other than asthma (Schmaling et al. 1999). Of course, as noted earlier, patients can and often do have both asthma and an anxiety disorder.

Psychological Factors in Asthma

Psychosomatic theories about asthma proposed by French and Alexander in 1939–1941 postulated that the central conflict involved unconscious dependency issues with the mother and fear of separation. However, these theories have little empirical support (Greenberg et al. 1996). No particular personality type is more susceptible to development of asthma. Asthma was once regarded as a classic psychosomatic disorder, and it is still widely believed that psychological factors (particularly anxiety) play an important role in the precipitation and aggravation of asthma.

Several psychosocial factors appear to increase the risk for development of asthma. One prospective study showed that subjects with low health-related quality of life had a higher likelihood of developing asthma 12 years later and had a higher prevalence of depression, difficulty relaxing, and sleep disturbances than did those who did not develop asthma (Lander et al. 2009). Risk of adult-onset asthma increases with increasing adversity in childhood independent of early-onset anxiety and depressive disorders, although both predict adult-onset asthma (Scott et al. 2008; Turyk et al. 2008).

Depression and anxiety are associated with worse medical outcomes in asthma. A prospective study found that a higher number of depressive symptoms correlated with an increased severity of asthma, lower quality of life, worse health outcomes, and increased risk of hospital admission due to asthma (Eisner et al. 2005). Another study reported an apparent dose-response relation between depressive symptoms and days of health-impaired quality of life in asthma patients in the past month. Depressive symptoms also were associated with more disability, life dissatisfaction, inadequate social supports, and increased risk behaviors in asthmatic patients (Strine et al. 2008). Youths with asthma and comorbid depressive disorders have significantly higher health care use and costs than do those with asthma alone (Richardson et al. 2008).

Similar to panic disorder, patients with asthma have a significant association between catastrophic cognitions and more asthma symptoms such as irritability, panic and fear, and rapid breathing (De Peuter et al. 2008; Giardino et al. 2002). Perceived discomfort, rather than actual bronchoconstriction, predicts use of bronchodilators (Schmaling et al. 1999). However, those with alexithymia have difficulty expressing emotions and perceiving physical symptoms and are at higher risk for near-fatal asthma attacks because they underestimate the severity of asthma exacerbations and delay seeking treatment (Serrano et al. 2006). In asthmatic adults, affective denial on the Levine Denial of Illness Scale was inversely correlated with adherence to inhaled asthma medications as monitored with a microelectronic monitor. Those with higher scores on the information avoidance subscale had suboptimal compliance with inhaled asthma medication. (McGann et al. 2008). Patients with difficult-to-control asthma were found to have significantly higher external locus of control scores, which may have interfered with adherence to the medical regimen, leading to a higher admission rate (Halimi et al. 2007). Asthmatic children with avoidant coping have poorer psychological functioning, and quality of life of both the patient and the mother was lower (Marsac et al. 2007). These studies may indicate that cognitive therapy and interventions focused on coping skills may affect outcomes with asthma patients because overreaction and underreaction to symptoms may affect quality of life and survival.

Psychological distress may provoke asthma attacks. A 27% increase in severity of asthma symptoms was reported in patients surveyed in New York City 5–9 weeks after the September 11, 2001, terrorist attacks (Centers for Disease Control and Prevention 2002), and posttraumatic stress disorder (PTSD) was a significant predictor of asthma symptom severity (Fagan et al. 2003).

Recent evidence is accumulating that witnessing or being a victim of physical or sexual abuse may be a risk factor in asthma morbidity (Kashiwagi et al. 2008; Subramanian et al. 2007). Among Puerto Rican children, the odds of having asthma were doubled if they had a history of physical or sexual abuse, but neighborhood violence and other stressful life events did not correlate with asthma (R.T. Cohen et al. 2008). Psychological factors and psychosocial problems in hospitalized asthma patients were a more powerful predictor of which patients required intubation than any other examined variable (e.g., smoking, infection, prior hospitalization) (LeSon and Gershwin 1996). Several psychological factors in asthma patients may be associated with asthma deaths. A case-control study involving 533 cases showed an increased risk of death associated with health behaviors such as poor adherence with follow-up visits and poor inhaler technique. Three independent psychosocial factors appeared to increase the odds of death: psychosis, financial problems, and learning difficulties. Two factors associated with reduced risk were sexual problems and prescription of antidepressant drugs. Surprisingly, factors such as bereavement, domestic abuse, family problems, and social isolation did not correlate with risk of asthma death (Sturdy et al. 2002).

Psychophysiological Mechanisms Mediating Asthma

From a physiological perspective, the vagus nerve is thought to mediate airway reactivity to emotion (Isenberg et al. 1992; B.D. Miller et al. 2009). The upper airways innervated by cholinergic neurons may be more affected by suggestion and emotion than are smaller airways (Lehrer et al. 1986). Research has shown that various emotions and types of stress can increase respiratory resistance in asthma (Ritz et al. 2000).

Acute and chronic stress has been reported to be correlated with several physiological measures in asthma patients, including increased salivary chromogranin A (Hoshino et al. 2008), decreased salivary alpha-amylase and cortisol (Wolf et al. 2008b), and increased interleukin 4 (IL-4), IL-5, and interferon-gamma, leading to an increase in asthma symptoms (Marin et al. 2009), decreased expression of beta$_2$-adrenergic receptor messenger ribonucleic acid (mRNA) and glucocorticoid receptor mRNA (G.E. Miller and Chen 2006), and other indices of anti-inflammatory response (G.E. Miller and Chen 2006; G.E. Miller et al. 2009). The clinical significance of these findings is not yet clearly established.

Psychological factors also may influence asthma through behavioral mechanisms. A large U.S. population-based study concluded that "Any degree of poor mental health appears to increase one's risk for asthma" (Chun et al. 2008). Psychological morbidity is associated with high levels of denial and delays in seeking medical care (D.A. Campbell et al. 1995; Miles et al. 1997), poor medication adherence (Cluley and Cochrane 2001; Put et al. 2000; Smith et al. 2006), and increased risk for smoking (Strine et al. 2008; M.O. Van De Ven et al. 2009). Psychopathology in persons with severe asthma is associated with increased hospitalization and outpatient and emergency department visits independent of asthma severity (Jones et al. 2008; Schneider et al. 2008; ten Brinke et al. 2001).

Interventions With Asthma Patients

In view of high levels of anxiety and depression in asthmatic patients, screening may be useful (Schneider et al. 2008). Screening and management of psychological symptoms in asthmatic patients may decrease the rate of clinic visits, hospitalization, and mortality and increase productivity at work (N. Schmitz et al. 2009). The Geriatric Depression Scale (GDS) may be more accurate in diagnosing depression than the short-form Center for Epidemiologic Studies Depression Scale (CESD-SF) because the CESD-SF is confounded by physical symptoms, unlike the GDS (Mancuso et al. 2008).

Many psychosocial adjuvant interventions have been studied in asthma, including cognitive-behavioral therapy (CBT), biofeedback, psychoeducation, hypnosis, stress management, symptom perception, and yoga (Kern-Buell et al. 2000; Lehrer et al. 2002, 2008; Yorke and Shuldham 2005). Patient education programs may reduce anxiety and improve self-management. Patient diaries of asthma attacks can be useful in determining triggers of attacks and the effect of the illness on social and academic development and family life (Weiss 1994). However, systematic reviews have concluded that the evidence base is not strong enough to draw any firm conclusions about the role of psychotherapeutic interventions in children (Yorke and Shuldham 2005) and adults (Yorke et al. 2006a) with asthma. In children with asthma, there have been many studies of family therapy (e.g., S.M. Ng et al. 2008), and a systematic review has been somewhat more supportive (Yorke and Shuldham 2005).

Although psychotropic drugs are frequently prescribed in asthma, the evidence base is very limited. Studies of antidepressant treatment in asthma patients have included small open trials of bupropion (Brown et al. 2007) and sertraline (Smoller et al. 1998) and a small randomized controlled trial of citalopram (Brown et al. 2005). No clinical trials of pharmacotherapy for anxiety in asthma have been reported.

Cystic Fibrosis

In the United States, cystic fibrosis (CF) affects more than 18,000 children younger than 18 years (1 in 2,500 births). CF is the most common hereditary disease in white children, and it is also seen in other races. Survival improved from a median age of 12 years in 1966 to 40 years by 2001 (Jaffe and Bush 2001), so adults living with CF are a relatively recent and growing population. (See also Chapter 34, "Pediatrics," for a discussion of CF in children.) More patients who did not develop lung problems until their 20s are receiving a diagnosis of CF (Widerman 2004).

Psychological Factors in Cystic Fibrosis

Several authors have described growing up with CF from a child's perspective. Knowing the key issues involved can enhance effectiveness of therapeutic interventions (Christian and D'Auria 1997; Hains et al. 1997; Llewellyn 1998).

Depression is more frequent in children and teenagers with CF than in healthy children and adversely affects family functioning (Quittner et al. 2008). Treatment adherence is challenging in both younger children and teenagers and may be influenced by psychological characteristics of the patients, as well as by caregiver and family traits (Szyndler et al. 2005; Ward et al. 2009; White et al. 2009). Having a child with CF is extremely stressful for parents, and anxiety and depression are common in caregivers (Hayes and Savage 2008; Ward et al. 2009).

In adults with CF, as with other chronic diseases, anxiety and depression are common and adversely affect treatment adherence and quality of life (Havermans et al. 2008; Quittner et al. 2008). One study showed that levels of anxiety and depression were not dependent on the severity of lung disease but on the CF patients' estimations of their disease and their level of perceived support (Wargnies et al. 2002). However, another study found that adults with CF did not have significant levels of depression, anxiety, or any other psychopathology, although lower anxiety correlated with better pulmonary function (D.L. Anderson et al. 2001). Adults with CF are resilient and have survived a disease to which others have succumbed.

Treatment adherence in adults with CF is better in those who cope via optimistic acceptance and hopefulness and worse in those who use avoidant strategies (J. Abbott et al. 2001). Additional potential stressors include chronic pancreatitis leading to malabsorption and the development of diabetes (Collins and Reynolds 2008) and chronic pain (Palermo et al. 2006). With CF patients living longer, patients are getting married, and their partners experience significant stress (Delelis et al. 2008). Infertility is common in adults with CF, but some are having children. Although disability is common, one study found that about half of subjects were working an average of 32 hours per week despite an average forced expiratory volume in 1 second of 31.9% (Burker et al. 2004b).

Interventions With Cystic Fibrosis Patients

Several psychological interventions in CF have been studied in clinical trials, including cognitive and behavior therapies; genetic counseling; biofeedback; and educational interventions to promote independence, adherence, knowledge, and quality of life. Overall, some evidence indicates that psychological interventions improve emotional outcomes in CF patients, but there have been no consistent benefits for lung function (Glasscoe and Quittner 2008). Novel interventions have included an interactive computer game to counter isolation and improve coping with the CF regimen (Duff et al. 2006) and weekly telemedicine for terminal CF patients for psychological support (Wilkinson et al. 2008). Finally, the CF care team may struggle with end-of-life care for terminal CF patients and have difficulty discussing death and dying, saying good-bye, and asking patients about their wishes regarding active or palliative care (Chapman et al. 2005). The psychiatrist can assist both patients and team members in better handling these issues (see Chapter 41, "Palliative Care").

Cystic Fibrosis and Lung Transplantation

Lung transplantation is the treatment of last resort for CF patients. Although CF patients on a waiting list for transplantation may experience a sense of displacement, disorder, and life being in limbo (Macdonald 2006), they have been reported to have lower levels of anxiety, be more likely to be working, and use more functional coping methods compared with other end-stage lung disease candidates (Burker et al. 2000). CF patients awaiting lung transplantation have better psychological quality of life if they use more active coping and less disengagement (Taylor et al. 2008). Nevertheless, neuropsychological deficits and depression are common (Crews et al. 2000).

Chronic Obstructive Pulmonary Disease

Almost 16 million Americans have chronic obstructive pulmonary disease (COPD): 14 million with chronic bronchitis and 2 million with emphysema. COPD ranks fourth as a cause of death in the United States after heart disease, cancer, and stroke. Cigarette smokers are 10 times as likely to die of COPD as nonsmokers.

COPD results in progressive declines in arterial oxygen, with carbon dioxide increasing late in the course of the disease. Hypoxia causes confusion, disorientation, altered consciousness, muscle twitching, tremor, and seizures. Mild hypoxia can be accompanied by irritability, mental slowing, and impairment of memory with poor reasoning and perseveration. Prolonged hypoxia can result in permanent memory deficits or dementia—that is, hypoxic encephalopathy. Chronic or severe hypoxia can also lead to extrapyramidal symptoms, pseudobulbar palsy, or visual agnosia. Patients with hypercapnia and respiratory acidosis may be lethargic and have auditory and visual hallucinations (Lishman 1987).

Comorbidity With Psychiatric Disorders

Psychiatric disorders are three times as prevalent in COPD patients as in the general population, with almost twice the rates of anxiety and depression in women as in men (Laurin et al. 2007). The Patient Health Questionnaire-9 appears to be a valid screening instrument for depression in COPD patients (Lamers et al. 2008). Both the World Health Organization Quality of Life-BREF instrument and the St. George's Respiratory Questionnaire have been shown to be reliable and valid in COPD patients (Liang et al. 2008).

Nicotine dependence is the most commonly associated psychiatric condition in COPD patients. More than 80% of COPD cases are associated with tobacco smoking (Tashkin et al. 2001). Alcohol abuse aggravates COPD because of a higher rate of severe community-acquired pneumonia, particularly aspiration pneumonia (Ewig and Torres 1999). Sexual dysfunction is also common in COPD (Ibanez et al. 2001). COPD patients have a high prevalence of hypogonadism, so checking testosterone levels may be prudent (Arver and Lehtihet 2009).

Major depression is also very common in patients with COPD, partly because of an increased prevalence in smokers (Aydin and Ulusahin 2001; Omachi et al. 2009; Yohannes et al. 2000). In one study, depression was found in 42% of the patients (Yohannes et al. 2000), yet only about one-fifth of COPD patients with major depression receive antidepressants. This is a worldwide phenomenon; depression was found to be very common in COPD in a population-based study in China (T. P. Ng et al. 2009) and in clinic patients in the Netherlands (van den Bemt et al. 2009) and in Wales (Lewis et al. 2007). A recent national multidisciplinary workshop concluded that although depression is very common in COPD, it remains underdiagnosed and ineffectively treated (Maurer et al. 2008).

Anxiety is also common in COPD (Aydin and Ulusahin 2001; Lewis et al. 2007; Yohannes et al. 2000). Like depression, anxiety disorders remain underdiagnosed and undertreated in COPD (Lewis et al. 2007; Maurer et al. 2008). As many as 44% of patients with severe COPD may have panic disorder, and the incidence of depression was linked to severity of panic symptoms (Potoczek et al. 2008). One group found that the prevalence of panic disorder was at least 10 times higher than in the general population and was due to increased sensitivity to inspiratory loads (Livermore et al. 2008). Whereas anxiety symptoms are linked to dyspnea, depressive symptoms are linked to dyspnea and decreased exercise capacity (Funk et al. 2009).

Cognitive dysfunction has long been recognized to be very common in hypoxemic COPD patients and is improved by supplemental oxygen. Most studies have been cross-sectional (e.g., Ozge et al. 2006), but a recent large population-based longitudinal cohort study found that COPD is associated with significant cognitive decline over time (Hung et al. 2009). Neuropsychological impairments in flexible problem solving and information sequencing have been observed (Emery et al. 2008). Anterior cerebral hypoperfusion has been identified on single photon emission computed tomography in hypoxemic COPD patients (Antonelli Incalzi et al. 2003).

Psychological Factors in COPD

As with other medical illnesses, measurement of physical symptoms in COPD may be confounded by psychological symptoms, and vice versa. Psychological distress in COPD amplifies dyspnea, usually without causing changes in objective pulmonary functions.

Depression and anxiety in COPD patients have led to lower exercise tolerance (Withers et al. 1999), noncompliance with treatment (Bosley et al. 1996), and increased disability (Aydin and Ulusahin 2001). Depression may adversely affect rehabilitation and contribute to difficulty ceasing tobacco use (Borson et al. 1998). Depression results in worse respiratory-specific and overall physical health-related quality of life (Cully et al. 2006; Omachi et al. 2009), is a risk factor for more COPD exacerbations and hospitalizations (Xu et al. 2008), and appears to be an independent predictor of mortality (Fan et al. 2007; Stage et al. 2005). Chronic steroid use may exacerbate depression, emotional lability, or irritability, which further strains interpersonal relationships. Anxiety has been found to be a risk factor in COPD for poorer health outcomes, smoking, and rehospitalization (Gudmundsson et al. 2005, 2006). Factors found to increase dropout in pulmonary rehabilitation include less confidence in treatment, lower fat-free mass, living alone, and smoking (M.J. Fischer et al. 2009).

Dependence on supplemental oxygen can be socially stigmatizing. Some cannot accept the need for oxygen because of denial about the illness. Others become psychologically dependent on oxygen, exceeding the amount prescribed, posing a risk of carbon dioxide retention, which leads to lethargy.

Interventions With COPD Patients

Psychotherapeutic, psychopharmacological, and rehabilitation intervention trials in COPD have been reviewed in detail elsewhere (Brenes 2003; Puhan et al. 2009). The first priority in the rehabilitation of patients with COPD is smoking cessation. Other interventions include pharmacotherapy, physical therapy, psychosocial interventions, nutritional therapy, and, for those who are hypoxemic, long-term oxygen therapy surgery. A small fraction of patients may benefit from bilateral lung volume reduction surgery (Wurtemberger and Hutter 2001).

The goals of treatment are to relieve symptoms, improve physical functioning via rehabilitation, and improve patients' coping skills (Small and Graydon 1992). Patients with dyspnea may avoid all activity and become homebound. Exercise may help build endurance and help patients learn to pace themselves. A treatment plan with realistic and attainable goals and rewards can counteract helplessness (Dudley et al. 1985). Pulmonary rehabilitation in COPD can increase patients' sense of control over their illness (Lacasse et al. 2002) and improves anxiety and depression (Coventry and Hind 2007).

Rose et al. (2002) reviewed 25 published studies of psychological treatments for reduction of anxiety in patients with COPD. Evidence is insufficient to recommend a specific psychological treatment for anxiety in COPD, but relaxation techniques are useful in motivated patients (Rose et al. 2002). Pharmacological treatments for anxiety and depression are discussed later in this chapter (see section "Psychopharmacology in Pulmonary Disease"). Although depression clearly appears associated with worse medical outcomes in COPD, a large retrospective study did not find that guideline-concordant treatment for depression reduced hospitalization or mortality in COPD (Jordan et al. 2009).

The evidence for the efficacy of CBT in COPD has been limited (Coventry and Gellatly 2008), but a recent randomized controlled trial found that both CBT and psychoeducation improved quality of life in COPD patients with depression or anxiety (Kunik et al. 2008).

Sarcoidosis

Sarcoidosis is characterized by noncaseating granulomatous involvement of lymph nodes, lymphatic channels in the lung, and other tissues. Sarcoidosis affects black patients more frequently than white patients in the United States (40 per 100,000 vs. 5 per 100,000). In Europe, Swedish and Danish patients have high prevalence rates (American Lung Association 2000). Onset of the illness is usually between ages 20 and 40. Diagnosis may be delayed by failure to recognize the slowly progressive symptoms until characteristic findings are recognized on a chest X ray. The disease often follows a relapsing and remitting course, with recovery in 80% of patients, but about 5% die from sarcoidosis. Patients often have a dry cough, shortness of breath, fatigue, and weight loss. Lesions can affect the skin, bones, joints, skeletal muscles, and heart. Fatal complications include progressive respiratory impairment, infection, cardiac disease, and renal failure.

Central Nervous System Sarcoidosis

Sarcoidosis may affect the central nervous system (CNS) in 5% of patients. Neurosarcoidosis may cause brain lesions, involve cranial nerves (especially VII), and cause peripheral neuropathies (and rarely choreoathetosis). Indirect evidence for the diagnosis comes from cerebrospinal fluid and magnetic resonance imaging (Stoudemire et al. 1983). Pituitary involvement may result in diabetes insipidus or the syndrome of inappropriate antidiuretic hormone secretion (SIADH), hypercalcemia, hyperprolactinemia, menstrual cycle changes, or hypogonadism (Bullman et al. 2000; Delaney 1977; Mino et al. 2000; Sharma 1975). There have been many case reports of neurosarcoidosis causing cognitive deficits, delirium (Mathews 1965; Silverstein et al. 1965), seizures (Thompson and Checkley 1981), dementia, mania, and psychosis (Hook 1954; Sabaawi et al. 1992; Suchenwirth and Dold 1969; Zerman 1952). Psychotic symptoms generally remit rapidly with steroids.

Psychological Factors in Sarcoidosis

Sarcoidosis rarely has been investigated from the psychological standpoint. A large study of members of the Dutch Sarcoidosis Society found that perceived stress was high and related to depressive symptoms, suggesting that addressing stress and depressive symptoms should be part of sarcoidosis management (De Vries and Drent 2004). In addition, psychiatric comorbidity was reported in 44% of Italian sarcoidosis patients, with major depression in 25%, panic disorder in 6.3%, bipolar disorder in 6.3%, generalized anxiety disorder in 5%, and obsessive-compulsive disorder in 1.3% (Goracci et al. 2008). Although sarcoidosis patients reported a higher magnitude of stressful life events, they had a lower capacity for coping with stress, possibly as a result of alexithymic characteristics (Yamada et al. 2003).

Quality of life in sarcoidosis patients has been related to objective pulmonary function measures (Güneyliolu et al. 2004), arthralgia, breathlessness, decreased exercise capacity, and fatigue (Michielsen et al. 2007). Depression is common and also associated with poorer quality of life (Yeager et al. 2005). Hoitsma et al. (2003) found that 72% of patients had pain, including arthralgia (53.8%), muscle pain (40.2%), headache (28%), and chest pain (26.9%), suggesting that pain management may be beneficial. Fatigue appears to be particularly problematic, yet a recent review found no clear relation between fatigue and clinical parameters of sarcoidosis (De Vries and Drent 2008). Longitudinal prospective studies of fatigue and its relation with depression are needed in this population (de Kleijn et al. 2009).

Pulmonary Fibrosis

The etiology of idiopathic pulmonary fibrosis is unknown, but the prevalence is approximately 3–5 per 100,000. Pulmonary fibrosis also may be caused by inhalation of a variety of agents (especially via occupational exposure), radiation, and rheumatological disorders, especially systemic sclerosis. There has been a recent shift in the view of idiopathic pulmonary fibrosis as solely an inflammatory condition to a primary fibrotic disease because of abnormal wound healing involving profibrogenic growth factors. This has led to a shift from use of anti-inflammatory medications to use of antifibrotic agents without significant effect on disease progression or quality of life (Abdelaziz et al. 2005; Allen and Spiteri 2002; Antoniu 2006).

Psychological factors have received surprisingly little attention in idiopathic pulmonary fibrosis. As with other chronic lung diseases, dyspnea, the subjective sense of breathlessness, is the most important factor in determining quality of life in idiopathic pulmonary fibrosis (De Vries et al. 2001; Martinez et al. 2000). Other important domains contributing to quality of life include disease symptoms, dependence, employment and finances, exhaustion, family, medical therapy, mental and spiritual well-being, mortality, sexual relationships, social participation, and sleep (Swigris et al. 2005). Poor sleep has been documented to be an important influence on emotional and physical functioning (Krishnan et al. 2008; Mermigkis et al. 2009).

Because median survival rates after diagnosis with idiopathic pulmonary fibrosis are less than 5 years, and current therapeutic options do not prolong survival, the goal is to find interventions that allow patients to be more active, be less anxious and depressed, have more control over the illness, and have improved quality of life (Swigris et al. 2008). A review of pulmonary rehabilitation for interstitial lung disease found only five studies. Although there was no indication that physical training improved survival, dyspnea was reduced and quality of life improved in all participants (Holland and Hill 2008). One small study specific to idiopathic pulmonary fibrosis patients showed similar results (Jastrzebski et al. 2008).

Because of lack of improvement in survival in idiopathic pulmonary fibrosis patients with medical therapy, lung transplantation remains the best treatment for end-stage idiopathic pulmonary fibrosis. Idiopathic pulmonary fibrosis is second only to COPD as an indication for lung transplantation; however, survival may be lower than for other lung diseases. Double lung transplant may offer higher 1- and 5-year survival but raises ethical questions because of the organ shortage.

Tuberculosis

The incidence of tuberculosis had been declining for more than 70 years but began to rise again in the United States, Western Europe, Asia, and Africa. Causes for this trend include the rise of AIDS, increasing substance abuse and homelessness, and the failure to fund public health systems. About one-third of the world's population, more than 2 billion people, is estimated to be infected with tuberculosis. About 14 million have active infection, 1.7 million deaths occur per year, and nearly 9.2 million new cases are diagnosed per year in the world (World Health Organization 2008). See Chapter 27, "Infectious Diseases," for a discussion of CNS tuberculosis.

Psychiatrists may be asked to make capacity determinations in patients who are nonadherent with tuberculosis treatment (O'Dowd et al. 1998). Evidence on behavioral interventions (other than direct observation) for improving long-term treatment adherence is limited, but several approaches may prove fruitful to foster adherence with tuberculosis and AIDS regimens (Munro et al. 2007). One survey of tuberculosis detainees showed that 81% had drug or alcohol abuse, 46% were homeless, and 28% had mental illness (Oscherwitz et al. 1997). Because alcoholic and drug-addicted patients are more susceptible to tuberculosis, access to adequate substance abuse treatment may be essential to achieving recovery from tuberculosis and preventing relapse (Sylla et al. 2007).

Psychiatrists also must be attuned to neuropsychiatric symptoms such as mania and psychosis during treatment with isoniazid (Alao and Yolles 1998), probably related to its being a weak but irreversible inhibitor of monoamine oxidase. No dietary restrictions are required, but it can interact with other drugs. Predisposing factors for psychiatric side effects of isoniazid include alcoholism, diabetes, hepatic insufficiency, old age, slow acetylation, and family and personal history of mental illness (Djibo and Lawan 2001). Pyridoxine deficiency also may play a role in the etiology of isoniazid-related psychosis. Psychiatric side effects also occur with several other tuberculosis drugs, most frequently with cycloserine, as well as with fluoroquinolones and ethionamide.

Psychiatric disorders are common in patients with tuberculosis, and psychiatric side effects are among the most common side effects resulting in withdrawal of one or more drugs from the treatment regimen in multidrug-resistant tuberculosis (Törün et al. 2005). In a Peruvian study of patients with multidrug-resistant tuberculosis, baseline levels of depression declined from 52.2% to 13.3% during multidrug-resistant tuberculosis treatment, whereas anxiety increased slightly from 8.7% to 12%. The incidence of psychosis during treatment was 12%. Psychiatric comorbidity did not contraindicate multidrug-resistant tuberculosis treatment or require discontinuation of cycloserine, except in one case (Vega et al. 2004). However, in a large U.S. study of patients who received treatment for multidrug-resistant tuberculosis, psychiatric disorder was an independent predictor of mortality (Franke et al. 2008).

Hyperventilation

Hyperventilation is a common presenting complaint in emergency departments leading to psychiatric consultation (Nguyen et al. 1992). These patients briefly experience an increase in the rate and depth of breathing and may have dizziness or syncope from the respiratory alkalosis and cerebral vasoconstriction that result. Symptoms of blurred vision, carpopedal spasm, myoclonic jerks, or paresthesias may frighten the patient or relatives and result in an emergency department visit.

The incidence of hyperventilation syndrome may be as high as 6%–11% in the general population (Lachman et al. 1992), especially in children, and hyperventilation syndrome may be recurrent. Medical illnesses that may be confused with hyperventilation syndrome include angina, arrhythmia, asthma (Demeter and Cordasco 1986; Kashiwagi et al. 2008), carbon monoxide poisoning (Skorodin et al. 1986), diabetic ketoacidosis (Treasure et al. 1987), pulmonary emboli (Hoegholm et al. 1987), epilepsy, hypoglycemia, ingestion of salicylates (Rognum et al. 1987), Meniere's disease, tetany (Hehrmann 1996), and vasovagal syncope. Neurological causes of hyperventilation also have been reported, including thalamic infarct (Scialdone 1990), Cheyne-Stokes breathing (Liippo et al. 1992), and traumatic vestibular hyperreactivity after whiplash injury (A.J. Fischer et al. 1995).

Medications reported to cause central hyperventilation include carbamazepine, salicylates, and topiramate. Central hyperventilation resolves promptly within a day or two after discontinuation of these drugs (Lasky and Brody 2000; Mizukami et al. 1990).

Psychiatric disorders to consider in hyperventilation syndrome include conversion disorder, histrionic personality disorder, hypochondriasis, the respiratory subtype of panic disorder, phobic disorders, and substance abuse (Abrams et al. 2006; Araki and Honma 1986). Hyperventilation syndrome also has occurred as part of mass psychogenic illness (Araki and Honma 1986). Estimates of the overlap between hyperventilation syndrome and panic disorder are between 35% and 83% (Cowley and Roy-Byrne 1987; de Ruiter et al. 1989; Hoes et al. 1987). The relation between hyperventilation syndrome and panic disorder is controversial.

Various treatments for hyperventilation syndrome have been used over the years, such as antidepressants (Saarijarvi and Lehtinen 1987), beta-blockers (L.L. Van De Ven et al. 1995), intravenous sedatives (Hirokawa et al. 1995), breathing retraining (DeGuire et al. 1992, 1996; Pinney et al. 1987), grief therapy (Paulley 1990), group therapy (Fensterheim and Wiegand 1991), and hypnosis (Conway et al. 1988).

Although having patients with acute hyperventilation rebreathe into a brown paper bag is a traditional technique used in the emergency department, it is dangerous and potentially fatal when mistakenly applied to patients with hypoxia or myocardial ischemia (Callaham 1989).

Vocal Cord Dysfunction

Vocal cord dysfunction (VCD) is a respiratory syndrome frequently confused with asthma, although they often occur together (Newman et al. 1995). It is not unusual for VCD to be misdiagnosed as steroid-resistant asthma (Thomas et al. 1999). VCD also may co-occur with hyperventilation syndrome. The syndrome of VCD was first described 200 years ago by Osler (Brugman 2003), yet it is still not well understood. The disorder may present in childhood, adolescence, or adulthood. Patients may appear in severe respiratory distress yet have relatively normal blood gas levels, or respiratory alkalosis from hyperventilation, only rarely presenting with hypoxemia. Unlike in asthma, wheezing in VCD will be loudest over the larynx and more pronounced in the inspiratory phase, but the chest is otherwise clear. Also unlike asthma, VCD attacks typically have rapid onset and equally rapid resolution. VCD may lead to frequent emergency department visits and hospitalizations, high doses of (ineffective) asthma medications, and unnecessary intubation or tracheotomy (Bahrainwala and Simon 2001; Ibrahim et al. 2007).

The differential diagnosis of VCD includes angioedema; asthma; factitious disorder; hyperventilation syndrome; iatrogenic, inflammatory, neoplastic, or neurological disorders (e.g., spasmodic dysphonia and laryngeal nerve injury); obsessive-compulsive disorder; personality disorder (dependent, histrionic, or mixed); PTSD; school phobia; and somatization disorder (Brugman 2003; Koufman and Block 2008; Lacy and McManis 1994). A multidisciplinary approach has been recommended, including specialists in allergy, psychiatry, pulmonary medicine, neurology, otolaryngology, and speech therapy (Nacci et al. 2007). Viewing the vocal cords via laryngoscopy allows a definitive diagnosis (Arndt and Voth 1996). Comorbid conditions in World Trade Center workers with VCD included acid reflux disease and allergic rhinitis (de la Hoz et al. 2008).

In most patients, VCD appears not to be a primary psychiatric disorder but rather a conditioned response, which may result in secondary anxiety. The onset of VCD is typically preceded by allergy, asthma, gastric reflux, irritant exposure (Perkner et al. 1998), or a dyspneic episode in athletes (Newsham et al. 2002). The psychiatric literature reflects referral bias capturing only part of the VCD spectrum. Psychiatrists are most likely to see those patients with VCD who develop panic attacks and phobic symptoms. Case reports and retrospective case series note strong dependency needs and fears of separation in patients with VCD and its acute precipitation following psychosocial stress.

Formal psychological testing in VCD patients at a tertiary-care center found high rates of conversion disorder and hypochondriasis, but a quarter had no evidence of any psychopathology. Comorbidities included asthma (65%), gastroesophageal reflux disease (51%), and history of abuse (38%) (Husein et al. 2008). Another study of tertiary-care VCD patients found that most had a history of childhood sexual abuse (Freedman et al. 1991), but this has not been replicated (Brugman 2003).

No empirically proven treatment for VCD is available, although antipanic pharmacotherapy, biofeedback, cognitive therapy, relaxation techniques, and speech therapy have been reported as helpful (Andrianopoulos et al. 2000; Brugman 2003; Earles et al. 2003). Benzodiazepines can be used to terminate a severe episode of VCD (Hicks et al. 2008).

Lung Cancer

Lung cancer is the most common cause of cancer death in the United States and the world (see also Chapter 23, "Oncology"). Smoking tobacco is the primary cause of most lung cancers (Strauss 1998). About 30% of all cancer mortality in the United States is due to lung cancer; it is the number one cancer diagnosis in men and the second most frequent cancer in women. Because 45% of patients present late with stage III disease, the 5-year survival rate is abysmally low: about 15% (Pearman 2008).

There has been a burgeoning literature on biological, psychological, and social aspects of lung cancer. Some studies and reviews indicate that psychological factors alter the incidence, course, or mortality of lung cancer (e.g., Chida et al. 2008; Faller and Bulzebruck 2002), whereas other studies do not support this association (e.g., Akechi et al. 2009). Some apparent associations disappear when other factors are adequately controlled (Nakaya et al. 2008). Publication bias, confounding by other clinical and demographic variables, and differences in study methods and patient populations make this literature difficult to interpret.

Symptoms of psychological distress are common in lung cancer. One study showed that newly diagnosed lung cancer patients had frequent insomnia (52%), loss of libido (48%), loss of interest in or ability to work (33%), concerns about their families (29%), and poor concentration (19%) (Ginsburg et al. 1995). Depression and anxiety are more frequent in patients with lung cancer than in those with breast cancer (Brintzenhofe-Szoc et al. 2009). In one study, type of lung cancer influenced the rate of depression (i.e., more frequent in small-cell cancer than in non-small-cell cancer); however, the most important risk factor was functional impairment (Hopwood and Stephens 2000). Suicide rates in cancer patients are twice those in the general population in the United States, with lung cancer having the highest standardized mortality ratio among cancers of various organs. Risk is highest in the first 5 years after diagnosis (Misono et al. 2008).

In patients with lung cancer, distress and quality of life vary depending on pretreatment psychosocial characteristics (e.g., Barlesi et al. 2006; Boehmer et al. 2007; Visser et al. 2006), specific chemotherapy agents given (e.g., Gralla and Thatcher 2004), cognitive and other side effects of chemotherapy and radiation (e.g., Whitney et al. 2008), marital relationship (Carmack Taylor et al. 2008; Zhang and Siminoff 2003), coping style (e.g., Wong and Fielding 2007), pain management (Akechi et al. 2001), and sexual functioning (Goodell 2007). Psychological distress is high in newly diagnosed lung cancer patients (Mohan et al. 2006), indicating the need for psychological support at the time of diagnosis (Lheureux et al. 2004). Management of symptoms associated with lung cancer such as anorexia, delirium, dyspnea, fatigue, and pain can improve quality of life (Bedor et al. 2005; Tishelman et al. 2005; Von Roenn and Paice 2005). Fatigue is more common at diagnosis with lung cancer than with most other cancers: 50% of those with inoperable non-small-cell cancer reported severe fatigue (Stone et al. 2000). Dyspnea is a subjective symptom even in lung cancer and is greater in patients with anxiety, fatigue, and poor coping (Henoch et al. 2008).

Given the high rate of dyspnea in lung cancer patients, one might expect that many patients would cease tobacco use. However, this is not the case, despite evidence that continued smoking after lung cancer diagnosis decreases treatment efficacy, increases complications, increases risk of recurrence and occurrence of another primary tumor, and decreases survival time. Lung cancer patients who are not ready to quit smoking or who are likely to relapse are more likely to be depressed, be fatalistic, have greater nicotine dependence, have less self-efficacy, have less education, and have relatives at home who also smoke (Schnoll et al. 2002; Walker et al. 2004).

Refusal of treatment for lung cancer is multifactorial, including distrust of medical authority, faith, fatalism, minimization of threats, and self-efficacy. Understanding the sources of resistance to treatment recommendations may help improve communication and engender trust during delivery of lung cancer care (Sharf et al. 2005). Denial is more often seen in lung cancer patients who are less educated, elderly, and male (Vos et al. 2008) but is not always maladaptive. Psychological factors also may influence response to treatment in other ways. Psychological distress influences chemotherapy-induced nausea (Takatsuki et al. 1998) and its response to treatment (Tsavaris et al. 2008).

Lung Transplantation

Indications and Contraindications

The first lung transplant was performed in 1963, but it was 20 years before the first successful operation in 1983 (Ochoa and Richardson 1999) (see also Chapter 31, "Organ Transplantation"). The most common indication is COPD (including alpha$_1$-antitrypsin deficiency), which accounts for about 45% of lung transplants (Hosenpud et al. 1998). Transplants are also performed for those with CF, idiopathic pulmonary fibrosis, Eisenmenger's syndrome, primary pulmonary hypertension, and several other pulmonary diseases (Etienne et al. 1997).

Exclusion criteria vary from one transplant center to another. Psychiatric factors that are considered to be absolute contraindications to lung transplantation include active alcoholism, drug abuse or cigarette use, severe psychiatric illness, and noncompliance with treatment (Aris et al. 1997; Paradowski 1997; Snell et al. 1993).

The four main approaches to lung transplantation are 1) single-lung transplantation, 2) bilateral sequential transplantation, 3) heart–lung transplantation, and 4) single-lobe donation from living donors (Arcasoy and Kotloff 1999). Living donor donation has been controversial because of the uncertainty regarding risks to the donor (Barr et al. 1998).

Medical and Surgical Outcomes

Patient survival in the United States at 1 year and 5 years after lung transplant is currently 83.8% and 52.3%, respectively. For comparison, the corresponding survival figures after heart transplant are 87.7% and 73.9% (United Network for Organ Sharing 2008). Some diagnoses confer better survival. Survival after lung and heart-lung transplant in CF may be as high as 90% at 1 year and 78% at 5 years (Haloun and Despins 2003).

For patients with CF and idiopathic pulmonary fibrosis, there appears to be increased survival relative to the natural history of the underlying illness. However, for patients with COPD, no survival advantage has been documented, although transplant improves quality of life and functional ability. Exercise capacity improves, with about 80% of recipients reporting no limitations in activity within 1 year of transplant. Quality of life remains stable for the first few years if the course is uncomplicated, but those who develop bronchiolitis obliterans show a sharp decline in quality of life. Despite improvements in exercise tolerance and quality of life, 40% or fewer of lung transplant recipients return to work. This finding may be a result of employer bias, a fear of losing health insurance or disability benefits, or a change in priorities after a life-threatening illness (Estenne and Hertz 2002; Paris et al. 1998).

Early complications after lung transplantation include primary graft failure, stenosis of the anastomosis, and a higher rate of infectious complications than in other solid organ transplantation (Christie et al. 1998; Kramer et al. 1993).

Psychological Factors and Quality of Life

One-quarter of patients awaiting lung transplantation may meet criteria for at least one anxiety or mood disorder (Parekh et al. 2003). Screening for depression among lung transplant candidates showed mild to moderate depressive symptoms in 56% (Najafizadeh et al. 2009). Patients showed more anxiety and depression the longer they were on the transplant list and expressed distress from wearing a beeper and fears that the transplant would come too late (Vermeulen et al. 2005). In both pre- and post-lung transplant patients, higher social support was associated with higher quality of life and lower depressive symptoms (Archonti et al. 2004). Candidates that used maladaptive coping styles (avoidance, disengagement, low solicitation of support, and rumination and venting emotions) were more likely to show emotional distress and disability and may benefit from psychotherapy and interventions to improve coping (Burker et al. 2004a).

About 37% of patients awaiting lung transplant have moderate to severe cognitive impairment that does not differ by specific disease. Higher partial pressure of oxygen (PO_2) values correlated with better executive function and attention, and lower partial pressure of carbon dioxide (PCO_2) values correlated with better executive function and attention and verbal memory. Verbal memory correlated with distance walked in 6 minutes (Parekh et al. 2005).

Most lung transplant recipients report significant improvement in general health, anxiety, depression, self-esteem, social functioning, and quality of life (Limbos et al. 2000), reaching a level equal to that of healthy control subjects, despite exercise capacity 30%–40% of normal (Tegtbur et al. 2004). Some recipients do experience emotional distress and disability, and their likelihood of doing so is influenced by coping style (Burker et al. 2005; Myaskovsky et al. 2003), PTSD (Köllner et al. 2003), social support (Myaskovsky et al. 2003), and pulmonary complications (Goetzmann et al. 2005), especially bronchiolitis obliterans (Goetzmann et al. 2006a, 2006b; Künsebeck et al. 2007). Social support also influences adherence with treatment posttransplant (Teichman et al. 2000). Patients became less compliant the further from the time of transplant, suggesting that periodic reeducation after transplantation may improve adherence. Quality of life in most patients begins to decline after 3–4 years (Vermeulen et al. 2003), with depressive symptoms increasing significantly in those with bronchiolitis obliterans (Fusar-Poli et al. 2007).

Psychological Interventions

Pretransplant assessment of affect (anxiety and depression), cognitive beliefs (sense of coherence and optimism), and social support may identify vulnerable candidates who may benefit from psychotherapy. Because depression affects adherence with immunosuppressants, treatment of depression is imperative. Telephone-based cognitive therapy and coping skills training have been shown to improve anxiety, depression, stress, optimism, social support, vitality, and quality of life (Blumenthal et al. 2006; Napolitano et al. 2002). A small randomized controlled trial in lung transplant candidates awaiting transplantation showed that a brief psychological intervention—quality-of-life therapy—was superior to supportive therapy in improving mood, social intimacy, and quality of life (Rodrigue et al. 2005). Although many transplant centers warn against having pets because of concerns about infection, one study found that more than half of the lung recipients owned pets and had significantly better life satisfaction, quality of life, and social support with no higher frequency of somatic complications than did those without pets (Irani et al. 2006).

Terminal Weaning

Patients with end-stage pulmonary disease caused by amyotrophic lateral sclerosis, COPD, CF, idiopathic pulmonary fibrosis, lung cancer, or other diseases may request terminal weaning. The term *terminal weaning* has been viewed by some as an oxymoron for several reasons. Although terminal implies that the withdrawal of ventilator support will inevitably end in death, patients do not always die shortly after discontinuation of ventilator support. In one study, 8% of patients survived and were discharged (M.L. Campbell 1994), although prediction has improved since then. The phrase "discontinuation of ventilator support" or "withdrawal of mechanical ventilation" is preferable when talking with the patient, family, and other health care professionals (Apelgren 2000; Daly et al. 1993).

Ethicists and legal experts concur that competent patients, or their surrogate decision makers when patients are not competent, have the right to refuse treatment, regardless of whether it is "lifesaving," and that there is no moral difference between not initiating treatment and withdrawing treatment in response to the patient's request. The patient or surrogate must be made aware that death is the expected outcome when ventilator support is discontinued and should make the decision only after due deliberation (Daly et al. 1993).

The patient's goals should guide the process of withdrawing ventilator support (J. Anderson and O'Brien 1995). If the patient shows ambivalence about terminal weaning, or it is unclear whether the patient has sufficient mental capacity to make a well-thought-out decision, a psychiatrist should be consulted. The first step in evaluation is to explore why the patient has requested discontinuation of ventilator support. Depression, delirium, and concerns about burdening the family require different interventions. In difficult cases, involvement of the hospital's ethics committee, chaplain, social worker, and legal counsel may be helpful. A brief delay (days) after the decision has been made to withdraw ventilator support may reassure staff and family that the patient made a decision that was not based on temporary frustration or discomfort.

Patients should be told that the weaning process may be stopped at any time if they wish. Evidence-based guidance is available (M.L. Campbell 2007). Withdrawal of the ventilator may follow the withdrawal of pressors, antibiotics, and enteral feeding (Brody et al. 1997). In a conscious patient, a gradual decrease in fraction of inspired oxygen (FIO_2), with decreased positive end-expiratory pressure (PEEP) and decrease in respiratory rate over several hours has been advocated (Grenvik 1983).

Adjunctive medication may alleviate distress. Opiates have been used to decrease anxiety, coughing, gasping, pain, or the sensation of shortness of breath and to provide sedation (Wilson et al. 1992). Documentation of the physician's intent in administering opiates is important to show that the medication is being used as a comfort measure and not to hasten death. One protocol suggests giving a bolus of 5–10 mg morphine intravenously followed by a drip of 2.5–5.0 mg/hour of morphine. Benzodiazepines may decrease anxiety and prevent myoclonus or twitching that may be unsettling to the family (Faber-Langendoen 1994). Phenobarbital may control twitching not relieved by benzodiazepines. Low-dose haloperidol may be used intravenously for anxiety not relieved by benzodiazepines or for delirium. One group observed that because opioids and sedatives decrease oxygen requirements, these drugs may prolong life, instead of hastening death (Bakker et al. 2008). Charting should include advance directives, code status, documentation of medications given and time of initiation of the ventilator withdrawal process, and whether the patient was extubated (Kirchhoff et al. 2004). The family should be educated prior to the procedure that the medications are used to prevent the patient from having physical distress and awareness of bodily events and may induce euphoria.

Psychiatric Side Effects of Pulmonary Drugs

Psychiatric side effects of pulmonary drugs are shown in Table 19–1 and noted in the following psychiatric syndrome sections. The adverse psychiatric effects of systemic corticosteroids are reviewed in Chapter 25, "Rheumatology," and the effects of antibiotics are reviewed in Chapter 27, "Infectious Diseases." Isoniazid and other drugs for tuberculosis were discussed earlier in this chapter. There have been reports of suicidality with montelukast and other leukotriene antagonists but insufficient data to prove that a causal relation exists (Manalai et al. 2009). In children, a variety of adverse psychiatric effects of montelukast have been reported, including nightmares and other sleep disorders, anxiety, and aggression (Wallerstedt et al. 2009).

Psychopharmacology in Pulmonary Disease

Anxiety

Anxiety in pulmonary patients may be caused by symptoms of lung disease such as breathlessness, bronchospasm, excessive secretions, or hypoxia, so the first step in treatment of anxiety is optimization of management of the patient's respiratory illness. Many drugs used to treat pulmonary disease may themselves cause anxiety (see Table 19–1). Theophylline can cause anxiety, nausea, tremor, and restlessness, especially at higher doses. Beta-adrenergic bronchodilators used in treatment of asthma or other obstructive lung disease can cause marked anxiety, tachycardia, and tremor, particularly in patients who overuse

TABLE 19–1. Psychiatric side effects of common pulmonary drugs

Anticholinergics	Auditory and visual hallucinations, anxiety, confusion, delirium, depersonalization, amnesia, paranoia
Antileukotrienes	Anxiety
Beta-agonists (selective)	Anxiety in susceptible patients
Beta-agonists (nonselective)	Anxiety, psychosis
Corticosteroids (inhaled)	None
Corticosteroids (systemic)	Depression, mania
Cycloserine	Agoraphobia, anxiety, depression, psychosis
Isoniazid	Amnesia, anxiety, depression, hallucinations, mania, psychosis
Theophylline	Anxiety, delirium, insomnia, mutism, restlessness, tremor

Source. Adapted from "Drugs That May Cause Psychiatric Symptoms" 2008.

their inhalers. Nonprescription asthma preparations contain nonselective sympathomimetics, which are even more likely to cause anxiety. At high doses, they may cause psychosis and seizures.

In anxious pulmonary patients with hypercapnia, buspirone is preferred for treatment of anxiety, but it may have a slow onset of action (Craven and Sutherland 1991). Buspirone may improve exercise tolerance and dyspnea, can be used safely in patients with sleep apnea (Mendelson et al. 1991), and can be combined with theophylline and terbutaline (Kiev and Domantay 1988).

In COPD patients who do not retain carbon dioxide, prudent doses of benzodiazepines may decrease breathlessness. In elderly or debilitated patients, shorter-acting benzodiazepines with no active metabolites, such as alprazolam, lorazepam, and oxazepam, are preferred. Zolpidem does not alter respiratory drive in COPD patients, but rebound insomnia or withdrawal similar to that with triazolam may result. Diazepam has no effect on breathlessness and may decrease exercise tolerance. Although some have advocated promethazine to decrease breathlessness and increase exercise tolerance in COPD, this drug is a phenothiazine and can cause akathisia, extrapyramidal effects, and neuroleptic malignant syndrome. Selective serotonin reuptake inhibitors (SSRIs) also may be helpful in treating panic symptoms and do not have pulmonary side effects. If panic does not respond to these measures, then neuroleptics may be effective in low doses. Beta-blockers should not be used for anxiety in asthma patients because of resulting bronchoconstriction.

Depression

When choosing an antidepressant, the side-effect profile and cytochrome P450 (CYP) interactions with pulmonary drugs should be considered. Among the SSRIs, sertraline, citalopram, and escitalopram have the lowest risk of interactions with pulmonary drugs, and SSRIs may decrease dyspnea and even increase arterial oxygen concentration in some patients (Ciraulo and Shader 1990; Smoller et al. 1998).

Many pulmonary patients may be taking other medications that can prolong the QT interval, so reviewing the electrocardiogram is prudent when considering treatment with a tricyclic antidepressant. In elderly patients or in patients with COPD or sleep apnea, nortriptyline or desipramine is preferred over the more sedating tertiary amines, which may cause delirium or hypotension. Protriptyline may be helpful in sleep apnea by increasing respiratory drive, but the half-life is very long (54–92 hours), three to four times longer than that of nortriptyline, with no evidence of greater efficacy compared with other tricyclics for sleep apnea (DeVane 1998).

Psychosis

Pulmonary patients may have primary psychotic disorders, such as bipolar disorder or schizophrenia, or may become psychotic because of medications such as beta-agonists, cycloserine, isoniazid, or corticosteroids. The incidence of steroid psychosis is dose related, seen in fewer than 1% of patients taking 40 mg or less of prednisone per day compared with 28% taking 80 mg daily (Boston Collaborative Drug Surveillance Program 1972).

Typical neuroleptics such as haloperidol at high doses may cause akathisia, laryngospasm, and paradoxical intercostal muscle movements that may cause restlessness and interfere with breathing. Tardive dyskinesia sometimes affects the diaphragm and other muscles used in breathing and in severe cases can result in respiratory insufficiency. For chronic treatment, newer drugs with lower incidence of extrapyramidal side effects may be preferred.

TABLE 19–2. Drug interactions between pulmonary and psychotropic drugs

Pulmonary drug	Psychotropic drug	Adverse effect
Isoniazid	TCAs	MAOI effect of isoniazid
Rifampin	Donepezil	Decreased donepezil effect
Rifampin	Diazepam	Induced diazepam metabolism
Rifampin	Valproate	Decreased valproate level
Rifampin	TCAs, MAOIs	Induced TCA, MAOI metabolism
Sympathomimetic drugs[a]	TCAs, MAOIs	Hypertensive crisis
Theophylline	Alprazolam	Decreased benzodiazepine effect
Theophylline	Carbamazepine	Decreased carbamazepine level
Theophylline	Clozapine	Increased theophylline level
Theophylline	Fluvoxamine	Increased theophylline level
Theophylline	Lithium	Reduced lithium level 20%–30%

Note. MAOI=monoamine oxidase inhibitor; TCA=tricyclic antidepressant.
[a]Epinephrine, ephedrine, pseudoephedrine.
Source. Adapted from Cozza et al. 2003.

Drug Interactions Between Psychotropic and Pulmonary Drugs

The psychiatrist should consider potential interactions when prescribing psychotropic medications to patients with pulmonary disease (Table 19–2). Theophylline levels may be reduced by 50%–80% by tobacco smoking. Nicotine gum does not have this effect. Polycyclic aromatic hydrocarbons in tobacco smoke may induce CYP isoenzymes 1A1, 1A2, and perhaps 2E1. If a patient quits smoking when admitted to the hospital, CYP1A2 induction rapidly declines, which can lead to increased effects of substrates, including caffeine, clozapine, fluvoxamine, olanzapine, tacrine, and theophylline. Likewise, when discharged patients resume smoking, these medications may need dosage adjustment. Inhaled corticosteroids are also influenced by smoking and may reach higher levels more quickly.

Alcohol can reduce clearance of theophylline as much as 30% for up to 24 hours. Most pulmonary medications do not affect lithium levels, except theophylline, which can lower lithium levels by 20%–30%. Patients with chronic pulmonary disease may develop right-sided heart failure and may receive diuretics that raise or lower lithium levels depending on choice of diuretic. Theophylline preparations administered concurrently with electroconvulsive therapy can prolong seizure duration, especially if the theophylline level is higher than the accepted therapeutic range, even if the level is below that typically associated with seizures (Peters et al. 1984).

Rifampin is a CYP3A4 substrate and so may compete with many psychotropic drugs, including the antidepressants amitriptyline, imipramine, fluoxetine, sertraline, bupropion, venlafaxine, and trazodone. Rifampin may compete through the same site with anticonvulsants (e.g., carbamazepine, tiagabine, and valproate) and with benzodiazepines, zolpidem, and haloperidol. Montelukast sodium may have similar interactions to those of rifampin because of metabolism via CYP3A4 and CYP2C9.

Fluvoxamine can increase sildenafil exposure by 40% and prolong the half-life by 19% ($P=0.9034$). Fluvoxamine can boost sodium nitroprusside–induced venodilation by 59% (Hesse et al. 2005).

Conclusion

In this chapter we have summarized the treatment of psychiatric conditions often seen in patients with lung disease. Diseases affecting the lungs occur across the life span. Some diseases, such as asthma and cystic fibrosis, often begin in childhood and may affect childhood developmental stages. Sarcoidosis may manifest in early to middle life, disrupting career and family life. Comorbid psychiatric conditions are also prevalent in conditions that begin between midlife and senescence, such as chronic bronchitis, emphysema, and pulmonary fibrosis. Hyperventilation syndrome and vocal cord dysfunction can have biological or psychological origins that need to be identified for effective treatment. Ultimately, the psychological aspects of lung disease determine to a large extent the quality of life and outcomes of patients with lung disease, including those with lung cancer and those that undergo lung transplantation. Finally, with the polypharmacy often required for treatment of lung disease, the psychiatrist must be aware of the ever-present risks of adverse interactions between pulmonary drugs and psychotropics.

References

Abbott J, Dodd M, Gee L, et al: Ways of coping with cystic fibrosis: implications for treatment adherence. Disabil Rehabil 23:315–324, 2001

Abdelaziz MM, Samman YS, Wali SO, et al: Treatment of idiopathic pulmonary fibrosis: is there anything new? Respirology 10:284–289, 2005

Abrams K, Rassovsky Y, Kushner MG: Evidence for respiratory and nonrespiratory subtypes in panic disorder. Depress Anxiety 23:474–481, 2006

Akechi T, Okamura H, Nishiwaki Y, et al: Psychiatric disorders and associated and predictive factors in patients with unresectable nonsmall cell lung carcinoma: a longitudinal study. Cancer 92:2609–2622, 2001

Akechi T, Okamura H, Okuyama T, et al: Psychosocial factors and survival after diagnosis of inoperable non-small cell lung cancer. Psychooncology 18:23–29, 2009

Alao AO, Yolles JC: Isoniazid-induced psychosis. Ann Pharmacother 32:889–891, 1998

Allen JT, Spiteri MA: Growth factors in idiopathic pulmonary fibrosis: relative roles. Respir Res 3:13, 2002

American Lung Association: Minority Lung Disease Data 2000. Available at: www.lungusa.org. Accessed January 2000.

American Psychiatric Association: Diagnostic and Statistical Manual of Mental Disorders, 4th Edition. Washington, DC, American Psychiatric Association, 1994

Anderson DL, Flume PA, Hardy KK: Psychological functioning of adults with cystic fibrosis. Chest 119:1079–1084, 2001

Anderson J, O'Brien M: Challenges for the future: the nurse's role in weaning patients from mechanical ventilation. Intensive Crit Care Nurs 11:2–5, 1995

Andrianopoulos MV, Gallivan GJ, Gallivan KH: PVCM, PVCD, EPL, and irritable larynx syndrome: what are we talking about and how do we treat it? J Voice 14:607–618, 2000

Antonelli Incalzi R, Marra C, Giordano A, et al: Cognitive impairment in chronic obstructive pulmonary disease—a neuropsychological and SPECT study. J Neurol 250:325–332, 2003

Antoniu SA: Perfenidone for the treatment of idiopathic pulmonary fibrosis. Expert Opin Investig Drugs 15:823–828, 2006

Apelgren KN: "Terminal" wean is the wrong term. Crit Care Med 28:3576–3577, 2000

Araki S, Honma T: Mass psychogenic systemic illness in school children in relation to the Tokyo photochemical smog. Arch Environ Health 41:159–162, 1986

Arcasoy SM, Kotloff RM: Lung transplantation. N Engl J Med 340:1081–1091, 1999

Archonti C, D'Amelio R, Klein T, et al: Physical quality of life and social support in patients on the waiting list and after a lung transplantation. Psychother Psychosom Med Psychol 54:17–22, 2004

Aris RM, Gilligan PH, Neuring IP, et al: The effect of panresistant bacteria in cystic fibrosis patients on lung transplant outcome. Am J Respir Crit Care Med 155:1699–1704, 1997

Arndt GA, Voth BR: Paradoxical vocal cord motion in the recovery room: a masquerader of pulmonary dysfunction. Can J Anaesth 43:1249–1251, 1996

Arver S, Lehtihet ML: Current guidelines for the diagnosis of testosterone deficiency. Front Horm Res 37:5–20, 2009

Aydin IO, Ulusahin A: Depression, anxiety comorbidity, and disability in tuberculosis and chronic obstructive pulmonary disease patients: applicability of GHQ-12. Gen Hosp Psychiatry 23:77–83, 2001

Bahrainwala AH, Simon MR: Wheezing and vocal cord dysfunction mimicking asthma. Curr Opin Pulm Med 7:8–13, 2001

Bakker J, Jansen TC, Lima A, et al: Why opioids and sedatives may prolong life rather than hasten death after ventilator withdrawal in critically ill patients. Am J Hosp Palliat Care 25:152–154, 2008

Barlesi F, Doddoli C, Loundou A, et al: Preoperative psychological global well being index (PGWBI) predicts postoperative quality of life for patients with non-small cell lung cancer managed with thoracic surgery. Eur J Cardiothorac Surg 30:548–553, 2006

Barnes PJ, Woolcock AJ: Difficult asthma. Eur Respir J 12:1209–1218, 1998

Barr ML, Schenkel FA, Cohen RG, et al: Recipient and donor outcomes in living related and unrelated lobar transplantation. Transplant Proc 30:2261–2263, 1998

Bedor M, Alexander C, Edelman MJ: Management of common symptoms of advanced lung cancer. Curr Treat Options Oncol 6:61–68, 2005

Blumenthal JA, Babyak MA, Keefe FJ, et al: Telephone-based coping skills training for patients awaiting lung transplantation. J Consult Clin Psychol 74:535–544, 2006

Boehmer S, Luszczynska A, Schwarzer R: Coping and quality of life after tumor surgery: personal and social resources promote different domains of quality of life. Anxiety Stress Coping 20:61–75, 2007

Borson S, Claypoole K, McDonald GJ: Depression and chronic obstructive pulmonary disease: treatment trials. Semin Clin Neuropsychiatry 3:115–130, 1998

Bosley CM, Corden ZM, Rees PJ, et al: Psychological factors associated with use of home nebulized therapy for COPD. Eur Respir J 9:2346–2350, 1996

Boston Collaborative Drug Surveillance Program: Acute adverse reaction to prednisone in relation to dosage. Clin Pharmacol Ther 13:694–697, 1972

Brenes GA: Anxiety and chronic obstructive pulmonary disease: prevalence, impact, and treatment. Psychosom Med 65:963–970, 2003

Brintzenhofe-Szoc KM, Levin TT, Li Y, et al: Mixed anxiety/depression symptoms in a large cancer cohort: prevalence by cancer type. Psychosomatics 50:383–391, 2009

Brody H, Campbell ML, Faber-Langendoen K, et al: Withdrawing intensive life-sustaining treatment—recommendations for compassionate clinical management. N Engl J Med 336:652–657, 1997

Brown ES, Vigil L, Khan DA, et al: A randomized trial of citalopram versus placebo in outpatients with asthma and major depressive disorder: a proof of concept study. Biol Psychiatry 58:865–870, 2005

Brown ES, Vornik LA, Khan DA, et al: Bupropion in the treatment of outpatients with asthma and major depressive disorder. Int J Psychiatry Med 37:23–28, 2007

Brugman SM: The many faces of vocal cord dysfunction: what 36 years of literature tell us. Am J Respir Crit Care Med 167:A588, 2003

Bullman C, Faust M, Hoffmann A, et al: Five cases with central diabetes insipidus and hypogonadism as first presentation of neurosarcoidosis. Eur J Endocrinol 142:365–372, 2000

Burker EJ, Carels RA, Thompson LF, et al: Quality of life in patients awaiting lung transplant: cystic fibrosis versus other end-stage lung diseases. Pediatr Pulmonol 30:453–460, 2000

Burker EJ, Evon DM, Sedway JA, et al: Appraisal and coping as predictors of psychological distress and self-reported physical disability before lung transplantation. Prog Transplant 14:222–232, 2004a

Burker EJH, Sedway J, Carone S: Psychological and educational factors: better predictors of work status than FEV1 in adults with cystic fibrosis. Pediatr Pulmonol 38:413–418, 2004b

Burker EJ, Evon DM, Sedway JA, et al: Religious and non-religious coping in lung transplant candidates: does adding God to the picture tell us more? J Behav Med 28.513–526, 2005

Callaham M: Hypoxic hazards of traditional paper bag rebreathing in hyperventilating patients. Ann Emerg Med 18:622–628, 1989

Campbell DA, Yellowlees PM, McLennan G, et al: Psychiatric and medical features of near fatal asthma. Thorax 50:254–259, 1995

Campbell ML: Terminal weaning: it's not simply "pulling the plug." Nursing 24:34–39, 1994

Campbell ML: How to withdraw mechanical ventilation: a systematic review of the literature. AACN Adv Crit Care 18:397–403, 2007

Carmack Taylor CL, Badr H, Lee JH, et al: Lung cancer patients and their spouses: psychological and relationship functioning within 1 month of treatment initiation. Ann Behav Med 36:129–140, 2008

Centers for Disease Control and Prevention: Self-reported increase in asthma severity after the September 11 attacks on the World Trade Center—Manhattan, New York, 2001. MMWR Morb Mortal Wkly Rep 51:781–784, 2002

Chapman E, Landy A, Lyon A, et al: End of life care for adult cystic fibrosis patients: facilitating a good enough death. J Cyst Fibros 4:249–257, 2005

Chida Y, Hamer M, Wardle S, et al: Do stress-related psychosocial factors contribute to cancer incidence and survival? Nat Clin Pract Oncol 5:466–475, 2008

Christian BJ, D'Auria JP: The child's eye: memories of growing up with cystic fibrosis. J Pediatr Nurs 12:3–12, 1997

Christie JD, Bavaria JE, Palevsky HI, et al: Primary graft failure following lung transplantation. Chest 114:51–60, 1998

Chun TH, Weitzen SH, Fritz GK: The asthma/mental health nexus in a population-based sample of the United States. Chest 34:1176–1182, 2008

Ciraulo DA, Shader RI: Fluoxetine drug-drug interactions II. J Clin Psychopharmacol 10:213–217, 1990

Cluley S, Cochrane GM: Psychological disorder in asthma is associated with poor control and poor adherence to inhaled steroids. Respir Med 95:37–39, 2001

Cohen RT, Canino GJ, Bird HR, et al: Violence, abuse, and asthma in Puerto Rican children. Am J Respir Crit Care Med 178:453–459, 2008

Collins S, Reynolds F: How do adults with cystic fibrosis cope following a diagnosis of diabetes? J Adv Nurs 64:478–487, 2008

Conway AV, Freeman LJ, Nixon PG: Hypnotic examination of trigger factors in the hyperventilation syndrome. Am J Clin Hypn 30:286–304, 1988

Coventry PA, Gellatly JL: Improving outcomes for COPD patients with mild-to-moderate anxiety and depression: a systematic review of cognitive behavioural therapy. Br J Health Psychol 13 (pt 3):381–400, 2008

Coventry PA, Hind D: Comprehensive pulmonary rehabilitation for anxiety and depression in adults with chronic obstructive pulmonary disease: systematic review and meta-analysis. J Psychosom Res 63:551–565, 2007

Cowley DS, Roy-Byrne PP: Hyperventilation and panic disorder. Am J Med 83:929–937, 1987

Cozza KL, Armstrong SC, Oesterheld JR: Drug Interaction Principles Pocket Guide. Washington, DC, American Psychiatric Publishing, 2003

Craven J, Sutherland A: Buspirone for anxiety disorders in patients with severe lung disease (letter). Lancet 338:249, 1991

Crews WD Jr, Jefferson AL, Broshek DK, et al: Neuropsychological sequelae in a series of patients with end-stage cystic fibrosis: lung transplant evaluation. Arch Clin Neuropsychol 15:59–70, 2000

Cully JA, Graham DP, Stanley MA, et al: Quality of life in patients with chronic obstructive pulmonary disease and comorbid anxiety or depression. Psychosomatics 47:312–319, 2006

Daly BJ, Newlon B, Montenegro HD, et al: Withdrawal of mechanical ventilation: ethical principles and guidelines for terminal weaning. Am J Crit Care 2:217–223, 1993

DeGuire S, Gevirtz R, Kawahara Y, et al: Hyperventilation syndrome and the assessment of treatment for functional cardiac symptoms. Am J Cardiol 70:673–677, 1992

DeGuire S, Gevirtz R, Hawkinson D, et al: Breathing retraining: a 3-year follow-up study of treatment for hyperventilation syndrome and associated functional cardiac symptoms. Biofeedback Self Regul 21:191–198, 1996

de Kleijn WP, De Vries J, Lower EE, et al: Fatigue in sarcoidosis: a systematic review. Curr Opin Pulm Med 15:499–506, 2009 de la Hoz RE, Shohet MR, Beinenfeld LA, et al: Vocal cord dysfunction in former World Trade Center (WTC) rescue and recovery workers and volunteers. Am J Ind Med 51:161–165, 2008

Delaney P: Neurologic manifestations in sarcoidosis: review of the literature, with a report of 23 cases. Ann Intern Med 87:336–345, 1977

Delelis G, Christophe V, Leroy S, et al: The effects of cystic fibrosis on couples: marital satisfaction, emotions, and coping strategies. Scand J Psychol 49:583–589, 2008

Demeter SL, Cordasco EM: Hyperventilation syndrome and asthma. Am J Med 81:989–994, 1986

De Peuter S, Lemaigre V, Van Diest I, et al: Illness-specific catastrophic thinking and overperception in asthma. Health Psychol 27:93–99, 2008

de Ruiter C, Garssen B, Rijken H, et al: The hyperventilation syndrome in panic disorder, agoraphobia and generalized anxiety disorder. Behav Res Ther 27:447–452, 1989

DeVane CL: Principles of pharmacokinetics and pharmacodynamics, in The American Psychiatric Press Textbook of Psychopharmacology, 2nd Edition. Edited by Schatzberg AF, Nemeroff CB. Washington, DC, American Psychiatric Press, 1998, pp 155–169

De Vries J, Drent M: Relationship between perceived stress and sarcoidosis in a Dutch patient population. Sarcoidosis Vasc Diffuse Lung Dis 21:57–63, 2004

De Vries J, Drent M: Quality of life and health status in sarcoidosis: a review of the literature. Clin Chest Med 29:525–532, 2008

De Vries J, Kessels BL, Drent M: Quality of life of idiopathic pulmonary fibrosis patients. Eur Respir J 17:954–961, 2001

Djibo A, Lawan A: Behavioral disorders after treatment with isoniazid [in French]. Bull Soc Pathol Exot 94:112–114, 2001

Drugs that may cause psychiatric symptoms. Med Lett Drugs Ther 50:100–103, 2008

Dudley DL, Sitzman J, Rugg M: Psychiatric aspects of patients with chronic obstructive pulmonary disease. Adv Psychosom Med 14:64–77, 1985

Duff A, Ball R, Wolfe S, et al: Betterland: an interactive CD-ROM guide for children with cystic fibrosis. Paediatr Nurs 18:30–33, 2006

Earles J, Kerr B, Kellar M: Psychophysiologic treatment of vocal cord dysfunction. Ann Allergy Asthma Immunol 90:669–671, 2003

Eisner MD, Katz PP, Lactao G, et al: Impact of depressive symptoms on adult asthma outcomes. Ann Allergy Asthma Immunol 94:566–574, 2005

Emery CF, Green MR, Suh S: Neuropsychiatric function in chronic lung disease: the role of pulmonary rehabilitation. Respir Care 53:1208–1216, 2008

Estenne M, Hertz MI: Bronchiolitis obliterans after human lung transplantation. Am J Respir Crit Care Med 166:440–444, 2002

Etienne B, Bertocchi M, Gamondes JP, et al: Successful double-lung transplantation for bronchioalveolar carcinoma. Chest 112:1423–1424, 1997

Ewig S, Torres A: Severe community-acquired pneumonia. Clin Chest Med 20:575–587, 1999

Faber-Langendoen K: The clinical management of dying patients receiving mechanical ventilation: a survey of physician practice. Chest 106:880–888, 1994

Fagan J, Galea S, Ahern J, et al: Relationship of self-reported asthma severity and urgent health care utilization to psychological sequelae of the September 11, 2001 terrorist attacks on the World Trade Center among New York City area residents. Psychosom Med 65:993–996, 2003

Faller H, Bulzebruck H: Coping and survival in lung cancer: a 10-year follow-up. Am J Psychiatry 159:2105–2107, 2002

Fan VS, Ramsey SD, Giardino ND, et al: Sex, depression, and risk of hospitalization and mortality in chronic obstructive pulmonary disease. Arch Intern Med 167:2345–2353, 2007

Fensterheim H, Wiegand B: Group treatment of the hyperventilation syndrome. Int J Group Psychother 41:399–403, 1991

Fischer AJ, Huygen PL, Folgering HT, et al: Vestibular hyperreactivity and hyperventilation after whiplash injury. J Neurol Sci 132:35–43, 1995

Fischer MJ, Scharloo M, Abbink JJ, et al: Drop-out and attendance in pulmonary rehabilitation: the role of clinical and psychosocial variables. Respir Med 103:1564–1571, 2009

Franke MF, Appleton SC, Bayona J, et al: Risk factors and mortality associated with default from multidrug-resistant tuberculosis treatment. Clin Infect Dis 46:1844–1851, 2008

Freedman MR, Rosenberg SJ, Schmaling KB: Childhood sexual abuse in patients with paradoxical vocal cord dysfunction. J Nerv Ment Dis 179:295–298, 1991

Funk GC, Kirchheiner K, Burghuber OC, et al: BODE index versus GOLD classification for explaining anxious and depressive symptoms in patients with COPD—a cross sectional study. Respir Res 10:1, 2009

Fusar-Poli P, Lazzaretti M, Ceruti M, et al: Depression after lung transplantation: causes and treatment. Lung 185:55–65, 2007

Giardino ND, Schmaling KB, Afari N: Relationship satisfaction moderates the association between catastrophic cognitions and asthma symptoms. J Asthma 39:749–756, 2002

Ginsburg ML, Quirt C, Ginsburg AD, et al: Psychiatric illness and psychosocial concerns of patients with newly diagnosed lung cancer. CMAJ 152:1961–1963, 1995

Glasscoe CA, Quittner AL: Psychological interventions for people with cystic fibrosis and their families. Cochrane Database Syst Rev (3):CD003148, 2008

Goetzmann L, Scheuer E, Naef R, et al: Psychosocial situation and physical health in 50 patients >1 year after lung transplantation. Chest 127:166–170, 2005

Goetzmann L, Klaghofer R, Wagner-Huber R, et al: Psychosocial need for counselling before and after a lung, liver or allogenic bone marrow transplant—results of a prospective study [in German]. Z Psychosom Med Psychother 52:230–242, 2006a

Goetzmann L, Klaghofer R, Wagner-Huber R, et al: Quality of life and psychosocial situation before and after a lung, liver or allogeneic bone marrow transplant. Swiss Med Wkly 136:281–290, 2006b

Goodell TT: Sexuality in chronic lung disease. Nurs Clin North Am 42:631–638, 2007

Goodwin RD, Jacobi F, Thefeld W: Mental disorders and asthma in the community. Arch Gen Psychiatry 60:1125–1130, 2003a

Goodwin RD, Pine DS, Hoven CW: Asthma and panic attacks among youth in the community. J Asthma 40:139–145, 2003b

Goracci A, Fagliolini A, Martinucci M, et al: Quality of life, anxiety and depression in sarcoidosis. Gen Hosp Psychiatry 30:441–445, 2008

Gralla RJ, Thatcher N: Quality of life assessment in advanced lung cancer: considerations for evaluation in patients receiving chemotherapy. Lung Cancer 46 (suppl 2):S41–S47, 2004

Greenberg DB, Halperin P, Kradin RL, et al: Internal medicine and medical subspecialties, in The American Psychiatric Press Textbook of Consultation-Liaison Psychiatry. Washington, DC, American Psychiatric Press, 1996, pp 565–566

Grenvik A: "Terminal weaning": discontinuance of life-support therapy in the terminally ill patient. Crit Care Med 11:394–395, 1983

Gudmundsson G, Gislason T, Janson C, et al: Risk factors for rehospitalisation in COPD: role of health status, anxiety and depression. Eur Respir J 26:414–419, 2005

Gudmundsson G, Gislason T, Janson C, et al: Depression, anxiety and health status after hospitalisation for COPD: a multicentre study in the Nordic countries. Respir Med 100:87–93, 2006

Güneyliolu D, Ozeker F, Bilgin S, et al: The influence of sarcoidosis on quality of life [in Turkish]. Tuberk Toraks 52:31–37, 2004

Hains AA, Davies WH, Behrens D, et al: Cognitive behavioral interventions for adolescents with cystic fibrosis. J Pediatr Psychol 22:669–687, 1997

Halimi L, Vachier I, Varrin M, et al: Interference of psychological factors in difficult-to-control asthma. Respir Med 101:154–161, 2007

Haloun A, Despins P: Lung and heart-lung transplantation in cystic fibrosis. Rev Pract 53:167–170, 2003

Havermans T, Colpaert K, Dupont LJ: Quality of life in patients with cystic fibrosis: association with anxiety and depression. J Cyst Fibros 7:581–584, 2008

Hayes CC, Savage E: Fathers' perspectives on the emotional impact of managing the care of their children with cystic fibrosis. J Pediatr Nurs 23:250–256, 2008

Hehrmann R: Hypocalcemic crisis: hypoparathyroidism—nonparathyroid origin—the most frequent form: hyperventilation syndrome [in German]. Fortschr Med 114:223–226, 1996

Henoch I, Bergman B, Gustafsson M, et al: Dyspnea experience in patients with lung cancer in palliative care. Eur J Oncol Nurs 12:86–96, 2008

Hesse C, Siedler H, Burhenne J, et al: Fluvoxamine affects sildenafil kinetics and dynamics. J Clin Psychopharmacol 25:589–592, 2005

Hicks M, Brugman SM, Katial R: Vocal cord dysfunction/paradoxical vocal fold motion. Prim Care 35:81–103, 2008

Hirokawa Y, Kondo T, Ohta Y, et al: Clinical characteristics and outcome of 508 patients with hyperventilation syndrome [in Japanese]. Nihon Kyobu Shikkan Gakkai Zasshi 33:940–946, 1995

Hoegholm A, Clementsen P, Mortensen SA: Syncope due to right atrial thromboembolism: diagnostic importance of two-dimensional echocardiography. Acta Cardiol 42:469–473, 1987

Hoes MJ, Colla P, Van Doorn P, et al: Hyperventilation and panic attacks. J Clin Psychiatry 48:435–437, 1987

Hoitsma E, DeVries J, van Santen-Hoeufft M, et al: Impact of pain in a Dutch sarcoidosis patient population. Sarcoidosis Vasc Diffuse Lung Dis 20:33–39, 2003

Holland A, Hill C: Physical training for interstitial lung disease. Cochrane Database Syst Rev (4):CD006322, 2008

Hook O: Sarcoidosis with involvement of the nervous system: report of nine cases. Arch Neurol Psychiatry 71:554–575, 1954

Hopwood P, Stephens RJ: Depression in patients with lung cancer: prevalence and risk factors derived from quality-of-life data. J Clin Oncol 18:893–903, 2000

Hosenpud JD, Bennett LE, Keck BM, et al: The Registry of the International Society for Heart and Lung Transplantation: fifteenth official report—1998. J Heart Lung Transplant 17:656–668, 1998

Hoshino K, Suzuki J, Yamauchi K, et al: Psychological stress evaluation of patients with bronchial asthma based on the chromogranin A level in saliva. J Asthma 45:596–599, 2008

Hung WW, Wisnivesky JP, Siu AL, et al: Cognitive decline among patients with chronic obstructive pulmonary disease. Am J Respir Crit Care Med 180:134–137, 2009

Husein OF, Husein TN, Gardner R, et al: Formal psychological testing in patients with paradoxical vocal fold dysfunction. Laryngoscope 118:740–747, 2008

Ibanez M, Aguilar JJ, Maderal MA, et al: Sexuality in chronic respiratory failure: coincidences and divergences between patients and primary caregiver. Respir Med 95:975–979, 2001

Ibrahim WH, Gheriani HA, Almohamed AA, et al: Paradoxical vocal cord motion disorder: past, present and future. Postgrad Med J 83:164–172, 2007

Irani S, Mahler C, Goetzmann L, et al: Lung transplant recipients holding companion animals: impact on physical health and quality of life. Am J Transplant 6:404–411, 2006

Isenberg SA, Lehrer PM, Hochron S: The effects of suggestion and emotional arousal on pulmonary function in asthma: a review and a hypothesis regarding vagal mediation. Psychosom Med 54:192–216, 1992

Jaffe A, Bush A: Cystic fibrosis: a review of the decade. Monaldi Arch Chest Dis 56:240–247, 2001

Jastrzebski D, Kozielski J, Zobrowska A: Pulmonary rehabilitation in patients with idiopathic pulmonary fibrosis with inspiratory muscle training [in Polish]. Pneumonol Alergol Pol 76:131–141, 2008

Jones IR, Ahmed N, Kelly M, et al: With an attack I associate it more with going into hospital: understandings of asthma and psychosocial stressors; are they related to use of services? Soc Sci Med 66:765–775, 2008

Jordan N, Lee TA, Valenstein M, et al: Effect of depression care on outcomes in COPD patients with depression. Chest 135:626–632, 2009

Kashiwagi H, Morimatsu Y, Kourogi H, et al: Two cases of bronchial asthma diagnosed as hyperventilation syndrome. Nihon Kokyuki Gakkai Zasshi 46:374–378, 2008

Katon W, Lozano P, Russo J, et al: The prevalence of DSM-IV anxiety and depressive disorders in youth with asthma compared with controls. J Adolesc Health 41:455–463, 2007

Kern-Buell CL, McGrady AV, Conran PB, et al: Asthma severity, psychophysiological indicators of arousal, and immune function in asthma patients undergoing biofeedback-assisted relaxation. Appl Psychophysiol Biofeedback 25:79–91, 2000

Kiev A, Domantay AG: A study of buspirone coprescribed with bronchodilators in 82 anxious ambulatory patients. J Asthma 25:281–284, 1988

Kirchhoff KT, Anumandla PR, Foth KT, et al: Documentation on withdrawal of life support in adult patients in the intensive care unit. Am J Crit Care 13:328–334, 2004

Köllner V, Einsle F, Schade I, et al: The influence of anxiety, depression and post traumatic stress disorder on quality of life after thoracic organ transplantation [in German]. Z Psychosom Med Psychother 49:262–274, 2003

Koufman JA, Block C: Differential diagnosis of paradoxical vocal fold movement. Am J Speech Lang Pathol 17:327–334, 2008

Kramer MR, Marshall SE, Starnes VA, et al: Infectious complications in heart-lung transplantation: analysis in 200 episodes. Arch Intern Med 153:2010–2016, 1993

Krishnan V, McCormack MC, Mathia SC, et al: Sleep quality and health related quality of life in idiopathic pulmonary fibrosis. Chest 134:693–698, 2008

Kunik ME, Veazey C, Cully JA, et al: COPD education and cognitive behavioral therapy group treatment for clinically significant symptoms of depression and anxiety in COPD patients: a randomized controlled trial. Psychol Med 38:385–396, 2008

Künsebeck HW, Kugler C, Fischer S, et al: Quality of life and bronchiolitis obliterans syndrome in patients after lung transplantation. Prog Transplant 17:136–141, 2007

Lacasse Y, Brosseau L, Milne S, et al: Pulmonary rehabilitation for chronic obstructive pulmonary disease. Cochrane Database Syst Rev (3):CD003793, 2002

Lachman A, Gielis O, Thys P, et al: Hyperventilation syndrome: current advances. Rev Mal Respir 9:277–285, 1992

Lacy TJ, McManis SE: Psychogenic stridor. Gen Hosp Psychiatry 16:213–223, 1994

Lamers F, Jonkers CC, Bosma H, et al: Summed score of the Patient Health Questionnaire-9 was a reliable and valid method for depression screening in chronically ill elderly patients. J Clin Epidemiol 61:679–687, 2008

Lander M, Cronquist A, Janson C, et al: Health-related quality of life predicts onset of asthma in a longitudinal population study. Respir Med 103:194–200, 2009

Lasky JA, Brody AR: Interstitial fibrosis and growth factors. Environ Health Perspect 108 (suppl 4):751–762, 2000

Laurin C, Lavoie KL, Bacon SL, et al: Sex differences in the prevalence of psychiatric disorders and psychological distress in patients with COPD. Chest 132:148–155, 2007

Lehrer PM, Hochron SM, McCann B, et al: Relaxation decreases large-airway but not small-airway asthma. J Psychosom Res 30:13–25, 1986

Lehrer P, Feldman J, Giardino N, et al: Psychological aspects of asthma. J Consult Clin Psychol 70:691–711, 2002

Lehrer PM, Karavidas MK, Lu SE, et al: Psychological treatment of comorbid asthma and panic disorder: a pilot study. J Anxiety Disord 22:671–683, 2008

LeSon S, Gershwin ME: Risk factors for asthmatic patients requiring intubation. J Asthma 33:27–35, 1996

Lewis KE, Annandale JA, Sykes RN, et al: Prevalence of anxiety and depression in patients with severe COPD: similar high levels with and without LTOT. COPD 4:305–312, 2007

Lheureux M, Raherison C, Vernejoux JM, et al: Quality of life in lung cancer: does disclosure of the diagnosis have an impact? Lung Cancer 43:175–182, 2004

Liang WM, Chen JJ, Chan CH, et al: An empirical comparison of the WHOQOL-BREF and the SGRQ among patients with COPD. Qual Life Res 17:793–800, 2008

Liippo K, Puolijoki H, Tala E: Periodic breathing imitating hyperventilation syndrome. Chest 102:638–639, 1992

Limbos MM, Joyce DP, Chan CK, et al: Psychological functioning and quality of life in lung transplant candidates and recipients. Chest 118:408–416, 2000

Lishman WA: Organic Psychiatry. London, England, Blackwell, 1987

Livermore N, Butler JE, Sharpe L, et al: Panic attacks and perception of inspiratory resistive loads in chronic obstructive pulmonary disease. Am J Respir Crit Care Med 178:7–12, 2008

Llewellyn K: CF and me: interview by Anna Sidey. Paediatr Nurs 10:21–22, 1998

Macdonald K: Living in limbo—patients with cystic fibrosis waiting for transplant. Br J Nurs 15:566–572, 2006

Manalai P, Woo JM, Postolache TT: Suicidality and montelukast. Expert Opin Drug Saf 8:273–282, 2009

Mancuso CA, Peterson MG, Charlson ME: Effects of depressive symptoms on health-related quality of life in asthma patients. J Gen Intern Med 15:301–310, 2000

Mancuso CA, Westermann H, Choi TN, et al: Psychological and somatic symptoms in screening for depression in asthma patients. J Asthma 45:221–225, 2008

Marin TJ, Chen E, Munch JA, et al: Double-exposure to acute stress and chronic family stress is associated with immune changes in children with asthma. Psychosom Med 71:378–384, 2009

Marsac ML, Funk JB, Nelson L: Coping styles, psychological functioning and quality of life in children with asthma. Child Care Health Dev 33:360–367, 2007

Martinez TY, Pereira CA, Dos Santos ML, et al: Evaluation of the short-form 36-item questionnaire to measure health-related quality of life in patients with idiopathic pulmonary fibrosis. Chest 117:1627–1632, 2000

Mathews WB: Sarcoidosis of the nervous system. J Neurol Neurosurg Psychiatry 28:23–29, 1965

Maurer J, Rebbapragada V, Borson S, et al: Anxiety and depression in COPD: current understanding, unanswered questions, and research needs. Chest 134 (4 suppl):43S–56S, 2008

McGann EF, Sexton D, Chyun DA: Denial and compliance in adults with asthma. Clin Nurs Res 17:151–170, 2008

Mendelson WB, Maczaj M, Holt J: Buspirone administration to sleep apnea patients. J Clin Psychopharmacol 11:71–72, 1991

Mermigkis C, Stagaki E, Amfilochiou A, et al: Sleep quality and associated daytime consequences in patients with idiopathic pulmonary fibrosis. Med Princ Pract 18:10–15, 2009

Michielsen HJ, Peros-Golubicic T, Drent M, et al: Relationship between symptoms and quality of life in sarcoidosis. Respiration 74:401–405, 2007

Miles JF, Garden GM, Tunnicliffe WS, et al: Psychological morbidity and coping skills in patients with brittle and non-brittle asthma: a case-control study. Clin Exp Allergy 27:1151–1159, 1997

Miller BD, Wood BL, Lim J, et al: Depressed children with asthma evidence increased airway resistance: "vagal bias" as a mechanism? J Allergy Clin Immunol 124:66–73, 2009

Miller GE, Chen E: Life stress and diminished expression of genes encoding glucocorticoid receptor and beta-2-adrenergic receptor in children with asthma. Proc Natl Acad Sci U S A 103:5496–5501, 2006

Miller GE, Gaudin A, Zysk E, et al: Parental support and cytokine activity in childhood asthma: the role of glucocorticoid sensitivity. J Allergy Clin Immunol 123:824–830, 2009

Mino M, Narita N, Ikeda H: A case of a pituitary mass in association with sarcoidosis. No To Shinkei 52:253–257, 2000

Misono S, Weiss NS, Fann JR, et al: Incidence of suicide in persons with cancer. J Clin Oncol 26:4731–4738, 2008

Mizukami K, Naito Y, Yoshida M, et al: Mental disorders induced by carbamazepine. Jpn J Psychiatry Neurol 44:59–63, 1990

Mohan A, Mohan C, Bhutani M, et al: Quality of life in newly diagnosed patients with lung cancer in a developing country: is it important? Eur J Cancer Care 15:293–298, 2006

Munro S, Lewin S, Swart T, et al: A review of health behaviour theories: how useful are these for developing interventions to promote long-term medication adherence for TB and HIV/AIDS? BMC Public Health 7:104, 2007

Myaskovsky L, Dew MA, Switzer GE, et al: Avoidant coping with health problems is related to poorer quality of life among lung transplant candidates. Prog Transplant 13:183–192, 2003

Nacci A, Fattori B, Ursino F, et al: Paradoxical vocal cord dysfunction: clinical experience and personal considerations. Acta Otorhinolaryngol Ital 27:248–254, 2007

Najafizadeh K, Ghorbani F, Rostami A, et al: Depression while on the lung transplantation waiting list. Ann Transplant 14:34–37, 2009

Nakaya N, Saito-Nakaya K, Akechi T, et al: Negative psychological aspects and survival in lung cancer patients. Psychooncology 17:466–473, 2008

Napolitano MA, Babyak MA, Palmer S, et al: Effects of a telephone-based psychosocial intervention for patients awaiting lung transplantation. Chest 122:1176–1184, 2002

National Center for Health Statistics: Vital and Health Statistics: Current Estimates From the National Health Interview Survey. U.S. Department of Health and Human Services, 1990–1993. Natl Vital Stat Rep 48(11):1–108, 2000

Newman KB, Mason UG 3rd, Schmaling KB: Clinical features of vocal cord dysfunction. Am J Respir Crit Care Med 152 (4 pt 1): 1382–1386, 1995

Newsham KR, Klaben BK, Miller VJ, et al: Paradoxical vocal-cord dysfunction: management in athletes. J Athl Train 37:325–328, 2002

Ng SM, Li AM, Lou VW, et al: Incorporating family therapy into asthma group intervention: a randomized waitlist-controlled trial. Fam Process 47:115–130, 2008

Ng TP, Niti M, Fones C, et al: Comorbid association of depression and COPD: a population-based study. Respir Med 103:895–901, 2009

Nguyen VQ, Byrd RP Jr, Fields CL, et al: DaCosta's syndrome: chronic symptomatic hyperventilation. J Ky Med Assoc 90:331–334, 1992

Ochoa LL, Richardson GW: The current status of lung transplantation: a nursing perspective. AACN Clin Issues 10:229–239, 1999

O'Dowd MA, Jaramillo J, Dubler N, et al: A noncompliant patient with fluctuating capacity. Gen Hosp Psychiatry 20:317–324, 1998

Omachi TA, Katz PP, Yelin EH, et al: Depression and health-related quality of life in chronic obstructive pulmonary disease. Am J Med 122:778.e9–e15, 2009

Oscherwitz T, Tulsky JP, Roger S, et al: Detention of persistently nonadherent patients with tuberculosis. JAMA 278:843–846, 1997

Ozge C, Ozge A, Unal O: Cognitive and functional deterioration in patients with severe COPD. Behav Neurol 17:121–130, 2006

Palermo TM, Harrison D, Koh JL: Effect of disease-related pain on the health-related quality of life of children and adolescents with cystic fibrosis. Clin J Pain 22:532–537, 2006

Paradowski LJ: Saprophytic fungal infections and lung transplantation revisited. J Heart Lung Transplant 16:524–531, 1997

Parekh PI, Blumenthal JA, Babyak MA, et al: Psychiatric disorder and quality of life in patients awaiting lung transplantation. Chest 124:1682–1688, 2003

Parekh PI, Blumenthal JA, Babyak MA, et al: Gas exchange and exercise capacity affect neurocognitive performance in patients with lung disease. Psychosom Med 67:425–432, 2005

Paris WP, Diercks M, Bright J, et al: Return to work after lung transplantation. J Heart Lung Transplant 17:430–436, 1998

Paulley JW: Hyperventilation. Recenti Prog Med 81:594–600, 1990

Pearman T: Psychosocial factors in lung cancer: quality of life, economic impact, and survivorship implications. J Psychosoc Oncol 26:69–80, 2008

Perkner JJ, Fennelly KP, Balkissoon R, et al: Irritant-associated vocal cord dysfunction. J Occup Environ Med 40:136–143, 1998

Peters SG, Wochos DN, Peterson GC: Status epilepticus as a complication of concurrent electroconvulsive and theophylline therapy. Mayo Clin Proc 59:568–570, 1984

Pinney S, Freeman LJ, Nixon PG: Role of the nurse counselor in managing patients with the hyperventilation syndrome. J R Soc Med 80:216–218, 1987

Potoczek A, Nizankowska-Mogilnicka E, Bochenek G, et al: Links between panic disorder, depression, defence mechanisms, coherence and family functioning in patients suffering from severe COPD [in Polish]. Psychiatr Pol 42:731–748, 2008

Puhan M, Scharplatz M, Troosters T, et al: Pulmonary rehabilitation following exacerbations of chronic obstructive pulmonary disease. Cochrane Database Syst Rev (1):CD005305, 2009

Put C, Van den Bergh O, Demedts M, et al: A study of the relationship among self-reported noncompliance, symptomatology, and psychological variables in patients with asthma. J Asthma 37:503–510, 2000

Quittner AL, Barker DH, Snell C, et al: Prevalence and impact of depression in cystic fibrosis. Curr Opin Pulm Med 14:582–588, 2008

Richardson LP, Russo JE, Lozano P, et al: The effect of comorbid anxiety and depressive disorders on health care utilization and costs among adolescents with asthma. Gen Hosp Psychiatry 30:398–406, 2008

Ritz T, Steptoe A, DeWilde S, et al: Emotions and stress increased respiratory resistance in asthma. Psychosom Med 62:402–412, 2000

Rodrigue JR, Baz MA, Widows MR, et al: A randomized evaluation of quality-of-life therapy with patients awaiting lung transplantation. Am J Transplant 5:2425–2432, 2005

Rognum TO, Olaisen B, Teige B: Hyperventilation syndrome: could acute salicylic acid poisoning be the cause? [in Norwegian]. Tidsskr Nor Laegforen 107:1043, 1050, 1987

Rose C, Wallace L, Dickson R, et al: The most effective psychologically based treatments to reduce anxiety and panic in patients with chronic obstructive pulmonary disease (COPD): a systematic review. Patient Educ Couns 47:311–318, 2002

Rosenkranz MA, Davidson RJ: Affective neural circuitry and mind-body influences in asthma. Neuroimage 47:972–980, 2009

Saarijarvi S, Lehtinen P: The hyperventilation syndrome treated with antidepressive agents. Duodecim 103:417–420, 1987

Sabaawi M, Gutierrez-Nunez J, Fragala MR: Neurosarcoidosis presenting as schizophreniform disorder. Int J Psychiatry Med 22:269–274, 1992

Schmaling KB, Niloofar A, Barnhart S, et al: Medical and psychiatric predictors of airway reactivity. Respir Care 44:1452–1457, 1999

Schmitz N, Wang J, Malla A, et al: The impact of psychological distress on functional disability in asthma: results from the Canadian community health survey. Psychosomatics 50:42–49, 2009

Schneider A, Löwe B, Meyer FJ, et al: Depression and panic disorder as predictors of health outcomes for patients with asthma in primary care. Respir Med 102:359–366, 2008

Schnoll RA, Malstrom M, James C, et al: Correlates of tobacco use among smokers and recent quitters diagnosed with cancer. Patient Educ Couns 46:137–145, 2002

Scialdone AM: Thalamic hemorrhage imitating hyperventilation. Ann Emerg Med 19:817–819, 1990

Scott KM, Von Korff M, Alonso J, et al: Childhood adversity, early-onset depressive/anxiety disorders, and adult-onset asthma. Psychosom Med 70:1035–1043, 2008

Serrano J, Plaxa V, Sureda B, et al: Alexithymia: a relevant psychological variable in near-fatal asthma. Eur Respir J 28:296–302, 2006

Sharf BF, Stelljes LA, Gordon HS: "A little bitty spot and I'm a big man": patients' perspectives on refusing diagnosis or treatment for lung cancer. Psychooncology 14:636–646, 2005

Sharma OP: Sarcoidosis: A Clinical Approach. Springfield, IL, Charles C Thomas, 1975

Silverstein A, Feuer M, Siltzback L: Neurologic sarcoidosis. Arch Neurol 12:1–11, 1965

Skorodin MS, King F, Sharp JT: Carbon monoxide poisoning presenting as hyperventilation syndrome. Ann Intern Med 105:631–632, 1986

Small SP, Graydon JE: Perceived uncertainty, physical symptoms, and negative mood in hospitalized patients with chronic obstructive pulmonary disease. Heart Lung 21:568–574, 1992

Smith A, Krishnan JA, Bilderback A, et al: Depressive symptoms and adherence to asthma therapy after hospital discharge. Chest 30:1034–1038, 2006

Smoller JW, Pollack MH, Systrom D, et al: Sertraline effects on dyspnea in patients with obstructive airways disease. Psychosomatics 39:24–29, 1998

Snell G, deHoyos A, Krajden M, et al: Pseudomonas capacia in lung transplantation recipients with cystic fibrosis. Chest 103:466–471, 1993

Stage KB, Middelboe T, Pisinger C: Depression and chronic obstructive pulmonary disease (COPD): impact on survival. Acta Psychiatr Scand 111:320–323, 2005

Stone P, Richards M, A'Hern R, et al: A study to investigate the prevalence, severity and correlates of fatigue among patients with cancer in comparison with a control group of volunteers without cancer. Ann Oncol 11:561–567, 2000

Stoudemire A, Linfors E, Houpt JL, et al: Central nervous system sarcoidosis. Gen Hosp Psychiatry 5:129–132, 1983

Strauss GM: Bronchogenic carcinoma, in Textbook of Pulmonary Disease, 6th Edition. Edited by Baum GL, Grapo JD, Celli BR. Philadelphia, PA, Lippincott-Raven, 1998, pp 1329–1381

Strine TW, Mokdad AH, Balluz LS, et al: Impact of depression and anxiety on quality of life, health behaviors, and asthma control among adults in the United States with asthma, 2006. J Asthma 45:123–133, 2008

Sturdy PM, Victor CR, Anderson HR, et al: Psychological, social and health behaviour risk factors for deaths certified as asthma: a national case-control study. Thorax 57:1034–1039, 2002

Subramanian SV, Ackerson LK, Subramanyam MA, et al: Domestic violence is associated with adult and childhood asthma prevalence in India. Int J Epidemiol 36:569–579, 2007

Suchenwirth R, Dold V: Functional psychoses in sarcoidosis. Verh Dtsch Ges Inn Med 75:757–759, 1969

Swigris JJ, Stewart AL, Gould MK, et al: Patients' perspectives on how idiopathic pulmonary fibrosis affects the quality of their lives. Health Qual Life Outcomes 3:61, 2005

Swigris JJ, Brown KK, Make BJ, et al: Pulmonary rehabilitation in idiopathic pulmonary fibrosis: a call for continued investigation. Repir Med 102:1675–1680, 2008

Sylla L, Bruce RD, Kamarulzaman A, et al: Integration and co-location of HIV/AIDS, tuberculosis and drug treatment services. Int J Drug Policy 18:306–312, 2007

Szyndler JE, Towns SJ, van Asperen PP, et al: Psychological and family functioning and quality of life in adolescents with cystic fibrosis. J Cyst Fibros 4:135–144, 2005

Takatsuki K, Kado T, Satouchi M, et al: Psychiatric studies of chemotherapy and chemotherapy-induced nausea and vomiting of patients with lung or thymic cancer. Gan To Kagaku Ryoho 25:403–408, 1998

Tashkin D, Kanner R, Bailey W, et al: Smoking cessation in patients with chronic obstructive pulmonary disease: a double-blind, placebo-controlled, randomised trial. Lancet 357:1571–1575, 2001

Taylor JL, Smith PJ, Babyak MA, et al: Coping and quality of life in patients waiting lung transplantation. J Psychosom Res 65:71–79, 2008

Tegtbur U, Sievers C, Busse MW, et al: Quality of life and exercise capacity in lung transplant recipients [in German]. Pneumologie 58:72–78, 2004

Teichman BJ, Burker EJ, Weiner M, et al: Factors associated with adherence to treatment regimens after lung transplantation. Prog Transplant 10:113–121, 2000

ten Brinke A, Ouwerkerk ME, Zwinderman AH, et al: Psychopathology in patients with severe asthma is associated with increased health utilization. Am J Respir Crit Care Med 163:1093–1096, 2001

ten Thoren C, Petermann F: Reviewing asthma and anxiety. Respir Med 94:409–415, 2000

Thomas PS, Geddes DM, Barnes PJ: Pseudo-steroid resistant asthma. Thorax 54:352–356, 1999

Thompson C, Checkley S: Short term memory deficit in a patient with cerebral sarcoidosis. Br J Psychiatry 139:160–161, 1981

Tishelman C, Degner LF, Rudman A, et al: Symptoms in patients with lung carcinoma: distinguishing distress from intensity. Cancer 104:2013–2021, 2005

Törün T, Güngör G, Ozmen I, et al: Side effects associated with the treatment of multidrug-resistant tuberculosis. Int J Tuberc Lung Dis 9:1373–1377, 2005

Treasure RA, Fowler PB, Millington HT, et al: Misdiagnosis of diabetic ketoacidosis as hyperventilation syndrome. BMJ (Clin Res Ed) 294:630, 1987

Tsavaris N, Kosmas C, Kopterides P, et al: Efficacy of tropisetron in patients with advanced non-small-cell lung cancer receiving adjuvant chemotherapy with carboplatin and taxanes. Eur J Cancer Care 17:167–173, 2008

Turyk ME, Hernandez E, Wright RJ, et al: Stressful life events and asthma in adolescents. Pediatr Allergy Immunol 19:255–263, 2008

United Network for Organ Sharing: 2008 Annual Report of the U.S. Organ Procurement and Transplantation Network and the Scientific Registry of Transplant Recipients: Transplant Data 1998–2007. Rockville, MD, U.S. Department of Health and Human Services, Health Resources and Services Administration, Healthcare Systems Bureau, Division of Transplantation, 2008. Available at: http://www.ustransplant.org/annual_reports/current/default.htm. Accessed November 27, 2009.

Van De Ven LL, Mouthan BJ, Hoes MJ: Treatment of the hyperventilation syndrome with bisoprodol: a placebo-controlled clinical trial. J Psychosom Res 39:1007–1013, 1995

Van De Ven MO, Engels RC, Sawyer SM: Asthma-specific predictors of smoking onset in adolescents with asthma: a longitudinal study. J Pediatr Psychol 34:118–128, 2009

van den Bemt L, Schermer T, Bor H, et al: The risk for depression comorbidity in patients with COPD. Chest 135:108–114, 2009

Van Lieshout RJ, Bienenstock J, MacQueen GM: A review of candidate pathways underlying association between asthma and major depressive disorder. Psychosom Med 71:187–195, 2009

Vega P, Sweetland A, Acha J, et al: Psychiatric issues in the management of patients with multidrug-resistant tuberculosis. Int J Tuberc Lung Dis 8:749–759, 2004

Vermeulen KM, Ouwens JP, van der Bij W, et al: Long-term quality of life in patients surviving at least 55 months after lung transplantation. Gen Hosp Psychiatry 25:95–102, 2003

Vermeulen KM, Bosma OH, Bij W, et al: Stress, psychological distress, and coping in patients on the waiting list for lung transplantation: an exploratory study. Transpl Int 18:954–959, 2005

Visser MR, van Lanschot JJ, van der Velden J, et al: Quality of life in newly diagnosed cancer patients waiting for surgery is seriously impaired. J Surg Oncol 93:571–577, 2006

Von Roenn JH, Paice JA: Control of common, non-pain cancer symptoms. Semin Oncol 32:200–210, 2005

Vos MS, Putter H, van Houwelingen HC, et al: Denial in lung cancer patients: a longitudinal study. Psychooncology 17:1163–1171, 2008

Walker MS, Larsen RJ, Zona DM, et al: Smoking urges and relapse among lung cancer patients: findings from a preliminary retrospective study. Prev Med 39:449–457, 2004

Wallerstedt SM, Brunlöf G, Sundström A, et al: Montelukast and psychiatric disorders in children. Pharmacoepidemiol Drug Saf 18:858–864, 2009

Ward C, Massie J, Glazner J, et al: Problem behaviours and parenting in preschool children with cystic fibrosis. Arch Dis Child 94:341–347, 2009

Wargnies E, Houze L, Vanneste J, et al: Depression, anxiety and coping strategies in adult patients with cystic fibrosis. Rev Mal Respir 19:39–43, 2002

Weiss ST: The origins of childhood asthma. Monaldi Arch Chest Dis 49:154–158, 1994

White T, Miller J, Smith GL, et al: Adherence and psychopathology in children and adolescents with cystic fibrosis. Eur Child Adolesc Psychiatry 18:96–104, 2009

Whitney KA, Lysaker PH, Steiner AR, et al: Is "chemobrain" a transient state? A prospective pilot study among persons with non-small cell lung cancer. J Support Oncol 6:313–321, 2008

Widerman E: The experience of receiving a diagnosis of cystic fibrosis after age 20: implications for social work. Soc Work Health Care 39:415–433, 2004

Wilkinson OM, Duncan-Skingle F, Pryor JA, et al: A feasibility study of home telemedicine for patients with cystic fibrosis awaiting transplantation. J Telemed Telecare 14:182–185, 2008

Wilson WC, Smedira NG, Fink C, et al: Ordering and administration of sedatives and analgesics during the withholding and withdrawal of life support from critically ill patients. JAMA 267:949–953, 1992

Withers NJ, Rudkin ST, White RJ: Anxiety and depression in severe chronic obstructive pulmonary disease: the effects of pulmonary rehabilitation. J Cardiopulm Rehabil 19:362–365, 1999

Wolf JM, Nicholis E, Chen E: Chronic stress, salivary control, and alpha-amylase in children with asthma and healthy children. Biol Psychol 78:20–28, 2008b

Wong WS, Fielding R: Quality of life and pain in Chinese lung cancer patients: is optimism a moderator or mediator? Qual Life Res 16:53–63, 2007

World Health Organization: Global Tuberculosis Control—Surveillance, Planning, Financing. WHO/HTM/TB/2008.393. Geneva, Switzerland, World Health Organization, 2008. Available at: http://www.who.int/tb/publications/global_report/2008/en/index.html. Accessed September 11, 2009.

Wurtemberger G, Hutter BO: The significance of health related quality of life for the evaluation of interventional measures in patients with COPD. Pneumologie 55:91–99, 2001

Xu W, Collet JP, Shapiro S, et al: Independent effect of depression and anxiety on chronic obstructive pulmonary disease exacerbations and hospitalizations. Am J Respir Crit Care Med 178:913–920, 2008

Yamada Y, Tatsumi K, Yamaguchi T, et al: Influence of stressful life events on the onset of sarcoidosis. Respirology 8:186–191, 2003

Yeager H, Rossman MD, Baughman RP, et al: Pulmonary and psychosocial findings at enrollment in the ACCESS study. Sarcoidosis Vasc Diffuse Lung Dis 22:147–153, 2005

Yohannes AM, Baldwin RC, Connolly MJ: Depression and anxiety in elderly outpatients with chronic obstructive pulmonary disease: prevalence, and validation of the BASDEC screening questionnaire. Int J Geriatr Psychiatry 15:1090–1096, 2000

Yorke J, Shuldham C: Family therapy for chronic asthma in children. Cochrane Database Syst Rev (2):CD000089, 2005

Yorke J, Fleming SL, Shuldham CM: Psychological interventions for adults with asthma. Cochrane Database Syst Rev (1): CD002982, 2006a

Zerman W: Die Meningoencephalitis. Nervenarzt 23:43–52, 1952

Zhang AY, Siminoff LA: Silence and cancer: why do families and patients fail to communicate? Health Commun 15:415–429, 2003

CHAPTER

20

Gastrointestinal Disorders

Catherine C. Crone, M.D.

Christopher R. Dobbelstein, M.D.

GASTROINTESTINAL (GI) DISORDERS cover a wide range of illnesses that span from mouth to anus and include the liver, pancreas, and gallbladder. Some disorders are uncommon, whereas others such as gastroesophageal reflux disorder (GERD), peptic ulcer, and irritable bowel syndrome (IBS) are common. Physical and psychological distress caused by GI disorders results in high rates of health care use, billions of dollars in annual health care costs, lost productivity, and reduced quality of life (QOL). Additionally, an interrelation between the brain and the gut adds to the complexity of care for many of these patients. Psychiatrists often encounter patients with concurrent GI disorders, and their presence may need to be factored into clinical evaluation and subsequent care plans. In this chapter, which is organized according to organ or GI region, we cover several GI disorders, both structural and functional in origin.

Functional Gastrointestinal Disorders

Patients often present to health care providers with various forms of GI distress that are found to lack specific structural or physiological etiologies. These represent *functional GI disorders,* a broad spectrum of symptom-defined diagnoses (e.g., globus, functional heartburn, functional dyspepsia, cyclic vomiting syndrome) with pathophysiology that is still not fully understood (Drossman 2006). A complex connection exists between the brain and the gut, with bidirectional communication pathways that involve the autonomic nervous system and the hypothalamic-pituitary-adrenal (HPA) axis. Disruptions along these pathways can result in functional GI problems.

The existence of the brain–gut axis is also thought to help explain how psychosocial factors, personality styles, and comorbid psychiatric disorders can influence the onset and course of various functional GI disorders, such as IBS, functional dyspepsia, and functional nausea and vomiting. Among patients with functional GI disorders, premorbid histories of traumatic events, particularly sexual and physical abuse, are often present. Neuroticism, hostility, maladaptive coping, and emotional hypersensitivity are personality traits that are commonly observed. Comorbid psychiatric syndromes, particularly depression, anxiety, and somatization, are also frequently noted.

Psychotropic medications and psychotherapy have had a role in the treatment of many functional GI disorders, although their mechanism of action is not truly known. For example, antidepressants can provide analgesic and autonomic effects in addition to their anxiolytic and antidepressant activities.

Because of the need for consistency in diagnosis of functional GI disorders, the Rome Criteria were developed and refined through an iterative consensus process. The most recent—Rome III Criteria—involved the work of clinicians and researchers from 18 countries around the world (Drossman 2006).

Oropharyngeal Disorders

Rumination Syndrome

Rumination syndrome involves repeated and effortless regurgitation of small amounts of food from the stomach, which are subsequently rechewed, reswallowed, or expelled (Papadopoulos and Mimidis 2007). This behavior is common among infants and developmentally disabled individuals but also can appear in children and adults of normal intelligence (Olden 2001). The problem is often mistaken for bulimia, GERD, or upper GI motility disorders, such as gastroparesis (Papadopoulos and Mimidis 2007). Nausea, heartburn, abdominal discomfort, weight loss, and bowel changes often accompany rumination syndrome. Limited case series suggest that comorbid psychiatric disorders, including bulimia nervosa, may be present in up to 20%–30% of patients (Malcolm et al. 1997; Olden 2001). Rumination also can develop following a stressful life event (Attri et al. 2008). Adults primarily seek out care because of societal discomfort with their behavior. Diagnosis is made by clinical assessment rather than invasive testing. Treatment centers on behavior therapy, including habit reversal, biofeedback, and relaxation techniques (Attri et al. 2008).

Burning Mouth Syndrome

Burning mouth syndrome is a chronic pain condition characterized by a persistent oral burning sensation without accompanying evidence of mucosal disturbance (Sardella 2007; Scala et al. 2003). Symptoms typically persist throughout the day, intensify late in the day, and may be relieved by eating or drinking. Xerostomia and dysgeusia often accompany the syndrome (Scala et al. 2003). Personal stressors, fatigue, or acidic foods worsen the burning sensation for most patients. The syndrome mainly affects middle-aged to elderly women, and the prevalence in the United States is estimated to be 0.7%–1.7% (Klasser et al. 2008). Onset of symptoms is usually spontaneous, although up to a third of patients may attribute onset to illness, medications, or dental procedures (Grushka et al. 2002; Klasser et al. 2008). Potential triggering medications include angiotensin-converting enzyme (ACE) inhibitors, angiotensin II receptor antagonists, antiretroviral agents, hormone replacement therapy, sertraline, fluoxetine, venlafaxine, and clonazepam (Levenson 2003; Salort Lorca et al. 2008). The underlying mechanism behind the syndrome is unknown, but some evidence suggests a neuropathic origin (Sardella 2007; Scala et al. 2003). Comorbid psychiatric disorders, including anxiety, depression, and hypochondriasis, have been identified in 40%–60% of patients, although it is unclear whether these are secondary to the condition itself (Bogetto et al. 1998). Clinical trials, most of which were small but some of which were placebo-controlled, reported partial or full remission of symptoms with oral or topical clonazepam, oral or topical capsaicin, amisulpride, paroxetine, sertraline, alpha-lipoic acid, and cognitive therapy (Bergdhal et al. 1995; Femiano and Scully 2002; Gremeau-Richard et al. 2004; Grushka et al. 1998; Maina et al. 2002; Mínguez Serra et al. 2007; Yamazaki et al. 2009; Zakrzewska et al. 2005). Recent case reports also noted success with olanzapine and electroconvulsive therapy (Sudas et al. 2008; Ueda et al. 2008).

Xerostomia

Xerostomia is a subjective complaint of dry mouth that may be associated with reduced saliva production. Among sampled populations, xerostomia has been found to be present in up to 30%; its presence predisposes patients to dental caries and oropharyngeal *Candida albicans* infections (Guggenheimer and Moore 2003). Adequate saliva production is needed to facilitate taste, speech, and swallowing. Patients with xerostomia may report accompanying difficulties with altered taste, dysgeusia, or dysphagia (Friedlander and Mahler 2001). Common causes include medications, autoimmune disorders (e.g., Sjögren's syndrome), radiation therapy, anxiety, depression, and other medical conditions (e.g., diabetes, HIV) (Guggenheimer and Moore 2003). Psychotropic medications (especially anticholinergic drugs) are often linked to xerostomia; included in this group are all antidepressants, benzodiazepines, typical and atypical antipsychotics, carbamazepine, and lithium (Clark 2003; Friedlander et al. 2004; Guggenheimer and Moore 2003). Interventions include medication change, avoidance of caffeine and alcohol, sips of water, ice chips, sugarless gum or candy, saliva substitutes, acupuncture, and cholinergic agents (e.g., pilocarpine, bethanechol) (Masters 2005; Schatzberg et al. 2007).

Dysphagia

Successful swallowing of liquids or foodstuffs requires a coordinated sequence of voluntary and involuntary neuromuscular contractions that moves a bolus from mouth to pharynx, to the esophagus, and finally to the stomach. Circumstances that interfere with this series of movements lead to dysphagia, which is estimated to affect 7%–10% of adults older than 50 years, with higher rates in hospitalized and nursing home patients (Spieker 2000). Dysphagia contributes to significant morbidity and mortality by causing malnutrition, esophageal rupture, aspiration, and aspiration pneumonia (Spieker 2000). Neurological disorders (i.e., cerebrovascular accident, multiple sclerosis, myasthenia gravis, Parkinson's disease) commonly cause dysphagia (Lind 2003). Medications also contribute to dysphagia by producing xerostomia, sedation, pharyngeal weakness, dystonia, or reflux (Palmer et al. 2000). Several patients have reported dysphagia from antipsychotic-induced dystonia, parkinsonism, and tardive dyskinesia (Dziewas et al. 2007; Nieves et al. 2007). With some, the dysphagia was the only sign of an underlying movement disorder (O'Neil and Remington 2003). Acute dystonia responds to intravenous diphenhydramine or benztropine, whereas dysphagia from drug-induced parkinsonism does not (Dziewas et al. 2007;

Garlow et al. 2006; O'Neil and Remington 2003). Rather, treatment requires discontinuing medication, lowering the dose, or switching to another agent (Dziewas et al. 2007). Tardive dyskinesia is also managed through these steps, but clonazepam is another option (Nieves et al. 2007; O'Neil and Remington 2003). Rarely, dysphagia is a manifestation of neuroleptic malignant syndrome or serotonin syndrome (Passmore et al. 2004; Shamash et al. 1994).

Globus Hystericus

Globus is the sensation of having a lump or mass in the throat that does not interfere with actual swallowing. Globus pharyngeus or hystericus represents a common benign disorder responsible for 4% of ear, nose, and throat referrals (Caylakli et al. 2006). Its course is variable, with most patients improving over time. The etiology of globus is unknown and may be multifactorial; various causes have been proposed, including cricopharyngeal spasm, lingual tonsil hypertrophy, thyroid nodules, cervical osteophytes, iron deficiency anemia, GERD, anxiety, and depression (Caylakli et al. 2006; Finkenbine and Miele 2004; Park et al. 2006). In one study of more than 100 patients who received a diagnosis of psychogenic globus, further evaluation detected physiological abnormalities in most patients (Leelamanit et al. 1996). A similar study in a smaller population yielded similar findings (Ravich et al. 1989). Treatment in those without evidence of physiological abnormalities primarily involves reassurance and psychotherapy, although antidepressants (e.g., tricyclic antidepressants [TCAs], monoamine oxidase inhibitors) have been reported to be effective for some cases (Bishop and Riley 1988; S.R. Brown et al. 1986; Finkenbine and Miele 2004). The role of anxiolytics is unclear, except for those with globus secondary to panic disorder (Finkenbine and Miele 2004).

Upper Gastrointestinal Disorders

Gastroesophageal Reflux Disorder

GERD is defined as a "condition which develops when the reflux of stomach contents causes troublesome symptoms and/or complications" (Vakil et al. 2006, p. 1903). When no reflux esophagitis is seen endoscopically but the patient is still symptomatic, it is called *nonerosive reflux disorder.* Chest pain identical to that of myocardial ischemia can be caused by GERD and is referred to as *reflux chest pain syndrome,* the most common cause of noncardiac chest pain (NCCP) (Cannon et al. 1994; Vakil et al. 2006). GERD adversely affects QOL and productivity (Camilleri et al. 2005; Moayyedi and Talley 2006). GERD is common in Western Europe and North America (prevalence = 10%–20%) but rare in the rest of the world (Dent et al. 2005).

The underlying mechanism of GERD is uncertain, but most experts believe that the increased frequency of transient lower esophageal sphincter relaxations is the most common cause (Moayyedi and Talley 2006). Higher frequency of transient lower esophageal sphincter relaxations increases exposure to gastric refluxate (Dent et al. 1980). However, the degree of esophageal injury present correlates poorly with the amount of acid exposure (Avidan et al. 2002). Esophageal mucosal hypersensitivity may play a role for some patients who show no evidence of macroscopic mucosal damage or abnormal reflux. These patients may experience pain even when a normal amount of acid contacts their esophagus (Rodriguez-Stanley et al. 1999). Central factors beyond mucosal hypersensitivity also may play a role. Prolonged stress leads to hypervigilance, increased symptom reporting, and health-care-seeking behavior. For example, GERD patients with a history of physical/sexual abuse are more likely to seek evaluation of their symptoms than are GERD patients without a history of abuse (Mizyed et al. 2009).

A study of NCCP patients that used esophageal evoked potentials showed that three subpopulations exist: 1) those with mucosal hypersensitivity (reduced pain threshold to electrical stimulus but normal cortical processing), 2) those with central factors (e.g., hypervigilance) mediating hypersensitivity (reduced pain threshold but delayed cortical processing), and 3) those without any esophageal hypersensitivity. They postulated that each group would need a different treatment strategy, with the first needing antinociceptive medications and the second needing psychotherapy (Hobson et al. 2006). It also should be noted that a large population-based study found that antidepressants (clomipramine and selective serotonin reuptake inhibitors [SSRIs]) are associated with an increased risk of reflux esophagitis (van Soest et al. 2007).

Several studies have shown higher prevalence of reflux symptoms among psychiatric patients (Mizyed et al. 2009). A case-control study comparing psychiatric inpatients with nonpsychiatric control subjects found that reflux symptoms were significantly more prevalent among the psychiatric patients, even after the study controlled for psychotropic drug use and smoking (Avidan et al. 2001). A population-based case-control study of more than 65,000 subjects found that individuals with anxiety had a 3.2-fold increased risk of severe reflux, those with depression had a 1.7-fold increased risk, and those with both anxiety and depression had a 2.8-fold increased risk (Jansson et al. 2007). A smaller population-based case-control study failed to show that anxiety and depression were risk factors for GERD (Eslick and Talley 2009).

Psychological stress influences the pathophysiology of GERD and plays a role in how patients respond to treatment. Several studies have shown that acute and chronic stress affects both subjective and objective outcomes in GERD (Mizyed et al. 2009). A small study found that experimentally induced stress increased reflux symptoms but did not increase objective measures of acid reflux (Bradley et al. 1993). A larger study showed similar results (Wright et al. 2005). Fass et al. (2008) compared 46 GERD patients with confirmed abnormal esophageal acid exposure with 10 control subjects; they found that GERD patients showed esophageal hypersensitivity to acid, and this hypersensitivity increased during experimental stress. Some studies have shown that patients with nonerosive reflux disorder are more likely than patients with erosive esophagitis to have psychological symptoms, but others disagree (Nojkov et al. 2008; Wu et al. 2007).

Regarding treatment response, one study showed that patients who had more severe GERD symptoms in association with psychological distress responded well to proton pump inhibitors (Nojkov et al. 2008). This finding is in contrast to two other studies that showed that depressed and anxious GERD patients were less likely to respond to proton pump inhibitors (K.J. Lee et al. 2009; Wiklund et al. 2006). Another study showed that patients with major depression reported less relief of GERD symptoms after antireflux surgery, despite having physiologically equivalent results (Kamolz et al. 2003).

Noncardiac Chest Pain

As previously noted, GERD can cause chest pain indistinguishable from that of cardiac ischemia and is the most common cause of NCCP (Cannon et al. 1994; Fass and Dickman 2006; Vakil et al. 2006). The annual prevalence in the general population is approximately 25% (Fass and Dickman 2006). Because NCCP usually persists over time and causes significant functional impairment, patients often continue to seek urgent medical care despite normal cardiac test results (Fass and Dickman 2006). Evidence suggests that NCCP is sometimes caused by esophageal hypersensitivity. Some patients experience chest pain during esophageal balloon distention, sensing the balloon at lower pressures than those felt by control subjects (Rao et al. 1996). Whether this is due to peripheral or central abnormal neural processes is currently under investigation, but treatment with visceral analgesics (such as TCAs, trazodone, or SSRIs; see below) has proven to be helpful (Chahal and Rao 2005; Fass and Dickman 2006). Psychiatric disorders, including panic disorder, other anxiety disorders, and major depression, tend to be more prevalent among NCCP patients compared with the general population (Fass and Dickman 2006). Compared with control subjects, NCCP patients tend to monitor more and use more problem-focused coping, behaviors associated with higher levels of anxiety and depression (Fass and Dickman 2006).

Functional Heartburn

Functional heartburn has been defined as burning retrosternal discomfort or pain in the absence of evidence that gastroesophageal acid reflux is the cause of the symptom and absence of histopathology-based esophageal motility disorder (Drossman 2006). Compared with control subjects, patients with functional heartburn have more somatization and lower pain thresholds during intraesophageal balloon distention (Shapiro et al. 2006). They also tend to have more atypical symptoms, more comorbid IBS, and more anxiety than do patients with GERD (S. Lee et al. 2009).

Treatment of GERD, Noncardiac Chest Pain, and Functional Heartburn

Case reports and a small study that used experimental stressors suggested a possible role for biofeedback and relaxation training for reduction of GERD symptoms (Gordon et al. 1983; McDonald-Haile et al. 1994). Cognitive therapy also has been proposed as a treatment for NCCP, and a method for conducting it has been described in detail (Salkovskis 1992). A randomized controlled trial in which this approach was used for NCCP showed that it was successful at decreasing the frequency of NCCP, even at 12-month follow-up. This effect, however, may have been mediated by the significant improvement in anxiety in these patients (van Peski-Oosterbaan et al. 1999). Another trial showed similar effects (Klimes et al. 1990). Hypnotherapy was effective for NCCP in a small randomized controlled trial that compared 12 hypnotherapy sessions with supportive therapy. Chest pain intensity but not frequency declined with hypnotherapy (Jones et al. 2006).

TCAs have been used to treat NCCP for many years, but it is unclear whether they exert their effect locally, as a visceral analgesic, or on the central nervous system (Fass and Dickman 2006). A small retrospective study of patients who received TCAs for NCCP reported that 81% had response or remission (Prakash and Clouse 1999b). Cannon et al. (1994) found that imipramine decreased chest pain in patients with normal coronary angiograms, although it did not reduce esophageal sensitivity to balloon distention. A small placebo-controlled trial found that trazodone reduced distress from esophageal symptoms, but it did not influence manometric parameters or actual symptoms (Clouse et al. 1987). Like TCAs, SSRIs also may have peripheral or central effects on NCCP, but their clinical utility remains unclear. A randomized placebo-controlled trial of sertraline for NCCP patients without major depression, panic disorder, or drug or alcohol abuse or dependence showed that sertraline was significantly helpful in decreasing subjective chest pain (Varia et al. 2000). On the contrary, compared with placebo, paroxetine failed to reduce pain scores significantly in NCCP patients without major depression or panic disorder (Doraiswamy et al. 2006). However, it should be kept in mind, as noted earlier, that antidepressants also can increase the risk of GERD.

Nausea and Vomiting

Hyperemesis Gravidarum

Nausea and vomiting of pregnancy affect up to 80% of pregnant women during their first trimester. When nausea and vomiting are severe and accompanied by ketonuria and weight loss, it is considered hyperemesis gravidarum (Bottomley and Bourne 2009; Gill and Einarson 2007). With an incidence rate of 0.5%–2%, hyperemesis gravidarum is the most common reason for hospitalization during the first trimester of pregnancy (T.M. Goodwin 2008). The etiology is unknown but may involve hormonal, infective, anatomical, and psychological factors (Bottomley and Bourne 2009; Kim et al. 2009). Although in the past, hyperemesis gravidarum was ascribed to psychological conflicts (e.g., ambivalence about pregnancy), there is a lack of evidence for this viewpoint (Kim et al. 2009). Rather, it appears that hyperemesis gravidarum causes significant emotional distress and reduced QOL (Gill and Einarson 2007). Some women will consider terminating the pregnancy to seek relief.

Management of hyperemesis gravidarum requires maintenance of adequate intravenous hydration and prevention of serious complications (e.g., Wernicke's encephalopathy, renal impairment, and Mallory-Weiss tears) (Chiossi et al. 2006; T.M. Goodwin 2008). Medications that have been effective include phenothiazines, metoclopramide, serotonin type 3 receptor (5-HT$_3$) antagonists, mirtazapine, benzodiazepines (diazepam), and vitamin B$_6$ (Bottomley and Bourne 2009; Gill and Einarson 2007; Guclu et al. 2005; Tasci et al. 2009). Treatment-resistant cases may require corticosteroids. Ginger has shown some benefits for nausea and vomiting of pregnancy, but no data are available for hyperemesis gravidarum (Boone and Shields 2005; Borrelli et al. 2005). See also Chapter 33, "Obstetrics and Gynecology."

Chemotherapy-Induced Nausea and Vomiting

Chemotherapy-induced nausea and vomiting affect 70%–80% of patients, influenced by specific type of chemotherapy, dose, schedule, route of administration, and patient-specific factors (Naeim et al. 2008). Severe chemotherapy-induced nausea and vomiting cause marked impairment in daily functioning and QOL and contribute to decisions to discontinue chemotherapy prematurely. Patients develop nausea and vomiting acutely within 24 hours after chemotherapy, or they develop a delayed response that may last for days (Feeney et al. 2007; Navari 2009). Risk factors for chemotherapy-induced nausea and vomiting include female gender, younger age, history of motion sickness or pregnancy-induced nausea, comorbid anxiety or depression, and low alcohol intake (Lohr 2008). Treatment typically relies on 5-HT$_3$ antagonists, dexamethasone, and neurokinin-1 antagonists (Lohr 2008; Naeim et al. 2008). A significant number of patients experience breakthrough or treatment-resistant chemotherapy-induced nausea and vomiting, requiring other adjunctive therapies. Lorazepam, metoclopramide, haloperidol, droperidol, and cannabinoids may be added (Lohr 2008). A few case reports (Pirl and Roth 2000; Srivastava et al. 2003) and Phase I and II trials support a role for olanzapine in both acute treatment of and prophylaxis against chemotherapy-induced nausea and vomiting (Navari et al. 2005, 2007; Passik et al. 2004). Two small open trials reported beneficial effects with gabapentin (Guttuso et al. 2003; Lohr 2008). A Cochrane review of 11 randomized trials concluded that acupuncture point stimulation reduced incidence of acute vomiting but not acute or delayed nausea (Ezzo et al. 2006). Electroacupuncture had the greatest effect. Acupressure studies are suggestive of benefits for acute nausea and delayed chemotherapy-induced nausea and vomiting (J. Lee et al. 2008).

Anticipatory Nausea and Vomiting

Anticipatory nausea and vomiting are conditioned responses to settings and circumstances primarily associated with actual episodes of nausea and vomiting. This condition is well recognized in the oncology literature, in which 10%–44% of patients may be affected, but anticipatory nausea and vomiting can develop with other causes of nausea and vomiting, such as pregnancy, gastroparesis, or cyclic vomiting syndrome (Aapro et al. 2005). Factors predictive of anticipatory nausea and vomiting include female gender, age younger than 50 years, susceptibility to motion sickness, nausea and vomiting after the last chemotherapy session, anxiety, hostility, depression, and subjective severity of and accompanying physical distress associated with the last chemotherapy session (Matteson et al. 2002). Expectations of experiencing nausea and vomiting also influence the likelihood of developing anticipatory nausea and vomiting (Hickok et al. 2001; Montgomery and Bovbjerg 2003). Compared with other types of nausea and vomiting, anticipatory nausea and vomiting do not respond to standard antiemetic agents. Benzodiazepines may be able to reduce the incidence of anticipatory nausea and vomiting, but behavioral interventions have proven to be the most effective approach (Matteson et al. 2002). Progressive muscle relaxation, systemic desensitization, hypnosis, and cognitive distraction with video games have been used in both adult and pediatric patient populations (Figueroa-Moseley et al. 2007; Mundy et al. 2003; Redd et al. 2001).

Functional Nausea and Vomiting

Functional nausea and vomiting refer to chronic nausea and vomiting without apparent cause. This condition was once referred to as "psychogenic" vomiting, but no evidence shows a direct link between psychiatric disorders and chronic unexplained nausea and vomiting (Olden and Chepyala 2008; Talley 2007). According to Rome III criteria, functional nausea and vomiting are divided into three specific conditions: chronic idiopathic nausea, functional vomiting, and cyclic vomiting syndrome (Olden and Chepyala 2008; Talley 2007). *Chronic idiopathic nausea* involves nausea that occurs several times a week, which is not usually accompanied by vomiting. *Functional vomiting* refers to unexplained vomiting that occurs at least once a week, is not cyclical, and lacks an organic basis. The epidemiology and pathophysiology of chronic idiopathic nausea and functional vomiting are currently unknown (Olden and Chepyala 2008). Two studies indicated that functional vomiting is often associated with a history of physical or sexual abuse or comorbid panic disorder (Olden and Crowell 2005; Olden et al. 2003). Management of chronic idiopathic nausea is purely symptomatic, and prokinetic and antiemetic medications are used. For functional vomiting, treatment requires nutritional support and reassurance (Olden and Chepyala 2008). A small retrospective study of patients with functional vomiting found significant benefit with low-dose TCAs, with half experiencing complete symptom remission (Prakash et al. 1998).

Cyclic vomiting syndrome is characterized by recurrent stereotypical bouts of severe nausea and vomiting. Once recognized only in children, cyclic vomiting syndrome also occurs in adults, primarily between ages 20 and 40 years (Abell et al. 2008; Sonje and Levenson 2009). Among children, the prevalence ranges from 0.03% to 1.9%. The syndrome typically manifests early in childhood and then either resolves in late childhood or adolescence or progresses to migraine headaches (Dulude et al. 2008; Sonje and Levenson 2009). The prevalence in adults is unknown, and the syndrome often goes undiagnosed for several years.

Cyclic vomiting syndrome consists of four phases: prodromal, emetic, recovery, and interepisode or well. During the prodromal phase, patients experience nausea, abdominal pain, pallor, lethargy, and anorexia lasting minutes to hours, followed by vomiting (emetic phase), which can persist for days. Recovery phase begins when vomiting ceases and hunger and food tolerance resume. Between episodes, patients are often symptom free or may have dyspeptic nausea. The clinical presentation of cyclic vomiting syndrome may be accompanied by fever, chills, sweating, diarrhea, neutrophilia, tachycardia, and elevated blood pressure, mimicking acute abdomen from other causes (Pareek et al. 2007). For many, certain triggers can set off an episode; triggers include infections, lack of sleep, psychologically stressful events (positive and negative), onset of a menstrual period, fasting, and certain foods. The pathogenesis of cyclic vomiting syndrome is unknown but may involve autonomic nervous system dysfunction, GI dysrhythmia, mitochondrial gene mutations, HPA axis defect, ion channelopathies, and chronic cannabis abuse (Abell et al. 2008). Comorbid migraine headache and family history of migraines are common. A higher-than-expected rate of psychiatric comorbidity (anxiety, panic attacks, depression) has been noted, but it is unclear if this represents a reaction to the stress of cyclic vomiting syndrome or an actual contributing factor (Abell et al. 2008; Fleisher et al. 2005; Tarbell 2008). Treatment is empirical and requires lifestyle adjustments, education, stress management, and reassurance, along with medications for prophylactic and acute use (Li et al. 2008). Prophylaxis primarily entails TCAs (amitriptyline), cyproheptadine, or propranolol (Chepyala et al. 2007; Li et al. 2008; Namin et al. 2007; Prakash and Clouse 1999a). L-carnitine, coenzyme Q10, low-estrogen contraceptives, anticonvulsants, and prokinetic agents also have been used. Acute periods of nausea and vomiting may require intravenous fluids, antiemetics, triptans, benzodiazepines (for sleep induction and anxiolysis), opioids, nonsteroidal anti-inflammatory drugs (NSAIDs), proton pump inhibitors, and histamine H_2-blockers.

Gastroparesis

Gastroparesis is a clinical disorder of delayed gastric emptying without evidence of mechanical obstruction. Symptoms are variable but often include nausea, vomiting, early satiety, abdominal bloating, and pain. Symptom severity does not necessarily correlate with the magnitude of delayed gastric emptying present (Khoo et al. 2009; Stapleton and Wo 2009). The prevalence of gastroparesis may be increasing in the United States and is responsible for causing reduced QOL, impaired nutrition, and interference with oral medication absorption (Khoo et al. 2009; Stapleton and Wo 2009). Gastroparesis may be idiopathic or associated with various conditions such as diabetes or other metabolic disturbances, surgery, chronic renal failure, connective tissue disorders, and neuromuscular disorders (Khoo et al. 2009; Patrick and Epstein 2008). Diabetes mellitus is considered to be the most common cause, although idiopathic gastroparesis has been nearly as common in some series (Hasler 2008). Most patients with idiopathic gastroparesis are young to middle-aged women, many with a history of acute gastroenteritis and/or viral syndrome (Patrick and Epstein 2008). Gastroparesis can also be caused by medications including opiates, TCAs, and lithium (Hasler 2008). The natural course of gastroparesis is one of relapsing and remitting symptoms (Khoo et al. 2009). Management may involve dietary changes, nutritional supplements, prokinetic agents (e.g., metoclopramide, domperidone, erythromycin, cisapride), antiemetics, botulinum injection, or paced gastric neurostimulation (Hasler 2008; Khoo et al. 2009). Metoclopramide is often prescribed but is increasingly recognized as a potential cause of tardive dyskinesia (Kenney et al. 2008). Although counterintuitive, TCAs were noted to be useful in a small group of diabetic patients with chronic vomiting unresponsive to prokinetic agents (Sawhney et al. 2007).

Dyspepsia and Peptic Ulcer Disease

Dyspepsia is characterized by chronic or recurrent pain or discomfort centered in the upper abdomen and may include early satiety and upper abdominal fullness (Talley et al. 2005a). Bloating and nausea also may occur but do not make the diagnosis by themselves (Talley et al. 2005a). *Functional dyspepsia,* as defined by the Rome III criteria, consists of "the presence of symptoms thought to originate in the gastroduodenal region, in the absence of any organic, systemic, or metabolic disease that is likely to explain the symptoms" (Tack et al. 2006b, p. 1466). The annual prevalence of dyspepsia in the United States and other Western countries is approximately 25%; if frequent heartburn is included, prevalence approaches 40% (Talley et al. 2005a). Approximately half of those with dyspepsia seek health care for their symptoms (Tack et al. 2006b).

The four major causes of dyspepsia are peptic ulcer disease, GERD, malignancy, and functional dyspepsia. Peptic ulcer disease is the cause of approximately 10% of all upper GI symptoms, and *Helicobacter pylori* is the main cause of peptic ulcer disease not resulting from NSAIDs (American Gastroenterological Association 2005). As the prevalence of *H. pylori* has dramatically declined in most of the Western world, so has the prevalence of peptic ulcer disease and gastric adenocarcinoma (Talley et al. 2005b). A meta-analysis of risk factors for serious peptic ulcer disease in North America showed that 48% of the risk was attributable to *H. pylori,* 24% was from NSAIDs, and 23% was from cigarette smoking (Kurata and Nogawa 1997). Risk factors differ in different parts of the world (Rosenstock et al. 2003). Tobacco is a risk factor for both gastric and duodenal peptic ulcer, and it delays duodenal ulcer healing (Kato et al. 1992; Reynolds et al. 1994; Rosenstock et al. 2003). Alcohol use in moderation has been shown to have either negligible or even protective effects on risk of peptic ulcer and gastritis, and it may improve or hinder the eradication of *H. pylori,* depending on the circumstances (Baena et al. 2002; Namiot et al. 2008; Taylor et al. 2005). Heavy drinking, however, increases the risk of peptic ulcer disease and gastritis (Levenstein 2000).

Evidence suggests an association between psychiatric disorders and increased risk of peptic ulcer disease. An epidemiological study of more than 43,000 subjects showed that all mood and anxiety disorders were significantly associated with peptic ulcer disease (especially generalized anxiety disorder and panic disorder), but alcohol and nicotine dependence mediated a portion of this association but not all of it (R.D. Goodwin et al. 2009). Intellectual and developmental disabilities predispose people to *H. pylori* infection, perhaps as a result of maladaptive behaviors. Their rate of infection is approximately twice that in the general population, and eradication is much more difficult (Kitchens et al. 2007).

Psychological factors have been postulated to play a role in causing peptic ulcer disease since the nineteenth century. Franz Alexander studied psychological factors' influence on GI disorders in the 1930s and included peptic ulcer disease as a classic psychosomatic disease in his 1950 book, *Psychosomatic Medicine: Its Principles and Applications* (Weiner 1991). Since then, numerous studies have confirmed that stressful life events, and perhaps personality characteristics, play a role in peptic ulcer disease (Levenstein 2000; Weiner 1991). Throughout history and in many different countries, both manmade and natural disasters have been associated with spikes in hospitalizations for peptic ulcer (Levenstein 2000). Case-control studies comparing patients with peptic ulcer disease with patients without peptic ulcer disease have noted greater likelihood of neuroticism, anxiety, guilt, stressful life events, and the perception of being under greater stress in reaction to life events in those with peptic ulcer disease (Christodoulou et al. 1983; Feldman et al. 1986). In a classic study, Weiner et al. (1957) successfully predicted which men in a large cohort of army draftees would have duodenal ulcers by combining psychological criteria with the biological criterion of high baseline pepsinogen secretion.

The prospective, longitudinal, population-based Alameda County Study identified various psychological risk factors for peptic ulcer disease, including depression, hostility, and lack of social connectedness (Levenstein et al. 1995). Adjustment for smoking, alcohol use, and other physiological variables weakened but did not eliminate these risk factors (Levenstein et al. 1995). The association between stress and peptic ulcer disease may be mediated by several factors. Lower socioeconomic status predisposes people to both stress and *H. pylori;* painful medical conditions are stressful and are associated with NSAID use; and smoking and heavy alcohol use are common in people experiencing stress. Despite all these potential mediators, a direct link between stress and peptic ulcer disease is still evident (Levenstein 2000).

Sometimes the association between psychological characteristics and peptic ulcer disease does not represent a causal relation (Jess and Eldrup 1994). One prospective case-control study concluded that the anxiety and neuroticism in peptic ulcer disease patients with *H. pylori* were caused by the duodenal ulcer, not vice versa (Wilhelmsen and Berstad 2004).

Given the consistent literature on the role of life stressors, personality, and psychopathology in the pathogenesis of peptic ulcer disease, it is not surprising that psychotherapeutic and psychopharmacological approaches have been investigated for treatment of peptic ulcer disease. Many of these studies were performed in the 1950s–1970s, before acid suppression and *H. pylori* eradication became the standard treatment. Randomized controlled trials of group psychotherapy have not found it helpful (Lööf et al. 1987; Wilhelmsen et al. 1994). TCAs were studied in the past and found to decrease gastric acid secretion and improve peptic ulcer healing (Andersen et al. 1984; Ries et al. 1984). Results were not consistent, however, and TCAs are no longer considered first-line therapy for peptic ulcer disease.

Functional Dyspepsia

Up to 70% of patients with dyspepsia have functional dyspepsia, and it negatively affects QOL (Talley et al. 2005b). The underlying pathophysiology remains unclear, but several possible mechanisms have been considered, one of which is hypersensitivity to gastric distention or acid exposure (Talley et al. 2005a). Functional brain imaging studies suggest that in patients with functional dyspepsia with gastric hypersensitivity, actual afferent input to the brain is increased (Vandenbergh et al. 2005; Vandenberghe et al. 2007). Functional brain imaging studies have also shown that the brains of patients with functional dyspepsia are different from those of control subjects at rest. Additionally, they have shown that endogenous pain modulation differs between functional dyspepsia patients and control subjects, regardless of whether patients have visceral hypersensitivity, and anxiety appears to play a role in this pain modulation (Van Oudenhove et al. 2010).

Many studies have shown that comorbidity between functional dyspepsia and psychiatric disorders, especially anxiety disorders, is high. Currently, it is unclear whether this reflects a causal relation between the two, a common predisposition, or anxiety-induced increased health-care-seeking behavior (Tack et al. 2006b). Case-control studies have reported that patients with functional dyspepsia have greater anxiety and depression, higher levels of other psychopathology, increased life stress, and reduced health-related QOL compared with healthy control subjects and duodenal ulcer patients (Haag et al. 2008; Haug et al. 1995). Various psychological factors also have been found to influence functional dyspepsia, such as history of abuse, sleep dysfunction, somatization, and other life stressors (Haug et al. 1995; Gathaiya et al. 2009; Talley et al. 2005a).

In general, both clinicians and questionnaire-based computer models do a poor job of distinguishing between functional and organic dyspepsia; thus, endoscopy must be used to distinguish between the two (Moayyedi et al. 2006). Reassurance and education are often all that are required to treat functional dyspepsia, but management can be difficult and requires frequent follow-ups (Talley et al. 2005a). Patients are often started on drugs that provide acid suppression, but at least 40% of patients fail to respond to medication (Monkemuller and Malfertheiner 2006; Talley et al. 2005b). Of patients with functional dyspepsia, 35% have been found to respond to placebo. Those with stable symptom patterns were less likely to respond, whereas those with inconsistent symptoms were more likely to respond (Talley et al. 2006).

Although psychotherapy and antidepressants are often used to treat functional dyspepsia, the benefits of these approaches are not yet established (American Gastroenterological Association 2005). Some empirical support exists for group therapy that uses relaxation techniques (Bates et al. 1988), cognitive therapy (Haug et al. 1994), psychodynamic-interpersonal psychotherapy (Hamilton et al. 2000), and hypnotherapy (Calvert et al. 2002). However, a Cochrane review including these studies concluded that "there is insufficient evidence to confirm the efficacy of psychological interventions for non-ulcer dyspepsia" (Soo et al. 2005, p. 6). Antidepressants may be prokinetic at the levels of both the enteric and the central nervous systems (Monkemuller and Malfertheiner 2006). However, small randomized controlled trials in healthy volunteers (Bouras et al. 2008; Choung et al. 2008) and patients with functional dyspepsia (Mertz et al. 1998) have provided little support that TCAs or mirtazapine would be helpful in functional dyspepsia, and a larger randomized controlled trial comparing venlafaxine with placebo also was not supportive (van Kerkhoven et al. 2008). The National Institute of Diabetes and Digestive and Kidney Diseases is currently conducting a randomized controlled trial to determine whether amitriptyline or escitalopram is helpful in treating functional dyspepsia. This study also aims to characterize the mechanism by which these medications may work, since gastric emptying, gastric accommodation, and gastric hypersensitivity will be measured (Talley et al. 2010).

Upper Gastrointestinal Bleeding and Serotonergic Medications

Abnormal bleeding associated with SSRIs is thought to be the result of depletion of platelet serotonin. Under normal circumstances, serotonin is released from platelets, promoting platelet aggregation, a necessary step in hemostasis. Because serotonin is not synthesized by platelets, the acquisition of adequate levels of serotonin depends on platelet receptor reuptake from plasma. This process is blocked by SSRIs and possibly by other antidepressants with moderate to high affinity for serotonin receptors (e.g., clomipramine, serotonin-norepinephrine reuptake inhibitors). Several case-control studies have sought to establish a particular link between SSRIs and increased risk of upper GI bleeding (de Abajo and García-Rodríguez 2008; de Abajo et al. 1999; Helin-Salmivaara et al. 2007; Kurdyak et al. 2005; Lewis et al. 2008; Opartny et al. 2008; Schalekamp et al. 2008; Tata et al. 2005; X. Vidal et al. 2008). Despite differences in study design and antidepressants, most studies suggest that there is a two- to threefold increased risk of hemorrhage (Dalton et al. 2006; Loke et al. 2008; Opartny et al. 2008). The absolute effect in healthy adults has been considered to be moderate, comparable with that of low-dose NSAIDs, but the risk is considered significantly greater among patients at increased risk for upper GI hemorrhage (i.e., patients who are elderly or who have concurrent NSAID use, thrombocytopenia, or history of upper GI bleeds) (Weinrieb et al. 2005; Yuan et al. 2006). For these patients, closer monitoring and greater care in selecting antidepressants and NSAIDs are suggested.

Lower Gastrointestinal Disorders

Inflammatory Bowel Disease: Ulcerative Colitis and Crohn's Disease

Inflammatory bowel disease (IBD) is a chronic relapsing and remitting bowel disorder that involves inflammation of the intestinal mucosa. Common symptoms include diarrhea, fever, and abdominal pain but also can involve bleeding, anorexia, weight loss, and fatigue (Irvine 2008). Ulcerative colitis and Crohn's disease are the two forms of IBD, which differ according to the extent of mucosal damage and GI tract involvement. For ulcerative colitis, the mucosal layer from rectum to colon may be affected, whereas Crohn's disease involves transmural inflammation of any portion of the GI tract. Complications of IBD result in bowel obstruction, perforation, malnutrition, fistulas, and ulcerations, along with increased risk for colon cancer.

The peak incidence for IBD onset ranges from ages 15 to 30 years; a second peak for Crohn's disease is between ages 50 and 80 years. Extraintestinal manifestations of IBD may be present in up to 40% of patients. Most often, this entails musculoskeletal, skin, or eye involvement. Less common is involvement of the cardiac, pulmonary, neurological (i.e., thromboembolism, sensorineural hearing loss), hematological, or renal systems (Williams et al. 2008).

Epidemiology of IBD

The incidence and prevalence of IBD are greatest in developed countries, including the United States, Canada, and Western Europe. In the past, less developed countries showed low incidence and prevalence rates for IBD, but this has changed over the past decade. Eastern Europe, South America, and Asia have shown progressive increases in their incidence of IBD. This increase is thought to be at least partly a result of the changes brought by modernization and development (e.g., diet, hygiene, pathogen exposure). Currently, prevalence rates for IBD range from 37 to 246 cases per 100,000 persons for ulcerative colitis to 26 to 199 cases per 100,000 persons for Crohn's disease (Mikocka-Walus et al. 2008b). Incidence rates for ulcerative colitis vary from 0.5 to 24.5 per 100,000 person-years, and rates for Crohn's disease vary from 0.1 to 16 per 100,000 person-years (Lakatos 2006). In the United States, IBD is estimated to affect approximately 1.5 million people (Shanahan and Bernstein 2009).

Pathophysiology of IBD

The underlying pathophysiology of IBD is not completely understood but appears to involve interactions between genetic, environmental, and immune factors. Approximately 5%–10% of IBD patients have at least one affected first-degree relative, and twin studies report a 50% concordance rate for Crohn's disease among monozygotic twins (Braus and Elliott 2009). In addition, more than 30 susceptibility genes for IBD have been identified (Noomen et al. 2009). Environmental factors also have been linked to IBD, although it is unclear if they affect only individuals already susceptible to IBD. Smoking increases the risk of developing Crohn's disease and worsens the course but serves a protective function in ulcerative colitis (Lakatos et al. 2007; Sainsbury and Heatley 2005). Appendectomies also appear to protect against development of ulcerative colitis in some studies (Andersson et al. 2001). In contrast, acute infectious gastroenteritis may increase the risk of developing IBD (Porter et al. 2008). Recent years have seen an increase in the focus on immune factors and their influence on IBD, with studies suggesting the presence of disruptions in the innate and adaptive immune system leading to altered responses to intestinal flora and chronic inflammation (Braus and Elliott 2009; Noomen et al. 2009).

Stress and IBD

Clinical observations and anecdotal reports have long suggested a relation between stress and IBD. A prospective longitudinal study of 60 ulcerative colitis patients in remission found that the number of stressful life events in the prior month was an independent determinant of time to relapse (Bitton et al. 2003). Another prospective study of 62 ulcerative colitis patients found that those with more long-term perceived stress had significantly increased risk of disease exacerbation (Levenstein et al. 2000). A smaller prospective study noted a significant relation between daily stress and IBD symptoms occurring the following month (Greene et al. 1994). Although these findings suggest a relation between stress and IBD disease activity, results have not been consistent across studies. In particular, studies involving mixed populations of IBD patients have tended to yield negative results, leading some to suggest that there may be enough differences between ulcerative colitis and Crohn's disease that they should not be studied together. Additional studies have failed to establish a relation between stress and IBD onset (Lerebours et al. 2007). Studies that used experimentally induced psychological stress and animal models of colitis have noted the development of altered intestinal mucosal permeability. This is considered the possible mechanism behind stress and increased risk of inflammation or relapse in IBD (Maunder 2005; Mawdsley and Rampton 2005).

Anxiety and Depression in IBD

Given that IBD is a chronic disorder that often involves significant morbidity, impaired functioning, and reduced QOL, the presence of anxiety and depression in this population is not surprising. Disease activity significantly influences the rates of anxiety and depression, which range from 29% to 35% during remission and rise to 80% for anxiety and 60% for depression during relapse (Mikocka-Walus et al. 2007). In general, Crohn's disease patients are considered to have a higher frequency of psychological disturbances than do ulcerative colitis patients (Caprilli et al. 2006; Sainsbury and Heatley 2005). This is thought to be due to the greater level of impairment and disability associated with Crohn's disease.

Some evidence indicates that depression and anxiety affect Crohn's disease. A small prospective study of Crohn's disease patients found that severity of depression was independently associated with current and future disease activity. Higher levels of anxiety also were associated with disease activity but were not independent of the effects of depression (Mardini et al. 2004). Another prospective study of IBD patients (mostly Crohn's disease) in remission reported that baseline depression scores were associated with the subsequent number of relapses and time to first relapse. Anxiety and low health-related QOL also were related to more frequent relapses (Mittermaier et al. 2004). In a study of 100 Crohn's disease patients who received infliximab, the presence of major depressive disorder was found to reduce the chance of achieving remission (Persoons et al. 2005). However, not all studies have confirmed a relation between psychological problems and number of relapses (Mikocka-Walus et al. 2008b).

IBD and Quality of Life

Compared with the general population, the QOL of IBD patients is significantly reduced, during both remission and active disease. Disease activity or severity is the strongest predictor of QOL among IBD patients (Han et al. 2005; Janke et al. 2005; Lix et al. 2008). Comorbid psychiatric disorders, psychological distress, socioeconomic status, educational level, and perceived quality of care also have been found to influence QOL (Irvine 2008; Sainsbury and Heatley 2005; van der Eijk et al. 2004; A. Vidal et al. 2008). Two disease-specific instruments have been developed to measure QOL in IBD patients: 1) the Inflammatory Bowel Disease Questionnaire, which was designed to measure subjective health status and has been well validated and translated into several languages (Guyatt et al. 1989), and 2) the Rating Form for IBD Patient Concerns (RFIPC), which measures psychosocial concomitants to illness, including effect of disease, sexual intimacy, and body stigma (Drossman et al. 1991).

Coping style also appears to influence QOL, as noted in cross-sectional studies of IBD patients. Concerns about disease reflected by the RFIPC total score were strongly influenced by the presence of depressive coping. Depressive coping, which represented a tendency toward irritability, self-pity, musing, and feelings of resignation, had a greater effect than either demographic or disease-related variables (Mussell et al. 2004). Among another group of IBD patients in remission, greater use of reaction formation and higher rates of somatization most closely and independently influenced health-related QOL (Hyphantis et al. 2010). Many IBD patients also have symptoms of functional GI disorders (Barratt et al. 2005; Minderhoud et al. 2004). Their presence has been noted to increase health care use and adversely affect health-related QOL (Farrokhyar et al. 2006). Some studies have noted that these patients experience reduced psychological well-being, with higher levels of anxiety and depression compared with patients with IBD alone (Mikocka-Walus et al. 2008a; Simren et al. 2002; Tanaka and Kazuma 2005)

Psychological and Pharmacological Interventions in IBD

Partly because of the recognition that stress influences IBD disease activity and partly because of reduced QOL in IBD, attempts have been made to use psychotherapeutic approaches to help this patient population. Clinical trials have used a variety of approaches, including short-term psychodynamic psychotherapy, relaxation training, supportive-expressive group therapy, cognitive-behavioral training, and patient education. Despite these efforts, the results have repeatedly failed to show a positive effect on disease activity, but there have been other benefits (von Wietersheim and Kessler 2006). A prospective randomized multicenter study found a trend for reduced hospital days among Crohn's disease patients who had participated in a course of psychodynamic therapy and relaxation training (Deter et al. 2007). Another large study reported significantly fewer hospital visits in IBD patients who participated in a patient-oriented self-management program (A.P. Kennedy et al. 2004). Other studies have reported improvement in depression scores, mental health scale scores of QOL measures, and patient satisfaction (Elsenbruch et al. 2005; Keller et al. 2004; Mussell et al. 2003; von Wietersheim and Kessler 2006; Waters et al. 2005).

Fewer data are available on the effectiveness of psychopharmacological agents in IBD. Case reports and a small open-label study described use of antidepressants for depression, panic disorder, and smoking cessation. Paroxetine, phenelzine, and bupropion were effective agents that also appeared to reduce IBD disease activity (Mikocka-Walus et al. 2006). Remission of Crohn's disease was described with phenelzine and bupropion, the latter of which may lower tumor necrosis factor–alpha levels (Brustholm et al. 2006; Kast and Altschuler 2005). This effect is similar to that of infliximab, a chimeric monoclonal antibody against tumor necrosis factor–alpha, which has proven therapeutic effectiveness in IBD. Nevertheless, depression remains undertreated in patients with Crohn's disease (Fuller-Thomson and Sulman 2006).

Irritable Bowel Syndrome

IBS is characterized by abdominal pain relieved by defecation and accompanied by changes in stool appearance or frequency. Efforts to refine the diagnostic criteria for IBS had led to the current Rome III criteria, which reflect the chronicity of symptoms along with the abdominal pain and change in bowel habits (Drossman 2006). Additional symptoms may include flatulence, bloating, stool urgency or straining, and a persistent sensation of incomplete bowel evacuation. IBS can be subdivided according to predominant bowel pattern: diarrhea, constipation, or alternating. Diagnosis is based on symptomatic history without the presence of accompanying alarm symptoms (e.g., fever, weight loss, rectal bleeding) that might reflect a more serious underlying GI condition. Comorbid medical conditions are common among IBS patients and include GERD, functional dyspepsia, chronic pelvic pain, interstitial cystitis, fibromyalgia, headache, backache, and sleep disturbance (Riedl et al. 2008; Talley 2006).

Epidemiology of IBS

IBS is the most common functional GI disorder and affects approximately 10%–15% of the general population. Western countries have a predominance of females with IBS, but this is not seen in Australia or Asian countries (Gwee 2005; Talley 2006). Despite the frequency of IBS, only 10%–25% of individuals seek medical treatment, yet they make up 25%–50% of all gastroenterology referrals. Currently, IBS care is estimated to account for $20 billion in direct and indirect costs (Brandt et al. 2009). IBS patients consume 50% more health care costs than do matched control subjects and lose an average of 8.5–22 days from work annually (Brandt et al. 2009, Maxion-Bergemann et al. 2006). QOL among IBS patients is significantly impaired compared with that in the general population.

Pathophysiology of IBS

Despite extensive efforts to study the pathophysiology of IBS, the exact mechanism behind the disorder remains unknown. Current evidence suggests a role for various factors, including abnormal GI motility, visceral hypersensitivity, altered stress responses, changes in serotonin signaling, psychological dysfunction, and inflammatory processes. These factors contribute to altered gut function likely via the brain–gut axis, which connects the central nervous system with the enteric nervous system. Interplay between these systems involves bidirectional communication through sympathetic and parasympathetic pathways, the HPA axis, sensory ganglia, and sites in the brain involved with attention, affect, and pain modulation. At present, no pathophysiological abnormalities are considered specific to all IBS patients.

Altered colonic motility has been observed among IBS patients, but motility changes may be present in other areas along the GI tract. Motility changes are not associated with severity of IBS symptoms, however. Autonomic dysfunction has been detected in some IBS patients, with increased sympathetic activity and decreased parasympathetic activity compared with control subjects, along with altered responses to psychological stress (Grover et al. 2009). Visceral hypersensitivity, the predisposition to having an exaggerated response to visceral stimuli, has been noted among

IBS patients, including lower pain thresholds to gut distention (Longstreth and Drossman 2002). Application of various stimuli, including food, stress, or bowel distention, shows altered sensitivity compared with healthy control subjects (Mertz et al. 1995; Murray et al. 2004; Simren et al. 2007). Differences in cortical processing of pain information have been noted in brain imaging studies (Simren et al. 2007). When rectal distention was used as a pain stimulus, IBS patients appeared to have increased cortical activity in the sensory areas, those involved with attention and affect, and subcortical regions associated with affect, arousal, and autonomic responses (Simren et al. 2007).

Among IBS patients, alterations in stress-mediated pathways have been noted in some studies. Increased corticotropin response to corticotropin-releasing factor and stress has been observed, along with changes in the HPA axis during both rest and stressful circumstances (Grover et al. 2009). Serotonin signaling in the gut is important for motility, secretion, vasodilatation, and visceral sensation. Most serotonin present in the gut is located in enterochromaffin cells, and reuptake of serotonin is achieved by serotonin reuptake transporter proteins (SERT). Among IBS patients, release of serotonin, serotonin signaling, and expression of SERT in the colonic mucosa have been reported to be disturbed in several studies (Mawe et al. 2006).

Psychological factors are known to affect the perception of GI symptoms and pain. Dorn et al. (2007) showed that increased colonic sensitivity was strongly influenced by the tendency to report pain and urgency rather than the actual presence of increased neurosensitivity. In the past, psychological factors have been viewed as influencing symptom distress and health-seeking behavior in IBS patients. Recent studies, however, suggest that psychological factors also may contribute directly to the etiopathogenesis of IBS. A population-based study evaluating the relation between psychological stress, fatigue, health anxiety, and illness and subsequent onset of abdominal pain noted an increased risk caused by psychological distress (Halder et al. 2002). Similarly, a large prospective population-based study reported that after results were adjusted for age, gender, and baseline abdominal pain, high levels of illness behavior, sleep problems, and somatic symptoms were independent predictors of IBS onset (Nicholl et al. 2008). Depression was found to be an independent predictor of developing postinfectious IBS in a study comparing patients with healthy control subjects (Dunlop et al. 2003). More life events and higher hypochondriasis scores were highly predictive of postinfectious IBS in another group of patients (Gwee et al. 1999).

Attention to the role of subclinical inflammatory changes in IBS has increased in recent years partly because of the recognition of the comorbidity between IBS and IBD. High rates of IBS-like symptoms have been reported among IBD patients in remission. Furthermore, it is not uncommon for IBS patients to have a premorbid history of acute bacterial gastroenteritis. Biopsies of GI tract tissue of IBS patients have identified qualitative and quantitative changes in inflammatory cell populations, including T cells, mast cells, and $CD3^+$ lymphocytes (Arebi et al. 2008). In addition, blood samples have shown elevated levels of inflammatory cytokines among patients with postinfectious IBS or diarrhea-predominant IBS (Liebregts et al. 2007).

IBS and Quality of Life

The QOL of IBS patients has been shown repeatedly to be worse than that in the general population. This decrement in QOL is also found when comparing IBS patients with those who have other chronic disorders such as asthma, migraine headache, and GERD (Frank et al. 2002). Even compared with more serious conditions such as diabetes mellitus and dialysis-dependent end-stage renal failure, IBS patients rate their QOL as worse on several factors such as energy level, pain, and role limitations (Gralnek et al. 2000). Studies also have sought to determine which differences among IBS patients influence QOL. Patients who do not seek medical care or are followed up by only primary care providers report better QOL than do those seen in secondary- and tertiary-care centers (Simren et al. 2004). This is consistent with findings that IBS symptom severity plays a significant role in QOL (Coffin et al. 2004; Sabate et al. 2008). The presence of accompanying extraintestinal symptoms (e.g., fatigue, sleep disturbance, sexual dysfunction) and psychological distress (e.g., hypochondriasis, anxiety) also contributes to reduced QOL (Rey et al. 2008; Sabate et al. 2008).

Psychiatric Comorbidity in IBS

The prevalence of comorbid Axis I disorders is estimated to range from 40% to 94% among IBS patients seen primarily in tertiary-care centers. Depression is the most common disorder, followed by anxiety and somatization disorders (Palsson and Drossman 2005). Bidirectional comorbidity exists between anxiety or depression and IBS because elevated rates of IBS have been detected among patients with anxiety and depressive disorders (Karling et al. 2007). Frequently, however, psychiatric disorders predate the onset of IBS symptoms. The presence of anxiety or depression among IBS patients is associated with more severe GI symptoms, greater functional impairment, and worse prognosis (Karling et al. 2007; S. Lee et al. 2009). Compared with IBS patients seen in secondary- or tertiary-care centers, patients who do not seek medical care do not have increased psychiatric comorbidity. However, some studies do show elevated rates of psychiatric disorders among IBS patients identified in community samples (Osterberg et al. 2000; Whitehead et al. 2002). Somatization disorder has been reported to be present in 25%–33% of IBS patients, with others showing a tendency to somatize (Choung et al. 2009; Whitehead et al. 2002). Differences in coping mechanisms or personality styles also have been noted, with elevated levels of catastrophizing and neuroticism (Palsson and Drossman 2005). Clinicians have long observed that IBS patients often have a history of physical or sexual abuse. The contribution of this abuse history to IBS remains unclear; it may increase vulnerability to anxiety, depression, somatization, or substance abuse; influence pain perception or coping; or promote seeking health care (Spiller et al. 2007). Limited data suggest that reduced pain coping or somatizing behavior may be present among IBS patients with abuse histories (Creed et al. 2005; Ringel et al. 2004).

Psychological Interventions in IBS

Recognition of the interaction between stress, psychopathology, and IBS has spurred studies examining the effects of various psychological interventions on IBS symptoms and QOL measures. Cognitive-behavioral therapy (CBT), psychodynamic therapy, hypnosis, and stress management or relaxation therapy all have been used in various clinical trials. A recent Cochrane review and meta-analysis concluded that evidence indicates that these interventions are superior to usual care or placement on a waiting list but not better than placebo (Zijdenbos et al. 2009). The meta-analysis was hampered by methodological quality, small sample sizes, group heterogeneity, and differences in outcome measures. Additional reviews and one other recent meta-analysis concluded that psychological therapies, particularly CBT and hypnosis, offer benefits for both IBS symptoms and accompanying psychosocial distress (Ford et al. 2009; Tan et al. 2005; Toner 2005; Wilson et al. 2006).

A considerable number of controlled clinical trials have used CBT, whether alone or as part of a more comprehensive treatment approach including other techniques. Among these, the largest and most methodologically sound study compared CBT with education in female patients with functional bowel disorders, including IBS. Outcome was measured with a composite score that incorporated aspects including bowel symptoms, QOL, and patient satisfaction. CBT produced a significantly greater treatment response than did education (70% vs. 37%) and was comparable to the response to desipramine therapy (Drossman et al. 2003). A recent randomized trial included two different versions of CBT, one self-administered and the other therapist-administered. Both forms of CBT were significantly superior to the control condition in the percentage of patients reporting adequate relief and improvement in IBS symptoms (Lackner et al. 2008). The sustainability of symptom improvements may be questionable, however; another study that followed up patients up to 12 months after CBT was added to standard antispasmodic therapy showed waning of improvements at 6 and 12 months (T. Kennedy et al. 2005). Positron emission tomography (PET) scans were used in another study to determine how CBT benefits IBS patients. Reduced baseline activity in the anterior cingulate gyrus and left medial temporal lobe was interpreted as reflecting reduced attention to visceral stimuli (Lackner et al. 2006).

Psychopharmacological Interventions in IBS

A recent systematic review and meta-analysis of both psychological interventions and antidepressants in IBS concluded that both approaches are effective, but the quality of evidence was greatest for antidepressant therapy. The estimated number needed to treat to prevent persistent IBS symptoms was 4 for both types of treatment (Ford et al. 2009). Antidepressants, specifically TCAs and SSRIs, have been used in several clinical trials involving IBS patients. Harris and Chang (2006) suggested that the rationale for trying antidepressants in IBS was threefold: frequent psychiatric comorbidity, central effects on pain modulation, and central or peripheral effects on visceral sensitivity and motor activity.

Most clinical trials that have used TCAs have used low dosages, although the choice of specific TCA has been quite variable (e.g., imipramine, amitriptyline, desipramine, doxepin, trimipramine). Although pooled results involving more than 500 patients in placebo-controlled trials showed significant benefits for IBS, a recent positive clinical trial involving imipramine was hampered by a considerable dropout rate resulting from side effects (Abdul-Baki et al. 2009; Ford et al. 2009). Another study used functional magnetic resonance imaging (MRI) to compare the effects of amitriptyline with those of placebo. Amitriptyline was associated with reduced pain-related activation of the anterior cingulate gyrus and left posterior parietal cortex during mental stress. These were considered areas involved in cognition and affect rather than sensory functions. This study suggested that TCAs work in the central nervous system to blunt pain and other symptoms exacerbated by stress in IBS patients (Morgan et al. 2005). The effectiveness of low-dose TCAs for functional bowel disorders was supported in a post hoc analysis of a randomized, placebo-controlled trial of desipramine. Clinical response to treatment was associated with detectable desipramine blood levels. However, no relation was established between clinical response and total desipramine dose or plasma drug level (Halpert et al. 2005).

Given that serotonin plays a significant role in control of gut function and pain pathways in the peripheral and enteric nervous systems, along with the presence of abnormal serotonin signaling and release in IBS, the choice of SSRIs is not surprising. Several randomized clinical trials have used paroxetine, fluoxetine, or citalopram. One double-blind randomized, placebo-controlled trial in IBS patients added paroxetine, 10–40 mg, to a high-fiber diet and noted significant improvement in overall well-being (Tabas et al. 2004). Another randomized controlled trial in constipation-predominant IBS patients found that compared with placebo, 20 mg of fluoxetine significantly reduced abdominal discomfort and bloating and resulted in improvements in stool consistency and bowel movement frequency; these benefits were independent of presence of depression (Vahedi et al. 2005). Several other studies did not show improvements in IBS symptoms with SSRIs (Masand et al. 2009; Talley et al. 2008). Differences in methodology, study population, and outcome measures have complicated attempts to compare these studies (Tack et al. 2006a). The evidence is less positive for SSRIs, but they do offer greater tolerability. Clear benefits from noradrenergic-serotonergic agents remains to be seen because a small open-label pilot study of duloxetine in IBS patients without depression was hampered by significant dropout as a result of adverse side effects (Brennan et al. 2009).

Liver Disorders

Hepatitis C

Epidemiology and Treatment of Hepatitis C Virus

Hepatitis C virus (HCV), the second most common bloodborne disease in the world, affects up to 2% of the world's population (Perry et al. 2008). In the United States, HCV is the leading indication for liver transplantation and is responsible for 8,000–10,000 deaths per year (Dienstag and McHutchinson 2006). Long-term consequences of infection include end-stage liver disease and hepatocellular cancer. Chronic HCV infection impairs QOL and may cause cognitive impairment independent of the presence of cirrhosis (Perry et al. 2008). Acute infection is often asymptomatic; therefore, many patients are unaware of being infected until they develop long-term consequences. The surreptitious nature of the disease makes screening patients at high risk for infection especially important. Intravenous drug use remains the greatest risk factor for HCV. Less commonly, transmission occurs by hemodialysis, blood transfusion, perinatal exposure, intranasal drug use, body piercing, tattooing, sexual contact, and receipt of an organ transplant from an HCV-positive donor (Ghany et al. 2009). Transmission via transfusion declined markedly following routine screening for HCV antibodies beginning in 1992.

Higher-than-average prevalence of HCV infection is found in adults with severe psychiatric disorders (Nelligan et al. 2008), whose prevalence is up to 11 times greater than that of the general population and is linked to comorbid substance abuse (Loftis et al. 2006). More than 90% of injection drug users may be infected with HCV. Incarceration, homelessness, HIV infection, and alcoholism are also associated with increased prevalence of HCV infection (Crone et al. 2006; Nyamathi et al. 2002).

Standard treatment for HCV involves the use of pegylated interferon-alpha and ribavirin (IFN therapy) for 24–48 weeks. Treatment response is measured by sustained virological response, and overall response rates are 54%–56%. Adherence to treatment is an important factor in achieving sustained virological response. Maintaining adherence is a challenge given the length of treatment and multiple side effects, including anemia, leukopenia, fatigue, anorexia, insomnia, cognitive impairment, autoimmune thyroiditis, and psychiatric symptoms. Intolerable side effects are a common reason that patients discontinue treatment prematurely. Efforts to optimize adherence through close monitoring and management of troubling side effects are necessary.

IFN-Induced Depression

IFN-induced depression has been reported to occur in 10%–40% of patients, depending on study design, diagnostic criteria, assessment methods, and study population (Schafer et al. 2007). The incidence of depression is also influenced by the dose and duration of IFN therapy. Depressive symptoms usually develop within the first 12 weeks of treatment and are often accompanied by irritability rather than dysphoria. Symptoms usually resolve within a short time after IFN therapy is ended. Because of its effects on treatment adherence, efforts have been made to identify which patients are at greatest risk for IFN-induced depression. Several studies have found that baseline subclinical or clinical depression increases the risk of developing IFN-induced depression (Capuron and Ravaud 1999; Martin-Santos et al. 2008; Raison et al. 2005a, 2005b; Reichenberg et al. 2005). In contrast, a history of depression or other psychiatric disorder has not proved to be a significant risk factor. The mechanism behind IFN-induced depression is unknown but may be linked to its ability to induce production of proinflammatory cytokines (e.g., interleukin-6), alter the serotonergic system, or activate the HPA axis (Asnis and De La Garza 2006; Malek-Ahmadi and Hilsabeck 2007).

Management of IFN-induced depression requires prompt identification, followed by initiation of antidepressant therapy. Prophylactic antidepressant therapy has been considered; most studies report reduced incidence and severity of depressive symptoms (Gleason et al. 2007; Kraus et al. 2005a; Morasco et al. 2007; Raison et al. 2007). Nonetheless, this approach lacks support for all patients, partly because of the risks associated with antidepressants (e.g., GI hemorrhage). Support does exist for starting antidepressant therapy in patients with baseline subclinical or clinical depression. SSRIs have been the primary choice and have been effective and well tolerated (Kraus et al. 2008; Schaefer et al. 2005). Mirtazapine is an option for patients with marked insomnia and/or anorexia (Crone et al. 2006). Bupropion and venlafaxine are also reasonable options. Psychostimulants are an alternative, especially for patients with severe fatigue and cognitive slowing, but should be avoided in patients who have HCV with a history of substance abuse. Tryptophan as monotherapy or add-on therapy was recently reported as effective for three patients (Schaefer et al. 2008). It is notable that depressive symptoms may not be equally responsive to pharmacotherapy, with fatigue and anorexia less responsive than mood and cognition (Raison et al. 2005a).

IFN-Induced Hypomania or Mania and Psychosis

Reports of mood lability and irritability are not uncommon with IFN therapy, but frank mania is infrequent and usually requires treatment termination. Most often, hypomania or mania appears to develop after weeks or months of treatment, but cases have been reported of mania appearing after marked dose reduction or abrupt discontinuation of IFN (Constant et al. 2005; Malik and Ravasia 2004; Onyike et al. 2004). The course of IFN-induced hypomania or mania is unclear, but most cases report resolution of symptoms after psychotropic medications are started and IFN therapy stopped. Reports of IFN-induced psychosis are rare (Bozikas et al. 2001; Hoffman et al. 2003; Tamam et al. 2003). Most are accompanied by significant mood disturbance. For hypomania, mania, and psychosis, atypical antipsychotics are likely the best option. Mood stabilizers are a consideration, but the risk of lithium-induced hypothyroidism and carbamazepine-induced hematological disturbances requires caution because they may aggravate similar problems caused by IFN therapy.

IFN-Induced Cognitive Impairment

Patients often report cognitive problems during IFN therapy, including difficulties with memory, concentration, and problem solving. IFN affects the frontal-subcortical system, producing problems with working memory and complex attention (Kraus et al. 2005b; Pawelczk et al. 2008; Perry et al. 2008). The effect depends on the dosage, duration, and route of administration of IFN. The means by which IFN causes cognitive dysfunction are unknown, although PET scans have detected hypometabolism in the prefrontal cortex (Juengling et al. 2000). Functional MRI shows activation of the anterior cingulate cortex, which may produce difficulties in error recognition or processing (Capuron et al. 2005). However, some investigators have been unable to identify objective evidence of cognitive impairment and hypothesize that symptoms are only subjective in nature (Fontana et al. 2007). Regardless, cognitive dysfunction appears to be independent of depressive symptoms and normally resolves after IFN is discontinued (Kraus et al. 2005b; Reichenberg et al. 2005). Frank delirium is rare.

IFN-Induced Fatigue

For many patients, fatigue is the most troubling side effect because of its persistence and overall effect on daily function. IFN-induced fatigue may be associated with alterations in the basal ganglia, including the nucleus accumbens and putamen (Capuron et al. 2007). Some patients may benefit from erythropoietin (if anemic) or thyroid hormone supplementation (if hypothyroid). SSRIs may not significantly lessen IFN-induced fatigue, but stimulants such as modafinil might be effective (Martin et al. 2007); however, data are lacking.

High-Risk Populations for IFN Therapy

Because of the need for treatment adherence and the frequency of psychiatric side effects, concerns have been raised about the ability of patients with preexisting psychiatric and/or substance abuse disorders to undergo successful IFN therapy. Fears about their inability to adhere to treatment and potentially higher risk for psychiatric side effects led many to be excluded from treatment. Subsequent studies involving high-risk populations showed that successful treatment was possible, even though some groups noted higher dropout rates and lower rates of virological response (Robaeys and Buntinx 2005; Schaefer et al. 2007; Sylvestre and Clements 2007). At this time, most treatment guidelines recommend that high-risk patients be assessed on a case-by-case basis and that treatment involve careful planning and coordination of care between mental health and hepatology providers (Ghany et al. 2009).

Hepatic Encephalopathy

Hepatic encephalopathy is a clinical condition characterized by disturbances of consciousness, mood, behavior, and cognition, which occur in the presence of acute or chronic liver disease. It is estimated to occur in 50%–70% of patients with cirrhosis and varies from mild cognitive impairment to gross confusion and disorientation to coma. The pathophysiology of hepatic encephalopathy is poorly understood but may involve ammonia, astrocyte swelling, and formation of reactive oxygen and nitric oxide species, all contributing to alterations in brain function (Haussinger and Schliess 2008; Lemberg and Fernandez 2009; Schliess et al. 2009). Other possible contributors include neurosteroids, endogenous benzodiazepine receptor ligands, inflammatory cytokines, manganese, mercaptans, and octanoic acid (Ahboucha and Butterworth 2008; Butterworth 2008; Rovira et al. 2008). Diagnosis of hepatic encephalopathy is by exclusion of other causes of mental status changes in patients with significant liver disease (e.g., infections, substance abuse, intracranial hemorrhage). Psychometric testing (e.g., Digit Symbol, Line Tracing, Trail-Making Tests/Parts A and B) can be helpful, especially when cognitive impairment is subtle (Crone et al. 2006). Electroencephalogram findings usually show generalized slowing; triphasic waves may be present but are not specific to hepatic encephalopathy (Kaplan 2004). Abnormal P300 event-related potentials reflect underlying impairments in cognitive processing (Saxena et al. 2001). Venous ammonia levels are elevated in many, but not all, patients.

Management of hepatic encephalopathy primarily involves correction of precipitating factors (e.g., infection, hyponatremia, acidosis or alkalosis, constipation, psychoactive medications, GI hemorrhage) (Sundaram and Shaikh 2009). Nonabsorbable disaccharides and nonantibiotics are routinely prescribed, but the evidence for efficacy is lacking (Als-Nielsen et al. 2004b). The benzodiazepine receptor antagonist flumazenil also has been used; two systematic reviews of the literature concluded that treatment of hepatic encephalopathy with flumazenil produced significant symptomatic improvement, but the benefit was short-lived, with no significant benefit on recovery or survival, and flumazenil may provoke withdrawal seizures in patients with benzodiazepine dependence (Als-Nielsen et al. 2004a; Goulenok et al. 2002). Other suggested treatments have included L-acetylcarnitine and ornithine aspartate, but evidence is insufficient to recommend their use (Sundaram and Shaikh 2009). See also Chapter 31, "Organ Transplantation."

Psychopharmacology in Liver Disease

In the face of hepatic dysfunction, added care is required when selecting and prescribing psychotropic drugs. No medications are absolutely contraindicated in patients with liver disease, but some carry a greater risk of significant hepatic toxicity (e.g., nefazodone), and some have a narrower therapeutic window (e.g., lithium, clozapine). Patients with liver disease who have hepatic encephalopathy are particularly sensitive to sedative-hypnotics (e.g., benzodiazepines, barbiturates). Hepatic dysfunction alters the absorption, distribution, metabolism, and excretion of most psychotropic agents. However, no specific biochemical test or marker can provide a direct measure of the degree of altered pharmacokinetics present in a selected patient. Rather, the Child-Pugh Scale (CPS) score can be used to provide a rough guideline for dosing medications (Table 20-1) (Albers et al. 1989; Crone et al. 2006). Among patients with CPS score A, mild hepatic failure or cirrhosis, most can tolerate 75%-100% of the usual starting dose of most psychotropic drugs. For patients with CPS score B, moderate hepatic failure or cirrhosis, a 50%-75% reduction in starting dose is warranted, along with smaller incremental dosing to compensate for a prolonged elimination half-life. Patients with CPS score B often can be successfully treated with 50% of the conventional dose of psychotropic medications. Among patients with CPS score C, severe hepatic failure or cirrhosis, cautious dosing and titration are needed, along with careful monitoring for potential drug-induced worsening of cognitive status (Crone et al. 2006; DiMartini et al. 2010). See also "Hepatic Disease" in Chapter 38, "Psychopharmacology."

TABLE 20-1. Child-Pugh Scale

Factor	1 Point	2 Points	3 Points
Serum bilirubin (μmol/L)	≤34	35-50	≥51
Serum albumin (g/dL)	>3.5	3.0-3.5	<3.0
Prothrombin time (s)	<4	4-6	>6
International normalized ratio (INR)	<1.7	1.7-2.3	>2.3
Ascites	None	Slight, medically controlled	Moderate-severe, poorly controlled
Encephalopathy	None	Stage 1-2	Stage 3-4
Total score[a]	5-6	7-9	10-15
Child-Pugh Scale score	A	B	C

[a]Combine scores together from all five factors.

Drug-Induced Liver Disease

Drug-induced liver disease spans from mild asymptomatic transaminase elevations to rare cases of fulminant hepatic failure. Most cases are idiosyncratic and therefore unpredictable, are not dose dependent, and develop after a variable time taking the drug in question. Fortunately, liver injury usually resolves after the drug is discontinued, but this may take up to a year. Risk factors for drug-induced liver disease include obesity, malnutrition, genetic polymorphisms, alcohol abuse, and adulthood (Hussaini and Farrington 2007; Navarro and Senior 2006). Women appear to be more susceptible to severe drug-induced liver disease (Hussaini and Farrington 2007). Patients with preexisting liver disease are not clearly at greater risk for drug-induced liver disease but have less hepatic reserve if injury occurs (Russo and Watkins 2004). There are three types of drug-induced liver disease: hepatocellular, cholestatic, and mixed. Hepatocellular damage causes a significant elevation in alanine aminotransferase relative to alkaline phosphatase, whereas the latter is increased with cholestatic injury. Most psychotropic medications present some risk of hepatotoxicity, but the risks are very low (Lucena et al. 2003; McIntyre et al. 2008; Norris et al. 2008). For most patients, routine monitoring of liver function tests while taking a particular drug is not recommended because of the idiosyncratic nature of drug-induced liver disease (Navarro and Senior 2006). Because it is unclear which patients may progress to severe liver injury, suspected medications should be discontinued in patients who develop alanine aminotransferase elevations three times the upper limit of normal, increases in bilirubin or international normalized ratio (INR), or symptoms of hepatic dysfunction (e.g., right upper quadrant pain, dark urine, pruritus, jaundice, nausea, anorexia) (Navarro and Senior 2006).

Pancreatic Disorders

Drug-Induced Pancreatitis

Drug-induced pancreatitis is a rare cause of acute pancreatitis, accounting for only 0.1%–2% of cases among the general population (Dhir et al. 2007). Timely recognition and diagnosis are needed to avoid serious consequences of acute pancreatitis (e.g., chronic pancreatitis, multiorgan failure, death) (Kaurich 2008). Patients with HIV, cancer, and Crohn's disease and those taking multiple medications are at greatest risk for drug-induced pancreatitis (Dhir et al. 2007). Most cases develop within a few weeks to months of starting a particular drug and are not dose related. The mechanism behind drug-induced pancreatitis is unclear (Kaurich 2008). Valproic acid is the psychotropic drug most often reported in cases of drug-induced pancreatitis, although the true incidence is 1 in 40,000 (Ben Salem et al. 2007; Gerstner et al. 2007; Zaccara et al. 2007). Transient asymptomatic hyperamylasemia, which occurs in 20% of adults taking valproic acid, does not increase the risk for pancreatitis (Zaccara et al. 2007). Rarely, pancreatitis has occurred with other anticonvulsants, including carbamazepine, gabapentin, lamotrigine, and topiramate (Jadresic 1994; Kaurich 2008; Soman and Swenson 1985; Zaccara et al. 2007). Among antipsychotic agents, clozapine and olanzapine have been associated with the most reported cases, fewer with risperidone and haloperidol, and more rarely with the other atypical antipsychotics (Cerulli 1999; Garlipp et al. 2002; Gropper and Jackson 2004; Hanft and Bourgeois 2004; Kahn and Bourgeois 2007; Koller et al. 2003; Reddymasu et al. 2006; Yang and McNeely 2002). Mirtazapine has been associated with several cases of drug-induced pancreatitis, and bupropion, venlafaxine, and SSRIs are occasionally causative agents (Hussain and Burke 2008; Kaurich 2008; Spigset et al. 2003).

Discontinuation of the offending drug usually results in resolution of pancreatitis within 10 days (Dhir et al. 2007). Following an episode of drug-induced pancreatitis, rechallenge with the same drug is discouraged because of the risk of recurrence. Substitution with another drug in the same class is an acceptable alternative (Dhir et al. 2007).

Pancreatic Cancer

Although pancreatic cancer represents only 2% of all cancer diagnoses in the United States, it is the fourth leading cause of cancer-related deaths (Boyd and Riba 2007; Cardenes et al. 2006). Mean survival is 1 year. Physical symptoms resulting from pancreatic cancer, including fatigue, weight loss, pain, and jaundice, tend to develop late (Hochster et al. 2006). As a result, most patients do not receive a diagnosis until they have advanced disease (Cardenes et al. 2006; Thomson et al. 2006). For decades, investigators have noted a higher-than-expected prevalence of depression among pancreatic cancer patients, even when compared with those who have other types of GI malignancies (Boyd and Riba 2007; Carney et al. 2003; Green and Austin 1993; Passik and Breitbart 1996). Furthermore, one-third to one-half of patients experience anxiety and depressive symptoms before receiving the diagnosis of pancreatic cancer (Passik and Breitbart 1996). The factors contributing to the relation between anxiety, depression, and pancreatic cancer are unknown. Various theories have been proposed, including a paraneoplastic syndrome (Makrilia et al. 2009). Pain is a frequent problem among pancreatic cancer patients and is also likely to contribute to depression (Kelsen et al. 1995). See also Chapter 23, "Oncology."

Conclusion

As noted at the beginning of this chapter, GI disorders span several organ systems responsible for helping to maintain physiological homeostasis through assistance with oral intake, digestion, absorption, and metabolism. Disorders affecting these organ systems produce considerable disruption in daily function, productivity, overall health, long-term survival, and QOL. Psychological distress secondary to GI disorders is perhaps not surprising, but it also may precede the onset of a GI disorder and possibly contribute to its development, clinical course, and subsequent treatment response. The effect of psychological factors or distress is particularly notable for functional GI disorders, which lack clear evidence of physiological or structural abnormalities. Increasing evidence indicates a strong link between the brain and the gut that helps to explain this interaction between psychological factors and GI disorders. Psychotherapeutic and psychopharmacological approaches can be beneficial to GI patients, even in the absence of clear psychopathology resulting from the effect on central brain-gut mechanisms.

References

Aapro MS, Molassiotis A, Olver I: Anticipatory nausea and vomiting. Support Care Cancer 13:117–121, 2005

Abdul-Baki H, El Hajj II, El Zahabi L, et al: A randomized controlled trial of imipramine in patients with irritable bowel syndrome. World J Gastroenterol 15:3636–3642, 2009

Abell TL, Adams KA, Boles RG, et al: Cyclic vomiting syndrome in adults. Neurogastroenterol Motil 20:269–284, 2008

Ahboucha S, Butterworth RF: The neurosteroid system: implication in the pathophysiology of hepatic encephalopathy. Neurochem Int 52:575–587, 2008

Albers I, Hartmann H, Bircher J, et al: Superiority of the Child-Pugh classification to quantitative liver function tests for assessing prognosis of liver cirrhosis. Scand J Gastroenterol 24:269–276, 1989

Als-Nielsen B, Gluud LL, Gluud C: Benzodiazepine receptor antagonists for hepatic encephalopathy. Cochrane Database Syst Rev (2):CD002798, 2004a

Als-Nielsen B, Gluud LL, Gluud C: Nonabsorbable disaccharides for hepatic encephalopathy. Cochrane Database Syst Rev (2):CD003044, 2004b

American Gastroenterological Association: American Gastroenterological Association medical position statement: evaluation of dyspepsia. Gastroenterology 129:1753–1755, 2005

Andersen OK, Bergsaker-Aspoy J, Halvorsen L, et al: Doxepin in the treatment of duodenal ulcer: a double-blind clinical study comparing doxepin and placebo. Scand J Gastroenterol 19:923–925, 1984

Andersson RE, Olaison G, Tysk C, et al: Appendectomy and protection against ulcerative colitis. N Engl J Med 344:808–814, 2001

Arebi N, Gurmany S, Bullas D, et al: Review article: the psychoneuroimmunology of irritable bowel syndrome: an exploration of interactions between psychological, neurological, and immunological observations. Aliment Pharmacol Ther 28:830–840, 2008

Asnis GM, De La Garza R: Interferon-induced depression in chronic hepatitis C: a review of its prevalence, risk factors, biology, and treatment approaches. J Clin Gastroenterol 40:322–335, 2006

Attri N, Ravipati M, Agrawal P, et al: Rumination syndrome: an emerging case scenario. South Med J 101:432–435, 2008

Avidan B, Sonnenberg A, Giblovich H, et al: Reflux symptoms are associated with psychiatric disease. Aliment Pharmacol Ther 15:1907–1912, 2001

Avidan B, Sonnenberg A, Schnell TG, et al: Acid reflux is a poor predictor for severity of erosive reflux esophagitis. Dig Dis Sci 47:2565–2573, 2002

Baena JM, Lopez C, Hidalgo A, et al: Relation between alcohol consumption and the success of Helicobacter pylori eradication therapy using omeprazole, clarithromycin and amoxicillin for 1 week. Eur J Gastroenterol Hepatol 14:291–296, 2002

Barratt HS, Kalantzis C, Polymeros D, et al: Functional symptoms in inflammatory bowel disease and their potential influence in misclassification of clinical status. Aliment Pharmacol Ther 21:141–147, 2005

Bates S, Sjoden P-O, Nyren O: Behavioral treatment of non-ulcer dyspepsia. Cognitive Behaviour Therapy 17:155–165, 1988

Ben Salem C, Biour M, Hmouda H, et al: Valproic acid-induced pancreatitis. J Gastroenterol 42:598–599, 2007

Bergdhal J, Anneroth G, Perris H: Cognitive therapy in the treatment of patients with resistant burning mouth syndrome: a controlled study. J Oral Pathol Med 24:213–215, 1995

Bishop LC, Riley WT: The psychiatric management of globus hystericus. Gen Hosp Psychiatry 10:214–219, 1988

Bitton A, Sewitch MJ, Peppercorn MA, et al: Psychosocial determinants of relapse in ulcerative colitis: a longitudinal study. Am J Gastroenterol 98:2203–2208, 2003

Bogetto F, Maina G, Ferro G, et al: Psychiatric comorbidity in patients with burning mouth syndrome. Psychosom Med 60:378–385, 1998

Boone SA, Shields KM: Treating pregnancy-related nausea and vomiting with ginger. Ann Pharmaother 39:1710–1713, 2005

Borrelli F, Capasso R, Aviello G, et al: Effectiveness and safety of ginger in the treatment of pregnancy-induced nausea and vomiting. Am Coll Obstet Gynecol 105:849–856, 2005

Bottomley C, Bourne T: Management strategies for hyperemesis. Best Pract Res Clin Obstet Gynaecol 23:549–564, 2009

Bouras EP, Talley NJ, Camilleri M, et al: Effects of amitriptyline on gastric sensorimotor function and postprandial symptoms in healthy individuals: a randomized, double-blind, placebo-controlled trial. Am J Gastroenterol 103:2043–2050, 2008

Boyd AD, Riba M: Depression and pancreatic cancer. J Natl Compr Canc Netw 5:113–116, 2007

Bozikas V, Petrikis P, Balla A, et al: An interferon-α-induced psychotic disorder in a patient with chronic hepatitis C. Eur Psychiatry 16:136–137, 2001

Bradley LA, Richter JE, Pulliam TJ, et al: The relationship between stress and symptoms of gastroesophageal reflux: the influence of psychological factors. Am J Gastroenterol 88:11–19, 1993

Brandt LJ, Chey WD, Orenstein AE, et al: An evidence-based systematic review on the management of irritable bowel syndrome. American College of Gastroenterology IBS Task Force. Am J Gastroenterol 104:S8–S35, 2009

Braus NA, Elliott DE: Advances in the pathogenesis and treatment of IBD. Clin Immunol 132:1–9, 2009

Brennan BP, Fogarty KV, Roberts JL, et al: Duloxetine in the treatment of irritable bowel syndrome: am open label pilot study. Hum Psychopharmacol Clin Exp 24:423–428, 2009

Brown SR, Schwartz JM, Summergrad P, et al: Globus hystericus syndrome responsive to antidepressants. Am J Psychiatry 143:917–918, 1986

Brustholm D, Ribeiro-dos-Santos R, Kast RE, et al: A new chapter opens in anti-inflammatory treatments: the antidepressant bupropion lowers production of tumor necrosis factor-alpha and interferon-gamma in mice. Int Immunopharmacol 6:903–907, 2006

Butterworth RF: Pathophysiology of hepatic encephalopathy: the concept of synergism. Hepatol Res 38 (suppl 1):S116–S121, 2008

Calvert EL, Houghton LA, Cooper P, et al: Long-term improvement in functional dyspepsia using hypnotherapy. Gastroenterology 123:1778–1785, 2002

Camilleri M, Dubois D, Coulie B, et al: Prevalence and socioeconomic impact of upper gastrointestinal disorders in the United States: results of the US Upper Gastrointestinal Study. Clin Gastroenterol Hepatol 3:543–552, 2005

Cannon RO, Quyyumi AA, Mincemoyer R, et al: Imipramine in patients with chest pain despite normal coronary angiograms. N Engl J Med 330:1411–1417, 1994

Caprilli R, Gassull MA, Escher JC, et al: European evidence-based consensus on the diagnosis and management of Crohn's disease: special situations. Gut 55 (suppl I):i36–i58, 2006

Capuron L, Ravaud A: Prediction of the depressive effects on interferon alfa therapy by the patient's initial affective state. N Engl J Med 340:1370, 1999

Capuron L, Pagnoni G, Demetrashvilli M, et al: Anterior cingulate activation and error processing during interferon-alpha treatment. Biol Psychiatry 58:190–196, 2005

Capuron L, Pagnoni G, Demetrashvilli MF, et al: Basal ganglia hypermetabolism and symptoms of fatigue during interferon-α therapy. Neuropsychopharmacology 32:2384–2392, 2007

Cardenes HR, Chiorean EG, DeWitt J, et al: Locally advanced pancreatic cancer: current therapeutic approach. Oncologist 11:612–623, 2006

Carney CP, Jones L, Woolson RF, et al: Relationship between depression and pancreatic cancer in the general population. Psychosom Med 65:884–888, 2003

Caylakli F, Yavuz H, Erkan AN, et al: Evaluation of patients with globus pharyngeus with barium swallow pharyngoesophagography. Laryngoscope 116:37–39, 2006

Cerulli TR: Clozapine-associated pancreatitis. Harv Rev Psychiatry 7:61–63, 1999

Chahal PS, Rao SS: Functional chest pain: nociception and visceral hyperalgesia. J Clin Gastroenterol 39:S204–S209, 2005

Chepyala P, Svoboda RP, Olden KW: Treatment of cyclic vomiting syndrome. Curr Treat Options Gastroenterol 10:273–282, 2007

Chiossi G, Neri I, Cavazzuti M, et al: Hyperemesis gravidarum complicated by Wernicke encephalopathy: background, case report, and review of the literature. Obstet Gynecol Survey 61:255–268, 2006

Choung RS, Cremonini F, Thapa P, et al: The effect of short-term, low-dose tricyclic and tetracyclic antidepressant treatment on satiation, postnutrient load gastrointestinal symptoms and gastric emptying: a double-blind, randomized, placebo-controlled trial. Neurogastroenterol Motil 20:220–227, 2008

Choung RS, Locke GR, Zinsmeister AR, et al: Psychosocial distress and somatic symptoms in community subjects with irritable bowel syndrome: a psychological component is the rule. Am J Gastroenterol 104:1772–1779, 2009

Christodoulou GN, Alevizos BH, Konstantakakis E: Peptic ulcer in adults: psychopathological, environmental, characterological and hereditary factors. Psychother Psychosom 39:55–62, 1983

Clark DB: Dental care for the patient with bipolar disorder. J Can Dent Assoc 69:20–24, 2003

Clouse RE, Lustman PJ, Eckert TC, et al: Low-dose trazodone for symptomatic patients with esophageal contraction abnormalities: a double-blind, placebo-controlled trial. Gastroenterology 92:1027–1036, 1987

Coffin B, Dapoigny M, Cloarec D, et al: Relationship between severity of symptoms and quality of life in 858 patients with irritable bowel syndrome. Gastroenterol Clin Biol 28:11–15, 2004

Constant A, Castera L, Dantzer R, et al: Mood alterations during interferon-alfa therapy in patients with chronic hepatitis C: evidence for an overlap between manic/hypomanic and depressive symptoms. J Clin Psychiatry 66:1050–1057, 2005

Creed F, Guthrie E, Ratcliffe J, et al: Reported sexual abuse predicts impaired functioning but a good response to psychological treatment in patients with severe irritable bowel syndrome. Psychosom Med 67:490–499, 2005

Crone CC, Gabriel GM, DiMartini A: An overview of psychiatric issues in liver disease for the consultation-liaison psychiatrist. Psychosomatics 47:188–205, 2006

Dalton SO, Sorenson HT, Johansen C: SSRIs and upper gastrointestinal bleeding: what is known and how should it influence prescribing? CNS Drugs 20:143–151, 2006

de Abajo FJ, García-Rodríguez LA: Risk of upper gastrointestinal tract bleeding associated with selective serotonin reuptake inhibitors and venlafaxine therapy: interaction with nonsteroidal anti-inflammatory drugs and effect of acid-suppressing agents. Arch Gen Psychiatry 65:795–803, 2008 de Abajo FJ, Rodríguez LA, Montero D: Association between selective serotonin reuptake inhibitors and upper gastrointestinal bleeding: population based case-control study. BMJ 319:1106–1109, 1999

Dent J, Dodds WJ, Friedman RH, et al: Mechanism of gastroesophageal reflux in recumbent asymptomatic human subjects. J Clin Invest 65:256–267, 1980

Dent J, El-Serag HB, Wallander M-A, et al: Epidemiology of gastro-esophageal reflux disease: a systematic review. Gut 54:710–717, 2005

Deter HC, Keller W, von Wietersheim J, et al: Psychological treatment may reduce the need for healthcare in patients with Crohn's disease. Inflamm Bowel Dis 13:745–752, 2007

Dhir R, Brown DK, Olden KW: Drug-induced pancreatitis: a practical review. Drugs Today (Barc) 43:499–507, 2007

Dienstag JL, McHutchinson JG: American Gastroenterological Association technical review on the management of hepatitis C. Gastroenterology 130:231–264, 2006

DiMartini AF, Crone CC, Fireman M: Organ transplantation, in Clinical Manual of Psychopharmacology in the Medically Ill. Edited by Ferrando SJ, Levenson JL, Owen JA. Arlington, VA, American Psychiatric Publishing, 2010, pp 469–499

Doraiswamy PM, Varia I, Hellegers C, et al: A randomized controlled trial of paroxetine for noncardiac chest pain. Psychopharmacol Bull 39:15–24, 2006

Dorn SD, Palsson OS, Thiwan SI, et al: Increased colonic pain sensitivity in irritable bowel syndrome is the result of an increased tendency to report pain rather than increased neurosensory sensitivity. Gut 56:1202–1209, 2007

Drossman DA (ed): Rome III: The Functional Gastrointestinal Disorders, 3rd Edition. McLean, VA, Degnon Associates, 2006

Drossman DA, Leserman J, Li ZM, et al: The rating form of IBD patient concerns: a new measure of health status. Psychosom Med 53:701–712, 1991

Drossman DA, Toner BB, Whitehead WE, et al: Cognitive-behavioral therapy versus education and desipramine versus placebo for moderate to severe functional bowel disorders. Gastroenterology 125:249–253, 2003

Dulude E, Desilets DJ, Boles RG: Up to Date—Cyclic Vomiting Syndrome 2008. Available at: http://www.uptodate.com. Accessed June 19, 2009.

Dunlop SP, Jenkins D, Neal KR, et al: Relative importance of enterochromaffin cell hyperplasia, anxiety, and depression in postinfectious IBS. Gastroenterology 125:1651–1659, 2003

Dziewas R, Warnecke T, Schnabel M, et al: Neuroleptic-induced dysphagia: case report and literature review. Dysphagia 22:63–67, 2007

Elsenbruch S, Langhorst J, Popkirowa K, et al: Effects of mind-body therapy on quality of life and neuroendocrine and cellular immune functions in patients with ulcerative colitis. Psychother Psychosom 74:277–287, 2005

Eslick GD, Talley NJ: Gastroesophageal reflux disease (GERD): risk factors, and impact on quality of life—a population-based study. J Clin Gastroenterol 43:111–117, 2009

Ezzo JM, Richardson MA, Vickers A, et al: Acupuncture-point stimulation for chemotherapy-induced nausea or vomiting. Cochrane Database Syst Rev (2):CD002285, 2006

Farrokhyar F, Marshall JK, Easterbrook B, et al: Functional gastrointestinal disorders and mood disorders in patients with inactive inflammatory bowel disease: prevalence and impact on health. Inflamm Bowel Dis 12:38–46, 2006

Fass R, Dickman R: Non-cardiac chest pain: an update. Neurogastroenterol Motil 18:408–417, 2006

Fass R, Naliboff BD, Fass SS, et al: The effect of auditory stress on perception of intraesophageal acid in patients with gastroesophageal reflux disease. Gastroenterology 134:696–705, 2008

Feeney K, Cain M, Nowak AK: Chemotherapy induced nausea and vomiting: prevention and treatment. Aust Fam Physician 36:702–706, 2007

Feldman M, Walker P, Green JL, et al: Life events stress and psychosocial factors in men with peptic ulcer disease: a multidimensional case-controlled study. Gastroenterology 91:1370–1379, 1986

Femiano F, Scully C: Burning mouth syndrome (BMS): double-blind controlled study of alpha lipoic acid (thioctic acid) therapy. J Oral Pathol Med 31:267–269, 2002

Figueroa-Moseley C, Jean-Pierre P, Roscoe JA, et al: Behavioral interventions in treating anticipatory nausea and vomiting. J Natl Compr Canc Netw 5:44–50, 2007

Finkenbine R, Miele VJ: Globus hystericus: a brief review. Gen Hosp Psychiatry 26:78–82, 2004

Fleisher DR, Gornowicz B, Adams K, et al: Cyclic vomiting syndrome in 41 adults: the illness, the patients, and problems of management. BMC Med 3:20, 2005

Fontana RJ, Bieliauskas LA, Lindsay KL, et al: Cognitive function does not worsen during pegylated interferon and ribavirin retreatment of chronic hepatitis C. Hepatology 45:1154–1163, 2007

Ford AC, Talley NJ, Schoenfeld PS, et al: Efficacy of antidepressants and psychological therapies in irritable bowel syndrome: systematic review and meta-analysis. Gut 58:367–378, 2009

Frank L, Kleinman L, Rentz A, et al: Health-related quality of life associated with irritable bowel syndrome: comparison with other chronic diseases. Clin Ther 24:675–689, 2002

Friedlander AH, Mahler ME: Major depressive disorder: psychopathology, medical management and dental implications. J Am Dent Assoc 132:629–638, 2001

Friedlander AH, Marder SR, Sung EC, et al: Panic disorder: psychopathology, medical management and dental implications. J Am Dent Assoc 135:771–778, 2004

Fuller-Thomson E, Sulman J: Depression and inflammatory bowel disease: findings from two nationally representative Canadian surveys. Inflamm Bowel Dis 12:697–707, 2006

Garlipp P, Rosenthal O, Haltenhof H, et al: The development of a clinical syndrome of asymptomatic pancreatitis and eosinophilia after treatment with clozapine in schizophrenia: implications for clinical care, recognition, and management. J Psychopharmacol 16:399–400, 2002

Garlow SJ, Purselle D, D'Orior B: Psychiatric emergencies, in Essentials of Clinical Psychopharmacology, 2nd Edition. Edited by Schatzberg AF, Nemeroff CB. Washington, DC, American Psychiatric Publishing, 2006, pp 707–724

Gathaiya N, Locke GR 3rd, Camilleri M, et al: Novel associations with dyspepsia: a community-based study of familial aggregation, sleep dysfunction and somatization. Neurogastroenterol Motil 21:922–e69, 2009

Gerstner T, Busing D, Bell N, et al: Valproic acid-induced pancreatitis: 16 new cases and a review of the literature. J Gastroenterol 42:38–48, 2007

Ghany MG, Strader DB, Thomas DL, et al: Diagnosis, management, and treatment of hepatitis C: an update. Hepatology 49:1335–1374, 2009

Gill SK, Einarson A: The safety of drugs for the treatment of nausea and vomiting of pregnancy. Expert Opin Drug Saf 6:685–694, 2007

Gleason OC, Fucci JC, Yates WR, et al: Preventing relapse of major depression during interferon-α therapy for hepatitis C: a pilot study. Dig Dis Sci 52:2557–2563, 2007

Goodwin RD, Keyes KM, Stein MB, et al: Peptic ulcer and mental disorders among adults in the community: the role of nicotine and alcohol use disorders. Psychosom Med 71:463–468, 2009

Goodwin TM: Hyperemesis gravidarum. Obstet Gynecol Clin N Am 35:401–417, 2008

Gordon A, Gordon E, Berelowitz M, et al: Biofeedback improvement of lower esophageal sphincter pressures and reflux symptoms. J Clin Gastroenterol 5:235–237, 1983

Goulenok C, Bernard B, Cadranel JF, et al: Flumazenil vs. placebo in hepatic encephalopathy in patients with cirrhosis: a meta-analysis. Aliment Pharmacol Ther 16:361–372, 2002

Gralnek IM, Hays RD, Kilbourne A, et al: The impact of irritable bowel syndrome on health-related quality of life. Gastroenterology 119:654–660, 2000

Green AI, Austin CP: Psychopathology of pancreatic cancer: a psychobiologic probe. Psychosomatics 34:208–221, 1993

Greene BR, Blanchard EB, Wan CK: Long-term monitoring of psychosocial stress and symptomatology in inflammatory bowel disease. Behav Res Ther 32:217–226, 1994

Gremeau-Richard C, Woda A, Navez ML, et al: Topical clonazepam in stomatodynia: a randomized placebo-controlled study. Pain 108:51–57, 2004

Gropper D, Jackson CW: Pancreatitis associated with quetiapine use. J Clin Psychopharmacol 24:343–345, 2004

Grover M, Herfarth H, Drossman DA: The functional-organic dichotomy: postinfectious irritable bowel syndrome and inflammatory bowel disease-irritable bowel syndrome. Clin Gastroenterol Hepatol 7:48–53, 2009

Grushka M, Epstein J, Mott A: An open-label, dose escalation pilot study of the effect of clonazepam in burning mouth syndrome. Oral Surg Oral Med Pathol Oral Radiol Endod 86:557–561, 1998

Grushka M, Epstein JB, Gorsky M: Burning mouth syndrome. Am Fam Physician 65:615–620, 2002

Guclu S, Gol M, Dogan E, et al: Mirtazapine use in resistant hyperemesis gravidarum: report of three cases and review of the literature. Arch Gynecol Obstet 272:298–300, 2005

Guggenheimer J, Moore PA: Xerostomia: etiology, recognition and treatment. J Am Dent Assoc 134:61–69, 2003

Guttuso T, Roscoe J, Griggs J: Effect of gabapentin on nausea induced by chemotherapy in breast cancer patients. Lancet 361:1703–1705, 2003

Guyatt G, Mitchell A, Irvine EJ, et al: A new measure of health status for clinical trials in inflammatory bowel disease Gastroenterology 96:804–810, 1989

Gwee KA: Irritable bowel syndrome in developing countries: a disorder of civilization or colonization? Neurogastoenterol Motil 17:317–324, 2005

Gwee KA, Leong YL, Graham C, et al: The role of psychological and biological factors in postinfective gut dysfunction. Gut 44:400–406, 1999

Haag S, Senf W, Hauser W, et al: Impairment of health-related quality of life in functional dyspepsia and chronic liver disease: the influence of depression and anxiety. Aliment Pharmacol Ther 27:561–571, 2008

Halder SLS, McBeth J, Silman AJ, et al: Psychosocial risk factors for the onset of abdominal pain: results from a large prospective population-based study. Int J Epidemiol 31:1219–1225, 2002

Halpert A, Dalton CB, Diamant NE, et al: Clinical response to tricyclic antidepressants in functional bowel disorders is not related to dosage. Am J Gastroenterol 100:664–671, 2005

Hamilton J, Guthrie E, Creed F, et al: A randomized controlled trial of psychotherapy in patients with chronic functional dyspepsia. Gastroenterology 119:661–669, 2000

Han SW, McColl E, Barton JR, et al: Predictors of quality of life in ulcerative colitis: the importance of symptoms and illness representations. Inflamm Bowel Dis 11:24–34, 2005

Hanft A, Bourgeois J: Risperidone and pancreatitis. J Am Acad Child Adolesc Psychiatry 43:1458–1459, 2004

Harris LA, Chang L: Irritable bowel syndrome: new and emerging therapies. Curr Opin Gastroenterol 22:128–135, 2006

Hasler WL: Management of gastroparesis. Expert Rev Gastroenterol Hepatol 2:411–423, 2008

Haug TT, Wilhelmsen I, Svebak S, et al: Psychotherapy in functional dyspepsia. J Psychosom Res 38:735–744, 1994

Haug TT, Wilhelmsen I, Berstad A, et al: Life events and stress in patients with functional dyspepsia compared with patients with duodenal ulcer and healthy controls. Scand J Gastroenterol 30:524–530, 1995

Haussinger D, Schliess F: Pathogenetic mechanisms of hepatic encephalopathy. Gut 57:1156–1165, 2008

Helin-Salmivaara A, Huttunen T, Gronroos JM, et al: Risk of serious upper gastrointestinal events with concurrent use of NSAIDs and SSRIs: a case-control study in the general population. Eur J Clin Pharmacol 63:403–408, 2007

Hickok JT, Roscoe JA, Morrow GR: The role of patients' expectations in the development of anticipatory nausea related to chemotherapy for cancer. J Pain Symptom Manage 22:843–850, 2001

Hobson AR, Furlong PL, Sarkar S, et al: Neurophysiologic assessment of esophageal sensory processing in noncardiac chest pain. Gastroenterology 130:80–88, 2006

Hochster HS, Haller DG, de Gramont A, et al: Consensus report of the International Society of Gastrointestinal Oncology on therapeutic progress in advanced pancreatic cancer. Cancer 107:678–685, 2006

Hoffman RG, Cohen MA, Alfonso CA, et al: Treatment of interferon-induced psychosis in patients with comorbid hepatitis C and HIV. Psychosomatics 44:417–420, 2003

Hussain A, Burke J: Mirtazapine associated with recurrent pancreatitis—a case report. J Psychopharmacol 22:336–337, 2008

Hussaini SH, Farrington EA: Idiosyncratic drug-induced liver injury: an overview. Expert Opin Drug Saf 6:673–684, 2007

Hyphantis TN, Tomenson B, Bai M, et al: Psychological distress, somatization, and defense mechanisms associated with quality of life in inflammatory bowel disease patients. Dig Dis Sci 55:724–732, 2010

Irvine EJ: Quality of life of patients with ulcerative colitis: past, present, and future. Inflamm Bowel Dis 14:554–556, 2008

Jadresic D: Acute pancreatitis associated with dual vigabatrin and lamotrigine therapy. Seizure 3:319, 1994

Janke KH, Klump B, Gregor M, et al: Determinants of life satisfaction in inflammatory bowel disease. Inflamm Bowel Dis 11:272–286, 2005

Jansson C, Nordenstedt H, Wallander M-A, et al: Severe gastroesophageal reflux symptoms in relation to anxiety, depression and coping in a population-based study. Aliment Pharmacol Ther 26:683–691, 2007

Jess P, Eldrup J: The personality patterns in patients with duodenal ulcer and ulcer-like dyspepsia and their relationship to the course of the diseases. Hvidovre Ulcer Project Group. J Intern Med 235:589–594, 1994

Jones H, Cooper P, Miller V, et al: Treatment of non-cardiac chest pain: a controlled trial of hypnotherapy. Gut 55:1381–1384, 2006

Juengling FD, Ebert D, Gut O, et al: Prefrontal cortical hypometabolism during low-dose interferon alpha treatment. Psychopharmacology 152:383–389, 2000

Kahn D, Bourgeois JA: Acute pancreatitis and diabetic ketoacidosis in a schizophrenic patient taking olanzapine. J Clin Psychopharmacol 4:397–399, 2007

Kamolz T, Granderath FA, Pointner R: Does major depression in patients with gastroesophageal reflux disease affect the outcome of laparoscopic antireflux surgery? Surg Endosc 17:55–60, 2003

Kaplan PW: The EEG in metabolic encephalopathy and coma. J Clin Neurophysiol 21:307–318, 2004

Karling P, Danielsson A, Adolfsson R, et al: No difference in symptoms of irritable bowel syndrome between healthy subjects and patients with recurrent depression in remission. Neurogastroenterol Motil 19:896–904, 2007

Kast RE, Altschuler EL: Anti-apoptosis function of TNF-α in chronic lymphocytic leukemia: lessons from Crohn's disease and the therapeutic potential of bupropion to lower TNF-α. Arch Immunol Ther Exp 53:143–147, 2005

Kato I, Nomura AM, Stemmermann GN, et al: A prospective study of gastric and duodenal ulcer and its relation to smoking, alcohol, and diet. Am J Epidemiol 135:521–530, 1992

Kaurich T: Drug-induced acute pancreatitis. Proc (Bayl Univ Med Cent) 21:77–81, 2008

Keller W, Pritsch M, von Wietersheim J, et al: Effect of psychotherapy and relaxation on the psychosocial and somatic course of Crohn's disease: main results of the German prospective multicenter psychotherapy treatment study on Crohn's disease. J Psychosom Res 56:687–696, 2004

Kelsen DP, Portenoy RK, Thaler HT, et al: Pain and depression in patients with newly diagnosed pancreas cancer. J Clin Oncol 13:748–755, 1995

Kennedy AP, Nelson E, Reeves D, et al: A randomized controlled trial to assess the effectiveness and cost of a patient oriented self management approach to chronic inflammatory bowel disease. Gut 53:1639–1645, 2004

Kennedy T, Jones R, Darnley S, et al: Cognitive behaviour therapy in addition to antispasmodic treatment for irritable bowel syndrome in primary care: randomised controlled trial. BMJ 331:435, 2005

Kenney C, Hunter C, Davidson A, et al: Metoclopramide, an increasingly recognized cause of tardive dyskinesia. J Clin Pharmacol 48:379–384, 2008

Khoo J, Rayner CK, Jones KL, et al: Pathophysiology and management of gastroparesis. Expert Rev Gastroenterol Hepatol 3:167–181, 2009

Kim DR, Connolly KR, Cristancho P, et al: Psychiatric consultation of patients with hyperemesis gravidarum. Arch Womens Ment Health 12:61–67, 2009

Kitchens DH, Binkley CJ, Wallace DL, et al: Helicobacter pylori infection in people who are intellectually and developmentally disabled: a review. Spec Care Dentist 27:127–133, 2007

Klasser GD, Fischer DJ, Epstein JB: Burning mouth syndrome: recognition, understanding, and management. Oral Maxillofacial Surg Clin N Am 20:255–271, 2008

Klimes I, Mayou RA, Pearce MJ, et al: Psychological treatment for atypical non-cardiac chest pain: a controlled evaluation. Psychol Med 20:605–611, 1990

Koller EA, Cross JT, Doraiswamy PM, et al: Pancreatitis associated with atypical antipsychotics: from the Food and Drug Administrations' Med Watch surveillance system and published reports. Pharmacotherapy 23:1123–1130, 2003

Kraus MR, Schäfer A, Al-Taie O, et al: Prophylactic SSRI during interferon alpha re-therapy in patients with chronic hepatitis C and a history of interferon-induced depression. J Viral Hepat 12:96–100, 2005a

Kraus MR, Schäfer A, Wibmann S, et al: Neurocognitive changes in patients with hepatitis C receiving interferon alfa-2b and ribavirin. Clin Pharmacol Ther 77:90–100, 2005b

Kraus MR, Schäfer A, Schottker K, et al: Therapy of interferon-induced depression in chronic hepatitis C with citalopram: a randomized, double-blind, placebo-controlled study. Gut 57:531–536, 2008

Kurata J, Nogawa A: Meta-analysis of risk factors for peptic ulcer: nonsteroidal anti-inflammatory drugs, Helicobacter pylori, and smoking. J Clin Gastroenterol 24:2–17, 1997

Kurdyak PA, Juurlink DN, Kopp A, et al: Antidepressants, warfarin, and the risk of hemorrhage. J Clin Psychopharmacol 25:561–564, 2005

Lackner JM, Lou Coad M, Mertz HR, et al: Cognitive therapy for irritable bowel syndrome is associated with reduced limbic activity, GI symptoms, and anxiety. Behav Res Ther 44:621–638, 2006

Lackner JM, Jaccard J, Krasner SS, et al: Self administered behavioral therapy for moderate to severe IBS: clinical efficacy, tolerability, feasibility. Clin Gastroenterol Hepatol 6:899–906, 2008

Lakatos PL: Recent trends in the epidemiology of inflammatory bowel diseases: up or down? World J Gastroenterol 12:6102–6108, 2006

Lakatos PL, Szamosi T, Lakatos L: Smoking in inflammatory bowel diseases: good, bad, or ugly? World J Gastroenterol 13:6134–6139, 2007

Lee J, Dodd M, Dibble S, et al: Review of acupressure studies for chemotherapy-induced nausea and vomiting control. J Pain Symptom Manage 36:529–544, 2008

Lee KJ, Kwon HC, Cheong JY, et al: Demographic, clinical, and psychological characteristics of the heartburn groups classified using the Rome III criteria and factors associated with the responsiveness to proton pump inhibitors in the gastroesophageal reflux disease group. Digestion 79:131–136, 2009

Lee S, Wu J, Ma YL, et al: Irritable bowel syndrome is strongly associated with generalized anxiety disorder: a community study. Aliment Pharmacol Ther 30:643–651, 2009

Leelamanit V, Geater A, Sinkitjaroenchai W: A study of 111 cases of globus hystericus. J Med Assoc Thai 79:460–467, 1996

Lemberg A, Fernandez MA: Hepatic encephalopathy, ammonia, glutamate, glutamine and oxidative stress. Ann Hepatol 8:95–102, 2009

Lerebours E, Gower-Rousseau C, Merle V, et al: Stressful life events as a risk factor for inflammatory bowel disease onset: a population-based case-control study. Am J Gastroenterol 102:122–131, 2007

Levenson JL: Burning mouth syndrome as a side effect of SSRIs. J Clin Psychiatry 64:336–337, 2003

Levenstein S: The very model of a modern etiology: a biopsychosocial view of peptic ulcer. Psychosom Med 62:176–185, 2000

Levenstein S, Kaplan GA, Smith M: Sociodemographic characteristics, life stressors, and peptic ulcer: a prospective study. J Clin Gastroenterol 21:185–192, 1995

Levenstein S, Prantera C, Varvo V, et al: Stress and exacerbation in ulcerative colitis: a prospective study of patients enrolled in remission. Am J Gastroenterol 95:1213–1220, 2000

Lewis JD, Strom BL, Localio AR, et al: Moderate and high affinity serotonin reuptake inhibitors increase the risk of upper gastrointestinal toxicity. Pharmacoepidemiol Drug Saf 17:328–335, 2008

Li BUK, Lefevre F, Chelimsky GG, et al: North American Society for Pediatric Gastroenterology, Hepatology, and Nutrition consensus statement on the diagnosis and management of cyclic vomiting syndrome. J Pediatr Gastroenterol Nutr 47:379–393, 2008

Liebregts T, Adams B, Bredlack C, et al: Immune activation in patients with irritable bowel syndrome. Curr Gastroenterol Rep 9:363–364, 2007

Lind CD: Dysphagia: evaluation and treatment. Gastroenterol Clin N Am 32:553–575, 2003

Lix LM, Graff LA, Wlaker JR, et al: Longitudinal study of quality of life and psychological functioning for active, fluctuating, and inactive disease patterns in inflammatory bowel disease. Inflamm Bowel Dis 14:1575–1584, 2008

Loftis JM, Mathews AM, Hauser P: Psychiatric and substance use disorders in individuals with hepatitis C: epidemiology and management. Drugs 66:155–174, 2006

Lohr L: Chemotherapy-induced nausea and vomiting. Cancer J 14:85–93, 2008

Loke YK, Trivedi AN, Singh S: Meta-analysis: gastrointestinal bleeding due to interaction between selective serotonin uptake inhibitors and non-steroidal anti-inflammatory drugs. Aliment Pharmacol Ther 27:31–40, 2008

Longstreth GF, Drossman DA: New developments in the diagnosis and treatment of irritable bowel syndrome. Curr Gastroenterol Rep 4:427–434, 2002

Lööf L, Adami HO, Bates S, et al: Psychological group counseling for the prevention of ulcer relapses: a controlled randomized trial in duodenal and prepyloric ulcer disease. J Clin Gastroenterol 9:400–407, 1987

Lucena MI, Caravajal A, Andrade RJ, et al: Antidepressant-induced hepatotoxicity. Expert Opin Drug Saf 2:249–262, 2003

Maina G, Vitalucci A, Gandolfo S, et al: Comparative efficacy of SSRIs and amisulpride in burning mouth syndrome: a single-blind study. J Clin Psychiatry 63:38–43, 2002

Makrilia N, Indeck B, Syrigos K, et al: Depression and pancreatic cancer: a poorly understood link. JOP 10:69–76, 2009

Malcolm A, Thumshirn MB, Camilleri M: Rumination syndrome. Mayo Clin Proc 72:646–652, 1997

Malek-Ahmadi P, Hilsabeck RC: Neuropsychiatric complications of interferons: classification, neurochemical bases, and management. Ann Clin Psychiatry 19:113–123, 2007

Malik AR, Ravasia S: Interferon-induced mania. Can J Psychiatry 49:867–868, 2004

Mardini HE, Kip KE, Wilson JW: Crohn's disease: a two-year prospective study of the association between psychological distress and disease activity. Dig Dis Sci 49:492–497, 2004

Martin KA, Krahn LE, Balan V, et al: Modafinil's use in combating interferon-induced fatigue. Dig Dis Sci 52:893–896, 2007

Martin-Santos R, Diez-Quevedo C, Castellvis P, et al: De novo depression and anxiety disorders and influence on adherence during peginterferon-alpha-2a and ribavirin treatment in patients with hepatitis C. Aliment Pharmacol Ther 27:257–265, 2008

Masand PS, Pae CU, Krulewicz S, et al: A double-blind, randomized, placebo-controlled trial of paroxetine controlled-release in irritable bowel syndrome. Psychosomatics 50:78–86, 2009

Masters KJ: Pilocarpine treatment of xerostomia induced by psychoactive medications. Am J Psychiatry 162:1023, 2005

Matteson S, Roscoe J, Hickok J, et al: The role of behavioral conditioning in the development of nausea. Am J Obstet Gynecol 186:S239–S243, 2002

Maunder RG: Evidence that stress contributes to inflammatory bowel disease: evaluation, synthesis, and future directions. Inflamm Bowel Dis 11:600–608, 2005

Mawdsley JE, Rampton DS: Psychological stress in IBD: new insights into pathogenic and therapeutic implications. Gut 54:1481–1491, 2005

Mawe GM, Coates MD, Moses PL: Review article: intestinal serotonin signaling in irritable bowel syndrome. Aliment Pharmacol Ther 23:1067–1076, 2006

Maxion-Bergemann S, Thielecke F, Abel F, et al: Costs of irritable bowel syndrome in the UK and US. Pharmacoeconomics 24:21–37, 2006

McDonald-Haile J, Bradley LA, Bailey MA, et al: Relaxation training reduces symptom reports and acid exposure in patients with gastroesophageal reflux disease. Gastroenterology 107:61–69, 1994

McIntyre RS, Panjwani ZD, Nguyen HT, et al: The hepatic safety profile of duloxetine: a review. Expert Opin Drug Metab Toxicol 4:281–285, 2008

Mertz H, Naliboff B, Munakata J, et al: Altered rectal perception is a biological marker of patients with irritable bowel syndrome. Gastroenterology 109:40–52, 1995

Mertz H, Fass R, Kodner F, et al: Effect of amitriptyline on symptoms, sleep, and visceral perception in patients with functional dyspepsia. Am J Gastroenterol 93:160–165, 1998

Mikocka-Walus AA, Turnbull DA, Moulding NT, et al: Antidepressants and inflammatory bowel disease: a systematic review. Clin Pract Epidemiol Ment Health 2:24, 2006

Mikocka-Walus AA, Turnbull DA, Moulding NT, et al: Controversies surrounding the comorbidity of depression and anxiety in inflammatory disease patients: a literature review. Inflamm Bowel Dis 13:225–234, 2007

Mikocka-Walus AA, Turnbull DA, Andrews JM, et al: Does psychological status influence clinical outcomes in patients with inflammatory bowel disease (IBD) and other chronic gastrointestinal diseases: an observational cohort prospective study. Biopsychosoc Med 2:11, 2008a

Mikocka-Walus AA, Turnbull DA, Andrews JM, et al: The effect of functional gastrointestinal disorders on psychological comorbidity and quality of life in patients with inflammatory bowel disease. Aliment Pharmacol Ther 28:475–483, 2008b

Minderhoud IM, Oldenburg B, Wismeijer JA, et al: IBS-like symptoms in patients with inflammatory bowel disease in remission: relationships with quality of life and coping behavior. Dig Dis Sci 49:469–474, 2004

Mínguez Serra MP, Salort Llorca C, Silvestre Donat FJ: Pharmacological treatment of burning mouth syndrome: a review and update. Med Oral Patol Oral Cir Bucal 12:E299–304, 2007

Mittermaier C, Dejaco C, Walhoer T, et al: Impact of depressive mood on relapse in patients with inflammatory bowel disease: a prospective 18-month follow-up study. Psychosom Med 66:79–84, 2004

Mizyed I, Fass SS, Fass R: Review article: gastro-esophageal reflux disease and psychological comorbidity. Aliment Pharmacol Ther 29:351–358, 2009

Moayyedi P, Talley NJ: Gastro-oesophageal reflux disease. Lancet 367:2086–2100, 2006

Moayyedi P, Talley NJ, Fennerty MB, et al: Can the clinical history distinguish between organic and functional dyspepsia? JAMA 295:1566–1576, 2006

Monkemuller K, Malfertheiner P: Drug treatment of functional dyspepsia. World J Gastroenterol 12:2694–2700, 2006

Montgomery GH, Bovbjerg DH: Expectations of chemotherapy-related nausea: emotional and experiential predictors. Ann Behav Med 25:48–54, 2003

Morasco BJ, Rifai MA, Loftis JM, et al: A randomized trial of paroxetine to prevent interferon-α-induced depression in patients with hepatitis C. J Affect Disord 103:83–90, 2007

Morgan V, Pickens D, Gautam S, et al: Amitriptyline reduces rectal pain related activation of the anterior cingulate cortex in patients with irritable bowel syndrome. Gut 54:601–607, 2005

Mundy EA, DuHamel KN, Montgomery GH: The efficacy of behavioral interventions for cancer treatment related side effects. Semin Clin Neuropsychiatry 8:253–275, 2003

Murray CD, Flynn J, Ratcliffe L, et al: Effects of acute physical and psychological stress on gut autonomic innervation in irritable bowel syndrome. Gastroenterology 127:1695–1703, 2004

Mussell M, Bocker U, Nagel N: Reducing psychological distress in patients with inflammatory bowel disease by cognitive-behavioral treatment: exploratory study of effectiveness. Scand J Gastroenterol 38:755–762, 2003

Mussell M, Bocker U, Nagel N, et al: Predictors of disease-related concerns and other aspects of health-related quality of life in outpatients with inflammatory bowel disease. Eur J Gastroenterol Hepatol 16:1273–1280, 2004

Naeim A, Dy SM, Lorenz KA: Evidence-based recommendations for cancer nausea and vomiting. J Clin Oncol 26:3903–3910, 2008

Namin F, Patel J, Lin Z, et al: Clinical, psychiatric and manometric profile of cyclic vomiting syndrome in adults and response to tricyclic therapy. Neurogastroenterol Motil 19:196–202, 2007

Namiot DB, Leszcynska K, Namiot Z, et al: Smoking and drinking habits are important predictors of Helicobacter pylori eradication. Adv Med Sci 53:310–315, 2008

Navari RM: Antiemetic control: toward a new standard of care for emetogenic chemotherapy. Expert Opin Pharmacother 10:629–644, 2009

Navari RM, Einhorn LH, Passik SD, et al: A phase II trial of olanzapine for the prevention of chemotherapy-induced nausea and vomiting: a Hoosier Oncology Group study. Support Care Cancer 13:529–534, 2005

Navari RM, Einhorn LH, Loehrer PJ, et al: A phase II trial of olanzapine, dexamethasone, and palonosetron for the prevention of chemotherapy-induced nausea and vomiting: a Hoosier Oncology Group study. Support Care Cancer 15:1285–1291, 2007

Navarro VJ, Senior JR: Drug-related hepatotoxicity. N Engl J Med 354:731–739, 2006

Nelligan JA, Loftis JM, Mathews AM, et al: Depression comorbidity and antidepressant use in veterans with chronic hepatitis C: results from a retrospective chart review. J Clin Psychiatry 69:810–816, 2008

Nicholl BI, Halder SL, Macfarlane GJ, et al: Psychosocial risk factors for new onset irritable bowel syndrome: results of a large prospective population-based study. Pain 137:147–155, 2008

Nieves JE, Stack KM, Harrison ME, et al: Dysphagia: a rare form of dyskinesia? J Psychiatr Pract 13:199–201, 2007

Nojkov B, Rubenstein JH, Adlis SA, et al: The influence of comorbid IBS and psychological distress on outcomes and quality of life following PPI therapy in patients with gastroesophageal reflux disease. Aliment Pharmacol Ther 27:473–482, 2008

Noomen CG, Hommes DW, Fidder HH: Update on genetics in inflammatory disease. Best Pract Res Clin Gastroenterol 23:233–243, 2009

Norris W, Paredes AH, Lewis JH: Drug-induced liver injury in 2007. Curr Opin Gastroenterol 24: 287–297, 2008

Nyamathi AM, Dixon EL, Robbins W, et al: Risk factors for hepatitis C virus infection among homeless adults. J Gen Intern Med 17:134–143, 2002

O'Neil JL, Remington TL: Drug-induced esophageal injuries and dysphagia. Ann Pharmacother 37:1675–1684, 2003

Olden KW: Rumination. Curr Treat Options Gastroenterol 4:351–358, 2001

Olden KW, Chepyala P: Functional nausea and vomiting. Nat Clin Pract Gastroenterol Hepatol 5:202–208, 2008

Olden KW, Crowell MD: Chronic nausea and vomiting: new insights and approach to treatment. Curr Treat Options Gastroenterol 8:305–310, 2005

Olden KW, Radam T, Crowell MD: Rome II functional vomiting is not associated with psychological disturbance (abstract). Am J Gastroenterol 98:S274, 2003

Onyike CU, Bonner JO, Lyketsos CG, et al: Mania during treatment of chronic hepatitis C with pegylated interferon and ribavirin. Am J Psychiatry 161:429–435, 2004

Opartny L, Delaney JA, Suissa S: Gastrointestinal hemorrhage risks of selective serotonin receptor antagonist therapy: a new look. Br J Clin Pharmacol 66:76–81, 2008

Osterberg E, Blomquist L, Krakau I, et al: A population study of irritable bowel syndrome and mental health. Scand J Gastroenterol 35:264–268, 2000

Palmer JB, Drennan JC, Baba M: Evaluation and treatment of swallowing impairments. Am Fam Physician 61:2453–2462, 2000

Palsson OS, Drossman DA: Psychiatric and psychological dysfunction in irritable bowel syndrome and the role of psychological treatments. Gastroenterol Clin N Am 34:281–303, 2005

Papadopoulos V, Mimidis K: The rumination syndrome in adults: a review of the pathophysiology, diagnosis and treatment. J Postgrad Med 53:203–206, 2007

Pareek N, Fleisher DR, Abell T: Cyclic vomiting syndrome: what a gastroenterologist needs to know. Am J Gastroenterol 102:2832–2840, 2007

Park KH, Choi SM, Kwon SU, et al: Diagnosis of laryngopharyngeal reflux among globus patients. Otolaryngol Head Neck Surg 134:81–85, 2006

Passik SD, Breitbart WS: Depression in patients with pancreatic carcinoma: diagnostic and treatment issues. Cancer 78:615–626, 1996

Passik SD, Navari RM, Jung SH, et al: A phase I trial of olanzapine (Zyprexa) for the prevention of delayed emesis in cancer patients: a Hoosier Oncology Group study. Cancer Invest 22:383–388, 2004

Passmore MJ, Devarajan S, Ghatavi K, et al: Serotonin syndrome with prolonged dysphagia. Can J Psychiatry 49:79–80, 2004

Patrick A, Epstein O: Review article: gastroparesis. Aliment Pharmacol Ther 27:724–740, 2008

Pawelczk T, Pawelczk A, Strzelecki D, et al: Pegylated interferon α and ribavirin therapy may induce working memory disturbances in chronic hepatitis C patients. Gen Hosp Psychiatry 30:501–508, 2008

Perry W, Hilsabeck RC, Hassanein TI: Cognitive dysfunction in chronic hepatitis C: a review. Dig Dis Sci 53:307–321, 2008

Persoons P, Vermiere S, Demyttenaere K, et al: The impact of major depressive disorder on the short- and long-term outcome of Crohn's disease treatment with infliximab. Aliment Pharmacol Ther 22:101–110, 2005

Pirl WF, Roth AJ: Remission of chemotherapy-induced emesis with concurrent olanzapine treatment: a case report. Psychooncology 9:84–87, 2000

Porter CK, Tribble DR, Aliaga PA, et al: Infectious gastroenteritis and risk of developing inflammatory bowel disease. Gastroenterology 135:781–786, 2008

Prakash C, Clouse RE: Cyclic vomiting syndrome in adults: clinical features and response to tricyclic antidepressants. Am J Gastroenterol 94:2855–2860, 1999a

Prakash C, Clouse RE: Long-term outcome from tricyclic antidepressant treatment of functional chest pain. Dig Dis Sci 44:2373–2379, 1999b

Prakash C, Lustman PJ, Freedland KE, et al: Tricyclic antidepressants for functional nausea and vomiting: clinical outcome in 37 patients. Dig Dis Sci 43:1951–1956, 1998

Raison CL, Borisov AS, Broadwell SD, et al: Depression during pegylated interferon-alpha plus ribavirin therapy: prevalence and prediction. J Clin Psychiatry 66:41–48, 2005a

Raison CL, Demetrashvili M, Capuron L, et al: Neuropsychiatric adverse effects of interferon-α: recognition and management. CNS Drugs 19:105–123, 2005b

Raison CL, Woolwine BJ, Demetrashvili MF, et al: Paroxetine for prevention of depressive symptoms induced by interferon-alpha and ribavirin for hepatitis C. Aliment Pharmacol 25:1163–1174, 2007

Rao SSC, Gregersen H, Hayek B, et al: Unexplained chest pain: the hypersensitive, hyperreactive, and poorly compliant esophagus. Ann Intern Med 124:950–958, 1996

Ravich WJ, Wilson RS, Jones B, et al: Psychogenic dysphagia and globus: reevaluation of 23 patients. Dysphagia 4:35–38, 1989

Redd WH, Montgomery GH, DuHamel KN: Behavioral intervention for cancer treatment. J Natl Cancer Inst 93:810–823, 2001

Reddymasu S, Bahta E, Levine S, et al: Elevated lipase and diabetic ketoacidosis associated with aripiprazole. JOP 7:303–305, 2006

Reichenberg A, Gorman JM, Dietrich DT: Interferon-induced depression and cognitive impairment in hepatitis C virus patients: a 72 week prospective study. AIDS 19 (suppl 3):S174–S178, 2005

Rey E, Garcis-Alonso MO, Moreno-Ortega M, et al: Determinants of quality of life in irritable bowel syndrome. J Clin Gastroenterol 42:1003–1009, 2008

Reynolds JC, Schoen RE, Maislin G, et al: Risk factors for delayed healing of duodenal ulcers treated with famotidine and ranitidine. Am J Gastroenterol 89:571–580, 1994

Riedl A, Schmidtmann M, Stengel A, et al: Somatic comorbidities of irritable bowel syndrome: a systematic analysis. J Psychosom Res 64:573–582, 2008

Ries RK, Gilbert DA, Katon W: Tricyclic antidepressant therapy for peptic ulcer disease. Arch Intern Med 144:566–569, 1984

Ringel Y, Whitehead WE, Toner BB, et al: Sexual and physical abuse is not associated with rectal hypersensitivity in patients with irritable bowel syndrome. Gut 53:838–842, 2004

Robaeys G, Buntinx F: Treatment of hepatitis C viral infections in substance abusers. Acta Gastroenterol Belg 68:55–67, 2005

Rodriguez-Stanley S, Robinson M, Earnest DL, et al: Esophageal hypersensitivity may be a major cause of heartburn. Am J Gastroenterol 94:628–631, 1999

Rosenstock S, Jorgensen T, Bonnevie O, et al: Risk factors for peptic ulcer disease: a population based prospective cohort study comprising 2416 Danish adults. Gut 52:186–193, 2003

Rovira A, Alonso J, Córdoba J: MR imaging findings in hepatic encephalopathy. AJNR Am J Neuroradiol 29:1612–1621, 2008

Russo MW, Watkins PB: Are patients with elevated liver tests at increased risk of drug-induced liver injury? (editorial) Gastroenterology 126:1477–1480, 2004

Sabate JM, Veyrac M, Mion F, et al: Relationship between rectal sensitivity, symptoms intensity and quality of life in patients with irritable bowel syndrome. Aliment Pharmacol Ther 24:484–490, 2008

Sainsbury A, Heatley RV: Review article: psychosocial factors in the quality of life of patients with inflammatory bowel disease. Aliment Pharmacol Ther 21:499–508, 2005

Salkovskis PM: Psychological treatment of noncardiac chest pain: the cognitive approach. Am J Med 92(5A):114S–121S, 1992

Salort Lorca CS, Paz MPM, Silvestre FJ: Drug-induced burning mouth syndrome: a new etiological diagnosis. Med Oral Patol Oral Cir Bucal 13:167–170, 2008

Sardella A: An up-to-date review on burning mouth syndrome. Minerva Stomatol 56:327–340, 2007

Sawhney MS, Prakash C, Lustman PJ, et al: Tricyclic antidepressants for chronic vomiting in diabetic patients. Dig Dis Sci 52:418–424, 2007

Saxena N, Bhatia M, Joshi YK, et al: Utility of P300 auditory event-related potential in detecting cognitive dysfunction in patients with cirrhosis of the liver. Neurol India 49:350–354, 2001

Scala A, Checci L, Montevecchi M, et al: Update on burning mouth syndrome: overview and patient management. Crit Rev Oral Biol Med 14:275–291, 2003

Schaefer M, Shwaiger M, Garkisch AS, et al: Prevention of interferon-alpha associated depression in psychiatric risk patients with chronic hepatitis C. J Hepatol 42:793–798, 2005

Schaefer M, Hinzpeter A, Mohmand A, et al: Hepatitis C treatment in "difficult-to-treat" psychiatric patients with pegylated interferon-alpha and ribavirin response and psychiatric side effects. Hepatology 46:991–998, 2007

Schaefer M, Winterer J, Sarkar R, et al: Three cases of successful tryptophan add-on or monotherapy of hepatitis C and IFN α-associated mood disorders. Psychosomatics 49:442–446, 2008

Schafer A, Wittchen HU, Seufert J, et al: Methodological approaches in the assessment of interferon-alfa-induced depression in patients with chronic hepatitis C: a critical review. Int J Methods Psych Res 16:186–201, 2007

Schalekamp T, Klungel OH, Souverein PC, et al: Increased bleeding risk with concurrent use of selective serotonin reuptake inhibitors and coumarins. Arch Intern Med 168:180–185, 2008

Schatzberg AF, Cole JO, DeBattista C: Antidepressants, in Manual of Clinical Psychopharmacology, 6th Edition. Washington, DC, American Psychiatric Publishing, 2007, pp 35–157

Schliess F, Gorg B, Haussinger D: RNA oxidation and zinc in hepatic encephalopathy and hyperammonemia. Metab Brain Dis 24:119–134, 2009

Shamash J, Miall L, Williams F, et al: Dysphagia in the neuroleptic malignant syndrome. Br J Psychiatry 164:849–850, 1994

Shanahan F, Bernstein CN: The evolving epidemiology of inflammatory bowel disease. Curr Opin Gastroenterol 25:301–305, 2009

Shapiro M, Green C, Bautista J, et al: Functional heartburn patients demonstrate traits of functional bowel disorder but lack a uniform increase of chemoreceptor sensitivity to acid. Am J Gastroenterol 101:1084–1091, 2006

Simren M, Axelsson J, Gillberg R, et al: Quality of life in inflammatory bowel disease in remission: the impact of IBS-like symptoms and associated psychological factors. Am J Gastroenterol 97:389–396, 2002

Simren M, Brazier J, Coremans G, et al: Quality of life costs in irritable bowel syndrome. Digestion 69:254–261, 2004

Simren M, Agerforz P, Bjornsson ES, et al: Nutrient-dependent enhancement of rectal sensitivity in irritable bowel syndrome (IBS). Neurogastroenterol Motil 19:20–29, 2007

Soman M, Swenson C: A possible case of carbamazepine-induced pancreatitis. Drug Intell Clin Pharm 19:925–927, 1985

Sonje S, Levenson JL: Cyclic vomiting syndrome, part 1. Prim Psychiatry 16:15–18, 2009

Soo S, Moayyedi P, Deeks J, et al: Psychological interventions for non-ulcer dyspepsia. Cochrane Database Syst Rev (2): CD002301, 2005

Spieker MR: Evaluating dysphagia. Am Fam Physician 61:3639–3648, 2000

Spigset O, Hagg S, Bate A: Hepatic injury and pancreatitis during treatment with serotonin reuptake inhibitors: data from the World Health Organization (WHO) database of adverse drug reactions. Int Clin Psychopharmacol 18:157–161, 2003

Spiller R, Aziz Q, Creed F, et al: Guidelines on the irritable bowel syndrome: mechanisms and practical management. Gut 56:1770–1798, 2007

Srivastava M, Brito-Dellan N, Davis MP, et al: Olanzapine as an antiemetic in refractory nausea and vomiting in advanced cancer. J Pain Symptom Manage 25:578–582, 2003

Stapleton J, Wo JM: Current treatment of nausea and vomiting associated with gastroparesis: antiemetics, prokinetics, tricyclics. Gastrointest Endosc Clin N Am 19:57–72, vi, 2009

Sudas S, Takagai S, Inoshima-Takahashi K, et al: Electroconvulsive therapy for burning mouth syndrome. Acta Psychiatr Scand 118:503–504, 2008

Sundaram V, Shaikh OS: Hepatic encephalopathy: pathophysiology and emerging therapies. Med Clin North Am 93:819–836, 2009

Sylvestre DL, Clements BJ: Adherence to hepatitis C treatment in recovering heroin users maintained on methadone. Eur J Gastroenterol Hepatol 19:741–747, 2007

Tabas G, Beaves M, Wang J, et al: Paroxetine to treat irritable bowel syndrome not responding to high fiber diet: a double-blind placebo-controlled trial. Am J Gastroenterol 99:914–920, 2004

Tack J, Fried M, Houghton JA: Systematic review: the efficacy of treatments for irritable bowel syndrome—a European perspective. Aliment Pharmacol Ther 24:183–205, 2006a

Tack J, Talley NJ, Camilleri M, et al: Functional gastroduodenal disorders. Gastroenterology 130:1466–1479, 2006b

Talley NJ: Irritable bowel syndrome. Intern Med J 36:724–728, 2006

Talley NJ: Functional nausea and vomiting. Aust Fam Physician 36:694–697, 2007

Talley NJ, Vakil N, Practice Parameters Committee of the American College of Gastroenterology: Guidelines for management of dyspepsia. Am J Gastroenterol 100:2324–2337, 2005a

Talley NJ, Vakil N, Moayyedi P: American Gastroenterological Association technical review on the evaluation of dyspepsia. Gastroenterology 129:1756–1780, 2005b

Talley NJ, Locke GR, Lahr BD, et al: Predictors of the placebo response in functional dyspepsia. Aliment Pharmacol Ther 23:923–936, 2006

Talley NJ, Kellow JE, Boyce P, et al: Antidepressant therapy (imipramine and citalopram) for irritable bowel syndrome: a double-blind, randomized, placebo-controlled trial. Dig Dis Sci 53:108–115, 2008

Talley NJ, Herrick L, Locke GR: Antidepressants in functional dyspepsia. Expert Rev Gastroenterol Hepatol 4:5–8, 2010

Tamam L, Yerdelen D, Ozpoyraz N: Psychosis associated with interferon-α therapy for chronic hepatitis B. Ann Pharmacother 37:384–387, 2003

Tan G, Hammond DC, Joseph G: Hypnosis and irritable bowel syndrome: a review of efficacy and mechanism of action. Am J Clin Hypn 47:161–178, 2005

Tanaka M, Kazuma K: Ulcerative colitis: factors affecting difficulties of life and psychological well being of patients in remission. J Clin Nurs 14:65–73, 2005

Tarbell S: Psychiatric symptomatology in children and adolescents with cyclic vomiting syndrome and their parents. Headache 48:259–266, 2008

Tasci Y, Demir B, Dilbaz S, et al: Use of diazepam for hyperemesis gravidarum. J Matern Fetal Neonatal Med 22:353–356, 2009

Tata LJ, Fortun PJ, Hubbard RB, et al: Does concurrent prescription of selective serotonin reuptake inhibitors and non-steroidal anti-inflammatory drugs substantially increase the risk of upper gastrointestinal bleeding? Aliment Pharmacol Ther 22:175–181, 2005

Taylor B, Rehm J, Gmel G: Moderate alcohol consumption and the gastrointestinal tract. Dig Dis 23:170–176, 2005

Thomson BN, Banting SW, Gibbs P: Pancreatic cancer—current management. Aust Fam Physician 35:212–217, 2006

Toner BB: Cognitive-behavioral treatment of irritable bowel syndrome. CNS Spectr 11:883–890, 2005

Ueda N, Kodama Y, Hori H, et al: Two cases of burning mouth syndrome treated with olanzapine. Psychiatry Clin Neurosci 62:359–361, 2008

Vahedi H, Merat S, Rashidioon A, et al: The effect of fluoxetine in patients with pain and constipation-predominant irritable bowel syndrome: a double-blind randomized-controlled study. Aliment Pharmacol Ther 22:381–385, 2005

Vakil N, van Zanten SV, Kahrilas P, et al: The Montreal definition and classification of gastroesophageal reflux disease: a global evidence-based consensus. Am J Gastroenterol 101:1900–1920, 2006

Vandenbergh J, DuPont P, Fischler B, et al: Regional brain activation during proximal stomach distention in humans: a positron emission tomography study. Gastroenterology 128:564–573, 2005

Vandenberghe J, Dupont P, Van Oudenhove L, et al: Regional cerebral blood flow during gastric balloon distention in functional dyspepsia. Gastroenterology 132:1684–1693, 2007

van der Eijk I, Vlachonikolis IG, Munkholm P, et al: The role of quality of care in health-related quality of life in patients with IBD. Inflamm Bowel Dis 10:392–398, 2004

van Kerkhoven LA, Laheij RJ, Aparicio N, et al: Effect of the antidepressant venlafaxine in functional dyspepsia: a randomized, double-blind, placebo-controlled trial. Clin Gastroenterol Hepatol 6:746–752, 2008

Van Oudenhove L, Vandenberghe J, Dupont P, et al: Abnormal regional brain activity during rest and (anticipated) gastric distension in functional dyspepsia and the role of anxiety: a H(2)(15)O-PET study. Am J Gastroenterol 105:913–924, 2010

van Peski-Oosterbaan AS, Spinhoven P, van Rood Y, et al: Cognitive-behavioral therapy for noncardiac chest pain: a randomized trial. Am J Med 106:424–429, 1999 van Soest EM, Dieleman JP, Siersema PD, et al: Tricyclic antidepressants and the risk of reflux esophagitis. Am J Gastroenterol 102:1870–1877, 2007

Varia I, Logue E, O'Connor C, et al: Randomized trial of sertraline in patients with unexplained chest pain of noncardiac origin. Am Heart J 140:367–372, 2000

Vidal A, Gomez-Gil E, Sans M, et al: Health-related quality of life in inflammatory bowel disease patients: the role of psychopathology and personality. Inflamm Bowel Dis 14:977–983, 2008

Vidal X, Ibanez L, Vendrell L, et al: Risk of upper gastrointestinal bleeding and the degree of serotonin reuptake inhibition by antidepressants: a case-control study. Drug Saf 31:159–168, 2008

von Wietersheim J, Kessler H: Psychotherapy with chronic inflammatory bowel disease patients: a review. Inflamm Bowel Dis 12:1175–1184, 2006

Waters BM, Jensen L, Fedorak RN: Effects of formal education for patients with inflammatory bowel disease: a randomized controlled trial. Can J Gastroenterol 19:235–244, 2005

Weiner H: From simplicity to complexity (1950–1990): the case of peptic ulceration, I: human studies. Psychosom Med 53:467–490, 1991

Weiner H, Thaler M, Reiser MF, et al: Etiology of duodenal ulcer, I: relation of specific psychological characteristics to rate of gastric secretion (serum pepsinogen). Psychosom Med 19:1–10, 1957

Weinrieb RM, Auriacombe M, Lynch KG, et al: Selective serotonin reuptake inhibitors and the risk of bleeding. Expert Opin Drug Saf 4:337–344, 2005

Whitehead WE, Palsson O, Jones KR: Systematic review of the comorbidity of irritable bowel syndrome and other disorders: what are the causes and implications? Gastroenterology 122:1140–1156, 2002

Wiklund I, Carlsson R, Carlsson J, et al: Psychological factors as a predictor of treatment response in patients with heartburn: a pooled analysis of clinical trials. Scand J Gastroenterol 41:288–293, 2006

Wilhelmsen I, Berstad A: Reduced relapse rate in duodenal ulcer disease leads to normalization of psychological distress: twelve-year follow-up. Scand J Gastroenterol 39:717–721, 2004

Wilhelmsen I, Haug TT, Ursin H, et al: Effect of short-term cognitive psychotherapy on recurrence of duodenal ulcer: a prospective randomized trial. Psychosom Med 56:440–448, 1994

Williams H, Walker D, Orchard TR: Extraintestinal manifestations of inflammatory bowel disease. Curr Gastroenterol Rep 10:597–605, 2008

Wilson S, Maddison T, Roberts L, et al: Systematic review: the effectiveness of hypnotherapy in the management of irritable bowel syndrome. Aliment Pharmacol Ther 24:769–780, 2006

Wright CE, Ebrecht M, Mitchell R, et al: The effect of psychological stress on symptom severity and perception in patients with gastro-oesophageal reflux. J Psychosom Res 59:415–424, 2005

Wu JCY, Cheung CMY, Wong VWS, et al: Distinct clinical characteristics between patients with nonerosive reflux disease and those with reflux esophagitis. Clin Gastroenterol Hepatol 5:690–695, 2007

Yamazaki Y, Hata H, Kitamori S, et al: An open-label, non-comparative dose escalation pilot study of the effect of paroxetine in treatment of burning mouth syndrome. Oral Surg Oral Med Oral Pathol Oral Radiol Endod 107:6–11, 2009

Yang SH, McNeely MJ: Rhabdomyolysis, pancreatitis, and hyperglycemia with ziprasidone. Am J Psychiatry 159:1435, 2002

Yuan Y, Tsoi K, Hunt RH: Selective serotonin reuptake inhibitors and risk of upper GI bleeding: confusion or confounding? Am J Med 119:719–727, 2006

Zaccara G, Franciotta D, Perucca E: Idiosyncratic adverse reactions to antiepileptic drugs. Epilepsia 48:1223–1244, 2007

Zakrzewska JM, Forssell H, Glenny AM: Interventions for the treatment of burning mouth syndrome. Cochrane Database Syst Rev (1):CD002779, 2005

Zijdenbos IL, de Wit NJ, van der Heijden GJ, et al: Psychological treatment for the management of irritable bowel syndrome. Cochrane Database Syst Rev (1):CD006442, 2009

CHAPTER 21

Renal Disease

Daniel Cukor, Ph.D.

Deborah Rosenthal-Asher, M.A.

Lewis M. Cohen, M.D.

James L. Levenson, M.D.

Paul L. Kimmel, M.D.

IN THIS CHAPTER we summarize the literature on psychiatric issues in chronic kidney disease (CKD) and end-stage renal disease (ESRD), including psychiatric disorders in renal disease patients, social support, sexual dysfunction, adherence, withdrawal from dialysis, renal psychiatric palliative care, psychotherapy and psychopharmacology, psychiatric adverse effects of renal drugs, and drug interactions. Renal transplantation is also discussed in Chapters 31, "Organ Transplantation," and 34, "Pediatrics," and hemodialysis for toxic ingestions is covered in Chapter 37, "Medical Toxicology." Electrolyte disorders are discussed in Chapter 22, "Endocrine and Metabolic Disorders."

As the techniques of dialysis and transplantation have advanced, ESRD patients are living longer, including those with more severe illnesses and comorbidities. As comorbid psychiatric disorders are widely prevalent among dialysis and renal transplant populations, mental health professionals can play a vital role in management, including intervention for mental health difficulties, promotion of compliance, as well as in palliative care for dying patients and those who wish to decline or discontinue dialysis.

Nephrology has recognized the need for psychiatric consultation since the initial development of kidney dialysis in the late 1960s and early 1970s. Nearly universal access to treatment followed passage of the 1972 End-Stage Renal Disease amendment to the Social Security Act, which provided government subsidy for dialysis. Subsequently, the population has steadily grown, aged, and become more severely ill (McBride 1995). Psychiatry's potential role in the collaborative care of patients with renal disease is increasing. Each year, approximately 80,000 Americans develop ESRD. Over 500,000 individuals are treated for ESRD (United States Renal Data System 2009). About 360,000 people are receiving maintenance dialysis, and 120,000 have a functioning kidney transplant. In 2006, the prevalent dialysis population was 354,754 patients (United States Renal Data System 2009). The number of patients starting renal replacement therapy in the United States continues to increase each year by 5%–7%. An additional 8 million individuals are estimated to have earlier stage CKD in the United States (United States Renal Data System 2009). The current annual cost for treating ESRD in the United States is approximately $21 billion, and the Medicare expenditure is about $16 billion for hemodialysis and $2 billion for transplantation (United States Renal Data System 2009).

The major causes of renal failure include diabetes, hypertension, generalized arteriosclerosis, lupus, AIDS, and primary renal diseases, such as chronic glomerulonephritis, chronic interstitial nephritis, polycystic kidney disease, and other hereditary and congenital disorders. In 1999, only 9% of dialysis patients were free of significant comorbid conditions. Of particular importance, diabetes is now found in almost half of ESRD cases. Diabetic patients are especially likely to have increased morbidity because of its plethora of microvascular and macrovascular complications (Lea and Nicholas 2002).

Renal transplantation is the treatment of choice for many patients, and if a transplant is successful, the patient's survival (United States Renal Data System 2009; Wolfe et al. 1999) and quality of life (Franke et al. 2003; Kimmel and Patel 2006; Laupacis et al. 1996) are improved over what they would have been with maintenance dialysis. A major issue in transplantation is the shortage of donor organs. Transplanted kidneys may come from a living donor or through organ donation following death. During the period from 1992 to 2002, the number of cadaveric transplants increased by only 16%, while living-related transplants increased by 68% (United States Renal Data System 2003). Recent data reveal that this trend has reversed, and the overall number of cadaveric kidney transplants decreased 1% and living donor transplants decreased 6% (United States Renal Data System 2009). Despite this, many more transplants are performed with cadaveric kidneys than with living-donor kidneys. More than 18,000 kidney transplants were performed in 2006 (United States Renal Data System 2009). Long-term kidney survival is greater with living donors (D.D. Koo et al. 1999). The critical shortage of cadaveric organs is leading many transplant programs to liberalize their requirements and to make use of kidneys from living unrelated donors, and from donors with more comorbid conditions.

Peritoneal dialysis and hemodialysis are the two forms of dialysis. In peritoneal dialysis, dialysate fluid is introduced and then removed from the peritoneal space through an indwelling catheter. The peritoneum serves as a semipermeable membrane, and fluid and wastes are removed together with dialysate. Peritoneal dialysis may be performed by a machine in the home at night (continuous cycling peritoneal dialysis [CCPD]), or manually at home four to six times per day (continuous ambulatory peritoneal dialysis [CAPD]). Only 8% of ESRD patients use peritoneal dialysis as the initial mode of renal replacement therapy (United States Renal Data System 2009). Hemodialysis may be conducted at the patient's home, but it usually takes place at outpatient dialysis units for 3- to 4-hour sessions typically held three times per week. Home dialysis requires the participation of another person, who must be available to assist with 12–15 hours of weekly treatment. There has been a great deal of recent interest in quotidian dialysis done nightly at home or frequently in a dialysis facility (Lockridge et al. 2001; Pierratos 2004). Data from uncontrolled studies suggest that this new approach may result in improved quality of life and health. Although patients have not been randomized to dialysis modalities, patients receiving peritoneal dialysis rate their care higher than do those receiving hemodialysis (Rubin et al. 2004).

Psychiatric Disorders in Renal Disease

In a study of psychiatric illness involving 200,000 U.S. dialysis patients, almost 10% had been hospitalized with a psychiatric diagnosis. A psychiatric syndrome was the primary reason for hospitalization of 25% of the subgroup (Kimmel et al. 1998b). Depression and other affective disorders were the most common diagnoses, followed by delirium and dementia. In a smaller scale study in an urban hemodialysis population, roughly 70% of the sample had at least one current Axis I diagnosis, as determined by the Structured Clinical Interview for the DSM (SCID) (Cukor et al. 2007). Depression and anxiety were the two most prevalent psychiatric disorders, followed by substance abuse and psychosis. Compared with other medical illnesses, the primary diagnosis of depression was more frequent in renal failure patients than in those with ischemic heart disease and cerebrovascular disease (Kimmel et al. 1998b).

Depression

Early studies of depression in ESRD reported prevalence rates ranging from 0% to 100%, reflecting widely variable definitions, criteria, and measurement methods (see recent review by Cukor et al. 2006). In the nephrology literature, there is a lack of clarity around the term depression and whether it refers to the affective symptom or the psychiatric disorder (L. Cohen 1996). In addition, the evaluation of depression is complicated by the fact that many of the somatic signs and symptoms of ESRD are very similar to signs of depression. Many uremic patients have diminished appetite, loss of energy, poor sleep, and diminished sexual interest (Kimmel 2002; Kimmel et al. 2007; Meyer and Hostetter 2007).

A variety of techniques have been used to improve the diagnostic accuracy of depression in patients with renal disease. Some ESRD research studies have relied exclusively on self-report instruments that determine the severity of the symptom, but have adjusted the scoring of the measure to account for somatic complaints (Craven et al. 1988; Kimmel et al. 1993; Smith et al. 1985). Other studies (Cukor et al. 2007; Finkelstein and Finkelstein 2000; Hedayati et al. 2006; Watnick et al. 2003) have combined self-report measures with a structured diagnostic interview based on DSM-IV-TR (American Psychiatric Association 2000) criteria or have used multiple measurement points across time (Boulware et al. 2006; Cukor et al. 2008b; Kimmel et al. 2000). There has been much less study of depression in patients with CKD before initiation of dialysis, but screening instruments have recently been validated in this population (Hedayati et al. 2009b).

Studies that have adjusted self-report measures to account for the somatic complaints of renal disease patients have generally produced consistent results across diverse racial samples. In a group of white Canadian hemodialysis patients, Craven et al. (1988) found that a Beck Depression Inventory (BDI) score of 15 or greater, as compared with the standard 10, had better sensitivity and specificity for the diagnosis of major depression in dialysis patients when the Diagnostic Interview Schedule (DIS) was utilized as the criterion for the diagnosis. Kimmel and colleagues (Kimmel 2001; Kimmel et al. 1996, 1998a) studied primarily African American ESRD patients in hemodialysis centers in Washington, DC. They found that about half of the patients scored greater than 10 on the BDI. When the more conservative cutoff of 15 was employed, about 25% of the patients screened positive (Kimmel et al. 2000).

One study (Watnick et al. 2005) validated the BDI and the Patient Health Questionnaire-9 (PHC-9) against SCID-diagnosed major depressive disorder and found that the optimal cutoff value was 16 for the BDI and 10 for the PHQ-9. Another study (Hedayati et al. 2006) compared the BDI and the Center for Epidemiologic Studies Depression Scale (CES-D) against the SCID in ESRD patients. The prevalence of major depression was 27% in their sample of ethnically diverse patients, including one-quarter of the subjects who were veterans. A BDI cutoff score of 14 and a CES-D score of 18 had the most predictive value. These studies indicate an emerging consensus that there is agreement between the BDI and clinician-administered diagnostic tools and that a BDI score of 14–16 is indicative of major depression in chronic hemodialysis patients. Recent data indicate that the prevalence of major depression is about 20% in CKD patients (Hedayati et al. 2009a).

Depression in patients with ESRD is a strong predictor of worse medical outcomes. Using time to death or hospitalization, Hedayati et al. (2008) found the diagnosis of major depression to be associated with a hazard ratio of 2.07 compared with nondepressed control subjects, after adjustment for other variables. Kimmel et al. (2000) found that tracking multiple measurements of depression produced a more robust association with mortality than any single measurement. Similarly, Boulware et al. (2006) demonstrated that associations with outcomes existed with multiple measurements of depression that did not exist with baseline data. Cukor et al. (2008b) reassessed SCID-diagnosed depressed and anxious ESRD patients after 16 months and noted a variety of clinical trajectories. The persistent course of depression was associated with significantly lower quality of life and more reported health problems compared with intermittent depression. These data suggest that a single measure of depression at a specific point in time might not be as meaningful as assessment of depression over a longer time span. Despite the high prevalence of depression in dialysis patients, there has been little study of the effectiveness of antidepressants. Selective serotonin reuptake inhibitors (SSRIs) are widely prescribed for depression in ESRD patients, but only two small short-term randomized controlled trials have shown some benefit of paroxetine (J.R. Koo et al. 2005) and fluoxetine (Blumenfield et al. 1997).

In addition to pharmacotherapy, psychotherapy is an appropriate intervention for depressed ESRD patients, but there are no reported controlled clinical trials of psychotherapy for depression specifically in renal patients (Rabindranath et al. 2005). Despite this lack of evidence, there are indications that psychotherapy, including cognitive-behavioral therapy (CBT), may be an effective intervention strategy (Cukor 2007). Cukor et al. (2007) found higher levels of depressogenic cognitive distortions in SCID-diagnosed depressed hemodialysis patients compared with nondepressed control subjects. One study in which renal transplant recipients were randomly assigned to either individual or group psychotherapy and compared with usual-care patients (Baines et al. 2004) showed that both individual and group psychotherapy were successful in reducing depressive symptoms.

Anxiety

Anxiety is a complicating comorbid diagnosis for many medical illnesses and often co-occurs with depression in ESRD populations (Cukor et al. 2007, 2008a, 2008b). There is relatively little anxiety research specific to ESRD patients, but it appears that an anxiety diagnosis is associated with diminished quality of life (Cukor et al. 2008a; Sareen et al. 2006). One early study (Nichols and Springford 1984) found that about one-third of patients experienced episodes of moderate anxiety during their first year of dialysis treatment. In a study that assessed psychiatric diagnoses in a sample of 70 predominately African American ESRD patients, about 45% had at least one anxiety disorder. The most common diagnoses identified were phobias and panic disorder (Cukor et al. 2008a). The prevalence of panic disorder was much higher than in community samples and may be related to hypervigilance to bodily sensations associated with hemodialysis or fears about the outcome of ESRD treatment.

Traumatic stress symptoms related to dialysis experiences, serious medical events, or other traumas are also common among hemodialysis patients (Tagay et al. 2007). Phobias to needles or the sight of blood are common in the general population (see Chapter 11, "Anxiety Disorders"), and such phobias are among the most commonly reported reasons that hemodialysis patients do not choose in-center dialysis instead of self-care treatment (McLaughlin et al.

2003). There are no published clinical trials of psychopharmacology or psychotherapy for anxiety in patients with ESRD and very few case reports regarding anxiety in this population.

Substance Abuse

Substance use disorders, such as cocaine or heroin dependence, can lead to CKD (Jaffe and Kimmel 2006; Norris et al. 2001). Substance use may also result in HIV infection, which can secondarily cause renal failure (Kimmel et al. 2003). In a sample of 145 hemodialysis patients, Hegde et al. (2000) found 28% to have difficulty with chronic alcoholism (Hegde et al. 2000). Those who abused alcohol had poorer nutrition than nonabusers, as demonstrated by serum albumin measurements. Another study found cocaine users to be less compliant with their dialysis attendance than nonusers (Obialo et al. 2008). Although additional research is needed regarding substance abuse and dialysis, substance abuse should be taken seriously and addressed with specialist care.

The Disruptive Dialysis Patient

To function well, dialysis units depend on the ability of their staff to provide appropriate patient care. There has been an increase in the number of reported disruptive patients within dialysis units (Hashmi and Moss 2008). Disruption on the unit may impact the individual, as in the case of noncompliance with treatment. A patient's disruptive behavior may also affect other patients receiving dialysis therapy. A disruptive patient may harm others by coming late to appointments, thus disrupting dialysis scheduling for others, or by threatening the staff (Hashmi and Moss 2008).

Withholding dialysis treatment from a disruptive patient must be carefully considered. While all patients should be treated equally and with respect, the balance between the welfare of a disruptive patient and the welfare of health care personnel or other patients should be maintained. If disruptive behavior affects only the patient him- or herself, the individual should not be refused dialysis treatment. For example, treatment cannot be denied to a patient who is noncompliant with his or her medical regimen but continues to want dialysis. For a disruptive patient who continually shows up late to appointments and does not abide by rules of the unit, moving the individual to a different shift or unit could be considered (Hashmi and Moss 2008). Verbal or physical abuse on the unit should not be tolerated, and the welfare of staff and other patients should not be compromised.

Suggested strategies for dealing with disruptive patients include attempting to first create a calm environment, approaching the patient directly about his or her behavior, using reflective listening techniques to help the patient feel understood, attempting to understand the reasons for the individual's responses and behavior, outlining specific goals the patient has for treatment, educating the patient about consequences that may result from his or her behavior (ideally through a behavioral contract), and referral to a skilled team member such as a psychologist or social worker (Goldman 2008; Hashmi and Moss 2008; Sukolsky 2004). Two helpful resources addressing dialysis-related disruptive behavior and conflict resolution are the Renal Physicians Association's "Clinical Practice Guideline on Shared Decision-Making in the Appropriate Initiation of and Withdrawal From Dialysis" (Galla 2000) and the Decreasing Dialysis Patient/Provider Conflict (DPC) project (see review by Goldman 2008).

Cognitive Disorders

Cognitive disorders are common in the ESRD patient population (Murray et al. 2006) and may be related to uremia, a variety of medical comorbidities (e.g., electrolyte disturbances, severe malnutrition, impaired metabolism, cerebrovascular disease), or adverse effects of treatment. Uremia is a clinical syndrome resulting from profound loss of renal function and has been associated with cognitive impairment, including difficulty with concentration, memory, and intellectual functioning (Pliskin et al. 1996; Souheaver et al. 1982; Williams et al. 2004). Signs and symptoms of uremia vary considerably, with severity presumably depending on both the magnitude and speed with which renal function is lost. Central nervous system symptoms may begin with mild cognitive dysfunction, fatigue, and headache, progressing to hypoactive delirium and, if untreated, coma. Restless legs syndrome, muscle cramps, and sleep disorders are also common in uremic patients (see Chapter 15, "Sleep Disorders"). Other common symptoms include pruritus, anorexia, nausea, and vomiting (Haddy et al. 2008; Meyer and Hostetter 2007; Weisbord et al. 2003). Anemia is another potential risk factor for compromised cognitive functioning in patients with kidney disease (Pereira et al. 2005). Reduced oxygen availability secondary to anemia may decrease cognitive function, especially in patients with other neurological or cerebrovascular diseases (Johnson et al. 1990).

The rate of cognitive decline and its relationship to CKD have not been well delineated. Kurella et al. (2004) assessed cognitive functioning in a sample of 80 CKD patients not requiring dialysis and 80 ESRD patients receiving hemodialysis. An association between stage of CKD and degree of cognitive impairment was found on measures of mental status, executive functioning, and verbal memory. Another study (Elias et al. 2009) also found an association between CKD severity and cognitive impairment. CKD patients with lower renal function as well as those with higher creatinine demonstrated decreased performance on visuospatial processing, attention, and planning abilities.

Dementia has been identified as a mortality risk factor in ESRD. Hypertension and diabetes, both highly prevalent among ESRD patients, are known risk factors for the development of dementia (Saczynski et al. 2008; Semplicini et al. 2006). One large study of hemodialysis patients (Kurella et al. 2006) found a 4% prevalence of dementia in the overall sample. Individuals diagnosed with dementia had a 1.48 times greater risk of death than those not diagnosed with dementia. Furthermore, those who were diagnosed with dementia were twice as likely to withdraw from treatment. Consistent with findings in the general population, age, race, education, diabetes, and cerebrovascular disease were found to be related to dementia.

Dialysis itself has been implicated as a causal factor in the dementia-like memory deficits observed in some patients. Dialysis dementia, or dialysis encephalopathy, is a distinct, progressive neurological disorder whose etiology remains controversial (Fraser and Arieff 1988). Not uncommon 30 years ago, it is now rare. Signs have included memory impairment, dysarthria, stuttering speech, depression, psychosis, asterixis, bizarre limb movements, and generalized tremulousness.

The wide use of recombinant human erythropoietin has improved many of the negative cognitive consequences previously associated with chronic anemia. Maintaining an optimal level of cognitive function is important for quality of life and is a prerequisite for successful adaptation to dialysis.

Social Support

ESRD patients can receive social support from family, friends, and individuals on the dialysis unit (e.g., physicians, social workers, nurses, other patients). Increased levels of social support may positively impact outcomes through various mechanisms, including decreased levels of depressive affect, increased patient perception of quality of life, increased access to health care, increased patient compliance with prescribed therapies, and physiological effects on the immune system (S.D. Cohen et al. 2007b). Higher levels of perceived social support are thought to have a positive influence on health outcomes, utilization of health care services, and compliance. Previous research has demonstrated that social support is related to improved health outcomes and lower mortality for ESRD patients (Christensen et al. 1994; S.D. Cohen et al. 2007b; Kimmel et al. 1998a; McClellan et al. 1991, 1993).

Sexual Dysfunction

The impact of hemodialysis on both male and female sexual functioning is well documented (Levy and Cohen 2001) but often not discussed openly with patients. One recent study reported that 43% of ESRD patients reported having a decreased interest in sex and 47% reported trouble getting aroused (Abdel-Kader et al. 2009). The relative roles of physical dysfunction, medical illness, medication effects, and psychological function in inducing sexual dysfunction in CKD patients have not been determined. A review by Palmer (2003) noted similarly high rates of sexual dysfunction in men and women with ESRD. The first line of treatment for sexual dysfunction is typically sildenafil, which appears to be safe in ESRD patients if they do not have contraindications to treatment (Palmer 2003; Seibel et al. 2002; Zarifian 1999). The subject of sexual performance is often sensitive, and both the patient's and the doctor's perceptions can be influenced by the interplay of cultural, age, gender, racial, religious, and emotional factors (see also Chapter 16, "Sexual Dysfunction").

Treatment Adherence

Clinical and behavioral indices of adherence in dialysis patients include dialysis attendance, interdialytic weight gain, and medication adherence. Lack of adherence to treatment regimens is believed to be a common cause of inadequate dialysis and poor outcome (Kaveh and Kimmel 2001). Many factors may contribute to nonadherence, including depression, anxiety, cognitive dysfunction, personality, the doctor–patient relationship, and financial difficulties. The rate of nonadherence among dialysis patients varies by country as well (Bleyer et al. 1999; Hecking et al. 2004). Common noncompliant behaviors include skipping or missing dialysis sessions and engaging in dietary and medication indiscretions. According to self-reports, 12% of dialysis patients miss one peritoneal dialysis exchange per week, and 5% skip two to three exchanges per week (United States Renal Data System 2009). To maintain optimal health, ESRD patients must adhere to their prescribed treatments. Patients are prescribed regimens for their medications, diet, fluid intake, exercise, medical appointments, and dialysis attendance. Measures of behavioral compliance are clinically meaningful and associated with hard outcomes (Kimmel et al. 1995, 1998a; Leggat 2005). A recent study that examined medication adherence in ESRD found that 37% of hemodialysis patients reported less than perfect adherence to the medication regimen and that increased depressive affect was associated with decreased medication adherence (Cukor et al. 2009). Because adherence was self-reported, the data may be an underestimation of the actual level of adherence, demonstrating the great need for addressing this issue in this population. Another study found that the median daily pill burden of an ESRD cohort was 19. In one-quarter of the subjects, it exceeded 25 pills per day. Phosphate binders accounted for about one-half of the daily pill burden, and 62% of the participants were noncompliant with the prescribed phosphate binder therapy (Chiu et al. 2009). A recent systematic review of studies of adherence to prescribed oral medications in adult chronic hemodialysis patients found that more than half of the included studies reported nonadherence rates of 50% or more, with a mean of 67% (Schmid et al. 2009).

The development of interventions to target adherence in this population is increasingly gaining attention in the literature. Some of these interventions are educational in nature, attempting to increase knowledge of the importance of adherence and the consequences of noncompliance. However, the efficacy of educational interventions that target adherence is questionable. One study found that the hemodialysis patients who demonstrated better knowledge about the importance of monitoring phosphorus levels in their dietary regimens were *less* compliant, as measured by biomarkers and interdialytic weight gain (Durose et al. 2004). Other interventions introduce psychological techniques such as CBT, social skills training, self-monitoring, and behavioral reinforcement to increase adherence (Nozaki et al. 2005; Sharp et al. 2005b; Tsay and Lee 2005). In a small randomized controlled trial of CBT to increase fluid adherence in hemodialysis patients, results demonstrated an increase in fluid adherence (as measured by interdialytic weight gain) at 10 weeks postbaseline (Sharp et al. 2005a). Another small study (Christensen et al. 2002) compared levels of adherence in hemodialysis patients who participated in a 7-week behavioral self-regulation intervention and matched control hemodialysis patients. The study showed that the intervention patients had higher adherence (as measured by interdialytic weight gain) 8 weeks after completing the intervention compared with the control patients. These studies suggest the potential value of implementing interventions to target adherence, but the studies to date have been small and of short duration and have had bias-prone study designs (Sharp et al. 2005b).

Withdrawal From Dialysis

Withdrawal from dialysis can be viewed as part of the life cycle of the ESRD patient and part of the dying process. In the United States, dialysis withdrawal has been more common among women and older patients and less common among African American and Asian patients (Kurella Tamura et al. 2010; Leggat et al. 1997; Munshi et al. 2001). Cognitive impairment has also been associated with the decision to withdraw (Chater et al. 2006).

The topic of dialysis withdrawal is commonly approached in the assessment of patient quality of life versus quantity of life (Hackett and Watnick 2007). Reasons for the decisions of individuals who choose not to initiate or continue dialysis have included concerns about being a burden to family members and mistrust of medical treatment (Ashby et al. 2005). However, withdrawal from dialysis is often appropriate for the dying dialysis patient. Many patients and families choose this option because it allows for a quicker death and the end of a patient's suffering (L.M. Cohen and Germain 2005; L.M. Cohen et al. 2003). The median time to death after stopping dialysis is 8 days (Catalano et al. 1996), and dialysis termination usually does not cause pain or discomfort (L.M. Cohen et al. 2000). Withdrawal typically results in lethargy progressing to coma and death. Psychiatrists can assist with determinations of patient capacity and the potential influence of depression or other psychosocial factors. One study that controlled for biomarkers and age found depression to be a unique predictor of withdrawal from dialysis treatment (McDade-Montez et al. 2006). Suicidality is a symptom of depression; thus, for a patient who is experiencing severe depression, the decision to withdraw from treatment should be postponed (Russ et al. 2007).

Renal Palliative Care

In providing better end-of-life care for this very ill population, L.M. Cohen et al. (2005) have advocated that attention be focused on the following issues:

1. *Early frank discussions concerning prognosis and goals of care*—Ideally, these discussions should include the family and should begin when options for care are discussed. The possibility of not starting dialysis, especially if the burdens of dialysis might outweigh the benefits, should be considered. Patients should also know that they have the option of stopping dialysis if their quality of life diminishes. Written advance directives can help focus the discussion, and do-not-resuscitate orders should be strongly considered when cardiopulmonary resuscitation is likely to be futile (Moss 2000).
2. *Attention to symptoms at all stages of the disease process*—Patients with ESRD have a high burden of symptoms, related to dialysis and their comorbid conditions (L.M. Cohen and Germain 2005; Weisbord et al. 2008).

3. *Early hospice referrals*—Such referrals can take place in the hospital, home, nursing home, or inpatient hospice unit. All patients who terminate dialysis should be offered referral to hospice.
4. *Maximal palliative care at the end of life*—This care includes aggressive pain control, spiritual and emotional support, and attention to the patient's terminal treatment preferences and goals. Utmost sensitivity is needed in making decisions about withholding or discontinuing care, and one needs to be alert to cultural biases, countertransference, and other complicating factors (Moss 1998, 2000). In a survey of American nephrologists, nearly 90% reported withholding dialysis at least once in the previous year, and more than 30% reported withholding it at least six times (Moss 2000; Singer 1992).

Psychotherapy in Dialysis Patients

As noted earlier in this chapter, there have been no randomized controlled trials of psychotherapy for depression in ESRD patients. Most trials of psychological intervention have aimed to improve adherence (see "Treatment Adherence" above). There are other recent small randomized controlled trials in dialysis patients showing that group therapy can improve quality of life (Lii et al. 2007) and that CBT can improve sleep disturbance (Chen et al. 2008). Although individual and group psychotherapies have been considered very helpful in ESRD for many years, the evidence base supporting such interventions remains very limited.

Psychopharmacology in Renal Disease

Antidepressants

Among the SSRIs, citalopram and sertraline would be expected to have the fewest potential interactions with other medications taken by patients with renal impairment. Paroxetine clearance is reduced in patients with renal insufficiency (Doyle et al. 1989). Some evidence suggests that dosage adjustments may not be needed for citalopram (Spigset et al. 2000) and fluoxetine (Finkelstein and Finkelstein 2000) in patients with renal insufficiency. While the longest experience has been with the tricyclic antidepressants (TCAs), patients with ESRD, especially those with diabetes, are often more sensitive to the side effects of TCAs. Hydroxylated metabolites of TCAs may be markedly elevated in patients with ESRD and responsible for some TCA side effects. Nortriptyline and desipramine are the preferred TCAs in renal failure because they are less likely to cause anticholinergic effects or orthostatic hypotension than other TCAs (Gillman 2007). Limited data are available on the use of newer antidepressants in patients with renal failure. The half-life of venlafaxine is prolonged in renal insufficiency; its clearance is reduced by over 50% in patients undergoing dialysis (Troy et al. 1994). Desvenlafaxine undergoes significant renal elimination requiring dosage reduction in moderate to severe renal impairment. Because antidepressants are typically metabolized by the liver and those metabolites are excreted by the kidney, it seems prudent to initially reduce the dose for all antidepressants to minimize the potential accumulation of active metabolites (S.D. Cohen et al. 2007a). Ordinary dosages however are frequently required in ESRD patients and are usually well tolerated.

Antipsychotics

Antipsychotics typically do not depend on renal elimination, with the exception of paliperidone, which is largely excreted unchanged in urine and thus requires dose reduction in patients with renal insufficiency (Vermeir et al. 2008). As with TCAs, adverse effects of antipsychotics may be amplified by medical comorbidities in ESRD patients, such as diabetes, hyperlipidemia, and cerebrovascular disease.

Anxiolytics and Sedative-Hypnotics

No clinical trials of pharmacotherapy for anxiety in ESRD patients have been published. The preferred benzodiazepines are those with inactive metabolites (e.g., lorazepam, oxazepam). Even so, the half-lives of lorazepam and oxazepam may rise significantly in patients with ESRD, and dosage reduction is required.

Mood Stabilizers

Lithium is almost entirely excreted by the kidneys. It is contraindicated in patients with acute renal failure. Some clinicians consider lithium relatively contraindicated in patients with stable renal insufficiency. If used, lithium should be conservatively dosed while monitoring renal function frequently. Despite these cautions and lithium's possible nephrotoxicity (discussed under "Renal Effects of Psychotropics" later in this chapter), there are some bipolar patients who do not respond to or tolerate the alternative mood stabilizers; for these patients, lithium is the only effective drug. Lithium is completely dialyzed and may be given as a single oral dose (300–600 mg) following hemodialysis treatment. Lithium levels should not be checked until at least 2–3 hours after dialysis because re-equilibration from tissue stores occurs in the immediate postdialysis period. The dose of gabapentin, pregabalin, lithium, and topiramate should be modified based on creatinine clearance (Ferrando et al. 2010).

Cholinesterase Inhibitors and Memantine

While the data are limited, dosage adjustment of donepezil and rivastigmine is probably unnecessary. Galantamine should be used cautiously in patients with moderate renal insufficiency and is not recommended in patients with severe renal insufficiency. Memantine requires dosage reduction in patients with severe renal insufficiency (Ferrando et al. 2010).

Renal Effects of Psychotropics

The syndrome of inappropriate antidiuretic hormone secretion (SIADH), resulting in hyponatremia, may be caused by many psychotropic drugs, especially carbamazepine and oxcarbazepine, but also SSRIs, TCAs, and antipsychotics. Hypernatremia due to nephrogenic diabetes insipidus (NDI) may be caused by lithium through inhibition of renal tubular water reabsorption. Most patients receiving lithium have polydipsia and polyuria, reflecting NDI. Lithium-induced NDI varies from mild polyuria to hyperosmolar coma, and sometimes has persisted long after lithium discontinuation. Amiloride is considered the treatment of choice for lithium-induced NDI, but it also has been treated with nonsteroidal anti-inflammatory drugs (NSAIDs), thiazides, and sodium restriction (Grunfeld and Rossier 2009). Some studies report that longer duration of lithium therapy is predictive of a decrease in estimated glomerular filtration, while others do not. Although chronic lithium use may result in nephropathic changes in 10%–20% of patients, including interstitial fibrosis, tubular atrophy, urinary casts, and, occasionally, glomerular sclerosis (Bendz et al. 1996), these histological changes are often not associated with impaired renal function. Progression of lithium nephrotoxicity to ESRD is rare (0.2%–0.7%) and requires lithium use for many years (Presne et al. 2003). Other factors besides lithium use that may contribute to such changes include age, episodes of lithium toxicity, other medications (analgesics, substance abuse) and the presence of comorbid disorders (hypertension, diabetes). Lithium nephrotoxicity is not strongly dose related (Freeman and Freeman 2006). One recent meta-analysis concluded that any lithium-induced effect on renal function is quantitatively small and probably clinically insignificant (Paul et al. 2009) and considered acceptable with yearly monitoring of renal function.

Urological Effects of Psychotropics

Drugs with significant anticholinergic activity, such as TCAs and antipsychotics (both low-potency typical agents and atypical agents), frequently cause urinary retention. Less commonly, urinary retention has been reported to occur with SSRIs, serotonin–norepinephrine reuptake inhibitors (SNRIs), and bupropion. Urinary incontinence and other lower urinary tract side effects are very common with clozapine (Jeong et al. 2008). Sexual side effects of psychotropic drugs are reviewed in Chapter 16, "Sexual Dysfunction."

Psychiatric Adverse Effects of Renal and Urological Agents

Anticholinergic agents commonly used to treat overactive bladder are associated with psychiatric adverse effects including cognitive impairment, confusion, fatigue and psychosis. Mild cognitive impairment was found in 80% of elderly patients receiving anticholinergics (Ancelin et al. 2006). Thiazide diuretics are a common cause of hyponatremia, which when severe can cause lethargy, stupor, confusion, psychosis, irritability, and seizures. The risk is increased further if the patient is also taking a psychotropic drug that causes hyponatremia, such as an SSRI (Rosner 2004) or carbamazepine (Ranta and Wooten 2004). Psychiatric adverse effects of other medications frequently used to treat patients with renal disease are covered elsewhere in this book: corticosteroids for autoimmune nephritis (Chapter 25, "Rheumatology"), antihypertensives (Chapter 18, "Heart Disease"), and immunosuppressants after renal transplant (Chapter 31, "Organ Transplantation").

Drug–Drug Interactions

A number of pharmacodynamic and pharmacokinetic drug interactions frequently occur between drugs prescribed for renal and urological disorders and psychotropic drugs. Anticholinergic side effects will be increased if anticholinergic psychotropic drugs are given to patients taking urinary antispasmodics. Like other anticholinergics, antispasmodics may block the benefits of cholinesterase inhibitors. As noted above, the hyponatremic effects of thiazide diuretics may be enhanced in combination with oxcarbazepine and carbamazepine, and to a lesser degree with SSRIs, TCAs, and antipsychotics (Ranta and Wooten 2004; Rosner 2004).

Diuretics variably affect lithium excretion, depending on the type of diuretic and the volume status of the patient. Thiazide diuretics may reduce lithium excretion, resulting in increased lithium levels. Acute administration of loop diuretics (e.g., furosemide, ethacrynic acid, bumetanide) increases lithium excretion causing a drop in lithium levels, but with chronic use, compensatory changes leave lithium levels somewhat unpredictable but usually not significantly changed. Carbonic anhydrase inhibitors (e.g., acetazolamide) and osmotic diuretics (e.g., mannitol) reduce lithium levels (Ferrando et al. 2010). Potassium-sparing diuretics (amiloride, triamterene, spironolactone) may increase lithium excretion. Furosemide and amiloride are considered to have the least effects on lithium excretion (Ferrando et al. 2010).

References

Abdel-Kader K, Unruh ML, Weisbord SD: Symptom burden, depression, and quality of life in chronic and end-stage kidney disease. Clin J Am Soc Nephrol 4:1057–1064, 2009

American Psychiatric Association: Diagnostic and Statistical Manual of Mental Disorders, 4th Edition, Text Revision. Washington, DC, American Psychiatric Association, 2000

Ancelin ML, Artero S, Portet F, et al: Nondegenerative mild cognitive impairment in elderly people and use of anticholinergic drugs: longitudinal cohort study. BMJ 332:455–459, 2006

Ashby M, op't Hoog C, Kellehear A, et al: Renal dialysis abatement: lessons from a social study. Palliat Med 19:389–396, 2005

Baines LS, Joseph JT, Jindal RM: Prospective randomized study of individual and group psychotherapy versus controls in recipients of renal transplants. Kidney Int 65:1937–1942, 2004

Bendz H, Sjödin I, Aurell M: Renal function on and off lithium in patients treated with lithium for 15 years or more. A controlled, prospective lithium withdrawal study. Nephrol Dial Transplant 11:457–460, 1996

Bleyer AJ, Hylander B, Sudo H, et al: An international study of patient compliance with hemodialysis. JAMA 281:1211–1213, 1999

Blumenfield M, Levy NB, Spinowitz B, et al: Fluoxetine in depressed patients on dialysis. Int J Psychiatry Med 27:71–80, 1997

Boulware LE, Liu Y, Fink NE, et al. Temporal relation among depression symptoms, cardiovascular disease events, and mortality in end-stage renal disease: contribution of reverse causality. Clin J Am Soc Nephrol 1:496–504, 2006

Catalano C, Goodship TH, Graham KA, et al: Withdrawal of renal replacement therapy in Newcastle upon Tyne: 1964–1993. Nephrol Dial Transplant 11:133–139, 1996

Chater S, Davison SN, Germain MJ, et al: Withdrawal from dialysis: a palliative care perspective. Clin Nephrol 66:364–372, 2006

Chen HY, Chiang CK, Wang HH, et al: Cognitive-behavioral therapy for sleep disturbance in patients undergoing peritoneal dialysis: a pilot randomized controlled trial. Am J Kidney Dis 52:314–323, 2008

Chiu YW, Teitelbaum I, Misra M, et al: Pill burden, adherence, hyperphosphatemia, and quality of life in maintenance dialysis patients. Clin J Am Soc Nephrol 4:1089–1096, 2009

Christensen AJ, Wiebe JS, Smith TW, et al: Predictors of survival among hemodialysis patients: effect of perceived family support. Health Psychol 13:521–525, 1994

Christensen AJ, Moran PJ, Wiebe JS, et al: Effect of a behavioral self-regulation intervention on patient adherence in hemodialysis. Health Psychol 21:393–397, 2002

Cohen L (ed): Renal disease, in The American Psychiatric Press Textbook of Consultation-Liaison Psychiatry. Washington, DC, American Psychiatric Press, 1996, pp 573–578

Cohen LM, Germain M, Poppel DM, et al: Dialysis discontinuation and palliative care. Am J Kidney Dis 36:140–144, 2000

Cohen LM, Germain MJ: The psychiatric landscape of withdrawal. Semin Dial 18:147–153, 2005

Cohen LM, Germain MJ, Poppel DM: Practical considerations in dialysis withdrawal: "to have that option is a blessing." JAMA 289:2113–2119, 2003

Cohen LM, Levy NB, Tessier EG, et al: Renal disease, in The American Psychiatric Press Textbook of Psychosomatic Medicine. Edited by Levenson JL. Arlington, VA, American Psychiatric Publishing, 2005, pp 483–493

Cohen SD, Norris L, Acquaviva K, et al: Screening, diagnosis, and treatment of depression in patients with end-stage renal disease. Clin J Am Soc Nephrol 2:1332–1342, 2007a

Cohen SD, Sharma T, Acquaviva K, et al: Social support and chronic kidney disease: an update. Adv Chronic Kidney Dis 14:335–344, 2007b

Craven JL, Rodin GM, Littlefield C: The Beck Depression Inventory as a screening device for major depression in renal dialysis patients. Int J Psychiatry Med 18:365–374, 1988

Cukor D: The hemodialysis center: a model for psychosocial intervention. Psychiatr Serv 58:711–712, 2007

Cukor D, Peterson RA, Cohen SD, et al: Depression in end-stage renal disease hemodialysis patients. Nat Clin Pract Nephrol 2:678–687, 2006

Cukor D, Coplan J, Brown C, et al: Depression and anxiety in urban hemodialysis patients. Clin J Am Soc Nephrol 2:484–490, 2007

Cukor D, Coplan J, Brown C, et al: Anxiety disorders in adults treated by hemodialysis: a single-center study. Am J Kidney Dis 52:128–136, 2008a

Cukor D, Coplan J, Brown C, et al: Course of depression and anxiety diagnosis in patients treated with hemodialysis: a 16-month follow-up. Clin J Am Soc Nephrol 3:1752–1758, 2008b

Cukor D, Rosenthal DS, Jindal RM, et al: Depression is an important contributor to low medication adherence in hemodialyzed patients and transplant recipients. Kidney Int 75:1223–1229, 2009

Doyle GD, Laher M, Kelly JG, et al: The pharmacokinetics of paroxetine in renal impairment. Acta Psychiatr Scand Suppl 350:89–90, 1989

Durose CL, Holdsworth M, Watson V, et al: Knowledge of dietary restrictions and the medical consequences of noncompliance by patients on hemodialysis are not predictive of dietary compliance. J Am Diet Assoc 104:35–41, 2004

Elias MF, Elias PK, Seliger SL, et al: Chronic kidney disease, creatinine and cognitive functioning. Nephrol Dial Transplant 24:2446–2452, 2009

Ferrando SJ, Levenson JL, Owen JA: Renal and urological disorders, in Clinical Manual of Psychopharmacology in the Medically Ill. Edited by Ferrando SJ, Levenson JL, Owen JA. Arlington, VA, American Psychiatric Publishing, 2010, pp 149–180

Finkelstein FO, Finkelstein SH: Depression in chronic dialysis patients: assessment and treatment. Nephrol Dial Transplant 15:1911–1913, 2000

Franke GH, Reimer J, Philipp T, et al: Aspects of quality of life through end-stage renal disease. Qual Life Res 12:103–115, 2003

Fraser CL, Arieff AI: Nervous system complications in uremia. Ann Intern Med 109:143–153, 1988

Freeman MP, Freeman SA: Lithium: clinical considerations in internal medicine. Am J Med 119:478–481, 2006

Galla JH (Renal Physicians Association/American Society of Nephrology Working Group): Clinical practice guideline on shared decision-making in the appropriate initiation of and withdrawal from dialysis. The Renal Physicians Association and the American Society of Nephrology. J Am Soc Nephrol 11:1340–1342, 2000

Gillman PK: Tricyclic antidepressant pharmacology and therapeutic drug interactions updated. Br J Pharmacol 151:737–748, 2007

Goldman RS: Medical director responsibilities regarding disruptive behavior in the dialysis center—leading effective conflict resolution. Semin Dial 21:245–249, 2008

Grunfeld JP, Rossier BC: Lithium nephrotoxicity revisited. Nat Rev Nephrol 5:270–276, 2009

Hackett AS, Watnick SG: Withdrawal from dialysis in end-stage renal disease: medical, social, and psychological issues. Semin Dial 20:86–90, 2007

Haddy FJ, Meyer TW, Hostetter TH: Uremia. N Engl J Med 358:95; author reply 95, 2008

Hashmi A, Moss AH: Treating difficult or disruptive dialysis patients: practical strategies based on ethical principles. Nat Clin Pract Nephrol 4:515–520, 2008

Hecking E, Bragg-Gresham JL, Rayner HC, et al: Haemodialysis prescription, adherence and nutritional indicators in five European countries: results from the Dialysis Outcomes and Practice Patterns Study (DOPPS). Nephrol Dial Transplant 19:100–107, 2004

Hedayati SS, Bosworth HB, Kuchibhatla M, et al: The predictive value of self-report scales compared with physician diagnosis of depression in hemodialysis patients. Kidney Int 69:1662–1668, 2006

Hedayati SS, Bosworth HB, Briley LP, et al: Death or hospitalization of patients on chronic hemodialysis is associated with a physician-based diagnosis of depression. Kidney Int 74:930–936, 2008

Hedayati SS, Minhajuddin AT, Toto RD, et al: Prevalence of major depressive episode in CKD. Am J Kidney Dis 54:424–432, 2009a

Hedayati SS, Minhajuddin AT, Toto RD, et al: Validation of depression screening scales in patients with CKD. Am J Kidney Dis 54:433–439, 2009b

Hegde A, Veis JH, Seidman A, et al: High prevalence of alcoholism in dialysis patients. Am J Kidney Dis 35:1039–1043, 2000

Jaffe JA, Kimmel PL: Chronic nephropathies of cocaine and heroin abuse: a critical review. Clin J Am Soc Nephrol 1:655–667, 2006

Jeong SH, Kim JH, Ahn YM, et al: A 2-year prospective follow-up study of lower urinary tract symptoms in patients treated with clozapine. J Clin Psychopharmacol 28:618–624, 2008

Johnson WJ, McCarthy JT, Yanagihara T, et al: Effects of recombinant human erythropoietin on cerebral and cutaneous blood flow and on blood coagulability. Kidney Int 38:919–924, 1990

Kaveh K, Kimmel PL: Compliance in hemodialysis patients: multidimensional measures in search of a gold standard. Am J Kidney Dis 37:244–266, 2001

Kimmel PL: Psychosocial factors in dialysis patients. Kidney Int 59:1599–1613, 2001

Kimmel PL: Depression in patients with chronic renal disease: what we know and what we need to know. J Psychosom Res 53:951–956, 2002

Kimmel PL, Patel SS: Quality of life in patients with chronic kidney disease: focus on end-stage renal disease treated with hemodialysis. Semin Nephrol 26:68–79, 2006

Kimmel PL, Weihs K, Peterson RA: Survival in hemodialysis patients: the role of depression. J Am Soc Nephrol 4:12–27, 1993

Kimmel PL, Peterson RA, Weihs KL, et al: Behavioral compliance with dialysis prescription in hemodialysis patients. J Am Soc Nephrol 5:1826–1834, 1995

Kimmel PL, Peterson RA, Weihs KL, et al: Psychologic functioning, quality of life, and behavioral compliance in patients beginning hemodialysis. J Am Soc Nephrol 7:2152–2159, 1996

Kimmel PL, Peterson RA, Weihs KL, et al: Psychosocial factors, behavioral compliance and survival in urban hemodialysis patients. Kidney Int 54:245–254, 1998a

Kimmel PL, Thamer M, Richard CM, et al: Psychiatric illness in patients with end-stage renal disease. Am J Med 105:214–221, 1998b

Kimmel PL, Peterson RA, Weihs KL, et al: Multiple measurements of depression predict mortality in a longitudinal study of chronic hemodialysis outpatients. Kidney Int 57:2093–2098, 2000

Kimmel PL, Barisoni L, Kopp JB: Pathogenesis and treatment of HIV-associated renal diseases: lessons from clinical and animal studies, molecular pathologic correlations, and genetic investigations. Ann Intern Med 139:214–226, 2003

Kimmel PL, Cukor D, Cohen SD, et al: Depression in end-stage renal disease patients: a critical review. Adv Chronic Kidney Dis 14:328–334, 2007

Koo DD, Welsh KI, McLaren AJ, et al: Cadaver versus living donor kidneys: impact of donor factors on antigen induction before transplantation. Kidney Int 56:1551–1559, 1999

Koo JR, Yoon JY, Joo MH, et al: Treatment of depression and effect of antidepression treatment on nutritional status in chronic hemodialysis patients. Am J Med Sci 329:1–5, 2005

Kurella M, Chertow GM, Luan J, et al: Cognitive impairment in chronic kidney disease. J Am Geriatr Soc 52:1863–1869, 2004

Kurella M, Mapes DL, Port FK, et al: Correlates and outcomes of dementia among dialysis patients: the Dialysis Outcomes and Practice Patterns Study. Nephrol Dial Transplant 21:2543–2548, 2006

Kurella Tamura M, Goldstein M, Perez-Stable E: Preferences for dialysis withdrawal and engagement in advance care planning within a diverse sample of dialysis patients. nephrology dialysis and transplantation. Nephrol Dial Transplant 25:237–242, 2010

Laupacis A, Keown P, Pus N, et al: A study of the quality of life and cost-utility of renal transplantation. Kidney Int 50:235–242, 1996

Lea JP, Nicholas SB: Diabetes mellitus and hypertension: key risk factors for kidney disease. J Natl Med Assoc 94 (8 suppl):7S–15S, 2002

Leggat JE Jr: Adherence with dialysis: a focus on mortality risk. Semin Dial 18:137–141, 2005

Leggat JE Jr, Bloembergen WE, Levine G, et al: An analysis of risk factors for withdrawal from dialysis before death. J Am Soc Nephrol 8:1755–1763, 1997

Levy NB, Cohen LM (eds): Central and peripheral nervous systems in uremia, in Textbook of Nephrology, 4th Edition. Edited by Massry SG, Glassock R. Philadelphia, PA, Williams & Wilkins, 2001, pp 1279–1282

Lii YC, Tsay SL, Wang TJ: Group intervention to improve quality of life in haemodialysis patients. J Clin Nurs 16:268–275, 2007

Lockridge RS Jr, Spencer M, Craft V, et al: Nocturnal home hemodialysis in North America. Adv Ren Replace Ther 8:250–256, 2001

McBride P: The development of hemodialysis and peritoneal dialysis, in Clinical Dialysis, 3rd Edition. Edited by Nissenson AR, Fine RN, Gentile DE. Norwalk, CT, Appleton & Lang, 1995, pp 6–18

McClellan WM, Anson C, Birkeli K, et al: Functional status and quality of life: predictors of early mortality among patients entering treatment for end stage renal disease. J Clin Epidemiol 44:83–89, 1991

McClellan WM, Stanwyck DJ, Anson CA: Social support and subsequent mortality among patients with end-stage renal disease. J Am Soc Nephrol 4:1028–1034, 1993

McDade-Montez EA, Christensen AJ, Cvengros JA, et al: The role of depression symptoms in dialysis withdrawal. Health Psychol 25:198–204, 2006

McLaughlin K, Manns B, Mortis G, et al: Why patients with ESRD do not select self-care dialysis as a treatment option. Am J Kidney Dis 41:380–385, 2003

Meyer TW, Hostetter TH: Uremia. N Engl J Med 357:1316–1325, 2007

Moss AH: "At least we do not feel guilty": managing conflict with families over dialysis discontinuation. Am J Kidney Dis 31:868–883, 1998

Moss AH: A new clinical practice guideline on initiation and withdrawal of dialysis that makes explicit the role of palliative medicine. J Palliat Med 3:253–260, 2000

Munshi SK, Vijayakumar N, Taub NA, et al: Outcome of renal replacement therapy in the very elderly. Nephrol Dial Transplant 16:128–133, 2001

Murray AM, Tupper DE, Knopman DS, et al: Cognitive impairment in hemodialysis patients is common. Neurology 67:216–223, 2006

Nichols KA, Springford V: The psycho-social stressors associated with survival by dialysis. Behav Res Ther 22:563–574, 1984

Norris KC, Thornhill-Joynes M, Robinson C, et al: Cocaine use, hypertension, and end-stage renal disease. Am J Kidney Dis 38:523–528, 2001

Nozaki C, Oka M, Chaboyer W: The effects of a cognitive behavioural therapy programme for self-care on haemodialysis patients. Int J Nurs Pract 11:228–236, 2005

Obialo CI, Bashir K, Goring S, et al: Dialysis "no-shows" on Saturdays: implications of the weekly hemodialysis schedules on nonadherence and outcomes. J Natl Med Assoc 100:412–419, 2008

Palmer BF: Sexual dysfunction in men and women with chronic kidney disease and end-stage kidney disease. Adv Ren Replace Ther 10:48–60, 2003

Paul R, Minay J, Cardwell C, et al: Meta-analysis of the effects of lithium usage on serum creatinine levels. J Psychopharmacol 2009 Apr 24 [Epub ahead of print]

Pereira AA, Weiner DE, Scott T, et al: Cognitive function in dialysis patients. Am J Kidney Dis 45:448–462, 2005

Pierratos A: Daily nocturnal home hemodialysis. Kidney Int 65:1975–1986, 2004

Pliskin NH, Yurk HM, Ho LT, et al: Neurocognitive function in chronic hemodialysis patients. Kidney Int 49:1435–1440, 1996

Presne C, Fakhouri F, Noel LH, et al: Lithium-induced nephropathy: rate of progression and prognostic factors. Kidney Int 64:585–592, 2003

Rabindranath KS, Daly C, Butler JA, et al: Psychosocial interventions for depression in dialysis patients. Cochrane Database Syst Rev (3):CD004542, 2005

Ranta A, Wooten GF: Hyponatremia due to an additive effect of carbamazepine and thiazide diuretics. Epilepsia 45:879, 2004

Rosner MH: Severe hyponatremia associated with the combined use of thiazide diuretics and selective serotonin reuptake inhibitors. Am J Med Sci 327:109–111, 2004

Rubin HR, Fink NE, Plantinga LC, et al: Patient ratings of dialysis care with peritoneal dialysis vs hemodialysis. JAMA 291:697–703, 2004

Russ AJ, Shim JK, Kaufman SR: The value of "life at any cost": talk about stopping kidney dialysis. Soc Sci Med 64:2236–2247, 2007

Saczynski JS, Jonsdottir MK, Garcia ME, et al: Cognitive impairment: an increasingly important complication of type 2 diabetes: the age, gene/environment susceptibility—Reykjavik study. Am J Epidemiol 168:1132–1139, 2008

Sareen J, Jacobi F, Cox BJ, et al: Disability and poor quality of life associated with comorbid anxiety disorders and physical conditions. Arch Intern Med 166:2109–2116, 2006

Schmid H, Hartmann B, Schiffl H: Adherence to prescribed oral medication in adult patients undergoing chronic hemodialysis: a critical review of the literature. Eur J Med Res 14:185–190, 2009

Seibel I, Poli De Figueiredo CE, Teloken C, et al: Efficacy of oral sildenafil in hemodialysis patients with erectile dysfunction. J Am Soc Nephrol 13:2770–2775, 2002

Semplicini A, Amodio P, Leonetti G, et al: Diagnostic tools for the study of vascular cognitive dysfunction in hypertension and antihypertensive drug research. Pharmacol Ther 109:274–283, 2006

Sharp J, Wild MR, Gumley AI, et al: A cognitive behavioral group approach to enhance adherence to hemodialysis fluid restrictions: a randomized controlled trial. Am J Kidney Dis 45:1046–1057, 2005a

Sharp J, Wild MR, Gumley AI: A systematic review of psychological interventions for the treatment of nonadherence to fluid-intake restrictions in people receiving hemodialysis. Am J Kidney Dis 45:15–27, 2005b

Singer PA: Nephrologists' experience with and attitudes towards decisions to forego dialysis. The End-Stage Renal Disease Network of New England. J Am Soc Nephrol 2:1235–1240, 1992

Smith MD, Hong BA, Robson AM: Diagnosis of depression in patients with end-stage renal disease. Comparative analysis. Am J Med 79:160–166, 1985

Souheaver GT, Ryan JJ, DeWolfe AS: Neuropsychological patterns in uremia. J Clin Psychol 38:490–496, 1982

Spigset O, Hagg S, Stegmayr B, et al: Citalopram pharmacokinetics in patients with chronic renal failure and the effect of haemodialysis. Eur J Clin Pharmacol 56:699–703, 2000

Sukolsky A: Patients who try our patience. Am J Kidney Dis 44:893–901, 2004

Tagay S, Kribben A, Hohenstein A, et al: Posttraumatic stress disorder in hemodialysis patients. Am J Kidney Dis 50:594–601, 2007

Troy SM, Schultz RW, Parker VD, et al: The effect of renal disease on the disposition of venlafaxine. Clin Pharmacol Ther 56:14–21, 1994

Tsay SL, Lee YC: Effects of an adaptation training programme for patients with end-stage renal disease. J Adv Nurs 50:39–46, 2005

United States Renal Data System: USRDS 2003 Annual Data Report: Atlas of End-Stage Renal Disease in the United States. Bethesda, MD, National Institutes of Health, National Institute of Diabetes and Digestive and Kidney Diseases, 2003

United States Renal Data System: USRDS 2008 Annual Data Report: Atlas of End-Stage Renal Disease in the United States. Bethesda, MD, National Institutes of Health, National Institute of Diabetes and Digestive and Kidney Diseases, 2009

Vermeir M, Naessens I, Remmerie B, et al: Absorption, metabolism, and excretion of paliperidone, a new monoaminergic antagonist, in humans. Drug Metab Dispos 36:769–779, 2008

Watnick S, Kirwin P, Mahnensmith R, et al: The prevalence and treatment of depression among patients starting dialysis. Am J Kidney Dis 41:105–110, 2003

Watnick S, Wang PL, Demadura T, et al: Validation of 2 depression screening tools in dialysis patients. Am J Kidney Dis 46:919–924, 2005

Weisbord SD, Carmody SS, Bruns FJ, et al: Symptom burden, quality of life, advance care planning and the potential value of palliative care in severely ill haemodialysis patients. Nephrol Dial Transplant 18:1345–1352, 2003

Weisbord SD, Bossola M, Fried LF, et al: Cultural comparison of symptoms in patients on maintenance hemodialysis. Hemodial Int 12:434–440, 2008

Williams MA, Sklar AH, Burright RG, et al: Temporal effects of dialysis on cognitive functioning in patients with ESRD. Am J Kidney Dis 43:705–711, 2004

Wolfe RA, Ashby VB, Milford EL, et al: Comparison of mortality in all patients on dialysis, patients on dialysis awaiting transplantation, and recipients of a first cadaveric transplant. N Engl J Med 341:1725–1730, 1999

Zarifian A: The role of Viagra in the treatment of male impotence in ESRD. ANNA J 26:242, 1999

CHAPTER

22

Endocrine and Metabolic Disorders

Ann Goebel-Fabbri, Ph.D.

Gail Musen, Ph.D.

James L. Levenson, M.D.

THE ONSET, COURSE, AND OUTCOMES of endocrine disorders traditionally have been linked to psychological and social factors. A growing body of neuroendocrine research has begun to illuminate important biological mechanisms underlying the interplay of psyche and soma, and there are important clinical ramifications of these connections. In this chapter, we focus primarily on these latter pragmatic issues. Diabetes mellitus is the most common endocrine condition and is now growing in epidemic proportions, so it has been given major emphasis. Other topics covered include disturbances in thyroid, parathyroid, adrenal, growth, prolactin, and gonadal hormones; pheochromocytomas; and metabolic disorders including electrolyte and acid-base disturbances, vitamin deficiencies, osteoporosis, and inherited disorders including the porphyrias.

Diabetes

Type 1 Diabetes

Type 1 diabetes is a chronic autoimmune disease that affects an estimated 500,000 to 1 million people in the United States. It is most commonly diagnosed in children and young adults, with peak onset occurring during puberty (i.e., ages 10–12 in girls and 12–14 in boys). (See also Chapter 34, "Pediatrics," for discussion of diabetes in pediatric populations.) The exact cause of type 1 diabetes is not known; however, it appears that genetic and environmental factors trigger an autoimmune response, which attacks the insulin-producing beta cells of the pancreas. Prolonged hyperglycemia can lead to the severe macro- and microvascular complications of diabetes, such as cardiovascular disease, retinopathy, nephropathy, and peripheral and autonomic neuropathy (Kahn et al. 2005).

The Diabetes Control and Complications Trial (DCCT), a 9-year multicenter intervention study in the United States, established that improvement in glycemic control delays the onset and slows the progression of diabetic complications (Diabetes Control and Complications Trial Research Group 1993). The DCCT's findings have informed and increased the complexity of what is now the standard treatment for type 1 diabetes. As such, treatment is aimed at lowering and stabilizing blood glucose to near normal levels through dietary control, exercise, blood glucose monitoring, and multiple daily insulin injections. Intensive blood glucose management for type 1 diabetes usually entails three or more insulin injections per day (or the use of a continuous insulin infusion pump)—with the goal of mirroring as closely as possible the physiological patterns of insulin release and near-normal blood glucose levels. Hemoglobin A_{1c} is a laboratory value reflective of average blood glucose concentrations over a 2- to 3-month period. It is used as the standard measure of diabetes self-care success and treatment effectiveness, with a typical target of as close to 7% as possible (normal range in people without diabetes is 4%–6%).

Type 2 Diabetes

Approximately 90%–95% (16 million in the United States) of all people with diabetes have type 2 diabetes, which encompasses a variety of abnormalities involving blood glucose metabolism. The hallmark of the disease is insulin resistance, in which the body requires progressively increased pancreatic insulin production to achieve normal glycemia. In patients with type 2 diabetes, the pancreas can no longer meet the need, and chronic hyperglycemia results. Risk factors for type 2 diabetes include obesity and sedentary lifestyle because both lead to insulin resistance. Onset of type 2 diabetes is typically during middle age, but with growing rates of obesity at younger ages, children and adolescents are starting to develop the disease at higher rates. Because they decrease insulin resistance, prescribed weight loss and regular exercise are first-line treatments for type 2 diabetes (Beaser 2001).

The United Kingdom Prospective Diabetes Study (UKPDS), the largest and longest prospective study of type 2 diabetes to date, found that for every 1-point reduction in hemoglobin A_{1c}, there was a corresponding 35% reduction in risk of diabetes complications. Successfully treating hypertension led to similar or greater reduction in cardiovascular complications (Krentz 1999; Matthews 1999). Treatment for type 2 diabetes is aimed at lowering and stabilizing blood glucose levels through weight loss (when applicable), dietary control, exercise, blood glucose monitoring, oral hypoglycemic medication, and treatment with insulin injections if insulin resistance and hyperglycemia persist.

Stress and Diabetes

There is conflicting evidence whether stress directly affects the onset of diabetes or its course (Helz and Templeton 1990; Mooy et al. 2000; Wales 1995). Stress hormones are involved in the body's counterregulatory response to insulin, so it is likely that stress plays a role in increasing blood glucose. Several studies have shown that glycemic control is poorer in people with diabetes who report more stress (Garay-Sevilla et al. 2000; Lloyd et al. 1999). However, it is not clear whether stress directly influences metabolic regulation or whether people under stress change their self-care behaviors. A recent meta-analysis found that psychosocial stressors, especially low social support, were significantly associated with poor metabolic control (Chida and Hamer 2008). In an effort to evaluate the effects of stress under controlled conditions, a few laboratory studies have been undertaken. Although some laboratory studies have suggested that psychological stress can impair glucose control in both type 1 (Moberg et al. 1994) and type 2 diabetes (Goetsch et al. 1993), other studies have not found this effect (Kemmer et al. 1986). Thus, it is not yet clear to what extent stressful events directly affect the physiology of glucose regulation.

Psychiatric Disorders and Diabetes Management

The publication of the DCCT and UKPDS studies established that intensive management of type 1 and type 2 diabetes improves long-term health outcomes in diabetes (Diabetes Control and Complications Trial Research Group 1993; Krentz 1999; Matthews 1999; UK Prospective Diabetes Study Group 1998a, 1998b). However, the goal of achieving near-normal blood glucose values requires a complex set of daily behaviors and problem solving. Many patients have difficulty sustaining the burden of self-care over time—the stress of coping with a chronic disease is a major risk factor for psychopathology and nonadherence to complex treatment recommendations. There is a growing literature examining the relation of type 1 and type 2 diabetes and psychiatric disorders, especially depression, anxiety, and eating disorders. In both types of diabetes, psychiatric disorders have been linked to treatment nonadherence, worse blood glucose control, and ultimately greater prevalence of micro- and macrovascular complications. Because disease outcomes in diabetes are so dependent on patient behaviors, attitudes, and cognitions, optimal treatment is multidisciplinary, including psychiatrists and other mental health professionals, and takes into account the psychology of individual patients, their support systems, and doctor–patient relationships.

Depression and Diabetes

The prevalence of depression in both type 1 and type 2 diabetes is two to three times higher than that found in the general population (Gendelman et al. 2009; Li et al. 2008). Several studies suggest that patients with depressive disorders appear to develop worse glycemic control and have a heightened risk of diabetes complications such as retinopathy, nephropathy, hypertension, cardiac disease, and sexual dysfunction (Ciechanowski et al. 2000; de Groot et al. 2001). However, it remains unclear if depression is a cause or an effect of poorer outcomes in diabetes. In a meta-analysis of 24 studies of depression, hyperglycemia, and diabetes, Lustman et al. (2000a) reported a consistently strong association between elevated hemoglobin A_{1c} values (indicating chronic hyperglycemia) and depression. They were unable to determine the direction of the association from their analyses, so it remains unclear whether hyperglycemia causes depressed mood or if hyperglycemia is a consequence of depression. Furthermore, Lustman et al. (2000a) noted that the relation may be a reciprocal one, in which hyperglycemia is provoked by depression as well as independently contributes to the exacerbation of depression.

Anxiety symptoms are also frequently reported by patients with diabetes and depression but may independently contribute to diminished quality of life in these patients (Collins et al. 2009). After accounting for depression, one study found that panic symptoms correlated with elevated hemoglobin A_{1c} levels, higher rates of complications, and lower self-rated functional health (Ludman et al. 2006).

Until recently, it was assumed that depression develops as a consequence of diabetes, with both psychosocial and biological mechanisms suggested to account for this excess prevalence. Although depression may be a result of complications and disease duration, it also has been found to occur relatively early in the course of type 1 diabetes before the onset of complications (Jacobson et al. 2002). Therefore, it does not appear that the increased rate of depression in diabetes can be explained solely by emotional reactions to a chronic disease with complications. Another meta-analysis, by de Groot et al. (2001), of studies of depression and diabetes indicated that an increase in depressive symptoms was consistently associated with an increase in severity and number of diabetes complications. Related research showed that the number of diabetes symptoms patients reported was directly related to the number of depressed symptoms patients reported; indeed, this association was stronger than the relation between diabetes symptoms and hemoglobin A_{1c} levels or diabetes complications themselves (Ludman et al. 2004). Depression may cause poorer outcomes in diabetes through biological and behavioral mechanisms because symptoms of depression such as decreased motivation, poor energy, and hopelessness likely interfere with adherence to diabetes treatment and lead to worse glycemic control (de Groot et al. 2001). Depression is associated with increased mortality in diabetes (Black et al. 2003; Katon et al. 2005).

Studies of type 2 diabetes are less clear with regard to the development of depression (Talbot and Nouwen 2000). The increased rates of depression seen in patients with type 2 diabetes appear in some instances to precede the onset of illness, thereby raising an entirely different hypothesis about the etiological relation—that is, that depressive disorders themselves may place patients at risk for developing type 2 diabetes. Katon (2003) proposed a complex model for the relation between depression and chronic medical diseases, which accounts for complex interactions of stress and adverse life events, overall self-care and healthy lifestyle activities, functional impairments, genetic risks, and biobehavioral risks. Support for these concepts derives in part from the fact that patients with depression can have alterations in the hypothalamic-pituitary axis, which lead to increased rates of cortisol production and other counterregulatory hormones, leading to insulin resistance (Musselman et al. 2003). Other biological mechanisms include alterations in central glucose transporter function and increased inflammatory activation (Cameron et al. 1984; Geringer 1990; Hudson et al. 1984). Depressed patients also decrease physical activity and increase cardiovascular risk factors by smoking and eating high-caloric and fatty foods, which place them at higher risk for developing type 2 diabetes (Marcus et al. 1992). In fact, a meta-analysis found that patients with premorbid major depression had a 37% increased risk of developing type 2 diabetes (Knol et al. 2006). The bidirectional relation between depression and type 2 diabetes was examined recently by Golden and colleagues (2008), who reported a modest association between premorbid symptoms of depression and newly diagnosed type 2 diabetes. They also reported a negative association between untreated diabetes and newly reported depression symptoms, whereas they found a positive association between treated diabetes and symptoms of depression.

Some investigators have suggested that the metabolic problems of diabetes (increased rates of hypoglycemia and hyperglycemia) could themselves play a causal role in the development of depression. There is increasing evidence that diabetes leads to changes in white matter in the brain (Dejgaard et al. 1991) and that these white matter abnormalities, if present in regions of the brain involved in affect regulation (e.g., the limbic system), may play a causal role in the development of depression (Jacobson et al. 2000). At this point, such white matter changes are of unknown etiology; however, they may be associated with accelerated vascular disease in diabetes. Indeed, history of cerebrovascular disease is significantly associated with depression in older adults with diabetes (Bruce et al. 2006).

Screening instruments such as the nine-item depression scale of the Patient Health Questionnaire (PHQ-9) (Kroenke et al. 2001) or the Beck Depression Inventory (BDI; Lustman et al. 2000b; Musselman et al. 2003) are useful in identifying patients with diabetes and depression. The PHQ-9 is currently one of the most widely used screening instruments in medical settings because it is brief and simple to use in routine clinical practice. Diabetes-specific measures of quality of life, such as the Problem Areas in Diabetes (PAID) Scale (Polonsky et al. 1995; Welch et al. 1997, 2003) and the Diabetes Quality of Life (DQOL) Measure (Jacobson 1996), also may be useful in screening patients who are overburdened by diabetes and may be at increased risk for depression.

Evidence is limited and somewhat contradictory about whether specific treatment of depression can lead to improvements in diabetes treatment adherence and improved glycemic control. Two small controlled studies have reported that nortriptyline and fluoxetine are effective treatments for depression in diabetes. However, nortriptyline improved mood but did not improve glucose regulation, whereas fluoxetine was associated with improvements in mood and a nonsignificant trend for improved hemoglobin A_{1c} levels (Lustman et al. 1997, 2000b). Sertraline maintenance treatment was recently found to lengthen the time to depression recurrence over placebo in patients with diabetes; hemoglobin A_{1c} also was found to improve slightly in relation to symptom improvement and deteriorate with depression recurrence (Lustman et al. 2006). Sertraline maintenance also was shown to decrease the risk of recurrence of depression in younger patients with diabetes (Williams et al. 2007). Compared with patients receiving diabetes education only, patients receiving cognitive-behavioral therapy (CBT) to address their depression symptoms showed significant improvements in hemoglobin A_{1c} levels (Lustman et al. 1998). A similar study showed improved mood in response to CBT but no change in hemoglobin A_{1c} levels during treatment or 1 year later (Georgiades et al. 2007). Rates of depression do not appear to differ among ethnic groups with diabetes, but fewer ethnic minority patients with diabetes report receiving appropriate treatment for depression (de Groot et al. 2006). It appears that standard treatments for depression not only lead to improvement in depressive symptoms but also may in some cases lead to better glycemic control. However, it remains unclear whether psychiatric treatment of depression in diabetes can improve psychological and biomedical outcomes.

The Pathways Study, a large-scale randomized trial, investigated an innovative approach to managing depression and diabetes in primary care clinics that provided enhanced education and support for antidepressant medication taking and behavioral problem solving. Patients receiving this intervention showed improvements in adequacy of medication dosing and improvements in depressive symptoms; however, no hemoglobin A_{1c} differences were observed between intervention patients and control subjects (Katon et al. 2004). Patients with fewer than two diabetes complications experienced the same improvement in depressive symptoms in the intervention and standard care groups; however, patients with multiple complications received more relief from their depression symptoms with the targeted intervention (Kinder et al. 2006). This intervention was shown to add no additional long-term cost to care and possibly to reduce health care costs for patients with multiple diabetes complications (Katon et al. 2008). A similar study, examining a subgroup of patients with diabetes in the Improving Mood—Promoting Access to Collaborative Treatment (IMPACT) trial, found that treating depression in older adults with diabetes contributed to significant clinical benefits to this cohort without adding to health care costs (Katon et al. 2006).

In summary, the high prevalence of depression and its adverse effects in diabetes, combined with clinically proven treatments, argue for aggressive identification and treatment of depression as early as possible in diabetes. Depression should always be suspected in patients who are having difficulty adapting to diabetes and show poor or worsening glycemic control.

Bipolar Disorder, Schizophrenia, and Diabetes

A number of studies have demonstrated a significantly increased prevalence of diabetes (mainly type 2) in bipolar disorder and schizophrenia. Patients with these disorders have diabetes rates of 10%–15%, which is between two and three times higher than rates in the general population (de Hert et al. 2009). The reasons for this added risk are unclear. Much of the association appears to be related to more obesity in both of these patient populations, which is associated with but not fully accounted for by weight gain associated with psychotropic drugs. It also may reflect the generally poor lifestyle choices of individuals with chronic psychiatric conditions—that is, they are quite sedentary, frequently smoke, and tend to overeat high-carbohydrate and high-fat foods (Newcomer 2006). In fact, both schizophrenia and bipolar patients have an equally high prevalence—about twice that in the general population—of modifiable cardiovascular risk factors, including smoking, obesity, metabolic syndrome, and diabetes (Birkenaes et al. 2007). With several of the atypical antipsychotics, the onset of diabetes may occur suddenly, with emergent ketoacidosis or hyperosmolar coma (Buse 2002; Geller and MacFadden 2003). The diabetes typically recedes once the antipsychotic medication is stopped, but it is likely that the sudden emergence of symptoms occurs in patients who already had glucose intolerance, for the increased risk of diabetes among individuals with schizophrenia precedes the use of the atypical agents (Dixon et al. 2000).

Several proposed mechanisms may help explain the association between antipsychotic treatment and diabetes; these include medication-induced weight gain, serotonin antagonism leading to decreasing insulin levels and corresponding hyperglycemia, and drug-induced leptin resistance (Buchholz et al. 2008). Family history of diabetes should be assessed prior to initiating treatment, and measurements of weight, blood glucose, and lipid levels should be taken at baseline and at periodic intervals throughout treatment. Patients also should be educated about the risks of developing diabetes and encouraged to monitor their weight (Henderson and Doraiswamy 2008). In patients with known diabetes, antipsychotics less likely to cause weight gain and glucose intolerance, such as perphenazine, molindone, aripiprazole, and ziprasidone, should be favored (Guo et al. 2007; Meyer et al. 2008; Van Winkel et al. 2008) (see Chapter 38, "Psychopharmacology," for a full discussion).

Eating Disorders and Diabetes

Despite its promise of reducing long-term complications of type 1 diabetes, a negative side of intensive diabetes management is weight gain (see also Chapter 14, "Eating Disorders"). During the first 6 years of the DCCT, patients in the intensively treated group gained an average of 10.45 pounds more than the patients in the standard treatment cohort, and 9-year follow-up data showed that this weight was hard to lose (Diabetes Control and Complications Trial Research Group 1988, 2001). A survey of patients' responses to the recommendations of the DCCT study documented that women with type 1 diabetes were especially concerned about tight glucose control causing weight gain (Thompson et al. 1996). It has been argued that the heightened attention to food portions, blood sugars, and risk of weight gain in intensive diabetes management parallels the obsessional thinking about food and body image characteristic of women with eating disorders, and this might place women with diabetes at heightened risk for developing eating disorders.

Disturbed eating behavior, usually mild in severity, is common among adolescent girls and young women in the general population; however, those with type 1 diabetes are more likely to have two or more disturbed eating behaviors than are their peers without diabetes (Colton et al. 2004). Olmsted and colleagues (2008) defined disturbed eating behavior as eating disorder symptoms not yet at the level of frequency or severity to merit a formal diagnosis, including dieting for weight loss, binge eating, or calorie purging through self-induced vomiting, laxative or diuretic use, excessive exercise, or insulin restriction in the case of type 1 diabetes. Studies of the natural history of disturbed eating behaviors in type 1 diabetes indicate that these behaviors persist and increase in severity over time as well as become more common into young adulthood (Colton et al. 2004; Peveler et al. 2005). Evidence suggests that women with type 1 diabetes are 2.4 times more at risk for developing an eating disorder and 1.9 times more at risk for developing subthreshold eating disorders than are women without diabetes (Jones et al. 2000).

Women with type 1 diabetes may use insulin manipulation (e.g., administering reduced insulin doses or omitting necessary doses altogether) as a means of caloric purging. Intentionally induced glycosuria is a powerful weight loss behavior and a symptom of eating disorders unique to type 1 diabetes. Questions such as "Do you ever change your insulin dose or skip insulin doses to influence your weight?" or "How often do you take less insulin than prescribed?" can be helpful in screening for insulin omission, especially when patients present with persistently elevated hemoglobin A_{1c} levels or unexplained diabetic ketoacidosis. Intermittent insulin omission or dose reduction for weight loss purposes has been found to be a common practice among women with type 1 diabetes. As many as 31% of women with type 1 diabetes report intentional insulin restriction, with rates of this disturbed eating behavior peaking in late adolescence and early adulthood (40% of women between ages 15 and 30 years) (Polonsky et al. 1994). This behavior, even at a subclinical level of severity, places women at heightened risk for medical complications of diabetes. Women reporting intentional insulin misuse had higher hemoglobin A_{1c} values (approximately 2 or more percentage points higher than values in similarly aged women without eating disorders), higher rates of hospital and emergency department visits, and higher rates of neuropathy and retinopathy than women who did not report insulin omission (Bryden et al. 1999; Polonsky et al. 1994; Rydall et al. 1997). The chronic hyperglycemia found in women with diabetes who intentionally omit or reduce their insulin doses places these women at much greater risk for frequent episodes of diabetic ketoacidosis and the long-term onset of macro- and microvascular complications of diabetes. Even subthreshold disturbed eating behaviors are strongly associated with significant medical and psychological consequences in the context of diabetes (Verrotti et al. 1999). In fact, endorsing insulin restriction alone was recently shown to increase mortality risk threefold over an 11-year follow-up period (Goebel-Fabbri et al. 2008).

Because obesity is a significant risk factor in type 2 diabetes, recurrent binge eating may increase the chances of developing it in part because of significantly higher body mass index (BMI) (Striegel-Moore et al. 2000). Initial studies of binge eating in type 2 diabetes relied on small, nonrepresentative samples. Kenardy et al. (1994) found that 14% of the patients with newly diagnosed type 2 diabetes experienced problems with binge eating compared with 4% of the age-, sex-, and weight-matched control group. Night eating symptoms also have been implicated for their association with obesity and poor diabetes control. One study found that patients reporting symptoms of night eating were more likely to be obese, have hemoglobin A_{1c} values higher than recommended targets, and have two or more diabetes complications (Morse et al. 2006). In the largest study of its kind to date, more than 5,000 patients with type 2 diabetes were evaluated to determine whether binge eating was related to weight loss after a 1-year intervention. Larger weight losses were observed in those patients who never endorsed binge eating or who reported that they were no longer binge eating at 1-year follow-up (Gorin et al. 2008). Thus, recurrent binge eating and symptoms of night eating syndrome can be expected to make it increasingly difficult to control diabetes and weight.

A multidisciplinary team approach, including an endocrinologist or a diabetologist, nurse educator, nutritionist with eating disorder and diabetes training, and mental health practitioner, is ideal for the treatment of comorbid eating disorders and diabetes (Kahn et al. 2005; Mitchell et al. 1997). Depending on the severity of the eating disorder and other comorbid psychopathology, a psychiatrist also may be needed for psychopharmacological evaluation and treatment. At this time, little research has examined treatment efficacy for eating disorders in the context of diabetes; however, a large research literature on treatment outcomes in bulimia nervosa supports the use of CBT in combination with antidepressant medications as the most effective treatment (Peterson and Mitchell 1999; B.T. Walsh and Devlin 1995). These approaches would need to be adapted slightly to address directly the role of insulin omission as the means of caloric purging.

Early in treatment, intensive glycemic management of diabetes is not an appropriate target for a person with diabetes and an eating disorder. As noted earlier, overly intensive diabetes management may actually aggravate obsessional thinking about food and weight in patients with eating disorders. The first goal should focus on medical stabilization. Gradually, the team can build toward increasing doses of insulin, increases in food intake, greater flexibility of meal plan, regularity of eating routine, and more frequent blood glucose monitoring.

Sexual Function and Diabetes

For information on diabetes and sexual function, see Chapter 16, "Sexual Dysfunction."

Cognitive Functioning and Diabetes

Several researchers have studied the effect of diabetes on cognitive functioning. Results from a meta-analysis of 31 studies published between 1980 and 2004 indicated that young and middle-aged diabetic adults, ages 18–50 years, performed significantly more poorly than did their nondiabetic peers on measures of intelligence, attention, psychomotor efficiency, cognitive flexibility, and visual perception (Brands et al. 2005). Effect sizes were largest on tasks that rely on general knowledge and on psychomotor efficiency. In general, performance on virtually all tasks requiring rapid responding or cognitive flexibility was affected to some degree, whereas effects on learning and memory function were modest, with small between-group differences.

The etiology of these neurocognitive differences remains unclear. Early studies emphasized the role of recurrent episodes of severe hypoglycemia (Bjorgaas et al. 1997; Deary et al. 1993; Frazekas 1989; Langan et al. 1991; Perros et al. 1997). Several studies, including the recent 18-year follow-up of more than 1,300 subjects from the DCCT, have found no cognitive effects associated with recurrent episodes of severe hypoglycemia (Austin and Deary 1999; Diabetes Control and Complications Trial Research Group 1996; Jacobson et al. 2007) but suggested that chronically elevated hemoglobin A_{1c} levels predict cognitive dysfunction and cognitive decline over time (Ferguson et al. 2003; Jacobson et al. 2006, 2007; Ryan 2006; Ryan et al. 2003).

Long-term exposure to hyperglycemia and related micro- and macrovascular damage also has been posited to heighten risk of cognitive decline and dementia in diabetes. In fact, two studies reported a 60%–100% increased risk for cognitive decline among patients with diabetes as compared with those without diabetes (Gregg and Brown 2003). This increased risk appears to be mediated primarily by an increase in vascular dementia rather than a heightened risk for Alzheimer's disease in diabetes (Gregg and Brown 2003).

Hypoglycemia in Diabetic and Nondiabetic Individuals

Hypoglycemia has been a popular explanation for anxiety symptoms, especially panic attacks, with past widespread use of 5-hour glucose tolerance tests for diagnosis and recommendations for dietary management with multiple small meals. This practice is no longer commonly recommended by physicians, but hypoglycemia is still a popular diagnosis among alternative medicine practitioners and many patients. Symptomatic hypoglycemia rarely occurs except in diabetic (mainly insulin-dependent) patients and patients with insulinomas. Although marked hypoglycemia does cause symptoms of adrenergic hyperactivity, they can be reliably distinguished by patients from panic attacks (Schweizer et al. 1986; Uhde et al. 1984).

However, insulin-induced hypoglycemia is an aversive experience, which has been reported to cause phobic anxiety—that is, a fear of hypoglycemia—in diabetic patients, leading to poorer diabetic control (Green et al. 2000).

Thyroid Disorders

Hyperthyroidism and hypothyroidism are accompanied by a variety of physiological, psychiatric, and cognitive symptoms. Patients with psychiatric disorders, especially depression, have elevated rates of thyroid disease (Farmer et al. 2008; Lobo-Escolar et al. 2008). In this section, we focus on cognitive and psychiatric symptoms associated with thyroid problems.

Hyperthyroidism

Hyperthyroidism is accompanied by a host of physiological symptoms, including nervousness, sweating, fatigue, heat intolerance, weight loss, and muscle weakness (Kornstein et al. 2000). The most common cause of hyperthyroidism (or thyrotoxicosis) is Graves' disease. Graves' disease is an autoimmune disorder that results in hyperthyroidism when thyroid-stimulating immunoglobulins (TSIs) bind to thyrotropin receptors and mimic thyrotropin. TSIs thereby stimulate the synthesis of hormones (thyroxine [T_4] and triiodothyronine [T_3]) while serum thyrotropin levels are very low or undetectable (Porterfield 1997). The factors that trigger this immune response are unknown. Patients with type 1 diabetes are at increased risk for Graves' disease. Some evidence shows that stress can precipitate Graves' disease (Santos et al. 2002; Yoshiuchi et al. 1998) and aggravate treated disease (Fukao et al. 2003).

Patients with Graves' disease often present with anxiety, hypomania, depression, and cognitive difficulties. Both physiological and psychiatric symptoms correlate poorly with thyroid hormone levels (Trzepacz et al. 1989). These symptoms typically resolve with antithyroid therapy (Alvarez et al. 1983; Kathmann et al. 1994) or with use of beta-blockers such as propranolol (Trzepacz et al. 1988b). However, in a study evaluating women with treated hyperthyroidism, mood and anxiety disorders still persisted (Bunevicius et al. 2005). Treatment options for Graves' disease include antithyroid medications, thyroidectomy, and radioactive iodine. Graves' disease patients have been reported to have difficulties with sustained attention and visuomotor speed tasks (Alvarez et al. 1983) and with memory and concentration (MacCrimmon et al. 1979). It is possible that the memory and concentration difficulties appear only after long-term thyroid dysregulation. We do know that without treatment for Graves' disease, psychiatric symptoms such as major depressive disorder, generalized anxiety disorder, and hypomania will persist (Trzepacz et al. 1988a). Affective psychosis (e.g., depression and mania) also can result from thyrotoxicosis (Brownlie et al. 2000).

Although thyroid disorders are known to affect behavior, the relation between thyroid hormones per se and brain function has not been well studied. Kathmann et al. (1994) investigated the effects of T_3 (the biologically active thyroid hormone) on brain performance in healthy subjects. When T_3 levels were experimentally elevated, subjects made subjective overestimates of time intervals and were able to increase their word fluency, in the absence of more global cognitive problems (Kathmann et al. 1994).

Anxiety and irritability are common in Graves' disease prior to treatment. Only a few studies (Bunevicius et al. 2005; Trzepacz et al. 1988b) have investigated the prevalence of psychiatric complaints in hyperthyroid patients and whether these complaints persist after treatment. R.A. Stern et al. (1996) conducted a survey of members of the National Graves' Disease Foundation to investigate patient self-report of psychiatric and cognitive symptoms. The most common symptoms reported were irritability (78%), shakiness (77%), and anxiety (72%). Slowed thinking was reported by 40%.

In addition to anxiety and cognitive difficulties, some patients with hyperthyroidism experience depression secondary to their medical condition. When patients are given antithyroid therapy, depressive symptoms often disappear. Thus, antithyroid therapy should be the first course of action in treating depression in these patients (Kathol et al. 1986). However, treatment for depression may be indicated if the symptoms are sufficiently problematic or persistent. Hyperthyroidism may present differently depending on the age of the patient. In younger patients, hyperthyroidism typically manifests as hyperactivity or anxious dysphoria (Bhatara and Sankar 1999), whereas in the elderly, it can manifest as apathy or depression, referred to as "apathetic hyperthyroidism" (Mooradian 2008).

Hypothyroidism

Hypothyroid patients often experience weakness, fatigue, somnolence, cold intolerance, weight gain, constipation, hair loss, hoarseness, stiffness, and muscle aches (Kornstein et al. 2000). The most common cause of hypothyroidism is autoimmune thyroiditis (Hashimoto's thyroiditis). Hypothyroidism can also be a side effect of lithium. Radioactive iodine, the most commonly used modality for treating hyperthyroidism (such as in Graves' disease), may cause hypothyroidism, which may go undiagnosed for several years after treatment for hyperthyroidism (New York Thyroid Center 2003).

The symptoms of hypothyroidism overlap with retarded depression, and the diagnosis is easy to miss in patients who already have a depression diagnosis. Physical signs of hypothyroidism include weakness, bradycardia, facial puffiness, weight gain, hair loss, hoarseness, and slowed speech (Kornstein et al. 2000). The best screening test for hypothyroidism is measurement of serum thyrotropin concentration, but an elevated thyrotropin level should be followed by a free T_4 determination to confirm the diagnosis. A serum thyrotropin determination will be misleading in the patient with secondary hypothyroidism caused by pituitary or hypothalamic disease. In such a patient, a free T_4 measurement usually will allow the clinician to make the appropriate diagnosis.

Severe hypothyroidism is relatively rare, although milder hypothyroidism is fairly common (Joffe and Levitt 1992). Hypothyroidism can be divided into three grades (Haggerty and Prange 1995). Grade 1 refers to patients with *overt* hypothyroidism who are usually symptomatic and have elevated serum thyrotropin and low serum free T_4 concentrations. Patients with *subclinical* hypothyroidism are classified as having grade 2 or 3; these patients typically have either mild or no symptoms of thyroid hormone deficiency. The laboratory features of grade 2 hypothyroidism are an elevated serum thyrotropin level and a serum free T_4 level within the normal range. Patients with grade 3 hypothyroidism have normal thyrotropin and free T_4 levels, and the diagnosis can be confirmed only by an exaggerated serum thyrotropin response to thyrotropin-releasing hormone (TRH). Subclinical hypothyroidism is fairly common, affecting 5%–10% of the population, mainly women, and occurs in 15%–20% of women older than 45 years. Subclinical hypothyroidism is particularly common in elderly women.

Cognitive Function

Hypothyroidism can impair memory function. It is not well understood whether this impairment is limited to memory or whether it extends to other cognitive skills such as attention, inhibition of irrelevant information, and task switching. One possibility is that cognitive inefficiency in hypothyroidism is a result of secondary depression. However, in some cases, cognitive problems are independent of depression. For example, Burmeister et al. (2001) found no relation between cognitive ability and level of depression in a group of hypothyroid patients (although patients in this study scored within normal limits on most aspects of cognition). This study suggests that patient perceptions of cognitive difficulty (rather than actual cognitive dysfunction) may be a result of depression, fatigue, or response bias.

Patients with subclinical hypothyroidism often show subtle signs of cognitive dysfunction on tests of memory that may improve after treatment (Baldini et al. 1997; Capet et al. 2000; Jensovsky et al. 2002). Furthermore, Miller et al. (2006, 2007) reported that hypothyroid-related memory dysfunction stems from retrieval deficits rather than any problems in encoding and storing the information. Although most hypothyroid patients who receive treatment are prescribed T_4, administration of both T_4 and T_3 may improve cognitive performance more than T_4 alone (Bunevicius et al. 1999). Other studies, however, do not support this observation (Sawka et al. 2003; J.P. Walsh et al. 2003). Mennemeier et al. (1993) reported that after thyroid treatment, some forms of cognition returned to normal levels (e.g., performance on the Object Assembly subtest of the Wechsler Adult Intelligence Scale and on the Peterson-Peterson task that assesses short-term memory), whereas other functions remained impaired (e.g., logical memory or paired-associate learning). Whether to treat subclinical hypothyroidism, however, remains controversial.

Depression

Hypothyroidism is a known cause of secondary depression. Almost all patients with hypothyroidism have some concurrent symptoms of depression (Haggerty and Prange 1995). In the early stages of hypothyroidism, circulating T_4 levels decline, whereas T_3 levels often remain in the normal range. The brain preferentially uses T_4, as compared with other body tissues, and is thus more sensitive than other areas of the body to lower levels of T_4 (Haggerty et al. 1990). This imbalance in thyroid hormones may contribute to mood disorder, and subclinical hypothyroidism is now recognized as a potential risk factor for depression (Haggerty and Prange 1995).

T_3 also has been used to augment the effects of antidepressants, suggesting a link between depression and thyroid function (Cooper-Kazaz et al. 2007). Interestingly, in the elderly, there does not appear to be a link between subclinical hypothyroidism and impaired cognition, depression, or anxiety (Gussekloo et al. 2004; Roberts et al. 2006).

Patients with bipolar disorder with either rapid-cycling or mixed episodes have particularly high rates of subclinical hypothyroidism. In one study, almost 40% of rapid-cycling or mixed-episode bipolar patients were found to have subclinical hypothyroidism (although lithium-induced thyroid dysfunction could have contributed) (Joffe et al. 1988). Every patient with rapid-cycling bipolar disorder should be evaluated for (subclinical) hypothyroidism and receive T_4 if thyrotropin levels are elevated. Some patients may benefit even if they are euthyroid (Haggerty and Prange 1995).

Psychosis

Untreated hypothyroidism can result in psychosis, so-called myxedema madness. This condition was fairly common—reported in up to 5% of all hypothyroid patients (Kudrjavcev 1978)—before the widespread use of modern thyroid function tests, but it is now rare. Psychotic symptoms typically remit when thyrotropin levels return to normal, although cognitive dysfunction may continue (Haggerty et al. 1986). Another rare possibility in hypothyroid patients is Hashimoto's encephalopathy, a delirium with psychosis, seizures, and focal neurological signs, associated with high serum antithyroid antibody concentrations, responsive to corticosteroids, and possibly thought to be an autoimmune disorder (Schiess and Pardo 2008).

Congenital Hypothyroidism

Congenital hypothyroidism usually occurs as a result of thyroid agenesis or dysgenesis, although inherited defects in thyroid hormone synthesis also may play a role. From a global perspective, iodine deficiency is the most common cause of congenital hypothyroidism. Newborns with untreated hypothyroidism develop the syndrome of cretinism, characterized by mental retardation, short stature, poor motor development, and a characteristic puffiness of the face and hands. Because early treatment is essential to prevent permanent mental retardation, all infants born in the United States are screened for hypothyroidism at birth (American Academy of Pediatrics et al. 2006). Treatment with thyroid hormones before age 3 months can result in normal intellectual development in most infants.

Parathyroid Disorders

Hyperparathyroidism

Hyperparathyroidism can cause bone disease, kidney stones, and hypercalcemia via oversecretion of parathyroid hormone (PTH). Symptoms of hypercalcemia include anorexia, thirst, frequent urination, lethargy, fatigue, muscle weakness, joint pain, constipation, and, when severe, depression and eventually coma.

The prevalence of hyperparathyroidism is 0.1%. It is three times more common in women than in men, and its prevalence increases with age. Hyperparathyroidism may occur as a consequence of radiation therapy to head and neck and is an underrecognized side effect of long-term lithium therapy. Cessation of lithium often does not correct the hyperparathyroidism, necessitating parathyroidectomy. Prior to 1970, more than 90% of patients with hyperparathyroidism presented with renal disease or bone disease. However, after the introduction of routine calcium screening, fewer than 20% of patients present with renal or bone disease, and more than 50% of patients present with no symptoms at all.

With mild hypercalcemia, patients may show personality changes, lack of spontaneity, and lack of initiative. Moderate hypercalcemia (serum calcium concentration = 10–14 mg/dL) may cause dysphoria, anhedonia, apathy, anxiety, irritability, and impairment of concentration and recent memory. In severe hypercalcemia (serum calcium concentration >14 mg/dL), confusion, disorientation, catatonia, agitation, paranoid ideation, delusions, auditory and visual hallucinations, and lethargy progressing to coma may occur. Verbal memory and logical abilities are also impaired. Psychiatric and/or neurocognitive symptoms were the sole presenting symptoms in 12% (16 of 136) of patients who subsequently underwent parathyroidectomy, and these tended to be the older patients (Casella et al. 2008). Another study found symptoms of depression in 23.4% of patients preparathyroidectomy, and 15.6% had anxiety, both of which declined after surgery (Weber et al. 2007). After treatment of hypercalcemia, psychiatric and cognitive symptoms disappear in most patients (Roman and Sosa 2007).

Hypoparathyroidism

Patients with hypoparathyroidism present with hypocalcemia causing increased neuromuscular irritability. Typical symptoms include paresthesias, muscle cramps, carpopedal spasm, and (less commonly) facial grimacing and seizures. Complications include calcification of the basal ganglia and pseudotumor cerebri. Psychiatric symptoms may include anxiety and emotional irritability and lability. Severe hypocalcemia causes tetany and seizures. Hypoparathyroidism is caused by inadequate parathyroid hormone secretion, most often as a result of parathyroid or thyroid surgery. Hypoparathyroidism is also common in the 22q11.2 deletion syndrome (velocardiofacial syndrome), in which schizophrenia and bipolar disorder are common in adults and mood, anxiety, attentional, and behavior disorders are common in children (Jolin et al. 2009).

Kowdley et al. (1999) showed that cognitive and neurological deficits are often present in patients with long-standing hypoparathyroidism (≥9 years). These deficits are thought to be related to the presence of intracranial calcification and thus irreversible (Kowdley et al. 1999).

Osteoporosis

Osteoporosis is a metabolic disturbance of bone resulting in low bone mass, reduced bone strength, and increased risk of fractures. Osteoporosis occurs most commonly in postmenopausal women. The association between depression and reduction in bone mineral density is well established in premenopausal women (Eskandari et al. 2007; Petronijevi et al. 2008), and some support exists for a similar association in older men (Laudisio et al. 2008; Mezuk et al. 2008). The relation between depression and osteoporosis is complex. Some of the association may be the result of antidepressants, especially selective serotonin reuptake inhibitors (SSRIs), which have been themselves associated with reduced bone mineral density and increased fracture risk (Haney et al. 2007; Mezuk et al. 2008; Ziere et al. 2008). Individuals with depression also tend to have other risk factors for low bone mass, including hypercortisolism (Altindag et al. 2007) and lifestyle factors (smoking, alcohol, physical inactivity). An increased risk of osteoporosis would be expected in patients receiving long-term augmentation of antidepressant therapy with T_3, but this has not been studied.

Adrenal Gland Disorders

Cushing's Syndrome

Cushing's syndrome results from abnormally high levels of cortisol and other glucocorticoids. The most common cause is the pharmacological use of corticosteroids, followed by excessive corticotropin secretion (most commonly by a pituitary tumor, referred to as Cushing's disease) and adrenal tumors. Symptoms and signs of Cushing's syndrome include truncal obesity and striae, diabetes, hypertension, hyperglycemia, muscle weakness, osteopenia, skin atrophy and bruising, increased susceptibility to infections, and gonadal dysfunction.

Cushing's syndrome patients commonly experience a range of psychiatric symptoms, including depression, anxiety, hypomania or frank mania, psychosis, and cognitive dysfunction (Arnaldi et al. 2003; Sonino et al. 2006), with rates varying widely across studies. Depression is the most prevalent psychiatric disturbance in Cushing's syndrome. A full depressive syndrome has been reported in 50%–80% of cases, accompanied by irritability, insomnia, crying, decreased energy and libido, poor concentration and memory, and suicidal ideation (Arnaldi et al. 2003). Although antidepressants are less effective than in regular major depressive disorder, they are helpful until definitive treatment of Cushing's syndrome can be provided. Mood symptoms generally improve with resolution of hypercortisolemia (Arnaldi et al. 2003).

Significant anxiety has been reported in up to 79% of cases (Loosen et al. 1992). There are many case reports of Cushing's syndrome patients presenting with a variety of psychotic symptoms, usually as part of a manic or depressive syndrome (Arnaldi et al. 2003), leading to misdiagnosis as bipolar disorder or a schizophrenia spectrum disorder. Mifepristone, a glucocorticoid receptor blocker, may be particularly useful in acute treatment of cortisol-induced psychosis (Johanssen and Allolio 2007).

Cognition may be impaired in patients with Cushing's syndrome. For example, Starkman et al. (2001) found that, compared with a healthy control group, Cushing's disease patients scored poorly on verbal and performance IQ measures and had lower memory quotients, with verbal skills the most affected. The deficits in cognitive function were not explained by depression (Starkman et al. 2001). The neocortex and the hippocampus are rich in glucocorticoid receptors (Sapolsky 2000; Starkman et al. 2001), so it is not surprising that learning and memory are affected in Cushing's syndrome. In fact, Cushing's disease causes reduction in hippocampal volume, reversible after cortisol levels return to normal. This effect is age dependent, such that the older the individual, the less plastic is the hippocampus and the less susceptible the patient is to recovery (Starkman et al. 1999). The data are mixed on whether cognitive deficits improve or persist after treatment of Cushing's syndrome (Arnaldi et al. 2003; Hook et al. 2007).

The primary treatment for corticotropin-dependent Cushing's syndrome is surgery with selective pituitary or ectopic corticotroph tumor resection. Second-line treatments include more radical surgery, radiation therapy (for Cushing's disease), medical therapy, and bilateral adrenalectomy.

Adrenal Insufficiency: Addison's Disease and Corticotropin Deficiency

Insufficient production of adrenal corticosteroids can be caused by several mechanisms. Primary adrenal insufficiency, or Addison's disease, results in deficient secretion of mineralocorticoids and glucocorticoids. The major causes of Addison's disease are autoimmune destruction of the adrenal cortex, tuberculosis, and human immunodeficiency virus. The most common cause of secondary adrenal insufficiency is suppression of corticotropin secretion by chronic glucocorticoid administration. Less common secondary causes include diseases that result in pituitary destruction. In secondary adrenal insufficiency, corticotropin levels are low, whereas in Addison's disease, the deficiency in cortisol results in an increase in corticotropin production. This increase in corticotropin can cause hyperpigmentation, particularly in sun-exposed skin, scars, and mucous membranes. The decrease in mineralocorticoid levels results in contraction of the extracellular volume, leading to postural hypotension. Individuals with adrenal insufficiency are prone to not only hypotension but also hypoglycemia when stressed or fasting. Although electrolytes can be normal in mild Addison's disease, hyponatremia and hyperkalemia are typical. Water intoxication with hyponatremia can occur if a water load is given because cortisol deficiency impairs the ability to increase free water clearance. Other manifestations of adrenal insufficiency include anemia, anorexia, nausea, vomiting, diarrhea, abdominal pain, weight loss, and muscle weakness.

Psychiatric symptoms such as apathy, social withdrawal, fatigue, anhedonia, poverty of thought, and negativism are common in patients with Addison's disease. A large Danish registry study found that patients with adrenal insufficiency had more than twice the number of psychiatric admissions for mood disorders than did patients with osteoarthritis (Thomsen et al. 2006). Nonspecific symptoms such as weakness, fatigue, and anorexia often appear before more specific findings, making it difficult to attribute the cause to adrenal insufficiency. Cognitive impairment, especially memory loss, is often present but ephemeral and varying in severity. During Addisonian crisis, patients may experience delirium, disorientation, confusion, and even psychosis (Anglin et al. 2006). Adrenal insufficiency is particularly likely to be misdiagnosed as primary major depression in patients with chronic medical illness who previously received high doses of corticosteroids, resulting in unrecognized secondary adrenal insufficiency. Another possible psychiatric misdiagnosis is anorexia nervosa.

Although the diagnosis of adrenal insufficiency may be suspected on the basis of a low serum cortisol level in the morning, definitive diagnosis requires a corticotropin stimulation test. This is typically performed with cosyntropin, a synthetic corticotropin analogue. An increase in the serum cortisol concentration to greater than 20 ng/dL following cosyntropin injection excludes the diagnosis of adrenal insufficiency.

The cause of depression in patients with Addison's disease is not clear. Regardless of the etiology of adrenal insufficiency, urgent treatment is indicated. Both glucocorticoid and mineralocorticoid replacement are usually necessary in the treatment of Addison's disease, whereas glucocorticoid replacement alone is sufficient in secondary adrenal insufficiency.

Adrenal insufficiency is also a feature in adrenoleukodystrophy, a rare, X-linked inherited metabolic disease, which also leads to leukoencephalic myeloneuropathy. Adult onset is rare but commonly presents with psychiatric symptoms, including mania, psychosis, and cognitive dysfunction (Rosebush et al. 1999).

Acromegaly

Acromegaly is a disease of excess growth hormone (GH) secretion. Deficiency of GH in children results in short stature, as discussed in Chapter 34, "Pediatrics." The most common cause of acromegaly is a GH-secreting adenoma of the anterior pituitary. These benign tumors account for 30% of all hormone-secreting pituitary adenomas (DeGroot et al. 2001). Clinical manifestations of acromegaly include headache, cranial nerve palsies, acral enlargement (frontal bossing), increased hand and foot size, prognathism, soft tissue overgrowth (macroglossia), glucose intolerance, and hypertension. Suprasellar extension of the tumor may cause visual field defects.

Psychiatric disturbances associated with acromegaly include mood disorders, anxiety, and personality change (Sievers et al. 2009a, 2009b). Psychiatric symptoms and impairment in quality of life in acromegaly have been attributed to the endocrine disorder itself and the psychosocial stress of disfigurement (T'Sjoen et al. 2007). Personality change described in acromegalic patients includes loss of initiative and spontaneity, with marked lability in mood (Pantanetti et al. 2002).

Treatment of acromegaly may include surgery, medication, and radiation. Surgery is usually the primary treatment for GH-secreting pituitary adenomas and may enhance the effectiveness of subsequent medical therapy. Medical management includes somatostatin analogues (e.g., octreotide), the GH receptor antagonist pegvisomant, dopamine agonists (e.g., bromocriptine), and radiation. In the past, high doses of bromocriptine were sometimes necessary to reduce levels of GH, which increased the risk of psychiatric adverse effects, including psychosis (Boyd 1995).

Pheochromocytoma

Pheochromocytomas are rare catecholamine-secreting tumors derived from the adrenal medulla and sympathetic ganglia. The clinical signs and symptoms result from the release of catecholamines, leading to increased heart rate, blood pressure, myocardial contractility, and vasoconstriction, resulting in paroxysmal hypertension, headache, palpitations, diaphoresis, anxiety, tremulousness, pallor (rarely flushing), chest and abdominal pain, and often nausea and vomiting (Manger 2009). Because these are nonspecific symptoms, pheochromocytomas may mimic anxiety disorders (especially panic disorder), migraine or cluster headaches, amphetamine or cocaine abuse, alcohol withdrawal, brain tumors, subarachnoid hemorrhage, neuroblastoma in children, or temporal lobe seizures (DeGroot et al. 2001). Of the patients tested for pheochromocytoma, fewer than 2% are found to have the tumor (Eisenhofer et al. 2008). Unexplained severe symptomatic paroxysmal hypertension, often referred to as "pseudopheochromocytoma," appears to be triggered by anxiety in many of these patients (Pickering and Clemow 2008).

Cases of classic panic attacks in patients with pheochromocytoma have been reported in both adults and children (Carre 1996; Prokhorova and Fritz 2002). Rarely, the initial psychiatric manifestation has been depression, posttraumatic stress disorder, or psychosis (Benabarre et al. 2005).

Antidepressants have been reported to have unmasked silent pheochromocytomas, presumably by inhibiting neuronal intake of circulating catecholamines.

There is still no consensus as to the "best test" for the diagnosis of pheochromocytoma. Some centers rely on 24-hour urine measurement of increased excretion of catecholamines or catecholamine metabolites, including vanillylmandelic acid (VMA) and metanephrines. Plasma metanephrine determinations have an extremely high sensitivity (approaching 99%) and overall specificity (in the 85%–90% range) (Lenders et al. 2002). The finding of elevated urinary catecholamine levels is not specific to pheochromocytoma and can lead to misdiagnosis. A variety of psychological and physiological stressors can elevate levels of urinary catecholamines. Urinary VMA levels can be elevated with ingestion of foods high in vanillin, including vanilla extract, bananas, coffee, nuts, and citrus fruits (Sheps et al. 1990). Elevated urinary VMA levels are the least specific indicator of pheochromocytoma, whereas elevated metanephrines are the most sensitive (T.A. Stern and Cremens 1998). Misdiagnosis of pheochromocytoma has been reported in patients with hypertension and raised urinary catecholamines who were taking clozapine (Krentz et al. 2001) or selegiline (Lefebvre et al. 1995).

Multiple cases of factitious pheochromocytoma have been reported and include cases involving intentional vanilla extract ingestion (T.A. Stern and Cremens 1998), phenylpropanolamine abuse (Hyams et al. 1985), surreptitious injection of catecholamines intravaginally (Spitzer et al. 1998), epinephrine injection (Keiser 1991), and conscious altering of autonomic function with Valsalva maneuvers (Kailasam et al. 1995).

The rare possibility of a pheochromocytoma should be considered in patients with panic attacks, headaches, and labile hypertension, particularly those who do not respond to treatment. It is not necessary to screen for pheochromocytoma in patients who have only psychiatric symptoms; elevated catecholamines are common and likely to be false-positive results. Some psychotropic drugs may cause hypertensive reactions that mimic pheochromocytoma, and in rare cases the drugs may be unmasking an unsuspected pheochromocytoma.

Hyperprolactinemia

Hyperprolactinemia is the most common pituitary hormone hypersecretion syndrome (Melmed 2001). The differential diagnosis of hyperprolactinemia includes pituitary adenomas, physiological causes (pregnancy and lactation), medication effects, chronic renal failure (via decreased peripheral prolactin clearance), primary hypothyroidism, and lesions of the pituitary stalk and the hypothalamus (e.g., hypothalamic tumors). Clinical signs in women include galactorrhea, menstrual irregularities, infertility, and decreased libido. Men present with diminished libido and rarely with galactorrhea.

Numerous studies and case reports identified an association between hyperprolactinemia and depression and anxiety, as well as resolution of symptoms with treatment of hyperprolactinemia (Kars et al. 2007), but sample sizes have been small. Fava et al. (1982) found that hyperprolactinemic patients reported a significant increase in symptoms of depression, anxiety, and hostility compared with amenorrheic and healthy control subjects. Another study found a surprisingly high prevalence of anxiety and a small increase in hostility yet no significant difference in depression (Reavley et al. 1997).

Medication-induced hyperprolactinemia has been associated with antipsychotics and, to a lesser extent, antidepressants. Conventional antipsychotic drugs block dopamine D_2 receptors on lactotroph cells and thus remove the main inhibitory influence on prolactin secretion (Wieck and Haddad 2003). Prolactin levels between 10 and 100 ng/L are typical in drug-induced hyperprolactinemia (Melmed 2001). Serum prolactin levels in patients taking therapeutic doses of typical antipsychotics are increased six- to tenfold from mean baseline prolactin levels (Arvanitis and Miller 1997).

Atypical antipsychotics vary with respect to their effects on prolactin. In most reports, clozapine, quetiapine, olanzapine, and ziprasidone either cause no increase in prolactin secretion or increase prolactin transiently, but sustained hyperprolactinemia can occur in patients taking risperidone and paliperidone. Haloperidol raises the serum prolactin concentration by an average of 17 ng/mL, while risperidone may raise it by 45–80 ng/mL, with larger increases in women than in men (David et al. 2000). Women taking prolactin-elevating antipsychotics and not receiving specific interventions to improve bone density showed evidence of ongoing bone demineralization over a year, while women taking prolactin-sparing antipsychotics had a modest overall increase in bone mineral density (Meaney and O'Keane 2007). A study of patients switched from risperidone to aripiprazole reported that previously elevated prolactin levels were reduced to within normal range in 1 week (Byerly et al. 2009), and hyperprolactinemia in patients taking haloperidol was reversed by the addition of adjunctive aripiprazole (Shim et al. 2007).

Antidepressants with serotonergic activity, including SSRIs, monoamine oxidase inhibitors, and some tricyclic antidepressants, can cause modest elevations of prolactin (Papakostas et al. 2006) and may further elevate prolactin levels in patients also taking prolactin-elevating antipsychotics (Wieck and Haddad 2003).

Women taking psychiatric medications that chronically elevate prolactin levels are at risk for premature bone loss secondary to hypoestrogenism. Patients taking prolactin-elevating antipsychotics should be educated about—and regularly monitored for—signs and symptoms of hyperprolactinemia (David et al. 2000; Haddad et al. 2001). No published trials have examined the effects of hormone replacement on bone mineral density in patients taking antipsychotics long term, but preliminary data suggest that active management of bone loss in those with antipsychotic-associated bone disease may halt or even reverse this process (O'Keane 2008).

In patients with mood disorders whose symptoms are unresponsive to treatment and who have galactorrhea and/or amenorrhea, hyperprolactinemia should be considered as a causal factor (Holroyd and Cohen 1990).

Gonadal Disorders

Perimenstrual Disorders and Menopause

For information on perimenstrual disorders and menopause, refer to Chapter 33, "Obstetrics and Gynecology."

Polycystic Ovary Syndrome

Polycystic ovary syndrome (PCOS) is a common disorder, affecting 5%–10% of women of childbearing age. Clinical manifestations include amenorrhea or oligomenorrhea, infrequent or absent ovulation, increased levels of testosterone, infertility, truncal obesity or weight gain, alopecia, hirsutism, acanthosis nigricans, hypertension, and insulin resistance. The cause of the disorder is unknown. The risk of developing PCOS is increased during treatment with valproate and seems to be higher in women with epilepsy than in women with bipolar disorders (Bilo and Meo 2008).

There are adverse psychosocial consequences of PCOS. Women with PCOS may complain they feel "abnormal or freakish" (Kitzinger and Willmott 2002), related to hirsutism, obesity, and altered reproductive function (Kitzinger and Willmott 2002). High rates of clinically significant anxiety and depression have been reported in women with PCOS (Benson et al. 2009b; Månsson et al. 2008; Tan et al. 2008). Psychological problems are common in women with hirsutism of any cause. Although these physical abnormalities may affect feelings of self-worth and femininity, some research suggests that psychological morbidity, such as depression, may be caused by neuroendocrine changes in PCOS (Benson et al. 2009a). Of course, both psychosocial and neuroendocrine factors may play a role. A recent self-report study found that three-quarters of women with PCOS worried about being childless; one-quarter had mild to moderate depression and one-quarter had clinical depression, but depression was not associated with infertility concern (Tan et al. 2008). The rate of bipolar disorder may be higher among women with PCOS than in the general population, independent of an association with valproate (Klipstein and Goldberg 2007). Although the causal link between psychological symptoms and PCOS is not resolved, their frequency points to the importance of screening all PCOS patients for psychiatric syndromes, especially depression.

Testosterone Deficiency

Testosterone deficiency in men can result from diseases affecting the testes, pituitary gland, or hypothalamus. Consequences of testosterone deficiency vary depending on the stage of sexual development. Testosterone production declines naturally with age, so that a relative testosterone deficiency occurs in older men. Hypogonadal disorders of the testes (primary hypogonadism) are most commonly caused by Klinefelter's syndrome, mumps orchitis, trauma, tumor, cancer chemotherapy, or immune testicular failure (see Chapter 28, "HIV/AIDS," for a discussion of hypotestosteronism in HIV infection). Pituitary lesions caused by tumors, hemochromatosis, sarcoidosis, or cranial irradiation can lead to secondary hypogonadism. The classic cause of hypothalamic hypogonadism is Kallmann's syndrome (hypogonadotropic hypogonadism with hyposmia, sensorineural hearing loss, oral clefts, micropenis, and cryptorchidism). Hypogonadism in childhood is characterized by failure of normal secondary sexual characteristics to develop and diminished muscle mass. In adult men, typical complaints are sexual dysfunction, diminished energy, decreased beard and body hair, muscle loss, and breast enlargement.

Decreasing testosterone levels as men age may be associated with changes in mood and cognition, but no clear relation between psychiatric syndromes and testosterone level has been established. One study found an adjusted hazard ratio for depression of 4.2 (95% confidence interval [CI] = 1.5–12.0; P = 0.008) in hypogonadal men (Shores et al. 2004). In a community sample of elderly men, free testosterone concentration in the lowest quintile was associated with a higher prevalence of depression (Almeida et al. 2008). The concept of a male climacteric and related mood, anxiety, and cognitive disorders is controversial.

Patients with Klinefelter's syndrome (XYY) are reported to have higher rates of mental retardation and a wide variety of psychiatric and behavioral symptoms, but these are a consequence primarily of the chromosomal abnormality rather than hypogonadism.

The evidence supporting testosterone replacement therapy in hypogonadal men is strong for body composition and sexual function. Questions remain about the value of testosterone replacement in age-related testosterone decline as well as in the treatment of depressive disorder in hypogonadal men. Testosterone does seem to improve mood, as well as sexual dysfunction and muscle strength, in hypogonadal men. However, results from multiple randomized controlled clinical trials are conflicting. Although data derived from androgen treatment trials and androgen replacement do not support testosterone treatment for major depressive disorder, the clinical impression is that, for some subthreshold depressive syndromes, testosterone may lead to antidepressant benefits (Amore et al. 2009). The risks associated with physiological doses of testosterone appear small. The possible increased risk of prostate cancer remains a concern, but little evidence is available to substantiate it.

Some studies have found that testosterone deficiency in women is associated with impaired sexual function, low energy, and depression, but others have found testosterone levels inversely related to depression (Morsink et al. 2007). What level represents deficiency and the indications, risks, and benefits of replacement are even less well defined than in men (see Chapter 16, "Sexual Dysfunction").

Other Metabolic Disorders

Electrolyte and Acid–Base Disturbances

Hyponatremia and Hypernatremia

Hyponatremia's principal manifestations are neuropsychiatric, and their severity is related to both the degree and the rapidity with which it develops. Patients may have lethargy, stupor, confusion, psychosis, irritability, and seizures. Hyponatremia has many different causes, but those of particular psychiatric relevance include the syndrome of inappropriate antidiuretic hormone secretion (SIADH), which can be caused by many psychotropic drugs (especially carbamazepine and oxcarbazepine but also SSRIs, tricyclic antidepressants, and antipsychotics), and psychogenic polydipsia. Polydipsia leading to hyponatremia in patients with schizophrenia is mediated by a reduced osmotic threshold for the release of vasopressin and by a defect in the osmoregulation of thirst. Acute-onset symptomatic hyponatremia may require emergent treatment with hypertonic (3%) saline. In chronic cases, correction should be gradual to minimize the risk of pontine myelinolysis, relying on fluid restriction and vasopressin receptor antagonists (Siegel 2008).

The signs of hypernatremia are also predominantly neuropsychiatric and include cognitive dysfunction, delirium, seizures, and lethargy progressing to stupor and coma. Similar symptoms are seen with any hyperosmolar state, such as extreme hyperglycemia. Hypernatremia is usually caused by dehydration, with significant total body water deficits. A rare cause is adipsia, the absence of thirst even in the presence of water depletion or sodium excess, usually caused by a hypothalamic lesion (which may result in other psychopathology) (Floris et al. 2008).

Hypokalemia and Hyperkalemia

Hypokalemia produces muscular weakness and fatigue and, if severe, may cause severe paralysis (hypokalemic periodic paralysis), but central nervous system functions typically are not affected. Nevertheless, patients with symptomatic hypokalemia sometimes receive the misdiagnosis of depression. Hypokalemia is very common in eating disorders (see Chapter 14, "Eating Disorders," for full discussion of the metabolic complications of eating disorders), chronic alcoholism, and alcohol withdrawal. The adverse effects of hyperkalemia are mainly cardiac, but severe muscle weakness also may occur.

Hypocalcemia and Hypercalcemia; Hypomagnesemia and Hypermagnesemia

Hypocalcemia and hypercalcemia were described earlier in this chapter in the "Parathyroid Disorders" section. Magnesium levels usually rise and fall in concert with calcium levels. Hypomagnesemia can cause anxiety, irritability, tetany, and seizures. Low magnesium levels are very common in alcoholic patients and in refeeding starving patients (including those with anorexia nervosa and catatonia). Cyclosporine causes hypomagnesemia, which can contribute to its neuropsychiatric side effects. Hypermagnesemia is much less common, usually resulting from excessive ingestion of magnesium-containing antacids or cathartics, and causes central nervous system depression.

Hypophosphatemia

Hypophosphatemia causes anxiety, hyperventilation, irritability, weakness, delirium, and, if severe, seizures, coma, and death, in addition to symptoms in many other organ systems. Hypophosphatemia occurs in the same settings as hypomagnesemia.

Acidosis and Alkalosis

Metabolic acidosis results in compensatory hyperventilation. When the acidosis is severe and acute, as in diabetic ketoacidosis, fatigue and delirium are present and may progress to stupor and coma. Acute metabolic acidosis is a complication of a wide variety of overdoses and toxic ingestions. Patients with chronic metabolic acidosis appear depressed, with prominent anorexia and fatigue. Patients with severe metabolic alkalosis present with apathy, confusion, and stupor. Respiratory acidosis results from ventilatory insufficiency, and respiratory alkalosis results from hyperventilation (see Chapter 19, "Lung Disease").

Vitamin Deficiencies

Deficiencies of vitamin B_{12} and folate are discussed in Chapter 24, "Hematology."

Pellagra, originally thought to be a deficiency of niacin, is now recognized to be a complex deficiency of multiple vitamins and amino acids. The classic triad of symptoms is dermatitis, dementia, and diarrhea, but irritability, anxiety, depression, apathy, and psychosis all have been reported (Prakash et al. 2008). Pellagra is now rare in the developed nations, but cases are still reported in anorexia nervosa, inflammatory bowel disease, and alcoholism.

Thiamine deficiency (beriberi) causes cardiac and neuropsychiatric syndromes, including peripheral neuropathy and Wernicke-Korsakoff encephalopathy. Wernicke's consists of vomiting, nystagmus, ophthalmoplegia, fever, ataxia, and confusion that can progress to coma and death. Korsakoff's is a dementia with amnesia, impaired ability to learn, confabulation, and often psychosis. Improvement usually occurs with thiamine replacement but may be slow. Giving intravenous glucose to a thiamine-deficient patient without coadministering thiamine may precipitate acute beriberi. Thiamine deficiency is well known and most frequent in alcoholic patients, but it also occurs in patients undergoing chronic dialysis, patients refeeding after starvation (including patients with anorexia nervosa), and individuals on fad diets.

Pyridoxine (vitamin B_6) deficiency causes peripheral neuropathy and neuropsychiatric disorders, including reports of seizures, migraine, chronic pain, depression, and psychosis. Homocysteine is elevated in B_6 deficiency and may play a role in accelerating vascular disease and dementia. Pyridoxine deficiency is common because many drugs act as its antagonist. Clinical trials of B_6 supplementation in healthy elderly and in cognitively impaired subjects to date have not shown improvements in mood or cognition.

Vitamin E deficiency can cause areflexia, ataxia, and decreased vibratory and proprioceptive sensation. Although several small studies have reported lower levels of vitamin E in major depression (e.g., Owen et al. 2005), a large epidemiological study in the elderly found no association between low vitamin E levels and depressive symptoms or major depression (Tiemeier et al. 2002). Clinical trials of vitamin E supplementation have not shown any benefit in cognitively impaired individuals.

Porphyrias

The porphyrias are a group of rare disorders of heme biosynthesis that can be inherited or acquired. Neuropsychiatric manifestations occur in the two neuroporphyrias (acute intermittent porphyria and plumboporphyria) and two neurocutaneous porphyrias (hereditary coproporphyria and variegate porphyria). Acute intermittent porphyria is the most common. Recurrent acute attacks are typical in all four, with variable manifestations. In acute porphyria, the cardinal signs are abdominal pain, peripheral neuropathy, and psychiatric symptoms, which can be the sole presenting symptoms, including anxiety, depression, psychosis, and delirium. Seizures, autonomic instability, dehydration, electrolyte imbalance, and dermatological changes also may occur. Symptoms may vary considerably among patients and in the same patient over time, and they can mimic symptoms of other psychiatric and medical disorders, making diagnosis a challenge. Stress has long been considered a precipitant of acute episodes, but data are lacking. The diagnosis is made by measuring porphyrins and their metabolites in stool and urine during an acute episode. Between episodes, porphyrin levels return to normal. Diagnosis is more likely to be made when the clinician has a high index of suspicion. The diagnosis may be especially difficult because neuropsychiatric symptoms may continue well after the end of an acute episode (Millward et al. 2005). Therapy is primarily supportive and includes identification of precipitants. Although barbiturates clearly can trigger attacks, evidence is inadequate regarding the role of other psychotropic drugs. A comprehensive rating of drugs' risk for porphyrinogenicity is available at http://www.drugs-porphyria.org.

Other Genetic Metabolic Disorders

Inborn errors of metabolism usually presenting in neonates or young children may in rare cases first present in adolescence or adulthood as a psychiatric disorder. Such a possibility may be suspected because of family history or because psychiatric symptoms present as part of a more complex clinical picture with systemic, cognitive, or motor signs (Sedel et al. 2007). Such a diagnostic possibility also should be considered when a psychiatric disorder presents atypically with subtle "organic" signs and responds poorly to standard treatments. Some of these disorders present with acute and recurrent attacks of confusion, which may be misdiagnosed as acute psychosis. Examples include urea cycle disorders (e.g., ornithine transcarbamylase deficiency) and homocysteine remethylation defects (e.g., hyperhomocysteinemia). Others may produce chronic psychiatric symptoms (e.g., catatonia, hallucinations), including the homocystinurias, Wilson's disease, adrenoleukodystrophy, and some lysosomal disorders (e.g., Gaucher's disease). Mild mental retardation and late-onset behavioral or personality changes may be a manifestation of the homocystinurias, cerebrotendinous xanthomatosis, monoamine oxidase A deficiency, succinic semialdehyde dehydrogenase deficiency, and creatine transporter deficiency. Recognition of such disorders in an adult with only psychiatric symptoms may be very difficult, but earlier recognition and specific intervention can avert irreversible nervous system (and other organ) injury.

Conclusion

Endocrine and metabolic disorders frequently occur in conjunction with common psychiatric conditions. The causal linkages and mechanisms vary widely. In some situations, the endocrine state manifests in part as a psychiatric condition. In other instances, the psychiatric condition may be a complex biopsychosocial and/or biological response to the endocrine disorder. Psychiatric conditions and their treatment may also increase risk of endocrine disorders. Moreover, treatment with psychotropic drugs can induce endocrinopathies. Consequently, understanding the ways in which these disorders intersect represents an important facet of knowledge for the practitioners treating psychiatric and/or endocrine disorders.

References

Almeida OP, Yeap BB, Hankey GJ, et al: Low free testosterone concentration as a potentially treatable cause of depressive symptoms in older men. Arch Gen Psychiatry 65:283–289, 2008

Altindag O, Altindag A, Asoglu M, et al: Relation of cortisol levels and bone mineral density among premenopausal women with major depression. Int J Clin Pract 61:416–420, 2007

Alvarez MA, Gomez A, Alavez E, et al: Attention disturbance in Graves' disease. Psychoneuroendocrinology 8:451–454, 1983

American Academy of Pediatrics, Rose SR, Section on Endocrinology and Committee on Genetics, et al: Update of newborn screening and therapy for congenital hypothyroidism. Pediatrics 117:2290–2303, 2006

Amore M, Scarlatti F, Quarta AL, et al: Partial androgen deficiency, depression and testosterone treatment in aging men. Aging Clin Exp Res 21:1–8, 2009

Anglin RE, Rosebush PI, Mazurek MF: The neuropsychiatric profile of Addison's disease: revisiting a forgotten phenomenon. J Neuropsychiatry Clin Neurosci 18:450–459, 2006

Arnaldi G, Angeli A, Atkinson AB, et al: Diagnosis and complications of Cushing's syndrome: a consensus statement. J Clin Endocrinol Metab 88:5593–5602, 2003

Arvanitis LA, Miller BG: Multiple fixed doses of "Seroquel" (quetiapine) in patients with acute exacerbation of schizophrenia: a comparison with haloperidol and placebo. The Seroquel Trial 13 Study Group. Biol Psychiatry 42:233–246, 1997

Austin EJ, Deary IJ: Effects of repeated hypoglycemia on cognitive function: a psychometrically validated reanalysis of the Diabetes Control and Complications Trial data. Diabetes Care 22:1273–1277, 1999

Baldini IM, Vita A, Mauri MC, et al: Psychopathological and cognitive features in subclinical hypothyroidism. Prog Neuropsychopharmacol Biol Psychiatry 21:925–935, 1997

Beaser RS: Joslin Diabetes Deskbook: A Guide for Primary Care Providers. Boston, MA, Joslin Diabetes Center, 2001

Benabarre A, Bosch X, Plana MT, et al: Relapsing paranoid psychosis as the first manifestation of pheochromocytoma. J Clin Psychiatry 66:949–950, 2005

Benson S, Arck PC, Tan S, et al: Disturbed stress responses in women with polycystic ovary syndrome. Psychoneuroendocrinology 34:727–735, 2009a

Benson S, Hahn S, Tan S, et al: Prevalence and implications of anxiety in polycystic ovary syndrome: results of an Internet-based survey in Germany. Hum Reprod 24:1446–1451, 2009b

Bhatara VS, Sankar R: Neuropsychiatric aspects of pediatric thyrotoxicosis. Indian J Pediatr 66:277–284, 1999

Bilo L, Meo R: Polycystic ovary syndrome in women using valproate: a review. Gynecol Endocrinol 24:562–570, 2008

Birkenaes AB, Opjordsmoen S, Brunborg C, et al: The level of cardiovascular risk factors in bipolar disorder equals that of schizophrenia: a comparative study. J Clin Psychiatry 68:917–923, 2007

Bjorgaas M, Gimse R, Vik T, et al: Cognitive function in type 1 diabetic children with and without episodes of hypoglycaemia. Acta Paediatr 86:148–153, 1997

Black SA, Markides KS, Ray LA: Depression predicts increased incidence of adverse health outcomes in older Mexican Americans with type 2 diabetes. Diabetes Care 26:2822–2828, 2003

Boyd A: Bromocriptine and psychosis: a literature review. Psychiatr Q 66:87–95, 1995

Brands AM, Biessels G, de Haan EH, et al: The effects of type 1 diabetes on cognitive performance: a meta-analysis. Diabetes Care 28:726–735, 2005

Brownlie BE, Rae AM, Walshe JW, et al: Psychoses associated with thyrotoxicosis—"thyrotoxic psychosis": a report of 18 cases, with statistical analysis of incidence. Eur J Endocrinol 142:438–444, 2000

Bruce DG, Casey G, Davis WA, et al: Vascular depression in older people with diabetes. Diabetologia 49:2828–2836, 2006

Bryden KS, Neil A, Mayou RA, et al: Eating habits, body weight, and insulin misuse: a longitudinal study of teenagers and young adults with type 1 diabetes. Diabetes Care 22:1956–1960, 1999

Buchholz S, Morrow AF, Coleman PL: Atypical antipsychotic-induced diabetes mellitus: an update on epidemiology and postulated mechanisms. Intern Med J 38:602–606, 2008

Bunevicius R, Kazanavicius G, Zalinkevicius R, et al: Effects of thyroxine as compared with thyroxine plus triiodothyronine in patients with hypothyroidism. N Engl J Med 340:424–429, 1999

Bunevicius R, Velickiene D, Prange AJ: Mood and anxiety disorders in women with treated hyperthyroidism and ophthalmopathy caused by Graves' disease. Gen Hosp Psychiatry 27:133–139, 2005

Burmeister LA, Ganguli M, Dodge HH, et al: Hypothyroidism and cognition: preliminary evidence for a specific defect in memory. Thyroid 11:1177–1185, 2001

Buse JB: Metabolic side effects of antipsychotics: focus on hyperglycemia and diabetes. J Clin Psychiatry 63 (suppl 4):37–41, 2002

Byerly MJ, Marcus RN, Tran QV, et al: Effects of aripiprazole on prolactin levels in subjects with schizophrenia during cross-titration with risperidone or olanzapine: analysis of a randomized, open-label study. Schizophr Res 107:218–222, 2009

Cameron O, Kronfol Z, Greden J, et al: Hypothalamic-pituitary-adrenocortical activity in patients with diabetes mellitus. Arch Gen Psychiatry 41:1090–1095, 1984

Capet C, Jego A, Denis P, et al: Is cognitive change related to hypothyroidism reversible with replacement therapy? Rev Med Interne 21:672–678, 2000

Carre A: Panic attack: viewpoint of the internist. Encephale 22 (spec no 5):11–12, 1996

Casella C, Pata G, Di Betta E, et al: [Neurological and psychiatric disorders in primary hyperparathyroidism: the role of parathyroidectomy]. Ann Ital Chir 79:157–161, 2008

Chida Y, Hamer M: An association of adverse psychosocial factors in diabetes mellitus: a meta-analytic review of longitudinal cohort studies. Diabetologia 51:2168–2178, 2008

Ciechanowski PS, Katon WJ, Russo JE: Depression and diabetes: impact of depressive symptoms on adherence, function, and costs. Arch Intern Med 160:3278–3285, 2000

Collins MM, Corcoran P, Perry IJ: Anxiety and depression symptoms in patients with diabetes. Diabet Med 26:153–161, 2009

Colton P, Olmsted M, Daneman D, et al: Disturbed eating behavior and eating disorders in preteen and early teenage girls with type 1 diabetes: a case-controlled study. Diabetes Care 27:1654–1659, 2004

Cooper-Kazaz R, Apter JT, Cohen R, et al: Combined treatment with sertraline and liothyronine in major depression: a randomized, double-blind, placebo-controlled trial. Arch Gen Psychiatry 64:679–688, 2007

David SR, Taylor CC, Kinon BJ, et al: The effects of olanzapine, risperidone, and haloperidol on plasma prolactin levels in patients with schizophrenia. Clin Ther 22:1085–1096, 2000

Deary IJ, Crawford JR, Hepburn DA, et al: Severe hypoglycemia and intelligence in adult patients with insulin-treated diabetes. Diabetes 42:341–344, 1993

de Groot M, Anderson RJ, Freedland KE, et al: Association of depression and diabetes complications: a meta analysis. Psychosom Med 63:619–630, 2001

de Groot M, Pinkerman B, Wagner J, et al: Depression treatment and satisfaction in a multicultural sample of type 1 and type 2 diabetic patients. Diabetes Care 29:549–553, 2006

DeGroot LJ, Jameson JL, Burger HG, et al: Endocrinology, 4th Edition. Philadelphia, PA, WB Saunders, 2001

De Hert M, Dekker JM, Wood D, et al: Cardiovascular disease and diabetes in people with severe mental illness position statement from the European Psychiatric Association (EPA), supported by the European Association for the Study of Diabetes (EASD) and the European Society of Cardiology (ESC). Eur Psychiatry 24:412–424, 2009

Dejgaard A, Gade A, Larsson H, et al: Evidence for diabetic encephalopathy. Diabet Med 8:162–167, 1991

Diabetes Control and Complications Trial Research Group: Weight gain associated with intensive therapy in the diabetes control and complications trial. Diabetes Care 11:567–573, 1988

Diabetes Control and Complications Trial Research Group: The effect of intensive treatment of diabetes on the development and progression of long-term complications in insulin-dependent diabetes mellitus. N Engl J Med 329:977–986, 1993

Diabetes Control and Complications Trial Research Group: Effects of intensive diabetes therapy on neuropsychological function in adults in the Diabetes Control and Complications Trial. Ann Intern Med 124:379–388, 1996

Diabetes Control and Complications Trial Research Group: Influence of intensive diabetes treatment on body weight and composition of adults with type 1 diabetes in the Diabetes Control and Complications Trial. Diabetes Care 24:1711–1721, 2001

Dixon L, Weiden P, Delahanty J, et al: Prevalence and correlates of diabetes in national schizophrenia samples. Schizophr Bull 26:903–912, 2000

Eisenhofer G, Sharabi Y, Pacak K: Unexplained symptomatic paroxysmal hypertension in pseudopheochromocytoma: a stress response disorder? Ann NY Acad Sci 1148:469–478, 2008

Eskandari F, Martinez PE, Torvik S, et al: Premenopausal, Osteoporosis Women, Alendronate, Depression (POWER) Study Group. Low bone mass in premenopausal women with depression. Arch Intern Med 167:2329–2336, 2007

Farmer A, Korszun A, Owen MJ, et al: Medical disorders in people with recurrent depression. Br J Psychiatry 192:351–355, 2008

Fava M, Fava GA, Kellner R, et al: Depression and hostility in hyperprolactinemia. Prog Neuropsychopharmacol Biol Psychiatry 6:479–482, 1982

Ferguson SC, Blane A, Perros P, et al: Cognitive ability and brain structure in type 1 diabetes: Relation to microangiopathy and preceding severe hypoglycemia. Diabetes 52:149–156, 2003

Floris G, Cannas A, Melis M, et al: Pathological gambling, delusional parasitosis and adipsia as a post-haemorrhagic syndrome: a case report. Neurocase 14:385–389, 2008

Frazekas F: Magnetic resonance signal abnormalities in asymptomatic individuals: their incidence and functional correlates. Eur Neurol 29:164–168, 1989

Fukao A, Takamatsu J, Murakami Y, et al: The relationship of psychological factors to the prognosis of hyperthyroidism in antithyroid drug-treated patients with Graves' disease. Clin Endocrinol (Oxf) 58:550–555, 2003

Garay-Sevilla ME, Malacara JM, Gonzalez-Contreras E, et al: Perceived psychological stress in diabetes mellitus type 2. Rev Invest Clin 52:241–245, 2000

Geller WK, MacFadden W: Diabetes and atypical neuroleptics. Am J Psychiatry 160:388, 2003

Gendelman N, Snell-Bergeon JK, McFann K, et al: Prevalence and correlates of depression in persons with and without type 1 diabetes. Diabetes Care 32:575–579, 2009

Georgiades A, Zucker N, Friedman KE, et al: Changes in depressive symptoms and glycemic control in diabetes mellitus. Psychosom Med 69:235–241, 2007

Geringer ED: Affective disorders and diabetes mellitus, in Neuropsychological and Behavioral Aspects of Diabetes. Edited by Holmes CS. New York, Springer, 1990, pp 239–272

Goebel-Fabbri AE, Fikkan J, Franko DL, et al: Insulin restriction and associated morbidity and mortality in women with type 1 diabetes. Diabetes Care 31:415–419, 2008

Goetsch VL, VanDorsten B, Pbert LA, et al: Acute effects of laboratory stress on blood glucose in noninsulin-dependent diabetes. Psychosom Med 55:492–496, 1993

Golden SH, Lazo M, Carnethon M, et al: Examining a bidirectional association between depressive symptoms and diabetes. JAMA 299:2751–2759, 2008

Gorin AA, Niemeier HM, Hogan P, et al: Binge eating and weight loss outcomes in overweight and obese individuals with type 2 diabetes: results from the Look AHEAD trial. Arch Gen Psychiatry 65:1447–1455, 2008

Green L, Feher M, Catalan J: Fears and phobias in people with diabetes. Diabetes Metab Res Rev 16:287–293, 2000

Gregg E, Brown A: Cognitive and physical disabilities and aging-related complications of diabetes. Clinical Diabetes 21:113–116, 2003

Guo JJ, Keck PE, Corey-Lisle PK, et al: Risk of diabetes mellitus associated with atypical antipsychotic use among Medicaid patients with bipolar disorder: a nested case-control study. Pharmacotherapy 27:27–35, 2007

Gussekloo J, van Exel E, de Craen AJ, et al: Thyroid status, disability and cognitive function, and survival in old age. JAMA 292:2591–2599, 2004

Haddad PM, Helleweil JS, Wieck A: Antipsychotic induced hyperprolactinaemia: a series of illustrative case reports. J Psychopharmacol 15:293–295, 2001

Haggerty JJ Jr, Prange AJ: Borderline hypothyroidism and depression. Annu Rev Med 46:37–46, 1995

Haggerty JJ Jr, Evans DL, Prange AJ Jr: Organic brain syndrome associated with marginal hypothyroidism. Am J Psychiatry 143:785–786, 1986

Haggerty JJ Jr, Garbutt JC, Evans DL, et al: Subclinical hypothyroidism: a review of neuropsychiatric aspects. Int J Psychiatry Med 20:193–208, 1990

Haney EM, Chan BK, Diem SJ, et al, for the Osteoporotic Fractures in Men Study Group: Association of low bone mineral density with selective serotonin reuptake inhibitor use by older men. Arch Intern Med 167:1246–1251, 2007

Helz JW, Templeton B: Evidence of the role of psychosocial factors in diabetes mellitus: a review. Am J Psychiatry 147:1275–1282, 1990

Henderson DC, Doraiswamy PM: Prolactin-related and metabolic adverse effects of atypical antipsychotic agents. J Clin Psychiatry 69 (suppl 1):32–44, 2008

Holroyd S, Cohen MJ: Treatment of hyperprolactinemia in major depression. Am J Psychiatry 147:810, 1990

Hook JN, Giordani B, Schteingart DE, et al: Patterns of cognitive change over time and relationship to age following successful treatment of Cushing's disease. J Int Neuropsychol Soc 13:21–29, 2007

Hudson J, Hudson M, Rothschild A, et al: Abnormal results of dexamethasone suppression test in non-depressed patients with diabetes mellitus. Arch Gen Psychiatry 41:1086–1089, 1984

Hyams JS, Leichtner AM, Breiner RG, et al: Pseudopheochromocytoma and cardiac arrest associated with phenylpropanolamine. JAMA 253:1609–1610, 1985

Jacobson AM: The psychological care of patients with insulin-dependent diabetes mellitus. N Engl J Med 334:1249–1253, 1996

Jacobson AM, Weinger K, Hill TC, et al: Brain functioning, cognition and psychiatric disorders in patients with type 1 diabetes. Diabetes 49 (suppl 1):537, 2000

Jacobson AM, Samson JA, Weinger K, et al: Diabetes, the brain, and behavior: is there a biological mechanism underlying the association between diabetes and depression? Int Rev Neurobiol 51:455–479, 2002

Jacobson AM, Ryan CM, Cleary PA, et al: Effects of intensive and conventional treatment on cognitive function 12 years after the completion of the Diabetes Control and Complications Trial (DCCT). Presented at the American Diabetes Association 66th Scientific Sessions, Washington, DC, June 9–13, 2006

Jacobson AM, Musen G, Ryan CM, et al: Long-term effect of diabetes and its treatment on cognitive function. N Engl J Med 356:1842–1852, 2007

Jensovsky J, Ruzicka E, Spackova N, et al: Changes of event related potential and cognitive processes in patients with subclinical hypothyroidism after thyroxine treatment. Endocr Regul 36:115–122, 2002

Joffe RT, Levitt AJ: Major depression and subclinical (grade 2) hypothyroidism. Psychoneuroendocrinology 17:215–221, 1992

Joffe RT, Kutcher S, MacDonald C: Thyroid function and bipolar affective disorder. Psychiatry Res 25:117–121, 1988

Johanssen S, Allolio B: Mifepristone (RU 486) in Cushing's syndrome. Eur J Endocrinol 157:561–569, 2007

Jolin EM, Weller RA, Jessani NR, et al: Affective disorders and other psychiatric diagnoses in children and adolescents with 22q11.2 deletion syndrome. J Affect Disord 119:177–180, 2009

Jones JM, Lawson ML, Daneman D, et al: Eating disorders in adolescent females with and without type 1 diabetes: cross sectional study. BMJ 320:1563–1566, 2000

Kahn CR, Weir GC, King GL, et al: Joslin's Diabetes Mellitus, 14th Edition. New York, Lippincott Williams & Wilkins, 2005

Kailasam MT, Parmer RJ, Stone RA, et al: Factitious pheochromocytoma: novel mimicry by Valsalva maneuver and clues to diagnosis. Am J Hypertens 8:651–655, 1995

Kars M, van der Klaauw AA, Onstein CS, et al: Quality of life is decreased in female patients treated for microprolactinoma. Eur J Endocrinol 157:133–139, 2007

Kathmann N, Kuisle U, Bommer M, et al: Effects of elevated triiodothyronine on cognitive performance and mood in healthy subjects. Neuropsychobiology 29:136–142, 1994

Kathol RG, Turner R, Delahunt J: Depression and anxiety associated with hyperthyroidism: response to antithyroid therapy. Psychosomatics 27:501–505, 1986

Katon WJ: Clinical and health services relationships between major depression, depressive symptoms, and general medical illness. Biol Psychiatry 54:216–226, 2003

Katon WJ, Von Korff M, Lin EH, et al: The Pathways Study: a randomized trial of collaborative care in patients with diabetes and depression. Arch Gen Psychiatry 61:1042–1049, 2004

Katon WJ, Rutter C, Simon G, et al: The association of comorbid depression with mortality in patients with type 2 diabetes. Diabetes Care 28:2668–2672, 2005

Katon W, Unutzer J, Fan MY, et al: Cost-effectiveness and net benefit of enhanced treatment of depression in older adults with diabetes and depression. Diabetes Care 29:265–270, 2006

Katon WJ, Russo JE, Von Korff M, et al: Long-term effects on medical costs of improving depression outcomes in patients with depression and diabetes. Diabetes Care 31:1155–1159, 2008

Keiser HR: Surreptitious self-administration of epinephrine resulting in a "pheochromocytoma." JAMA 266:1553–1555, 1991

Kemmer FW, Bisping R, Steingruber HJ, et al: Psychological stress and metabolic control in patients with type I diabetes mellitus. N Engl J Med 314:1078–1084, 1986

Kenardy J, Mensch M, Bowen K, et al: A comparison of eating behaviors in newly diagnosed NIDDM patients and case-matched control subjects. Diabetes Care 17:1197–1199, 1994

Kinder LS, Katon WJ, Ludman E, et al: Improving depression care in patients with diabetes and multiple complications. J Gen Intern Med 21:1036–1041, 2006

Kitzinger C, Willmott J: "The thief of womanhood": women's experience of polycystic ovarian syndrome. Soc Sci Med 54:349–361, 2002

Klipstein KG, Goldberg JF: Screening for bipolar disorder in women with polycystic ovary syndrome: a pilot study. J Affect Disord 91:205–209, 2006

Knol MJ, Twisk JW, Beekman AT, et al: Depression as a risk factor for the onset of type 2 diabetes mellitus: a meta-analysis. Diabetologia 49:837–845, 2006

Kornstein SG, Sholar EF, Gardner DG: Endocrine disorders, in Psychiatric Care of the Medical Patient, 2nd Edition. Edited by Stoudemire A, Fogel BS, Greenberg D. New York, Oxford University Press, 2000, pp 801–819

Kowdley KV, Coull BM, Orwoll ES: Cognitive impairment and intracranial calcification in chronic hypoparathyroidism. Am J Med Sci 317:273–277, 1999

Krentz AJ: UKPDS and beyond: into the next millennium. United Kingdom Prospective Diabetes Study. Diabetes Obes Metab 1:13–22, 1999

Krentz AJ, Mikhail S, Cantrell P, et al: Pseudophaeochromocytoma syndrome associated with clozapine. BMJ 322:1213, 2001

Kroenke K, Spitzer RL, Williams JB: The PHQ-9: validity of a brief depression severity measure. J Gen Intern Med 16:606–613, 2001

Kudrjavcev T: Neurologic complications of thyroid dysfunction. Adv Neurol 19:619–636, 1978

Langan SJ, Deary IJ, Hepburn DA, et al: Cumulative cognitive impairment following recurrent severe hypoglycaemia in adult patients with insulin-treated diabetes mellitus. Diabetologia 34:337–344, 1991

Laudisio A, Marzetti E, Cocchi A, et al: Association of depressive symptoms with bone mineral density in older men: a population-based study. Int J Geriatr Psychiatry 23:1119–1126, 2008

Lefebvre H, Noblet C, Moore N, et al: Pseudo-phaeochromocytoma after multiple drug interactions involving the selective monoamine oxidase inhibitor selegiline. Clin Endocrinol (Oxf) 42:95–98, 1995

Lenders JW, Pacak K, Walther MM, et al: Biochemical diagnosis of pheochromocytoma: which test is best? JAMA 287:1427–1434, 2002

Li C, Ford ES, Strine TW, et al: Prevalence of depression among U.S. adults with diabetes: findings from the behavioral risk factor surveillance system. Diabetes Care 31:105–107, 2008

Lloyd CE, Dyer PH, Lancashire RJ, et al: Association between stress and glycemic control in adults with type 1 (insulin-dependent) diabetes. Diabetes Care 22:1278–1283, 1999

Lobo-Escolar A, Saz P, Marcos G, et al, for ZARADEMP Workgroup: Somatic and psychiatric comorbidity in the general elderly population: results from the ZARADEMP Project. J Psychosom Res 65:347–355, 2008

Loosen PT, Chambliss B, DeBold CR, et al: Psychiatric phenomenology in Cushing's disease. Pharmacopsychiatry 25:192–198, 1992

Ludman EJ, Katon W, Russo J, et al: Depression and diabetes symptom burden. Gen Hosp Psychiatry 26:430–436, 2004

Ludman EJ, Katon W, Russo J, et al: Panic episodes among patients with diabetes. Gen Hosp Psychiatry 28:475–481, 2006

Lustman PJ, Griffith LS, Clouse RE, et al: Effects of nortriptyline on depression and glycemic control in diabetes: results of a double-blind, placebo-controlled trial. Psychosom Med 59:241–250, 1997

Lustman PJ, Griffith LS, Freedland KE, et al: Cognitive behavior therapy for depression in type 2 diabetes mellitus: a randomized, controlled trial. Ann Intern Med 129:613–621, 1998

Lustman PJ, Anderson RJ, Freedland KE, et al: Depression and poor glycemic control: a meta-analytic review of the literature. Diabetes Care 23:934–942, 2000a

Lustman PJ, Freedland KE, Griffith LS, et al: Fluoxetine for depression in diabetes: a randomized double-blind placebo-controlled trial. Diabetes Care 23:618–623, 2000b

Lustman PJ, Clouse RE, Nix BD, et al: Sertraline for prevention of depression recurrence in diabetes mellitus: a randomized, double-blind, placebo-controlled trial. Arch Gen Psychiatry 63:521–529, 2006

MacCrimmon DJ, Wallace JE, Goldberg WM, et al: Emotional disturbance and cognitive deficits in hyperthyroidism. Psychosom Med 41:331–340, 1979

Manger WM: The protean manifestations of pheochromocytoma. Horm Metab Res 41:658–663, 2009

Månsson M, Holte J, Landin-Wilhelmsen K, et al: Women with polycystic ovary syndrome are often depressed or anxious—a case control study. Psychoneuroendocrinology 33:1132–1138, 2008

Marcus MD, Wing RR, Guare J, et al: Lifetime prevalence of major depression and its effect on treatment outcome in obese type II diabetic patients. Diabetes Care 15:253–255, 1992

Matthews DR: The natural history of diabetes-related complications: the UKPDS experience. United Kingdom Prospective Diabetes Study. Diabetes Obes Metab 1 (suppl 2):S7–S13, 1999

Meaney AM, O'Keane V: Bone mineral density changes over a year in young females with schizophrenia: relationship to medication and endocrine variables. Schizophr Res 93:136–143, 2007

Melmed S: Disorders of the anterior pituitary and hypothalamus, in Principles of Internal Medicine, 15th Edition. Edited by Braunwald E, Fauci AS, Kasper DL, et al. New York, McGraw-Hill, 2001, pp 2029–2051

Mennemeier M, Garner RD, Heilman KM: Memory, mood and measurement in hypothyroidism. J Clin Exp Neuropsychol 15:822–831, 1993

Meyer JM, Davis VG, Goff DC, et al: Change in metabolic syndrome parameters with antipsychotic treatment in the

CATIE Schizophrenia Trial: prospective data from phase 1. Schizophr Res 101:273–286, 2008

Mezuk B, Eaton WW, Golden SH, et al: Depression, antidepressants, and bone mineral density in a population-based cohort. J Gerontol A Biol Sci Med Sci 63:1410–1415, 2008

Miller KJ, Parsons TD, Whybrow PC, et al: Memory improvement with treatment of hypothyroidism. Int J Neurosci 116:895–906, 2006

Miller KJ, Parsons TD, Whybrow PC, et al: Verbal memory retrieval deficits associated with untreated hypothyroidism. J Neuropsychiatry Clin Neurosci 19:132–136, 2007

Millward LM, Kelly P, King A, Peters TJ: Anxiety and depression in the acute porphyrias. J Inherit Metab Dis 28:1099–1107, 2005

Mitchell JE, Pomeroy C, Adson DE: Managing medical complications, in Handbook for Treatment of Eating Disorders. Editor by Garner D, Garfinkel P. New York, Guilford, 1997, pp 383–393

Moberg E, Kollind M, Lins PE, et al: Acute mental stress impairs insulin sensitivity in IDDM patients. Diabetologia 37:247–251, 1994

Mooradian AD: Asymptomatic hyperthyroidism in older adults: is it a distinct clinical and laboratory entity? Drugs Aging 25:371–380, 2008

Mooy JM, de Vries H, Grootenhuis PA, et al: Major stressful life events in relation to prevalence of undetected type 2 diabetes: the Hoorn Study. Diabetes Care 23:197–201, 2000

Morse SA, Ciechanowski PS, Katon WJ, et al: Isn't this just bedtime snacking? The potential adverse effects of night-eating symptoms on treatment adherence and outcomes in patients with diabetes. Diabetes Care 29:1800–1804, 2006

Morsink LF, Vogelzangs N, Nicklas BJ, et al: Associations between sex steroid hormone levels and depressive symptoms in elderly men and women: results from the Health ABC study. Health ABC study. Psychoneuroendocrinology 32:874–883, 2007

Musselman DL, Betan E, Larsen H, et al: Relationship of depression to diabetes types 1 and 2: epidemiology, biology, and treatment. Biol Psychiatry 54:317–329, 2003

Newcomer JW: Medical risk in patients with bipolar disorder and schizophrenia. J Clin Psychiatry 67 (suppl 9):25–30, 2006

New York Thyroid Center: Overview of thyroid disorders. 2003. Available at: http://cpmcnet.columbia.edu/dept/thyroid/disorders.html. Accessed August 2004.

O'Keane V: Antipsychotic-induced hyperprolactinaemia, hypogonadism and osteoporosis in the treatment of schizophrenia. J Psychopharmacol 22 (2 suppl):70–75, 2008

Olmsted MP, Colton PA, Daneman D, et al: Prediction of the onset of disturbed eating behavior in adolescent girls with type 1 diabetes. Diabetes Care 31:1978–1982, 2008

Owen AJ, Batterham MJ, Probst YC, et al: Low plasma vitamin E levels in major depression: diet or disease? Eur J Clin Nutr 59:304–306, 2005

Pantanetti P, Sonino N, Arnaldi G, et al: Self image and quality of life in acromegaly. Pituitary 5:17–19, 2002

Papakostas GI, Miller KK, Petersen T, et al: Serum prolactin levels among outpatients with major depressive disorder during the acute phase of treatment with fluoxetine. J Clin Psychiatry 67:952–957, 2006

Perros P, Deary IJ, Sellar RJ, et al: Brain abnormalities demonstrated by magnetic resonance imaging in adult IDDM patients with and without a history of recurrent severe hypoglycemia. Diabetes Care 20:1013–1018, 1997

Peterson CB, Mitchell JE: Psychosocial and pharmacological treatment of eating disorders: a review of research findings. J Clin Psychol 55:685–697, 1999

Petronijevi M, Petronijevi N, Ivkovi M, et al: Low bone mineral density and high bone metabolism turnover in premenopausal women with unipolar depression. Bone 42:582–590, 2008

Peveler RC, Bryden KS, Neil HA, et al: The relationship of disordered eating habits and attitudes to clinical outcomes in young adult females with type 1 diabetes. Diabetes Care 28:84–88, 2005

Pickering TG, Clemow L: Paroxysmal hypertension: the role of stress and psychological factors. J Clin Hypertens (Greenwich) 10:575–581, 2008

Polonsky WH, Anderson BJ, Lohrer PA, et al: Insulin omission in women with IDDM. Diabetes Care 17:1178–1185, 1994

Polonsky WH, Anderson BJ, Lohrer PA, et al: Assessment of diabetes-related distress. Diabetes Care 18:754–760, 1995

Porterfield SP: Endocrine Physiology. St. Louis, MO, Mosby—Year Book, 1997

Prakash R, Gandotra S, Singh LK, et al: Rapid resolution of delusional parasitosis in pellagra with niacin augmentation therapy. Gen Hosp Psychiatry 30:581–584, 2008

Prokhorova M, Fritz S: Case of a 73-year-old man with dementia and a likely pheochromocytoma mistaken for an anxiety disorder. Psychosomatics 43:82, 2002

Reavley A, Fisher AD, Owen D, et al: Psychological distress in patients with hyperprolactinaemia. Clin Endocrinol (Oxf) 47:343–348, 1997

Roberts LM, Pattison H, Roalfe A, et al: Is subclinical thyroid dysfunction in the elderly associated with depression or cognitive dysfunction? Ann Intern Med 145:573–581, 2006

Roman S, Sosa JA: Psychiatric and cognitive aspects of primary hyperparathyroidism. Curr Opin Oncol 19:1–5, 2007

Rosebush PI, Garside S, Levinson AJ, et al: The neuropsychiatry of adult-onset adrenoleukodystrophy. J Neuropsychiatry Clin Neurosci 11:315–327, 1999

Ryan CM: Diabetes and brain damage: more (or less) than meets the eye? Diabetologia 49:2229–2233, 2006

Ryan C, Geckle M, Orchard T: Cognitive efficiency declines over time in adults with type 1 diabetes: effects of micro- and macrovascular complications. Diabetologia 46:940–948, 2003

Rydall AC, Rodin GM, Olmsted MP, et al: Disordered eating behavior and microvascular complications in young women with insulin-dependent diabetes mellitus. N Engl J Med 336:1849–1854, 1997

Santos AM, Nobre EL, Garcia e Costa, et al: Graves' disease and stress [in Portuguese]. Acta Med Port 15:423–427, 2002

Sapolsky RM: Glucocorticoids and hippocampal atrophy in neuropsychiatric disorders. Arch Gen Psychiatry 57:925–935, 2000

Sawka AM, Gerstein HC, Marriott MJ, et al: Does a combination regimen of thyroxine (T_4) and 3,5,3'-triiodothyronine improve depressive symptoms better than T_4 alone in patients with hypothyroidism? Results of a double-blind, randomized, controlled trial. J Clin Endocrinol Metab 88:4551–4555, 2003

Schiess N, Pardo CA: Hashimoto's encephalopathy. Ann N Y Acad Sci 1142:254–265, 2008

Schweizer E, Winokur A, Rickels K: Insulin-induced hypoglycemia and panic attacks. Am J Psychiatry 143:654–655, 1986

Sedel F, Baumann N, Turpin JC, et al: Psychiatric manifestations revealing inborn errors of metabolism in adolescents and adults. J Inherit Metab Dis 30:631–641, 2007

Shim JC, Shin JG, Kelly DL, et al: Adjunctive treatment with a dopamine partial agonist, aripiprazole, for antipsychotic-induced hyperprolactinemia: a placebo-controlled trial. Am J Psychiatry 164:1404–1410, 2007

Siegel AJ: Hyponatremia in psychiatric patients: update on evaluation and management. Harv Rev Psychiatry16:13–24, 2008

Sievers C, Dimopoulou C, Pfister H, et al: Prevalence of mental disorders in acromegaly: a cross-sectional study in 81 acromegalic patients. Clin Endocrinol (Oxf) 71:691–701, 2009a

Sievers C, Ising M, Pfister H, et al: Personality in patients with pituitary adenomas is characterized by increased anxiety-related traits: comparison of 70 acromegalic patients with patients with non-functioning pituitary adenomas and age- and gender-matched controls. Eur J Endocrinol 160:367–373, 2009b

Sheps SG, Jiang NS, Klee GG, et al: Recent developments in the diagnosis and treatment of pheochromocytoma. Mayo Clin Proc 65:88–95, 1990

Shores MM, Sloan KL, Matsumoto AM, et al: Increased incidence of diagnosed depressive illness in hypogonadal older men. Arch Gen Psychiatry 61:162–167, 2004

Sonino N, Bonnini S, Fallo F, et al: Personality characteristics and quality of life in patients treated for Cushing's syndrome. Clin Endocrinol (Oxf) 64:314–318, 2006

Spitzer D, Bongartz D, Ittel TH, et al: Simulation of a pheochromocytoma—Munchausen syndrome. Eur J Med Res 3:549–553, 1998

Starkman MN, Giordani B, Gebarski SS, et al: Decrease in cortisol reverses human hippocampal atrophy following treatment of Cushing's disease. Biol Psychiatry 46:1595–1602, 1999

Starkman MN, Giordani B, Berent S, et al: Elevated cortisol levels in Cushing's disease are associated with cognitive decrements. Psychosom Med 63:985–993, 2001

Stern RA, Robinson B, Thorner AR, et al: A survey study of neuropsychiatric complaints in patients with Graves' disease. J Neuropsychiatry Clin Neurosci 8:181, 1996

Stern TA, Cremens CM: Factitious pheochromocytoma. Psychosomatics 39:283–287, 1998

Striegel-Moore RH, Wilfley DE, Pike KM, et al: Recurrent binge eating in black American women. Arch Fam Med 9:83–87, 2000

Talbot F, Nouwen A: A review of the relationship between depression and diabetes in adults: is there a link? Diabetes Care 23:1556–1562, 2000

Tan S, Hahn S, Benson S, et al: Psychological implications of infertility in women with polycystic ovary syndrome. Hum Reprod 23:2064–2071, 2008

Thompson CJ, Cummings JF, Chalmers J, et al: How have patients reacted to the implications of the DCCT? Diabetes Care 19:876–879, 1996

Thomsen AF, Kvist TK, Andersen PK, et al: The risk of affective disorders in patients with adrenocortical insufficiency. Psychoneuroendocrinology 31:614–622, 2006

Tiemeier H, Hofman A, Kiliaan AJ, et al: Vitamin E and depressive symptoms are not related. The Rotterdam Study. J Affect Disord 72:79–83, 2002

Trzepacz PT, McCue M, Klein I, et al: A psychiatric and neuropsychological study of patients with untreated Graves' disease. Gen Hosp Psychiatry 10:49–55, 1988a

Trzepacz PT, McCue M, Klein I, et al: Psychiatric and neuropsychological response to propranolol in Graves' disease. Biol Psychiatry 23:678–688, 1988b

Trzepacz PT, Klein I, Roberts M, et al: Graves' disease: an analysis of thyroid hormone levels and hyperthyroid signs and symptoms. Am J Med 87:558–561, 1989

T'Sjoen G, Bex M, Maiter D, et al: Health-related quality of life in acromegalic subjects: data from AcroBel, the Belgian registry on acromegaly. Eur J Endocrinol 157:411–417, 2007

Uhde TW, Vittone BJ, Post RM: Glucose tolerance testing in panic disorder. Am J Psychiatry 141:1461–1463, 1984

UK Prospective Diabetes Study (UKPDS) Group: Effect of intensive blood-glucose control with metformin on complications in overweight patients with type 2 diabetes (UKPDS 34). Lancet 352:854–865, 1998a

UK Prospective Diabetes Study (UKPDS) Group: Intensive blood-glucose control with sulphonylureas or insulin compared with conventional treatment and risk of complications in patients with type 2 diabetes (UKPDS 33). Lancet 352:837–853, 1998b

Van Winkel R, De Hert M, Wampers M, et al: Major changes in glucose metabolism, including new-onset diabetes, within 3 months after initiation of or switch to atypical antipsychotic medication in patients with schizophrenia and schizoaffective disorder. J Clin Psychiatry 69:472–479, 2008

Verrotti A, Catino M, De Luca FA, et al: Eating disorders in adolescents with type 1 diabetes mellitus. Acta Diabetol 36:21–25, 1999

Wales JK: Does psychological stress cause diabetes? Diabet Med 12:109–112, 1995

Walsh BT, Devlin MJ: Pharmacotherapy of bulimia nervosa and binge eating disorder. Addict Behav 20:757–764, 1995

Walsh JP, Shiels L, Lim EM, et al: Combined thyroxine/liothyronine treatment does not improve well-being, quality of life, or cognitive function compared to thyroxine alone: a randomized controlled trial in patients with primary hypothyroidism. J Clin Endocrinol Metab 88:4543–4550, 2003

Weber T, Keller M, Hense I, et al: Effect of parathyroidectomy on quality of life and neuropsychological symptoms in primary hyperparathyroidism. World J Surg 31:1202–1209, 2007

Welch GW, Jacobson AM, Polonsky WH: The Problem Areas in Diabetes scale: an evaluation of its clinical utility. Diabetes Care 20:760–766, 1997

Welch G, Weinger K, Anderson B, et al: Responsiveness of the Problem Areas in Diabetes (PAID) questionnaire. Diabet Med 20:69–72, 2003

Wieck A, Haddad PM: Antipsychotic-induced hyperprolactinaemia in women: pathophysiology, severity and consequences: selective literature review. Br J Psychiatry 182:199–204, 2003

Williams MM, Clouse RE, Nix BD, et al: Efficacy of sertraline in prevention of depression recurrence in older versus younger adults with diabetes. Diabetes Care 30:801–806, 2007

Yoshiuchi K, Kumano H, Nomura S, et al: Stressful life events and smoking were associated with Graves' disease in women, but not in men. Psychosom Med 60:182–185, 1998

Ziere G, Dieleman JP, van der Cammen TJ, et al: Selective serotonin reuptake inhibiting antidepressants are associated with an increased risk of nonvertebral fractures. J Clin Psychopharmacol 28:411–417, 2008

CHAPTER

23

Oncology

Mary Jane Massie, M.D.

Kimberley Miller, M.D., F.R.C.P.C.

CANCER IS A MAJOR PUBLIC health problem in the United States, Canada, and other developed nations. In 2010, more than 1.5 million new cases of invasive cancer are expected to be diagnosed in the United States, and more than half a million people are expected to die of cancer (American Cancer Society 2010). Although one in four deaths is now caused by cancer, death rates from many cancers, including those of the prostate, breast, colon, and rectum, continue to decline because of new adjuvant therapies and the use of targeted therapies that attack cancer cells, leaving healthy cells intact. However, as the death rate decreases and the population ages, more people will be living with cancer, with an anticipated doubling from 1.3 million to 2.6 million between the years 2000 and 2050. Although only modest cancer-specific survival differences are evident for black and white patients receiving comparable treatment for similar-stage cancer, black patients still carry a higher burden because they often receive diagnoses at a later stage and have poorer survival within each stage. Unfortunately, black and Hispanic women and women younger than 60 years and older than 70 years often do not receive irradiation after limited resection for early-stage breast cancer, which leads to a higher local recurrence rate and possibly higher mortality (Friedman et al. 2008). Differences in exposure to risk factors, access to high-quality screening and treatment, stage at presentation, and mortality from other diseases represent the primary targets of research and interventions designed to reduce disparities in cancer outcomes (Bach et al. 2002).

The 2007 Institute of Medicine (IOM) report, *Cancer Care for the Whole Patient: Meeting Psychosocial Health Needs,* drew attention to the importance of health care providers discussing psychosocial issues with patients, recognizing psychiatric syndromes, linking patients to psychosocial health care providers, and following up on a plan to address patients' psychosocial needs.

In this chapter, we review psychological factors in cancer risk and progression, the most frequently encountered psychiatric disorders (depression, anxiety, and delirium) in adult cancer patients, psychiatric issues in specific cancers, psychiatric aspects of cancer treatments, psychiatric interventions in cancer patients, survivor issues, and cancer patients' use of complementary and alternative medicine treatments. See Chapter 34, "Pediatrics," for additional coverage of cancer in children.

Psychological Factors Affecting Cancer Risk and Progression

Studies examining the role that stress or psychological factors play in cancer onset, progression, and survival are numerous and have yielded conflicting results in all areas. Methodological differences, including study design and definitions of type of distress, as well as publication bias and the presence of multiple confounding factors are some of the limitations evident and contribute to many reviews recommending use of caution when interpreting

The authors gratefully acknowledge Isabel Sulimanoff's assistance in the preparation of this chapter.

results. It also has been found that in community-based cohorts, study participants with cancer history may overestimate the association between distress and subsequent cancer mortality (Hamer et al. 2009). Although a recent review concluded that psychosocial factors have an adverse effect on cancer incidence and survival, it also noted that approximately 70% of studies reported a null effect (Chida et al. 2008). Another review of 70 studies did not find any psychological factors that convincingly influenced cancer development but "could not totally dismiss" helplessness and repression contributing to an unfavorable prognosis (Garssen 2004). More often than not, associations, rather than clear causality, are identified in studying psychological factors and cancer outcomes.

Although retrospective and case-control studies have suggested an association between severe stressors and cancer risk, larger prospective studies often have not found such an association. In 1,011 of 8,736 randomly selected Danish patients who subsequently developed cancer, the accumulation of stressful life events was associated with an unhealthy lifestyle but not an increase in cancer incidence (Bergelt et al. 2006). Similarly, certain personality traits have not been found to affect cancer risk directly or indirectly (through influence on health behavior) (Bleiker et al. 2008; Hansen et al. 2005). A prospective cohort study of 19,730 adults, with an average follow-up of 9 years, did not detect a significant association between anger control or negative affect and risk of breast cancer, melanoma, or total cancers but did identify weak associations in prostate (hazards ratio [HR] = 1.17), colorectal (HR = 1.14), and lung cancer (HR = 1.24) (White et al. 2007). In evaluating the effect of psychological distress on cancer outcome, some have suggested that associations between patients' self-ratings on distress scales and survival may reflect patients' perception of their disease status rather than a causal effect of distress on the cancer process (Groenvold et al. 2007). Attempts to control for disease status have yielded both positive (Groenvold et al. 2007) and negative (Coates et al. 2000) results in linking distress with cancer outcome.

The evidence associating depression with cancer incidence is weaker than that for cancer progression (Spiegel and Giese-Davis 2003), although the literature has included contradictory and inconclusive results in both. Depressive symptoms were associated with a higher-than-normal frequency of cancer and twice as high a risk for death from cancer in an early large epidemiological study (Persky et al. 1987; Shekelle et al. 1981). Later epidemiological studies and a meta-analysis did not find statistically or clinically significant associations (Archer et al. 2008; Gallo et al. 2000; McGee et al. 1994). A review of depressive symptoms and the prospective incidence of colorectal adenomas and cancer in more than 80,000 women enrolled in the Nurses' Health Study showed that women with the highest levels of depressive symptoms had elevated risk of colon cancer but not colorectal adenomas (Kroenke et al. 2005). A "small and marginally significant association" (relative risk [RR] = 1.12) between depression and subsequent overall cancer risk was found in a 2007 review, which included 13 studies (Oerlemans et al. 2007).

Mixed results also have been found when examining the possible link between depression and cancer mortality (Coyne et al. 2007; Garssen and Goodkin 1999; Watson et al. 1999). A population-based epidemiological study that included data on 10,025 patients followed up over an 8-year period found that those with cancer and depression had a higher risk of death from all causes than did those with either condition alone (Onitilo et al. 2006). Although depression did not affect survival in pancreatic cancer (Sheibani-Rad and Velanovich 2006), Steel et al.'s (2007) prospective study of 101 patients with hepatobiliary cancer showed that patients with depression, which was present in one-third of patients, had a significantly shorter survival time. Declines in natural killer cell activity were associated with shorter survival (Steel et al. 2007). In a comprehensive review of the effect of the comorbidity of cancer and depression, Archer et al. (2008) concluded that both behavioral (e.g., smoking, alcohol use in head and neck cancer) and biological factors (e.g., cytokines and the stress-hormone axis) contribute to the negative effect. Lutgendorf et al. (2008) reported significant correlation between interleukin-6, cortisol, and vegetative components of depression in women with advanced-stage ovarian cancer. Depression also may affect the course of illness in patients with cancer through its effect on poorer pain control, poorer treatment adherence, and less desire for life-sustaining therapy. Although it remains unclear if alleviating cancer patients' psychological distress will prolong their survival, it is prudent to intervene to improve quality of life and ensure optimal treatment adherence.

Psychiatric Disorders in Cancer Patients

A person's ability to manage a cancer diagnosis and treatment commonly changes over the course of the illness and depends on medical, psychological, and social factors: the disease itself (i.e., site, symptoms, clinical course, prognosis, type of treatments required); the prior level of adjustment; the threat that cancer poses to attaining age-appropriate developmental tasks and goals (i.e., adolescence, career, family, retirement); cultural, spiritual, and religious attitudes; the presence of emotionally supportive persons; the potential for physical and psychological rehabilitation; the patient's own personality and coping style; and experience with loss.

Depression

Depressive symptoms in the cancer patient may occur as part of adjustment to different phases of illness (e.g., diagnosis, initiation and completion of treatment, survivorship, recurrence, palliation) or be caused by the cancer itself (e.g., primary or secondary brain tumors) and its related symptoms (e.g., fatigue or pain) and treatments (e.g., exogenous cytokines, corticosteroids). Those with a preexisting history of major depression are at increased risk for a depressive recurrence during their cancer experience. In other words, depressive symptoms may represent a normal reaction, a psychiatric disorder, or a somatic consequence of cancer or its treatment.

Cancer is associated with a rate of depression that is higher than that in the general population and at least as high as the rate associated with other serious medical illnesses (Massie 2004). In patients with cancer, depression has been studied with a range of assessment methods (Härter et al. 2001; Trask 2004), including self-report, brief screening instruments, and structured clinical interviews. Reports of prevalence of depression in cancer are highly variable, given the lack of standardization of methodology and diagnostic criteria used. In more than 150 studies, Massie (2004) found that major depression occurred in 0%–38% of cancer patients and that depression spectrum syndromes occurred in 0%–58%. A clinical rule of thumb is that 25% of cancer patients will likely be depressed enough at some point in the course of disease to warrant evaluation and treatment.

Emotional distress is often not recognized by oncology professionals (Söllner et al. 2001), resulting in distress screening initiatives being developed in many countries. These typically advocate for a two-stage process, involving an initial self-report scale, followed by a diagnostic interview (which remains the gold standard in assessing depression) for those patients reaching a predetermined cutoff score on the screening instrument. The single-item Distress Thermometer compares favorably (Jacobsen et al. 2005) with multiple-item measures, including the 18-item version of the Brief Symptom Inventory (BSI-18; Derogatis 2000) and the 14-item Hospital Anxiety and Depression Scale (Zigmond and Snaith 1983), all of which have been evaluated and identified as useful in screening for distress in cancer patients. Other instruments to screen for distress specific to cancer patients also have been developed (e.g., Herschbach et al. 2004).

Many of the somatic symptoms caused by cancer or its treatment overlap with the diagnostic criteria for major depression, including disturbances in sleep, appetite, energy, psychomotor activity, and concentration. Emphasis on exploring the psychological symptoms of depression (depressed mood, anhedonia, guilt, worthlessness, hopelessness, helplessness, and suicidal ideation) may be a helpful clinical approach. Hypoactive delirium may resemble depression because the patient may be less engaged, may be less motivated to participate in his or her care, and may even voice suicidal ideation. Differentiating between delirium and depression is extremely important, given the differences in causes, risks, and interventions. See Chapter 5, "Delirium," for a more thorough review. Poorly controlled pain, fatigue, or anorexia-cachexia syndrome also may present with a depressive component.

In cancer patients, risk factors for the development of depression have been found to include younger age, poor social support, and advanced disease. The predominance of women developing major depression seen in the general population does not consistently occur in the oncology setting (Pirl 2004; Rodin et al. 2007a; Strong et al. 2007). The role of specific tumor sites in contributing to emotional distress has conflicting results. Strong et al. (2007) did not find cancer diagnosis to be a predictor for distress, whereas Carlson et al. (2004) found that patients with Hodgkin's disease or lung, pancreatic, head and neck, and brain cancer were most distressed, which is consistent with another large study examining distress by cancer site (Zabora et al. 2001). A strong relation has been found between disease burden (especially pain and fatigue), perceived social support, and insecure attachment style in patients with metastatic cancer (Rodin et al. 2007b). A study in 2,595 early-stage breast cancer patients found that stressful life events, less optimism, ambivalence over expressing negative emotions, sleep disturbance, and poorer social functioning better predicted risk for depression than did cancer-related variables (Bardwell et al. 2006). Biopsychosocial risk factors most commonly associated with depression in cancer are listed in Table 23–1.

Several barriers to the diagnosis of depression in cancer patients exist (Greenberg 2004). At the physician level, difficulty distinguishing somatic symptoms related to cancer and its treatment from depression, as well as uncertainty about the effectiveness of psychosocial interventions, may contribute to fewer referrals for psychosocial services. Lack of access to and poor patient awareness of psychosocial services are additional barriers. At the patient level, reluctance to report depressive symptoms may be related to a fear of psychiatric medication side effects, stigma about psychosocial support, perceived repercussions of expressing "negativity" on the course of the cancer, and social and cultural differences in expression of distress (Söllner et al. 2001). Recognizing and treating depression are essential not only for the patient but also for the patient's

TABLE 23–1. Biopsychosocial risk factors most commonly associated with depression in cancer

Biological	Psychological	Social
Younger age	Relationships	Low supports
Family history of depression	Perceived low supports	Poorer social functioning
Personal history of depression	Anxious or avoidant attachment	Recent loss
Cancer-related factors	Attitudes	Stressful life events
Advanced disease	Less optimism	History of trauma or abuse
Low performance status	Ambivalence in expressing emotions	Substance use disorder
Physical burden (pain, fatigue)	Low self-esteem	
Tumor site (?pancreas, head and neck, lung, brain, Hodgkin's disease)		
Treatment (see Table 23–2)		

loved ones. A recent multinational study of cancer patients and their children showed that depression in a parent (the cancer patient or the patient's partner) is significantly associated with impairment in family functioning (Schmitt et al. 2008).

Suicide and Desire for Hastened Death

Although suicide accounts for a very low number of deaths in cancer patients, an elevated risk has been consistently found. In the United States, a large retrospective cohort study comparing cancer patients with the general population reported that patients with cancer had nearly twice the incidence of suicide (Misono et al. 2008). Higher suicide rates were associated with male gender, white race, and older age at diagnosis. Highest suicide rates were observed in cancers of the respiratory system, stomach, and head and neck. In the United Kingdom, almost 8% of 2,924 outpatient cancer patients had thoughts of being "better off dead" or of hurting themselves in some way in the previous 2 weeks (Walker et al. 2008). Clinically significant emotional distress and substantial pain (and, to a lesser extent, older age) were associated with these thoughts. Desire for hastened death has been positively associated with hopelessness, depression, and higher physical distress and negatively with physical functioning, spiritual well-being, social support, and self-esteem (Chochinov et al. 1998; Rodin et al. 2007c). Those closer to death have been found to express desire for hastened death more commonly (17%) than do those with a prognosis of greater than 6 months (2%) (Chochinov et al. 1998; Rodin et al. 2007c). Understanding the complex contributing factors in a patient with desire for hastened death can aid in differentiating a depressive illness from a desire to have control over intolerable symptoms, or even death acceptance (see also Chapter 9, "Suicidality," and Chapter 41, "Palliative Care").

Anxiety

Anxiety is a normal response to threat, uncertainty, and loss of control. It is common as patients face the existential plight of cancer and the specific threats of deformity, abandonment, pain, or death. The diagnosis and treatment of cancer are stressful and often traumatic. After the initial shock and disbelief of diagnosis, patients typically feel anxious and irritable. They may experience anorexia, insomnia, and difficulty with concentration because they are distracted by intrusive thoughts about their prognosis. Often this acute anxiety dissipates as a treatment plan is established and prognosis clarified. Anxiety is common at crisis points such as the start of a new treatment or the diagnosis of recurrence or illness progression, but it also occurs before routine follow-up visits without evidence of disease.

Specific phobias, panic disorder with or without agoraphobia, generalized anxiety disorder, and posttraumatic stress disorder (PTSD) are the most commonly reported anxiety disorders in cancer patients (Roy-Byrne et al. 2008), and patients frequently present with anxious symptoms in the context of adjustment disorders. In a cross-sectional observational study of 178 patients with cancer, almost half had significant anxiety symptoms, but the rate of anxiety disorders was 18%, comparable to that in the general population. In this study, female gender and poor support systems were correlated with anxiety disorders (Stark et al. 2002). In 1,408 testicular cancer survivors, anxiety disorders correlated with younger age at follow-up, relapse anxiety, psychiatric treatment, peripheral neuropathy, alcohol abuse, economic problems, and sexual dysfunction (Dahl et al. 2005).

Some forms of anxiety can affect a patient's adherence to treatment. Patients with claustrophobia may have difficulty tolerating magnetic resonance imaging (MRI) scans, radiation therapy, or placement in isolation because of neutropenia. Needle phobia and other health-related phobias (see Chapter 11, "Anxiety Disorders") may delay or prevent patient adherence to recommended chemotherapeutic and/or surgical treatments.

PTSD has been reported to occur in 4%–6% of cancer patients (Kangas et al. 2002; Mehnert and Koch 2007), with more patients experiencing subsyndromal episodes of intrusive thoughts, avoidance, or hypervigilance (Jim and Jacobsen 2008). Intrusive thoughts in cancer patients may be focused on past events, including disclosure of diagnosis and traumatic treatment experiences, or on anticipatory fears of cancer recurrence. Reminders of the traumas of cancer can provoke anxiety and physiological arousal. A sample of women 2 years after diagnosis of stages I to III breast cancer had heightened arousal (as measured by skin conductance, heart rate, and facial muscle electrical activity) during mental imagery of the traumatic event as they listened to their own narrative of their two most stressful experiences associated with breast cancer. Breast cancer–specific posttraumatic stress symptoms were noted in 24%, but only 9% reported full PTSD. Those with the strongest responses had current PTSD, and most had comorbid major depressive disorder (Pitman et al. 2001).

Risk factors for posttraumatic stress in cancer patients include perception of cancer as threatening, trauma history, younger age, less social support, and more difficult interactions with medical staff (Jim and Jacobsen 2008). Medical sequelae of cancer treatment (e.g., paresthesias because of nerve injury) may act as a trigger for traumatic memories of treatment (Kornblith et al. 2004).The importance of exploring both patient and caregiver distress was highlighted in a study of 168 non–genetically related patient-caregiver dyads, in which the presence of anxiety disorder in one partner (patient or caregiver) was associated with a greater likelihood of anxiety disorder in the other (Bambauer et al. 2006). In recent years, improved antiemetic treatments have reduced the number of patients who vomit as a result of chemotherapy, but nausea is still common (Hickok et al. 2003). Anxiety related to nausea and vomiting from highly emetogenic chemotherapy may develop into a conditioned response, which may persist after cessation of treatment (Bovbjerg 2006).

Evaluation of acute anxiety in cancer patients includes consideration of conditions that mimic anxiety disorders. Antipsychotics, as well as antiemetic phenothiazines (prochlorperazine, perphenazine, promethazine) or metoclopramide, may cause akathisia. Akathisia's inner feeling of restlessness is frequently misperceived by patients and misdiagnosed by caregivers as anxiety. The abrupt onset of anxiety and dyspnea may signal pulmonary emboli, which are common among cancer patients. Hypoxia related to primary or secondary lung cancer may cause significant anxiety. The experience of severe, intermittent, or uncontrolled pain is associated with acute and chronic anxiety, and the patient's confidence that he or she has the analgesics to control pain alleviates anxiety. Furthermore, anxiety amplifies pain, and the drive behind additional requests for analgesia may be anxiety rather than somatic pain (see also Chapter 11, "Anxiety Disorders," and Chapter 36, "Pain").

Mania

In cancer patients, corticosteroids are the most common reason for hypomania or mania (corticosteroid psychiatric side effects are discussed in detail in Chapter 25, "Rheumatology"). Steroids are commonly given as a component of chemotherapy for lymphoma and multiple myeloma, as an antiemetic or to prevent hypersensitivity reactions with chemotherapy, to reduce cerebral or spinal edema, or to prevent cerebral edema during cranial radiation therapy. Lower doses of corticosteroids also may be used in palliative care to improve appetite, energy, and general well-being. Full-blown manic episodes are rare. In a study of dexamethasone prophylaxis for emesis caused by chemotherapy, the psychological symptoms most commonly reported by patients were insomnia and agitation (Vardy et al. 2006). Although it is more commonly associated with depression, interferon-alpha also has been associated with mania and mixed affective syndromes (Greenberg et al. 2000). Diencephalic tumors are a rare cause of secondary mania (see also Chapter 10, "Psychosis, Mania, and Catatonia").

Delirium

The prevalence of delirium in cancer patients has been reported as 5%–30%, as up to 25%–50% on hospital admission, and as high as 85% in the terminal stages of illness. Advanced age, possible preexisting dementia, and malnutrition are predisposing factors for delirium in cancer, and potential precipitants include intracranial disease, medications, and systemic disease (e.g., organ failure, infection, and hematological or metabolic abnormalities). One study found that a median of three (range=1–6) precipitants contributed to a delirious episode (Lawlor 2002). In a review of hospitalized cancer patients, daily doses of benzodiazepines greater than 2 mg of lorazepam equivalents, corticosteroids greater than 15 mg of dexamethasone equivalents, or opioids greater than 90 mg of morphine equivalents were associated with an increased risk of delirium (Gaudreau et al. 2005). A follow-up study to evaluate the risk of these medications found that opioids affected longitudinal risk of delirium but corticosteroids and benzodiazepines did not (Gaudreau et al. 2007). Delirium is associated with greater morbidity and mortality in patients and greater distress in patients, their families, and caregivers.

Early symptoms of delirium are often unrecognized or misdiagnosed by medical or nursing staff because of fluctuation in presentation, presence of a hypoactive subtype of delirium, and lack of mental status examination of the patient. Delirium is frequently misdiagnosed as dementia, depression, anxiety, or other psychiatric disorders. Early recognition of delirium is essential because the etiology may be a treatable complication of cancer or its treatment. In addition to the general causes of delirium (see Chapter 5, "Delirium"), there are particular considerations in cancer patients. Primary brain tumor and brain metastases (especially common with lung and breast cancer) can cause delirium. Immunosuppressed cancer patients, particularly those with hematological malignancies, are at high risk for opportunistic infections. Head and neck cancer patients undergoing surgery are at high risk for delirium because of their older age and high prevalence of alcohol abuse and withdrawal. Several antineoplastic agents (e.g., cytarabine, methotrexate, ifosfamide, asparaginase, procarbazine, and fluorouracil) and immunotherapeutic agents (e.g., interferon and interleukins) can cause delirium and other alterations in mental status (Table 23-2) (Kannarkat et al. 2007; Minisini et al. 2008). Some antibiotics (e.g., quinolones) and antifungals (e.g., amphotericin B), as well as opioids, anticholinergics, and nutritional deficiencies, can cause delirium. Hypercalcemia causes delirium in patients with bone metastases or ectopic parathyroid hormone production. Hyperviscosity syndrome with lymphoma, Waldenström's macroglobulinemia, and myeloma are unusual causes of delirium. Thromboembolic events involving the central nervous system (CNS) also may contribute to acute, subacute, or delayed mental status changes. L-Asparaginase, thalidomide, tamoxifen, and erythropoietin all have been associated with the development of cerebral venous thrombosis (Minisini et al. 2008). Rare autoimmune encephalopathies resulting from paraneoplastic syndromes (Lieberman and Schold 2002) manifest with cognitive impairment and delirium. Limbic encephalopathy (or encephalitis) is a specific type of autoimmune encephalopathy most often reported with small-cell carcinoma of the lung but uncommonly with many other malignancies. Limbic encephalopathy may present with impaired memory, fluctuating mood, and seizures (Kung et al. 2002), as well as a wide variety of psychiatric symptoms including anxiety, depression, schizophreniform or manic psychosis, and personality change (Foster and Caplan 2009) (see also Chapter 32, "Neurology and Neurosurgery").

Chapter 5, "Delirium," and Chapter 41, "Palliative Care," review the general management of delirium. Of special note in the oncology setting is the use of methylene blue (50 mg slow intravenous push or orally every 4–6 hours until recovery) to treat ifosfamide-induced encephalopathy, although controlled trials are lacking (Brunello et al. 2007).

Interplay of Physical and Psychological Symptoms in Cancer Patients

Pain

Pain is a highly prevalent symptom in cancer, and for those not experiencing pain, it is often a commonly feared future symptom. Pain may be a sign of progression of disease, which can contribute to significant distress. Depression and anxiety are very common in cancer patients with severe pain. In a recent systematic review of cancer pain and depression, a statistically significant association between pain and depression was found in 9 of 14 studies, although none of the studies examined a causal relation (Laird et al. 2009). Pain intensity and its effect on enjoyment of life were related to depression.

The psychiatric symptoms of patients who are in significant pain should initially be considered a consequence of uncontrolled pain. Acute anxiety, depression with despair (especially when the patient believes the pain means disease progression), agitation, irritability, lack of cooperation, anger, and insomnia all may accompany pain. Such symptoms usually should not be diagnosed as a psychiatric disorder unless they persist after pain is adequately controlled. Although antidepressants have been studied more often in the nonmalignant pain population, their use as adjuvant analgesics in the management of neuropathic pain in cancer has been recommended, especially for those with comorbid depression. The tricyclic antidepressants (TCAs) and the serotonin–norepinephrine reuptake inhibitors (SNRIs) venlafaxine and duloxetine are most effective, with a possible role for bupropion (McDonald and Portenoy 2006). No evidence indicates increased risk of abuse or addiction in cancer patients receiving opioids. In fact, many patients associate the narcotics with the unpleasant aspects of the illness and avoid them after their recovery (pain management is discussed in full in Chapter 36, "Pain").

Cancer-Related Fatigue

Cancer-related fatigue refers to a pervasive feeling of tiredness, weakness, or lack of energy, related to cancer or its treatment, that is not relieved by rest. Anticancer treatments, including surgery, chemotherapy, radiation, bio-

TABLE 23–2. Neuropsychiatric side effects of common chemotherapeutic agents

Hormones

Corticosteroids

- Mild to severe insomnia, hyperactivity, anxiety, depression, psychosis with prominent manic features

Tamoxifen

- Sleep disorder, irritability

Biologicals

Cytokines

- Encephalopathy

Interferon-alpha

- Depression, suicidality, mania, psychosis
- Delirium, akathisia
- Seizures

Interleukin-2

- Dysphoria, delirium, psychosis
- Seizures

Chemotherapy agents

L-Asparaginase

- Somnolence, lethargy, delirium, depression

Chlorambucil

- Hallucinations, lethargy, seizures, stupor, coma

Capecitabine

- Multifocal leukoencephalopathy
- Cerebellar ataxia
- Reversible neuromuscular syndrome: trismus, slurred speech, confusion, ocular abnormalities

Cisplatin

- Encephalopathy (rare), sensory neuropathy

Cytarabine

- Delirium, seizures
- Leukoencephalopathy

5-Fluorouracil

- Fatigue, rare seizure or confusion, cerebellar syndrome

Gemcitabine

- Fatigue

Ifosfamide

- Lethargy, seizures, drunkenness, cerebellar signs, delirium, hallucinations

Methotrexate

- Intrathecal regimens: possible leukoencephalopathy (acute and delayed forms)
- High dose: possible transient delirium

Procarbazine

- Somnolence, depression, delirium, psychosis, cerebellar disorder

TABLE 23–2. Neuropsychiatric side effects of common chemotherapeutic agents *(continued)*

Taxanes

- Sensory neuropathy, fatigue, depression

Thalidomide

- Fatigue, reversible dementia

Vincristine, vinblastine, vinorelbine

- Depression, fatigue, encephalopathy

Multikinase inhibitors

Sorafenib, sunitinib, bevacizumab

- Posterior leukoencephalopathy syndrome

logical response modifiers, hormones, and hematopoietic stem cell transplants, all may contribute to cancer-related fatigue. Prue et al. (2006) reported that 39%–90% of patients who are undergoing cancer treatment and 19%–38% of patients who have completed active treatment will experience fatigue. Common causes of cancer-related fatigue are listed in Table 23–3. Proposed neurobiological mechanisms have been reviewed by others (Levy 2008; Ryan et al. 2007; Schubert et al. 2007) and include serotonin dysregulation, abnormalities in the hypothalamic-pituitary-adrenal (HPA) axis, circadian rhythm disruption, muscle metabolism or adenosine triphosphate dysregulation, vagal afferent nerve activation, and prolonged inflammatory response involving cytokines (Stone and Minton 2008). Comorbid conditions including anemia, cachexia, pain, depression, and sleep disorders also may contribute to cancer-related fatigue.

Psychiatrists play an important role in the treatment of comorbid psychiatric illnesses while being aware of the potential contribution of sedative-hypnotics and other psychotropic medications to cancer-related fatigue. A recent Cochrane review (Minton et al. 2008) examining drug therapy for cancer-related fatigue found that methylphenidate was superior to placebo, but only two studies, combining 264 patients, met criteria for inclusion, highlighting the relative dearth of evidence in this area. Preliminary results from four studies, including a large randomized, placebo-controlled, double-blind trial of 642 patients, showed the benefit and safety of modafinil in the treatment of cancer-related fatigue (Cooper et al. 2009). Some patients who have persistent fatigue with progressive disease or after cancer treatment respond well to low-dose psychostimulants such as methylphenidate or modafinil and do not need increased doses over time (Carroll et al. 2007). Data are conflicting about the usefulness of exercise programs and psychosocial interventions to decrease cancer-related fatigue. A Cochrane review identified lim-

TABLE 23–3. Causes of cancer-related fatigue

Cancer treatment
- Interferon
- Chemotherapy
- Irradiation

Pain

Anemia

Nutritional deficits

Hormonal imbalance
- Thyroid
- Estrogen
- Androgens

Immune response

Cytokine release

Drug effects
- Opioids
- Sedatives

Psychiatric disorders
- Sleep disruption
- Depression

TABLE 23–4. Causes of cancer anorexia–cachexia syndrome

Gastrointestinal dysfunction
- Mechanical obstruction from tumors of mouth, esophagus, stomach, gastrointestinal tract
- Extrinsic pressure from metastatic disease

Anticancer treatment
- Change in food smell or taste (food aversions): dysosmia, dysgensia
- Nausea, vomiting, mucositis

Altered (hyper) metabolism
- Carbohydrate
- Lipid
- Protein

Host response to cancer
- Cytokine production
  - Tumor necrosis factor, interleukin-1, interleukin-6, interferon

Psychological factors
- Depression
- Anxiety
- Preexisting eating disorder
- Conditioned responses

ited evidence that psychosocial interventions improve cancer-related fatigue during cancer treatment. However, interventions specifically targeting fatigue have yielded more positive results, through assisting patients with their coping and activity management as well as educating them about fatigue (Goedendorp 2009). A meta-analytic review showed that psychosocial interventions may be most useful when applied after the completion of cancer therapy, and exercise interventions may be most useful when applied concurrent with therapy (Kangas et al. 2008). Segal et al. (2009) found in a randomized controlled trial that resistance and aerobic exercise mitigated fatigue in men with prostate cancer who were receiving radiotherapy. Dy et al. (2008) described evidence-based recommendations for screening for, treating, and following up cancer fatigue, anorexia, depression, and dyspnea.

Anorexia–Cachexia Syndrome

Cachexia in cancer patients is debilitating and life-threatening. It is associated with anorexia, fat and muscle wasting, weakness, decreased quality of life, and psychological distress. The causes of cachexia are gastrointestinal (GI) dysfunction, altered metabolism and host response to cancer (cytokine production), hormone production by tumors, and anticancer treatments (Bennani-Baiti and Davis 2008; Inui 2002) (Table 23–4). Anorexia–cachexia drug treatment trials and laboratory-based studies have been summarized by others (Loprinzi et al. 2007).

Anorexia may be the result of depression or anxiety. Preexisting eating disorders complicate nutritional management in cancer patients. Treatments of anorexia and cachexia in cancer patients are shown in Table 23–5.

Psychiatric Issues in Specific Cancers

Prostate Cancer

The prostate is the most common site of cancer in men in the United States. In 2010, an estimated 217,730 new cases will be diagnosed (American Cancer Society 2010). No high-risk prostate cancer–specific genes have been identified; however, *BRCA2* confers a risk of prostate cancer that is 20 times that of the general population (Foulkes 2008). In general, although the reaction of men with prostate cancer depends on age, marital status, recent losses, and social support, older men are less likely to seek or accept intervention for emotional distress.

Routine screening for prostate cancer with the serum prostate-specific antigen (PSA) test has “a modest effect on

TABLE 23–5. Treatment of cancer anorexia–cachexia syndrome

Hypercaloric feeding (enteral and parenteral nutrition)

Does not increase skeletal muscle mass

Useful for nutritional support for patients with potentially therapy-responsive cancer

Drugs

Amino acids; adenosine triphosphate

Corticosteroids

- Increase sense of well-being
- Useful adjunct for pain control
- Decrease nausea
- May cause osteoporosis, muscle weakness, immunosuppression, delirium
- No demonstrated effects on body weight

Progestational agents

- Megestrol acetate
  - Increases body weight (fat) gain
  - Increases appetite and sense of well-being
  - Can cause thromboembolic phenomena, edema, hyperglycemia, hypertension, adrenal insufficiency (if abrupt discontinuation)
  - Does not affect survival
- Medroxyprogesterone acetate
  - Increases appetite and body weight
  - Available in depot and oral suspension

Antiserotonergic agents

- Cyproheptadine
  - Increases appetite; does not prevent weight loss
- Ondansetron
  - Does not prevent weight loss

Prokinetic agents

- Metoclopramide
  - Treatment for chemotherapy-induced emesis
  - May relieve anorexia
- Cannabinoids
  - Dronabinol (Marinol)
  - May improve mood and appetite
  - Minimally effective in increasing body weight
  - Can cause euphoria, dizziness

Emerging drugs

Melatonin, thalidomide

Nonsteroidal anti-inflammatory drugs (prostaglandin inhibitors)

Testosterone

Educational and behavioral approaches

prostate cancer mortality" and a substantial risk of overdiagnosis and treatment (Barry 2009). A recent study of anxiety in 1,781 Swedish men who had elevated PSA levels showed that severe anxiety while waiting for PSA results affected only a small group of susceptible men (Carlsson et al. 2007). Anxiety surrounding each PSA test may be greater in spouses than in patients (Kornblith et al. 1994).

It is difficult to distinguish indolent forms of prostate cancer that will not affect the quality or length of patients' survival from more lethal varieties. It is also difficult to assess the relative risk of treatment complications that may significantly impair quality of life. Controversy among clinicians about primary treatment for early-stage cancer (nerve-sparing radical prostatectomy vs. radiation therapy) or active surveillance creates uncertainty and makes treatment decisions difficult. Counseling assists patients with these choices by considering the extent of disease, age of patient, life expectancy, expense, and geography, and the choices are often based on the potential side effects (e.g., impotence, urinary incontinence, and bowel problems). In general, men undergoing surgery, older men, and men with less serious disease have less mental distress (Litwin et al. 2002).

Men who are reluctant to participate in individual therapy may agree to participate in national psychoeducational or support groups (US Too, Man to Man, MaleCare) and may use other sources of information about the illness, treatment options, and maintenance of good quality of life (Roth et al. 2008). However, many men describe participation in support groups as stigmatizing (B.A. Weber and Sherwill-Navarro 2005). Because many men and their partners develop sexual difficulties in response to erectile dysfunction, which occurs in many men after prostatectomy, radiation treatment, and hormonal therapies, sex therapy for the couple aimed at exploring new sexual possibilities and restoring intimacy can be helpful (Wittmann et al. 2009).

In prostate cancer patients, the most important risk factor for the development of major depressive disorder is a history of depression (Ingram et al. 2003; Pirl et al. 2002). Androgen deprivation therapy by orchiectomy or chronic administration of gonadotropin-releasing hormone agonists may cause hot flashes, reduced libido, erectile dysfunction, fatigue, anemia, decreased muscle mass, and osteoporosis. Men with prostate cancer who received androgen deprivation therapy reported poorer quality of life compared with men who underwent any prostate cancer treatment without hormonal treatment (Wei et al. 2002). A recent prospective cohort study showed that anxiety about cancer "independently and robustly" predicted earlier start of androgen deprivation therapy in older men with biochemical recurrence, although life expectancy may not change and quality of life may be negatively affected (Dale et al. 2009). Analysis of a sample culled from tumor registries of more than 50,000 men who had survived at least 5 years found that the risk of developing a depressive or cognitive disorder diagnosis after androgen deprivation therapy was no higher than in men who had not received androgen deprivation therapy when tumor characteristics, age, and other factors were controlled (Shahinian et al. 2006). However, the incidence of suicide in older men with prostate cancer has been reported to be 4.24 times that of an age- and gender-specific cohort (Llorente et al. 2005). In this study, depression, recent cancer diagnosis, pain, and foreign birth were risk factors for suicide. Fatigue, a common side effect of irradiation for prostate cancer, may be helped by resistance and aerobic exercise (Segal et al. 2009).

Breast Cancer

Breast cancer is the most common cancer in women, second only to lung cancer in cancer deaths in women. In 2010, an estimated 207,090 new cases of invasive breast cancer and more than 54,000 new cases of in situ breast cancer will be diagnosed in the United States. More than 40,000 men and women are expected to die of breast cancer in 2010 (American Cancer Society 2010). The number of women diagnosed with breast cancer has decreased as a result of the decline in the use of hormone replacement therapy in postmenopausal women, and the modest improvement in the death rate is probably attributable to successful treatment of cancers diagnosed at an early stage (Robbins and Clark 2007). More than 85% of women diagnosed with stage I cancers (small cancers confined to the breast) will be alive 5 years later. Survival drops dramatically when cancers are diagnosed at later stages.

Although only 5% of breast cancer occurs in women younger than 40 years, a disproportionately large number of younger women seek psychiatric consultation regarding treatment options; sexual side effects of treatments; fertility concerns; self- and body-image issues; prophylactic contralateral mastectomy; genetic testing; and the effects of cancer on relationships, children, and career.

Treatment and Side Effects

The treatments of breast cancer include surgery, irradiation, chemotherapy, antiestrogen therapy (tamoxifen; raloxifene; aromatase inhibitors such as anastrazole, letrozole, and exemestane), and zoledronic acid, a bisphosphonate. Local control is still critical; the size, location, and aggressiveness of the tumor usually dictate the initial surgery (mastectomy vs. limited resection). Use of sentinel-node mapping reduces, but does not eliminate, the risk of developing unsightly and, at times, disabling lymphedema. Although many women now have a choice between mastectomy and limited resection, mastectomy is preferred by an increasing number of women because it offers "peace of mind" and avoidance of irradiation (Collins et al. 2009; Throckmorton 2009). Natural tissue or silicone or saline implant breast reconstruction techniques provide satisfactory to excellent results for women eligible for reconstruction (Cordeiro 2008). Involvement of the patient's husband or partner in preoperative medical appointments, in viewing of the scar, and in discussions about resuming sexual activity is helpful for optimal recovery. Phantom breast syndrome, distinct from postmastectomy pain syndrome, has been described in breast cancer patients who have undergone mastectomies. Spyropoulou et al. (2008) recently found that 22.9% of 105 women after modified radical mastectomy experienced phantom breast syndrome, which was associated with higher Zung Self-Rating Depression Scale scores and younger age.

Chemotherapy with alkylating agents can cause alopecia, ovarian failure, premature menopause (Schover 2008), decline in cognitive function, and weight gain (Hayes 2007). Taxanes can cause painful and disabling peripheral neuropathy, arthralgia or myalgia, and depression (Thornton et al. 2008). Antiestrogen therapy is prescribed over a period of years and may cause insomnia, hot flashes, irritability, and depression in some women (Duffy et al. 1999). Despite early concerns, a large placebo-controlled retrospective cohort study of women with breast cancer concluded that tamoxifen does not increase the risk for developing depression (Lee et al. 2007). An individual patient pooled analysis found that newer antidepressants and gabapentin reduced hot flashes within 4 weeks of initiating treatment by 3%–41% compared with placebo. Venlafaxine (75 mg/day) and paroxetine (10–25 mg/day) are more effective than sertraline (50–100 mg/day) or fluoxetine (20 mg/day) (Henry et al. 2008). However, because tamoxifen requires metabolism by cytochrome P450 (CYP) 2D6 to its active metabolite, paroxetine, fluoxetine, duloxetine, bupropion, and other CYP 2D6 inhibitors should be avoided during tamoxifen therapy (Goetz et al. 2007). Gabapentin (900–2,400 mg/day) reduced hot flashes by 35%–38% compared with placebo. Other options for hot flashes include clonidine, which is less effective, and megestrol acetate, whose safety in this population is unclear. Hot flashes are also an issue for men on androgen deprivation treatment regimens, although much less evidence exists to guide treatment decisions. Zoledronic acid, which is used both to prevent osteoporosis and to treat bone metastases, can cause bone pain, arthralgia, and emotionally devastating osteonecrosis of the jaw. Aromatase inhibitors, which interfere with the body's ability to produce estrogen, are used to treat breast cancer in postmenopausal women; however, they cause loss of bone density, which is a significant problem for women who already have osteoporosis or osteopenia,

Many women undergoing chemotherapy report difficulty with concentration and memory, but these reports do not correlate consistently with persistent deficits on neuropsychological testing (see "Survivor Issues" section later in this chapter).

Psychological distress is common at the conclusion of breast cancer treatment. Women who had more physical symptoms or side effects from treatment have great post-treatment distress (Jim et al. 2007). Many feel vulnerable and less protected when not being seen regularly by their oncologist; thus, increased physician visits and emotional support at this time are often beneficial. Ganz et al. (1996) found that survivors appear to attain maximum recovery from the physical and emotional trauma at 1 year after breast surgery. Sexual problems are important to address after acute treatment (see Chapter 16, "Sexual Dysfunction").

The emotional burden of breast cancer treatment is high, particularly for young women who hope to become pregnant. Although evidence indicates that breast cancer diagnosed during lactation increases the risk of death from breast cancer (Stensheim et al. 2009), no evidence indicates that pregnancy affects the outcome of breast cancer. However, continuation or elective termination of pregnancy is a consideration for some who receive their diagnosis very early in a pregnancy and are unwilling to postpone treatment with teratogenic alkylating agents. Most young women, even women who are considered to have a good prognosis and are likely cured by initial treatments, ponder the ramifications of adoption or future childbearing, taking into account the unpredictability of disease recurrence or progression.

Breast Cancer in Men

Breast cancer in men is rare, and in one cross-sectional survey of 161 men, the prevalence of anxiety and depressive symptoms was low (Brain et al. 2006). However, use of avoidant coping strategies, negative body image, feelings of fear and uncertainty, and unmet informational needs were risk factors for traumatic stress symptoms. Men, like women, may benefit from counseling and support.

Genetics

The two most significant risk factors for breast cancer are increasing age and family history. Fewer than 10% of breast cancers result from hereditary mutations in single dominant genes. However, women with mutations in *BRCA1* and *BRCA2* genes have a 30 times greater risk of developing breast cancer compared with the risk in other women (Antoniou et al. 2003). Of all ovarian cancer, 10% is a result of *BRCA1* and *BRCA2* mutations. The risk of developing contralateral breast cancer in *BRCA1* and *BRCA2* mutation carriers is high at 3% per year, leading to referral of women for MRI and consideration of prophylactic mastectomy (Foulkes 2008). Now that gene testing is available, women who likely have a hereditary predisposition are first referred for consultation with a clinical geneticist, which includes preparing a pedigree, documenting cancer diagnoses, estimating cancer risks, and discussing options for genetic testing and cancer screening and prevention (Robson and Offit 2002). Women who have positive test results for a gene mutation are advised to enroll in a high-risk surveillance clinic where they will receive information about chemoprevention and the potential effectiveness of risk-reducing surgery. Bilateral prophylactic mastectomy is associated with a greater than 90% reduction in the incidence of breast cancer in women with a family history of breast cancer (Hartmann et al. 1999). Risk-reducing salpingo-oophorectomy, usually performed laparoscopically as an ambulatory procedure, reduces breast cancer risk by 50% in *BRCA1* mutation carriers and prevents 80% of ovarian cancer in women with *BRCA1* and *BRCA2* mutations (B.L. Weber et al. 2000).

In some cancer centers, psychiatric consultation is an essential part of the evaluation process. The components of a thorough evaluation of women considering prophylactic surgery have been described (Massie and Greenberg 2005). Some women at high risk choose to have prophylactic mastectomy or risk-reducing salpingo-oophorectomy in the absence of genetic testing. In this case, psychiatric evaluation should be a standard component of the surgical evaluation. The women who later express regret about having had prophylactic mastectomy are those who feel that the decision to have surgery was driven by their surgeon (Payne et al. 2000). A prospective study of women who underwent bilateral mastectomy showed that anxiety decreased after surgery and social activities improved. Sexual pleasure was rated lower 1 year after surgery, and nearly half of the 90 women studied were more self-conscious and felt less sexually attractive (Brandberg et al. 2008). Similarly, mental distress is reduced in women who have risk-reducing salpingo-oophorectomy; however, somatic morbidity (i.e., osteoporosis, palpitations, pain, and stiffness) is increased (Michelsen et al. 2009).

Colorectal Cancer

Although screening can detect precancerous polyps, an estimated 102,900 cases of colon cancer and 39,670 cases of rectal cancer are expected to be diagnosed in the United States in 2010, and more than 51,000 people will die of colorectal cancer (American Cancer Society 2010). Only 39% of colorectal cancers are diagnosed at an early stage, and surgical resection is the only curative therapy. A patient's adjustment is closely related to the type and extent of surgery, the presence or absence of a stoma and an ostomy, and the partner's adjustment. Psychosocial adjustment to colon cancer can be complicated by anorexia, nausea and vomiting, weight loss, abdominal discomfort, diarrhea, and constipation. Concerns about body image, sexual functioning, fatigue, pain, and odor can lead to social withdrawal (Bernhard et al. 1999; Sahay et al. 2000). In patients with liver metastases, serum interleukin-2R, a cytokine, may be an independent predictor of depression (Allen-Mersh et al. 1998). Confusion occurs in 1% of colon cancer patients in the last 6 months of life but in 28% in the last 3 days. Significant financial burden occurs in the 3–6 months before death (McCarthy et al. 2000).

A recent prospective survey of 1,822 colorectal cancer patients found a low prevalence of global psychological distress at 6 (8.3%) and 12 (6.7%) months postdiagnosis (Lynch et al. 2008). In another survey of colorectal cancer survivors, noncancer comorbid disorders and low-income status had more influence on quality of life than did stage or time since diagnosis. Compared with an age-matched population, long-term survivors reported higher quality-of-life scores, but they had higher rates of depression. Frequent bowel movements and chronic recurrent diarrhea were a problem for many (Ramsey et al. 2002) (see Chapter 30, "Surgery," for a discussion of ostomies). Many self-help groups provide vital education and coping skills for these patients and their families.

Lung Cancer

An estimated 222,520 new cases of lung and bronchus cancer are expected to be diagnosed in the United States in 2010, and 157,300 deaths are expected to occur (American Cancer Society 2010). Lung cancer accounts for 28% of all cancer deaths. Although it is the most preventable of all cancers, with 87% of cases linked to cigarette smoking, lung cancer is difficult to diagnose early. In a study of 4,496 cancer patients, including patients with 14 different primary tumor sites, those with lung cancer had the highest rate of distress on the BSI (Zabora et al. 2001). About one-fifth of patients with non-small-cell lung cancer (NSCLC) have depressed mood at the time of diagnosis, and their depression tends to persist. In one study, depression following the diagnosis or resection of operable NSCLC predicted depression 1 year later (Uchitomi et al. 2003). At the time of diagnosis, many tumors are inoperable. In unresectable NSCLC, self-reported anxiety and depression at baseline were found to predict subsequent psychological distress (Akechi et al. 2001). In one study of 145 survivors of NSCLC who had been disease-free for 5 or more years, most were hopeful. Half viewed their cancer experience as contributing to positive life changes (Sarna et al. 2002).

Depressive symptoms and difficulty concentrating are more common at diagnosis of small-cell lung cancer than with NSCLC. Small-cell lung cancer, more than any other tumor, is associated with paraneoplastic syndromes such as Cushing's syndrome, hyponatremia, and autoimmune encephalopathy. Because pulmonary emboli are common during treatment, dyspnea and anxiety should be evaluated carefully. Hypoxia due to preexisting chronic obstructive pulmonary disease and postradiation hypothyroidism may contribute to cognitive dysfunction. Postthoracotomy neuralgic pain is common.

Patients with small-cell lung cancer may receive prophylactic cranial radiation because the risk of brain metastases is 50% over 2 years. Isolated brain lesions may be removed surgically, but cranial radiation is common once the metastasis is noted. Some cognitive deficits have been noted in long-term survivors of small-cell cancer regardless of whether they received cranial radiation. Leukoencephalopathy has occurred after treatment for small-cell cancer as a result of the combination of chemotherapy and radiation, but changes in chemotherapy have reduced this risk.

Many smokers with cancer and smoking partners of cancer patients experience guilt, but many continue to smoke. Continued smoking is associated with decreased survival, development of a secondary primary cancer, and increased risk of developing or exacerbating other medical conditions. Chemotherapy and radiation are likely to produce more complications and greater morbidity among smokers than among nonsmokers (Sanderson et al. 2002). Although some health care providers are hesitant to raise the issue of smoking cessation during the stress of initial diagnosis, the literature supports early antismoking intervention with patients and their family members (Sanderson et al. 2002). However, in terminal lung cancer, if the patient derives pleasure from smoking, cessation interventions are not indicated. For further review of lung cancer, see Chapter 19, "Lung Disease."

Ovarian Cancer

The second most frequent gynecological cancer among women in the United States, ovarian cancer, is the fifth most frequent cause of cancer death in women and has the highest mortality rate of all gynecological cancers (American Cancer Society 2010). Annually, more than 21,000 new cases of ovarian cancer are diagnosed, and nearly 14,000 deaths result. Ovarian cancer usually has an insidious onset and progression; 70% of cases are stage II to IV at time of diagnosis. The 5-year survival rate is only 46% overall.

Because cancer antigen (CA) 125 levels often rise before symptoms appear, patients' emotions often rise and fall with the report of the CA 125 level. Kornblith et al. (1995) found that more than 60% of ovarian cancer patients described being worried, tired, sad, and in pain. In one prospective study, persistent anxiety was present in nearly one-quarter of women who had received an ovarian cancer diagnosis, predictors being neuroticism and marital status (Goncalves et al. 2008). In a prospective study of 63 ovarian cancer patients, a reduction in depression and an increase in anxiety were found 3 months after the completion of chemotherapy (Hipkins et al. 2004). Factors associated with anxiety included poor perceived social support, increased intrusive thoughts, and younger age. Patients report difficulties with sexual desire, response, and communication after gynecological cancer treatment (see Chapter 16, "Sexual Dysfunction"). Infertility concerns are vital for younger women, who require information about fertility and emotional support to make treatment decisions and to cope with those choices.

Melanoma

More than 68,000 Americans are expected to be diagnosed with melanoma in 2010 (American Cancer Society 2010). It is the most aggressive and fatal form of skin cancer, which may result in scarring or lymphedema from lymph node sampling, and affects mobility if lower extremities are involved. Fawzy et al. (2003) reported that a short-term focused psychological treatment could diminish distress and prolong survival. The intervention was associated with survival benefit after 6 years, but the benefit weakened after 10 years. A replication study in 262 Danish melanoma patients showed no prolonged survival after 6 years (Boesen et al. 2007).

Advanced disease may be treated with interferon-alpha, the side effects of which include fatigue, anxiety, insomnia, depression, and rarely mania (Kirkwood et al. 2002). Paroxetine started at the time interferon-alpha is started has been shown to reduce the incidence of depression (Musselman et al. 2001). Because melanoma commonly metastasizes to the brain, changes in personality or other new neurological symptoms should always prompt the clinician to consider CNS imaging.

Head and Neck Cancers

Head and neck cancers are highly distressing (Zabora et al. 2001) and, together with their treatments, often result in facial disfigurement and loss of ability to speak, eat, taste, or swallow. With more than 60% of patients with head and neck cancers surviving longer than 5 years, quality-of-life issues become paramount (American Cancer Society 2010). Disfigurement is associated with reduced quality of life and increased depression but is subjectively experienced and less related to objective ratings of disfigurement (M.R. Katz et al. 2000). Distress may be higher in those patients whose identity is closely tied to body image or ability to communicate. Treatment is daunting and leads to mucositis, pain, dysphagia, xerostomia, and sticky saliva, all of which make eating difficult and affect social functioning. Feeding tubes and tracheotomies are often necessary. Hypothyroidism is common following radiation treatment to the neck. Cranial radiation for nasopharyngeal cancer has been associated with the development of radionecrosis, resulting in structural and functional brain changes (Cheung et al. 2003), with consequent cognitive dysfunction. Memory, language, motor performance, and executive functions may become impaired.

Head and neck cancer patients often have comorbid substance use disorders, putting them at high risk for alcohol and nicotine withdrawal if admitted to the hospital. Underlying comorbid psychiatric illness and maladaptive coping styles often accompany substance use, which will affect psychosocial intervention. Guilt about the role substance use has in the development of their cancer may contribute to distress. A link between human papillomavirus, a sexually transmitted disease, and tonsillar cancer has been shown, which may add further to feelings of self-blame regarding behavior.

Pancreatic Cancer

Pancreatic cancer is one of the leading causes of cancer deaths, and 80% of cases are unresectable at diagnosis, with a 5-year survival rate of 6% (American Cancer Society 2010). Receiving this information at the time of diagnosis can be a devastating psychological blow and most certainly contributes to high rates of distress and depression seen in these patients. However, several earlier small studies have found that up to 50% of pancreatic cancer patients manifested psychiatric symptoms at least 6 months prior to their cancer diagnosis (Fras et al. 1967; Green and Austin 1993; Joffe et al. 1986), suggesting that there may be a direct tumor-induced effect. One clinical study reported that depressive thoughts were more common in people with pancreatic cancer than in those with gastric cancer (Holland et al. 1986), and a retrospective cohort study found that depression preceded pancreatic cancer more often than other GI malignancies (odds ratio [OR] = 4.6) (Carney et al. 2003). One study of 130 patients with newly diagnosed pancreatic cancer found that 38% had scores higher than 15 on the Beck Depression Inventory. Depression was more common in those who had pain (Kelsen et al. 1995). Larger prospective studies examining distress by cancer site did find pancreatic cancer to be highly distressing but no more so than other tumor sites with high symptom burden and poor prognosis, such as lung and brain cancer (Carlson et al. 2004; Zabora et al. 2001).

The signs and symptoms of pancreatic cancer are typically vague and nonspecific and may include abdominal pain, anorexia and weight loss, fatigue, and jaundice. Symptoms of upper abdominal disease occur in 25% of patients 6 months before diagnosis. Anorexia, early satiety, and back pain are features of progressive disease, and diabetes also may develop. Management of pain and discomfort includes palliative chemotherapy and/or radiotherapy, opiates, celiac blocks, stenting procedures, pancreatic enzymes to relieve cramping associated with pancreatic insufficiency, and prevention and treatment of constipation and diarrhea. Antidepressants and psychostimulants may be used to treat depression and fatigue.

Psychiatric Aspects of Cancer Treatments

Chemotherapy

The neuropsychiatric side effects of common chemotherapeutic agents are listed in Table 23–2. Most chemotherapy agents are metabolized by CYP 3A4, so careful consideration of drug-drug interactions involving this enzyme is warranted. St. John's wort and modafinil both induce CYP 3A4 and therefore may render chemotherapy less effective, whereas fluoxetine and fluvoxamine both inhibit CYP 3A4 and may increase the level of chemotherapy-related toxicity. Because of its mild inhibition of monoamine oxidase (MAO), procarbazine may contribute to serotonin syndrome if prescribed in combination with a selective serotonin reuptake inhibitors (SSRI) or SNRI antidepressant. See "Survivor Issues" section later in this chapter for discussion of cognitive impairment related to chemotherapy.

Tamoxifen is used in the prevention of breast cancer recurrence, as well as in the metastatic setting, in women with both invasive and noninvasive breast cancers. Inconsistent reports implicate it in the development of depression. In fact, in the noncancer population, the use of tamoxifen recently has been recommended as a third-line augmentation strategy in the treatment of acute mania by the Canadian Network for Mood and Anxiety Treatments (CANMAT), in conjunction with the International Society for Bipolar Disorders (ISBD) (Yatham et al. 2009).

Antidepressants are frequently prescribed to breast cancer patients taking tamoxifen for management of depression and hot flashes. Reports of interactions between tamoxifen and antidepressants have led to concern about antidepressant prescribing (Henry et al. 2008). Tamoxifen is metabolized to its most active metabolite, 4-hydroxy-*N*-desmethyl-tamoxifen (endoxifen), through CYP 2D6. Breast cancer patients with decreased metabolism, through genetic variation (e.g., poor metabolizer genotype) or potent CYP 2D6 inhibition with medications, have been found to have shorter time to recurrence and worse relapse-free survival. Because of this risk, recommendations have been made by some to avoid the use of potent CYP 2D6 inhibitors, such as fluoxetine or paroxetine, and to use weaker or noninhibitors, such as citalopram. Patients who are unable to tolerate or who are nonresponsive to the weaker CYP 2D6 inhibitors may benefit from a discussion between the oncologist and psychiatrist to establish the best overall treatment for them.

Radiation

Radiation treatment usually requires a patient to remain absolutely still on a flat table for 5–10 minutes daily, 5 days a week, so that a prescribed dose can be applied to a specific site over 2–9 weeks. Patients worry that they cannot remain still either because of claustrophobia or because of inadequate pain control. Fatigue continues to increase during the month following radiation treatment but then begins to diminish. Nausea and vomiting from radiation treatment, more severe when viscera are irradiated, are reduced by serotonin type 3 (5-HT_3) receptor antagonists such as ondansetron. Irradiation for gynecological cancers can cause severe side effects, such as vaginal atrophy, that can interfere with sexual function. Effective use of vaginal dilators, estrogen creams, and vaginal moisturizers for these painful and persistent problems has been described by others (A. Katz 2009). Brain irradiation causes more profound fatigue than does treatment of other sites. Concomitant dexamethasone reduces cerebral edema, but late sequelae of brain radiation, including focal radiation necrosis or leukoencephalopathy, may appear. Newer methods to reduce the volume of brain that requires radiation may decrease these risks.

Hematopoietic Stem Cell Transplant

Hematopoietic stem cell transplant (SCT) broadly includes bone marrow transplants (BMTs) and SCTs from peripheral or umbilical cord blood. Allogeneic transplantation uses donor stem cells, so the patient has a risk of developing graft-versus-host disease (GVHD), whereas autologous transplantation uses the patient's own cells, thereby eliminating this risk.

Although most patients note an improved quality of life physically, psychologically, and socially in the years following their transplant, a review of 22 prospective reports found that a significant minority experience ongoing anxiety and/or depressive symptoms (5%–40%), fatigue, sexual dysfunction, and fertility concerns (Mosher et al. 2009). The psychological stress of hematopoietic SCT begins when transplant is first considered. Although outcomes have improved with the use of autologous hematopoietic SCT, approximately 40% of patients who receive allogeneic hematopoietic SCT die from related complications (Copelan 2006).

An important part of the pretransplant planning is to evaluate and shore up the patient's social support that is of vital importance both while the patient is in isolation and after discharge. During high-dose chemotherapy and irradiation, visitors are limited to avoid infection. Patients often experience nausea, vomiting, mucositis, and fatigue. During this time, psychiatric disorders are extremely common, especially adjustment disorder with anxiety and depression (Khan et al. 2007). GVHD is not generally associated with occurrence of mental disorders (Sasaki et al. 2000), although when severe, it may result in delirium.

The transplant itself is anticlimactic compared with the pretransplant regimen and the anxious period involved in awaiting recovery from pancytopenia. Hypervigilant patients keep charts of their cell counts, anticipating the day of "probable" recovery; others request medications to "sleep through the experience," a passive attitude antithetical to caregivers, who want these patients to participate in self-care.

After a prolonged period of dependence, patients are often very fearful as they anticipate hospital discharge and must assume greater roles in self-care. Persistent fatigue is a major problem when patients resume normal activities at home and work. Chronic anxiety and depression are the most common psychiatric sequelae, and psychological adjustment is particularly difficult for those patients who have delayed or disrupted important developmental life tasks. In the years following hematopoietic SCT, spouses or partners experience similar psychological effects (depressive symptoms, sleep and sexual problems) but less social support, dyadic satisfaction, and spiritual well-being and more loneliness than do their survivor partners, highlighting the attention required for spousal evaluation and psychosocial support (Bishop et al. 2007).

In general, successful adaptation to BMT is associated with the ability to use information about illness and treatment, coupled with the ability to delegate control and authority temporarily and to trust the staff.

Cancer Surgery

See Chapter 30, "Surgery," for a general discussion of the emotional aspects of surgery and Chapter 33, "Obstetrics and Gynecology," for a discussion of gynecological surgery.

Psychiatric Interventions in Cancer

Small sample sizes, high attrition rates contributing to selection bias, and confounding factors are common in both nonpharmacological and pharmacological intervention studies in cancer patients. We acknowledge these limitations and review psychiatric management of the cancer patient.

Psychotherapy

Providing psychotherapeutic support for the cancer patient involves tailoring the intervention to the patient's individual biopsychosocial needs. Exploration of patients' understanding and meaning of their illness and prognosis, concurrent stressors, and current level of supports helps to develop an individualized psychosocial intervention plan. Flexibility in scheduling of patients and in choice of psychotherapeutic model is required. In the clinical setting, an eclectic approach may be undertaken that uses elements of different models of psychotherapy and is related to the chief concerns at the time of treatment. Many cancer patients will confront issues related to loss of control; uncertainty; and fear of future dependency, suffering, and death. Psychotherapy supports patients in navigating these challenges through individual, couples, family, or group interventions by offering a supportive, validating, and nonjudgmental presence; providing realistic reassurance; and emphasizing prior strengths and coping.

Although studies are limited by small sample sizes, confounding factors, and high withdrawal rates with related selection bias, evidence has shown the benefit of psychosocial treatments in reducing emotional distress and improving quality of life (Meyer and Mark 1995; Osborn et al. 2006; Sheard and Maguire 1999).

However, interpretation of the studies may affect conclusions drawn, leading some to suggest that psychosocial interventions do not clearly show a benefit (Coyne et al. 2006). Weaknesses regarding the evidence base include the presence of inconsistent findings in the literature; the quality of the studies; the lack of studies of certain demographic, disease, and treatment factors; and the lack of research on patients with clinically significant levels of distress (Jacobsen and Jim 2008). Alternatively, a meta-analysis of six studies, including incurable cancer patients, found improvement in depression scores in non-clinically depressed samples but no improvement in those with a diagnosis of depression (Akechi et al. 2008). The inherent challenges of implementing a randomized controlled trial in seriously ill cancer patients include high attrition rates, inability to implement standard randomization design, and heterogeneity of patient samples (Moorey et al. 2009).

Educational and behavioral training, through either group or individual psychotherapy, reduces distress in cancer patients (Fawzy et al. 1995; Newell et al. 2002). Cognitive and behavioral models can be tailored to the specific tumor type (Tatrow and Montgomery 2006).

Group therapy and self-help groups facilitate the sharing of information and support coping strategies among cancer patients facing similar situations. In a group setting, patients can glean practical tips and see the range of normal reactions to illness, as well as adaptive coping styles and strategies that make adjustment to illness easier. Group therapy helps to decrease the sense of isolation and alienation as the patient and family see that they are not alone adjusting to illness. Groups are often disease specific or targeted for patients at the same stage of illness. Spiegel et al. (1989) developed supportive-expressive group therapy led by trained professionals for women with breast cancer. The goals of supportive-expressive psychotherapy are to help patients with existential concerns and disease-related emotions, to deepen social support and physician-patient relationships, and to provide symptom control. The therapist challenges patients' tendency to withdraw from the implications of having metastatic breast cancer. Such groups relieve distress while reducing avoidance of the implications of the diagnosis. This strategy improves mood and pain perception, especially in the most distressed (Goodwin et al. 2001).

In the advanced or terminally ill cancer population, existential, life narrative, dignity-conserving, and meaning-centered interventions may be considered. Driven by previous research indicating the role meaning has in reducing depression and hopelessness, Breitbart et al. (2010) developed a meaning-centered group psychotherapy. When compared with supportive group psychotherapy, meaning-centered group psychotherapy showed significantly greater improvement in spiritual well-being and sense of meaning (Breitbart et al. 2010). Legacy documents created during a 1-hour interview with a terminally ill patient reduce suffering and depressed mood (Chochinov et al. 2005) (see Chapter 41, "Palliative Care").

More recent studies have shown the potential to prevent anxiety or depressive illness in cancer patients. Supportive-expressive group therapy plus relaxation therapy prevented depressive disorders in 227 metastatic breast cancer patients, compared with relaxation therapy alone (Kissane et al. 2007). A study of 465 mixed cancer patients, free of anxiety or depressive disorder, stratified patients by risk of developing either disorder. High-risk patients were less likely to develop an anxiety or a depressive disorder following a brief (three-session) cognitive-behavioral intervention compared with those who received usual care (OR = 0.54); no effect was seen in low-risk patients (Pitceathly et al. 2009).

Earlier studies of the effect of psychosocial interventions suggested that they could prolong survival (Fawzy et al. 1993, 2003; Spiegel et al. 1989). Replication studies, which have been methodologically more rigorous, have failed to find any survival benefit (Boesen et al. 2007; Goodwin et al. 2001; Kissane et al. 2007; Spiegel et al. 2007), suggesting that future trials should focus on improving quality of life, easing suffering, and optimizing coping (Kissane 2009). Three meta-analyses and one systematic review have not found a survival benefit conferred by psychotherapy (Chow et al. 2004; Edwards et al. 2008; Newell et al. 2002; Smedslund and Ringdal 2004). Some psychological intervention trials in cancer have shown improved survival, but most have not; however, essentially all have reported improvements in psychological well-being.

Psychopharmacology

Choosing a psychotropic medication for a cancer patient requires consideration of a patient's medical comorbidities, potential drug interactions, route of administration, onset of action required with related patient prognostic information, somatic symptom profile (e.g., pain, insomnia, agitation, hot flashes), and adverse-effect profile of the intended psychotropic medication. In cancer patients with thrombocytopenia, intramuscular (IM) injections and restraints should be avoided. Patients who are unable to take medications orally because of mucositis or those with GI obstruction may require alternative routes of administration (see "Alternative Routes" section of Chapter 38, "Psychopharmacology"). Mirtazapine, olanzapine, and risperidone all have orally disintegrating forms. In addition, low albumin levels and ascites may occur in the cancer patient, affecting the volume of distribution of drugs.

Depression

Earlier reports suggested that antidepressants increased one's risk for developing cancer; however, this concern has been dismissed (Theoharides and Konstantinidou 2003). Although antidepressants are commonly used in the clinical setting, the evidence for their use in depressed cancer patients is somewhat limited, with few trials studying patients with major depression (Rodin et al. 2007a; Williams and Dale 2006). Seven placebo-controlled trials have shown benefit in cases of depression or depressive symptoms when fluoxetine, paroxetine, and mianserin were used. However, other placebo-controlled studies have shown no difference in depression when fluoxetine, paroxetine, desipramine, and sertraline were used compared with placebo (Owen and Ferrando 2010).

The SSRIs and SNRIs are often first-line treatments because of clinical experience, safety, and tolerability. Some cancer patients may already be experiencing GI symptoms from their disease or treatment, which may worsen if SSRIs or SNRIs are added. Patients with carcinoid tumors may have elevated levels of serotonin and, therefore, may be less able to tolerate the SSRIs or SNRIs. Because GI bleeding has been reported with SSRIs, caution is advised when prescribing these agents to cancer patients with thrombocytopenia. All of the SSRIs, as well as venlafaxine and mirtazapine, have been associated with hyponatremia. Monitoring of electrolytes is advisable, especially in cancer patients who have additional risk factors (e.g. those receiving vincristine, those with small-cell lung cancer). Some antidepressants also may alleviate hot flashes, as previously described (see "Breast Cancer" subsection). SNRIs (venlafaxine and duloxetine) may improve neuropathic pain caused by cancer treatments.

Mirtazapine has a high affinity for histaminic H_1 receptors and antagonizes 5-HT_2 and 5-HT_3 receptors, possibly contributing to its properties of anxiolysis, sedation, appetite stimulation, and antiemesis. These properties may be advantageous in anorexic-cachectic depressed cancer patients or those experiencing nausea or vomiting from chemotherapy but are less desirable in patients with weight gain from steroids or chemotherapy or those with significant fatigue or sedation. Small studies in which mirtazapine was used have shown improvement in anxiety, depression, and insomnia, with mixed results in nausea (Cankurtaran et al. 2008; Kim et al. 2008). Side effects include constipation, drowsiness, and, rarely, reversible neutropenia, all considerations when treating the depressed cancer patient.

Bupropion may improve sexual function and fatigue in cancer patients. Its stimulating properties make it useful in lethargic patients, but because of its association with increased seizure risk, it should be used with caution in patients who are malnourished or who have a history of seizures or brain tumor. It tends to be weight neutral or to contribute to weight loss, so this agent may not be the preferred choice in depressed cachectic patients. Bupropion may assist in smoking cessation, especially in patients with lung or head and neck cancers.

The TCAs may be used to treat comorbid neuropathic pain caused by chemotherapy and surgery, usually at lower doses than are indicated in depression. Nortriptyline and desipramine have more favorable side-effect profiles compared with amitriptyline, with fewer anticholinergic symptoms.

Psychostimulants can promote a sense of well-being, treat depression, decrease fatigue, stimulate appetite, and improve cognitive function. Psychostimulants are used in cancer pain as an adjuvant to potentiate the analgesic effects of opioids and are commonly used to counteract opioid-induced sedation (Rozans et al. 2002). Because their onset of action occurs within days, rather than weeks as with antidepressants, psychostimulants are often the preferred choice in terminally ill patients. Four out of five non-placebo-controlled studies, together with case series and reports, have shown improved mood in 73%–100% of cancer patients, but well-designed placebo-controlled studies are needed (Orr and Taylor 2007). Side effects may include insomnia, agitation, and, rarely, psychosis. They may stimulate the cardiovascular system, so caution is advised when treating patients with hypertension or arrhythmias. (See also Chapter 8, "Depression.")

Mood stabilizers and antipsychotics generally can be continued during cancer treatment. However, complications of chemotherapy, including vomiting, diarrhea, dehydration, and renal insufficiency, may raise lithium levels, and symptoms of toxicity, nausea, diarrhea, and confusion may be misattributed to chemotherapy. Antipsychotics (e.g., haloperidol, olanzapine) may improve nausea and vomiting in cancer patients. Metabolic parameters should be monitored in patients prescribed steroids and atypical antipsychotics, given their risk of causing hyperglycemia, although this is much less of a concern when the cancer is advanced. Patients may be at risk for QT prolongation if prescribed antipsychotics, antibiotics, TCAs, tacrolimus, tamoxifen, octreotide, and ondansetron (Strevel et al. 2007). Cancer patients also may have other risk factors for QT prolongation, including dehydration, hypomagnesemia, hypocalcemia, and hypokalemia. Although close monitoring, collaboration with the treating oncologist, and a thorough risk-benefit analysis must occur, continuation of clozapine during chemotherapy has not resulted in any reports of associated agranulocytosis (Frieri et al. 2008). See also Chapter 10, "Psychosis, Mania, and Catatonia."

Anxiety

Before initiating treatment with a benzodiazepine, all patients should be screened for depressive symptoms and for specific anxiety disorders such as PTSD and generalized anxiety disorder because of treatment implications. When anxiety is a manifestation of a primary depressive disorder, treatment should be an antidepressant with, or instead of, a benzodiazepine.

Benzodiazepines are frequently given to patients for acute anxiety and/or insomnia and may be prescribed to augment antiemetics during chemotherapy. Dosing depends on the patient's tolerance and the drug's duration of action. Lorazepam and alprazolam are favored in the acute setting because of their rapid onset of action and benefit on an as-needed basis. Buspirone and antidepressants are alternatives for longer treatment of anxiety. Low doses of antipsychotics are useful in patients who are unresponsive to or intolerant of benzodiazepines or in patients who have severe anxiety and agitation. If patients have been taking a benzodiazepine chronically, they may experience withdrawal if the dose is not tapered. Benzodiazepines and opiates may have an additive effect on reducing respiratory drive, contributing to respiratory depression, so caution is advised when using this combination. See also Chapter 11, "Anxiety Disorders."

Delirium

See Chapter 5, "Delirium," for a discussion of psychopharmacological treatment of delirium and Chapter 41, "Palliative Care," for a discussion of terminal delirium.

Electroconvulsive Therapy

Although the use of electroconvulsive therapy (ECT) in patients with brain tumor was once believed to be contraindicated because of the risk of brain herniation, numerous case reports have described safe and effective use of ECT in such patients (Patkar et al. 2000). (See Chapter 40, "Electroconvulsive Therapy.")

Survivor Issues

Advances in cancer treatment over the past 30 years have led to a rapidly growing population of more than 9 million long-term survivors in the United States, many of them children and young adults. The long-term adjustment of many appears to be largely unimpaired (Kornblith et al. 2004). Some cured cancer patients have delayed medical complications (e.g., organ failure, CNS dysfunction, infertility, secondary malignancies, and decreased physical stamina) and psychological concerns, including fears of termination of treatment; preoccupation with the threat of disease recurrence; pervasive awareness of mortality and a sense of greater vulnerability to illness; difficulty with reentry into normal life; persistent guilt; difficult adjustment to physical losses and handicaps that lead to problems with peer acceptance and social integration; diminished self-esteem or confidence; perceived loss of employment opportunity or mobility; and fear of job and insurance discrimination. Concerns about infertility, often understandably submerged at the time of diagnosis and treatment, reappear when treatment concludes. Several elements are necessary to achieve optimal outcome for cancer survivors: access to state-of the-art cancer care; active participation or engagement in one's care (active coping); use of social support (or perception that support is available); and a sense of meaning or purpose in life (Rowland and Massie 2010). Cancer survivors with unmet psychosocial needs are more likely to use complementary and alternative medicine (see following section) (Mao et al. 2008).

The survivor's cognitive functioning is also a concern. Some children and adults who have undergone bone marrow transplant or who have been treated for a brain tumor have residual deficits with neuropsychological impairment, including compromised motor and cognitive test performance (Meyers and Brown 2006; Phipps et al. 2008).

Some adult patients who have received chemotherapy and/or hormonal therapy for solid tumors reported cognitive changes. These changes in attention, concentration, memory, and processing speed may affect functioning, are often subtle, and have been challenging to study (Vardy et al. 2008). Possible biological and neural mechanisms that contribute to cognitive changes in patients undergoing chemotherapy include direct neurotoxic effects, changes in neurotransmitter levels, hormonal changes, immune dysregulation, cytokine release, and blood clotting in CNS vessels (Ahles and Saykin 2007). Some treatment-induced changes in neurochemical brain function may be mediated by genetic predisposition (Ahles et al. 2003). Cognitive dysfunction has been found to be independent of depression and fatigue (Correa and Ahles 2008). In one study, breast cancer survivors who participated in a cognitive-behavioral treatment aimed at improving ability to compensate for cognitive dysfunction associated with adjuvant chemotherapy rated the therapy as helpful in improving their ability to compensate for memory problems (Ferguson et al. 2007).

Potential resources include the National Coalition of Cancer Survivorship, the Office of Cancer Survivorship of the National Cancer Institute, and the organizations whose Web sites are shown in Table 23-6.

Complementary and Alternative Medicine

More than 50% of cancer patients use complementary and alternative medicine (CAM) therapies after their diagnosis, during or after standard cancer treatment for symptom management, and for promotion of "general overall health" (Vapiwala et al. 2006). In one study of 2,198 women unaffected by breast cancer, nearly half of the women used CAM with the goal of preventing breast cancer (Myers et al. 2008). A recent survey of more than 4,000 cancer survivors showed that the most commonly used complementary methods were prayer or spiritual practice, relaxation, faith or spiritual healing, and nutritional supplements or vitamins (Gansler et al. 2008). Some complementary therapies (acupuncture; relaxation; yoga; meditation; massage; tai chi; biofeedback; music, art, movement, and aroma therapies) are offered as adjuncts to traditional cancer care aimed at increasing quality of life and decreasing symptoms, with no promise of cure. A course of four sessions of aromatherapy massage has been shown to decrease anxiety and depression in the short term but had no beneficial long-term effects on anxiety, depression, pain, nausea, vomiting, or global quality of life (Wilkinson et al. 2007). Alternative therapies such as shark cartilage, colonics, herbal remedies, and high-dose vitamin therapies do not improve quality of life and may be harmful. Some remedies are highly toxic (Markman 2002). Laetrile, now banned in

TABLE 23–6. Organizations (and their Web sites) that provide accurate information for cancer patients and health professionals

National Cancer Institute: http://www.cancer.gov/cancer_information

1-800-4-CANCER: telephone number to get answers to cancer-related questions

National Comprehensive Cancer Network: http://www.nccn.com

Memorial Sloan-Kettering Cancer Center: www.mskcc.org/aboutherbs (about herbs, botanicals, and other products)

American Cancer Society: http://www.cancer.org

American Society of Clinical Oncology: http://www.asco.org

People Living With Cancer: http://www.plwc.org

Fertile Hope: http://www.fertilehope.org

Young Survival Coalition: http//www.youngsurvival.org

the United States, contains cyanide; chaparral tea causes liver damage; and Ma huang, also now banned in the United States, contains ephedrine, a CNS stimulant. Because ginger, garlic, ginseng, and ginkgo have antiplatelet effects, patients are cautioned about their use preoperatively and when thrombocytopenic. Soy and red clover are mildly estrogenic and may stimulate hormonally sensitive cancers (Wesa et al. 2008). Although the number of studies of the use of CAM techniques in people with cancer is increasing, benefits are often inconsistent and may be related to methodological flaws (Jane et al. 2008). No CAM technique or preparation has been shown to cause tumor regression. Several Web sites (e.g., www.mskcc.org/aboutherbs) provide unbiased scientific reviews about complementary therapies and potential drug interactions and adverse effects of herbal and botanical agents relevant to cancer patients (Wesa et al. 2008). See also "Complementary Medicines" section of Chapter 38, "Psychopharmacology."

In the United States, 83 million people use alternative therapies for malignant and nonmalignant disorders, and 70%–90% do not inform their doctors about these treatments (Gertz and Bauer 2001), in part because doctors often do not ask—or make negative remarks—about CAM. A study of women with newly diagnosed early-stage breast cancer found that 28% used alternative medicine (Burstein et al. 1999). Interestingly, the use of alternative medicine was independently associated with depression, fear of recurrence of cancer, lower scores for mental health and sexual satisfaction, and more physical symptoms, suggesting that those who seek alternative medicine therapies may be experiencing more anxiety, depression, or physical symptoms. Those taking alternative medications may be more in need of but less open to psychiatric consultation. However, a study conducted in Austria in cancer patients at the end of active cancer treatment showed that patients who used CAM were those who had a more active coping style. They were as compliant with standard cancer treatment and more interested in receiving psycho-oncological support than were patients not using CAM (Söllner et al. 2000).

Most patients who elect to use untried or unproven therapies do so in a desperate search for a cure or for a more acceptable quality of life. The clinician must openly communicate about patients' needs and their attitudes toward CAM and find a balance between condoning unproven or harmful treatment and preserving the patients' hope.

References

Ahles TA, Saykin AJ: Candidate mechanisms for chemotherapy-induced cognitive changes. Nat Rev Cancer 7:192–201, 2007

Ahles TA, Saykin AJ, Noll WW, et al: The relationship of the APOE genotype to neuropsychological performance in long-term cancer survivors treated with standard dose chemotherapy. Psychooncology 12:612–619, 2003

Akechi T, Okamura H, Nishiwaki Y, et al: Psychiatric disorder and associated and predictive facts in patients with unresectable nonsmall cell lung carcinoma: a longitudinal study. Cancer 92:2609–2622, 2001

Akechi T, Okuyama T, Onishi J, et al: Psychotherapy for depression among incurable cancer patients. Cochrane Database Syst Rev (2):CD005537, 2008

Allen-Mersh TG, Glover C, Fordy C, et al: Relation between depression and circulating immune products in patients with advanced colorectal cancer. J R Soc Med 91:408–413, 1998

American Cancer Society: Cancer Facts & Figures 2010 [Internet]. Atlanta, GA, American Cancer Society, 2010. Available at: http://www.cancer.org/docroot/STT/stt_0.asp. Accessed June 4, 2010.

American Psychiatric Association: Diagnostic and Statistical Manual of Mental Disorders, 4th Edition, Text Revision. Washington, DC, American Psychiatric Association, 2000

Antoniou A, Pharoah PD, Narod S, et al: Average risks of breast and ovarian cancer associated with BRCA1 or BRCA2 mutations detected in case series unselected for family history: a combined analysis of 22 studies. Am J Hum Genet 72:1117–1130, 2003

Archer J, Hutchison I, Korszun A: Mood and malignancy: head and neck cancer and depression. J Oral Pathol Med 37:255–270, 2008

Bach PB, Schrag D, Brawley OW, et al: Survival of blacks and whites after a cancer diagnosis. JAMA 287:2106–2113, 2002

Bambauer KZ, Zhang B, Maciejewski PK, et al: Mutuality and specificity of mental disorders in advanced cancer patients and caregivers. Soc Psychiatry Psychiatr Epidemiol 41:819–824, 2006

Bardwell WA, Natarajan L, Dimsdale JE, et al: Objective cancer-related variables are not associated with depressive symptoms in women treated for early stage breast cancer. J Clin Oncol 24:2420–2427, 2006

Barry MJ: Screening for prostate cancer—the controversy that refuses to die. N Engl J Med 360:1351–1354, 2009

Bennani-Baiti N, Davis MP: Cytokines and cancer anorexia cachexia syndrome. Am J Hosp Palliat Care 25:407–411, 2008

Bergelt C, Prescott E, Grønbaek M, et al: Stressful life events and cancer risk. Br J Cancer 95:1579–1581, 2006

Bernhard J, Hurny C, Maibach R, et al: Quality of life as subjective experience: reframing of perception in patients with colon cancer undergoing radical resection with or without adjuvant chemotherapy. Ann Oncol 10:775–782, 1999

Bishop MM, Beaumont JL, Hahn EA, et al: Late effects of cancer and hematopoietic stem cell transplantation on spouses or partners compared with survivors and survivor-matched controls. J Clin Oncol 25:1403–1411, 2007

Bleiker EMA, Hendriks JHCL, Otten JDM, et al: Personality factors and breast cancer risk: a 13-year follow-up. J Natl Cancer Inst 100:213–218, 2008

Boesen EH, Boesen SH, Frederiksen K, et al: Survival after a psychoeducational intervention for patients with cutaneous malignant melanoma: a replication study. J Clin Oncol 25:5698–5703, 2007

Bovbjerg DH: The continuing problem of post chemotherapy nausea and vomiting: contributions of classical conditioning. Auton Neurosci 129:92–98, 2006

Brain K, Williams B, Iredale R, et al: Psychological distress in men with breast cancer. J Clin Oncol 24:95–101, 2006

Brandberg Y, Sandelin K, Erikson S, et al: Psychological reactions, quality of life, and body image after bilateral prophylactic mastectomy in women at high risk for breast cancer: a prospective 1-year follow-up study. J Clin Oncol 26:3943–3949, 2008

Breitbart W, Rosenfeld B, Gibson C, et al: Meaning-centered group psychotherapy for patients with advanced cancer: a pilot randomized controlled trial. Psychooncology 19:21–28, 2010

Brunello A, Basso U, Rosi E, et al: Ifosfamide-related encephalopathy in elderly patients: report of five cases and review of the literature. Drugs Aging 24:967–973, 2007

Burstein HJ, Gelber S, Guadagnoli E, et al: Use of alternative medicine by women with early stage breast cancer. N Engl J Med 340:1733–1739, 1999

Cankurtaran ES, Ozlap E, Soygur H, et al: Mirtazapine improves sleep and lowers anxiety and depression in cancer patients: superiority over imipramine. Support Care Cancer 16:1291–1298, 2008

Carlson LE, Angen M, Cullum J, et al: High levels of untreated distress and fatigue in cancer patients. Br J Cancer 90:2297–2304, 2004

Carlsson S, Aus G, Wessman C, et al: Anxiety associated with prostate cancer screening with special reference to men with a positive screening test (elevated PSA)—results from a prospective population-based, randomized study. Eur J Cancer 43:2109–2116, 2007

Carney CP, Jones L, Woolson RF, et al: Relationship between depression and pancreatic cancer in the general population. Psychosom Med 65:884–888, 2003

Carroll JK, Kohli S, Mustian KM, et al: Pharmacologic treatment of cancer-related fatigue. Oncologist 12 (suppl 1):43–51, 2007

Cheung MC, Chan AS, Law SC, et al: Impact of radionecrosis on cognitive dysfunction in patients after radiotherapy for nasopharyngeal carcinoma. Cancer 97:2019–2026, 2003

Chida Y, Hamer M, Wardle J, et al: Do stress-related psychosocial factors contribute to cancer incidence and survival? Nat Clin Pract Oncol 5:466–475, 2008

Chochinov HM, Wilson KG, Enns M, et al: Depression, hopelessness, and suicidal ideation in the terminally ill. Psychosomatics 39:366–370, 1998

Chochinov HM, Hack T, Hassard T, et al: Dignity therapy: a novel psychotherapeutic intervention for patients near the end of life. J Clin Oncol 23:5520–5525, 2005

Chow E, Tsao M, Harth T: Does psychosocial intervention improve survival in cancer? A meta-analysis. Palliat Med 18:25–31, 2004

Coates AS, Hurny C, Peterson HF, et al: Quality-of-life scores predict outcome in metastatic but not early breast cancer. International Breast Cancer Study Group. J Clin Oncol 18:3768–3774, 2000

Collins ED, Moore CP, Clay KF, et al: Can women with early stage breast cancer make an informed decision for mastectomy? J Clin Oncol 27:519–525, 2009

Cooper MR, Bird HM, Steinberg M: Efficacy and safety of modafinil in the treatment of cancer-related fatigue. Ann Pharmacother 43:721–725, 2009

Copelan EA: Hematopoietic stem-cell transplantation. N Engl J Med 354:1813–1826, 2006

Cordeiro PG: Breast reconstruction after surgery for breast cancer. N Engl J Med 359:1590–1601, 2008

Correa DD, Ahles TA: Neurocognitive changes in cancer survivors. Cancer J 14:396–400, 2008

Coyne JC, Lepore SJ, Palmer SC: Efficacy of psychosocial interventions in cancer care: evidence is weaker than it first looks. Ann Behav Med 32:104–110, 2006

Coyne JC, Pajak TF, Harris J, et al: Emotional well-being does not predict survival in head and neck cancer patients. Cancer 110:2568–2575, 2007

Dahl AA, Haaland CF, Mykletun A, et al: Study of anxiety disorder and depression in long-term survivors of testicular cancer. J Clin Oncol 23:2389–2395, 2005

Dale W, Hemmerich J, Bylow K, et al: Patient anxiety about prostate cancer independently predicts early initiation of androgen deprivation therapy for biochemical cancer recurrence in older men: a prospective cohort study. J Clin Oncol 27:1557–1563, 2009

Derogatis LR: Brief Symptom Inventory 18. Minneapolis, MN, National Computer Systems, 2000

Duffy LS, Greenberg DB, Younger J, et al: Iatrogenic acute estrogen deficiency and psychiatric syndromes in breast cancer patients. Psychosomatics 40:304–308, 1999

Dy SM, Lorenz KA, Naeim A, et al: Evidence-based recommendations for cancer fatigue, anorexia, depression and dyspnea. J Clin Oncol 26:3886–3895, 2008

Edwards AGK, Hulbert-Williams N, Neal RD: Psychological interventions for women with metastatic breast cancer. Cochrane Database Syst Rev (3):CD004253, 2008

Fawzy FI, Fawzy N, Hun CS, et al: Malignant melanoma: effects of an early structured psychiatric intervention, coping and affective state on recurrence and survival 6 years later. Arch Gen Psychiatry 50:681–689, 1993

Fawzy FI, Fawzy NW, Arndt LA, et al: Critical review of psychosocial interventions in cancer care. Arch Gen Psychiatry 52:100–113, 1995

Fawzy FI, Canada AL, Fawzy NW: Effects of a brief, structured psychiatric intervention on survival and recurrence at 10-year follow-up. Arch Gen Psychiatry 60:100–103, 2003

Ferguson RJ, Ahles TA, Saykin AJ, et al: Cognitive-behavioral management of chemotherapy-related cognitive change. Psychooncology 16:772–777, 2007

Foster AR, Caplan JP: Paraneoplastic limbic encephalitis. Psychosomatics 50:108–113, 2009

Foulkes WD: Inherited susceptibility to common cancers. N Engl J Med 349:2143–2153, 2008

Fras I, Litin EM, Pearson JS: Comparison of psychiatric symptoms in carcinoma of the pancreas with those in some other intra-abdominal neoplasms. Am J Psychiatry 123:1553–1562, 1967

Friedman RA, He Y, Winer EP, et al: Trends in racial and age disparities in definitive local therapy of early stage breast cancer. J Clin Oncol 27:713–719, 2008

Frieri T, Barzega G, Badà A, et al: Maintaining clozapine treatment during chemotherapy for non-Hodgkin's lymphoma. Prog Neuropsychopharmacol Biol Psychiatry 32:1611–1612, 2008

Gallo JJ, Amernian HK, Ford DE, et al: Major depression and cancer: the 13-year follow-up of the Baltimore Epidemiologic Catchment Area sample (United States). Cancer Causes Control 11:751–758, 2000

Gansler T, Kaw C, Crammer C, et al: A population-based study of prevalence of complementary methods use by cancer survivors: a report from the American Cancer Society's studies of cancer survivors. Cancer 113:1048–1057, 2008

Ganz PA, Coscarelli A, Fred C, et al: Breast cancer survivors: psychosocial concerns and quality of life. Breast Cancer Res Treat 38:183–199, 1996

Garssen B: Psychological factors and cancer development: evidence after 30 years of research. Clin Psychol Rev 24:315–338, 2004

Garssen B, Goodkin K: On the role of immunological factors as mediators between psychosocial factors and cancer progression. Psychiatry Res 85:51–61, 1999

Gaudreau JD, Gagnon P, Roy MA, et al: Association between psychoactive medications and delirium in hospitalized patients: a critical review. Psychosomatics 46:302–316, 2005

Gaudreau JD, Gagnon P, Roy MA, et al: Opioid medications and longitudinal risk of delirium in hospitalized cancer patients. Cancer 109:2365–2373, 2007

Gertz MA, Bauer BA: Caring (really) for patients who use alternative therapies for cancer. J Clin Oncol 19:4346–4349, 2001

Goedendorp MM, Gielissen MF, Verhagen CA, et al: Psychosocial interventions for reducing fatigue during cancer treatment in adults. Cochrane Database Syst Rev (1):CD006953, 2009

Goetz MP, Knox SK, Suman VJ, et al: The impact of cytochrome P450 2D6 metabolism in women receiving adjuvant tamoxifen. Breast Cancer Res Treat 101:113–121, 2007

Goncalves V, Jayson G, Tarrier N: A longitudinal investigation of psychological morbidity in patients with ovarian cancer. Br J Cancer 99:1794–1801, 2008

Goodwin PJ, Leszcz M, Ennis M, et al: The effects of group psychosocial support on survival in metastatic breast cancer. N Engl J Med 345:1719–1726, 2001

Green AI, Austin CP: Psychopathology of pancreatic cancer: a psychobiological probe (review). Psychosomatics 34:208–221, 1993

Greenberg DB: Barriers to the treatment of depression in cancer patients. J Natl Cancer Inst Monogr 32:127–135, 2004

Greenberg DB, Jonasch E, Gadd MA, et al: Adjuvant therapy of melanoma with interferon alpha 2b associated with mania and bipolar syndromes. Cancer 89:356–362, 2000

Groenvold M, Petersen MA, Idler E, et al: Psychological distress and fatigue predicted recurrence and survival in primary breast cancer patients. Breast Cancer Res Treat 105:209–219, 2007

Hamer M, Chida Y, Molloy G: Psychological distress and cancer mortality. J Psychosom Res 66:255–258, 2009

Hansen PE, Floderus B, Frederiksen K, et al: Personality traits, health behavior, and risk for cancer: a prospective study of a Swedish twin cohort. Cancer 103:1082–1091, 2005

Härter M, Reuter K, Aschenbrenner A, et al: Psychiatric disorders and associated factors in cancer: results of an interview study with patients in inpatient, rehabilitation and outpatient treatment. Eur J Cancer 37:1385–1393, 2001

Hartmann LC, Schaid DJ, Woods JE, et al: Efficacy of bilateral prophylactic mastectomy in women with a family history of breast cancer. N Engl J Med 340:77–84, 1999

Hayes DF: Follow-up of patients with early breast cancer. N Engl J Med 356:2505–2513, 2007

Henry NL, Stearns V, Flockhart DA, et al: Drug interactions and pharmacogenomics in the treatment of breast cancer and depression. Am J Psychiatry 165:1251–1255, 2008

Herschbach P, Keller M, Knight L, et al: Psychological problems of cancer patients: a cancer distress screening with a cancer-specific questionnaire. Br J Cancer 91:504–511, 2004

Hickok JT, Roscoe JA, Morrow GR, et al: Nausea and emesis remain significant problems of chemotherapy despite prophylaxis with 5-hydroxytryptamine-3 antiemetics. Cancer 97:2880–2886, 2003

Hipkins J, Whitworth M, Tarrier N, et al: Social support, anxiety and depression after chemotherapy for ovarian cancer: a prospective study. Br J Health Psychol 9:569–581, 2004

Holland JC, Korzun AH, Tross S, et al: Comparative psychological disturbance in patients with pancreatic and gastric cancer. Am J Psychiatry 143:982–986, 1986

Ingram D, Browne G, Reyno L, et al: Prevalence, correlates and cost of anxiety and affective disorder in men with prostate cancer one year after initial assessment (abstract #523). Psychooncology 12:S1–S277, 2003

Institute of Medicine: Cancer Care for the Whole Patient: Meeting Psychosocial Health Needs. Washington, DC, National Academies Press, 2007

Inui A: Cancer anorexia-cachexia syndrome. CA Cancer J Clin 52:72–91, 2002

Jacobsen PB, Jim HS: Psychosocial interventions for anxiety and depression in adult cancer patients: achievements and challenges. CA Cancer J Clin 58:214–230, 2008

Jacobsen PB, Donovan KA, Trask PC, et al: Screening for psychologic distress in ambulatory cancer patients. Cancer 103:1494–1502, 2005

Jane SW, Wilkie DJ, Gallucci BB, et al: Systematic review of massage intervention for adult patients with cancer: a methodological perspective. Cancer Nurs 31:E24–E35, 2008

Jim HS, Jacobsen PB: Posttraumatic stress and posttraumatic growth in cancer survivorship: a review. Cancer J 14:414–419, 2008

Jim HS, Andrykowski MA, Munster PN, et al: Physical symptoms/side effects during breast cancer treatment predict posttreatment distress. Ann Behav Med 34:200–208, 2007

Joffe RT, Rubinow DR, Denicoff KD, et al: Depression and carcinoma of the pancreas. Gen Hosp Psychiatry 8:241–245, 1986

Kangas M, Henry JL, Bryant RA: Posttraumatic stress disorder following cancer: a conceptual and empirical review. Clin Psychol Rev 22:499–524, 2002

Kangas M, Bovbjerg DH, Montgomery GH: Cancer-related fatigue: a systematic and meta-analytic review of non-pharmacological therapies for cancer patients. Psychol Bull 134:700–741, 2008

Kannarkat G, Lasher EE, Schiff D: Neurologic complications of chemotherapy agents. Curr Opin Neurol 20:719–725, 2007

Katz A: Interventions for sexuality after pelvic radiation therapy and gynecological cancer. Cancer J 15:45–47, 2009

Katz MR, Irish JC, Devins GM, et al: Reliability and validity of an observer-rated disfigurement scale for head and neck cancer patients. Head Neck 22:132–141, 2000

Kelsen DP, Portenoy RK, Thaler HT, et al: Pain and depression in patients with newly diagnosed pancreas cancer. J Clin Oncol 13:748–755, 1995

Khan AG, Irfan M, Shamsi TS, et al: Psychiatric disorders in bone marrow transplant patients. J Coll Physicians Surg Pak 17:98–100, 2007

Kim SW, Shin IL, Kim JM, et al: Effectiveness of mirtazapine for nausea and insomnia in cancer patients with depression. Psychiatry Clin Neurosci 62:75–83, 2008

Kirkwood JM, Bender C, Agarwala S, et al: Mechanisms and management of toxicities associated with high-dose interferon alfa-2b therapy. J Clin Oncol 20:3703–3718, 2002

Kissane D: Beyond the psychotherapy and survival debate: the challenge of social disparity, depression and treatment adherence in psychosocial care. Psychooncology 18:1–5, 2009

Kissane D, Grabsch B, Clarke DM, et al: Supportive-expressive group therapy for women with metastatic breast cancer: survival and psychosocial outcome from a randomized controlled trial. Psychooncology 16:277–286, 2007

Kornblith AB, Herr HW, Ofman US, et al: Quality of life of patients with prostate cancer and their spouses: the value of a database in clinical care. Cancer 73:2791–2802, 1994

Kornblith AB, Thaler HT, Wong G, et al: Quality of life of women with ovarian cancer. Gynecol Oncol 59:231–242, 1995

Kornblith AB, Herndon JE II, Weiss RB, et al: Long-term adjustment of survivors of early stage breast carcinoma, 20 years after adjuvant chemotherapy. Cancer 98:679–689, 2004

Kroenke CH, Bennett GG, Fuchs C, et al: Depressive symptoms and prospective incidence of colorectal cancer in women. Am J Epidemiol 162:839–848, 2005

Kung S, Mueller PS, Yonas EG, et al: Delirium resulting from paraneoplastic limbic encephalitis caused by Hodgkin's disease. Psychosomatics 43:498–501, 2002

Laird BJA, Boyd AC, Colvin LA, et al: Are cancer pain and depression interdependent? A systematic review. Psychooncology 18:459–464, 2009

Lawlor PG: The panorama of opioid-related cognitive dysfunction in patients with cancer: a critical literature appraisal. Cancer 94:1836–1853, 2002

Lee KC, Ray GT, Hunkeler EM, et al: Tamoxifen treatment and new-onset depression in breast cancer patients. Psychosomatics 48:205–210, 2007

Levy MR: Cancer fatigue: a neurobiological review for psychiatrists. Psychosomatics 49:283–291, 2008

Lieberman FS, Schold SC: Distant effects of cancer on the nervous system. Oncology 16:1539–1548, 2002

Litwin MS, Lubeck DP, Spitalny GM, et al: Mental health in men treated for early stage prostate carcinoma. Cancer 95:54–60, 2002

Llorente MD, Burke M, Gregory GR, et al: Prostate cancer: a significant risk factor for late-life suicide. Am J Geriatr Psychiatry 13:195–201, 2005

Loprinzi CL, Barton DL, Jatoi A, et al: Symptom control trials: a 20 year experience. J Support Oncol 5:119–125, 2007

Lutgendorf SK, Weinrib AZ, Penedo F, et al: Interleukin-6, cortisol, and depressive symptoms in ovarian cancer patients. J Clin Oncol 26:4820–4827, 2008

Lynch BM, Steginga SK, Hawkes AL, et al: Describing and predicting psychological distress after colorectal cancer. Cancer 112:1363–1370, 2008

Mao JJ, Palmer SC, Straton JB, et al: Cancer survivors with unmet needs were more likely to use complementary and alternative medicine. J Cancer Surviv 2:116–124, 2008

Markman M: Safety issues in using complementary and alterative medicine. J Clin Oncol 20:S39–S41, 2002

Massie MJ: Prevalence of depression in patients with cancer. J Natl Cancer Inst Monogr 32:57–71, 2004

Massie MJ, Greenberg DB: Oncology, in The American Psychiatric Publishing Textbook of Psychosomatic Medicine. Edited by Levenson JL. Washington, DC, American Psychiatric Publishing, 2005, pp 517–534

McCarthy EP, Phillips RS, Zhong Z, et al: Dying with cancer: patients' function, symptoms, and care preferences as death approaches. J Am Geriatr Soc 48:S110–S121, 2000

McDonald AA, Portenoy RK: How to use antidepressants and anticonvulsants as adjuvant analgesics in the treatment of neuropathic cancer pain. J Support Oncol 4:43–52, 2006

McGee R, Williams S, Elwood M: Depression and the development of cancer: a meta-analysis. Soc Sci Med 38:187–192, 1994

Mehnert A, Koch U: Prevalence of acute and post-traumatic stress disorder and comorbid mental disorders in breast cancer patients during primary care: a prospective study. Psychooncology 16:181–188, 2007

Meyer TJ, Mark MM: Effects of psychosocial interventions with adult cancer patients: a meta-analysis of randomized experiments. Health Psychol 14:101–108, 1995

Meyers CA, Brown PD: Role and relevance of neurocognitive assessment in clinical trials of patients with CNS tumors. J Clin Oncol 24:1305–1309, 2006

Michelsen TM, Dorum A, Dahl AA: A controlled study of mental distress and somatic complaints after risk-reducing salpingo-oophorectomy in women at risk for hereditary breast ovarian cancer. Gynecol Oncol 113:128–133, 2009

Minisini AM, Pauletto G, Andreetta C, et al: Anticancer drugs and central nervous system: clinical issues for patients and physicians. Cancer Lett 267:1–9, 2008

Minton O, Stone P, Richardson A, et al: Drug therapy for the management of cancer related fatigue. Cochrane Database Syst Rev (1):CD006704, 2008

Misono S, Weiss NS, Fann JR, et al: Incidence of suicide in persons with cancer. J Clin Oncol 26:4731–4738, 2008

Moorey S, Cort E, Kapari M, et al: A cluster randomized controlled trial of cognitive behaviour therapy for common mental disorders in patients with advanced cancer. Psychol Med 39:713–723, 2009

Mosher CE, Redd WH, Rini CM, et al: Physical, psychological, and social sequelae following hematopoietic stem cell transplantation: a review of the literature. Psychooncology 18:113–127, 2009

Musselman DL, Lawson DH, Gumnick JF, et al: Paroxetine for the prevention of depression induced by high-dose interferon alfa. N Engl J Med 344:961–966, 2001

Myers CD, Jacobsen PB, Huang Y, et al: Familial and perceived risk of breast cancer in relation to use of complementary medicine. Cancer Epidemiol Biomarkers Prev 17:1527–1534, 2008

Newell SA, Sanson-Fisher RW, Savolainen NJ: Systematic review of psychological therapies for cancer patients: overview and recommendations for future research. J Natl Cancer Inst 94:558–584, 2002

Oerlemans MEJ, van den Akker M, Schuurman AG, et al: A meta-analysis on depression and subsequent cancer risk. Clin Pract Epidemiol Ment Health 3:29, 2007

Onitilo AA, Nietert PJ, Egede LE: Effect of depression on all-cause mortality in adults with cancer and differential effects by cancer site. Gen Hosp Psychiatry 28:396–402, 2006

Orr K, Taylor D: Psychostimulants in the treatment of depression: a review of the literature. CNS Drugs 21:239–257, 2007

Osborn RL, Demoncada AC, Feuerstein M: Psychosocial interventions for depression, anxiety and quality of life in cancer survivors: meta-analyses. Int J Psychiatry Med 36:13–34, 2006

Owen JA, Ferrando SJ: Oncology, in Clinical Manual of Psychopharmacology in the Medically Ill. Edited by Ferrando SJ, Levenson JL, Owen JA. Washington, DC, American Psychiatric Publishing, 2010, pp 237–269

Patkar AA, Hill KP, Weinstein SP, et al: ECT in the presence of brain tumor and increased intracranial pressure: evaluation and reduction of risk. J ECT 16:189–197, 2000

Payne DK, Biggs C, Tran KN, et al: Women's regrets after bilateral prophylactic mastectomy. Ann Surg Oncol 7:150–154, 2000

Persky VW, Kempthorne-Rawson J, Shekelle RB: Personality and risk of cancer: 20 year follow-up of the Western Electric Study. Psychosom Med 49:435–449, 1987

Phipps S, Rai SN, Leung W, et al: Cognitive and academic consequences of stem-cell transplantation in children. J Clin Oncol 26:2027–2033, 2008

Pirl WF: Evidence report on the occurrence, assessment, and treatment of depression in cancer patients. J Natl Cancer Inst Monogr 32:32–39, 2004

Pirl WF, Siegel GI, Goode MJ, et al: Depression in men receiving androgen deprivation therapy for prostate cancer: a pilot study. Psychooncology 11:518–523, 2002

Pitceathly C, Maguire P, Fletcher I, et al: Can a brief psychological intervention prevent anxiety or depressive disorders in cancer patients? A randomized controlled trial. Ann Oncol 20:928–934, 2009

Pitman RK, Lanes DM, Williston SK, et al: Psychophysiologic assessment of post-traumatic stress disorder in breast cancer patients. Psychosomatics 42:133–140, 2001

Prue G, Rankin J, Allen J, et al: Cancer-related fatigue: a critical appraisal. Eur J Cancer 42:846–863, 2006

Ramsey SD, Berry K, Moinpour C, et al: Quality of life in long term survivors of colorectal cancer. Am J Gastroenterol 97:1228–1234, 2002

Robbins AS, Clark CA: Regional changes in hormone replacement therapy use and breast cancer incidence in California from 2001 to 2004. J Clin Oncol 25:3437–3439, 2007

Robson ME, Offit K: Considerations in genetic counseling for inherited breast cancer predisposition. Semin Radiat Oncol 12:362–370, 2002

Rodin G, Lloyd N, Katz M, et al: The treatment of depression in cancer patients: a systematic review. Support Care Cancer 15:123–136, 2007a

Rodin G, Walsh A, Zimmerman C, et al: The contribution of attachment security and social support to depressive symptoms in patients with metastatic cancer. Psychooncology 16:1–12, 2007b

Rodin G, Zimmerman C, Rydall A, et al: The desire for hastened death in patients with metastatic cancer. J Pain Symptom Manage 33:661–675, 2007c

Roth AJ, Weinberger MI, Nelson CJ: Prostate cancer: psychosocial implications and management. Future Oncol 4:561–568, 2008

Rowland JH, Massie MJ: Breast cancer, in Psycho-Oncology, 2nd Edition. Edited by Holland J. New York, Oxford University Press, 2010, pp 177–186

Roy-Byrne PP, Davidson KW, Kessler RC, et al: Anxiety disorders and comorbid medical illness. Gen Hosp Psychiatry 30:208–225, 2008

Rozans M, Dreisbach A, Lertora JJ, et al: Palliative uses of methylphenidate in patients with cancer: a review. J Clin Oncol 20:335–339, 2002

Ryan JL, Carroll JK, Ryan EP, et al: Mechanisms of cancer-related fatigue. Oncologist 12:22–34, 2007

Sahay TB, Gray RE, Fitch M: A qualitative study of patient perspectives on colorectal cancer. Cancer Pract 8:38–44, 2000

Sanderson L, Patten CH, Ebbert JO: Tobacco use outcomes among patients with lung cancer treated for nicotine dependence. J Clin Oncol 20:3461–3469, 2002

Sarna L, Padilla G, Holmes C, et al: Quality of life of long-term survivors on non-small-cell lung cancer. J Clin Oncol 20:2920–2929, 2002

Sasaki T, Akaho R, Sakamaki H, et al: Mental disturbances during isolation in bone marrow transplant patients with leukemia. Bone Marrow Transplant 25:315–318, 2000

Schmitt F, Piha J, Helenius H, et al: Multinational study of cancer patients and their children: factors associated with family functioning. J Clin Oncol 26:5877–5883, 2008

Schover LR: Premature ovarian failure and its consequences: vasomotor symptoms, sexuality, and fertility. J Clin Oncol 26:753–758, 2008

Schubert C, Hong S, Natarajan L, et al: The association between fatigue and inflammatory marker levels in cancer patients: a quantitative review. Brain Behav Immun 21:413–427, 2007

Segal RJ, Reid RD, Courneya KS, et al: Randomized controlled trial of resistance or aerobic exercise in men receiving radiation therapy for prostate cancer. J Clin Oncol 27:344–351, 2009

Shahinian VB, Yong-Fang K, Freeman JL, et al: Risk of androgen deprivation syndrome in men receiving androgen deprivation for prostate cancer. Arch Intern Med 166:465–471, 2006

Sheard T, Maguire P: The effect of psychological interventions on anxiety and depression in cancer patients: results of two meta-analyses. Br J Cancer 80:1770–1780, 1999

Sheibani-Rad S, Velanovich V: Effects of depression on the survival of pancreatic adenocarcinoma. Pancreas 32:58–61, 2006

Shekelle RB, Raynor WJ, Ostfeld AM, et al: Psychological depression and 17-year risk of death from cancer. Psychosom Med 43:117–125, 1981

Smedslund G, Ringdal G: Meta-analysis of the effects of psychological interventions on survival time in cancer patients. J Psychosom Res 57:123–131, 2004

Söllner W, Maislinger S, DeVries A, et al: Use of complementary and alternative medicine by cancer patients is not associated with perceived distress or poor compliance with standard treatment but with active coping behavior: a survey. Cancer 89:873–880, 2000

Söllner W, DeVries A, Steixner E, et al: How successful are oncologists in identifying patient distress, perceived social support, and need for psychosocial counselling? Br J Cancer 84:179–185, 2001

Spiegel D, Giese-Davis J: Depression and cancer: mechanisms and disease progression. Biol Psychiatry 54:269–282, 2003

Spiegel D, Bloom JR, Kramer HJC, et al: Effect of psychosocial treatment on survival of patients with metastatic breast cancer. Lancet 14:88–89, 1989

Spiegel D, Butler LD, Giese-Davis J, et al: Effects of supportive-expressive group therapy on survival of patients with metastatic breast cancer: a randomized prospective trial. Cancer 110:1130–1138, 2007

Spyropoulou AC, Papageorgiou C, Markopoulos C, et al: Depressive symptomatology correlates with phantom breast syndrome in mastectomized women. Eur Arch Psychiatry Clin Neurosci 258:165–170, 2008

Stark D, Kiely M, Smith A, et al: Anxiety disorders in cancer patients: their nature, associations, and relation to quality of life. J Clin Oncol 20:3137–3148, 2002

Steel JL, Geller DA, Gamblin TC, et al: Depression, immunity, and survival in patients with hepatobiliary cancer. J Clin Oncol 25:2397–2405, 2007

Stensheim H, Moller B, van Dijk T, et al: Cause-specific survival for women diagnosed with cancer during pregnancy or lactation: a registry-based cohort study. J Clin Oncol 27:45–51, 2009

Stone PC, Minton O: Cancer-related fatigue. Eur J Cancer 44:1097–1104, 2008

Strevel EL, Ing DI, Siu LL: Molecularly targeted oncology therapeutics and prolongation of the QT interval. J Clin Oncol 25:3362–3371, 2007

Strong V, Waters R, Hibberd C, et al: Emotional distress in cancer patients: the Edinburgh Cancer Centre symptom study. Br J Cancer 96:868–874, 2007

Tatrow K, Montgomery GH: Cognitive behavioral therapy techniques for distress and pain in breast cancer patients: a meta-analysis. J Behav Med 29:17–27, 2006

Theoharides T, Konstantinidou A: Antidepressants and risk of cancer: a case of misguided associations and priorities. J Clin Psychopharmacol 23:1–4, 2003

Thornton LM, Carson WE 3rd, Shapiro CL, et al: Delayed emotional recovery after taxane-based chemotherapy. Cancer 113:638–647, 2008

Throckmorton AD: When informed, all women do not prefer breast conservation. J Clin Oncol 27:484–486, 2009

Trask PC: Assessment of depression in cancer patients. J Natl Cancer Inst Monogr 32:80–92, 2004

Uchitomi Y, Mikami I, Nagai K, et al: Depression and psychological distress in patients during the year after curative resection of non-small-cell lung cancer. J Clin Oncol 21:69–77, 2003

Vapiwala N, Mick R, Hampshire MK, et al: Patient initiation of complementary and alternative medical therapies (CAM) following cancer diagnosis. Cancer J 12:467–474, 2006

Vardy J, Chiew KS, Galica J, et al: Side effects associated with the use of dexamethasone for prophylaxis of delayed emesis after moderately emetogenic chemotherapy. Br J Cancer 94:1011–1015, 2006

Vardy J, Wefel JS, Ahles T, et al: Cancer and cancer-therapy related cognitive dysfunction: an international perspective from the Venice cognitive workshop. Ann Oncol 19:623–629, 2008

Walker J, Waters RA, Murray G, et al: Better off dead: suicidal thoughts in cancer patients. J Clin Oncol 26:4725–4730, 2008

Watson M, Haviland JS, Greer S, et al: Influence of psychological response on survival in breast cancer: a population-based cohort study. Lancet 354:1331–1336, 1999

Weber BA, Sherwill-Navarro P: Psychosocial consequences of prostate cancer: 30 years of research. Geriatr Nurs 26:166–175, 2005

Weber BL, Punzalan C, Eisen A, et al: Ovarian cancer risk reduction after bilateral prophylactic oophorectomy (BPO) in BRCA1 and BRCA2 mutation carriers (abstract). Am J Hum Genet 67(suppl):59, 2000

Wei JT, Dunn RL, Sandler HM, et al: Comprehensive comparison of health related quality of life after contemporary therapies for localized prostate cancer. J Clin Oncol 20:557–566, 2002

Wesa K, Gubili J, Cassileth B: Integrative oncology: complementary therapies for cancer survivors. Hematol Oncol Clin N Am 22:343–353, 2008

White VM, English DR, Coates H, et al: Is cancer risk associated with anger control and negative affect? Findings from a prospective cohort study. Psychosom Med 69:667–674, 2007

Wilkinson SM, Love SB, Westcombe AM, et al: Effectiveness of aromatherapy massage in the management of anxiety and depression in patients with cancer: a multicenter randomized controlled trial. J Clin Oncol 25:532–539, 2007

Williams S, Dale J: The effectiveness of treatment for depression/depressive symptoms in adults with cancer: a systematic review. Br J Cancer 94:372–390, 2006

Wittmann D, Northouse L, Foley S, et al: The psychosocial aspects of sexual recovery after prostate cancer treatment. Int J Impot Res 21:99–106, 2009

Yatham LN, Kennedy SH, Schaffer A, et al: Canadian Network for Mood and Anxiety Treatments (CANMAT) and International Society for Bipolar Disorders (ISBD) collaborative update of CANMAT guidelines for the management of patients with bipolar disorder: update 2009. Bipolar Disord 11:225–255, 2009

Zabora J, BrintzenhofeSzoc K, Curbow B, et al: The prevalence of psychological distress by cancer site. Psychooncology 10:19–28, 2001

Zigmond AS, Snaith RP: The Hospital Anxiety and Depression Scale. Acta Psychiatr Scand 67:361–370, 1983

CHAPTER

24

Hematology

Madeleine Becker, M.D., M.A.

David J. Axelrod, M.D., J.D.

Olu Oyesanmi, M.D., M.P.H.

Dimitri D. Markov, M.D.

Elaine Martin, M.D.

Elisabeth J. Shakin Kunkel, M.D.

THE CONSULTATION psychiatrist is frequently called on to assess patients in medical settings who have primary or secondary hematological disorders. Our review addresses psychiatric issues that are specific to patients who have selected hematological disorders, including iron, B_{12}, or folate deficiency; sickle cell disease; hemophilia; and thalassemia. We discuss the diseases, their unique psychiatric manifestations, and approaches to management. Fear of blood transfusions and psychological factors affecting clotting are described. Finally, hematological side effects of psychotropic medications and their drug interactions are reviewed.

Iron Deficiency Anemia

Iron is a component of hemoglobin and is essential to red blood cell production. Iron deficiency anemia (IDA), an advanced state of iron deficiency, causes a hypochromic microcytic anemia characterized by low or absent iron stores and low iron serum concentration, low transferrin saturation, low serum ferritin, elevated free erythrocyte porphyrin, elevated transferrin, and low hemoglobin concentration (Dorland's Illustrated Medical Dictionary 2003). IDA may manifest with a variety of physical and neuropsychiatric symptoms.

IDA is the most common nutrient deficiency in the world; however, its prevalence and etiology vary by race, sex, geography, and socioeconomic status. Prevalence is 3% in toddlers ages 1–2 years, 2%–5% in adolescent girls, 2% in adult men, 9%–12% in white women, and about 20% in African American and Mexican American women (Killip et al. 2007; Looker et al. 1997). The World Health Organization (WHO) estimates that 43% of nonpregnant women of reproductive age in developing countries and 12% in industrialized countries are anemic. This number increases to 56% and 18%, respectively, by the third trimester of pregnancy (Milman 2006).

The most common etiology of IDA is blood loss. In men and in postmenopausal women, chronic bleeding from the gastrointestinal tract is the most common cause of IDA. Peptic ulcer, hiatal hernia, gastritis, hemorrhoids, vascular anomalies, and neoplasms are the most common causes of gastrointestinal bleeding in adults. Causes of chronic blood loss also include colon cancer, colonic diverticulae, periampullary tumors, leiomyomas, adenomas, and other malignant or benign neoplasms of the intestine (Coban et al. 2003).

Unsupplemented milk diets do not contain adequate amounts of iron for infants. During the first year of life, iron demands are increased, and milk products are poor sources of iron; prolonged breast feeding or bottle feeding of infants frequently leads to IDA unless there is iron supplementation. Premature infants are at even greater risk of

IDA. Children experience a higher risk during rapid growth periods. The low iron supply in the American diet has put young women and children at higher risk of IDA (Hallberg et al. 1995).

IDA is highly prevalent in pregnant women as the result of iron loss from diversion of iron to the fetus and from blood loss during delivery. Daily iron demand dramatically increases during pregnancy and continues through to term. Breast-feeding leads to additional iron diversion to the baby. For these reasons, IDA continues or worsens for a significant percentage of women during the postpartum period (Milman 2006).

Intestinal malabsorption of iron is an uncommon cause of iron deficiency except after gastrointestinal surgery and in malabsorption syndromes such as celiac disease (Annibale et al. 2003). In malabsorption syndromes, IDA may take years to develop due to the indolent nature of iron loss.

Clinical Manifestations

IDA occasionally results in severe anemia, with some patients having blood hemoglobin levels below 4 g/dL. Severe IDA is associated with all of the various symptoms of anemia (resulting from both hypoxia and the body's response to hypoxia), including tachycardia, palpitations, pounding in the ears, headache, light-headedness, angina, and retinal hemorrhages and exudates. Less severe anemia presents with fatigue, weakness, headache, irritability, and exercise intolerance. Glossal pain, dry mouth, atrophy of tongue papillae, and alopecia may be more specific to IDA (Trost et al. 2006). Physical findings include pallor, glossitis (smooth red tongue), stomatitis, and angular cheilitis.

Neuropsychiatric Manifestations

Neuropsychiatric symptoms of IDA include depression, developmental delay, cognitive deficits, restless legs syndrome, and fatigue. IDA may affect visual and auditory functions. IDA leads to decreased work and exercise performance as well as neurological dysfunction (Cook and Skikne 1989). IDA may result in cognitive and motor developmental delays in infants and young children (Booth and Aukett 1997). The pathophysiology of these behavioral deficits is not well understood (Lozoff 1988). Even school-age children and adolescents with iron deficiency (with or without anemia) have been shown to have lower standardized math scores compared with children with normal iron status (Halterman et al. 2001).

In adults, IDA impairs cognitive function, limits activity, and causes work paucity (Beard et al. 2005). Women who have IDA are more likely to have postpartum fatigue (K.A. Lee and Zaffke 1999). Mild anemia is independently associated with worse selective attention performance and disease-specific quality-of-life ratings (Lucca et al. 2008). Mildly anemic elderly patients (not limited to those with IDA) score significantly worse than nonanemic control subjects on multiple cognitive, functional, mood, and quality-of-life measures (Lucca et al. 2008).

Patients with IDA may crave both food items and nonfood substances. Pica and particularly pagophagia (craving ice) are specific symptoms that reportedly occur in 50% of patients with IDA (Rector 1989; R.D. Reynolds et al. 1968). The mechanism by which IDA produces pica is unknown.

Motor impairment, cognitive dysfunction, and restless legs syndrome probably result from iron deficiency in the central nervous system (CNS) (Krieger and Schroeder 2001). Early studies demonstrated that IDA plays a role in restless legs syndrome and that treatment with iron improves the syndrome (Krieger and Schroeder 2001; O'Keeffe et al. 1994). The severity of restless legs syndrome correlates with serum ferritin levels (Sun et al. 1998). Iron deficiency is also a risk factor for neuroleptic malignant syndrome (Rosebush and Mazurek 1991) and may aggravate akathisia and other extrapyramidal movement disorders.

Diagnosis and Treatment

IDA often is discovered incidentally through screening laboratory tests. IDA is a microcytic, hypochromic anemia. Plasma iron concentration and serum ferritin concentration are low, and iron-binding capacity is increased. Ferritin is the single best test. The classic laboratory findings occur consistently only when IDA is far advanced, is unaccompanied by complicating factors (such as infection or cancer), and is untreated (via transfusions or administration of parenteral iron).

Patients should be educated to maintain a diversified diet with adequate iron. Recovery from IDA almost always requires iron supplementation. Therapy should be initiated immediately. Iron can be replaced orally, parenterally, or (rarely) via blood transfusion. Oral iron is preferred. The adult dosage provides 150–200 mg elemental iron daily, taken in 3–4 doses 1 hour before meals. Poor tolerance to oral iron, poor absorption of iron, iron need in excess of the amount that can be taken orally, or noncompliance may necessitate intravenous therapy. Intravenous iron is effective and safe and is usually indicated in instances when hemoglobin is consistently less than 10 g/dL despite oral therapy (Schaefer et al. 2006). Symptom improvement after iron repletion is often realized quickly. Headache, fatigue, paresthesias, and pica rapidly resolve (Rector 1989). There are conflicting data as to whether oral iron improves cognitive development in infants (Lozoff et al. 1982; Walter et al. 1983). The prognosis of IDA is excellent when the cause of iron deficiency is benign.

Vitamin B_{12} and Folate Deficiency

Vitamin B_{12} deficiency and folate deficiency have similar consequences on the nervous system and lead to megaloblastic anemia (E. Reynolds 2006). Both B_{12} and folate are cofactors for the conversion of homocysteine to methionine. Deficiency of either B_{12} or folate correlates with high homocysteine levels, which is a risk factor for cardiovascular disease, stroke, dementia, and Alzheimer's disease (Carmel et al. 2003; Ravaglia et al. 2005; E. Reynolds 2006; Seshadri et al. 2002). Both high homocysteine levels and deficiencies of B_{12} and folate are also associated with depression (Bottiglieri et al. 2000; Kim et al. 2008b).

Vitamin B_{12} Deficiency

Vitamin B_{12} (cobalamin) is found primarily in meat and dairy products. B_{12} is a necessary coenzyme and cofactor in various reactions, including DNA synthesis and the synthesis of methionine from homocysteine. In the duodenum, vitamin B_{12} binds to intrinsic factor. Intrinsic factor is released by parietal cells, which are located in the fundus and body of the stomach. The B_{12} complex is then absorbed in the terminal ileum. There is usually enough B_{12} stored in the liver to supply daily requirements for up to 2–5 years; therefore, it typically takes years to develop B_{12} deficiency (Andres et al. 2004). In the elderly, the prevalence of B_{12} deficiency, including mild and subclinical cases, may exceed 20% (Andres et al. 2004; Loikas et al. 2007).

Pernicious anemia is the most common cause of B_{12} deficiency (Toh et al. 1997). Pernicious anemia is an autoimmune disorder resulting in the loss of parietal cells in the stomach and subsequent loss of intrinsic factor production, which is necessary for B_{12} absorption. Pernicious anemia frequently is associated with other autoimmune disorders, including thyroiditis, diabetes mellitus, Addison's disease, Graves' disease, vitiligo, myasthenia gravis, Lambert-Eaton myasthenic syndrome, and hypoparathyroidism (Carmel et al. 2003; Toh et al. 1997).

Dietary B_{12} deficiency is rare but may occur in strict vegans. B_{12} deficiency also can occur in children who are exclusively breast-fed and whose mothers are vegetarians (Chalouhi et al. 2008). In the elderly, deficiency usually is secondary to malabsorption due to gastric atrophy or pernicious anemia (Andres et al. 2009). Food or oral cobalamin malabsorption may be caused by *Helicobacter pylori* infection, intestinal overgrowth due to antibiotics, chronic use of metformin (Bauman et al. 2000; K.W. Liu et al. 2006) or antacids, H_2 receptor antagonists, proton pump inhibitors (Valuck and Ruscin 2004), alcoholism, pancreatic failure, and Sjögren's syndrome. Vitamin B_{12} malabsorption also may result from gastrectomy, gastric bypass surgery (Malinowski 2006; Vargas-Ruiz et al. 2008), ileal diseases or resection, Crohn's disease, blind loops, and infection with *Diphyllobothrium latum* or HIV (Andres et al. 2004).

Clinical Manifestations

The most common clinical manifestations of B_{12} deficiency are macrocytic anemia and neuropsychiatric symptoms. Hematological manifestations of B_{12} deficiency include megaloblastic anemia, macrocytosis with hypersegmented polymorphonuclear leukocytes, thrombocytopenia, leukopenia, pancytopenia or (rarely) hemolytic anemia, and thrombotic microangiopathy. Gastrointestinal manifestations include intestinal metaplasia, diarrhea, jaundice, and increased lactate dehydrogenase and bilirubin levels. Vaginal atrophy may also occur (Andres et al. 2004; Toh et al. 1997).

Neuropsychiatric Manifestations

Neuropsychiatric manifestations are common in vitamin B_{12} deficiency, especially in the elderly (Andres et al. 2004). The hematological and neuropsychiatric symptoms of B_{12} deficiency are often disassociated, and neuropsychiatric symptoms may precede hematological signs (E. Reynolds 2006). Symmetrical peripheral neuropathy occurs frequently, with paresthesias and numbness. Subacute combined degeneration of the spinal cord is less common (E. Reynolds 2006). Subacute combined degeneration encompasses both posterior column disruption (resulting in loss of vibration and position sense and ataxia with a positive Romberg's sign) and lateral column disruption (causing weakness, spasticity, and extensor plantar responses) (Toh et al. 1997). Rare manifestations of B_{12} deficiency include optic neuritis, optic atrophy, and incontinence. Psychiatric symptoms may include mood changes, including depression (Kim et al. 2008b), psychosis, cognitive impairment, and obsessive-compulsive disorder (Bauman et al. 2000; Fava et al. 1997; K.W. Liu et al. 2006; Valuck and Ruscin 2004). B_{12} deficiency appears to be a risk factor for dementia (Andres et al. 2004). In children, vitamin B_{12} deficiency may cause irritability, failure to thrive, apathy, anorexia, abnormal movements, and developmental regression, which generally respond to supplementation. Long-term cognitive and developmental retardation are most dependent on the duration of the deficiency and the severity of symptoms (Chalouhi et al. 2008).

Diagnosis and Treatment

A low normal serum vitamin B_{12} level in the presence of megaloblastic cells (with or without anemia and/or the typical neuropsychiatric findings) should lead to further investigation for B_{12} deficiency. There is no "gold standard," and there are different normal values for cobalamin levels; however, a deficiency is usually defined as a B_{12} level of less than 150 ng/L (Andres et al. 2004). Elevated serum methylmalonic acid and elevated serum total homocysteine can help establish whether deficiency exists (Carmel et al. 2003). Tests for intrinsic factor antibody and serum gastrin and a Schilling test may be helpful in diagnosing pernicious anemia. Differentiating the causes of B_{12} deficiency yields important clinical information and can guide diagnosis and treatment (Carmel et al. 2003).

Daily injections of 1,000 mcg of hydroxycobalamin or cyanocobalamin are recommended for 1 week, followed by weekly injections of 1 mg for 4 weeks, and then maintenance doses every 1–3 months, depending on the severity of deficiency (Andres et al. 2009). Clinical evidence suggests that oral B_{12} replacement also is effective as a second-line therapy (Andres et al. 2009). Remission is typically achieved within weeks, but continued maintenance therapy is recommended to fully replete body stores and to maintain longer periods of remission. Significant improvement of neuropsychiatric function has been shown after B_{12} administration (Andres et al. 2009); the degree of recovery is correlated with symptom severity before treatment (E. Reynolds 2006). Administration of folate, without B_{12}, will reverse the hematological abnormalities, but if there is an unrecognized B_{12} deficiency, neurological impairment may progress further, sometimes leading to irreversible deficits (E. Reynolds 2006). There is no evidence that B_{12} injections provide any benefit for symptoms of fatigue or depression in patients who have normal B_{12} levels.

Folic Acid Deficiency

Folic acid is found in both animal products and leafy green vegetables. Folate is important in mood and cognition, brain growth, and cell differentiation, development, and repair. These mechanisms are likely mediated through nucleotide synthesis and DNA transcription and integrity (Carmel et al. 2003). Adequate folate levels may protect against certain cancers, birth defects (Lucock 2004), and dementia (Wang et al. 2001), presumably by lowering homocysteine (Ravaglia et al. 2005).

Inadequate diet, alcoholism, chronic illness, drugs (e.g., phenytoin, valproic acid, lamotrigine, and barbiturates, trimethoprim/sulfamethoxazole, oral contraceptives, and methotrexate), and malabsorption all can cause folate deficiency (E.H. Reynolds 2002). Deficiency is more common in the elderly (E. Reynolds 2006). Low folate levels are more prevalent in psychiatric inpatients than in patients without psychiatric illness, even after controlling for drug and alcohol abuse (Lerner et al. 2006). Folate deficiency has been reported in up to one-third of psychiatric patients and is especially prevalent in those with depression (Bottiglieri et al. 2000; Carney et al. 1990). It is unclear how much of folate deficiency can be attributed to the use of psychotropic medications, especially antiepileptic drugs, which are known to decrease folate levels.

Clinical Manifestations

Symptoms of folate deficiency are similar to those of B_{12} deficiency; however, subacute combined degeneration of the spinal cord is specific to B_{12} deficiency and depression is more common in folate deficiency (E. Reynolds 2006). The megaloblastic anemia in folate deficiency is identical to that seen in B_{12} deficiency. Folate deficiency is invariably accompanied by a raised plasma homocysteine level (Bottiglieri et al. 2000; Jacques et al. 1999), which carries an increased risk of cardiovascular disease, dementia (Kim et al. 2008a; Malouf et al. 2003; Ravaglia et al. 2005), and depression (Bottiglieri et al. 2000; Fava et al. 1997; Kim et al. 2008b).

Insufficient folate during conception and early pregnancy may result in neural tube defects. Since 1998, the U.S. Food and Drug Administration has mandated fortification of grains with folate to help lower women's risk of having a pregnancy affected by neural tube defects. This action has led to a reduction in neural tube defects and an improvement of blood folate status and homocysteine levels in adults in the United States (Choumenkovitch et al. 2001, 2002; Dietrich et al. 2005; Jacques et al. 1999).

Diagnosis and Treatment

Low red blood cell folate combined with high plasma homocysteine is a good standard for the diagnosis of folate deficiency and is more accurate than measuring serum folate alone. Full treatment response to folate takes many months (E. Reynolds 2006). Although there are no clear guidelines for the dose or duration of folate therapy, treatment is recommended for at least 6 months; clinical improvement is usually seen within the first few months (E. Reynolds 2006). Dose recommendations vary, but at least 0.4 mg daily is recommended for women of childbearing age (U.S. Preventive Services Task Force 1996), although higher doses are probably more effective. Usually, 1 mg daily is prescribed to pregnant women and women trying to conceive to decrease the risk of neural tube defects (Wald 2004; Wald et al. 2001). To lower the homocysteine level, 0.8 mg daily is typically required (Homocysteine Lowering Trialists' Collaboration 2005). To treat folate deficiency, 1 mg daily until hematological recovery is generally recommended (Kunkel et al. 2000).

The relationship of vitamin deficiency to depression and dementia is complex and probably bidirectional. Depression has been associated with low baseline levels of both folate and B_{12} (Kim et al. 2008b). In depressed patients, low folate levels were correlated with higher levels of depression, and these patients were less likely to respond to antidepressants (Fava et al. 1997; Papakostas et al. 2004). Supplementation of fluoxetine with folic acid improved antidepressant response, especially in women, although improvement was attributed to the concurrent decrease in plasma homocysteine levels rather than to increased plasma folate levels (Coppen et al. 2000). A large randomized, placebo-controlled trial in older men, however, showed no difference in depressive symptoms among subjects who received B_{12}, folic acid and B_6 supplementation compared with those who received placebo (Ford et al. 2008).

There is increasing interest in the possibility that elevated homocysteine levels are linked to cognitive impairment and dementia. Researchers have debated whether supplementation of either folate or B_{12}, which can lower homocysteine levels, has any effect on cognition or the development of dementia (Clarke et al. 2008). Findings to date have been inconsistent. Low baseline folate levels and an exaggerated decline in folate levels were predictive of dementia (Kim et al. 2008a). Multiple studies have shown that folic acid supplementation increases blood folate and decreases homocysteine (Durga et al. 2007; Jacques et al. 1999). Most studies found that a higher intake of folate, but not of the other B vitamins, is related to a lower risk of Alzheimer's dementia (Luchsinger et al. 2007; Ravaglia et al. 2005) and to better cognitive functioning (Durga et al. 2007). Other investigators found no association between dietary intake of folate or B_{12} and the later development of Alzheimer's disease (Morris et al. 2006). Several large reviews show that supplementation of either folic acid or B_{12} does not have a significant effect on cognition in individuals with either normal or impaired cognitive functioning (Balk et al. 2007; Malouf et al. 2003). Until more definitive information is available regarding the benefits of supplementation, it is prudent to consider checking folic acid and B_{12} levels in elderly patients and in patients with depression or dementia and supplementing as needed.

Sickle Cell Disease

Sickle cell disease (SCD) is the most common hemoglobinopathy. The disease is a classic example of a balanced polymorphism; the asymptomatic sickle cell trait provides a selective advantage against malaria, while the homozygous disease has devastating consequences. SCD includes the homozygous disease of sickle cell anemia (SCA), sickle cell–beta thalassemia, sickle cell–hemoglobin C, and other SCD variants. Sickle cell trait has insignificant clinical consequences.

SCD occurs primarily in those of African descent, but also afflicts people of Mediterranean, Asian, and Middle Eastern origin. More than 70,000 Americans suffer from SCD. Among African Americans, the prevalence is approximately 1 in 300; 8% carry the trait. Medical advances have transformed the disease from a pediatric illness into one that chronically extends into adulthood. Life expectancy over the past 35 years has increased, from a mean of age 14 years in the 1970s to close to age 50 years today (Platt et al. 1994).

The vaso-occlusive crisis is the hallmark of SCD. These recurrent crises, or severe pain episodes, are the cause of acute episodes of severe pain and represent the most common reason patients seek medical care. Extremes of temperature, infectious illness, dehydration, and physical exertion may precipitate crises, but the majority of crises occur without an identifiable cause. Vaso-occlusion produces acute pain in the short term and end-organ damage in the long term. Vaso-occlusion potentially affects all organ systems but leads to particular damage in bones, kidneys, lungs, eyes, and brain. Many patients suffer from chronic pain as a result of avascular necrosis, leg ulcers, or poorly understood chronic pain syndromes. The neuropsychiatric manifestations of SCD can be divided into three main categories: 1) depression and anxiety resulting from living with a chronic stigmatizing disease associated with unpredictable, painful crises and high morbidity and mortality; 2) problems related to living with chronic and acute pain (often undertreated), control of which involves long-term use of analgesics, potentially leading to opioid dependency, addiction, and pseudoaddiction; and 3) CNS damage resulting from cerebral vascular accidents, primarily during childhood. These issues are further complicated by poor psychosocial circumstances and the learned helplessness of many patients.

A significant problem with obtaining psychiatric treatment in patients with SCD is that African Americans in general are often reluctant to obtain help for mental health issues and may attempt to overcome mental health problems through self-reliance and determination (Snowden 2001). In addition, lack of psychosocial resources may put SCD patients at higher risk for poor adaptation to SCD (Burlew et al. 2000). There may be additional barriers to accessing care in patients with lower socioeconomic status. In conclusion, psychological and psychiatric complications in patients with SCD are common and contribute to functional impairment and reduced quality of life. Psychological and psychiatric care improves outcomes and should be a routine component of comprehensive SCD care.

Depression and Anxiety

As with many chronic diseases, depression and anxiety are common in adult patients with SCD. The prevalence of depression approaches 30% in SCD (Jenerette et al. 2005; Levenson et al. 2008). Anxiety disorders occur in about 7% of patients (Levenson et al. 2008). Depression and anxiety predict more daily pain and poorer physical and psychosocial quality of life in adults with SCD and account for more of the variance in all domains of quality of life than does hemoglobin type (Levenson et al. 2008). Studies assessing depression and anxiety in children with SCD have yielded mixed results (Benton et al. 2007). However, children with SCD have a higher prevalence of excessive fatigue, physical complaints, impaired self-esteem, morbid ideation, and feelings of hopelessness (Anie 2005; Yang et al. 1994). These feelings arise in the context of frequent hospitalizations, chronic absences from school, and inability to experience a normal childhood like other children.

The stigma associated with SCD significantly contributes to anxiety and depression (Jenerette et al. 2005). Adults with SCD face physical deformities, the stigma of chronic opioid use and/or mental illness, and biases related to race. The strain of facing these stigmas may have a variety of negative psychological consequences. Physical deformities result from delayed growth and development as a consequence of chronic hemolysis and chronic vaso-occlusion. In comparison with control subjects, pediatric SCD patients weigh less, are shorter, and have delayed puberty (Cepeda et al. 2000). For adolescents, these physical differences may lead to problems with self-esteem, heightened self-consciousness, dissatisfaction with body image, and social isolation (Morgan and Jackson 1986). Participation in athletics is limited due to short stature and fear of initiating a vaso-occlusive crisis. School performance suffers when hospitalizations cause multiple missed school days. Accordingly, adolescents often experience hopelessness and social withdrawal (Hurtig and Park 1989). In the United States, the stigma of SCD is compounded by the disease's predominance in an ethnic minority that already is vulnerable to racial prejudice and stereotyping (Jacob and American Pain Society 2001).

Chronic and Acute Pain and Opioid Use

Patients with SCD most commonly seek medical care for treatment of their pain. In the Pain in Sickle Cell Epidemiologic Study (PiSCES), a prospective cohort study in which adults with SCD completed daily diaries for up to 6 months, patients reported experiencing pain on more than 50% of days, and 29% reported pain on more than 95% of days. Subjects reported having sickle cell crises on 16% of days, but they sought urgent health care for crisis pain on only 3.5% of days (Smith et al. 2008). Previous studies reported a much lower frequency of painful crises; however, those studies used health care utilization as a proxy for crisis (e.g., the classic 1991 study, which reported that the average adult SCD patient experiences 0.8 episodes of vaso-occlusive severe pain episodes per year [Platt et al. 1991]) rather than obtaining patient self-reports. Patients live with the uncertainty of never knowing when the next severe pain episode will occur. Both the nature of the pain (which has been reported to be as severe as childbirth [Ballas 1998]) and its unpredictable onset can be psychologically debilitating.

Over the last 15 years, opioid treatment has gained mainstream acceptance for the treatment of SCD pain. Opioids help control pain, improve functional capacity, and decrease hospitalizations in patients with SCD (Brookoff and Polomano 1992). Chronic opioid use may result in tolerance, physiological dependence as well as substance dependence, and abuse. There is concern among authors that cognitive deficits may occur with opioid use in patients with chronic pain; however, studies have not revealed consistent evidence to support this claim (Chapman et al. 2002; see also Chapter 36, "Pain").

Substance dependence and addiction behaviors are difficult to define in any chronic pain condition. The few studies that address addiction in SCD report a low prevalence. Despite the lack of evidence in the medical literature for addiction in SCD, medical practitioners often overestimate the prevalence of addiction (Labbe et al. 2005). In surveys of health care practitioners, 63% of nurses believed that addiction was prevalent in SCD (Pack-Mabien et al. 2001), and 53% of emergency department physicians and 23% of hematologists thought that more than 20% of SCD patients were addicted (Shapiro et al. 1997). Some of this misconception results from failure to understand the difference between physiological tolerance and opioid dependence.

Due to skepticism and fear of introducing iatrogenic addiction, medical practitioners may undertreat pain in patients with SCD (Labbe et al. 2005). As a result of undertreatment, patients may develop a pseudoaddiction, where addiction-like behaviors occur as a result of inadequate pain management (Weissman and Haddox 1989). Some SCD patients may seek out illegal narcotics as a way to manage their painful crises. This behavior can lead to long-term problems with true addiction and illicit substance abuse (Alao et al. 2003). Some patients may inappropriately use opioids to help with nonpain symptoms such as insomnia, depression, and anxiety. In the PiSCES study, 31.4% of adult SCD patients were found to abuse alcohol. Although the alcoholic patients did not use more opioids than the nonalcoholic patients, they reported more pain relief from opioids. Alcohol-abusing patients also showed lower use of health care resources and, unexpectedly, reported better overall physical quality of life (Levenson et al. 2007).

Central Nervous System Damage

Brain injury from SCD complications begins early in life and is associated with neurocognitive dysfunction. An estimated 25%–33% of children with SCD have CNS effects from the disease (Schatz and McClellan 2006). Seizures occur in 12%–14% of pediatric patients with SCD and often herald stroke (Adams 1994; J.E. Liu et al. 1994). Cerebrovascular accidents occur in 10%–15% of children with SCA. These children demonstrate intellectual deficits ranging from borderline to moderate mental retardation, reduced language function, and problems with adjustment (Hariman et al. 1991). Cognitive deficits in children with SCD can result in intellectual impairment and educational problems, as well as problems with attention and concentration, and may lead to dementia later in life (Anie 2005). SCD patients have been found to have lower scores in language skills and auditory discrimination as early as kindergarten; thus, deficits cannot be attributed to school absences (Steen et al. 2002).

Hemophilia

Hemophilia is a bleeding disorder caused by a deficiency of the coagulation factors essential for blood clotting. Hemophilia A (factor VIII deficiency) and hemophilia B (factor IX deficiency) are the most well-known inherited bleeding disorders. Hemophilia A and B are X-linked diseases and mainly affect males. Female carriers can experience excessive bleeding, as they may have half the normal amount of clotting factors. Hemophilia A and B are clinically indistinguishable from one another.

Disease severity is related to the plasma concentrations of the clotting factors. Classification into severe, moderate, and mild hemophilia is useful for predicting bleeding tendency and prognosis, as well as for guiding treatment (Bolton-Maggs and Pasi 2003; Casey and Brown 2003; Manco-Johnson 2005). Patients with severe hemophilia (<1% clotting factor) typically bleed spontaneously into joints, muscles, soft tissues, and body cavities. During the neonatal period, especially during the first week of life, the risk of intracranial hemorrhage is estimated to be between 1% and 4%. Most children are asymptomatic until they start crawling or walking. Affected children may bruise easily and bleed following minor injuries. Families of these children may inappropriately be suspected of child abuse. By 4 years of age, many children with hemophilia have experienced a bleed into a joint.

Since the 1960s, the availability of purified factor VIII has allowed for home-based infusions, improved quality of life, and increased the life expectancy of patients with severe hemophilia. This has reduced the frequency of recurrent bleeds into large joints and muscles, with resultant fewer complications of joint injury and chronic pain. *Moderate* hemophilia (1%–5% clotting factor) is typically diagnosed by 5 years of age; bleeding episodes in patients with moderate hemophilia occur less frequently. *Mild* hemophilia (>5% clotting factor) is usually diagnosed later, following trauma, tooth extraction, or surgery. Bleeding episodes in patients with mild hemophilia typically occur secondary to trauma; spontaneous bleeding is rare (Bolton-Maggs and Pasi 2003; Manco-Johnson 2005; White et al. 2001). In the early 1980s, more than 80% of patients with severe hemophilia who were older than 10 years were infected with viral illnesses, including HIV, hepatitis B, and hepatitis C. Beginning in the 1990s, the use of recombinant clotting factors almost eliminated the risk of transmitting viral infections (since there remains a small risk with transfusions). Advances in the treatment of hemophilia have resulted in effective prevention and control of bleeding. Nowadays, patients with severe hemophilia are much less likely to experience bleeding and its associated complications (Bolton-Maggs and Pasi 2003; Manco-Johnson 2005).

The extent of psychiatric disorders in patients with hemophilia is unknown. Higher rates of anxiety disorders have been reported in children and adolescents with hemophilia compared with those with asthma (who also have increased rates of anxiety) (Bussing and Burket 1993). Children with hemophilia must attain developmental milestones while dealing with chronic disease and must confront different disease-related stressors at different ages of development. While facing chronic pain, disability, social ostracism, and job and insurance discrimination, adults living with hemophilia strive for a healthy identity, autonomy, and a good quality of life (Spilsbury 2004).

Physicians who fear inducing drug dependence with opiates are reluctant to prescribe opiates, despite the severe pain associated with joint bleeds. Even adult patients without drug dependence report concern about potential narcotic addiction (Elander and Barry 2003). In actual practice, opiate analgesics may be used safely in patients with hemophilia. It is important to address patient concerns about becoming opiate dependent in order to provide adequate analgesia (Kunkel et al. 2000).

Individual, group, and family psychotherapy are useful psychotherapeutic modalities. Caution is needed in prescribing psychotropic agents to individuals with hemophilia. For older patients with impaired liver function from viral hepatitis, dosages of antidepressants, antipsychotics, or opiate analgesics should be reduced. Several psychotropic agents may increase the risk of bleeding, and caution must be exercised when prescribing those agents to hemophiliacs (Casey and Brown 2003; Gerstner et al. 2006; see "Hematological Side Effects and Drug Interactions of Psychotropic Agents" later in this chapter).

Hemophiliacs who developed AIDS face many additional stressors: opportunistic infections, physical wasting, declining health, chronic pain, CNS complications, frequent monitoring of viral load and CD4+ cell counts, medication side effects, and disclosure of HIV status, resulting in further social ostracism and insurance discrimination. After a loved one's death from AIDS, bereaved families may need extensive psychological counseling and support. A study in Japan found that 7–9 years after their loved one's death, bereaved family members reported continuing deep sorrow and grief about their loss, as well as resentment, regret, anger, guilt, and anxiety over discrimination. Additionally, up to 70% of bereaved family members reported restricting their daily activities due to stigma of HIV or fear of discrimination, and up to half of bereaved family members continued suffering from mental health problems (Mizota et al. 2006).

When caring for HIV-infected hemophiliacs, health care workers may experience anxiety about exposure to HIV and guilt about having unknowingly administered hepatitis and HIV-infected clotting factors to patients in the 1980s (before safe clotting factors became available). Health care providers are faced with complex ethical and medical dilemmas when caring for HIV-infected hemophiliacs. Examples include whether to disclose HIV status to an HIV-positive child or teenager when the patient's parents oppose the disclosure, and whether to breach the confidentiality of a sexually active hepatitis or HIV-positive hemophiliac in order to inform their sexual partners of the potential risk of contracting hepatitis or HIV (Kulkarni et al. 2001).

Thalassemia

Thalassemia, originally termed *thalassa anemia* ("anemia by the sea") due to its link to the Mediterranean region, is an inherited autosomal recessive blood disease (Lorey et al. 1996; Vichinsky et al. 2005) caused by a mutation in one of the globin chains of hemoglobin. Normal adult hemoglobin is a tetramer composed of two alpha-like and two beta-like globin chains. Adult hemoglobin consists primarily of hemoglobin A ($\alpha_2\beta_2$), with small amounts of hemoglobin A_2 ($\alpha_2\delta_2$) and hemoglobin F ($\alpha_2\gamma_2$). A mutation in either chain results in either decreased (α+ or β+) or absent (α° or β°) production of the affected globin chain and a proportional excess of the other chain. These excess globin chains are unstable and precipitate within red blood cells, leading to various clinical manifestations. As of about 1999, 200 beta-globin and 30 alpha-globin mutations have been identified, resulting in considerable clinical variability among the different types of thalassemias (Olivieri 1999). The thalassemias are named according to the globin chain affected by a mutation. Patients with alpha-thalassemia have a mutation in the gene encoding alpha-globin. In beta-thalassemia, there is a mutation in the gene encoding beta-globin (Cunningham 2008).

Demographics

In recent years there has been a dramatic change in the demographics of those affected with thalassemia. Once considered a fatal childhood illness, thalassemia now is considered a chronic adult disease. Due to advances in treatment, the median life span of patients with thalassemia is approaching 40 years of age in North America and other developed countries (Vichinsky et al. 2005). Increased survival as well as changes in immigration have drastically changed the ethnicity and age distribution of patients with thalassemia in North America (Vichinsky et al. 2005). According to the Thalassemia Clinical Research Network (TCRN) of the National Heart, Lung, and Blood Institute, in 1973 only 2% of thalassemics were age 25 years or older. By 2002, 36% of the thalassemic population was older than 25 years. There has been a decline in Mediterranean-origin patients due to declining immigration from these regions as well as the introduction of genetic counseling programs and prenatal screening. Asian patients now account for at least 50% of the thalassemic population in North America due to an increase in Asian immigration to the United States (Vichinsky et al. 2005).

Clinical Manifestations

Because the thalassemias are such a heterogeneous group of disorders, clinical manifestations usually are discussed for the group as a whole. Removal of damaged red blood cells results in splenomegaly, which leads to increased trapping of red blood cells and worsening anemia. Increased but ineffective erythropoiesis can cause bony deformities, resulting in severe disfigurement of the pelvis, spine, and skull (Olivieri 1999); facial deformities, including frontal bossing, overgrowth of the maxillae, and a prominent malar eminence (Raiola et al. 2003); and shortening of the limbs. Iron deposition may cause endocrine (hypogonadism, secondary amenorrhea, short stature) and cardiac (arrhythmias, congestive heart failure) complications (Cunningham 2008). A more comprehensive look at classification of specific clinical manifestations can be found in Cunningham (2008).

Alpha-Thalassemia

Silent carriers (α+) manifest no clinical symptoms. In alpha-thalassemia *trait,* patients generally do not have symptoms but may have microcytosis, hypochromia and are at risk of later carrying a baby with a more severe alpha-thalassemia *syndrome* (Rappaport et al. 2004). In hemoglobin H disease, patients suffer from symptomatic anemia with microcytosis and hypochromia. It is usually mild, but some patients may develop severe hemolytic anemia with hepatosplenomegaly.

Beta-Thalassemia

Silent carriers (β+) are clinically asymptomatic. In beta-thalassemia *minor,* patients have mild anemia, microcytosis, and hypochromia. In beta-thalassemia *intermedia,* patients may infrequently require red blood cell transfusions. Patients with beta-thalassemia *major* have severe anemia and hepatosplenomegaly and may require more than eight red blood cell transfusions per year. Without treatment, these patients will die in childhood (Cunningham 2008). Patients with beta-thalassemia intermedia and major are at risk for transient ischemic attacks and silent brain infarcts (Armstrong 2005).

Treatment

In severe forms of thalassemia, patients require red blood cell transfusions to avoid growth retardation, congestive heart failure, severe bony defects, and endocrinopathies (Schrier and Angelucci 2005). Transfusions are generally based on the severity of the anemia (Olivieri 1999). During pregnancy, rapid growth periods, and infection-associated aplastic crises, more frequent transfusions may be necessary (Borgna-Pignatti 2007; Nassar et al. 2006). Globally and prior to available screening, transfusions carried a risk of red blood cell alloimmunization and transmission of HIV and hepatitis B and C (Schrier and Angelucci 2005).

Regular red blood cell transfusions are associated with iron overload and/or hemosiderosis (Schrier and Angelucci 2005), which may result in cirrhosis, diabetes mellitus, hypothyroidism, hypoparathyroidism, growth failure, sexual immaturity, and cardiac dysfunction (Olivieri 1999). In order to prevent hemosiderosis, patients are treated with iron chelators, usually deferoxamine infusion or oral deferasirox. Currently, the only curative treatment is bone marrow transplant. Gene therapy seems promising but currently is still investigational (Olivieri 1999; Schrier and Angelucci 2005).

Psychosocial Aspects

Prior to the advent of effective therapies and early diagnosis, severely affected individuals rarely survived past early adulthood. Thalassemia may cause psychological problems, as it is an early-onset chronic illness. Frequent hospitalizations, long-term medication use, and a restricted social life are common (Ghanizadeh et al. 2006). Few studies have formally examined the psychosocial issues faced by adults; most of the literature focuses on children and their families. Common issues in children include denial and acting out, body image concerns, depression, anxiety, and impaired self-esteem (Shakin and Thompson 1991). Patients with thalassemia have an increased risk of developing psychosocial disturbances, especially in regard to physical appearance (bony deformities, delayed or absent sexual development, and/or growth retardation), which may result in poor self-esteem (Vardaki et al. 2004).

The incidence of psychiatric disorders varies widely among patients with thalassemia. Most studies cite depression as the most common psychiatric diagnosis in patients with thalassemia. Fifty percent of patients suffer from a depressed mood, and 60% or more report irritability and anger (Ghanizadeh et al. 2006). Psychological sources of depression include the impact of chronic disease and treatment, poor self-esteem related to physical appearance, impaired fertility, and loss of peers or siblings with the disease (Bush et al. 1998; Telfer et al. 2005).

Depression also may be due to organic causes, such as zinc deficiency (Jeejeebhoy 2007; Maes et al. 1994; Nowak et al. 2005) resulting from regular deferoxamine injections (Lanskowsky et al. 2000; Lukens 1993). Several studies have found that patients with major depression have significantly lower serum zinc levels (Manser et al. 1989; McLoughlin and Hodge 1990; Moafi et al. 2008; Nowak and Szewczyk 2002), although this has not been linked specifically to thalassemia.

Frequent transfusions, hospitalizations, and overnight chelator infusions disrupt daily activities. Schooling can be adversely affected from frequent absences due to illness (Di Palma et al. 1998). Children with thalassemia may have lower mean verbal IQ scores than unaffected children (Sherman et al. 1985). Several studies have found that thalassemic children have impaired abstract reasoning and deficits in attention and memory (Monastero et al. 2000; Zafeiriou et al. 2006). They also suffer from problems with visual-spatial skills and executive functioning (Monastero et al. 2000). Likewise, one study found that adults with beta-thalassemia major exhibited impairments on tests of abstract reasoning, attention/processing speed, language abilities, memory, and visual-constructional skills (Armstrong 2005). Cognitive deficits could be a result of chronic anemia. Alternatively, treatment complications such as iron deposits in the brain from multiple transfusions may contribute to cognitive deficits, which are more pronounced in hemosiderotic patients (Armstrong 2005). Patients with beta-thalassemia intermedia/major also are at risk for transient ischemic attacks and silent brain infarctions, which also may result in neurocognitive deficits (Armstrong 2005).

Most literature supports a multidisciplinary approach to treatment. In places where medical care is combined with psychosocial support, patients show improved social integration and acceptance. They are more likely to finish school and to go on to higher education (McAnarney 1985). Many are able to establish relationships with peers, marry, and start a family (Politis et al. 1990; Psihogios et al. 2002).

Psychiatric illness has been found to have a significant impact on compliance; one study found psychiatric disorders present in 68% of patients who were noncompliant with deferoxamine, but in only 10% of compliant patients (Beratis 1989).

Both psychosocial support and improved doctor–patient communication have been shown to increase compliance with treatment (Bush et al. 1998). It has been recommended that patients receive an annual assessment of their psychological life as part of their routine medical care (Ratip et al. 1995; Tsiantis 1990). Other recommendations include group meetings, support groups for families, patient education, and encouragement of self-management (Masera et al. 1990). It has been found that children with a limited understanding of their disease have poorer psychiatric adjustment (Sherman et al. 1985). It has been recommended that thalassemia clinics be organized so as to minimize disruption to daily activities, such as schooling and employment, by scheduling treatments during evenings or weekends (Telfer et al. 2005).

Fear of Blood Transfusions

In the early 1980s, many patients were infected with transfusion-transmitted HIV and hepatitis viruses. At this time, the risk for transfusion-related hepatitis C infection was as high as 1 in 200 units, and in some cities, the risk for transfusion-related HIV infection was as high as 1 in 100 units. By 1997, the risk for transfusion-related infection had decreased to 1 in 100,000 units for hepatitis C and 1 in 680,000 units for HIV. Due to careful screening and testing of blood donors, improved ability to detect bloodborne pathogens, as well as technology to inactivate viruses in blood products, the blood supply in the United States is now safer than it has ever been, and the risk for transfusion-related viral infection is lower than ever (AuBuchon et al. 1997). Despite improvements in transfusion safety, however, concern persists among the general public. Even though physicians and experts view blood transfusion risks as low, substantial proportions of the population perceive transfusions as risky and are not willing to receive allogeneic blood. Some question the safety of blood transfusions and overestimate the likelihood of contracting transfusion-related HIV infection (Slovic 1987). Even though transfusions of blood are perceived as beneficial, the fear of contracting HIV and the perception that the blood supply is not safe remains the dominant concern for those who decline allogeneic blood transfusions. Instead of viewing risk as a unidimensional probability-based variable, people's perception of the risk varies with their life experiences, beliefs, values, trust, worldviews, gender, skin color, personal characteristics, and cognitive abilities (Finucane et al. 2000; D. Lee 2006). People differ in their beliefs about what is risky for them, and physicians need to balance the need for blood products with a reasonable discussion of the risks associated with the administration of blood products or with the refusal of such treatment. Some patients' fears of transfusion are unrelated to the fear of infection; fear of blood and fear of needles are some of the most common phobias (Bienvenu and Eaton 1998).

Psychological Factors Affecting Clotting Disorders

In healthy individuals, psychological states such as major depression and anxiety may trigger the formation of blood clots (possibly via release of fibrinogen or von Willebrand's factor) and fibrinolysis (possibly via release of tissue-type plasminogen activator) (von Kanel et al. 2001). In patients with atherosclerosis and impaired endothelial cell function, procoagulant responses to acute psychosocial stressors may be more important than anticoagulant mechanisms and therefore promote a hypercoagulable state (von Kanel et al. 2001). A reduction in fibrinolytic capacity and an increase in procoagulant molecules (i.e., coagulation factor VIII or fibrinogen) have been reported in individuals with persistent psychosocial stressors such as job strain, general life stress, depression or hopelessness, anxiety, neuroticism, negative affect, and low socioeconomic status (Chida and Hamer 2008; Geiser et al. 2008; Thrall et al. 2007; von Kanel et al. 2001, 2004a, 2004b, 2005, 2006). Among patients with anxiety (e.g., panic disorder with agoraphobia or social phobia), fibrinolysis and the coagulation cascade may be activated toward a more hypercoagulable state (Geiser et al. 2008). In individuals without cardiovascular disease, depression may activate the inflammation and coagulation cascade system, which may lead to thrombosis. A positive correlation between markers of thrombosis and depression was demonstrated in patients with major depressive disorder who did not have any cardiovascular disease (Panagiotakos et al. 2004). Patients with major depression and anxiety disorders are at increased risk of thrombosis, which can predispose them to coronary artery disease (Geiser et al. 2008; Kop et al. 1998; Panagiotakos et al. 2004; Thrall et al. 2007).

Hematological Side Effects and Drug Interactions of Psychotropic Agents

Antipsychotics

Various psychotropics and their potential hematological side effects are listed in Table 24–1; potential interactions with anticoagulants are listed in Table 24–2. Antipsychotic agents with no reported hematological side effects include aripiprazole and ziprasidone. Hematological adverse effects of antipsychotics include agranulocytosis, aplastic anemia, neutropenia, eosinophilia, and thrombocytopenia.

Agranulocytosis is rare except with clozapine, but it is the most common and most serious hematological side effect of the antipsychotics (Buckley and Meltzer 1995; Flanagan and Dunk 2008; Gareri et al. 2008; Rajagopal 2005; Sedky et al. 2005). Low-potency antipsychotics have a higher frequency of agranulocytosis than high-potency ones. Clozapine causes agranulocytosis in 0.8% of patients (Flanagan and Dunk 2008; Guzelcan and Scholte 2006; Opgen-Rhein and Dettling 2008). The highest risk of clozapine-induced agranulocytosis is present during the first 6 months of treatment and then decreases significantly. The case fatality rate of clozapine-induced agranulocytosis is estimated as 4.2%–16%, depending on whether a granulocyte colony-stimulating factor (G-CSF) is used (Schulte 2006). A weekly white blood cell (WBC) count is necessary to detect and monitor for clozapine-induced agranulocytosis (Opgen-Rhein and Dettling 2008). A WBC count lower than 2,000/mm^3 or an absolute neutrophil count (ANC) lower than 1,000/mm^3 is an indication for immediate cessation of clozapine. Stopping clozapine usually leads to recovery in WBC counts within 3 weeks (Berk et al. 2007; Folkenberg 1990; Opgen-Rhein and Dettling 2008). The mortality risk associated with agranulocytosis is significantly increased if infection occurs before the drug is stopped (Gerson and Meltzer 1992; McEvoy et al. 2006). Because clozapine causes bone marrow suppression, G-CSF therapy may help restore normal bone marrow production (Gerson and Meltzer 1992; Lieberman and Alvir 1992; Sedky and Lippmann 2006). Patients with history of clozapine-induced agranulocytosis should be closely monitored in cases of reintroduction. However, the level of risk following reintroduction of clozapine is currently unknown.

Antidepressants

Selective serotonin reuptake inhibitors (SSRIs) inhibit platelet function and have been associated with bruising and bleeding, especially with concomitant use of aspirin or nonsteroidal anti-inflammatory drugs (NSAIDs) (Andreasen et al. 2006; de Abajo et al. 2006; Goldberg 1998; Mort et al. 2006; Turner et al. 2007; Wessinger et al. 2006). SSRIs increase CNS 5-hydroxytryptamine (5-HT; serotonin) and reduce 5-HT in platelets (leading to reduced platelet aggregation). Platelets normally release serotonin at the site of a vascular tear, leading to further platelet aggregation and vasodilatation and permitting the sealing of the tear without thrombosis of the vessel (Hourani and Cusack 1991).

Especially in the elderly, bleeding from the upper gastrointestinal tract may occur at a frequency ranging from 1 in 100 to 1 in 1,000 patient-years of exposure to drugs, such as the SSRIs, that have high affinity to 5-HT (de Abajo et al. 2006). The likelihood of gastrointestinal bleeding with SSRIs is similar to low dose NSAIDs (Weinrieb et al. 2005). Caution is advised in patients at high risk of gastrointestinal bleeding, for whom clinicians may consider prescribing an antidepressant with low serotonin reuptake inhibition. Patients who are at risk for gastrointestinal hemorrhage and who are taking antidepressants with high serotonin reuptake inhibition should generally use smaller doses or avoid aspirin and NSAIDs (Loke et al. 2008; Mansour et al. 2006; Serebruany 2006; Weinrieb et al. 2005). Whereas some studies have reported no associated risk of increased gastrointestinal bleeding in patients taking both SSRIs and NSAIDs (Schalekamp et al. 2008; Vidal et al. 2008), others have reported an increased risk of gastrointestinal bleeding among this group of patients (Loke et al. 2008; Weinrieb et al. 2005). Although the evidence to date indicates that SSRIs do not cause intracranial bleeding (Ramasubbu 2004), there is one report that patients taking SSRIs along with statins had a higher risk for subarachnoid hemorrhage-related vasospasm (Singhal et al. 2005). Pharmacovigilance is prudent when SSRIs are used in patients at high risk for hemorrhagic and vasoconstrictive stroke (Ramasubbu 2004).

Although some reviews have concluded there is no increased risk from combining SSRIs with warfarin (Kurdyak et al. 2005), there have been case reports of bleeding with concomitant use of warfarin and the SSRIs. Among the SSRIs, fluoxetine is the most commonly reported offending agent (Skop and Brown 1996). The interactions between warfarin and antidepressants can have potentially serious consequences, resulting from either platelet inhibition or inhibition of the cytochrome P450 (CYP) system. Of the antidepressants, fluoxetine, fluvoxamine, and paroxetine appear to have the highest potential for interactions (Duncan et al. 1998; Halperin and Reber 2007), while citalopram and sertraline may be relatively less likely to interact with warfarin (Duncan et al. 1998) (see also Chapter 38, "Psychopharmacology," Table 38–2 [Drugs with clinically significant pharmacokinetic interactions]).

Agranulocytosis due to tricyclic antidepressants (TCAs) is a rare, idiosyncratic condition caused by direct bone mar-

TABLE 24–1. Psychotropic medications and hematological side effects

Psychotropic agent	Hematological side effects
Antipsychotics	
Conventional agents	Agranulocytosis, anemia (aplastic, hemolytic), eosinophilia, leukopenia, thrombocytopenia
Atypical agents	
Clozapine	Agranulocytosis (1%–2%), eosinophilia, leukocytosis, leukopenia, thrombocytopenia
Other atypicals	Anemia, leukopenia, thrombocytopenia
Antidepressants	
Tricyclic antidepressants	Agranulocytosis, eosinophilia, leukopenia, thrombocytopenia
Serotonin-norepinephrine reuptake inhibitors	Impaired platelet aggregation
Monoamine oxidase inhibitors	
Tranylcypromine	Thrombocytopenia
Selective serotonin reuptake inhibitors	Impaired platelet aggregation
Serotonin$_2$ receptor antagonism with serotonin reuptake blockade	
Trazodone	Agranulocytosis
Alpha$_2$ antagonism plus serotonin$_2$ and serotonin3 antagonism	
Mirtazapine	Agranulocytosis, thrombocytopenia
Benzodiazepines	Agranulocytosis (reported but not proven)
Mood stabilizers	
Carbamazepine	Agranulocytosis, anemia, eosinophilia, leukocytosis, leukopenia, pure red cell aplasia, thrombocytopenia
Gabapentin	Leukopenia, neutropenia
Lamotrigine	Agranulocytosis, anemia, neutropenia, pancytopenia, pure red cell aplasia, thrombocytopenia
Lithium	Leukocytosis, thrombocytosis
Phenytoin	Agranulocytosis, granulocytopenia, leukopenia, pancytopenia (with or without bone marrow suppression), thrombocytopenia
Tiagabine	Ecchymosis
Topiramate	Anemia, thrombocytopenia
Valproic acid	Pure red cell aplasia, thrombocytopenia
Zonisamide	Anemia, leukopenia

Note. Some of the reports are based on single cases, and therefore validity is not certain.

Sources. Data from Cimo et al. 1977; Damiani and Christensen 2000; Derbyshire and Martin 2004; Fadul et al. 2002; Lexi-Drugs 2007; Micromedex 2007; Mosby Drug Consult 2007; Opgen-Rhein and Dettling 2008; Physicians' Desk Reference 2007; Stahl 1998.

Reprinted and adapted with permission from Saunders/Elsevier: (1) Shakin EJ, Thompson TL: "Psychiatric Aspects of Hematologic Disorders," in *Medical-Psychiatric Practice,* Volume 1. Edited by Stoudemire A, Fogel BS. Washington, DC, American Psychiatric Press, 1991, pp. 193–242 (Shakin and Thompson 1991); (2) Shakin EJ, Thompson TL: "Hematologic Disorders," in *Psychiatric Care of the Medical Patient.* Edited by Stoudemire A, Fogel BS, Oxford University Press, 1993, pp. 691–712 (Shakin and Thompson 1993); (3) Kunkel EJS, Thompson TL, Oyesanmi O: "Hematologic Disorders," in *Psychiatric Care of the Medical Patient,* 2nd Edition. Edited by Stoudemire A, Fogel BS, Greenberg D. New York, Oxford University Press, 2000, pp. 835–856 (Kunkel et al. 2000).

TABLE 24–2. Psychotropic medications and their possible interactions with anticoagulants

Psychotropic agent	Interaction with anticoagulant
Antidepressants	
Tricyclic antidepressants	Increased bleeding with warfarin anticoagulants[a]
Selective serotonin reuptake inhibitors	Increased INR with warfarin (fluvoxamine, fluoxetine, paroxetine)
Mood stabilizers	
Carbamazepine (CBZ)	Reduced INR with warfarin; CBZ increases metabolism of warfarin by inducing hepatic metabolism Warfarin decreases effect of CBZ
Anticonvulsants	
Phenobarbital	Reduces INR by inducing hepatic metabolism

Note. Some of the reports are based on single cases, and therefore validity is not certain.
[a]Although some reports suggest that imipramine may alter the anticoagulant effect of warfarin by unknown mechanism, a more recent study (Yoo et al. 2009) concluded that there is no allosteric effect or competition between both drugs. Until additional information is presented, it may be advisable to monitor the International Normalized Ratio (INR) and clinical response if both drugs are to be administered.
Sources. Data from Buckley and Meltzer 1995; Jenkins and Hansen 1995; Physicians' Desk Reference 2007; Rosse et al. 1989.
Reprinted and adapted with permission from Saunders/Elsevier: (1) Shakin EJ, Thompson TL: "Psychiatric Aspects of Hematologic Disorders," in *Medical-Psychiatric Practice,* Volume 1. Edited by Stoudemire A, Fogel BS. Washington, DC, American Psychiatric Press, 1991, pp. 193–242 (Shakin and Thompson 1991); (2) Shakin EJ, Thompson TL: "Hematologic Disorders," in *Psychiatric Care of the Medical Patient.* Edited by Stoudemire A, Fogel BS, Oxford University Press, 1993, pp. 691–712 (Shakin and Thompson 1993); (3) Kunkel EJS, Thompson TL, Oyesanmi O: "Hematologic Disorders," in *Psychiatric Care of the Medical Patient,* 2nd Edition. Edited by Stoudemire A, Fogel BS, Greenberg D. New York, Oxford University Press, 2000, pp. 835–856 (Kunkel et al. 2000).

row toxicity, with a lower frequency than is reported for antipsychotics (Oyesanmi et al. 1999). Agranulocytosis has been associated with imipramine (Albertini and Penders 1978; Gravenor 1986), clomipramine (Alderman et al. 1993; Gravenor et al. 1986; Souhami et al. 1976), and desipramine (Crammer and Elkes 1967; Hardin and Conrath 1982). Clomipramine-induced agranulocytosis may be treated with recombinant G-CSF (Hunt and Resnick 1993).

Benzodiazepines

Agranulocytosis has rarely been reported with the benzodiazepines, but no causal relationship has been established. There is no relationship between the daily dose or total cumulative dose and the occurrence of hematological side effects (Moss 1980).

Lithium

Lithium stimulates leukocytosis with a true proliferative response. In patients on lithium therapy for cluster headaches, Medina and colleagues (Albertini and Penders 1978; Medina et al. 1980) documented increases in the number of platelets and in platelet serotonin and histamine levels. In the past, because of its hematological side effects, lithium therapy was considered for persistent leukopenia and thrombocytopenia following chemotherapy or radiotherapy; however, more effective therapies are now available.

Anticonvulsants and Mood Stabilizers

Carbamazepine should be avoided in patients with a history of bone marrow depression. Carbamazepine produces a transient reduction in WBC count in approximately 10% of patients during the first 4 months of treatment (Rall and Schleifer 1980). Very rarely it can cause potentially fatal agranulocytosis and aplastic anemia. Agranulocytosis results from direct toxicity to the bone marrow (Sedky and Lippmann 2006). A baseline complete blood count (CBC) is always advised before starting carbamazepine. Carbamazepine should be discontinued if the WBC count drops below 3,500/mm^3. Administration of lithium and carbamazepine concurrently may lower the risk of carbamazepine-induced neutropenia, because lithium stimulates WBC production, predominantly neutrophils (Kramlinger and Post 1990). Carbamazepine induces its own metabolism. Thus, after taking the drug for a period of time, the amount of carbamazepine in the blood will suddenly decrease. Because carbamazepine induces CYP1A2, 2C, and 3A4, it reduces the anticoagulant effect of warfarin, so both the carbamazepine level and the international normalized ratio will need to be monitored frequently when both drugs are used (Herman et al. 2006; Whiskey and Taylor 2007).

Valproate-induced increases in red blood cell mean corpuscular volume (MCV) and mean corpuscular hemoglobin concentration (MCHC) have been postulated to result from alterations in erythrocyte membrane phospholipids (Ozkara et al. 1993). Potentially fatal hematopoietic complications such as neutropenia, thrombocytopenia, and macrocytic anemia have been associated with valproate (Acharya and Bussel 2000; Dulcan et al. 1995; Nasreddine and Beydoun 2008). Lamotrigine also may cause agranulocytosis (de Camargo and Bode 1999; Fadul et al. 2002). All anticonvulsants should be discontinued if the WBC count drops below 3,000/mm^3 (Ramsay 1994).

Acetylcholinesterase Inhibitors

Donepezil is associated with anemia, thrombocythemia, thrombocytopenia, ecchymosis, and eosinophilia. The mechanism for the hematological side effects is unknown. Purpura occurs in up to 2% of patients on tacrine. Only one case of agranulocytosis has been reported with tacrine (Micromedex 2007). Rivastigmine has been reported to cause anemia, and galantamine can cause epistaxis, purpura, and thrombocytopenia (Mosby Drug Consult 2007).

Conclusion

Iron deficiency anemia primarily is associated with changes in mood and cognition. Vitamin B_{12} deficiency is associated with problems in cognition, mood, psychosis, and (less commonly) anxiety. Folate deficiency primarily is associated with problems in mood. Patients who have sickle cell disease, a disease of chronic pain, experience difficulties with depression, anxiety, and stigma and are at risk for substance abuse and dependence. Patients with hemophilia have benefited from advances in treatment; however, their morbidity and mortality were compromised if they received blood products contaminated with HIV, hepatitis B, or hepatitis C. Depression is the most common psychiatric diagnosis associated with thalassemia. Some psychiatric disorders are associated with hypercoagulable states as well.

Most of the commonly used psychotropic medications have uncommon but potentially important hematological side effects or may interact with the anticoagulants used in medically ill patients. In this group of patients, hematological side effects may affect quality of life and contribute to medication noncompliance. When the administration of potentially interacting psychotropic drugs cannot be avoided, these side effects may be reduced by monitoring clinical response and serum drug levels. Psychiatrists who practice psychosomatic medicine should expect to encounter patients with the problems addressed in this chapter, which are frequently seen in medical settings.

References

Acharya S, Bussel JB: Hematologic toxicity of sodium valproate. J Pediatr Hematol Oncol 22:62–65, 2000

Adams RJ: Neurological complications, in Sickle Cell Disease: Basic Principles and Clinical Practice. Edited by Mohandas N, Steinberg MH. New York, Raven, 1994, pp 560–621

Alao AO, Westmoreland N, Jindal S: Drug addiction in sickle cell disease: case report. Int J Psychiatry Med 33:97–101, 2003

Albertini RS, Penders TM: Agranulocytosis associated with tricyclics. J Clin Psychiatry 39:483–485, 1978

Alderman CP, Atchison MM, McNeece JI: Concurrent agranulocytosis and hepatitis secondary to clomipramine therapy. Br J Psychiatry 162:688–689, 1993

Andreasen JJ, Riis A, Hjortdal VE, et al: Effect of selective serotonin reuptake inhibitors on requirement for allogeneic red blood cell transfusion following coronary artery bypass surgery. Am J Cardiovasc Drugs 6:243–250, 2006

Andres E, Loukili NH, Noel E, et al: Vitamin B12 (cobalamin) deficiency in elderly patients. CMAJ 171:251–259, 2004

Andres E, Dali-Youcef N, Vogel T, et al: Oral cobalamin (vitamin B12) treatment: an update. Int J Lab Hematol 31:1–8, 2009

Anie KA: Psychological complications in sickle cell disease. Br J Haematol 129:723–729, 2005

Annibale B, Capurso G, Delle Fave G: The stomach and iron deficiency anaemia: a forgotten link. Dig Liver Dis 35:288–295, 2003

Armstrong FD: Thalassemia and learning: neurocognitive functioning in children. Ann N Y Acad Sci 1054:283–289, 2005

AuBuchon JP, Birkmeyer JD, Busch MP: Safety of the blood supply in the United States: opportunities and controversies. Ann Intern Med 127:904–909, 1997

Balk EM, Raman G, Tatsioni A, et al: Vitamin B6, B12, and folic acid supplementation and cognitive function: a systematic review of randomized trials. Arch Intern Med 167:21–30, 2007

Ballas SK: Sickle Cell Pain: Progress in Pain Research and Management. Seattle, WA, IASP Press, 1998

Bauman WA, Shaw S, Jayatilleke E, et al: Increased intake of calcium reverses vitamin B12 malabsorption induced by metformin. Diabetes Care 23:1227–1231, 2000

Beard JL, Hendricks MK, Perez EM, et al: Maternal iron deficiency anemia affects postpartum emotions and cognition. J Nutr 135:267–272, 2005

Benton TD, Ifeagwu JA, Smith-Whitley K: Anxiety and depression in children and adolescents with sickle cell disease. Curr Psychiatry Rep 9:114–121, 2007

Beratis S: Noncompliance with iron chelation therapy in patients with beta thalassaemia. J Psychosom Res 33:739–745, 1989

Berk M, Fitzsimons J, Lambert T, et al: Monitoring the safe use of clozapine: a consensus view from Victoria, Australia. CNS Drugs 21:117–127, 2007

Bienvenu OJ, Eaton WW: The epidemiology of blood-injection-injury phobia. Psychol Med 28:1129–1136, 1998

Bolton-Maggs PH, Pasi KJ: Haemophilias A and B. Lancet 361:1801–1809, 2003

Booth IW, Aukett MA: Iron deficiency anaemia in infancy and early childhood. Arch Dis Child 76:549–553; discussion 553–554, 1997

Borgna-Pignatti C: Modern treatment of thalassaemia intermedia. Br J Haematology 138:291–304, 2007

Bottiglieri T, Laundy M, Crellin R, et al: Homocysteine, folate, methylation, and monoamine metabolism in depression. J Neurol Neurosurg Psychiatry 69:228–232, 2000

Brookoff D, Polomano R: Treating sickle cell pain like cancer pain. Ann Intern Med 116:364–368, 1992

Buckley PF, Meltzer HY: Treatment of schizophrenia, in Textbook of Psychopharmacology. Edited by Schatzberg AF, Nemeroff CB. Washington, DC, American Psychiatric Press, 1995, pp 615–639

Burlew K, Telfair J, Colangelo L, et al: Factors that influence adolescent adaptation to sickle cell disease. J Pediatr Psychol 25:287–299, 2000

Bush S, Mandel FS, Giardina PJ: Future orientation and life expectations of adolescents and young adults with thalassemia major. Ann N Y Acad Sci 850:361–369, 1998

Bussing R, Burket RC: Anxiety and intrafamilial stress in children with hemophilia after the HIV crisis. J Am Acad Child Adolesc Psychiatry 32:562–567, 1993

Carmel R, Green R, Rosenblatt DS, et al: Update on cobalamin, folate, and homocysteine. Hematology Am Soc Hematol Educ Program 62–81, 2003

Carney MW, Chary TK, Laundy M, et al: Red cell folate concentrations in psychiatric patients. J Affect Disord 19:207–213, 1990

Casey RL, Brown RT: Psychological aspects of hematologic diseases. Child Adolesc Psychiatr Clin N Am 12:567–584, 2003

Cepeda ML, Allen FH, Cepeda NJ, et al: Physical growth, sexual maturation, body image and sickle cell disease. J Natl Med Assoc 92:10–14, 2000

Chalouhi C, Faesch S, Anthoine-Milhomme MC, et al: Neurological consequences of vitamin B12 deficiency and its treatment. Pediatr Emerg Care 24:538–541, 2008

Chapman SL, Byas-Smith MG, Reed BA: Effects of intermediate- and long-term use of opioids on cognition in patients with chronic pain. Clin J Pain 18 (4 suppl):S83–S90, 2002

Chida Y, Hamer M: Chronic psychosocial factors and acute physiological responses to laboratory-induced stress in healthy populations: a quantitative review of 30 years of investigations. Psychol Bull 134:829–885, 2008

Choumenkovitch SF, Jacques PF, Nadeau MR, et al: Folic acid fortification increases red blood cell folate concentrations in the Framingham study. J Nutr 131:3277–3280, 2001

Choumenkovitch SF, Selhub J, Wilson PW, et al: Folic acid intake from fortification in United States exceeds predictions. J Nutr 132:2792–2798, 2002

Cimo PL, Pisciotta AV, Desai RG, et al: Detection of drug-dependent antibodies by the 51Cr platelet lysis test: documentation of immune thrombocytopenia induced by diphenylhydantoin, diazepam, and sulfisoxazole. Am J Hematol 2:65–72, 1977

Clarke R, Sherliker P, Hin H, et al: Folate and vitamin B12 status in relation to cognitive impairment and anaemia in the setting of voluntary fortification in the UK. Br J Nutr 100:1054–1059, 2008

Coban E, Timuragaoglu A, Meric M: Iron deficiency anemia in the elderly: prevalence and endoscopic evaluation of the gastrointestinal tract in outpatients. Acta Haematol 110:25–28, 2003

Cook JD, Skikne BS: Iron deficiency: definition and diagnosis. J Intern Med 226:349–355, 1989

Coppen A, Bailey J: Enhancement of the antidepressant action of fluoxetine by folic acid: a randomised, placebo controlled trial. J Affect Disord 60:121–130, 2000

Crammer JL, Elkes A: Agranulocytosis after desipramine. Lancet 1(7481):105–106, 1967

Cunningham MJ: Update on thalassemia: clinical care and complications. Pediatr Clin North Am 55:447–460, ix, 2008

Damiani JT, Christensen RC: Lamotrigine-associated neutropenia in a geriatric patient. Am J Geriatr Psychiatry 8:346, 2000

de Abajo FJ, Montero D, Rodriguez LA, et al: Antidepressants and risk of upper gastrointestinal bleeding. Basic Clin Pharmacol Toxicol 98:304–310, 2006

de Camargo OA, Bode H: Agranulocytosis associated with lamotrigine. BMJ (Clin Res) 318:1179, 1999

Derbyshire E, Martin D: Neutropenia occurring after starting gabapentin for neuropathic pain. Clin Oncol (R Coll Radiol) 16:575–576, 2004

Di Palma A, Vullo C, Zani B, et al: Psychosocial integration of adolescents and young adults with thalassemia major. Ann N Y Acad Sci 850:355–360, 1998

Dietrich M, Brown CJ, Block G: The effect of folate fortification of cereal-grain products on blood folate status, dietary folate intake, and dietary folate sources among adult non-supplement users in the United States. J Am Coll Nutr 24:266–274, 2005

Dorland's Illustrated Medical Dictionary, 30th Edition. Philadelphia, PA, WB Saunders, 2003

Dulcan MK, Bregman JD, Weller BE, et al: Treatment of childhood and adolescent disorders, in Textbook of Psychopharmacology. Edited by Schatzberg AF, Nemeroff CB. Washington, DC, American Psychiatric Press, 1995, pp 680–697

Duncan D, Sayal K, McConnell H, et al: Antidepressant interactions with warfarin. Int Clin Psychopharmacol 13:87–94, 1998

Durga J, van Boxtel MP, Schouten EG, et al: Effect of 3-year folic acid supplementation on cognitive function in older adults in the FACIT trial: a randomised, double blind, controlled trial. Lancet 369:208–216, 2007

Elander J, Barry T: Analgesic use and pain coping among patients with haemophilia. Haemophilia 9:202–213, 2003

Fadul CE, Meyer LP, Jobst BC, et al: Agranulocytosis associated with lamotrigine in a patient with low-grade glioma. Epilepsia 43:199–200, 2002

Fava M, Borus JS, Alpert JE, et al: Folate, vitamin B12, and homocysteine in major depressive disorder. Am J Psychiatry 154:426–428, 1997

Finucane ML, Slovic P, Mertz CK: Public perception of the risk of blood transfusion. Transfusion 40:1017–1022, 2000

Flanagan RJ, Dunk L: Haematological toxicity of drugs used in psychiatry. Hum Psychopharmacol 23 (suppl 1):27–41, 2008

Folkenberg J: New schizophrenia drug; balancing hope with safety. FDA Consumer, June 1990. Available at: http://findarticles.com/p/articles/mi_m1370/is_n5_v24/ai_9155643. Accessed August 2010.

Ford AH, Flicker L, Thomas J, et al: Vitamins B12, B6, and folic acid for onset of depressive symptoms in older men: results from a 2-year placebo-controlled randomized trial. J Clin Psychiatry 69:1203–1209, 2008

Gareri P, De Fazio P, Russo E, et al: The safety of clozapine in the elderly. Exp Opin Drug Saf 7:525–538, 2008

Geiser F, Meier C, Wegener I, et al: Association between anxiety and factors of coagulation and fibrinolysis. Psychother Psychosom 77:377–383, 2008

Gerson SL, Meltzer H: Mechanisms of clozapine-induced agranulocytosis. Drug Saf 7 (suppl 1):17–25, 1992

Gerstner T, Teich M, Bell N, et al: Valproate-associated coagulopathies are frequent and variable in children. Epilepsia 47:1136–1143, 2006

Ghanizadeh A, Khajavian S, Ashkani H: Prevalence of psychiatric disorders, depression, and suicidal behavior in child and adolescent with thalassemia major. J Pediatr Hematol Oncol 28:781–784, 2006

Goldberg RJ: Selective serotonin reuptake inhibitors: infrequent medical adverse effects. Arch Fam Med 7:78–84, 1998

Gravenor DS, Leclerc JR, Blake G: Tricyclic antidepressant agranulocytosis. Can J Psychiatry 31:661, 1986

Guzelcan Y, Scholte WF: Clozapine-induced agranulocytosis: genetic risk factors and an immunologic explanatory model [in Dutch]. Tijdschrift Voor Psychiatrie 48:295–302, 2006

Hallberg L, Hulthen L, Bengtsson C, et al: Iron balance in menstruating women. Eur J Clin Nutr 49:200–207, 1995

Halperin D, Reber G: Influence of antidepressants on hemostasis. Dialogues Clin Neurosci 9:47–59, 2007

Halterman JS, Kaczorowski JM, Aligne CA, et al: Iron deficiency and cognitive achievement among school-aged children and adolescents in the United States. Pediatrics 107:1381–1386, 2001

Hardin TC, Conrath FC: Desipramine-induced agranulocytosis. A case report. Drug Intell Clin Pharm 16:62–63, 1982

Hariman LM, Griffith ER, Hurtig AL, et al: Functional outcomes of children with sickle-cell disease affected by stroke. Arch Phys Med Rehab 72:498–502, 1991

Herman D, Locatelli I, Grabnar I, et al: The influence of co-treatment with carbamazepine, amiodarone and statins on warfarin metabolism and maintenance dose. Eur J Clin Pharmacol 62:291–296, 2006

Homocysteine Lowering Trialists' Collaboration: Dose-dependent effects of folic acid on blood concentrations of homocysteine: a meta-analysis of the randomized trials. Am J Clin Nutr 82:806–812, 2005

Hourani SM, Cusack NJ: Pharmacological receptors on blood platelets. Pharmacol Rev 43:243–298, 1991

Hunt KA, Resnick MP: Clomipramine-induced agranulocytosis and its treatment with G-CSF. Am J Psychiatry 150:522–523, 1993

Hurtig AL, Park KB: Adjustment and coping in adolescents with sickle cell disease. Ann N Y Acad Sci 565:172–182, 1989

Jacob E, American Pain Society: Pain management in sickle cell disease. Pain Manage Nurs 2:121–131, 2001

Jacques PF, Selhub J, Bostom AG, et al: The effect of folic acid fortification on plasma folate and total homocysteine concentrations. N Engl J Med 340:1449–1454, 1999

Jeejeebhoy KN: Human zinc deficiency. Nutr Clin Pract 22:65–67, 2007

Jenerette C, Funk M, Murdaugh C: Sickle cell disease: a stigmatizing condition that may lead to depression. Issues Ment Health Nurs 26:1081–1101, 2005

Jenkins SC, Hansen MR: A Pocket Reference for Psychiatrist, 2nd Edition. Washington, DC, American Psychiatric Press, 1995

Killip S, Bennett JM, Chambers MD: Iron deficiency anemia. Am Fam Physician 75:671–678, 2007

Kim JM, Stewart R, Kim SW, et al: Changes in folate, vitamin B12 and homocysteine associated with incident dementia. J Neurol Neurosurg Psychiatry 79:864–868, 2008a

Kim JM, Stewart R, Kim SW, et al: Predictive value of folate, vitamin B12 and homocysteine levels in late-life depression. Br J Psychiatry 192:268–274, 2008b

Kop WJ, Hamulyak K, Pernot C, et al: Relationship of blood coagulation and fibrinolysis to vital exhaustion. Psychosom Med 60:352–358, 1998

Kramlinger KG, Post RM: Addition of lithium carbonate to carbamazepine: hematological and thyroid effects. Am J Psychiatry 147:615–620, 1990

Krieger J, Schroeder C: Iron, brain and restless legs syndrome. Sleep Med Rev 5:277–286, 2001

Kulkarni R, Scott-Emuakpor AB, Brody H, et al: Nondisclosure of human immunodeficiency virus and hepatitis C virus coinfection in a patient with hemophilia: medical and ethical considerations. J Pediatr Hematol Oncol 23:153–158, 2001

Kunkel EJ, Thompson TL, Abdelgheni MB, et al: Hematologic disorders, in Psychiatric Care of the Medical Patient, 2nd Edition. Edited by Stoudemire A, Fogel BS, Greenberg DB. New York, Oxford University Press, 2000, pp 833–856

Kurdyak PA, Juurlink DN, Kopp A, et al: Antidepressants, warfarin, and the risk of hemorrhage. J Clin Psychopharmacol 25:561–564, 2005

Labbe E, Herbert D, Haynes J: Physicians' attitude and practices in sickle cell disease pain management. J Palliat Care 21:246–251, 2005

Lanskowsky P: Hemolytic anemia, in Manual of Pediatric Hematology and Oncology. Edited by Lanskowsky P. San Diego, CA, Academic Press, 2000, pp 137–201

Lee D: Perception of blood transfusion risk. Transfus Med Rev 20:141–148, 2006

Lee KA, Zaffke ME: Longitudinal changes in fatigue and energy during pregnancy and the postpartum period. J Obstet Gynecol Neonatal Nurs 28:183–191, 1999

Lerner V, Kanevsky M, Dwolatzky T, et al: Vitamin B12 and folate serum levels in newly admitted psychiatric patients. Clin Nutr 25:60–67, 2006

Lexi-Drugs [computer program]. Hudson, OH, Lexi-Comp, Inc., 2007

Levenson JL, McClish DK, Dahman BA, et al: Alcohol abuse in sickle cell disease: the Pisces Project. Am J Addict 16:383–388, 2007

Levenson JL, McClish DK, Dahman BA, et al: Depression and anxiety in adults with sickle cell disease: the PiSCES project. Psychosom Med 70:192–196, 2008

Lieberman JA, Alvir JM: A report of clozapine-induced agranulocytosis in the United States: incidence and risk factors. Drug Saf 7 (suppl 1):1–2, 1992

Liu JE, Gzesh DJ, Ballas SK: The spectrum of epilepsy in sickle cell anemia. J Neurol Sci 123:6–10, 1994

Liu KW, Dai LK, Jean W: Metformin-related vitamin B12 deficiency. Age Ageing 35:200–201, 2006

Loikas S, Koskinen P, Irjala K, et al: Vitamin B12 deficiency in the aged: a population-based study. Age Ageing 36:177–183, 2007

Loke YK, Trivedi AN, Singh S: Meta-analysis: gastrointestinal bleeding due to interaction between selective serotonin uptake inhibitors and non-steroidal anti-inflammatory drugs. Aliment Pharmacol Ther 27:31–40, 2008

Looker AC, Dallman PR, Carroll MD, et al: Prevalence of iron deficiency in the United States. JAMA 277:973–976, 1997

Lorey FW, Arnopp J, Cunningham GC: Distribution of hemoglobinopathy variants by ethnicity in a multiethnic state. Genet Epidemiol 13:501–512, 1996

Lozoff B: Behavioral alterations in iron deficiency. Adv Pediatr 35:331–359, 1988

Lozoff B, Brittenham GM, Viteri FE, et al: The effects of short term oral iron therapy on developmental deficits in iron-deficient anemic infants. J Pediatr 100:351–357, 1982

Lucca U, Tettamanti M, Mosconi P, et al: Association of mild anemia with cognitive, functional, mood and quality of life outcomes in the elderly: the "health and anemia" study. PLoS ONE 3:e1920, 2008

Luchsinger JA, Tang MX, Miller J, et al: Relation of higher folate intake to lower risk of Alzheimer disease in the elderly. Arch Neurol 64:86–92, 2007

Lucock M: Is folic acid the ultimate functional food component for disease prevention? BMJ (Clin Res) 328:211–214, 2004

Lukens JN: Thalassemias and related disorders: quantitative disorders of hemoglobin synthesis, in Wintrobe's Clinical Hematology, 9th Edition, Vol 1. Edited by Lee GR, Bithell TC, Foerster J, et al. Philadelphia, PA, Lea & Febiger, 1993, pp 1102–1145

Maes M, D'Haese PC, Scharpe S, et al: Hypozincemia in depression. J Affect Disord 31:135–140, 1994

Malinowski SS: Nutritional and metabolic complications of bariatric surgery. Am J Med Sci 331:219–225, 2006

Malouf M, Grimley EJ, Areosa SA: Folic acid with or without vitamin B12 for cognition and dementia. Cochrane Database Syst Rev (4):CD004514, 2003

Manco-Johnson M: Hemophilia management: optimizing treatment based on patient needs. Curr Opin Pediatr 17:3–6, 2005

Manser WW, Khan MA, Hasan Z: Trace element studies in Karachi populations, part III: blood copper, zinc, magnesium and lead levels in psychiatric patients with disturbed behaviour. J Pak Med Assoc 39:235–238, 1989

Mansour A, Pearce M, Johnson B, et al: Which patients taking SSRIs are at greatest risk of bleeding? J Fam Pract 55:206–208, 2006

Masera G, Monguzzi W, Tornotti G, et al: Psychosocial support in thalassemia major: Monza Center's experience. Haematologica 75 (suppl 5):181–190, 1990

McAnarney ER: Social maturation. A challenge for handicapped and chronically ill adolescents. J Adolesc Health Care 6:90–101, 1985

McEvoy JP, Lieberman JA, Stroup TS, et al: Effectiveness of clozapine versus olanzapine, quetiapine, and risperidone in patients with chronic schizophrenia who did not respond to prior atypical antipsychotic treatment. Am J Psychiatry 163:600–610, 2006

McLoughlin IJ, Hodge JS: Zinc in depressive disorder. Acta Psychiatr Scand 82:451–453, 1990

Medina JL, Fareed J, Diamond S: Lithium carbonate therapy for cluster headache: changes in number of platelets, and serotonin and histamine levels. Arch Neurol 37:559–563, 1980

Micromedex Healthcare Series [Internet database]. Greenwood Village, CO, Thomson Reuters (Healthcare), 2007

Milman N: Iron and pregnancy—a delicate balance. Ann Hematol 85:559–565, 2006

Mizota Y, Ozawa M, Yamazaki Y, et al: Psychosocial problems of bereaved families of HIV-infected hemophiliacs in Japan. Soc Sci Med 62:2397–2410, 2006

Moafi A, Mobaraki G, Taheri SS, et al: Zinc in thalassemic patients and its relation with depression. Biol Trace Elem Res 123:8–13, 2008

Monastero R, Monastero G, Ciaccio C, et al: Cognitive deficits in beta-thalassemia major. Acta Neurol Scand 102:162–168, 2000

Morgan SA, Jackson J: Psychological and social concomitants of sickle cell anemia in adolescents. J Pediatr Psychol 11:429–440, 1986

Morris MC, Evans DA, Schneider JA, et al: Dietary folate and vitamins B-12 and B-6 not associated with incident Alzheimer's disease. J Alzheimers Dis 9:435–443, 2006

Mort JR, Aparasu RR, Baer RK: Interaction between selective serotonin reuptake inhibitors and nonsteroidal anti-inflammatory drugs: review of the literature. Pharmacother 26:1307–1313, 2006

Mosby Drug Consult. St. Louis, MO, Mosby, 2007

Moss RA: Drug-induced immune thrombocytopenia. Am J Hematol 9:439–446, 1980

Nasreddine W, Beydoun A: Valproate-induced thrombocytopenia: a prospective monotherapy study. Epilepsia 49:438–445, 2008

Nassar AH, Usta IM, Rechdan JB, et al: Pregnancy in patients with beta-thalassemia intermedia: outcome of mothers and newborns. Am J Hematol 81:499–502, 2006

Nowak G, Szewczyk B: Mechanisms contributing to antidepressant zinc actions. Pol J Pharmacol 54:587–592, 2002

Nowak G, Szewczyk B, Pilc A: Zinc and depression: an update. Pharmacol Rep 57:713–718, 2005

O'Keeffe ST, Gavin K, Lavan JN: Iron status and restless legs syndrome in the elderly. Age Ageing 23:200–203, 1994

Olivieri NF: The beta-thalassemias. N Engl J Med 341:99–109, 1999

Opgen-Rhein C, Dettling M: Clozapine-induced agranulocytosis and its genetic determinants. Pharmacogenomics 9:1101–1111, 2008

Oyesanmi O, Kunkel EJ, Monti DA, et al: Hematologic side effects of psychotropics. Psychosomatics 40:414–421, 1999

Ozkara C, Dreifuss FE, Apperson Hansen C: Changes in red blood cells with valproate therapy. Acta Neurol Scand 88:210–212, 1993

Pack-Mabien A, Labbe E, Herbert D, et al: Nurses' attitudes and practices in sickle cell pain management. Appl Nurs Res 14:187–192, 2001

Panagiotakos DB, Pitsavos C, Chrysohoou C, et al: Inflammation, coagulation, and depressive symptomatology in cardiovascular disease-free people: the ATTICA study. Eur Heart J 25:492–499, 2004

Papakostas GI, Petersen T, Mischoulon D, et al: Serum folate, vitamin B12, and homocysteine in major depressive disorder, part 2: predictors of relapse during the continuation phase of pharmacotherapy. J Clin Psychiatry 65:1096–1098, 2004

Physicians' Desk Reference, 61st Edition. Montvale, NJ, Medical Economics, 2007

Platt OS, Thorington BD, Brambilla DJ, et al: Pain in sickle cell disease: rates and risk factors. N Engl J Med 325:11–16, 1991

Platt OS, Brambilla DJ, Rosse WF, et al: Mortality in sickle cell disease. Life expectancy and risk factors for early death. N Engl J Med 330:1639–1644, 1994

Politis C, Di Palma A, Fisfis M, et al: Social integration of the older thalassaemic patient. Arch Dis Child 65:984–986, 1990

Psihogios V, Rodda C, Reid E, et al: Reproductive health in individuals with homozygous beta-thalassemia: knowledge, attitudes, and behavior. Fertil Steril 77:119–127, 2002

Raiola G, Galati MC, De Sanctis V, et al: Growth and puberty in thalassemia major. J Pediatr Endocrinol Metab 16 (suppl 2): 259–266, 2003

Rajagopal S: Clozapine, agranulocytosis, and benign ethnic neutropenia. Postgrad Med J 81:545–546, 2005

Rall TW, Schleifer LS: Drugs effective in the therapy of the epilepsies, in The Pharmacological Basis of Therapeutics, 6th Edition. Edited by Gilman AG, Goldman LG, Gilman A. New York, Macmillan, 1980, pp 448–474

Ramasubbu R: Cerebrovascular effects of selective serotonin reuptake inhibitors: a systematic review. J Clin Psychiatry 65: 1642–1653, 2004

Ramsay RE: Clinical efficacy and safety of gabapentin. Neurology 44 (6 suppl 5):S23–3S0; discussion S31–S32, 1994

Rappaport VJ, Velazquez M, Williams K: Hemoglobinopathies in pregnancy. Obstet Gynecol Clin North Am 31:287–317, vi, 2004

Ratip S, Skuse D, Porter J, et al: Psychosocial and clinical burden of thalassaemia intermedia and its implications for prenatal diagnosis. Arch Dis Child 72:408–412, 1995

Ravaglia G, Forti P, Maioli F, et al: Homocysteine and folate as risk factors for dementia and Alzheimer disease. Am J Clin Nutr 82:636–643, 2005

Rector WG Jr: Pica: its frequency and significance in patients with iron-deficiency anemia due to chronic gastrointestinal blood loss. J Gen Intern Med 4:512–513, 1989

Reynolds EH: Benefits and risks of folic acid to the nervous system. J Neurol Neurosurg Psychiatry 72:567–571, 2002

Reynolds E: Vitamin B12, folic acid, and the nervous system. Lancet Neurol 5:949–960, 2006

Reynolds RD, Binder HJ, Miller MB, et al: Pagophagia and iron deficiency anemia. Ann Intern Med 69:435–440, 1968

Rosebush P, Mazurek MF: Serum iron and neuroleptic malignant syndrome. Lancet 338:149–151, 1991

Rosse RB, Giese AA, Deutsch SI, et al: Hematological measures of potential relevance to psychiatrists, in Concise Guide to Laboratory and Diagnostic Testing in Psychiatry. Washington, DC, American Psychiatric Press, 1989, pp 31–35

Schaefer RM, Huch R, Krafft A, Anemia Working Group: The iron letter—an update on the treatment of iron deficiency anemia [in German]. Praxis 95:357–364, 2006

Schalekamp T, Klungel OH, Souverein PC, et al: Increased bleeding risk with concurrent use of selective serotonin reuptake inhibitors and coumarins. Arch Intern Med 168:180–185, 2008

Schatz J, McClellan CB: Sickle cell disease as a neurodevelopmental disorder. Ment Retard Dev Disabil Res Rev 12:200–207, 2006

Schrier SL, Angelucci E: New strategies in the treatment of the thalassemias. Annu Rev Med 56:157–171, 2005

Schulte PF: Risk of clozapine-associated agranulocytosis and mandatory white blood cell monitoring. Ann Pharmacother 40:683–688, 2006

Sedky K, Lippmann S: Psychotropic medications and leukopenia. Curr Drug Targets 7:1191–1194, 2006

Sedky K, Shaughnessy R, Hughes T, et al: Clozapine-induced agranulocytosis after 11 years of treatment. Am J Psychiatry 162:814, 2005

Serebruany VL: Selective serotonin reuptake inhibitors and increased bleeding risk: are we missing something? Am J Med 119:113–116, 2006

Seshadri S, Beiser A, Selhub J, et al: Plasma homocysteine as a risk factor for dementia and Alzheimer's disease. N Engl J Med 346:476–483, 2002

Shakin EJ, Thompson TL: Psychiatric aspects of hematologic disorders, in Medical-Psychiatric Practice. Edited by Stoudemire A, Fogel BS. Washington, DC, American Psychiatric Press, 1991, pp 193–242

Shakin EJ, Thompson TL: Hematologic disorders, in Psychiatric Care of the Medical Patient. Edited by Stoudemire A, Fogel BS. New York, Oxford University Press, 1993, pp 691–712

Shapiro BS, Benjamin LJ, Payne R, et al: Sickle cell-related pain: perceptions of medical practitioners. J Pain Symptom Manage 14:168–174, 1997

Sherman M, Koch D, Giardina P, et al: Thalassemic children's understanding of illness: a study of cognitive and emotional factors. Ann N Y Acad Sci 445:327–336, 1985

Singhal AB, Topcuoglu MA, Dorer DJ, et al: SSRI and statin use increases the risk for vasospasm after subarachnoid hemorrhage. Neurology 64:1008–1013, 2005

Skop BP, Brown TM: Potential vascular and bleeding complications of treatment with selective serotonin reuptake inhibitors. Psychosomatics 37:12–16, 1996

Slovic P: Perception of risk. Science 236:280–285, 1987

Smith WR, Penberthy LT, Bovbjerg VE, et al: Daily assessment of pain in adults with sickle cell disease. Ann Intern Med 148:94–101, 2008

Snowden LR: Barriers to effective mental health services for African Americans. Ment Health Serv Res 3:181–187, 2001

Souhami RL, Ashton CR, Lee-Potter JP: Agranulocytosis and systemic candidiasis following clomipramine therapy. Postgrad Med J 52:472–474, 1976

Spilsbury M: Models for psychosocial services in the developed and developing world. Haemophilia 10 (suppl 4):25–29, 2004

Stahl SM: Basic psychopharmacology of antidepressants, part 1: antidepressants have seven distinct mechanisms of action. J Clin Psychiatry 59 (suppl 4):5–14, 1998

Steen RG, Hu XJ, Elliott VE, et al: Kindergarten readiness skills in children with sickle cell disease: evidence of early neurocognitive damage? J Child Neurology 17:111–116, 2002

Sun ER, Chen CA, Ho G, et al: Iron and the restless legs syndrome. Sleep 21:371–377, 1998

Telfer P, Constantinidou G, Andreou P, et al: Quality of life in thalassemia. Ann N Y Acad Sci 1054:273–282, 2005

Thrall G, Lane D, Carroll D, et al: A systematic review of the effects of acute psychological stress and physical activity on haemorheology, coagulation, fibrinolysis and platelet reactivity: implications for the pathogenesis of acute coronary syndromes. Thromb Res 120:819–847, 2007

Toh BH, van Driel IR, Gleeson PA: Pernicious anemia. N Engl J Med 337:1441–1448, 1997

Trost LB, Bergfeld WF, Calogeras E: The diagnosis and treatment of iron deficiency and its potential relationship to hair loss. J Am Acad Dermatol 54:824–844, 2006

Tsiantis J: Family reactions and relationships in thalassemia. Ann N Y Acad Sci 612:451–461, 1990

Turner MS, May DB, Arthur RR, et al: Clinical impact of selective serotonin reuptake inhibitors therapy with bleeding risks. J Intern Med 261:205–213, 2007

U.S. Preventive Services Task Force: Guide to Clinical Preventative Services, 2nd Edition. Baltimore, MD, Williams & Wilkins, 1996. Available at: http://odphp.osophs.dhhs.gov/pubs/guidecps/. Accessed December 22, 2009.

Valuck RJ, Ruscin JM: A case-control study on adverse effects: H2 blocker or proton pump inhibitor use and risk of vitamin B12 deficiency in older adults. J Clin Epidemiol 57:422–428, 2004

Vardaki MA, Philalithis AE, Vlachonikolis I: Factors associated with the attitudes and expectations of patients suffering from B-thalassaemia: a cross-sectional study. Scandinavian Journal of Caring Sciences 18:177–187, 2004

Vargas-Ruiz AG, Hernandez-Rivera G, Herrera MF: Prevalence of iron, folate, and vitamin B12 deficiency anemia after laparoscopic Roux-en-Y gastric bypass. Obes Surg 18:288–293, 2008

Vichinsky EP, MacKlin EA, Waye JS, et al: Changes in the epidemiology of thalassemia in North America: a new minority disease. Pediatrics 116:e818–e825, 2005

Vidal X, Ibanez L, Vendrell L, et al: Risk of upper gastrointestinal bleeding and the degree of serotonin reuptake inhibition by antidepressants: a case-control study. Spanish-Italian Collaborative Group for the Epidemiology of Gastrointestinal Bleeding. Drug Saf 31:159–168, 2008

von Kanel R, Mills PJ, Fainman C, et al: Effects of psychological stress and psychiatric disorders on blood coagulation and fibrinolysis: a biobehavioral pathway to coronary artery disease? Psychosom Med 63:531–544, 2001

von Kanel R, Dimsdale JE, Adler KA, et al: Effects of depressive symptoms and anxiety on hemostatic responses to acute mental stress and recovery in the elderly. Psychiatry Res 126:253–264, 2004a

von Kanel R, Kudielka BM, Schulze R, et al: Hypercoagulability in working men and women with high levels of panic-like anxiety. Psychother Psychosom 73:353–360, 2004b

von Kanel R, Kudielka BM, Preckel D, et al: Opposite effect of negative and positive affect on stress procoagulant reactivity. Physiol Behav 86:61–68, 2005

von Kanel R, Hepp U, Buddeberg C, et al: Altered blood coagulation in patients with posttraumatic stress disorder. Psychosom Med 68:598–604, 2006

Wald NJ: Folic acid and the prevention of neural-tube defects. N Engl J Med 350:101–103, 2004

Wald NJ, Law MR, Morris JK, et al: Quantifying the effect of folic acid. Lancet 358:2069–2073, 2001

Walter T, Kovalskys J, Stekel A: Effect of mild iron deficiency on infant mental development scores. J Pediatr 102:519–522, 1983

Wang HX, Wahlin A, Basun H, et al: Vitamin B(12) and folate in relation to the development of Alzheimer's disease. Neurology 56:1188–1194, 2001

Weinrieb RM, Auriacombe M, Lynch KG, et al: A critical review of selective serotonin reuptake inhibitor-associated bleeding: balancing the risk of treating hepatitis C-infected patients. J Clin Psychiatry 64:1502–1510, 2003

Weinrieb RM, Auriacombe M, Lynch KG, et al: Selective serotonin re-uptake inhibitors and the risk of bleeding. Exp Opin Drug Saf 4:337–344, 2005

Weissman DE, Haddox JD: Opioid pseudoaddiction—an iatrogenic syndrome. Pain 36:363–366, 1989

Wessinger S, Kaplan M, Choi L, et al: Increased use of selective serotonin reuptake inhibitors in patients admitted with gastrointestinal haemorrhage: a multicentre retrospective analysis. Aliment Pharmacol Ther 23:937–944, 2006

Whiskey E, Taylor D: Restarting clozapine after neutropenia: evaluating the possibilities and practicalities. CNS Drugs 21:25–35, 2007

White GC 2nd, Rosendaal F, Aledort LM, et al: Definitions in hemophilia: recommendation of the scientific subcommittee on factor VIII and factor IX of the scientific and standardization committee of the International Society on Thrombosis and Haemostasis. Thromb Haemost 85:560, 2001

Yang YM, Cepeda M, Price C, et al: Depression in children and adolescents with sickle-cell disease. Arch Pediatr Adolesc Med 148:457–460, 1994

Yoo MJ, Smith QR, Hage DS: Studies of imipramine binding to human serum albumin by high-performance affinity chromatography. J Chromatogr B Analyt Technol Biomed Life Sci 877:1149–1154, 2009

Zafeiriou DI, Economou M, Athanasiou-Metaxa M: Neurological complications in beta-thalassemia. Brain Dev 28:477–481, 2006

CHAPTER 25

Rheumatology

James L. Levenson, M.D.

Chris Dickens, M.B.B.S., Ph.D.

Michael R. Irwin, M.D.

RHEUMATOLOGICAL DISORDERS are an overlapping group of conditions that are characterized by chronic inflammation involving connective tissues and organs. The disorders arise as the result of autoimmune processes, and the various diseases are differentiated on the basis of the clinical presentation and the patterns of immune disturbance.

In this chapter we describe aspects of the rheumatological disorders that are likely to be relevant to a clinician working in the field of psychosomatic medicine. Most of the chapter is devoted to rheumatoid arthritis (RA) and systemic lupus erythematosus (SLE), because these disorders are likely to be encountered most commonly; other disorders, including osteoarthritis, Sjögren's syndrome, systemic sclerosis, temporal arteritis, polymyositis, polyarteritis nodosa, Behçet's syndrome, and Wegener's granulomatosis, are also discussed. Psychiatric side effects of medications used in treating rheumatological disorders are addressed as well. Fibromyalgia is covered in Chapter 26, "Chronic Fatigue and Fibromyalgia Syndromes."

General Principles of Diagnosis and Assessment

Detecting Central Nervous System Involvement in Rheumatological Disorders

Although many clinical signs and symptoms, as well as laboratory test results, are suggestive of neuropsychiatric involvement, none is diagnostic. Psychiatric diagnosis is primarily based on a constellation of clinical signs and symptoms, and possibly laboratory test results and neuroimaging findings, which should be viewed as corroboratory or exclusionary of comorbid conditions and secondary causes of neuropsychiatric symptoms.

Mental Status Examination and Neuropsychological Testing

The mental status examination is the most sensitive and least expensive tool available for detecting and tracking neuropsychiatric status in patients with rheumatological disorders. Neuropsychological testing provides a more detailed, sensitive assessment of cognitive function, but it is not specific. For example, even in the absence of any rheumatological disorder, neuropsychological testing often detects subtle cognitive abnormalities; consequently, such findings are not necessarily diagnostic of active neuropsychiatric rheumatological disease.

Laboratory Tests

No laboratory test, or set of tests, is considered diagnostic of neuropsychiatric involvement in rheumatological disorders. Nevertheless, laboratory studies serve two purposes. First, they help rule out possible infection, as well as other complications of rheumatological disorders or their treatment that can present with neuropsychiatric symptoms. Second, positive laboratory results can be used to confirm the presence of rheumatological disease activity. Although neuropsychiatric involvement can pursue a clinical course somewhat independent of flares in other organs, high disease activity increases the likelihood of central nervous system (CNS) involvement because the pathogenesis is shared. However, the absence of systemic disease activity does not preclude primary CNS involvement. Moreover, for certain neuropsychiatric symptoms, particularly fatigue and cognitive dysfunction, systemic disease activity seems to have little, if any, correlation with their severity (Waterloo et al. 2002).

Laboratory tests also can be useful in evaluating the basis for changes in psychiatric symptoms in rheumatology patients with a history of a primary psychiatric illness such as schizophrenia or major depression. Primary psychiatric disorders do not cause elevations in erythrocyte sedimentation rate (ESR), C reactive protein, or other markers of inflammation. Accordingly, if the psychiatric symptoms temporally coincide with a markedly increased ESR, then medical etiologies, particularly infection and CNS involvement, must be strongly considered.

When rheumatology patients present with acute changes in neuropsychiatric symptoms, lumbar puncture is indicated to rule out CNS infection and to assess the degree of disease activity in the CNS. In patients without CNS infection, cerebrospinal fluid (CSF) pleocytosis and increased CSF protein are suggestive of CNS involvement by lupus or other rheumatological disease. In addition, CSF studies should include oligoclonal bands, which are present in only a few disorders, including neurosyphilis, Lyme disease, multiple sclerosis, Sjögren's syndrome, and CNS SLE. Several other CSF tests have been associated with neuropsychiatric SLE but are not widely available or timely (Cohen et al. 2004).

Electroencephalogram

In patients with rheumatological disorders who also have neuropsychiatric symptoms, the electroencephalogram (EEG) often has abnormal findings but seldom is useful as a diagnostic tool (Waterloo et al. 1999), except in identifying subclinical seizure activity or differentiating hypoactive delirium (diffuse slowing on EEG) from depression (normal EEG).

Neuroimaging

Although magnetic resonance imaging (MRI) is the best available imaging technique for identifying focal neurological lesions in patients with rheumatological disorders and neuropsychiatric symptoms, it is inherently limited because it detects only structural lesions, whereas the pathophysiology of the neuropsychiatric problems is often functional. Also, MRI cannot reliably differentiate active from chronic lesions resulting from a previous neuropsychiatric insult (Sabbadini et al. 1999).

Detecting, Diagnosing, and Quantifying Psychiatric Symptoms and Disorders

Despite their high prevalence and significant effect on the patient's illness and overall quality of life, psychiatric disorders are often not fully recognized or treated in patients with rheumatological disorders. Clinicians who focus primarily on the physical aspects of disease may fail to recognize, diagnose, and treat psychiatric disorders. For example, the presence of overlapping symptoms between depression and rheumatological disorders (e.g., fatigue, weight loss, insomnia, and lack of appetite) may lead the clinician to attribute these symptoms to the rheumatological disorder, rather than recognizing the presence of comorbid depression (Copsey Spring et al. 2007). Moreover, treatment of depression may be deferred if clinicians hold the misconception that depression is secondary to the pain and disability, rather than understanding that the presence of comorbid depression can exacerbate such symptoms in rheumatological disorders.

Self-rated questionnaires may be used by rheumatologists or specialist nurses to screen for possible cases of psychiatric disorder, with the recognition that some questionnaires (Beck Depression Inventory [BDI] and the Center for Epidemiologic Studies Depression Scale [CES-D]) tend to overestimate the prevalence of depression in medically ill populations because of their prominent inclusion of somatic symptoms that occur in medical illness including rheumatological disorders (Callahan et al. 1991). Scales that have little somatic content, such as the Geriatric Depression Scale (Sheikh and Yesavage 1989), the Hospital Anxiety and Depression Scale (HADS; Zigmond and Snaith 1983), or disease-specific instruments (Smedstad et al. 1995), may aid accurate diagnosis of depression in such patients (see also Covic et al. 2009 and Chapter 8, "Depression"). With additional training in the clinical assessment of mood-specific symptoms and related somatic symptoms, the diagnosis of depression can be made, with the initiation of antidepressant treatment when indicated; referral to psychiatric specialists can occur for complicated cases.

Complex cases will require more detailed assessment by a psychosomatic medicine specialist. In addition to assessing the patient's current mental state, the psychiatrist should explore the development of psychiatric symptoms and how these relate to the recent disease state and changes in treatment, availability of social support, psychosocial stresses resulting from pain and disability, and stresses independent of the illness. Inquiries about maladaptive coping strategies for physical symptoms (e.g., "I just lie down and wait for my symptoms to ease"; "I simply avoid activities that cause me pain") can identify fruitful targets for psychological interventions. Assessing psychiatric history and family history will help identify which patients are most vulnerable to developing depression and other psychiatric disorders. Finally, investigating the patient's personal beliefs about the illness, such as the perceived causes, possible outcomes, and likelihood of controlling disease progression through treatment, can identify psychological factors that may facilitate recovery or perpetuate the sick role, thus influencing adherence with and response to treatment and health-related quality of life.

General Principles of Treatment

Primary Neuropsychiatric Involvement

When rheumatological diseases affect the CNS, the primary treatment is *corticosteroids* when the pathophysiology is thought to be neuronal injury or inflammation resulting from autoantibodies and *anticoagulants* when hypercoagulability is involved (e.g., the anticardiolipin antibody syndrome). When corticosteroids are ineffective, other immunosuppressive agents may be helpful.

Primary Psychiatric Disorders

The gold standard of behavioral approaches, cognitive-behavioral therapy (CBT), attempts to change maladaptive ways of thinking and feeling in response to the illness with an extensive range of strategies, including biofeedback and relaxation training, cognitive restructuring and distraction, and activity pacing. Most studies have focused on the management of pain. A recent review of 25 randomized clinical trials that tested psychosocial treatments for RA underscored the effectiveness of CBT in increasing efficacy in coping with pain and in reducing pain, physical disability, and depressive symptoms (Astin et al. 2002). However, findings show substantial variability across outcome measures. For example, among RA patients, Parker et al. (2003) found that CBT added no further benefit to the treatment of depression, as compared with pharmacological treatment alone. In contrast, an intervention (e.g., mindfulness meditation) that specifically targeted affective disturbances by way of attention to regulation of negative affective responses to stress and/or encouragement of positive engagement in daily life was found to produce consistent improvements in depressive symptoms, particularly in those RA patients who were vulnerable to depression and had reported a history of depression (Zautra et al. 2008). Such therapies may reduce pain and improve functioning (Bradley et al. 1987; Sharpe et al. 2001), with some evidence that such behavioral improvements are co-occurring with decreases in cellular markers of inflammation (Zautra et al. 2008).

Whereas pharmacological interventions are more often used to treat depression, the adjunctive use of psychological interventions should be considered in patients with rheumatological disorders who have psychiatric problems, given the positive effects of such interventions on overlapping symptoms of pain and fatigue. Given the salience of these complaints and their effect on disease activity and treatment adherence, rheumatologists, specialist nurses, and physical or occupational therapists might apply cognitive-behavioral principles to optimize patients' care. For example, as a matter of routine, newly diagnosed patients should be educated about the disease and its likely course—an approach that can facilitate adherence. Subjects with severe advanced disease might benefit from psychological adjuncts to physical management. Between these two extremes, maintaining an awareness of the importance of psychological processes in determining illness behavior might help the rheumatologist identify, treat, and make referrals for problems appropriately.

For the treatment of depressive disorders in rheumatological patients, many antidepressants are currently available to clinicians. Although their efficacy in adult populations is widely recognized, few antidepressant studies have specifically targeted rheumatological patients. One study found that sertraline had strong effects on depression outcomes as compared with a group of untreated RA patients who were clinically followed up (Parker et al. 2003). Furthermore, basic studies have suggested that activation of serotonin receptors has potent anti-inflammatory effects (Yu et al. 2008), although the clinical translational implications of these findings for the treatment of depression in RA patients are not known. Current evidence indicates that all antidepressants have approximately equal efficacy in the treatment of depression, but they do differ in their analgesic efficacy, tolerability, and potential drug interactions.

Tricyclic antidepressants (TCAs) have long been recognized to have analgesic benefits, even at low doses (e.g., 25 mg of amitriptyline) and independent of whether depression is present. In higher doses, tolerability and safety are poor, particularly in the elderly. Selective serotonin reuptake inhibitors (SSRIs) have comparable antidepressant efficacy but less analgesic efficacy. Serotonin-norepinephrine reuptake inhibitors (SNRIs) possess more analgesic potential than do SSRIs. The only randomized, placebo-controlled trials reporting analgesic efficacy of antidepressants in rheumatological disorders have been of TCAs (e.g., Ash et al. 1999; Grace et al. 1985). (See Chapter 36, "Pain.") Drug interactions may occur, although this is generally not a problem with first- and second-line treatments for RA.

Treatment of anxiety, mania, psychosis, delirium, and pain in rheumatological disorders is similar to their treatment in other medical diseases, following the principles reviewed in other chapters in this book (Chapter 5, "Delirium"; Chapter 10, "Psychosis, Mania, and Catatonia"; Chapter 11, "Anxiety Disorders"; Chapter 36, "Pain").

Rheumatoid Arthritis

RA affects approximately 0.8% of the population (range= 0.3%–2.1%), with women being affected approximately three times more frequently than men. It is a chronic disorder characterized by persistent inflammatory synovitis. Although any synovial joint can be affected, the disease typically involves peripheral small joints in a symmetrical pattern. Inflammation of the synovium can result in destruction of joint cartilage and bony erosions, which can eventually result in destruction of the joint. Extra-articular manifestations are common, with some degree of extra-articular involvement being found in most patients. These extra-articular manifestations vary widely among patients but may include systemic symptoms (e.g., anorexia, weight loss, myalgia); more localized abnormalities such as rheumatoid nodules; or involvement of the cardiovascular system (e.g., vasculitis, pericarditis), respiratory system (e.g., pleural effusions, pulmonary fibrosis), or CNS (e.g., spinal cord compression, peripheral neuropathy). The typical course of RA is prolonged, characterized by relapses and remissions. As the disease advances, progressive joint destruction results in limitations to joint movements, joint instability and deformities that increase pain, and functional disability.

The main aims of treatment of RA are 1) analgesia, 2) reduction of inflammation, 3) joint protection, 4) maintenance of functional ability, and 5) reduction of systemic manifestations. Pharmacological management of RA involves several different types of drug treatment:

- Nonsteroidal anti-inflammatory drugs (NSAIDs) control symptoms and signs of local inflammation, although they do not appear to alter the eventual course of the disease.
- Several drugs alter the course of the disease by reducing the inflammatory component of RA (e.g., methotrexate, antimalarials, minocycline, and sulfasalazine); gold and penicillamine are almost never used anymore.
- Corticosteroids can be used to reduce signs of inflammation by systemic administration (oral or parenteral) or by local injection.
- Currently available biological response modifiers include the anti-tumor necrosis factor (TNF)-alpha therapies—namely, etanercept (Enbrel), infliximab (Remicade), adalimumab (Humira), and an interleukin-1 (IL-1) receptor antagonist, anakinra (Kineret) (Olsen and Stein 2004).
- Immunosuppressive agents (azathioprine, leflunomide, cyclosporine, and cyclophosphamide) also reduce inflammation in RA, but because of toxicity, their use is limited to patients who do not respond to other treatments.

Neuropsychiatric Disorders in Rheumatological Disease

Epidemiology of Neuropsychiatric Disorders in RA

Neuropsychiatric disorders are common in patients with rheumatological diseases, as they are in most chronic illness populations. In a recent cross-sectional population survey in 17 countries with more than 85,000 participating adults, the presence of a mental disorder was assessed by a structured diagnostic interview in persons with and without arthritis (He et al. 2008). Findings from this large and diverse population sample indicated that depression was about twice as likely to occur in persons with arthritis compared with those without (odds ratio [OR] = 1.9; 95% confidence interval [CI] = 1.7 to 2.1) with similar increased risk for dysthymia (OR = 2.4; 95% CI = 2.0 to 2.7), anxiety disorders (OR = 1.9; 95% CI = 1.8 to 2.3), and possibly alcohol dependence, although the prevalence of alcohol abuse or dependence was fairly low (He et al. 2008). In a nationwide cohort study from Sweden with follow-up over three decades, individuals with rheumatological diseases had a higher risk of psychiatric disorders than did the general population, with a standardized incidence ratio of 1.45 for RA (Sundquist et al. 2008). Finally, according to standardized research interviews, it is estimated that nearly one-fifth of patients with RA have a psychiatric disorder, most often a depressive disorder.

Etiology of Neuropsychiatric Manifestations in RA

Neuropsychiatric manifestations in RA can arise through several processes, including direct CNS involvement, emotional reactions to chronic illness, and possibly secondary effects of the illness (e.g., the CNS effects of inflammatory cytokines).

Involvement of the central nervous system in RA. Despite its multisystem manifestations, neurological complications in RA are not common. When CNS involvement is present, the most common form is peripheral neuropathy. Direct involvement of the CNS is rare. Atlanto-axial subluxation may occur, resulting in transverse myelitis, and is the most widely recognized CNS complication of RA.

Vasculitis in RA can involve cerebral vessels, resulting in cerebral ischemia or infarction, and has been associated with acute and chronic brain syndromes (Ando et al. 1995; Kurne et al. 2009; Zolcinski et al. 2008). Treatment with corticosteroids usually can alleviate vasculitis and edema, with resultant improvement in symptoms, but impairment from the infarction is permanent.

Psychiatric disorders as an emotional reaction to chronic illness. Given the well-recognized association between chronic psychosocial stress and depression (G.W. Brown and Harris 1989), it is thought that the burden of chronic physical symptoms along with personal losses resulting from RA and its associated disability contribute to the increased risk of depression in RA patients. Albers et al. (1999) found that in 89% of RA patients, the disease adversely affected at least one domain of socioeconomic functioning (e.g., work, income, required rest time during day, leisure activity, transport mobility, housing, social dependency), with 58% experiencing adverse effects in at least three domains. Other social effects to consider are loss of personal ambitions, loss of social role, loss of future financial security, relationship disturbances, and body image concerns. Social support that might help to offset the stress of RA may be less available because of limited mobility. Furthermore, RA patients may have fewer coping resources available to deal with comorbid illnesses and stresses unrelated to RA. Finally, such chronic psychosocial and interpersonal stressors are known to increase cellular and molecular markers of inflammation (Davis et al. 2008; Pace et al. 2006), which might contribute to a worsening of disease activity and a further exacerbation of disease-related stress. Indeed, chronic negative events are associated with increases in the cellular production of the inflammatory cytokine interleukin-6 (IL-6) in RA patients, which leads to increases in symptoms of fatigue independent of pain severity (Davis et al. 2008). However, such stress-induced activation of inflammatory signaling appears to be blocked by treatments that antagonize production of inflammatory cytokines (e.g., use of TNF-alpha antagonists such as infliximab, etanercept, or adalimumab) (Motivala et al. 2008).

Psychiatric symptoms as consequences of RA and associated inflammation. Animal models, cell culture data, and anti-inflammatory cytokine antagonist treatments provide converging evidence that dysregulation of the proinflammatory cytokine network underlies synovial inflammation in patients with RA. Indeed, proinflammatory cytokines show potent additive effects; TNF-alpha strongly induces production of IL-1 and IL-6, which promotes a cascade of processes, such as leukocyte infiltration of synovial tissue, collagenase and prostaglandin E production, and bone resorption.

Basic research on neural immune signaling has shown that peripheral proinflammatory cytokines exert potent effects on neural processes that lead to a constellation of behavior changes, including abnormal sleep, depressed mood, and social withdrawal (Miller et al. 2009). Experimentally induced immune activation is associated with depressed mood, fatigue, and increases in pain sensitivity (Eisenberger et al. 2009; Reichenberg et al. 2001). These findings may be particularly relevant for RA patients because the use of medications that block peripheral proinflammatory cytokine activity (e.g., TNF antagonists) is associated with a lower prevalence of major depressive and anxiety disorders independent of clinical status (Uguz et al. 2009). Likewise, in an open study, infliximab induced acute (within hours) improvement in sleep as measured by polysomnography (Zamarron et al. 2004). Together, these data raise the possibility that inflammatory responses may initiate and perpetuate behavioral complications in RA. Alternatively, targeting inflammatory mechanisms may represent a novel strategy to ameliorate depressive symptoms in RA; for example, etanercept has been found to reduce depressive symptoms in patients with psoriasis (Tyring et al. 2006). Finally, in animal studies of "sickness behaviors," novel antidepressant drugs that target the inflammatory signaling pathways that are activated in RA (e.g., stress-activated/mitogen-activated protein kinases [SAPK/MAPK]) may work jointly to reverse the behavioral symptoms and to reduce the inflammation found in RA (Malemud and Miller 2008).

Reciprocal Associations Between Psychiatric Symptoms and Clinical Disease

Depression and Clinical State

Numerous studies have examined the associations of depression with the physical symptoms of RA. Older cross-sectional studies that used self-report measures showed that levels of depressive symptoms are associated with the severity of the pain experienced (Frank et al. 1988; Hurwicz and Berkanovic 1993; Peck et al. 1989; Smedstad et al. 1995; Wolfe 1999) and the degree of functional disability (G.K. Brown et al. 1989; Hurwicz and Berkanovic 1993; Pow 1987; Smedstad et al. 1996; Wolfe 1999). Some of the associations observed might be attributable to the use of depression measures such as the BDI, in which physical symptoms associated with the RA itself—for example, disturbed sleep, fatigue, and loss of appetite—are rated as indicators of depression. Exclusion of these somatic items leaves smaller but still significant associations between depression and the physical symptoms of RA (Peck et al. 1989).

Few longitudinal studies have examined the reciprocal associations between depression and changes in the severity of RA symptoms. Wolfe and Hawley (1993) found that changes in depression were associated with changes in pain and disability, although only 17% of the variance in depression was accounted for by these two variables, indicating that the degree of association was weak. However, in a recent study involving more than 22,000 patients with RA followed up for nearly 10 years, self-reported increases in depression were primarily predicted by symptoms of pain and fatigue (Wolfe and Michaud 2009).

The literature just cited indicates that psychological symptoms, particularly depression, are most marked in patients with worse pain and disability, although the strength of this association is modest at best. However, it is possible that these studies underestimate the strength of the association of physical symptoms and psychological problems. The measures used to assess physical state are generic assessments of functional ability. If depression is related to loss of function, the value or meaning of the lost activity to the individual could be important. In other words, generic measures provide a broad overview of function but may not be sensitive to what is important to the individual. Katz and Yelin (1995) performed an extremely detailed prospective longitudinal study of women with RA. Subjects were followed up for 4 years to identify aspects of functioning that predicted the development of depression in the final year of the study. Although generic measures of function predicted a fourfold increase in depression, a 10% loss in activities that the individuals had identified as being important to them resulted in a sevenfold increase in depression in the subsequent year.

Furthermore, the vast majority of the research performed in this area has focused on ambulatory outpatients, probably for a combination of ethical and convenience reasons. The association between physical and psychiatric symptoms may be weak because of the mild to moderate nature of the symptoms in many of the patients studied. Mindham et al. (1981) conducted a prospective study involving a small number of patients with RA. They confirmed the positive association between symptoms of RA and the development of psychiatric symptoms considered to be of "pathological severity," but this association was weak and nonspecific in most of their patients. Only in subjects with the most severe and disabling RA did they find an association between symptoms of RA and the development of several psychiatric symptoms together, indicating the development of a psychiatric disorder. Thus, the association between symptoms of RA and psychological symptoms may become more pronounced in subjects with the most severe disease.

Role of Cognitive Appraisal Mechanisms

The way RA patients think about their illness is crucial to understanding the association of depression with pain and disability. Depression is associated with increased worry about illness and conviction of severe disease. Depressed RA patients perceive their illness as being more serious and feel hopeless about a cure compared with nondepressed RA patients (H. Murphy et al. 1999). Furthermore, depressed patients are more likely to have cognitive distortions relating to the RA (Smith et al. 1988). These associations remain significant in RA patients even after the extent of disease and pain levels are controlled, indicating that the association between depression and negative appraisals of health status is not simply the result of depressed people having more severe illness.

The way people think about or understand their illness is also important because it influences the way RA patients cope with the illness. According to Leventhal's model, individuals hold personal representations and beliefs about their health and any threat posed to it (Leventhal et al. 1997). These personal representations have both cognitive and emotional components, are based on a lay knowledge or understanding of health and illness, and thus may significantly differ from those of the consulting clinician. Patients' perceptions of a health threat initiate the use of coping strategies, the results of which are then appraised and may result in a change in the representations or a revision of the strategy. Coping strategies may be broadly described as adaptive if they result in normalization of a patient's life—that is, minimizing symptom effect—or maladaptive if they result in increased dependency. Depression is associated with impairment of general coping, especially at high levels of pain (G.K. Brown et al. 1989; Hurwicz and Berkanovic 1993).

Thus, psychiatric disorders, particularly depression, appear to be associated with a more negative appraisal of the illness and impairment in ability to cope with the illness. As such, these cognitive appraisal mechanisms may act as mediators in the association between the physical symptoms of RA and psychiatric disorders. It should be recognized, however, that the amount of variance in depression accounted for by perceived control, coping ability, and cognitive distortions is small, with the majority being unexplained (Persson et al. 1999).

Other Psychosocial Factors Contributing to Psychiatric Symptoms

Several other psychosocial and behavioral factors that may predispose any RA patient toward psychiatric problems have been suggested.

Neuroticism. Some individuals are predisposed to experience and react to stress, including health stress, in a negative way. People with such negative affectivity, or *neuroticism,* have been shown to be more sensitive to physical sensations (Larsen 1992), interpret physical sensations as threatening (Larsen 1992), experience more emotional distress regardless of the environment (Ormel and Wohlfart 1991), and choose less effective coping strategies (Bolger and Zuckerman 1995). The importance of neuroticism has been confirmed in patients with RA. In a prospective study, RA patients completed daily reports on joint pain and mood for a period of 75 days. Those scoring higher on neuroticism experienced more chronic distress, regardless of their pain intensity (Affleck et al. 1992). Another prospective study found neuroticism to be the most effective predictor of anxiety and depressed mood in RA patients after 3 and 5 years, irrespective of other psychosocial and medical factors assessed (Evers et al. 2002).

Social support. It is recognized that social support is associated with health and good quality of life in the general population. Some studies have found that social support benefits patients with RA. In patients with RA, social support and its actual or perceived availability have been shown to be associated with use of more adaptive coping strategies (Holtzman et al. 2004), greater perception of ability to control the disease (Spitzer et al. 1995), and less psychological distress (Zyrianova et al. 2006). Not all social contacts are supportive, however, and critical or punishing comments are associated with increased psychological distress (Griffin et al. 2001).

RA has an adverse effect on the availability of social support to its patients, however. Patients with RA have been shown to have reduced social networks and social support (Fyrand et al. 2001). This disruption of social support appears to be greatest in those with disease of longest duration with the most severe functional disability, possibly caused by a significant reduction in the availability of important others to patients with RA (S. Murphy et al. 1988). That may be why longitudinal studies have found that social support's benefits are short term in RA (Demange et al. 2004; Strating et al. 2006). Importantly, such subjective social isolation may drive increases in inflammation and contribute to disease activity. Among socially isolated older adults who report high levels of loneliness, the expression of inflammatory response genes increases, which is driven in part by a reduced glucocorticoid receptor sensitivity and a failure of endogenous glucocorticoids to downregulate the inflammatory response (Cole et al. 2007).

Social stresses. Social stresses are recognized as being potent causes of depression in the general population. Particularly important in causing depression are those stresses in which the degree of threat to the individual is great—so-called severe events and marked difficulties (G.W. Brown and Harris 1979). As indicated previously, in addition to the burden of the symptoms, RA patients experience considerable hardship in association with their chronic illness. Social stresses independent of those of RA are also likely to contribute to the development of depression in RA patients, however. In fact, among ambulatory outpatients, the stresses independent of RA may well have a greater importance in predicting depression than do the RA-related stresses (Dickens et al. 2003). The findings of this study indicate that in patients with mild to moderate arthritis, RA-related life difficulties cause psychological distress that does not amount to a full-blown psychiatric disorder, perhaps because the degree of threat is not marked. The combination of RA-related and RA-independent stresses, however, is sufficient to cause a depressive disorder. Clearly, in subjects with the most severe, disabling arthritis, the situation is likely to be different, with RA-related difficulties alone being a sufficiently potent stress to result in depressive disorder (Mindham et al. 1981).

In 27 independent studies involving more than 3,000 RA patients, stress, defined as minor hassles and life events lasting hours or days, was associated with subsequent increases in disease activity (Straub et al. 2005). In addition, some studies have suggested that social stresses might play an important part in triggering the onset of RA in adults (e.g., Baker and Brewerton 1981). Whereas some studies used unreliable retrospective measures that could be contaminated by the RA patients' effort to explain the onset of their disease, Conway et al. (1994) used a structured life event interview (e.g., Life Events and Difficulties Schedule; G.W. Brown and Harris 1989) to evaluate the associations between negative life event and RA disease onset. However, among 60 consecutive outpatients with RA, no evidence showed an increase in stressful events in the 12 months preceding the onset of RA, although conclusions from this study were constrained by the use of normative data rather than an experimental control group.

Sleep disturbance. Sleep disturbance is thought to contribute to pain, fatigue, and depressed mood in patients with RA, and several studies showed that subjective sleep complaints correlate with fatigue, functional disability, greater joint pain, and more depressive symptoms in these patients (Moldofsky 2001). Indeed, sleep difficulties, pain, depressed mood, and fatigue appear to cluster in RA; depression is associated with greater pain, whereas sleep difficulties are associated with fatigue, depression, and pain (Drewes et al. 1998; Frank et al. 1988; Nicassio et al. 2002). However, the relation between sleep disturbance and other symptoms is complex. For example, sleep disturbance may be a symptom of depression, or it may precipitate feelings of depression because it interferes with normal activities. Alternatively, both sleep disturbance and depression may be manifestations of an underlying biological disturbance such as an increase in inflammatory activity, which may alter CNS function, as noted previously. For example, sleep loss induces increases in the production of inflammatory markers (Irwin et al. 2006, 2008), which then promote symptoms such as pain, fatigue, and affective disturbance. In turn, nocturnal elevations of proinflammatory cytokines and pain might recursively initiate further difficulties with sleep (Irwin et al. 2008), leading to a feed-forward vicious circle with progressive deterioration in clinical outcomes.

Effect of Mental Disorders on Inflammatory Processes

The mechanisms by which depression influences pain and disability are also poorly understood. Depression, psychological stress, and sleep disturbance have all been shown to result in increases in cellular and molecular markers of inflammation, including increases in inflammatory signaling pathways such as nuclear factor kappa-B (Irwin et al. 2006, 2008; Pace et al. 2006). Furthermore, increases in the cellular production of inflammatory cytokines correlate with self-reported fatigue in RA patients, independent of pain (Davis et al. 2008). Finally, behavioral interventions that target negative affective and emotion regulation have been found to produce improvements in depression and pain outcomes, which are coupled with a downregulation of cellular production of inflammatory markers (Zautra et al. 2008). Moreover, in another controlled trial of a CBT intervention for patients in an early stage of RA, those receiving adjunctive CBT showed improvement in C reactive protein (but not ESR) immediately after therapy compared with those receiving the control condition, but this effect was lost by 6 months (Sharpe et al. 2001). It remains unclear whether this improvement was a direct effect of the CBT on inflammatory activity or a result of behavior-mediating factors, which seems more likely, such as improved compliance with treatment in the intensively followed-up group. Indeed, depression in patients with rheumatological disorders is a strong predictor of poor medication and treatment adherence (Julian et al. 2009).

Psychiatric disorders, particularly anxiety and depression, are associated with more negative illness cognitions in RA. As a result of these negative illness cognitions, health-seeking behaviors and health care use may increase as they do in other medical patients. Depressed RA patients are more likely to report physical symptoms (H. Murphy et al. 1999), less likely to be reassured by a doctor, and less likely to comply with medications (DiMatteo et al. 2000). We know that there is an immense variation in the health care costs among subjects that is not directly related to the severity of RA (Lubeck et al. 1986). Depression has been shown to contribute to these hitherto unexplained costs (Joyce et al. 2009). The effect of depression on indirect (social) costs is likely to be even greater (Yelin et al. 1979).

Osteoarthritis

Osteoarthritis is the most common joint disease, with the idiopathic form being the most prevalent. Secondary osteoarthritis arises most frequently as the result of trauma (acute or chronic), although it also may occur in a variety of metabolic and endocrine disorders. The prevalence of osteoarthritis increases sharply with age: fewer than 2% of women younger than 45 years are affected, compared with 30% of those between 45 and 64 years of age and 68% of those older than 65 years.

The pattern of joint involvement varies with age and sex; osteoarthritis involving the hip is more common in older men, whereas involvement of the interphalangeal joints and of the first metacarpophalangeal joint is more common in elderly women. Previous joint overload—in particular, repetitive incidences, as in vocational injuries—has a considerable influence on the distribution of joint involvement. Clinically affected joints are painful, especially on movement, and are stiff after a period of inactivity. In later stages of the disease, movements are limited, and joint instability may occur, which is exacerbated by atrophy of muscles adjacent to the affected joint.

There has been less research interest in the causes, prevalence, and effect of psychological disorders in osteoarthritis compared with RA and SLE. Because direct involvement of the CNS is not a feature of primary osteoarthritis, one can conclude that psychological disorders in patients with this disorder arise either as a reaction to the pain, disability, and life difficulties related to the osteoarthritis or for reasons independent of the osteoarthritis. Nevertheless, data implicate psychological stress in worsening the severity of pain symptoms in osteoarthritis patients, particularly among those who report higher levels of depressive symptoms (Zautra et al. 2004).

Research on depression in osteoarthritis has shown findings very similar to those in RA. The prevalence of depression is significantly increased in patients with osteoarthritis, and increased pain, poor social support, and stressful life events are predictors of more depression in patients with osteoarthritis (Rosemann et al. 2007a; Sale et al. 2008). Depression in osteoarthritis patients leads to greater activity limitations, poorer quality of life, and increased health care utilization (Machado et al. 2008; Rosemann et al. 2007b).

Few intervention studies have examined the efficacy of antidepressants and psychological therapies in osteoarthritis. Those that have been performed suggest that both antidepressants and CBT are efficacious in the treatment of depression in patients with osteoarthritis and that improvement in depression is associated with reduced pain and disability from the disease (Lin et al. 2003). A randomized trial is ongoing to evaluate the effectiveness of combined pharmacological and nonpharmacological therapies to target depression and pain in osteoarthritis (Lin 2008).

Systemic Lupus Erythematosus

SLE is an autoimmune disorder of unknown cause characterized by immune dysregulation with tissue damage caused by pathogenic autoantibodies, immune complexes, and T lymphocytes. Approximately 90% of cases are in women, usually of childbearing age. The incidence is 2.4 per 100,000 across genders and race, 9.2 for black women, and 3.5 for white women; and prevalence rates are 90 per 100,000 for white women and 280 per 100,000 for black women. Asian people are also more often affected than white people. At onset, SLE may involve one or multiple organ systems. Common clinical manifestations include cutaneous lesions (e.g., photosensitivity, malar or discoid rash, oral ulcers), constitutional symptoms (e.g., fatigue, weight loss, fevers), arthralgias and frank arthritis, serositis (e.g., pericarditis or pleuritis), renal disease, neuropsychiatric disorders, and hematological disorders (e.g., anemia, leukopenia). Autoantibodies are detectable at presentation in most cases.

The spectrum of treatment options in SLE is similar to that in RA: namely, NSAIDs, antimalarials (e.g., hydroxychloroquine), corticosteroids, and other immunosuppressants (e.g., azathioprine, mycophenolate mofetil, methotrexate, cyclophosphamide). The role of biological response modifiers is currently under investigation, but none is currently approved for this indication. In addition, anticoagulants are used in SLE patients who have antiphospholipid antibodies if the patients have a history of arterial or venous thrombosis. The rate of 20-year survival has been reported to be 50%–70% (Lahita 2004) but is improving with newer immunosuppressive treatments.

Neuropsychiatric Manifestations in Systemic Lupus Erythematosus

Neuropsychiatric symptoms of SLE were first reported in 1872 by Kaposi (1872). Depending on the diagnostic methodology used, neuropsychiatric manifestations have a prevalence of up to 90% (Ainiala et al. 2001b), ranging from stroke, seizures, headaches, neuropathy, transverse myelitis, and movement disorders to cognitive deficits, depression, mania, anxiety, psychosis, and delirium. CNS involvement is a major cause of morbidity in SLE, second only to renal failure as a cause of mortality. The pathogenesis of neuropsychiatric syndromes in SLE is complex. For a more detailed review of psychiatric aspects of SLE, see Cohen et al. (2004).

Pathogenesis of Neuropsychiatric Syndromes in SLE

Psychiatric syndromes in SLE can be caused by 1) direct CNS involvement; 2) infection, other systemic illness, or drug-induced side effects; 3) reaction to chronic illness; or 4) comorbid primary psychiatric illness.

Direct pathophysiological central nervous system effects. Two major antibody-mediated mechanisms of CNS injury have been proposed: neuronal injury and microvasculopathy (Scolding and Joseph 2002). Autoantibodies may directly damage neurons by either causing cell death or transiently and reversibly impairing neuronal function. Antibody-mediated microvasculopathy seems to involve two processes: either endothelial damage (Wierzbicki 2000) or coagulation disturbances resulting from the prothrombotic effects of antiphospholipid (including anticardiolipin) antibodies (Gharavi 2001), both culminating in ischemia or infarction. These two pathogenic mechanisms may be mutually reinforcing, perpetuating the disease process. Microvascular endothelial injury in the CNS may increase the permeability of the blood–brain barrier, leading to influx of autoantibodies and further CNS damage. In addition, antibodies against the *N*-methyl-D-aspartate (NMDA) receptor may play a role in some manifestations of CNS lupus (Kowal et al. 2006).

Autoimmune antibodies seem to play a much larger role in direct CNS involvement (Jennekens and Kater 2002) than does immune complex deposition. Antiribosomal-P antibodies have been associated with psychosis (Isshi and Hirohata 1998) and severe depression (Arnett et al. 1996), but not consistently (Gerli et al. 2002). Antibodies against endothelial cells have been associated with psychosis and mood disorders (Conti et al. 2004). Antineuronal antibodies have been associated with psychosis, depression, delirium, coma, and cognitive dysfunction (West et al. 1995). However, these are not proven causal relationships. In contrast, antiphospholipid antibodies (e.g., anticardiolipin) cause focal deficits (strokes) and cognitive dysfunction (Levine et al. 2002; West et al. 1995). Cytokines also appear to be involved in the pathogenesis of neuropsychiatric SLE, although their role remains unclear.

With the possible exception of cognitive dysfunction, all the major psychiatric manifestations of SLE (i.e., psychosis, depression, mania, anxiety, and delirium) show a degree of reversibility, as does coma. Even the cognitive deficits sometimes respond to corticosteroids (Denburg et al. 1994; Hanly et al. 1997). Because psychiatric syndromes tend to resolve within 2–3 weeks with corticosteroid treatment (Denburg et al. 1994), they are probably caused by reversible or transient mechanisms rather than irreversible neuronal death. The reversibility of psychiatric dysfunction stands in contrast to most focal neurological events, which often have no more reversibility than atherosclerotic stroke and are associated with fixed lesions on neuroimaging. Similarly, in some individuals, the progressive nature of the cognitive impairment (Hanly et al. 1997), often with cerebral atrophy, suggests cumulative irreversible CNS damage.

Risk factors for direct CNS involvement in SLE include cutaneous vasculitis and antiphospholipid syndrome and its manifestations, especially arterial thromboses (Karassa et al. 2000). Patients with mainly articular manifestations or discoid rash have a much lower risk of neuropsychiatric lupus, as do those few who are antinuclear antibody (ANA)–negative and those with drug-induced SLE. Antiphospholipid antibodies may be the single strongest marker of CNS risk because they are associated with stroke, cognitive dysfunction, and epilepsy (Herranz et al. 1994; Sabet et al. 1998).

Psychological effects of coping with SLE. Coping with SLE is particularly challenging because lupus is a chronic, often debilitating multisystem illness, and its course is unpredictable. Because SLE can involve almost any organ system or include vague systemic symptoms, the diagnosis is often elusive. The inability to make a diagnosis may erode the patient's confidence in the medical system, and when no etiology can be found, the physician may deem the illness psychogenic. Given that SLE can affect many organ systems, patients may worry that the illness pervades their entire body, even when the disease is limited. The diffuse nature of SLE distinguishes it from most other chronic, recurrent diseases, such as asthma or inflammatory bowel disease, which are primarily limited to one organ. SLE patients are often under the care of an entourage of specialists, which may fragment care. One of the most stressful aspects of SLE is its unpredictable course, with sudden exacerbations, remissions, and variable prognoses, resulting in a profound loss of control, as well as a loss of ability to plan for the future.

Psychological reactions to having SLE are common and include grief, depression, anxiety, regression, denial, and invalidism. A feeling of isolation is reinforced by public ignorance about lupus. People with SLE may become socially withdrawn, especially if they are self-conscious about their appearance. Women with a malar rash or discoid lesions may feel branded as if by the "scarlet letter." The most prevalent fears of SLE patients are worsening disease, disability, and death. In particular, patients fear cognitive impairment, stroke, renal failure, and becoming a burden on their families (Liang et al. 1984). Although negative reactions to having SLE are common, at least 50% of patients experience positive reactions at some point during their illness (Liang et al. 1984).

Stress and SLE. Although stress may cause a lupus flare, it is also likely, if not inevitable, that lupus flares cause stress. Several studies have provided support for stress-induced immune dysregulation in SLE (for review, see Cohen et al. 2004). Daily stress in patients with SLE has been correlated positively with ANAs and anti-double-stranded DNA antibodies (Pawlak et al. 2003) and resulted in worsening of SLE symptoms (Peralta-Ramírez et al. 2004) and cognitive dysfunction (Peralta-Ramírez et al. 2006).

Whether stress precipitates onset or exacerbation of SLE symptoms has received relatively little study. Only one controlled study has reported that 20 patients hospitalized for SLE had significantly greater stress prior to the onset of their illness than did the seriously ill hospitalized control subjects (Otto and Mackay 1967). A more recent prospective study found no effect of stressful life events on SLE disease activity of symptoms (Peralta-Ramírez et al. 2004).

Classification of Neuropsychiatric Disorders in SLE

The literature on neuropsychiatric SLE has been plagued by terminology that has been imprecise and unstandardized. Terms such as *lupus cerebritis* have obfuscated our understanding because they imply a pathogenesis (inflammation) that remains unproven. Furthermore, because there is no gold standard for the diagnosis of neuropsychiatric SLE, ascertaining which conditions are direct CNS manifestations of SLE and which are a reaction to illness or a coincidental disorder has been controversial. To rectify these problems, the American College of Rheumatology (ACR) convened a committee to develop a standardized nomenclature for neuropsychiatric SLE, and guidelines were published in 1999 (American College of Rheumatology Ad Hoc Committee 1999). The guidelines defined neuropsychiatric lupus as "the neurological syndromes of the central, peripheral, and autonomic nervous systems, and the psychiatric syndromes observed in patients with SLE in which other causes have been excluded." Psychiatric disorders included psychosis, acute confusional state, cognitive dysfunction, anxiety disorder, and mood disorders. Overall, the ACR criteria significantly broadened the spectrum of syndromes that can be considered neuropsychiatric SLE (American College of Rheumatology Ad Hoc Committee 1999). The criteria have good sensitivity but low specificity (Ainiala et al. 2001a), making them better suited for identifying all possible cases of neuropsychiatric SLE. A large international collaborative cohort study of 572 patients newly diagnosed with SLE reported that whereas 28% of patients experienced at least one ACR-defined neuropsychiatric event around the time of diagnosis, only a minority of these events were attributable to SLE (Hanly et al. 2007). A more fundamental problem with the ACR classification system is that it is difficult to apply clinically. To diagnose neuropsychiatric SLE as the cause of the psychiatric symptoms, one must exclude a primary psychiatric disorder. In contrast, in DSM-IV-TR (American Psychiatric Association 2000), a primary psychiatric disorder cannot be diagnosed unless medical disorders and substance use are ruled out as etiologies. Whereas medical disorders and substance use can be easily excluded, no clinical criteria or laboratory tests are available for excluding primary psychiatric disorders. For example, if a patient with SLE becomes depressed, it is unclear how one would rule out primary depression as the cause.

Cognitive dysfunction is the most common neuropsychiatric disorder in patients with SLE, occurring in up to 80% of patients (Ainiala et al. 2001a; Denburg et al. 1994). On neuropsychological testing, even patients who have never had overt neuropsychiatric symptoms are often found to have cognitive impairment. Patients with anticardiolipin antibodies have a three- to fourfold increased risk of cognitive impairment, which is often progressive (Hanly et al. 1997). Cognitive impairment may be associated with lymphocytotoxic antibodies, CSF antineuronal antibodies, and pathological findings such as microinfarcts and cortical atrophy. Although cognitive dysfunction often fluctuates and is reversible (Hanly et al. 1997), presumably when attributable to edema and inflammation, it tends to be irreversible when secondary to multiple infarcts and may culminate in dementia.

Depression is the second most common neuropsychiatric disorder in SLE. The reported prevalence of depression has varied widely, depending on the diagnostic criteria, patient population, and study design. When structured interviews were used, the prevalence of depression in SLE was approximately 50% (Bachen et al. 2009). Depression may be a preexisting primary psychiatric disorder; an iatrogenically induced illness, particularly from corticosteroids; a reaction to having a chronic disease; and, possibly, a direct CNS manifestation of lupus. Kozora et al. (2006) found that patients with SLE (both those with neuropsychiatric SLE and those with nonneuropsychiatric SLE) showed higher symptoms of depression, higher levels of fatigue, greater pain, and more perceived cognitive problems. However, only patients with neuropsychiatric SLE had significant correlations among depression, fatigue, and pain. Neither the nonneuropsychiatric SLE patients nor the control subjects showed significant associations among these behavioral measures. One study has suggested that psychiatric symptoms (e.g., depression) are correlated with a reduction in regional cerebral blood flow in the posterior cingulate gyrus and thalamus (gross structural lesions were ruled out by brain MRI) (Oda et al. 2005). Nevertheless, the question of whether depression is a direct manifestation of CNS SLE or a reaction to the stress and multiple losses associated with having a chronic debilitating illness remains unresolved (for a review of the evidence, see Cohen et al. 2004). Diagnosing depression in SLE is confounded by the overlap between depressive symptoms and those associated with SLE or its treatment. Hypothyroidism should be ruled out because it can mimic depression and is more common in SLE than in the general population.

Anxiety is quite common in SLE patients, often as a reaction to the illness. The question of whether anxiety is attributable to direct CNS involvement in SLE or simply a reaction to chronic illness remains controversial, as with depression. In patients with SLE, the most common cause of mania is corticosteroid therapy. Psychosis in SLE patients can be a manifestation of direct CNS involvement, and in some but not all studies, it has been linked to antiribosomal-P antibodies. Distinguishing psychosis caused by CNS lupus from corticosteroid-induced psychosis presents a major diagnostic challenge (see section titled "Corticosteroid-Induced Psychiatric Symptoms" below). Delirium, referred to as "acute confusional state" in the ACR criteria, is common in severe SLE and is a result of CNS lupus, medication, or medical disorders, as shown in Table 25-1. Personality changes have been reported in SLE patients whose disease has damaged the frontal or temporal lobes, and symptoms are typical of those resulting from pathology in those brain regions.

TABLE 25–1. Secondary medical and psychiatric causes of neuropsychiatric symptoms in systemic lupus erythematosus and other rheumatological disorders

CNS infections
Systemic infections
Renal failure (e.g., due to lupus nephritis or vasculitis involving the renal artery)
Fluid or electrolyte disturbance
Hypertensive encephalopathy
Hypoxemia
Fever
CNS tumor (e.g., cerebral lymphoma because of immunosuppression)
Medication side effects (see Tables 25–2 and 25–3)
Comorbid medical illness
Psychiatric symptoms in reaction to illness
Comorbid psychiatric illness

Note. CNS=central nervous system.

Prevalence of Neuropsychiatric Disorders in SLE

Estimates of the prevalence of neuropsychiatric disorders in SLE have ranged from 17% to 91% (Ainiala et al. 2001a; Bachen et al. 2009; Brey et al. 2002; Cohen et al. 2004). This variation is a consequence of multiple factors: 1) lack of standardized terminology, 2) changing terminology over time, 3) differences in diagnostic methods, 4) variations in which disease entities are considered direct manifestations of CNS SLE versus reactions to a chronic unpredictable illness, 5) differences in study populations, 6) differences in specialties of the investigators, 7) inclusion or exclusion of mild psychiatric symptoms, and 8) inclusion or exclusion of particular CNS neurological disorders, as well as the arbitrariness of separating these disorders from psychiatric disorders.

The ACR nomenclature was used in two studies—a cross-sectional Finnish population-based study (Ainala et al. 2001a) and a cohort study of predominantly Mexican American persons (Brey et al. 2002)—that examined the prevalence of neuropsychiatric syndromes in outpatients with SLE. Overall, 80%–91% of patients had at least one neuropsychiatric disorder, and the prevalence rates in the two studies were similar for individual neuropsychiatric syndromes. Cognitive dysfunction was the most common neuropsychiatric condition, occurring in 79%–80% of patients; however, fewer than a third of those patients had moderate to severe impairment. Indeed, in a nationwide study from Sweden with a follow-up for more than three decades, patients with SLE showed a significantly increased risk for subsequent psychiatric disorder (e.g., standardized incidence ratio=2.38), which was primarily due to an increased risk of dementia and delirium (Sundquist et al. 2008). In the Finnish (Ainala et al. 2001a) and Mexican American (Brey et al. 2002) studies, major depression occurred in 28%–39%, mania or mixed episodes in 3%–4%, anxiety in 13%–24%, and psychosis in 0%–5%. A recent U.S. cohort study that used the Composite International Diagnostic Interview in white women with SLE found that 65% of the participants received a lifetime mood or anxiety diagnosis. Major depression (47%), specific phobia (24%), panic disorder (16%), obsessive-compulsive disorder (9%), and bipolar I disorder (6%) were all more common than in other white women (Bachen et al. 2009). Acute confusional state occurred in 7% of the Finnish patients with SLE; it was not reported in the Mexican American cohort. Although comparable prevalence studies have not been reported for acutely ill inpatients with neuropsychiatric SLE, the incidence of psychosis and delirium is likely to be substantially higher.

Laboratory Detection of Central Nervous System Disease Activity in Systemic Lupus Erythematosus

The general principles of treatment discussed earlier in this chapter are applicable to neuropsychiatric SLE, but relevant laboratory tests are specific to SLE. In SLE, complement levels (C3, C4, CH_{50}) and anti-DNA antibodies are elevated during disease flares (West et al. 1995). Serum ANA titers need not be obtained in SLE because they do not seem to correlate with systemic or CNS lupus activity. Testing for antiphospholipid antibodies (including lupus anticoagulant and anticardiolipin) is crucial, particularly in patients with focal symptoms, because the results may determine treatment and prognosis (Levine et al. 2002). Unlike antiphospholipid antibody–negative patients, those with antiphospholipid syndrome are treated primarily with anticoagulation rather than corticosteroid or cytotoxic therapy. As noted earlier, antiribosomal-P, antineuronal, and antiendothelial cell antibodies have been linked to psychosis and/or depression, but their usefulness is limited by their low positive predictive value (Arnett et al. 1996; Gerli et al. 2002).

Corticosteroid-Induced Psychiatric Symptoms in Systemic Lupus Erythematosus

Corticosteroids have been shown to cause a variety of psychiatric syndromes. However, such symptoms in SLE patients are usually not attributable to corticosteroids. First, severe psychiatric syndromes were reported historically in SLE prior to the introduction of corticosteroids and occur in SLE patients who have not received corticosteroids. Second, psychiatric symptoms in SLE are more frequent and severe than in other disorders treated with comparable doses of corticosteroids. Third, psychiatric symptoms in SLE are often ameliorated, not worsened, by maintenance or an increase in high-dose corticosteroids. In contrast, a reduction in steroid dosage often does not alleviate psychiatric symptoms and may exacerbate them.

Distinguishing corticosteroid-induced psychiatric reactions from flares of CNS lupus is one of the most challenging aspects of treating SLE. Helpful distinguishing features are summarized in Table 25–2 (Kohen et al. 1993). Given the risk of untreated CNS lupus and the likelihood that corticosteroids will alleviate such flares and only temporarily exacerbate corticosteroid-induced psychiatric reactions, an empirical initiation or increase of corticosteroids is often the most prudent intervention (Denburg et al. 1994). (Corticosteroid-induced psychiatric reactions are discussed later in this chapter in the section "Secondary Causes of Neuropsychiatric Symptoms in Rheumatological Disorders.")

TABLE 25–2. Differentiation of CNS lupus flares from corticosteroid-induced psychiatric reactions

	Active primary CNS lupus	Corticosteroid-induced psychiatric reaction
Onset	After decrease in corticosteroid dosage or during ongoing low-dose treatment	Generally <2 weeks after increase in corticosteroid dosage (~90% within 6 weeks)
Corticosteroid dosage	Variable	Rare if <40 mg/day, common if >60 mg/day
Psychiatric symptoms	Psychosis, delirium> mood disorders, cognitive impairment (new onset)	Mania, mixed states, or depression (often with psychotic features) >> delirium, psychosis
SLE symptoms	Often present; may coincide with onset of psychiatric symptoms	Often present but precede onset of psychiatric symptoms
Laboratory tests	Increases in indices of inflammation	No specific laboratory findings
Response to corticosteroids	Improvement	Exacerbation of symptoms
Response to decreased corticosteroid dosage	Exacerbation	Improvement

Note. CNS = central nervous system; SLE = systemic lupus erythematosus.
Source. Adapted from Kohen M, Asheron RA, Gharavi AE, et al.: "Lupus Psychosis: Differentiation From the Steroid-Induced State." *Clinical and Experimental Rheumatology* 11:323–326, 1993. Used with permission.

Differential Diagnosis of Psychiatric Disorders in Systemic Lupus Erythematosus

Other Medical Disorders

A wide variety of diseases can mimic neuropsychiatric SLE. One group of diseases, associated with a medium to high ANA titer (>1:160), includes Sjögren's syndrome and mixed or undifferentiated connective tissue disease. A second group of diseases, associated with a low ANA titer (<1:160), includes multiple sclerosis and, less commonly, ANA-positive RA, sarcoidosis, and hepatitis C. A third group of diseases, characterized by a negative ANA, also may be mistaken for CNS lupus. This group includes polyarteritis nodosa, microscopic angiitis, Wegener's granulomatosis, chronic fatigue syndrome, fibromyalgia, temporal arteritis, and Behçet's syndrome.

Psychotropic Drug–Induced Lupus

Patients who are receiving antipsychotic drugs, particularly chlorpromazine, may have positive ANAs and antiphospholipid antibodies; most of these patients do not develop signs of an autoantibody-associated disease. Compared with other (nonpsychiatric) drugs known to cause a symptomatic lupuslike syndrome, chlorpromazine and carbamazepine carry low risk, and several other psychotropics (divalproex, other anticonvulsants, and lithium) have very low risk. CNS involvement is usually absent in drug-induced lupus. Laboratory findings may include mild cytopenia and elevated ESR and ANA titers. Antihistone antibodies are positive in up to 95% but are not pathognomonic of drug-induced lupus. After discontinuation of the drug, symptoms and antibody titers decline usually over a period of weeks; however, the recovery can be relatively slow and may require a year (Vedove et al. 2009).

Somatization Disorder ("Psychogenic Pseudolupus")

SLE can be misdiagnosed in "somatizing" patients with multisystem complaints and mildly positive tests for ANAs, which are common in young women.

Factitious SLE

Factitious SLE appears to be rare, but several cases have been reported (Tlacuilo-Parra et al. 2000). Patients have simulated hematuria by pricking a finger surreptitiously to add trace amounts of blood to urine specimens, injected themselves with feces or other contaminants to cause infections, or applied rouge to their cheeks to simulate a malar rash. One patient feigned proteinuria by inserting a packet of protein into her bladder. These patients had no serological evidence of an autoimmune disorder.

Pregnancy in Women With Systemic Lupus Erythematosus

Pregnancy is safe for both mother and fetus in most women with inactive and stable SLE. Pregnancy is considered high risk if the woman has active disease (especially nephritis), hypertension, or specific antibodies (Khamashta 2006). Some patients with antiphospholipid syndrome have been advised to forgo reproduction because of the risk of thrombosis, preeclampsia, and fetal demise (now much less common because of anticoagulation therapy). Family tension may escalate when a patient wants to (or her partner wants her to) risk jeopardizing her health by becoming pregnant, despite admonitions about possible worsening renal or heart failure, hypertension, or stroke.

Sjögren's Syndrome

Sjögren's syndrome is characterized by lymphocytic infiltration of the exocrine glands. It can occur alone (primary Sjögren's) or in association with another autoimmune rheumatic disease. It is associated with a medium to high ANA titer (>1:160) and positive anti-SSA and/or anti-SSB antibodies. Many patients with primary Sjögren's make multiple autoantibodies, including rheumatoid factor and antiphospholipid antibodies. Some will go on to develop lymphoma. Although Sjögren's syndrome may be difficult to distinguish from CNS SLE (and the two syndromes may overlap), establishing a specific diagnosis is less crucial clinically because the treatment is the same. The most common symptoms result from drying of the eyes, mouth, and upper respiratory and urogenital tracts, but systemic manifestations can occur in up to one-third of patients. In general, these extraglandular manifestations are rare in secondary Sjögren's syndrome but relatively common in primary Sjögren's syndrome.

Neurological involvement has been reported in 20%–40% of cases, with both CNS and peripheral manifestations common (Delalande et al. 2004; Lafitte et al. 2001; Segal et al. 2008). Unlike SLE, CNS involvement is not correlated with titers of autoantibodies (Delalande et al. 2004). The nature of CNS involvement can be focal (e.g., cerebellar ataxia, vertigo, ophthalmoplegia, cranial nerve involvement) or diffuse (e.g., encephalopathy, aseptic meningoencephalitis, dementia, or psychiatric manifestations). Focal lesions may be visible on MRI. CNS involvement is most often manifested in subcortical dysfunction (Lafitte et al. 2001). A relatively high rate of affective and cognitive symptoms, as well as abnormal fatigue, headache, and poorly characterized pain, is noted in patients with Sjögren's syndrome (Harboe et al. 2009; Segal et al. 2008). The exact prevalence of psychiatric complications is not clear because most studies have investigated small populations with limited questionnaire methods. Psychological distress and quality of life in Sjögren's syndrome appear to be a function of the amount of fatigue and pain rather than degree of dryness (Champey et al. 2006).

Systemic Sclerosis (Scleroderma)

Systemic sclerosis is a chronic disorder of unknown etiology. The condition is characterized by thickening of the skin as a result of the accumulation of fibrotic connective tissue and damage to the microvasculature. Multiple body systems can be involved, including the gastrointestinal tract, heart, lungs, and kidneys. Of all the connective tissue disorders, systemic sclerosis is considered to be the least likely to cause CNS damage. CNS involvement in systemic sclerosis is rare, and most neurological complications of scleroderma are peripheral neuropathies.

Psychiatric symptoms are common, with between one-third and two-thirds reporting symptoms of depression (Thombs et al. 2007). Depression and anxiety symptoms are common (Mozzetta et al. 2008). High rates of depressive symptoms in systemic sclerosis are not a result of bias related to the reporting of somatic symptoms (Thombs et al. 2008). Symptoms of anxiety, hostility, somatization, and sensitivity have been shown to be higher in those with systemic sclerosis than in healthy control subjects (Angelopoulos et al. 2001). Body image dissatisfaction is common and in one study was greater than in patients with severe burn injuries (Benrud-Larson et al. 2003), but psychological distress has not always been found related to the extent of skin involvement (van Lankveld et al. 2007). As in many other chronic diseases, impaired psychological functioning is associated with poorer health-related quality of life (Hyphantis et al. 2007).

No known treatment is available to prevent progression of scleroderma (although some medications alleviate symptoms), and the prognosis can be poor because of renal failure and pulmonary hypertension. Some patients have severe pain secondary to digital ischemia. Fatigue, pain, and concern about prognosis and disfigurement (skin thickening, discoloration, and telangiectasias on face) are common in patients with scleroderma.

Temporal (Giant Cell) Arteritis

Temporal (giant cell) arteritis, a granulomatous arteritis of unknown etiology, predominantly affects those older than 60 years. Although almost any large artery may be involved, most of the clinical features arise because of involvement of the carotid artery and its branches. Extradural arteries are most commonly involved, leading to the typical clinical picture of headache, superficial pain, or sensitivity in skin overlying inflamed vessels (e.g., pain on combing hair). Pain overlying the temporal artery with loss of pulsations is characteristic of temporal arteritis. Pain in the face, mouth, and jaw may occur, the latter characteristically being worse on eating (jaw claudication). Visual problems occur in 25% of untreated patients, and avoidable blindness may occur if treatment with corticosteroids is delayed. In 50% of patients, pain and tenderness occur in the proximal limb muscles without signs of joint effusion, which constitutes the diagnosis of polymyalgia rheumatica. Systemic features such as weight loss and malaise can occur. Such patients may be given the misdiagnosis of fibromyalgia, but new onset later in life and an elevated ESR point toward polymyalgia rheumatica.

Neuropsychiatric manifestations of temporal arteritis arise because of the involvement of arteries supplying blood to the CNS. The insults to the CNS in temporal arteritis can be ischemic (either permanent or transient) or hemorrhagic. The clinical characteristics of the presentation depend on the nature and extent of the brain areas affected. Resultant impairments can be focal (e.g., cerebrovascular accidents leading to specific motor or sensory deficit) or diffuse, resulting in impairment of consciousness. Visual hallucinations (Charles Bonnet syndrome) are a sign of optic ischemia and if not quickly treated progress to permanent visual loss (Nesher et al. 2001). Most psychiatric symptoms in patients with temporal arteritis are a result of corticosteroid therapy (Fauchais et al. 2002).

Treatment with high-dose corticosteroids is commenced as soon as the diagnosis has been made on clinical grounds, before results of arterial biopsy are available, to prevent progression of the disease, resulting in irreversible blindness or other serious CNS damage.

Polymyositis

Polymyositis is a disease of unknown etiology that results in inflammation of the muscles. Dermatomyositis is a related condition that includes inflammation of the skin as well. The disease can occur on its own or as part of other rheumatological diseases. The clinical picture is typically that of symmetrical, proximal muscle weakness. Involvement of heart (arrhythmias, cardiac failure), gastrointestinal tract (dysphagia, reflux, constipation), and respiratory muscles (breathlessness and respiratory failure) can occur. Vasculitis can occur, rarely affecting the CNS and resulting in neuropsychiatric manifestations, including seizures, cognitive dysfunction, and depression (Ramanan et al. 2001). As with SLE and temporal arteritis, the clinical features of neuropsychiatric involvement secondary to vasculitis depend on the site and extent of the vasculitic lesions. In 20% of patients, an underlying malignancy is present (most commonly, bronchus, breast, stomach, or ovary). Thus, neuropsychiatric manifestations also may occur as the result of secondary spread of malignancy to the CNS.

Polyarteritis Nodosa

Polyarteritis nodosa is a necrotizing arteritis affecting small and medium-sized vessels, often related to hepatitis B virus infection, typically presenting with systemic symptoms (e.g., fatigue, fever, arthralgias) and signs of multisystem involvement (e.g., hypertension, renal insufficiency, neurological dysfunction, abdominal pain). Asymmetric polyneuropathy is common. Direct involvement of the CNS is less rare than previously thought. Small cerebral infarcts are the most common neuroradiological findings, although intracranial aneurysms and intracranial hemorrhage have been reported. There have been case reports of psychosis in polyarteritis nodosa with cerebral vasculitis (e.g., Kohlhaas et al. 2007).

Behçet's Syndrome

Behçet's syndrome is an idiopathic inflammatory disorder with incidence primarily in Asia and highest incidence in Turkey. In Europe, most cases are in Turkish immigrants. The most common symptoms include oral and genital ulcers, uveitis, and skin lesions. Behçet's can be life-threatening. Neuropsychiatric involvement occurs in 10%–25% of cases (Houman et al. 2007; Tohmé et al. 2009). The most common neurological manifestations include meningoencephalitis (and/or myelitis), brain stem syndromes, and vascular thrombosis. Personality change, psychiatric disorders, movement disorders, and dementia may develop. Depression and anxiety are very common, with one study finding significant symptoms of depression in half of the patients (Taner et al. 2007). Cognitive dysfunction has been found in patients with Behçet's syndrome without overt neurological involvement (Erberk-Ozen et al. 2006; Monastero et al. 2004). Differential diagnosis includes other autoimmune disorders, multiple sclerosis, and herpes simplex infections. Brain imaging and CSF studies have abnormal but not specific results. Acute neuropsychiatric symptoms respond to corticosteroids, but chronic progressive CNS disease does not.

Wegener's Granulomatosis

Wegener's granulomatosis, an uncommon disorder of unknown etiology, is characterized by a granulomatous vasculitis, predominantly affecting the upper and lower respiratory tracts together with glomerulonephritis. Necrotizing vasculitis is the hallmark of this disorder, involving both small arteries and veins. As the result of vasculitis and granuloma formation, virtually any organ in the body can be involved, including the brain and CNS. Literature relating to the neuropsychiatric manifestations is sparse.

Secondary Causes of Neuropsychiatric Symptoms in Rheumatological Disorders

Infection, Other Central Nervous System or Systemic Illness, and Drug-Induced Side Effects

Neuropsychiatric symptoms are often secondary to complications of the rheumatological disorder or its treatment, especially infection. Because some rheumatological disorders or their treatments can be associated with immune dysregulation or immunosuppression, these disorders predispose individuals to CNS and systemic infections. These infections can simulate direct involvement of the CNS by the primary disease process as in, for example, neuropsychiatric lupus. Infections causing these secondary neuropsychiatric complications include cryptococcal, tubercular, and meningococcal infections and *Listeria* meningitis; herpes encephalitis; neurosyphilis; CNS nocardiosis; toxoplasmosis; brain abscesses; and progressive multifocal leukoencephalopathy (see also Chapter 27, "Infectious Diseases"). Other etiologies of neuropsychiatric manifestations in rheumatological disorders include uremia, hypertensive encephalopathy, cerebral lymphoma, and medication side effects, as well as comorbid medical or psychiatric disorders and psychological reactions to illness (see Tables 25–1 and 25–3).

Corticosteroid-Induced Psychiatric Syndromes

Corticosteroids have psychiatric adverse effects, including mania, depression, mixed states, psychosis, anxiety, insomnia, and delirium. A previous psychiatric reaction to corticosteroids does not necessarily predict recurrent reactions with subsequent steroids. Mild psychiatric side effects include insomnia, hyperexcitability, mood lability, mild euphoria, irritability, anxiety, agitation, and racing thoughts. Mood disorders, including depression and mania, are the most common psychiatric reaction to corticosteroids. Patients may experience both mania and depression during a single course of corticosteroid therapy. Affective symptoms are often accompanied by psychotic symptoms. The psychiatric symptoms induced by corticosteroids most often resemble those of bipolar disorder, with manic symptoms most often encountered with high-dose, short-term administration and depression most often seen with chronic therapy (Bolanos et al. 2004). Delirium and psychosis (without mood symptoms) are less common. Cognitive dysfunction also has been reported. The most common

TABLE 25–3. Psychiatric side effects of medications used in treating rheumatological disorders

Medication	Psychiatric side effects
NSAIDs (high dose)	Depression, anxiety, paranoia, hallucinations, hostility, confusion, delirium, reduced concentration
Sulfasalazine	Insomnia, depression, hallucinations
Corticosteroids	Mood lability, euphoria, irritability, anxiety, insomnia, mania, depression, psychosis, delirium, cognitive disturbance
Gold	None reported
Penicillamine	None reported
Leflunomide	Anxiety
Azathioprine	Delirium
Mycophenolate mofetil	Anxiety, depression, sedation (all rare)
Cyclophosphamide	Delirium (at high doses) (rare)
Methotrexate	Delirium (at high doses) (rare)
Cyclosporine	Anxiety, delirium, visual hallucinations
Tacrolimus	Anxiety, delirium, insomnia, restlessness
Immunoglobulin (intravenous)	Delirium, agitation
LJP-394[a]	None reported
Hydroxychloroquine	Confusion, psychosis, mania, depression, nightmares, anxiety, aggression, delirium

Note. NSAIDs=nonsteroidal anti-inflammatory drugs.
[a]B-cell tolerogen–anti-double-stranded DNA antibodies.

symptoms in children are agitation and sleep disturbances (Tavassoli et al. 2008).

The incidence of corticosteroid-induced psychiatric symptoms is dose related: 1.3% in patients receiving less than 40 mg/day of prednisone, 4.6% in those receiving 41–80 mg/day, and 18.4% in those receiving greater than 80 mg/day (Boston Collaborative Drug Surveillance Program 1972). For most patients, the onset of psychiatric symptoms is within the first 2 weeks (and in 90%, within the first 6 weeks) of initiating or increasing corticosteroid treatment. In children, psychiatric side effects are also dose related, most often occurring at either prescribed or inadvertent high doses (Tavassoli et al. 2008).

The preferred treatment for corticosteroid-induced psychiatric reactions is tapering of corticosteroids, if possible, resulting in greater than 90% response rate. However, rapid tapering or discontinuation of corticosteroids also can induce psychiatric reactions by precipitating a flare of the rheumatological disease, iatrogenic adrenal insufficiency, or possibly corticosteroid-withdrawal syndrome. Corticosteroid-withdrawal syndrome is manifested by headache, fever, myalgias, arthralgias, weakness, anorexia, nausea, weight loss, and orthostatic hypotension and sometimes depression, anxiety, agitation, or psychosis (Margolin et al. 2007; Mercadante et al. 2007). Symptoms respond to an increase or a resumption of corticosteroid dosage. Adjunctive treatment with antipsychotics, antidepressants, and mood stabilizers can be helpful, depending on the particular psychiatric symptom constellation.

Other drugs used in treating rheumatological disorders may cause psychiatric side effects, especially hydroxychloroquine (see Table 25–3).

References

Affleck G, Tennen H, Urrows S, et al: Neuroticism and the pain-mood relation in rheumatoid arthritis: insights from a prospective daily study. J Consult Clin Psychol 60:119–126, 1992

Ainiala H, Hietaharju A, Loukkola J, et al: Validity of the American College of Rheumatology criteria for neuropsychiatric lupus syndromes: a population-based evaluation. Arthritis Care Res 45:419–423, 2001a

Ainiala H, Loukkola J, Peltola J, et al: The prevalence of neuropsychiatric syndromes in systemic lupus erythematosus. Neurology 57:496–500, 2001b

Albers JM, Kuper HH, van Riel PL, et al: Socio-economic consequences of rheumatoid arthritis in the first years of the disease. Rheumatology (Oxf) 38:423–430, 1999

American College of Rheumatology Ad Hoc Committee on Neuropsychiatric Lupus Nomenclature: Nomenclature and case definitions for neuropsychiatric lupus syndromes. Arthritis Rheum 42:599–608, 1999

American Psychiatric Association: Diagnostic and Statistical Manual of Mental Disorders, 4th Edition, Text Revision. Washington, DC, American Psychiatric Association, 2000

Ando Y, Kai S, Uyama E, et al: Involvement of the central nervous system in rheumatoid arthritis: its clinical manifestations and analysis by magnetic resonance imaging. Intern Med 34:188–191, 1995

Angelopoulos NV, Drosos AA, Moutsopoulos HM: Psychiatric symptoms associated with scleroderma. Psychother Psychosom 70:145–150, 2001

Arnett FC, Reveille JD, Moutsopoulos HM, et al: Ribosomal P autoantibodies in systemic lupus erythematosus: frequencies in different ethnic groups and clinical and immunogenetic associations. Arthritis Rheum 39:1833–1839, 1996

Ash G, Dickens CM, Creed FH, et al: The effects of dothiepin on subjects with rheumatoid arthritis and depression. Rheumatology (Oxford) 38:959–967, 1999

Astin JA, Beckner W, Soeken K, et al: Psychological interventions for rheumatoid arthritis: a meta-analysis of randomized controlled trials. Arthritis Rheum 47:291–302, 2002

Bachen EA, Chesney MA, Criswell LA: Prevalence of mood and anxiety disorders in women with systemic lupus erythematosus. Arthritis Rheum 61:822–829, 2009

Baker GHB, Brewerton DA: Rheumatoid arthritis: a psychiatric assessment. BMJ 282:2014, 1981

Benrud-Larson LM, Heinburg LJ, Boling C, et al: Body image dissatisfaction among women with scleroderma and relationship to psychosocial function. Health Psychol 22:130–139, 2003

Bolanos SH, Khan DA, Hanczyc M, et al: Assessment of mood states in patients receiving long-term corticosteroid therapy and in controls with patient-rated and clinician-rated scales. Ann Allergy Asthma Immunol 92:500–505, 2004

Bolger N, Zuckerman A: A framework for studying personality in the stress process. J Pers Soc Psychol 69:890–902, 1995

Boston Collaborative Drug Surveillance Program: Acute adverse reactions to prednisone in relation to dosage. Clin Pharmacol Ther 13:694–698, 1972

Bradley LA, Young LD, Anderson KO, et al: Effects of psychological therapy on pain behavior of rheumatoid arthritis patients: treatment outcome and six-month follow-up. Arthritis Rheum 30:1105–1114, 1987

Brey RL, Holliday SL, Saklad AR, et al: Neuropsychiatric syndromes in lupus: prevalence using standardized definitions. Neurology 58:1214–1220, 2002

Brown GK, Nicassio PM, Wallston KA: Pain coping strategies and depression in rheumatoid arthritis. J Clin Psychol 57:652–657, 1989

Brown GW, Harris T: Social Origins of Depression: A Study of Psychiatric Disorder in Women. London, Tavistock, 1979

Brown GW, Harris TO: Life Events and Illness. New York, Guilford, 1989

Callahan LF, Kaplan MR, Pincus T: The Beck Depression Inventory, Center for Epidemiological Studies Depression Scale (CES-D), and General Well-Being Schedule depression subscale in rheumatoid arthritis. Arthritis Care Res 4:3–11, 1991

Champey J, Corruble E, Gottenberg JE, et al: Quality of life and psychological status in patients with primary Sjögren's syndrome and sicca symptoms without autoimmune features. Arthritis Rheum 55:451–457, 2006

Cohen W, Roberts WN, Levenson JL: Psychiatric aspects of SLE, in Systemic Lupus Erythematosus. Edited by Lahita R. San Diego, CA, Elsevier, 2004, pp 785–825

Cole SW, Hawkley LC, Arevalo JM, et al: Social regulation of gene expression in human leukocytes. Genome Biol 8:R189, 2007

Conti F, Alessandri C, Bompane D, et al: Autoantibody profile in systemic lupus erythematosus with psychiatric manifestations: a role for anti-endothelial-cell antibodies. Arthritis Res Ther 6:R366–R372, 2004

Conway S, Creed FH, Symmons DPM: Life events and the onset of rheumatoid arthritis. J Psychosom Res 38:837–847, 1994

Copsey Spring TR, Yanni LM, Levenson JL: A shot in the dark: failing to recognize the link between physical and mental illness. J Gen Intern Med 22:677–680, 2007

Covic T, Pallant JF, Tennant A, et al: Variability in depression prevalence in early rheumatoid arthritis: a comparison of the CES-D and HAD-D Scales. BMC Musculoskelet Disord 10:18, 2009

Davis MC, Zautra AJ, Younger J, et al: Chronic stress and regulation of cellular markers of inflammation in rheumatoid arthritis: implications for fatigue. Brain Behav Immun 22:24–32, 2008

Delalande S, de Seze J, Fauchais AL, et al: Neurologic manifestations in primary Sjögren syndrome: a study of 82 patients. Medicine (Baltimore) 83:280–291, 2004

Demange V, Guillemin F, Baumann M, et al: Are there more than cross-sectional relationships of social support and support networks with functional limitations and psychological distress in early rheumatoid arthritis? The European Research on Incapacitating Diseases and Social Support Longitudinal Study. Arthritis Rheum 51:782–791, 2004

Denburg SD, Carbotte RM, Denburg JA: Corticosteroids and neuropsychological functioning in patients with systemic lupus erythematosus. Arthritis Rheum 37:1311–1320, 1994

Dickens C, Jackson J, Tomenson B, et al: Associations of depression in rheumatoid arthritis. Psychosomatics 44:209–215, 2003

DiMatteo MR, Lepper HS, Croghan TW: Depression is a risk factor for noncompliance with medical treatment: meta-analysis of the effects of anxiety and depression on patient adherence. Arch Intern Med 160:2101–2107, 2000

Drewes AM, Svendsen L, Taagholt SJ, et al: Sleep in rheumatoid arthritis: a comparison with healthy subjects and studies of sleep/wake interactions. Br J Rheumatol 37:71–81, 1998

Eisenberger NI, Inagaki TK, Rameson LT, et al: An fMRI study of cytokine-induced depressed mood and social pain: the role of sex differences. Neuroimage 47:881–890, 2009

Erberk-Ozen N, Birol A, Boratav C, et al: Executive dysfunctions and depression in Behçet's disease without explicit neurological involvement. Psychiatry Clin Neurosci 60:465–472, 2006

Evers AW, Kraaimaat FW, Geenen R, et al: Longterm predictors of anxiety and depressed mood in early rheumatoid arthritis: a 3 and 5 year followup. J Rheumatol 29:2327–2336, 2002

Fauchais AL, Boivin V, Hachulla E, et al: Psychiatric complications of corticoid therapy in the elderly over 65 years of age treated for Horton disease [in French]. Rev Med Interne 23:828–833, 2002

Frank RG, Beck NC, Parker JC, et al: Depression in rheumatoid arthritis. J Rheumatol 15:920–925, 1988

Fyrand L, Moum T, Finset A, et al: Social support in female patients with rheumatoid arthritis compared with healthy controls. Psychol Health 6:429–439, 2001

Gerli R, Caponi L, Tincani A, et al: Clinical and serological associations of ribosomal P autoantibodies in systemic lupus erythematosus: prospective evaluation in a large cohort of Italian patients. Rheumatology (Oxf) 41:1357–1366, 2002

Gharavi AE: Anticardiolipin syndrome: antiphospholipid syndrome. Clin Med 1:14–17, 2001

Grace EM, Bellamy N, Kassam Y, et al: Controlled, double-blind, randomized trial of amitriptyline in relieving articular pain and tenderness in patients with rheumatoid arthritis. Curr Med Res Opin 9:426–429, 1985

Griffin KW, Friend R, Kaell AT, et al: Distress and disease status among patients with rheumatoid arthritis: roles of coping styles and perceived responses from support providers. Ann Behav Med 23:133–138, 2001

Hanly JG, Cassell K, Fisk JD: Cognitive function in systemic lupus erythematosus: results of a 5-year prospective study. Arthritis Rheum 40:1542–1543, 1997

Hanly JG, Urowitz MB, Sanchez-Guerrero J, et al: Neuropsychiatric events at the time of diagnosis of systemic lupus erythematosus: an international inception cohort study. Arthritis Rheum 56:265–273, 2007

Harboe E, Tjensvoll AB, Vefring HK, et al: Fatigue in primary Sjögren's syndrome—a link to sickness behaviour in animals? Brain Behav Immun 23:1104–1108, 2009

He Y, Zhang M, Lin EH, et al: Mental disorders among persons with arthritis: results from the World Mental Health Surveys. Psychol Med 38:1639–1650, 2008

Herranz MT, Rivier G, Khamashta MA, et al: Association between antiphospholipid antibodies and epilepsy in patients with systemic lupus erythematosus. Arthritis Rheum 37:568–571, 1994

Holtzman S, Newth S, Delongis A: The role of social support in coping with daily pain among patients with rheumatoid arthritis. J Health Psychol 9:677–695, 2004

Houman MH, Neffati H, Braham A, et al: Behçet's disease in Tunisia. Demographic, clinical and genetic aspects in 260 patients. Clin Exp Rheumatol 25 (4 suppl 45):S58–S64, 2007

Hurwicz ML, Berkanovic E: The stress process in rheumatoid arthritis. J Rheumatol 20:1836–1844, 1993

Hyphantis TN, Tsifetaki N, Siafaka V, et al: The impact of psychological functioning upon systemic sclerosis patients' quality of life. Semin Arthritis Rheum 37:81–92, 2007

Irwin MR, Wang M, Campomayor CO, et al: Sleep deprivation and activation of morning levels of cellular and genomic markers of inflammation. Arch Intern Med 166:1756–1762, 2006

Irwin MR, Wang M, Ribeiro D, et al: Sleep loss activates cellular inflammatory signaling. Biol Psychiatry 64:538–540, 2008

Isshi K, Hirohata S: Differential roles of antiribosomal P antibody and antineuronal antibody in the pathogenesis of central nervous system involvement in systemic lupus erythematosus. Arthritis Rheum 41:1819–1827, 1998

Jennekens FGI, Kater L: The central nervous system in systemic lupus erythematosus, part 2: pathogenic mechanisms of clinical syndromes: a literature investigation. Rheumatology 41:619–630, 2002

Joyce AT, Smith P, Khandker R, et al: Hidden cost of rheumatoid arthritis (RA): estimating cost of comorbid cardiovascular disease and depression among patients with RA. J Rheumatol 36:743–752, 2009

Julian LJ, Yelin E, Yazdany J, et al: Depression, medication adherence, and service utilization in systemic lupus erythematosus. Arthritis Rheum 61:240–246, 2009

Kaposi M: Neue beitrage zur Kenntnis des lupus erythematosus. Archiv fur Dermatologie und Syphilis 4:36–79, 1872

Karassa FB, Ioannidis JPA, Touloumi G, et al: Risk factors for central nervous system involvement in systemic lupus erythematosus. QJM 93:169–174, 2000

Katz PP, Yelin EH: The development of depressive symptoms among women with rheumatoid arthritis: the role of function. Arthritis Rheum 38:49–56, 1995

Khamashta MA: Systemic lupus erythematosus and pregnancy. Best Pract Res Clin Rheumatol 20:685–694, 2006

Kohen M, Asheron RA, Gharavi AE, et al: Lupus psychosis: differentiation from the steroid-induced state. Clin Exp Rheumatol 11:323–326, 1993

Kohlhaas K, Brechmann T, Vorgerd M: Hepatitis B associated polyarteritis nodosa with cerebral vasculitis [in German]. Dtsch Med Wochenschr 132(34–35):1748–1752, 2007

Kowal C, Degiorgio LA, Lee JY, et al: Human lupus autoantibodies against NMDA receptors mediate cognitive impairment. Proc Natl Acad Sci U S A 103:19854–19859, 2006

Kozora E, Ellison MC, West S: Depression, fatigue, and pain in systemic lupus erythematosus (SLE): relationship to the American College of Rheumatology SLE neuropsychological battery. Arthritis Rheum 55:628–635, 2006

Kurne A, Karabudak R, Karadag O, et al: An unusual central nervous system involvement in rheumatoid arthritis: combination of pachymeningitis and cerebral vasculitis. Rheumatol Int 29:1349–1353, 2009

Lafitte C, Amoura Z, Cacoub P, et al: Neurological complications of primary Sjögren's syndrome. J Neurol 248:577–584, 2001

Lahita R (ed): Systemic Lupus Erythematosus. San Diego, CA, Elsevier, 2004

Larsen RJ: Neuroticism and selective encoding and recall of symptoms: evidence from a combined concurrent retrospective study. J Pers Soc Psychol 62:480–488, 1992

Leventhal H, Benyamini Y, Brownlee S, et al: Illness representations: theory and measurement, in Perceptions of Health and Illness. Edited by Petrie KJ, Weinman JA. Amsterdam, The Netherlands, Harwood Academic Publishers, 1997, pp 19–46

Levine JS, Branch DW, Rauch J: The antiphospholipid syndrome. N Engl J Med 346:752–763, 2002

Liang MH, Rogers M, Larson M, et al: The psychosocial impact of systemic lupus erythematosus and rheumatoid arthritis. Arthritis Rheum 27:13–19, 1984

Lin EH: Depression and osteoarthritis. Am J Med 121:S16–S19, 2008

Lin E, Katon W, Von Korff M, et al: Effects of improving depression care on pain and functional outcomes among older adults with arthritis. JAMA 290:2428–2434, 2003

Lubeck DP, Spitz PW, Fries JF, et al: A multicenter study of annual health service utilization and costs in rheumatoid arthritis. Arthritis Rheum 29:488–493, 1986

Machado GP, Gignac MA, Badley EM: Participation restrictions among older adults with osteoarthritis: a mediated model of physical symptoms, activity limitations, and depression. Arthritis Rheum 59:129–135, 2008

Malemud CJ, Miller AH: Pro-inflammatory cytokine-induced SAPK/MAPK and JAK/STAT in rheumatoid arthritis and the new anti-depression drugs. Expert Opin Ther Targets 12:171–183, 2008

Margolin L, Cope DK, Bakst-Sisser R, et al: The steroid withdrawal syndrome: a review of the implications, etiology, and treatments. J Pain Symptom Manage 33:224–228, 2007

Mercadante S, Villari P, Intravaia G: Withdrawal acute psychosis after corticosteroid discontinuation. J Pain Symptom Manage 34:118–119, 2007

Miller AH, Maletic V, Raison CL: Inflammation and its discontents: the role of cytokines in the pathophysiology of major depression. Biol Psychiatry 65:732–741, 2009

Mindham RH, Bagshaw A, James SA, et al: Factors associated with the appearance of psychiatric symptoms in rheumatoid arthritis. J Psychosom Res 25:429–435, 1981

Moldofsky H: Sleep and pain. Sleep Med Rev 5:385–396, 2001

Monastero R, Camarda C, Pipia C, et al: Cognitive impairment in Behçet's disease patients without overt neurological involvement. J Neurol Sci 220(1–2):99–104, 2004

Motivala SJ, Khanna D, FitzGerald J, et al: Stress activation of cellular markers of inflammation in rheumatoid arthritis: protective effects of tumor necrosis factor alpha antagonists. Arthritis Rheum 58:376–383, 2008

Mozzetta A, Antinone V, Alfani S, et al: Mental health in patients with systemic sclerosis: a controlled investigation. J Eur Acad Dermatol Venereol 22:336–340, 2008

Murphy H, Dickens C, Creed F, et al: Depression, illness perception and coping in rheumatoid arthritis. J Psychosom Res 46:155–164, 1999

Murphy S, Creed F, Jayson MI: Psychiatric disorder and illness behaviour in rheumatoid arthritis. Br J Rheumatol 27:357–363, 1988

Nesher G, Nesher R, Rozenman Y, et al: Visual hallucinations in giant cell arteritis: association with visual loss. J Rheumatol 28:2046–2048, 2001

Nicassio PM, Moxham EG, Schuman CE, et al: The contribution of pain, reported sleep quality, and depressive symptoms to fatigue in fibromyalgia. Pain 100:271–279, 2002

Oda K, Matsushima E, Okubo Y, et al: Abnormal regional cerebral blood flow in systemic lupus erythematosus patients with psychiatric symptoms. J Clin Psychiatry 66:907–913, 2005

Olsen NJ, Stein CM: New drugs for rheumatoid arthritis. N Engl J Med 350:2167–2179, 2004

Ormel J, Wohlfart T: How neuroticism, long-term difficulties and life situation change influence psychological distress: a longitudinal model. J Pers Soc Psychol 60:744–755, 1991

Otto R, Mackay IR: Psycho-social and emotional disturbance in systemic lupus erythematosus. Med J Aust 2:488–493, 1967

Pace TW, Mletzko TC, Alagbe O, et al: Increased stress-induced inflammatory responses in male patients with major depression and increased early life stress. Am J Psychiatry 163:1630–1633, 2006

Parker JC, Smarr KL, Slaughter JR, et al: Management of depression in rheumatoid arthritis: a combined pharmacologic and cognitive-behavioral approach. Arthritis Rheum 49:766–777, 2003

Pawlak C, Witte T, Heiken H, et al: Flares in patients with systemic lupus erythematosus are associated with daily psychological stress. Psychother Psychosom 72:159–165, 2003

Peck JR, Smith TW, Ward JR, et al: Disability and depression in rheumatoid arthritis: a multi-trait, multi-method investigation. Arthritis Rheum 32:1100–1106, 1989

Peralta-Ramirez MI, Jimenez-Alonso J, Godoy-Garcia JF, et al: The effects of daily stress and stressful life events on the clinical symptomatology of patients with lupus erythematosus. Psychosom Med 66:788–794, 2004

Peralta-Ramirez MI, Coin-Mejias MA, Jimenez-Alonso J, et al: Stress as a predictor of cognitive functioning in lupus. Lupus 15:858–864, 2006

Persson LO, Berglund K, Sahlberg D: Psychological factors in chronic rheumatic diseases—a review: the case of rheumatoid arthritis, current research and some problems. Scand J Rheumatol 28:137–144, 1999

Pow J: The role of psychological influences in rheumatoid arthritis. J Psychosom Res 31:223–229, 1987

Ramanan AV, Sawhney S, Murray KJ: Central nervous system complications in two cases of juvenile onset dermatomyositis. Rheumatology (Oxford) 40:1293–1298, 2001

Reichenberg A, Yirmiya R, Schuld A, et al: Cytokine-associated emotional and cognitive disturbances in humans. Arch Gen Psychiatry 58:445–452, 2001

Rosemann T, Backenstrass M, Joest K, et al: Predictors of depression in a sample of 1,021 primary care patients with osteoarthritis. Arthritis Rheum 57:415–422, 2007a

Rosemann T, Gensichen J, Sauer N, et al: The impact of concomitant depression on quality of life and health service utilisation in patients with osteoarthritis. Rheumatol Int 27:859–863, 2007b

Sabbadini MG, Manfredi AA, Bozzolo E, et al: Central nervous system involvement in systemic lupus erythematosus patients without overt neuropsychiatric manifestations. Lupus 8:1–2, 1999

Sabet A, Sibbitt WL, Stidley CA, et al: Neurometabolite markers of cerebral injury in the antiphospholipid antibody syndrome of SLE. Stroke 29:2254–2260, 1998

Sale JE, Gignac M, Hawker G: The relationship between disease symptoms, life events, coping and treatment, and depression among older adults with osteoarthritis. J Rheumatol 35:335–342, 2008

Segal B, Thomas W, Rogers T, et al: Prevalence, severity, and predictors of fatigue in subjects with primary Sjögren's syndrome. Arthritis Rheum 59:1780–1787, 2008

Scolding NJ, Joseph FG: The neuropathology and pathogenesis of systemic lupus erythematosus. Neuropathol Appl Neurobiol 28:173–189, 2002

Sharpe L, Sensky T, Timberlake N, et al: A blind, randomized, controlled trial of cognitive-behavioural intervention for patients with recent onset rheumatoid arthritis: preventing psychological and physical morbidity. Pain 89:275–283, 2001

Sheikh JI, Yesavage J: Geriatric Depression Scale (GDS): recent evidence and development of a shorter version. Clin Gerontol 9:37–43, 1989

Smedstad LM, Vaglum P, Kvien TK, et al: The relationship between self-reported pain and sociodemographic variables, anxiety, and depressive symptoms in rheumatoid arthritis. J Rheumatol 22:514–520, 1995

Smedstad LM, Moum T, Vaglum P, et al: The impact of early rheumatoid arthritis on psychological distress: a comparison between 238 patients with RA and 116 matched controls. Scand J Rheumatol 25:377–382, 1996

Smith TW, Peck JR, Milano RA, et al: Cognitive distortion in rheumatoid arthritis: relation to depression and disability. J Consult Clin Psychol 56:412–416, 1988

Spitzer A, Bar-Tal Y, Golander H: Social support: how does it really work? J Adv Nurs 22:850–854, 1995

Strating MM, Suurmeijer TP, van Schuur WH: Disability, social support, and distress in rheumatoid arthritis: results from a 13-year prospective study. Arthritis Rheum 55:736–744, 2006

Straub RH, Dhabhar FS, Bijlsma JW, et al: How psychological stress via hormones and nerve fibers may exacerbate rheumatoid arthritis. Arthritis Rheum 52:16–26, 2005

Sundquist K, Li X, Hemminki K, et al: Subsequent risk of hospitalization for neuropsychiatric disorders in patients with rheumatic diseases: a nationwide study from Sweden. Arch Gen Psychiatry 65:501–507, 2008

Taner E, Cosar B, Burhanoglu S, et al: Depression and anxiety in patients with Behçet's disease compared with that in patients with psoriasis. Int J Dermatol 46:1118–1124, 2007

Tavassoli N, Montastruc-Fournier J, Montastruc JL: Psychiatric adverse drug reactions to glucocorticoids in children and adolescents: a much higher risk with elevated doses. French Association of Regional Pharmacovigilance Centres. Br J Clin Pharmacol 66:566–567, 2008

Thombs BD, Taillefer SS, Hudson M, et al: Depression in patients with systemic sclerosis: a systematic review of the evidence. Arthritis Rheum 57:1089–1097, 2007

Thombs BD, Hudson M, Taillefer SS, et al: Prevalence and clinical correlates of symptoms of depression in patients with systemic sclerosis. Canadian Scleroderma Research Group. Arthritis Rheum 59:504–509, 2008

Tlacuilo-Parra JA, Guevara-Gutierrez E, Garcia-De La Torre I: Factitious disorders mimicking systemic lupus erythematosus. Clin Exp Rheumatol 18:89–93, 2000

Tohmé A, Koussa S, Haddad-Zébouni S, et al: [Neurological manifestations of Behçet's disease: 22 cases among 170 patients]. Presse Med 38:701–709, 2009

Tyring S, Gottlieb A, Papp K, et al: Etanercept and clinical outcomes, fatigue, and depression in psoriasis: double-blind placebo-controlled randomised phase III trial. Lancet 367:29–35, 2006

Uguz F, Akman C, Kucuksarac S, et al: Anti-tumor necrosis factor-alpha therapy is associated with less frequent mood and anxiety disorders in patients with rheumatoid arthritis. Psychiatry Clin Neurosci 63:50–55, 2009

van Lankveld WG, Vonk MC, Teunissen H, et al: Appearance self-esteem in systemic sclerosis—subjective experience of skin deformity and its relationship with physician-assessed skin involvement, disease status and psychological variables. Rheumatology (Oxford) 46:872–876, 2007

Vedove CD, Del Giglio M, Schena D, et al: Drug-induced lupus erythematosus. Arch Dermatol Res 301:99–105, 2009

Waterloo K, Omdal R, Jacobsen EA, et al: Cerebral computed tomography and electroencephalography compared with neuropsychological findings in systemic lupus erythematosus. J Neurol 246:706–711, 1999

Waterloo K, Omdal R, Husby G, et al: Neuropsychological function in systemic lupus erythematosus: a five-year longitudinal study. Rheumatology 41:411–415, 2002

West SG, Emlen W, Wener MH, et al: Neuropsychiatric lupus erythematosus: a prospective study on the value of diagnostic tests. Am J Med 99:153–163, 1995

Wierzbicki AS: Lipids, cardiovascular disease and atherosclerosis in systemic lupus erythematosus. Lupus 9:194–201, 2000

Wolfe F: Psychological distress and rheumatic disease. Scand J Rheumatol 28:131–136, 1999

Wolfe F, Hawley DJ: The relationship between clinical activity and depression in rheumatoid arthritis. J Rheumatol 20:2032–2037, 1993

Wolfe F, Michaud K: Predicting depression in rheumatoid arthritis: the signal importance of pain extent and fatigue, and comorbidity. Arthritis Rheum 61:667–673, 2009

Yelin EH, Feshbach DM, Meenan RF, et al: Social problems, services and policy for persons with chronic disease: the case of rheumatoid arthritis. Soc Sci Med [Med Econ] 13C:13–20, 1979

Yu B, Becnel J, Zerfaoui M, et al: Serotonin 5-hydroxytryptamine(2A) receptor activation suppresses tumor necrosis factor-alpha-induced inflammation with extraordinary potency. J Pharmacol Exp Ther 327:316–323, 2008

Zamarron F, Maceiras F, Mera A, et al: Effects of the first infliximab infusion on sleep and alertness in patients with active rheumatoid arthritis. Ann Rheum Dis 63:88–90, 2004

Zautra AJ, Yocum DC, Villanueva I, et al: Immune activation and depression in women with rheumatoid arthritis. J Rheumatol 31:457–463, 2004

Zautra AJ, Davis MC, Reich JW, et al: Comparison of cognitive behavioral and mindfulness meditation interventions on adaptation to rheumatoid arthritis for patients with and without history of recurrent depression. J Consult Clin Psychol 76:408–421, 2008

Zigmond AS, Snaith RP: The Hospital Anxiety and Depression Scale. Acta Psychiatr Scand 67:361–370, 1983

Zolcinski M, Bazan-Socha S, Zwolinska G, et al: Central nervous system involvement as a major manifestation of rheumatoid arthritis. Rheumatol Int 28:281–283, 2008

Zyrianova Y, Kelly BD, Gallagher C, et al: Depression and anxiety in rheumatoid arthritis: the role of perceived social support. Ir J Med Sci 175:32–36, 2006

CHAPTER 26

Chronic Fatigue and Fibromyalgia Syndromes

Michael C. Sharpe, M.A., M.D., F.R.C.P., F.R.C.Psych.
Patrick G. O'Malley, M.D., M.P.H., F.A.C.P.

IN THIS CHAPTER, WE REVIEW two symptom-defined somatic syndromes: chronic fatigue syndrome (CFS) and fibromyalgia syndrome (FMS). The central feature of CFS is the symptom of severe chronic, disabling fatigue that is typically exacerbated by exertion and unexplained by any other medical condition. The central feature of FMS is widespread pain with localized tenderness that is similarly unexplained by any other diagnosis. Although these syndromes have different historical origins, it is increasingly recognized that they have much in common (Sullivan et al. 2002). Therefore, in this chapter we will consider them together.

CFS, FMS, and other symptom-defined somatic syndromes are conditions whose homes both in medicine (as functional syndromes) and in psychiatry (as somatoform disorders) are rather temporary structures located in unfashionable areas of their respective communities. These so-called functional somatic syndromes (Wessely et al. 1999) are, however, of central concern to psychosomatic medicine. Other functional or medically unexplained syndromes covered elsewhere in this volume include noncardiac chest pain (see Chapter 18, "Heart Disease"), hyperventilation syndrome (see Chapter 19, "Lung Disease"), irritable bowel and functional upper gastrointestinal disorders (see Chapter 20, "Gastrointestinal Disorders"), idiopathic pruritus (see Chapter 29, "Dermatology"), migraine (see Chapter 32, "Neurology and Neurosurgery"), chronic pelvic pain and vulvodynia (see Chapter 33, "Obstetrics and Gynecology"), and several other pain syndromes (see Chapter 36, "Pain"). Somatization is also discussed in Chapter 12, "Somatization and Somatoform Disorders."

General Issues

Symptom or Disorder?

Although CFS and FMS are often regarded as discrete conditions, the severity of their core symptoms of fatigue and pain is continuously distributed in the general population (Croft et al. 1996; Pawlikowska et al. 1994); the case definitions can therefore be regarded as simply defining clinically significant cutoff points on these severity continua.

Organic or Psychogenic?

The history of CFS and FMS has been notorious for sometimes bitter disputes about whether these disorders are "organic" or "psychogenic" (Asbring and Narvanen 2003). The extreme organic position argues that they eventually will be found to be as firmly based in disease pathology as any other medical condition, whereas the extreme psychogenic view is that these syndromes are really pseudodiseases, not rooted in biology but rather mere social constructions based on the psychological amplification of normal somatic sensations such as tiredness and pain. Neither of these extreme positions can be satisfactorily sustained by

We are grateful to the following for helpful comments on earlier versions of the chapter: Dr. Peter White, Dr. Leslie Arnold, Professor Simon Wessely, Professor Gijs Belijenberg, Professor Dan Clauw, and Dr. Robert Perry.

the evidence or indeed is helpful in managing patients. The extreme organic view encourages the doctor to endlessly seek pathology while the patient adopts the life of the helpless invalid. The extreme psychological view encourages the doctor to dismiss the patient's physical symptoms and paradoxically can also lead to a defensive entrenchment of the patient's belief that he or she has an untreatable disease (Hadler 1996b). An etiologically neutral and integrated perspective that both recognizes the reality of the physical symptoms and acknowledges the contribution of biological, psychological, and social factors offers the best basis for effective clinical practice (Engel 1977).

Medical or Psychiatric?

In parallel with the debate about etiology is an argument about whether these conditions are most appropriately regarded as "medical" or as "psychiatric" illnesses. For a given set of symptoms, the appropriate medical diagnosis might be CFS (chronic fatigue and immune dysfunction syndrome; myalgic encephalomyelitis or encephalopathy—see "History" subsection in the following section, "The Syndromes") or FMS, whereas for the very same symptoms the appropriate psychiatric diagnosis might be an anxiety, mood, or somatoform disorder. Which is correct? We argue that neither alone is an adequate description of the illness and that both should be used. Proper use of the DSM-IV-TR (American Psychiatric Association 2000) axes allows the patient to be given both a medical (Axis III) and a psychiatric (Axis I) diagnosis. Consequently, the best diagnosis may be, for example, FMS *and* generalized anxiety disorder (GAD). Ultimately, however, a classification that avoids the need for two separate diagnoses for the same symptoms is desirable. Achieving this will be a challenge for the authors of the forthcoming DSM-V (Mayou et al. 2003).

The Syndromes

Chronic Fatigue Syndrome

History

CFS is not a new illness. A very similar, if not identical, condition was described as *neurasthenia* over 100 years ago and probably existed long before that (Wessely 1990). However, the term *chronic fatigue syndrome* was coined as recently as 1988 to describe a condition characterized by chronic disabling fatigue accompanied by many other somatic symptoms (Holmes et al. 1988). The authors of this early definition anticipated that a specific disease cause, possibly infectious, would be found, but an etiology has so far not been established.

CFS has subsumed a multitude of previous terms used to describe patients with similar symptoms. These include *chronic Epstein-Barr virus infection* (see Chapter 27, "Infectious Diseases"), *myalgic encephalomyelitis, neurasthenia* (still a specific diagnosis in ICD-10 [World Health Organization 1992]), and *postviral fatigue syndrome.* Arguments persist about the appropriateness of subsuming all of these diagnoses under the umbrella term *CFS.* Patient advocacy groups in particular have been very vocal in arguing that the name *CFS* is an inadequate description of their illness and that a name such as *myalgic encephalomyelitis* or *encephalopathy* or *chronic fatigue and immune dysfunction syndrome,* which emphasizes a biological pathology, is more appropriate. The introduction of the new terminology of CFS has, however, had the important advantage for researchers of being clearly operationally defined and consequently has provided a firm basis for replicable scientific research.

Definition

Several operational diagnostic criteria for CFS have been published. The first case definition (noted in the preceding subsection, "History"), by Holmes et al. (1988), was excessively cumbersome and restrictive. Furthermore, it was found that requiring multiple somatic symptoms selected patients who were more—rather than less—likely to also meet criteria for a psychiatric diagnoses, which, combined with the strict psychiatric exclusions, made the condition very rare. Consequently, simpler and less exclusive Australian (Lloyd et al. 1988) and British (Oxford) (Sharpe et al. 1991) case definitions were constructed. The currently most widely used criteria (shown in Table 26-1) are based on an international consensus case definition published in 1994 (Fukuda et al. 1994) that has since been further clarified (Reeves et al. 2003). Finally, it should be remembered that all of these definitions have been constructed by committees with the primary aim of aiding research. Consequently, clinical practice should not be too rigidly bound by them.

Clinical Features

The core symptoms of CFS are fatigue exacerbated by exercise, and subjective cognitive impairment; in addition, disrupted and unrefreshing sleep is almost universally described, with some degree of widespread pain also common (Prins et al. 2006). Patients often report marked fluctuations in their fatigue that occur from week to week and even from day to day. Few patients are so disabled that they cannot attend an outpatient consultation, although some describe difficulty walking and require the aid of wheelchairs and other appliances. A minority remain bedridden, unable to visit the clinic, and represent an important and neglected group.

The symptom of fatigue is subjective. The correlation between the feeling of fatigue and objectively measured decrements in performance has long been known to be

TABLE 26–1. Diagnostic criteria for chronic fatigue syndrome

Inclusion criteria

1. Clinically evaluated, medically unexplained fatigue of at least 6 months' duration that is
   - Of new onset (not lifelong)
   - Not the result of ongoing exertion
   - Not substantially alleviated by rest
   - Associated with a substantial reduction in previous level of activities
2. Presence of four or more of the following symptoms:
   - Subjective memory impairment
   - Sore throat
   - Tender lymph nodes
   - Muscle pain
   - Joint pain
   - Headache
   - Unrefreshing sleep
   - Postexertional malaise lasting more than 24 hours

Exclusion criteria

Active, unresolved, or suspected medical disease

Psychotic, melancholic, or bipolar depression (but not uncomplicated major depression)

Psychotic disorders

Dementia, anorexia or bulimia nervosa

Alcohol or other substance misuse

Severe obesity

Source. Adapted from Fukuda et al. 1994.

weak (Welford 1953). Hence, if a patient with CFS is asked to perform exercise tests, he or she may not show the expected objective decrement in performance but instead may report greater subjective effort and increased fatigue, both at the time of the test and over the following days (Wallman and Sacco 2007). Similarly, standard neuropsychological testing usually yields normal results but is often accompanied by a report of greater effort (Vercoulen et al. 1998). Some evidence indicates that more complex cognitive tests do show deficits in functioning, including reduced attention, motor speed, and working memory, although these usually appear less severe than expected from the severity of the patient's subjective complaints (Dickson et al. 2009; Majer et al. 2008; Wearden and Appleby 1996).

In summary, the core clinical features of CFS are subjective physical and mental fatigue exacerbated by physical and mental effort. Although some may interpret this subjectivity as evidence of exaggeration of disability, it can also be seen as reflecting the essentially sensory nature of this condition.

Fibromyalgia

History

More than 100 years ago, Gowers (1904) coined the term *fibrositis* to describe a chronic widespread pain thought to be caused by inflammation of muscles. However, as with CFS, specific disease pathology in muscle has not subsequently been confirmed. Other terms, such as *chronic widespread pain* (CWP) and *myofascial pain syndrome,* have been used to describe the condition. In 1990, the American College of Rheumatology adopted the operationally defined and descriptive term *fibromyalgia* as an alternative to *fibrositis* (Wolfe et al. 1990). As with CFS, the new case definition has facilitated replicable research and has been widely adopted.

Definition

The American College of Rheumatology criteria specify widespread pain of at least 3 months' duration and tenderness at 11 or more of 18 specific sites on the body. They are shown in Table 26–2.

A particular feature of the FMS criteria is the specification of specific examination findings as well as of symptoms. A standardized method of eliciting these "tender points" has been defined (i.e., the application of pressure with the thumb pad perpendicular to each defined site with increasing force by approximately 1 kg/second until 4 kg of pressure is achieved, which usually leads to whitening of the thumbnail bed). Despite the apparent precision of this clinical sign, both the specificity of the locations and the uniqueness of the proposed tender points to FMS have been questioned (Croft et al. 1996; Wolfe 1997).

Clinical Features

The core features of fibromyalgia are chronic widespread pain and musculoskeletal tenderness (muscles; ligaments and tendons). Pain occurs typically in all four quadrants of the body and the axial skeleton but also can be regional. Fatigue, sleep disturbance, and subjective cognitive impairment (memory and concentration) are common associations. As with CFS, the report of pain is essentially a subjective phenomenon and may not be reflected in attempts to assess physical and mental performance objectively.

Patients have a range of associated disability, although most patients are able to attend outpatient services. The symptoms of FMS overlap considerably with those of other rheumatological conditions, creating a diagnostic dilemma for the clinician faced with a patient who has an

TABLE 26–2. American College of Rheumatology 1990 criteria for fibromyalgia

1. History of widespread pain. Pain in the right and left sides of the body, pain above and below the waist, axial skeletal pain (cervical spine or anterior chest or thoracic spine or low back). In this definition, shoulder and buttock pain is considered as pain for each involved side. Low back pain is considered lower-segment pain.
2. Pain, on digital palpation, must be present in at least 11 of 18 specified tender point sites. Digital palpation should be performed with an approximate force of 4 kg. For a tender point to be considered positive, the patient must state that the palpation was painful. Tender is not to be considered painful.

Source. Adapted from Wolfe et al. 1990.

undifferentiated constellation of chronic musculoskeletal symptoms (see subsection "Identification of Medical and Psychiatric Conditions" later in this chapter).

Primary or Secondary?

Both CFS and FMS are typically diagnosed when the patient has no evidence of another general medical condition. This makes it easy to define the symptoms as unexplained by another condition. However, similar symptoms are also found in patients with other medical diagnoses. For example, symptoms of FMS have been reported in patients with systemic lupus erythematosus (Buskila et al. 2003) and rheumatoid arthritis (Wolfe et al. 1984), and symptoms of CFS have been reported in disease-free cancer patients (Servaes et al. 2002) and in patients with multiple sclerosis (Vercoulen et al. 1996a). The terms *primary* (occurring in the absence of another condition) and *secondary* (accompanying a medical condition) have been used to describe these findings. The terminology is, however, confusing and arguably more a matter of differential diagnosis than of comorbidity (see subsection "Association With Other Symptom-Defined Syndromes" later in this section). It is best avoided.

Same or Different?

Pain and fatigue tend to co-occur in the general population (Creavin et al. 2010). Furthermore, there is an overlap in the symptoms of patients with a diagnosis of FMS and those with a diagnosis of CFS. Put simply, CFS is fatigue with pain, and FMS is pain with fatigue. A latent class analysis of the symptoms of more than 600 patients failed to identify separate syndromes (Sullivan et al. 2002). Not only are the symptoms similar, but a patient who has received the diagnosis of one of these conditions is also likely to meet the diagnostic criteria for the other. Of 163 consecutive female patients with CFS enrolled at a tertiary care clinic, more than a third also met criteria for FMS (Ciccone and Natelson 2003). Consequently, most authorities now accept that important similarities exist between CFS and FMS (Aaron and Buchwald 2003; Wessely et al. 1999). One potential difference between CFS and FMS is the presence of so-called tender points in the former. However, tender points also are often found in patients with CFS. Whether these conditions will be found ultimately to be distinct entities, overlapping conditions, or just aspects of the same condition currently remains both unclear and controversial.

Association With Other Symptom-Defined Syndromes

Studies that have assessed the comorbidity of CFS and FMS with other symptom-defined syndromes (also known as medically unexplained symptoms or functional somatic syndromes) also have found high rates of migraine, irritable bowel syndrome, pelvic pain, and temporomandibular joint pain (Aggarwal et al. 2006; Kanaan et al. 2007; Kato et al. 2006). These syndromes, like CFS and FMS, are also associated with high lifetime rates of comorbid mood and anxiety disorders (Hudson and Pope 1994). Other similarities are also seen between CFS, FMS, and these disorders, such as a female predominance, association with childhood abuse, and response to similar treatments. This observation raises the possibility not only that CFS and FMS are similar but also that all the functional syndromes have more in common than previously thought by the specialists who diagnose them (Sullivan et al. 2002; Wessely et al. 1999). It has been further suggested that these syndromes, along with mood and anxiety disorders, share a common psychological and central nervous system (CNS) pathophysiology (Clauw and Chrousos 1997) and indeed genes (Kato et al. 2009).

Association With Psychiatric Disorders

In clinical practice, many (but not all) patients who have received a diagnosis of CFS or FMS also meet criteria for a psychiatric diagnosis. Most will meet criteria for a depression or an anxiety syndrome. Those who do not are likely to meet DSM criteria for a somatoform disorder or for the ICD-10 diagnosis of neurasthenia (Sharpe 1996). The more somatic symptoms the patient has, the more likely is a diagnosis of depression or anxiety disorder (Skapinakis et al. 2003). However, the precise prevalence rates of psychiatric disorders reported vary and will depend on a number of factors: compared with a community sample, patients attending clinics are likely to be more disabled and distressed and therefore to have more depression and anxiety. Some symptoms (such as fatigue, sleep disturbance, and poor concentration) overlap with the symptoms of depression and anxiety, and the observed prevalence of psychiatric disorders will depend on whether all symptoms are counted toward a diagnosis of psychiatric disorder or whether those considered medically explained by CFS or FMS are excluded. Finally, it has been argued that atypical presentations of depression (Van Hoof et al. 2003) and anxiety (Kushner and Beitman 1990) are common in these groups, adding further uncertainty to the estimates quoted in the following subsections.

Depression

Fatigue is strongly associated with depression. The international World Health Organization (WHO) study of more than 5,000 primary care patients in several countries (Sartorius et al. 1993) found that 67% of the patients meeting criteria for CFS (defined from survey data) also had an ICD-10 depressive syndrome (Skapinakis 2000). A study of clinic attenders with CFS reported that more than 25% had a current DSM major depression diagnosis and 50%–75% had a lifetime diagnosis (Afari and Buchwald 2003). Population studies have also found an elevated prevalence, although a lower rate than in some clinic-based studies (Taylor et al. 2003).

Chronic pain is also strongly associated with depression in the general population (Ohayon and Schatzberg 2003; see also Chapter 36, "Pain"). In FMS, a study of attenders at a specialist clinic reported that 32% had a depressive disorder (22% with major depression) (Epstein et al. 1999). An increased prevalence of lifetime and family history of major depression also has been reported in FMS (Hudson and Pope 1996). As with CFS, the prevalence of depression is probably lower in patients with FMS in the general population (Clauw and Crofford 2003).

Generalized Anxiety Disorder, Panic Disorder, and Posttraumatic Stress Disorder

Anxiety disorders have been relatively neglected as associations with CFS and FMS. One study reported finding GAD in as many as half of the clinic patients with CFS or FMS when the hierarchical rules that subsume it under major depression were suspended (Fischler et al. 1997).

Panic disorder is especially common in patients with medically unexplained symptoms. A prevalence of 13% was reported in one study of CFS (Manu et al. 1991), and the prevalence was 7% in clinic patients with FMS (Epstein et al. 1999). Panic disorder, which may present with predominantly somatic symptoms (Chen et al. 2009), should be suspected when the reported somatic symptoms are markedly episodic.

The prevalence of posttraumatic stress disorder (PTSD) has been reported to be higher in patients with CFS (Taylor and Jason 2001), and much higher in those with FMS (Roy-Byrne et al. 2004), than in the general population. PTSD is associated with reports of previous abuse (see "Abuse" under the "Etiology" section later in this chapter).

Somatoform Disorders

Somatoform disorders are descriptive diagnoses primarily defined by somatic symptoms that are not explained by a medical condition. Hence, replacing a diagnosis of CFS or FMS with a somatoform one may simply be to relabel it. Furthermore, the choice of diagnosis depends on one's beliefs about the nature of these conditions. If one regards CFS and FMS as medical conditions, then the symptoms will not be counted toward a diagnosis of a somatoform disorder, whereas if one regards CFS and FMS as medically unexplained syndromes, then they will be (Johnson et al. 1996). Some patients will meet the criteria for hypochondriasis because of persistent anxious concern about the nature of their illness. Others may meet the criteria for somatization disorder because of a long history of multiple symptoms (Martin et al. 2007). Patients with FMS are likely to meet criteria for pain disorder as described in DSM-IV. Finally, most of the patients with CFS or FMS who do not meet the criteria for anxiety, depression, or these more specific disorders will fit the undemanding criteria for a diagnosis of undifferentiated somatoform disorder.

Summary

If sought, diagnoses of depressive and anxiety disorders can be commonly made in patients with CFS and FMS. There is some suggestion that anxiety is associated more with pain, and depression with fatigue (Kurtze and Svebak 2001). This association with psychiatric disorders appears not to be explained simply by overlapping symptoms, because it remains high even when fatigue is excluded from the diagnostic criteria for major depression (Kruesi et al. 1989). Neither can the occurrence of depression or anxiety disorders be attributed entirely to referral bias because the rate is still elevated, although less so, in community cases (Kato et al. 2006; Nater et al. 2009). It does not appear that depression can be explained entirely as a reaction to disability, because it has been found to be more common than in patients with disabling rheumatoid arthritis (Katon et al. 1991; Walker et al. 1997). However, despite the robustness of the association, many patients with CFS and FMS are not found to have depressive and anxiety syndromes, even after detailed assessment (Henningsen et al. 2003). Whether it is appropriate to give these people a diagnosis of a somatoform disorder rather then CFS or FMS is controversial.

It has been proposed that depression, anxiety, CFS, and FMS have shared risk factors. These may include both genetics (Kato et al. 2009) and adverse experiences such as abuse and victimization (Van Houdenhove et al. 2001a).

The lack of acceptance by others of the suffering associated with these medically ambiguous conditions may also contribute to emotional distress (Lehman et al. 2002).

The relation between symptom syndromes defined by psychiatry and those of CFS and FMS defined by general medicine is an intimate and complex one. It can be conceived of either as psychiatric comorbidity with a general medical condition or alternatively as different perspectives on the same condition. Whichever view one takes, the importance of making the psychiatric diagnosis lies in its implications for treatment.

Epidemiology

Prevalence of Fatigue and Chronic Fatigue Syndrome

Fatigue is common, but CFS as currently defined is relatively rare. A large survey of 90,000 residents in Wichita, Kansas, which used rigorous assessment and exclusion criteria, found that 6% of the population reported fatigue of more than 1 month's duration, but only 235 per 100,000 (or 0.2%) met criteria for CFS (Reyes et al. 2003). It should be noted, however, that the application of the current diagnostic criteria (Fukuda et al. 1994) excluded numerous patients, mainly because of diagnoses of rheumatoid arthritis and psychiatric disorder. A more recent study found that 1% of the Dutch population endorsed symptoms of CFS on a self-report measure, most of whom had not sought medical attention (van't Leven et al. 2010).

Prevalence of Pain and Fibromyalgia Syndrome

Studies of the prevalence of pain and FMS have reported similar findings (Makela 1999). Chronic pain is common and has been reported in as much as 10% of the general population (Croft et al. 1993), whereas FMS defined according to the American College of Rheumatology criteria has an estimated prevalence of only 2% (Wolfe et al. 1995) to 4% (K.P. White et al. 1999). The observation that FMS appears to be more common than CFS (Bazelmans et al. 1997) may indicate that chronic pain states are more common than chronic fatigue states or, alternatively, may simply reflect the requirement in the CFS diagnostic criteria for a longer duration and greater disability (see Tables 26-1 and 26-2).

Associations

Gender

Both CFS and FMS are more common in women. The female-to-male ratio for CFS has been reported to be about 4:1 (Reyes et al. 2003) and for FMS, 8:1 (Wolfe et al. 1995), although this increased female preponderance in FMS may reflect a greater frequency of tender points rather than more frequent pain (Clauw and Crofford 2003).

Age

The most common age at onset for both CFS and FMS is between 30 and 50 years, although patients who present with FMS are on average 10 years older (Reyes et al. 2003; K.P. White et al. 1999). These syndromes are also diagnosed, although controversially, in children. An epidemiological study from the United Kingdom found a prevalence of CFS of only 0.002% in 5- to 15-year-olds (Chalder et al. 2003). CFS and FMS are also diagnosed in the elderly, but the frequency of other chronic medical conditions complicates the differential diagnosis.

Socioeconomic Status

Both CFS and FMS are more prevalent in persons who are of lower socioeconomic status and in those who have received less education (Jason et al. 1999; K.P. White et al. 1999). CFS is 50% more common in semiskilled and unskilled workers than in professionals.

International and Cross-Cultural Studies

It is often noted that the diagnoses of CFS and FMS are almost entirely restricted to Western nations, whereas the symptoms of fatigue and pain are universal. It is unclear to what extent this reflects differing epidemiology or simply different diagnostic practice. For example, in France fatigue may be diagnosed as a condition called *spasmophilia.* In the Far East, neurasthenia remains a popular diagnosis and accordingly is still listed in the ICD-10 diagnostic classification. The WHO Collaborative Study of Psychological Problems in General Health Care conducted in 14 countries reported wide variations in the prevalence of both persistent pain (including both medically explained and medically unexplained pain) and fatigue (Gureje et al. 2001; World Health Organization 1995).

Disability and Work

CFS and FMS are both associated with substantial self-reported loss of function and substantial work disability (Assefi et al. 2003). Unemployment in patients with CFS and FMS attending specialist services in the United States is as high as 50% (Bombardier and Buchwald 1996).

Prognosis

The prognosis for patients with CFS or FMS is variable; these illnesses typically have a chronic but fluctuating course. Rehabilitative therapy improves the outcome, however (see subsection "Specialist Nonpharmacological Treatments" later in this chapter).

Prospective studies of CFS and FMS in the general population have reported that in about half the cases, the syndrome is in partial or complete remission by 2–3 years after diagnosis (Granges et al. 1994; Nisenbaum et al. 2003). Poor outcome in CFS and FMS is predicted by longer illness duration, more severe symptoms, older age, depression, and lack of social support (van der Werf et al. 2002), and in CFS by a strong belief in physical causes (Cairns and Hotopf 2005). Severely disabled patients attending specialist clinics have a particularly poor prognosis for recovery (Hill et al. 1999; Wolfe et al. 1997).

Etiology

The etiology of CFS and FMS remains unknown. While a wide range of etiological factors have been proposed, none has been unequivocally established. The available evidence may be summarized as suggesting that a combination of environmental factors and individual vulnerability initiates a series of biological, psychological, and social processes that lead to the development of CFS or FMS (Table 26–3). These factors are discussed in the following subsections as predisposing, precipitating, and perpetuating factors. It is worth mentioning that, with notable exceptions, the preponderance of research in this area is based on small case-control studies (typically 10–20 patients per case and control group) with insufficient power to control for confounding variables, thereby limiting our ability to draw strong causal inferences about any of the findings reported below.

Predisposing Factors

Biological Factors: Genetics

Modest evidence from family and twin studies suggests that genetic factors play a part in predisposing individuals to CFS and to FMS. In a study of 146 female-female twins, one of whom had CFS, the concordance was 55% in monozygotic and 20% in dizygotic twins (Buchwald et al. 2001), suggesting both moderate heritability and the importance of environmental factors. In FMS, a similar familial clustering has been reported (Buskila and Neumann 1997). Claims for the role of specific genes in the etiology of these conditions remain unproven (Kaiser 2006).

Psychological and Social Factors

Personality and activity. Clinicians often claim a predisposing "obsessional" personality type, but this theory has been little studied. The clinical observation that CFS and FMS patients lead abnormally active lives or have high levels of exercise before becoming ill does have some empirical support (Harvey et al. 2008a; Van Houdenhove et al. 2001b).

Previous psychiatric illness. A long-term cohort study has confirmed that persons with a prior history of depression or anxiety are more likely to develop CFS (Harvey et al. 2008b), suggesting that either the psychiatric illness itself or a shared risk factor such as genetics (Kato et al. 2009) predisposes individuals to CFS.

Abuse. Childhood and adult neglect, abuse, and maltreatment have been reported to be more common in CFS and FMS (Heim et al. 2006; Paras et al. 2009) than in comparison groups. A recent study found that people who reported abuse had six times the risk of CFS (Paras et al. 2009). Both psychological and biological etiological mechanisms for the etiological role of trauma have been suggested.

Social status. Low social status and lower levels of education are risk factors for both CFS and FMS (see subsection "Socioeconomic Status" in the "Epidemiology" section earlier in this chapter).

Precipitating Factors

Precipitating factors trigger the illness in vulnerable persons.

Biological Factors

Infection. There is some evidence that infection can precipitate CFS, and some, but less, evidence indicates that infection also may trigger FMS (Rea et al. 1999). Specific infections have been found to be associated with the subsequent development of CFS in 10%–40% of patients. These infections are Epstein-Barr virus (P.D. White et al. 2001), Q fever (Ayres et al. 1998), viral meningitis (Hotopf et al. 1996), viral hepatitis (Berelowitz et al. 1995), and parvovirus (Kerr and Mattey 2008). The etiological mechanism to explain this association remains unclear but may include stress, immunological factors, and an acute reduction in activity (P.D. White et al. 2001) (see "Perpetuating Factors" later in this section).

Injury. The role of physical injury in the etiology of CFS and FMS has been controversial, in part because of the implications for legal liability and compensation. Limited evidence indicates that both conditions may be precipitated by injury, particularly to the neck. If a link exists, it is stronger for FMS (Al Allaf et al. 2002).

Psychological and Social Factors: Life Stress

Clinical experience indicates that patients often report the onset of CFS and FMS as occurring during or after a stress-

TABLE 26–3. Possible etiological factors to consider in a formulation of chronic fatigue syndrome or fibromyalgia syndrome

	Predisposing	Precipitating	Perpetuating
Biological	Genetics	Acute infection, disease, or injury	Neuroendocrine changes Immunological changes Deconditioning Sleep disorder
Psychological	Personality Depression or anxiety	Perceived stress	Depression Fixed disease attribution Catastrophizing Low self-efficacy Avoidance of activity
Social	Lack of support	Life events	Illness-reinforcing information Lack of legitimacy of illness Social or work stress Occupational and financial factors

ful period in their lives. The evidence for life stress or life events being a precipitant of FMS and CFS is, however, both limited and retrospective (Anderberg et al. 2000; Theorell et al. 1999). One of the best studies so far published examined 64 patients and a similar number of matched control subjects. An excess of severe life events and difficulties was found in the CFS patients for the year prior to onset. More specifically, a certain type of life event called a *dilemma* (defined as an event when the person had to choose between two equally undesirable responses to circumstances) was found in one-third of the patients with CFS and none of the control subjects (Hatcher and House 2003).

Perpetuating Factors

Perpetuating factors are those that maintain a condition once it is established. They are clinically the most important because they are potential targets for treatment.

Biological Factors

Chronic infection. There has been much interest in the potential role of ongoing infection and in associated immunological factors, especially in CFS. It was previously thought that chronic Epstein-Barr virus was a cause of CFS, but that hypothesis has been rejected. There have been numerous reports of evidence of chronic infection with other agents in both CFS and FMS, the most recent being with a xenotropic murine leukemia-related virus (XMRV) (Lombardi et al. 2009). None has so far been substantiated.

Immunological factors. Immunological factors, especially cytokines, also have been much investigated in CFS and FMS, not only because of the possible triggering effect of infection but also because administration of immune active agents, such as interferons, is recognized as a cause of fatigue and myalgia (Vial and Descotes 1994) and because similar symptoms in conditions such as hepatitis C have been associated with changes in measured cytokines (Thompson and Barkhuizen 2003). Various minor immune abnormalities, mainly mild degrees of activation, have been reported in patients with CFS and FMS. However, a systematic review found no evidence of any consistent immune abnormality in CFS (Lyall et al. 2003). The hypothesis that CFS is associated with immune activation therefore remains tantalizing but unproven.

Myopathic or biochemical abnormalities and physiological deconditioning. The bulk of evidence indicates that there are no proven pathological or biochemical abnormalities of muscle or muscle metabolism, either at rest or with exercise, other than those expected with deconditioning. *Deconditioning* describes the physiological changes that lead to the loss of tolerance of activity after prolonged rest (e.g., as a result of pain). It has been found in many, but not all, patients with CFS (Bazelmans et al. 2001; Fulcher and White 2000) and also in those with FMS (Valim et al. 2002). Deconditioning offers one biological explanation for exercise-induced fatigue and worsening or persistent muscle pain in patients with CFS and FMS and also provides a rationale for treatment with graded activity (see subsection "Specialist Nonpharmacological Treatments" later in this chapter).

Sleep abnormalities. Patients with CFS and FMS typically complain of unrefreshing and broken sleep, a symptom that has been objectively confirmed with polysomnography. Abnormalities in sleep have been claimed to be of major etiological importance, especially in FMS. Early work (Moldofsky et al. 1975) reported a specific sleep electroencephalogram abnormality of alpha wave intrusion into slow-wave sleep (so-called alpha–delta sleep) and suggested that this was a cause of the myalgia. However, attempts to replicate this finding in both CFS and FMS have produced inconsistent results, and its specificity to chronic pain remains unclear (Rains and Penzien 2003). A number of other abnormalities in sleep variables have been reported in recent years in CFS and FMS, but no clear and consistent differences are apparent.

Neuroendocrine changes. One of the best-supported biological abnormalities associated with both CFS and FMS is changes in the level and response of neuroendocrine stress hormones. A repeated observation has been of a tendency to low blood levels of cortisol and a poor cortisol response to stress (Parker et al. 2001). This finding differs from what would be expected in depression (in which blood levels of cortisol are typically elevated) but is similar to that reported in other stress-induced and anxiety states. It is not known whether this is a primary abnormality or merely a consequence of inactivity or sleep disruption. Low cortisol has been reported to be associated with a history of childhood trauma (Heim et al. 2009). Although there is evidence that cortisol levels can be raised by successful cognitive-behavioral therapy (CBT) treatment (Roberts et al. 2009), low cortisol at baseline predicts a poorer response to CBT (Roberts et al. 2010).

Patients with FMS may also have an elevated level of substance P in their cerebrospinal fluid (Russell et al. 1994). A similar finding has been made in patients with other chronic pain syndromes such as osteoarthritis. However, elevated substance P has not been found in CFS patients (Evengard et al. 1998).

Blood pressure regulation. Failure to maintain blood pressure when assuming erect posture (orthostatic intolerance) and particularly a pattern in which the heart rate increases abnormally (postural orthostatic tachycardia syndrome) have been reported in both CFS (Rowe et al. 1995) and FMS (Bou-Holaigah et al. 1997). These findings have been interpreted as indicating abnormal autonomic nervous system function (Newton et al. 2009). However, postural hypotension commonly occurs in healthy persons after prolonged inactivity (Sandler and Vernikos 1986), and its specificity to CFS and FMS remains unclear.

CNS structure. The brains of patients with CFS and FMS are probably structurally normal, although a reduction in gray matter has been reported in both CFS (de Lange et al. 2005) and FMS (Burgmer et al. 2009). However, this apparent difference in amount of gray matter has been reported to disappear after controlling for depression (Hsu et al. 2009). Interestingly, the reduction in gray matter also appears to be at least partially reversed by treatment with CBT (de Lange et al. 2008).

CNS function. The use of functional brain imaging has great potential to elucidate the biology of these conditions but remains in its infancy. There is, however, accumulating evidence of abnormally increased activation of pain systems in patients with fibromyalgia in response to painful stimuli (Pujol et al. 2009) and even with only the anticipation of a painful stimulus (Schweinhardt et al. 2008). These findings are consistent with a "symptom amplification" model of these syndromes.

An early single photon emission computed tomography (SPECT) study (Costa et al. 1995) and a positron emission tomography (PET) study (Tirelli et al. 1998) reported reduced brain stem perfusion in patients with CFS. However, another study that found fewer differences when CFS patients were compared with depressed patients reminds us of the need for careful control for variables such as depression (Machale et al. 2000). As with pain, more widespread cerebral activation is seen in CFS patients than in control subjects when performing a fatiguing cognitive task (Cook et al. 2007).

Although tantalizing, these imaging findings must be regarded as preliminary. Furthermore, evidence of changes in brain activation or brain reorganization must not be taken to mean that the symptoms are necessarily based in fixed neurological pathology; behavioral rehabilitation and drug therapy can potentially reverse such changes (Flor 2003).

Psychological and Social Factors

There is strong evidence that psychological and behavioral factors play a major role in perpetuating CFS and FMS.

Illness beliefs. One of the most striking aspects of the presentation of CFS and FMS to clinicians involves the often strong beliefs many patients hold about the cause of their illness. Three categories of illness beliefs are considered here: 1) cause of symptoms (attributions), 2) significance of symptoms (catastrophizing), and 3) what one can do despite having symptoms (self-efficacy).

Although the causes of CFS and FMS are unknown, many patients, and especially those seen in specialist clinics, often strongly attribute their symptoms to a physical disease (Neerinckx et al. 2000). A systematic review of prognostic studies in CFS found that such strong attributions predicted a poorer outcome (Cairns and Hotopf 2005). The mechanism of this effect is unclear. It may be that such an attribution favors a focusing of attention on symptoms, more passive coping, and greater inactivity (Heijmans 1998) or, alternatively, that such an attribution leads to nonparticipation in potentially effective psychological and behavioral treatment.

Catastrophizing is a tendency to make excessively negative predictions about symptoms, such as "If I do more, my pain or fatigue will keep getting worse and worse." Catastrophizing has been observed in patients with CFS (Nijs et al. 2008) and FMS (Hassett et al. 2000) and is associated with increased symptom vigilance, avoidance of activity, and more severe disability. Furthermore, a reduction in the belief that activity is damaging is associated with recovery during rehabilitative therapy (Deale et al. 1998), suggesting that it may be a critical psychological target for effective rehabilitation.

Self-efficacy—the belief that one can do something, despite symptoms—has been found both to be low and to be associated with more severe disability in patients with CFS (Findley et al. 1998), FMS (Buckelew et al. 1996), and chronic pain (Asghari and Nicholas 2001). Self-efficacy is therefore another potential target for treatment that aims to improve function.

Behavioral factors. Patients cope with their symptoms in different ways. The way in which a patient copes will be influenced by his or her illness beliefs (Silver et al. 2002). Of particular interest is a style of coping through avoidance of any activity that the patient fears will lead to an exacerbation of symptoms. This fear-avoidance phenomenon is well described in chronic pain patients (Philips 1987) and also has been observed in patients with CFS (Afari et al. 2000; Nater et al. 2006) and FMS (Davis et al. 2001). Objective assessment also confirms that patients with CFS and FMS show reduced overall activity, with most patients oscillating between activity and rest, and a quarter being more pervasively inactive. This reduced activity produces deconditioning; gradually increasing activity is a target for treatment.

Another potentially important coping behavior is the focusing of attention on symptoms—so-called symptom focusing or symptom vigilance (Roelofs et al. 2003). This behavior is, not surprisingly, associated with catastrophizing beliefs and greater perceived symptom intensity; it offers another target for treatment.

Social factors. Patients' beliefs about their illness and associated coping behavior will be influenced by the information they receive. One striking social aspect of CFS and FMS is the high level of activity of patient support and advocacy organizations, which communicate mainly over the Internet (Ross 1999). Studies from the United Kingdom have reported that patients who are members of a self-help group have poorer outcomes than those who are not, despite similar illness duration and disability (Sharpe et al. 1992), as well as a poorer response to rehabilitation (Bentall et al. 2002). It is not known whether this association reflects self-selection into such groups or the effect of the group on patients' beliefs, coping, and willingness to engage in rehabilitation. Some patients reported negative experiences related to having the legitimacy of their illness repeatedly questioned by doctors and others, a process that probably drives some patients to join defensively focused advocacy organizations. Perhaps unsurprisingly, the acquisition of a disability pension is also associated with a worse prognosis (Wigers 1996).

Summary

The available evidence suggests that patients are predisposed to develop CFS and FMS by some combination of genetics, previous experience including childhood trauma, and possibly lack of social support. Many patients with CFS have a history of preceding infection, and many patients with FMS point to an accident, injury, or trauma as the triggering event. Others can identify no precipitant. Most research has been into those factors associated with established illness, so-called perpetuating factors, because these are both clearly more accessible to study and more relevant to treatment of established cases. Many biological factors have been investigated, with interest initially being directed at peripheral nerves and muscles and subsequently focusing on the functioning of the CNS and its neuroendocrine and autonomic outputs. Tantalizing findings have suggested—but have not yet established—a role for immune factors and possibly for ongoing infection. The physiological effects of inactivity seem to be important. Substantial evidence indicates the importance of psychological and behavioral factors, especially the fear of exacerbating symptoms and the associated avoidance of activity in both CFS and FMS. Social factors are more difficult to study but often are of striking importance clinically.

Models of Chronic Fatigue and Fibromyalgia Syndromes

The findings discussed in the previous section can be amalgamated into explanatory models. Three main models can be discerned that correspond approximately to biological, psychological, and social perspectives, although, in reality, all three are probably relevant.

Biological Model

It is well known that the immune system, the CNS, and the endocrine system interact and also have reciprocal relations with sleep and activity. It is thus possible to construct a tentative biological model in which these systems interact to perpetuate the illness (Moldofsky 1995). There seems to be stronger evidence for the role of infection in triggering CFS and for the role of trauma in FMS. However, it is unclear whether these represent real differences or simply differences in the hypotheses pursued by researchers.

Psychological Model

Whatever the biological aspects of these conditions, psychological models assume that the symptoms and disability are perpetuated, at least in part, by psychological and behavioral factors (Deary et al. 2007). Biological factors are not excluded from this model but are assumed to be either only partially responsible for the illness or largely reversible (Surawy et al. 1995). The cognitive-behavioral models for chronic pain and CFS have much in common (Philips 1987). Both emphasize the importance of fear of symptoms leading to a focusing on the symptoms, helplessness, and avoidance of activity. This model provides the rationale for behavioral and cognitive-behavioral approaches to rehabilitation (see section "Management" later in this chapter).

Social Model

The social model emphasizes the role of social factors in shaping illness. A fight for the legitimacy of the syndrome as a chronic medical condition is central (Banks and Prior 2001). Patient advocacy has been strongly hostile to psychological and psychiatric involvement, probably because it is seen as undermining legitimacy. The social model proposes that patient organizations, while providing valuable social support, can also reinforce patients' illness beliefs, medical care, and disability payment seeking in ways that are not conducive to recovery (Shorter 1997).

Diagnostic Evaluation

Effective management of patients with possible CFS or FMS requires that 1) alternative medical and psychiatric diagnoses are considered and 2) all patients receive an adequately comprehensive assessment.

Identification of Medical and Psychiatric Conditions

Medical Differential Diagnosis

The medical differential diagnosis for CFS and FMS is a long one because so many diseases can present with pain and/or fatigue (Sharpe and Wilks 2002; Yunus 2002; Table 26–4). Both a physical and a mental status examination must be performed in every case to determine the presence of alternative medical and psychiatric diagnoses. As with many chronic diseases, particularly rheumatological conditions, time is often the principal arbiter because these conditions evolve clinically. For symptoms in general, 75% of the patients presenting to primary care improve within 2–4 weeks (Kroenke 2003). Thus, it makes sense to rely on an initial 4- to 6-week wait to clarify whether the symptoms will persist (Kroenke and Jackson 1998). For persistent symptoms, most of the common medical disorders can be diagnosed from a standard history, physical examination, and basic laboratory studies.

Routine investigations. Initial investigation depends on the clinical signs, symptoms, and temporal nature of symptoms. When symptom duration exceeds 4–6 weeks, an initial basic screening workup is appropriate. If there are no specific indications for special investigations, the following have been found to be adequate as screening tests: thyrotropin, erythrocyte sedimentation rate (sensitive for any condition with systemic inflammation), complete blood count, basic chemistries, and withdrawal of some medications (particularly statins or 3-hydroxy-3-methylglutaryl coenzyme A reductase inhibitors; typical resolution of symptoms in 4–6 weeks).

Special investigations. Special investigations should be carried out only if clearly indicated by the history or examination. Immunological and virological tests are generally unhelpful as routine investigations and remain research tools. Sleep studies can be useful in excluding other diagnoses (especially when the fatigue is characterized by sleepiness), including sleep apnea, narcolepsy, nocturnal myoclonus, and periodic leg movements during sleep (see Chapter 15, "Sleep Disorders"). Once symptoms become chronic (duration greater than 3 months) and remain unexplained, the general approach is to avoid excessive testing, establish regular follow-up, screen for depressive and anxiety disorders, and focus on symptom management.

Medical misdiagnosis. Physicians who are concerned about missing a serious medical diagnosis can be reassured that in most cases, the primary care physician's initial judgment in this regard is likely to be accurate (Khan et

TABLE 26–4. Medical differential diagnosis for patients with chronic fatigue syndrome (CFS) and fibromyalgia syndrome (FMS)

Relative frequency	Diagnoses	Syndrome	Differentiating clinical features	Initial workup
Very common (~1 per 100)	Thyroid disorders	CFS, FMS	Hypothyroidism: cold intolerance, slowed relaxation phase of reflexes, weight gain, elevated cholesterol Hyperthyroidism: heat intolerance, tremor, weight loss	Thyrotropin
	Medications (statins)	CFS, FMS	Symptom resolution with withdrawal of medication	Creatine kinase, aldolase
	Sleep apnea	CFS, FMS	Daytime somnolence, motor vehicle accidents, witnessed nighttime apnea and snoring, hypertension	Sleep study
	Spinal stenosis	FMS	History of osteoarthritis, degenerative disc disease, back pain with radiculopathy, sensory and/or motor deficits, pseudoclaudication	Nerve conduction study, electromyogram, magnetic resonance imaging of spine if neurological deficits
	Anemia	CFS	Pallor	Complete blood cell count
Common (~1 per 1,000)	Chronic infection: HIV, hepatitis C, endocarditis, osteomyelitis, Lyme disease, occult abscess	CFS, FMS	Infection-specific risk factors and signs (e.g., sexual habits, diabetes, fevers, murmur)	Serology, erythrocyte sedimentation rate, liver function tests, serial blood cultures, bone scan, indium scan
	Polymyalgia rheumatica	FMS	Age >60 years	Erythrocyte sedimentation rate
	Cancer	CFS	Pallor, anemia, anorexia, weight loss, cachexia	Complete blood cell count, albumin, age-appropriate cancer screening studies
	Pulmonary condition: asthma, obstructive lung disease, interstitial lung disease	CFS	Shortness of breath, prominent exertional symptoms, smoking history, hypoxia	Chest X ray, pulmonary function tests, oxygenation saturation with exercise
	Rheumatoid arthritis	FMS	Symmetric synovitis, morning stiffness	Rheumatoid factor
	Inflammatory bowel disease (Crohn's)	CFS	Diarrhea, weight loss, fever, anemia	Serial fecal occult blood with endoscopy if positive
Uncommon (~1 per 2,500–100,000)	Systemic lupus	FMS	Malar rash, joint pain	Antinuclear antibody, double-stranded DNA
	Polymyositis, dermatomyositis, myopathy	CFS, FMS	Proximal muscle weakness	Antinuclear antibody, creatine kinase, aldolase

TABLE 26–4. Medical differential diagnosis for patients with chronic fatigue syndrome (CFS) and fibromyalgia syndrome (FMS) *(continued)*

Relative frequency	Diagnoses	Syndrome	Differentiating clinical features	Initial workup
	Myasthenia gravis, multiple sclerosis	CFS	Neurological findings: extinguishing strength with repetitive movements, ptosis, swallowing difficulties, optic neuritis, sensory deficits	Tensilon test, acetylcholine receptor antibodies, magnetic resonance imaging of brain
	Narcolepsy	CFS	Drop attacks, falling asleep during daily activities	Sleep study
	Symptomatic hyperparathyroidism	CFS	Bone pain, nephrolithiasis, pancreatitis, renal insufficiency	Serum calcium and parathyroid hormone

al. 2003). However, there is some evidence that CFS and FMS may be overdiagnosed by primary care physicians (Fitzcharles and Boulos 2003); evaluating psychiatrists should feel able to request second medical opinions.

Psychiatric Differential Diagnosis

Underdiagnosis and undertreatment of psychiatric disorders are common (Torres-Harding et al. 2002), probably reflecting a focus of the initial medical assessment on the patient's somatic symptoms and a tendency to disregard mood changes as a consequence of those symptoms. The most important psychiatric diagnoses to consider are depressive and anxiety disorders because of their frequency and their implications for treatment. Depression may be masked and require an expert assessment if it is to be detected. Panic attacks with agoraphobia may cause intermittent severe fatigue and disability. Somatoform disorders are common but have fewer implications for management. A diagnosis of somatization disorder indicates a poorer prognosis, and hypochondriasis indicates special attention to repeated reassurance seeking, which may perpetuate fears of undiagnosed disease (Sharpe and Williams 2001).

Assessment of the Illness

Other than to make diagnoses, the aims of the assessment are to 1) establish a collaborative relationship with the patient, 2) elicit the patient's own understanding of his or her illness and how he or she copes with it and 3) identify current family and social factors such as employment and litigation that may complicate management. It is important to inquire fully about the patient's understanding of his or her illness (e.g., "What do you think is wrong with you?" or "What do you think the cause is?"). Patients may be fearful that their symptoms indicate a progressive, not-yet-diagnosed disease or that exertion will cause a long-term worsening of their condition. A formulation that identifies potential predisposing, precipitating, and perpetuating factors (see Table 26–3) is valuable both in providing an individualized explanation to the patient and for targeting interventions.

Management

Diagnosis, Formulation, and Management Plan

Forming a Therapeutic Relationship With the Patient

It is important to see the consultation from the patient's perspective. He or she may have already seen many other doctors and may have experienced problematic interactions with them (Asbring and Narvanen 2003). These doctors may have offered overly biomedical or overly psychological explanations or even dismissed the patient completely.

Explaining Psychiatric Involvement

It is helpful to explain to the patient why he or she is seeing a psychiatrist. A psychiatrist's involvement in management may be interpreted by the patient as indicating that his or her condition is considered to be "all in his or her head." It is therefore often best to begin with an assessment of the physical symptoms and only then to introduce a discussion of psychological factors. This can be done in a nonblaming and normalizing way; for example: "You have clearly had a terrible time that has been made worse by not being believed. It is entirely understandable that this has gotten you down." It is generally unhelpful to force a psychiatric diagnosis on an unwilling patient. It is also important to explain that treatments commonly associated with psychiatry (particularly antidepressants and CBT) do not necessarily imply that the person is mentally ill; rather, they can be seen as ways of normalizing brain and bodily functions in conditions that are exacerbated by stress (Sharpe and Carson 2001).

Giving the Diagnosis

Some controversy exists about whether giving patients a diagnosis of CFS or FMS is helpful or harmful (Huibers and Wessely 2006). Some who believe that a positive diagnosis is helpful argue that it enables patients to both conceptualize their illness and communicate about it (Sharpe 1998). Others who are concerned about the potentially harmful effect of diagnosis argue that it medicalizes and pathologizes symptoms in a way that can exacerbate social and occupational disability (Hadler 1996a). It is our clinical experience that a positive diagnosis, linked to a clear explanation of the potential reversibility of symptoms and a management plan to achieve this, is not only a positive intervention but also an essential starting point from which to plan effective management.

Offering an Explanation

The explanation offered should ideally be scientifically accurate, acceptable to the patient, and congruent with the management plan. It can be explained that although the specific causes of CFS or FMS remain unknown, a combination of vulnerability and environmental stress that have changed the function of the brain and endocrine system is most likely. One such explanation is that the illness is a disorder of brain *function* rather than *structure*—that is, a functional nervous disorder (Stone et al. 2002).

Explaining the Management Plan

The management plan should be explained to the patient as following from the etiological formulation, focusing on illness-perpetuating factors and consisting of elements intended to 1) relieve symptoms such as depression, pain, and sleep disturbance with agents such as antidepressants; 2) assist the patient's efforts at coping by stabilizing activity and retraining the body to function effectively (graded exercise, CBT); and 3) assist the patient in managing the social and financial aspects of his or her illness and, when possible, remaining in or returning to employment (problem solving).

General Measures

Providing Advice on Symptom Management

One of the most important interventions the clinician can make is to encourage and guide patients in the active self-management of the illness. Such advice will include the importance of being realistic about what they are able to accomplish right now without giving up hope for improvement in the future. It should involve advice on the pros and cons of self-medication, particularly with analgesics, and also might require a discussion of the potential benefits and risks associated with seeking treatment from other practitioners, both conventional and alternative. The overall aim is to encourage patients to feel that they can do things to manage the condition themselves, to accept the reality of their illness while still planning positively for the future, and to be cautious about seeking potentially harmful and expensive treatments.

Managing Activity and Avoidance

Once a patient's pattern of activity has been stabilized and large fluctuations between excessive rest and unsustainable activity reduced, very gradual increases in activity can be advised. It is critical, however, to distinguish between carefully graded increases carried out in collaboration with the patient and a forced or overambitious exercise regimen.

Managing Occupational and Social Factors

Patients who continue working despite illness may become overstressed by the effort of doing this. Those who have left work because of illness may have become inactive and demoralized. These situations require a problem-solving approach to consider how to manage work demands, achieve a graded return to work, or plan an alternative career. Ongoing litigation regarding the illness is potentially a complicating factor because it reinforces (and may reward) the patient for remaining symptomatic and disabled.

Pharmacotherapy

Most pharmacological treatment studies in CFS and FMS have focused on antidepressants, although various other agents have been advocated.

Antidepressants

Antidepressant drug treatment is indicated by the fact that 1) many patients with CFS or FMS have depressive and anxiety syndromes and 2) these agents can reduce pain and improve sleep, even in the absence of depression. Overall there is good evidence for the short-term efficacy of antidepressants in FMS (Hauser et al. 2009a) but less evidence in CFS.

The tricyclic antidepressants (TCAs) are more effective than the selective serotonin reuptake inhibitors (SSRIs) for relieving pain and for inducing sleep. Small doses (e.g., 25–50 mg of amitriptyline) are often adequate for these purposes, whereas full doses are required to treat major depression.

Cyclobenzaprine, a tricyclic agent chemically similar to amitriptyline but used as a "muscle relaxant" rather than as an antidepressant, has been found to be effective in improving symptoms in FMS, especially pain and sleep disturbance (Tofferi et al. 2004).

SSRIs are generally better tolerated than TCAs. However, in CFS, fluoxetine was found in a large trial to be no more effective than placebo (Vercoulen et al. 1996b), and in FMS, the benefit of SSRIs was reported to be small (Hauser et al. 2009a).

The dual-action serotonin-norepinephrine reuptake inhibitors (SNRIs) such as venlafaxine, duloxetine, and milnacipran are also of benefit in fibromyalgia but may be less effective than TCAs in relieving pain (Hauser et al. 2009a). Other antidepressant agents may also be of value. For example, there is some evidence for the value of mirtazapine in CFS (Stubhaug et al. 2008).

Other Pharmacological Agents

Patients with CFS or FMS frequently take nonsteroidal anti-inflammatory drugs (NSAIDs) to relieve pain. No evidence from clinical trials indicates that NSAIDs are effective when used alone, although they may be of some benefit in FMS when combined with amitriptyline (Kroenke et al. 2009).

Opiates are occasionally used for pain relief in CFS and FMS. There is some evidence for the efficacy of tramadol (Bennett et al. 2003) but not for other opiates. Adverse effects, including dependence, are major concerns with opiate use.

As with opiates, great caution is required with benzodiazepines because of the risk of dependence in patients with chronic conditions. TCAs are probably preferable to benzodiazepines for treating insomnia, and the chronic use of benzodiazepines should be reserved for patients with intractable anxiety.

Given the finding of low serum cortisol, it is not surprising that corticosteroids have been tried as a treatment. Prednisone was found to be ineffective in FMS (Clark et al. 1985). Hydrocortisone was reported to produce some benefit in CFS but was not recommended because of the long-term risks of adrenal suppression (Cleare et al. 1999). In CFS, fludrocortisone has been used in patients with orthostatic hypotension but has not been found to be of value (Rowe et al. 2001).

Serotonin$_3$ receptor antagonists (e.g., ondansetron, tropisetron) have analgesic effects (Kranzler et al. 2002). A randomized, placebo-controlled double-blind trial in FMS found short-term benefit only with the lowest dosage (5 mg/day) (Farber et al. 2001). Trials of longer duration are needed.

Gabapentin and pregabalin both appear to be effective in reducing pain and other symptoms in fibromyalgia but do not suit all patients (Hauser et al. 2009b).

Stimulating medications such as bupropion, methylphenidate, dextroamphetamine, modafinil, and amantadine have all been reported to have value for other fatigue states (e.g., in multiple sclerosis) and have been advocated for use in CFS, but the evidence for their efficacy in CFS is very limited. Like opiates and benzodiazepines, stimulants pose a risk of dependence and abuse.

Summary

Caution is required when prescribing pharmacological therapy for CFS and FMS. The mainstay of drug treatment continues to be the so-called antidepressant drugs, which may be helpful for mood, pain, and sleep (but not fatigue), and which have limited effect on overall outcome. TCAs are preferred for nighttime sedation and pain, but greater tolerability may mean that an SSRI or an SNRI is preferable as first-line treatment. Although patients often receive low doses of antidepressants, higher doses may be required to achieve a therapeutic response. The increased interest in pharmacological treatment of functional syndromes in the past few years will likely expand future treatment options. However, the available evidence suggests that drug therapy currently has a limited role in the management of these conditions.

Specialist Nonpharmacological Treatments

If the patient does not respond to or requires a more active treatment than that described above, referral for specialist therapy should be considered. For most patients, a rehabilitative outpatient program based on appropriately planned increases in activity, either as graded exercise therapy (GET) or as CBT, is indicated. Some patients may require inpatient multidisciplinary rehabilitation, although evidence of its efficacy is inadequate (Karjalainen et al. 2000).

Graded Exercise Therapy

GET is a structured progressive exercise program administered and carefully monitored by an exercise therapist. It also may be given in individual or group form, but the evidence is best for individually administered treatment (Fulcher and White 1998).

GET follows the basic principles of exercise prescription for healthy individuals, adapted to the patient's current capacity. The initial exercise intensity and duration are determined on an individual basis and may be done by heart rate monitoring. Most patients can begin at an intensity of 40% of their maximum aerobic capacity, which approximately equates to 50% of their estimated individual heart rate reserve added to their resting heart rate (e.g., if the maximum heart rate is 180 beats per minute [bpm] and the resting heart rate is 80 bpm, the heart rate reserve is 100 bpm, and the exercise target heart rate is 80 + (0.5 × 100) = 130 bpm). This heart rate should not be exceeded; if it is, the patient should stop exercising for 1–2 minutes and then resume. Patients who are very disabled, or who have extremely low exercise tolerance to begin with, should begin with 2 weeks of stretching alone without aerobic activity and then should adopt alternate-day aerobic exercise before building up frequency, duration, and then intensity. The important principle is to calculate exercise capacity conservatively to start with, as well as to ensure that the patient will try that which is proposed.

At each clinic visit, joint planning of the exercise prescription for the following 1–2 weeks is completed. The initial aim is to establish a regular pattern of exercise (usually walking), with exercise 5 days/week. Home exercise sessions should initially last between 5 and 15 minutes, depending on ability and exercise tolerance. The duration is increased by 1–2 minutes/week up to a maximum of 30 minutes per homework session. Then the intensity of exercise can be increased to a target heart rate of 60% and then 70% of the patient's heart rate reserve added to his or her resting heart rate. Patients will respond differently; some will take a lot longer to adapt to each new level, whereas others will have to be held back, particularly those who have been active sports participants in the past. Those patients who are inclined to overexert themselves in an attempt to speed up the recovery process should be monitored carefully because this can be a contributing factor in nonrecovery or relapse.

GET has been found in systematic reviews to be of benefit in both CFS and FMS. In FMS, there is strong evidence (from a systematic review of 34 studies) that supervised aerobic exercise is of value in relieving symptoms and disability (Busch et al. 2007). In CFS, a systematic review of five studies found exercise to be better than comparison treatments in improving fatigue and disability. However, there were a number of dropouts from treatment, suggesting that exercise approaches may have limited acceptability (Edmonds et al. 2004). Of particular interest was a trial of brief simple education about the physiology and rationale of exercise that found this intervention to be as effective as CBT (Powell et al. 2001). A subsequent trial of this approach found that the benefit was not sustained, however (Wearden et al. 2010).

Cognitive-Behavioral Therapy

CBT is not a single treatment, and there are a variety of types (Williams 2003). Here, we refer to a collaborative psychologically informed type of rehabilitation that aims to achieve both graded increases in activity and changes in unhelpful beliefs and concerns about symptoms. It also may include problem solving for life and occupational dilemmas. It can be given in an individual or a group form, although more evidence exists for the efficacy of individual therapy (Sharpe 1997).

The procedure is 1) to elicit the patient's own illness model, appraisal of his or her situation and the ways in which he or she copes; 2) to introduce the possibility of alternatives; and 3) to help the patient select the beliefs and coping behaviors that are most helpful to him or her by conducting behavioral experiments. The key question for the behavioral experiment is "Is it possible for me to make changes in my behavior that will allow me to achieve my goals?" The patient is encouraged to think of the illness as a real one but one that is reversible by his or her own efforts rather than (as many patients do) as a fixed disease only alterable by medical intervention. The evidence that the patient can make changes and achieve goals acts as a test of these alternative hypotheses. Problem solving is used to address relevant occupational and interpersonal difficulties. A typical therapy takes place over 14 sessions (the first 90 minutes, the rest 50 minutes), the first 4 sessions being weekly and thereafter biweekly over 5 months.

In CFS, individually administered CBT has been tested in trials that together have included more than 1,000 patients. CBT has been found to be moderately effective and safe (Price et al. 2008). It is acceptable to most patients if explained adequately, but early dropouts may occur in routine practice (Scheeres et al. 2008).

Although CBT is an established treatment for chronic pain, a systematic review suggests that its efficacy is modest (Eccleston et al. 2009; see also Chapter 36, "Pain"). While it is reported to be of value in clinical practice (Bennett and Nelson 2006), randomized evaluations of the type of intensive individual CBT shown to be effective in CFS are required in FMS.

Patients Who Do Not Respond to Treatment

Most patients respond to some degree to rehabilitative therapies, but many will achieve only partial improvement, and some will fail to improve at all. In such cases, the management is the same as that for other chronic conditions—to maximize functioning and quality of life while minimizing the risk of iatrogenic harm. Although it is desirable that all patients should have a trial of rehabilitative treatment, a balance has to be struck between treatment and acceptance of chronic illness. Many physicians are reluctant to accept chronic disability in these patients, perhaps because the physicians do not regard these conditions as true diseases. However, pushing patients beyond their capabilities may only demoralize them and may even cause them to retreat further into invalidism. For such patients, regular supportive long-term follow-up from a single physician is often the best form of management.

Conclusion

Although peripheral to both internal medicine and psychiatry, functional somatic syndromes such as CFS and FMS are both common and core to the practice of psychosomatic medicine. A willingness and an ability to integrate biological, psychological, and social factors are essential in order to achieve an adequate understanding of these syndromes and to implement effective management. The challenge that these syndromes present to narrow biomedical and psychopathological perspectives of illness makes them a potential Trojan horse for those who seek to persuade others of the benefits of a much greater integration of medical and psychiatric theory and practice in achieving our core aim: to help our patients.

References

Aaron LA, Buchwald D: Chronic diffuse musculoskeletal pain, fibromyalgia and co-morbid unexplained clinical conditions: Bailliere's best practice and research. Clin Rheumatol 17:563–574, 2003

Afari N, Buchwald D: Chronic fatigue syndrome: a review. Am J Psychiatry 160:221–236, 2003

Afari N, Schmaling KB, Herrell R, et al: Coping strategies in twins with chronic fatigue and chronic fatigue syndrome. J Psychosom Res 48:547–554, 2000

Aggarwal VR, McBeth J, Zakrzewska JM, et al: The epidemiology of chronic syndromes that are frequently unexplained: do they have common associated factors? Int J Epidemiol 35:468–476, 2006

Al Allaf AW, Dunbar KL, Hallum NS, et al: A case-control study examining the role of physical trauma in the onset of fibromyalgia syndrome. Rheumatology (Oxford) 41:450–453, 2002

American Psychiatric Association: Diagnostic and Statistical Manual of Mental Disorders, 4th Edition, Text Revision. Washington, DC, American Psychiatric Association, 2000

Anderberg UM, Marteinsdottir I, Theorell T, et al: The impact of life events in female patients with fibromyalgia and in female healthy controls. Eur Psychiatry 15:295–301, 2000

Asbring P, Narvanen AL: Ideal versus reality: physicians' perspectives on patients with chronic fatigue syndrome (CFS) and fibromyalgia. Soc Sci Med 57:711–720, 2003

Asghari A, Nicholas MK: Pain self-efficacy beliefs and pain behaviour: a prospective study. Pain 94:85–100, 2001

Assefi NP, Coy TV, Uslan D, et al: Financial, occupational, and personal consequences of disability in patients with chronic fatigue syndrome and fibromyalgia compared to other fatiguing conditions. J Rheumatol 30:804–808, 2003

Ayres JG, Flint N, Smith EG, et al: Post-infection fatigue syndrome following Q fever. Q J Med 91:105–123, 1998

Banks J, Prior L: Doing things with illness: the micro politics of the CFS clinic. Soc Sci Med 52:11–23, 2001

Bazelmans E, Vercoulen JH, Galama JMD, et al: Prevalence of chronic fatigue syndrome and primary fibromyalgia syndrome (PFS) in the Netherlands. Ned Tijdschr Geneeskd 141:1520–1523, 1997

Bazelmans E, Bleijenberg G, Van der Meer JW, et al: Is physical deconditioning a perpetuating factor in chronic fatigue syndrome? A controlled study on maximal exercise performance and relations with fatigue, impairment and physical activity. Psychol Med 31:107–114, 2001

Bennett R, Nelson D: Cognitive behavioral therapy for fibromyalgia. Nat Clin Pract Rheumatol 2:416–424, 2006

Bennett RM, Kamin M, Karim R, et al: Tramadol and acetaminophen combination tablets in the treatment of fibromyalgia pain: a double-blind, randomized, placebo-controlled study. Am J Med 114:537–545, 2003

Bentall RP, Powell P, Nye FJ, et al: Predictors of response to treatment for chronic fatigue syndrome. Br J Psychiatry 181:248–252, 2002

Berelowitz GJ, Burgess AP, Thanabalasingham T, et al: Post-hepatitis syndrome revisited. J Viral Hepat 2:133–138, 1995

Bombardier CH, Buchwald D: Chronic fatigue, chronic fatigue syndrome, and fibromyalgia: disability and health-care use. Med Care 34:924–930, 1996

Bou-Holaigah I, Calkins H, Flynn JA, et al: Provocation of hypotension and pain during upright tilt table testing in adults with fibromyalgia. Clin Exp Rheumatol 15:239–246, 1997

Buchwald D, Herrell R, Ashton S, et al: A twin study of chronic fatigue. Psychosom Med 63:936–943, 2001

Buckelew SP, Huyser B, Hewett JE, et al: Self-efficacy predicting outcome among fibromyalgia subjects. Arthritis Care Res 9:97–104, 1996

Burgmer M, Gaubitz M, Konrad C, et al: Decreased gray matter volumes in the cingulo-frontal cortex and the amygdala in patients with fibromyalgia. Psychosom Med 71:566–573, 2009

Busch AJ, Barber KA, Overend TJ, et al: Exercise for treating fibromyalgia syndrome. Cochrane Database Syst Rev (4): CD003786, 2007

Buskila D, Neumann L: Fibromyalgia syndrome (FM) and nonarticular tenderness in relatives of patients with FM. J Rheumatol 24:941–944, 1997

Buskila D, Press J, Abu-Shakra M: Fibromyalgia in systemic lupus erythematosus: prevalence and clinical implications. Clin Rev Allergy Immunol 25:25–28, 2003

Cairns R, Hotopf M: A systematic review describing the prognosis of chronic fatigue syndrome. Occup Med (Lond) 55:20–31, 2005

Chalder T, Goodman R, Wessely S, et al: Epidemiology of chronic fatigue syndrome and self reported myalgic encephalomyelitis in 5–15 year olds: cross sectional study. BMJ 327:654–655, 2003

Chen J, Tsuchiya M, Kawakami N, et al: Non-fearful vs fearful panic attacks: a general population study from the National Comorbidity Survey. J Affect Disord 112:273–278, 2009

Ciccone DS, Natelson BH: Comorbid illness in women with chronic fatigue syndrome: a test of the single-syndrome hypothesis. Psychosom Med 65:268–275, 2003

Clark SR, Tindall E, Bennett RM: A double blind crossover trial of prednisone versus placebo in the treatment of fibrositis. J Rheumatol 12:980–983, 1985

Clauw DJ, Chrousos GP: Chronic pain and fatigue syndromes: overlapping clinical and neuroendocrine features and potential pathogenic mechanisms. Neuroimmunomodulation 4:134–153, 1997

Clauw DJ, Crofford LJ: Chronic widespread pain and fibromyalgia: what we know, and what we need to know. Bailliere's best practice and research. Clin Rheumatol 17:685–701, 2003

Cleare AJ, Heap E, Malhi GS, et al: Low-dose hydrocortisone in chronic fatigue syndrome: a randomised crossover trial. Lancet 353:455–458, 1999

Cook DB, O'Connor PJ, Lange G, et al: Functional neuroimaging correlates of mental fatigue induced by cognition among chronic fatigue syndrome patients and controls. Neuroimage 36:108–122, 2007

Costa DC, Tannock C, Brostoff J: Brainstem perfusion is impaired in chronic fatigue syndrome. Q J Med 88:767–773, 1995

Creavin ST, Dunn KM, Mallen CD, et al: Co-occurrence and associations of pain and fatigue in a community sample of Dutch adults. Eur J Pain 14:327–334, 2010

Croft P, Rigby AS, Boswell R, et al: The prevalence of chronic widespread pain in the general population. J Rheumatol 20:710–713, 1993

Croft P, Burt J, Schollum J, et al: More pain, more tender points: is fibromyalgia just one end of a continuous spectrum? Ann Rheum Dis 55:482–485, 1996

Davis MC, Zautra AJ, Reich JW: Vulnerability to stress among women in chronic pain from fibromyalgia and osteoarthritis. Ann Behav Med 23:215–226, 2001

Deale A, Chalder T, Wessely S: Illness beliefs and treatment outcome in chronic fatigue syndrome. J Psychosom Res 45:77–83, 1998

de Lange FP, Kalkman JS, Bleijenberg G, et al: Gray matter volume reduction in the chronic fatigue syndrome. Neuroimage 26:777–781, 2005

de Lange FP, Koers A, Kalkman JS, et al: Increase in prefrontal cortical volume following cognitive behavioural therapy in patients with chronic fatigue syndrome. Brain 131(pt 8): 2172–2180, 2008

Deary V, Chalder T, Sharpe M: The cognitive behavioural model of medically unexplained symptoms: a theoretical and empirical review. Clin Psychol Rev 27:781–797, 2007

Dickson A, Toft A, O'Carroll RE: Neuropsychological functioning, illness perception, mood and quality of life in chronic fatigue syndrome, autoimmune thyroid disease and healthy participants. Psychol Med 39:1567–1576, 2009

Eccleston C, Williams AC, Morley S: Psychological therapies for the management of chronic pain (excluding headache) in adults. Cochrane Database Syst Rev (2):CD007407, 2009

Edmonds M, McGuire H, Price J: Exercise therapy for chronic fatigue syndrome. Cochrane Database Syst Rev (3):CD003200, 2004

Engel GL: The need for a new medical model: a challenge for biomedicine. Science 196:129–196, 1977

Epstein SA, Kay G, Clauw D, et al: Psychiatric disorders in patients with fibromyalgia: a multicenter investigation. Psychosomatics 40:57–63, 1999

Evengard B, Nilsson CG, Lindh G, et al: Chronic fatigue syndrome differs from fibromyalgia: no evidence for elevated substance P levels in cerebrospinal fluid of patients with chronic fatigue syndrome. Pain 78:153–155, 1998

Farber L, Stratz TH, Bruckle W, et al: Short-term treatment of primary fibromyalgia with the 5-HT3-receptor antagonist tropisetron: results of a randomized, double-blind, placebo-controlled multicenter trial in 418 patients. Int J Clin Pharmacol Res 21:1–13, 2001

Findley JC, Kerns R, Weinberg LD, et al: Self-efficacy as a psychological moderator of chronic fatigue syndrome. J Behav Med 21:351–362, 1998

Fischler B, Cluydts R, De Gucht Y, et al: Generalized anxiety disorder in chronic fatigue syndrome. Acta Psychiatr Scand 95:405–413, 1997

Fitzcharles MA, Boulos P: Inaccuracy in the diagnosis of fibromyalgia syndrome: analysis of referrals. Rheumatology (Oxford) 42:263–267, 2003

Flor H: Cortical reorganisation and chronic pain: implications for rehabilitation. J Rehabil Med 41 (suppl):66–72, 2003

Fukuda K, Straus SE, Hickie I, et al: The chronic fatigue syndrome: a comprehensive approach to its definition and study. International Chronic Fatigue Syndrome Study Group. Ann Intern Med 121:953–959, 1994

Fulcher KY, White PD: Chronic fatigue syndrome: a description of graded exercise treatment. Physiotherapy 84:223–226, 1998

Fulcher KY, White PD: Strength and physiological response to exercise in patients with chronic fatigue syndrome. J Neurol Neurosurg Psychiatry 69:302–307, 2000

Gowers WR: A lecture on lumbago: its lessons and analogues. BMJ 1:117–121, 1904

Granges G, Zilko P, Littlejohn GO: Fibromyalgia syndrome: assessment of the severity of the condition 2 years after diagnosis. J Rheumatol 21:523–529, 1994

Gureje O, Simon GE, Von Korff M: A cross-national study of the course of persistent pain in primary care. Pain 92:195–200, 2001

Hadler NM: Fibromyalgia, chronic fatigue, and other iatrogenic diagnostic algorithms: do some labels escalate illness in vulnerable patients? Postgrad Med 102:161–162, 1996a

Hadler NM: If you have to prove you are ill, you can't get well: the object lesson of fibromyalgia. Spine 21:2397–2400, 1996b

Harvey SB, Wadsworth M, Wessely S, et al: Etiology of chronic fatigue syndrome: testing popular hypotheses using a national birth cohort study. Psychosom Med 70:488–495, 2008a

Harvey SB, Wadsworth M, Wessely S, et al: The relationship between prior psychiatric disorder and chronic fatigue: evidence from a national birth cohort study. Psychol Med 38:933–940, 2008b

Hassett AL, Cone JD, Patella SJ, et al: The role of catastrophizing in the pain and depression of women with fibromyalgia syndrome. Arthritis Rheum 43:2493–2500, 2000

Hatcher S, House A: Life events, difficulties and dilemmas in the onset of chronic fatigue syndrome: a case-control study. Psychol Med 33:1185–1192, 2003

Hauser W, Bernardy K, Uceyler N, et al: Treatment of fibromyalgia syndrome with antidepressants: a meta-analysis. JAMA 301:198–209, 2009a

Hauser W, Bernardy K, Uceyler N, et al: Treatment of fibromyalgia syndrome with gabapentin and pregabalin: a meta-analysis of randomized controlled trials. Pain 145:69–81, 2009b

Heijmans MJ: Coping and adaptive outcome in chronic fatigue syndrome: importance of illness cognitions. J Psychosom Res 45:39–51, 1998

Heim C, Wagner D, Maloney E, et al: Early adverse experience and risk for chronic fatigue syndrome: results from a population-based study. Arch Gen Psychiatry 63:1258–1266, 2006

Heim C, Nater UM, Maloney E, et al: Childhood trauma and risk for chronic fatigue syndrome: association with neuroendocrine dysfunction. Arch Gen Psychiatry 66:72–80, 2009

Henningsen P, Zimmermann T, Sattel H: Medically unexplained physical symptoms, anxiety, and depression: a meta-analytic review. Psychosom Med 65:528–533, 2003

Hill NF, Tiersky LA, Scavalla VR, et al: Natural history of severe chronic fatigue syndrome. Arch Phys Med Rehabil 80:1090–1094, 1999

Holmes GP, Kaplan JE, Gantz NM, et al: Chronic fatigue syndrome: a working case definition. Ann Intern Med 108:387–389, 1988

Hotopf MH, Noah N, Wessely S: Chronic fatigue and minor psychiatric morbidity after viral meningitis: a controlled study. J Neurol Neurosurg Psychiatry 60:504–509, 1996

Hsu MC, Harris RE, Sundgren PC, et al: No consistent difference in gray matter volume between individuals with fibromyalgia and age-matched healthy subjects when controlling for affective disorder. Pain 143:262–267, 2009

Hudson JI, Pope HG: The concept of affective spectrum disorder: relationship to fibromyalgia and other syndromes of chronic fatigue and chronic muscle pain. Baillieres Clin Rheumatol 8:839–856, 1994

Hudson JI, Pope HG Jr: The relationship between fibromyalgia and major depressive disorder. Rheum Dis Clin North Am 22:285–303, 1996

Huibers MJ, Wessely S: The act of diagnosis: pros and cons of labelling chronic fatigue syndrome. Psychol Med 36:895–900, 2006

Jason LA, Richman JA, Rademaker AW, et al: A community-based study of chronic fatigue syndrome. Arch Intern Med 159: 2129–2137, 1999

Johnson SK, DeLuca J, Natelson BH: Assessing somatization disorder in the chronic fatigue syndrome. Psychosom Med 58:50–57, 1996

Kaiser J: Biomedicine. Genes and chronic fatigue: how strong is the evidence? Science 312:669–671, 2006

Kanaan RA, Lepine JP, Wessely SC: The association or otherwise of the functional somatic syndromes. Psychosom Med 69:855–859, 2007

Karjalainen K, Malmivaara A, van Tulder M, et al: Multidisciplinary rehabilitation for fibromyalgia and musculoskeletal pain in working age adults. Cochrane Database Syst Rev (2):CD001984, 2000

Kato K, Sullivan PF, Evengard B, et al: Chronic widespread pain and its comorbidities: a population-based study. Arch Intern Med 166:1649–1654, 2006

Kato K, Sullivan PF, Evengard B, et al: A population-based twin study of functional somatic syndromes. Psychol Med 39:497–505, 2009

Katon W, Buchwald DS, Simon GE, et al: Psychiatric illness in patients with chronic fatigue and rheumatoid arthritis. J Gen Intern Med 6:277–285, 1991

Kerr JR, Mattey DL: Preexisting psychological stress predicts acute and chronic fatigue and arthritis following symptomatic parvovirus B19 infection. Clin Infect Dis 46(9):e83–e87, 2008

Khan AA, Khan A, Harezlak J, et al: Somatic symptoms in primary care: etiology and outcome. Psychosomatics 44:471–478, 2003

Kranzler JD, Gendreau JF, Rao SG: The psychopharmacology of fibromyalgia: a drug development perspective. Psychopharmacol Bull 36:165–213, 2002

Kroenke K: Patients presenting with somatic complaints: epidemiology, psychiatric comorbidity and management. Int J Methods Psychiatr Res 12:34–43, 2003

Kroenke K, Jackson JL: Outcome in general medical patients presenting with common symptoms: a prospective study with a 2-week and a 3-month follow-up. Fam Pract 15:398–403, 1998

Kroenke K, Krebs EE, Bair MJ: Pharmacotherapy of chronic pain: a synthesis of recommendations from systematic reviews. Gen Hosp Psychiatry 31:206–219, 2009

Kruesi MJ, Dale JK, Straus SE: Psychiatric diagnoses in patients who have chronic fatigue syndrome. J Clin Psychiatry 50:53–56, 1989

Kurtze N, Svebak S: Fatigue and patterns of pain in fibromyalgia: correlations with anxiety, depression and co-morbidity in a female county sample. Br J Med Psychol 74:523–537, 2001

Kushner MG, Beitman BD: Panic attacks without fear: an overview. Behav Res Ther 28:469–479, 1990

Lehman AM, Lehman DR, Hemphill KJ, et al: Illness experience, depression, and anxiety in chronic fatigue syndrome. J Psychosom Res 52:461–465, 2002

Lloyd AR, Wakefield D, Boughton CR, et al: What is myalgic encephalomyelitis? Lancet 1(8597):1286–1287, 1988

Lombardi VC, Ruscetti FW, Das Gupta J, et al: Detection of an infectious retrovirus, XMRV, in blood cells of patients with chronic fatigue syndrome. Science 326:585–589, 2009

Lyall M, Peakman M, Wessely S: A systematic review and critical evaluation of the immunology of chronic fatigue syndrome. J Psychosom Res 55:79–90, 2003

Machale SM, Lawrie SM, Cavanagh JT, et al: Cerebral perfusion in chronic fatigue syndrome and depression. Br J Psychiatry 176:550–556, 2000

Majer M, Welberg LA, Capuron L, et al: Neuropsychological performance in persons with chronic fatigue syndrome: results from a population-based study. Psychosom Med 70:829–836, 2008

Makela MO: Is fibromyalgia a distinct clinical entity? The epidemiologist's evidence. Baillieres Best Pract Res Clin Rheumatol 13:415–419, 1999

Manu P, Matthews DA, Lane TJ: Panic disorder among patients with chronic fatigue. South Med J 84:451–456, 1991

Martin A, Chalder T, Rief W, et al: The relationship between chronic fatigue and somatization syndrome: a general population survey. J Psychosom Res 63:147–156, 2007

Mayou R, Levenson J, Sharpe M: Somatoform disorders in DSM-V. Psychosomatics 44:449–451, 2003

Moldofsky H: Sleep, neuroimmune and neuroendocrine functions in fibromyalgia and chronic fatigue syndrome. Adv Neuroimmunol 5:39–56, 1995

Moldofsky H, Scarisbrick P, England R, et al: Musculoskeletal symptoms and non-REM sleep disturbances in patients with fibrositis syndrome and healthy subjects. Psychosom Med 37:341–351, 1975

Nater UM, Wagner D, Solomon L, et al: Coping styles in people with chronic fatigue syndrome identified from the general population of Wichita, KS. J Psychosom Res 60:567–573, 2006

Nater UM, Lin JM, Maloney EM, et al: Psychiatric comorbidity in persons with chronic fatigue syndrome identified from the Georgia population. Psychosom Med 71:557–565, 2009

Neerinckx E, Van Houdenhove B, Lysens R, et al: Attributions in chronic fatigue syndrome and fibromyalgia syndrome in tertiary care. J Rheumatol 27:1051–1055, 2000

Newton JL, Sheth A, Shin J, et al: Lower ambulatory blood pressure in chronic fatigue syndrome. Psychosom Med 71:361–365, 2009

Nijs J, Van de Putte K, Louckx F, et al: Exercise performance and chronic pain in chronic fatigue syndrome: the role of pain catastrophizing. Pain Med 9:1164–1172, 2008

Nisenbaum R, Jones JF, Unger ER, et al: A population-based study of the clinical course of chronic fatigue syndrome. Health Qual Life Outcomes 1:49, 2003

Ohayon MM, Schatzberg AF: Using chronic pain to predict depressive morbidity in the general population. Arch Gen Psychiatry 60:39–47, 2003

Paras ML, Murad MH, Chen LP, et al: Sexual abuse and lifetime diagnosis of somatic disorders: a systematic review and meta-analysis. JAMA 302:550–561, 2009

Parker AJ, Wessely S, Cleare AJ: The neuroendocrinology of chronic fatigue syndrome and fibromyalgia. Psychol Med 31:1331–1345, 2001

Pawlikowska T, Chalder T, Hirsch SR, et al: Population based study of fatigue and psychological distress. BMJ 308:763–766, 1994

Philips HC: Avoidance behaviour and its role in sustaining chronic pain. Behav Res Ther 25:273–279, 1987

Powell P, Bentall RP, Nye FJ, et al: Randomised controlled trial of patient education to encourage graded exercise in chronic fatigue syndrome. BMJ 322:387–390, 2001

Price JR, Mitchell E, Tidy E, et al: Cognitive behaviour therapy for chronic fatigue syndrome in adults. Cochrane Database Syst Rev (3):CD001027, 2008

Prins JB, Van der Meer JW, Bleijenberg G: Chronic fatigue syndrome. Lancet 367:346–355, 2006

Pujol J, Lopez-Sola M, Ortiz H, et al: Mapping brain response to pain in fibromyalgia patients using temporal analysis of FMRI. PLoS One 4(4):e5224, 2009

Rains JC, Penzien DB: Sleep and chronic pain: challenges to the alpha-EEG sleep pattern as a pain specific sleep anomaly. J Psychosom Res 54:77–83, 2003

Rea T, Russo J, Katon W, et al: A prospective study of tender points and fibromyalgia during and after an acute viral infection. Arch Intern Med 159:865–870, 1999

Reeves WC, Lloyd A, Vernon SD, et al: Identification of ambiguities in the 1994 chronic fatigue syndrome research case definition and recommendations for resolution. BMC Health Serv Res 3:25, 2003

Reyes M, Nisenbaum R, Hoaglin DC, et al: Prevalence and incidence of chronic fatigue syndrome in Wichita, Kansas. Arch Intern Med 163:1530–1536, 2003

Roberts AD, Papadopoulos AS, Wessely S, et al: Salivary cortisol output before and after cognitive behavioural therapy for chronic fatigue syndrome. J Affect Disord 115:280–286, 2009

Roberts AD, Charler ML, Papadopoulos A, et al: Does hypocortisolism predict a poor response to cognitive behavioural therapy in chronic fatigue syndrome? Psychol Med 40:515–522, 2010

Roelofs J, Peters ML, McCracken L, et al: The pain vigilance and awareness questionnaire (PVAQ): further psychometric evaluation in fibromyalgia and other chronic pain syndromes. Pain 101:299–306, 2003

Ross SE: Memes as infectious agents in psychosomatic illness. Ann Intern Med 131:867–871, 1999

Rowe PC, Bou Holaigah I, Kan JS, et al: Is neurally mediated hypotension an unrecognised cause of chronic fatigue? Lancet 345:623–624, 1995

Rowe PC, Calkins H, DeBusk K, et al: Fludrocortisone acetate to treat neurally mediated hypotension in chronic fatigue syndrome: a randomized controlled trial. JAMA 285:52–59, 2001

Roy-Byrne P, Smith WR, Goldberg J, et al: Post-traumatic stress disorder among patients with chronic pain and chronic fatigue. Psychol Med 34:363–368, 2004

Russell IJ, Orr MD, Littman B, et al: Elevated cerebrospinal fluid levels of substance P in patients with the fibromyalgia syndrome. Arthritis Rheum 37:1593–1601, 1994

Sandler H, Vernikos J: Inactivity: Physiological Effects. London, Academic Press, 1986

Sartorius N, Ustun TB, Costa e Silva JA, et al: An international study of psychological problems in primary care: preliminary report from the World Health Organization collaborative project on psychological problems in general health care. Arch Gen Psychiatry 50:819–824, 1993

Scheeres K, Wensing M, Knoop H, et al: Implementing cognitive behavioral therapy for chronic fatigue syndrome in a mental

health center: a benchmarking evaluation. J Consult Clin Psychol 76:163–171, 2008
Schweinhardt P, Sauro KM, Bushnell MC: Fibromyalgia: a disorder of the brain? Neuroscientist 14:415–421, 2008
Servaes P, Prins J, Verhagen S, et al: Fatigue after breast cancer and in chronic fatigue syndrome: similarities and differences. J Psychosom Res 52:453–459, 2002
Sharpe M: Chronic fatigue syndrome. Psychiatr Clin North Am 19:549–574, 1996
Sharpe M: Cognitive behavior therapy for functional somatic complaints: the example of chronic fatigue syndrome. Psychosomatics 38:356–362, 1997
Sharpe M: Doctors' diagnoses and patients' perceptions: lessons from chronic fatigue syndrome. Gen Hosp Psychiatry 20:335–338, 1998
Sharpe M, Carson A: Unexplained somatic symptoms, functional syndromes, and somatization: do we need a paradigm shift? Ann Intern Med 134(9 pt 2):926–930, 2001
Sharpe M, Wilks D: ABC of psychological medicine: fatigue. BMJ 325:480–483, 2002
Sharpe M, Williams A: Treating patients with hypochondriasis and somatoform pain disorder, in Psychological Approaches to Pain Management. Edited by Turk DC, Gatchel RJ. New York, Guilford, 2001, pp 515–533
Sharpe M, Archard LC, Banatvala JE, et al: A report—chronic fatigue syndrome: guidelines for research. J R Soc Med 84:118–121, 1991
Sharpe M, Hawton KE, Seagroatt V, et al: Patients who present with fatigue: a follow up of referrals to an infectious diseases clinic. BMJ 305:147–152, 1992
Shorter E: Somatization and chronic pain in historic perspective. Clin Orthop 336:52–60, 1997
Silver A, Haeney M, Vijayadurai P, et al: The role of fear of physical movement and activity in chronic fatigue syndrome. J Psychosom Res 52:485–493, 2002
Skapinakis P: Clarifying the relationship between unexplained chronic fatigue and psychiatric morbidity: results from a community survey in Great Britain. Am J Psychiatry 157:1492–1498, 2000
Skapinakis P, Lewis G, Mavreas V: Unexplained fatigue syndromes in a multinational primary care sample: specificity of definition and prevalence and distinctiveness from depression and generalized anxiety. Am J Psychiatry 160:785–787, 2003
Stone J, Wojcik W, Durrance D, et al: What should we say to patients with symptoms unexplained by disease? The number needed to offend. BMJ 325:1449–1450, 2002
Stubhaug B, Lie SA, Ursin H, et al: Cognitive-behavioural therapy v mirtazapine for chronic fatigue and neurasthenia: randomised placebo-controlled trial. Br J Psychiatry 192:217–223, 2008
Sullivan PF, Smith W, Buchwald D: Latent class analysis of symptoms associated with chronic fatigue syndrome and fibromyalgia. Psychol Med 32:881–888, 2002
Surawy C, Hackmann A, Hawton KE, et al: Chronic fatigue syndrome: a cognitive approach. Behav Res Ther 33:535–544, 1995
Taylor RR, Jason LA: Sexual abuse, physical abuse, chronic fatigue, and chronic fatigue syndrome: a community-based study. J Nerv Ment Dis 189:709–715, 2001
Taylor RR, Jason LA, Jahn SC: Chronic fatigue and sociodemographic characteristics as predictors of psychiatric disorders in a community-based sample. Psychosom Med 65:896–901, 2003
Theorell T, Blomkvist V, Lindh G, et al: Critical life events, infections, and symptoms during the year preceding chronic fatigue syndrome (CFS): an examination of CFS patients and subjects with a nonspecific life crisis. Psychosom Med 61:304–310, 1999
Thompson ME, Barkhuizen A: Fibromyalgia, hepatitis C infection, and the cytokine connection. Curr Pain Headache Rep 7:342–347, 2003
Tirelli U, Chierichetti F, Tavio M, et al: Brain positron emission tomography (PET) in chronic fatigue syndrome: preliminary data. Am J Med 105:54S–58S, 1998
Tofferi J, Jackson JL, O'Malley PG: Treatment of fibromyalgia with cyclobenzaprine: a meta-analysis. Arthritis Rheum 51:9–13, 2004
Torres-Harding SR, Jason LA, Cane V, et al: Physicians' diagnoses of psychiatric disorders for people with chronic fatigue syndrome. Int J Psychiatry Med 32:109–124, 2002
Valim V, Oliveira LM, Suda AL, et al: Peak oxygen uptake and ventilatory anaerobic threshold in fibromyalgia. J Rheumatol 29:353–357, 2002
van der Werf SP, de Vree B, Alberts M, et al: Natural course and predicting self-reported improvement in patients with chronic fatigue syndrome with a relatively short illness duration. J Psychosom Res 53:749–753, 2002
Van Hoof E, Cluydts R, De Meirleir K: Atypical depression as a secondary symptom in chronic fatigue syndrome. Med Hypotheses 61:52–55, 2003
Van Houdenhove B, Neerinckx E, Lysens R, et al: Victimization in chronic fatigue syndrome and fibromyalgia in tertiary care: a controlled study on prevalence and characteristics. Psychosom 42:21–28, 2001a
Van Houdenhove B, Neerinckx E, Onghena P, et al: Premorbid overactive lifestyle in chronic fatigue syndrome and fibromyalgia: an etiological factor or proof of good citizenship? J Psychosom Res 51:571–576, 2001b
van't Leven M, Zielhuis GA, van der Meer JW, et al: Fatigue and chronic fatigue syndrome-like complaints in the general population. Eur J Public Health 20:251–257, 2010
Vercoulen JH, Hommes OR, Swanink CM, et al: The measurement of fatigue in patients with multiple sclerosis: a multidimensional comparison with patients with chronic fatigue syndrome and healthy subjects. Arch Neurol 53:642–649, 1996a
Vercoulen JH, Swanink CM, Zitman FG, et al: Randomized, double-blind, placebo-controlled study of fluoxetine in chronic fatigue syndrome. Lancet 347:858–861, 1996b
Vercoulen JH, Bazelmans E, Swanink CM, et al: Evaluating neuropsychological impairment in chronic fatigue syndrome. J Clin Exp Neuropsychol 20:144–156, 1998

Vial T, Descotes J: Clinical toxicity of the interferons. Drug Saf 10:115–150, 1994

Walker EA, Keegan D, Gardner G, et al: Psychosocial factors in fibromyalgia compared with rheumatoid arthritis, I: sexual, physical, and emotional abuse and neglect. Psychosom Med 59:572–577, 1997

Wallman KE, Sacco P: Sense of effort during a fatiguing exercise protocol in chronic fatigue syndrome. Res Sports Med 15:47–59, 2007

Wearden AJ, Appleby J: Research on cognitive complaints and cognitive functioning in patients with chronic fatigue syndrome (CFS): what conclusions can we draw? J Psychosom Res 41:197–211, 1996

Wearden AJ, Dowrick C, Chew-Graham C, et al: Nurse led, home based self help treatment for patients in primary care with chronic fatigue syndrome: randomised controlled trial. Fatigue Intervention by Nurses Evaluation (FINE) trial writing group and the FINE trial group. BMJ 340:c1777, 2010

Welford AT: The psychologist's problem in measuring fatigue, in Fatigue. Edited by Floyd WF, Welford AT. London, HK Lewis, 1953, pp 183–191

Wessely S: Old wine in new bottles: neurasthenia and M.E. Psychol Med 20:35–53, 1990

Wessely S, Nimnuan C, Sharpe M: Functional somatic syndromes: one or many? Lancet 354:936–939, 1999

White KP, Speechley M, Harth M, et al: The London Fibromyalgia Epidemiology Study: the prevalence of fibromyalgia syndrome in London, Ontario. J Rheumatol 26:1570–1576, 1999

White PD, Thomas JM, Kangro HO, et al: Predictions and associations of fatigue syndromes and mood disorders that occur after infectious mononucleosis. Lancet 358:1946–1954, 2001

Wigers SH: Fibromyalgia outcome: the predictive values of symptom duration, physical activity, disability pension, and critical life events—a 4.5 year prospective study. J Psychosom Res 41:235–243, 1996

Williams DA: Psychological and behavioural therapies in fibromyalgia and related syndromes. Baillieres Best Pract Res Clin Rheumatol 17:649–665, 2003

Wolfe F: The relation between tender points and fibromyalgia symptom variables: evidence that fibromyalgia is not a discrete disorder in the clinic. Ann Rheum Dis 56:268–271, 1997

Wolfe F, Cathey MA, Kleinheksel SM: Fibrositis (fibromyalgia) in rheumatoid arthritis. J Rheumatol 11:814–818, 1984

Wolfe F, Smythe HA, Yunus MB, et al: The American College of Rheumatology 1990 criteria for the classification of fibromyalgia: report of the Multicenter Criteria Committee. Arthritis Rheum 33:160–172, 1990

Wolfe F, Ross K, Anderson JA, et al: The prevalence and characteristics of fibromyalgia in the general population. Arthritis Rheum 38:19–28, 1995

Wolfe F, Anderson J, Harkness D, et al: Health status and disease severity in fibromyalgia: results of a six-center longitudinal study. Arthritis Rheum 40:1571–1579, 1997

World Health Organization: International Statistical Classification of Diseases and Related Health Problems, 10th Revision. Geneva, World Health Organization, 1992

World Health Organization: Mental Illness in General Health Care: An International Study. Chichester, Wiley, 1995

Yunus MB: A comprehensive medical evaluation of patients with fibromyalgia syndrome. Rheum Dis Clin North Am 28:201–205, 2002

CHAPTER 27

Infectious Diseases

James L. Levenson, M.D.

PSYCHIATRIC SYMPTOMS ARE part of the clinical presentation of many systemic and central nervous system (CNS) infectious processes. Rapid cultural and economic changes affecting regional and international mobility, sexuality, and other behaviors have led to worldwide spread of new epidemics (e.g., human immunodeficiency virus [HIV], severe acute respiratory syndrome [SARS]; Cheng et al. 2004) and more limited spread of previously geographically isolated diseases (e.g., cysticercosis). Infectious diseases have been considered as contributing to the pathogenesis of psychiatric disorders (e.g., viral antibodies in schizophrenia). Associations between specific infections and a subset of psychiatric syndromes (e.g., pediatric autoimmune neuropsychiatric disorder associated with streptococcal infection [PANDAS]) provide intriguing models of etiology. Controversy surrounds some attributions of psychopathology to infectious pathophysiology (e.g., Lyme disease).

Consulting psychiatrists should carefully consider relevant aspects of patients' histories, including immune status, regions of origin and residence, travel, high-risk sexual behaviors, occupation, and recreational activities. Physicians must consider which infectious diseases are endemic in the practice area and in the areas where the patient has traveled or resided. Similar neuropsychiatric symptoms might suggest possible Lyme disease in a hiker in the northeastern United States and neurocysticercosis in an immigrant from Central America.

Many brain diseases or injuries, as well as the effects of aging, render patients more vulnerable to neuropsychiatric effects of even minor metabolic or toxic insults and similarly to adverse effects of even limited infectious diseases. For example, a simple upper respiratory or bladder infection may cause only discomfort in an otherwise healthy individual but agitation, irritability, and frank delirium in the elderly, especially in patients who also have dementia. The reasons that older age and brain disease would make patients vulnerable to delirium with minor infections are not understood but may involve changes in immune function and the blood–brain barrier.

Psychological factors may significantly affect the risk for and course of infectious diseases, with HIV as the most studied example (see Chapter 28, "HIV/AIDS"). Psychological factors have been shown to influence other infectious diseases as well, from the common cold (Takkouche et al. 2001) to hepatitis B and C infection (Osher et al. 2003). One mechanism for such effects is through poor sleep (Cohen et al. 2009).

This chapter is divided into bacterial, viral, fungal, and parasitic infections, followed by psychiatric side effects of antimicrobial drugs and their interactions with psychotropic medications, and finally a discussion of fears of infectious disease and psychiatric aspects of immunization. HIV and AIDS are covered in Chapter 28. In the current chapter, we focus on psychiatric aspects of all other infectious diseases.

Occult Infections

Occult infections, irrespective of location, by definition are concealed or mysterious, often requiring diligent detective work. Such infections may occur essentially anywhere in the body (Table 27–1). Psychiatric symptoms may result from even a small focus of chronic infection. The psychiatric symptoms most likely to be present are subtle cognitive dysfunction or mood change (e.g., irritability) consistent with a mild encephalopathy, but depression, psychosis, and delirium also may occur.

The diagnosis is suggested by secondary signs of infection, specifically temperature dysregulation, or increases

TABLE 27–1. Occult infections that may cause psychiatric symptoms

Sinusitis
Chronic otitis
Abscess (e.g., dental, lung, intra-abdominal, retroperitoneal, perirectal)
Bronchiectasis
Endocarditis
Cholecystitis
Parasitosis
Urinary tract infection
Pelvic inflammatory disease
Osteomyelitis
Subclinical systemic infections (e.g., HIV, tuberculosis)

in white blood cell count, granulocyte count, or sedimentation rate. A careful history and physical examination may identify overlooked clues to guide the search (e.g., chronic toothache or lymphadenopathy). If repeat history and physical examination are not fruitful, other studies may be needed (e.g., chest X rays, computed tomography [CT] scans, ultrasounds).

Bacterial Infections

Bacteremia and Sepsis

Bacteremia literally means entry of bacteria into the bloodstream, whereas *sepsis* refers to the systemic inflammatory response to bacteremia. Systemic symptoms of sepsis, including CNS symptoms, result from many different mechanisms, including bacterial toxins, release of cytokines, hyperthermia, shock (poor perfusion), acute renal insufficiency, pulmonary failure ("shock lung"), coagulopathy, disruption of the blood–brain barrier, and spread of the organism into the CNS and other organs. An acute change in mental status may be the first sign of impending sepsis and may precede the development of fever. Any patient who has an abrupt change in mental status in concert with a shaking chill should be presumed to have a high risk for impending sepsis.

Septic encephalopathy occurs more frequently than is generally assumed. Its severity is associated with the severity of overall illness, and it is often part of multiorgan failure (Siami et al. 2008). Standard treatment is broad-spectrum antibiotics at first and is then tailored to the identified organism and its antimicrobial susceptibilities. Symptoms of posttraumatic stress disorder recently have been recognized as very common following septic shock. Although the role of corticosteroids in septic shock remains controversial, one group has reported studies showing that stress doses of hydrocortisone lead to a significant reduction of posttraumatic stress disorder symptoms in long-term survivors (Schelling et al. 2006).

Toxic Shock Syndrome

Toxic shock syndrome (TSS) typically occurs in otherwise healthy people with intact immune systems, caused by either *Streptococcus pyogenes* (most often) or *Staphylococcus aureus*. TSS generally manifests with rapid onset of fever, rash, and hypotension (shock). There may be a prodromal period of 2–3 days of malaise, myalgia, and chills followed by confusion and lethargy. TSS should be suspected in any patient with a recent wound who acutely develops unexplained pain, lethargy, and confusion and may occur even when a surgical wound appears not to be inflamed.

Pediatric Autoimmune Neuropsychiatric Disorder Associated With Streptococcal Infection

PANDAS is not a diagnosis but an acronym for the clinical characteristics of a subgroup of children whose obsessive-compulsive and tic disorders seem to have been triggered by an infection with group A beta-hemolytic streptococci (GABHS). The syndrome is defined by early childhood onset of symptoms; an episodic course characterized by abrupt onset of symptoms with frequent relapses and remissions; association with neurological signs, especially tics; and temporal association with GABHS infections (most commonly pharyngitis). The best way to show the association between recent GABHS infection and PANDAS symptoms is to document a rapid rise in antistreptococcal (ASO) titers associated with symptom onset or exacerbation and a decrease in titers associated with symptom resolution or improvement. Children with PANDAS also may have behavioral symptoms (e.g., attention deficits and hyperactivity) (Swedo et al. 1998). GABHS may play a role in some cases of Tourette's syndrome as well.

In addition to ASO titers, a throat culture should be obtained, keeping in mind that some children who have GABHS infection may not have a sore throat (Swedo et al. 1998). Prompt antibiotic treatment may prevent the expected rise in ASO titers, and children with uncomplicated streptococcal infections treated with antibiotics appear to have no increased risk for PANDAS (Perrin et al. 2004). In children with recurrent streptococcal infections, antibiotic prophylaxis to prevent neuropsychiatric symptoms has yielded mixed results. One double-blind, placebo-controlled trial found no benefit over placebo in preventing PANDAS exacerbations (Garvey et al. 1999), but another trial found that either penicillin or azithromycin was able to lower rates of recurrent streptococcal infections and to decrease PANDAS exacerbations (Snider et al. 2005). Even though one study found that the severity of obsessive-compulsive symptoms diminished by 45%–58% following treatment with either plasma exchange or intravenous immunoglobulin (Perlmutter et al. 1999), immunomodulatory therapies are not recommended as routine treatment of PANDAS.

PANDAS has been and remains a controversial concept (Shulman 2009). It must be emphasized that most cases of obsessive-compulsive disorder (OCD) and tic disorders in children are unrelated to streptococcal infection. Even in children meeting PANDAS criteria, most exacerbations of OCD or tic symptoms are not due to GABHS infection (Kurlan et al. 2008). The failure of immune markers to correlate with clinical exacerbations of PANDAS challenges the autoimmune theory of its etiology (Singer et al. 2008). Outside of specialty centers, inadequate diagnostic evaluation has led to unwarranted antibiotic and immunomodulatory medications in children with OCD or tics (Gabbay et al. 2008).

Bacterial Endocarditis

Bacterial endocarditis may cause neuropsychiatric symptoms at all stages of the disease via focal, systemic, and CNS disease processes. Endocardial infections are focal infections that usually occur on one of the valves of the heart. Rheumatic heart disease was originally the typical cause of the predisposing cardiac abnormality. Its incidence has decreased, whereas the incidence of senescent valvular disease, prosthetic valve placement, and intravenous drug use has increased, thus changing the risk factors in the developed world. Malaise and fatigue may represent early symptoms before progression of the infection is evident. CNS symptoms are related to 1) occlusion of cerebral arteries by septic emboli; 2) expansion, leakage, or rupture of mycotic aneurysms; and 3) direct infection of meninges or brain abscess. Neuropsychiatric deficits resulting from septic emboli will reflect which cerebral vessels have been affected. The most common psychiatric symptoms are those of diffuse encephalopathy, which may occur at any stage of infection. Their onset may be insidious to acute, paralleling the course of the endocarditis (chronic, subacute, acute).

Diagnosis is based on clinical history and physical examination, particularly looking for new or changing heart murmurs, signs of microembolism (splinter hemorrhages, retinal hemorrhages, microscopic hematuria), and positive blood cultures in a patient with fever. Cardiac echocardiography is important for evaluation of valvular abnormalities.

Rocky Mountain Spotted Fever

The etiological agent for Rocky Mountain spotted fever (RMSF) is *Rickettsia rickettsii.* RMSF is a tickborne disease with a seasonal distribution paralleling human contact with ticks, peaking May through September. Its name is misleading because half of the U.S. cases are in the South Atlantic region, and rickettsial spotted fevers occur worldwide. RMSF typically (although not invariably) includes fever and a rash characterized by erythematous macules that later progress to maculopapular lesions with central petechiae. Initially appearing as a nonspecific severe febrile illness, the diagnosis is seldom suspected until the rash appears. Only half of RMSF patients report exposure to ticks. *R. rickettsii* causes a diffuse vasculitis in many organs. CNS involvement occurs in 25% of cases and includes lethargy, confusion, and occasionally fulminant delirium. Subtle changes such as irritability, personality changes, and apathy may occur before the rash, particularly in children. Abnormalities on brain imaging may show focal lesions, but 80% of RMSF patients with normal scans have symptoms of encephalopathy as well (Bonawitz et al. 1997). Because mortality is high in untreated patients, a provisional clinical diagnosis (e.g., fever, rash in the appropriate season, and geographic setting) is sufficient to initiate definitive antimicrobial therapy.

Typhus Fevers

Typhus fevers are caused by two species of *Rickettsia. R. prowazekii* is the cause of mouseborne and squirrelborne typhus. *R. typhi* is the cause of fleaborne typhus. Mouseborne typhus usually occurs in epidemics related to war or famine when communal hygiene deteriorates. Fleaborne typhus is associated with fleas found on rodents. The annual disease frequency in the United States was 2,000–5,000 cases in the 1940s. It is now fewer than 100, with most in Texas. This dramatic change is a result of rat control programs. Clinical manifestations, diagnosis, and treatment of typhus are similar to those of RMSF. The psychiatric manifestations are confusion, lethargy, and particularly headache in a febrile illness with rash. The delirium of typhus and typhoid has been classically described as having a peculiar preoccupied nature, with patients picking at the bedclothes and imaginary objects (Verghese 1985). In fact, the word *typhus* in Greek means "cloud" or "mist," a term Hippocrates used to describe clouded mental status in patients with unremitting fevers.

Typhoid Fever

Typhoid fever is an enteric fever caused by salmonellae. The incidence of typhoid fever has steadily declined in the United States over the last century primarily because of improved sanitation. Typhoid fever is still endemic in many places in the world. Most of the cases in the United States are acquired outside the country, most often in Mexico and India.

Abdominal pain, headache, and fever are the classic presentation. However, when typhoid fever is endemic or not treated promptly, psychiatric symptoms may appear. *Salmonella typhi* enters a bacteremic phase, and the typhoid bacilli can localize in the CNS. The high fever and electrolyte imbalances also may cause encephalopathy, with delirium reported in up to 75% of the cases in some parts of the world (Aghanwa and Morakinyo 2001) and very infrequently (2%) in others (Parry et al. 2002). Mental symptoms such as indifference, listlessness, and dullness are common at presentation. Published cases have described persistent psychiatric symptoms, including irritability, personality change, and psychosis (Parry et al. 2002), but most survivors completely recover following treatment.

Tetanus

Tetanus is uncommon in the United States but remains internationally significant. *Clostridium tetani* produces a potent neurotoxin called *tetanospasmin,* which is the cause of tetanus. The greatest risk factor for tetanus remains lack of up-to-date immunization. Infections generally occur because an open wound comes into contact with soil contaminated with spores from *C. tetani.* After initial inoculation, tetanospasmin is disseminated via blood, lymph, and nerves and produces symptoms by binding to receptors at the neuromuscular junction.

The classic symptom is muscle stiffness, particularly in the muscles of mastication, thus the descriptive term *lockjaw.* If the muscle stiffness extends across the entire face, risus sardonicus occurs, an expression of continuous grimace. Also, stiffness may progress to the entire body if left untreated.

Tetanospasmin may enter the CNS, causing encephalopathic symptoms. Diagnosis is based on the clinical manifestations and a history of likely exposure. On initial presentation, patients with tetanus have been given misdiagnoses of an anxiety disorder or a conversion disorder (Treadway and Prange 1967), although more commonly, a conversion disorder is mistakenly thought to be possible tetanus (Barnes and Ware 1993). If the patient had received neuroleptics or antiemetics, one could easily mistake the symptoms as drug-induced acute dystonia.

Brucellosis

Brucellosis is a worldwide zoonosis caused by species of *Brucella,* gram-negative intracellular coccobacilli. They infect many animals, but most human cases are acquired from consumption of unpasteurized dairy products from sheep or goats. It has become rare in developed countries (about 100 cases per year in the United States) but is likely underdiagnosed because of the nonspecificity of symptoms. Brucellosis can occur at any age, with insidious or abrupt onset, affecting any organ system, and hence is notorious for mimicking other diseases. Signs of acute brucellosis include fever, diaphoresis, headache, and myalgia. Chronic brucellosis is not always preceded by acute symptoms. Its manifestations include fatigue, depression, subtle cognitive dysfunction, and multiple chronic pains (Eren et al. 2006), so it is not surprising that patients' symptoms are frequently misdiagnosed as primary psychiatric illness (Sacks and Van Rensbueg 1976). Protean complications in many different organs have been reported. CNS involvement occurs in 5%–18% of cases and may present as meningitis, psychosis, or cranial nerve dysfunction (Bodur et al. 2003; Yetkin et al. 2006). Diagnosis is confirmed by isolation of the organism or serological testing.

Syphilis

Syphilis is a chronic systemic disease caused by the spirochetal bacterium *Treponema pallidum.* Although *T. pallidum* was not identified until 1905, syphilis was described in the medical literature before the sixteenth century. A hundred years ago, syphilis was the leading diagnosis in psychiatric inpatients; the incidence declined as the antibiotic era began. The rates of syphilis have been increasing over the past decade, in part related to the global pandemic of HIV infection.

The clinical manifestations are varied and mimic those of other diseases. Syphilis was the original "great imitator." In adults, syphilis passes through several stages. *Primary syphilis* develops first as a small papule at the site of inoculation that develops into an ulcer called a chancre. If left untreated, the chancre will disappear, but about 6–24 weeks after the initial infection, *secondary syphilis* occurs with a variety of symptoms. During this stage, multiple organ systems, including the CNS, may become involved. Most symptoms are constitutional (malaise, fatigue, anorexia, and weight loss). Skin, gastrointestinal tract, lymphatics, bones, kidneys, and eyes all may be affected. Most syphilitic meningitis occurs within the first year of infection. Symptoms of headache, stiff neck, nausea, and vomiting prevail, and focal neurological findings may be present. Often, signs and symptoms of secondary syphilis disappear, and the infection becomes latent.

Tertiary syphilis refers to infection years to decades after initial infection. It has been divided into three types: late benign syphilis (gummatous), cardiovascular syphilis, and neurosyphilis. Gummatous and cardiovascular forms were very prevalent before antibiotics; neurosyphilis is now the predominant form of tertiary syphilis (Gliatto and Caroff 2001).

Neurosyphilis is divided into asymptomatic, meningeal, meningovascular, and parenchymatous forms. Meningeal syphilis may occur early in the course (as noted earlier in this subsection) or late. Meningovascular syphilis typically occurs 4–7 years after infection. Presenting symptoms of neurosyphilis include changes in memory and personality, dizziness, and other encephalopathic symptoms that can mimic atherosclerotic disease (e.g., transient ischemic attack, multi-infarct dementia). Parenchymatous neurosyphilis syndromes are tabes dorsalis and general paresis. Tabes dorsalis occurs 20–25 years after infection and results from demyelination of the posterior columns and dorsal roots. Paresthesias, Argyll Robertson pupils (pupils that accommodate but do not react to light), impotence, incontinence, and truncal ataxia may develop. General paresis is an insidious dementia that can include seizures and personality deterioration. This form of syphilis presents 15–20 years after infection and—if untreated—may be fatal.

Diagnosis relies on serological testing. However, in primary and secondary syphilis, dark-field microscopy of material from chancres, condylomata, and mucous patches usually identifies many organisms.

Except in populations in which syphilis is common, it is not cost-effective to screen all new psychiatric patients for syphilis (Roberts et al. 1992); screening should focus on patients with unexplained cognitive dysfunction or other neurological symptoms accompanying the psychopathology. The most frequently used tests and their sensitivities are shown in Table 27–2.

Serological testing is based on two types of antibody response to the syphilitic infection: nontreponemal antibodies and antitreponemal antibodies. The Venereal Disease Research Laboratory (VDRL) and the rapid plasma reagin (RPR) are the most commonly used tests that detect nontreponemal (nonspecific) antibodies. The reactivity of these tests depends on the stage of the disease. In secondary syphilis and early latent syphilis, the nontreponemal tests show reactivity 95%–100% of the time. However, the reactivity in primary syphilis and tertiary syphilis is 76% and 70%, respectively. The fluorescent treponemal antibody absorption (FTA-ABS) test is more sensitive and more specific. This test is used to confirm the diagnosis when syphilis is suspected and a nontreponemal test was nonreactive and to confirm a positive nontreponemal test result. The FTA-ABS test is not used as a screening test because its false-positive rate is as high as 1%. Another treponemal test is the microhemagglutination assay of *T. pallidum* (MHA-TP). This assay is used as a confirmatory test, typically after a positive RPR test result (Hicks 2004).

False-positive nontreponemal tests (i.e., positive VDRL or RPR and negative FTA-ABS and no clinical evidence of disease) are divided into acute (those that revert to normal in less than 6 months) and chronic (those that persist for longer than 6 months). Acute false-positive results occur after some immunizations, during acute infections, and during pregnancy. Chronic false-positive results occur in individuals with autoimmune disease (e.g., lupus), in narcotic-addicted persons, in persons with leprosy, and in the elderly.

Intravenous penicillin G is the recommended treatment for all forms of neurosyphilis (Jay 2006). If a definitive diagnosis cannot be made, it is prudent to treat presumptively. In some patients with dementia due to neurosyphilis, the infection appears to have "burned out," and they show no clinical response to penicillin G. Multiple case reports but no controlled trials have addressed treatment of psychiatric symptoms associated with neurosyphilis. A recent review (Sanchez and Zisselman 2007) and case reports (Taycan et al. 2006; Turan et al. 2007) recommended use of a typical or an atypical antipsychotic to treat psychosis in patients with neurosyphilis. An anticonvulsant such as divalproex sodium also was recommended for agitation and mood stabilization.

Lyme Disease

Lyme disease is caused by the spirochete *Borrelia burgdorferi*, which is transmitted by deer ticks. The risk of contracting Lyme disease from a single tick bite is 3% (Nadelman et al. 2001). Lyme disease occurs worldwide; it is the most common tickborne disease in the United States, with four times as many cases as reported in Europe. Disease onset is marked by erythema migrans, a characteristic (more than 90% of cases) large spreading rash with central clearing. Acute disseminated disease includes fatigue, arthralgia, headache, fever, and stiff neck. If untreated, Lyme disease may disseminate to other organs and produce subacute or chronic disease. Neurological symptoms occur in about 15% and may include cranial neuropathies (most often, the facial nerve), meningitis, or painful radiculopathy. If still untreated, patients may develop chronic neuroborreliosis, including a mild sensory radiculopathy, cognitive dysfunction, or depression. Typical symptoms of chronic Lyme encephalopathy include difficulty with concentration and memory, fatigue, daytime hypersomnolence, irritability, and depression. Very rarely, Lyme disease has included chronic encephalomyelitis. Although these chronic syn-

TABLE 27–2. Sensitivity (%) of diagnostic tests of serum[a] in different stages of syphilis

	Screening[b]		Confirmatory[c]	
Stage of disease	**RPR or VDRL**	**FTA-ABS**	**TPI**	**MHA-TP**
Primary	75	85	40	80
Secondary and early latent	95–100	100	98	100
Late latent and tertiary	70	99	95	98

Note. FTA-ABS=fluorescent treponemal antibody absorption; MHA-TP=microhemagglutination assay of *Treponema pallidum;* RPR=rapid plasma reagin; TPI=*Treponema pallidum* immunofluorescence assay; VDRL=Venereal Disease Research Laboratory.
[a]Sensitivity and specificity cannot be determined on cerebrospinal fluid because no gold standard exists.
[b]Detects nontreponemal antibodies.
[c]Detects treponemal antibodies. Typically, a laboratory performs one of these tests when a screening test result is positive.

dromes are not distinctive, they are almost always preceded by the classic early symptoms of Lyme disease, such as erythema migrans, arthritis, cranial neuropathy, or radiculopathy (Feder et al. 2007).

The clear relation between another spirochetal disease, syphilis, and psychopathology makes the possibility that *B. burgdorferi* can cause psychiatric syndromes an area of interest and controversy. Many different psychiatric symptoms have been reported to be associated with Lyme disease, including depression, mania, delirium, dementia, psychosis, obsessions or compulsions, panic attacks, catatonia, and personality change (Tager and Fallon 2001). However, association does not allow one to infer causation by Lyme. Evaluation of patients with Lyme disease at 10- to 20-year follow-up showed no significant differences in symptoms or neuropsychological testing compared with control subjects without Lyme disease. Although symptoms such as pain, fatigue, and difficulty with daily activities are common in patients who received treatment for Lyme disease years earlier, the frequencies of such symptoms are similar in control subjects without Lyme disease (Seltzer et al. 2000). Studies of whether children have cognitive sequelae after treated Lyme disease have had mixed results (McAuliffe et al. 2008; Vázquez et al. 2003).

The differential diagnosis of neuroborreliosis in a patient presenting with fatigue, depression, and/or impaired cognition includes fibromyalgia, chronic fatigue syndrome, other infections (e.g., babesiosis or ehrlichiosis), somatoform disorders, depression, autoimmune diseases, and multiple sclerosis (Tager and Fallon 2001).

Unfortunately, Lyme disease has been grossly overdiagnosed in patients with nonspecific cognitive, affective, or other psychiatric symptoms. As noted earlier in this section, numerous reports in the literature attribute a wide variety of psychiatric symptoms to neuroborreliosis on the basis of positive serological testing. As explained later in this section, this is inappropriate. Adverse consequences of overdiagnosis include reinforcement of somatization and creation of invalidism. Overdiagnosis leads to overtreatment. The diagnosis of an infection that can be treated with antibiotics can be very appealing to patients for whom depression or somatoform disorder is an unacceptable diagnosis, but this leads to inappropriate diagnostic procedures and inappropriate extended prescription of antibiotics for a putative chronic CNS infection. Chronic antibiotic prescription is not benign and may lead to secondary infections, antibiotic resistance, and drug toxicity (Feder et al. 2007). Even in patients with classic symptomatic Lyme disease confirmed by serological testing, persisting symptoms are usually explained by some illness other than chronic borreliosis if these patients have received adequate antibiotic therapy (Kalish et al. 2001; Seltzer et al. 2000).

Diagnosis is based on the characteristic clinical features. Serological testing (enzyme-linked immunosorbent assay followed by Western blot) can support the diagnosis but should never be the primary basis. False-negative and false-positive results are common with serological testing. Even a true-positive test result simply indicates that the patient has had Lyme disease at some point in life, but no conclusion about current disease activity or extent of infection can be drawn on that basis alone. In chronic neuroborreliosis, increased cerebrospinal fluid (CSF) protein and antibody to the organism occur in more than 50% of the patients. Electroencephalogram (EEG) findings are typically normal, whereas magnetic resonance imaging (MRI) shows nonspecific white matter lesions in about 25%. Neuropsychological assessment is useful in measuring cognitive dysfunction, but the findings are not specific (Ravdin et al. 1996).

Treatment is straightforward for acute Lyme disease (see Wormser et al. 2006). Neither serological testing nor antibiotic treatment is cost-effective in patients who have a low probability of having the disease (e.g., nonspecific symptoms, low incidence region) (Nichol et al. 1998). Multiple controlled trials have found no benefit of extended intravenous or oral antibiotics in patients with well-documented, previously treated Lyme disease who had persistent pain, neurocognitive symptoms, dysesthesias, or fatigue (Kaplan et al. 2003; Klempner et al. 2001; Krupp et al. 2003; Oksi et al. 2007). The only exception is a recent, very small placebo-controlled trial (n=37) of 10 weeks of intravenous ceftriaxone in patients with at least 3 weeks of prior intravenous antibiotics, which showed moderate generalized cognitive improvement at week 12, but it was not sustained to week 24 (Fallon et al. 2008). The consensus of experts is that chronic antibiotic therapy is not indicated for persistent neuropsychiatric symptoms in patients who received adequate treatment for Lyme disease (Feder et al. 2007).

Leptospirosis

Leptospirosis is another protean spirochetal disease. It was previously thought of as a rural tropical disease, but it occurs globally in rural and urban areas. The organism is spread through the urine of many species of mammals. Most leptospirosis infections resemble influenza and are relatively benign. The more severe form of leptospirosis is a multiorgan disease affecting liver, kidneys, lung, and brain (meningoencephalitis, aseptic meningitis). Confusion and delirium are common, and leptospirosis has presented with mania and psychosis (Semiz et al. 2005).

Bacterial Meningitis

Bacterial meningitis is an acute illness associated with significant morbidity and mortality. Psychiatric symptoms play an important role in its presentation. Irrespective of the organism, most cases of bacterial meningitis result from hematogenous spread of bacteria from a primary site to the subarachnoid space. Once the organism crosses the blood-brain barrier at the choroid plexus and enters the subarachnoid space, host defenses become activated. Psychiatric symptoms may result by several mechanisms, including toxic effects of the organism, mediators of inflammation, cerebral edema, and hypoxia.

The classic sign of meningeal inflammation is nuchal rigidity. Headache, nausea, vomiting, confusion, lethargy, and apathy also may occur. Psychiatric symptoms are the result of encephalopathy. As in other infections, encephalopathy may initially present as subtle changes in personality, mood, motivation, or mentation. Symptom severity generally correlates with the magnitude of the host's immune response. When the patient cannot mount a full inflammatory response, the classic symptoms may not occur. In infants, the elderly, or immunocompromised patients, the only clinical signs may be irritability or minor changes in mentation or personality. Even after good recovery from bacterial meningitis, some patients may have subtle cognitive impairment (van de Beek et al. 2002).

Once clinically suspected, the diagnosis is usually confirmed by examination of the CSF, which typically shows pleocytosis, low glucose, high protein, and evidence of the offending organism on appropriate staining. Although neuroimaging is routinely performed to rule out other CNS processes, it rarely establishes the diagnosis of bacterial meningitis.

Cat-Scratch Disease

Cat-scratch disease (CSD), which is caused by *Bartonella henselae,* usually presents as self-limiting lymphadenopathy in young people following a cat scratch or bite. Encephalopathy is one of the common complications, with almost all cases reported in children. Patients with CSD encephalopathy present with combative behavior, lethargy, and seizures, and significant fever may be absent. Diagnosis is made by serology and/or biopsy of skin or lymph node.

Bacterial Brain Abscess

The portals of entry for organisms causing brain abscesses are similar to those in bacterial meningitis. In fact, brain abscesses frequently occur as a complication of bacterial meningitis, although they also are a frequent complication of infective endocarditis. The classic triad of headache, fever, and focal neurological deficits has been described for the diagnosis of brain abscess, but these symptoms occur in fewer than half of the patients who have a brain abscess. Seizures are common. Various psychiatric symptoms may occur, depending on the size and location of the abscess, the degree of irritation of the organism, and the extent of the inflammatory response.

Mortality rates have markedly declined as a result of improved neuroimaging and antimicrobials, but morbidity remains high. Neuroimaging can show focal abscesses in the CNS with very good sensitivity. Effective treatment includes empirical antibiotics that cross the blood-brain barrier, with primary excision or aspiration of the abscess usually required. After successful treatment of the infection, psychiatric symptoms may persist.

Tuberculous Meningitis

Tuberculosis (TB) incidence is at an all-time low in the United States but remains a major world health problem, endemic in many developing countries. Extensively drug-resistant TB has been reported in 49 countries worldwide. Where AIDS is prevalent, the epidemiology of TB has markedly changed. TB now represents the most common serious HIV-related complication worldwide. In countries where TB is not endemic, the diagnosis of tuberculous meningitis is often not considered because the clinical manifestations are often nonspecific. Early diagnosis of tuberculous meningitis is essential because delay in treatment is associated with high morbidity and mortality. Tuberculous meningitis is caused by bacilli discharged from small tuberculous lesions adjacent to the meninges. These small tuberculous lesions arise early via hematogenous spread following a primary pulmonary infection or as a consequence of reactivation.

Early symptoms of tuberculous meningitis are nonspecific and include low-grade fever, generalized malaise, fatigue, and mild headache. Over the course of a week, progression to high-grade fever, severe nuchal rigidity, confusion, and delirium occurs. Persons with HIV, the elderly, substance abusers, and others with impaired immunity are more likely to present without nuchal rigidity and headache. In such patients, the symptoms will tend to be most nonspecific, with a higher risk of missing the correct diagnosis while attributing the symptoms to more common diagnoses such as alcohol withdrawal.

Confirming the diagnosis can be difficult. The organisms are difficult to detect in the CSF, so diligent search is needed to identify them when present. Early in the course when symptoms are mild, CSF glucose may be unchanged and protein only marginally elevated. As the disease progresses, glucose declines drastically, and protein becomes markedly elevated, with white blood cell counts typically between 50 and 200 cells/mm^3 (predominantly lymphocytes). Later complications include cerebral vasculitis and cranial nerve involvement. Diffuse meningeal involvement by TB may be seen on MRI.

Strong suspicion of tuberculous meningitis calls for early multidrug treatment. In many parts of the world today, including the United States, multidrug-resistant TB is present, requiring different drug combinations.

Whipple's Disease

Whipple's disease is a rare infection, caused by the bacterium *Tropheryma whipplei.* Most patients experience arthralgia, diarrhea, and weight loss. Neurological involvement has been reported in 6%–63% of patients, may occur without intestinal involvement, and can mimic almost any neurological syndrome. Psychiatric symptoms (e.g., depression, personality change) are present in about half of the patients with neurological involvement. Cognitive deficits are even more common and may extend to dementia. Whipple's disease is treated with antibiotics, but patients with neurological involvement have a poor prognosis (Fenollar et al. 2007).

Viral Infections

The overwhelming majority of viral infections are asymptomatic or mild and do not receive medical attention. Many viruses are difficult to detect, most infections are difficult to treat, and none are cured by treatment. Viruses can produce psychiatric symptoms by primary CNS involvement, from secondary effects of immune activation, or indirectly from systemic effects. One serious sequela of several viral infections is acute disseminated encephalomyelitis; patients with this condition can present with encephalopathy, acute psychosis, seizures, and other CNS dysfunction. Active demyelination is widespread, and the disease may be difficult to distinguish from multiple sclerosis. Residual cognitive dysfunction may occur (Jacobs et al. 2004). Despite viral syndromes' ubiquity and frequent nonspecificity, it is important for psychiatrists to know particular viral syndromes.

Epstein-Barr Virus

Epstein-Barr virus (EBV), one of the herpesviruses, commonly causes infectious mononucleosis ("mono") in children and young adults. The prodromal stage of infectious mononucleosis is characterized by headache, fatigue, and malaise, with progression to fever, sore throat, and lymphadenopathy. Diagnosis is based on the combination of typical clinical symptoms and a positive heterophil antibody test (Monospot) result. Because the Monospot test is an antibody measure, it may have false-negative results in immunosuppressed patients. Most cases completely resolve, although some may take several months. Fatigue commonly persists for a few months, but this can occur with other viral infections as well (Hickie et al. 2006). In the rare, more severe form of infectious mononucleosis, anemia, leukopenia, eosinophilia, thrombocytopenia, pneumonitis, hepatosplenomegaly, uveitis, and an abnormal pattern of serum globulins may occur. EBV also can cause acute encephalitis and other neurological syndromes.

Because EBV may persist lifelong in a latent state following acute infection, periodic reactivation may occur. Patients with reactivated EBV infection typically report overwhelming fatigue, malaise, depression, low-grade fever, lymphadenopathy, and other nonspecific symptoms, essentially the picture of the chronic fatigue syndrome. However, only a small fraction of chronic fatigue symptoms are attributable to EBV infection. In the past, patients with chronic fatigue and depression (and sometimes their physicians) pursued an explanation in chronic EBV infection, erroneously confirming this after a positive Monospot test result. It was erroneous because the test result remains positive long after complete resolution of uncomplicated infectious mononucleosis in youths, and most adults have had the infection. (See analogous discussion in "Lyme Disease" earlier in this chapter.)

Cytomegalovirus

Like EBV, cytomegalovirus (CMV) is a herpesvirus with the ability to develop a lifelong latency in the host with possible reactivation. Seroprevalence in adults has been reported to be between 40% and 100%. Most CMV infections are subclinical and occur across a broader age group than does EBV. In adults, CMV can produce a syndrome identical to infectious mononucleosis, except that heterophil antibody testing is negative in CMV, and a sore throat is usually absent. CMV also may cause hepatitis, retinitis, colonitis, and pneumonitis. CMV can cause encephalitis in immunocompromised patients (especially posttransplant and AIDS) and rarely in immunocompetent patients. Following patient recovery, CMV has been implicated as a cause of depression or dementia. Seropositive transplant recipients are at risk for reactivation of infection, and seronegative transplant recipients are at risk for a more serious primary CMV infection if the graft is seropositive. Prophylactic therapy has reduced posttransplant CMV infections but also delayed their appearance. Without prophylaxis, the symptoms of CMV reactivation usually occur between the first and fourth month after transplantation.

Viral Meningoencephalitis

Most viruses that cause encephalitis cause meningitis as well. Enteroviruses, mumps, and lymphocytic choriomeningitis primarily affect the meninges, with enteroviruses responsible for most identifiable cases. Patients with viral meningitis (often referred to as aseptic meningitis) present with headache, fever, nuchal rigidity, malaise, drowsiness, nausea, and photophobia. Typically, the CSF shows pleocytosis, elevated protein, and no evidence of an organism. Treatment for aseptic meningitis is generally supportive.

In viral encephalitis, psychiatric symptoms are very common in the acute phase and frequent after recovery (Arciniegas and Anderson 2004; Caroff et al. 2001). Occasionally, patients with viral encephalitis may initially present with psychopathology without neurological symptoms. Caroff et al. (2001) reviewed 108 published cases of psychiatric presentation, classified as psychosis (35%), catatonia (33%), psychotic depression (16%), or mania (11%). Patients in such cases often receive misdiagnosis and inappropriate treatment, and Caroff et al. (2001) noted that patients with viral encephalitis are more vulnerable to adverse effects of neuroleptics, including extrapyramidal side effects, catatonia, and neuroleptic malignant syndrome.

For those who survive viral encephalitis, outcomes vary from complete recovery to serious neuropsychiatric sequelae. Psychiatric sequelae, especially mood disorders, are common following recovery from acute viral encephalitis and constitute a major cause of disability. Depression, hypomania, irritability, and disinhibition of anger, aggression, or sexuality have been frequently noted months after recovery, and psychosis occurs rarely. Depressive symptoms may respond to treatment with antidepressants or stimulants (Neel 2000). Hypomania, irritability, and disinhibition have benefited from neuroleptics, mood stabilizers including lithium, and electroconvulsive therapy (Ferrando et al. 2010; Monnet 2003). Specific viruses are discussed below.

Arboviruses

Arboviruses (short for arthropod-borne viruses) are the most common cause of viral encephalitis worldwide. Of the arbovirus diseases, Japanese encephalitis is the most common worldwide and annually causes 10,000 deaths in Asia. In the United States, the major types are St. Louis encephalitis, eastern equine encephalomyelitis, western equine encephalomyelitis, California encephalitis, and West Nile virus. Most arboviruses are mosquito-borne. Arboviral encephalitis typically appears in the summer or fall in children (Japanese encephalitis) or young adults (West Nile virus and St. Louis encephalitis), with abrupt onset of fever, headache, nausea, photophobia, and vomiting, and may be fatal. Reduced level of consciousness, flaccid paralysis resembling poliomyelitis, parkinsonism, and seizures are common (Solomon 2004). Persistent depression is very common after West Nile infection (Murray et al. 2007) Although no specific treatment is available for arboviral encephalitis, rapid diagnosis is important for public health measures, mosquito control, and, ideally, vaccines.

Dengue. Dengue, another disease caused by an arbovirus, is transmitted by mosquitoes, endemic in 100 countries, and encountered in temperate developed countries mainly in travelers and new immigrants (Castleberry and Mahon 2003). The virus causes three syndromes: the relatively more benign dengue fever, which is a painful influenza-like illness, and the serious forms, hemorrhagic dengue and dengue shock syndrome, which are rare in travelers. Neuropsychiatric symptoms were noted in 14% of the tourists who returned to France with dengue (Badiaga et al. 2003). CNS involvement has been reported in 3%–21% of cases of dengue, and in the more serious endemic dengue infections, encephalitis is common, with confusion, delirium, and seizures (Domingues et al. 2008; Wasay et al. 2008).

Herpes Simplex Virus

Herpes encephalitis is the most common cause of sporadic fatal encephalitis worldwide, with more than 90% caused by herpes simplex type 1 virus. Symptoms may include hypomania, personality change, dysphasia, seizures, autonomic dysfunction, ataxia, delirium, psychosis, and focal neurological symptoms. Herpes simplex virus (HSV) encephalitis differs from arboviral encephalitis by causing more unilateral and focal findings, with a predilection for temporoparietal areas of the brain. HSV encephalitis is more likely to cause focal seizures, olfactory hallucinations, and personality change. HSV is the most common identified cause of viral encephalitis simulating a primary psychiatric disorder (Arciniegas and Anderson 2004; Caroff et al. 2001). One possible sequela of HSV encephalitis is the Klüver-Bucy syndrome, which includes oral touching compulsions, hypersexuality, amnesia, placidity, agnosia, and hyperphagia. CSF typically shows pleocytosis, red blood cells (because of the hemorrhagic nature of HSV encephalitis), and elevated protein. Glucose is usually normal. EEG is a sensitive (but not specific) diagnostic test, showing periodic temporal spikes and slow waves as opposed to more diffuse changes usually seen in other forms of viral encephalitis. MRI may show diffuse inflammation, particularly in the temporoparietal areas. The gold standard for diagnosis had been brain biopsy, but detection of HSV DNA by polymerase chain reaction is now the standard. Diagnosis based on symptoms and signs alone misses 50% of the cases.

Rapid diagnosis is essential because only early treatment improves outcome. HSV encephalitis is treated with intravenous acyclovir, which itself can cause neuropsychiatric adverse effects (see Table 27-3 later in this chapter). No well-defined treatments are available for the associated cognitive and neuropsychiatric symptoms, but case reports describe success with anticonvulsants such as carbamazepine (especially in patients with comorbid seizures), atypical antipsychotics, selective serotonin reuptake inhibitors, stimulants, clonidine, and cholinesterase inhibitors (Ferrando et al. 2010).

Varicella/Herpes Zoster

The varicella/herpes zoster virus causes chickenpox in children and herpes zoster in adults. Most cases of encephalopathy in children with varicella infection have been due to Reye's syndrome, although the virus itself can cause encephalitis. Zoster-associated encephalitis typically presents in adults with delirium within days after the appearance of the rash. The most common neurological sequela of herpes zoster is postherpetic neuralgia (see Chapter 36, "Pain"). Depression and anxiety are common in postherpetic neuralgia (Volpi et al. 2008) and may influence the choice of treatment for the neuropathic pain (e.g., tricyclic or serotonin-norepinephrine reuptake inhibitor antidepressant vs. anticonvulsant). Weeks or months after recovery from herpes zoster, encephalitis or arteritis may appear (mostly in immunosuppressed patients). The arteritis may affect large vessels, producing strokelike symptoms, or small vessels, producing headache, altered mental status, fever, seizures, and focal deficits (Gilden et al. 2000).

Measles

Measles can cause postinfectious encephalomyelitis, subacute measles encephalitis, and subacute sclerosing panencephalitis (SSPE). SSPE typically occurs 7–10 years after measles infection, presenting with cognitive dysfunction, behavior change, headache, and myoclonic jerks (Garg 2008). Most cases are in children or adolescents, but cases beginning in middle age have been reported.

Tickborne Encephalitis

Tickborne encephalitis (TBE) is an important human infection of the CNS throughout Europe and parts of Asia, caused by a virus (TBEV) mainly transmitted by tick bites and rarely by unpasteurized milk (Kaiser 2008). TBE presents as meningitis or meningoencephalitis. Neurological and psychiatric sequelae, including motor, affective, cognitive, and personality changes, are common in adults. No specific treatment for TBE is known, but it can be prevented by active immunization.

Postencephalitis Syndromes

Following recovery from acute viral encephalitis, psychiatric sequelae are common and constitute a major cause of disability, especially mood disorders. Depression, amnestic disorders, hypomania, irritability, and disinhibition of anger, aggression, or sexuality have been frequently noted months after recovery, and psychosis occurs rarely. Depressive symptoms may respond to treatment with antidepressants or stimulants. Hypomania, irritability, and disinhibition have benefited from mood stabilizers and antipsychotics, and behavior modification also may be helpful for aggressive and sexual behaviors.

The global pandemic encephalitis in 1917–1929 known as *encephalitis lethargica* (von Economo's disease) had an acute encephalitic phase during which lethargy, psychosis, and catatonia were common. This period was followed by a chronic postencephalitic syndrome, including parkinsonism, mania, depression, and apathy in adults and conduct disorder, emotional lability, and tics in children, with relatively little cognitive impairment (Cummings et al. 2001; Vilensky et al. 2007). Sporadic similar cases continue to be reported (Dale et al. 2007; Raghav et al. 2007). Whether encephalitis lethargica was a postinfluenzal phenomenon remains controversial (Mortimer 2009).

Viral Hepatitis

Some viruses—including hepatitis A, B, and C; EBV; and CMV—cause acute or chronic hepatitis (see also Chapter 20, "Gastrointestinal Disorders"). Hepatitis C infection is very common in the chronically mentally ill (Himelhoch et al. 2009). Fatigue, malaise, and anorexia are usually prominent in viral hepatitis and may lead to a misdiagnosis of depression. However, fatigue in chronic hepatitis is more closely correlated with depression and other psychological factors than is severity of hepatitis (McDonald et al. 2002). Depression is frequently comorbid, especially in the chronic forms of hepatitis B (Kunkel et al. 2000) and hepatitis C infection (Nelligan et al. 2008), but whether the etiology of depression in hepatitis C infection is really viral has been questioned (Wessely and Pariante 2002). Subtle cognitive dysfunction not attributable to depression, substance abuse, or hepatic encephalopathy has been documented in hepatitis C infection, and the virus has been identified in brain, suggesting that cerebral infection also may occur (Weissenborn et al. 2009).

Complicating the diagnostic picture further, treatment with interferon causes depression itself in 20%–40% of patients and depressive symptoms in as many as two-thirds receiving long-term interferon treatment (Neri et al. 2006). Depression has been the most common adverse effect leading to cessation of interferon treatment. Depression reduces adherence to antiviral therapy (Martín-Santos et al. 2008) and is associated with a poorer antiviral response (Fontana et al. 2008). Depression associated with hepatitis or interferon is amenable to treatment with antidepressants (Kraus et al. 2008), allowing continuation of interferon in most patients. Therefore, depression should not be considered a contraindication to interferon therapy. Dosing should be adjusted downward if the patient has impaired liver function.

Rabies

Rabies is a viral infection of mammals transmitted by bite. In the United States, nondomesticated animals (i.e., bats, raccoons) account for most cases of rabies because domesticated animals are vaccinated. Worldwide, human mortality from endemic canine rabies is estimated to be about 55,000 deaths annually, with more than 31,000 deaths in Asia alone, mostly children (Dodet et al. 2008). Transmission to humans is rare in developed countries, but rabies has been misdiagnosed as an anxiety disorder (Centers for Disease Control 1991) or alcohol withdrawal (Centers for Disease Control and Prevention 1998).

The usual incubation period is 20–60 days but can vary from several days to years. Initial symptoms are nonspecific and include generalized anxiety, fever, depression, hyperesthesia, and dysesthesia, especially at the site of inoculation. In one U.S. case, "mild personality changes" preceded more suggestive symptoms such as unsteady gait and slurred speech by more than a week (Centers for Disease Control and Prevention 2003). The rabies virus has a proclivity for attacking the limbic system; thus, delusions may result. The initial phase is followed by an excitatory phase, when the classic symptom of hydrophobia may occur. Hydrophobia is an aversion to swallowing liquids (not a phobia of water) secondary to the spasmodic contractions of the muscles of swallowing and respiration, resulting in pain and aspiration. The final phase is a progressive, general flaccid paralysis that progresses relentlessly to death. Both rabies and the rabies vaccine may cause delirium (Leung et al. 2003).

No effective treatment exists for rabies once symptoms are evident. After a bite by an infected animal, the rabies vaccine should be given as soon as possible because outcome is related to the proximity in time to the bite.

Prion Diseases

Prions are proteinaceous agents that cause spongiform changes in the brain. Prion diseases are rare and universally fatal, with an incubation period of months to years—hence the term *slow viruses* (see also Chapter 32, "Neurology and Neurosurgery"). Kuru occurs only in Papua, New Guinea. It is spread by the cannibalistic consumption of dead relatives during mourning rituals. Scrapie is a spongiform encephalopathy found in sheep. Although known to have been present in Great Britain for almost three centuries, scrapie has never been shown to cause disease in humans. Bovine spongiform encephalopathy ("mad cow disease") appears to have been transmitted to cattle by the practice of feeding cattle recycled sheep by-products.

Creutzfeldt-Jakob disease (CJD) occurs sporadically (i.e., sporadic CJD [sCJD]) and sometimes familially in humans, with a mean age at onset around 60 years. It also has been transmitted by intracerebral electrodes, grafts of dura mater, corneal transplants, human growth hormone, and gonadotropin, but iatrogenic transmission is now rare. sCJD is a severe dementia accompanied by psychosis, affective lability, and dramatic myoclonus that rapidly progresses to rigid mutism and then death. A retrospective review of 126 cases of sCJD found that 26% had psychiatric symptoms at presentation and 80% within the first 100 days of illness—most commonly, sleep disturbances, psychotic symptoms, and depression (Wall et al. 2005). Young patients with sCJD present with psychiatric symptoms similar to those seen in patients with new-variant CJD (nvCJD) (see next paragraph) but progress more rapidly to severe dementia than in nvCJD (Boesenberg et al. 2005).

nvCJD was initially reported mainly in Great Britain but now has been found in many other countries and has distinct differences from CJD. nvCJD patients are considerably younger than sCJD patients, with an average age at onset of about 30, and the disease progresses less rapidly. In most cases of nvCJD, psychiatric symptoms, including depression, irritability, anxiety, and apathy, appear several months before any neurological symptoms (Spencer et al. 2002). Bovine spongiform encephalopathy and nvCJD are caused by the same prion strain, but the disease can be transmitted through the same iatrogenic routes as sCJD, years after initial exposure. Detection of the 14-3-3 protein in CSF supports the diagnosis of sCJD but is not as sensitive or specific as initially thought and is insensitive for nvCJD. The EEG usually has abnormal results in both forms of CJD, but definitive diagnosis requires brain biopsy.

Fatal familial insomnia is an even rarer prion disease in which progressive insomnia (and sometimes behavior change) (Raggi et al. 2009) appears months before any cognitive, autonomic, or motor symptoms develop. Despite its name, the disease also occurs through sporadic mutation. Patients with this disorder initially may be given misdiagnoses of mood, anxiety, or somatoform disorders.

Fungal Infections

The frequency of fungal infection has increased steadily over the last three decades, coincident with the growing number of immunocompromised patients who are surviving longer than in the past. An aging population, an increased number of malignancies, the spread of AIDS, the use of immunosuppressive and cytotoxic drugs, the use of intravenous catheters, hyperalimentation, illicit drug use, extensive surgery, and the development of burn units also have contributed to the increased frequency of fungal infection. CNS symptom development depends on the size and shape of the fungi. The smallest fungi have access to the cerebral microcirculation and infect the subarachnoid space. Large hyphae obstruct large and intermediate arteries, giving rise to extensive infarctions (e.g., aspergillosis). Fungi with pseudohyphae occlude small blood vessels, producing small infarctions and microabscesses (e.g., *Candida*). Most fungi are opportunistic (as in aspergillosis, mucormycosis, and candidiasis), whereas others are pathogenic (as in coccidioidomycosis and cryptococcosis) irrespective of the host's defenses. Most systemic fungal infections are treated with amphotericin B, which can cause neuropsychiatric side effects (see Table 27-3 later in this chapter).

Aspergillosis

Aspergillus, an opportunistic organism, infects only debilitated patients. *Aspergillus* genus is commonly found in soil. In aspergillosis, CNS involvement usually follows infection of the lungs or gastrointestinal tract. Symptoms of confusion, headache, and lethargy often accompany focal neurological signs.

Cryptococcosis

Cryptococcosis is an infection caused by *Cryptococcus* species, a pathogen distributed worldwide, found in bird excreta, the soil, and other animals. *Cryptococcus* may act as a solo pathogen, but in up to 85% of cases, it is associated with another illness, especially AIDS. The portal of entry is usually the respiratory tract from which hematogenous spread occurs, although at the time of presentation, pulmonary infection may not be evident.

Cryptococcus is the most common form of fungal meningitis. It is typically insidious in onset and slowly progressive. Headache is present in up to 75% of the cases, varying from mild and episodic to progressively incapacitating and constant. Other signs include cerebellar, cranial nerve, and motor deficits; irritability; psychosis; and lethargy, which may progress to coma. Remission and relapse are common in untreated patients. Isolation of the fungi provides definitive diagnosis. Serological testing of patients with cryptococcal meningitis identifies cryptococcal antigen in serum, CSF, or both 90% of the time. Treatment is typically a prolonged course of an antifungal agent.

Coccidioidomycosis

Coccidioidomycosis is restricted to warm, dry areas such as the southwestern United States, Mexico, and parts of South America (particularly Argentina and Paraguay). Its spores are inhaled in infected dust. Initial infection produces a mild febrile illness, often followed by pulmonary symptoms. Dissemination beyond the lung is relatively rare, and the CNS is not the most common extrapulmonary site. When it does occur, CNS infection is typically insidious in onset, 1-3 months after initial infection, with headache associated with confusion, restlessness, hallucinations, lethargy, and transient focal signs.

Histoplasmosis

Histoplasmosis is a common respiratory infection found throughout the world and is especially common in the central United States. *Histoplasma capsulatum* is inhaled with dust contaminated with chicken, bird, or bat excreta. Most infections are asymptomatic and involve the lungs or the reticuloendothelial system. The CNS is involved in 5%-10% of patients with progressive disseminated histoplasmosis. Most but not all are immunocompromised. CNS histoplasmosis may cause chronic meningitis, focal brain lesions, stroke due to infected emboli, and diffuse encephalitis (Saccente 2008).

Blastomycosis

Blastomyces dermatitidis is an uncommon mycotic infection that rarely causes CNS infections, mainly in immunocompromised patients. Blastomycosis is coendemic with histoplasmosis in the central United States. The most common CNS manifestations are stiff neck and headache, eventually progressing to confusion and lethargy.

Mucormycosis

Mucormycosis refers to any infection caused by a member of the family *Mucoraceae,* opportunistic fungi found in common bread and fruit molds. Mucormycosis is notorious for causing an acute fulminant infection in diabetic patients and patients with neutropenia. *Mucor* directly invades tissue and disseminates by attacking contiguous structures. Any diabetic patient with a purulent, febrile infection of the face or nose should be emergently evaluated for mucormycosis because it may rapidly erode into the orbit and cerebrum in a matter of hours. Early mild encephalopathy may quickly progress to severe delirium. Aggressive debridement and intravenous antifungal medication are required.

Candidiasis

Candida causes limited local infections (cutaneous, vaginal, oral) in immune-competent hosts, typically after broad-spectrum antibiotics. Disseminated candidiasis occurs only in immunocompromised patients. Psychiatric symptoms occur from the toxic effects of fungemia or from direct invasion of the CNS. Cerebral lesions generally occur late in the course of disseminated candidiasis. *Candida* may cause meningitis, microabscesses, macroabscesses, or vasculitis in the CNS. The nonspecific signs include confusion, drowsiness, lethargy, and headache. Sometimes *Candida* can be cultured from blood or CSF, but most cases of CNS candidiasis are not discovered until autopsy. Suggestive neuroimaging findings and isolation of *Candida* from a non-CNS site in an immunocompromised patient should prompt treatment with appropriate antifungal agents.

An alternative medicine belief is that occult systemic *Candida* infection is the cause of a wide array of somatic and psychological symptoms. There is no scientific support for this theory or its advocated treatments.

Parasitic Infections

Neurocysticercosis

One of the world's most common parasitic infections—neurocysticercosis—is an infection of the CNS caused by the larval form (cysticerci) of *Taenia solium,* also known as the pork tapeworm. For neurocysticercosis to occur, a human must ingest the tapeworm's eggs, from contact with infected swine or humans. Once ingested, the eggs hematogenously spread to the CNS and other sites. Cysticercosis is endemic in the developing nations. A Venezuelan study found that cysticercosis infection was much more common in psychiatric inpatients, especially those with mental retardation, than in healthy control subjects (Meza et al. 2005). In the United States, it is usually reported in immigrants from Latin America and has been reportedly found in 10% of the patients with seizures presenting to an emergency department in Los Angeles, California, and in 6% in an emergency department in New Mexico (Ong et al. 2002). However, infected food handlers may transmit it to people who have no contact with pork or other contaminated foods.

A high percentage of neurocysticercosis infections remain asymptomatic. Cerebral involvement may produce seizures, stroke, or hydrocephalus; neurocysticercosis is the leading cause of seizures in adults in endemic areas. Psychiatric symptoms are frequently reported and include depression and psychosis (Mahajan et al. 2004). Neurocysticercosis is a common cause of dementia in developing nations (Jha and Patel 2004), but the cognitive decline may be reversible (Ramirez-Bermudez et al. 2005).

Between clinical history, neuroimaging, and serology, a presumptive diagnosis of neurocysticercosis usually can be made. Definitive diagnosis of neurocysticercosis is through biopsy, but this is usually impractical. Treatment of neurocysticercosis has involved anticonvulsants, steroids, antihelminthics, and shunting for hydrocephalus. However, antihelminthic drugs in neurocysticercosis may actually aggravate neuropsychiatric symptoms, and their use in some forms of the disease is controversial.

Toxoplasmosis

Toxoplasmosis refers to the disease caused by *Toxoplasma gondii,* a parasite ubiquitously affecting all mammals, some birds, and probably some reptiles. Latent infection is common, but in immunosuppressed individuals, particularly those with AIDS, the parasite may preferentially infect the CNS, resulting in a wide range of clinical presentations. Mass lesions mimicking tumor or abscess are most common, but psychosis has been reported as a presenting symptom (Donnet et al. 1991). Effective antibiotic therapy can produce rapid remission of active infection but must be continued throughout life to prevent recurrence. Some data have supported the hypothesis that maternal or patient toxoplasmosis exposure might be a risk factor for schizophrenia (e.g., Niebuhr et al. 2008). However, one randomized trial found no benefits of trimethoprim as adjuvant treatment in Ethiopian schizophrenic patients, almost 90% of whom were positive for the *T. gondii* antibody (Shibre et al. 2009).

Trypanosomiasis

The family of protozoa *Trypanosomatidae* causes two different syndromes: African trypanosomiasis (sleeping sickness) and American trypanosomiasis (Chagas' disease). African trypanosomiasis, which occurs in several sub-Saharan African countries, is caused by a subspecies of *Trypanosoma brucei* and is transmitted to humans and animals by the bite of the tsetse fly. The illness begins with a lesion at the site of the fly bite, headache, fever, malaise, weight loss, and myalgia and is often misdiagnosed as malaria. Later, the parasite crosses the blood-brain barrier and causes encephalitis with neuropsychiatric, motor, and sensory abnormalities (Blum et al. 2006; Kennedy 2006), with usually fatal outcome. Sleeping sickness is a disturbance of the sleep-wake cycle with bouts of fatigue progressing to daytime somnolence and nighttime insomnia. Meningoencephalitis may develop with prominent somnolence—hence the name *sleeping sickness*. Africans living in other countries have received misdiagnoses of primary psychiatric disorders (Bedat-Millet et al. 2000). The drug used to treat late-stage disease is very toxic, with an often-fatal encephalopathy the most feared complication of treatment (Blum et al. 2001); for this reason, early detection—permitting less toxic treatment—is important.

American trypanosomiasis, or Chagas' disease, is caused by *Trypanosoma cruzi*, which is carried by insects ("kissing bugs" or "assassin bugs") in Latin America. More than 100,000 persons chronically infected with Chagas' disease now live in the United States. Transmission is so inefficient that years of exposure are required to acquire the infection, and most infections are quiescent. Following immunosuppression, reactivated disease may present as meningoencephalitis. In immunocompetent patients, manifestations of CNS Chagas' disease are nonspecific and minor (Wackermann et al. 2008).

On brain imaging, the lesions are indistinguishable from those of toxoplasmosis, and the organism is often not identifiable in blood. Reactivated Chagas' disease should be suspected in immunosuppressed immigrants from endemic areas of Latin America, especially in presumed cases of toxoplasmosis not responsive to chemotherapy.

Malaria

Malaria remains a major cause of morbidity in tropical nations, especially in young children and pregnant women. In other parts of the world, cases occur in immigrants and travelers to malarial areas. *Plasmodium* species are transmitted to humans by the bite of mosquitoes.

Relapsing fever typifies malaria, and with temperatures commonly in excess of 41°C (105°F), delirium is common. *Plasmodium falciparum* causes cerebral malaria, the most catastrophic complication of malaria, with a mortality rate of 15%–20%. Cerebral malaria begins with disorientation, mild stupor, agitation, and psychosis and rapidly progresses to seizures and coma (Mishra and Newton 2009). Some but not all children and adults who survive cerebral malaria have persistent cognitive deficits in attention, memory, visuospatial skills, language, and executive functions (Kihara et al. 2006). Anxiety and depression are common after recovery (Dugbartey et al. 1998), but they are more likely a result of psychological and social stress associated with severe illness (Weiss 1985). More severe neuropsychiatric signs, including psychosis in fully recovered (aparasitemic) cerebral malaria, are most likely attributable to pharmacotherapeutic agents. Antimalarial drugs commonly cause psychiatric side effects (see Table 27–3 later in this chapter). Mefloquine in chemoprophylaxis doses causes severe CNS side effects (e.g., psychosis, seizures) in 0.1% and other adverse psychiatric symptoms (e.g., nightmares, depression, irritability) in 0.02%–0.5%. Vivid dreams occur in 15%–25% (Freedman 2008). Mefloquine's psychiatric adverse effects are more common in patients who have had cerebral malaria.

Schistosomiasis

Schistosomiasis is an infection caused by blood flukes (trematodes) of the genus *Schistosoma*. Infection by the larval stage usually occurs while the individual is swimming in infected freshwater. The infection affects about 200 million people in 74 countries (*Schistosoma japonicum* in the Far East; *Schistosoma mansoni* and *Schistosoma haematobium* in Africa). Most infections are asymptomatic. CNS symptoms are uncommon, but once the worms mature and the eggs have been laid, CNS involvement may be observed with any of the clinical forms of schistosomal infection. Eggs in the CNS may induce a granulomatous reaction, but in most cases, eggs in the CNS are clinically silent. Neurological complications of cerebral schistosomiasis include delirium, seizures, dysphasia, visual field impairment, focal motor deficits, and ataxia. Brain tumor–like masses in neuroschistosomiasis can present with increased intracranial pressure, headache, nausea and vomiting, and seizures (Carod-Artal 2008). In advanced disease with *S. mansoni* or *S. haematobium,* portal hypertension is a serious complication, with hepatic encephalopathy.

Trichinosis

Trichinosis is a worldwide disease caused by the ingestion of *Trichinella* larvae encysted in the muscles of infected animals. They are most commonly found in pork in the United States and Europe, but 150 species of mammals from all latitudes may acquire the infection. Trichinosis has become rare in most developed nations but still occurs in ethnic groups that prefer raw or undercooked pork or wild animals, such as boar, polar bear, or walrus. Typical symptoms of infection include a febrile illness with myalgias and diarrhea, accompanied by marked eosinophilia. CNS involvement occurs in 10%–20% through a variety of mechanisms, including obstruction, toxicity, inflammation, vasculitis, and allergic reactions such as headache, delirium, insomnia, meningoencephalitis, and seizures. Neuropsychiatric sequelae and chronic fatigue are common after infection (Nemet et al. 2009), and residual cognitive dysfunction may occur (Harms et al. 1993). CT or MRI scans show multiple small hypodense lesions with ringlike enhancement with contrast. A muscle biopsy is usually diagnostic. Treatment in severe cases requires corticosteroids for the inflammation and antihelminthic drugs to kill *Trichinella.*

Amebiasis

Several amebas cause human disease, and all are ubiquitous in the environment worldwide. CNS infection with amebas is rare in the United States. Primary amebic meningoencephalitis is produced by *Naegleria fowleri* in healthy young individuals engaged in water sports. Its course is acute and fulminant, with headache, nausea, confusion, and stiff neck followed by coma and death within days. Granulomatous amebic encephalitis, caused by *Balamuthia mandrillaris* and some species of *Acanthamoeba,* usually occurs in debilitated, immunosuppressed (especially in cases of AIDS), or malnourished individuals. The course is more chronic, with personality changes, confusion, and irritability, eventually progressing to seizures and death (Schuster et al. 2009).

Drugs for Infectious Diseases: Adverse Psychiatric Effects and Drug Interactions

That antibiotics can cause delirium and other psychiatric symptoms is not well appreciated. The best-documented psychiatric side effects of drugs for infectious diseases are listed in Table 27–3 (antiretroviral drugs are discussed in Chapter 28, "HIV/AIDS"). Delirium and psychosis have been particularly associated with quinolones (e.g., ciprofloxacin), procaine penicillin, antimalarial and other antiparasitic drugs (especially mefloquine), and the antituberculous drug cycloserine. The most common adverse effect causing discontinuation of interferon is depression. Metronidazole and tinidazole can cause disulfiram-like reactions after alcohol ingestion. More detailed review is available elsewhere (Ferrando et al. 2010).

Table 27–4 shows selected well-established interactions between antimicrobial and psychotropic drugs. Drug interactions between antibiotics and nonpsychiatric drugs also may present risk in psychiatric practice. Erythromycin (and similar antibiotics such as clarithromycin) and ketoconazole (and similar antifungals) may cause QT interval prolongation and ventricular arrhythmias when given to a patient taking other QT-prolonging drugs, including tricyclic antidepressants and many antipsychotics. Linezolid is an irreversible monoamine oxidase-A inhibitor and therefore may cause serotonin syndrome if taken with serotonergic antidepressants and hypertensive crisis if taken with sympathomimetics or meperidine. Isoniazid is a weaker monoamine oxidase inhibitor. Details regarding antibiotics' effects on psychiatric drugs via cytochrome P450 interactions can be found elsewhere (Ferrando et al. 2010).

Fears of Infectious Disease

Infectious diseases historically have been, and remain, frightening. In the epidemic of SARS, both affected patients and health care workers experienced fears of the illness and fears of contagion to family and friends, sometimes resulting in posttraumatic stress disorder (Sim et al. 2004). Quarantined patients struggled with loneliness, isolation, and stigmatization, and they feared the effect of their absence on those who depend on them (Maunder et al. 2003). Feared, stigmatized infected individuals may delay seeking care and remain undetected (Person et al. 2004). Widespread panic may occur in the event of a human avian influenza outbreak, pointing to the need for psychologically informed public health measures (Lau et al. 2007).

Both individual and group reactions to real or imagined threats of infectious diseases also may include hysterical and phobic behaviors. Anxiety about acquiring a feared disease may lead to conversion symptoms, hypochondriacal preoccupation, and unnecessary avoidance behaviors. Contamination obsessions and washing compulsions are among the most frequent symptoms in OCD. Delusional fears or beliefs that one is infected also occur in psychotic disorders, including schizophrenia, psychotic depression, and delusional disorder, somatic type (e.g., delusions of intestinal parasitosis); however, it is important to consider that a patient with a delusion of infection may actually be infected. Unrealistic fears of infection are especially likely with venereal diseases (particularly HIV), serious outbreaks (e.g., meningococcal meningitis on campus), and infectious threats given heavy media coverage (e.g., bacterial food contamination, bovine spongiform encephalopathy, SARS, anthrax, smallpox). Of course, how much vigilance and which precautions are optimal may be uncertain even among experts, but the early years of the

TABLE 27–3. Psychiatric side effects of drugs for infectious diseases (excluding antiretroviral drugs)

Drug	Side effects
Antibacterial	
Cephalosporins	Euphoria, delusions, depersonalization, illusions
Dapsone	Insomnia, agitation, hallucinations, mania, depression
Procaine penicillin[a]	Delirium, psychosis, agitation, depersonalization, fear of imminent death, hallucinations (probably due to procaine)
Quinolones[a]	Psychosis, paranoia, mania, agitation, Tourette-like syndrome
Trimethoprim-sulfamethoxazole	Delirium, psychosis
Gentamicin	Delirium, psychosis
Clarithromycin	Delirium, mania
Antituberculous	
Cycloserine[a]	Agitation, depression, psychosis, anxiety
Isoniazid	Psychosis, mania
Ethionamide	Depression, hallucinations
Antiviral	
Acyclovir, ganciclovir	Psychosis, delirium, depression, anxiety
Amantadine[a]	Psychosis, delirium
Oseltamivir, zanamivir	Psychosis, delirium
Interferon-alpha[a]	Irritability, depression, agitation, paranoia
Interleukin-2	Psychosis, delirium
Antiparasitic	
Antimalarials[a] (especially mefloquine)	Confusion, psychosis, mania, depression, anxiety, aggression, delirium
Metronidazole	Depression, delirium, disulfiram-like reactions
Thiabendazole	Psychosis
Antifungal	
Amphotericin	Delirium, psychosis, depression

Note. See also Brown and Stoudemire 1998.
[a]More significant (more frequent and/or better established) effects.
Source. Adapted from Abouesh A, Stone C, Hobbs WR: "Antimicrobial-Induced Mania (Antiomania): A Review of Spontaneous Reports." *Journal of Clinical Psychopharmacology* 22:71–81, 2002; "Drugs That May Cause Psychiatric Symptoms." *Medical Letter* 44:59–62, 2002.

AIDS epidemic were a clear example of the potential for widespread irrational behaviors among the public, health care professionals, and officials.

At times, mass outbreaks of symptoms occur, falsely attributed to a supposed toxic exposure (e.g., bacterial food poisoning or toxic fumes) or infectious disease. There have been hundreds of reports in the literature of such outbreaks of "mass psychogenic" or "mass sociogenic" illness, and they tend to follow trends in societal concerns (e.g., bioterrorism) (Bartholomew and Wessely 2002). They are most likely to occur in groups of young people in close quarters, such as students at schools or military recruits. Some aspects of "germ panic" have become socially normative (Tomes 2000)—for example, inappropriate use of antibiotics such as ciprofloxacin during the anthrax scare and the widespread overuse of antiseptic soaps, mouthwashes, sprays, and cleaning agents. A related phobia of fever in their children remains prevalent among parents (Crocetti et al. 2001).

Psychiatric Aspects of Immunizations

A growing body of research has indicated that psychological factors can influence the antibody response to vaccination. Several studies have convincingly shown that psychological stress suppresses the secondary (but not primary) antibody response to immunization (Cohen et al. 2001). More recent studies have shown reduced antibody re-

TABLE 27–4. Selected antimicrobial–psychotropic drug interactions

Antimicrobial	Effect on psychiatric drug
Antimalarials	Increase phenothiazine level
Azoles	Increase alprazolam, midazolam levels
	Increase buspirone level
Clarithromycin, erythromycin	Increase alprazolam, midazolam levels
	Increase carbamazepine level
	Increase buspirone level
	Increase clozapine level
Quinolones	Increase clozapine level
	Increase benzodiazepine level
	Decrease benzodiazepine effect via GABA receptor
Isoniazid	Increase haloperidol level
	Increase carbamazepine level
	With disulfiram, causes ataxia
Linezolid	Serotonin syndrome with serotonergic drugs

Note. GABA = γ-aminobutyric acid.
Source. Adapted from Cozza KL, Armstrong SC, Oesterheld JR: *Concise Guide to Drug Interaction Principles for Medical Practice,* 2nd Edition. Washington, DC, American Psychiatric Publishing, 2003; Hansten PD, Horn JR: *Drug Interactions and Management.* Vancouver, WA, Applied Therapeutics, 1997.

sponse of influenza vaccine in subjects who are unmarried or have bereavement, loneliness, or neuroticism (Moynihan et al. 2004; Phillips et al. 2005, 2006; Pressman et al. 2005).

Mass outbreaks of psychogenic symptoms similar to those described earlier in this chapter have been reported several times following vaccinations (Clements 2003). In developed countries, the public's fears of vaccine-preventable diseases have waned, and awareness of potential adverse effects of the vaccines has increased, which is threatening vaccine acceptance (Amanna and Slifka 2005). The media and Web sites have disseminated much disinformation about vaccination risks, adding to the tendency toward phobic avoidance of immunization. Rare, serious CNS adverse effects, including acute disseminated encephalomyelitis (see section "Viral Infections" earlier in this chapter; see also Huynh et al. 2008), can occur after a variety of vaccinations. However, extensive research to date does not support the widely publicized fears that measles-mumps-rubella vaccination causes encephalitis or autism (Demicheli et al. 2005; Doja and Roberts 2006). The data also do not support the hypothesis that exposure to thimerosal, a mercury-containing preservative in some vaccines, causes neuropsychological deficits (Thompson et al. 2007).

References

Aghanwa HS, Morakinyo O: Correlates of psychiatric morbidity in typhoid fever in a Nigerian general hospital setting. Gen Hosp Psychiatry 23:158–162, 2001

Amanna I, Slifka MK: Public fear of vaccination: separating fact from fiction. Viral Immunol 18:307–315, 2005

Arciniegas DB, Anderson CA: Viral encephalitis: neuropsychiatric and neurobehavioral aspects. Curr Psychiatry Rep 6:372–379, 2004

Badiaga S, Barrau K, Brouqui P, et al: Imported Dengue in French University Hospitals: a 6-year survey. Infectio-Sud Group. J Travel Med 10:286–289, 2003

Barnes V, Ware MR: Tetanus, pseudotetanus, or conversion disorder: a diagnostic dilemma? South Med J 86:591–592, 1993

Bartholomew RE, Wessely S: Protean nature of mass sociogenic illness: from possessed nuns to chemical and biological terrorism fears. Br J Psychiatry 180:300–306, 2002

Bedat-Millet AL, Charpentier S, Monge-Strauss MF, et al: Psychiatric presentation of human African trypanosomiasis: overview of diagnostic pitfalls, interest of difluoromethylornithine treatment and contribution of magnetic resonance imaging. Rev Neurol (Paris) 156:505–509, 2000

Blum J, Nkunku S, Burri C: Clinical description of encephalopathic syndromes and risk factors for their occurrence and outcome during melarsoprol treatment of human African trypanosomiasis. Trop Med Int Health 6:390–400, 2001

Blum J, Schmid C, Burri C: Clinical aspects of 2541 patients with second stage human African trypanosomiasis. Acta Trop 97:55–64, 2006

Bodur H, Erbay A, Akinci E, et al: Neurobrucellosis in an endemic area of brucellosis. Scand J Infect Dis 35:94–97, 2003

Boesenberg C, Schulz-Schaeffer WJ, Meissner B, et al: Clinical course in young patients with sporadic Creutzfeldt-Jakob disease. Ann Neurol 58:533–543, 2005

Bonawitz C, Castillo M, Mukherji SK: Comparison of CT and MR features with clinical outcome in patients with Rocky Mountain spotted fever. Am J Neuroradiol 18:459–464, 1997

Brown TM, Stoudemire A: Psychiatric Side Effects of Prescription and Over-the-Counter Medications: Recognition and Management. Washington, DC, American Psychiatric Publishing, 1998

Carod-Artal FJ: Neurological complications of Schistosoma infection. Trans R Soc Trop Med Hyg 102:107–116, 2008

Caroff SN, Mann SC, Glittoo MF, et al: Psychiatric manifestations of acute viral encephalitis. Psychiatr Ann 31:193–204, 2001

Castleberry JS, Mahon CR: Dengue fever in the Western Hemisphere. Clin Lab Sci 16:34–38, 2003

Centers for Disease Control: Human rabies—Texas, Arkansas, and Georgia, 1991. MMWR Morb Mortal Wkly Rep 40:765–769, 1991

Centers for Disease Control and Prevention: Human rabies: Texas and New Jersey, 1997. MMWR Morb Mortal Wkly Rep 47:1–5, 1998

Centers for Disease Control and Prevention: First human death associated with raccoon rabies—Virginia, 2003. MMWR Morb Mortal Wkly Rep 52:1102–1103, 2003

Cheng SK, Tsang JS, Ku KH, et al: Psychiatric complications in patients with severe acute respiratory syndrome (SARS) during the acute treatment phase: a series of 10 cases. Br J Psychiatry 184:359–360, 2004

Clements CJ: Mass psychogenic illness after vaccination. Drug Saf 26:599–604, 2003

Cohen S, Miller GE, Rabin BS: Psychological stress and antibody response to immunization: a critical review of the human literature. Psychosom Med 63:7–18, 2001

Cohen S, Doyle WJ, Alper CM, et al: Sleep habits and susceptibility to the common cold. Arch Intern Med 169:62–67, 2009

Crocetti M, Moghbeli N, Serwint J: Fever phobia revisited: have parental misconceptions about fever changed in 20 years? Pediatrics 107:1241–1246, 2001

Cummings JL, Chow T, Masterman D: Encephalitis lethargica: lessons for neuropsychiatry. Psychiatr Ann 31:165–169, 2001

Dale RC, Webster R, Gill D: Contemporary encephalitis lethargica presenting with agitated catatonia, stereotypy, and dystonia-parkinsonism. Mov Disord 22:2281–2284, 2007

Demicheli V, Jefferson T, Rivetti A, et al: Vaccines for measles, mumps and rubella in children. Cochrane Database Syst Rev (4):CD004407, 2005

Dodet B, Goswami A, Gunasekera A, et al: Rabies awareness in eight Asian countries. Vaccine 26:6344–6348, 2008

Doja A, Roberts W: Immunizations and autism: a review of the literature. Can J Neurol Sci 33:341–346, 2006

Domingues RB, Kuster GW, Onuki-Castro FL, et al: Involvement of the central nervous system in patients with dengue virus infection. J Neurol Sci 267:36–40, 2008

Donnet A, Harle JR, Cherif AA, et al: Acute psychiatric pathology disclosing subcortical lesion in neuro-AIDS. Encephale 17:79–81, 1991

Dugbartey AT, Dugbartey MT, Apedo MY: Delayed neuropsychiatric effects of malaria in Ghana. J Nerv Ment Dis 186:183–186, 1998

Eren S, Bayam G, Ergönül O, et al: Cognitive and emotional changes in neurobrucellosis. J Infect 53:184–189, 2006

Fallon BA, Keilp JG, Corbera KM, et al: A randomized, placebo-controlled trial of repeated IV antibiotic therapy for Lyme encephalopathy. Neurology 70:992–1003, 2008

Feder HM Jr, Johnson BJ, O'Connell S, et al: A critical appraisal of "chronic Lyme disease." Ad Hoc International Lyme Disease Group. N Engl J Med 357:1422–1430, 2007

Fenollar F, Puéchal X, Raoult D: Whipple's disease. N Engl J Med 356:55–66, 2007

Ferrando SJ, Levenson JL, Owen JA: Infectious diseases, in Clinical Manual of Psychopharmacology in the Medically Ill. Edited by Ferrando SJ, Levenson JL, Owen JA. Arlington, VA, American Psychiatric Publishing, 2010, pp 371–404

Fontana RJ, Kronfol Z, Lindsay KL, et al: Changes in mood states and biomarkers during peginterferon and ribavirin treatment of chronic hepatitis C.; HALT-C Trial Group. Am J Gastroenterol 103:2766–2775, 2008

Freedman DO: Clinical practice: malaria prevention in short-term travelers. N Engl J Med 359:603–612, 2008

Gabbay V, Coffey BJ, Babb JS, et al: Pediatric autoimmune neuropsychiatric disorders associated with streptococcus: comparison of diagnosis and treatment in the community and at a specialty clinic. Pediatrics 122:273–278, 2008

Garg RK: Subacute sclerosing panencephalitis. J Neurol 255:1861–1871, 2008

Garvey MA, Perlmutter SJ, Allen AJ, et al: A pilot study of penicillin prophylaxis for neuropsychiatric exacerbations triggered by streptococcal infections. Biol Psychiatry 45:1564–1571, 1999

Gilden DH, Klienschmidt-DeMasters BK, LaGuardia JJ, et al: Neurologic complications of the reactivation of varicella-zoster virus. N Engl J Med 342:635–645, 2000

Gliatto MF, Caroff SN: Neurosyphilis: a history and clinical review. Psychiatr Ann 31:153–161, 2001

Harms G, Binz P, Feldmeier H, et al: Trichinosis: a prospective controlled study of patients ten years after acute infection. Clin Infect Dis 17:637–643, 1993

Hickie I, Davenport T, Wakefield D, et al, and the Infection Outcomes Study Group: Post-infective and chronic fatigue syndromes precipitated by viral and non-viral pathogens: prospective cohort study. BMJ 333:575, 2006

Hicks CB: Serologic testing for syphilis. UpToDate Online 12.2, 2004. Available at: http://patients.uptodate.com. Accessed July 2004.

Himelhoch S, McCarthy JF, Ganoczy D, et al: Understanding associations between serious mental illness and hepatitis C virus among veterans: a national multivariate analysis. Psychosomatics 50:30–37, 2009

Huynh W, Cordato DJ, Kehdi E, et al: Post-vaccination encephalomyelitis: literature review and illustrative case. J Clin Neurosci 15:1315–1322, 2008

Jacobs RK, Anderson VA, Neale JL, et al: Neuropsychological outcome after acute disseminated encephalomyelitis: impact of age at illness onset. Pediatr Neurol 31:191–197, 2004

Jay CA: Treatment of neurosyphilis. Curr Treat Options Neurol 8:185–192, 2006

Jha S, Patel R: Some observations on the spectrum of dementia. Neurol India 52:213–214, 2004

Kaiser R: Tick-borne encephalitis. Infect Dis Clin North Am 22:561–575, 2008

Kalish RA, Kaplan RF, Taylor E, et al: Evaluation of study patients with Lyme disease: 10–20 year follow-up. J Infect Dis 183:453–460, 2001

Kaplan RF, Trevino RP, Johnson GM, et al: Cognitive function in post-treatment Lyme disease: do additional antibiotics help? Neurology 60:1916–1922, 2003

Kennedy PG: Human African trypanosomiasis-neurological aspects. J Neurol 253:411–416, 2006

Kihara M, Carter JA, Newton CR: The effect of Plasmodium falciparum on cognition: a systematic review. Trop Med Int Health 11:386–397, 2006

Klempner MS, Hu LT, Evans J, et al: Two controlled trials of antibiotic treatment in patients with persistent symptoms and a history of Lyme disease. N Engl J Med 344:85–92, 2001

Kraus MR, Schäfer A, Schöttker K, et al: Therapy of interferon-induced depression in chronic hepatitis C with citalopram: a randomised, double-blind, placebo-controlled study. Gut 57:531–536, 2008

Krupp LB, Hyman LG, Grimson R, et al: Study and treatment of post Lyme disease (STOP-LD): a randomized double masked clinical trial. Neurology 60:1923–1930, 2003

Kunkel EJ, Kim JS, Hann HW, et al: Depression in Korean immigrants with hepatitis B and related liver diseases. Psychosomatics 41:472–480, 2000

Kurlan R, Johnson D, Kaplan EL, and the Tourette Syndrome Study Group: Streptococcal infection and exacerbations of childhood tics and obsessive-compulsive symptoms: a prospective blinded cohort study. Pediatrics 121:1188–1197, 2008

Lau JT, Kim JH, Tsui H, et al: Perceptions related to human avian influenza and their associations with anticipated psychological and behavioral responses at the onset of outbreak in the Hong Kong Chinese general population. Am J Infect Control 35:38–49, 2007

Leung AM, Kennedy R, Levenson JL: Rabies exposure and psychosis. Psychosomatics 44:336–338, 2003

Mahajan SK, Machhan PC, Sood BR, et al: Neurocysticercosis presenting with psychosis. J Assoc Physicians India 52:663–665, 2004

Martín-Santos R, Díez-Quevedo C, Castellví P, et al: De novo depression and anxiety disorders and influence on adherence during peginterferon-alpha-2a and ribavirin treatment in patients with hepatitis C. Aliment Pharmacol Ther 27:257–265, 2008

Maunder R, Hunter J, Vincent L, et al: The immediate psychological and occupational impact of the 2003 SARS outbreak in a teaching hospital. CMAJ 168:1245–1251, 2003

McAuliffe P, Brassard MR, Fallon B: Memory and executive functions in adolescents with posttreatment Lyme disease. Appl Neuropsychol 15:208–219, 2008

McDonald J, Jayasuriya J, Bindley P, et al: Fatigue and psychological disorders in chronic hepatitis C. J Gastroenterol Hepatol 17:171–176, 2002

Meza NW, Rossi NE, Galeazzi TN, et al: Cysticercosis in chronic psychiatric inpatients from a Venezuelan community. Am J Trop Med Hyg 73:504–509, 2005

Mishra SK, Newton CR: Diagnosis and management of the neurological complications of falciparum malaria. Nat Rev Neurol 5:189–198, 2009

Monnet FP: Behavioural disturbances following Japanese B encephalitis. Eur Psychiatry 18:269–273, 2003

Mortimer PP: Was encephalitis lethargica a post-influenzal or some other phenomenon? Time to re-examine the problem. Epidemiol Infect 137:449–455, 2009

Moynihan JA, Larson MR, Treanor J, et al: Psychosocial factors and the response to influenza vaccination in older adults. Psychosom Med 66:950–953, 2004

Murray KO, Resnick M, Miller V: Depression after infection with West Nile virus. Emerg Infect Dis 13:479–481, 2007

Nadelman RB, Nowakowski J, Fish D, et al: Prophylaxis with single-dose doxycycline for the prevention of Lyme disease after an Ixodes scapularis tick bite. N Engl J Med 345:79–84, 2001

Neel JL: Neuropsychiatric sequelae in a case of St. Louis encephalitis. Gen Hosp Psychiatry 22:126–128, 2000

Nelligan JA, Loftis JM, Matthews AM, et al: Depression comorbidity and antidepressant use in veterans with chronic hepatitis C: results from a retrospective chart review. J Clin Psychiatry 69:810–816, 2008

Nemet C, Rogozea L, Dejica R: Results of the follow-up of the former trichinosis patients from Brasov County—Romania. Vet Parasitol 159:320–323, 2009

Neri S, Pulvirenti D, Bertino G: Psychiatric symptoms induced by antiviral therapy in chronic hepatitis C: comparison between interferon-alpha-2a and interferon-alpha-2b. Clin Drug Investig 26:655–662, 2006

Nichol G, Dennis DT, Steere AC, et al: Test-treatment strategies for patients suspected of having Lyme disease: a cost-effectiveness analysis. Ann Intern Med 128:37–48, 1998

Niebuhr DW, Millikan AM, Cowan DN, et al: Selected infectious agents and risk of schizophrenia among U.S. military personnel. Am J Psychiatry 165:99–106, 2008

Oksi J, Nikoskelainen J, Hiekkanen H, et al: Duration of antibiotic treatment in disseminated Lyme borreliosis: a double-blind, randomized, placebo-controlled, multicenter clinical study. Eur J Clin Microbiol Infect Dis 26:571–581, 2007

Ong S, Talan DA, Moran GJ, et al: Neurocysticercosis in radiographically imaged seizure patients in U.S. emergency departments. Emerg Infect Dis 8:608–613, 2002

Osher FC, Goldberg RW, McNary SW, et al: Substance abuse and the transmission of hepatitis C among persons with severe mental illness. Five-Site Health and Risk Study Research Committee. Psychiatr Serv 54:842–847, 2003

Parry CM, Hien TT, Dougan G, et al: Typhoid fever. N Engl J Med 347:1770–1782, 2002

Perlmutter SJ, Leitman SF, Garvey MA, et al: Therapeutic plasma exchange and intravenous immunoglobulin for obsessive-compulsive disorder and tic disorders in childhood. Lancet 354:1153–1158, 1999

Perrin EM, Murphy ML, Casey JR, et al: Does group A beta-hemolytic streptococcal infection increase risk for behavioral and neuropsychiatric symptoms in children? Arch Pediatr Adolesc Med 158:848–856, 2004

Person B, Sy F, Holton K, et al: Fear and stigma: the epidemic within the SARS outbreak. Emerg Infect Dis 10:358–363, 2004

Phillips AC, Carroll D, Burns VE, et al: Neuroticism, cortisol reactivity, and antibody response to vaccination. Psychophysiology 42:232–238, 2005

Phillips AC, Carroll D, Burns VE, et al: Bereavement and marriage are associated with antibody response to influenza vaccination in the elderly. Brain Behav Immun 20:279–289, 2006

Pressman SD, Cohen S, Miller GE, et al: Loneliness, social network size, and immune response to influenza vaccination in college freshmen. Health Psychol 24:297–306, 2005

Raggi A, Perani D, Giaccone G, et al: The behavioural features of fatal familial insomnia: a new Italian case with pathological verification. Sleep Med 10:581–585, 2009

Raghav S, Seneviratne J, McKelvie PA, et al: Sporadic encephalitis lethargica. J Clin Neurosci 14:696–700, 2007

Ramirez-Bermudez J, Higuera J, Sosa AL, et al: Is dementia reversible in patients with neurocysticercosis? J Neurol Neurosurg Psychiatry 7:1164–1166, 2005

Ravdin LD, Hilton E, Primeau M, et al: Memory functioning in Lyme borreliosis. J Clin Psychiatry 57:281–286, 1996

Roberts MC, Emsley RA, Jordaan GP: Screening for syphilis and neurosyphilis in acute psychiatric admissions. S Afr Med J 82:16–18, 1992

Saccente M: Central nervous system histoplasmosis. Curr Treat Options Neurol 10:161–167, 2008

Sacks N, Van Rensbueg AJ: Clinical aspects of chronic brucellosis. S Afr Med J 50:725–728, 1976

Sanchez FM, Zisselman MH: Treatment of psychiatric symptoms associated with neurosyphilis. Psychosomatics 48:440–445, 2007

Schelling G, Roozendaal B, Krauseneck T, et al: Efficacy of hydrocortisone in preventing posttraumatic stress disorder following critical illness and major surgery. Ann N Y Acad Sci 1071:46–53, 2006

Schuster FL, Yagi S, Gavali S, et al: Under the radar: balamuthia amebic encephalitis. Clin Infect Dis 48:879–887, 2009

Seltzer EG, Gerber MA, Cartter ML, et al: Long-term outcomes of persons with Lyme disease. JAMA 283:609–616, 2000

Semiz UB, Turhan V, Basoglu C, et al: Leptospirosis presenting with mania and psychosis: four consecutive cases seen in a military hospital in Turkey. Int J Psychiatry Med 35:299–305, 2005

Shibre T, Alem A, Abdulahi A, et al: Trimethoprim as adjuvant treatment in schizophrenia: a double-blind, randomized, placebo-controlled clinical trial. Schizophr Bull June 16, 2009 [Epub ahead of print]

Shulman ST: Pediatric autoimmune neuropsychiatric disorders associated with streptococci (PANDAS): update. Curr Opin Pediatr 21:127–130, 2009

Siami S, Annane D, Sharshar T: The encephalopathy in sepsis. Crit Care Clin 24:67–82, 2008

Sim K, Chong PN, Chan YU, et al: Severe acute respiratory syndrome-rated psychiatric and posttraumatic morbidities and coping responses in medical staff within a primary health care setting in Singapore. J Clin Psychiatry 65:1120–1127, 2004

Singer HS, Gause C, Morris C, and the Tourette Syndrome Study Group: Serial immune markers do not correlate with clinical exacerbations in pediatric autoimmune neuropsychiatric disorders associated with streptococcal infections. Pediatrics 121:1198–1205, 2008

Snider LA, Lougee L, Slattery M, et al: Antibiotic prophylaxis with azithromycin or penicillin for childhood-onset neuropsychiatric disorders. Biol Psychiatry 57:788–792, 2005

Solomon T: Flavivirus encephalitis. N Engl J Med 351:370–378, 2004

Spencer MD, Knight RS, Will RG: First hundred cases of variant Creutzfeldt-Jakob disease: retrospective case note review of early psychiatric and neurological features. BMJ 324:1479–1482, 2002

Swedo SE, Susan E, Leonard HL, et al: Pediatric autoimmune neuropsychiatric disorders associated with streptococcal infections: clinical description of the first 50 cases. Am J Psychiatry 155:264–271, 1998

Tager FA, Fallon BA: Psychiatric and cognitive features of Lyme disease. Psychiatr Ann 31:172–181, 2001

Takkouche B, Regueira C, Gestal-Otero JJ: A cohort study of stress and the common cold. Epidemiology 12:345–349, 2001

Taycan O, Uur M, Ozmen M: Quetiapine vs. risperidone in treating psychosis in neurosyphilis: a case report. Gen Hosp Psychiatry 8:359–361, 2006

Thompson WW, Price C, Goodson B, et al, and the Vaccine Safety Datalink Team: Early thimerosal exposure and neuropsychological outcomes at 7 to 10 years. N Engl J Med 357:1281–1292, 2007

Tomes N: The making of a germ panic, then and now. Am J Public Health 90:191–198, 2000

Treadway CR, Prange AJ Jr: Tetanus mimicking psychophysiologic reaction: occurrence after dental extraction. JAMA 200:891–892, 1967

Turan S, Emul M, Duran A, et al: Effectiveness of olanzapine in neurosyphilis related organic psychosis: a case report. J Psychopharmacol 21:556–558, 2007

van de Beek D, Schmand B, de Gans J, et al: Cognitive impairment in adults with good recovery after bacterial meningitis. J Infect Dis 186:1047–1052, 2002

Vázquez M, Sparrow SS, Shapiro ED: Long-term neuropsychologic and health outcomes of children with facial nerve palsy attributable to Lyme disease. Pediatrics 112:e93–e97, 2003

Verghese A: The "typhoid state" revisited. Am J Med 79:370–372, 1985

Vilensky JA, Foley P, Gilman S: Children and encephalitis lethargica: a historical review. Pediatr Neurol 37:79–84, 2007

Volpi A, Gatti A, Pica F, et al: Clinical and psychosocial correlates of post-herpetic neuralgia. J Med Virol 80:1646–1652, 2008

Wackermann PV, Fernandes RM, Elias J Jr, et al: Involvement of the central nervous system in the chronic form of Chagas' disease. J Neurol Sci 269:152–157, 2008

Wall CA, Rummans TA, Aksamit AJ, et al: Psychiatric manifestations of Creutzfeldt-Jakob disease: a 25-year analysis. J Neuropsychiatry Clin Neurosci 17:489–495, 2005

Wasay M, Channa R, Jumani M, et al: Encephalitis and myelitis associated with dengue viral infection clinical and neuroimaging features. Clin Neurol Neurosurg 110:635–640, 2008

Weiss MG: The interrelationship of tropical disease and mental disorder: conceptual framework and literature review (Part I: malaria). Cult Med Psychiatry 9:121–200, 1985

Weissenborn K, Tryc AB, Heeren M, et al: Hepatitis C virus infection and the brain. Metab Brain Dis 24:197–210, 2009

Wessely S, Pariante C: Fatigue, depression and chronic hepatitis C infection. Psychol Med 32:1–10, 2002

Wormser GP, Dattwyler RJ, Shapiro ED, et al: The clinical assessment, treatment, and prevention of Lyme disease, human granulocytic anaplasmosis, and babesiosis: clinical practice guidelines by the Infectious Diseases Society of America. Clin Infect Dis 43:1089–1134, 2006

Yetkin MA, Bulut C, Erdinc FS, et al: Evaluation of the clinical presentations in neurobrucellosis. Int J Infect Dis 10:446–452, 2006

CHAPTER

28

HIV/AIDS

Crystal C. Watkins, M.D., Ph.D.

Niccolo D. Della Penna, M.D.

Andrew A. Angelino, M.D.

Glenn J. Treisman, M.D., Ph.D.

SOON AFTER THE HUMAN immunodeficiency virus (HIV) epidemic began in the early 1980s, neurologists described several HIV-related central nervous system (CNS) syndromes. Psychiatrists and other mental health professionals initially focused on grief, loss, and supportive psychotherapy but soon recognized some specific psychiatric conditions, including acquired immunodeficiency syndrome (AIDS) dementia; AIDS mania; increased rates of major depression; and psychiatric consequences of CNS involvement with HIV, opportunistic infections, and neoplasms.

Decades later, it is apparent that psychiatric issues play a central role in the HIV epidemic. HIV is transmitted almost entirely by specific risk behaviors and in high-risk populations targeted for education and prevention since the mid-1980s. Because of this, HIV, at least in the developed countries, has become a condition predominantly of vulnerable people with certain risk factors. Transfusion recipients and homosexual men who were unaware of the risk of HIV were the early patients, whereas many current individuals are aware of the risks but are at increased jeopardy because of addictions, personality vulnerabilities, mood disorders, impulse-control disorders, cognitive impairment, social isolation and disenfranchisement, or other barriers to behavior change. HIV-infected patients with psychiatric illness may have great difficulty in modifying risk behaviors. Psychiatric disorders also can adversely affect the treatment of HIV infection primarily through undermining adherence because taking medications as prescribed is critical to successful treatment. Thus, the same psychiatric disorders that prevented patients from reducing their risk prevent them from obtaining benefit from their treatment. Untreated patients with high viral loads are more infectious, leading to an increased potential for spread of the HIV epidemic.

In this chapter, we address those conditions commonly seen in HIV, including those that increase risk for HIV or are barriers to HIV treatment. The introductory part of the chapter is a medical overview of HIV disease. In the second part, we consider neuropsychiatric and medical complications associated with HIV, and we include psychiatric conditions associated with HIV in the third part. Additional details about psychiatric disorders and treatment issues can be found in the American Psychiatric Association's "Practice Guideline for the Treatment of Patients With HIV/AIDS" (Forstein et al. 2006).

Medical Overview of HIV Infection and AIDS

HIV was originally recognized through a series of cases of young homosexual men with *Pneumocystis carinii* pneumonia in the early 1980s in California. It later became clear that these patients had severe immune system compromise and were vulnerable to infections commonly seen in other immunocompromised individuals. Current global statistics suggest that 400,000 infants are born each year with HIV infection, and some estimate that 7,400 new infections occur each day, with one individual being infected about every 10 seconds (UNAIDS Joint United Nations Programme on HIV/AIDS 2008).

In the United States, as of December 31, 2001, 807,075 adults and adolescents had been reported as having AIDS, with current estimates suggested around 1 million. Of these, 462,653 (57%) have died. The number of people estimated to be living with HIV/AIDS worldwide has declined from 42 million people in 2002 to 33 million people in 2007, with an estimated 2.7 million people acquiring the infection in 2007 (Centers for Disease Control and Prevention 2006). An estimated 20 million individuals have died from HIV worldwide. The number of new cases of HIV infection has remained steady. The prevalence and mortality rates have slowly declined since 1996, in large part because of the introduction of highly active antiretroviral therapy (HAART). There has been a subsequent reduction in viral load and an increase in CD4 cell counts in many HIV-positive patients who received HAART.

Some populations within the United States are at increased risk for infection. Homosexual men have reduced their risk substantially but as a group continue to have high seroprevalence. Blood product screening has made transfusion risk negligible. Vertical transmission risk from mother to fetus, which occurs in up to 30% of live births without intervention, is influenced by delivery type, severity of HIV disease, and the availability of preventive antiviral treatment. The frequency of vertical transmission in the developed countries has decreased dramatically in the last decade as a result of education efforts focused on avoiding breast-feeding. However, vertical transmission remains a significant problem in many other parts of the world and in some subpopulations in the United States and other developed countries. Unfortunately, psychiatric disorders continue to make many vulnerable patients unable to access or benefit from prevention efforts. For example, injection drug users and their sexual partners are currently the population with the greatest risk for infection. The introduction of crystal methamphetamines into the gay community has increased high-risk sexual behaviors that expose methamphetamine users to HIV. The Internet also has emerged as a tool for anonymous sexual activity and permits access to an expanded sexual network where people can be vulnerable to infection.

Patients who have comorbid mental illness or substance abuse are likely to have poor medical and antiretroviral adherence and therefore would fail treatment or may be excluded from treatment (Mellins et al. 2009). The primary reason for excluding them from antiretroviral drug treatment is that inconsistent adherence breeds viral resistance, rendering treatment ineffective and increasing public health risk. Additionally, resources are often scarce in HIV clinics, and patients who are less likely to remain adherent are the least likely to receive effective treatment. These patients include injection drug users, mentally ill patients, and other patients at high risk for poor outcomes. Therefore, the ability to provide adequate psychiatric care to HIV-infected patients is critical for effective treatment of HIV. Psychiatric disorders compromise the ability to take medications, adhere to treatment, practice safer sexual behaviors, and stop using injection drugs.

HIV is a retrovirus; it contains ribonucleic acid (RNA) strands that must be transcribed into deoxyribonucleic acid (DNA) by the action of an enzyme called reverse transcriptase, an enzyme not present in uninfected cells. The mechanism of viral infection within the cell is illustrated in Figure 28–1. The viral particles contain the enzyme, two viral RNA molecules, and accessory proteins. Viral particles bind to the surface of cells expressing CD4 antigens at the CD4 protein with the help of a second cell surface protein called CCR5. After the virus is internalized, the protein coat dissolves to release the two viral strands and the viral reverse transcriptase enzyme, which then uses the deoxynucleotides present in the cell to make a DNA strand from the viral RNA. The strands are moved to the nucleus where they are spliced into the DNA by a viral enzyme called integrase. If the cell is activated, the DNA template rapidly makes a huge number of viral RNA strands, which then use the cell's own machinery to make and process viral proteins. A viral protease finally cleaves the proteins and allows mature infectious particles to leave the cell. These steps do not occur within normal human cells and are therefore optimal targets for antiviral drugs. Drugs that interfere with binding (binding inhibitors), internalization (fusion inhibitors), reverse transcription (nucleotide and nonnucleotide reverse trancriptase inhibitors, also known as NRTIs or nucs and NNRTIs or nonnucs, respectively), integrase activity (integrase inhibitors), and viral protease (protease inhibitors) are all currently on the market. Successful treatment with several drugs at once reduces virus production to undetectable levels and should extend life into the normal range for most patients.

Because reverse transcriptase is a somewhat sloppy enzyme, many viral mutations occur. All possible single point mutations probably occur in a single day of uninhibited viral infection. This means that missed medication doses can lead to the rapid development of drug-resistant virus strains. Antiviral drug resistance has become one of the major problems in the epidemic in the United States. Psychiatric disorders are known to interfere with successful medical treatment and lead to increased HIV-related mortality. Successful treatment of psychiatric disorders leads to improved outcome. Collaborative care by psychiatry in the HIV clinic facilitates successful treatment of HIV infection.

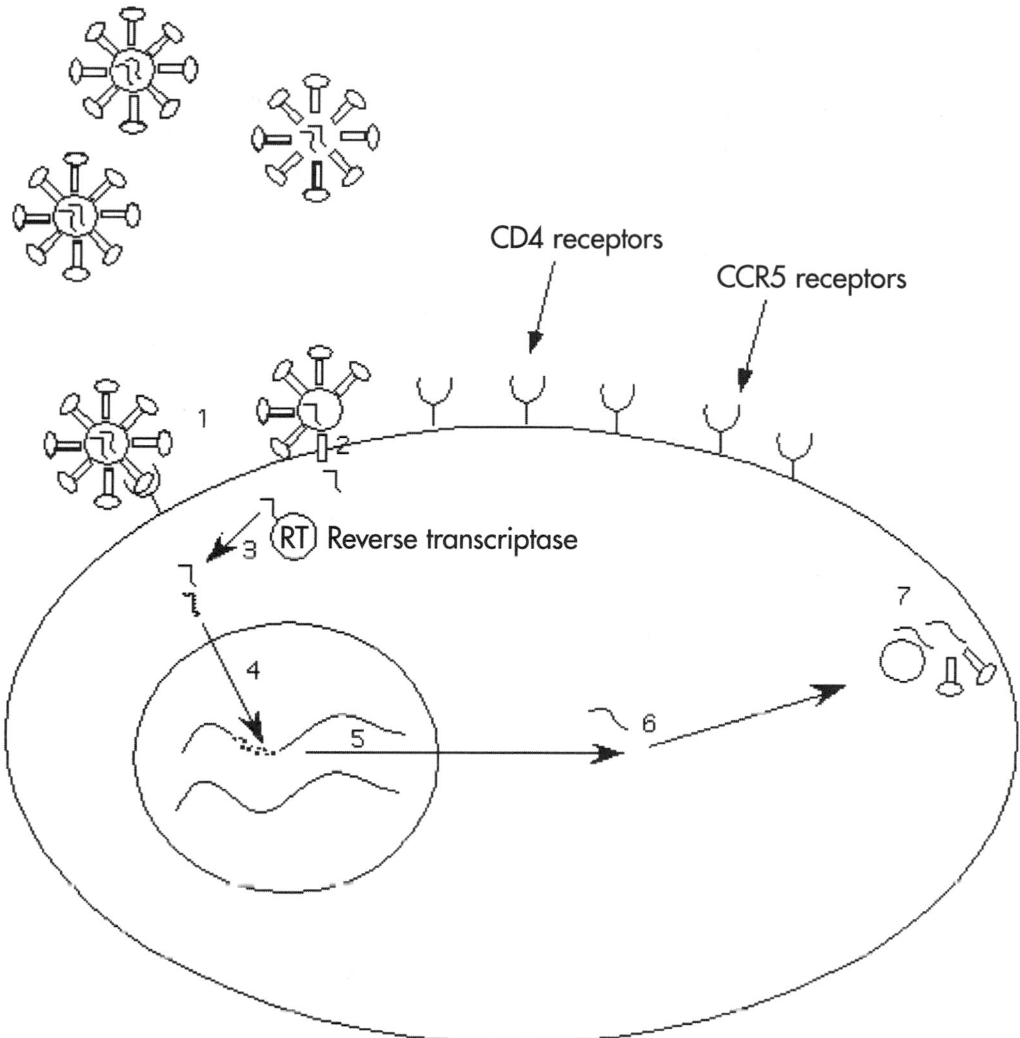

1 Viral binding to cell surface receptors
(entry inhibitors)
2 Internalization of viral content
(fusion inhibitors)
3 Reverse transcriptase makes viral DNA
(nucleotide and nonnucleotide reverse trancriptase inhibitors)
4 Viral integration into host genome
(integrase inhibitors)
5 Transcription of DNA to RNA
6 Translation of viral RNA to protein components
7 Protein processing, cleavage, viral assembly, and budding
(protease inhibitors)

FIGURE 28–1. HIV infection and replication.
Viral particles covered with gp120, a recognition glycoprotein, bind to CD4 receptors and then to the co-receptor. A protein unfolds as a result of the bonding and facilitates fusion of the viral particle with the CD4 cell. The viral envelope dissolves and releases the viral RNA and several viral enzymes, including reverse transcriptase. The RNA is used as the template to make a viral DNA strand, which is integrated into the human DNA by the action of an enzyme called integrase. When the cell is activated, viral RNA is made from the integrated DNA and usurps the cell's machinery to make more viral RNA and viral proteins. These are further processed and then packaged as immature viral particles. Further processing by viral enzymes allows the viral particle to become a mature infectious virion.

The Internet and HIV

The Internet has become a major mechanism to disseminate information about rapidly changing areas of medicine. HIV is one of the most rapidly evolving areas of treatment, and Dr. John Bartlett was one of the first clinicians to recognize the online potential of rapid dissemination of new HIV-related information. He began a Web site at Johns Hopkins University (www.hopkins-aids.edu) that has become a reference point for HIV care. About the same time, the first commercial online HIV medical information site was launched by Dr. Jeff Drezner (a psychiatrist) as Medscape (www.medscape.com), one of the pioneering Web information sources in medicine (R. Chaisson, personal communication, September 2009). Medscape went on to become a source for general medical information and a model for other Web sites. Other later Web sites were devoted to reducing risk-related behaviors for HIV prevention, providing information about access to treatment and care, and providing information about the latest changes in treatment recommendations.

Unfortunately, the Internet is also a conduit for anonymous sexual encounters and high-risk behavior promoting erotic material. Some studies estimate that up to 16 million men and women have gone online to find love and companionship and to solicit sex (Madden and Lenhart 2006; Rebchook et al. 2006). Whether the Internet is a mediator or moderator of behavior in populations at risk for HIV is not well understood. Distinct from encounters initiated on the Internet or a traditional social scene, risk-taking individuals will still engage in high-risk sexual acts (McKirnan et al. 2007). At the same time, individuals who solicit sexual partners online have been shown to be more likely to have a sexually transmitted disease (STD) history, to participate in more unsafe sexual behaviors, and to have considerably more sexual partners compared with those who do not pursue Internet sexual partners (Liau et al. 2006; Rebchook et al. 2006; Tashima et al. 2003). A particular chat room was linked to a 1999 outbreak of syphilis among men having sex with men (Klausner et al. 2000), and cases of acute HIV infection occurred after meeting a sexual partner in another Internet chat room (Tashima et al. 2003). The anonymity of being able to connect sexually with partners from alternative social networks is also suggested to generate a hybrid of high- and low-risk persons that usually would not intermingle. This subsequent extension and interaction of sexual networks can propagate transmission of HIV and other STDs (Rebchook et al. 2006).

Creative new approaches are needed to combat STDs and HIV transmission via the Internet. The Centers for Disease Control and Prevention assembled an international panel of HIV disease experts to discuss how to use the Internet to promote HIV prevention efforts and educate others about the disease transmission risks of sexual partnering online.

Effect of Psychiatric Disorders on HIV Medication Adherence

The single most important factor affecting outcome of HIV treatment is the patient's ability to adhere to a prescribed regimen. A study of HIV-infected prisoners reported that under directly observed therapy in a prison setting, 85% of the individuals developed undetectable viral loads, with prisoners taking approximately 93% of doses (Kirkland et al. 2002). In contrast, British community studies found that only 42% of treatment-naive patients taking antiretroviral medications attained undetectable viral loads (Lee and Monteiro 2003). Antiretroviral adherence rates between 54% and 76% have been reported in other general clinic or community samples (Liu et al. 2001; McNabb et al. 2001; Paterson et al. 2000; Wagner and Ghosh-Dastidar 2002), including groups of patients with serious mental illness (Beyer et al. 2007; Wagner et al. 2003).

Psychiatric factors associated with nonadherence include dementia, depression, psychosis, aversive life experience, personality factors, and substance use (Mellins et al. 2009). Many studies have shown decreased adherence to HAART attributable to depression (Campos et al. 2010; Koenig et al. 2008). Treatment of depression is associated with improved outcomes (Kumar and Encinosa 2009). Psychotic patients may refuse medications, deny their illness, or be too disorganized to manage adherence. Patients with dementia may forget doses and appointments. Aversive life experiences, such as sexual abuse in childhood (Meade et al. 2009), are associated with poor adherence. Personality vulnerabilities also have strong positive and negative effects on medication adherence. Substance use disorders, particularly alcohol abuse (Conen et al. 2009), contribute profoundly to poor medication adherence (Malta et al. 2008). Treatment of addictions can improve adherence and outcome (Roux et al. 2008). Constant and consistent coaching of patients at each visit is imperative, including clarifying goals of treatment (both short- and long-term) and anticipating misunderstandings. It is also useful over time to positively reinforce compliance with treatment.

Neuropsychiatric and Medical Complications of HIV Infection

Opportunistic infection rates have dramatically decreased over the last two decades and are covered in Chapter 27, "Infectious Diseases." Here we review some specifics related to HIV infection.

Toxoplasmosis

Infection with *Toxoplasma gondii* generally occurs in 30% of patients with fewer than 100 CD4 cells/mm^3 (Kaplan et al. 2009). In AIDS patients, toxoplasmosis is the most common reason for intracranial masses, affecting between 2% and 4% of the AIDS population. Symptoms of CNS infection are fever, change in level of alertness, headache, confusion, focal neurological signs (approximately 80% of cases), and partial or generalized seizures (approximately 30% of cases). Computed tomography (CT) usually shows multiple bilateral, ring-enhancing lesions in the basal ganglia or at the gray-white matter junction. Magnetic resonance imaging (MRI) is more sensitive than CT and is the preferred technique for individuals without focal neurological deficits (Kupfer et al. 1990).

Treatment is usually empirical, based on clinical and imaging findings, and consists of pyrimethamine and leucovorin plus sulfadiazine or clindamycin. Clinical and radiological improvement is seen in more than 85% of the patients by day 7 (Kaplan et al. 2009). Acute treatment (6 weeks) has been followed by continuous prophylaxis to prevent relapse. Recent studies suggest that HIV-infected adult patients receiving effective HAART can safely discontinue primary and secondary prophylaxis against toxoplasmic encephalitis if their CD4$^+$ T cell count has been greater than 200 cells/mm^3 for more than 3 months (Miro et al. 2006).

The use of trimethoprim-sulfamethoxazole as prophylaxis has reduced the incidence of *T. gondii* infection in HIV. Patients with hypersensitivity to sulfa drugs may use pyrimethamine plus dapsone.

Cytomegalovirus

Cytomegalovirus (CMV) infection is found at autopsy in about 30%–50% of brains from HIV-infected patients (Jellinger et al. 2000). However, the development of clinically evident CMV encephalitis is fairly rare and most often occurs in patients with CD4 cell counts less than 50 cells/mm^3. Short-term memory is especially impaired in CMV encephalitis in HIV-infected patients, mimicking Korsakoff's syndrome (Pirskanen-Matell et al. 2009). CMV infection of another organ, such as retina, blood, adrenal glands, or gastrointestinal tract, is often found at the time of encephalitis diagnosis. CMV encephalitis in AIDS may progress gradually as a dementia with focal deficits (Holland et al. 1994) or rapidly as a fatal delirium (Kalayjian et al. 1993). Treatment is mostly supportive. Ganciclovir and foscarnet may be prescribed but are of questionable benefit.

Cryptococcal Meningitis

Although meningitis caused by *Cryptococcus neoformans* is rare in immunocompetent persons, it is a devastating illness that has occurred in approximately 8%–10% of AIDS patients in the United States and in up to 30% of AIDS patients in other parts of the world (Powderly 2000). More recent published incidence estimates range from 0.04% to 12% per year among persons with HIV in various regions (Park et al. 2009). Patients generally present with fever and delirium. Meningeal signs are not universally seen. Seizures and focal neurological deficits occur in about 10% of patients, and intracranial pressure is elevated in about 50% of patients. The 3-month case fatality rate is estimated to be 9% in high-income countries, 55% in low- and middle-income ones, and 70% in sub-Saharan Africa (Park et al. 2009).

Treatment of cryptococcal meningitis in HIV requires amphotericin B. Patients who survive must receive prophylaxis against recurrence. Prophylaxis can be prescribed as oral fluconazole or intermittent intravenous amphotericin B. Some authors suggest that patients who receive HAART for 6 months with a rise in CD4 cell count to greater than 100 cells/mm^3 may terminate secondary prophylaxis (E. Martinez et al. 2000). Although earlier trials did not show a survival benefit from primary prophylaxis for *C. neoformans,* a prospective, multicenter trial of low-dose fluconazole showed significant survival benefit in HIV-infected patients with severe immune deficiency (Chetchotisakd et al. 2004).

Progressive Multifocal Leukoencephalopathy

Progressive multifocal leukoencephalopathy (PML) is a demyelinating disease of white matter in immunocompromised patients. First described in cancer patients, the causative agent is a polyomavirus, named *JC virus* after a patient. Its transmission route is unclear but may be respiratory, and there is no clear clinical syndrome of acute infection. Prior to the implementation of HAART in 1996, the prevalence of PML in AIDS was between 1% and 10%, and AIDS patients account for almost three-quarters of PML cases reported in the United States (Engsig et al. 2009). The incidence rate of PML has been reduced by almost 50% with widespread use of HAART (Engsig et al. 2009; Sacktor 2002). The risk of PML remains significant in AIDS patients with fewer than 100 CD4 cells/mm^3.

The clinical syndrome consists of multiple focal neurological deficits, such as mono- or hemiparetic limb weakness, dysarthria, gait disturbances, sensory deficits, and progressive dementia, with eventual coma and death. Occasionally, seizures or visual losses may occur. A Brazilian study found that the most common clinical manifestations were focal weakness (75%), speech disturbances (58%), visual disturbances (42%), cognitive dysfunction (42%), and impaired coordination (42%) (Vidal et al. 2008). Usually, no fever or headache occurs.

The pathology of PML consists of demyelination and death of astrocytes and oligodendroglia. MRI is more useful than CT in diagnosis; multiple areas of attenuated signal are seen on T2 images, primarily in the white matter of brain, although gray matter, brain stem, cerebellar, and spinal cord lesions are possible. Cerebrospinal fluid (CSF) studies are generally unhelpful, except for polymerase chain reaction evaluation for the presence of JC virus, which is sensitive and specific. Brain biopsy provides the definitive diagnosis but is rarely used. Trials of the antiviral agents cytarabine, cidofovir, and topotecan for the treatment of PML in HIV-infected patients have been largely unsuccessful, probably because the acute infection with JC virus occurs many years before PML develops.

Central Nervous System Neoplasms

Lymphoma is the most common neoplasm seen in AIDS patients, affecting between 0.6% and 3%. AIDS is the most common condition associated with primary CNS lymphoma. The patient is generally afebrile; may develop a single lesion with focal neurological signs or small, multifocal lesions; and most commonly presents with mental status change. Seizures occur in about 15% of these patients. CNS lymphoma manifests late in the course of HIV infection and is associated with a very poor prognosis.

CNS lymphoma is at times misdiagnosed as toxoplasmosis, HIV dementia, or other encephalopathy. CT scan of the brain may be normal or show one or multiple hypodense or patchy, nodular enhancing lesions. MRI generally shows enhanced lesions that may be difficult to differentiate from CNS toxoplasmosis, but thallium single photon emission computed tomography (SPECT) and positron emission tomography (PET) scanning may help differentiate the two disorders. CSF studies may be normal or show a moderate monocytosis; cytology studies report lymphoma cells in fewer than 5% of patients. Brain biopsy is required for confirmation of the diagnosis of CNS lymphoma. Because this procedure carries some morbidity, clinicians should strongly consider the possibility of lymphoma in afebrile patients with a negative toxoplasma immunoglobulin G (IgG) screening test result, patients with a single lesion, and patients whose symptoms do not respond to empirical therapy for toxoplasmosis as indicated by clinical examination and repeat MRI. The differential diagnosis of CNS neoplasm also includes metastatic Kaposi's sarcoma and primary glial tumors.

Lymphoma may respond in part to radiation therapy, thus alleviating high intracranial pressure and its associated symptoms. Chemotherapy is generally adjunctive for lymphoma. CNS lymphoma had a grim prognosis with an average survival of 3–5 months prior to the advent of HAART. In the post-HAART era, there appears to be a distinction between the onset and prognosis of systemic lymphoma and that of CNS non-Hodgkin's lymphoma, with an overall marked improvement in survival. HIV-related lymphomas arising in the periphery are in a less advanced stage and manifest earlier in the disease, whereas CNS lymphomas still carry a poor prognosis and manifest late in the disease course (Robotin et al. 2004).

Fatigue

Fatigue is a very common symptom in HIV-infected patients, which is often overlooked, improperly assessed, or inadequately investigated. It is associated with poor quality of life and impaired physical functioning (Marcellin et al. 2007; Pence et al. 2008). Estimates of prevalence of fatigue in patients infected with HIV range from 10% to 38% in early infection to 40% to 60% in AIDS cases (Sullivan and Dworkin 2003) and even higher in some samples (Pence et al. 2008). Fatigue may be mild and annoying, or it may be severe enough to impair function. A scale specific to HIV-related fatigue has been published (Pence et al. 2008). Fatigue is a nonspecific symptom and may have a single or multifactorial etiology. In a sample of ambulatory AIDS patients, fatigue significantly correlated with anemia and pain (Breitbart et al. 1998). In addition to disease causes, fatigue may be a side effect of medications, including HAART. Fatigue is one of the most common side effects of protease inhibitors and may be a reason for nonadherence (Duran et al. 2001).

Fatigue also may be the result of substance abuse, depression, or other psychiatric disorders. HIV-infected patients with major depression are much more likely to complain of fatigue than are patients without depression (Sullivan and Dworkin 2003; Voss et al. 2007). HIV wasting syndrome, chronic diarrhea, and testosterone deficiency are all associated with fatigue. Low serum testosterone level has been found among symptomatic AIDS patients, especially those with HIV wasting syndrome (Knapp et al. 2008). HIV-infected men with wasting syndrome treated with testosterone experienced significant improvements in fatigue, energy, mood, and quality of life compared with HIV-infected individuals who received placebo (Knapp et al. 2008). Another study showed that the testosterone-treated group had a profound amelioration of fatigue symptoms, even greater than in the fluoxetine-treated group (Rabkin et al. 2004). Hypotestosteronism is most likely in advanced AIDS (Kopicko et al. 1999; Rabkin et al. 2004) but also may be caused by medications (e.g., fluconazole, ketoconazole, or ganciclovir) (Wagner et al. 1995).

In many HIV-positive patients, the fatigue has no clear etiology, and empirical treatment is reasonable. Testosterone may be a successful treatment for fatigue in HIV-infected men, even when depressive symptoms are present

(Kong and Edmonds 2003). HIV-infected women taking testosterone for 18 months appear to have significant improvement in quality of life as well as an increase in skeletal muscle mass and bone mineral density without a change in body weight (Dolan Looby et al. 2009).

More activating antidepressants may be better tolerated by fatigued depressed patients. Some authors have reported that stimulants may be useful in treating fatigue and depression in HIV, as discussed later in this chapter. Care must be exercised in using stimulants in patients with histories of substance abuse, although risk of abuse loses relevance in terminal AIDS.

Psychiatric Conditions Associated With HIV

Delirium

Prevalence and Clinical Presentation

Delirium occurs frequently in patients with advanced HIV infection (Angelino and Treisman 2008; Bialer et al. 1991). One study found that 46% of the AIDS patients at a skilled nursing facility had at least one episode of delirium (Uldall and Berghuis 1997). More subtle delirium is common in compromised patients, although assessment can be difficult. In addition, delirium has been shown to be a marker for decreased survival in patients with AIDS (Uldall et al. 2000b). Hospitalized patients with AIDS also were found to have increased mortality if delirium complicated their hospital course (Uldall et al. 2000a). Delirium also occurs in children with AIDS (Hatherill and Flisher 2009).

The clinical presentation of delirium in HIV-infected patients is the same as in non-HIV-infected individuals and is characterized by inattention, disorganized thinking or confusion, and fluctuations in level of consciousness. Emotional changes are common and often unpredictable, and hallucinations and delusions are frequently seen. The syndrome has an acute or a subacute onset and remits fairly rapidly once the underlying etiology is treated. If untreated, patients have a marked increased risk of mortality, with estimates of about 20% in hospitalized patients.

Differential Diagnosis

Aside from general risk factors such as older age, multiple medical problems, multiple medications, impaired visual acuity, and previous episodes of delirium, patients with HIV-associated dementia are at increased risk to develop delirium. The differential diagnosis of delirium includes HIV-associated dementia (especially with AIDS mania), minor cognitive-motor disorder, major depression, bipolar disorder, panic disorder, and schizophrenia. Delirium usually can be differentiated on the basis of its rapid onset, fluctuating level of consciousness, and link to medical etiology.

Etiology

The cause of delirium should be aggressively sought. The approach to determining cause is similar to that for delirium in general (see Chapter 5, "Delirium"). Particular considerations in HIV-positive patients include hypoxia with *P. carinii* pneumonia, malnutrition, CNS infections and neoplasms, systemic infections (e.g., mycobacteria, CMV, bacterial sepsis), HIV nephropathy, substance intoxication and withdrawal, medication toxicity, and polypharmacy. Variations in hydration or electrolyte status also may profoundly affect patients with HIV who already have cerebral compromise. HIV infection itself also may produce an acute encephalopathy similar to that reported with CMV (Vlassova et al. 2009).

Treatment

Management of delirium in HIV is very similar to that for delirium in general (see Chapter 5, "Delirium"), including identification and removal of the underlying cause (when possible), nonpharmacological reorientation and environmental interventions, and pharmacotherapy. Low doses of high-potency antipsychotic agents, such as haloperidol, usually are effective. Newer atypical antipsychotics are currently being used with some success, but those with more anticholinergic activity may worsen the condition. Benzodiazepines should be used with caution because they may contribute to delirium in some patients but are of particular use in alcohol or benzodiazepine withdrawal deliria. Physical restraint may be necessary if the patient becomes violent but should be used only when alternatives are inadequate because restraint may worsen delirium.

Treatment with antipsychotic medication requires awareness of the higher susceptibility of patients with HIV to neuroleptic-induced extrapyramidal symptoms (EPS), even with exposure to drugs with low potential for inducing EPS (D.V. Kelly et al. 2002; Meyer et al. 1998). Increased susceptibility to EPS has been particularly notable with use of conventional antipsychotic medications and has limited the dosage that can be used to treat patients (Sewell et al. 1994). Patients with AIDS-related psychosis are more sensitive to EPS and respond to lower than standard doses of antipsychotics (Dolder et al. 2004; Sewell et al. 1994). Extreme sensitivity to EPS is encountered in patients with HIV dementia (Dolder et al. 2004). Marked neuronal degeneration in the basal ganglia of patients with HIV (Ferrando and Wapenyi 2002; Itoh et al. 2000), with accompanying dopaminergic neuron destruction or alteration, may explain these findings. Dyslipidemia and hyperglycemia are also potential side effects when using antipsychotics in the setting of antiretroviral therapy (Oh and Hegele 2007).

To date, only one randomized controlled trial in delirious patients with AIDS has documented efficacy of low-dose haloperidol and chlorpromazine. Lorazepam was ineffective and was associated with significant adverse effects (Breitbart et al. 1996). Lorazepam was reported to be useful in cases of AIDS-associated psychosis with catatonia, however (Scamvougeras and Rosebush 1992). Case reports indicate that molindone and ziprasidone are of benefit for HIV-associated psychosis and have minimal EPS (Fernandez and Levy 1993; Leso and Schwartz 2002).

If indicated, typical neuroleptic medications should be used at the lowest dosage and for the briefest duration possible. Atypical antipsychotics are generally preferred because of lower risk for EPS. Terminal delirium in HIV, as in other terminal diseases, is more refractory to treatment.

Dementia

Prevalence

Early in the AIDS epidemic, some patients presented with rapidly progressive neurocognitive disturbances, which led to an intensive search for etiology. Several CNS opportunistic conditions were identified, including CMV encephalitis, PML, cerebral toxoplasmosis, cryptococcal meningitis, and CNS lymphoma. However, a subset of patients remained for which no identifiable pathogen could be found, and it was deduced that HIV itself was the causative factor behind the dementia. Autopsy studies of AIDS patients with dementia found characteristic white matter changes and demyelinization, microglial nodules, multinucleated giant cells, and perivascular infiltrates but a marked absence of HIV within neurons. This has led to the current theories of neuronal loss through the action of macrophages and microglial cells and/or through activation of cytokines and chemokines that trigger abnormal neuronal pruning. It appears that basal ganglia and nigrostriatal structures are affected early in the dementia process, with diffuse neuronal losses following. Typical late findings show an approximate 40% reduction in frontal and temporal neurons. Analyses of CSF (Gallo et al. 1989; Laverda et al. 1994) and autopsy material (Tyor et al. 1992; Wesselingh et al. 1994) also have shown aberrant production of specific cytokines in patients with HIV-associated dementia.

In 1986, HIV-associated dementia was reported in up to two-thirds of AIDS patients (Navia et al. 1986), but it is less frequent now in patients receiving HAART. It became one of the leading causes of dementia in persons younger than 60 years (McArthur et al. 1993). However, its frequency among patients with otherwise asymptomatic HIV infection or CD4 cell count greater than 500 cells/mm^3 is probably less than 5% in a community sample (Handelsman et al. 1992; Krikorian et al. 1990; Maj et al. 1994; McKegney et al. 1990; Wilkie et al. 1990). In the Multicenter AIDS Cohort Study (Sacktor et al. 2001), the incidence of HIV-associated dementia declined 50% from 1990–1992 to 1996–1998, a period during which effective antiretroviral therapy was used (Sacktor 2002; Sacktor et al. 2001).

With the widespread use of HAART in developing countries in the mid 1990s, there was a dramatic decrease in the rates of AIDS dementia (Bhaskaran et al. 2008), with cases usually associated with specific risk factors, including higher HIV RNA viral load, lower educational level, older age, anemia, illicit drug use, and female gender. In the post-HAART era, minor cognitive–motor disorder and depression are more predictive of severity of HIV-associated dementia (Dunlop et al. 2002; Sevigny et al. 2004; Stern et al. 2001). HIV-associated dementia generally occurs in patients who have had a CD4 cell count nadir of less than 200/mm^3. With patients living longer with HAART, there is some concern that AIDS dementia prevalence will increase in association with the length of infection, or with residual virus confined to the CNS (Letendre et al. 2008). However, the overall incidence and prevalence rates of HIV dementia in the post-HAART era vary greatly by geography, treatment, and risk factors studied, as well as by whether patients are sampled in the community, a clinic, or a hospital. Studies from 1996 to 2002 in Italy estimated rates of cognitive impairment and dementia as 55% and 10%, respectively (Tozzi et al. 2005). In the country of Georgia, an estimated 25% of HIV/AIDS patients have developed dementia from the disease (Bolokadze et al. 2008). Of the women in Puerto Rico who were identified as "at risk" for development of dementia because of their HIV status, 49% had cognitive impairment, and 29% had dementia (Wojna et al. 2006). This is in contrast to what is observed in hospitalized HIV/AIDS patients in Kenya, where dementia is rarely detected (Jowi et al. 2007). The factors that contribute to the variance of prevalence and incidence rates, whether related to the disease, environment, or diagnostic tools used, require further investigation.

Pathophysiology

Although mechanisms of neuronal death in HIV-associated dementia have been unclear (McArthur et al. 1989; Wiley et al. 1991), the prevailing theories involve infection of the virus in brain macrophages and activated microglia in the CNS (Gonzalez-Scarano and Martin-Garcia 2005; Kaul 2009). Neurons, astrocytes, and oligodendrocytes do not appear to be directly infected by the virus. A cascade of chemokines and cytokines mediated by activated microglial cells leads to cell death through decreased arborization of neurons.

Assessment

Clinically, HIV dementia presents with the typical triad of symptoms seen in other subcortical dementias—memory and psychomotor speed impairments, depressive symptoms, and movement disorders. Initially, patients may notice slight problems with reading, comprehension, memory, and mathematical skills, but these symptoms are subtle, so they may be overlooked or discounted as being caused by fatigue and illness. Patients with early dementia usually will show impairments in timed trials, such as a timed oral Trail-Making Test or grooved pegboard. Cognitive screening tools have been recently reviewed (Skinner et al. 2009). A useful bedside screening tool, the Modified HIV Dementia Scale, has been shown to be the most specific and valid assessment tool and can be administered serially to document disease progression (Davis et al. 2002). Later, patients develop more global dementia, with marked impairments in naming, language, and praxis.

Motor symptoms are also often subtle in the early stages and include occasional stumbling while walking or running; slowing of fine repetitive movements, such as playing the piano or typing; and slight tremor. On examination, patients will have impaired saccadic eye movements, dysdiadochokinesia, hyperreflexia, and, especially in later stages, frontal release signs. In late stages, motor symptoms may be quite severe, with marked difficulty in smooth limb movements, especially in the lower extremities. Impairments on tests of psychomotor speed in patients at the time of AIDS diagnosis with no memory complaints have been shown to predict development of HIV-associated dementia up to 2 years later (Dunlop et al. 2002; Sevigny et al. 2004). Rate of progression is variable and may cause mild dysfunction over a long period or rapid progression with severe impairment (Price and Brew 1988). Parkinsonian features are common in HIV-associated dementia, and clinical correlates between HIV and parkinsonism have been identified (Koutsilieri et al. 2002; Mirsattari et al. 1998). Parkinsonian features may be provoked by dopamine antagonists (Hriso et al. 1991), opportunistic infections including toxoplasmosis (P. Maggi et al. 2000), or CNS infection with HIV itself (Mirsattari et al. 1998).

Apathy is a common early symptom of HIV-associated dementia, often causing noticeable withdrawal by the patient from social activity. A frank depressive syndrome also commonly develops, typically with irritable mood and anhedonia instead of sadness and crying spells. Sleep disturbances and weight loss are common. Restlessness and anxiety may occur. Psychosis develops in a significant number of patients, typically with paranoid thoughts and hallucinations. In about 5%–8% of patients, a syndrome known as AIDS mania develops (see subsection "Bipolar Disorder" later in this chapter). Overall, HIV-associated dementia is rapidly progressive, usually ending in death within 2 years. Because of impulsive behavior and emotional lability, HIV-associated dementia has been suggested as a strong risk factor for suicide (Alfonso and Cohen 1994).

Diagnosis

Typical findings on MRI of patients with advanced HIV-associated dementia include significant white matter lesions, as well as cortical and subcortical atrophy (Descamps et al. 2008; Roc et al. 2007). These abnormalities may appear as discreet foci, as patchy regions of confluent involvement, or as diffuse parenchymal involvement (Descamps et al. 2008; Roc et al. 2007). Partial improvement of MRI signal abnormalities (Olsen et al. 1988) and worsening of atrophy and white matter lesions (Post et al. 1992) have been reported in small reviews of patients taking zidovudine. MRI also has been suggested to be of utility in monitoring HIV-associated dementia treatment with HAART (Thurnher et al. 2000).

Various functional neuroimaging techniques, including PET (Rottenberg et al. 1996), SPECT (Harris et al. 1994; Rosci et al. 1996), and magnetic resonance spectroscopy (MRS) (Barker et al. 1995; Chang et al. 1999; Lopez-Villegas et al. 1997), have shown alterations in cerebral blood flow and metabolic patterns in the brains of individuals infected with HIV. Most of these studies were done in patients with dementia or other cognitive impairment, but other MRS investigations showed abnormalities in patients with no cognitive deficit (Chang et al. 1999; Meyerhoff et al. 1999; Suwanwelaa et al. 2000). Increased brain activation on functional MRI during working memory was found in patients with early HIV cognitive disturbance (Chang et al. 2001). Further studies showed increased activation on functional MRI in HIV-positive patients that predated clinical signs or deficits on cognitive tests (Ernst et al. 2002).

HIV-associated dementia also may develop in the presence of milder immunosuppression (Dore et al. 1999). The rates of HIV-associated dementia have declined but not to the same extent that other AIDS-defining illnesses have declined, suggesting that CNS eradication of HIV is becoming more challenging with current antiretroviral regimens. It has been proposed that increasing resistance to HAART regimens may be linked to this possible evolution. In the Multicenter AIDS Cohort Study (1990–1998; Sacktor et al. 2001), the proportion of cases of HIV-associated dementia in patients with CD4 cell counts between 201 and 350 cells/mm^3 was higher in 1996–1998 compared with the early 1990s. This suggests that screening for HIV-associated dementia should be extended to patients with CD4 cell counts less than 350 cells/mm^3 (McArthur 2004). The extended survival that antiretroviral regimens have offered patients also may increase their vulnerability to developing dementia rather than dying secondary to other fulminant complications (McArthur 2004).

Treatment

Controlled trials for HIV-associated dementia through 2008 have been reviewed elsewhere (Clifford 2000; Uthman and Abdulmalik 2008). Intensification of antiretroviral therapy and associated control of viral load are associated with significantly lower risk for progression to HIV-associated dementia (Letendre et al. 2007). Furthermore, HAART improves cognitive impairment in patients with HIV-associated dementia (Letendre et al. 2007; Robinson-Papp et al. 2009).

Controversy exists regarding the duration of treatment and outcome of dementia. The long-term effect of HAART on the course of HIV-associated dementia remains undetermined, with some evidence of ongoing HIV-related cognitive damage despite more than 3 years of potent antiretroviral treatment (Joska et al. 2010; Tozzi et al. 2001). The only other controlled trial of antiretroviral drugs compared effective antiviral therapy with and without added high-dose abacavir (Brew et al. 2007), but the study did not detect further cognitive improvement.

At first, it was believed that only antiretroviral agents with good penetration into the CNS would be useful in treating HIV-associated dementia with associated reduction of CSF HIV RNA levels (Halman and Rourke 2000), but later efforts indicated that HAART in many different combinations, including those with poor CNS levels, could provide some relief. Drugs that cross well into CSF include nucleoside reverse transcriptase inhibitors (zidovudine, stavudine, and abacavir) and the nonnucleoside nevirapine. Despite these theoretical considerations, little evidence suggests an improved outcome for any particular antiretroviral regimen (Clifford 2000). However, the observation of increased proportions of patients with HIV-associated dementia compared with other AIDS-defining illnesses (Dore et al. 1999; Masliah et al. 2000) suggests that HAART may not be as effective for treating HIV-associated dementia.

Various clinical trials have evaluated neuroprotective medications for HIV-associated dementia, including nimodipine (Navia et al. 1998), antioxidants (The Dana Consortium on the Therapy of HIV Dementia and Related Cognitive Disorders 1997, 1998), a platelet-activating factor antagonist (Schifitto et al. 1999), peptide T (Heseltine et al. 1998), and memantine (Schifitto et al. 2007), but none were shown to be efficacious.

Use of dopamine receptor agonists in pediatric patients with HIV and parkinsonian features has led to improvement in motor function (Mintz et al. 1996), yet results of similar medications in adults have been less fruitful (Kieburtz et al. 1991). Psychostimulants have been shown to improve cognitive performance in patients with HIV (Brown 1995; Hinkin et al. 2001), but others have noted apparent acceleration of HIV-associated dementia following psychostimulant use (Czub et al. 2001; Nath et al. 2001). There have not been more recent reported clinical trials with dopamine agonists or stimulants.

Risperidone and clozapine have been described in case reports of HIV-associated dementia with psychosis, with significant improvement in psychotic symptoms and few EPS (Dettling et al. 1998; Zilikis et al. 1998).

Quality care for patients with HIV-associated dementia is to ensure an optimal HAART regimen and to treat associated symptoms aggressively. Depression can be treated with standard antidepressants, and, in some cases, methylphenidate or other stimulants may be useful in treatment of apathy.

Minor Cognitive–Motor Disorder

Clinical Presentation and Prevalence

HIV-associated dementia is a late-stage disorder, whereas minor cognitive–motor disorder (or mild neurocognitive disorder) is a less severe syndrome seen in earlier HIV infection. The symptoms of minor cognitive–motor disorder are often overlooked because they may be very subtle, but they are essentially mild manifestations of the same symptoms seen in HIV-associated dementia (cognitive and motor slowing). Patients with this disorder may present with a singular minor complaint, such as taking longer to read a novel, dysfunction when performing fine-motor tasks such as playing the piano, an increased tendency to stumble or trip, or making more mistakes when balancing the checkbook. Minor cognitive–motor disorder is now regarded as part of the spectrum of HIV-associated dementia, and its description in the literature has fallen out of use.

Prevalence data for minor cognitive–motor disorder are variable, often suggesting up to 60% prevalence by late-stage AIDS (Sevigny et al. 2004). Prevalence in earlier stages is not well defined. Whether minor cognitive–motor disorder inevitably leads to HIV-associated dementia is uncertain. It appears that some patients may continue to have minor problems, whereas others will progress to frank dementia. This question is now confounded by the effects of HAART; data from earlier in the epidemic cannot be reasonably compared with current data.

Treatment

No controlled treatment data are available specifically for minor cognitive–motor disorder.

Major Depression

Prevalence

Depression is a significant problem among persons with HIV and AIDS. The estimated prevalence of major depressive disorder (MDD) in HIV-infected patients has been reported as 19%–43% (Cysique et al. 2007; Gibbie et al. 2007). The question of whether the incidence or prevalence of major depression is increasing in HIV-infected patients has been a controversial topic (Ciesla and Roberts 2001). Several factors complicate this issue. First, identification of MDD rather than depressive symptoms is a methodological barrier to cross-sample comparison. Additionally, populations at risk for HIV infection, including homosexual men and patients with substance use disorders, have elevated rates of major depression. A meta-analysis of 10 studies comparing HIV-positive and at-risk HIV-negative patients found a twofold increase in the prevalence of major depression in patients infected with HIV (Ciesla and Roberts 2001). Studies have shown that depression has a negative effect on patient adherence to treatment (Dimatteo et al. 2000; Mello et al. 2010), quality of life (Lenz and Demal 2000; Meltzer-Brody and Davidson 2000), and treatment outcome (J. Holmes and House 2000).

Lyketsos et al. (1993b) reported an association between depression and HIV infection as early as 1993 and speculated that major depression was a risk factor for developing HIV. Studies have shown prevalence rates of major depression among individuals with HIV of 15%–40%, depending on the setting and risk group studied (American Psychiatric Association 2000b; Rabkin et al. 2004). However, the prevalence exceeds 50% in individuals with HIV seeking psychiatric treatment (American Psychiatric Association 2000b). Major depression is a risk factor for HIV infection (McDermott et al. 1994) by virtue of its effect on behavior, intensification of substance abuse, exacerbation of self-destructive behaviors, and promotion of poor partner choice in relationships. HIV-negative persons with higher scores on screening instruments for general psychological distress were found to have increased risk behaviors for HIV acquisition (Hartgers et al. 1992). Distress symptoms in AIDS patients have been found to correlate with poor performance, decreased global quality of life, and presence of HIV-related medical conditions but not with CD4 cell count (Vogl et al. 1999). A sevenfold increase was found in the lifetime prevalence of mood disorders among patients without substance use disorders presenting for HIV screening (Perry et al. 1990).

Risk Factors

Major depression also is a risk factor for various behavioral disturbances that may increase exposure to HIV infection (W.D. Johnson et al. 2008). In this way, depression can be seen as a vector of HIV transmission (Angelino and Treisman 2001). Depression not only serves as a risk for perpetuation of the HIV epidemic (Himelhoch and Medoff 2005) but also is a complication preventing effective treatment. It has been clearly shown to hinder effective treatment of HIV infection (Sledjeski et al. 2005; van Servellen et al. 2002). Patients with major depression are at increased risk for disease progression and mortality (Alciati et al. 2007; Ickovics et al. 2001).

HIV increases the risk of developing major depression through a variety of mechanisms, including direct injury to subcortical areas of brain, chronic stress, worsening social isolation, and intense demoralization.

Direct evidence for a relation between worsening HIV disease and the development of major depression is supported by several studies, particularly the Multicenter AIDS Cohort Study. This study showed that rates of depression increased 2.5-fold as CD4 cells declined to fewer than $200/mm^3$ just before patients developed AIDS (Lyketsos et al. 1996a), suggesting that lower CD4 cell counts predict increased rates of depression. Major depression is associated with decreased killer T cell activity (Alciati et al. 2007) and lower CD4 cell counts in people living with HIV (Sledjeski et al. 2005).

Patients with AIDS have been recognized as a group with a high risk for psychological distress (Himelhoch et al. 2007a; Lyketsos et al. 1996b). High prevalence rates of suicide have been reported among HIV-infected patients (Carrico et al. 2007; Sherr et al. 2008). Factors associated with HIV and suicide include depression, hopelessness, alcohol abuse, poor social support, low self-esteem, and history of psychiatric disorder (Carrico et al. 2007; Sherr et al. 2008). Recent diagnosis of HIV or presence of pain also is associated with increased suicidal thoughts (Andraghetti et al. 2001; Louhivuori and Hakama 1979). The course of HIV has been purported to affect the prevalence of suicidal thoughts and behavior (Rabkin et al. 1993), and stage of HIV infection also may alter the potential for suicidal behavior and other psychiatric symptoms (Lyketsos et al. 1994) (see also Chapter 9, "Suicidality").

Taken together, these lines of evidence indicate that HIV is a risk factor for depression and that depression is a risk factor for HIV and its morbidity, underlining the importance of recognition and treatment of depression in HIV-infected patients.

Differential Diagnosis

The diagnosis of major depression in the HIV clinic is complicated by the high frequency of depressive symptoms that are associated with these other problems. Despite this, studies of HIV-positive patients with major depression have shown that its response to treatment is similar to that expected in other populations.

The differential diagnosis of depression in HIV includes nonpathological states of grief and mourning (sometimes made quite severe by the vulnerabilities of the person) and a variety of psychological and physiological disturbances. Patients with complaints of depressive syndromes can have dysthymia, dementia, delirium, demoralization, intoxication, withdrawal, CNS injury or infection, malnutrition, wasting syndromes, medication side effects, and a variety of other conditions. HIV-associated dementia and other HIV-related CNS conditions can produce a flat, apathetic state that is often misdiagnosed as depression. Cocaine withdrawal produces a depressive syndrome, and hypoactive delirium can be mistaken for depression. CNS syphilis, a condition that had become quite rare prior to the HIV epidemic, has been reappearing and remains "the great imitator," as it was originally described.

HIV-infected patients with major depression frequently present to internists and family practitioners with multiple somatic symptoms. These include (but are not limited to) headache, gastrointestinal disturbances, inexplicable musculoskeletal or visceral pain, cardiac symptoms, dizziness, tinnitus, weakness, and anesthesia. Neurovegetative symptoms are especially common. Patients report slowed thought processes, with impairments in concentration and short-term memory and occasionally generalized confusion. Given the burdens of HIV, the medical problems associated with the disease, and the side effects of medications, depression may be very low on the list of considered causes of the patient's complaints. Even patients complaining of depressive symptoms may have their depression overlooked or discounted because of the presence of a plethora of other diagnoses. Nonspecific somatic symptoms are often the result of depression rather than HIV infection in patients whose infection is early and asymptomatic. Depression is most likely to be missed when symptoms are attributed to HIV-associated dementia, fatigue, demoralization and disenfranchisement, wasting syndrome, or substance abuse. Care should be taken in distinguishing between major depression and demoralization (i.e., adjustment disorder) in patients with HIV. Approximately one-half of the patients presenting to an urban HIV clinic with depressive complaints were found to have demoralization alone (Lyketsos et al. 1994). The ability to report feeling fairly normal when distracted from thinking about the precipitating event or circumstance causing distress is a hallmark of demoralization.

As an example, fatigue has been found to be more associated with depression than with HIV disease progression. Worsening of fatigue and insomnia at 6-month follow-up was highly correlated with worsening depression but not with CD4 cell count, change in CD4 cell count, or disease progression by Centers for Disease Control and Prevention category (Leserman et al. 2008). These findings support the notion that somatic symptoms generally suggestive of depression should trigger a full psychiatric evaluation. In later-stage HIV infection, various illnesses are common, often moving depression down on the differential diagnosis list. Somatic symptoms always should be evaluated carefully and considered in context (i.e., either with other indicators of progression of HIV disease or with other indicators of depression).

Certain HIV-related medical conditions and medications can cause depressive symptoms. These include CNS infections, such as toxoplasmosis, cryptococcal meningitis, lymphoma, and syphilis. Some investigators have found significant rates of depressive symptoms, including low mood, poor appetite with loss of weight, decreased libido, and fatigue, among male HIV-positive patients with low testosterone levels (Rabkin et al. 2006). Several drugs used in patients with HIV, including efavirenz, interferon, metoclopramide, sulfonamides, anabolic steroids, and corticosteroids, have been reported to produce depression. These depressive symptoms often respond to withdrawal of the offending drug; when they do not respond to withdrawal of the drug or when the drug must be continued, the symptoms should be treated as major depression with appropriate antidepressant medication.

Routine screening for depression in people with HIV can effectively identify cases. Both the nine-item depression scale of the Patient Health Questionnaire (PHQ-9) and the PHQ-2 (see Chapter 1, "Psychiatric Assessment and Consultation," and Chapter 8, "Depression") have been valid and reliable (Hirshfield et al. 2008; Mao et al. 2009).

Treatment

Pharmacotherapy. Treatment with HAART was associated with significant improvement in symptoms of depression but did not necessarily have a causal relation (Ferrando and Freyberg 2008; Himelhoch and Medoff 2005). Several studies reported efficacy of various antidepressants in HIV-infected patients, but no single antidepressant has been found superior in treating HIV-infected patients as a group. As with all depressed patients, nonadherence is the most common reason for ineffective drug treatment, and adverse effects are the most common reason for nonadherence. Because HIV-infected patients are likely to be more sensitive to side effects, antidepressants should be started at subtherapeutic dose and raised slowly.

For a detailed review of the pharmacological treatment of major depression in HIV, see the article by Ferrando and Freyberg (2008). There are methodological limitations in interpreting clinical trial outcomes, including variable stage of infection, wide-ranging durations of treatment, overrepresentation of gay and bisexual males, and underrepresentation of injection drug users and women. Inclusion and outcome criteria also have been variable, and high placebo response rates have been seen (up to 50%).

One early double-blind study reported a favorable response to imipramine; 74% of the patients responded, compared with 30% taking placebo (Rabkin et al. 1994a). Another study found a favorable response to imipramine but showed a slightly higher placebo response (Manning et al. 1990). Attrition from the imipramine group was significant; 30% discontinued it by 6 months, most often because of side effects. Clomipramine and imipramine might have anti-inflammatory and neuroprotective effects by modulating glial cell activation in the CNS (Hwang et al. 2008). However, anticholinergic and other adverse effects of the tricyclic antidepressants (TCAs) make them difficult to use in patients with AIDS. Open-label trials of fluoxetine, sertraline, and paroxetine in various stages of HIV illness reported response rates (including affective and somatic depressive symptoms) between 70% and 90%, and all the medications were well tolerated (Ferrando and Freyberg 2008; Rabkin et al. 1994b). One double-blind, placebo-controlled study of fluoxetine found significant response (Rabkin et al. 1999a). Another similarly designed trial in HIV-infected users of intravenous cocaine and opioids showed significant reduction in depressive symptoms with fluoxetine compared with placebo (Batki et al. 1993).

Supportive group psychotherapy and fluoxetine were found to be superior to placebo plus group therapy for a population of homosexual or bisexual men with HIV, and patients with more severe symptoms tended to achieve greater benefits from medication (Himelhoch et al. 2007b; Zisook et al. 1998). In a comparison of paroxetine and imipramine, both drugs were superior to placebo in patients with HIV and major depression (Elliott et al. 1998). Small open-label trials of venlafaxine, mirtazapine, and nefazodone in patients with major depression and HIV found that response rates were higher than 70%, and few side effects occurred (Elliott and Roy-Byrne 2000; Elliott et al. 1999; Fernandez and Levy 1997).

Fewer specific studies of the treatment of major depression have been conducted in HIV-positive women. In a comparison between fluoxetine and desipramine in women with AIDS, rates of response were 53% and 75%, respectively (Schwartz and McDaniel 1999). A separate trial comparing women taking fluoxetine and sertraline showed response rates of 78% and 75%, respectively (Ferrando et al. 1999).

Major depression in HIV-positive men with testosterone deficiency has been effectively treated with intramuscular testosterone in clinical trials (with 79% response in mood symptoms) (Rabkin et al. 1999b, 2004, 2006) and was replicated in a double-blind, controlled trial (Rabkin et al. 2000b). Dehydroepiandrosterone, a precursor to testosterone, improved mood symptoms during an open-label phase but not during a placebo-controlled discontinuation phase (Rabkin et al. 2000a).

Psychostimulants also have been evaluated for treatment of fatigue, cognitive impairment, and depression in patients with HIV. Open-label trials report an 85% mood response rate in patients with HIV-associated dementia taking methylphenidate (V.F. Holmes et al. 1989) and a 95% mood response rate in men with AIDS taking dextroamphetamine (Wagner et al. 1997). A double-blind trial showed that patients with AIDS and major depression, subthreshold major depression, or dysthymia had a significant response to dextroamphetamine compared with placebo (Wagner and Rabkin 2000). Double-blind comparison of methylphenidate, pemoline, and placebo in patients with HIV (most with AIDS) found improvement in both depressive symptoms and fatigue (Breitbart et al. 2001). No known reports document abuse of prescription stimulants in patients with HIV (Ferrando and Wapenyi 2002).

St. John's wort is often used by patients as alternative antidepressant treatment, but it may lower serum levels of protease inhibitors (Di et al. 2008; "St. John's Wort and HAART" 2000) (see also Chapter 38, "Psychopharmacology"), and patients receiving any HIV treatment should be advised not to take it. *S*-Adenosylmethionine also has been studied in patients with HIV and major depression, with preliminary suggestion of antidepressant efficacy (Shippy et al. 2004).

The side effects of certain antidepressants can render them advantageous or disadvantageous in particular patients with HIV. For example, selective serotonin reuptake inhibitors are best avoided in patients with chronic diarrhea. Sedating antidepressants should be avoided in patients with weakness, lethargy, orthostasis, or other risk for falls. TCAs should be avoided with oral candidiasis because of the aggravating effect of dry mouth on thrush. In cases of anorexia or cachexia, antidepressants with appetite-stimulating effects are best selected.

An important issue is the interaction of antidepressants and HAART medications. Potential interactions are designated in Table 38-2 in Chapter 38, "Psychopharmacology." Two points deserve emphasis. First, particularly because depression is associated with reductions in adherence to HAART, the risks of untreated depression must be measured against those of potential medication interactions. Second, the clinical significance of some of these drug-drug interactions has not yet been clearly established (i.e., dose adjustments are probably not required). This is likely because both antidepressants and HAART, unlike drugs such as warfarin or digoxin, have wide therapeutic indices. Finally, no evidence indicates that antidepressants cause fluctuations in CD4 cell counts (Kumar and Encinosa 2009; Schroecksnadel et al. 2008).

Psychotherapy. The literature on the use of psychotherapy for treatment of depression in HIV-infected patients is extensive, but clinical trial data are sparse. One study showed that interpersonal psychotherapy and supportive psychotherapy with adjunctive use of imipramine were superior to cognitive-behavioral therapy (CBT) or supportive psychotherapy without antidepressants in treating symptoms of depression and improving Karnofsky performance scores (Himelhoch et al. 2007b; Markowitz et al. 1998). Group CBT used alone or in combination with medication also has shown efficacy for HIV-infected patients. Improvements have been reported as well for HIV-positive patients receiving group CBT either as a single treatment modality or combined with medication (Antoni et al. 1991; J. Kelly 1998; Lutgendorf et al. 1997; Safren et al. 2009). Quality of life in women with AIDS also improved after group-based cognitive-behavioral interventions (Berg et al. 2008; Lechner et al. 2003).

A wide range of intrapsychic or interpersonal issues may be the focus of psychotherapy. Supportive psychotherapy can help patients with major depression who interpret their suffering to be a sign of weakness in the face of adversity. These patients often believe that they should pull themselves out of depression and get frustrated when they fail. Education about the disease and nature of their depression, encouragement, and therapeutic optimism all may be helpful. Other issues that arise in psychotherapy include guilt over acquiring HIV; guilt over infecting others; and anger at the source of disease, at oneself, or at God. The diagnosis of HIV infection may lead to precipitous revelation of hidden sexual or drug abuse behavior, eliciting shame and self-loathing. The stigma of HIV may lead to rejection or abandonment by loved ones, and shunning by wider society, making patients feel like lepers. Despite the development of HAART, some patients become hopeless and nihilistic and forgo HIV treatment.

Bipolar Disorder

Prevalence and Clinical Presentation

Patients with preexisting bipolar disorder may experience exacerbations because of the stresses of HIV illness. Perhaps the additional presence of CNS inflammation or degeneration secondary to HIV may also worsen underlying bipolar disorder, and new-onset mania could be a result of the organic insult itself. The first report of mania associated with HIV was in 1984 (Hoffman 1984). Numerous case reports and case series since then have described mania in HIV-infected patients (Lyketsos et al. 1997; Nakimuli-Mpungu et al. 2008).

The prevalence of mania has been found to be increased in patients with AIDS compared with the general population (Atkinson et al. 2009). One report indicated a 17-month prevalence of 1.4% in those with HIV and 8.0% in patients with AIDS, which was 10 times the expected 6-month prevalence in the general population (Lyketsos et al. 1993a). In this group, late-onset patients were less likely to have a personal or family history of mood disorder. Another study among inpatients reported a 29-month prevalence of secondary mania of 1.2% in patients with HIV and 4.3% in those with AIDS (Ellen et al. 1999).

Some have suggested that mania should be subdivided into primary and secondary types, with patients who have the secondary type showing close temporal proximity to an organic insult, no history of illness, essentially negative family history, and late age at onset (Ellen et al. 1999; Nakimuli-Mpungu et al. 2006). Secondary mania includes those cases caused by HIV brain disease itself (Nakimuli-Mpungu et al. 2006, 2008; Robinson 2006), those due to antiretroviral drugs (O'Dowd and McKegney, 1988), and those due to other HIV-related conditions (e.g., cryptococcal meningitis) or medications. Concurrent or subsequent cognitive impairment has been reported among cases of HIV-related mania (Lyketsos et al. 1997; Nakimuli-Mpungu et al. 2008). However, cases without such deficits also have been reported. An increased risk of HIV-associated dementia and cognitive slowing was found in one group of patients with secondary HIV mania, with cognitive decline prior to onset of mania (Lyketsos et al. 1997). In addition, the secondary mania associated with HIV is associated with low CD4 cell count (Nakimuli-Mpungu et al. 2006, 2008), often lower than 100 cells/mm^3. The incidence of secondary mania, like that of HIV-associated dementia, appears to have declined since the widespread use of HAART (Ferrando and Freyberg 2008).

AIDS mania seems to have a clinical profile somewhat different from that of primary mania (Ellen et al. 1999; Lyketsos et al. 1993a, 1997). Irritable mood is often a prominent feature, but elevated mood can be observed. Sometimes prominent psychomotor slowing accompanying the cognitive slowing of AIDS dementia will replace the expected hyperactivity of mania, which complicates the differential diagnosis. AIDS mania is usually quite severe in its presentation and malignant in its course. In one series, patients with late-onset mania (presumed to have AIDS mania) had a greater total number of manic symptoms than did early-onset patients. Late-onset patients also were more commonly irritable and less commonly hyperverbal. AIDS mania seems to be more chronic than episodic, with infrequent spontaneous remissions, and usually relapses with cessation of treatment. Because of their cognitive deficits, patients have little functional reserve to begin with and are less able to pursue treatment independently or consistently.

One presentation of mania, either early or late, is the delusional belief that one has discovered a cure for HIV or has been cured. Although this belief may serve to cheer otherwise demoralized patients, it also may result in the resumption of high-risk behavior and lead to the spread of HIV and exposure to other infections. When euphoria is a prominent symptom in otherwise debilitated late-stage patients, caregivers may question whether to deprive patients of the illusion of happiness. It is the often-devastating effects of the other symptoms of mania that tip the balance toward treatment.

Neuroradiological correlates of secondary HIV mania have been attempted, but the results have been conflicting. Some studies indicate that findings on neuroimaging are not of any clinical significance (Ellen et al. 1999). Abnormal MRI scans have been reported, however (Kieburtz et al. 1991).

Treatment

Treatment of secondary HIV or AIDS mania has not been systematically studied to date, and the optimal treatment remains unclear. Reports often have indicated a particular resistance of manic symptoms to treatment. Others have noted few differences in response in the treatment of secondary HIV mania compared with bipolar disorder (Ellen et al. 1999). The treatment of mania in early-stage HIV infection is not substantially different from the standard treatment of bipolar disorder with mood stabilizers and antipsychotics. As HIV infection advances, with lower CD4 cell counts, more medical complications, more CNS involvement, and greater overall physiological vulnerability, changes in treatment may be required. Treatment with traditional antimanic agents can be very difficult in patients with advanced disease. AIDS mania patients may respond to monotherapy with antipsychotic agents such as risperidone (A. Singh et al. 1997) or mood stabilizers such as carbamazepine (Ellen et al. 1999). Late-stage patients are sensitive to side effects of antipsychotics, especially EPS, as noted earlier in this chapter (see "Treatment" subsection of "Delirium" section). Thus, the dose of antipsychotic required may be much lower than that customarily used for mania. The more advanced these patients' HIV and/or dementia, the more sensitive they are to small dosage increases. These patients are also very sensitive to anticholinergic side effects, including delirium.

There has been considerable experience with traditional mood-stabilizing agents in selected AIDS mania patients, but with relatively little published literature. One case report of lithium use in secondary HIV mania showed control of symptoms at a dose of 1,200 mg/day (Tanquary 1993). Lithium use has been problematic for several reasons, including side effects of cognitive slowing, nausea, diarrhea, and polyuria resulting in dehydration, all of which may already plague HIV-infected patients. The major problem with lithium in AIDS patients has been rapid fluctuations in blood level, especially in the hospital, despite previously stable doses. Anecdotal reports describe problems with administering lithium and valproic acid because of subsequent delirium (Angelino and Treisman 2001).

Valproic acid has been used with success, titrated to the usual therapeutic serum levels of 50–100 μg/L. Enteric-coated valproic acid is better tolerated in many patients. A study of valproic acid in the treatment of HIV-associated mania reported that it was well tolerated and led to significant improvement in manic symptoms, with doses up to 1,750 mg/day and serum levels greater than 50 μg/L (Halman et al. 1993). Another report documented reduction in symptoms with levels of 93 and 110 μg/L (RachBeisel and Weintraub 1997). Concern has been raised over hepatotoxicity in patients with HIV taking valproic acid (Cozza et al. 2000) and potential interactions with antiretroviral therapy (Sheehan et al. 2006). In cases of severe hepatic insufficiency (e.g., *Mycobacterium avium* complex [MAC] infiltration with portal hypertension), valproic acid probably should be avoided, but this has not been studied. Valproic acid also can affect hematopoietic function, so white blood cell and platelet counts must be monitored.

Carbamazepine also was reported to be effective in the treatment of HIV mania in a placebo-controlled trial (Vlassova et al. 2009). However, concerns exist regarding the potential for synergistic bone marrow suppression in combination with antiviral medications and HIV itself. It also may lower serum levels of protease inhibitors (Ferrando and Freyberg 2008). Lamotrigine may be ideal as monotherapy because it is well tolerated in the elderly and is efficacious in treating bipolar disorder (Angelino and Treisman 2008). Potential drug interactions between anticonvulsant mood stabilizers and HAART are shown in Chapter 38, "Psychopharmacology."

The treatment of psychosis in HIV-related mania with risperidone has shown significant improvement (A. Singh et al. 1997). Two case reports note potential drug interactions when combined with the cytochrome P450 2D6 inhibitor ritonavir, including EPS (D.V. Kelly et al. 2002) and a reversible coma from risperidone toxicity (Jover et al. 2002). Olanzapine has been anecdotally reported to be effective in HIV-associated mania (Ferrando and Wapenyi 2002). Remoxipride was found to be effective in HIV-related mania but was subsequently withdrawn because of reports of aplastic anemia (Scurlock et al. 1995). Atypical antipsychotics have the advantage of lower risk of tardive dyskinesia, but this is not an important issue for patients with end-stage AIDS.

Reduction of the risk of EPS is a noteworthy consideration in selecting an antipsychotic, in addition to other factors including affordability. The common side effect of significant weight gain with some atypical antipsychotics is less problematic for patients with HIV who are cachectic.

One case report showed rapid clinical improvement of HIV-associated manic symptoms with clonazepam, allowing reduction of antipsychotic dosage (Budman and Vandersall 1990). No unacceptable side effects were reported, but treatment with benzodiazepines is less useful in maintenance treatment because of tolerance, abuse liability, and cognitive impairment.

Schizophrenia

Prevalence and Clinical Presentation

The literature on patients with severe and chronic mental illnesses, primarily schizophrenia and bipolar disorder, reports HIV prevalence rates of between 2% and 20% in both inpatient and outpatient samples (De Hert et al. 2009; Senn and Carey 2008). Investigators have noted that clinicians working with patients with schizophrenia were often unaware of their increased risk for acquiring HIV and made little effort to screen for seropositivity (Cournos et al. 1991, 2005). Perhaps this is because schizophrenic patients traditionally have been seen as markedly hyposexual because of the illness itself and antipsychotic drugs. However, many schizophrenic patients are sexually active (Cournos et al. 1994), often with higher-risk partners (Kalichman et al. 1994); seldom use condoms (Cournos et al. 1994); and do not otherwise practice safe sex. Substance abuse is very common in schizophrenic patients, including during sexual activity (Cournos et al. 1994; Forney et al. 2007). Patients with schizophrenia have significantly less knowledge about HIV infection and transmission than do persons without schizophrenia (Kalichman et al. 1994; J.A. Kelly et al. 1992). Even increased knowledge about HIV in schizophrenic patients may not lead to decreased risk behaviors (McKinnon et al. 1996). Cumulatively, these factors help explain the increased risk of HIV infection in schizophrenic patients (Cournos et al. 1991, 2005). Suicidality is increased in patients with both schizophrenia and HIV infection. For all these reasons, clinicians should evaluate schizophrenic patients for risk behaviors and for their knowledge about HIV. A validated screening tool—the "Risk Behaviors Questionnaire"—is available (Volavka et al. 1992).

Treatment

Treatment of schizophrenia in HIV-infected patients follows the same basic principles as for other patients with schizophrenia—namely, control of symptoms with medications and psychosocial support and rehabilitation. Close collaboration with HIV providers is strongly suggested, so that HIV treatment can be coordinated. Schizophrenic patients are very likely to have difficulties accessing care, affording medication, and adhering to complex HAART regimens. Educational interventions have promoted safer sexual practices (Jacobs and Bobek 1991; Leucht et al. 2007) and may decrease risk behaviors (Carmen and Brady 1990; Kalichman et al. 1995).

Haloperidol is effective in treating psychotic symptoms of schizophrenia in patients with HIV (Mauri et al. 1997). Patients with HIV may be highly sensitive to the EPS of antipsychotic medications, as already noted. Molindone was reported to be of benefit for psychosis and agitation with few EPS in patients with HIV (Fernandez and Levy 1993). Clozapine also has shown efficacy in treating HIV-associated psychosis in patients with drug-induced parkinsonism (Lera and Zirulnik 1999). Risperidone also has been reported to be effective (A. Singh et al. 1997). However, in one study, two-thirds of patients with schizophrenia and AIDS who received antipsychotic medication did not continue taking antipsychotics (Bagchi et al. 2004). Drug interactions between antipsychotics and HAART are discussed in Chapter 38, "Psychopharmacology."

Substance Abuse and Addiction

Substance abuse is a primary vector for the spread of HIV for those who use injection drugs and their sexual partners and those who are disinhibited by intoxication or driven by addiction to unsafe sexual practices. Patients with substance use disorders may not seek health care or may be excluded from or discriminated against in health care settings. In addition, intoxication and the behaviors necessary to obtain drugs interfere with access to, and effectiveness of, health care.

Triple diagnosis refers to a patient with a dual diagnosis (substance abuse and psychiatric disorder) who also has HIV, and such patients are overrepresented in HIV-infected populations. One study found that as many as 44% of the new entrants to the HIV medical clinic at the Johns Hopkins Hospital had an active substance use disorder. Of these patients, 24% had both a current substance use disorder and another nonsubstance-related Axis I diagnosis (Lyketsos et al. 1994). The Criminal Justice Drug Abuse and Treatment studies show the strongest correlation between comorbid substance abuse and mental illness for risk of contracting HIV (Pearson et al. 2008; Treisman et al. 2001).

In the United States at the end of 2008, the proportion of injection drug users with AIDS had declined to 19% from 24% in 2001 (Centers for Disease Control and Prevention 2008). Even among noninjection drug users, substance abuse plays a major, albeit more subtle, role in HIV transmission. Addiction and high-risk sexual behavior have been linked across a wide range of settings. Addiction has been shown to promote unsafe sexual practices by disinhibition, prostitution, needle sharing, and concentrating patients at high risk into networks of HIV dissemination. Specific drugs have been implicated in different routes of transmission. The advent of drugs that can be rapidly absorbed without injection did not decrease HIV transmission as many had hoped, although it did diminish needle sharing in some groups. This was because the advent of smokable cocaine (crack) and later smokable amphetamine (crystal methamphetamine, crystal meth) led to increased use of these substances. The dramatic increase in the use of crystal methamphetamine is partly a result of the ease of manufacture, the length of time the drug produces intoxication, and the low cost of the drug.

Crack cocaine abusers are more likely to engage in prostitution to obtain money for drugs (Edwards et al. 2006). Men who use crack cocaine are more likely to engage in unprotected anal sex with casual male contacts (Schönnesson et al. 2008). Additionally, methamphetamine has been linked to an upsurge in sexually transmitted HIV in homosexual men who use the drug in conjunction with sildenafil, particularly in group settings (Semple et al. 2009). Methamphetamine increases sexual drive, decreases caution, and increases the desire for intense sexual experiences. Both cocaine and amphetamines are thought to work through the release of dopamine, and dopamine has been shown to increase the uptake of HIV viral particles by macrophages (Gaskill et al. 2009). Alcohol intoxication also can lead to risky sexual behaviors by way of cognitive impairment and disinhibition (Pearson et al. 2008). All of these drugs have been shown to affect medication adherence, the crucial factor in both successful treatment and successful prevention. Poorer medication adherence leads to higher viral loads, making viral transmission more likely, and to the development of resistant virus, increasing the risk of treatment failure. The transmission of resistant virus is also likely to be increased by substance abuse and has become a major problem in HIV treatment.

Neuropsychological testing of drug abusers with and without HIV indicates that substance use can contribute to the cognitive decline of HIV-associated dementia (Pakesch et al. 1992). Substance use may augment HIV replication in the CNS and increase HIV encephalopathy in early AIDS (Kenedi et al. 2008; Kibayashi et al. 1996). For example, cocaine abuse augments HIV replication in vitro (Kenedi et al. 2008) and also increases permeability of the blood-brain barrier to HIV (Zhang et al. 1998).

Treatment

Substance abuse can be successfully treated in those at risk for HIV. One of the most extensively studied interventions in risk reduction is methadone maintenance, which resulted in sustained reductions in HIV risk and lower incidence of HIV infection (Davstad et al. 2009). Linked programs providing model care for HIV-infected patients with triple (i.e., HIV, substance abuse, and psychiatric) diagnoses have shown promising results. Methadone can be linked to directly observed therapy for HIV, which has been shown to improve outcome. Model programs of fully integrated care providing HIV treatment, substance abuse treatment, and psychiatric treatment have been shown to improve outcome as well (Himelhoch et al. 2007a).

Substance Use Disorders and Interaction With HIV Treatment

The medical sequelae of chronic substance abuse accelerate the process of immunocompromise and amplify the burdens of HIV infection. Injection drug users are at higher risk for developing bacterial infections such as pneumonia, sepsis, and endocarditis. Tuberculosis, STDs, viral hepatitis, coinfection with human CD4 cell lymphotrophic virus, and lymphomas also occur more commonly in injection drug users with HIV than in other patients with HIV. HIV-infected injection drug users are at higher risk for fungal or bacterial infections of the CNS. Alcohol abuse is immunosuppressive and increases risk for bacterial infections, tuberculosis, and dementia. Heroin may worsen HIV-associated nephropathy.

Important drug interactions occur between abused substances and antiretroviral and antibiotic drugs. Rifampin increases the elimination of methadone and may result in withdrawal symptoms. Decreased plasma levels of methadone also occur with concurrent administration of ritonavir, nelfinavir, efavirenz, and nevirapine (Kharasch et al. 2008a, 2008b). Patients in a methadone program will be unlikely to take medications that have caused withdrawal.

Posttraumatic Stress Disorder

Posttraumatic stress disorder (PTSD) and its symptoms occur at greatly increased rates in HIV-infected patients (A. Martinez et al. 2002). Of the HIV-infected women attending county medical clinics, 42% met diagnostic criteria for PTSD (Cottler et al. 2001) with a lifetime prevalence of 40% (Martin and Kagee 2008). Minority women (Hien et al. 2010) and women prisoners (Hutton et al. 2001; Lewis 2005) are particularly at risk for both PTSD and HIV. Male veterans with a diagnosis of PTSD are at increased risk for HIV infection, especially if they are substance abusers (Fuller et al. 2009; Hoff et al. 1997). PTSD symptoms are associated with high-risk behaviors, including prostitution, choosing other high-risk sexual partners, injection drug use, and unsafe sexual practices (Martin and Kagee 2008). Among the HIV-infected female partners of male drug users, those who had a history of rape or being assaulted were more likely to engage in high-risk HIV behaviors (Hien et al. 2010). These studies are cross-sectional and cannot determine causality. PTSD from early-life trauma may predispose an individual to engage in high-risk sexual or drug behavior. On the other hand, risk behaviors such as prostitution and drug abuse increase exposure to trauma and thus the likelihood of developing PTSD. Finally, HIV infection itself may be the cause of PTSD (Boarts et al. 2009). Rates of PTSD in response to HIV infection are higher than those in response to other debilitating illnesses (Fauerbach et al. 1997), including cancer (Alter et al. 1996). In one study, about 30% of persons recently diagnosed with HIV subsequently developed PTSD, with half of the cases appearing within 1 month of HIV diagnosis (B. Kelly et al. 1998). Prior PTSD increased the risk for PTSD in response to HIV diagnosis. Even asymptomatic HIV-infected individuals have high levels of PTSD symptoms (Botha 1996), and occupational exposure to HIV also has resulted in PTSD (Worthington et al. 2006).

PTSD in at-risk or HIV-infected individuals is significant for several reasons. PTSD has high rates of psychiatric comorbidity (up to 80%), most often depression (Leserman et al. 2008), and cocaine and opioid abuse (Kessler et al. 1995), which are also risks for HIV (Lyketsos and Federman 1995). HIV-infected persons with PTSD have higher levels of pain (Tsao et al. 2004). PTSD symptoms in HIV-positive patients predicted lower CD4 cell counts (Fincham et al. 2008; Leserman et al. 2008) and lower CD4-to-CD8 T cell ratios (Kimerling et al. 1999). This may represent faster HIV disease progression, generally associated with stressful life events (Leserman et al. 2008).

Persons at risk for HIV and HIV-infected individuals should be routinely screened for PTSD and psychiatric comorbidities, with treatment targeted accordingly. Failure to do so in this very high-risk population has serious consequences, both for this population's welfare and for public health.

Issues of Personality in Patients Infected With HIV

A disturbing trend in the HIV epidemic has been the persistence of modifiable risk factors among persons who are HIV infected. Such individuals, who report high rates of sexual and/or drug risk behaviors, include HIV-infected drug users (Latkin et al. 2009), patients presenting at HIV primary care clinics for medical treatment (Beyer et al. 2007), and HIV-infected men who have sex with other men (Fox et al. 2009). The fact that knowledge of HIV and its transmission is insufficient to deter these individuals from engaging in HIV risk behaviors suggests that certain personality characteristics may enhance a person's tendency to engage in such behaviors.

Traditional approaches in risk reduction counseling emphasize the avoidance of negative consequences in the future, such as condom use during sexual intercourse to prevent STDs. Such educational approaches have proved ineffective for individuals with certain personality characteristics (Vlassova et al. 2009). Effective prevention and treatment programs for HIV-infected individuals must consider specific personality factors. In this section, we outline the role of personality characteristics and personality disorders in the risk of acquiring HIV and highlight specific interventions to reduce the risk of HIV that are formulated for individuals whose personality characteristics place them at increased risk.

Implications of Personality for HIV Risk Behavior

Our clinical experience suggests that unstable extroverts are the most prone to engage in practices that place them at risk for HIV. We estimate that in the psychiatry service of the Johns Hopkins AIDS clinic (a referral-biased sample), about 60% of our patients present with this blend of extroversion and emotional instability. These individuals are preoccupied by, and act on, their feelings, which are labile, leading to unpredictable and inconsistent behavior. Most striking is the inconsistency between thought and action. Regardless of intellectual ability or knowledge of HIV, unstable extroverts can engage in extremely risky behavior. Past experience and future consequences have little importance in decision making for the individual who is ruled by feeling; the present is paramount. Their primary goal is to achieve immediate pleasure or removal of pain, regardless of circumstances. As part of their emotional instability, they experience intense fluctuations in mood. It is difficult for them to tolerate painful affects; they want to escape or avoid feelings as quickly as possible. They are motivated to pursue pleasurable experiences, however risky, to eliminate negative moods.

Unstable extroverts are more likely to engage in behavior that places them at risk for HIV infection and are more likely to pursue sex promiscuously. They are less likely to plan and carry condoms and more likely to have unprotected vaginal or anal sex. They are more fixed on the reward of sex and remarkably inattentive to the STD they may acquire if they do not use a condom. Unstable extroverts are also less likely to accept the diminution of pleasure associated with the use of condoms or, once aroused, to interrupt the "heat of the moment" to use condoms. Similarly, unstable extroverts are more vulnerable to alcohol and drug abuse. They are drawn to alcohol and drugs as a quick route to pleasure. They are more likely to experiment with different kinds of drugs and to use greater quantities. Unstable extroverts are also more likely to become injection drug users.

The second most common personality type that we have observed, which may represent about 25% of our patients, is that of the stable extrovert. Stable extroverts are also present oriented and pleasure seeking; however, their emotions are not as intense, as easily provoked, or as mercurial. Hence they are not as strongly driven to achieve pleasure. Stable extroverts may be at risk because they are too optimistic or sanguine to believe that they will become infected with HIV.

Introverted personalities appear to be less common among our psychiatric patients. Their focus on the future, avoidance of negative consequences, and preference for cognition over feeling render them more likely to engage in protective and preventive behaviors. HIV risk for introverts is determined by the dimension of emotional instability–stability. About 14% of our patients present with a blend of introversion and instability. Unstable introverts are anxious, moody, and pessimistic. Typically, these patients seek drugs and/or sex not for pleasure, but for relief or distraction from pain. They are concerned about the future and adverse outcomes but believe that they have little control over their fates. Stable introverts constitute the remaining 1% of patients. These patients, with their controlled, even-tempered personalities, are least likely to engage in risky or hedonistic behaviors. Typically, these individuals are HIV positive as a result of a blood transfusion or an occupational needle stick. These percentages of personality styles are illustrative of one center's experience and may not be generalizable.

Personality Disorders in HIV

Prevalence rates of personality disorders among HIV-infected patients (19%–36%) and individuals at risk for HIV (15%–20%) (Hansen et al. 2009) are high and significantly exceed rates found in the general population (10%) (J.G. Johnson et al. 1995). The most common personality disorders among HIV-infected patients are antisocial and borderline types (Bennett et al. 2009). Antisocial personality disorder is the most common (Perkins et al. 1993) and is a risk factor for HIV infection (Weissman 1993). Individuals with personality disorder, particularly antisocial personality disorder, have high rates of substance abuse and are more likely to inject drugs and share needles compared with those without an Axis II diagnosis (Hansen et al. 2009). Approximately half of drug abusers may meet criteria for a diagnosis of antisocial personality disorder. Individuals with antisocial personality disorder are also more likely to have higher numbers of lifetime sexual partners, engage in unprotected anal sex, and contract STDs compared with individuals without antisocial personality disorder (Ladd and Petry 2003).

In our AIDS clinic, patients are characterized along the dimensions of extraversion–introversion and emotional stability–instability rather than in the discrete categories provided by DSM's Axis II for several reasons. First, it is easier for staff to determine where a patient falls along two dimensions than to evaluate the many criteria for personality disorders. Second, it is simpler to design intervention strategies for two dimensions. Third, a diagnosis of antisocial or borderline personality disorder can be stigmatizing, particularly in a general medical clinic. Finally, a classification system based on a continuum approach may be a better predictor of HIV risk behavior than are DSM-IV-TR Axis II categories (American Psychiatric Association 2000a; Tourian et al. 1997).

Effect of Personality on Medication Adherence

Identifying factors that influence adherence in HIV disease is important in improving overall health outcomes (Koenig et al. 2008; Murri et al. 2009). Adherence is especially challenging in HIV, which carries all of the components of low adherence, long duration of treatment, preventive rather than curative treatment, asymptomatic periods, and frequent and complex medication dosing (Koenig et al. 2008; Murri et al. 2009).

Our clinical experience suggests that nonadherence is more common among our extraverted or unstable patients. The same personality characteristics that place them at risk for HIV also reduce their ability to adhere to demanding drug regimens. Specifically, their present-time orientation, combined with reward-seeking behavior, makes it more difficult to tolerate side effects from drugs whose benefits may not be immediately apparent. It is also difficult for feeling-driven individuals to maintain consistent, well-ordered routines, so following frequent, rigid dosing schedules is problematic. Our unstable extroverted patients usually intend to follow the schedule, but their chaotic and mercurial emotions interfere and disrupt daily routines. For example, a patient may report that he felt very upset and nihilistic after a fight with a family member and missed several doses of his antiretroviral medicines. Missing doses of HAART can increase the chance of HIV resistance developing.

Treatment Implications

We have found that a cognitive-behavioral approach is most effective in treating patients who present with extroverted and/or emotionally unstable personalities. Five principles guide our care:

1. *Focus on thoughts, not feelings.* Individuals with unstable extroverted personalities often do not recognize the extent to which their actions are driven by feelings of the moment.
2. *Use a behavioral contract for all patients to build consistency.* The contract outlines goals for treatment and responsibilities and expectations of both the patient and the providers.
3. *Emphasize constructive rewards.* Positive outcomes, not adverse consequences, are salient to extroverts. Most of the patients have already experienced negative consequences from their behavior. Exhortations to use condoms to avoid STDs are unpersuasive. More success has been achieved with extroverts by eroticizing the use of condoms (Tanner and Pollack 1988) or by incorporating novel techniques into sexual repertoires (Abramson and Pinkerton 1995). Similarly, the rewards of abstaining from drugs or alcohol are emphasized, such as having money to buy clothing, having a stable home, or maintaining positive relationships with children. In building adherence to antiretroviral therapies, the focus is on the rewards of an increased CD4 cell count and reduced viral load rather than on the avoidance of illness. Use of the viral load as a strategy to build adherence can increase acceptance in all patients but is especially effective in reward-driven extroverts.
4. *Use relapse prevention techniques.* The relapse prevention model, originally developed for treatment of substance abuse behavior, is an effective method for changing habitual ways of behaving.
5. *Develop a coordinated treatment plan.* The mental health professional coordinates with the medical care provider, supplying information about a patient's personality and how it influences behavior. Both professionals work in tandem to develop behavioral contracts to reduce HIV risk behaviors and build medication adherence.

Psychosocial Interventions to Prevent HIV Transmission

In intervention studies of men who have sex with other men (still the largest subgroup in terms of new HIV infections in the United States), many psychosocial interventions have shown a decrease in either risk behaviors or infection (Dilley et al. 2002; Fox et al. 2009; W.D. Johnson et al. 2002, 2008). A meta-analysis examining the effect of HIV prevention strategies found that psychosocial interventions can lead to sexual risk reduction among drug users (Semaan et al. 2002), as did a separate large study of cocaine-dependent patients (Woody et al. 2003). Studied interventions have included stress management and relaxation techniques, group counseling, education, cognitive training, negotiation skills training, psychotherapy directed at emotional distress reduction, relapse prevention models of high-risk behavior reduction, education directed at eroticizing safer sex, assertiveness training, and peer education in bars. All of these interventions showed a modest effect on either risk behavior or HIV infection. Although most studies focused on men who have sex with other men, the results have been similar in heterosexually transmitted HIV, women, injection drug users, and adolescents (DiClemente et al. 2008). It is unclear from the data what the best intervention is and how to stratify the interventions. The HIV notification rates for men having sex with men, which declined in the second half of the 1990s, have shown a slight increase beginning in 2000 (Sullivan et al. 2009). This is an indication that effective preventive interventions need to be studied further and implemented worldwide.

Mental Health Care for Patients With HIV Infection

Patients with HIV infection are underserved with regard to mental health. This is critical because psychiatric disorders increase the risk for HIV and have a negative effect on HIV treatment. Although model clinics exist, in which treatment for HIV, substance abuse, and psychiatric illness is integrated, these clinics are exceptional. Psychiatric disorders are underrecognized and undertreated in patients with many chronic medical conditions, but HIV-infected patients are especially likely to be impoverished, disenfranchised, vulnerable, and members of underserved minorities, all of which further decrease the likelihood that they will receive adequate treatment. Integrated expert care by psychiatrists and other mental health professionals should be a high priority both to promote effective treatment of HIV infection and to stem the tide of an epidemic that spreads through modifiable behaviors.

Conclusion

The interrelations between HIV/AIDS and psychiatry are myriad and complex. In a sense, psychiatric disorders can be seen as vectors of HIV transmission, through associated high-risk behaviors. They also complicate the treatment of HIV infection. HIV causes several psychiatric conditions and exacerbates many others. Comorbid psychopathology, including major depression, schizophrenia, addictions, personality vulnerabilities such as unstable extroversion, and the effects of traumatic life experiences, is highly prevalent in patients with HIV/AIDS. Each of these problems has the potential to sabotage treatment for HIV infection and its many complications. Yet there is a profound shortage of funding and availability of psychiatric care in HIV clinics. Our experience in caring for HIV patients is that by developing a comprehensive diagnostic formulation on which to base treatment, even many of the most difficult patients can be successfully treated.

With the advent of HAART, we have seen terminal patients who have undergone nearly miraculous recoveries only to find themselves unprepared to meet the challenges of facing life again—of pressing on in the face of the daily burdens of ongoing treatment, side effects, stigma, and continuing injury. To assist them with this monumental task is a great challenge, but we have the lessons from the field of psychiatry that have helped patients shoulder similar burdens from chronic mental illness. At the heart of our work, we try to impart hope for the future, therapeutic optimism, advocacy, sanctuary, and rehabilitation.

References

Abramson PR, Pinkerton SD: With Pleasure: Thoughts on the Nature of Human Sexuality. New York, Oxford University Press, 1995

Alciati A, Gallo L, Monforte AD, et al: Major depression related immunological changes and combination antiretroviral therapy in HIV-seropositive patients. Hum Psychopharmacol 22:33–40, 2007

Alfonso CA, Cohen MA: HIV-dementia and suicide. Gen Hosp Psychiatry 16:45–46, 1994

Alter CL, Pelcovitz D, Axelrod A, et al: Identification of PTSD in cancer survivors. Psychosomatics 37:137–143, 1996

American Psychiatric Association: Diagnostic and Statistical Manual of Mental Disorders, 4th Edition, Text Revision. Washington, DC, American Psychiatric Association, 2000a

American Psychiatric Association, Work Group on HIV/AIDS: Practice guideline for the treatment of patients with HIV/AIDS. Am J Psychiatry 157 (11 suppl):1–62, 2000b

Andraghetti R, Foran S, Colebunders R, et al: Euthanasia: from the perspective of HIV infected persons in Europe. HIV Med 2:3–10, 2001

Angelino AF, Treisman GJ: Management of psychiatric disorders in patients infected with human immunodeficiency virus. Clin Infect Dis 33:847–856, 2001

Angelino AF, Treisman GJ: Issues in co-morbid severe mental illnesses in HIV infected individuals. Int Rev Psychiatry 20:95–101, 2008

Antoni MH, Baggett L, Ironson G, et al: Cognitive-behavioral stress management buffers distress responses and immunologic changes following notification of HIV-1 seropositivity. J Consult Clin Psychol 59:906–915, 1991

Atkinson JH, Higgins JA, Vigil O, et al: Psychiatric context of acute/early HIV infection: the NIMH Multisite Acute HIV Infection Study: IV. AIDS Behav 13:1061–1067, 2009

Bagchi A, Sambamoorthi U, McSpiritt E, et al: Use of antipsychotic medications among HIV-infected individuals with schizophrenia. Schizophr Res 71:435–444, 2004

Barker PB, Lee RR, McArthur JC: AIDS dementia complex: evaluation with proton MR spectroscopic imaging. Radiology 195:58–64, 1995

Batki SL, Manfredi LB, Murphy JM, et al: Randomized, placebo-controlled trial of paroxetine versus imipramine in depression in HIV-infected injection drug users. Abstract (PO-B16-1685) presented at International Conference on AIDS, Berlin, Germany, June 1993

Bennett WR, Joesch JM, Mazur M, et al: Characteristics of HIV-positive patients treated in a psychiatric emergency department. Psychiatr Serv 60:398–401, 2009

Berg C, Raminani S, Greer J, et al: Participants' perspectives on cognitive-behavioral therapy for adherence and depression in HIV. Psychother Res 18:271–280, 2008

Beyer JL, Taylor L, Gersing KR, et al: Prevalence of HIV infection in a general psychiatric outpatient population. Psychosomatics 48:31–37, 2007

Bhaskaran K, Mussini C, Antinori A, et al: Changes in the incidence and predictors of human immunodeficiency virus-associated dementia in the era of highly active antiretroviral therapy. Ann Neurol 63:213–221, 2008

Bialer PA, Wallack JJ, Snyder SL: Psychiatric diagnosis in HIV-spectrum disorders. Psychiatr Med 9:361–375, 1991

Boarts JM, Buckley-Fischer BA, Armelie AP, et al: The impact of HIV diagnosis-related vs. non-diagnosis related trauma on PTSD, depression, medication adherence, and HIV disease markers. J Evid Based Soc Work 6:4–16, 2009

Bolokadze N, Gabunia P, Ezugbaia M, et al: Neurological complications in patients with HIV/AIDS. Georgian Med News (165):34–38, 2008

Botha KIT: Posttraumatic stress disorder and illness behaviour in HIV+ patients. Psychol Rep 79:843–845, 1996

Breitbart W, Marotta R, Platt M, et al: A double-blind trial of haloperidol, chlorpromazine and lorazepam in the treatment of delirium in hospitalized AIDS patients. Am J Psychiatry 153:231–237, 1996

Breitbart W, McDonald MV, Rosenfeld B, et al: Fatigue in ambulatory AIDS patients. J Pain Symptom Manage 15:159–167, 1998

Breitbart W, Rosenfeld B, Kaim M, et al: A randomized, double-blind, placebo-controlled trial of psychostimulants for the treatment of fatigue in ambulatory patients with human immunodeficiency virus disease. Arch Intern Med 161:411–420, 2001

Brew BJ, Halman M, Catalan J, et al: Factors in AIDS dementia complex trial design: results and lessons from the abacavir trial. PLoS Clin Trials 2(3):e13, 2007

Brown GR: The use of methylphenidate for cognitive decline associated with HIV disease. Int J Psychiatry 25:21–37, 1995

Budman CL, Vandersall TA: Clonazepam treatment of acute mania in an AIDS patient. J Clin Psychiatry 51:212, 1990

Campos LN, Guimarães MD, Remien RH: Anxiety and depression symptoms as risk factors for non-adherence to antiretroviral therapy in Brazil. AIDS Behav 14:289–299, 2010

Carmen E, Brady SM: AIDS risk and prevention in the chronic mentally ill. Hosp Community Psychiatry 41:652–657, 1990

Carrico AW, Johnson MO, Morin SF, et al: Correlates of suicidal ideation among HIV-positive persons. AIDS 21:1199–1203, 2007

Centers for Disease Control and Prevention: HIV/AIDS Surveillance Report, 2006. Available at: http://www.cdc.gov. Accessed May 2009.

Centers for Disease Control and Prevention: Diagnoses of HIV Infection and AIDS in the United States and Dependent Areas, 2008 (HIV Surveillance Report, Vol 20). Available at: http://www.cdc.gov/hiv/surveillance/resources/reports/2008report/index.htm. Accessed June 2010.

Chang L, Ernst T, Leonido-Yee M, et al: Cerebral metabolite abnormalities correlate with clinical severity of HIV-1 cognitive motor complex. Neurology 52:100–108, 1999

Chang L, Speck O, Miller E, et al: Neural correlates of attention and working memory deficits in HIV patients. Neurology 57:1001–1007, 2001

Chetchotisakd P, Sungkanuparph S, Thinkhamrop B, et al: A multicentre, randomized, double-blind, placebo-controlled trial of primary cryptococcal meningitis prophylaxis in HIV-infected patients with severe immune deficiency. HIV Med 5:140–143, 2004

Ciesla JA, Roberts JE: Meta-analysis of the relationship between HIV infection and risk for depressive disorders. Am J Psychiatry 158:725–730, 2001

Clifford DB: Human immunodeficiency virus-associated dementia. Arch Neurol 57:321–324, 2000

Conen A, Fehr J, Glass TR, et al: Self-reported alcohol consumption and its association with adherence and outcome of antiretroviral therapy in the Swiss HIV Cohort Study. Antivir Ther 14:349–357, 2009

Cottler LB, Nishith P, Compton WM III: Gender differences in risk factors for trauma exposure and post-traumatic stress disorder among inner-city drug abusers in and out of treatment. Compr Psychiatry 42:111–117, 2001

Cournos F, Empfield M, Horwath E, et al: HIV seroprevalence among patients admitted to two psychiatric hospitals. Am J Psychiatry 48:1225–1230, 1991

Cournos F, Guido JR, Coomaraswamy S, et al: Sexual activity and risk of HIV infection among patients with schizophrenia. Am J Psychiatry 151:228–232, 1994

Cournos F, McKinnon K, Sullivan G: Schizophrenia and comorbid human immunodeficiency virus or hepatitis C virus. J Clin Psychiatry 66 (suppl 6):27–33, 2005

Cozza KL, Swanton EJ, Humphreys CW: Hepatotoxicity with combination of valproic acid, ritonavir, and nevirapine: a case report. Psychosomatics 41:452–453, 2000

Cysique LA, Deutsch R, Atkinson JH, et al: Incident major depression does not affect neuropsychological functioning in HIV-infected men. J Int Neuropsychol Soc 13:1–11, 2007

Czub S, Koutsilieri E, Sopper S, et al: Enhancement of CNS pathology in early simian immunodeficiency virus infection by dopaminergic drugs. Acta Neuropathol 101:85–91, 2001

Dana Consortium on the Therapy of HIV Dementia and Related Cognitive Disorders: Safety and tolerability of the antioxidant OPC-14117 in HIV-associated cognitive impairment. Neurology 49:142–146, 1997

Dana Consortium on the Therapy of HIV Dementia and Related Cognitive Disorders: A randomized, double-blind, placebo-controlled trial of deprenyl and thioctic acid in human immunodeficiency virus-associated cognitive impairment. Neurology 50:645–651, 1998

Davis HF, Skolasky R Jr, Selnes OA, et al: Assessing HIV-associated dementia: modified HIV Dementia Scale versus the grooved pegboard. AIDS Reader 12:29–31, 38, 2002

Davstad I, Stenbacka M, Leifman A, et al: An 18-year follow-up of patients admitted to methadone treatment for the first time. J Addict Dis 28:39–52, 2009

De Hert M, Wampers M, Van Eyck D, et al: Prevalence of HIV and hepatitis C infection among patients with schizophrenia. Schizophr Res 108:307–308, 2009

Descamps M, Hyare H, Stebbing J, et al: Magnetic resonance imaging and spectroscopy of the brain in HIV disease. J HIV Ther 13:55–58, 2008

Dettling M, Muller-Oerlinghausen B, Britsch P: Clozapine treatment of HIV-associated psychosis: too much bone marrow toxicity? Pharmacopsychiatry 31:156–157, 1998

Di YM, Li CG, Xue CC, et al: Clinical drugs that interact with St. John's wort and implication in drug development. Curr Pharm Des 14:1723–1742, 2008

DiClemente RJ, Crittenden CP, Rose E, et al: Psychosocial predictors of HIV-associated sexual behaviors and the efficacy of prevention interventions in adolescents at-risk for HIV infection: what works and what doesn't work? Psychosom Med 70:598–605, 2008

Dilley JW, Woods WJ, Sabatino J, et al: Changing sexual behavior among gay male repeat testers for HIV: a randomized, controlled trial of a single-session intervention. J Acquir Immune Defic Syndr 30:177–186, 2002

Dimatteo MR, Lepper HS, Croghan TW: Depression is a risk factor for noncompliance with medical treatment: meta-analysis of the effects of anxiety and depression on patient adherence. Arch Intern Med 160:2101–2107, 2000

Dolan Looby SE, Collins M, Lee H, et al: Effects of long-term testosterone administration in HIV-infected women: a randomized, placebo-controlled trial. AIDS 23:951–959, 2009

Dolder CR, Patterson TL, Jeste DV: HIV, psychosis and aging: past, present and future. AIDS 18 (suppl 1):S35–S42, 2004

Dore GJ, Correll PK, Li Y, et al: Changes to AIDS dementia complex in the era of highly active antiretroviral therapy. AIDS 13:1249–1253, 1999

Dunlop O, Bjørklund R, Bruun JN, et al: Early psychomotor slowing predicts the development of HIV dementia and autopsy-verified HIV encephalitis. Acta Neurol Scand 105:270–275, 2002

Duran S, Spire B, Raffi F, et al: Self-reported symptoms after initiation of a protease inhibitor in HIV-infected patients and their impact on adherence to HAART. HIV Clin Trials 2:38–45, 2001

Edwards JM, Halpern CT, Wechsberg WM: Correlates of exchanging sex for drugs or money among women who use crack cocaine. AIDS Educ Prev 18:420–429, 2006

Ellen SR, Judd FK, Mijch AM, et al: Secondary mania in patients with HIV infection. Aust N Z J Psychiatry 33:353–360, 1999

Elliott AJ, Roy-Byrne PP: Mirtazapine for depression in patients with human immunodeficiency virus (letter). J Clin Psychopharmacol 20:265–267, 2000

Elliott AJ, Uldall KK, Bergam K, et al: Randomized, placebo-controlled trial of paroxetine versus imipramine in depressed HIV-positive outpatients. Am J Psychiatry 155:367–372, 1998

Elliott AJ, Russo J, Bergam K, et al: Antidepressant efficacy in HIV-seropositive outpatients with major depressive disorder: an open trial of nefazodone. J Clin Psychiatry 60:226–231, 1999

Engsig FN, Hansen AB, Omland LH, et al: Incidence, clinical presentation and outcome of progressive multifocal leukoencephalopathy in HIV-infected patients during the highly active antiretroviral therapy era: a nationwide cohort study. J Infect Dis 199:77–83, 2009

Ernst T, Chang L, Jovicich J, et al: Abnormal brain activation on functional MRI in cognitively asymptomatic HIV patients. Neurology 59:1343–1349, 2002

Fauerbach JA, Lawrence J, Haythornthwaite J, et al: Preburn psychiatric history affects post-trauma morbidity. Psychosomatics 38:374–385, 1997

Fernandez F, Levy JK: The use of molindone in the treatment of psychotic and delirious patients infected with the human immunodeficiency virus: case reports. Gen Hosp Psychiatry 15:31–35, 1993

Fernandez F, Levy J: Efficacy of venlafaxine in HIV-depressive disorders. Psychosomatics 38:173–174, 1997

Ferrando SJ, Freyberg Z: Treatment of depression in HIV positive individuals: a critical review. Int Rev Psychiatry 20:61–71, 2008

Ferrando S, Wapenyi K: Psychopharmacological treatment of patients with HIV and AIDS. Psychiatr Q 73:33–49, 2002

Ferrando SJ, Rabkin JG, de Moore G, et al: Antidepressant treatment of depression in HIV+ women. J Clin Psychiatry 60:741–746, 1999

Fincham D, Smit J, Carey P, et al: The relationship between behavioural inhibition, anxiety disorders, depression and CD4 counts in HIV-positive adults: a cross-sectional controlled study. AIDS Care 20:1279–1283, 2008

Forney JC, Lombardo S, Toro PA: Diagnostic and other correlates of HIV risk behaviors in a probability sample of homeless adults. Psychiatr Serv 58:92–99, 2007

Forstein M, Cournos F, Douaihy A, et al: Guideline Watch: Practice Guideline for the Treatment of Patients With HIV/AIDS. Arlington, VA, American Psychiatric Association, 2006. Available at: http://www.psychiatryonline.com/content.aspx?aid=147976. Accessed May 13, 2009.

Fox J, White PJ, Macdonald N, et al: Reductions in HIV transmission risk behaviour following diagnosis of primary HIV infection: a cohort of high-risk men who have sex with men. HIV Med 10:432–438, 2009

Fuller BE, Loftis JM, Rodriguez VL, et al: Psychiatric and substance use disorders comorbidities in veterans with hepatitis C virus and HIV coinfection. Curr Opin Psychiatry 22:401–408, 2009

Gallo P, Piccinno MG, Krzalic L, et al: Tumor necrosis factor alpha (TNF alpha) and neurological diseases: failure in detecting TNF alpha in the cerebrospinal fluid from patients with multiple sclerosis, AIDS dementia complex, and brain tumours. J Neuroimmunol 23:41–44, 1989

Gaskill PJ, Calderon TM, Luers AJ, et al: Human immunodeficiency virus (HIV) infection of human macrophages is increased by dopamine: a bridge between HIV-associated neurologic disorders and drug abuse. Am J Pathol 175:1148–1159, 2009

Gibbie T, Hay M, Hutchison CW, et al: Depression, social support and adherence to highly active antiretroviral therapy in people living with HIV/AIDS. Sex Health 4:227–232, 2007

Gonzalez-Scarano F, Martin-Garcia J: The neuropathogenesis of AIDS. Nat Rev Immunol 5:69–81, 2005

Halman M, Rourke SB: HAART and neuropsychological impairment: neuroscience in HIV infection, Edinburgh 22–24 June 2000 (abstract 03). J Neurovirol 6:246, 2000

Halman MM, Worth JL, Sanders KM, et al: Anticonvulsant use in the treatment of manic syndromes in patients with HIV-1 infection. J Clin Neuropsychiatry Clin Neurosci 5:430–434, 1993

Handelsman L, Aronson M, Maurer G, et al: Neuropsychological and neurological manifestations of HIV-1 dementia in drug users. J Neuropsychiatry Clin Neurosci 4:21–28, 1992

Hansen NB, Cavanaugh CE, Vaughan EL, et al: The influence of personality disorder indication, social support, and grief on alcohol and cocaine use among HIV-positive adults coping with AIDS-related bereavement. AIDS Behav 13:375–384, 2009

Harris GJ, Pearlson GD, McArthur JC, et al: Altered cortical blood flow in HIV-seropositive individuals with and without dementia: a single photon emission computed tomography study. AIDS 8:495–499, 1994

Hartgers C, Van Den Hoek JAR, Coutinho RA, et al: Psychopathology, stress and HIV-risk injecting behaviour among drug users. Br J Addict 87:857–865, 1992

Hatherill S, Flisher A: Delirium in Children With HIV/AIDS. J Child Neurol 24:879–883, 2009

Heseltine PNR, Goodkin K, Atkinson JH, et al: Randomized double-blind placebo-controlled trial of peptide T for HIV-associated cognitive impairment. Arch Neurol 55:41–51, 1998

Hien DA, Campbell AN, Killeen T, et al: The impact of trauma-focused group therapy upon HIV sexual risk behaviors in the NIDA Clinical Trials Network "Women and trauma" multisite study. AIDS Behav 14:421–430, 2010]

Himelhoch S, Medoff DR: Efficacy of antidepressant medication among HIV-positive individuals with depression: a systematic review and meta-analysis. AIDS Patient Care STDS 19:813–822, 2005

Himelhoch S, McCarthy JF, Ganoczy D, et al: Understanding associations between serious mental illness and HIV among patients in the VA Health System. Psychiatr Serv 58:1165–1172, 2007a

Himelhoch S, Medoff DR, Oyeniyi G: Efficacy of group psychotherapy to reduce depressive symptoms among HIV-infected individuals: a systematic review and meta-analysis. AIDS Patient Care STDS 21:732–739, 2007b

Hinkin CH, Castellon SA, Hardy DJ, et al: Methylphenidate improves HIV-1-associated cognitive slowing. J Neuropsychiatry Clin Neurosci 13:248–254, 2001

Hirshfield S, Wolitski RJ, Chiasson MA, et al: Screening for depressive symptoms in an online sample of men who have sex with men. AIDS Care 20:904–910, 2008

Hoff RA, Beam-Goulet J, Rosenheck RA: Mental disorder as a risk factor for human immunodeficiency virus infection in a sample of veterans. J Nerv Ment Dis 185:556–560, 1997

Hoffman RS: Neuropsychiatric complications of AIDS. Psychosomatics 25:393–400, 1984

Holland NR, Power C, Mathews VP, et al: Cytomegalovirus encephalitis in acquired immunodeficiency syndrome (AIDS). Neurology 44:507–514, 1994

Holmes J, House A: Psychiatric illness predicts poor outcome after surgery for hip fracture: a prospective cohort study. Psychol Med 30:921–929, 2000

Holmes VF, Fernandez F, Levy JK: Psychostimulant response in AIDS-related complex patients. J Clin Psychiatry 50:5–8, 1989

Hriso E, Kuhn T, Masdeu JC, et al: Extrapyramidal symptoms due to dopamine-blocking agents in patients with AIDS encephalopathy. Am J Psychiatry 148:1558–1561, 1991

Hutton HE, Treisman GJ, Hunt WR, et al: HIV risk behaviors and their relationship to posttraumatic stress disorder among women prisoners. Psychiatr Serv 52:508–513, 2001

Hwang J, Zheng LT, Ock J, et al: Inhibition of glial inflammatory activation and neurotoxicity by tricyclic antidepressants. Neuropharmacology 55:826–834, 2008

Ickovics JR, Hamburger ME, Vlahov D, et al: Mortality, CD4 cell count decline, and depressive symptoms among HIV-seropositive women: longitudinal analysis from the HIV epidemiology research study. JAMA 285:1466–1474, 2001

Itoh K, Mehraein P, Weis S: Neuronal damage of the substantia nigra in HIV-1 infected brains. Acta Neuropathol (Berl) 99:376–384, 2000

Jacobs P, Bobek SC: Sexual needs of the schizophrenic client. Perspect Psychiatr Care 27:15–20, 1991

Jellinger KA, Setinek U, Drlicek M, et al: Neuropathology and general autopsy findings in AIDS during the last 15 years. Acta Neuropathol 100:213–220, 2000

Johnson JG, Williams JBW, Rabkin JG, et al: Axis I psychiatric symptomatology associated with HIV infection and personality disorder. Am J Psychiatry 152:551–554, 1995

Johnson WD, Hedges LV, Ramirez G, et al: HIV prevention research for men who have sex with men: a systematic review and meta-analysis. J Acquir Immune Defic Syndr 30 (suppl 1):S118–S129, 2002

Johnson WD, Diaz RM, Flanders WD, et al: Behavioral interventions to reduce risk for sexual transmission of HIV among men who have sex with men. Cochrane Database Syst Rev (3):CD001230, 2008

Joska JA, Gouse H, Paul RH, et al: Does highly active antiretroviral therapy improve neurocognitive function? A systematic review. J Neurovirol 16:101–114, 2010

Jover F, Cuadrado JM, Andreu L, et al: Reversible coma caused by risperidone-ritonavir interaction. Clin Neuropharmacol 25:251–253, 2002

Jowi JO, Mativo PM, Musoke SS: Clinical and laboratory characteristics of hospitalised patients with neurological manifestations of HIV/AIDS at the Nairobi hospital. East Afr Med J 84:67–76, 2007

Kalayjian RC, Cohen ML, Bonomo RA, et al: Cytomegalovirus ventriculoencephalitis in AIDS: a syndrome with distinct clinical and pathologic features. Medicine (Baltimore) 72:67–77, 1993

Kalichman SC, Sikkema KJ, Kelly JA, et al: Factors associated with risk for HIV infection among chronic mentally ill adults. Am J Psychiatry 15:221–227, 1994

Kalichman SC, Sikkema KJ, Kelly JA, et al: Use of a brief behavioral skills intervention to prevent HIV infection among chronic mentally ill adults. Psychiatr Serv 46:275–280, 1995

Kaplan JE, Benson C, Holmes KH, et al: Guidelines for prevention and treatment of opportunistic infections in HIV-infected adults and adolescents: recommendations from CDC, the National Institutes of Health, and the HIV Medicine Association of the Infectious Diseases Society of America. MMWR Recomm Rep 58(RR-4):1–207, 2009

Kaul M: HIV-1 associated dementia: update on pathological mechanisms and therapeutic approaches. Curr Opin Neurol 22:315–320, 2009

Kelly B, Raphael B, Judd F, et al: Posttraumatic stress disorder in response to HIV infection. Gen Hosp Psychiatry 20:345–352, 1998

Kelly DV, Béïque LC, Bowmer MI: Extrapyramidal symptoms with ritonavir/indinavir plus risperidone. Ann Pharmacother 36:827–830, 2002

Kelly J: Group psychotherapy for persons with HIV and AIDS-related illnesses. Int J Group Psychother 98:143–162, 1998

Kelly JA, Murphy DA, Bahn GR, et al: AIDS/HIV risk behaviour among the chronic mentally ill. Am J Psychiatry 149:886–889, 1992

Kenedi CA, Joynt KE, Goforth HW: Comorbid HIV encephalopathy and cocaine use as a risk factor for new-onset seizure disorders. CNS Spectr 13:230–234, 2008

Kessler RC, Sonega A, Bromer E: Posttraumatic stress disorder in the National Comorbidity Survey. Arch Gen Psychiatry 52:1048–1060, 1995

Kharasch ED, Bedynek PS, Park S, et al: Mechanism of ritonavir changes in methadone pharmacokinetics and pharmacodynamics, I: evidence against CYP3A mediation of methadone clearance. Clin Pharmacol Ther 84:497–505, 2008a

Kharasch ED, Bedynek PS, Walker A, et al: Mechanism of ritonavir changes in methadone pharmacokinetics and pharmacodynamics, II: ritonavir effects on CYP3A and P-glycoprotein activities. Clin Pharmacol Ther 84:506–512, 2008b

Kibayashi K, Mastri AR, Hirsch CS: Neuropathology of human immunodeficiency virus infection at different disease stages. Hum Pathol 27:637–642, 1996

Kieburtz KD, Epstein LG, Gelbard HA, et al: Excitotoxicity and dopaminergic dysfunction in the acquired immunodeficiency syndrome dementia complex: therapeutic implications. Arch Neurol 48:1281–1284, 1991

Kimerling R, Calhoun KS, Forehand R, et al: Traumatic stress in HIV-infected women. AIDS Educ Prev 11:321–330, 1999

Kirkland LR, Fischl MA, Tashima KT, et al: Response to lamivudine-zidovudine plus abacavir twice daily in antiretroviral-naive, incarcerated patients with HIV infection taking directly observed treatment. Clin Infect Dis 34:511–518, 2002

Klausner JD, Wolf W, Fischer-Ponce L, et al: Tracing a syphilis outbreak through cyberspace. JAMA 284:447–449, 2000

Knapp PE, Storer TW, Herbst KL, et al: Effects of a supraphysiological dose of testosterone on physical function, muscle performance, mood, and fatigue in men with HIV-associated weight loss. Am J Physiol Endocrinol Metab 294:E1135–E1143, 2008

Koenig LJ, Pals SL, Bush T, et al: Randomized controlled trial of an intervention to prevent adherence failure among HIV-infected patients initiating antiretroviral therapy. Health Psychol 27:159–169, 2008

Kong A, Edmonds P: Testosterone therapy in HIV wasting syndrome: systematic review and meta-analysis. Lancet Infect Dis 4:187–188, 2003

Kopicko JJ, Momodu I, Adedokun A, et al: Characteristics of HIV-infected men with low serum testosterone levels. Int J STD AIDS 10:817–820, 1999

Koutsilieri E, Sopper S, Scheller C, et al: Parkinsonism in HIV dementia. J Neural Transm 109:767–775, 2002

Krikorian R, Wrobel AJ, Meinecke C, et al: Cognitive deficits associated with human immunodeficiency virus encephalopathy. J Neuropsychiatry Clin Neurosci 2:256–260, 1990

Kumar V, Encinosa W: Effects of antidepressant treatment on antiretroviral regimen adherence among depressed HIV-infected patients. Psychiatr Q 80:131–141, 2009

Kupfer MC, Zee CS, Colletti PM, et al: MRI evaluation of AIDS-related encephalopathy: toxoplasmosis vs. lymphoma. Magn Reson Imaging 8:51–57, 1990

Ladd GT, Petry NM: Antisocial personality in treatment-seeking cocaine abusers: psychosocial functioning and HIV risk. J Subst Abuse Treat 24:323–330, 2003

Latkin CA, Kuramoto SJ, Davey-Rothwell MA, et al: Social norms, social networks, and HIV risk behavior among injection drug users. AIDS Behav May 23, 2009 [Epub ahead of print]

Laverda AM, Gallo P, De Rossi A, et al: Cerebrospinal fluid analysis in HIV-1-infected children: immunological and virological findings before and after AZT therapy. Acta Paediatr 83:1038–1042, 1994

Lechner SC, Antoni MH, Lydston D, et al: Cognitive-behavioral interventions improve quality of life in women with AIDS. J Psychosom Res 54:253–261, 2003

Lee R, Monteiro EF: Third regional audit of antiretroviral prescribing in HIV patients. Yorkshire Audit Group for HIV Related Diseases. Int J STD AIDS 14:58–60, 2003

Lenz G, Demal U: Quality of life in depression and anxiety disorders: an exploratory follow-up after intensive cognitive-behavior therapy. Psychopathology 33:297–302, 2000

Lera G, Zirulnik J: Pilot study with clozapine in patients with HIV-associated psychosis and drug-induced parkinsonism. Mov Disord 14:128–131, 1999

Leserman J, Barroso J, Pence BW, et al: Trauma, stressful life events and depression predict HIV-related fatigue. AIDS Care 20:1258–1265, 2008

Leso L, Schwartz TL: Ziprasidone treatment of delirium. Psychosomatics 43:61–62, 2002

Letendre SL, van den Brande G, Hermes A, et al: Lopinavir with ritonavir reduces the HIV RNA level in cerebrospinal fluid. Clin Infect Dis 45(11), October 19, 2007 [Epub ahead of print]

Letendre S, Marquie-Beck J, Capparelli E, et al: Validation of the CNS Penetration-Effectiveness rank for quantifying antiretroviral penetration into the central nervous system. Arch Neurol 65:65–70, 2008

Leucht S, Burkard T, Henderson J, et al: Physical illness and schizophrenia: a review of the literature. Acta Psychiatr Scand 116:317–333, 2007

Lewis CF: Post-traumatic stress disorder in HIV-positive incarcerated women. J Am Acad Psychiatry Law 33:455–464, 2005

Liau A, Millett G, Marks G: Meta-analytic examination of online sex-seeking and sexual risk behavior among men who have sex with men. Sex Transm Dis 33:576–584, 2006

Liu H, Golin CE, Miller LG, et al: A comparison study of multiple measures of adherence to HIV protease inhibitors. Ann Intern Med 134:968–977, 2001

Lopez-Villegas D, Lenkinski RE, Frank I: Biochemical changes in the frontal lobe of HIV-infected individuals detected by magnetic resonance spectroscopy. Proc Natl Acad Sci U S A 94:9854–9859, 1997

Louhivuori KA, Hakama M: Risk of suicide among cancer patients. Am J Epidemiol 109:50–65, 1979

Lutgendorf S, Antoni MH, Ironson G, et al: Cognitive-behavioral stress management decreases dysphoric mood and herpes simplex virus-type 2 antibody titers in symptomatic HIV-seropositive gay men. J Consult Clin Psychol 65:31–43, 1997

Lyketsos CG, Federman EB: Psychiatric disorders and HIV infection: impact on one another. Epidemiol Rev 17:152–164, 1995

Lyketsos CG, Hanson AL, Fishman M, et al: Manic syndrome early and late in the course of HIV. Am J Psychiatry 150:326–327, 1993a

Lyketsos CG, Hoover DR, Guccione M, et al: Depressive symptoms as predictors of medical outcomes in HIV infection: Multicenter AIDS Cohort Study. JAMA 270:2563–2567, 1993b

Lyketsos CG, Hanson A, Fishman M, et al: Screening for psychiatric morbidity in a medical outpatient clinic for HIV infection: the need for a psychiatric presence. Int J Psychiatry Med 24:103–113, 1994

Lyketsos CG, Hoover DR, Guccione M, et al: Changes in depressive symptoms as AIDS develops. Am J Psychiatry 153:1430–1437, 1996a

Lyketsos CG, Hutton H, Fishman M, et al: Psychiatric morbidity on entry to an HIV primary care clinic. AIDS 10:1033–1039, 1996b

Lyketsos CG, Schwartz J, Fishman M, et al: AIDS mania. J Neuropsychiatry Clin Neurosci 9:277–279, 1997

Madden M, Lenhart A: Online dating: report prepared by the Pew Internet and American Life Project. March 2006. Available at: http://www.pewinternet.com/Reports/2006/Online-Dating.aspx?r=1. Accessed May 2010.

Maggi P, de Mari M, Moramarco A, et al: Parkinsonism in a patient with AIDS and cerebral opportunistic granulomatous lesions. Neurol Sci 21:173–176, 2000

Maj M, Satz P, Janssen R, et al: WHO Neuropsychiatric AIDS Study, cross-sectional phase II: neuropsychological and neurological findings. Arch Gen Psychiatry 51:51–61, 1994

Malta M, Strathdee SA, Magnanini MM, et al: Adherence to antiretroviral therapy for human immunodeficiency virus/acquired immune deficiency syndrome among drug users: a systematic review. Addiction 103:1242–1257, 2008

Manning D, Jacobsberg L, Erhart S, et al: The efficacy of imipramine in the treatment of HIV-related depression. Abstract (Th.B.32) presented at the International Conference on AIDS, San Francisco, CA, June 20–23, 1990

Mao L, Kidd MR, Rogers G, et al: Social factors associated with major depressive disorder in homosexually active, gay men attending general practices in urban Australia. Aust N Z J Public Health 33:83–86, 2009

Marcellin F, Préau M, Ravaux I, et al: Self-reported fatigue and depressive symptoms as main indicators of the quality of life (QOL) of patients living with HIV and hepatitis C: implications for clinical management and future research. HIV Clin Trials 8:320–327, 2007

Markowitz JC, Kocsis JH, Fishman B, et al: Treatment of depressive symptoms in human immunodeficiency virus-positive patients. Arch Gen Psychiatry 55:452–457, 1998

Martin L, Kagee A: Lifetime and HIV-related PTSD among persons recently diagnosed with HIV. AIDS Behav Dec 12, 2008 [Epub ahead of print]

Martinez A, Israelski D, Walker C, et al: Posttraumatic stress disorder in women attending human immunodeficiency virus outpatient clinics. AIDS Patient Care STDS 16:283–291, 2002

Martinez E, Garcia-Viejo MA, Marcos MA, et al: Discontinuation of secondary prophylaxis for cryptococcal meningitis in HIV-infected patients responding to highly active antiretroviral therapy. AIDS 14:2615–2617, 2000

Masliah E, De Teresa RM, Mallory RE, et al: Changes in pathological findings at autopsy in AIDS cases for the last 15 years. AIDS 14:69–74, 2000

Mauri MC, Fabiano L, Bravin S, et al: Schizophrenic patients before and after HIV infection: a case-control study. Encephale 23:437–441, 1997

McArthur J: HIV dementia: an evolving disease. J Neuroimmunol 157:3–10, 2004

McArthur JC, Becker PS, Parisi JE, et al: Neuropathological changes in early HIV dementia. Ann Neurol 26:681–684, 1989

McArthur JC, Hoover DR, Bacellar H, et al: Dementia in AIDS patients: incidence and risk factors. Multicenter AIDS Cohort Study. Neurology 43:2245–2252, 1993

McDermott BE, Sautter FJ, Winstead DK, et al: Diagnosis, health beliefs, and risk of HIV infection in psychiatric patients. Hosp Community Psychiatry 45:580–585, 1994

McKegney FP, O'Dowd MA, Feiner C, et al: A prospective comparison of neuropsychologic function in HIV-seropositive and seronegative methadone-maintained patients. AIDS 4:565–569, 1990

McKinnon K, Cournos F, Sugden R, et al: The relative contributions of psychiatric symptoms and AIDS knowledge to HIV risk behaviors among people with severe mental illness. J Clin Psychiatry 57:506–513, 1996

McKirnan D, Houston E, Tolou-Shams M: Is the Web the culprit? Cognitive escape and Internet sexual risk among gay and bisexual men. AIDS Behav 11:151–160, 2007

McNabb J, Ross JW, Abriola K, et al: Adherence to highly active antiretroviral therapy predicts outcome at an inner-city human immunodeficiency virus clinic. Clin Infect Dis 33:700–705, 2001

Meade CS, Hansen NB, Kochman A, et al: Utilization of medical treatments and adherence to antiretroviral therapy among HIV-positive adults with histories of childhood sexual abuse. AIDS Patient Care STDS 23:259–266, 2009

Mellins CA, Havens JF, McDonnell C, et al: Adherence to antiretroviral medications and medical care in HIV-infected adults diagnosed with mental and substance abuse disorders. AIDS Care 21:168–177, 2009

Mello VA, Segurado AA, Malbergier A: Depression in women living with HIV: clinical and psychosocial correlates. Arch Womens Ment Health 13:193–199, 2010

Meltzer-Brody S, Davidson JR: Completeness of response and quality of life in mood and anxiety disorders. Depress Anxiety 12 (suppl 1):95–101, 2000

Meyer JM, Marsh J, Simpson G: Differential sensitivities to risperidone and olanzapine in a human immunodeficiency virus patient. Biol Psychiatry 44:791–794, 1998

Meyerhoff DJ, Bloomer C, Cardenas V, et al: Elevated subcortical choline metabolites in cognitively and clinically asymptomatic HIV+ patients. Neurology 52:995–1003, 1999

Mintz M, Tardieu M, Hoyt L, et al: Levodopa therapy improves motor function in HIV-infected children with extrapyramidal syndromes. Neurology 47:1583–1585, 1996

Miro JM, Lopez JC, Podzamczer D, et al: Discontinuation of primary and secondary toxoplasma gondii prophylaxis is safe in HIV-infected patients after immunological restoration with highly active antiretroviral therapy: results of an open, randomized, multicenter clinical trial. Clin Infect Dis 43:79–89, 2006

Mirsattari SM, Power C, Nath A: Parkinsonism with HIV infection. Mov Disord 13:684–689, 1998

Murri R, Guaraldi G, Lupoli P, et al: Rate and predictors of self-chosen drug discontinuations in highly active antiretroviral therapy-treated HIV-positive individuals. AIDS Patient Care STDS 23:35–39, 2009

Nakimuli-Mpungu E, Musisi S, Mpungu SK, et al: Primary mania versus HIV-related secondary mania in Uganda. Am J Psychiatry 163:1349–1354, 2006

Nakimuli-Mpungu E, Musisi S, Kiwuwa Mpungu S, et al: Early onset versus late-onset HIV-related secondary mania in Uganda. Psychosomatics 49:530–534, 2008

Nath A, Maragos WF, Avison MJ, et al: Acceleration of HIV dementia with methamphetamine and cocaine. J Neurovirol 7:66–71, 2001

Navia BA, Jordan BD, Price RW: The AIDS dementia complex, I: clinical features. Ann Neurol 19:517–524, 1986

Navia BA, Dafni U, Simpson D, et al (for the AIDS Clinical Trials Group): A phase I/II trial of nimodipine for HIV-related neurologic complications. Neurology 51:221–228, 1998

O'Dowd MA, McKegney FP: Manic syndrome associated with zidovudine (letter). JAMA 260:3587, 1988

Oh J, Hegele RA: HIV-associated dyslipidaemia: pathogenesis and treatment. Lancet Infect Dis 7:787–796, 2007

Olsen WL, Longo FM, Mills CM, et al: White matter disease in AIDS: findings at MR imaging. Radiology 169:445–448, 1988

Pakesch G, Loimer N, Grunberger J, et al: Neuropsychological findings and psychiatric symptoms in HIV-1 infected and non-infected drug users. Psychiatry Res 41:163–177, 1992

Park BJ, Wannemuehler KA, Marston BJ, et al: Estimation of the current global burden of cryptococcal meningitis among persons living with HIV/AIDS. AIDS 23:525–530, 2009

Paterson DL, Swindells S, Mohn J, et al: Adherence to protease inhibitor therapy and outcomes in patients with HIV infection. Ann Intern Med 133:21–30, 2000

Pearson FS, Cleland CM, Chaple M, et al: Substance use, mental health problems, and behavior at risk for HIV: evidence from CJDATS. J Psychoactive Drugs 40:459–469, 2008

Pence BW, Barroso J, Leserman J, et al: Measuring fatigue in people living with HIV/AIDS: psychometric characteristics of the HIV related fatigue scale. AIDS Care 20:829–837, 2008

Perkins DO, Davidson EJ, Leserman J, et al: Personality disorder in patients infected with HIV: a controlled study with implications for clinical care. Am J Psychiatry 150:309–315, 1993

Perry S, Jacobsberg LD, Fishman B, et al: Psychiatric diagnosis before serological testing for the human immunodeficiency virus. Am J Psychiatry 147:89–93, 1990

Pirskanen-Matell R, Grützmeier S, Nennesmo I, et al: Impairment of short-term memory and Korsakoff syndrome are common in AIDS patients with cytomegalovirus encephalitis. Eur J Neurol 16:48–53, 2009

Post MJD, Levin BE, Berger JR, et al: Sequential cranial MR findings of asymptomatic and neurologically symptomatic HIV+ subjects. Am J Neuroradiol 13:359–370, 1992

Powderly WG: Cryptococcal meningitis in HIV-infected patients. Curr Infect Dis Rep 2:352–357, 2000

Price RW, Brew BJ: The AIDS dementia complex. J Infect Dis 158:1079–1083, 1988

Rabkin JG, Remien R, Katoff L, et al: Suicidality in AIDS long-term survivors: what is the evidence? AIDS Care 5:401–411, 1993

Rabkin JG, Rabkin R, Harrison W, et al: Effect of imipramine on mood and enumerative measures of immune status in depressed patients with HIV illness. Am J Psychiatry 151:516–523, 1994a

Rabkin JG, Rabkin R, Wagner G: Effects of fluoxetine on mood and immune status in depressed patients with HIV illness. J Clin Psychiatry 55:92–97, 1994b

Rabkin JG, Wagner GJ, Rabkin R: Fluoxetine treatment for depression in patients with HIV and AIDS: a randomized, placebo-controlled trial. Am J Psychiatry 156:101–107, 1999a

Rabkin JG, Wagner GJ, Rabkin R: Testosterone therapy for human immunodeficiency virus-positive men with and without hypogonadism. J Clin Psychopharmacol 19:19–27, 1999b

Rabkin JG, Ferrando SJ, Wagner G, et al: DHEA treatment of men and women with HIV infection. Psychoneuroendocrinology 25:53–68, 2000a

Rabkin JG, Wagner GJ, Rabkin R: A double-blind, placebo-controlled trial of testosterone therapy for HIV-positive men with hypogonadal symptoms. Arch Gen Psychiatry 57:141–147, 2000b

Rabkin JG, Wagner GJ, McElhiney MC, et al: Testosterone versus fluoxetine for depression and fatigue in HIV/AIDS: a placebo-controlled trial. J Clin Psychopharmacol 24:379–385, 2004

Rabkin JG, McElhiney MC, Rabkin R, et al: Placebo-controlled trial of dehydroepiandrosterone (DHEA) for treatment of nonmajor depression in patients with HIV/AIDS. Am J Psychiatry 163:59–66, 2006

RachBeisel JA, Weintraub E: Valproic acid treatment of AIDS-related mania. J Clin Psychiatry 58:406–407, 1997

Rebchook GM, Kegeles SM, Huebner D, et al: Translating research into practice: the dissemination and initial implementation of an evidence-based HIV prevention program. AIDS Educ Prev 18 (4 suppl A):119–136, 2006

Robinson RG: Primary mania versus secondary mania of HIV/AIDS in Uganda. Am J Psychiatry 163:1309–1311, 2006

Robinson-Papp J, Elliott KJ, Simpson DM: HIV-related neurocognitive impairment in the HAART era. Curr HIV/AIDS Rep 6:146–152, 2009

Robotin MC, Law MG, Milliken S, et al: Clinical features and predictors of survival of AIDS-related non-Hodgkin's lymphoma in a population-based case series in Sydney, Australia. HIV Med 5:377–384, 2004

Roc AC, Ances BM, Chawla S, et al: Detection of human immunodeficiency virus induced inflammation and oxidative stress in lenticular nuclei with magnetic resonance spectroscopy despite antiretroviral therapy. Arch Neurol 64:1249–1257, 2007

Rosci MA, Pignorini F, Bernabei A, et al: Methods for detecting early signs of AIDS dementia complex in asymptomatic subjects: a quantitative tomography study of 18 cases. AIDS 6:1309–1316, 1996

Rottenberg DA, Sidtis JJ, Strother SC, et al: Abnormal cerebral glucose metabolism in HIV-1 seropositive subjects with and without dementia. J Nucl Med 37:1133–1141, 1996

Roux P, Carrieri MP, Villes V, et al: The impact of methadone or buprenorphine treatment and ongoing injection on highly active antiretroviral therapy (HAART) adherence: evidence from the MANIF2000 cohort study. Addiction 103:1828–1836, 2008

Sacktor N: The epidemiology of human immunodeficiency virus-associated neurological disease in the era of highly active antiretroviral therapy. J Neuroviral 2:115–121, 2002

Sacktor N, Lyles RH, Skolasky R, et al: HIV-associated neurologic disease incidence changes: Multicenter AIDS Cohort Study, 1990–1998. Neurology 56:257–260, 2001

Safren SA, O'Cleirigh C, Tan JY, et al: A randomized controlled trial of cognitive behavioral therapy for adherence and depression (CBT-AD) in HIV-infected individuals. Health Psychol 28:1–10, 2009

Scamvougeras A, Rosebush PI: AIDS-related psychosis with catatonia responding to low-dose lorazepam. J Clin Psychiatry 53:414–415, 1992

Schifitto G, Sacktor N, Marder K, et al (for the Neurological AIDS Research Consortium): Randomized, placebo-controlled trial of the PAF antagonist lexipafant in HIV-associated cognitive impairment. Neurology 53:391–396, 1999

Schifitto G, Navia BA, Yiannoutsos CT, et al: Memantine and HIV-associated cognitive impairment: a neuropsychological and proton magnetic resonance spectroscopy study. AIDS 21:1877–1886, 2007

Schönnesson LN, Atkinson J, Williams ML, et al: A cluster analysis of drug use and sexual HIV risks and their correlates in a sample of African-American crack cocaine smokers with HIV infection. Drug Alcohol Depend 97:44–53, 2008

Schroecksnadel K, Sarcletti M, Winkler C, et al: Quality of life and immune activation in patients with HIV-infection. Brain Behav Immun 22:881–889, 2008

Schwartz JAJ, McDaniel JS: Double-blind comparison of fluoxetine and desipramine in the treatment of depressed women with advanced HIV disease: a pilot study. Depress Anxiety 9:70–74, 1999

Scurlock H, Singh A, Catalan J: Atypical antipsychotic drugs in the treatment of manic syndromes in patients with HIV-1 infection. J Psychopharmacol 9:151–154, 1995

Semaan S, Des Jarlais DC, Sogolow E, et al: A meta-analysis of the effect of HIV prevention interventions on the sex behaviors of drug users in the United States. J Acquir Immune Defic Syndr 30 (suppl 1):S73–S93, 2002

Semple SJ, Zians J, Strathdee SA, et al: Sexual marathons and methamphetamine use among HIV-positive men who have sex with men. Arch Sex Behav 38:583–590, 2009

Senn TE, Carey MP: HIV, STD, and sexual risk reduction for individuals with a severe mental illness: review of the intervention literature. Curr Psychiatry Rev 4:87–100, 2008

Sevigny JJ, Albert SM, McDermott MP, et al: Evaluation of HIV RNA and markers of immune activation as predictors of HIV-associated dementia. Neurology 63:2084–2090, 2004

Sewell DD, Jeste DV, McAdams LA, et al: Neuroleptic treatment of HIV-associated psychosis. HNRC group. Neuropsychopharmacology 10:223–229, 1994

Sheehan NL, Brouillette MJ, Delisle MS, et al: Possible interaction between lopinavir/ritonavir and valproic acid exacerbates bipolar disorder. Ann Pharmacother 40:147–150, 2006

Sherr L, Lampe F, Fisher M, et al: Suicidal ideation in UK HIV clinic attenders. AIDS 22:1651–1658, 2008

Shippy RA, Mendez D, Jones K, et al: S-adenosylmethionine (SAM-e) for the treatment of depression in people living with HIV/AIDS. BMC Psychiatry 4:38, 2004

Singh A, Golledge H, Catalan J: Treatment of HIV-related psychotic disorders with risperidone: a series of 21 cases. J Psychosom Res 42:489–493, 1997

Skinner S, Adewale AJ, DeBlock L, et al: Neurocognitive screening tools in HIV/AIDS: comparative performance among patients exposed to antiretroviral therapy. HIV Med 10:246–252, 2009

Sledjeski EM, Delahanty DL, Bogart LM: Incidence and impact of posttraumatic stress disorder and comorbid depression on adherence to HAART and CD4+ counts in people living with HIV. AIDS Patient Care STDs 19:728–736, 2005

St. John's wort and HAART. AIDS Patient Care STDS 14:281–283, 2000

Stern Y, McDermott MP, Albert S, et al: Factors associated with incident human immunodeficiency virus-dementia. Arch Neurol 58:473–479, 2001

Sullivan PS, Dworkin MS: Prevalence and correlates of fatigue among patients with HIV infection. J Pain Symptom Manage 25:329–333, 2003

Sullivan PS, Hamouda O, Delpech V, et al: Reemergence of the HIV epidemic among men who have sex with men in North America, Western Europe, and Australia, 1996–2005. Ann Epidemiol 19:423–431, 2009

Suwanwelaa N, Phanuphak P, Phanthumchinda K, et al: Magnetic resonance spectroscopy of the brain in neurologically asymptomatic HIV-infected patients. Magn Reson Imaging 18:859–865, 2000

Tanner WM, Pollack RH: The effect of condom use and erotic instructions on attitudes towards condoms. J Sex Res 25:537–541, 1988

Tanquary J: Lithium neurotoxicity at therapeutic levels in an AIDS patient. J Nerv Ment Dis 181:519–520, 1993

Tashima K, Alt E, Harwell J, et al: Internet sex-seeking leads to acute HIV infection: a report of two cases. Int J STD AIDS 14:285–286, 2003

Thurnher MM, Schindler EG, Thurnher SA, et al: Highly active antiretroviral therapy for patients with AIDS dementia complex: effect on MR imaging findings and clinical course. Am J Neuroradiol 21:670–678, 2000

Tourian K, Alterman A, Metzger D, et al: Validity of three measures of antisociality in predicting HIV risk behaviors in methadone-maintenance patients. Drug Alcohol Depend 47:99–107, 1997

Tozzi V, Balestra P, Galgani S, et al: Changes in neurocognitive performance in a cohort of patients treated with HAART for 3 years. J Acquir Immune Defic Syndr Hum Retrovirol 28:19–27, 2001

Tozzi V, Balestra P, Lorenzini P, et al: Prevalence and risk factors for human immunodeficiency virus-associated neurocognitive impairment, 1996 to 2002: results from an urban observational cohort. J Neurovirol 11:265–273, 2005

Treisman GJ, Angelino AF, Hutton HE: Psychiatric issues in the management of patients with HIV infection. JAMA 286:2857–2864, 2001

Tsao JC, Dobalian A, Naliboff BD: Panic disorder and pain in a national sample of persons living with HIV. Pain 109:172–180, 2004

Tyor WR, Glass JD, Griffin JW, et al: Cytokine expression in the brain during the acquired immunodeficiency syndrome. Ann Neurol 31:349–360, 1992

Uldall KK, Berghuis JP: Delirium in AIDS patients: recognition and medication factors. AIDS Patient Care STDS 11:435–441, 1997

Uldall KK, Harris VL, Lalonde B: Outcomes associated with delirium in acutely hospitalized acquired immune deficiency syndrome patients. Compr Psychiatry 41:88–91, 2000a

Uldall KK, Ryan R, Berghuis JP, et al: Association between delirium and death in AIDS patients. AIDS Patient Care STDS 14:95–100, 2000b

UNAIDS Joint United Nations Programme on HIV/AIDS: Report on the Global AIDS Epidemic. August 2008. Available at: http://viewer.zmags.com/publication/ad3eab7c#/ad3eab7c/1. Accessed May 2009.

Uthman OA, Abdulmalik JO: Adjunctive therapies for AIDS dementia complex. Cochrane Database Syst Rev (3):CD006496, 2008

van Servellen G, Chang B, Garcia L, et al: Individual and system level factors associated with treatment nonadherence in human immunodeficiency virus-infected men and women. AIDS Patient Care STDS 16:269–281, 2002

Vidal JE, Penalva de Oliveira AC, Fink MC, et al: AIDS-related progressive multifocal leukoencephalopathy: a retrospective study in a referral center in São Paulo, Brazil. Rev Inst Med Trop Sao Paulo 50:209–212, 2008

Vlassova N, Angelino AF, Treisman GJ: Update on mental health issues in patients with HIV infection. Curr Infect Dis Rep 11:163–169, 2009

Vogl D, Rosenfeld B, Breitbart W, et al: Symptom prevalence, characteristics, and distress in AIDS outpatients. J Pain Symptom Manage 18:253–262, 1999

Volavka J, Convit A, O'Donnell J, et al: Assessment of risk behaviors for HIV infection among psychiatric inpatients. Hosp Community Psychiatry 43:482–485, 1992

Voss J, Portillo CJ, Holzemer WL, et al: Symptom cluster of fatigue and depression in HIV/AIDS. J Prev Interv Community 33:19–34, 2007

Wagner GJ, Ghosh-Dastidar B: Electronic monitoring: adherence assessment or intervention? HIV Clin Trials 3:45–51, 2002

Wagner GJ, Rabkin R: Effects of dextroamphetamine on depression and fatigue in men with HIV: a double-blind, placebo-controlled trial. J Clin Psychiatry 61:436–440, 2000

Wagner G, Rabkin J, Rabkin R: Illness stage, concurrent medications, and other correlates of low testosterone in men with HIV illness. J Acquir Immune Defic Syndr Hum Retrovirol 8:204–207, 1995

Wagner GJ, Rabkin JG, Rabkin R: Dextroamphetamine as a treatment for depression and low energy in AIDS patients: a pilot study. J Psychosom Res 42:407–411, 1997

Wagner GJ, Kanouse DE, Koegel P, et al: Adherence to HIV antiretrovirals among persons with serious mental illness. AIDS Patient Care STDS 17:179–186, 2003

Weissman MM: The epidemiology of personality disorders: a 1990 update. J Personal Disord 7(suppl):44–62, 1993

Wesselingh SL, Glass J, McArthur JC, et al: Cytokine dysregulation in HIV-associated neurological disease. Adv Neuroimmunol 4:199–206, 1994

Wiley CA, Masliah E, Morey M, et al: Neocortical damage during HIV infection. Ann Neurol 29:651–657, 1991

Wilkie FL, Eisdorfer C, Morgan R, et al: Cognition in early human immunodeficiency virus infection. Arch Neurol 41:433–440, 1990

Wojna V, Skolasky RL, Hechavarría R, et al: Prevalence of human immunodeficiency virus-associated cognitive impairment in a group of Hispanic women at risk for neurological impairment. J Neurovirol 12:356–364, 2006

Woody GE, Gallop R, Luborsky L, et al: HIV risk reduction in the National Institute on Drug Abuse Cocaine Collaborative Treatment Study. J Acquir Immune Defic Syndr 33:82–87, 2003

Worthington MG, Ross JJ, Bergeron EK: Posttraumatic stress disorder after occupational HIV exposure: two cases and a literature review. Infect Control Hosp Epidemiol 27:215–217, 2006

Zhang L, Looney D, Taub D, et al: Cocaine opens the blood-brain barrier to HIV-1 invasion. J Neurovirol 4:619–626, 1998

Zilikis N, Nimatoudis I, Kiosses V, et al: Treatment with risperidone of an acute psychotic episode in a patient with AIDS. Gen Hosp Psychiatry 20:384–385, 1998

Zisook S, Peterkin J, Goggin KJ, et al: Treatment of major depression in HIV-seropositive men. J Clin Psychiatry 59:217–224, 1998

CHAPTER 29

Dermatology

Madhulika A. Gupta, M.D., F.R.C.P.C.

James L. Levenson, M.D.

DERMATOLOGICAL DISORDERS are associated with psychiatric and psychosocial comorbidity in 25%–30% of cases (Gupta and Gupta 1996). The skin is the largest organ of the body and functions as a social, psychological, and metabolically active biological interface between the individual and the environment. Beginning at birth, the skin functions as a powerful organ of communication—at the social, psychological, and biological levels. The skin and its appendages are well innervated with a dense network of afferent sensory nerves and efferent autonomic nerves. The afferent sensory nerves convey sensations for touch, pain, itch, temperature, and other physical stimuli. The efferent autonomic—mainly sympathetic—nerves play a role in maintaining cutaneous homeostasis by regulating vasomotor and pilomotor functions and the activity of the apocrine and eccrine sweat glands. Stimulation of the skin, which is richly innervated and has bilateral communication with the central nervous system (CNS), serves as a means of regulating affect and coping with intense emotional states.

As an organ of communication, the skin plays a vital role in attachment, starting in infancy. Freud observed that during early development, the ego was rooted in the body, especially the skin. Bodily sensations and experiences, both internal and from the surface of the body, form the core around which the ego develops. The skin reacts to emotional states such as extreme fear, anxiety, and embarrassment with blanching, increased perspiration, flushing, and blushing. In addition, even minimal flaws in the overall appearance of the skin can have a profound effect on the body image of the individual, especially in adolescents, and can result in body image pathology.

The impact of psychological stress on the skin is not necessarily primarily mediated by the CNS but instead appears to be mediated by a local stress response system in the skin that further interacts with the CNS. The skin (Arck et al. 2006) is both a target and a source of key stress mediators, such as corticotropin-releasing hormone (CRH) and the proopiomelanocortin (POMC)-derived peptides, cortisol, catecholamines, prolactin, substance P, and nerve growth factor. An equivalent of the central hypothalamic-pituitary-adrenal (HPA) axis is activated in the skin in response to stress (Slominski et al. 2000). The skin's responses to acute stress include an enhanced skin immune function with increased intracutaneous migration of immunocompetent cells, while chronic stress may suppress cutaneous immunity. Acute psychological stress, which is associated with increased glucocorticoid levels, adversely affects recovery of skin barrier function after tape stripping and may exacerbate barrier-mediated dermatoses such as psoriasis and atopic dermatitis (Choi et al. 2005; Garg et al. 2001). Acute stress is associated with increased mast cell activation and degranulation with release of histamine. The mast cell is an important regulator of neurogenic inflammation during the stress response and plays an important role in various stress-mediated dermatoses. Chronic stress can reduce the immune response to vaccines, slow wound healing, and reactivate latent viral infections such as herpesviruses. Dermatology and psychiatry interface at both basic and clinical levels; this chapter reviews the clinical aspects of psychocutaneous disorders.

Classification

Psychodermatological disorders have been generally divided into two major categories (Gupta and Gupta 1996; Koblenzer 1987; Medansky and Handler 1981):

1. *Dermatological manifestations of psychiatric disorders* (Table 29–1)—This category also includes the self-induced dermatoses. A subgroup of disorders (i.e., the mucocutaneous dysesthesias, idiopathic pruritus, prurigo nodularis, and lichen simplex chronicus) can be loosely classified as "functional dermatological disorders," as their primary cause remains unclear; however, these disorders are strongly influenced by psychosomatic factors.
2. *Psychological factors in dermatological disorders*—This category includes a wide range of skin conditions and has been further separated into three subcategories:
   a. Disorders that have a primary dermatopathological basis but may be influenced in part by psychological factors—for example, psoriasis, atopic dermatitis, urticaria and angioedema, alopecia areata, and acne. Most of the disorders in this group are exacerbated by psychological stress and are associated with psychiatric comorbidity. A wide range of other dermatological disorders, such as viral infections of the skin (e.g., viral warts) and other immunologically mediated skin disorders such as vitiligo, may be exacerbated by psychological stress.
   b. Disorders and states that represent an accentuated physiological response, such as hyperhidrosis and blushing.
   c. Disorders that result in an emotional reaction primarily as a result of cosmetic disfigurement and/or the social stigma associated with the disease.

   These three subcategories are not mutually exclusive, and some dermatological disorders may fall into more than one subgroup.

TABLE 29–1. Dermatological manifestations of psychiatric disorders

Delusions

- Delusions of parasitosis
- Delusions of bromhidrosis (delusional belief that a foul odor is being emitted)
- Delusions of disfigurement

Hallucinations

- Tactile or haptic hallucinations

Distorted perceptions

- Amplified or dysesthetic cutaneous pain
- Intractable pruritus

Conversion and dissociation

- Unexplained sensory syndromes (e.g., involving cutaneous pain or numbness)
- Unexplained pruritic states
- Idiopathic urticaria and angioedema
- Self-induced dermatoses (e.g., dermatitis artefacta, trichotillomania)
- "Psychogenic purpura"

Obsessions and compulsions

- Compulsive hand washing
- Compulsive rubbing or picking of the skin
- Self-excoriation
- Hair plucking or trichotillomania
- Onychophagia and onychotillomania

Anxiety and panic

- Unexplained profuse perspiration, night sweats
- Flushing reactions
- Urticarial reactions

Body image misperceptions related to the skin

- Dermatological complaints about imagined or slight "flaws" of the skin
- Concern about skin lesion out of proportion to its clinical severity

General Guidelines for Management of the Psychocutaneous Patient

Standard psychiatric therapies are used to treat psychiatric comorbidity in the dermatology patient. Psychiatric drugs are generally used for one of three purposes: 1) management of dermatological manifestations of primary psychiatric disorders, 2) management of psychiatric disorders that are comorbid with primary dermatological disorders, and 3) provision of certain desired pharmacological properties of psychotropic agents (e.g., the antihistaminic effect of doxepin), even in the absence of a comorbid psychiatric disorder. Currently, no orally administered psychotropic agents are approved by the U.S. Food and Drug Administration (FDA) for the treatment of a primary dermatological disorder; 5% topical doxepin cream is FDA approved for short-term (up to 8 days) management of moderate pruritus in adults with conditions such as atopic dermatitis.

In diagnosis and management of comorbid psychopathology, there are some special considerations in patients with skin diseases. Certain dermatological disorders, such as atopic dermatitis, acne, and psoriasis, have been associated with a high prevalence of suicidal ideation, which may not always be commensurate with the clinical severity of the skin disorder. Suicidal ideation has been reported among patients with a wide range of dermatological conditions (at rates of 6.2%–8.6%) (Picardi et al. 2006) and is especially prevalent in patients with severe pruritus and cosmetically disfiguring skin conditions (Gupta et al. 2005). Body dysmorphic disorder (BDD) may be overtly or covertly comorbid with skin diseases and can impair functional outcomes, contribute to treatment resistance, and increase suicide risk. Disease-related stress and daily hassles from the impact of the skin condition on the patient's quality of life, as well as other psychosocial stressors such as major life events, have been associated with exacerbation of the dermatological disorder in up to 70% of cases of psoriasis, atopic dermatitis, chronic idiopathic urticaria, and acne. Even minor lesions in easily visible body regions or the genital area can lead to significant disease-related stress and should be treated aggressively. Pediatric and adolescent patients should be asked about appearance-related teasing and bullying (Magin et al. 2008), as this can significantly contribute to psychological morbidity. Pruritus (itching), the most common symptom of skin disorders, interferes with sleep and is associated with increased psychiatric comorbidity (Weisshaar et al. 2008), making it an important target of treatment. Some patients with posttraumatic stress and dissociative symptoms (especially those secondary to childhood neglect and emotional and sexual abuse) may excessively manipulate or excoriate their skin in an effort to regulate emotions (see "Self-Induced Dermatoses" later in this chapter) (Gupta 2006), and the cutaneous self-injury can in turn exacerbate comorbid dermatological conditions such as psoriasis.

Dermatological Manifestations of Psychiatric Disorders

Delusional Parasitosis

Delusional parasitosis (delusions of infestation) is classified as a *delusional disorder, somatic type,* and is characterized by a fixed false belief that one is infested by parasites or insects that is maintained despite negative clinical and laboratory findings (Bishop 1983). Delusional parasitosis is rarely seen by general psychiatrists but is common in dermatological practice. The mean age at onset is the mid-50s to 60s, with an equal sex distribution in patients younger than 50 years and a female-to-male ratio of 3:1 in patients ages 50 years and older (Lyell 1983). Patients with delusional parasitosis typically present the doctor with alleged parasite specimens in a pill bottle, matchbox, adhesive tape, or plastic bag (Lepping and Freudenmann 2008). Such patients tend to treat their skin by scratching and may use disinfectants, repellants, pesticides, and antimicrobials. They may consult exterminators or entomologists, repeatedly launder clothing and linens, and discard possessions and even pets (fearing them as the source). Tactile and olfactory hallucinations related to the delusional theme may be present. Patients with delusional parasitosis often complain of *formication*—cutaneous sensations of crawling, stinging, and/or biting. Belief of infestation may extend to any body orifice—for example, the nares (Walling and Swick 2008), oral cavity (Maeda et al. 1998), or orbit (Sherman et al. 1998). In contrast to schizophrenia, apart from the impact of the delusion, the patient's thought processes, behavior, and functioning are not obviously odd or bizarre. Delusional parasitosis has been reported to lead to *folie a dèux* (shared psychotic disorder), in which the belief in the patient's infestation comes to be shared by a significant other (Trabert 1999). This has been reported to occur in 5%–15% of cases of delusional parasitosis (Lepping and Freudenmann 2008). Although most cases of delusional parasitosis appear to represent a primary delusional disorder, some have been considered secondary to other psychiatric disorders—for example, schizophrenia, obsessive-compulsive disorder (OCD), or psychotic depression—or medical disorders—for example, structural brain disease, delirium, dementia, endocrinopathy (e.g., hypothyroidism), vitamin deficiency (B_{12} deficiency and pellagra), neuropathies, uremia, hepatic encephalopathy, and other toxic states, especially abuse of amphetamines or cocaine (Lepping and Freudenmann 2008). Of course, it is important not to make the diagnosis of delusional parasitosis prematurely; some patients really do have infestations (e.g., scabies, lice).

Management

Appropriate dermatological and medical examinations and investigations are required to rule out dermatological disease and secondary causes of delusional parasitosis. Because patients with delusional parasitosis do not view themselves as having a psychiatric disorder, they are usually unwilling to be referred to a psychiatrist. Consequently, treatment is best carried out with a psychiatrist providing consultation and liaison to a dermatologist (Harth et al. 2009). Patients present with firmly held beliefs that they have an infestation or infection or "Morgellons disease" (Harth et al. 2010a). The biggest challenge in the pharmacotherapy of delusional parasitosis is convincing the patient to take a psychiatric drug. Delusional parasitosis is often difficult to manage even in a dermatological setting because of limited response to antipsychotic medications and problems with adherence to treatment recommendations (Ahmad and Ramsay 2009). Psychotherapy is of little help, and the clinician should focus on developing a therapeutic relationship (which is likely to enhance adherence to psychopharmacology) rather than emphasizing the delusional nature of the complaint. The dermatologist should be advised to listen to the patient's stories, ask about how the condition has affected the patient's life, and attempt to prevent harm (e.g., determine whether the patient is using pesticides). Socially isolated (often elderly) patients with relative sensory deprivation can misinterpret cutaneous sensations; such patients may benefit from increased social support and sensory stimulation.

Both typical and atypical antipsychotics have been effective in delusional parasitosis (Freudenmann and Lepping 2008; Kenchaiah et al. 2010), although there are no randomized controlled trials (RCTs). An antipsychotic with antihistaminic and sedative properties may be helpful in ameliorating anxiety and pruritus. A recent review of antipsychotic treatment in primary and secondary delusional parasitosis noted that risperidone and olanzapine have been the most widely used atypical antipsychotics and have resulted in full or partial remission in 69% and 72% of cases, respectively (Freudenmann and Lepping 2008). There is an extensive dermatological literature on the use of pimozide, but no evidence demonstrates the superiority of pimozide over other antipsychotics for delusional parasitosis. Pimozide is generally started at 1 mg/day and increased by 1 mg every 5–7 days to a maximum of 4 mg/day (C.S. Lee 2008). Sudden deaths have been reported with pimozide and are thought to be due to ventricular arrhythmias caused by QTc prolongation. Additive effects on QTc prolongation should be anticipated if pimozide is administered concomitantly with tricyclic antidepressants (TCAs) or cytochrome P450 (CYP) 3A4 inhibitors (e.g., fluoxetine, azole antifungals, macrolide antibiotics, grapefruit juice). Secondary delusional parasitosis is more likely than primary delusional parasitosis to respond to antipsychotics (78% vs. 59% trend) (Freudenmann and Lepping 2008). Selective serotonin reuptake inhibitors (SSRIs) have sometimes been helpful in patients whose parasite sensations have been more obsessional than delusional (Fellner and Majeed 2009).

Cutaneous Body Image Disorders

Cutaneous body image (Gupta et al. 2004), defined as an individual's mental perception of the appearance of his or her integument (skin, hair, and nails), is an important core dermatological construct. This is relevant both in cosmetically disfiguring skin disorders, where cutaneous body image dissatisfaction can have a profound impact on quality of life, and in situations where the cutaneous body image is distorted, as in BDD. Cutaneous body image dissatisfaction has been associated with increased risk for suicide (Cotterill and Cunliffe 1997). Patients with BDD, which usually begins during adolescence, present to dermatologists with complaints about imagined or slight "flaws" of the face or head (e.g., hair thinning, wrinkles, very minimal acne, scars, vascular markings, paleness or redness of the complexion, swelling or facial asymmetry, excessive facial hair) or concerns about the shape, size, or some other aspect of the nose, eyes, eyelids, eyebrows, ears, mouth, lips, teeth, jaw, chin, or cheeks. BDD patients may also excessively pick their skin (Phillips and Taub 1995). Reported rates of BDD in cosmetic surgery and dermatology settings range from 6% to 15% of patients (American Psychiatric Association 2000); a Polish survey of 118 dermatologists reported that almost 18% were currently treating a BDD patient (Szepietowski et al. 2008), and a Turkish study (Kaymak et al. 2009) of university students reported higher BDD-related symptom scores among students with a wide range of skin diseases, including acne (which was present in the majority of cases). The diagnosis *delusional disorder, somatic type,* should be considered if the preoccupation with an imagined defect in appearance reaches delusional proportions. If obsessional preoccupation about the appearance is associated with compulsive behaviors (e.g., compulsive mirror checking), a diagnosis of OCD may be appropriate (American Psychiatric Association 2000).

Patient dissatisfaction with cutaneous body image is often the primary consideration in deciding whether to institute treatment in skin disorders such as acne, where BDD may be comorbid in more than one-third of cases in some centers (Bowe et al. 2007). In a study of 200 BDD patients (Phillips et al. 2006), 25% reported BDD-related tanning (i.e., tanning motivated by a desire to improve a perceived defect in one's appearance). In 84% of the tanners with BDD, the skin was the body area of chief concern; 26% of the tanners with BDD had attempted suicide, and 52% had received dermatological treatment, which was usually ineffective for their symptoms. Tanners were more likely than nontanners to compulsively pick their skin (Phillips et al. 2006).

Anorexia nervosa and *bulimia nervosa* can initially present as dermatological complaints (Gupta et al. 1987a) resulting from malnutrition (e.g., lanugo-like body hair, carotenodermia, perniosis) and bingeing and purging (hand calluses, gingivitis, flare-ups of acne), as well as increased cutaneous body image concerns. In a cross-sectional study (Gupta and Gupta 2001a) examining concerns about various aspects of skin appearance among young adult (<30 years) eating disorder patients ($n=32$) and nonclinical control subjects ($n=34$), it was observed that 81% of the eating disorder patients, versus 56% of control subjects, reported dissatisfaction with the appearance of their skin ($P=0.03$).

The cutaneous attributes of greatest concern among the eating disorder patients were those that are also associated with aging and photodamage (e.g., "darkness" under the eyes, freckles, fine wrinkles, and patchy hyperpigmentation) in addition to dryness and roughness of the skin, which are often secondary to the eating disorder. Starvation in eating disorders has been associated with pruritus (Gupta et al. 1992), and rapid refeeding can lead to a flare-up of acne, mostly likely because of rising androgen levels (Gupta and Gupta 2001b). It has been advised that anorexia nervosa should be considered in all patients with low body weight and pruritus (J. F. Morgan and Lacey 1999). As patients with eating disorders often tend to minimize or deny their symptoms, the dermatological signs may be the first clinical clue that the patient has an eating disorder.

Management

BDD may occur on its own or be comorbid with other dermatological disorders. If the BDD is not addressed, the patient is likely to remain dissatisfied with dermatological treatment outcomes. Treatments for BDD include SSRI antidepressants and cognitive-behavior therapy (CBT) (Phillips et al. 2002).

Self-Induced Dermatoses

Dermatitis Artefacta

Dermatitis artefacta describes cutaneous lesions that are wholly self-inflicted; however, the patient typically denies the self-inflicted nature of the lesions (Fabisch 1980; Gupta et al. 1987b; Nielsen et al. 2005). The median age has been reported as 39 years (range 18–60 years), with about three-fourths of adult cases in women (Nielsen et al. 2005; Verraes-Derancourt et al. 2006) and a similar female preponderance in children (Saez-de-Ocariz et al. 2004). The lesions in dermatitis artefacta have a wide range of features and may present as purpura, blisters, ulcers, erythema, sinuses, edema, or nodules, depending on the means employed to create them; thus, they can mimic a wide range of cutaneous disorders. Cutaneous ulcers and excoriations are the most common types of lesions, and 35%–90% of patients have multiple lesions (Nielsen et al. 2005; Saez-de-Ocariz et al. 2004; Verraes-Derancourt et al. 2006). The lesions typically occur in regions that are accessible by hand; they may occur at the site of an old scar or surgical wound or appear suddenly in previously normal skin. Facial and periocular skin and the upper limbs are the most common sites (Saez-de-Ocariz et al. 2004; Ugurlu et al. 1999). Self-inflicted lesions are often bizarre, with sharp geometric borders surrounded by normal-looking skin. Full-thickness skin loss or severe scarring from self-inflicted lesions may necessitate extensive plastic surgery or amputation (Gupta et al. 1987b). Like patients with other factitious disorders, patients with dermatitis artefacta typically consult numerous physicians and are treated unsuccessfully with multiple medications before the correct diagnosis is made (Ugurlu et al. 1999).

Psychiatric comorbidity. A personality disorder characterized by very immature coping mechanisms is often observed in which the self-induced lesions serve as "an appeal for help." In the pediatric population, many cases may be associated with mental retardation (Saez-de-Ocariz et al. 2004), and Munchausen's syndrome by proxy should be ruled out (Harth et al. 2010b). Dissociative disorders, which are often underrecognized, should also be considered—especially when a patient denies any memory of self-inducing the lesions—as well as posttraumatic stress disorder (PTSD) with prominent dissociative symptoms (Gupta 2006). Dermatitis artefacta may co-occur in mood, anxiety, and psychotic disorders, as well as in malingering (Cohen and Vardy 2006). The clinician should always rule out an underlying dermatological disorder in the patient suspected of having dermatitis artefacta, as a patient may self-excoriate a primary dermatological lesion and create secondary artifactual lesions (Ahmad and Ramsay 2008).

Management. Early diagnosis is important, as this may prevent unnecessary surgery and chronic morbidity (Gupta and Gupta 1996). Patients with dermatitis artefacta typically are not able to describe how their lesions evolved, and the lesions heal if occlusive dressing or a plaster dressing is used. Most authors recommend a supportive and empathic approach to the patient, avoiding direct discussion or confrontation regarding the self-inflicted nature of the lesions. Patients typically refuse to see a psychiatrist; however, nursing staff can play an important role in the psychosocial assessment and management of the patient (Nielsen et al. 2005). Once a satisfactory therapeutic alliance has been established, a more insight-oriented psychotherapeutic approach may be used (Fabisch 1980). A major psychosocial stressor such as illness, accident, or bereavement may precede dermatitis artefacta in about 20%–30% of cases, and recovery may occur through mobilization of social support for the patient. Other helpful adjunctive therapies that have been used include relaxation exercises and a course of antianxiety or antidepressant medications if indicated (Fabisch 1980; Nielsen et al. 2005).

Neurotic or Psychogenic Excoriation, Acne Excoriée, Onychophagia, and Onychotillomania

In neurotic or psychogenic excoriation, lesions are produced as a result of repetitive self-excoriation that may be initiated by an itch or other cutaneous dysesthesia or through the urge to excoriate an acne pimple or other irregularity on the skin. Unlike patients with dermatitis artefacta, patients with neurotic excoriation typically acknowledge the self-inflicted nature of their lesions (Freunsgaard 1984). Self-excoriation can initiate and perpetuate the "itch-scratch cycle," and in some cases the self-excoriative behavior can become a true compulsive ritual (Hatch et al. 1992). The lesions in neurotic excoriation are usually a few centimeters in diameter, may range in number from a few to several hundred, and are weeping, crusted, or scarred with postinflammatory hypo- or hyperpigmentation. Unlike lesions in dermatitis artefacta, the lesions in neurotic excoriation do not mimic those of other cutaneous disorders. The repetitive self-excoriation may exacerbate a preexisting dermatosis (e.g., in acne excoriée). Onychophagia involves repetitive nail biting; onychotillomania refers to compulsive peeling of the nail and surrounding skin.

Psychiatric comorbidity. The psychiatric disorders most commonly associated with neurotic or psychogenic excoriation or "pathological skin picking" (Arnold et al. 2001; Calikusu et al. 2003; Freunsgaard 1984; Grant and Odlaug 2009; Gupta et al. 1987b; Hatch et al. 1992; Mutasim and Adams 2009) include OCD, personality disorders, major depressive disorder, and bipolar disorder, as well as BDD, PTSD, and dissociative disorders where the self-excoriation and/or nail biting or picking often serve as a means of self-regulating intense emotional states. Psychosocial stressors precede neurotic excoriation in 33%–98% of cases (Freunsgaard 1984; Gupta et al. 1987b). Neurotic excoriation may follow physical disability from illness or aging in persons with strongly compulsive personality traits (Gupta et al. 1986).

Management. The patient should be fully investigated for other systemic and local causes of pruritus. An empathic and supportive approach in psychotherapy (Freunsgaard 1984) has been reported to be more effective than insight-oriented psychotherapy, which can exacerbate symptoms. Several small trials suggest the efficacy of SSRIs in cutaneous excoriation (skin picking), including clomipramine 50–100 mg/day (Gupta et al. 1986), fluoxetine (up to 80 mg/day) (Simeon et al. 1997), sertraline (up to 200 mg) (Kalivas et al. 1996), and fluvoxamine (Arnold et al. 1999), with little correlation with presence of, or improvement in, psychiatric comorbidity. There have also been case reports of the efficacy of doxepin (30–75 mg/day) (Harris et al. 1987), olanzapine (2.5–5.0 mg/day) (Blanch et al. 2004; Gupta and Gupta 2000), aripiprazole augmentation of fluoxetine (Curtis and Richards 2007), and naltrexone (50 mg at bedtime) (Smith and Pittelkow 1989).

Trichotillomania

Trichotillomania refers to nonscarring alopecia as a result of self-plucking of hair. The hair of the scalp (especially the crown and parietal regions), eyebrows, eyelashes, beard, or pubic area can be affected (Gupta and Gupta 1996; Koo and Lee 2008). Trichotillomania occurring solely during sleep has been reported (Murphy et al. 2007). Patients deny that their alopecia is self-induced in 43% of cases (Christenson et al. 1991a). In one-third of cases, the extracted hair may be chewed or swallowed (Grant and Odlaug 2008), and the trichophagia can lead to trichobezoars, which may cause gastrointestinal complications such as obstruction and acute pancreatitis. An affected area in trichotillomania is rarely completely devoid of hair, and hairs of various lengths are usually partially distributed over the area of alopecia. Histopathological examination may be necessary to confirm the diagnosis. Trichotillomania should be distinguished from benign hair pulling, which can be associated with thumb sucking and nail biting in children.

Psychiatric comorbidity. Trichotillomania is a heterogeneous disorder (Duke et al. 2010; Lochner et al. 2010). It is classified as an impulse-control disorder in both DSM-IV-TR (American Psychiatric Association 2000) and ICD-10 (World Health Organization 1992). In trichotillomania, the hair pulling helps to regulate emotions by decreasing negative ones such as boredom, sadness, anger, and tension and increasing positive ones such as relief and calm (Diefenbach et al. 2008). Although an extensive literature classifies trichotillomania as an obsessive-compulsive spectrum disorder, brain imaging studies of trichotillomania (Rauch et al. 2007) do not support this. Trichotillomania has been associated with a history of psychological trauma (e.g., bereavement) and PTSD (Gershuny et al. 2006), high dissociation scores (Gupta et al. 2000; Lochner et al. 2004), and depression. Trichotillomania may be a feature of mental retardation, eating disorders, and personality disorders in which patients tend to be highly dissociated.

Management. The three major treatments studied in trichotillomania are habit-reversal therapy, SSRIs, and clomipramine (Bloch et al. 2007). A systematic review of these interventions in seven blinded, randomized clinical trials in which the primary outcome measure was mean change in trichotillomania severity revealed that habit-reversal therapy was superior to both SSRIs and clomipramine. Clomipramine, but not SSRIs, was more effective than placebo (Bloch et al. 2007). A 10-week controlled trial found clomipramine (100–250 mg/day) to be more effective than desipramine (150–200 mg/day) in trichotillomania (Swedo et al. 1989). A 12-week RCT involving 25 trichotillomania patients reported that olanzapine, at an average dose of about 10 mg daily, was significantly more effective than placebo in decreasing ratings of psychological morbidity except for hair pulling (Van Ameringen et al. 2010). Some open-label and case studies report the efficacy of mood stabilizers such as lithium (Christenson et al. 1991b), topiramate (Lochner et al. 2006), and oxcarbazepine (Leombruni and Gastaldi 2010). Group therapy in clinical trials has not been effective (Diefenbach et al. 2006). It is possible that treatments will be more effective when the underlying issues of trauma and dissociation in trichotillomania are addressed.

Functional Dermatological Disorders

Mucocutaneous Dysesthesias

The mucocutaneous dysesthesias represent a heterogeneous group of disorders that involve unexplained cutaneous pain and other sensory syndromes. One form is "scalp dysesthesia" (Hoss and Segal 1998), in which patients (women are most often affected) present with complaints of pruritus, pain, trichodynia, and burning and/or stinging sensations of the scalp without objective physical findings. Other such localized dysesthesias without objective physical findings include vulvodynia, scrotodynia, atypical facial pain, and "burning mouth syndrome" or glossodynia (Abetz and Savage 2009; Eli et al. 1994; Hampf et al. 1987; Lamey and Lamb 1988; McKay 1994). Commonly associated psychiatric disorders include depressive and somatoform disorders, PTSD, and dissociative states (Gupta and Gupta 2006).

Management

Various psychotherapeutic interventions including hypnosis and eye movement desensitization and reprocessing (EMDR) (Gupta and Gupta 2002) may be helpful when the cutaneous symptom represents a conversion disorder, a dissociative state, or a sensory flashback in PTSD. The mucocutaneous dysesthesias are usually treated with the same agents used for the treatment of neuropathic pain, such as TCAs, serotonin-norepinephrine reuptake inhibitors (SNRIs), or anticonvulsants, but controlled clinical trials are lacking (Haefner et al. 2005; Zakrzewska et al. 2005; see also Chapter 36, "Pain"). Scalp dysesthesia and other idiopathic pruritic conditions may respond to antihistaminic TCAs such as amitriptyline and doxepin (Hoss and Segal 1998).

Idiopathic Pruritus

Psychosomatic Aspects of Pruritus

Pruritus, or itching, is an unpleasant sensation that elicits a desire to scratch, which leads to inflammation and stimulation of cutaneous nerve fibers, which in turn leads to more itching and scratching and perpetuation of the itch-scratch cycle. Scratching leads to problems with skin barrier function, lichenification, and prurigo formation. Pruritus, the most common symptom of skin disorders (Weisshaar et al. 2008), may occur with or without visible skin lesions. Pruritus may be a feature of a systemic disease in 10%–50% of cases (e.g., hepatic or renal failure, HIV), especially in advanced age, or may occur as a drug side effect (e.g., opioids). The pathophysiology of pruritus is not well understood, and it is unclear why it is worse at night. Itch is mediated by both peripheral (e.g., histamine, proteinases, substance P, opioid peptides, neurotrophins such as nerve growth factor) and CNS factors (Yosipovitch and Ishiuji 2009). Perception of pruritus, irrespective of etiology, can be modulated by psychological factors. Recent stressful life events and anxiety and/or depressive symptoms have been correlated with an increased ability to experience itching. Persons with mental distress were found to be twice as likely to experience itching as those without (Dalgard et al. 2007).

Chronic Idiopathic Pruritus

Whereas pruritus is a common symptom of many dermatological and systemic diseases, the cause in chronic pruritus is often not identifiable. Such idiopathic pruritus is typically experienced on a daily basis, especially at night and in the evening, resulting in most having difficulty falling asleep. Generalized idiopathic pruritus mainly involves the legs, arms, and back. The most common focal presentations of idiopathic pruritus are pruritus ani, vulvae, and scroti. Idiopathic pruritus may be described as crawling, tickling, stinging, or burning (T-J Goon et al. 2007; Yosipovitch et al. 2002). In one study, patients with idiopathic pruritus described the itching as unbearable (73%), bothersome (72%), annoying (67%), and/or worrisome (45%) (T-J Goon et al. 2007). Psychiatric symptoms are common in idiopathic pruritus, and idiopathic pruritus is common in psychiatric patients: two Israeli studies in psychiatric inpatients reported a prevalence of 32% (Mazeh et al. 2008) and 42% (Kretzmer et al. 2008), respectively. In the latter study, patients without adequate social support and those without regular employment showed higher rates of idiopathic pruritus (Kretzmer et al. 2008). It is not surprising that depression is common among patients with idiopathic pruritus, especially given the condition's chronicity and associated sleep disturbance (Sheehan-Dare et al. 1990). Idiopathic pruritus was more frequent in patients with high trait anger (Kretzmer et al. 2008) and dissociation (Gupta and Gupta 2006; Gupta et al. 2000). However, not all patients with idiopathic pruritus have psychopathology or high life stress, and idiopathic pruritus should be considered as a functional disorder rather than a psychogenic one.

Management. New onset of unexplained pruritus should lead to evaluation for occult medical disease before considering it to be idiopathic pruritus. Idiopathic pruritus represents a heterogeneous condition and may be a symptom of psychophysiological arousal in the psychiatric patient. Treatment of the underlying psychiatric disorder should therefore help the pruritus. For focal idiopathic pruritus (e.g., pruritus ani, vulvae, scroti), topical treatments are used. For both generalized and focal idiopathic pruritus, the most commonly prescribed oral medications are antihistamines, which usually provide some short-term relief. TCAs, especially doxepin, can relieve chronic idiopathic pruritus. Paroxetine has also been reported to be helpful (Zylicz et al. 2003). Opiate receptor antagonists and anticonvulsants (e.g., gabapentin, pregabalin, carbamazepine) have been suggested as possible remedies (Lynde et al. 2008). Behavioral treatment such as habit reversal training and CBT may also be helpful in interrupting the itch-scratch cycle, and there are reports of the benefits of hypnosis.

Prurigo Nodularis

Prurigo nodularis (Koo and Lee 2008) is a chronic skin condition characterized by intensely pruritic hard dome-shaped papules or nodules with central scale-crust. Patients may present with a few hundred lesions, usually in a symmetric distribution, with predominance on the extensor surfaces of the limbs. It is thought that the lesions of prurigo are caused by chronic and severe scratching and rubbing; however, the morphology of the lesions is not easily explained (Koo and Lee 2008), and the etiology of prurigo nodularis remains unknown (M.R. Lee and Shumack 2005). Histologically, there is hypertrophy and proliferation of dermal nerves and marked increase in calcitonin gene-related peptide and substance P immunoreactivity. These neuropeptides may mediate the cutaneous neurogenic inflammation and pruritus in prurigo nodularis (M.R. Lee and Shumack 2005).

Psychiatric Comorbidity

Psychosocial factors such as anxiety and depression may be a primary factor or secondary to the itch in prurigo nodularis (M.R. Lee and Shumack 2005), and psychosocial stress is a factor among 33% of patients (Harth et al. 2009). When compared with psoriasis patients, prurigo nodularis patients had the same degree of alexithymia, somatization symptoms, hypochondriasis, anxiety, and depression, with 18% cases of anxiety and 22% cases of depression (Schneider et al. 2006).

Management

Treatment involves interruption of the itch-scratch cycle, which is typically difficult (M.R. Lee and Shumack 2005). Among psychiatric therapies, relaxation techniques such as autogenic training and progressive muscle relaxation may be helpful (Harth et al. 2009). Strongly antihistaminic psychotropic agents such as doxepin (10–75 mg at night) may reduce pruritus (M.R. Lee and Shumack 2005). It should be noted that the first-line treatments for prurigo nodularis involve standard dermatological therapies such as corticosteroids.

Lichen Simplex Chronicus

Lichen simplex chronicus (LSC) is characterized by hyperpigmented, lichenified, leathery plaques that result from habitual scratching and rubbing of the skin (Koo and Lee 2008). LSC is most frequently observed in older adults. The plaques of LSC have a predilection for the nuchal and occipital area in women and for the scrotum and perineal area in men. The scratching can begin unconsciously and evolves into a compulsive ritual, which may lead to lichenification of the skin (Konuk et al. 2007). Peripheral neuropathy may play a role in some patients (Solak et al. 2009).

Psychiatric Comorbidity

Psychosocial stressors, OCD, depression, and high levels of dissociation have all been associated with LSC (Konuk et al. 2007; Koo and Lee 2008). LSC is associated with arousals from Stage II non-rapid eye movement (REM) sleep due to scratching and a lower percentage of time spent in Stages III and IV sleep (Koca et al. 2006). This in turn can lead to nonrestorative sleep and daytime fatigue.

Management

Treatment involves interruption of the itch-scratch cycle. Counseling and support for underlying psychosocial stressors, SSRI antidepressants, and doxepin (Koo and Lee 2008) may be useful adjunctive therapies.

Psychogenic Purpura

Psychogenic purpura, also referred to as "autoerythrocyte sensitization syndrome" and Gardner-Diamond syndrome, is a poorly understood condition that presents as spontaneous, painful ecchymotic bruising. The condition mainly affects adult women, with a few cases affecting men and children. In addition to dermatological symptoms, menorrhagia, epistaxis, and gingival and gastrointestinal bleeding (Ivanov et al. 2009; Puetz and Fete 2005) have been described in two-thirds of patients (Ratnoff 1989). Severe emotional stress and other psychological factors (Ivanov et al. 2009; Ratnoff 1980, 1989) have been observed in the majority of cases; however, there is a marked heterogeneity of psychological findings, and the exact role of psychological factors in psychogenic purpura remains unclear. Some of the reported psychological associations (Ivanov et al. 2009; Ratnoff 1980) include conversion reaction, hysterical or masochistic personality, depression, anxiety, difficulty in dealing with hostile feelings, and religious stigmata.

Gardner and Diamond (1955), who described four cases, postulated that patients become sensitized to their own red blood cells. Subcutaneous injection of autologous red blood cells and hemolysate has been shown to reproduce the lesions, suggesting an underlying autoimmune process. Overall, fewer than 200 cases have been described in the literature (Ivanov et al. 2009). In their review of the literature, Puetz and Fete (2005) observed that most case studies of Gardner-Diamond syndrome have not reported detailed results of screening for von Willebrand's disease or platelet dysfunction and that patients in whom platelet aggregation studies have been reported have been found to have a platelet function disorder.

Psychiatric Aspects of Selected Dermatological Disorders

Atopic Dermatitis

Atopic dermatitis, which is a form of eczema (Kang et al. 2008), is a chronic relapsing dermatitis associated with intense pruritus, which is a hallmark of atopic dermatitis. Most prevalence data are derived from school-age children, with a 10%–20% estimated prevalence in the United States, which has been on the rise over the past decades. Pruritus in atopic dermatitis is often worse in the evening and can interfere with nighttime sleep. The rubbing and scratching in response to the pruritus, which typically further exacerbates the atopic dermatitis, can result in excoriations with or without hemorrhagic crusts, and produces lichenified plaques and prurigo nodularis. As a result of repeated rubbing and scratching, lichen simplex chronicus (thickened and leathery skin with exaggerated skin markings) may develop. Atopic dermatitis can occur at any age; however, up to 90% of cases have their onset before the age of 5 years, and usually not before the age of 2 months. Atopic dermatitis has a partially genetic basis with variable expression that is influenced by environmental factors. Atopic dermatitis is often associated with a personal or family history of atopy (i.e., xerosis), asthma, and/or allergic rhinitis. Typically, there are three stages—infantile, childhood, and adulthood—and periods of disease quiescence can occur between these stages. With increasing age, atopic dermatitis typically presents as chronic inflammation and lichenification and tends to localize in the flexural regions; atopic dermatitis skin is characterized by severe dryness with an impaired barrier function of the stratum corneum. Psychoneuroimmunological factors play an important role in the pathogenesis of atopic dermatitis (Steinhoff and Steinhoff 2009).

Stress

The onset or exacerbation of atopic dermatitis often follows stressful life events (Picardi and Abeni 2001). Divorce or separation of parents and severe disease of a family member have been identified as events that particularly increase risk (Bockelbrink et al. 2006). In children, stress as a risk factor for atopic dermatitis interacts with environmental variables such as sweating (Langan et al. 2006; Williams et al. 2004). Two small studies, one in adults (Buske-Kirschbaum et al. 2002) and one in children (Buske-Kirschbaum et al. 1997), have demonstrated a hyporesponsive HPA axis, as evidenced by a blunted cortisol response to a stressor, in patients with atopic dermatitis compared with healthy control subjects.

Psychosocial and Psychiatric Factors

Atopic individuals with emotional problems may develop a vicious cycle between anxiety/depression and dermatological symptoms. Pruritus severity has been directly correlated with the severity of depression in atopic dermatitis (Gupta et al. 1994). Suicidal ideation has been reported among 2.1% of mild to moderately affected adult atopic dermatitis patients in one U.S. sample (Gupta and Gupta 1998); however, a Japanese study of patients ages 15–49 years reported a suicidal ideation prevalence of 0.21%, 6%, and 19.6%, respectively, for patients with mild, moderate, and severe atopic dermatitis (Kimata 2006). Atopic dermatitis patients have also been found to have higher state and trait anxiety and greater psychophysiological reactivity that cannot be attributed solely to increased disease activity (Seiffert et al. 2005). Data from a German population-based administrative database showed a significant association between atopic eczema and attention-deficit/hyperactivity disorder (ADHD) (odds ratio [OR] = 1.54; 95% confidence interval [CI] = 1.06–2.22; P = 0.02) among the 6- to 17-year age group (Schmitt et al. 2009). The authors noted that because of the cross-sectional study design, it remains unclear whether the observed association is due to shared etiological factors or whether the symptoms of atopic dermatitis (e.g., itching, sleep impairment) and disease-related psychosocial factors might exacerbate ADHD symptoms in a subgroup of patients (Schmitt et al. 2009).

In one direction of causality, anxiety and depression are frequently a consequence of the disorder. The misery of living with atopic dermatitis may have a profoundly negative effect on health-related quality of life of children and their families. Intractable itching causes significant insomnia, and sleep deprivation then leads to fatigue, mood lability, and impaired functioning. Teasing and bullying related to contagion, and use of teasing as an instrument of social exclusion, can lead to significant psychological sequelae in the child and adolescent with atopic dermatitis (Magin et al. 2008). Similar embarrassment in adults promotes social isolation. The social stigma of a visible skin disease, frequent visits to doctors, and the need to constantly apply messy topical remedies all add to the burden of disease. Lifestyle restrictions in more severe cases can be significant and include limitations on clothing, staying with friends, owning pets, and engaging in swimming or sports. The impairment of quality of life caused by childhood atopic dermatitis has been shown to be greater than or equal to that caused by asthma or diabetes (Lewis-Jones 2006).

In the other direction of causality, anxiety and depression also aggravate atopic dermatitis. This may occur via several possible mechanisms, including modulation of pruritus perception (Gupta et al. 1994), perturbation of epidermal permeability barrier homeostasis (Garg et al. 2001), or acceleration of immune responses (Hashizume et al. 2005).

There is an extensive literature on emotional dysfunction and disturbed child-family relationships in childhood atopic dermatitis (Howlett 1999). Early theories hypothesized inadequate holding and caressing of the infant and maternal rejection and neglect, but later literature focused on increased symptoms in the child, such as dependency, clinginess, and sleep difficulties, with mothers who were stressed and lacking in social support (Howlett 1999). Parents are often reluctant to discipline their child for fear that this could provoke distress and precipitate scratching. Furthermore, parents and sometimes medical professionals may focus more on the care of the skin disorder than on the emotional and developmental needs of the child with atopic dermatitis (Howlett 1999).

Management

Psychotherapy. At least 47 different medical, psychological, and environmental interventions for atopic dermatitis have been studied in clinical trials (Hoare et al. 2000). A wide variety of psychotherapeutic treatments have been advocated to interrupt the vicious cycle of itching and scratching in atopic dermatitis, including psychological, behavioral, and psychoeducational therapies. There have been several RCTs of psychological and educational interventions (including relaxation training, habit reversal training, cognitive-behavioral techniques, and stress management training) as an adjunct to conventional therapy for children with atopic eczema to enhance the effectiveness of topical therapy, but the evidence base remains limited regarding their efficacy (Ersser et al. 2007). RCTs have also shown that interventions directed toward the parents of the child with atopic dermatitis can decrease the severity of the skin disease (Ersser et al. 2007).

Psychopharmacology. Pharmacotherapy of atopic dermatitis should aim to interrupt the itch-scratch cycle and optimize nighttime sleep. Topical doxepin (5% cream) is effective in the treatment of pruritus in atopic dermatitis (Drake and Millikan 1995) and is FDA approved for short-term treatment in adults but not children. Low-dose oral doxepin (e.g., starting at 10 mg at bedtime) is helpful in adults because of its antihistaminic and sedative properties (Kelsay 2006), with dose increases based on response and side effects. There have also been reports suggesting some benefit from bupropion (Modell et al. 2002), mirtazapine (Hundley and Yosipovitch 2004; Mahtani et al. 2005), and trimipramine (Savin et al. 1979). Sedating antidepressants may be beneficial in part through promoting sleep. The strongly antihistaminic antidepressants doxepin, trimipramine, and amitriptyline may also be effective because of their strong anticholinergic properties, as the eccrine sweat glands in atopic dermatitis have been found to be hypersensitive to acetylcholine. There are no established guidelines for the treatment of sleep disturbance in atopic dermatitis (Kelsay 2006). A small short-term RCT of the benzodiazepine nitrazepam did not significantly reduce nocturnal scratching (Ebata et al. 1998), and benzodiazepine withdrawal may further exacerbate pruritus.

Psoriasis

Psoriasis (Van de Kerkhof and Schalkwijk 2008) is a chronic and recurrent inflammatory disorder characterized by circumscribed erythematous, dry, scaling plaques that are usually covered by silvery white adherent scales. The lesions are typically symmetrical; have a predilection for the scalp, nails, extensor surfaces of the limbs, hands and feet, and sacral and genital regions; and are associated with pruritus. Psoriasis is influenced by both genetic and environmental factors, with about 70% concordance rate in monozygotic twins. In addition to psychosocial stress, other risk factors and comorbidities in psoriasis include cigarette smoking, alcohol consumption, obesity, diabetes, hypertension, and hyperlipidemia (Gottlieb et al. 2008). The worldwide prevalence of psoriasis is 2%. Psoriasis can occur at any age; in approximately 75% of patients, the onset is before age 40 years. In contrast to atopic dermatitis, psoriasis is uncommon (about 1%) in individuals younger than 16 years. More than one-third of patients have severe disease, and 5%–30% have psoriatic arthritis. Visibility of lesions, presence of lesions in the genital area, degree of scaling, and pruritus severity have the greatest impact on patient quality of life (Gupta et al. 1989).

Lithium-induced psoriasis can appear within a few months but usually occurs within the first few years of treatment. The absolute increased risk is quite small (Brauchli et al. 2009). Psoriasis precipitated or exacerbated by lithium is typically resistant to conventional antipsoriatic treatments. When the psoriasis becomes intractable, lithium must be discontinued, and the psoriasis usually remits within a few months. A small RCT showed that inositol supplements have a significant beneficial effect on psoriasis patients taking lithium (Allan et al. 2004). Beta-blockers such as propranolol (often used to treat lithium-induced tremors) have also been associated with psoriasis, but a recent population-based study does not support this (Brauchli et al. 2009).

Stress

Stress has long been reported to trigger psoriasis. Uncontrolled studies have reported very high rates of stressful life events preceding the onset of the illness; for example, in one study, antecedent stressful life events were reported by 50% of children and 43% of adults (Raychaudhuri and Gross 2000). However, perception and recall biases influence such rates. In a case-control study comparing 560 psoriasis patients and 690 patients with new diagnoses of other skin conditions, psoriasis patients were more than twice as likely as the control patients to have experienced stressful life events within 1 year prior to onset of their psoriasis (Naldi et al. 2005). A prospective study of psoriasis patients found that at times of higher daily stress, patients experienced more severe psoriasis and significantly more itching (Verhoeven et al. 2009a). However, not all studies have supported the belief that stressful life events precipitate psoriasis (Picardi et al. 2003a). Ultimately, however, most patients who report episodes of psoriasis precipitated by stress describe disease-related stress resulting from the cosmetic disfigurement and social stigma of psoriasis, rather than stressful major life events or nonspecific distress.

Psychosocial and Psychiatric Factors

There is an extensive literature on psychosocial and psychiatric comorbidity in psoriasis (Fortune et al. 2005; Gupta and Gupta 2003). In general, psychological factors, including perceived health, perceptions of stigmatization, and depression, are stronger determinants of disability in patients with psoriasis than are disease severity, location, and duration (Fortune et al. 2005; Kirby et al. 2001). The impact of psoriasis on both physical and mental health-related quality of life has been found to be comparable to the impact of conditions such as cancer, diabetes, arthritis, hypertension, depression, and heart disease (Rapp et al. 1999). Many studies have reported the presence of symptoms of depressive and anxiety disorders, which occur largely in reaction to the cosmetic disfigurement and social stigma associated with psoriasis and anticipatory anxiety about the reaction of others. Patients' cognitive and behavioral patterns of worrying and scratching have been shown to influence their vulnerability to the impact of stress on psoriasis in a prospective study (Verhoeven et al. 2009b). Some of the psychological reactions associated with feelings of stigmatization include shame, decreased self-esteem and increased self-consciousness, social anxiety, and social phobia. A study of 2,490 Vietnam war veterans reported an odds ratio of 4.7 (95% CI=1.9–11.7) for comorbidity of psoriasis and chronic PTSD (Boscarino 2004).

A review of the literature indicates a 10%–58% prevalence of depression in psoriasis (Fortune et al. 2005). Suicidal ideation has been reported among 2.5%–10% of psoriasis patients (Gupta and Gupta 1998; Picardi et al. 2006). Several but not all studies have reported a direct correlation between severity of psoriasis and severity of depressive symptoms (Fortune et al. 2005; Gupta et al. 1994). However, even clinically mild psoriasis may lead to stigmatization and depression in some patients. Improvement in depression has been shown to be associated with improvement in psoriasis (Gupta et al. 1988; Sampogna et al. 2007). Several recent studies (Bassukas et al. 2008; Tyring et al. 2006) have reported significant improvement in psychological comorbidity in psoriasis patients treated with biological response modifiers.

Management

Psychotherapy. Psychotherapy should be considered in patients whose psoriasis is stress-reactive (Harth et al. 2009), because stress associated with daily hassles can in turn result in flare-ups of the psoriasis (Gupta et al. 1989), and psychological distress can undermine the effectiveness of medical therapies. For example, psoriasis patients with high levels of pathological worrying were almost half as likely as low-worrying patients to achieve improvement with psoralen plus ultraviolet A (PUVA) photochemotherapy, after other dermatological, psychological, and demographic factors were controlled for (Fortune et al. 2003). Obesity, moderately heavy alcohol use, and tobacco smoking have been associated with poor response to dermatological therapies (Gottlieb et al. 2008) and need to be managed. There are a number of specific targets for psychological interventions, including interpersonal dependency or an inordinate need to gain the approval of others, and difficulty with the expression of anger, which have been associated with greater stress reactivity of the psoriasis (Gupta et al. 1989). Psychological consequences of psoriasis such as social isolation, sedentary lifestyle, and comorbid depressive illness promote other psoriasis risk factors such as substance abuse and obesity (Skolnick and Alexander 2006). Regular support groups aimed at addressing feelings regarding the impact of psoriasis on quality of life, reducing feelings of isolation, and enhancing coping skills and self-efficiency can be a helpful adjunct to standard therapies (Abel et al. 1990). Various interventions have been reported to be effective; these include group psychotherapy for psychoeducation, mindfulness meditation–based stress reduction (Kabat-Zinn et al. 1998), CBT that provides support and targets negative patterns of thinking (Fortune et al. 2005), cognitive-behavioral stress management, relaxation training and symptom control imagery training (Zachariae et al. 1996), hypnosis (Tausk and Whitmore 1999), and EMDR (Gupta and Gupta 2002).

Psychopharmacology. The association between psoriasis and metabolic syndrome (Gottlieb et al. 2008) has important implications for the choice of psychotherapeutic agents. Treatment of depressive symptoms may reduce pruritus and insomnia in psoriasis. In a placebo-controlled trial, the reversible monoamine oxidase inhibitor (MAOI) moclobemide (currently not available in the United States) reduced psoriasis severity and anxiety (Alpsoy et al. 1998). In a small open-label trial, bupropion induced improvement in psoriasis, with return to baseline levels after its discontinuation (Modell et al. 2002), and paroxetine was reported to be effective in two cases with both depression and psoriasis (Luís Blay 2006).

Urticaria and Angioedema

Urticaria (Grattan and Black 2008), or hives, is characterized by transient (usually lasting less than 24 hours) mucosal or skin swellings due to plasma leakage. The superficial swellings are *wheals*; the deep swellings in the dermis and subcutaneous or submucosal tissue are termed *angioedema* and typically last for 2–3 days. Angioedema can also be a feature of anaphylaxis if the throat is involved. The wheals of urticaria are characteristically pruritic, and the angioedema is often painful. Urticaria has a spectrum of clinical presentations, ranging from occasional localized wheals to widespread recurrent whealing and angioedema affecting the skin, mouth, and/or genitalia. Urticaria is found worldwide, is more common in women, and can occur at any age, with an estimated prevalence of 1%–5% (Grattan and Black 2008). All urticarias are acute initially and termed chronic when they occur over a period of 6 weeks or longer. Chronic urticaria may be a manifestation of an underlying autoimmune disorder. Mast cell degranulation with release of histamine is central to the development of urticaria. The underlying etiology is not identifiable in about 70% of cases of chronic urticaria. Psychogenic factors are reported to be important in around 50% of cases of chronic urticaria (Gupta 2009). "Adrenergic urticaria," which presents as "halo-hives" or papules surrounded by blanched vasoconstricted skin, is an entity that is largely stress induced (Haustein 1990); the symptoms can be provoked by injection of epinephrine or norepinephrine and treated with propranolol (Haustein 1990).

Stress

Severe emotional stress may exacerbate urticarial reactions, regardless of the primary cause. There is an extensive body of literature on stress and urticaria that is more than 30 years old (Gupta 2009). Stress so often seemed a precipitant to angioedema that for many years clinicians referred to the disorder as *angioneurotic edema*. However, the evidence base for this belief about stress inducing urticaria is somewhat limited. In one study of 48 patients (Czubalski and Rudzki 1977), exacerbation by emotional factors occurred in 77% of patients with cholinergic urticaria and 82% of patients with dermographism, but did not occur in cold urticaria. Urticaria had been referred to as an "emotional allergy" in the earlier literature, and two forms of psychogenic urticaria were described (Panconesi and Hautmann 1996, p. 418): 1) an "acute emotional form" that follows specific events with a clear cause–effect relationship; and 2) a "chronic recurrent form" that "seems to be structured deeply on a psychodynamic basis as a psychosomatic disease." Panconesi and Hautmann (1996) further noted that in specific immunological tests, immunoglobulin E (IgE)–dependent induction is evident in only a minority (<20%) of cases. A review of the literature indicates that stressful major life events have been reported to precede the onset of urticaria in 30%–81% of patients (Gupta 2009). Stressors have ranged from catastrophic and traumatic major life events such as earthquakes, bereavement, or accidents to chronic and prolonged stressors such as family and marital problems or problems at work (Gupta 2009). One possible mediator in the relationship between stress and urticaria is dehydroepiandrosterone sulfate (DHEAS), which plays an important role in modulating the vulnerability of the organism to the negative effects of stress (J.F. Morgan et al. 2004). Some patients with chronic urticaria have been shown to have lower serum levels of DHEAS during the active period of the disease (Kasperska-Zajac et al. 2008), and low DHEAS levels were associated with greater psychological distress, as exemplified by higher anxiety and depression scores (Brzoza et al. 2008).

Psychosocial and Psychiatric Factors

Recent studies in Turkey and Germany have shown 48%–60% prevalence of Axis I diagnoses in chronic urticaria patients, with depressive disorders and OCD most common (Ozkan et al. 2007; Staubach et al. 2006; Uguz et al. 2008). A Turkish study using the Minnesota Multiphasic Personality Inventory found a diverse range of psychopathological traits (including high scores for hypochondriasis, depression, hysteria, psychopathic deviance, paranoia, psychasthenia, schizophrenia, and social introversion) which did not correlate with the duration of chronic urticaria (Pasaoglu et al. 2006). Pruritus in chronic urticaria has a significant adverse effect on quality of life and has been directly correlated with the severity of comorbid depression (Gupta et al. 1994). Sixty-two percent of chronic urticaria patients reported that pruritus interfered with sleep, and itch scores were significantly higher in chronic urticaria patients who were also depressed (Yosipovitch et al. 2002). Insomnia has been reported to be the most important symptom associated with onset of chronic urticaria and a mediator of the relationship with stress (Yang et al. 2005). The role of PTSD, often chronic, tends to be underrecognized as a contributing factor in some cases of chronic urticaria (Gupta 2009); a study of 100 chronic urticaria patients and controls with allergies reported an odds ratio of 1.89 for PTSD among the chronic urticaria patients versus the controls (Chung et al. 2010).

Management

Psychotherapy. There is an extensive literature on the effect of hypnotic suggestion on urticaria. Hypnosis is known to be able to influence cutaneous blood flow and other autonomic functions that are not under conscious control (Shenefelt 2000). For example, hypnotized volunteers have been shown to have a significantly decreased flare reaction to the histamine prick test (Shenefelt 2000). In one small pre-post controlled study of hypnosis for chronic idiopathic urticaria, hypnosis in combination with relaxation techniques reduced pruritus but not the number of wheals, although at follow-up 5–14 months after therapy, 40% were free of hives and most of the rest reported improvement (Shertzer and Lookingbill 1987). The impact of chronic urticaria on patient quality of life (Poon et al. 1999) should be addressed. Individual and group psychotherapy and stress management may be useful adjunctive therapies.

Psychopharmacology. In interpreting the chronic urticaria treatment literature, one must first recognize the very high rate of response to placebo (Rudzki et al. 1970). The less-sedating second-generation antihistamines (loratadine, fexofenadine, and cetirizine) are the first-line antihistaminic agents, and diphenhydramine is useful if itching is causing sleep disturbance. A low dose of a sedating antihistaminic antidepressant such as doxepin is helpful for pruritus in chronic urticaria, especially because pruritus interferes with sleep (Yosipovitch et al. 2002). Two small randomized trials of doxepin have demonstrated its efficacy at dosages of 10 mg three times daily (Greene et al. 1985) and 25 mg three times daily (Goldsobel et al. 1986). Doxepin may provide more than symptomatic relief, by reducing the urticarial reaction itself (Rao et al. 1988). Combined H_1 plus H_2 antihistamine therapy may be more effective than H_1 antihistamines alone for urticaria, as dermal blood vessels possess both H_1 and H_2 histamine receptors, and the TCAs doxepin, trimipramine, and amitriptyline are potent histamine H_1 and H_2 receptor antagonists. There are also case reports of the benefits of mirtazapine (Bigatà et al. 2005) and SSRIs (Gupta and Gupta 1995, 2001c) in chronic urticaria.

Alopecia Areata

Alopecia areata (Sperling 2008) is a nonscarring alopecia that typically presents as round or oval patches of nonscarring hair loss involving the scalp; other presentations include alopecia totalis (loss of all scalp hair) and alopecia universalis (loss of all scalp and body hair). Alopecia areata is postulated to be an autoimmune disease, with the average lifetime risk of developing alopecia areata estimated to be 1.5%. A concordance rate of 55% was found among monozygotic twins, suggesting the role of both genetic and environmental factors in its pathogenesis. Alopecia areata tends to have an unpredictable course and may improve spontaneously without any active treatment. The hair follicle is richly innervated and is both a source and a target of numerous cytokines, neuropeptides, and other neuroimmune factors. Like the skin, the hair follicle has a functionally organized HPA axis equivalent, and increased expression of corticotropin-releasing factor (CRF), adrenocorticotropic hormone (ACTH), and alpha-melanocyte-stimulating hormone (α-MSH) has been reported in hair follicles from alopecia areata patients (Tobin and Peters 2009). Substance P, a central stress-associated neuropeptide in the skin, regulates hair growth and perifollicular inflammation and plays an important role in alopecia areata (Tobin and Peters 2009).

Stress

There are conflicting conclusions regarding the role of stress in alopecia areata (Picardi and Abeni 2001; Picardi et al. 2003b). In one study, only 6.7% of alopecia areata patients reported a severely disturbing event 6 months before the onset of symptoms, but no patient reported a coincidence of alopecia areata with a stressful event (Van der Steen et al. 1992). In contrast, in a recent case-control study, significantly more alopecia areata patients than control patients experienced total lifetime (OR = 2.46; 95% CI = 1.15–5.28) and early childhood emotionally and physically traumatic events (OR = 2.16; 95% CI = 1.15–4.06) (Willemsen et al. 2009). Yet another study (Manolache and Benea 2007) reported that 68.9% of alopecia areata patients identified a stressful life event during the prior year, compared with 22.2% of dermatological control subjects with non-stress-related skin conditions (P=0.005). Almost half of the stressful events were family related (e.g., death of a family member, family disputes). Alopecia areata patients who consider their disease to be stress reactive have higher depression scores (Gupta et al. 1997).

Psychosocial and Psychiatric Factors

Alopecia areata patients often have a high prevalence of psychiatric comorbidity, which often does not necessarily have a direct temporal association with the onset, exacerbation, or severity of dermatological symptoms (Gupta and Gupta 1996). High rates of psychiatric comorbidity are also found in pediatric alopecia areata patients (Ghanizadeh 2008). However, the extent of alopecia areata is an important predictor of psychological distress, with 40% of women with alopecia areata attributing marriage breakup to alopecia areata and 63% reporting career-related problems as a result of alopecia areata (Hunt and McHale 2005). Loss of eyebrows and eyelashes has been associated with core identity issues in alopecia areata patients (Hunt and McHale 2005). Overall prevalence of psychiatric comorbidity has been reported to range from 23% to 93% (Gupta and Gupta 1996), and the prevalence of suicidal ideation in alopecia areata as 0% to 2%. Koo et al. (1994) reported an overall 23.3% prevalence of at least one psychiatric disorder, with 8.8% major depression, 18.2% generalized anxiety disorder, and 4.4% paranoid disorder. In a small study, 66% of alopecia areata patients presented with psychiatric comorbidity, mainly adjustment disorders, generalized anxiety disorder, and depressive episodes (Ruiz-Doblado et al. 2003). Picardi et al. (2003b) compared 21 patients with recent onset of alopecia areata and 102 dermatology control subjects and found that alopecia areata was associated with high avoidance in attachment relationships and poor social support.

Management

Psychotherapy. Objective evaluation of the efficacy of psychosocial therapies in alopecia areata is difficult because alopecia areata patients can experience remission of symptoms without active therapies (Delamere et al. 2008). A small open trial in patients with treatment-refractory alopecia areata used a hypnotherapeutic approach combining symptom-oriented suggestions with suggestions to improve self-esteem. Significant scalp hair growth occurred in 12 of 21 patients, and all patients had a significant decrease in scores for anxiety and depression (Willemsen and Vanderlinden 2008). Psychotherapy may help the patient's mental state but may not affect the alopecia areata, and self-help and support groups can help the patient cope with the psychosocial impact of alopecia areata (Beard 1986).

Psychopharmacology. The literature on the use of psychotropic agents in alopecia areata is inconclusive. A 2008 Cochrane review of treatment for alopecia areata concluded that very few treatments of any kind have been well evaluated in randomized trials (Delamere et al. 2008). In a double-blind, placebo-controlled study of 13 patients with alopecia areata, 5 of 7 patients taking imipramine, but none receiving placebo, had significant hair regrowth after 6 months (Perini et al. 1994), and reduction of alopecia did not correlate with alleviation of depressive symptoms. In a case series of 7 women with alopecia areata, a 3-month course of citalopram led to objective clinical improvement in alopecia in 6 of the 7 women, in addition to improvement in the anxiety and depression scores (Ruiz-Doblado et al. 1999). A 3-month randomized, double-blind, placebo-controlled study of paroxetine in 13 alopecia areata patients reported "complete regrowth of hair" in 2 patients and "partial regrowth" in 4, while 1 patient from the placebo group had "an almost complete regrowth of hair" (Cipriani et al. 2001, p. 601).

Acne

Acne vulgaris (Zaenglein and Thiboutot 2008) is a multifactorial disorder of the pilosebaceous unit characterized by comedones (whiteheads and blackheads), papules, pustules, nodules, cysts, and scars; it affects the face, neck, upper trunk, and upper arms. Acne vulgaris has a peak incidence during adolescence, affects 85% of individuals 12–24 years of age, and continues on into later life in 12% of women and 3% of men. Androgens from the gonads and adrenal glands affect sebum secretion and play a key role in the pathogenesis of acne. Endocrine disorders associated with high androgen levels are associated with increased risk for acne. Acne excoriée and acne excoriée des jeunes filles, which often have significant psychiatric comorbidity, develop when acne comedones and papules are excoriated by the patient, often young women, leaving crusted erosions that may scar.

Stress

Psychosocial stress can lead to exacerbations of acne in more than 60% of cases (Chiu et al. 2003; Harth et al. 2009). On the other hand, having to cope with the cosmetic disfigurement associated with acne can be a significant source of stress for some patients. The impact of acne on quality of life and acne-related stress often does not correlate directly with the clinical severity of the condition (Gupta and Gupta 2001b).

Psychosocial and Psychiatric Factors

Psychiatric and psychosocial comorbidity is one of the most disabling features of acne and is sometimes the most important factor in deciding whether to institute dermatological therapies. The extent of psychiatric morbidity in acne, including the prevalence of suicidal ideation, is not consistently related to the clinical severity of the skin condition. Bullying and teasing related to the cosmetic effects of acne can be a problem for a significant minority of adolescent acne patients (Magin et al. 2008), which in turn can lead to anxiety, poor self-esteem, acting out, or aggression. In a study of 18-year-old Norwegian high school students, those adolescents who had acne reported "significantly more depressive symptoms, lower self-attitude, more feelings of uselessness, fewer feelings of pride, lower self-worth, and lower body satisfaction" (Dalgard et al. 2008, p. 750). A cross-sectional survey of 9,567 12- to 18-year-olds in New Zealand revealed that self-reported "problem acne" was associated with approximately twice the frequency of depressive symptoms, anxiety, and suicide attempts. The association of acne with suicide attempts remained after controlling for depressive symptoms and anxiety (OR=1.50, 95% CI=1.21–1.86) (Purvis et al. 2006). The prevalence of suicidal ideation among acne patients has been reported to be 5%–7% (Gupta and Gupta 1998; Picardi et al. 2006).

Acne and eating disorders often coexist, patients with both are very sensitive about and preoccupied with their appearance. Acne is also one of the dermatological manifestations of eating disorders (Strumia 2005). Binge eating is often associated with acne flare-ups, and starvation, which can result in lower androgen levels, may improve acne. Acne is a major concern among patients with BDD, and dermatological treatments are the most frequently sought after and received nonpsychiatric treatments in BDD, the most common being topical acne agents (Crerand et al. 2005). In a study of acne patients ages 16–35 years, 36.7% of patients with clinically "minimal to nonexistent acne" and 32.9% of patients with clinically mild acne met criteria for BDD (Bowe et al. 2007). Those requiring systemic isotretinoin therapy were twice as likely to have BDD as those who never used it (Bowe et al. 2007).

The peak incidence of acne is during the mid-teens, a life stage when the individual is dealing with the social challenges of adolescence and is normally sensitive about his or her appearance and body image. This is also the age when mood and anxiety disorders, BDD, eating disorders, and schizophrenia often become symptomatic. The association of acne with depressive symptoms and BDD, and the higher prevalence of suicidal behavior in this age group, therefore does not necessarily imply a direct causal relationship with acne. Social isolation, difficulties in interpersonal relationships, and body image concerns, which may be a consequence of a psychiatric disorder, are often instead attributed to acne, both by the adolescent patients and sometimes by their parents, who may not be ready to acknowledge the possibility that their child has a mental disorder.

Isotretinoin and Psychiatric Side Effects

Isotretinoin, which is generally used to treat severe acne, has been associated with depression, psychosis, suicide, and aggressive behaviors (Physicians' Desk Reference 2008), an association first reported by the FDA in 1998 (Nightingale 1998) and followed in 2002 by an additional warning regarding aggressive and/or violent behaviors. In 2005, the FDA reported that it continues to assess reports of suicide and suicide attempts associated with the use of isotretinoin. However, the general consensus at present is that the relationship between psychiatric side effects and isotretinoin is unclear, with little support from controlled trial data (Marqueling and Zane 2005; Strahan and Raimer 2006). However, individual cases have been reported in which the relationship between depression and isotretinoin use was confirmed by rechallenge with isotretinoin (Scheinman et al. 1990). A recent Canadian case-crossover study reported a doubling of risk for depression in those exposed to isotretinoin (Azoulay et al. 2008). Overall, improvement in acne with isotretinoin is associated with an improvement in depression scores. Patients who develop depression with isotretinoin may have previously used the drug with no adverse psychiatric effects (Scheinman et al. 1990). The current guidelines for prescribing isotretinoin (Accutane is one of the trade names) in the United States state that "prior to initiation of Accutane therapy, patients and family members should be asked about any history of psychiatric disorder, and at each visit during therapy, patients should be assessed for symptoms of depression, mood disturbance, psychosis, or aggression to determine if further evaluation may be necessary" (Physicians' Desk Reference 2008, p. 2608). Discontinuation of isotretinoin is not necessarily associated with a remission of the psychiatric symptoms. The decision to continue isotretinoin in a patient who has experienced a psychiatric reaction should be based on the risk-benefit ratio for the particular patient.

Management

Psychotherapy. Acne can lead to problems with socialization, self-esteem, anger, and body image that can be addressed in psychotherapy (Fried and Wechsler 2006). When adolescent acne is untreated, some of these problems may persist into later life, when acne is no longer a problem. BDD patients, who typically express concern about clinically mild acne, tend to resist any psychological explanation for their skin concerns. Some patients pick their skin and self-excoriate their acne to regulate emotions (e.g., in PTSD); underlying trauma issues should be addressed in therapy after the patient is adequately stabilized. Cognitive-behavioral therapies and hypnosis have been used in *acne excoriée* (Shenefelt 2003). Because a significant number of adolescents with eating disorders also develop acne, it is important for the clinician to be aware of this association and to evaluate the potential impact of acne on the patient's body image and eating behavior.

Psychopharmacology. Psychotropic medications in acne patients are directed at underlying psychiatric pathology. Some patients on isotretinoin who develop depression may require standard antidepressant agents. There are some case studies of failure of hormonal contraceptives in patients using isotretinoin who self-medicate depression with St. John's wort, which is a CYP 3A4 inducer and thus increases the metabolism of some hormonal contraceptives. Case reports attest to the benefits of a wide variety of psychotropic agents for acne, including paroxetine (Moussavian 2001) and olanzapine for *acne excoriée* (Gupta and Gupta 2000), but there are no controlled clinical trials.

Cutaneous Reactions to Psychopharmacological Agents

Adverse cutaneous drug reactions (ACDRs) can be divided into common (usually relatively benign) ACDRs (Table 29–2), rare life-threatening ACDRs (Table 29–3), and precipitation or aggravation of a primary dermatological disorder (Litt 2004; Warnock and Morris 2002a, 2002b, 2003).

Common Adverse Cutaneous Drug Reactions

Common ACDRs include pruritus, exanthematous rashes, urticaria with or without angioedema, fixed drug eruptions, photosensitivity reactions, drug-induced pigmentation, and alopecia.

TABLE 29–2. Most common cutaneous drug reactions to psychotherapeutic agents

Pruritus and exanthematous rashes
Urticaria with or without angioedema
Fixed drug eruptions
Photosensitivity reactions
Drug-induced pigmentation
Alopecia

Pruritus is the most common ACDR, encountered with all antipsychotics, antidepressants, and mood stabilizers, and is usually secondary to other ACDRs.

Exanthematous rashes (morbilliform or maculopapular eruptions) can occur with all antipsychotics, antidepressants, and mood stabilizers. The rash usually occurs within the first 3–14 days of starting the drug and may subside without discontinuation of the causative agent. A rash accompanied by painful skin lesions, mucosal lesions, or sore throat may represent the early stages of one of the more severe and life-threatening ACDRs, such as Stevens-Johnson syndrome.

Urticaria with or without *angioedema* is the second most common ACDR after pruritus; it occurs within minutes to hours—but sometimes as late as several days—after starting the drug and can lead to laryngeal angioedema and anaphylaxis. Urticaria can occur with all antipsychotics, antidepressants, and anticonvulsants.

Fixed drug eruptions, which can theoretically occur with any drug, characteristically present as sharply demarcated, solitary or occasionally multiple lesions. Eruptions occur within a few to 24 hours after ingestion of the drug and resolve within several weeks of drug discontinuation.

Drug-induced photosensitivity can present either as phototoxicity (an exaggerated sunburn restricted to sun-exposed skin) or as photoallergy (a more generalized eruption triggered by sun exposure when a person is on certain drugs). Drug-induced photosensitivity tends to involve only sun-exposed skin, although there may be exceptions. Photosensitivity reactions can be caused by any of the antipsychotics but are much more frequently associated with chlorpromazine (3% incidence). Photosensitivity also occurs with many antidepressants, anticonvulsants, and sedative-hypnotics. Patients should be advised regarding the use of sunscreen and minimization of sun exposure in those instances where the medication has to be continued. Photosensitivity caused by psychotropic drugs may interfere with PUVA and ultraviolet B (UVB) phototherapy for psoriasis and other pruritic dermatoses.

TABLE 29–3. Severe and life-threatening cutaneous drug reactions to psychotherapeutic agents

Erythema multiforme
Stevens-Johnson syndrome
Toxic epidermal necrolysis
Drug hypersensitivity syndrome (also drug eruption with eosinophilia and systemic symptoms [DRESS])
Exfoliative dermatitis
Drug hypersensitivity vasculitis

Drug-induced pigmentation, which may involve the skin and eyes (retina, lens, and cornea), has been reported after long-term (>6 months) high-dose (>500 mg/day) use of low-potency typical antipsychotics, especially chlorpromazine and thioridazine. Pigmentary changes have been associated with some antidepressants, including various TCAs, all SSRIs, venlafaxine (hypopigmentation), and several anticonvulsants (also changes in hair color and texture).

Alopecia has been frequently reported with lithium (>5%) and valproic acid (>5%) and less frequently with the other mood stabilizers. Alopecia has also been associated with most antidepressants and several antipsychotics. Hair loss may occur rapidly or a few months after the drug is started, with recovery generally 2–18 months after drug discontinuation.

Severe and Life-Threatening Adverse Cutaneous Drug Reactions

Severe and life-threatening skin reactions (see Table 29–3) are most often associated with anticonvulsants and include erythema multiforme, Stevens-Johnson syndrome, toxic epidermal necrolysis (TEN), drug hypersensitivity syndrome or drug eruption with eosinophilia and systemic symptoms (DRESS), exfoliative dermatitis, and vasculitis (Litt 2004; Warnock and Morris 2002a, 2002b, 2003). Erythema multiforme, Stevens-Johnson syndrome, and TEN lie on a continuum of increasing severity. About 16% of Stevens-Johnson syndrome/TEN cases have been associated with short-term use of anticonvulsant drugs, with greatest risk for development of TEN within the first 8 weeks of initiating therapy. Use of multiple anticonvulsants and higher dosages increases the risk. Treatment of severe reactions should include immediate discontinuation of the drug and emergency dermatology consult. Patients typically require fluid and nutritional support as well as infection and pain control, which may involve management in an intensive care or burn unit.

Erythema multiforme occurs within days of starting the drug and may present as a polymorphous eruption, with pathognomonic "target lesions" typically involving the extremities and palmoplantar surfaces. The potential for evolution to more serious Stevens-Johnson syndrome and TEN should always be considered. Although rarely associated with antipsychotics and antidepressants, it is most commonly associated with carbamazepine, valproic acid, lamotrigine, gabapentin, and oxcarbazepine.

Stevens-Johnson syndrome usually occurs within the first few weeks after drug exposure and presents as flu-like symptoms followed by mucocutaneous lesions; it has a mortality rate as high as 5% due to loss of the cutaneous barrier and sepsis. Bullous lesions can involve mucosal surfaces, including the eyes, mouth, and genital tract. Stevens-Johnson syndrome is most frequently associated with the same anticonvulsants as erythema multiforme.

Toxic epidermal necrolysis is considered to be an extreme variant of Stevens-Johnson syndrome, resulting in epidermal detachment in excess of 30% of patients, occurring within the first 2 months of treatment, with a mortality rate as high as 45% due to sepsis. In 80% of TEN cases, a strong association is made with specific medications (versus a 50% association with specific medications in Stevens-Johnson syndrome), most often anticonvulsants.

Drug hypersensitivity syndrome (drug eruption with eosinophilia and systemic symptoms, or DRESS) characteristically occurs 1–8 weeks after starting drug treatment, presenting as a drug eruption with fever, eosinophilia, lymphadenopathy, and multiple organ involvement. Treatment involves immediate discontinuation of the suspected drug, systemic steroids, and antihistamines. The mortality rate is 10% if symptoms are unrecognized or untreated. The rash can range from a simple exanthem to TEN and is almost exclusively associated with anticonvulsants.

Exfoliative dermatitis presents as a widespread rash characterized by desquamation, pruritic erythema, fever, and lymphadenopathy within the first few weeks of drug therapy, with a good prognosis if the causative agent is withdrawn immediately. It has been reported with antipsychotics, most TCAs and other antidepressants, mood stabilizers, lithium, sedatives, and hypnotics.

Drug hypersensitivity vasculitis, characterized by inflammation and necrosis of the walls of blood vessels, occurs within a few weeks of starting a drug. Lesions (e.g., palpable purpura) are primarily localized on the lower third of the legs and ankles. It has been associated rarely with clozapine, maprotiline, trazodone, carbamazepine, lithium, phenobarbital, pentobarbital, diazepam, and chlordiazepoxide.

Drug-Induced Precipitation or Aggravation of a Primary Dermatological Disorder

A number of primary dermatological disorders (Litt 2004; Warnock and Morris 2002a, 2002b, 2003) may be precipitated or exacerbated by a psychotropic drug, including acne, psoriasis, seborrheic dermatitis, hyperhidrosis, and porphyria. Acne has been associated with most antidepressants, lithium, anticonvulsants, and antipsychotics. It is well recognized that lithium can precipitate or exacerbate psoriasis. Lithium-induced psoriasis can occur within a few months but usually occurs within the first few years of treatment. Psoriasis precipitated or exacerbated by lithium is typically resistant to conventional antipsoriatic treatments and usually there is no family history of psoriasis. When psoriasis becomes intractable, lithium must be discontinued, and remission usually follows within a few months. Anticonvulsants, atypical antipsychotics, and SSRIs have been less commonly reported to precipitate or aggravate psoriasis. Seborrheic dermatitis is very common in patients on long-term phenothiazines and also has been reported with other antipsychotics, lithium, and anticonvulsants. Hyperhidrosis, often manifested as night sweats, is common with SSRIs, SNRIs, bupropion, and MAOIs. Sweating is mediated by the sympathetic cholinergic innervation of the eccrine sweat glands; however, the more anticholinergic TCAs have also caused hyperhidrosis, and therefore switching to a more anticholinergic antidepressant is not necessarily helpful. Hyperhidrosis has also been reported with antipsychotics and anticonvulsants. Porphyria may be exacerbated by certain drugs (e.g., carbamazepine, valproic acid, and many sedative-hypnotics (especially barbiturates), resulting in acute dermatological, neuropsychiatric, and abdominal pain symptoms. Chlorpromazine, although photosensitizing, is considered to be "safe" and actually was approved by the FDA for use in acute intermittent porphyria.

Interactions Between Dermatology Drugs and Psychopharmacological Agents

Most pharmacokinetic interactions (Litt 2004) between dermatological and psychotropic drugs result from inhibition of CYP-mediated drug metabolism, mainly involving the CYP 2D6 and 3A4 isoenzymes. Selected interactions are listed in Table 29-4.

Conclusion

Psychodermatological disorders are usually classified either as dermatological manifestations of a primary psychiatric disorder—for example, delusional or body image pathology presenting as a dermatological complaint—or as psychological factors in a primary dermatological disorder (e.g., psoriasis, atopic dermatitis) that is exacerbated by psychosocial stress and that often is comorbid with psychiatric morbidity (e.g., depression, anxiety). Psychological trauma and dissociative symptoms are often factors in the self-induced dermatoses. Factors that increase psychiatric morbidity (including suicide risk) in the dermatology patient include pruritus and sleep difficulties, disease-related stress (largely due to the cosmetic disfigurement), social stigma associated with the skin disorder, and (in the pediatric age group) appearance-related bullying. The a high prevalence of suicidal ideation among dermatology patients is not consistently related to the clinical severity of the skin condition. Covert body dysmorphic disorder can also increase suicide risk and treatment resistance. Standard psychopharmacological agents, with adequate clinical monitoring, may be used to treat psychiatric comorbidity in dermatological disorders. Severe and life-threatening dermatological reactions to psychotropic agents (e.g., Stevens-Johnson syndrome, toxic epidermal necrolysis) are most frequently associated with the mood-stabilizing anticonvulsants, with the greatest risk of development during the first 2 months of therapy. Assessment and treatment of the dermatology patient should follow a biopsychosocial model. The psychiatrist should thoroughly address and

TABLE 29-4. Selected dermatological drug-psychotherapeutic drug pharmacokinetic interactions

Medication used in dermatology	Effects on CYP isoenzymes	Effects on psychotropic drug levels
Azole antifungals (oral formulations only) Itraconazole Ketaconazole Macrolide antibiotics Clarithromycin Erythromycin Cyclosporine (both substrate and inhibitor of CYP 3A4)	Inhibition of CYP 3A4	Benzodiazepine serum levels for agents that undergo hepatic oxidative metabolism (e.g., alprazolam, triazolam) may increase. Buspirone levels are increased. Carbamazepine levels are increased. Pimozide levels are increased.
Terbinafine	Inhibition of CYP 2D6	Antidepressant serum levels may increase for CYP 2D6 substrates (e.g., tricyclic antidepressants, paroxetine, venlafaxine, atomoxetine). Antipsychotic serum levels may increase for CYP 2D6 substrates (e.g., phenothiazines, haloperidol, risperidone, olanzapine, clozapine, aripiprazole).

Note. CYP = cytochrome P450.

manage any pruritus and sleep difficulties the patient may be experiencing and should recommend aggressive dermatological treatment of even clinically mild skin disease that is cosmetically disfiguring or stigmatizing.

References

Abel EA, Moore US, Glathe JP: Psoriasis patient support group and self-care efficacy as an adjunct to day care center treatment. Int J Dermatol 29:640–643, 1990

Abetz LM, Savage NW: Burning mouth syndrome and psychological disorders. Aust Dent J 54:84–93, 2009

Ahmad K, Ramsay B: Misdiagnosis of dermatitis artefacta: how did we get it wrong? Clin Exp Dermatol 34:113–114, 2008

Ahmad K, Ramsay B: Delusional parasitosis: lessons learnt. Acta Derm Venereol 89:165–168, 2009

Allan SJ, Kavanagh GM, Herd RM, et al: The effect of inositol supplements on the psoriasis of patients taking lithium: a randomized, placebo-controlled trial. Br J Dermatol 150:966–969, 2004

Alpsoy E, Ozcan E, Cetin L, et al: Is the efficacy of topical corticosteroid therapy for psoriasis vulgaris enhanced by concurrent moclobemide therapy? A double-blind, placebo-controlled study. J Am Acad Dermatol 38:197–200, 1998

American Psychiatric Association: Diagnostic and Statistical Manual of Mental Disorders, 4th Edition, Text Revision. Washington, DC, American Psychiatric Association, 2000

Arck PC, Slominski A, Theoharides TC, et al: Neuroimmunology of stress: skin takes center stage. J Invest Dermatol 126:1697–1704, 2006

Arnold LM, Mutasim DF, Dwight MM, et al: An open clinical trial of fluvoxamine treatment of psychogenic excoriation. J Clin Psychopharmacol 19:15–18, 1999

Arnold LM, Auchenbach MB, McElroy SL: Psychogenic excoriation. Clinical features, proposed diagnostic criteria and approaches to treatment. CNS Drugs 15:351–359, 2001

Azoulay L, Blais L, Koren G, et al: Isotretinoin and the risk of depression in patients with acne vulgaris: a case-crossover study. J Clin Psychiatry 69:526–532, 2008

Bassukas ID, Hyphantis T, Gamvroulia C, et al: Infliximab for patients with plaque psoriasis and severe psychiatric comorbidity. J Eur Acad Dermatol Venereol 22:257–258, 2008

Beard HO: Social and psychological implications of alopecia areata. J Am Acad Dermatol 14:697–700, 1986

Bigatà X, Sais G, Soler F: Severe chronic urticaria: response to mirtazapine. J Am Acad Dermatol 53:916–917, 2005

Bishop ER Jr: Monosymptomatic hypochondriacal syndromes in dermatology. J Am Acad Dermatol 9:152–158, 1983

Blanch J, Grimalt F, Massana G, et al: Efficacy of olanzapine in the treatment of psychogenic excoriation. Br J Dermatol 151:714–716, 2004

Bloch MH, Landeros-Weisenberger A, Dombrowski P, et al: Systematic review: pharmacological and behavioral treatment for trichotillomania. Biol Psychiatry 62:839–846, 2007

Bockelbrink A, Heinrich J, Schäfer I, et al: Atopic eczema in children: another harmful sequel of divorce. The LISA Study Group. Allergy 61:1397–1402, 2006

Boscarino JA: Posttraumatic stress disorder and physical illness. Ann N Y Acad Sci 1032:141–153, 2004

Bowe WP, Leyden JJ, Crerand CE, et al: Body dysmorphic disorder symptoms among patients with acne vulgaris. J Am Acad Dermatol 57:222–230, 2007

Brauchli YB, Jick SS, Curtin F, et al: Lithium, antipsychotics, and risk of psoriasis. J Clin Psychopharmacol 29:134–140, 2009

Brzoza Z, Kasperska-Zajac A, Badura-Brzoza K, et al: Decline in dehydroepiandrosterone sulfate observed in chronic urticaria is associated with psychological distress. Psychosom Med 70:723–728, 2008

Buske-Kirschbaum A, Jobst S, Wustmans A, et al: Attenuated free cortisol response to psychosocial stress in children with atopic dermatitis. Psychosom Med 59:419–426, 1997

Buske-Kirschbaum A, Geiben A, Hollig H, et al: Altered responsiveness of the hypothalamus-pituitary-adrenal axis and the sympathetic adrenomedullary system of stress in patients with atopic dermatitis. J Clin Endocrinol Metab 87:4245–4251, 2002

Calikusu C, Yucel B, Polat A, et al: The relation of psychogenic excoriation with psychiatric disorders: a comparative study. Compr Psychiatry 44:256–261, 2003

Chiu A, Chon SY, Kimball AB: The response of skin disease to stress: changes in the severity of acne vulgaris as affected by examination stress. Arch Dermatol 139:897–900, 2003

Choi EH, Brown BE, Crumrine D, et al: Mechanisms by which psychological stress alters cutaneous permeability barrier homeostasis and stratum corneum integrity. J Invest Dermatol 124:587–595, 2005

Christenson GA, Mackenzie TB, Mitchell JE: Characteristics of 60 adult chronic hair pullers. Am J Psychiatry 148:365–370, 1991a

Christenson GA, Popkin MK, MacKenzie TB, et al: Lithium treatment of chronic hair pulling. J Clin Psychiatry 52:116–120, 1991b

Chung MC, Symons C, Gilliam J, et al: The relationship between posttraumatic stress disorder, psychiatric comorbidity, and personality traits among patients with chronic idiopathic urticaria. Compr Psychiatry 51:55–63, 2010

Cipriani R, Perini GI, Rampinelli S: Paroxetine in alopecia areata. Int J Dermatol 40:600–601, 2001

Cohen AD, Vardy DA: Dermatitis artefacta in soldiers. Mil Med 171:497–499, 2006

Cotterill JA, Cunliffe WJ: Suicide in dermatological patients. Br J Dermatol 137:246–250, 1997

Crerand CE, Phillips KA, Menard W, et al: Nonpsychiatric medical treatment of body dysmorphic disorder. Psychosomatics 46:549–555, 2005

Curtis AR, Richards RW: The treatment of psychogenic excoriation and obsessive compulsive disorder using aripiprazole and fluoxetine. Ann Clin Psychiatry 19:199–200, 2007

Czubalski K, Rudzki E: Neuropsychic factors in physical urticaria. Dermatologica 154:1–4, 1977

Dalgard F, Lien L, Dalen I: Itch in the community: associations with psychosocial factors among adults. J Eur Acad Dermatol Venereol 21:1215–1219, 2007

Dalgard F, Gieler U, Holm JØ, et al: Self-esteem and body satisfaction among late adolescents with acne: results from a population survey. J Am Acad Dermatol 59:746–751, 2008

Delamere FM, Sladden MM, Dobbins HM, et al: Interventions for alopecia areata. Cochrane Database Syst Rev (2):CD004413, 2008

Diefenbach GJ, Tolin DF, Hannan S, et al: Group treatment for trichotillomania: behavior therapy versus supportive therapy. Behav Ther 37:353–363, 2006

Diefenbach GJ, Tolin DF, Meunier S, et al: Emotion regulation and trichotillomania: a comparison of clinical and nonclinical hair pulling. J Behav Ther 39:32–41, 2008

Drake LA, Millikan LE: The antipruritic effect of 5% doxepin cream in patients with eczematous dermatitis. Doxepin Study Group. Arch Dermatol 131:1403–1408, 1995

Duke DC, Keeley ML, Geffken GR, et al: Trichotillomania: a current review. Clin Psychol Rev 30:181–193, 2010

Ebata T, Izumi H, Aizawa H, et al: Effects of nitrazepam on nocturnal scratching in adults with atopic dermatitis: a double-blind placebo-controlled crossover study. Br J Dermatol 138:631–634, 1998

Eli I, Baht R, Littner MM, et al: Detection of psychopathologic trends in glossodynia patients. Psychosom Med 56:389–394, 1994

Ersser SJ, Latter S, Sibley A, et al: Psychological and educational interventions for atopic eczema in children. Cochrane Database Syst Rev (3):CD004054, 2007

Fabisch W: Psychiatric aspects of dermatitis artefacta. Br J Dermatol 102:29–34, 1980

Fellner MJ, Majeed MH: Tales of bugs, delusions of parasitosis, and what to do. Clin Dermatol 27:135–138, 2009

Fortune DG, Richards HL, Kirby B, et al: Psychological distress impairs clearance of psoriasis in patients treated with photochemotherapy. Arch Dermatol 139:752–756, 2003

Fortune DG, Richards HL, Griffiths CE: Psychologic factors in psoriasis: consequences, mechanisms, and interventions. Dermatol Clin 23:681–694, 2005

Freudenmann RW, Lepping P: Second-generation antipsychotics in primary and secondary delusional parasitosis. J Clin Psychopharmacol 28:500–508, 2008

Freunsgaard K: Neurotic excoriations: a controlled psychiatric examination. Acta Psychiatr Scand Suppl 312:1–52, 1984

Fried RG, Wechsler A: Psychological problems in the acne patient. Dermatol Ther 19:237–240, 2006

Gardner FM, Diamond LK: Autoerythrocyte sensitization: a form of purpura producing painful bruising following autosensitization to red blood cells in certain women. Blood 10:675–690, 1955

Garg A, Chren MM, Sands LP, et al: Psychological stress perturbs epidermal permeability barrier homeostasis: implications for the pathogenesis of stress-associated skin disorders. Arch Dermatol 137:53–59, 2001

Gershuny BS, Keuthen NJ, Gentes EL, et al: Current posttraumatic stress disorder and history of trauma in trichotillomania. J Clin Psychol 62:1521–1529, 2006

Ghanizadeh A: Comorbidity of psychiatric disorders in children and adolescents with alopecia areata in a child and adolescent psychiatry clinical sample. Int J Dermatol 47:1118–1120, 2008

Goldsobel AB, Rohr AS, Siegel SC, et al: Efficacy of doxepin in the treatment of chronic idiopathic urticaria. J Allergy Clin Immunol 78(5 pt 1):867–873, 1986

Gottlieb AB, Chao C, Dann F: Psoriasis comorbidities. J Dermatolog Treat 19:5–21, 2008

Grant JE, Odlaug BL: Clinical characteristics of trichotillomania with trichophagia. Compr Psychiatry 49:579–584, 2008

Grant JE, Odlaug BL: Update on pathological skin picking. Curr Psychiatry Rep 11:283–288, 2009

Grattan CEH, Black AK: Urticaria and angioedema, in Dermatology, 2nd Edition, Vol 1. Edited by Bolognia JL, Jorizzo JL, Rapini RP. London, Mosby Elsevier, 2008, pp 261–276

Greene SL, Reed CE, Schroeter AL: Double-blind crossover study comparing doxepin with diphenhydramine for the treatment of chronic urticaria. J Am Acad Dermatol 12:669–675, 1985

Gupta MA: Somatization disorders in dermatology. Int Rev Psychiatry 18:41–47, 2006

Gupta MA: Stress and urticaria, in Neuroimmunology of the Skin: Basic Science to Clinical Practice. Edited by Granstein RD, Luger T. Berlin Heidelberg, Springer-Verlag, 2009, pp 209–217

Gupta MA, Gupta AK: Chronic idiopathic urticaria associated with panic disorder: a syndrome responsive to selective serotonin reuptake inhibitor antidepressants? Cutis 56:53–54, 1995

Gupta MA, Gupta AK: Psychodermatology: an update. J Am Acad Dermatol 34:1030–1046, 1996

Gupta MA, Gupta AK: Depression and suicidal ideation in dermatology patients with acne, alopecia areata, atopic dermatitis and psoriasis. Br J Dermatol 139:846–850, 1998

Gupta MA, Gupta AK: Olanzapine is effective in the management of some self-induced dermatoses: three case reports. Cutis 66:143–146, 2000

Gupta MA, Gupta AK: Dissatisfaction with skin appearance among patients with eating disorders and non-clinical controls. Br J Dermatol 145:110–113, 2001a

Gupta MA, Gupta AK: The psychological comorbidity in acne. Clin Dermatol 19:360–363, 2001b

Gupta MA, Gupta AK: The use of antidepressant drugs in dermatology. J Eur Acad Dermatol Venereol 15:512–518, 2001c

Gupta MA, Gupta AK: Use of eye movement desensitization and reprocessing (EMDR) in the treatment of dermatologic disorders. J Cutan Med Surg 6:415–421, 2002

Gupta MA, Gupta AK: Psychiatric and psychological co-morbidity in patients with dermatologic disorders: epidemiology and management. Am J Clin Dermatol 4:833–842, 2003

Gupta MA, Gupta AK: Medically unexplained cutaneous sensory symptoms may represent somatoform dissociation: an empirical study. J Psychosom Res 60:131–136, 2006

Gupta MA, Gupta AK, Haberman HF: Neurotic excoriations: a review and some new perspectives. Compr Psychiatry 27:381–386, 1986

Gupta MA, Gupta AK, Haberman HF: Dermatologic signs in anorexia nervosa and bulimia nervosa. Arch Dermatol 123:1386–1390, 1987a

Gupta MA, Gupta AK, Haberman HF: The self-inflicted dermatoses: a critical review. Gen Hosp Psychiatry 9:45–52, 1987b

Gupta MA, Gupta AK, Kirkby S, et al: Pruritus in psoriasis: a prospective study of some psychiatric and dermatologic correlates. Arch Dermatol 124:1052–1057, 1988

Gupta MA, Gupta AK, Kirkby S, et al: A psychocutaneous profile of psoriasis patients who are stress reactors: a study of 127 patients. Gen Hosp Psychiatry 11:166–173, 1989

Gupta MA, Gupta AK, Voorhees JJ: Starvation-associated pruritus: a clinical feature of eating disorders. J Am Acad Dermatol 27:118–120, 1992

Gupta MA, Gupta AK, Schork NJ, et al: Depression modulates pruritus perception. A study of pruritis in psoriasis, atopic dermatitis, and chronic idiopathic urticaria. Psychosom Med 56:36–40, 1994

Gupta MA, Gupta AK, Watteel GN: Stress and alopecia areata: a psychodermatologic study. Acta Derm Venereol 77:296–298, 1997

Gupta MA, Gupta AK, Chandarana PC, et al: Dissociative symptoms and self-induced dermatoses: a preliminary empirical study (abstract). Psychosom Med 62:116, 2000

Gupta MA, Gupta AK, Johnson AM: Cutaneous body image: empirical validation of a dermatologic construct. J Invest Dermatol 123:405–406, 2004

Gupta MA, Gupta AK, Ellis CN, et al: Psychiatric evaluation of the dermatology patient. Dermatol Clin 23:591–599, 2005

Haefner HK, Collins ME, Davis GD, et al: The vulvodynia guideline. J Low Genit Tract Dis 9:40–51, 2005

Hampf G, Vikkula J, Ylipaavalniemi P, et al: Psychiatric disorders in orofacial dysaesthesia. Int J Oral Maxillofac Surg 16:402–407, 1987

Harris BA, Sherertz EF, Flowers FP: Improvement of chronic neurotic excoriations with oral doxepin therapy. Int J Dermatol 26:541–543, 1987

Harth W, Gieler U, Kusnir D, et al: Clinical Management in Psychodermatology. Berlin Heidelberg, Springer-Verlag, 2009

Harth W, Hermes B, Freudenmann RW: Morgellons in dermatology. J Dtsch Dermatol Ges 8:234–242, 2010a

Harth W, Klaus-Michael T, Gieler U: Factitious disorders in dermatology. J Dtsch Dermatol Ges 8:361–373, 2010b

Hashizume H, Horibe T, Ohshima A, et al: Anxiety accelerates T-helper 2-tilted immune responses in patients with atopic dermatitis. Br J Dermatol 152:1161–1164, 2005

Hatch ML, Paradis C, Freidman S, et al: Obsessive-compulsive disorder in patients with chronic pruritic conditions: case studies and discussion. J Am Acad Dermatol 26:549–551, 1992

Haustein UF: Adrenergic urticaria and adrenergic pruritus. Acta Derm Venereol 70:82–84, 1990

Hoare C, Li Wan Po A, Williams H: Systematic review of treatments for atopic eczema. Health Technol Assess 4:1–191, 2000

Hoss D, Segal S: Scalp dysesthesia. Arch Dermatol 134:327–330, 1998

Howlett S: Emotional dysfunction, child-family relationships and childhood atopic dermatitis. Br J Dermatol 140:381–384, 1999

Hundley JL, Yosipovitch G: Mirtazapine for reducing nocturnal itch in patients with chronic pruritus: a pilot study. J Am Acad Dermatol 50:889–891, 2004

Hunt N, McHale S: The psychological impact of alopecia. BMJ 331:951–953, 2005

Ivanov OL, Lvov AN, Michenko AV, et al: Autoerythrocyte sensitization syndrome (Gardner-Diamond syndrome): review of the literature. J Eur Acad Derm Venereol 23:499–504, 2009

Kabat-Zinn J, Wheeler E, Light T, et al: Influence of a mindfulness meditation-based stress reduction intervention on rates of skin clearing in patients with moderate to severe psoriasis undergoing phototherapy (UVB) and photochemotherapy (PUVA). Psychosom Med 60:625–632, 1998

Kalivas J, Kalivas L, Gilman D, et al: Sertraline in the treatment of neurotic excoriations and related disorders. Arch Dermatol 132:589–590, 1996

Kang K, Poster AM, Nedorost ST, et al: Atopic dermatitis, in Dermatology, 2nd Edition, Vol 1. Edited by Bolognia JL, Jorizzo JL, Rapini RP. London, Mosby Elsevier, 2008, pp 181–195

Kasperska-Zajac A, Brzoza Z, Rogala B: Lower serum dehydroepiandrosterone sulphate concentration in chronic idiopathic urticaria: a secondary transient phenomenon? Br J Dermatol 159:743–744, 2008

Kaymak Y, Taner E, Simsek I: Body dysmorphic disorder in university students with skin diseases compared with healthy controls. Acta Derm Venereol 89:281–284, 2009

Kelsay K: Management of sleep disturbance associated with atopic dermatitis. J Allergy Clin Immunol 118:198–201, 2006

Kenchaiah BK, Kumar S, Tharyan P: Atypical antipsychotics in delusional parasitosis: a retrospective case series of 20 patients. International J Dermatol 49:95–100, 2010

Kimata H: Prevalence of suicidal ideation in patients with atopic dermatitis. Suicide Life Threat Behav 36:120–124, 2006

Kirby B, Richards HL, Woo P, et al: Physical and psychologic measures are necessary to assess overall psoriasis severity. J Am Acad Dermatol 45:72–76, 2001

Koblenzer CS: Psychocutaneous Disease. Orlando, FL, Grune & Stratton, 1987

Koca R, Altin R, Konuk N, et al: Sleep disturbance in patients with lichen simplex chronicus and its relationship to nocturnal scratching: a case control study. South Med J 99:482–485, 2006

Konuk N, Koca R, Atik L, et al: Psychopathology, depression and dissociative experiences in patients with lichen simplex chronicus. Gen Hosp Psychiatry 29:232–235, 2007

Koo J, Lee CS: Psychocutaneous disease, in Dermatology, 2nd Edition, Vol 1. Edited by Bolognia JL, Jorizzo JL, Rapini RP. London, Mosby Elsevier, 2008, pp 105–114

Koo JY, Shellow WV, Hallman CP, et al: Alopecia areata and increased prevalence of psychiatric disorders. Int J Dermatol 33:849–850, 1994

Kretzmer GE, Gelkopf M, Kretzmer G, et al: Idiopathic pruritus in psychiatric inpatients: an explorative study. Gen Hosp Psychiatry 30:344–348, 2008

Lamey PJ, Lamb AB: Prospective study of aetiological factors in burning mouth syndrome. Br Med J (Clin Res Ed) 296:1243–1246, 1988

Langan SM, Bourke JF, Silcocks P, et al: An exploratory prospective observational study of environmental factors exacerbating atopic eczema in children. Br J Dermatol 154:979–980, 2006

Lee CS: Delusions of parasitosis. Dermatol Ther 21:2–7, 2008

Lee MR, Shumack S: Prurigo nodularis: a review. Australas J Dermatol 46:211–220, 2005

Leombruni P, Gastaldi F: Oxcarbazepine for the treatment of trichotillomania. Clin Neuropharmacol 33:107–108, 2010

Lepping P, Freudenmann RW: Delusional parasitosis: a new pathway for diagnosis and treatment. Clin Exp Dermatol 33:113–117, 2008

Lewis-Jones S: Quality of life and childhood atopic dermatitis: the misery of living with childhood eczema. Int J Clin Pract 60:984–992, 2006

Litt JZ: Litt's Drug Eruption Reference Manual Including Drug Interactions. New York, Taylor & Francis, 2004

Lochner C, Seedat S, Hemmings SMJ, et al: Dissociative experiences in obsessive-compulsive disorder and trichotillomania: clinical and genetic findings. Compr Psychiatry 45:384–391, 2004

Lochner C, Seedat S, Niehaus DJ, et al: Topiramate in the treatment of trichotillomania: an open-label pilot study. Int Clin Psychopharmacol 21:255–259, 2006

Lochner C, Seedat S, Stein DJ: Chronic hair-pulling: phenomenology-based subtypes. J Anxiety Disord. 24:196–202, 2010

Luís Blay S: Depression and psoriasis comorbidity. Treatment with paroxetine: two case reports. Ann Clin Psychiatry 18:271–272, 2006

Lyell A: The Michelson Lecture. Delusions of parasitosis. Br J Dermatol 108:485–499, 1983

Lynde CB, Kraft JN, Lynde CW: Novel agents for intractable itch. Skin Therapy Lett 13:6–9, 2008

Maeda K, Yamamoto Y, Yasuda M, et al: Delusions of oral parasitosis. Prog Neuropsychopharmacol Biol Psychiatry 22:243–248, 1998

Magin P, Adams J, Heading G, et al: Experiences of appearance-related teasing and bullying in skin diseases and their psychological sequelae: results of a qualitative study. Scan J Caring Sci 22:430–436, 2008

Mahtani R, Parekh N, Mangat I, et al: Alleviating the itch-scratch cycle in atopic dermatitis. Psychosomatics 46:373–374, 2005

Manolache L, Benea V: Stress in patients with alopecia areata and vitiligo. J Eur Acad Dermatol Venereol 21:921–928, 2007

Marqueling AL, Zane LT: Depression and suicidal behavior in acne patients treated with isotretinoin: a systematic review. Semin Cutan Med Surg 24:92–102, 2005

Mazeh D, Melamed Y, Cholostoy A, et al: Itching in the psychiatric ward. Acta Derm Venereol 88:128–131, 2008

McKay M: Vulvodynia, scrotodynia, and other chronic dysesthesias of the anogenital region (including pruritus ani), in Itch: Mechanisms and Management of Pruritus. Edited by Bernhard JD. New York, McGraw-Hill, 1994, pp 161–183

Medansky RS, Handler RM: Dermatopsychosomatics: classification, physiology, and therapeutic approaches. J Am Acad Dermatol 5:125–136, 1981

Modell JG, Boyce S, Taylor E, et al: Treatment of atopic dermatitis and psoriasis vulgaris with bupropion SR: a pilot study. Psychosom Med 64:835–840, 2002

Morgan CA 3rd, Southwick S, Hazlett G, et al: Relationships among plasma dehydroepiandrosterone sulfate and cortisol levels, symptoms of dissociation, and objective performance in humans exposed to acute stress. Arch Gen Psychiatry 61:819–825, 2004

Morgan JF, Lacey JH: Scratching and fasting: a study of pruritus and anorexia nervosa. Br J Dermatol 140:453–456, 1999

Moussavian H: Improvement of acne in depressed patients treated with paroxetine. J Am Acad Child Adolesc Psychiatry 40:505–506, 2001

Murphy C, Redenius R, O'Neill E, et al: Sleep-isolated trichotillomania: a survey of dermatologists. J Clin Sleep Med 3:719–721, 2007

Mutasim DF, Adams BB: The psychiatric profile of patients with psychogenic excoriation. J Am Acad Dermatol 61:611–613, 2009

Naldi L, Chatenoud L, Linder D, et al: Cigarette smoking, body mass index, and stressful life events as risk factors for psoriasis: results from an Italian case-control study. J Invest Dermatol 125:61–66, 2005

Nielsen K, Jeppesen M, Simmelsgaard L, et al: Self-inflicted skin diseases. A retrospective analysis of 57 patients with dermatitis artefacta seen in a dermatology department. Acta Derm Venereol 85:512–515, 2005

Nightingale SL: From the Food and Drug Administration. JAMA 279:984, 1998

Ozkan M, Oflaz SB, Kocaman N, et al: Psychiatric morbidity and quality of life in patients with chronic idiopathic urticaria. Ann Allergy Asthma Immunol 99:29–33, 2007

Panconesi E, Hautmann G: Psychophysiology of stress in dermatology. The psychobiologic pattern of psychosomatics. Dermatol Clin 14:399–421, 1996

Pasaoglu G, Bavbek S, Tugcu H, et al: Psychological status of patients with chronic urticaria. J Dermatol 33:765–771, 2006

Perini G, Zara M, Cipriani R, et al: Imipramine in alopecia areata: a double-blind, placebo-controlled study. Psychother Psychosom 61:195–198, 1994

Phillips KA, Taub SL: Skin picking as a symptom of body dysmorphic disorder. Psychopharmacol Bull 31:278–288, 1995

Phillips KA, Albertini RS, Rasmussen SA: A randomized placebo-controlled trial of fluoxetine in body dysmorphic disorder. Arch Gen Psychiatry 59:381–388, 2002

Phillips KA, Conroy M, Dufresne RG, et al: Tanning in body dysmorphic disorder. Psychiatr Q 77:129–138, 2006

Physicians' Desk Reference: Physicians' Desk Reference 2009, 63rd Edition. New York, Thomson Reuters, 2008

Picardi A, Abeni D: Stressful life events and skin diseases: disentangling evidence from myth. Psychother Psychosom 70:118–136, 2001

Picardi A, Pasquini P, Cattaruzza MS, et al: Only limited support for a role of psychosomatic factors in psoriasis: results from a case-control study. J Psychosom Res 55:189–196, 2003a

Picardi A, Pasquini P, Cattaruzza MS, et al: Psychosomatic factors in first-onset alopecia areata. Psychosomatics 44:374–381, 2003b

Picardi A, Mazzotti E, Pasquini P: Prevalence and correlates of suicidal ideation among patients with skin diseases. J Am Acad Dermatol 54:420–426, 2006

Poon E, Seed PT, Greaves MW, et al: The extent and nature of disability in different urticarial conditions. Br J Dermatol 140:667–671, 1999

Puetz J, Fete T: Platelet function disorder in Gardner-Diamond syndrome. A case report and review of the literature. J Pediatr Hematol Oncol 27:323–325, 2005

Purvis D, Robinson E, Merry S, et al: Acne, anxiety, depression and suicide in teenagers: a cross-sectional survey of New Zealand secondary school students. J Paediatr Child Health 42:793–796, 2006

Rao KS, Menon PK, Hilman BC, et al: Duration of the suppressive effect of tricyclic antidepressants on histamine-induced wheal-and-flare in human skin. J Allergy Clin Immunol 82(5 pt 1):752–757, 1988

Rapp SR, Feldman SR, Exum ML, et al: Psoriasis causes as much disability as other major medical diseases. J Am Acad Dermatol 41(3 pt 1):401–407, 1999

Ratnoff OD: The psychogenic purpuras: a review of autoerythrocyte sensitization, autosensitization to DNA, "hysterical" and factitial bleeding, and the religious stigmata. Semin Hematol 17:192–213, 1980

Ratnoff OD: Psychogenic purpura (autoerythrocyte sensitization): an unsolved dilemma. Am J Med 87(3N):16N–21N, 1989

Rauch SL, Wright CI, Savage CR, et al: Brain activation during implicit sequence learning in individuals with trichotillomania. Psychiatry Res 154:233–240, 2007

Raychaudhuri SP, Gross J: A comparative study of pediatric onset psoriasis with adult onset psoriasis. Pediatr Dermatol 17:174–178, 2000

Rudzki E, Borkowski W, Czubalski K: The suggestive effect of placebo on the intensity of chronic urticaria. Acta Allergol 25:70–73, 1970

Ruiz-Doblado S, Carrizosa A, García-Hernández MJ, et al: Selective serotonin reuptake inhibitors (SSRIs) and alopecia areata. Int J Dermatol 38:798–799, 1999

Ruiz-Doblado S, Carrizosa A, García-Hernández MJ: Alopecia areata: psychiatric comorbidity and adjustment to illness. Int J Dermatol 42:434–437, 2003

Saez-de-Ocariz M, Orozco-Covarrubias L, Mora-Magaña I, et al: Dermatitis artefacta in pediatric patients: experience of the National Institute of Pediatrics. Pediatric Dermatol 21:205–211, 2004

Sampogna F, Tabolli S, Abeni D, et al: The impact of changes in clinical severity on psychiatric morbidity in patients with psoriasis: a follow-up study. IDI Multipurpose Psoriasis Research on Vital Experiences (IMPROVE) Investigators. Br J Dermatol 157:508–513, 2007

Savin JA, Paterson WD, Adam K, et al: Effects of trimeprazine and trimipramine on nocturnal scratching in patients with atopic eczema. Arch Dermatol 115:313–315, 1979

Scheinman PL, Peck GL, Rubinow DR, et al: Acute depression from isotretinoin. J Am Acad Dermatol 22(6 pt 1):1112–1114, 1990

Schmitt J, Romanos M, Schmitt NM, et al.: Atopic eczema and attention-deficit/hyperactivity disorder in a population-based sample of children and adolescents. J Am Med Assoc 301:724–728, 2009

Schneider G, Hockmann J, Ständer S, et al: Psychological factors in prurigo nodularis in comparison with psoriasis vulgaris: results of a case-control study. Br J Dermatol 154:61–66, 2006

Seiffert K, Hilbert E, Schaechinger H, et al: Psychophysiological reactivity under mental stress in atopic dermatitis. Dermatology 210:286–293, 2005

Sheehan-Dare RA, Henderson MJ, Cotterill JA: Anxiety and depression in patients with chronic urticaria and generalized pruritus. Br J Dermatol 123:769–774, 1990

Shenefelt PD: Hypnosis in dermatology. Arch Dermatol 136:393–399, 2000

Shenefelt PD: Biofeedback, cognitive behavioral methods and hypnosis in dermatology: is it all in your mind? Dermatol Ther 16:114–122, 2003

Sherman MD, Holland GN, Holsclaw DS, et al: Delusions of ocular parasitosis. Am J Ophthalmol 125:852–856, 1998

Shertzer CL, Lookingbill DP: Effects of relaxation therapy and hypnotizability in chronic urticaria. Arch Dermatol 123:913–916, 1987

Simeon D, Stein DJ, Gross S, et al: A double-blind trial of fluoxetine in pathologic skin picking. J Clin Psychiatry 58:341–347, 1997

Skolnick AH, Alexander ZJ: Psychiatric implications of psoriasis. JAMA 295:2249–2250, 2006

Slominski A, Wortsman J, Luger T, et al: Corticotropin releasing hormone and proopiomelanocortin involvement in the cutaneous response to stress. Physiol Rev 80:979–1020, 2000

Smith KC, Pittelkow MR: Naltrexone for neurotic excoriations. J Am Acad Dermatol 20(5 pt 1):860–861, 1989

Sperling LC: Alopecias, in Dermatology, 2nd Edition, Vol 1. Edited by Bolognia JL, Jorizzo JL, Rapini RP. London, Mosby Elsevier, 2008, pp 987–1005

Solak O, Kulac M, Yaman M, et al: Lichen simplex chronicus as a symptom of neuropathy. Clin Exp Dermatol 34:476–480, 2009

Staubach P, Eckhardt-Henn A, Dechene M, et al: Quality of life in patients with chronic urticaria is differentially impaired and determined by psychiatric comorbidity. Br J Dermatol 154:294–298, 2006

Steinhoff A, Steinhoff M: Neuroimmunology of atopic dermatitis, in Neuroimmunology of the Skin: Basic Science to Clinical Practice. Edited by Granstein RD, Luger T. Berlin Heidelberg, Springer-Verlag, 2009, pp 197–207

Strahan JE, Raimer S: Isotretinoin and the controversy of psychiatric adverse effects. Int J Dermatol 45:789–799, 2006

Strumia R. Dermatologic signs in patients with eating disorders. Am J Clin Dermatol 6:165–73, 2005

Swedo SE, Leonard HL, Rapoport JL, et al: A double-blind comparison of clomipramine and desipramine in the treatment of trichotillomania (hair pulling). N Engl J Med 321:497–501, 1989

Szepietowski JC, Salomon J, Pacan P, et al: Body dysmorphic disorder and dermatologists. J Eur Acad Dermatol Venereol 22:795–799, 2008

T-J Goon A, Yosipovitch G, Chan YH, et al: Clinical characteristics of generalized idiopathic pruritus in patients from a tertiary referral center in Singapore. Int J Dermatol 46:1023–1026, 2007

Tausk F, Whitmore SE: A pilot study of hypnosis in the treatment of patients with psoriasis. Psychother Psychosom 68:221–225, 1999

Tobin DJ, Peters EM: Neurobiology of hair, in Neuroimmunology of the Skin: Basic Science to Clinical Practice. Edited by Granstein RD, Luger T. Berlin Heidelberg, Springer-Verlag, 2009, pp 139–157

Trabert W: Shared psychotic disorder in delusional parasitosis. Psychopathology 32:30–34, 1999

Tyring S, Gottlieb A, Papp K, et al: Etanercept and clinical outcomes, fatigue, and depression in psoriasis: double-blind placebo controlled randomized phase III trial. Lancet 367:29–35, 2006

Ugurlu S, Bartley GB, Otley CC, et al: Factitious disease of periocular and facial skin. Am J Ophthalmology 127:196–201, 1999

Uguz F, Engin B, Yilmaz E: Axis I and Axis II diagnoses in patients with chronic idiopathic urticaria. J Psychosom Res 64:225–229, 2008

Van Ameringen M, Mancini C, Patterson B, et al: A randomized, double-blind, placebo-controlled trial of olanzapine in the treatment of trichotillomania. J Clin Psychiatry 2010 Apr 20 [Epub ahead of print]

Van de Kerkhof PCM, Schalkwijk J: Psoriasis, in Dermatology, 2nd Edition, Vol 1. Edited by Bolognia JL, Jorizzo JL, Rapini RP. London, Mosby Elsevier, 2008, pp 115–135

Van der Steen P, Boezeman J, Duller P, et al: Can alopecia areata be triggered by emotional stress? An uncontrolled evaluation of 178 patients with extensive hair loss. Acta Derm Venereol 72:279–280, 1992

Verhoeven EW, Kraaimaat FW, de Jong EM, et al: Effect of daily stressors on psoriasis: a prospective study. J Invest Dermatol 129:2075–2077, 2009a

Verhoeven EW, Kraaimaat FW, de Jong EM, et al: Individual differences in the effect of daily stressors on psoriasis: a prospective study. Br J Dermatol 161:295–299, 2009b

Verraes-Derancourt S, Derancourt C, Poot F, et al: Dermatitis artefacta: retrospective study in 31 patients [in French]. Ann Dermatol Venereol 133:235–238, 2006

Walling HW, Swick BL: Intranasal formication correlates with diagnosis of delusions of parasitosis. J Am Acad Dermatol 58 (2 suppl):S35–S36, 2008

Warnock JK, Morris DW: Adverse cutaneous reactions to antidepressants. Am J Clin Dermatol 3:329–339, 2002a

Warnock JK, Morris DW: Adverse cutaneous reactions to antipsychotics. Am J Clin Dermatol 3:629–636, 2002b

Warnock JK, Morris DW: Adverse cutaneous reactions to mood stabilizers. Am J Clin Dermatol 4:21–30, 2003

Weisshaar E, Fleischer AB Jr, Bernhard JD: Pruritus and dysesthesia, in Dermatology, 2nd Edition, Vol 1. Edited by Bolognia JL, Jorizzo JL, Rapini RP. London, Mosby Elsevier, 2008, pp 91–104

Willemsen R, Vanderlinden J: Hypnotic approaches to alopecia areata. Int J Clin Exp Hypnosis 56:318–333, 2008

Willemsen R, Vanderlinden J, Roseeuw D, et al: Increased history of childhood and lifetime traumatic events among adults with alopecia areata. J Am Acad Dermatol 60:388–393, 2009

Williams JR, Burr ML, Williams HC: Factors influencing atopic dermatitis: a questionnaire survey of schoolchildren's perceptions. Br J Dermatol 150:1154–1161, 2004

World Health Organization: The ICD-10 Classification of Mental and Behavioural Disorders: Clinical Descriptions and Diagnostic Guidelines. Geneva, World Health Organization, 1992

Yang HY, Sun CC, Wu YC, et al: Stress, insomnia, and chronic idiopathic urticaria: a case-control study. J Formos Med Assoc 104:254–263, 2005

Yosipovitch G, Ishiuji Y: Neurophysiology of itch, in Neuroimmunology of the Skin: Basic Science to Clinical Practice. Edited by Granstein RD, Luger T. Berlin Heidelberg, Springer-Verlag, 2009, pp 179–186

Yosipovitch G, Ansari N, Goon A, et al: Clinical characteristics of pruritus in chronic idiopathic urticaria. Br J Dermatol 147:32–36, 2002

Zachariae R, Oster H, Bjerring P, et al: Effects of psychologic intervention on psoriasis: a preliminary report. J Am Acad Dermatol 34:1008–1015, 1996

Zaenglein AL, Thiboutot DM: Acne vulgaris, in Dermatology, 2nd Edition, Vol 1. Edited by Bolognia JL, Jorizzo JL, Rapini RP. London, Mosby Elsevier, 2008, pp 495–508

Zakrzewska JM, Forssell H, Glenny AM: Interventions for the treatment of burning mouth syndrome. Cochrane Database Syst Rev (1):CD002779, 2005

Zylicz Z, Krajnik M, Sorge AA, et al: Paroxetine in the treatment of severe non-dermatological pruritus: a randomized, controlled trial. J Pain Symptom Manage 26:1105–1112, 2003

CHAPTER 30

Surgery

Pauline S. Powers, M.D.

Carlos A. Santana, M.D.

SURGICAL PATIENTS OFTEN have preexisting psychiatric disorders, and a range of psychosocial problems may become evident after surgery. The prevalence of psychiatric problems in surgical patients has been estimated to be as high as 50% (Strain 1982) and is known to be particularly high in certain specialized surgical units, such as burn and trauma centers. Although surgeons are less likely to refer patients to psychiatrists than are other physicians, there is evidence that rates of referrals for both consultation and liaison services are increasing across medical specialties and that during the last 20 years, the most frequent reasons for referral have begun to change from suicide attempts and a history of psychosis to depression and other current psychiatric symptoms (Devasagayam and Clarke 2008; Sloan and Kirsh 2008). Another important trend has been a global increase in reports of consultation-liaison service use. For example, a review of 3,608 consecutive referrals to hospital consultation-liaison psychiatry units conducted by the European Study on Quality Assurance in Consultation-Liaison Psychiatry and Psychosomatics in Spain reported that the main sources of referrals were internal medicine (17.5%,), traumatology (7.5), and general surgery (7.3%) (Valdés et al. 2000).

In the hospital, psychiatrists provide consultations for patients on general surgical floors, but they are more likely to provide liaison services to specialized surgical units such as burn units or organ transplant programs. Consultations for general surgical patients often involve preoperative issues such as consent for surgery, fear of anesthesia or surgery, or management of preexisting psychiatric disorders during hospitalization. Postoperative hospital consultations are often initiated for assessment and treatment of delirium or behavior problems. On specialized surgical units, the psychiatrist is more likely to provide classic liaison services, including teaching members of an interdisciplinary team to recognize and manage various psychiatric and psychological problems unique to the unit.

General Issues

Open, Closed, and Random Systems

The general surgical unit and specialized units often have significant differences in operational style. Systems theory can be helpful in understanding these differences (Luhmann and Knodt 1995). An *open system* has regular members who belong to the system and flexible rules about entering and leaving the system. In a *closed system,* only certain individuals can come into and go out of the system, and "outsiders" are excluded from the system. In *random systems,* individuals move into and out of the system at random, with few rules about how entry and exit occur.

Most general surgical units are open systems, and some poorly functioning ones are random systems. Specialized units, such as burn units, are often closed systems with very rigid rules about entering or leaving the system. Because hospital consultations usually involve one to three sessions, it is important that the consultant be able to move easily into and out of the system. This is possible in the open systems typically present on general surgical floors. However, communication with the consultee may require significant effort on the part of the consultant, who may have to track down the consulting surgeon (who may be in the operating room all day); this problem is accentuated on a ward that tends toward randomness. In contrast, the psychiatrist who provides liaison to a closed specialized unit will need to be well known to the team and be a regular attendee at team meetings. Communication within the closed system may be easier because all members are likely to accept recommendations from another member of the team.

Outpatient Consultation-Liaison Services

In the outpatient department, the psychiatrist may be an integral part of a specialized team. For example, bariatric surgery teams typically rely on a presurgical psychiatric assessment of patients to determine whether the patient is an appropriate candidate for surgery; the psychiatrist also may participate in the long-term follow-up of the patient after bariatric surgery. This type of psychiatric consultation requires detailed knowledge of the unique risks and benefits of the proposed surgery.

The dramatic rise in outpatient surgery, in which the patient may arrive only a few hours before the operation and leave a few hours later, has complicated identification of perisurgical psychiatric problems. This relatively new development in surgery has occurred at the same time that it has been recognized that patients so often present with multiple physical and psychiatric disorders, whether in the inpatient, outpatient, or ambulatory surgery setting. A recent proposal is to reenvision consultation-liaison psychiatry as one means of providing integrated care for the multiple and complex needs of patients (G.C. Smith 2009). This would entail integrating quantitative methods (e.g., utilizing results of randomized clinical trials) and qualitative methods (e.g., assessment and treatment of psychodynamic conflicts) and devising effective methods of communication between all health care personnel. Such a systematic approach might resolve the issues related to identification of psychiatric problems among ambulatory surgery patients because the patient would be part of a well-informed system in which key problems are known and incorporated into an integrated treatment plan.

Transference and Countertransference

Transference and countertransference issues are important, irrespective of the site of the surgical intervention. *Transference* is defined as the set of emotional reactions that a patient has toward the surgeon: these reactions are shaped by previous relationships with important people in the life of the patient and may facilitate or inhibit the relationship with the surgeon. Relationships with parents and others in authority typically influence current reactions to the surgeon. For example, a surgical candidate who has had a trusting relationship with parents and positive experiences with physicians is likely to approach surgery calmly and to be able to discuss options openly with the surgeon. However, a patient who grew up with harsh, controlling, and demanding parents, and who also has had negative interactions with physicians, is more likely to be suspicious of the surgeon and fearful of the surgery. Recognition of the likely source of the patient's reactions to the surgeon is the key to managing these reactions. For example, if a new patient is suspicious and unduly fearful of a usually safe surgical procedure, it may be helpful to give the patient time to discuss the procedure with a trusted partner or friend and then offer to explain the procedure to this person while the patient is present.

Surgeons, like other physicians, may have countertransference reactions to their patients. Clues to negative countertransferential reactions to the patient include feelings of anger, irritability, sadness, or boredom. In these situations, it is often helpful for the surgeon to ask him- or herself: "Why am I [angry, sad, or bored or overly involved] with this patient?" The answer may be that the patient has elicited feelings related to another situation in the surgeon's life. Recognition of this fact usually allows the surgeon to refocus on the patient. An example might be an overly solicitous response to a woman shot by an abusive husband; it might be that in this situation, the surgeon was reminded of his own abusive father. Another example is the surgeon who is angry because a patient fails to improve after multiple back surgeries. This reaction may relate to the surgeon's unrecognized and unrealistic grandiose belief that she can conquer any problem.

Staff Coping Mechanisms

Certain surgical situations, such as traumas and burns, particularly among children, elicit powerful emotional responses from the surgeons and nurses working with these patients and their families. Jones (2001) poignantly described the reaction of a patient and her husband to life-threatening surgery and commented that the "impact of physical illness is such that there is potential for the seriously ill to saturate health workers in anxiety and raw feelings" (p. 459). To protect themselves emotionally, the surgeon or nurse may ignore the emotional needs of the patient (and family) and focus solely on the physical aspects of care.

To be able to function effectively, the surgeon must be able to maintain defense mechanisms, including, when appropriate, isolation of affect, denial, humor, and suppression. Treatment team members, including psychiatrists, psychologists, and chaplains, may be able to cope more effectively with the feelings emanating from the patient because they do not have to perform surgery. Although surgeons are often blamed for not attending to the emotional needs of their patients, it may be that it is not usually possible both to empathize fully with the feelings of the patient and to maintain the objectivity needed to perform surgery. Thus, the emotional needs of both the surgeon and the patient must be respected.

Several recent reports have recognized the stresses experienced by surgeons, particularly when there is an intraoperative death (Taylor et al. 2008) or when palliative surgical care is required. One report (Bradley and Brasel 2007) describes a core competency program in effective interpersonal and communication skills for surgical residents. Case examples and appropriate wording and actions are described for four areas of surgical practice: preoperative counseling, presentation of a devastating diagnosis or poor prognosis, discussion of error, and discussion of death.

Role of the Family

The effect of the family on the patient's experience with surgery and on long-term recovery is known to be very important. Qualitative research methods including narratives have been used to understand the experience of the family during the perioperative period (e.g., Pai et al. 2008). A consistent theme from these reports is that knowing is better than not knowing. Another theme is that families want much more information than was initially realized. For example, one study (Kocyildirim et al. 2007) found that 17 parents who viewed videotapes of their child's cardiac surgery procedure were not distressed by the videotape, found it useful in understanding exactly what happened to their child, and reported that it made it easier to share the experience with other family members and friends. Recent research has also begun to describe responses of family members other than parents. A case series of siblings of children who undergo bone marrow transplant (Wilkins and Woodgate 2007) showed they have definite ideas about how health care professionals should support them. One specific example was that they want to be included in the definition of "family." Finally, it is clear that a more comprehensive view of the role of the family is emerging globally: the three studies cited in this paragraph are from India, the United Kingdom, and Canada.

General Conceptual Model

To conceptualize the problems requiring psychiatric intervention, the perioperative period can be divided into preoperative, intraoperative, and postoperative periods. Although these periods are considered separately because special strategies and different personnel may be required in each, the connection between preoperatively identified psychiatric problems and outcome of surgery has been a topic widely studied. For example, in a study of patients with severe low back pain who underwent surgery, low presurgical neuroticism scores were associated with better postoperative functional improvement (Hagg et al. 2003). In another study of patients with gastroesophageal reflux disorder undergoing laparoscopic antireflux surgery (Kamolz et al. 2003), all the patients had normalized physiological findings after surgery, but the patients with comorbid major depression had significantly more symptoms of postoperative dysphagia and had less improvement in quality of life than did the patients without depression.

Psychiatry is often consulted in the preoperative period around the issues of consent for treatment or refusal of surgery and may be consulted at any time when the patient threatens to sign out against medical advice (AMA). Preexisting psychiatric disorders and their management often are also the reason for psychiatric consultation. Fear of surgery, anesthesia, needles, or machines may result in preoperative panic and necessitate urgent psychiatric intervention.

With the emergence of outpatient surgery and use of drugs that induce a lighter stage of anesthesia, some patients may recall events from the intraoperative period. Psychiatric consultation may be needed to assist the patient in coping with these memories.

In the postoperative period, delirium (including withdrawal from various substances) is a very common cause for consultation. Agitation and management problems are also common. Patients who were admitted because of trauma (including burns) may begin to develop symptoms of posttraumatic stress disorder (PTSD).

General Preoperative Issues

Capacity and Consent

Informed consent is required prior to the performance of any surgical procedure. In this process, surgeons provide patients with information necessary to make an autonomous decision about whether to have surgery and ensure that patients are aware of the risks, benefits, and alternatives. The ethical practice of surgery requires a patient's voluntary informed consent. Valid informed surgical consent includes principles of volunteerism, disclosure, understanding, and capacity for decision making (del Carmen and Joffe 2005). In some instances, however, direct consent is impossible, and surgeons seek permission from surrogates or guidance from written advance directives. Informed consent and decision making are at the core of the preoperative period. The communication of factual information understandable to the patient is the responsibility of the surgeon. It should include diagnosis, reasons that the operation is thought to be the treatment of choice, and expected risks and benefits and their probabilities. Alternatives and their consequences, as well as financial costs, also should be discussed. Informed consent is not merely the provision of information; it also involves ascertaining that patients have an adequate understanding of the procedure they are to undergo. Asking patients to describe, in their own words, the procedure they are about to have is a way the surgeon can assess whether patients have sufficient health literacy to understand the procedures to be performed and the risks, benefits, and alternatives to surgery. Competent patients have a right to decide whether to accept or reject proposed surgery. A psychiatric consultant cannot legally declare a patient incompetent, but he or she can evaluate the medical–legal elements of the decision-making capacity of the patient. Examiners must be aware of the legal standards governing determination of competence in their jurisdiction.

The assessment also includes a determination of the cause of the patient's limitation (i.e., the nature of the mental disorder) and the recommendations for treatment, if treatment is possible. The general principles regarding legal and ethical aspects of capacity and consent are discussed in Chapter 2, "Legal Issues," and Chapter 3, "Ethical Issues."

Preoperative Psychiatric Evaluation

The preoperative period is the time to obtain a psychiatric history. Patients with a history of anxiety disorder, depression, bipolar disorder, or psychosis are at risk for experiencing symptoms of these disorders during the postoperative period. Knowing what medications have been effective or not tolerated in the past is obviously valuable. Certain personality disorders and traits are known to predispose to behavior problems during the postoperative period.

When a surgeon requests a psychiatric consultation, the consultant should establish the urgency. Surgical patients seldom initiate or request a psychiatric consultation themselves and may even assume an adversarial attitude toward the consultant.

Although one of the most common reasons for the underreferral of surgical inpatients for psychiatric evaluation is lack of recognition (or dismissal) of psychological distress by the surgical team, this may be changing. Recent articles originating with surgical and anesthesia teams are exploring issues related to preoperative anxiety and depression (e.g., Perks et al. 2009). In some cases, surgical inpatients have felt the need to refer themselves for psychiatric evaluation of anxiety, although the surgical staff did not consider their anxiety sufficient to warrant a consultation (Fulop and Strain 1985). On the other hand, inappropriate or premature psychiatric consultation sometimes occurs when a patient expresses normal feelings (e.g., starts to cry) that the surgeon finds uncomfortable. One of the psychiatrist's major tasks is establishing a relationship with the referring surgeon, who may or may not be knowledgeable about psychiatric issues.

Psychiatric Disorders in the Perioperative Period

Depression

The proportion of patients taking antidepressants who undergo surgery is reported to be 35% (Scher and Anwar 1999). Preoperative executive dysfunction and depressive symptoms are predictive of postoperative delirium among noncardiac surgical patients (P.J. Smith et al. 2009). Brander et al. (2003) found that the most severe cases of chronic postsurgical pain after 1 year appeared in those patients with the most severe levels of preoperative depression. Undoubtedly, depression can emerge from the experience of pain. However, in the study of Hinrichs-Rocker et al. (2009), it is suggested that depression, at least in severe cases, represents a risk factor for the development of chronic postsurgical pain.

The question of whether to discontinue a psychiatric drug prior to surgery is both common and complex. The evidence base concerning this issue is thin at best and mostly composed of case reports. Practical and ethical considerations compound the lack of answers and make controlled methodologically sound trials unlikely. In the past, when monoamine oxidase inhibitors (MAOIs) were more frequently prescribed, it was common to discontinue antidepressants prior to general anesthesia. This is no longer the case, since MAOIs can be continued with relative safety prior to surgery by use of specific anesthetic techniques and/or substitution of a reversible MAOI (M.S. Smith et al. 1996). In a study of 80 depressed patients who were scheduled to undergo orthopedic surgery under general anesthesia, Kudoh et al. (2002) concluded that antidepressants administered to depressed patients should be continued. Their group further reported that whereas discontinuation of antidepressants did not increase the incidence of hypotension or arrhythmias during anesthesia, discontinuation did increase the symptoms of depression and delirium. One expert consensus report (Huyse et al. 2006) concluded that the decision of whether to stop a psychotropic drug prior to surgery should be individualized, taking into account the surgical procedure, the patient's condition (e.g., diagnosis, comorbidities, stability), the choice of anesthetic agents, the length of preoperative fasting, and the risks of discontinuation (e.g., withdrawal, relapse). They recommended that MAOIs and tricyclic antidepressants (TCAs) be discontinued in patients prior to surgery and that selective serotonin reuptake inhibitors (SSRIs) be continued in patients who are mentally and physically stable. Other experts caution against discontinuation and advise that the safest course of action in the vast majority of cases is to continue the psychotropic drug until the time of surgery, with particular attention to the medications that have the potential to cause a withdrawal syndrome (Nobe and Kehlet 2000).

Schizophrenia

The management of schizophrenic patients requiring surgery can be difficult. Bizarre behavior and communication expression by schizophrenic patients can confuse and upset surgeons, nurses, and other patients, eliciting fear, anger, and nontherapeutic responses. Patients with paranoid delusions may refuse surgery because of psychotic misperception of the surgeon's intentions. Schizophrenic patients also often have deficits in the processing of cognitive or sensory information and concrete reasoning. These deficits may complicate the consent process and the patient's ability to cooperate with treatment, requiring the staff to make changes in management (Adler and Griffith 1991).

Schizophrenic patients are impaired in their biological response to stress and are at increased risk of medical illnesses such as cardiovascular and respiratory diseases as well as diabetes (Goldman 1999). Aside from difficulties with communication, these patients will also present challenges related to concomitant pathology associated with chronic schizophrenia, such as abnormalities of the endocrine, immune, and cardiovascular system. In addition, there may be interactions between antipsychotic and anesthetic drugs. Lanctot et al. (1998) suggested that 21% of patients receiving antipsychotics had a serious side effect such as extrapyramidal symptoms, sedation, or hypotension and disturbances of the cardiovascular and autonomic nervous systems. Nearly half of schizophrenic patients have comorbid medical conditions owing to adverse affects of antipsychotic drugs and poor self-care such as increased smoking or alcohol abuse (Goldman 1999). Pain insensitivity, which may occur in patients with schizophrenia, can have life-threatening consequences. Pain insensitivity can delay the diagnosis and treatment of illness in schizophrenic patients and is partly responsible for many postoperative complications (Herz and Marder 2002). Patients with chronic schizophrenia should continue their antipsychotics preoperatively to minimize exacerbation or relapse of their illness (Kudoh et al. 2004).

Bipolar Disorder

The stress of surgery may psychologically and physiologically destabilize bipolar disorder, and acute relapse into mania in the postoperative period can be extremely disruptive to care, as well as potentially life-threatening. The bipolar spectrum also includes hypomanic periods that may occur even if the patient is receiving pharmacotherapy or other somatic treatments. Use of lithium, anticonvulsants, antidepressants, and most antipsychotics is precluded for periods without oral intake in the perioperative period, during which parenteral haloperidol serves as the primary vehicle substitute for mood stabilization. Abrupt discontinuation of anticonvulsant mood stabilizers risks causing seizures. Lithium is difficult to use safely during periods of rapid fluid shifts (e.g., after cardiac surgery and acute burns).

Preoperative Fears

An emerging literature has begun to systematically assess the nature and etiology of common preoperative fears, including fears of surgery, anesthesia, needles, and medical machines. Several new psychological instruments have been developed that assess parameters not previously measured. For example, the Perioperative Adult Child Behavioral Interaction Scale (PACBIS; Sadhasivam et al. 2009) is a real-time tool that measures perioperative behaviors of both children and their parents. Strategies to decrease anxiety are being studied; novel approaches being used (particularly among children) include clowns (Cantó et al. 2008) and music (Walworth et al. 2008). Large and more sophisticated randomized controlled trials (RCTs) are now available. Provision of information often decreases anxiety about surgery; however, with the emergence of day surgery, it has become more difficult to provide such information, because the patient may arrive just before surgery. This problem has been widely recognized, and various solutions are being tested.

Although the preoperative period has been the most widely studied in terms of fears, one interesting study looked at fears 6 weeks after surgery (Oude Voshaar et al. 2006). Among 291 older patients with hip fractures, cognitive impairment and fear of falling at 6 weeks was associated with poorer functional outcome at 6 months postsurgery, leading the authors to suggest that a psychiatric assessment might be most appropriate for this type of patient at discharge rather than at admission.

Fear of Surgery and Anesthesia

Nearly a quarter-century ago, Regal et al. (1985) systematically assessed 150 patients before surgery and found that 54% were anxious or very anxious. Many patients were anxious about the anesthesia: patients often feared that the anesthetic would prematurely wear off or that they would not wake up from the anesthesia. Two decades ago, van Wijk and Smalhout (1990) found that nearly one-third of patients were afraid of anesthesia, as distinct from the operation itself. Since these landmark studies, it has been consistently shown that appropriate provision of information in an empathic relationship can reduce preoperative anxiety and length of hospital stay (Koivula et al. 2002; Ng et al. 2004). Efforts to alleviate preoperative anxiety may result in decreased postoperative pain, but this is less certain (Rolfson et al. 2009; Vaughn et al. 2007). Timing the delivery of information is even more important today than it was in the past, because day surgeries afford fewer opportunities to provide information. It is also now clearly recognized that the same methods of providing information do not work for everyone. For example, Fitzgerald and Elder (2008) found that a brief one-page informational handout was most effective in reducing the fears of patients who had undergone no previous surgery and who were younger than 40 years and less effective in older patients with a history of surgery.

Treatment of Preoperative Anxiety

Preoperative anxiety has been treated with antianxiety medications, particularly benzodiazepines. A Cochrane Database review of premedication for anxiety in adult day surgery (A.F. Smith and Pittaway 2003) concluded that use of benzodiazepines does not delay discharge after adult outpatient surgery but that less is known about the actual clinical benefit of these medications for preoperative anxiety. Since that review, Pekcan et al. (2005) reported that in comparison with placebo, premedication with oral diazepam (10 mg) in the evening before surgery and midazolam (1.5 mg) at least 15 minutes before surgery resulted in lower preoperative anxiety as well as a reduction in the usual postoperative increase in cortisol. Among women undergoing abdominal hysterectomy, diazepam-treated patients had lower postoperative anxiety and lower incidence of surgical wound infection compared with those receiving placebo (Levandovski et al. 2008). One RCT (C.C. Chen et al. 2008) of 80 women undergoing gynecological surgery found that presurgical administration of 30 mg of mirtazapine plus dexamethasone was associated with a reduction in preoperative anxiety and reduced the risk of postoperative nausea and vomiting compared with presurgical administration of dexamethasone alone. Other medications have also shown promise, including gabapentin (Ménigaux et al. 2005) and clonidine (Caumo 2009). Although several studies have concluded that benzodiazepines (especially midazolam) reduce anxiety, particularly among pediatric dental and oral surgery patients, a Cochrane Database review (Matharu and Ashley 2005) was unable to reach a definitive conclusion on which was the most effective drug or method of sedation for anxious children.

Although providing information and social support may be more time-consuming than prescribing an antianxiety agent, it may be more effective than medication in reducing preoperative anxiety and is likely to have postoperative benefits as well.

Children and Preoperative Anxiety

It is estimated that as many as 4 million children undergo anesthesia and surgery annually in the United States, and as many as 40%–60% experience significant anxiety before surgery. It has been postulated that postoperative outcome may be influenced by preoperative anxiety. Kain et al. (1996, 2002) emphasized the importance of educating parents about the possible negative behavioral responses that children may have after surgery. Figure 30–1 illustrates changes in the number of negative behavioral responses after surgery as a function of time. At 2 weeks postoperatively, most children had one to three negative behavioral responses, but only 7.6% had seven or more negative responses. By 1 year, only 7.3% of children had one to three negative responses, and no subjects had more than four negative responses.

In a comparison of four different means of relieving preoperative anxiety in children, Kain et al. (2007) found that the ADVANCE method (a family-centered behavioral approach) was superior to parental presence during induction of anesthesia, oral midazolam, and a control condition (usual care). A careful evidence-based review (Chundamala et al. 2009) also concluded that contrary to popular belief, parental presence does not usually relieve anxiety in either the child or the parent; these reviewers suggested that premedication with midazolam may be helpful, as well as distractions such as "clown doctors" (Vagnoli et al. 2005). Rawlinson and Short (2007) have reviewed books that may help children prepare for surgery. For example, *Going to the Hospital,* by Ann Civardi (2005), is recommended for children ages 2–4 years to help prepare them for undergoing anesthesia, and *Chris Gets Ear Tubes,* by Betty Pace (1987), is recommended for children ages 5–7 years to help prepare them for going to the hospital (or ambulatory surgery center).

Although there is great interest in whether preoperative patient-related factors in children are associated with an increase in emergent delirium following surgery and anesthesia, results of studies are conflicting. One review concluded that intense preoperative anxiety (both in children and in their parents), younger age, and less adaptability to environmental changes may contribute to postanesthesia agitation (Vlajkovic and Sindjelic 2007).

Fear of Needles, Blood, and Medical Equipment

Fear of needles is common and may first arise in the preoperative period. Estimates of the prevalence of needle phobia have ranged from 10% to 21% (Hamilton 1995; Nir et al. 2003), but probably about 8%–10% of adults have unreasonable fears of needles that interfere with treatment. Needle phobia appears to be partly inherited (especially the vasovagal response that may result in fainting) and partly

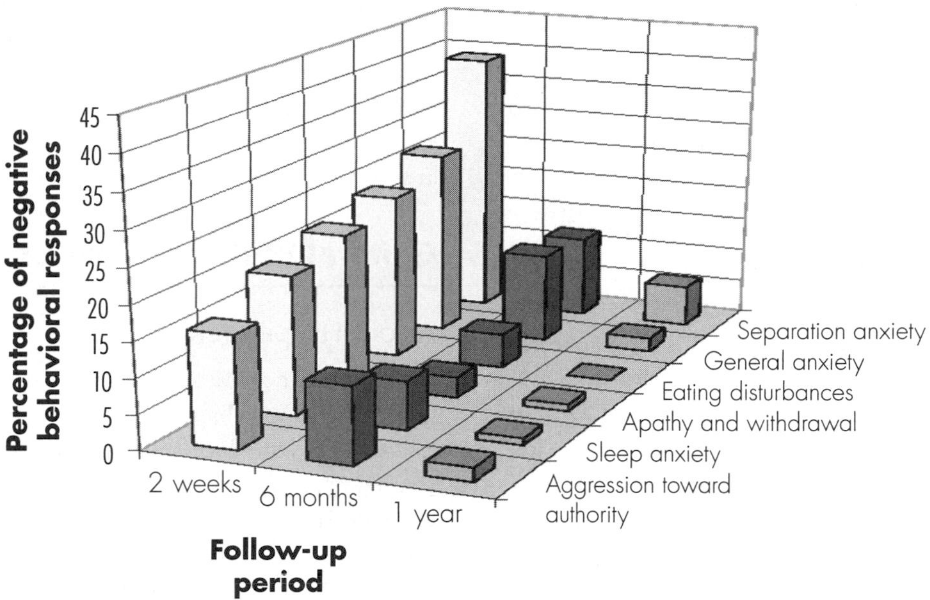

FIGURE 30–1. Decreases in postoperative negative behavioral symptoms in children shown as a function of time.
Source. Reprinted from Kain ZN, Mayes LC, O'Connor TZ, et al.: "Preoperative Anxiety in Children: Predictors and Outcomes." *Archives of Pediatrics and Adolescent Medicine* 150:1238–1245, 1996. Copyright 1996, American Medical Association. Used with permission.

learned from conditioned responses, including past fainting spells when injected or after watching others being vaccinated (Hamilton 1995; Neale et al. 1994; Nir et al. 2003). Individuals who experience disgust in response to needles may be more likely to faint (Page 2002). Initial treatments for needle phobia have been primarily described in case reports and included behavioral strategies (exposure techniques and participant modeling), empathy from treating professionals, and anesthesia. In a small controlled trial in children and adults receiving chemotherapy, needles and syringes decorated with butterflies were compared with standard needles and syringes (Kettwich et al. 2007). These devices reduced aversion, anxiety, fear, and overall stress in 76% of children and 92% of adults.

Fear of blood is closely related to fear of needles. There may be a genetic component to these fears as well. In a study of 541 monozygotic twins and 388 dizygotic twins in the Virginia Twin Registry, unreasonable fears of blood, needles, hospitals, and illness were correlated and showed family aggregation (Neale et al. 1994). A recent review of treatments for blood, injury, and injection phobias concluded that data for effective treatment are limited and that exposure techniques might result in the greatest improvements (Ayala et al. 2009). Some patients are fearful of contracting HIV or hepatitis virus from blood transfusions (now a very rare occurrence) or from needles contaminated with blood (although this should never occur, except in very poor countries); correcting misconceptions and providing accurate information can be reassuring.

Blood refusal is common and is usually related to religious beliefs or fear of blood-borne infections. Because Jehovah's Witnesses and others have refused blood transfusions, there has been a rigorous pursuit of alternatives. Many surgeries previously thought to require transfusions are now routinely done without them. A recent review (Hughes et al. 2008) found that increased morbidity and mortality is rarely observed in patients with a hemoglobin concentration greater than 7 g/dL, and the acute hemoglobin threshold for cardiovascular collapse may be as low as 3–6 g/dL. Various other strategies (such as intravascular volume expanders) may eventually permit even fewer transfusions.

If the patient refuses blood, a careful psychiatric assessment may be needed to determine why the patient is refusing and whether the patient is competent to refuse treatment. For anxious patients, cognitive-behavioral interventions and benzodiazepines are helpful. If the patient is a child and the parents refuse transfusion on the basis of the parents' beliefs, legal and ethical consultation should be obtained, but the decision is usually to transfuse the child.

Fear of medical equipment is also common. Claustrophobia in a closed magnetic resonance imaging (MRI) device is the best described and may result in inability to obtain a scan. Use of an open MRI was shown to result in successful scans in 94% of 50 patients with claustrophobia who had been unable to tolerate the closed MRI (Spouse and Gedroyc 2000). A plan to devise an open positron emission tomography scanner has been described (Yamaya et al. 2008) that may reduce patient stress and permit doctors and nurses to assist patients during scanning. Various coping strategies for the claustrophobia, including patient education and various relaxation techniques, are often helpful but have not been systematically investigated.

Intraoperative Issues—Anesthesia and Awareness With Recall

In 1992, Ghoneim and Block stated: "It is a sobering commentary that after 145 years it is not always possible to determine with certainty whether an anesthetized patient is conscious during surgery" (p. 296). This is still true more than 15 years later, despite multiple efforts to determine whether the patient is conscious. During the past decade, several large studies have concluded that a small percentage of adult patients, between 0.1% and 0.6%, can explicitly recall events that occurred during surgery (for a review, see Errando et al. 2008 and Samuelsson et al. 2007). Although this is a small percentage, given the many surgical procedures performed, a large number of patients are involved. Errando et al. (2008) used the following definition of awareness with recall (AWR): "when the patient (spontaneously or at interview) stated or remembered that he or she had been awake at a time when consciousness was not intended" (p. 179). The incidence of AWR in a large study of 928 children was 0.6% (Blussé et al. 2009), which may be higher than among adults. Several factors are known to influence the likelihood of AWR, including type of anesthesia, type of preanesthetic, and depth of anesthesia. A new method to assess the depth of anesthesia—the bispectral index (BIS), developed from a processed electroencephalogram—was initially thought to offer promise in terms of determining a depth of anesthesia that was both safe and decreased the likelihood of AWR. However, in a careful comparative study of 2,000 patients randomly assigned to BIS-guided anesthesia or end-tidal anesthetic gas (ETAG), there was no difference in incidence of AWR between the two groups even when the anesthesia was in the target range for each procedure (Avidan et al. 2008).

It has been recognized that during surgery there can be sensory, emotional, and cognitive symptoms associated with awareness and that after surgery there can be early or late psychiatric symptoms. A few patients with AWR have severe lasting psychiatric symptoms often closely associated with PTSD (Samuelsson et al. 2007).

At this time, it is not possible to prevent all cases of intraoperative awareness (and it may be even more difficult as day surgery becomes more common, because a lighter stage of anesthesia is used). Preoperative preparation of the patient for the unlikely possibility of AWR may be helpful. It is always prudent for the surgical and anesthesia team to avoid inappropriate comments that may be remembered by the patient. If AWR occurs, a psychiatrist should be consulted in the immediate postoperative period and follow-up care arranged to ensure that appropriate treatment is provided if symptoms persist.

General Postoperative Issues

Alcohol Dependence

Chronic alcohol misuse is more common in surgical patients than in psychiatric or neurological patients. Almost half of all trauma beds are occupied by patients who were injured while under the influence of alcohol (Gentilello et al. 1995; Spies et al. 1996). In addition to the life-threatening complications of the alcohol withdrawal syndrome, the rate of morbidity and mortality resulting from infections, cardiopulmonary insufficiency, and bleeding disorders is two to four times greater in patients with chronic alcoholism (Spies et al. 1997). The development of an alcohol withdrawal syndrome can change a normal postoperative course into a life-threatening situation in which the patient requires intensive care unit (ICU) treatment.

Nearly 50% of patients hospitalized in trauma centers have an alcohol-related injury (Soderstrom 2005). Compared with trauma patients who are not intoxicated at the time of injury, intoxicated trauma patients are more likely to suffer another injury within 28 months (Rivara et al. 1993). In one study, patients admitted to trauma centers with a blood alcohol concentration (BAC) greater than zero died from subsequent injury at nearly twice the rate as that in a cohort of patients with negative BAC tests (Dischinger et al. 2001). Methods for screening medical/surgical patients for alcohol misuse are discussed in Chapter 17, "Substance-Related Disorders."

An alcohol-related history is frequently unobtainable in trauma patients because of their injuries (which may include closed head injury) and subsequent endotracheal intubation. Laboratory tests with sufficient sensitivity and specificity may assist in the diagnosis and possible prevention of complications (Sillanaukee 1996). If an ordinary alcohol history is not obtainable, the biological marker known as carbohydrate-deficient transferrin is a useful alternative. The carbohydrate-deficient transferrin correlates with alcohol consumption in surgical patients (Tønnesen et al. 1999).

Chronic alcohol intake may produce either enhanced or reduced sensitivity to anesthetics. The net effect varies with the amount of alcohol used, the relative affinity of alcohol and other drugs for the microsomal enzymes, and the severity of any underlying liver injury (Lieber 1995).

Alcohol dependence is often complicated by disorders such as cirrhosis, seizures, pancreatitis, polyneuropathy, cardiomyopathy, and/or other psychiatric conditions. It seems obvious that surgical interventions in an alcoholic patient with one or more of these disorders may be associated with increased morbidity and mortality. An increased risk of complications is seen after both minor and major surgery, as well as after elective and emergency procedures. In general, the risk of postoperative infections is related to decreased immune function and enhanced stress response to surgical trauma. This enhanced stress response is characterized by a greater release of stress hormones and catecholamines in patients with alcoholism compared with control subjects (Moesgaard and Lykkegaard-Nielsen 1989; Tønnesen et al. 1992). Alcoholic patients are at risk for excessive surgical blood loss secondary to coagulopathy from liver disease and platelet dysfunction. Many alcoholic patients are chronically malnourished, which retards wound healing.

Opioid Dependence

There is no evidence to suggest that provision of appropriate doses of opiates for postoperative pain in the hospital creates addiction, yet some patients who fear becoming dependent decline or underuse postoperative opiates. If a surgical patient is receiving methadone maintenance, the dose used for maintenance should be continued throughout the surgical hospitalization. If the opioid-dependent patient does not have an established maintenance regimen, control of withdrawal can, in most cases, be achieved with methadone dosages of 10–30 mg/day. Once-daily dosing is usually sufficient to prevent withdrawal, but the total daily dose can be split into two or three doses to prevent breakthrough symptoms and maximize pain management. If anesthesia is necessary, the anesthesiologist obviously should be provided with the history of the patient's opioid dependence. Pentazocine or other mixed agonist–antagonists such as buprenorphine are contraindicated for analgesia, as they can cause or worsen withdrawal because they compete with other opiates and block their effect, mainly at the mu opioid receptors.

Postoperative opiate-dependent patients require higher doses of opiates to control surgical pain because of tolerance. When such patients are given only "normal" doses, they complain of not receiving enough and often are considered to be inappropriately "drug-seeking" when in fact they are being undermedicated. See also Chapters 17 ("Substance-Related Disorders"), 31 ("Organ Transplantation"), and 36 ("Pain").

Postoperative Delirium

Both surgical advances and increases in the elderly population have resulted in more operations in patients who have serious comorbid illnesses that increase the risk for postoperative delirium. The rise in day surgeries also complicates full recognition of risk factors, but efforts are being made to address this issue with the development of rapid screening methods. It has long been suspected that postoperative delirium may either reflect preexisting undetected dementia or be a risk factor for postoperative development of dementia, particularly in older patients.

Postoperative delirium is common; however, the incidence depends on patient variables as well as the type of surgery. In one large study of patients 50 years and older undergoing an operation requiring a postoperative ICU stay, 44% developed delirium that began a mean of 2 days after surgery and had a mean duration of 4 days (Robinson et al. 2009). This percentage is significantly higher than that in younger patients who do not require an ICU stay.

Risk Factors and Preoperative Screening Strategies

Risk factors for postoperative delirium include patient variables and surgical variables. Presurgical patient risk factors for postoperative delirium include dementia, older age, cognitive impairment (especially executive function), and depression (Greene et al. 2009; Kazmierski et al. 2008; Robinson et al. 2009) as well as the underlying illness requiring surgery and various other comorbid conditions (including substance use disorders). "Frailty" among older patients undergoing surgery has been found to be associated with postoperative complications (Dasgupta et al. 2009). Surgical risks include type of surgery and type of anesthetic as well as the experience and skill of the surgeon, anesthesiologist, consultants, nursing team, and hospital support system. Methods for screening and diagnosing delirium are reviewed in Chapter 5, "Delirium."

Consequences of Postoperative Delirium

Delirium in the surgical trauma patient is independently associated with more days requiring mechanical ventilation, longer ICU and hospital stays (Lat et al. 2009), and higher early mortality rates (e.g., Robinson et al. 2009).

Treatment of Postoperative Delirium

There are several recent reports of various medications for postoperative delirium. Cholinesterase inhibitors have been ineffective (Gamberini et al. 2009; Sampson et al. 2007). Traditionally, the antipsychotics (particularly haloperidol in the past and more recently the atypical antipsychotics) have been utilized for management of behavioral symptoms that are disruptive to required care in postsurgical patients who develop delirium. The evidence for the effectiveness of antipsychotics is slender, but their use is widely practiced.

Prevention of Postoperative Delirium

Despite the cautions regarding cardiac risk with antipsychotic medication, it may be that in some circumstances the benefits outweigh the risk, especially since delirium following surgery can be very hazardous. RCTs in surgical patients have shown that low-dose haloperidol may prevent postoperative delirium (Kaneko et al. 1999) or reduce its severity and duration (Kalisvaart et al. 2005). An RCT in cardiac surgery patients found that 1 mg risperidone given preoperatively reduced the incidence of postoperative delirium significantly (11.1% in risperidone group vs. 31.7% in placebo group) (Prakanrattana and Prapaitrakool 2007). Other possible preventive measures are being considered as well, including bright light therapy immediately after surgery (Taguchi et al. 2007) and preoperative tryptophan (Robinson et al. 2008).

Quite compelling, however, are the reports indicating that reduction of risk for postoperative delirium is more likely to be achieved with a team approach that includes geriatric nurses and consultants working together to reduce the many potential risks (Gurlit and Möllmann 2008; Marcantonio et al. 2001) even though this is easier to accomplish in a hospital setting than in ambulatory care. For further discussion of delirium and its management, see Chapter 5, "Delirium."

Posttraumatic Stress Disorder in the Postoperative Period

In the surgical arena, PTSD has been best studied in trauma patients (especially burn patients) and motor vehicle accident victims (E. Klein et al. 2003), but several studies have shown that a significant percentage of patients also develop PTSD following cardiac surgery or neurosurgery (Powell et al. 2002; Stoll et al. 2000). Although full syndromal PTSD develops in 18%–40% of adult patients after trauma, many more develop some of the symptoms of PTSD. Children who experience traumatic disfiguring injuries seem to be at particular risk, with up to 82% having some symptoms of PTSD 1 month after the trauma (Rusch et al. 2002). Quality of life is significantly impaired in patients who develop PTSD posttrauma or postsurgery compared with patients who do not develop PTSD (Zatzick et al. 2002).

Several studies have tried to identify factors that predict the emergence of PTSD (for a review, see Tedstone and Tarrier 2003). As expected, better prior emotional adjustment and social support are relatively protective. However, contrary to expectation, the severity of the injury, or the severity of the illness requiring surgery, is not clearly correlated with the emergence of PTSD. Also, alcohol intoxication or concussion at the time of the trauma seems to decrease the likelihood of PTSD (perhaps because memory for the event is impaired). Furthermore, some patients with no apparent predisposing factors develop PTSD. The course of PTSD is not completely clear, but symptoms usually appear within the first week after a trauma and increase in intensity over the next 3 months. Perhaps the best predictor of PTSD at 1 year is the presence of symptoms during the acute hospitalization after a trauma (McKibben et al. 2008; Zatzick et al. 2002). Although most studies show that symptoms decrease by 1 year, many patients continue to meet full criteria, and many more still have symptoms.

Diagnosis of acute stress disorder, PTSD's predecessor, can be difficult in surgical trauma or postoperative patients who manifest symptoms of delirium. For the diagnosis of PTSD, the duration criterion is often not met in hospitalized patients because of relatively brief hospital stays. Almost all patients who meet full criteria will have nightmares, but among patients with only some symptoms, the cluster of symptoms likely to be affected varies. For example, female burn victims with facial burns have been reported to have predominantly avoidance and emotional numbness symptoms (Fukunishi 1999), whereas reexperiencing and startle symptoms are more likely in other burn patients (Ehde et al. 1999).

In the United States, 20% of general hospital ICU survivors have symptoms consistent with a diagnosis of PTSD (Davydow et al. 2008). The National Comorbidity Survey data (Kessler 1995) suggested that more than 50% of individuals who are symptomatic at 12 months will remain symptomatic at the 5-year posttrauma time point. A more recent report found that among burn patients, once PTSD is established, it usually persists (McKibben et al. 2008). Thus, early PTSD screening and intervention may have the potential to mitigate chronic PTSD after injury.

Treatment of PTSD in medical settings is covered in Chapter 11, "Anxiety Disorders." Few studies of treatment of PTSD have been done specifically in surgical patients, but general principles appear applicable. Cognitive-behavioral therapy has been shown to be more effective than a wait-list control condition or supportive psychotherapy for PTSD among motor vehicle accident survivors (Blanchard et al. 2003). There is general agreement (although not much evidence) that psychotherapy should be the primary treatment of trauma-related PTSD in children and that the SSRIs should be adjunctive (Putnam and Hulsmann 2002).

Postoperative Pain

There have been dramatic advances in the understanding and treatment of postoperative pain, as evidenced by a significant increase in RCTs (75 during the past 10 years, 73 of these in English) (National Center for Biotechnology Information database [www.ncbi.nlm.nih.gov]; accessed September 30, 2009). Many of these studies focused on pain relief measures instituted by anesthesiologists (e.g., "Postoperative pain and analgesic requirements after anesthesia with sevoflurane, desflurane, or propofol," by Fassoulaki et al. 2008) and on the use of patient-controlled analgesia (PCA). A Cochrane Database review of PCA (Hudcova et al. 2006) reported on a meta-analysis of 55 studies involving 2,003 patients assigned to PCA compared with 1,838 patients assigned to conventional "as needed" pain relief. Patients assigned to PCA used higher amounts of opioids than did control patients and had more pruritus but a similar pattern of other adverse events. The groups did not differ in length of hospital stay, but the PCA group had better pain control and greater patient satisfaction compared with the conventional as-needed pain relief group.

Despite these encouraging findings, significant misunderstandings about opioids and other pain-relieving measures persist. Although there have been improvements in the management of uncomplicated postoperative pain, this is often not the case if the operation occurred for an illness that has enduring chronic pain, or in patients who have a history of substance use disorders. There have been valiant attempts on the part of various legislative bodies to improve the knowledge base of physicians about pain management; for example, in California, physician licensees are required to take an 8-hour course in pain management. Nonetheless, erroneous beliefs about pain medication continue (especially in regard to a patient who requires more pain medication than the usual uncomplicated patient). It is worth remembering, however, that a dramatic rise in misuse of pain medications (Substance Abuse and Mental Health Services Administration Health Information Network [www.samhsa.gov/shin]; accessed September 30, 2009) among people with substance use disorders occurred at roughly the same time as the Joint Commission on Accreditation of Health Care Organizations implemented its new standards of pain management in 2001 (see Summers 2001 for a review of the development of these guidelines). Thus, the physician managing postoperative pain must consider many factors, including the nature of the surgery, the usual range of requirements for pain medication (which vary widely among patients), the presence of underlying chronic pain, any history of a substance use disorder, and current vulnerability to relapse (if the patient is in remission from misuse of pain medications).

Body Image and Surgery

Body image is the inner mental experience of one's body, with a neurological substrate, also influenced by prior life events and interactions within important relationships. All of the senses contribute to body image, but touch and kinesthesia may be the most important. Whereas body image develops throughout life, the changes that occur during childhood, and particularly during adolescence, are relatively enduring. Nonetheless, there can be wide fluctuations in the experiencing of one's body. Adaptations to the new realities of the body (including aging, trauma, and surgical alteration) can occur, but a host of factors influence how readily these changes are incorporated. In three important surgical areas, body image is key to patient outcome: 1) amputation and the phenomenon of phantom limb pain; 2) change in body image that may occur after trauma or surgery, including cosmetic surgery; and 3) body image concerns in bariatric surgery patients.

Phantom limb is the experience of feeling as if an amputated part is still present. It was first described by Ambrose Paré (1649), a seventeenth-century surgeon. In the United States, approximately 134,000 surgical amputations occur annually (Zanni and Wick 2008). Many amputees experience phantom limb sensations, which range from pleasant warmth to discomfort (pain, paresthesias, itching). Chronic phantom limb pain occurs in up to 85% of amputees and is a cause of significant disability and impaired quality of life (see Brodie et al. 2007 for summary). Many previous studies of phantom limb have been complicated by a failure to distinguish between stump pain and various types of phantom limb phenomena (C. Richardson et al. 2006). Multiple interacting factors contribute to distressing phantom limb sensations and pain, including a previous history of pain and passive coping styles (C. Richardson et al. 2007).

The exact etiology of the phantom limb experience and the pain that often accompanies it is complex and poorly understood. Phantom limb pain is considered to be an example of neuropathic, rather than nociceptive, pain (see Chapter 36, "Pain"). This conceptualization underlies ingenious treatment strategies such as "mirror therapy" (Brodie et al. 2007; Chan et al. 2007; Darnall 2009) and the "rubber hand illusion" technique (Ehrsson et al. 2008), as well as the pharmacological options discussed in Chapter 36, "Pain."

There are also patients who request that a healthy limb be amputated. There are several case reports and one case series (First 2005) of a group of 52 patients, 17 of whom did have amputations (either from their own efforts or after enlisting the assistance of a surgeon), and many felt better afterward. This has been called "body integrity identity disorder" and may be an extreme type of body image disturbance. It might also be an unusual variant of body dysmorphic disorder. Consultation-liaison psychiatrists might be asked to evaluate a patient with this problem, which in some ways appears to be the opposite of phantom limb phenomenon.

In addition to amputations, body image can change after trauma or surgery. Trauma, as in the case of burn injuries, may cause dramatic changes in the body that require significant adaptation and integration of these changes into a new body image. However, the ease with which such integration occurs is influenced more by premorbid adjustment and stage of development than by the actual percentage of total body surface area (TBSA) burned.

The literature on body image in obesity is extensive. Stunkard and Burt (1967) studied body image in obese individuals who had lost significant weight. They found that these patients often misperceived themselves as still large and frequently had negative attitudes toward this misperception. The definition of body image in patients with eating disorders has evolved to divide body image into perceptual and attitudinal aspects. Most current studies of body image following bariatric surgery focus on one part of the attitudinal aspect of body image called *body satisfaction.*

General Determinants of Functional Outcome

Functional outcome includes the ability to carry out the activities of daily living, the ability to function in one's usual role, and satisfaction with life. These areas are currently being explored under the category of quality of life. Perhaps the most interesting finding is that the actual severity of the underlying trauma or surgery does not necessarily determine quality of life. For example, the percentage TBSA burned does not directly correlate with the likelihood of PTSD, nor does the size of a scar necessarily correlate with posttraumatic adjustment. It has been repeatedly reported that an adequate social support system is positively correlated with postsurgical and posttraumatic adaptation.

A confluence of factors determines functional outcome. These factors include the condition requiring surgical intervention, presurgical psychiatric status, and surgical strategy. Other factors that may improve outcome include preparation of the patient and family for surgery, detection and management of preoperative fears, respectful attitude of the surgeon and operating room personnel during surgery, detection and appropriate treatment of pain, and detection and management of various psychiatric problems following surgery, including delirium and PTSD.

Specific Topics in Surgery

Burn Trauma

The experience of being seriously burned and the treatment that follows for the survivors is one of the most frightening and painful known to humanity. Perhaps because of this, several important concepts in medicine have been learned from the study of burn victims. For example, Erich Lindemann (1944/1994) described the evaluation and treatment of survivors, friends, and relatives of people who died in the Coconut Grove fire. He identified five major symptoms of normal grief: somatic distress, preoccupation with the image of the deceased, guilt, hostile reactions, and loss of patterns of conduct. These concepts continue to influence the management of normal and pathological acute grief in burn units and elsewhere.

Imbus and Zawacki (1977) opened an ethical debate over prolongation of life that continues today. An unusual aspect of burns is that even mortally burned patients often have a lucid period that lasts for a few hours during which patients can participate in making decisions about their own care. For every severely burned patient, these investigators searched the literature to determine whether cases of survival had been reported, and, if not, they offered the patients a choice between a full therapeutic regimen and palliative care. They concluded that the mortality rate did not change but that this strategy increased the autonomy of patients and increased the empathy that they received. This report ignited a controversy that has grown to encompass all critical care: when is treatment futile, and who should decide?

The American Burn Association (2007) reports that an estimated 500,000 people a year receive treatment for burns in the United States. There are approximately 4,000 burn-related deaths annually, with 3,500 of these from residential fires. In 2007, there were 40,000 hospitalizations for burn injuries, which included 25,000 admissions to 125 hospitals with specialized burn centers. The percentage of patients admitted to specialized burn centers has progressively increased, from about 50% in 2004 to 60% in 2007. Burn centers now average 200 admissions per year, whereas other U.S. hospitals average fewer than 3 burn admissions per year. Interdisciplinary specialized burn centers are staffed by physicians, nurses, physical and occupational therapists, pain specialists, mental health professionals, social workers, and chaplains. Typically, the burn center is directed by either a general surgeon or a plastic surgeon. Burn Center Verification is an accreditation process intended to enhance the quality of care at specialized burn centers. Since the inception of this program in 1995, 70 centers have met the rigorous requirements for participation. Other important developments include establishment of the American Burn Association National Burn Repository (ABA-NBR), which (as of 2005) included data for more than 31,000 adult patients admitted to these 70 burn centers, and the National Institute on Disability and Rehabilitation Research Burn Model System Database, which included data for 3,400 patients alive at discharge who have consented to follow-up data collection (M.B. Klein et al. 2007).

Psychiatric Disorders Among Burn Patients

Many burn patients have preexisting psychiatric disorders, the most common of which are substance use disorders and mood disorders. The classic studies of adults by Andreasen et al. (1972) and of children by Bernstein (1976) led to the recognition that psychiatric problems are very common among burn patients. A study using ABA-NBR data reported that 12.3% of patients admitted to the burn centers had psychiatric disorders. Of these, alcohol abuse accounted for 5.8%, drug abuse for 3.3%, dementia for 0.3%, and other psychiatric disorders for 2.9% (Thombs et al. 2007). These percentages are significantly lower than those found in other reports, and this study had some notable limitations; for example, not all patients in the ABA-NBR were evaluated by mental health professionals, ICD-9-CM (World Health Organization 1978) codes were utilized rather than DSM criteria, and personality disorders were not considered. By contrast, a recent study at one burn center found that two-thirds of burn survivors had a history of lifetime psychiatric disorders and that those with such a history were more likely to have postburn psychiatric problems (Dyster-Aas et al. 2008). Nonetheless, in the study by Thombs et al. (2007), after controlling for demographic and burn injury characteristics, it was found that preexisting alcohol abuse was a significant predictor of mortality in the burn unit and that preexisting dementia, psychiatric diagnosis, alcohol abuse, and drug abuse were all significantly associated with increased length of hospital stay. Many smaller studies from single burn centers have found that many patients have preexisting maladaptive coping mechanisms or dysfunctional families, and these factors are known to predispose to poorer functional outcomes.

There have been several recent attempts to understand, quantify, and modulate the multiple interacting negative factors that may worsen functional status and quality of life in patients who have had significant burns. A recent consensus summit of burn rehabilitation clinicians from the United States and Canada addressed 15 key topic areas pertinent to clinical burn rehabilitation (Richard et al. 2009). Another group from England and Australia (Falder et al. 2009) identified seven core domains of outcome for adult burn survivors, four of which are particularly relevant to psychiatric assessment and treatment: 1) sensory and pain, 2) psychological function (PTSD and depression), 3) community participation (social integration), and 4) perceived quality of life. In their extensive review, Falder et al. (2009) evaluated questionnaires and instruments that have been used to diagnose the common psychiatric complications following burn injuries. For example, they noted that PTSD symptoms that occur in the acute phase of treatment are associated with poorer long-term psychological recovery. Methods of assessing PTSD discussed include clinician-administered instruments (Clinician-Administered PTSD Scale; Structured Clinical Interview for DSM) and self-report measures (Impact of Events Scale; Davidson Trauma Scale). The validity and reliability of these instruments in assessing burn patients are clearly described. Regarding depression, the authors noted that very careful assessment of patients who are in the acute phase of treatment is required to accurately distinguish symptoms of depression from physiological symptoms related to the burn injuries (Falder et al. 2009). Use of the recommendations from this review is likely to be very helpful in guiding future research in terms of identifying adult patients with the most common psychiatric complications of burn injuries.

A unique psychopathological topic in burn care is self-immolation, discussed below. The meaning and psychological importance of burn scars (particularly of the face, hands, and genital area) have been studied as well. Equally important in burn care is the delirium that frequently occurs during the acute-care phase. Psychiatric consultants also have described effective methods for the management of pain in burn patients. One method of conceptualizing the psychiatric problems seen in burn patients is to envision a time sequence from preexisting psychiatric problems to problems that develop after the patient leaves the hospital. Thus, there are preexisting psychiatric disorders and psychosocial problems (including those that have resolved but may be rekindled by the trauma), problems that occur at the time of the injury, problems that emerge during acute hospitalization, and psychiatric disorders that develop after discharge from the hospital.

Burns and substance use disorders. Preinjury substance use disorders are common among burn victims. One study found that among 727 deaths from fires, blood alcohol assays were positive in 29%, with a mean blood ethanol level of 193.9 mg/dL; 14.6% of the victims studied had positive results for other substances of abuse (Barillo and Goode 1996). Although 40% of the fatalities were in people younger than 11 years or older than 70 years, 75% of the drug-positive and 58% of the ethanol-positive fatalities were in people between the ages of 21 and 50 years. The authors concluded that substance use disorders are a particular risk factor for death from fires in the middle-aged sector of the population.

Among patients who survive to be treated, several studies have attempted to identify the prevalence of alcohol intoxication, alcohol abuse, or alcohol dependence. One study (J.D. Jones et al. 1991) found that 27% were intoxicated at the time of the burn, and 90% of these were then identified as having an alcohol abuse diagnosis compared with 11% of the nonintoxicated burn patients. Other reports estimated the prevalence of alcohol abuse and dependence in patients with burn injuries as between 6% and 11% (Powers et al. 1994; Tabares and Peck 1997). The Alcohol Use Disorders Identification Test (developed by the World Health Organization; J. B. Saunders et al. 1993) was more effective in identifying at-risk drinkers than blood alcohol level among a group of 123 burn patients (Albright et al. 2009). Steenkamp et al. (1994) found that 57% of the patients had evidence of alcohol problems on the Michigan Alcoholism Screening Test, and of these patients, 57% thought that the use of alcohol had contributed to the accident.

Among burn patients who are identified as having alcohol or drug problems, referral for treatment occurs in fewer than half of the patients (Powers et al. 1994), and among those who are referred, fewer than half accept treatment (Tabares and Peck 1997). Denial is a key defense mechanism in patients with substance use disorders, but the crisis of a burn trauma may be an opportunity to broach this defense. Psychiatrists (and other mental health consultants) on the burn unit are often in a unique position to help burn patients relinquish the denial that prevents appropriate treatment. Alcohol use has been found to be associated with increased percentage TBSA burned, an increased likelihood of death, longer length of hospital stay, and, consequently, increased medical costs (J. D. Jones et al. 1991; Powers et al. 1994). Silver et al. (2008) found that even after controlling for age, sex, and percentage TBSA burned, patients with admission blood alcohol levels above 30 mg/dL had longer durations of mechanical ventilation, longer lengths of stay in the ICU, and higher hospital charges compared with patients with undetectable blood alcohol levels. The reasons for these deleterious consequences are the subject of intense study at present. For example, ethanol exposure prior to burn injury in mice is associated with elevated proinflammatory cytokines (interleukin 6 [IL-6] and tumor necrosis factor–alpha [TNF-α]) and aberrant inflammatory responses (Bird and Kovacs 2008). In a recent review, Choudhry and Chaudry (2008) suggested that alcohol intoxication before burn injury suppresses intestinal immune defense, impairs gut barrier functions, and increases bacterial growth, all of which may contribute to postinjury infections.

Withdrawal symptoms from alcohol dependence may be difficult to distinguish from other causes of delirium. Given that many patients who were intoxicated when burned are nondependent binge drinkers (Albright et al. 2009), alcohol withdrawal is less common than one otherwise might predict. The relevant literature regarding the appropriate treatment when alcohol dependence is suspected is limited to a few case reports and case series. The best approach in a burn unit may be a standard withdrawal protocol with a relatively long-acting benzodiazepine (e.g., chlordiazepoxide). Because 90% of intoxicated burn patients abuse alcohol, and because the development of alcohol withdrawal can be particularly dangerous in a burn patient, a liberal approach to prescribing the withdrawal regimen among patients suspected of alcohol dependence is probably the safest course of treatment. Although intermittent administration of benzodiazepines, especially the short-acting ones such as lorazepam, has been advocated, this may not be wise because the complex phenomenology of the acute phase of burn care may obscure the presence of withdrawal symptoms. Haloperidol is frequently added to the regimen for psychotic symptoms during withdrawal but should not be used alone.

Even though burn patients have a high rate of preexisting drug abuse, withdrawal from narcotics is less likely because most patients require narcotic treatment for pain. However, it is helpful to remember that burn patients with preexisting opioid dependence may require a larger dose of narcotics to suppress pain, and this larger dose should be provided.

Self-inflicted burn injuries. The frequency of self-immolation varies widely from nation to nation; the reasons for self-immolation also vary. In a study in Iran, for example, 27% of suicide cases were the result of self-immolation, and 71% of these cases were in females. Suicide by self-immolation was more prevalent in provinces with severe postwar problems and in the Kurdish ethnic group. Self-immolation was more likely to be associated with unemployment but not with psychiatric disorders or lack of access to care (Ahmadi et al. 2008). By contrast, a report from Turkey indicated that 87.5% of self-inflicted burn injuries were in men, and that 62.5% of these men had psychiatric disorders (Uygur et al. 2009). A study in Zimbabwe reported that 22% of adult burn patients had self-immolated; most were married women, and the most common reason for self-immolation was conflict in a love relationship (Mzezewa et al. 2000).

In the United States, the frequency of self-inflicted injuries among patients who are admitted to a burn center ranges from 0.07% to 9% (Daniels et al. 1991; Scully and Hutcherson 1983). Although political and cultural motivations for self-immolation predominate in some cultures, in the United States, most severely burned patients who have self-injured have a preexisting Axis I psychiatric disorder, usually a psychotic disorder (Mulholland et al. 2008). Compared with patients who have been assaulted, patients with self-inflicted burn injuries are more likely to be male, to have a larger percentage TBSA burned, and to have a longer mean length of hospital stay (Reiland et al. 2006). Substance abuse appears to increase the likelihood of a severe self-inflicted injury. Not all of these patients are actually suicidal; for example, patients with schizophrenia may be responding to command hallucinations.

Among patients who have inflicted less severe burns, personality disorders are common (Cameron et al. 1997), especially borderline personality disorder. The patient may continue to self-injure in the hospital and thereby pose a difficult management problem. The psychiatric consultant is often able to defuse these problems with judicious use of behavioral strategies known to be helpful for patients with borderline personality disorder (Wiechman et al. 2000). Close supervision may be required to prevent further self-harm when the patient moves from an ICU to a unit with less nursing supervision.

Patients with self-inflicted burns often elicit intense countertransference reactions from the entire staff, including the psychiatric team. It is helpful to remember that most patients (at least in the United States) with self-inflicted burns have a chronic mental illness, and that appropriate psychiatric care may not have been available to or effective for the patients. Burn center teams understand chronic medical illness and the need for expert treatment, and this "medical model" analogy may help them better understand and empathize with a patient who has chronic mental illness and who has a self-inflicted burn injury.

PTSD in burn patients. PTSD occurs in a significant minority of patients who have been burned. Estimates range from 21% to 45% (for a review, see Yu and Dimsdale 1999). A study by Zatzick et al. (2007) found that more than 20% of trauma survivors had symptoms of PTSD 12 months after acute inpatient care, and in a large prospective multisite cohort study of major burn injury survivors, psychological stress was common and tended to persist (Fauerbach et al. 2007). The difficulties in estimating frequency are often related to the confounding effects of delirium and mild traumatic brain injury and to the duration criterion requirement of 1 month. Many patients are discharged from the hospital before a month elapses, and less severely injured patients may not be seen again; thus, the diagnosis of PTSD may be missed. Nonetheless, many patients do develop the full syndrome of PTSD, and many more have symptoms in the reexperiencing cluster (particularly nightmares [Low et al. 2006]) even though they do not meet full criteria. Some patients also have PTSD symptoms related to their treatment, especially in regard to the extreme pain inflicted during debridement and dressing changes. Recent work has shown that acute pain is associated with long-term negative effects, including depression, suicidal ideation, and PTSD for as long as 2 years after the burn injury (Wiechman Askay and Patterson 2008). Some patients also remember psychotic experiences from the delirium that often occurs during the acute phase of treatment, and these memories may elicit symptoms of PTSD.

Several attempts have been made to identify factors that predispose to the emergence of PTSD in burn patients, but clarity has yet to be achieved. Fauerbach et al. (2000) found that the personality characteristic of neuroticism increased risk and that high extroversion was protective. Six independent risk and protective factors for PTSD were identified from assessments of 127 burn victims trapped in a ballroom fire (Maes et al. 2001). The odds of developing PTSD were increased with the number of previous traumas, a history of simple phobia, and a sense of loss of control. In contrast, odds were decreased with a sense of control, alcohol consumption, and alcohol intoxication. In a study of 90 patients hospitalized for severe burns, Van Loey et al. (2008) found that those who attributed the injury to individuals not close to them and who were unforgiving were more likely to have PTSD. Gaylord et al. (2009) found that there was no difference in risk for PTSD between military personnel and civilians who suffered burn injuries; in this study, factors that predicted PTSD were percentage TBSA burned and scores on the Injury Severity Score.

Efforts are under way to determine the factors that increase risk of development of PTSD and modify these factors during the acute treatment phase in the hospital. In the large prospective multisite study described earlier (Fauerbach et al. 2007), it was found that a very high percentage of the burn injury patients (34%) experienced acute stress reactions that included feelings of "alienation" and anxiety in the hospital. Although in a few (12%), there was a change in the nature of the symptoms, the percentage of affected individuals remained high for at least 2 years, resulting in significant impairment in function and quality of life. In a prospective study by this same group (McKibben et al. 2008), the prevalence of in-hospital acute stress disorder in 178 patients was 23.6%, and 35.1%, 33.3%, 28.6%, and 25.4% of the participants met PTSD criteria at 1, 6, 12, and 24 months, respectively. Although not well studied, treatment of PTSD in burn patients is likely to be similar to treatment of PTSD in other patients (see Chapter 11, "Anxiety Disorders"). Thus far, reports of various medications for burn patients with PTSD have not yielded consistently helpful results. Increasing patients' sense of control and alleviating pain, especially during the acute phase of treatment in the burn center, may decrease the likelihood of emergent and enduring stress and anxiety symptoms.

Delirium and psychosis in burn patients. Delirium during the acute care of severely burned patients is common, although this topic has not been well studied. In one unpublished report, one-fourth of the burn patients were noted to be psychotic during their initial acute hospitalization. Most of these patients had delirium related to sepsis, pain medication, or other organic factors (Powers 1996). Other causes of delirium in burn patients include hypoxia from smoke inhalation, massive fluid shifts, and electrolyte imbalance, especially hyponatremia and hypophosphatemia. The psychotic symptoms that occur most often include hallucinations (often visual and not always distressing) and delusions. The delusions are often paranoid and frequently involve nursing care personnel. Because patients with delirium are disoriented, they frequently misinterpret events and may then suspect treatment personnel of malevolent intent. It is often difficult to distinguish between pain, agitation, anxiety, and confusion in the ICU, and the psychiatric consultant is invaluable in this differentiation. The principles of treatment of delirium in the burn unit are the same as described earlier for postoperative delirium (see subsection "Postoperative Delirium" earlier in this chapter; also see Chapter 5, "Delirium"). As the population ages and with continuing advances in burn care, many older patients will survive who are more vulnerable to delirium and will require the expertise of psychiatric consultants (Keck et al. 2009).

Burn Pain Management

Pain in burn care arises from both the pain from various procedures, including dressing changes and wound debridement, and the background pain of the injury itself. The key concept in managing pain on the burn unit is to recognize that it is often undertreated, and this can result in worsening delirium, anxiety, and other management problems. Symptoms resulting from acute distress in the burn center may endure for years after discharge. Depression, anxiety (and associated disorders such as PTSD), and pain influence one another and can result in long-term functional and psychological impairment and poorer quality of life (Ullrich et al. 2009). There is also a bidirectional relationship between sleep and pain. Patients with major burns who had insomnia at hospital discharge had significantly increased pain severity during long-term follow-up (M.T. Smith et al. 2008).

Pain is undertreated for many reasons, but the most important reasons are an unrealistic fear of addiction (both by the patient and by the physician) and fear of respiratory compromise (which, at least in the intensive care portion of most burn centers, can be adequately managed by competent nursing staff). Management of burn care pain requires a flexible therapeutic plan with frequent reassessment. Burn wound debridement (in which the eschar is removed) is an excruciatingly painful procedure, and various techniques are now available to alleviate much of the pain. When sharp debridement (involving use of a scalpel) is needed, general anesthesia offers the greatest relief of pain and also may facilitate a more thorough debridement (Powers et al. 1993) and may help avoid some of the distress associated with long term psychological and functional impairments. Parenteral narcotics, especially intravenous morphine, are often preferable for blunt debridement (in which scalpels are not used) and dressing changes. A common error is not waiting the 10–15 minutes required for adequate distribution after intravenous injection of the opioid before beginning blunt debridement. Intramuscular injections are often contraindicated because they may add to the pain, and sufficient injection sites may not be available.

The background pain of burn injuries is best managed with oral narcotics whenever possible. Fentanyl is often helpful for intermittent pain because it is short acting and will allow the patient to be awake to participate in rehabilitation, but morphine is the gold standard and can be flexibly utilized (Connard-Ballard 2009; P. Richardson and Mustard 2009). Meperidine is usually contraindicated because it is relatively ineffective orally and may aggravate delirium. Benzodiazepines are often used to promote sedation and reduce anxiety, but the optimal dose is not known. They are often used inappropriately to treat pain. If pain is adequately managed and the patient has anticipatory anxiety, use of benzodiazepines may then be very helpful. Although many different strategies—including music, relaxation therapy, and maybe virtual reality techniques—may also contribute to the alleviation of pain, they should be adjunctive to the appropriate flexible use of opioids.

Treatment of Burns in Children

Several psychosocial research teams have been particularly interested in the treatment of burned children (Martin-Herz et al. 2003; Stoddard et al. 2002). These groups have emphasized the importance of the developmental stage of the burned child and the need for careful age-appropriate assessment and treatment of pain and anxiety. Emerging studies indicate that appropriate management of pain partially predicts the long-term outcome for the child. For example, Saxe et al. (2005) found that two pathways to PTSD are common among burned children and account for 60% of the variance in PTSD. The first pathway is from size of the burn and level of pain following the burn to the child's level of acute separation anxiety and then to PTSD. The second pathway is from the size of the burn to the child's level of acute dissociation following the burn and then to PTSD. Another study by Wollgarten-Hadamek et al. (2009) found that school-age children (ages 9–16 years) who had suffered moderate or severe burn injuries in infancy had alterations in sensory and pain processing. Because early

TABLE 30–1. Guidelines for pain and anxiety management in children with burns

Patient category	Background pain	Background anxiety	Procedural pain	Procedural anxiety	Transition to next clinical state
Category 1: mechanically ventilated acute	Morphine sulfate intravenous infusion	Midazolam intravenous infusion	Morphine sulfate intravenous bolus	Midazolam intravenous bolus	Wean infusions 10%–20% per day, and substitute nonmechanically ventilated guideline
Category 2: nonmechanically ventilated acute	Scheduled enteral morphine sulfate	Scheduled enteral lorazepam	Morphine sulfate enteral or intravenous bolus	Lorazepam intravenous or enteral bolus	Wean scheduled drugs 10%–20% per day, and substitute chronic guideline
Category 3: chronic acute	Scheduled enteral morphine sulfate	Scheduled enteral lorazepam	Morphine sulfate enteral bolus	Lorazepam enteral bolus	Wean scheduled and bolus drugs 10%–20% per day to outpatient requirements and pruritus medications
Category 4: reconstructive surgical	Scheduled enteral morphine sulfate	Scheduled enteral lorazepam	Morphine sulfate enteral bolus	Lorazepam enteral bolus	Wean scheduled and bolus drugs to outpatient requirements

Source. Reprinted from Stoddard FJ, Sheridan RL, Saxe GN, et al.: "Treatment of Pain in Acutely Burned Children." *Journal of Burn Care and Rehabilitation* 23:135–156, 2002. Copyright 2002, Lippincott Williams & Wilkins. Used with permission.

traumatic and painful injuries can induce long-term alterations, management of acute pain in children in a burn center is crucial.

A guideline has been proposed for the management of pain and anxiety in children (Stoddard et al. 2002). It is based on intensity of care, whether the pain is background or procedural pain, and stage in the hospital (see Table 30–1). In designing this guideline, the focus was on safe, effective medications; a limited formulary; and nursing strategies to assess pain (with age-appropriate ratings). The guideline also was designed to contain explicit recommendations. The authors used this guideline in a series of 125 pediatric patients and reported excellent to adequate control of both pain and anxiety in most patients most of the time (Stoddard et al. 2002). One major advantage of the guideline is that the most-recommended drugs (morphine and lorazepam) are well known to most physicians. Only the use of intravenous infusion of midazolam for background anxiety in mechanically ventilated acutely ill pediatric patients would require an anesthesiologist or a critical care specialist.

Although psychological treatments of pain may ultimately prove to be effective for children, the evidence for these treatments is scant. Hanson et al. (2008) reviewed 900 citations for nonpharmacological treatments in children utilizing the U.S. Preventive Services Task Force criteria, and only seven were considered fair or good. Some of the strategies being considered—for example, music and virtual reality strategies—may eventually prove to be helpful adjunctive techniques.

Several studies have attempted to assess outcome in burned children including the reports noted above. One important confounding factor is that many children who are burned have preexisting psychiatric and psychosocial problems that influence long-term outcome. A study from the United Kingdom (James-Ellison et al. 2009) found that among children younger than 3 years who sustained burns (most of whom were thought to have accidental injuries), about one-third had been referred to Social Services by their sixth birthday, and 9.7% had been abused or neglected, compared with 1.4% of control subjects. A study from the Netherlands (Liber et al. 2008) found that adolescents with a history of childhood burns who used more passive coping methods had increased behavioral problems and more symptoms of depression. A better understanding of the long-term course of burned children will require multisite studies with larger numbers of children sharing similar characteristics.

Psychiatric Practice Guideline for Adults With Acute Burns

Although the evidence base is sparse, consensus guidelines have been developed for several areas of burn care, and a guideline has been proposed for the management of psychiatric disorders in adult burn patients during their initial hospitalization (Powers 2002). Figure 30–2 is a revision of this algorithm designed to incorporate recent findings and to guide the clinician in assessment and management of burn patients with psychiatric problems. A major difference is that it is now widely recognized that nearly all patients and their families benefit from having more information and that for most, participation in the planning and treatment process facilitates recovery. One example of this approach, which has been termed "family inclusive care," is described by Sacco et al. (2009).

Facial Disfigurement and Scars

The adaptation to facial disfigurement depends, in part, on the age at which the disfigurement occurs. Children with congenital disfigurement often encounter significant developmental difficulties and are frequently stigmatized by peers, adults, and health care personnel. These problems may be incorporated into an enduring negative sense of self. If the child has a strong social support system and receives well-informed physiological and psychological care, these problems can be mitigated.

The adjustment to facial disfigurement also depends on the patient's preexisting personality and mental defense mechanisms. In his classic book about scarred burn victims, Bernstein (1976) described variables critical to adaptation, including adaptive versus maladaptive defenses; active coping versus passive surrender; loving exchange versus rage; leading and co-managing treatment versus resisting treatment; and denial versus overawareness. For example, a patient who participates in managing his or her own care; who has a flexible, extensive repertoire of mental defense mechanisms; and who has loving exchanges with friends and family is more likely to make a successful adjustment to facial disfigurement.

Irrespective of the cause of facial disfigurement, the objective nature of the disfigurement may not correlate with the patient's self-perception. In a study of 50 patients who received extensive multidisciplinary treatment from birth to age 18 years for cleft palate, no correlation was found between the objective measure of the residual deformities and the patient's subjective judgment of the remaining deformity (Vegter and Hage 2001). Thus, the subjective self-assessment of the deformity is probably more important than the actual nature of the deformity in determining quality of life. There has been little work done to identify effective treatments for the stress and stigmatization that occur with facial disfigurement. A workshop hosted by the Centers for Disease Control and Prevention identified research on the psychosocial outcomes of children with orofacial clefts as a priority (Yazdy et al. 2007). Using a specially designed assessment questionnaire, the Cleft Evaluation Profile, researchers have found that children with orofacial clefts are often teased and that their self-confidence suffers as a result (Noor and Musa 2007). Despite these promising beginnings, research is needed to determine the efficacy of various psychosocial interventions.

Scars that develop after burn injuries can be very extensive. Scar tissue is different from normal skin and has an aberrant color, a rough surface texture, increased thickness, and decreased pliability and may be associated with pain or pruritus. Assessment of the various treatments for scars (including surgical treatments) has been limited by the lack of any systematic approach to the evaluation of scars (Idriss and Maibach 2009). There is also a marked lack of large, well-designed RCTs of the currently available scar reduction treatments. However, even when better physiological treatments of scars are available, the subjective experience of the scar appears to be more important than the actual physical characteristics of the scar. Sarwer et al. (1998) reported that a subset of patients who underwent surgical revision of their scars had a level of dissatisfaction consistent with body dysmorphic disorder.

Despite the recognition that the *emotional* experience of the facial disfigurement is one of the primary determinants of quality of life, research is only now beginning to assess the problem. Brown et al. (2008) interviewed 24 women with facial scars and identified 44 themes related to quality of life. They classified these themes into five main areas: 1) physical comfort and functioning, 2) acceptability to self and others, 3) social functioning, 4) confidence in the nature and management of the scarring, and 5) emotional well-being.

Pelvic Surgery

Hysterectomy

In patients who have undergone hysterectomy, four stages in the experience have been described (H.J. Krouse 1990):

1. The recognition/exploration stage centers on the discovery of symptoms and diagnosis.
2. The crisis/climax stage occurs when treatment is initiated.
3. The adaptation stage occurs after treatment.
4. The resolution/disorganization stage concerns the long-term sequelae.

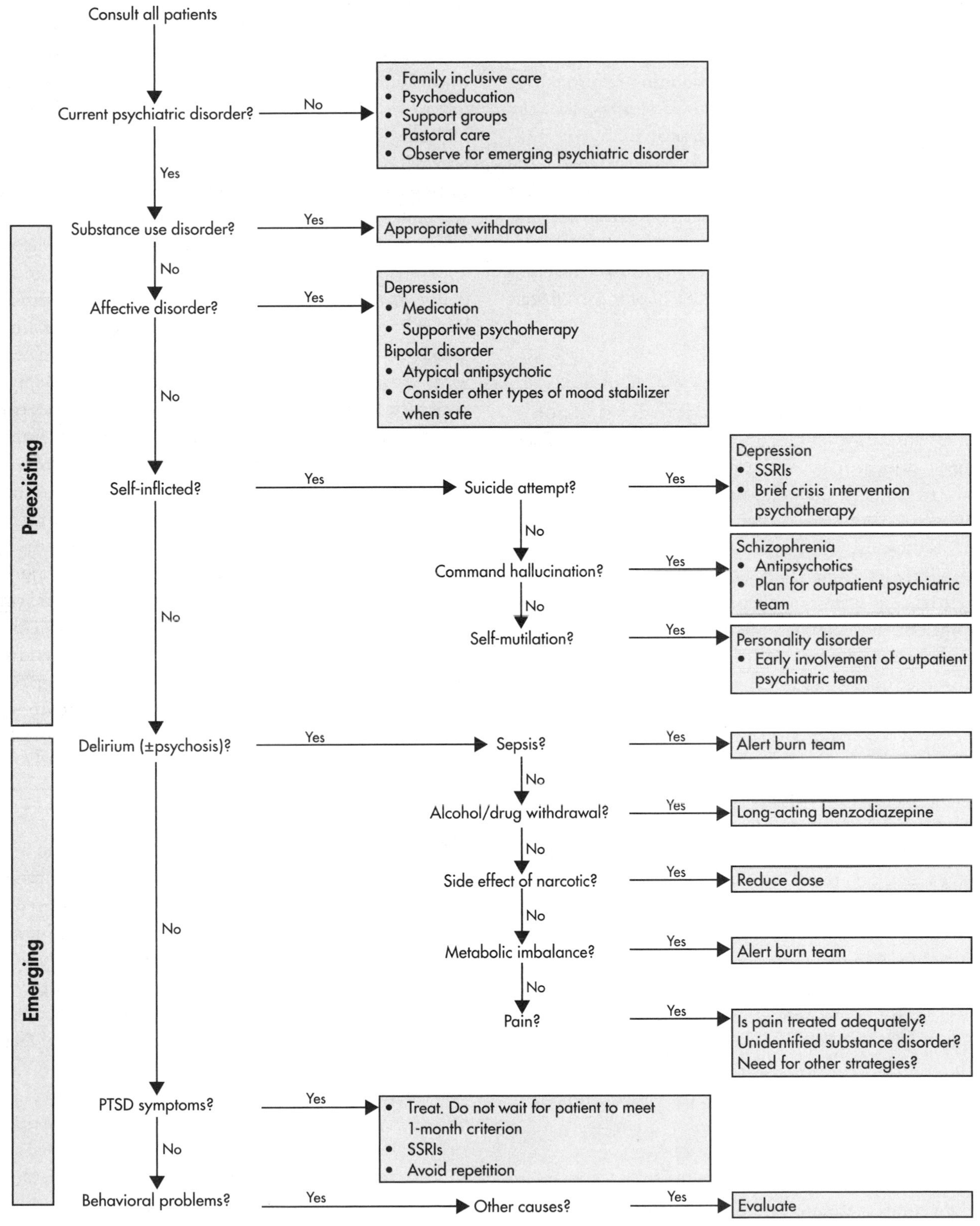

FIGURE 30–2. Algorithm for the initial psychiatric assessment of the burn patient during the initial acute hospitalization.

Note. PTSD=posttraumatic stress disorder; SSRIs=selective serotonin reuptake inhibitors.

Guilt, embarrassment, anxiety, isolation, fear, and denial of the disease are hallmarks of the first stage of the hysterectomy experience, whereas anxiety, depression, altered body image, and concerns about changing relationships characterize the second stage. Many women associate the uterus with femininity, the sex drive, sexual attractiveness, and status as a wife or mother. Thus, for some women, a hysterectomy leads to impaired self-image and self-esteem. If concerns about the quality of the marital relationship and the deleterious effect of surgery on sexual functioning arise, they must be addressed. Anxiety and depression are common and should be addressed (see also Chapter 33, "Obstetrics and Gynecology").

Gynecological Cancer

Gynecological cancer treatment leads to deterioration of sexual functioning in 30%–35% of patients in terms of sexual motivation, arousal, and orgasm. Prognostic variables include previous sexual behavior, partner-related factors, availability of education and counseling, dyspareunia, postcoital bleeding, estrogen deprivation, and vaginal stenosis or shortening. The magnitude of the surgery and psychosocial factors (including presurgical body image, pretreatment libidinal level, anxiety, attitude toward sex role, and age) contribute to postsurgical adjustment (Weigman-Schultz and van de Wiel 1992; see also Chapter 16, "Sexual Dysfunction").

Prostatectomy

In prostatectomy, the frequency of postsurgical impotence and incontinence dramatically affects quality of life. Libman et al. (1991) reported that prostatectomy often has a negative effect on erectile function, particularly in older men. Rossignol et al. (1991) evaluated the effect of radical prostatectomy in 429 patients and found that those men who were satisfied with their postsurgical sexual life were younger and had normal sexual function prior to the surgery. Braslis et al. (1995) concluded that despite fairly drastic complications (incontinence and impotence) and associated distress, radical prostatectomy is a well-accepted procedure (see also Chapter 16, "Sexual Dysfunction").

Ostomies

There has been a steady increase in the number of people surviving colorectal cancer at least 5 years following diagnosis (American Cancer Society 2007). Many of these survivors will receive intestinal stomas as part of their treatment; however, patients with stomas face many problems, both physical and psychosocial. In colostomy patients, Wade (1990) reported that physical symptoms such as fatigue, nausea, diarrhea, flatulence, urinary incontinence, and stoma complications were associated with higher levels of distress. A study by Kelly (1991) found that malfunction of the stoma, skin damage, and poor healing of the perianal wound add their toll to an already trying situation and interfere with functioning and, sometimes, identity. Accidental leakage, or the fear thereof, may limit activity or travel. Several bothersome aspects of caring for ostomies, with resulting changes in daily routines, troublesome side effects, and embarrassing accidental leakage, further stress the patient's resilience and coping skills (Thomas et al. 1988).

Systematically reviewed studies of colorectal cancer patients with and without a stoma have reported significantly higher rates of depression, suicidal thoughts, feelings of loneliness, low self-esteem, and sexual problems in persons with a stoma (Sprangers et al. 1995). The increasing survival rates and acknowledgment of the difficulties experienced by these patients have led to a call for more emphasis on addressing social and psychological concerns (Simmons et al. 2007). Anxiety and embarrassment over a stoma may lead to an alteration in lifestyle and overall self-image (Nugent et al. 1999), and sexuality and intimacy concerns merit special attention (R.S. Krouse et al. 2009). The majority of patients experience sexual dysfunction after rectal cancer surgery as the result of damage to the autonomic plexus that occurs during surgery and radiotherapy (Hendren et al. 2005; Marijnen et al. 2005; see also Chapter 16, "Sexual Dysfunction"). Successful adjustment to colostomy depends on education for ostomy self-care, psychosocial support to help accept the changes in body image, and a social support network (Piwonka and Merino 1999).

Management Strategies After Pelvic Surgery

Pelvic surgery is often associated with pain, changes in body image, self-image distortions, and fear of becoming dependent or abandoned. Patients also fear possible sexual and reproductive changes. Patients undergoing these types of surgery are at risk for poor psychosocial outcome in terms of psychological distress, limitation of activities, and sexual adjustment. Patients and physicians may feel uncomfortable discussing sexual matters, and concerns about sexual functioning may be minimized. This may create severe distress postoperatively. Patients should be fully informed about the sexual effects of surgery, provided ample opportunity to ask questions, and provided assistance in coping with the aftermath of the surgery (see also Chapter 16, "Sexual Dysfunction").

Bariatric Surgery

Extreme obesity is defined as a body mass index (BMI) greater than 40 kg/m^2. BMI is a calculated number (attained by dividing weight in kilograms by height in meters squared) and does not provide information about composition. Results from the 2005–2006 National Health and Nutrition Examination Survey (NHANES) revealed a significant increase in the number of extremely obese adults in the United States, with 5.9% of the population affected. Although the overall percentage of overweight and obese adults is stabilizing and may be decreasing, the percentage of extremely obese adults has increased since the 2003–2004 survey. Extreme obesity is also called *morbid obesity* because it is associated with high premature morbidity and mortality, most commonly as a result of complications of type 2 diabetes mellitus, hypertension, hyperlipidemia, or sleep apnea. Although multiple treatments have been tried for extreme obesity, including cognitive-behavioral strategies, very low calorie diets, and pharmacological treatments, bariatric surgery is clearly the most effective, both in terms of weight loss achieved and weight loss maintenance. For example, in the detailed Cochrane Database review of surgical treatments for obesity (Colquitt et al. 2009), six studies (three RCTs and three prospective cohort studies) compared surgical procedures against nonsurgical treatments (including diet, pharmacotherapy, behavioral therapy, and no treatment). These studies found clinically (and statistically) significant greater weight loss after surgery (compared with other interventions) that was maintained at follow-up ranging from 18 months to 10 years. In the Swedish Obese Subjects Study (Sjöström 2008) of 1,845 surgical patients compared with 1,660 control patients, weight loss at 2 years was 23.4% in the surgical patients versus a 0.1% gain in the control patients. At the 10-year follow-up of 655 surgical patients and 621 control patients, weight loss was 19.7% among the surgical patients versus a gain of 1.3% in the control patents.

The current weight criterion for bariatric (or obesity) surgery is a BMI greater than 40 or a BMI greater than 35 with life-threatening comorbidities (American Medical Association 2003; National Heart, Lung, and Blood Institute 2000; National Institute of Diabetes and Digestive and Kidney Diseases 2009). Although there have been studies demonstrating that extremely obese adolescents can lose weight with bariatric surgery, the long-term effects of surgery on their physical and cognitive development remains unclear. As less invasive surgical strategies have been devised, there has been a dramatic rise in the number of obese patients who have had bariatric surgery; for example, one report (Nguyen et al. 2005) estimated a 450% increase between 1998 and 2002 in the United States.

Bariatric surgery works in one of two ways: 1) by restricting a patient's ability to eat (restrictive procedures) and 2) by interfering with absorption of ingested food (malabsorptive procedures). The three most commonly performed operations are the Roux-en-Y gastric bypass, adjustable gastric banding, and the biliopancreatic bypass with duodenal switch. The Roux-en-Y gastric bypass combines restriction and malabsorption principles and results in greater weight loss than gastric banding, a restrictive procedure. The restrictive element of the Roux-en-Y gastric bypass involves creation of a small gastric pouch with a small outlet; the malabsorptive element involves bypass of the distal stomach, the entire duodenum, and about 20–40 cm of the proximal jejunum. The biliopancreatic bypass with duodenal switch involves removing a large portion of the stomach (to restrict meal sizes), rerouting food away from much of the small intestine (to prevent absorption of food), and rerouting bile, which impairs digestion. Both the gastric bypass and gastric banding are now often performed as laparoscopic procedures typically requiring very brief hospital stays.

Pories (2008) summarized the improvements that have occurred with bariatric surgery during the past decade. There are now multiple RCTs demonstrating that bariatric surgery produces durable, very significant weight loss with full and long-term remission of type 2 diabetes in the majority of patients. For example, in a report by Dixon et al. (2008), surgical intervention resulted in a remission rate for type 2 diabetes mellitus of 73% (vs. 13% with nonsurgical intervention). Other complications of severe obesity such as hypertension, obstructive sleep apnea, and lipid abnormalities also improve following surgery, but not as dramatically as type 2 diabetes. In terms of some of these other comorbidities, the large prospective-cohort Swedish Obese Subjects Study described earlier (Sjöström 2008) found that significantly greater proportions of people who received surgery (compared with nonsurgical control subjects) showed recovery from their diabetes, hypertension, and hypertriglyceridemia (recovery rates of 72%, 24%, and 62%, respectively) at the 2-year follow-up. However, at the 10-year follow-up, only 36% had maintained recovery from their diabetes. Even though it is clear that surgery confers an advantage in remission (although not necessarily a cure) of various comorbidities, it is not completely clear whether one surgical procedure is more effective than another. Part of the difficulty in ascertaining the comparative efficacy of procedures is that the reports of the various comorbidities are presented differently, patients are assessed over different time periods, and the quality of the reports differ widely.

Evidence from the Cochrane review indicates that there is less weight loss following gastric banding than following gastric bypass (Colquitt et al. 2009). Seven RCTs comparing gastric bypass against vertical banded gastroplasty were reviewed. Five of the seven reported percentage excess weight loss at 1 year and percentage excess weight loss at follow-up ranging from 18 months to 5 years. Percentage weight loss at 1 year ranged between 62.9% and 78% for gastric bypass procedures and between 44% and 62.9% for gastric banding. At the latest follow-up, percentage excess weight loss ranged from 66% to 84% for gastric bypass and from 37% to 59.8% for gastric banding.

Extremely obese patients present significant surgical risks; nonetheless, there has also been a marked improvement in the safety of bariatric surgery, with significantly lower complication rates. In the large 10-year Swedish Obese Subjects Study (Sjöström 2008), 90-day mortality following date of surgery (and comparison dates for the control subjects) was 5 deaths among the 2,010 surgical patients and 2 deaths among the 2,037 control patients. At 10-year follow-up, there had been 101 (5%) deaths in the surgical group versus 129 (6.3%) in the control group. Thus, there was a statistically significant decrease in all-cause mortality at follow-up in bariatric surgery patients compared with patients receiving conventional treatments. The possible complications of gastric bypass are more severe than those of gastric banding. For example, although perioperative death is uncommon, it is more likely with gastric bypass than with gastric banding. Early complications such as wound infection, ulcer, and abscess occur rarely with either procedure but are more common with gastric bypass (for a review, see Colquitt et al. 2009). Late complications such as postoperative cholecystectomy are similar between gastric bypass and gastric banding procedures. Figure 30–3 illustrates the Roux-en-Y gastric bypass, and Figure 30–4 is an illustration of a laparoscopic version of gastric banding.

Psychiatric and Psychosocial Aspects

Recent studies have documented a high prevalence of psychiatric disorders among extremely obese patients who present for bariatric surgery. The prevalence of Axis I diagnoses among candidates for bariatric surgery is high. Two recent relatively large studies (Mauri et al. 2008; Rosenberger et al. 2006) utilized the well-validated Structured Clinical Interview for DSM-IV Axis I Diagnoses (SCID-I) to examine the prevalence of Axis I psychiatric disorders in severely obese bariatric surgery candidates. The lifetime prevalence of Axis I diagnoses was very similar in the two studies (36.8% in Rosenberger et al. [2006] vs. 37.6% in Mauri et al. [2008]), and current Axis I diagnosis rate was also very similar (24.1% vs. 20.9%). In both studies, the most common Axis I diagnoses were affective disorders, followed by anxiety disorders and then eating disorders. Interestingly, alcohol and other substance use disorders

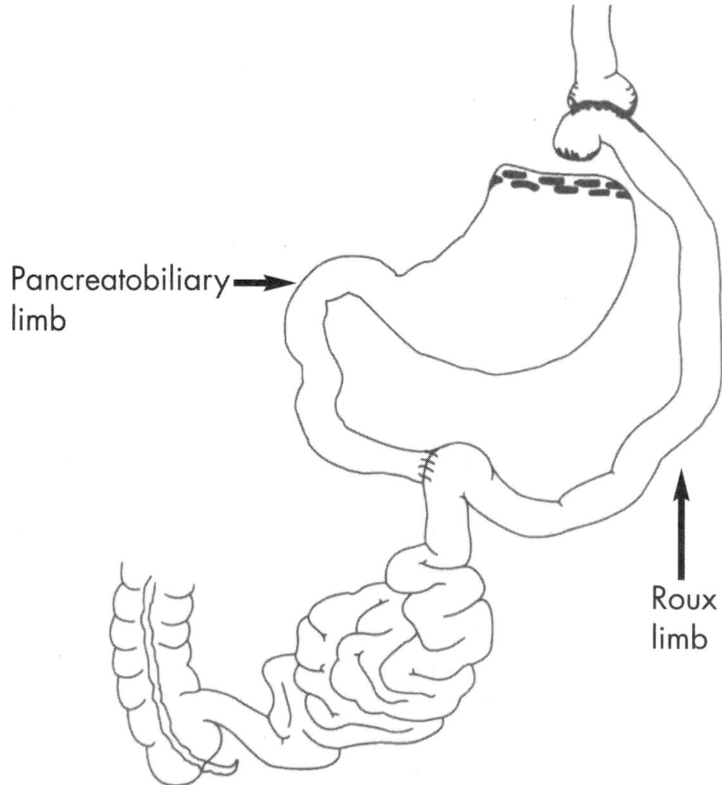

FIGURE 30–3. Diagram of Roux-en-Y gastric bypass.

Source. Reprinted from Neven K, Dymek M, leGrange D, et al.: "The Effects of Roux-en-Y Gastric Bypass Surgery on Body Image." *Obesity Surgery* 12:265–269, 2002. Copyright 2002, Springer Science. Used with permission.

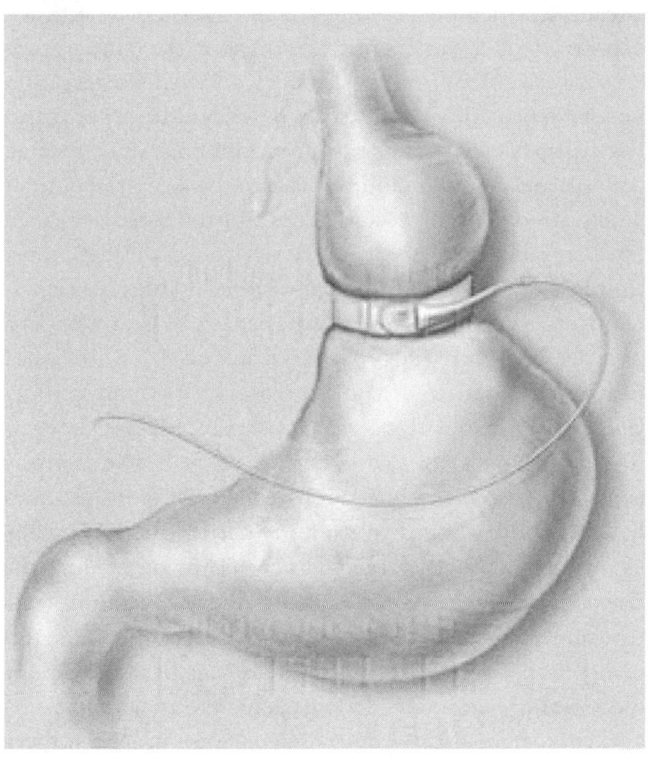

FIGURE 30–4. Diagram of laparoscopic adjustable gastric banding (LAGB) with the LAP-BAND system (INAMED Health, Santa Barbara, CA).

were uncommon in these two studies. This may be because physicians identify patients with substance use disorders and do not refer them for surgery, or it may be that patients do not reveal substance use disorders during the initial evaluation. In the study by Mauri et al. (2008), prevalence of Axis II diagnoses was also determined, with 19.5% meeting criteria for at least one Axis II diagnosis; almost all fell into the Cluster C category, including avoidant, dependent, and obsessive-compulsive personality disorders. Also using the SCID-I, Kalarchian et al. (2007) assessed 288 bariatric surgery candidates and found a lifetime Axis I diagnosis prevalence of 66.3% and a current Axis I prevalence of 37.8%. This group also found that Axis I psychiatric diagnoses were associated with greater obesity and lower functional health status (using the Medical Outcomes Study 36-item Short-Form Health Survey).

One way that psychiatric disorders can contribute to severe obesity is through weight gain caused by various psychotropic medications, particularly the antipsychotics. Most antidepressants and anticonvulsants can also cause substantial weight gain in a minority of patients taking them.

There have been early attempts to determine the effect that the presence or absence of presurgical psychiatric disorders or other negative psychosocial factors have on the outcome of bariatric surgery. Although some consensus is developing for the effect of presurgical eating disorders on outcome, the effect of other psychiatric conditions remains unclear. Data available are primarily from retrospective studies or from small single-site studies. For example, in a retrospective study (Fujioka et al. 2008) of 121 patients undergoing Roux-en-Y gastric bypass, 32% had a presurgical diagnosis of binge-eating disorder, and 17% had a history of sexual abuse; weight loss at 12 months among the sexually abused group was less than expected, but no effect of binge-eating disorder at 12 months was detected. In another study involving follow-up of 220 female patients after laparoscopic gastric banding (Kinzl et al. 2006), a mail questionnaire was returned by 140 patients; results suggested a less successful outcome in terms of weight loss in those patients who had two or more psychiatric disorders (particularly adjustment disorders, depression, and /or personality disorders).

In a careful recent study assessing quality of life following bariatric surgery, Kolotkin et al. (2009) compared 2-year outcomes among 308 patients who underwent gastric bypass surgery, 253 people who sought (but did not undergo) surgery, and 272 population-based obese individuals. At 2 years, mean weight loss was 34.2% for the gastric bypass patient group, and 1.4% for the group who did not undergo gastric bypass; there was a gain of 0.5% for the population-based group. Effect size changes for physical and weight-related quality of life were very large for the gastric bypass group and small to medium for the other two groups. Effect size changes for the psychosocial aspects of quality of life were moderate to large for the gastric bypass group and small for the two comparison groups. However, this study did not determine the effect of preexisting psychiatric diagnoses on outcome.

Eating Disorders and Bariatric Surgery

Presurgical eating disorders are common. The three careful studies cited earlier utilizing the SCID-I and SCID-II (Kalarchian et al. 2007; Mauri et al. 2008; Rosenberger et al. 2006) found a lifetime prevalence of eating disorders of 13.8%, 29.5%, and 12.8%, respectively. In all three studies, binge-eating disorder was by far the most common diagnosis (9.2%, 27.1%, and 11%), followed by much lower rates of bulimia nervosa and eating disorder not otherwise specified (other than binge-eating disorder). A complicating factor is that many more patients appear to have disordered eating behavior that is not identified as diagnostic of an eating disorder in DSM-IV (American Psychiatric Association 1994). For example, there are a number of other abnormal eating patterns that are more common among candidates for bariatric surgery. For example, night eating syndrome (for which diagnostic consensus may soon occur [Stunkard et al. 2009]) probably is present in up to 9% of patients presenting for bariatric surgery (Allison et al. 2006). Other abnormal eating patterns also are common including binge eating that does not meet full criteria for binge-eating disorder, preferences for high-sugar or high-fat foods, specific food "addictions," compulsive eating, emotional eating, lack of restraint in regard to portion size, and grazing (defined as a pattern of repeated episodes of eating small quantities of food over a long period of time, associated with feelings of loss of control). Although the term *grazing* is descriptive (and was initially used by R. Saunders 2004), it also has negative connotations. One important theme emerging from the literature is that among candidates for bariatric surgery, anxiety seems to be a consistent theme in patients with disordered eating or formal eating disorders.

There have been several reports indicating that patients with regular binge eating (not necessarily meeting current research criteria for binge-eating disorder) have weight loss and psychosocial outcomes similar to those without regular binge eating at early follow-up (e.g., White et al. 2006). A recent prospective study of 199 bariatric surgery patients (E. Chen et al. 2009) found that presurgical compensatory behavior (e.g., purging) was a small but significant predictor of lower BMI at 6 months postsurgery but not at 1 year postsurgery. The authors noted that these findings contradict the current clinical guidelines and thus should be interpreted with caution.

Ophthalmological Surgery

Cataract Surgery

Early reports by psychiatric consultants of "black patch" psychosis following cataract surgery ushered in studies of complications following eye surgery (Weisman and Hackett 1958). The initial reports focused on the sensory deprivation that occurred after bilateral cataract removal and led to recommendations that only one eye be operated on at a time. Subsequently, "black patch" psychosis was identified as a postoperative delirium that was relatively uncommon. Milstein et al. (2002) found that following cataract surgery, 4.4% of 296 patients had an immediate postoperative delirium. Factors found to be statistically associated with postoperative delirium included very old age (82 years compared with 73 years) and frequent preoperative use of benzodiazepines.

Cataract is a major public health problem, especially in developing countries: 47.8% of total blindness in the world is due to cataracts (Resnikoff et al. 2004). The number of cataract surgeries performed has increased dramatically in the past few years, in part because of an increase in the number of aging individuals. Risk factors for the development of cataracts include smoking, steroid use, diabetes, ultraviolet ray exposure, and aging. In addition, the consent process for cataract surgery, satisfaction with surgery, and postsurgery quality-of-life issues have come under scrutiny. Practice guidelines stress the importance of fully informed consent and positive communication between the patient and the treatment team (Canadian Ophthalmological Society Cataract Surgery Clinical Practice Guideline Expert Committee 2008). The key indication for surgery is interference with activities of daily life caused by cataracts. In a prospective study (Pager 2004), improvement in visual function in a patient did not correlate with overall satisfaction. Satisfaction with surgery appears to be closely related to expectations prior to surgery, which should be carefully explored during the consent process. Quality-of-life issues have been investigated, and among patients with clinically significant cataracts, surgery has been shown to reduce the risk of falls by 34% over 1 year and to reduce the annual fracture rate from 8% to 3% in women older than 75 years (Harwood et al. 2005). Another study found that the rate of motor vehicle accidents decreased in a group who had surgery compared with a group who chose not to have surgery (Owsley et al. 2002).

Stigma and Eye Abnormalities

Facial expression and eye contact are critically important in interpersonal relationships. Thus, abnormalities are likely to significantly influence quality of life. Several studies have confirmed this. For example, Bullock et al. (2001) showed pictures of patients with blepharoptosis and dermatochalasis to subjects without such abnormalities and asked them to rate the person in the picture on several dimensions, including friendliness, trustworthiness, mental illness, and happiness. After surgical correction of these eye abnormalities, the ratings of the pictures by the healthy subjects improved significantly.

In another study, patients with serious childhood-onset strabismus (before age 5 years) were evaluated prior to corrective surgery at ages 15–25 years (Menon et al. 2002). Eighty-five percent of the males and 75% of the females reported social problems caused by their continuous squint; they had been ridiculed at school and work, they had greater difficulty obtaining employment, and many avoided social activities. After corrective surgery, more than 90% reported improved self-confidence and self-esteem.

Eye Removal

Self-removal of the eye (autoenucleation), also termed *oedipism,* is a form of self-mutilation that occurs very uncommonly (Shiwach 1998). When it does, the patient is usually psychotic and often has religious preoccupations associated with a literal interpretation of the Bible ("and if thy right eye offend thee, pluck it out, and cast it from thee"; Matthew 5:28–30). Most reported cases have occurred in patients diagnosed with schizophrenia; however, cases of autoenucleation resulting from substance-induced psychosis, bipolar mania, obsessive-compulsive disorder, PTSD, and major depressive disorder have also been reported. Conjoint management of the patient by ophthalmologists and psychiatrists is crucial, especially because some patients reinjure themselves later. A review of 50 cases found a high (39%) incidence of bilateral autoenucleation (Dilly and Imes 2001). It is important to emphasize the need for treatment of the underlying psychiatric condition and close observation to prevent further harm.

Cosmetic Surgery

In an era and a culture in which people have increased interest in physical attractiveness, cosmetic surgery has dramatically increased. According to data from the American Society for Aesthetic Plastic Surgery (2009), nearly 10 million surgical and nonsurgical cosmetic procedures were performed in the United States in 2009, and Americans spent nearly $10.5 billion on cosmetic procedures. The most common surgical cosmetic procedures were breast augmentation, lipoplasty, blepharoplasty, rhinoplasty, and abdominoplasty. Women had more than 90% of the cosmetic procedures. Early studies of cosmetic surgery found that patients with psychiatric problems were common among cosmetic surgery candidates. More recent studies suggest that because more people consider cosmetic surgery a reasonable choice, the percentage of applicants with psychiatric disorders may be relatively lower. Most patients do well with cosmetic surgery, although it is thought that so-called type changes (e.g., rhinoplasty) require more extensive psychological adjustments than do restorative changes (e.g., face-lifts) (Castle et al. 2002).

Age at the time of cosmetic surgery is also important; it may be easier to incorporate changes into body image during childhood or adolescence. Cosmetic surgery is usually helpful in adolescents with a true defect if they are selected carefully and if genuine informed consent is obtained before surgery (McGrath and Mukerji 2000).

Because quality of life is significantly influenced by body image, a philosophical question raised by the increased number of aesthetic surgeries is whether cosmetic surgery should be considered medically necessary. The focus on possible negative body image changes after lifesaving surgeries for illnesses such as breast cancer has resulted in trials comparing the effectiveness (in terms of survival) of less disfiguring surgeries with that of more radical approaches. A persuasive argument can be made that improvements in body image and self-esteem may dramatically improve quality of life; this point of view is supported by many studies (e.g., Litner et al. 2008; Sabino Neto et al. 2008; Stuerz et al. 2008).

Preoperative Assessment

Even though the percentage of patients with psychiatric disorders may be lower among patients seeking aesthetic surgery than in previous decades, the percentage is probably still higher than among most other surgical candidates. Several research groups have attempted to determine which patients should not have cosmetic surgery at all and which patients should have psychiatric treatment before aesthetic surgery. A series of questions designed to detect psychiatric problems has been proposed (Grossbart and Sarwer 1999). One problem in determining who is likely to benefit from cosmetic surgery is that no widespread accepted method is available for determining patient satisfaction with the surgical results. Ching et al. (2003) reviewed the literature and suggested specific measures of body image and quality of life likely to provide valid evidence concerning the question of who should receive surgery. Most patient dissatisfaction with aesthetic surgery is based on failures of communication and patient selection criteria (Ward 1998). It is very important for the surgeon to have a clear idea of the patient's expectations regarding surgical outcome. When the patient's expectations are unrealistic and the surgeon feels he or she cannot meet those expectations, surgery should be refused. Taking a careful psychosocial history is an essential part of patient selection and is a way to establish rapport and ensure that the right operation is performed on the right patient. Blackburn and Blackburn (2008) have devised a method for assessing various parameters found to be relevant in determining whether the proposed surgery is likely to be successful and satisfactory to the patient. A template for taking a history is provided with the acronym *SAGA*, which stands for **S**ensitization (the patient's sensitivity to the deformity arising from internal or external sources), **A**esthetic self-assessment (the patient's own private evaluation of the feature about which he or she has a complaint), peer **G**roup comparison (how a patient compares the feature to the same feature in other people), and **A**voidance behavior (strategies used by the patient to camouflage or avoid exposure of the feature of complaint).

Body Dysmorphic Disorder

Body dysmorphic disorder (BDD) is reviewed in detail in Chapter 12, "Somatization and Somatoform Disorders." Also known as dysmorphophobia, BDD has been called the disorder of imagined ugliness. Patients with BDD often present to cosmetic surgeons for correction of trivial or nonexistent defects. Preoccupations commonly involve the face or head, although any body part can be the focus of concern (Phillips and Diaz 1997). In cosmetic surgery settings, BDD rates of 6%–15% have been reported. Surgical treatment outcomes are poor, especially after multiple operations on the same body part, and patients are often dissatisfied with their treatment and register complaints against their physicians (Fakuda 1977; Phillips and Dufresne 2000). BDD occasionally first makes its appearance after cosmetic surgery (Tignol et al. 2007) and may result in malpractice litigation (Nachshoni and Kotler 2007). It is important for the surgeon to explain to patients with BDD that rather than having a significant dermatological or surgical problem, they have a body image problem consisting of being overly concerned about and affected by how they think they look. They should also be told that BDD is a known and treatable disorder that many people have. In general, it is more fruitful to focus on the distress and impairment that the concerns about appearance are causing the patient than to focus on the patient's actual appearance, and doing so may facilitate referral to a mental health professional.

Conclusion

Psychiatric problems occur in many surgical patients. We have discussed common problems that occur during the preoperative, intraoperative, and postoperative periods. Preoperatively, issues around capacity and consent are important, as well as planning for the surgical and postoperative management of psychiatric disorders known to be present. Preoperative anxiety is common, and appropriate treatment can improve postoperative recovery. Psychiatric reactions to intraoperative recall can often be ameliorated through careful preparation for surgery. Postoperatively, delirium is a key issue and is often associated with alcohol or drug withdrawal syndromes. Postoperative pain, problems related to discontinuation of ventilator support, and PTSD are common reasons for psychiatric intervention. An awareness of specific issues that can arise in burn care, pelvic surgery, bariatric surgery, ophthalmological surgery, and cosmetic surgery is also important. In the past few years, there have been significant advances both in the identification of psychosocial problems among surgical patients and in methods of assessing severity of symptoms and change with treatment. Large controlled trials evaluating various treatments are beginning to emerge. In addition, there is now a global interest in psychiatric issues related to surgery, as reflected by the marked increase in research studies addressing this topic.

References

Adler LE, Griffith JM: Concurrent medical illness in the schizophrenic patient: epidemiology, diagnosis, and management. Schizophr Res 4:91–107, 1991

Ahmadi A, Mohammadi R, Stavrinos D, et al: Self-immolation in Iran. J Burn Care Res 29:451–460, 2008

Albright JM, Kovacs EJ, Gamelli RL, et al: Implications of formal alcohol screening in burn patients. J Burn Care Res 30:62–69, 2009

Allison KC, Wadden TA, Sarwer DB, et al: Night eating syndrome and binge eating disorder among persons seeking bariatric surgery: prevalence and related features. Obesity (Silver Spring) 14:77S–82S, 2006

American Burn Association: Burn Incidence and Treatment in the US: 2007 Fact Sheet. Chicago, IL, American Burn Association, 2007. Available at: www.ameriburn.org/resources_factsheet.php. Accessed June 23, 2009.

American Cancer Society: Cancer Facts and Figures 2007. Atlanta, GA, American Cancer Society, 2007

American Medical Association: Assessment and Management of Adult Obesity: A Primer for Physicians (Roadmaps for Clinical Practice: Case Studies in Disease Prevention and Health Promotion). Chicago, IL, American Medical Association, November 2003. Available at: http://www.ama-assn.org/ama/pub/physician-resources/public-health/general-resources-health-care-professionals/roadmaps-clinical-practice-series/assessment-management-adult-obesity.shtml. Accessed June 1, 2010.

American Psychiatric Association: Diagnostic and Statistical Manual of Mental Disorders, 4th Edition. Washington, DC, American Psychiatric Association, 1994

American Society for Aesthetic Plastic Surgery: Quick Facts: Highlights of the ASAPS 2009 Statistics on Cosmetic Surgery. Garden Grove, CA, 2009. Available at: http://www.surgery.org/sites/default/files/2009quickfacts.pdf. Accessed June 2010.

Andreasen NJ, Noyes R Jr, Hartford CE, et al: Management of emotional reactions in seriously burned adults. N Engl J Med 286:65–69, 1972

Avidan MS, Zhang L, Burnside BA, et al: Anesthesia awareness and the bispectral index. N Engl J Med 13:1097–1108, 2008

Ayala ES, Meuret AE, Ritz T: Treatments for blood-injury-injection phobia: a critical review of current evidence. J Psychiatr Res 43:1235–1242, 2009

Barillo DJ, Goode R: Substance abuse in victims of fire. J Burn Care Rehabil 17:71–76, 1996

Bernstein NR: Emotional Care of the Facially Burned and Disfigured. Boston, MA, Little, Brown, 1976

Bird MD, Kovacs EJ: Organ-specific inflammation following acute ethanol and burn injury. Leukoc Biol 84:607–613, 2008

Blackburn VF, Blackburn AV: Taking a history in aesthetic surgery: SAGA—the surgeon's tool for patient selection. J Plast Reconstr Aesthet Surg 61:723–729, 2008

Blanchard EB, Hickling EJ, Devineni T, et al: A controlled evaluation of cognitive behavioural therapy for posttraumatic stress in motor vehicle accident survivors. Behav Res Ther 41:79–96, 2003

Blussé van Oud-Alblas HJ, van Dijk M, Liu C, et al: Intraoperative awareness during paediatric anaesthesia. Br J Anaesth 102:104–110, 2009

Bradley CT, Brasel KJ: Core competencies in palliative care for surgeons: interpersonal and communication skills. Am J Hosp Palliat Care 24:499–507, 2007

Brander VA, Stulberg SD, Adams AD, et al: Predicting total knee replacement pain: a prospective, observational study. Clin Orthop Relat Res 416:27–36, 2003

Braslis KG, Santa-Cruz C, Brickman AL, et al: Quality of life 12 months after radical prostatectomy. Br J Urol 75:48–53, 1995

Brodie EE, Whyte A, Niven CA: Analgesia through the looking-glass? A randomized controlled trial investigating the effect of viewing a "virtual" limb upon phantom limb pain, sensation and movement. Eur J Pain 11:428–436, 2007

Brown BC, McKenna SP, Siddhi K, et al: The hidden cost of skin scars: quality of life after skin scarring. J Plast Reconstr Aesthet Surg 61:1049–1058, 2008

Bullock JD, Warwar RE, Bienenfeld DG, et al: Psychosocial implications of blepharoptosis and dermatochalasis. Trans Am Ophthalmol Soc 99:65–71, 2001

Cameron DR, Pegg SP, Muller M: Self-inflicted burns. Burns 23:519–521, 1997

Cantó MA, Quiles JM, Vallejo OG, et al: Evaluation of the effect of hospital clown's performance about anxiety in children subjected to surgical intervention. Cir Pediatr 21:195–198, 2008

Castle DJ, Honigman RJ, Phillips KA: Does cosmetic surgery improve psychosocial wellbeing? Med J Aust 176:601–604, 2002

Caumo W, Levandovski R, Hidalgo MP: Preoperative anxiolytic effect of melatonin and clonidine on postoperative pain and morphine consumption in patients undergoing abdominal hysterectomy: a double-blind, randomized, placebo-controlled study. J Pain 10:100–108, 2009

Chan BL, Witt R, Charrow AP, et al: Mirror therapy for phantom limb pain. N Engl J Med 357:2206–2207

Chen CC, Lin CS, Ko YP, et al: Premedication with mirtazapine reduces preoperative anxiety and postoperative nausea and vomiting. Anesth Analg 106:109–113, 2008

Chen E, Roehrig M, Herbozo S, et al: Compensatory eating behaviors and gastric bypass surgery outcome. Int J Eat Disord 42:363–366, 2009

Ching S, Thoma A, McCabe RE, et al: Measuring outcomes in aesthetic surgery: a comprehensive review of the literature. Plast Reconstr Surg 111:469–480, 2003

Choudhry MA, Chaudry IH: Alcohol, burn injury, and the intestine. J Emerg Trauma Shock 1:81–87, 2008

Chundamala J, Wright JG, Kemp SM: An evidence-based review of parental presence during anesthesia induction and parent/child anxiety. Can J Anaesth 56:57–70, 2009

Civardi A: Going to the Hospital (Usborne First Experiences), Revised Edition. Tulsa, OK, Educational Development Corporation, December 2005

Colquitt JL, Picot J, Loveman E, et al: Surgery for obesity. Cochrane Database Syst Rev (2):CD003641, 2009

Connard-Ballard PA: Understanding and managing burn pain: Part 2. Am J Nurs 109:54–62, 2009

Daniels SM, Fenley JD, Powers PS, et al: Self-inflicted burns: a ten-year retrospective study. J Burn Care Rehabil 12:144–147, 1991

Darnall BD: Self-delivered home-based mirror therapy for lower limb phantom pain. Am J Phys Med Rehabil 88:78–81, 2009

Dasgupta M, Rolfson DB, Stolee P, et al: Frailty is associated with postoperative complications in older adults with medical problems. Arch Gerontol Geriatr 48:78–83, 2009

Davydow DS, Gifford JM, Desai SV, et al: Posttraumatic stress disorder in general intensive care unit survivors: a systematic review. Gen Hosp Psychiatry 30:421–443, 2008

del Carmen MG, Joffe S: Informed consent for medical treatment and research: a review. Oncologist 10:636–641, 2005

Devasagayam D, Clarke D: Changes in inpatient consultation-liaison psychiatry service delivery over a 7-year period. Australas Psychiatry 16:418–422, 2008

Dilly JS, Imes RK: Autoenucleation of a blind eye. J Neuroophthalmol 21:30–31, 2001

Dixon JB, O'Brien PE, Playfair J, et al: Adjustable gastric banding and conventional therapy for type 2 diabetes: a randomized controlled trial. JAMA 23:316–323, 2008

Dischinger PC, Mitchell KA, Kufera JA, et al: A longitudinal study of former trauma center patients: the association between toxicology status and subsequent injury mortality. J Trauma 51:877–886, 2001

Dyster-Aas J, Willebrand M, Wikehult B, et al: Major depression and posttraumatic stress disorder symptoms following severe burn injury in relation to lifetime psychiatric morbidity. J Trauma 64:1349–1356, 2008

Ehde DM, Patterson DR, Wiechman SA, et al: Post-traumatic stress symptoms and distress following acute burn injury. Burns 25:587–592, 1999

Ehrsson HH, Rosen B, Stockselius A, et al: Upper limb amputees can be induced to experience a rubber hand as their own. Brain 131:3443–3452, 2008

Errando CL, Sigl JC, Robles M, et al: Awareness with recall during general anesthesia: a prospective observational evaluation of 4001 patients. Br J Anaesth 101:178–185, 2008

Falder S, Browne A, Edgar D, et al: Core outcomes for adult burn survivors: a clinical overview. Burns 35:618–641, 2009

Fakuda O: Statistical analysis of dysmorphophobia in outpatient clinic. Jpn J Plast Reconstruct Surg 20:569–577, 1977

Fassoulaki A, Melemeni A, Paraskeva A, et al: Postoperative pain and analgesic requirements after anesthesia with sevoflurane, desflurane or propofol. Anesth Analg 107:1715–1719, 2008

Fauerbach JA, Lawrence JW, Schmidt CW Jr, et al: Personality predictors of injury-related posttraumatic stress disorder. J Nerv Ment Dis 188:510–517, 2000

Fauerbach JA, McKibben J, Bienvenu J, et al: Psychological distress after major burn injury. Psychosom Med 69:473–482, 2007

First MB: Desire for amputation of a limb: paraphilia, psychosis, or a new type of identity disorder. Psychol Med 35:919–928, 2005

Fitzgerald BM, Elder J: Will a 1-page informational handout decrease patients' most common fears of anesthesia and surgery? J Surg Educ 65:359–363, 2008

Fujioka K, Yan E, Wang HJ, et al: Evaluating preoperative weight loss, binge eating disorder, and sexual abuse history on Roux-en-Y gastric bypass outcome. Surg Obes Relat Dis 4:137–143, 2008

Fukunishi I: Relationship of cosmetic disfigurement to the severity of posttraumatic stress disorder in burn injury or digital amputation. Psychother Psychosom 68:82–86, 1999

Fulop G, Strain JJ: Medical and surgical inpatients who referred themselves for psychiatric consultation. Gen Hosp Psychiatry 7:267–271, 1985

Gamberini M, Bollinger D, Lurati Buse GA: Rivastigmine for the prevention of postoperative delirium in elderly patients undergoing elective cardiac surgery—a randomized controlled trial. Crit Care Med 37:1762–1768, 2009

Gaylord KM, Holcomb JB, Zolezzi ME: A comparison of posttraumatic stress disorder between combat casualties and civilians treated at a military burn center. J Trauma 66 (4 suppl):S191–S195, 2009

Gentilello LM, Donovan DM, Dunn CW, et al: Alcohol interventions in trauma centers: current practice and future directions. JAMA 274:1043–1048, 1995

Ghoneim MM, Block RI: Learning and consciousness during general anesthesia. Anesthesiology 76:279–305, 1992

Goldman LS: Medical illness in patients with schizophrenia. J Clin Psychiatry 60 (suppl 21):10–15, 1999

Greene NH, Attix DK, Weldon BC, et al: Measures of executive function and depression identify patients at risk for postoperative delirium. Anesthesology 110:788–795, 2009

Grossbart TA, Sarwer DB: Cosmetic surgery: surgical tools—psychosocial goals. Semin Cutan Med Surg 18:101–111, 1999

Gurlit S, Möllmann M: How to prevent perioperative delirium in the elderly? Z Gerontol Geriatr 41:447–452, 2008

Hagg O, Fritzell P, Ekselius L, et al: Predictors of outcome in fusion surgery for chronic low back pain: a report from the Swedish Lumbar Spine Study. Eur Spine J 12:22–33, 2003

Hamilton JG: Needle phobia: a neglected diagnosis. J Fam Pract 41:169–175, 1995

Hanson MD, Gauld M, Walthen CN, et al: Nonpharmacological interventions for acute wound care distress in pediatric patients with burn injury: a systematic review. J Burn Care Res 29:730–741, 2008

Harwood RH, Foss AJ, Osborn F, et al: Falls and health status in elderly women following first eye cataract surgery: a randomized controlled trial. Br J Ophthalmol 89:53–59, 2005

Hendren SK, O'Connor BL, Liu M, et al. Prevalence of male and female sexual dysfunction is high following surgery of rectal cancer. Ann Surg 242:212–213, 2005

Herz MI, Marder SR: Schizophrenia: Comprehensive Treatment and Management. Philadelphia, PA, Lippincott Williams & Wilkins, 2002

Hinrichs-Rocker A, Schulz K, Järvinen I, et al: Psychosocial predictors and correlates for chronic post-surgical pain (CPSP)—a systemic review. Eur J Pain 13:719–730, 2009

Hudcova J, McNicol E, Quah C, et al: Patient controlled opioid analgesia versus conventional opioid analgesia for postoperative pain. Cochrane Database Syst Rev (4):CD003348, 2006

Hughes DB, Ullery BW, Barie PS: The contemporary approach to the care of Jehovah's Witnesses. J Trauma 65:237–247, 2008

Huyse FJ, Touw DJ, vanSchijndel RS, et al: Psychotropic drugs and the perioperative period: a proposal for a guideline in elective surgery. Psychosomatics 47:8–22, 2006

Idriss N, Maibach HI: Scar assessment scales: a dermatologic overview. Skin Res Technol 15:1–5, 2009

Imbus SH, Zawacki BE: Autonomy for burned patients when survival is unprecedented. N Engl J Med 297:308–311, 1977

James-Ellison M, Barnes P, Maddocks A, et al: Social health outcomes following thermal injuries: a retrospective matched cohort study. Arch Dis Child 94:663–667, 2009

Jones A: A psychoanalytically informed conversation with a woman and her husband following major surgery for cancer of her neck and torso. J Adv Nurs 35:459–467, 2001

Jones JD, Barber B, Engrav L, et al: Alcohol use and burn injury. J Burn Care Rehabil 12:148–152, 1991

Kain ZN, Mayes LC, O'Connor TZ, et al: Preoperative anxiety in children: predictors and outcomes. Arch Pediatr Adolesc Med 150:1238–1245, 1996

Kain ZN, Caldwell-Andrews A, Wang SM: Psychological preparation of the patient and pediatric surgical patient. Anesthesiol Clin North Am 20:29–44, 2002

Kain ZN, Caldwell-Andrews AA, Mayes LC, et al: Family-centered preparation for surgery improves perioperative outcomes in children: a randomized controlled trial. Anesthesiology 106:65–74, 2007

Kalarchian MA, Marcus MD, Levine MD, et al: Psychiatric disorders among bariatric surgery candidates: relationship to obesity and functional health status. Am J Psychiatry 164:328–334, 2007

Kalisvaart KJ, de Jonghe JF, Bogaards MJ, et al: Haloperidol prophylaxis for elderly hip-surgery patients at risk for delirium: a randomized placebo-controlled study. J Am Geriatr Soc 53:1658–1666, 2005

Kamolz T, Granderath FA, Pointner R: Does major depression in patients with gastroesophageal reflux disease affect the outcome of laparoscopic antireflux surgery? Surg Endosc 17:55–60, 2003

Kaneko T, Cai J, Ishikura T, et al: Prophylactic consecutive administration of haloperidol can reduce the occurrence of postoperative delirium in gastrointestinal surgery. Yonago Acta Med 42:179–184, 1999

Kazmierski J, Kowman M, Banach M, et al: Clinical utility and use of DSM-IV and ICD-10 criteria and the Memorial Delirium Assessment Scale in establishing a diagnosis of delirium after cardiac surgery. Psychosomatics 49:73–76, 2008

Keck M, Lumenta DB, Andel H, et al: Burn treatment in the elderly. Burns 35:1071–1079, 2009

Kelly MP: Coping with an ileostomy. Soc Sci Med 33:115–125, 1991

Kessler RC, Sonnega A, Bromet E, et al: Posttraumatic stress disorder in the National Comorbidity Survey. Arch Gen Psychiatry 52:1048–1060, 1995

Kettwich SC, Sibbitt WL Jr, Brandt JR, et al: Needle phobia and stress-reducing medical devices in pediatric and adult chemotherapy patients. J Pediatr Oncol Nurs 24:20–28, 2007

Kinzl JF, Schrattenecker M, Traweger C, et al: Psychosocial predictors of weight loss after bariatric surgery. Obes Surg 16:1609–1614, 2006

Klein E, Koren D, Arnon I, et al: Sleep complaints are not corroborated by objective sleep measures in post-traumatic stress disorder: a 1-year prospective study in survivors of motor vehicle crashes. J Sleep Res 12:35–41, 2003

Klein MB, Lezotte DL, Fauerbach JA, et al: The National Institute on Disability and Rehabilitation Research model system database: a tool for the multicenter study of the outcome of burn injury. J Burn Care Res 28:84–96, 2007

Kocyildirim E, Franck LS, Elliott MJ: Intra-operative imaging in paediatric cardiac surgery: the reactions of parents who requested and watched a video of the surgery performed on their child. Cardiol Young 17:407–413, 2007

Koivula M, Tarkka MT, Tarkka M, et al: Fear and in-hospital social support for coronary artery bypass grafting patients on the day before surgery. Int J Nurs Stud 39:415–427, 2002

Kolotkin RL, Crosby RD, Gress RE, et al: Two-year changes in health-related quality of life in gastric bypass patients compared with severely obese controls. Surg Obes Relat Dis 5:250–256, 2009

Krouse HJ: Psychological adjustment of women to gynecologic cancers. NAACOGS Clin Issu Perinat Womens Health Nurs 1:495–512, 1990

Krouse RS, Herrinton LJ, Grant M, et al: Health related quality of life among long-term rectal cancer survivors with an ostomy: manifestation by sex. J Clin Oncol 27:4664–4670, 2009

Kudoh A, Katagai H, Takazawa T: Antidepressant treatment for chronic depressed patients should not be discontinued prior to anesthesia. Can J Anaesth 49:132–136, 2002

Kudoh A, Katagai H, Takazawa T: Effect of preoperative discontinuation of antipsychotics in schizophrenic patients on outcome during and after anesthesia. Eur J Anaesth 21:414–416, 2004

Lanctot KL, Best TS, Mittman N, et al: Efficacy and safety of neuroleptics in behavioral disorders associated with dementia. J Clin Psychiatry 59:550–561, 1998

Lat I, McMillian W, Taylor S, et al: The impact of delirium on clinical outcomes in mechanically ventilated surgical and trauma patients. Crit Care Med 37:1898–1905, 2009

Levandovski R, Ferreira MB, Hidalgo MP, et al: Impact of preoperative anxiolytic on surgical site infection in patients undergoing abdominal hysterectomy. Am J Infect Control 36:718–726, 2008

Liber JM, Faber AW, Treffers PD, et al: Coping style, personality and adolescent adjustment 10 years post-burn. Burns 34:775–782, 2008

Libman E, Fichten CS, Rothenberg P, et al: Prostatectomy and inguinal hernia repair: a comparison of the sexual consequences. J Sex Marital Ther 17:27–34, 1991

Lieber CS: Medical disorders of alcoholism. N Engl J Med 333: 1058–1065, 1995

Lindemann E: Symptomatology and management of acute grief (1944). Am J Psychiatry 151 (suppl 6):155–160, 1994

Litner JA, Rotenberg BW, Dennis M, et al: Impact of cosmetic facial surgery on satisfaction with appearance and quality of life. Arch Facial Plast Surg 10:79–83, 2008

Low AJ, Dyster-Aas J, Kildal M, et al: The presence of nightmares as a screening tool for symptoms of posttraumatic stress disorder in burn survivors. J Burn Care Res 27:727–733, 2006

Luhmann N, Knodt EM: Social Systems (Writing Science). Translated by Bedrara J, Baeder D. Stanford, CA, Stanford University Press, 1995

Maes M, Delmeire L, Mylle J, et al: Risk and preventive factors of post-traumatic stress disorder (PTSD): alcohol consumption and intoxication prior to a traumatic event diminishes the relative risk to develop PTSD in response to that trauma. J Affect Disord 63:113–121, 2001

Marcantonio ER, Flacker JM, Wright RJ, et al: Reducing delirium after hip fracture: a randomized trial. J Am Geriatr Soc 49:516–522, 2001

Marijnen CA, van de Velde CJ, Putter H, et al: Impact of short term preoperative radiotherapy on health related quality of life and sexual dysfunction in primary rectal cancer: report of a multicenter randomized trial. J Clin Oncol 23:1847–1858, 2005

Martin-Herz SP, Patterson DR, Honari S, et al: Pediatric pain control practices of North American Burn Centers. J Burn Care Rehabil 24:26–36, 2003

Matharu LM, Ashley PF: Sedation of anxious children undergoing dental treatment. Cochrane Database Syst Rev (2): CD003877, 2005

Mauri M, Rucci P, Calderone A, et al: Axis I and II disorders and quality of life in bariatric surgery candidates. J Clin Psychiatry 69:295–301, 2008

McGrath MH, Mukerji S: Plastic surgery and the teenage patient. J Pediatr Adolesc Gynecol 13:105–118, 2000

McKibben JB, Bresnick MG, Wiechman Askay SA, et al: Acute stress disorder and posttraumatic stress disorder: a prospective study of prevalence, course, and predictors in a sample with major burn injuries. J Burn Care Res 29:22–35, 2008

Ménigaux C, Adam F, Guignard B, et al: Preoperative gabapentin decreases anxiety and improves early functional recovery from knee surgery. Anesth Analg 100:1394–1399, 2005

Menon V, Saha J, Tandon R, et al: Study of the psychosocial aspects of strabismus. J Pediatr Ophthalmol Strabismus 39:203–208, 2002

Milstein A, Pollack A, Kleinman G, et al: Confusion/delirium following cataract surgery: an incidence study of 1-year duration. Int Psychogeriatr 14:301–306, 2002

Moesgaard F, Lykkegaard-Nielsen M: Preoperative cell-mediated immunity and duration of antibiotic prophylaxis in relation to postoperative infectious complications: a controlled trial in biliary, gastroduodenal and colorectal surgery. Acta Chir Scand 155:281–286, 1989

Mulholland R, Green L, Longstaff C, et al: Deliberate self-harm by burning: a retrospective case controlled study. J Burn Care Res 29:644–649, 2008

Mzezewa S, Jonsson K, Aberg M, et al: A prospective study of suicidal burns admitted to the Harare burns unit. Burns 26:460–464, 2000

Nachshoni T, Kotler M: Legal and medical aspects of body dysmorphic disorder. Med Law 26:721–735, 2007

National Heart, Lung, and Blood Institute: The Practical Guide: Identification, Evaluation, and Treatment of Overweight and Obesity in Adults (NIH Publ No. 00-4084). Bethesda, MD, U.S. Department of Health and Human Services, National Institutes of Health, National Heart, Lung, and Blood Institute, October 2000. Available at: http://www.nhlbi.nih.gov/guidelines/obesity/prctgd_c.pdf. Accessed June 1, 2010.

National Institute of Diabetes and Digestive and Kidney Diseases: Bariatric Surgery for Severe Obesity (NIH Publication No. 08-4006). Bethesda, MD, National Institute of Diabetes and Digestive and Kidney Diseases (NIDDK) Weight control Information Network (WIN), March 2009. Available at: http://win.niddk.nih.gov/publications/gastric.htm.

Neale MC, Walters EE, Eaves LJ, et al: Genetics of blood-injury fears and phobias: a population-based twin study. Am J Med Genet 54:326–334, 1994

Neven K, Dymek M, leGrange D, et al: The effects of Roux-en-Y gastric bypass surgery on body image. Obes Surg 12:265–269, 2002

Ng SK, Chau AW, Leung WK: The effect of pre-operative information in relieving anxiety in oral surgery patients. Community Dent Oral Epidemiol 32:227–235, 2004

Nguyen NT, Root J, Zainabadi K, et al: Accelerated growth of bariatric surgery with the introduction of minimally invasive surgery. Arch Surg 140:1198–1202, 2005

Nir Y, Paz A, Sabo E, et al: Fear of injections in young adults: prevalence and associations. Am J Trop Med Hyg 68:341–344, 2003

Nobe DW, Kehlet H: Risks of interrupting drug treatment before surgery. BMJ 321:719–720, 2000

Noor SN, Musa S: Assessment of patients' level of satisfaction with cleft treatment using the Cleft Evaluation Profile. Cleft Palate Craniofac J 44:292–303, 2007

Nugent KP, Daniels P, Stewart B, et al: Quality of life in stoma patients. Dis Colon Rectum 42:1569–1574, 1999

Oude Voshaar RC, Banerjee S, Horan M, et al: Fear of falling more important than pain and depression for functional recovery after surgery for hip fracture in older people. Psychol Med 36:1635–1645, 2006

Owsley C, McGwin G Jr, Sloane M, et al: Impact of cataract surgery on motor vehicle crash involvement by older adults. JAMA 288:841–849, 2002

Pace B: Chris Gets Ear Tubes. Washington, DC, Kendall Green Publications/Gallaudet University Press, 1987

Page AC: The role of disgust in faintness elicited by blood and injection stimuli. J Anxiety Disord 17:45–58, 2002

Pager CK: Assessment of visual satisfaction and function after cataract surgery. J Cataract Refract Surg 30:2510–2516, 2004

Pai MS, Bhaduri A, Jain AG, et al: The experiences of mothers of pediatric surgery children—a qualitative analysis. J Pediatr Nurs 23:479–489, 2008

Paré A: The Works of That Famous Chirurgion, Ambrose Parey, translated out of the Latin and compared with the French by T. Johnson. London, England, Cotes, 1649

Pekcan M, Celebioglu B, Demir B, et al: The effect of premedication on preoperative anxiety. Middle East J Anesthesiolol 18:421–433, 2005

Perks A, Chakravarti S, Manninen P: Preoperative anxiety in neurosurgical patients. Neurosurg Anesthesiol 21:127–130, 2009

Phillips KA, Diaz SF: Gender differences in body dysmorphic disorder. J Nerv Ment Dis 185:570–577, 1997

Phillips KA, Dufresne RG: Body dysmorphic disorder: a guide for dermatologists and cosmetic surgeons. Am J Clin Dermatol 1:235–243, 2000

Piwonka MA, Merino JM: A multidimensional modeling of predictors influencing the adjustment to a colostomy. J Wound Ostomy Continence Nurs 26:298–305, 1999

Pories WJ: Bariatric surgery: risks and rewards. J Clin Endocrinol Metab 93 (11 suppl 1):S89–S96, 2008

Powell J, Kitchen N, Heslin J, et al: Psychosocial outcomes at three and nine months after good neurological recovery from aneurysmal subarachnoid haemorrhage: predictors and prognosis. J Neurol Neurosurg Psychiatry 72:772–781, 2002

Powers PS: Psychosis in hospitalized burn patients: a two year prospective study. Paper presented at the Ninth Annual Regional Burn Seminar, Charleston, SC, December 1996

Powers PS: Practice guideline for psychiatric disorders. Paper presented at the 15th Regional Burn Meeting, Lexington, KY, December 2002

Powers PS, Cruse CW, Daniels S, et al: Safety and efficacy of debridement under anesthesia in patients with burns. J Burn Care Rehabil 14(2 pt 1):176–180, 1993

Powers PS, Stevens B, Arias F, et al: Alcohol disorders among patients with burns: crisis and opportunity. J Burn Care Rehabil 15:386–391, 1994

Prakanrattana U, Prapaitrakool S: Efficacy of risperidone for prevention of postoperative delirium in cardiac surgery. Anaesth Intensive Care 35:714–719, 2007

Putnam FW, Hulsmann JE: Pharmacotherapy for survivors of childhood trauma. Semin Clin Neuropsychiatry 7:129–136, 2002

Rawlinson SC, Short JA: The representation of anaesthesia in children's literature. Anaesthesia 62:1033–1038, 2007

Regal H, Rose W, Hahnel S, et al: Evaluation of psychological stress before general anesthesia. Psychiatr Neurol Med Psychol (Leipz) 37:151–155, 1985

Reiland A, Hovater M, McGwin G Jr, et al: The epidemiology of intentional burns. J Burn Care Res 27:276–280, 2006

Resnikoff S, Pascolini D, Etya'ale D, et al: Global data on visual impairment in the year 2002. Bull World Health Organ 82:844–851, 2004

Richard R, Baryza MJ, Carr JA, et al: Burn rehabilitation and research: proceedings of a consensus summit. J Burn Care Res 30:543–573, 2009

Richardson C, Glenn S, Nurmikko T, et al: Incidence of phantom phenomena including phantom limb pain 6 months after major lower limb amputation in patients with peripheral vascular disease. Clin J Pain 22:353–358, 2006

Richardson C, Glenn S, Horgan M, et al: A prospective study of factors associated with the presence of phantom limb pain six months after major lower limb amputation in patients with peripheral vascular disease. J Pain 8:793–801, 2007

Richardson P, Mustard L: The management of pain in the burns unit. Burns 35:921–936, 2009

Rivara FP, Koepsell TD, Jurkovich GJ, et al: The effects of alcohol abuse on readmission for trauma. JAMA 270:4–6, 1993

Robinson TN, Raeburn CD, Angles EM, et al: Low tryptophan levels are associated with postoperative delirium in the elderly. Am J Surg 196:670–674, 2008

Robinson TN, Raeburn CD, Tran ZV, et al: Postoperative delirium in the elderly: risk factors and outcomes. Ann Surg 249:173–178, 2009

Rolfson O, Dahlberg LE, Nilsson JA, et al: Variables determining outcome in hip replacement surgery. J Bone Joint Surg Br 91:57–61, 2009

Rosenberger PH, Henderson KE, Grilo CM: Psychiatric disorder comorbidity and association with eating disorders in bariatric surgery patients: a cross-sectional study using structured interview-based diagnosis. J Clin Psychiatry 67:1080–1085, 2006

Rossignol G, Leandri P, Gautier JR, et al: Radical retropubic prostatectomy: complications and quality of life (429 cases, 1983–1989). Eur Urol 19:186–191, 1991

Rusch MD, Gould LJ, Dzwierzynski WW, et al: Psychological impact of traumatic injuries: what the surgeon can do. Plast Reconstr Surg 109:18–24, 2002

Sabino Neto M, Demattê MF, Freire M, et al: Self-esteem and functional capacity outcomes following reduction mammaplasty. Aesthet Surg J 28:417–420, 2008

Sacco TL, Stapleton MF, Ingersoll GL: Support groups facilitated by families of former patients: creating family inclusive critical care units. Crit Care Nurse 29:36–45, 2009

Sadhasivam S, Cohen LL, Szabova A, et al: Real-time assessment of perioperative behaviors and prediction of perioperative outcomes. Anesth Analog 108:822–826, 2009

Sampson EL, Raven PR, Ndhlovu PN, et al: A randomized, double-blind, placebo-controlled trial of donepezil hydrochloride (Aricept) for reducing the incidence of postoperative delirium after elective total hip replacement. Int J Geriatr Psychiatry 22:343–349, 2007

Samuelsson P, Brudin L, Sandin RH: Late psychological symptoms after awareness among consecutively included surgical patients. Anesthesiology 106:26–32, 2007

Sarwer DB, Whitaker LA, Pertschuk MJ, et al: Body image concerns of reconstructive surgery patients: an underrecognized problem. Ann Plast Surg 40:403–407, 1998

Saunders JB, Aasland OG, Babor TF, et al: Development of the alcohol use disorders identification test (AUDIT): WHO collaborative project on early detection of persons with harmful alcohol consumption—II. Addiction 88:791–804, 1993

Saunders R: "Grazing": a high-risk behavior. Obes Surg 14:98–102, 2004

Saxe GN, Stoddard F, Hall E, et al: Pathways to PTSD, part I: children with burns. Am J Psychiatry 162:1299–1304, 2005

Scher CS, Anwar M: The self-reporting of psychiatric medications in patients scheduled for elective surgery. J Clin Anesth 11:619–621, 1999

Scully JH, Hutcherson R: Suicide by burning. Am J Psychiatry 140:905–906, 1983

Shiwach RS: Autoenucleation—a culture-specific phenomenon: a case series and review. Compr Psychiatry 39:318–322, 1998

Sillanaukee P: Laboratory markers of alcohol abuse. Alcohol Alcohol 31:613–616, 1996

Silver GM, Albright JM, Schermer CR, et al: Adverse clinical outcomes associated with elevated blood alcohol levels at the time of burn injury. J Burn Care Res 29:784–789, 2008

Simmons K, Smith JA, Bob KA, et al: Adjustment to colostomy: stoma acceptance, stoma care self-efficacy and interpersonal relationships. J Adv Nurs 60:627–635, 2007

Sjöström L: Bariatric surgery and reduction in morbidity and mortality experiences from the SOS study. Int J Obesity (Lond) 32:S93–S97, 2008

Sloan EP, Kirsh S: Characteristics of obstetrical inpatients referred to a consultation-liaison psychiatry service in a tertiary-level university hospital. Arch Womens Ment Health 11:327–333, 2008

Smith AF, Pittaway AJ: Premedication for anxiety in adult day surgery. Cochrane Database Syst Rev (1):CD002192, 2003

Smith GC: From consultation-liaison psychiatry to integrated care for multiple and complex needs. Aust N Z J Psychiatry 43:1–12, 2009

Smith MS, Muir H, Hall R: Perioperative management of drug therapy: clinical considerations. Drugs 51:238–259, 1996

Smith MT, Klick B, Kozachik S, et al: Sleep onset insomnia symptoms during hospitalization for major burn injury predict chronic pain. Pain 15:497–506, 2008

Smith PJ, Attix DK, Weldon BC, et al: Executive function and depression as independent risk factors for postoperative delirium. Anesthesiology 110:781–787, 2009

Soderstrom CA: Substance-abuse interventions-setting the stage for discussion. J Trauma 59:S77–S79, 2005

Spies CD, Neuner B, Neumann T, et al: Intercurrent complications in chronic alcoholic men admitted to the intensive care unit following trauma. Intensive Care Med 22:286–293, 1996

Spies CD, Spies KP, Zinke S, et al: Alcoholism and carcinoma change the intracellular pH and activate platelet Na+/H+ exchange in men. Alcohol Clin Exp Res 21:1653–1660, 1997

Spouse E, Gedroyc WM: MRI of the claustrophobic patient: interventionally configured magnets. Br J Radiol 73:146–151, 2000

Sprangers MA, Taal BG, Aaronson NK, et al: Quality of life in colorectal cancer. Stoma vs nonstoma patients. Dis Colon Rectum 38:361–369, 1995

Steenkamp WC, Botha NJ, Van der Merwe AE: The prevalence of alcohol dependence in burned adult patients. Burns 20:522–525, 1994

Stoddard FJ, Sheridan RL, Saxe GN, et al: Treatment of pain in acutely burned children. J Burn Care Rehabil 23:135–156, 2002

Stoll C, Schelling G, Goetz AE, et al: Health-related quality of life and post-traumatic stress disorder in patients after cardiac surgery and intensive care treatment. J Thorac Cardiovasc Surg 120:505–512, 2000

Strain JJ: Needs for psychiatry in the general hospital. Hosp Community Psychiatry 33:996–1001, 1982

Stuerz K, Piza H, Niermann K, et al: Psychosocial impact of abdominoplasty. Obes Surg 18:34–38, 2008

Stunkard A, Burt V: Obesity and the body image, II: age at onset of disturbances in the body image. Am J Psychiatry 123:1443–1447, 1967

Stunkard AJ, Allison KC, Geliebter A, et al: Development of criteria for a diagnosis: lessons from the night eating syndrome. Compr Psychiatry 50:391–399, 2009

Summers S: Evidence-based practice, part 3: acute pain management of the perianesthesia patient. J Perianesth Nurs 16:112–120, 2001

Tabares R, Peck MD: Chemical dependency in patients with burn injuries: a fortress of denial. J Burn Care Rehabil 18:283–286, 1997

Taguchi T, Yano M, Kido Y: Influence of bright light therapy on postoperative patients: a pilot study. Intensive Crit Care Nurs 23:289–297, 2007

Taylor D, Hassan MA, Luterman A, et al: Unexpected intraoperative patient death: the imperatives of family and surgeon-centered care. Arch Surg 143:807, 2008

Tedstone JE, Tarrier N: Posttraumatic stress disorder following medical illness and treatment. Clin Psychol Rev 23:409–448, 2003

Thomas C, Turner P, Madden F: Coping and the outcome of stoma surgery. J Psychosom Res 32:457–467, 1988

Thombs BD, Singh VA, Halonen J, et al: The effects of preexisting medical comorbidities on mortality and length of hospital stay in acute burn injury. Ann Surg 245:629–634, 2007

Tignol J, Biraben-Gotzamanis L, Martin-Guehl C, et al: Body dysmorphic disorder and cosmetic surgery: evolution of 24 subjects with a minimal defect in appearance 5 years after their request for cosmetic surgery. Eur Psychiatry 22:520–524, 2007

Tønnesen H, Petersen KR, Hojgaard L, et al: Postoperative morbidity among symptom-free alcohol misusers. Lancet 340:334–337, 1992

Tønnesen H, Carstensen M, Maina P: Is carbohydrate deficient transferrin a useful marker of harmful alcohol intake among surgical patients? Eur J Surg 165:522–527, 1999

Ullrich PM, Askay SW, Patterson DR: Pain, depression, and physical functioning following burn injury. Rehabil Psychol 54:211–216, 2009

Uygur F, Sever C, Oksuz S, et al: Profile of self-inflicted burn patients treated at a tertiary burn center in Istanbul. J Burn Care Res 30:427–431, 2009

Vagnoli L, Caprilli S, Robiglio BA, et al: Clown doctors as a treatment for preoperative anxiety in children: a randomized prospective study. Pediatrics 116:e563–e567, 2005

Valdés M, de Pablo J, Campos R, et al: Multinational European project and multicenter Spanish study of quality improvement of assistance on consultation-liaison psychiatry in general hospital: clinical profile in Spain. Medical Clin (Barc) 25:690–694, 2000

Van Loey NE, van Son MJ, van der Heijden PG, et al: PTSD in persons with burns: an exploratory study examining relationships with attributed responsibility, negative and positive emotional states. Burns 34:1082–1089, 2008

van Wijk MG, Smalhout B: A postoperative analysis of the patient's view of anaesthesia in a Netherlands teaching hospital. Anaesthesia 45:679–682, 1990

Vaughn F, Wichowski H, Bosworth G: Does preoperative anxiety level predict postoperative pain? AORN J 85:589–604, 2007

Vegter F, Hage JJ: Lack of correlation between objective and subjective evaluation of residual stigmata in cleft patients. Ann Plast Surg 46:625–629, 2001

Vlajkovic GP, Sindjelic RP: Emergence delirium in children: many questions, few answers. Anesth Analg 104:84–91, 2007

Wade BE: Colostomy patients: psychological adjustment at 10 weeks and 1 year after surgery in districts which employed stoma-care nurses and districts which did not. J Adv Nurs 15:1297–1304, 1990

Walworth D, Rumana CS, Nguyen J, et al: Effects of music therapy sessions on quality of life indicators, medications administered and hospital length of stay for patients undergoing elective surgical procedures for brain. J Music Ther 45:349–359, 2008

Ward CM: Consenting and consulting for cosmetic surgery. Br J Plast Surg 51:547–550, 1998

Weigman-Schultz WCM, van de Wiel HBM: Sexual rehabilitation after gynecological cancer. J Educ Ther 18:286–293, 1992

Weisman AD, Hackett TP: Psychosis after eye surgery: establishment of a specific doctor–patient relation in the prevention and treatment of "black-patch delirium." N Engl J Med 258:1284–1289, 1958

White MA, Masheb RM, Rothschild BS, et al: The prognostic significance of regular binge eating in extremely obese gastric bypass patients: 12-month postoperative outcomes. J Clin Psychiatry 67:1928–1935, 2006

Wiechman Askay S, Patterson DR: What are the psychiatric sequelae of burn pain? Curr Pain Headache Rep 12:94–97, 2008

Wiechman SA, Ehde DM, Wilson BL, et al: The management of self-inflicted burn injuries and disruptive behavior for patients with borderline personality disorder. J Burn Care Rehabil 21:310–317, 2000

Wilkins KL, Woodgate RL: Supporting siblings through the pediatric bone marrow transplant trajectory: perspectives of siblings of bone marrow transplant recipients. Cancer Nurs 3:E29–E34, 2007

Wollgarten-Hadamek I, Hohmeister J, Demirakea S, et al: Do burn injuries during infancy affect pain and sensory sensitivity in later childhood? Pain 141:165–172, 2009

World Health Organization: International Classification of Diseases, 9th Revision, Clinical Modification. Ann Arbor, MI, Commission on Professional and Hospital Activities, 1978

Yamaya T, Inaniwa T, Minohara S, et al: A proposal of an open PET geometry. Phys Med Biol 53:757–773, 2008

Yazdy MM, Honein MA, Rasmussen SA, et al: Priorities for future public health research in orofacial clefts. Cleft Palate Craniofac J 44:351–357, 2007

Yu BH, Dimsdale JE: Posttraumatic stress disorder in patients with burn injuries. J Burn Care Rehabil 20:426–433, 1999

Zanni GR, Wick JY: Understanding amputation. Consult Pharm 23:944–948, 2008

Zatzick DF, Jurkovich GJ, Gentilello L, et al: Posttraumatic stress, problem drinking, and functional outcomes after injury. Arch Surg 137:200–205, 2002

Zatzick DF, Rivara FP, Nathen AB, et al: A nationwide study of post-traumatic stress after hospitalization for physical injury. Psychol Med 37:1469–1480, 2007

CHAPTER

31

Organ Transplantation

Andrea F. DiMartini, M.D.

Jorge Luis Sotelo, M.D.

Mary Amanda Dew, Ph.D.

THE BENEFIT OF SOLID ORGAN transplantation was realized in 1954, when Dr. Joseph E. Murray performed the first successful kidney transplant, with the patient's identical twin as donor. However, for most patients an identical-twin donor was not an option, and more than a decade passed before immunosuppressive medications were available to conquer the immunological barrier. In 1967, the first successful liver transplant was performed, followed a year later by the first successful heart transplant. Yet despite the fact that the surgical challenges of solid organ transplantation had been overcome, it was not until the early 1980s, with the advent of improved immunosuppression, that organ transplantation changed from an experimental procedure to a standard of care for many types of end-stage organ disease.

In that decade, the National Organ Transplant Act established the framework for a national system of organ transplantation, and the United Network for Organ Sharing (UNOS) was awarded the contract with the U.S. Department of Health and Human Services to administer the nation's only Organ Procurement and Transplantation Network (OPTN) (United Network of Organ Sharing 2009). In addition to facilitating organ matching and allocation, UNOS collects data about every transplant performed in the United States and maintains information on every organ type (e.g., wait-list counts, survival rates) in an extensive database available on the OPTN Web site (www.OPTN.org) (United Network of Organ Sharing 2009).

Although immunological barriers still exist for transplant recipients, the greatest obstacle to receiving a transplant is the shortage of donated organs. The number of wait-listed individuals has increased far beyond the availability of donated organs. Currently, there are more than 100,000 persons active on the U.S. waiting list. As illustrated in Figure 31-1, the numbers of wait-listed patients for kidney transplantation (the most common transplant performed) have increased steadily between 2004 and 2008 (United Network of Organ Sharing 2009). By contrast, the numbers of patients waiting for liver, heart, lung, and pancreas transplants increased only marginally during the same period (see Figure 31-1). Additionally, the numbers of patients receiving transplants in 2008 for each solid organ type (United Network of Organ Sharing 2009) ranged from a low of 437 for isolated pancreas, 1,478 for lung, 2,163 for heart, and 6,318 for liver, to a high of 16,514 for kidney.

For some transplant types (e.g., kidney, liver, and more rarely lung transplantation), living organ donation has become an option to address the organ shortage (see subsection "Living Donor Transplantation" later in this chapter). In 2001 the number of living donors exceeded the number of deceased donors (6,526 vs. 6,081) for the first time, with the majority being kidney donors (United Network of Organ Sharing 2009). However, following two highly publicized U.S. liver donor deaths, the numbers of partial hepatectomy living liver donors decreased from a peak of 520 in 2001 to approximately 250 per year in 2008. Without an identified living donor, transplant candidates may wait years for an organ. The median wait-listed time depends on the organ type and the recipient's blood type and severity of illness at the time of listing. For most major organ types, more than 40% of U.S. wait-listed candidates waited 2 years or more for an organ (United Network of Organ Sharing

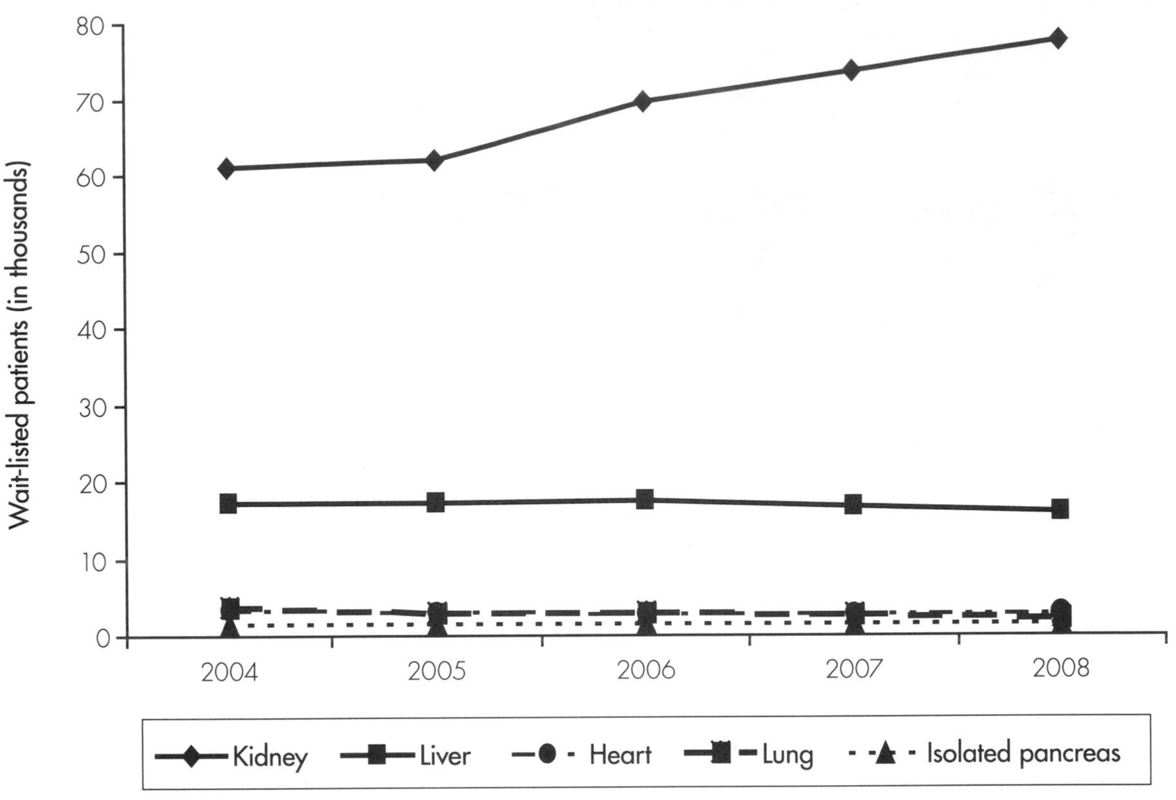

FIGURE 31–1. Year-end numbers of wait-listed patients, by organ type: 2004–2008.

Source. United Network of Organ Sharing (UNOS; www.optn.org) 2009.

2009). Although only 0.5% become medically unsuitable and are removed from the waiting list, 2% refuse transplant after being wait-listed, and 12%–20% die while on the waiting list (United Network of Organ Sharing 2009).

Following transplantation, living-donor liver and living-donor kidney recipients experience the highest long-term survival rates (76% alive at 10 years' posttransplantation) (see Figure 31–2). Recipients of deceased-donor kidneys, livers, and hearts have somewhat lower 10-year survival (61%, 59%, and 53%, respectively), and lung and intestine recipients have the poorest 10-year survival (41% and 26%, respectively) (United Network of Organ Sharing 2009). These data are from transplants performed more than 10 years ago, so advances in technology, immunosuppression, and medical care will most likely provide better survival rates for current recipients. Overall graft survival rates are significantly lower than patient survival rates (e.g., 43% for kidney graft survival and 52% for liver graft survival after 10 years), which means that many transplant recipients may have to face a second transplant 5–10 years after their first (United Network of Organ Sharing 2009).

These stark facts highlight the enormous stresses facing transplant candidates, transplant recipients, and their caregivers. These issues have also created a particular environment in which hospitals must evaluate, treat, and select patients for organ transplantation. The scarcity of donated organs has driven efforts to select candidates believed to have the best chance for optimal posttransplant outcomes. Additionally, the organ shortage has increasingly led to consideration of living kidney donors and, more recently, living liver donors (and, more rarely, living lung donors) as transplantation options.

Pretransplant psychosocial evaluations are commonly requested to assist in candidate and donor selection, and psychiatric consultation is often needed for clinical input during the pre- and posttransplant phases. Although a wide body of knowledge has been developed in the clinical care of transplant candidates and recipients, little longitudinal research is available to answer questions about long-term outcomes or the impact of psychiatric factors (assessed pretransplant and/or in the early years posttransplantation) on outcomes. Research primarily has focused on kidney, heart, and liver transplantation, which in combination currently account for almost 90% of transplants performed in the United States.

In this chapter, we outline the essential areas of the field for psychosomatic medicine specialists and other mental health clinicians involved in the care of transplant patients—pretransplant assessment and candidate selection, emotional and psychological aspects of the trans-

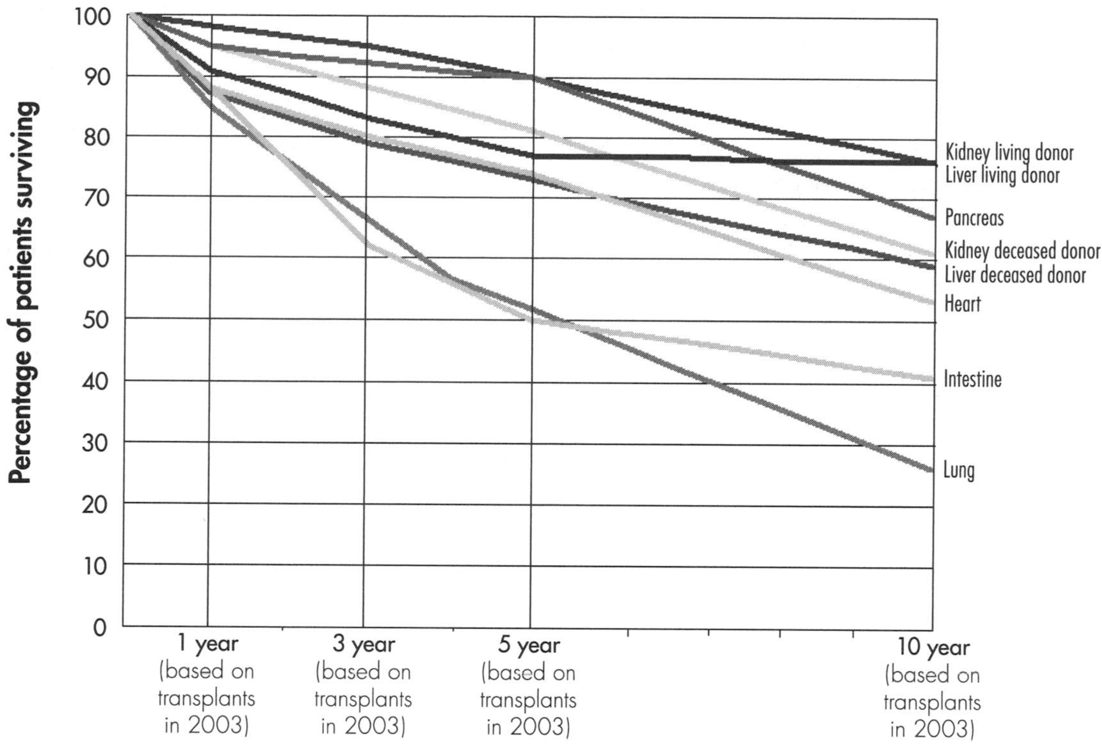

FIGURE 31–2. Survival rates of transplant recipients, by organ type.

Source. Data from 2006 Annual Report of the U.S. Organ Procurement and Transplantation Network and the Scientific Registry of Transplant Recipients: Transplant Data 1996–2005. Health Resources and Services Administration, Healthcare Systems Bureau, Division of Transplantation, Rockville, MD, 2006. Available at: http://www.ustransplant.org/annual_Reports/archives/2006/default.htm.

plant process, therapeutic issues, patients with complex or controversial features, psychopharmacological treatment, and neuropsychiatric side effects of immunosuppressive medications. Special pretransplantation topics of emerging importance to psychosomatic medicine specialists are also discussed (i.e., hepatic encephalopathy, ventricular assist devices in heart transplantation, tobacco use, and living donors). The neuropsychiatric sequelae of end-stage organ disease are not covered in this chapter, because those aspects are addressed in the respective chapters on each organ system. Specific transplantation issues are also discussed in Chapter 18, "Heart Disease"; Chapter 19, "Lung Disease"; Chapter 20, "Gastrointestinal Disorders"; Chapter 21, "Renal Disease"; and Chapter 34, "Pediatrics."

Pretransplantation Issues

Psychosocial/Psychiatric Assessment

Pretransplant psychosocial evaluations have been a traditional role of the psychiatric consultation team in the transplantation process. These evaluations are frequently used to assist in the determination of a candidate's eligibility for transplantation and to identify psychiatric and/or psychosocial problems and needs that must to be addressed to prepare the candidate and family for transplantation. These evaluations are also critical for the identification of psychiatric, behavioral, and psychosocial risk factors that may portend poor transplant outcomes (Crone and Wise 1999; Dew et al. 2000b).

Transplant programs will often refer for evaluation candidates with a known history of psychiatric problems or those who are identified during the initial clinical interviews with the transplant team as having such problems. Pretransplant psychosocial evaluations are also usually requested for patients with substance use disorders (including tobacco) and other poor health conditions and behaviors (e.g., obesity, noncompliance).

Although a truly comprehensive assessment of a potential transplant candidate would require a full psychiatric consultation, the current high numbers of candidates preclude this. To handle the increasing volume of evaluations, some centers employ screening batteries of patient-rated measures to identify candidates with elevated levels of psychological distress, who then undergo a full psychiatric evaluation. Screening instruments can provide baseline cognitive, affective, and psychosocial ratings for candidates; use of these instruments maximizes staff resources and minimizes costs. For example, using this strategy, Jowsey et al. (2002) identified 20%–44% of liver transplant candidates who had mild to severe symptoms on a range of measures, which prompted a higher level of evaluation.

Emerging evidence shows that preoperatively assessed psychosocial variables can predict posttransplantation psychiatric adjustment among recipients of most organ types (Dew et al. 2000b). These variables are increasingly being investigated as contributing to medical outcomes as well, although a consistent predictive effect has not yet been demonstrated (Dew et al. 2000b). Thus, psychosocial assessment of transplant candidates provides an opportunity to identify potential problems and intervene prior to transplantation, with the goal of improving posttransplant outcomes. Transplant programs vary considerably in their psychosocial assessment criteria and procedures (see Olbrisch and Levenson 1995 for a review of methodological and philosophical issues); in general, however, psychosocial evaluations have 10 objectives (although a given assessment may not include all 10), as enumerated in Table 31–1 (see Levenson and Olbrisch 2000).

Because information on all of these domains may not be obtainable during a single clinical interview, a follow-up reassessment may be necessary to clarify relevant issues, solidify a working relationship with the patient and family, and resolve problems. A multidisciplinary approach is often used with input from psychiatrists, psychologists, psychiatric nurse clinical specialists, addiction specialists, social workers, transplant surgeons, and transplant coordinators to construct a comprehensive picture of the patient and develop a coordinated treatment plan. As with any psychiatric evaluation, verbal feedback provided to the patient and family will serve to reiterate the expectations of the transplant team and the requirements of the patient for listing if indicated. Some centers also use written "contracts" to formalize these recommendations (Cupples and Steslowe 2001; Stowe and Kotz 2001). In difficult cases, these contracts serve to document expectations, thereby minimizing misinterpretation. Written contracts outline a treatment plan that can be referred to with each follow-up appointment. These contracts are particularly useful with transplant candidates who have alcohol or substance abuse/dependence problems, specifying the transplant program's requirements for addiction treatment, monitoring of adherence (e.g., documented random negative blood alcohol levels), and length of abstinence (see subsection "Alcohol and Other Substance Use Disorders" later in this chapter).

Psychosocial Instruments and Measures

Transplant-specific (e.g., Psychosocial Assessment of Candidates for Transplant [Olbrisch et al. 1989], Transplant Evaluation Rating Scale [Twillman et al. 1993]), disease-specific (e.g., Miller Health Attitude Scale for cardiac disease [Miller et al. 1981], Quality of Life Questionnaire—Chronic Lung Disease [Guyatt et al. 1987]), and disorder-specific (e.g., High Risk Alcohol Relapse Scale for alcoholism [Yates et al. 1993]) instruments have been used to evaluate transplant candidates and monitor their posttransplant recovery. These instruments have been used in conjunction with general instruments for rating behavior, coping, cognitive and affective states, and quality of life. Psychosocial instruments can be used to identify individuals who require further assessment (as described earlier) or to pursue evaluation of patients already identified as requiring additional screening. The evaluator's purpose for using such instruments will determine the type and specificity of the instruments chosen; for instance, in the subsection "Hepatic Encephalopathy" later in this chapter, we discuss the use of neuropsychiatric tests to aid in the identification of cognitive impairment. Some instruments are more applicable to transplant populations than others. For example, although there are many instruments and measures for assessing alcoholism, none of these instruments are tailored to transplant candidates; they are focused on general issues of detection and treatment of addiction rather than on issues important in evaluating appropriateness for transplantation. Formal cognitive testing may be appropriate to delineate cognitive deficits, taking into consideration the potential contribution of deficits that may be transient and related to the current degree of illness (e.g., delirium; see subsection "Cognitive Disorders and Delirium" later in this chapter).

Because psychosocial selection criteria differ significantly by program and organ type, development and use of structured evaluation instruments may help to direct and standardize the transplant selection protocols used nationally. The Structured Interview for Renal Transplantation (SIRT; Mori et al. 2000) is a structured yet flexible interview tool designed to guide the clinician efficiently through a comprehensive interview of pertinent information for potential renal transplant candidates. Use of the SIRT requires sound clinical judgment, but the instrument can also be used for training clinicians; the structure of the instrument could be appropriate for research purposes as well (Mori et al. 2000). This instrument is not scored, nor are there ratings for transplant candidacy. Two other instruments commonly used to assess candidates for transplantation are the Psychosocial Assessment of Candidates for Transplantation (PACT) and the Transplant Evaluation Rating Scale (TERS). Different from structured interviews with specific items or questions, these instruments can serve as heuristic tools to aid clinicians in considering and integrating the data gathered from their interviews in the candidacy determination.

TABLE 31–1. Goals of psychosocial screening

1. Assess coping skills; intervene with patients who appear to be unable to cope effectively.
2. Diagnose comorbid psychiatric conditions; provide for pre- and posttransplant monitoring and treatment.
3. Determine the candidate's capacity to understand the transplant process and to provide informed consent.
4. Evaluate the candidate's ability to collaborate with the transplant team and to adhere to treatment.
5. Assess substance use/abuse history, recovery, and ability to maintain long-term abstinence.
6. Identify health behaviors that may influence posttransplant morbidity and mortality (e.g., tobacco use, poor eating or exercise habits) and evaluate the candidate's ability to modify these behaviors over the long term.
7. Help the transplant team to understand the patient better as a person.
8. Evaluate the level of social support available to the candidate for pre- and posttransplant phases (including stable family/others committed to assisting the candidate, adequate insurance and financial resources, and logistical support).
9. Determine the psychosocial needs of the patient and family and plan for services during the waiting, recovery, and rehabilitation phases of the transplant process.
10. Establish baseline measures of mental functioning in order to be able to monitor postoperative changes.

Source. Adapted from Levenson J, Olbrisch ME: "Psychosocial Screening and Selection of Candidates for Organ Transplantation," in *The Transplant Patient.* Cambridge, UK, Cambridge University Press, 2000, p. 23. Used with permission.

The PACT was the first published psychosocial structured instrument specifically designed for screening candidates for transplantation (Olbrisch et al. 1989). It provides an overall score and subscale scores for psychological health (psychopathology, risk for psychopathology, stable personality factors), lifestyle factors (healthy lifestyle, ability to sustain change in lifestyle, adherence, drug and alcohol use), social support (support system stability and availability), and patient educability and understanding of the transplant process. The PACT can be completed in only a few minutes by the consultant following the evaluation but requires scoring by a skilled clinician, without which the instrument's predictive power could be diminished (Presberg et al. 1995). The final rating for candidate acceptability is made by the clinician, with the freedom to weigh individual item ratings variably (Presberg et al. 1995). Thus, a single area, such as alcohol abuse, could be assigned greater weight and could thereby disproportionately influence the final rating.

The PACT has been used to predict mortality in bone marrow recipients (independent of age, gender, or diagnosis), as well as to predict hospital lengths of stay following liver transplantation (Levenson et al. 1994). Its "risk for psychopathology" subscale identifies psychopathology that may require referral and treatment after liver, heart, and bone marrow transplantation (Levenson et al. 1994).

The TERS is used to rate patients' level of adjustment in 10 areas of psychosocial functioning: prior psychiatric history, current psychiatric diagnoses, substance use/abuse, adherence, health behaviors, quality of family support, prior history of coping, coping with disease and treatment, quality of affect, and mental status (Twillman et al. 1993). In one study, the TERS was significantly correlated with several clinician-reported outcome variables (e.g., adherence, health behaviors, substance use), with particularly high correlations between pretransplant TERS scores and posttransplant substance use (r=0.64) (Twillman et al. 1993). The instrument requires administration by a skilled clinician to maintain accuracy (Presberg et al. 1995). The TERS summary score is derived from a mathematical formula in which individual item scores are multiplied by theoretical, predetermined weightings.

Although individual candidates do not always easily fit within one of the three categories of each item on the TERS, the TERS has more items than the PACT, a feature that may prove useful in future research (Presberg et al. 1995). However, the PACT is the more flexible of the two instruments, both in the range of rating individual items and in the manner in which the summary score is determined (Presberg et al. 1995). Together, these instruments are useful in the organization of patient information and can be helpful both as tools for increasing the evaluator's understanding of the candidate and for research purposes.

Maldonado et al. (2008) recently developed a comprehensive standardized psychosocial assessment using data obtained from clinical interview, collateral sources, and a specific structured battery of instruments to create a rating scale for minimal psychosocial listing criteria for transplant candidacy. Their Stanford Integrated Psychosocial Assessment for Transplant (SIPAT) has not yet been validated (Maldonado et al. 2008). The SIPAT can be used either as a stand-alone scale with cutoff scores for minimal listing criteria or as a comprehensive battery including standardized tests.

Unique Role of the Psychiatric Consultant

Unlike in most psychiatric interviews, the psychiatrist performing the pretransplant assessment while identifying the needs of the transplant candidate will also be proposing what psychiatric issues, if any, the candidate needs to address to become a transplantation candidate. These requirements may be specific to transplantation, and the psychiatric consultant must be candid with the patient about his or her role of providing consultative advice to the transplant team on psychiatric recommendations for candidacy. Careful delineation of specific transplant-related expectations, explanation of the importance of these requirements to the success of transplantation, and exploration of the implications of these criteria for the individual candidate serve to establish a meaningful dialogue with the patient from which the therapeutic alliance necessary for future intervention can develop.

For the clinician, the seemingly reverse nature of this role can be uncomfortable or even anxiety provoking. This is especially true if the clinician is not recommending the candidate for transplantation. Fortunately, many programs do not reject patients outright for psychosocial reasons; rather, they offer such patients the opportunity to work to bring their problematic areas into alignment with the recommendations (i.e., through addiction counseling, behavioral changes, psychiatric treatment, identification of appropriate social supports) and then undergo reevaluation for candidacy. In these cases, the psychiatric consultant can often function as an advocate for the patient and assist in referral for appropriate treatment if indicated. Nevertheless, some patients will be unable to comply with the specified transplant requirements or will not survive to complete their efforts to meet candidacy requirements.

Philosophical, moral, ethical, legal, and therapeutic dilemmas are inherent in the role of transplant psychiatrist, as conflicting team opinions present themselves in the course of work with potential transplant candidates. Team discussions and consultation with other colleagues are the rule in complicated cases. In these instances, team discussions not only aid in resolving candidacy quandaries but also can help alleviate team members' anxiety and discomfort over declining a patient for transplantation. Group or team debriefing may also be desirable, and occasionally consultation with the ethics committee (or consult service), risk management, and/or the legal department of the hospital is needed (e.g., when a candidate is challenging candidacy requirements or the candidacy decision of the transplant team). Thorough documentation is essential in order to delineate the issues involved, the expectations of the team for transplantation candidacy, and the efforts to work with the patient.

Psychological and Psychiatric Issues in Organ Transplantation

Psychiatric Symptoms and Disorders in Transplant Patients

Similar to other medically ill populations, transplant candidates and recipients experience a significant amount of psychological distress and are at heightened risk of developing psychiatric disorders. The prevalence rates of major depression range from 4% to 28% in liver transplant patients, 0% to 58% in heart transplant patients, and 0.4% to 20% in kidney transplant patients (Dew 2003; Dew et al. 2000b). The range of rates for anxiety disorders appears to be 3%–33% (Dew 2003; Dew et al. 2000b), but there are not enough studies to identify rates for specific types of anxiety disorders. One investigation found that 10% of a cohort of heart or lung transplant recipients experienced posttraumatic stress disorder (PTSD) related to their transplant experience (Köllner et al. 2002). In a prospective study of 191 heart transplant recipients, the cumulative prevalence rates for psychiatric disorders during the 3 years posttransplantation were 38% for any disorder, including 25% with major depression, 21% with adjustment disorders, and 17% with PTSD (Dew et al. 2001a). PTSD related to transplant was limited almost exclusively to the first year after transplantation. In this group of heart recipients, there was a clustering of cases of major depression in the first year, and the cumulative rate of major depression was greater than the rate of any anxiety disorders. Factors that increased the cumulative risk for psychiatric disorders included a pretransplant psychiatric history, a longer period of hospitalization, female gender, greater impairments in physical functioning, and fewer social supports (Dew et al. 2001a). These risk factors were additive, and therefore the cumulative risk of a psychiatric disorder increased along with the number of risk factors. A recent review of depression in lung transplant recipients found that depression rates were high in the transplant candidates, with an improvement in the short term associated with better quality of life. In the long term (>3 years), however, decline in functional status was associated with a dramatic increase in depressive symptomatology. this review also revealed that comorbid personality disorders, poor coping strategies, life stressors, physical complications, corticosteroid use, male gender in the short term after transplantation, and lack of psychosocial support all contributed to depression in lung transplant recipients (Fusar-Poli et al. 2007).

Several studies have suggested an association between psychiatric disorders and transplant health outcomes, although the results have been mixed. A study of wait-listed liver transplant candidates found that candidates whose Beck Depression Inventory (BDI) scores were higher than 10 (64% of patients) were significantly more likely than nondepressed candidates to die while awaiting transplantation (Singh et al. 1997). The higher BDI scores were due more to affective than to somatic symptoms. However, for candidates who reached transplantation, pretransplant depression was not associated with poorer posttransplant survival (Singh et al. 1997). These results were not affected by the severity of and complications from liver disease, or by patients' social support, employment, or education (Singh et al. 1997). A study of lung transplant recipients found that those with a pretransplant psychiatric history (anxiety and/or depressive disorders) were more likely than those without such a history to be alive 1 year after transplantation (Woodman et al. 1999). However, in a study of 191 heart transplant recipients, a DSM-III-R (American Psychiatric Association 1987) diagnosis of PTSD (with the traumatic event being transplant related) was associated with higher mortality (odds ratio = 13.74) (Dew and Kormos 1999). Another study of heart transplant recipients found that patients with ischemic cardiomyopathy and high self-rated depression scores pretransplant had significantly higher posttransplant mortality compared with the low-depression group after adjustment for sociodemographic and somatic symptoms (Zipfel et al. 2002). Havik et al. (2007) followed 147 heart transplant patients for a period of 5 years and found that depressive symptoms (as measured on the BDI) were common, that they increased the risk of mortality, and that the risk remained significant even after adjustment for somatic and lifestyle factors. Although causal directions cannot be inferred from these data, studies in other medically ill populations have demonstrated the substantial contribution of depression and anxiety to health outcomes (see Chapter 8, "Depression," and Chapter 11, "Anxiety Disorders"). Whether treating these disorders will affect patient outcomes is unclear. However, the role of the psychiatrist in evaluating, diagnosing, and treating psychiatric disorders both pre- and posttransplantation is critical.

Adaptation to Transplantation

Transplant candidates typically experience a series of adaptive challenges as they proceed through evaluation, waiting, perioperative management, postoperative recuperation, and long-term adaptation to life with a transplant (Dew et al. 2007b; Olbrisch et al. 2002) (see Figure 31-3). With chronic illness, there can be progressive debility and gradual loss of vitality and of physical and social functioning. Patients may progressively lose their ability to work, participate in social/family activities, and drive and may even require assistance with activities of daily living. With these losses of functioning will come the loss of important roles in the family (e.g., breadwinner, parent, spouse, caregiver). Adapting to these changes can elicit anxiety, depression, anger, avoidance, and denial and requires the working through of grief (Olbrisch et al. 2002). Patients may express their distress or ambivalence by missing appointments/procedures or failing to complete requirements for transplant listing. Patients who are wait-listed may develop contraindications to transplantation (e.g., infection, serious stroke, progressive organ dysfunction), and both patients and families should be made aware that a candidate's eligibility can change over time for many reasons (Stevenson 2002). During this phase, psychiatrists may provide counseling to patients and families to help them navigate these transitions and prepare for either transplantation or death.

The summons for transplantation can evoke a mixture of elation and great fear. Patients can develop anxiety related to anticipation of the call from the transplant team. Patients may experience a panic attack when they are called for transplantation, and some—due to anxiety, fear, ambivalence, or not feeling ready—may even decline the offer of an organ.

Much of illness behavior depends on the coping strategies and personality style of the individual. In our experience, the adaptive styles of adult transplant recipients often depend on whether patients' pretransplant illness experience was chronic or acute, as delineated in the following broadly generalized profiles.

Patients who have dealt with chronic illness for years may adapt psychologically to the sick role and can develop coping strategies that perpetuate a dependency on being ill (Olbrisch et al. 2002). For these patients, transplantation may psychologically represent a transition from one state of illness to another, and such patients can have difficulty adjusting to or transitioning into a "state of health." They often complain that the transplant team is expecting too fast a recovery from them, and they may describe feeling pressured to get better. Some patients may develop unexplained chronic pain or other somatic complaints or may begin to evidence nonadherence with transplant team directives.

For patients with good premorbid functioning who become acutely ill, with only a short period of pretransplant infirmity, the transplant can be an unwelcome event. These patients can experience a heightened sense of vulnerability, and they may deny the seriousness of their medical situation (Olbrisch et al. 2002). These patients often wish to return to normal functioning as quickly as possible posttransplantation, and they may in fact recover more

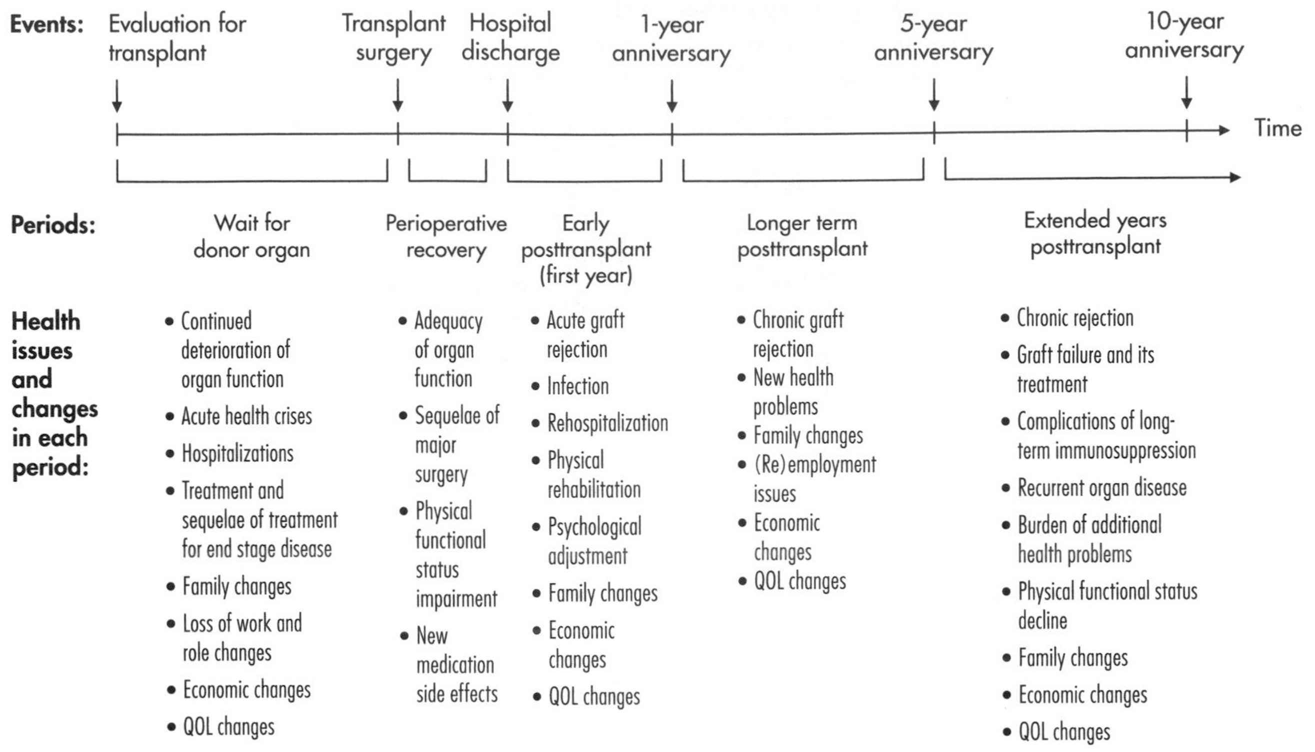

FIGURE 31–3. Organ transplant timeline: critical events, time periods, and health and psychosocial issues.
QOL=quality of life.
Source. Reprinted from Dew MA, DiMartini AF, Kormos RL: "Organ Transplantation, Stress of," in *Encyclopedia of Stress,* 2nd Edition, Vol 3. Edited by Fink G. Oxford, UK, Academic Press/Elsevier, 2007, pp. 35–44. Copyright 2007, Elsevier Inc. Used with permission.

rapidly than the transplant team expects; however, they may suffer later as the result of pushing themselves too much (e.g., returning to work before they are physically ready). They may resent being a transplant recipient, with all of the restrictions and regimens inherent in that role, and may act out their anger or denial in episodes of nonadherence (Olbrisch et al. 2002).

Treatment Modalities

A prospective study of kidney transplant recipients demonstrated that individual psychotherapy was effective in resolving transplant-related emotional problems, with significant reductions in BDI scores after therapy (Baines et al. 2002). Three recurring psychological themes were expressed by patients in this study: 1) fear of organ rejection, 2) feelings of paradoxical loss after surgery despite successful transplantation, and 3) psychological adaptation to the new kidney (Baines et al. 2002).

In addition to traditional therapies and pharmacotherapy, various innovative strategies have been employed to deal with specific issues of transplantation and also to address logistical and staffing resource issues. At the University of Toronto, a mentoring program was developed for heart transplant recipients. Mentorship by an already transplanted recipient augmented patient care by providing information and support from a peer perspective (Wright et al. 2001). The four topics most commonly discussed between mentors and mentees were postoperative complications (70%), medications (70%), wait on the transplant list (70%), and the surgery itself (50%) (Wright et al. 2001). Participants less frequently discussed psychiatric topics such as anxiety (40%) and depression (10%) and personal topics such as sexual relations (20%) and marital problems (10%). The program was well received, and patients were very satisfied with the experience. To increase patient satisfaction with the mentor program, Wright et al. (2001) recommend early introduction of a mentor and matching of mentors with mentees according to demographics and clinical course.

Group therapy for organ transplantation patients and family members has also been successfully used. At the Toronto Hospital Multi-Organ Transplantation Program, group psychotherapy is organized along three dimensions: course of illness (pre- vs. posttransplantation), homogeneous versus heterogeneous group membership (e.g., separate groups for patients and caregivers vs. integrated groups, organ-specific groups vs. cross-organ groups), and group focus (issue-specific vs. unstructured) (Abbey and

Farrow 1998). Increasing levels of group therapy intensity are used, depending on the needs of the patient. Educational groups are mandatory for pretransplant candidates to prepare them for transplantation. From these groups, candidates at risk for psychosocial problems are referred to supportive and psychoeducational groups. Interpersonal and supportive-expressive psychotherapy groups are available to those who require them and have the psychological capacity to benefit from them. Group therapy participants report decreases in negative affect, increases in positive affect and happiness, less illness intrusiveness, and improved quality of life (Abbey and Farrow 1998). Transplant coordinators also report that patients in group therapy require less contact, both in clinic and by telephone for social support (Abbey and Farrow 1998).

Dew et al. (2004) developed an innovative strategy for managing the logistical problem of recipients living at a distance from the transplant program. These researchers designed and evaluated an Internet-based psychosocial intervention for heart transplant recipients and their families. This multifaceted Web-based intervention included stress and medical regimen management workshops, monitored discussion groups, access to electronic communication with the transplant team, and information on transplant-related health issues (Dew et al. 2004). Compared with heart recipients without access to the Web site, intervention patients reported significant reductions in depressive and anxiety symptoms and improved quality of life in the social functioning domain; in addition, caregivers of intervention patients reported significant declines in anxiety and hostility symptoms ($P<0.05$). Mental health and quality-of-life benefits were greater among more frequent users of the Web site. The subgroup using the Web site's medical regimen workshop showed significantly better adherence at follow-up than did all other patients in attending clinic appointments, completing blood work, and following diet (Dew et al. 2004). Dew and colleagues concluded that a Web-based intervention could improve follow-up care, adherence, and mental health in patients and families as they adjust to heart transplantation.

Patients With Complex or Controversial Psychosocial and Psychiatric Issues

The stringency of selection criteria for transplantation appears to depend on the type of organ transplant being considered, and transplant programs often have strongly formed beliefs about the suitability of candidates with certain types of mental illness. Cardiac transplant programs are more likely than liver transplant programs to consider psychosocial issues as contraindications, and liver transplant programs in turn are more stringent than kidney transplant programs (Corley et al. 1998; Levenson and Olbrisch 1993). These differences may be attributable to the relative availability of specific types of organs (Yates et al. 1993); alternatively, the extent of experience with specific organ transplants may allow programs to feel more comfortable with less stringent criteria (e.g., kidney transplantation, with more than three decades of experience and more than 300,000 kidney transplants performed in the United States) (United Network of Organ Sharing 2009). In addition, for kidney transplantation, cost-effectiveness research has clearly demonstrated the long-term cost savings of kidney transplantation relative to dialysis (Eggers 1992). With such unequivocal evidence, insurance payers have a strong financial incentive to refer patients early for preemptive transplantation, before the high costs of dialysis begin to accumulate (Eggers 1992). In such a setting, psychosocial factors may have less impact on transplantation candidacy. Other issues influencing the selection process include moral and ethical beliefs, societal views, personal beliefs, and even financial constraints.

Although increasing numbers of poor prognostic indicators during the perioperative period may increase risk for nonadherence posttransplantation (Dew et al. 1996; see subsection "Posttransplant Regimen Adherence" below), it should be emphasized that candidates with any one of these features are not categorically poor recipients or that patients without any of these features do not categorically make the best candidates. What little research is available provides some support for clinical assumptions that patients with certain personality disorders, substance use disorders, poor coping skills, poor adherence, and poor social supports can have worse posttransplant outcomes. Nevertheless, case reports have demonstrated that even some patients who might seem inappropriate for transplant (e.g., patients with active psychosis or with severe personality disorders) (Carlson et al. 2000; DiMartini and Twillman 1994) can undergo transplantation and maintain adequate adherence after the procedure. Such patients should be carefully assessed pretransplant with optimization of their pretransplant condition and ongoing psychiatric monitoring and treatment posttransplantation. Prospective longitudinal studies are needed to clarify pretransplant factors that contribute to increased risk of poor outcomes (both psychological and medical) and the contribution of posttransplant factors on outcomes as well.

Posttransplant Regimen Adherence

Lifelong immunosuppression is a prerequisite for good graft function, and nonadherence with immunosuppressive medication is often associated with late acute rejection episodes, chronic rejection, graft loss, and death. It might be assumed that transplant patients, in general, constitute a highly motivated group and that their adherence levels would be high. Unfortunately, like other patients living with chronic disease, many organ recipients experience difficulty in maintaining high levels of adherence to the multiple components of their regimen (Dew et al. 2007a; Laederach-Hofmann and Bunzel 2000). A recent study compared heart and lung transplant recipients during the first 2 years posttransplant and found that rates of persistent nonadherence (i.e., nonadherence at ≥2 consecutive assessments—a span of approximately 6 months) regarding immunosuppressant medication, diet, and smoking were lower in lung recipients than in heart recipients. Relying on public health insurance and having poor caregiver support increased nonadherence risk in both groups of patients (Dew et al. 2008b). In a recent meta-analysis involving nearly 150 studies of all organ types, the average nonadherence rates ranged from 1–4 cases per 100 patients annually for substance use (including tobacco, alcohol, and illicit drugs) to 19–25 cases per 100 patients annually for a variety of areas of nonadherence (e.g., immunosuppressant medication, diet, exercise, and other transplant health care requirements) (Dew et al. 2007a). Medication nonadherence was especially high, and clinicians can expect to see 23 nonadherent patients for every 100 individuals seen during a given year of follow-up (Dew et al. 2007a). Immunosuppressant nonadherence was also highest in kidney recipients (36 cases per 100 patients annually vs. 7–15 cases for other organs) (Dew et al. 2007a).

Nonadherence to immunosuppressive medication is of particular concern, given these medications' role in preventing graft rejection, related morbidities, and mortality. With organ transplantation, nonadherence impairs both life quality and life span, as it is a major risk factor for graft-rejection episodes and may be responsible for up to 25% of deaths after the initial recovery period (Bunzel and Laederach-Hofmann 2000). Nonadherence leads to waste, as it reduces the potential benefits of therapy and adds to the costs of treating avoidable consequent morbidity. Graft loss from nonadherence is also tragic, given the large numbers of patients on the waiting lists. The global assessment of posttransplant regimen adherence is difficult, and patients can manifest varying degrees of adherence to medical recommendations. Moreover, the medical recommendations pertain to a multifaceted regimen of care. For transplant recipients, adherence to immunosuppressive medications is typically the chief area of focus. Yet the occurrence of clinically measurable events such as rejection episodes, organ loss, or death underrepresents the true amount of medication nonadherence, as some patients who are only partially adherent have not yet experienced a clinically adverse event (Bunzel and Laederach-Hofmann 2000; De Geest et al. 1995). Although such "subclinical" nonadherence is undetectable as a medical event, it is important as an indicator of those patients having difficulty following their medical regimens (Feinstein 1990).

Some research has examined correlates and outcomes of nonadherence. For example, several reports have found associations between nonadherence to both immunosuppressive medications and other aspects of the medical regimen and increased risk of morbidity and mortality in transplant recipients (De Geest et al. 1995; Dew and Kormos 1999; Dew et al. 1996; Paris et al. 1994). In terms of risk factors for nonadherence, Dew et al. (1996) carried out a "dose-response" analysis of specific factors found to contribute to nonadherence to medications in a preliminary regression analysis. A "dose" variable was created by determining how many of these six psychosocial risk factors—anxiety, anxiety-hostility, poor support from caregivers, poor support from friends, failure to use active cognitive coping strategies, and use of avoidance coping strategies—a recipient possessed. The logistic regression model showed a strong dose effect, in that if 0 to 1 psychosocial risk factor was present, the probability of having postoperative adherence difficulties was less than 30%. With 2–3 factors present, the probability rose to about 50%, and if 4 or more risk factors were present, more than 80% of patients encountered significant adherence difficulties. This means that if predictors cumulate, adherence problems are likely to rise dramatically.

From a research standpoint, we continue to have limited understanding of the full range of risk factors for posttransplantation adherence problems (Dew et al. 2007a). One review, which warrants further investigation, found a higher rate of nonadherence among U.S. patients compared with their European counterparts, which may be related to the differences in the health care systems of these regions, among other sociocultural factors (Denhaerynck et al. 2006). However, clinical observation of any given patient will quickly reveal that there can be many reasons for nonadherence, and an attempt to identify, understand, and correct the reasons is the first step in improving adherence. Patients may require ongoing or remedial education about the need for lifelong adherence to immunosuppressive medication. Often, the symptoms of chronic rejection are silent, and recipients may not recognize that they are developing complications, as they do not initially feel any adverse effects from discontinuing their medications. Discomfort with medication side effects should be elicited and alleviated if possible. Unfortunately, if the nonadherence results in acute or chronic graft rejection, the treatment typically requires an increase in the dosage of the primary calcineurin-inhibiting immunosuppressive medication and/or addition of other immunosuppressive medications including monoclonal antibodies, steroids, mycophenolate mofetil, or sirolimus, which tend to create or exacerbate neuropsychiatric medication side effects (see the section "Neuropsychiatric Side Effects of Immunosuppressive Agents" later in this chapter). Problems with insurance prescription coverage or other financial issues should be assessed. Additionally, depression has been implicated in cases of nonadherence, and mood symptoms should be elicited and treated (see Table 31–2). Some studies have determined that psychiatric problems that persist after transplantation are highly associated with nonadherence (Paris et al. 1994; Phipps 1997). In an extensive literature review of posttransplant adherence for all organ types, Bunzel and Laederach-Hofmann (2000) found that anxiety disorders and, in particular, untreated major depression were significantly associated with nonadherence. In a study of 125 heart transplant recipients (P.A. Shapiro et al. 1995), adherence problems were associated with a history of substance abuse (P=0.0007). Cukor et al. (2008) found that among patients who had undergone renal transplantation, those patients who perceived that they had control over their outcomes (internal locus of control) were less depressed compared with those who attributed their outcomes to chance. The belief that health was controlled by chance correlated significantly with depressive affect. In a follow-up study, these investigators found that depression was a significant predictor of nonadherence to medications in both posttransplant and end-stage renal disease patients on hemodialysis, although hemodialysis patients were more depressed and reported lower medication adherence (Cukor et al. 2009).

In comparison with adherence in adults, adherence in pediatric transplant recipients can be complicated by the additional factors of developmental stage, attempts at autonomy/individuation, parental control/support, and parental stress. Dew et al. (2009) found (across all organ types) that nonadherence to clinic appointment and tests was the most common type of nonadherence in pediatric patients, at 12.9 cases per 100 patients annually. The rate of nonadherence to immunosuppressive medications was 6 cases per 100 patients annually. Older age of the child, worse family functioning (e.g., greater parental distress, lower family cohesion), and poorer psychological status of the child (e.g., poorer behavioral functioning, greater distress) were significantly but only modestly correlated with poorer adherence (Dew et al. 2009).

In an attempt to develop a clinically useful measure of adherence, Stuber et al. (2008) recently investigated children and adolescent liver transplant recipients using a unique method to evaluate immunosuppressive medication levels. They calculated the standard deviation (SD) of tacrolimus blood levels over a 1 year period and found that rather than a one-time "snapshot" or a single abnormal blood level, a threshold value SD of 2.5 in the tacrolimus level over the year predicted rejection episodes (Stuber et al. 2008). Tacrolimus SDs were also significantly related to poor quality-of-life measures across domains of physical, social, and school functioning among adolescent liver transplant recipients. Nonadherent adolescents reported poorer health perceptions, lower self-esteem, and more limitations in social and school activities (Fredericks 2008). Better knowledge of medication regimens, using a pillbox to organize medications, and parental involvement in medication administration all contributed to improved adherence among adolescent renal transplant candidates (Zelikovsky et al. 2008). The reader is also referred to Chapter 34, "Pediatrics," for additional information on health regimen compliance in adolescents.

Surprisingly, the literature on techniques to improve posttransplant compliance is scant and has focused primarily on medication adherence and not on other forms of nonadherence (e.g., diet, substance abuse, health monitoring). A systematic review of the literature on interventions intended to improve medication adherence in transplant patients found only 12 intervention studies, only 5 of

TABLE 31–2. Recommendations to clinicians for assessing adherence of transplant recipients

Inquire about patients' adherence routinely both early posttransplant and in ensuing years.

Recognize that posttransplant adherence involves multiple activities:

- Taking medication.
- Attending clinic appointments.
- Completing required tests.
- Adhering to lifestyle requirements (e.g., diet, exercise).
- Avoiding alcohol, illicit drugs, and tobacco.

Collect evidence from multiple sources: the patient, spouse/significant other/family, transplant coordinator, laboratory data, and pharmacy records.

Inquire about correlates of nonadherence (e.g., psychological distress/psychiatric disorders, patient/family supports, insurance/financial issues).

Consider psychological, characterological, and other behavioral factors and coping strategies possibly playing a role in nonadherence.

Solutions may require multifaceted interventions to address not only nonadherence but these other contributory factors.

Source. Adapted from Dew et al. 2009.

which used randomized controlled trial designs. These studies were hampered by differences in the definition of nonadherence, lack of sufficient detail to replicate the study, and small sample sizes. A combination of cognitive, educational, counseling, and psychological interventions at the patient, health care provider, setting, and system levels was found more likely to be effective in the long term (De Bleser 2009).

Alcohol and Other Substance Use Disorders

Compared with other solid organ transplant candidates, liver transplant (LTX) candidates more often require psychiatric consultation for substance addiction assessment, due to the prevalence of alcoholic liver disease (ALD) and viral hepatitis transmitted through contaminated needles. An estimated 50% of LTX recipients have a pre-LTX history of alcohol and/or drug abuse/dependence (DiMartini et al. 2002). A survey of 69 U.S. liver transplantation programs found that 83% of programs have a psychiatrist or addiction medicine specialist routinely see each patient with ALD during the evaluation phase (Everhart and Beresford 1997). In the optimal situation, the psychiatric clinician is an integral member of the transplant clinical care team and can integrate the addiction treatment plan into the patient's pre- and posttransplant care. The Cleveland Clinic Foundation has formed a chemical dependence transplant team to assess, treat, and monitor transplant patients with addictive disorders (Stowe and Kotz 2001). This program is a model for the integration of such services.

Psychiatric consultation provides a thorough evaluation of the candidate's addiction history, the candidate's understanding of his/her addiction (especially in the context of his/her health and need for transplantation, stability in recovery, and need for further or ongoing addiction treatment), and the presence of other psychiatric disorders. Family and social support for the candidate's continued abstinence both pre- and posttransplantation must also be evaluated. In one study of LTX candidates, those with a history of substance abuse revealed significantly more distress, less adaptive coping styles, and more character pathology than their counterparts (Stilley et al. 1999). Because these features may heighten the potential for relapse, periodic reassessment by the psychiatric consultant provides follow-up on the candidate's progress in recovery, including verifying ongoing participation in rehabilitation as well as monitoring for psychological and affective distress and poor coping styles with therapeutic interventions targeting these problems as they arise. Documentation of treatment participation is desirable, as is random toxicological screening for alcohol and other substances. These measures are especially important for patients early in recovery and for those with a short period of abstinence, denial over their problem, resistance to seeking treatment, or poor social support for continuing abstinence. One study of pretransplant wait-listed ALD candidates found that 15% of candidates had used alcohol at some point after the initial transplant evaluation (Weinrieb 2003).

One-year post-LTX drinking rates (i.e., the percentage who used any alcohol by 1 year post-LTX) range from 8% to 37% (DiMartini 2000b; Everson et al. 1997), with cumulative rates estimated at 30%–40% by 5 years post-LTX (Lucey 1999). Rates of pathological drinking, defined as drinking that results in physical injury or alcohol dependence, are 10%–15% (Everson et al. 1997; Fireman 2000). In one study, 15% of LTX recipients had their first drink within the first 6 months post-LTX, a finding that highlights the importance of early and intensive clinical follow-up to identify alcohol use at its onset (DiMartini et al. 2001). In a meta-analysis of 50 studies of LTX recipients, the average alcohol relapse rates were 5.6 cases per 100 patients per year for any alcohol use and 2.5 cases per 100 patients per year for heavy alcohol use (Dew et al. 2008a). From this same meta-analysis, the rates of relapse to illicit drug use averaged 3.7 cases per 100 patients per year. Interestingly, this rate was significantly lower in liver recipients versus other organ recipients (1.9 vs. 6.1 cases). Although these rates of alcohol or drug use during any given year may appear relatively low, they are cumulative over time (Dew et al. 2008a). Other studies suggest that the rate of alcohol use may attenuate with the passage of time post-LTX (Berlakovich et al. 1994; Campbell et al. 1993); nevertheless, dependent drinking can begin years post-LTX (DiMartini 2000a).

Consistent predictors of posttransplant alcohol use have been difficult to identify. This may be due to the heterogeneity of the ALD transplant population and the potential selection bias whereby the most stable candidates are chosen, making this population different from the general alcohol-abusing/dependent populations (DiMartini et al. 2002). For example, a pretransplant history of illicit drug use has not been consistently associated with increased risk for posttransplant alcohol relapse in ALD recipients (Coffman et al. 1997; DiMartini et al. 2002; Fireman 2000; Foster et al. 1997; Newton 1999), possibly because many ALD recipients had discontinued their drug use many years prior to transplantation (Coffman et al. 1997). In one of the few prospective studies to examine posttransplant alcohol use, a pretransplant history of alcohol dependence, a family history of alcoholism, and prior rehabilitation experience (thought to be a marker for those with more severe addiction) were all found to be associated with posttransplant alcohol use ($P<0.05$). A prior history of other substance use was associated with a higher (but non-statistically significant) risk of posttransplant drinking (DiMartini 2000b). Similarly, a meta-analysis of LTX studies showed little correlation between demographics and most pretransplant characteristics, although poorer social support, a family alcohol history, and less than 6 months' pretransplant abstinence were associated with relapse (Dew et al. 2008a).

Compared with LTX candidates with alcohol dependence, LTX candidates with polysubstance dependence are more likely to have multiple prior addiction treatments; more likely to be diagnosed with personality disorders, especially Cluster B type (antisocial, narcissistic, histrionic, borderline); and less likely to have stable housing, a consistent work history, or stable social support (Fireman 2000). Yet despite evidence that this specific population could be at higher risk for relapse, there are few published outcome studies addressing the issue of posttransplant nonalcohol substance use. Most studies have investigated the rates of relapse only in ALD recipients who also had a nonalcohol substance use disorder. One of the few studies to investigate all patients with a pre-LTX addiction history found not only that patients with a pre-LTX history of polysubstance use disorders had a higher relapse rate compared with those with alcohol dependence alone (38% vs. 20%) but also that the majority of polysubstance users demonstrated ongoing post-LTX substance use (Fireman 2000). Studies investigating all transplant recipients are needed to identify the true posttransplant rates of other substance use.

After transplantation, maintaining an open, nonjudgmental dialogue with transplant recipients appears to be the most effective way to identify alcohol and/or other substance use in the posttransplant period, and most recipients are open to discussing their substance use habits with the transplant team (DiMartini et al. 2001; Weinrieb et al. 2000). A review of liver enzymes and biopsy results and a candid discussion of the damage caused by alcohol and other substances provide an opportunity to explore the patient's denial of the consequences of their use. Even in the most difficult cases, patients wish to maintain their health and are willing to listen to advice and recommendations on addiction treatment. In our experience, the transplant team has established a powerful emotional bond with the recipient. Many patients who have resumed substance use were relieved to learn that the transplant team would not abandon them. On the other hand, it is important not to condone or dismiss small amounts of alcohol or other substance use. What may seem supportive can be distorted by the patient with an addiction and become an excuse to use more regularly. In the case of alcohol use, we have found that few patients with alcoholism can drink "socially" posttransplantation (Tringali et al. 1996) and that those who take their first drink often consume moderate to heavy amounts of alcohol (DiMartini et al. 2002). Therefore, total alcohol abstinence is recommended for these patients.

Medications that may reduce cravings and potentially diminish relapse risk for alcohol (e.g., acamprosate, ondansetron, naltrexone) or opioids (e.g., naltrexone) have not been studied in transplant patients. One study that attempted to use naltrexone in actively alcohol-relapsing LTX recipients found that patients were reluctant to use naltrexone as a result of its potential, albeit small, risk of hepatotoxicity (Weinrieb et al. 2001). Naltrexone can be a direct hepatotoxin at dosages higher than recommended (>300 mg/day) and is not recommended for patients with active hepatitis or liver failure. Disulfiram has been used in nontransplant populations to provide a negative reinforcement to drinking alcohol. This agent blocks the oxidation of alcohol, resulting in an accumulation of acetaldehyde, and can create severe nausea, vomiting, and hemodynamic instability. It requires hepatic metabolism for conversion into an active drug. A metabolite of disulfiram is an inhibitor of cytochrome P450 (CYP) 3A4 (Madan et al. 1998), and posttransplantation may interfere with immunosuppressive medication metabolism. Use of disulfiram in transplant recipients could place these individuals at risk for serious harm and is not recommended. In nontransplant patients, selective serotonin reuptake inhibitors (SSRIs) and tricyclic antidepressants (TCAs) can stabilize mood and improve abstinence rates in depressed relapsing alcoholic individuals (Cornelius et al. 2003) and may be the most appropriate pharmacological interventions for transplant recipients if concurrent mood symptoms are present. Anecdotally, acamprosate has been safely used in a number of LTX recipients, with some success in decreasing cravings and alcohol use. It is renally excreted; thus, the dosage may need to be adjusted in renal insufficiency.

Methadone-Maintained Candidates

Transplant program acceptance of opioid-dependent patients receiving methadone maintenance treatment (MMT) is a controversial issue. Several studies have examined candidate selection processes and posttransplant outcomes for this population.

In a survey of U.S. liver transplantation programs (Koch and Banys 2001), of the 56% of programs that reported accepting patients for evaluation who were taking methadone, a surprising 32% required patients to discontinue their methadone use prior to transplantation. Of even more concern was the overall lack of experience with such patients (i.e., only 10% of the programs had treated more than five MMT patients). Although there are no studies of pretransplant methadone cessation in LTX patients, there exists an abundance of evidence showing that tapering methadone in stable methadone-maintained patients results in relapse to illicit opiate use in up to 82% of these individuals (Ball and Ross 1991). In our opinion, an attempt to taper a recovering opiate addict from methadone should not be made at a time when the patient is struggling with the stresses and pain associated with end-stage liver disease. Until data to the contrary emerge, requiring methadone tapering in stable opiate-dependent patients as a prerequisite for transplant candidacy could be considered unethical. This strategy potentially heightens the risk for relapse, and those that relapse would be denied transplantation.

In regard to posttransplant outcomes of MMT patients, Koch and Banys (2001) found that of the approximately 180 transplant patients on methadone maintenance at the time of the survey, relapse to illicit opiate use was reported for less than 10% of patients. Similar to other reports of nonadherence in transplant patients (see subsection "Posttransplant Regimen Adherence" earlier in this chapter), approximately 26% of MMT patients had adherence difficulties with immunosuppressive medications (Koch and Banys 2001). However, it was not reported whether those who used illicit drugs were also among those who had problems with adherence. In general, the transplant programs did not consider that the nonadherence necessarily affected outcomes, and the transplant coordinator's impressions were that only 7 of 180 patients had poor outcomes (Koch and Banys 2001). In two small series of MMT LTX recipients (5 in each), overall long-term patient and graft survival were found to be comparable to those of other LTX recipients at the transplant centers, with none of the MMT patients evidencing posttransplant nonadherence or illicit drug use (Hails and Kanchana 2000; Kanchana et al. 2002). Liu et al. (2003), in a study of the largest single cohort (N=36) of MMT LTX recipients to date, concluded that patient and graft survival were comparable to national averages (they did not use a control group, however). Although four patients (11%) reported isolated episodes of heroin use posttransplantation, relapses were not considered to have resulted in poorer outcomes.

An important clinical consideration is pain management for patients on MMT prior to transplantation. These patients may require higher-than-average doses of narcotic analgesics perioperatively, and the transplant team may need to be alerted to this issue. In one specific example, patients on MMT in whom methadone was also used as the posthospitalization pain medication required an average methadone dose increase of 60% posttransplantation, presumably to adjust for chronic downregulation of mu opioid pain receptors from chronic methadone exposure (Weinrieb et al. 2004) and improvement in metabolism after transplantation. Many clinicians consider methadone to be a useful choice for pain management rather than introducing another narcotic that may inadvertently precipitate a relapse. However, methadone dose increases, if not reduced to the prior pretransplant dose, may need to be renegotiated with the MMT program at the point the patient transitions back to the program's care. These issues and coordination of temporary leave from the MMT program, the timing of return, and whether the transplant recipient will need to return for daily doses or may be allowed "carry-outs" (especially useful for avoiding contact with other people while immunosuppressed) are important considerations for the psychosomatic medicine specialist to address.

Thus, the descriptive studies demonstrate that MMT transplant recipients can successfully undergo transplantation and do well; however, the lack of control groups makes it difficult to prove that MMT patients' rates of complications and survival are no different from those of transplant recipients in general. Although the small numbers of MMT candidates and recipients preclude large-scale prospective studies, a case-control study conducted by M.J. Gordon et al. (1986) found that posttransplant patient and graft survival rates in the 20 heroin-addicted kidney recipients were similar to those in the control group. The leading cause of death (infection) was the same in both groups. In the study group, only one patient returned to heroin use. Two other study patients who were not suspected of using heroin lost their grafts as a result of medication nonadherence, whereas no patient in the control group lost a graft as a result of nonadherence (M.J. Gordon et al. 1986). In summary, the data to date justify neither automatic exclusion of MMT patients from transplantation nor any requirement that such patients be tapered off methadone prior to transplant.

Personality Disorders

Personality disorders are characterized by persisting and inflexible maladaptive patterns of subjective experience and behavior that may create emotional distress and interfere with the individual's interpersonal relationships and social functioning. The requirements of successful transplantation can be too difficult for such an individual, as the process requires a series of adaptations to changes in physical and social functioning and significant ability to work constructively with both caregivers and the transplant team. By identifying personality traits and disorders, the psychiatrist can potentially predict patterns of behavior, recommend treatment, develop a behavioral plan with the team to work constructively with the patient, and render an opinion as to the candidate's ability to proceed with transplantation. Patients with personality disorders can require excessive amounts of time from the transplant team, which raises the issue of resource allocation as a potential selection criterion (Carlson et al. 2000). Not surprisingly, a majority of programs (50%–60% across organ types) consider personality disorders to be a relative contraindication to transplantation (Levenson and Olbrisch 1993). Yet all personality disorders should not be viewed similarly, as the behavioral and coping styles of different personality disorders can present varying degrees of concordance with the needs of transplantation. For example, the need for structure and orderliness of a candidate with obsessive-compulsive personality disorder would be more adaptive to the demands of transplantation than the coping style of a patient with borderline personality disorder.

The incidence of personality disorders in transplant populations is similar to that in the general population, ranging from 10% to 26% (Chacko et al. 1996; Dobbels et al. 2000), although in some cohorts estimates have been as high as 33% (in a cohort of heart and lung transplant recipients) (Stilley et al. 2005) or even 57% (predominantly in those with a history of substance abuse) (Stilley et al. 1997). However, the identification of personality disorders depends on the definition and measurement methods used. Unfortunately, studies investigating personality disorders and transplantation outcomes have not distinguished among the various personality disorder types (perhaps because of the low prevalence of each type), which makes generalizations difficult. Nevertheless, case reports of patients with severe character pathology demonstrate the extent of adherence problems that can arise from these disorders, resulting in significant morbidity and recipient death (Surman and Purtilo 1992; Weitzner et al. 1999). The disturbances in interpersonal relationships that can occur with personality disorders also can decrease the likelihood that patients will have stable and reliable social supports during the pre- and posttransplant phases (Yates et al. 1998). Of the personality disorders, borderline personality disorder is considered to represent the highest risk for posttransplant nonadherence (Bunzel and Laederach-Hofmann 2000).

Whereas sociopathy has not consistently been associated with substance relapse in the addiction literature (Vaillant 1997), a survey of transplant programs in the United States revealed that 4 of 14 programs (29%) would reject a candidate with comorbid antisocial personality disorder and alcohol dependence (Snyder et al. 1996). In a study of 73 ALD transplant candidates, patients with severe personality disorders had higher rates of divorce, higher rates of comorbid drug abuse/dependence, lower IQs, higher scores on indicators of emotional impairment, and were more likely, although not significantly so, to return to drug use during the pretransplant follow-up period (Yates et al. 1998). However, of this cohort, 3 patients with serious personality disorders underwent liver transplantation and did not relapse or become nonadherent in the early postoperative phase (Yates et al. 1998). In contrast, another study of 91 patients transplanted for ALD and followed for up to 3 years identified 18 patients exhibiting antisocial behavior (Coffman et al. 1997). Of those with antisocial behavior, 50% returned to either alcohol (n=6) or prescription narcotic addiction (n=3) posttransplantation, which was significantly higher than the 19.8% alcohol use by the total group (Coffman et al. 1997). In a prospective study of 125 heart transplant recipients, personality disorders were associated with posttransplant adherence problems (P=0.007) (P.A. Shapiro et al. 1995). Although personality disorders were not associated with survival, those individuals with personality disorders tended to have more graft rejection (P=0.06) (P.A. Shapiro et al. 1995). Using the Type D (for "distressed") personality construct (based on two broad and stable personality traits—negative affectivity and social inhibition), Denollet et al. (2007) found significantly higher rates of mortality and early allograft rejection in heart recipients with Type D personality. However, without any posttransplant psychological or compliance measures, the contribution of this personality type or psychological distress to outcomes was speculative (Denollet and Kupper 2007). Using a cross-sectional design to study heart transplant recipients (average of 7 years posttransplant), Pedersen et al. (2006) also found that those with Type D personality were more likely to have worse physical and mental health-related quality of life (3 and 6 times greater risk, respectively), suggesting that this personality construct has important implications for identifying those who may need additional psychosocial support and intervention.

Although not identified as specific personality disorder styles, various coping and behavioral styles have also been shown to influence survival. A study by Chacko et al. (1996) of survival after heart transplantation found that whereas the presence of clinician-rated Axis II disorders (26% of the group) was not associated with survival time, health behaviors, maladjustment, and coping styles represented some of the strongest predictors of survival. Using the same measure of health behavior and coping (Millon Behavioral Health Inventory [Millon et al. 1982]), Coffman and Brandwin (1999) found that wait-listed heart transplant candidates with high scores on the Life Threat Reactivity subscale had significantly higher mortality before transplantation (42% vs. 18%; P=0.0001) but not after transplantation. These investigators suggested that one possible explanation was that the detrimental psychological traits of the high-risk group were ameliorated by surviving to be transplanted (Coffman and Brandwin 1999).

Patients with personality disorders do best with ongoing pre- and posttransplant psychotherapy, specifically cognitive and behavioral interventions to promote adherence with the care regimen and to establish a working alliance with transplant team members (Dobbels et al. 2000). These patients should be given clear and consistent instructions on rules and requirements of transplantation, reinforced by regular outpatient appointments. A limited number of transplant center staff should maintain contact with the patient, and staff should communicate regularly among themselves and the outpatient psychiatric team (Carlson et al. 2000) to coordinate care and to reduce opportunities for cognitive distortions and splitting by the patient. A formal written contract can document the expectations of the transplant team and serve as a therapeutic treatment plan whereby the patient and team agree to work together toward common goals for the transplant recipient's health (Dobbels et al. 2000).

Psychotic Disorders

Although chronic and active psychosis is thought by many to be incompatible with successful transplantation, case reports of carefully selected patients with psychosis demonstrate that such patients can successfully undergo transplantation and survive after the procedure (DiMartini and Twillman 1994; Krahn et al. 1998). A survey of transplant psychiatrists at national and international transplant programs identified only 35 cases of pretransplant psychotic disorders in transplant recipients from 12 transplant centers (Coffman and Crone 2002), suggesting that such patients are highly underrepresented among transplant recipients. Results of this survey confirmed previously expressed stipulations that patients with psychotic disorders be carefully screened before acceptance. Candidates should have demonstrated good adherence to both medical and psychiatric follow-up requirements; possess adequate social supports, especially in-residence support; and be capable of establishing a working relationship with the transplant team. In this survey (Coffman and Crone 2002), risk factors for problems with adherence after transplantation included antisocial or borderline personality disorder features, a history of assault, living alone, positive psychotic symptoms, and a family history of schizophrenia. Posttransplant nonadherence with nonpsychiatric medications was found in 20% of patients (7 of 35), and noncompliance with laboratory tests was found in 17% (6 of 35 patients) (Coffman and Crone 2002); however, these numbers are similar to percentages of medication and laboratory testing nonadherence in general transplant populations. Overall, nonadherence resulted in rejection episodes in 5 patients (14%) and in reduced graft function or loss in 4 patients (12%) (Coffman and Crone 2002). Thirty-seven percent of patients experienced psychotic or manic episodes posttransplantation (not necessarily associated with immunosuppression), 20% attempted suicide (with two completed suicides), 20% experienced severe depression or catatonia, 5.7% committed assaults, 5.7% were arrested for disorderly conduct, and 8.6% required psychiatric commitment (Coffman and Crone 2002).

Although concerns have been raised in regard to the potential of immunosuppressive medications to produce or exacerbate psychotic symptoms, patients with a prior psychiatric history are not necessarily more susceptible to "steroid psychosis" than are patients without such a history (R.C. Hall et al. 1979), and appropriate use of antipsychotic medication is usually adequate to manage these symptoms if they emerge. Because transplant teams often overlook the early postoperative reinstitution of antipsychotic medications, it is essential that the psychiatrist devote careful attention to this issue during the immediate postoperative phase. If quick reintegration of the patient into his or her pretransplant outpatient psychiatric treatment regimen is not possible because of infirmity, interim in-home psychiatric follow-up care should be instituted.

Intestinal Transplantation

Isolated small bowel transplantation and multivisceral transplantation including the bowel are still relatively uncommon procedures, yet with improvements in therapies and longer survival, they are becoming a standard treatment for patients with intestinal failure and parenteral nutrition dependency (Fishbein 2009; Langnas 2004). Candidates for intestinal transplantation typically have experienced complications such as repeated episodes of sepsis or dehydration, early liver disease, or loss of central venous access (Fishbein 2009). For parenteral nutrition–dependent patients without complications who seek to improve their quality of life, the decision to transplant is controversial, and data on posttransplant improvement in patient quality of life are limited (Fishbein 2009). UNOS reported a 5-year survival of only 50% for those transplanted after 2001 ($n=353$) (Langnas 2004), and the 5-year survival of patients treated with total parenteral nutrition is only 63%, even at experienced centers (Fishbein 2009). An international conference in 2003 found that only 28 centers had performed one or more intestinal transplants in the 2 prior years, with the majority of recipients younger than 18 years (Langnas 2004). Perhaps because of small numbers and poor long-term survival, few studies have investigated outcomes beyond the immediate postoperative course and survival. Earlier studies on the psychiatric characteristics of the patient population showed them to be a complex group, often with character pathology and drug and/or alcohol dependence histories and with iatrogenic dependence on high-dose narcotics (DiMartini et al. 1996b). Some of these features could be ascribed to the difficulties of living with a chronic debilitating illness prior to transplantation, the severity and extent of the transplant surgery, and the prolonged posttransplantation hospitalizations marked by frequent setbacks.

Patients and their caregivers should be prepared for long and frequent hospitalizations, especially during the first years following transplantation (DiMartini et al. 1996b), although substantial reductions in the initial hospitalization and need for readmission have occurred in recent years (Langnas 2004; O'Keefe et al. 2007). Studies of quality of life among adults in the first years following intestinal transplantation show that patients can be weaned from nutritional support and achieve improvements in anxiety, depression, cognition, stress, parenting, digestive and urinary function, control of impulsivity, medical compliance, quality of social relations, and leisure and recreation (DiMartini et al. 1998; O'Keefe et al. 2007). For candidates or recipients without adequate gut absorption, the use of psychotropics without parenteral formulations is challenging, and other nonenteral routes of administration may need to be considered (Thompson and DiMartini 1999; see also "Alternative Routes of Administration" in Chapter 38, "Psychopharmacology"). Weaning from high-dose narcotics following successful transplantation may be difficult (DiMartini et al. 1996b). Information on the long-term psychological outcomes and functioning of intestinal transplant recipients is lacking.

Special Issues During the Pretransplant Phase

Cognitive Disorders and Delirium

Through the pre- to posttransplant phases, patients frequently experience cognitive dysfunction ranging from subclinical or mild symptoms to frank delirium. Impairment in cognitive function often results from physiological consequences of end-stage organ disease but may also be secondary to other comorbid disease processes (e.g., central nervous system [CNS] vascular disease from diabetes or hypertension), damage from prior alcohol or drug exposures, or previous structural damage to the brain (e.g., head trauma). Persistent cognitive deficits during the pretransplant phase indicate a preexisting dementia or static cognitive impairment. While a fluctuating course suggests a potentially reversible delirium, in some cases such encephalopathy can be chronic and persisting. Gathering information on symptom history over time is important. An electroencephalogram can aid in the diagnosis, especially if the symptoms are subtle or mostly behavioral in nature and not as readily identifiable as encephalopathy (although mild generalized slowing may also be seen in dementia), and imaging may be beneficial to evaluate evidence of structural damage (e.g., small-vessel disease, prior strokes, edema [as seen in some cases of hepatic encephalopathy]). Aggressive treatment of delirium and its causes should be pursued, with subsequent reassessment of cognition. The reversibility or progression of deficits may in part depend on age, the homeostatic reserve of the brain, prior CNS insults, and the ability to withstand future transplant-related stressors (e.g., prolonged anesthesia, use of cardiac bypass, hemodynamic fluctuations, posttransplant immunosuppressive medications). While the restoration of normal organ function and physiology after transplantation may be expected to correct reversible cognitive impairments, such deficits may take months to years to resolve and may not resolve completely (Arria et al. 1991; DiMartini and Chopra 2009; Kramer 1996; O'Carroll et al. 2003; Rovira et al. 2007).

In heart failure, low cardiac output and CNS hypoperfusion from reduced cerebral blood flow can contribute to cognitive impairment. Even in the absence of acute cerebrovascular events, impaired cerebrovascular reactivity and ischemia may result. CNS microemboli are common in preheart transplant patients especially for those on ventricular assist devices. In renal disease, accumulation of metabolic products (e.g., urea, uric acid, others), in addition to hormonal elevations, electrolyte imbalances, malnutrition, and decreased GABA and glycine activity, contributes to encephalopathy. Removal of uremic toxins by hemodialysis, correction of electrolyte imbalances and anemia, and treatment of malnutrition can diminish symptoms and improve cognition. For patients with end-stage lung disease, hypoxia and hypercapnia may cause mild to severe cognitive deficits, particularly in executive functions, attention, and memory (Parekh et al. 2005). Oxygen therapy may improve cognitive function for some lung candidates, and these patients can benefit from lung transplantation, but the extent to which these deficits are reversible is unclear (Parekh et al. 2005). Hepatic encephalopathy and adverse events related to ventricular assist devices are two specific areas considered in detail below.

Hepatic Encephalopathy

Hepatic encephalopathy (HE), a neuropsychiatric syndrome commonly encountered in LTX candidates, is characterized by a constellation of signs and symptoms, such as alteration of consciousness (including stupor or coma), cognitive impairment, confusion/disorientation, affective/emotional dysregulation, psychosis, behavioral disturbances, bioregulatory disturbances, and physical signs such as asterixis. (Hepatic encephalopathy is also addressed in Chapter 20, "Gastrointestinal Disorders.") Identification of HE is important, because its symptoms directly affect patient quality and quantity of life; fulminant HE is associated with intracranial hypertension, cerebral edema, and death pretransplant (Ferenci et al. 2002). Efforts to define HE have emphasized that it reflects a continuum of symptoms. Even subclinical HE is clinically important, because it can impair patient safety (Schomerus et al. 1981) and is associated with persistent cognitive deficits post-LTX (Tarter et al. 1990). Eighty-five percent of patients with subclinical HE were found to be either of questionable fitness or unfit to drive on psychometric testing of driving capacity, and in on-road testing one third performed unacceptably (Schomerus et al. 1981; Wein et al. 2004). By definition, subclinical HE is not identifiable on a typical clinical examination; detection may require additional neuropsychological tests of psychomotor speed, praxis, concentration, and attention. The Trail Making Test (A and B) and the Digit Symbol and Block Design tests from the Wechsler Adult Intelligence Scale—Revised are commonly used to identify subclinical HE impairment. Hepatic disease severity is strongly correlated with impairment in performance on tasks of immediate memory, delayed memory, and attention (Meyer et al. 2006). Whereas the prognostic significance of HE is well known, the long-term impact of subclinical encephalopathy on cognitive functioning requires further investigation.

The predominant strategy for treating HE involves reducing the production and absorption of ammonia from the intestinal tract, although a variety of compounds and metabolites (e.g., mercaptans, false neurotransmitters, manganese, endogenous benzodiazepines, increased concentrations of CNS gamma-aminobutyric acid [GABA]) have also been implicated in HE (Chung and Podolsky 2001; Riordan and Williams 1997). Psychiatric consultants should be familiar with ammonia-reducing strategies, because they are often the clinicians who must recognize and monitor HE symptoms, identify whether patients are being treated for HE, and make recommendations regarding the need for initiating or improving treatment. HE can be precipitated by gastrointestinal hemorrhage, uremia, use of some psychoactive medications or diuretics, dietary indiscretions, dehydration, or electrolyte imbalance (Chung and Podolsky 2001; Riordan and Williams 1997), and these problems should be corrected first. Additionally, patients who undergo shunting procedures to relieve portal hypertension will be at increased risk for ammonia buildup with subsequent HE, and they and their caregivers should be educated on monitoring for signs and symptoms of HE. In one study of patients following treatment with transjugular intrahepatic portosystemic shunting, 45% experienced HE, with more than half exhibiting moderate to severe symptoms (Riggio et al. 2008). Refractory HE may require reduction of the shunt diameter (Riggio et al. 2008). Treatment should strive to normalize ammonia levels, despite the fact that blood ammonia levels are not well correlated with symptoms of HE (Riordan and Williams 1997). Treatment strategies include administration of a nonabsorbable disaccharide, lactulose, that acts as an osmotic laxative to flush out ammonia; adherence to a protein-restricted diet to decrease the production of ammonia from protein; and prescription of nonabsorbable antibiotics to reduce intestinal bacteria that convert protein to ammonia. Some patients require all three treatments simultaneously. Medications that can contribute to symptoms of encephalopathy—anticholinergic drugs, tranquilizers, and sedatives—should be avoided.

Ventricular Assist Devices in Heart Transplantation

Progress in the development of implantable left ventricular assist devices (LVADs) has dramatically improved both the physical and the psychological health of potential cardiac transplant candidates. (Left ventricular assist devices are also discussed in Chapter 18, "Heart Disease.") The new LVADs consist of a mechanical pump implanted in the abdomen with conduits from the apex of the left ventricle to the device, and from the device to the ascending aorta. Blood returning from the lungs to the left side of the heart exits through the left ventricular apex into the LVAD pumping chamber. Blood is then actively pumped through the LVAD outflow valve into the ascending aorta. One transcutaneous line carries an electrical cable to an external battery pack and electronic controls, which are worn on a shoulder holster or belt.

Prior to the use of LVADs, the need for prolonged inotrope infusions before transplantation could lead to very lengthy hospitalizations for cardiac transplant candidates. These patients would become deconditioned and were at risk for deep vein thrombosis, pulmonary emboli, multiple organ dysfunction, and sudden cardiac death. However, experience with newer LVADs reveals improvement in mechanical/electrical failure rates and lessened risks for thromboembolism (Rose et al. 2001a, 2001b). Patients on LVADs can achieve better hepatic, renal, cerebral, and peripheral perfusion, leading to improvement in overall physical function, exercise tolerance, and well-being (Goldstein et al. 1998; Morrone et al. 1996). These devices are now portable, permitting discharge from the hospital before transplantation and a generally acceptable quality of life (Dew et al. 2000a; Frazier 1993; Loisance et al. 1994). Patients on LVADs can undergo physical and physiological rehabilitation, develop exercise tolerance, and rebuild muscle mass, thus stabilizing their cardiac condition (Goldstein et al. 1998; McCarthy 2002; Morrone et al. 1996). The lack of mobility restriction means that patients often can return to work and engage in activities such as dancing and driving (Catanese et al. 1996). With the urgency for transplantation diminished, the transplant team can wait for an optimal donor organ. LVADs are now used as "destination" therapy as well as to bridge patients to transplantation. Thus, some patients who may not desire transplantation or who do not meet criteria for transplantation may receive LVADs for permanent support.

However, there continue to be risks and drawbacks associated with either temporary or permanent LVAD therapy. The logistics of arranging outpatient care require a well-trained medical team whose members are available at all times, resulting in significant patient, caregiver, and medical system burden. All persons involved in the patient's care must receive extensive training, arrangements for outpatient housing or maintenance at home must be coordinated, and local emergency paramedical personnel must also be trained. Infection can occur in more than 60% of LVAD recipients (Genovese et al. 2009; S.M. Gordon et al. 2001); in one study of patients with permanent LVADs, 41% of deaths were related to infection (Rose et al. 2001b). Cardiovascular complications, bleeding, and reoperations have also been found to be prevalent adverse events (Genovese et al. 2009). Not surprisingly, in a study of recipients of ventricular assist devices (including both LVADs and biventricular assist devices), the most common concern expressed by patients was risk of infection (52%) (Dew et al. 2000a). In addition, 52% had difficulty sleeping because of the driveline, 46% had pain at the driveline site, 40% worried about device malfunction, and 32% were bothered by device-related noise (Dew et al. 2000a). Finally, although patients on LVADs have improved cerebral perfusion, they are at high risk for microembolic events. While many of the microembolic events are clinically silent (Thoennissen et al. 2005), the chronic effect of such silent microembolic events on cognitive function may be significant over time, and periodic neuropsychological or cognitive testing may be helpful (Komoda et al. 2005). The risk of such events appears to be lower with the newer generation of LVADs, but given that implantation periods have lengthened, routine care of LVAD recipients must continue to consider their cognitive status and the identification of any developing deficits.

In posttransplantation comparisons with heart recipients who did not receive a ventricular assist device (VAD; either biventricular or left ventricular assist device), patients who were bridged to transplantation with a VAD showed similar improvements in physical functioning and emotional well-being, significantly lower rates of anxiety, but poorer cognitive status (Dew et al. 2001b). The cognitive impairments observed in these VAD recipients were believed to be attributable to neurological events (e.g., microemboli, strokes) that occurred during the period of VAD support, and these events occurred at a higher rate among VAD recipients relative to non-VAD patients during the waiting period before transplantation. Although mild, these impairments appeared to persist during the first year following transplantation and were associated with reduced likelihood of returning to employment (Dew et al. 2001b).

Tobacco Use and Transplantation

Tobacco use by transplant candidates and recipients has received surprisingly little attention. Even in lung and heart transplantation, tobacco use is not routinely reported. Two meta-analyses of posttransplantation adherence show tobacco use rates of 3.4% of patients per year in the general transplant population and 10% of patients per year for transplant recipients with substance use histories (Dew et al. 2007a, 2008a). Tobacco use coupled with immunosuppressive therapy, which also increases cancer risk (Nabel 1999), may result in higher rates of cancer posttransplantation. In addition to increased risk for oropharyngeal and lung cancers, tobacco suppresses immunity and can aggravate many disease states, resulting in higher rates of infections, vascular thrombosis, and atherosclerosis. Atherosclerosis is especially problematic for transplant recipients already at risk for hypertension, hyperlipidemia, and hyperglycemia induced by immunosuppressive medication.

Studies of heart transplant recipients have reported that 26%–50% of smokers resumed smoking after transplantation (Bell and Van Triget 1991; Nagele et al. 1997). Compared with nonsmokers, smokers had higher rates of vasculopathy and of malignancies (Nagele et al. 1997); they also had significantly worse survival, with none of the smokers surviving more than 11.5 years after transplantation (vs. 80% of the nonsmokers surviving). When patients were grouped by carboxyhemoglobin level, investigators found that no patients with a level higher than 2.5% were surviving 4 years after transplantation (Nagele et al. 1997). In this cohort, smoking appeared to be much more important than other classical risk factors (Nagele et al. 1997). Similarly, a study of LTX recipients found a higher rate of vascular complications among patients with a history of smoking (17.8% vs. 8% among patients without such a history; $P=0.02$); furthermore, having quit smoking 2 years prior to transplantation reduced the incidence of vascular complications by 58% (Pungpapong et al. 2002). For ALD LTX recipients in one study, the rates of oropharyngeal cancer and lung cancer were 25 and 3.7 times higher, respectively, than rates in the general nontransplant population matched for age and gender (Jain et al. 2000), presumably as a result of tobacco use.

A cross-sectional retrospective study of renal transplant recipients identified cigarette smoking as a factor in the progression of kidney disease (Zitt et al. 2007). Compared with nonsmokers, smokers (22% of the cohort) had more cardiovascular events, graft failure (33% vs. 21%), and diabetes and showed a fourfold increase in the probability of arteriopathy. Relatively small doses of tobacco use (average of 3 pack years) induced abnormal renal vascular intimal thickening in the allograft (Zitt et al. 2007). In a prospective study of ALD LTX recipients, 53% were found to be using tobacco after transplantation (DiMartini et al. 2002). A study of 60 heart transplant recipients reported that 3 patients had resumed smoking within 6 months following transplantation and that all 3 had also relapsed to drug or alcohol abuse (Paris et al. 1994). Another study of heart transplant recipients found that elevated posttransplant anxiety was associated with a higher risk of resuming smoking (Dew et al. 1996).

Programs vary in whether they consider tobacco use to be a contraindication to transplantation. However, given that tobacco use is a modifiable risk factor that has demonstrated significant and negative effects on both patient and graft outcomes and survival, psychosomatic medicine specialists should make tobacco use a routine part of their assessment, plan for monitoring pre- and posttransplant, and provide smoking cessation assistance when necessary. Cessation of tobacco use (both smoked and smokeless) prior to transplantation is strongly recommended, given the high risk that pretransplant users will resume use posttransplantation. Treatments for smoking cessation include bupropion, nicotine replacement (patches, gum, lozenges, and aerosolized formulations), and behavioral therapies (Hurt et al. 1997; Jorenby et al. 1999). Nicotine replacement strategies have been safely used in patients with advanced liver and lung disease, but severe renal disease may affect nicotine clearance. Nicotine replacement is relatively contraindicated in serious heart disease due to the potential for worsening angina, increasing heart rate, and possibly exacerbating arrhythmias. When nicotine replacement has been combined with bupropion, cases of severe hypertension have been reported, so careful monitoring of blood pressure is indicated. Bupropion should be used cautiously in transplant recipients, who are already at increased risk for seizures from immunosuppressive medications, specifically during the early posttransplant period, when immunosuppressive levels are higher. Nortriptyline has a cessation success rate similar to that of bupropion in non-ill smokers (S.M. Hall et al. 1998), but its anticholinergic effects may increase risk for delirium. Nortriptyline's alpha-adrenergic, antiarrhythmic, and negative inotropic effects are tolerated post–heart transplant (Kay et al. 1991; P.A. Shapiro 1991) but should be carefully monitored in heart transplant candidates. Varenicline is eliminated by renal clearance, so dosage reductions are necessary for patients with renal insufficiency or on dialysis. Its side effects of nausea and vomiting may be problematic in transplant patients.

Living Donor Transplantation

Despite the physical risks, discomfort and pain, expense and inconvenience, and potential psychological consequences of donating an organ, an increasing number of people are becoming donors, and transplant programs are considering living donation as one solution to the organ shortage. Kidneys and portions of the liver, lung, pancreas, intestine, and even the heart (through a domino procedure in which a heart-lung recipient donates his or her heart) are donated for transplantation (Oaks et al. 1994; Rodrigue et al. 2001; Taguchi and Suita 2002).

Donation of an organ—putting one's life at risk to help another—is an incredibly generous and altruistic gift. Yet the evaluation of such donors is a complex process requiring assessment of the circumstances and motives of the donor, the dynamics of the relationship between donor and recipient, the severity of the recipient's illness, and family and societal forces. Current practice guidelines require a psychosocial evaluation for each potential donor, to thoroughly examine these and other issues (Table 31–3) (Dew et al. 2007c; Olbrisch et al. 2001; Surman 2002). All U.S. centers' living donor medical evaluation protocols include predonation psychosocial assessments, although the specifics of these evaluations and who performs them vary among centers. These assessments are designed to screen out potential donors with significant psychiatric morbidity (including substance abuse/dependence) and those unwilling or unable to give informed consent for donation (due to the presence of coercion, likely financial gain, and/or impaired cognitive/intellectual capacity). This screening process, combined with rigorous medical evaluation, ensures that living donors are very healthy before donation. Additionally, donors must be fully willing, independently motivated, and completely informed about the surgery. Yet for all donors, and liver donors in particular, long-term sequelae that may affect the donor's future health, functioning, and even ability to obtain health insurance (due to the presence of a preexisting condition) are not known.

Living liver donation is a much more surgically complex and invasive procedure than kidney donation and is therefore potentially more dangerous. Adult-to-adult living donor liver transplantation (LDLT) is a relatively new procedure in the United States, preceded by adult-to-child transplants. Whereas only 9 such procedures had been performed in the United States prior to 1998, in 2001 more than 400 adult-to-adult LDLTs were performed. Although mortality rates have been less than 1% for both kidney and liver donors (both adult-to-adult and to children) (Brown et al. 2003; Najarian et al. 1992), about one-third of liver donors have complications, with serious complications occurring in 14% of donors (Brown et al. 2003; Grewal et al. 1998; Tan et al. 2007b). There have been consensus recom-

TABLE 31–3. Areas of assessment for living donor evaluation

Reasons for donation
Relationship between donor and recipient
Donor's knowledge about the surgery
Motivation
Ambivalence
Evidence of coercion/inducement
Attitudes of significant others toward the donation
Availability of support
Financial resources
Work- and/or school-related issues (if applicable)
Donor's psychological health, including the following:
Psychiatric disorders
Personality disorders
Coping resources/style
Pain syndromes
Prior psychological trauma/abuse
Substance use

mendations that all potential live liver donors be evaluated by an independent physician advocate (i.e., not a member of the transplant team responsible for the recipient's care) as part of the informed consent process (Abecassis et al. 2000; Conti et al. 2002) to avoid conflicts of interest. However, in only 50% of programs does a physician who is not part of the transplant team evaluate the potential donor (Brown et al. 2003).

Kidney donors should expect to miss 4–6 weeks of work and liver donors 8–12 weeks of work, especially if their jobs involve heavy lifting. Since the late 1990s, laparoscopic donor nephrectomy has been increasingly used, a procedure that results in less postoperative pain, shorter hospital stays, overall quicker recovery times, and more favorable cosmetic results. Future research may show that this approach has psychosocial benefits as well. Living lung donation is a much less frequent procedure, with fewer than 10 such donations performed per year since 2004 in the United States. While no lung donor deaths have been reported, nearly 20% of lung donors will have perioperative complications following lobectomy and will lose 10%–20% of their predonation lung functioning even after 1 year postdonation (Sano et al. 2009; Tan et al. 2007a).

Living donors almost uniformly express no regret at having donated, would donate again if that were possible, and report deep feelings of gratification at being able to help another person (Dew et al. 2007c). Moreover, generic health-related quality of life assessments show that—at least in the early years postdonation—donors' well-being, on average, meets or exceeds that reported in the general population (Beavers et al. 2001; Chan et al. 2006; Diaz et al. 2002). Nevertheless, a growing body of qualitative and small cohort studies suggests that a significant proportion of donors experience major health and psychosocial difficulties. For example, up to 78% of donors experience high psychological distress and/or meet diagnostic criteria for mood or anxiety disorders (Beavers et al. 2001; Coffman and Jowsey 2006; Dew et al. 2007c; Erim et al. 2006, 2007; Fukunishi et al. 2001; Hsu et al. 2006; Jowsey and Schneekloth 2008), up to 33% report that their health is poorer after donation (Chan et al. 2006; Humar et al. 2005; Kim-Schluger et al. 2002; Kusakabe et al. 2008; Walter et al. 2006), up to 50% worry about the lasting effects on their health (Morimoto et al. 1993; Trotter et al. 2001), and over 25% have financial hardships with prominent concerns about current and future insurance status (Dew et al. 2007c; Yang et al. 2007). In one study that examined outcomes of parent-to-child liver donation, psychological testing was found to be useful in identifying families that were more likely to experience problems postdonation (Goldman 1993). Although donor outcomes were reported as good, with donors experiencing increased self-esteem and satisfaction, marital dissolution occurred in 2 of the 20 families following donation (Goldman 1993). More alarming is the finding from a large multicenter study that three donors had attempted suicide, with one completed suicide following donation (Trotter et al. 2007). Trotter et al. (2007) estimated the suicide rate in liver donors at 2 per 1,000 donors, although the contribution of the donation to these events is unclear.

A U.S. live organ donor consensus group recommended the development of a living donor registry to collect demographic, clinical, and outcome information on all living organ donors. The rationale for the development of such a registry included concern for donor well-being, limitations of current knowledge regarding the long-term consequences of donation, the potential to evaluate the impact of changes in criteria for donor eligibility on the outcome of donors, and the need within the transplant community to develop mechanisms to provide for quality assurance assessments (Abecassis et al. 2000). A large multicenter study of adult-to-adult living liver donor outcomes, commissioned by the National Institute of Diabetes and Digestive and Kidney Diseases, is under way and should help provide answers to these questions ("Adult-to-Adult Living Donor Liver Transplantation Cohort Study [A2ALL]" 2003). Similarly, a multicenter study was recently commissioned by the National Institute of Allergy and Infectious Diseases to examine emotional and medical outcomes of kidney and lung donors (RELIVE: Renal and Lung Donors Evaluation and Study); this study will be collecting data through 2011.

For all donor types, the issue of donor financial hardship is becoming an increasingly prominent concern. Although the recipients' insurance covers the evaluation and immediate postoperative medical care, donors frequently report out-of-pocket costs, and some may have significant long-term difficulties in obtaining or retaining health and life insurance (Dew et al. 2007c; Nissing and Hayashi 2005; Yang et al. 2007).

Japan has extensive experience with living liver donation as a result of cultural beliefs (lack of acceptance of brain death criteria) that hamper cadaveric donation. This created an environment in which living liver donation was necessary for LTX programs to exist. Of the almost 2,000 LDLTs performed in Japan there are no reported donor deaths (Umeshita et al. 2003). Fukunishi et al. (2001) first reported on psychiatric outcomes in LDLT donors and recipients, identifying post-LTX psychiatric disorders (excluding delirium) in 37% of LDLT recipients and "paradoxical reactions" (including guilt about receiving donation, avoidant coping behaviors, and psychological distress) in 34% of recipients, despite favorable medical outcomes for both recipient and donor. Ten percent of liver donors experienced major depression within the first month after donation. Fukunishi et al. (2003) speculated that before donation, the stronger sense of duty of adult children donating to their parents masked their true concerns and fears. Following donation, these concerns manifested as anxiety, fear, and pain. The prevalence of psychiatric disorders was higher in LDLT recipients than in a comparison group of living-donor kidney recipients, suggesting a potential greater need for psychiatric evaluation and care of LDLT patients.

Altruistic donors—those donating to an unknown recipient—pose one of the most complex challenges to transplant evaluation. In these cases, the psychosocial evaluation has particular importance in determining the suitability of the donor, and some believe that the medical standards for such donors should be higher (Friedman 2002). Altruistic donors are commonly viewed with some skepticism and are evaluated with greater caution than related donors. A detailed evaluation is critical, both to understand the motives and psychological meaning of the donation to the donor and to identify any financial or other types of compensation expected for the donation. A study of nondirected donors reported that 21% were excluded for psychological reasons (Matas et al. 2000). Psychological outcomes of altruistic liver donors are unknown.

Posttransplant Organ Function and Pharmacological Considerations

While many transplant-specific psychological stresses can be appropriately managed with psychotherapeutic techniques, pharmacotherapy is an essential treatment component in the psychiatric care of these patients. Given the high prevalence of psychiatric disorders in transplant candidates and recipients and the potential for untreated psychiatric disorders to influence outcomes, including adherence, pharmacological treatment is often required. Unfortunately, psychotropic medications are often not provided because of concerns about patients' medical fragility and the potential risks of psychotropic medications. The fact that psychiatric symptoms may evolve from complex, intertwined psychological and physiological processes should not preclude treatment. Although the treatment of transplant candidates and recipients can be complicated, a thorough knowledge of psychotropic pharmacokinetics in specific types of end-stage organ failure, coupled with careful attention to medication dosing, side effects, and drug interactions, can provide the necessary foundation for pharmacological management. End-stage organ disease alters most aspects of drug pharmacokinetics, including absorption, bioavailability, metabolism, and clearance. For a full review of the changes in pharmacokinetics of psychotropic drugs in general and in hepatic, renal, bowel, heart, and lung disease in particular, the reader is referred to Chapter 38, "Psychopharmacology"; see also Robinson and Levenson 2001 and Trzepacz et al. 2000. Here we discuss the important aspects of pharmacokinetics in the newly transplanted patient during the posttransplant recovery period (see DiMartini et al. 2010 for further pharmacological considerations in transplant patients).

Although organ function may deteriorate slowly over time before transplantation, following transplantation, for the majority of recipients, the newly transplanted organ functions immediately, so that normal physiological parameters are quickly restored and pharmacokinetic abnormalities resolve. Within the first month following transplantation for patients who have stable liver or kidney function, the clearance and steady-state volume of distribution of drugs can be similar to that in healthy volunteers (Hebert et al. 2003). Many transplant recipients can be treated with normal therapeutic drug dosing once they have recovered from immediate postoperative complications (e.g., delirium, sedation, intestinal paralysis). With the resumption of normal organ function after transplantation, any psychotropic medications prescribed at lower dosages prior to transplant to accommodate diminished metabolism or elimination may need to be adjusted to higher levels.

For some transplant recipients, however, the transplanted organ does not assume normal autonomous physiological function immediately, or the organ may slowly regain normal function over time. Studies examining posttransplantation pharmacokinetics have been mostly conducted in liver and kidney recipients due to the relevance of these organs to drug pharmacokinetics. Additionally, these studies have focused exclusively on immunosuppressive medications due to the need to achieve and maintain stable immunosuppressive medication levels to prevent organ rejection, the ability to monitor serum levels, and the narrow therapeutic range of these drugs. However, these data provide general guidelines on medication prescribing for specific types of posttransplant organ dysfunction.

Delayed Graft Function

Several graft-specific outcomes relevant to pharmacokinetics and patient outcomes in particular deserve definition. Primary nonfunction (PNF), an infrequent but life-threatening complication (3%–4% of renal and liver recipients), is defined as immediate primary graft failure that results in death or requires retransplantation within 30 days of the transplant and thus is less relevant to psychotropic pharmacokinetics.

The most common allograft complication affecting pharmacokinetics in the immediate posttransplantation period is delayed graft function (DGF). DGF prolongs hospitalization, may result in chronic graft impairment, and makes the management of immunosuppressive therapy more difficult (Shoskes and Cecka 1998). DGF occurs in 10%–25% of liver and kidney recipients, although rates can reach 50% of cases if marginal organs are counted (Angelico 2005; Shoskes and Cecka 1998; U.S. Renal Data System 2008). Liver recipients with DGF may require one-half of the typical immunosuppressive medication dose, and dosing requirements may not correlate with body weight, suggesting that in the early posttransplant period, metabolic capacity rather than volume of distribution is the critical factor in pharmacokinetics (Hebert et al. 2003; Luck et al. 2004). In addition, liver recipients with DGF can develop hyperbilirubinemia, ascites, and portal hypertension, further altering pharmacokinetic parameters. For kidney transplant recipients, DGF is defined as the recipient requiring dialysis within the first week of transplant. For kidney recipients, DGF alters pharmacokinetics by mechanisms that increase the free fraction of parent drugs and renally excreted metabolites (Shaw et al. 1998). Severe or acute impairment in renal function after transplant can result in immunosuppressive levels 3–6 times higher than those in nonimpaired recipients for renally excreted drugs and their metabolites (Bullingham et al. 1998; Shaw et al. 1998). DGF also affects the binding of drugs to plasma proteins even in the absence of hypoalbuminemia (Shaw et al. 1998). DGF does not result in poorer absorption of immunosuppressants (Browne et al. 2003). Perturbed pharmacokinetics can normalize over months, with improving metabolic and renal functions (Bullingham et al. 1998; Shaw et al. 1998).

Acute and Chronic Organ Rejection

Acute cellular rejection occurs in 20%–70% of LTX recipients, typically within the first 3 weeks posttransplant, resulting in transient graft dysfunction. Bilirubin and alkaline phosphatase levels rise initially, followed by elevations in liver enzymes (alanine aminotransferase and aspartate aminotransferase). Recipients may experience fever, malaise, liver tenderness, and occasionally ascites and mental status changes. Sixty-five percent to 80% of cases are effectively treated with high-dose steroids or high-dose steroid bolus followed by a rapid taper over 5–7 days, and most episodes do not lead to clinically significant alteration in liver histology or architecture (Lake 2003). About 15% of cases require additional antibody treatments such as monoclonal therapy or antithymocyte globulin (Lake 2003), and these medications can cause serious neuropsychological side effects (see section "Neuropsychiatric Side Effects of Immunosuppressive Agents" later in this chapter). Chronic graft rejection occurring in 5%–10% of liver recipients, manifests as gradual obliteration of small bile ducts and microvascular changes, and tends to respond poorly to treatment. Patients may experience jaundice and have treatment-resistant pruritus. Persistently elevated serum alkaline phosphatase and bilirubin levels occur early on, but loss of liver synthetic function may not occur until very late in the course (Lake 2003).

Twenty-five percent to 60% of kidney recipients will experience acute rejection, most often within the first 6 months after transplantation. Rejection may not be recognized without a biopsy, and in fact 25%–30% of kidney recipients with stable or improving renal function can actually be in an episode of undetected rejection (Rush et al. 1998; R. Shapiro et al. 2001). Treatment of an identified rejection episode typically restores prerejection functioning; however, subclinical rejection that remains undetected can result in gradually worsening renal function over time with eventual graft loss (Rush et al. 1998).

Nearly 50% of heart transplant recipients will experience an episode of acute rejection (either humoral or cellular) within the first posttransplant year. With rejection some heart recipients may develop unstable symptoms (increasing central venous pressure or pulmonary capillary wedge pressure, decreasing ejection fraction, arrhythmias, hypotension, or even shock). Even with unstable symptoms, rejection can be effectively treated in 50%–60% of cases with the addition of steroids without the need for monoclonal antibodies therapy (Michaels et al. 2003; Park et al. 1999). Persistent hemodynamic changes occur less often. Sinus node dysfunction or atrioventricular block requiring permanent pacing occurs in up to 19% of heart recipients and may be associated with rejection (Collins et al. 2003). By 5 years posttransplant, nearly 70% of those with humoral rejection will develop early coronary artery disease (Michaels et al. 2003).

If the episode of graft rejection is acute and resolves quickly, no specific change to psychotropic dosages would be required. This is true across all organ types. Chronic rejection tends to evolve over time, with a gradual decrease in organ function and subsequent loss of metabolic/elimination capacity. For all organ types, chronic graft rejection is potentially reversible in the early stages but not once chronic dysfunction has set in and progressive graft failure occurs. In these cases, pharmacokinetics may be seen as similar to the pretransplant state. With all organ types, care must be taken in the choice of medication (see Chapter 38, "Psychopharmacology," for types of organ failure and medication choices), and additional attention must be paid to potential hemodynamic instability in heart candidates with rejection.

General Issues

In addition to DGF or acute rejection, some recipients will have transient physiological abnormalities in the weeks following transplant that could also affect pharmacokinetics (e.g., liver congestion and/or renal hypoperfusion in heart recipients, fluid overload in renal recipients, and resolving hepatorenal syndrome in liver recipients). The mechanisms causing these derangements are complex and can include perioperative hemodynamic and fluid instability or graft-related factors such as graft harvesting, ischemic or reperfusion injury, or the use of marginal organs. Thus, in addition to the status of the transplanted organ, evaluation of the recipients' total physiological status is important in drug consideration and dosing.

Finally, for all organ types, calcineurin-inhibiting immunosuppressive medications in chronic use are nephrotoxic. While there may be cumulative causes for renal failure in organ recipients, chronic use of immunosuppressive medications results in renal failure for 10%–20% of recipients by 5 years posttransplant (Ojo et al. 2003). Thus, the quality of renal function should always be considered with medication usage, particularly for long-term transplant recipients and especially if the medication chosen requires renal clearance.

Neuropsychiatric Side Effects of Immunosuppressive Agents

Advances in our understanding of immunology and the development of newer strategies for immunosuppression may significantly reduce the need for—if not obviate completely—long-term maintenance immunosuppression. In the future, transplant recipients of all organ types may require immunosuppressive medication dosages only one or two times a week, or not at all (Starzl 2002). This achievement would remove the final obstacle to long-term successful outcomes for transplant recipients, given that the majority of long-term morbidity and mortality is due to chronic immunosuppression (e.g., infections, renal failure, cancer). Additionally, reduced requirements for immunosuppressive medication would aid in medication adherence and relieve some of the financial burden of long-term immunosuppression. However, for now, transplant recipients will continue to require immunosuppressive therapy and to be subject to their potential neurotoxic and neuropsychiatric side effects. Psychiatrists should be familiar with the signs, symptoms, differential diagnosis, neuroimaging findings, and management of immunosuppressive neurotoxicity and secondary psychiatric disorders in solid organ recipients (Strouse et al. 1998) (see DiMartini et al. 2010 for further discussion of neuropsychiatric side effects of immunosuppressant medications).

Calcineurin-Inhibiting Immunosuppressive Medications

Cyclosporine

Cyclosporine (Gengraf, Neoral, Sandimmune), a lipophilic polypeptide derived from the fungus *Tolypocladium inflatum,* is used as a primary immunosuppressive agent. Side effects are usually mild and include tremor, restlessness, and headache (Wijdicks et al. 1999). A smaller proportion of patients (12%) experience more serious neurotoxicity characterized by acute confusional states, psychosis, seizures, speech apraxia, cortical blindness, and coma (de Groen et al. 1987; Wijdicks et al. 1995, 1996; S.E. Wilson et al. 1988). A higher incidence (33%) of serious neurotoxic side effects was reported in one study of 52 LTX recipients. Seizures were experienced by 25%; less commonly reported effects included central pontine myelinolysis, delirium, cerebral abscess, and psychosis (Adams et al. 1987).

More recent evidence suggests that earlier reports of serious neurological side effects may have been attributable to intravenous administration and higher dosages (Wijdicks et al. 1999). The use of the oral form of cyclosporine (Neoral) results in fewer serious neurological side effects (Wijdicks et al. 1999). Cyclosporine trough levels correlate poorly with cyclosporine neurotoxicity (Wijdicks et al. 1999), although in most studies symptoms resolved when the cyclosporine was discontinued and subsequently reinstated at a lower dosage (Wijdicks et al. 1999). Anticonvulsants can successfully treat cyclosporine-induced seizures but are not required long-term (Wijdicks et al. 1996), and seizures may cease with reduction or discontinuation of cyclosporine. A few patients with serious clinical neurotoxic side effects have been found to have diffuse white matter abnormalities, predominantly in the occipitoparietal region, on computed tomography (CT) scanning (de Groen et al. 1987; Gijtenbeek et al. 1999; Wijdicks et al. 1995) (see discussion of posterior reversible [leuko]encephalopathy syndrome [PRES] in "Tacrolimus" subsection below). In one case, symptoms of cyclosporine-induced cortical blindness resolved with drug discontinuation, although pathological evidence of CNS demyelination persisted for months afterward (S.E. Wilson et al. 1988).

Several mechanisms may contribute to the CNS neurotoxicity of cyclosporine. Hypocholesterolemia has been found in a high percentage of patients with serious neurotoxicity (de Groen et al. 1987; Wijdicks et al. 1995). Hypocholesterolemia may increase the intracellular transport of cyclosporine by upregulating low-density lipoprotein receptors (Wijdicks et al. 1995). Access of cyclosporine to brain tissue may be particularly high in the white matter, with a relatively high density of low-density lipoprotein receptors (Wijdicks et al. 1995). In addition to hypocholesterolemia, other factors that may contribute to cyclosporine neurotoxicity include hypertension, hypomagnesemia, and the vasoactive agent endothelin (Gijtenbeek et al. 1999).

Tacrolimus

Tacrolimus (FK506, Prograf), a macrolide produced by *Streptomyces tsukubaensis,* is used as primary immunosuppressive therapy, as rescue therapy for patients who fail to respond to cyclosporine, and as treatment for graft-versus-host disease. It is more potent and possibly less toxic than cyclosporine, although the neuropsychiatric side effects appear to be similar (DiMartini et al. 1991; Freise et al. 1991). As with cyclosporine, neuropsychiatric side effects are more common with intravenous administration and diminish with oral administration and dosage reduction. Common symptoms include tremulousness, headache, restlessness, insomnia, vivid dreams, hyperesthesias, anxiety, and agitation (Fung et al. 1991). Cognitive impairment, coma, seizures, dysarthria, and delirium occur less often (8.4%) and are associated with higher plasma levels (DiMartini et al. 1997; Fung et al. 1991). Tacrolimus can produce symptoms of akathisia (Bernstein and Daviss 1992). However, a prospective study of 25 renal transplant recipients found no correlation between tacrolimus plasma levels and scores on an akathisia rating scale, although higher plasma levels were associated with higher levels of subjective restlessness, tension, and autonomic and cognitive symptoms of anxiety (DiMartini et al. 1996a).

Tacrolimus has low aqueous solubility and cannot be detected in the cerebrospinal fluid of patients with suspected neurotoxicity (Venkataramanan et al. 1991). However, because tacrolimus has been identified in the brain tissue of animals, it is believed to cross the blood-brain barrier in humans. In addition, more serious neurotoxic side effects (e.g., focal neurological abnormalities, speech disturbances, hemiplegia, and cortical blindness) may occur from higher CNS levels in patients who have a disrupted blood-brain barrier (Eidelman et al. 1991). In a study of 294 consecutive transplant recipients on tacrolimus, those with preexisting CNS damage (e.g., from stroke, multiple sclerosis) were at higher risk for neurotoxic side effects (Eidelman et al. 1991). As described above with cyclosporine, both drugs are associated with an uncommon clinico-neuro-radiological syndrome termed posterior reversible (leuko)encephalopathy syndrome (PRES) involving demyelination (particularly in the parieto-occipital region and centrum semiovale) (Ahn et al. 2003; Bartynski and Boardman 2007; Small et al. 1996). PRES typically occurs early postoperatively but can also occur years later. The clinical presentation can be varied and includes mental status changes, focal neurological symptoms, or generalized seizures without a clear metabolic etiology. Thus, moderate to serious symptoms of neurotoxicity warrant investigation with radiological imaging. Characteristic neuroradiological abnormalities (low attenuation of white matter on CT scan or hyperintense lesions on T2-weighted magnetic resonance imaging [MRI] images) are most commonly seen in the cortical and subcortical white matter, typically involving the posterior lobes (parietal and/or occipital), although cases have been reported involving the anterior brain, cerebellum, and brain stem (Bartynski and Boardman 2007). MRI may be better than CT at identifying the radiographic changes seen with PRES (DiMartini et al. 2008). Like other serious neurotoxic side effects, this syndrome is not associated with the absolute serum level of tacrolimus but does resolve on discontinuation of the drug (Small et al. 1996). The mechanism of tacrolimus neurotoxicity is unclear but may include direct activity at the CNS neuronal level (Dawson and Dawson 1994), an immune-mediated cause (J.R. Wilson et al. 1994), or vasogenic edema (Ahn et al. 2003; Bartynski and Boardman 2007). Multifocal sensorimotor polyneuropathy can occur from long-term immunosuppressive medication use and may require either lowering of the dose if possible or medication treatment for painful peripheral neuropathy.

Other Agents for Adjunctive Immunosuppression or Treatment of Rejection

Corticosteroids

Although chronic corticosteroid use has become less essential in immunosuppression for most patients posttransplantation, high dosages of corticosteroids are still employed in the early postoperative phase and also as "pulsed" dosages to treat acute rejection. Behavioral and psychiatric side effects are common, but conclusions regarding the incidence or characteristics of these effects—or the specific dosages required to cause such effects—are not well established. We have observed that some recipients and clinicians may not recognize the energizing and euphoric effects of steroids and may believe that a setback has occurred when patients report loss of energy and motivation and a less ebullient mood after the steroids used early postsurgery are tapered and discontinued. Serious psychiatric side effects occur infrequently (5%–6%) (Kershner and Wang-Cheng 1989; Lewis and Smith 1983) and include a wide range of cognitive, affective, psychotic, and behavioral symptoms (R.C. Hall et al. 1979; Kershner and Wang-Cheng 1989; Lewis and Smith 1983; Varney et al. 1984). These side effects are reviewed elsewhere in this volume, particularly in Chapter 8, "Depression"; Chapter 10, "Psychosis, Mania, and Catatonia"; Chapter 22, "Endocrine and Metabolic Disorders"; and Chapter 25, "Rheumatology."

Sirolimus

Sirolimus (SRL, rapamycin, Rapamune), a macrocyclic lactone isolated from *Streptomyces hygroscopicus,* is a recent addition to the posttransplant immunosuppressive armamentarium but is not commonly used as primary therapy. The side-effect profile of sirolimus so far does not include neurotoxicity (Watson et al. 1999), perhaps because sirolimus does not block calcineurin (Sindhi et al. 2001). However, a systematic evaluation of sirolimus neurotoxicity has yet to be conducted.

Azathioprine

Azathioprine (Imuran) is a purine analog first used in organ transplantation in 1968. It is primarily used as an adjunctive immunosuppressive agent and is less widely used today because of the availability of alternative agents. Specific neuropsychiatric side effects have not been reported for this agent. Several reports of depressive symptoms in patients receiving azathioprine have been confounded by the concurrent use of other medications (specifically cyclosporine and prednisone) that may have contributed to mood disturbance. Nevertheless, caution is recommended when using azathioprine in patients with a history of depression.

Mycophenolate Mofetil

Few neuropsychiatric symptoms have been reported with mycophenolate mofetil (CellCept), a relatively new immunosuppressant promoted as an improvement over azathioprine. Adverse CNS events (>3% to <20% incidence) include anxiety, depression, delirium, seizures, agitation, hypertonia, paresthesias, neuropathy, psychosis, and somnolence (Roche Pharmaceuticals 2003); however, because the patients in whom these symptoms occurred were being treated with mycophenolate mofetil in combination with cyclosporine and corticosteroids, the precise contribution of mycophenolate mofetil to the symptoms is difficult to interpret.

Monoclonal Antibodies

Monoclonal antibodies to T cells are used for induction immunosuppression or adjunctive therapy when a recipient is experiencing an episode of rejection. Neuropsychiatric side effects, including headache, weakness, dizziness, tremor, and anxiety, are generally mild. Muromonab-CD3 (OKT-3) is an exception, frequently causing more severe headache, tremor, agitation, and depression. It may also cause cerebral edema and encephalopathy with confusion, disorientation, hallucinations, and seizures (Alloway et al. 1998). Rituximab has been associated with progressive multifocal leukoencephalopathy (Kranick et al. 2007).

Drug Interactions Between Psychotropic and Immunosuppressive Medications

Many of the immunosuppressive medications (e.g., tacrolimus, cyclosporine, and mycophenolate mofetil) are metabolized by CYP 3A4; thus, concurrent use of psychotropic medications that strongly inhibit 3A4 should be avoided. Specific CYP 3A4 inhibitors capable of interacting adversely with immunosuppressive medications, in decreasing order of inhibition, are as follows: fluvoxamine, nefazodone > fluoxetine > sertraline, TCAs, paroxetine > venlafaxine (see also Table 38–1 in Chapter 38, "Psychopharmacology"). There are case reports in which nefazodone has caused toxic tacrolimus levels (Campo et al. 1998) and a 70% increase in the trough plasma level of cyclosporine (Helms-Smith et al. 1996). In a study in which fluoxetine and TCAs were used to treat depressed transplant recipients, no difference in cyclosporine blood level–dosage ratios and dose-response relationships was found between those treated and those not treated with antidepressants (Strouse et al. 1996). This finding suggests that antidepressants with less CYP 3A4 inhibition may not have clinically meaningful drug interactions with these immunosuppressive medications.

Several side effects relevant to immunosuppressant and psychotropic medication combinations deserve mention. Gastrointestinal symptoms (e.g., nausea, vomiting, diarrhea) are common adverse effects of immunosuppressant medications in more than 60% of patients, and additional requirements for supplemental magnesium may aggravate these symptoms (Pescovitz and Navarro 2001). The choice of a psychotropic drug should take into consideration these symptoms, especially prior to administering psychotropics with similar adverse effects (e.g., SSRIs, venlafaxine). Immunosuppressants have significant metabolic side effects (e.g., weight gain, glucose intolerance, hyperlipidemia). Similarly, these side effects must be considered when psychotropic medications with similar effects (e.g., atypical antipsychotics) are to be used. Psychotropic medications with minimal metabolic side effects should be considered.

It is possible that psychotropic medications may alter immune function. Some psychotropic medications induce a variety of neuroendocrine and cellular actions that could have immunological effects, yet this area has not been well investigated (Surman 1993). For example, lithium has been shown to enhance neutrophil migration, increase phagocytosis by macrophages, and amplify mitogen stimulation of lymphocytes (Surman 1993). Although the role of these effects in allograft function is not known, lithium has been used to increase the number of peripheral neutrophils (Ballin et al. 1998) to reduce neutropenia. The modulatory effects of psychotropic drugs on the immune system are largely unexplored but may provide valuable information for the future care of transplant patients (see Kradin and Surman 2000 for a complete review).

References

Abbey S, Farrow S: Group therapy and organ transplantation. Int J Group Psychother 48:163–185, 1998

Abecassis M, Adams M, Adams P, et al: The Live Organ Donor Consensus Group: consensus statement on the live organ donor. JAMA 284:2919–2926, 2000

Adams DH, Ponsford S, Gunson B, et al: Neurological complications following liver transplantation. Lancet 1(8539):949–951, 1987

Adult-to-adult living donor liver transplantation cohort study (A2ALL). Hepatology 38:792, 2003

Ahn KJ, Lee JW, Hahn ST, et al: Diffusion-weighted MRI and ADC mapping in FK506 neurotoxicity. Br J Radiol 76:916–919, 2003

Alloway RR, Holt C, Somerville KT: Solid organ transplant, in Pharmacotherapy Self-Assessment Program, 3rd Edition. Kansas City, MO, American College of Clinical Pharmacy, 1998, pp 219–272

American Psychiatric Association: Diagnostic and Statistical Manual of Mental Disorders, 3rd Edition, Revised. Washington, DC, American Psychiatric Association, 1987

Angelico M: Donor liver steatosis and graft selection for liver transplantation: a short review. Eur Rev Med Pharmacol Sci 9:295–297, 2005

Arria AM, Tarter RE, Starzl TE, et al: Improvement in cognitive functioning of alcoholics following orthotopic liver transplantation. Alcohol Clin Exp Res 15:956–962, 1991

Baines LS, Joseph JT, Jindal RM: Emotional issues after kidney transplantation: a prospective psychotherapeutic study. Clin Transplant 16:455–460, 2002

Ball J, Ross A: The Effectiveness of Methadone Maintenance Treatment. New York, Springer-Verlag, 1991

Ballin A, Lehman D, Sirota P, et al: Increased number of peripheral blood CD34+ cells in lithium-treated patients. Br J Haematol 100:219–221, 1998

Bartynski WS, Boardman JF: Distinct Imaging patterns and lesion distribution in posterior reversible encephalopathy syndrome. Am J Neuroradiol 28:1320–1327, 2007

Beavers KL, Sandler RS, Fair JH, et al: The living donor experience: donor health assessment and outcomes after living donor liver transplantation. Liver Transpl 7:943–947, 2001

Bell M, Van Triget P: Addictive behavior patterns in cardiac transplant patients (abstract). J Heart Lung Transplant 10:158, 1991

Berlakovich G, Steininger R, Herbst F: Efficacy of liver transplantation for alcoholic cirrhosis with respect to recidivism and compliance. Transplantation 58:560–565, 1994

Bernstein L, Daviss S: Organic anxiety disorder with symptoms of akathisia in a patient treated with the immunosuppressant FK506. Gen Hosp Psychiatry 14:210–211, 1992

Brown RS Jr, Russo MW, Lai M: A survey of liver transplantation from living adult donors in the United States. N Engl J Med 348:818–825, 2003

Browne BJ, Op't Holt C, Emovon OE: Delayed graft function may not adversely affect short-term renal allograft outcome. Clin Transplant 17 (suppl 9):35–38, 2003

Bullingham RES, Nicholls AJ, Kamm BR: Clinical pharmacokinetics of mycophenolate mofetil. Clin Pharmacokinet 34:429–455, 1998

Bunzel B, Laederach-Hofmann K: Solid organ transplantation: are there predictors for posttransplant noncompliance? A literature overview. Transplantation 70:711–716, 2000

Campbell D, Beresford T, Merion R, et al: Alcohol relapse following liver transplantation for alcoholic cirrhosis: long term follow-up. Proceedings of the American Society of Transplant Surgeons (May):A131, 1993

Campo JV, Smith C, Perel JM: Tacrolimus toxic reaction associated with the use of nefazodone: paroxetine as an alternative agent. Arch Gen Psychiatry 55:1050–1052, 1998

Carlson J, Potter L, Pennington S, et al: Liver transplantation in a patient at psychosocial risk. Prog Transplant 10:209–214, 2000

Catanese KA, Goldstein DJ, Williams DL, et al: Outpatient left ventricular assist device support: a new destination rather than a bridge. Ann Thorac Surg 62:646–652, 1996

Chacko RC, Harper RG, Gotto J, et al: Psychiatric interview and psychometric predictors of cardiac transplant survival. Am J Psychiatry 153:1607–1612, 1996

Chan SC, Liu CL, Lo CM et al: Donor quality of life before and after adult-to-adult right liver live donor liver transplantation. Liver Transpl 12:1529–1536, 2006

Chung RT, Podolsky DK: Cirrhosis and its complications, in Harrison's Principles of Internal Medicine, 15th Edition. Edited by Braunwald E, Fauci AS, Isselbacher KJ, et al. New York, McGraw-Hill, 2001, pp 1754–1766

Coffman KL, Brandwin M: The Millon Behavioral Health Inventory Life Threat Reactivity Scale as a predictor of mortality in patients awaiting heart transplantation. Psychosomatics 40:44–49, 1999

Coffman K, Crone C: Rational guidelines for transplantation in patients with psychotic disorders. Current Opinion in Organ Transplantation 7:385–388, 2002

Coffman KL, Jowsey S: Psychiatric issues in living liver donors: safeguarding the rescuers. Curr Opin Organ Transplant 11:199–205, 2006

Coffman KL, Hoffman A, Sher L, et al: Treatment of the postoperative alcoholic liver transplant recipient with other addictions. Liver Transpl Surg 3:322–327, 1997

Collins KK, Thiagarajan RR, Chin C, et al: Atrial tachyarrhythmias and permanent pacing after pediatric heart transplantation. J Heart Lung Transplant 22:1126–1133, 2003

Conti DJ, Delmonico FL, Dubler N, et al: New York State Committee on Quality Improvement in Living Liver Donation: A Report to New York State Transplant Council and New York State Department of Health, December 2002. Available at: http://www.health.state.ny.us. Accessed January 14, 2004.

Corley MC, Westerberg N, Elswick RK Jr, et al: Rationing organs using psychosocial and lifestyle criteria. Res Nurs Health 21:327–337, 1998

Cornelius JR, Bukstein O, Salloum I, et al: Alcohol and psychiatric comorbidity. Recent Dev Alcohol 16:361–374, 2003

Crone CC, Wise TN: Psychiatric aspects of transplantation: evaluation and selection of candidates. Crit Care Nurse 19:79–87, 1999

Cukor D, Newville H, Jindal R: Depression and immunosuppressive medication adherence in kidney transplant patients. Gen Hosp Psychiatry 30:386–387, 2008

Cukor D, Rosenthal DS, Jindal RM, et al: Depression is an important contributor to low medication adherence in hemodialyzed patients and transplant recipients. Kidney Int 75:1223–1229, 2009

Cupples SA, Steslowe B: Use of behavioral contingency contracting with heart transplant candidates. Prog Transplant 11:137–144, 2001

Dawson TM, Dawson VL: Nitric oxide: actions and pathologic roles. Neuroscience (preview issue):9–20, 1994

De Bleser L, Matteson M, Dobbels F, et al: Interventions to improve medication-adherence after transplantation: a systematic review. Transpl Int 22:780–797, 2009

De Geest S, Borgermans L, Gemoets H: Incidence, determinants, and consequences of subclinical noncompliance with immunosuppressive therapy in renal transplant recipients. Transplantation 59:340–347, 1995

de Groen PC, Aksamit AJ, Rakela J, et al: Central nervous system toxicity after liver transplantation: the role of cyclosporine and cholesterol. N Engl J Med 317:861–866, 1987

Denhaerynck K, Desmyttere A, Dobbels F, et al: Nonadherence with immunosuppressive drugs: U.S. compared with European kidney transplant recipients. Prog Transplant 16:206–214, 2006

Denollet J, Kupper N: Type-D personality, depression, and cardiac prognosis: cortisol dysregulation as a mediating mechanism. J Psychosom Res 62:607–609, 2007

Denollet J, Holmes RVF, Vrints CJ, et al: Unfavorable outcome of heart transplantation in recipients with type D personality. J Heart Lung Transplant 26:152–158, 2007

Dew MA: Anxiety and depression following transplantation. Presented at the Contemporary Forums Conference on Advances in Transplantation, Chicago, IL, September 2003

Dew M, Kormos R: Early posttransplant medical compliance and mental health predict physical morbidity and mortality one to three years after heart transplantation. J Heart Lung Transplant 18:549–562, 1999

Dew MA, Roth LH, Thompson ME, et al: Medical compliance and its predictors in the first year after heart transplantation. J Heart Lung Transplant 15:631–645, 1996

Dew MA, Kormos RL, Winowich S, et al: Human factors issues in ventricular assist device recipients and their family caregivers. ASAIO J 46:367–373, 2000a

Dew MA, Switzer GE, DiMartini AF, et al: Psychosocial assessments and outcomes in organ transplantation. Prog Transplant 10:239–259, 2000b

Dew MA, Kormos RL, DiMartini AF, et al: Prevalence and risk of depression and anxiety-related disorders during the first three years after heart transplantation. Psychosomatics 42:300–313, 2001a

Dew MA, Kormos RL, Winowich S, et al: Quality of life outcomes after heart transplantation in individuals bridged to transplant with ventricular assist devices. J Heart Lung Transplant 20:1199–1212, 2001b

Dew MA, Goycoolea JM, Harris RC, et al: An Internet-based intervention to improve psychosocial outcomes in heart transplant recipients and family caregivers: development and evaluation. J Heart Lung Transplant 23:745–758, 2004

Dew MA, DiMartini A, De Vito Dabbs A, et al: Rates and risk factors for nonadherence to the medical regimen after adult solid organ transplantation. Transplantation 83:858–873, 2007a

Dew MA, DiMartini AF, Kormos RL: Organ transplantation, stress of, in Encyclopedia of Stress, 2nd Edition, Vol 3. Edited by Fink G. Oxford, UK, Academic Press/Elsevier, 2007b, pp 35–44

Dew MA, Switzer GE, DiMartini AF, et al: Psychosocial aspects of living organ donation, in Living Donor Organ Transplantation. Edited by Tan HP, Marcos A, Shapiro R. New York, Taylor & Francis, 2007c, pp 7–26

Dew MA, DiMartini AF, Steel J, et al: Meta-analysis of risk for relapse to substance use after transplantation of the liver or other solid organs. Liver Transpl 14:159–172, 2008a

Dew MA, DiMartini AF, Dabbs A, et al: Adherence to the medical regimen during the first two years after lung transplantation. Transplantation 85:193–202, 2008b

Dew MA, Dabbs AD, Myaskovsky L, et al: Meta-analysis of medical regimen adherence outcomes in pediatric solid organ transplantation. Transplantation 88:736–746, 2009

Diaz GC, Renz JF, Mudge C, et al: Donor health assessment after living-donor liver transplantation. Ann Surg 236:120–126, 2002

DiMartini A: Monitoring alcohol use following liver transplantation. Presented at the Research Society on Alcoholism, Symposium on Liver Transplantation for the Alcohol Dependent Patient. Denver, CO, June 2000a

DiMartini A: Psychosocial variables for predicting outcomes after liver transplantation for alcoholic liver disease. Presented at the Alcohol Induced Liver Disease: The Role of Transplantation conference, University of Massachusetts Medical Center, October 20, 2000b

DiMartini A, Chopra K: The importance of hepatic encephalopathy: pre- and post-transplant. Liver Transpl 15:121–123, 2009

DiMartini A, Twillman R: Organ transplantation in paranoid schizophrenia. Psychosomatics 35:159–161, 1994

DiMartini A, Pajer K, Trzepacz P, et al: Psychiatric morbidity in liver transplant patients. Transplant Proc 23:3179–3180, 1991

DiMartini AF, Trzepacz PT, Daviss SR: Prospective study of FK506 side effects: anxiety or akathisia? Biol Psychiatry 40:407–411, 1996a

DiMartini A, Fitzgerald MG, Magil J, et al: Psychiatric evaluations of small intestinal transplant patients. Gen Hosp Psychiatry 18:25S–29S, 1996b

DiMartini AF, Trzepacz PT, Pager K, et al: Neuropsychiatric side effects of FK506 vs. cyclosporine A: first-week postoperative findings. Psychosomatics 38:565–569, 1997

DiMartini AF, Rovera GM, Graham T, et al: Quality of life after small intestinal transplantation and among home parenteral nutrition patients. JPEN J Parenter Enteral Nutr 22:357–362, 1998

DiMartini A, Day N, Dew M, et al: Alcohol use following liver transplantation: a comparison of follow-up methods. Psychosomatics 42:55–62, 2001

DiMartini A, Weinrieb R, Fireman M: Liver transplantation in patients with alcohol and other substance use disorders. Psychiatr Clin North Am 25:195–209, 2002

DiMartini A, Fontes P, Dew MA, et al: Age, MELD score and organ functioning predict post-transplant tacrolimus neurotoxicity. Liver Transpl 14:815–822, 2008

DiMartini A, Crone C, Fireman M: Organ transplantation, in Clinical Manual of Pharmacology in the Medically Ill. Edited by Ferrando SJ, Levenson JL, Owen JA. Arlington, VA, American Psychiatric Publishing, 2010, pp 469–499

Dobbels F, Put C, Vanhaecke J: Personality disorders: a challenge for transplantation. Prog Transplant 10:226–232, 2000

Eggers P: Comparison of treatment costs between dialysis and transplantation. Semin Nephrol 12:284–289, 1992

Eidelman BH, Abu-Elmagd K, Wilson J, et al: Neurologic complications of FK 506. Transplant Proc 23:3175–3178, 1991

Erim Y, Beckmann M, Valentin-Gamazo C, et al: Quality of life and psychiatric complications after adult living donor liver transplantation. Liver Transpl 12:1782–1790, 2006

Erim Y, Beckmann M, Kroencke S, et al: Psychological strain in urgent indications for living donor liver transplantation. Liver Transpl 13:886–895, 2007

Everhart JE, Beresford TP: Liver transplantation for alcoholic liver disease: a survey of transplantation programs in the United States. Liver Transpl Surg 3:220–226, 1997

Everson G, Bharadhwaj G, House R, et al: Long-term follow-up of patients with alcoholic liver disease who underwent hepatic transplantation. Liver Transpl Surg 3:263–274, 1997

Feinstein AR: On white-coat effects and the electronic monitoring of compliance. Arch Intern Med 150:1377–1378, 1990

Ferenci P, Lockwood A, Mullen K, et al: Hepatic encephalopathy—definition, nomenclature, diagnosis, and quantification: final report of the working party at the 11th World Congresses of Gastroenterology, Vienna, 1998. Hepatology 35:716–721, 2002

Fireman M: Outcome of liver transplantation in patients with alcohol and polysubstance dependence. Presented at Research Society on Alcoholism: Symposium on Liver Transplantation for the Alcohol Dependent Patient. Denver, CO, June 2000

Fishbein TM: Intestinal transplantation. N Engl J Med 361:998–1008, 2009

Foster P, Fabrega F, Karademir S, et al: Prediction of abstinence from ethanol in alcoholic recipients following liver transplantation. Hepatology 25:1469–1477, 1997

Frazier OH: Chronic left ventricular support with a vented electric assist device. Ann Thorac Surg 55:273–275, 1993

Fredericks EM, Magee JC, Opipari-Arrigan L, et al: Adherence and health-related quality of life in adolescent liver transplant recipients. Pediatr Transplant 12:289–299, 2008

Freise CE, Rowley H, Lake J, et al: Similar clinical presentation of neurotoxicity following FK506 and cyclosporine in a liver transplant recipient. Transplant Proc 23:3173–3174, 1991

Friedman L: All donations should not be treated equally. Journal of Law, Medicine, and Ethics 30:448–451, 2002

Fukunishi I, Sugawara Y, Takayama T, et al: Psychiatric disorders before and after living-related transplantation. Psychosomatics 42:337–343, 2001

Fukunishi I, Sugawara Y, Makuuchi M, et al: Pain in liver donors. Psychosomatics 44:172–173, 2003

Fung JJ, Alessiani M, Abu-Elmagd K, et al: Adverse effects associated with the use of FK506. Transplant Proc 23:3105–3108, 1991

Fusar-Poli P, Lazzaretti M, Ceruti M, et al: Depression after lung transplantation: causes and treatment. Lung 185:55–65, 2007

Genovese EA, Dew MA, Teuteberg JJ, et al: Incidence and patterns of adverse event onset during the first 60 days after ventricular assist device implantation. Ann Thorac Surg 88:1162–1170, 2009

Gijtenbeek HJ, van den Bent MJ, Vecht CJ: Cyclosporine neurotoxicity: a review. J Neurol 246:339–346, 1999

Goldman LS: Liver transplantation using living donors: preliminary donor psychiatric outcomes. Psychosomatics 34:235–240, 1993

Goldstein DJ, Oz MC, Rose EA: Implantable left ventricular assist devices. N Engl J Med 339:1522–1533, 1998

Gordon MJ, White R, Matas AJ, et al: Renal transplantation in patients with a history of heroin abuse. Transplantation 42:556–557, 1986

Gordon SM, Schmitt SK, Jacobs M, et al: Nosocomial bloodstream infections in patients with implantable left ventricular assist devices. Ann Thorac Surg 72:725–730, 2001

Grewal HP, Thistlewaite JR Jr, Loss GE, et al: Complications in 100 living-liver donors. Ann Surg 228:214–219, 1998

Guyatt GH, Berman LB, Townsend M, et al: A measure of quality of life for clinical trials in chronic lung disease. Thorax 42:773–778, 1987

Hails KC, Kanchana T: Outcome of liver transplants for patients on methadone. Poster presentation, American Psychiatric Association Annual Meeting, Chicago, IL, May 2000

Hall RC, Popkin MK, Stickney SK, et al: Presentation of the steroid psychoses. J Nerv Ment Dis 167:229–236, 1979

Hall SM, Reus VI, Munoz RF, et al: Nortriptyline and cognitive-behavioral therapy in the treatment of cigarette smoking. Arch Gen Psychiatry 55:683–690, 1998

Havik OE, Siversten B, Relbo A, et al: Depressive symptoms and all-cause mortality after heart transplantation. Transplantation 84:97–103, 2007

Helms-Smith KM, Curtis SL, Hatton RC: Apparent interaction between nefazodone and cyclosporine (letter). Ann Intern Med 125:424, 1996

Hebert MF, Wacher VJ, Roberts JP, et al: Pharmacokinetics of cyclosporine pre- and post-liver transplantation. J Clin Pharmacol 43:38–42, 2003

Hsu HT, Hwang SL, Lee PH, et al: Impact of liver donation on quality of life and physical and psychological distress. Transplant Proc 38:2102–2105, 2006

Humar A, Carolan E, Ibrahim H, et al: A comparison of surgical outcomes and quality of life surveys in right lobe vs. left lateral segment liver donors. Am J Transplant 5:805–809, 2005

Hurt RD, Sachs DP, Glover ED, et al: A comparison of sustained-release bupropion and placebo for smoking cessation. N Engl J Med 337:1195–1202, 1997

Jain A, DiMartini A, Kashyap R, et al: Long-term follow-up after liver transplantation for alcoholic liver disease under tacrolimus. Transplantation 70:1335–1342, 2000

Jorenby DE, Leischow SJ, Nides MA, et al: A controlled trial of sustained-release bupropion, a nicotine patch, or both for smoking cessation. N Engl J Med 340:685–691, 1999

Jowsey SG, Taylor M, Trenerry MR: Special topics in transplantation: psychometric screening of transplant candidates. Oral presentation at the annual Academy of Psychosomatic Medicine meeting, Tucson, AZ, November 2002

Jowsey SG, Schneekloth TD: Psychosocial factors in living organ donation: clinical and ethical challenges. Transplant Rev 22:192–195, 2008

Kanchana T, Kaul V, Manzarbeitia C, et al: Transplantation for patients on methadone maintenance. Liver Transpl 8:778–782, 2002

Kay J, Bienenfeld D, Slomowitz M, et al: Use of tricyclic antidepressants in recipients of heart transplants. Psychosomatics 32:165–170, 1991

Kershner P, Wang-Cheng R: Psychiatric side effects of steroid therapy. Psychosomatics 30:135–139, 1989

Kim-Schluger L, Florman SS, Schiano T, et al: Quality of life after lobectomy for adult liver transplantation. Transplantation 73:1593–1597, 2002

Koch M, Banys P: Liver transplantation and opioid dependence. JAMA 285:1056–1058, 2001

Komoda T, Drews T, Sakuraba S, et al: Executive cognitive dysfunction without stroke after long-term mechanical circulatory support. ASAIO J 51:764–768, 2005

Kradin R, Surman O: Psychoneuroimmunology and organ transplantation: theory and practice, in The Transplant Patient. Edited by Trzepacz P, DiMartini A. Cambridge, UK, Cambridge University Press, 2000, pp 255–274

Krahn LE, Santoscoy G, Van Loon JA: A schizophrenic patient's attempt to resume dialysis following renal transplantation. Psychosomatics 39:470–473, 1998

Kramer L, Madl C, Stockenhuber F, et al: Beneficial effect of renal transplantation on cognitive brain function. Kidney Int 49:833–838, 1996

Kranick SM, Mowry EM, Rosenfeld MR: Progressive multifocal leukoencephalopathy after rituximab in a case of non-Hodgkin lymphoma. Neurology 69:704–706 2007

Köllner V, Schade I, Maulhardt T, et al: Posttraumatic stress disorder and quality of life after heart or lung transplantation. Transplant Proc 34:2192–2193, 2002

Kusakabe T, Irie S, Ito N, et al: Feelings of living donors about adult-to-adult living donor liver transplantation. Gastroenterol Nurs 31:263–272, 2008

Laederach-Hofmann K, Bunzel B: Noncompliance in organ transplant recipients: a literature review. Gen Hosp Psychiatry 22:412–424, 2000

Lake JR: Liver transplantation, in Current Diagnosis and Treatment in Gastroenterology, 2nd Edition. Edited by Friedman SL, McQuaid KR, Grendell JH. New York, McGraw-Hill, 2003, pp 813–834

Langnas AN: Advances in small intestine transplantation. Transplantation 77:S75–S78, 2004

Levenson JL, Olbrisch ME: Psychosocial evaluation of organ transplant candidates: a comparative survey of process, criteria, and outcomes in heart, liver and kidney transplantation. Psychosomatics 34:314–323, 1993

Levenson J, Olbrisch ME: Psychosocial screening and selection of candidates for organ transplantation, in The Transplant Patient. Edited by Trzepacz PT, DiMartini AF. Cambridge, UK, Cambridge University Press, 2000, pp 21–41

Levenson JL, Best A, Presberg B, et al: Psychosocial Assessment of Candidates for Transplantation (PACT) as a predictor of transplant outcome. Oral presentation at the 41st Annual Meeting of the Academy of Psychosomatic Medicine. Phoenix, AZ, November 19, 1994

Lewis DA, Smith RE: Steroid-induced psychiatric syndromes: a report of 14 cases and a review of the literature. J Affect Disord 5:319–332, 1983

Liu L, Schiano T, Lau N, et al: Survival and risk of recidivism in methadone-dependent patients undergoing liver transplantation. Am J Transplant 3:1273–1277, 2003

Loisance DY, Deleuze PH, Mazzucotelli JP, et al: Clinical implantation of the wearable Baxter Novacor ventricular assist system. Ann Thorac Surg 58:551–554, 1994

Lucey M: Liver transplantation for alcoholic liver disease: a progress report. Graft 2:S73–S79, 1999

Luck R, Boger J, Kuse E, et al: Achieving adequate cyclosporine exposure in liver transplant recipients: a novel strategy for monitoring and dosing using intravenous therapy. Liver Transpl 10:686–691, 2004

Madan A, Parkinson A, Faiman MD: Identification of the human P-450 enzymes responsible for the sulfoxidation and thionooxidation of diethyldithiocarbamate methyl ester: role of P-450 enzymes in disulfiram bioactivation. Alcohol Clin Exp Res 22:1212–1219, 1998

Maldonado J, Plante R, David E: The Stanford Integrated Psychosocial Assessment for Transplantation (SIPAT). Oral presentation at the Academy of Psychosomatic Medicine annual meeting, Miami, FL, November 22, 2008

Matas AJ, Garvey CA, Jacobs CL, et al: Nondirected donation of kidneys from living donors. N Engl J Med 343:433–436, 2000

McCarthy PM: Implantable left ventricular assist device bridge-to-transplantation: natural selection, or is this the natural selection? J Am Coll Cardiol 39:1255–1237, 2002

Meyer T, Eshelman A, Abouljoud M: Neuropsychological changes in a large sample of liver transplant candidates. Transplant Proc 38:3559–3560, 2006

Michaels PJ, Espejo ML, Kobashigawa J, et al: Humoral rejection in cardiac transplantation: risk factors, hemodynamic consequences and relationship to transplant coronary artery disease. J Heart Lung Transplant 22:58–69, 2003

Miller P, Wikoff R, McMahon M, et al: Development of a health attitude scale. Nurs Res 31:132–136, 1981

Millon T, Green C, Meagher R: Millon Behavioral Health Inventory Manual, 3rd Edition. Minneapolis, MN, National Computer Systems, 1982

Mori DL, Gallagher P, Milne J: The Structured Interview for Renal Transplantation—SIRT. Psychosomatics 41:393–406, 2000

Morimoto T, Yamaoka T, Tanaka K, et al: Quality of life among donors of liver transplants to relatives. N Engl J Med 329:363–364, 1993

Morrone TM, Buck LA, Catanese KA, et al: Early progressive mobilization of patients with left ventricular assist devices is safe and optimizes recovery before heart transplantation. J Heart Lung Transplant 15:423–429, 1996

Nabel GJ: A transformed view of cyclosporine. Nature 397:471–472, 1999

Nagele H, Kalmar P, Rodiger W: Smoking after heart transplantation: an underestimated hazard? Eur J Cardiothorac Surg 12:70–74, 1997

Najarian JS, Chavers BM, McHugh LE: 20 years or more of follow-up of living kidney donors. Lancet 340:807–810, 1992

Newton SE: Recidivism and return to work posttransplant. J Subst Abuse Treat 17:103–108, 1999

Nissing MH, Hayashi PH: Right hepatic lobe donation adversely affects donor life insurability up to one year after donation. Liver Transpl 11:843–847, 2005

Oaks TE, Aravot D, Dennis C, et al: Domino heart transplantation: the Papworth experience. J Heart Lung Transplant 13:433–437, 1994

O'Carroll RE, Couston M, Cossar J, et al: Psychological outcome and quality of life following liver transplantation: a prospective, national, single-center study. Liver Transpl 9:712–720, 2003

Ojo AO, Held PJ, Port KP, et al: Chronic renal failure after transplantation of a nonrenal organ. N Engl J Med 349:931–940, 2003

O'Keefe SJ, Emerling M, Koritsky D, et al: Nutrition and quality of life following small intestinal transplantation. Am J Gastroenterol 102:1093–1100, 2007

Olbrisch ME, Levenson J: Psychosocial assessment of organ transplant candidates: current status of methodological and philosophical issues. Psychosomatics 36:236–243, 1995

Olbrisch ME, Levenson JL, Hamer R: The PACT: a rating scale for the study of clinical decision making in psychosocial screening of organ transplant candidates. Clin Transplant 3:164–169, 1989

Olbrisch ME, Benedict SM, Haller DL, et al: Psychosocial assessment of living organ donors: clinical and ethical considerations. Prog Transplant 11:40–49, 2001

Olbrisch ME, Benedict SM, Ashe K, et al: Psychological assessment and care of organ transplant patients. J Consult Clin Psychol 70:771–783, 2002

Parekh PI, Blumenthal JA, Babyak MA, et al: Gas exchange and exercise capacity affect neurocognitive performance in patients with lung disease. Psychosom Med 67:425–432, 2005

Paris W, Muchmore J, Pribil A, et al: Study of the relative incidences of psychosocial factors before and after heart transplantation and the influence of posttransplantation psychosocial factors on heart transplantation outcome. J Heart Lung Transplant 13:424–432, 1994

Park MH, Starling RC, Ratliff NB, et al: Oral steroid pulse without taper for the treatment of asymptomatic moderate cardiac allograft rejection. J Heart Lung Transplant 18:1224–1227, 1999

Pedersen SS, Holkamp PG, Caliskan K, et al: Type D personality is associated with impaired health-related quality of life 7 years following heart transplantation. J Psychosom Res 61:791–795, 2006

Pescovitz MD, Navarro MT: Immunosuppressive therapy and post-transplantation diarrhea. Clin Transplantation 15 (suppl 4): 23–28, 2001

Phipps L: Psychiatric evaluation and outcomes in candidates for heart transplantation. Clin Invest Med 20:388–395, 1997

Presberg BA, Levenson JL, Olbrisch ME, et al: Rating scales for the psychosocial evaluation of organ transplant candidates: comparison of the PACT and TERS with bone marrow transplant patients. Psychosomatics 36:458–461, 1995

Pungpapong S, Manzarbeitia C, Ortiz J, et al: Cigarette smoking is associated with an increased incidence of vascular complications after liver transplantation. Liver Transplant 8:582–587, 2002

Riggio O, Angeloni S, Salvatori FM, et al: Incidence, natural history, and risk factors of hepatic encephalopathy after transjugular intrahepatic portosystemic shunt with polytetrafluoroethylene-covered stent grafts. Am J Gastroenterol 103:2738–2746, 2008

Riordan SM, Williams R: Treatment of hepatic encephalopathy. N Engl J Med 337:473–479, 1997

Robinson MJ, Levenson JL: Psychopharmacology in transplant patients, in Biopsychosocial Perspectives on Transplantation. Edited by Rodrigue JR. New York, Kluwer Academic/Plenum, 2001, pp 151–172

Roche Pharmaceuticals: CellCept (mycophenolate mofetil) product information. Nutley, NJ, Roche Laboratories, 2003

Rodrigue JR, Bonk V, Jackson S: Psychological considerations of living organ donation, in Biopsychosocial Perspectives on Transplantation. Edited by Rodrigue JR. New York, Kluwer Academic/Plenum Publishers, 2001, pp 59–70

Rose EA, Gelijns AC, Moskowitz AJ, et al: Long-term use of a left ventricular assist device for end-stage heart failure. N Engl J Med 345:1435–1493, 2001a

Rose EA, Gelijns AC, Moskowitz AJ, et al: Randomized Evaluation of Mechanical Assistance for the Treatment of Congestive Heart Failure (REMATCH) Study Group: long-term mechanical left ventricular assistance for end-stage heart failure. N Engl J Med 345:1435–1443, 2001b

Rovira A, Minguez B, Aymerich FX, et al: Decreased white matter lesion volume and improved cognitive function after liver transplantation. Hepatology 46:1485–1490, 2007

Rush D, Nickerson P, Gough J, et al: Beneficial effects of treatment of early subclinical rejection: a randomized study. Am Soc Nephrol 9:2129–2134, 1998

Sano Y, Oto T, Yamane M, et al: Donor outcome after living-donor lobar lung donation: 93 donor lobectomies in a single-center experience. J Heart Lung Transplant 28:S135, 2009

Schomerus H, Hamster W, Blunck H, et al: Latent portosystemic encephalopathy, I: nature of cerebral functional defects and their effect on fitness to drive. Dig Dis Sci 26:622–630, 1981

Shapiro PA: Nortriptyline treatment of depressed cardiac transplant recipients. Am J Psychiatry 148:371–373, 1991

Shapiro PA, Williams DL, Foray AT, et al: Psychosocial evaluation and prediction of compliance problems and morbidity after heart transplantation. Transplantation 60:1462–1466, 1995

Shapiro R, Randhawa P, Jordan ML, et al: An analysis of early renal transplant protocol biopsies: the high incidence of subclinical tubulitis. Am J Transplant 1:47–50, 2001

Shaw LM, Mick R, Nowak I, et al: Pharmacokinetics of mycophenolic acid in renal transplant patients with delayed graft function. J Clin Pharmacol 38:268–275, 1998

Shoskes DA, Cecka JM: Deleterious effects of delayed graft function in cadaveric renal transplant recipients independent of acute rejection. Transplantation 66:1697–1701, 1998

Sindhi R, Webber S, Venkataramanan R, et al: Sirolimus for rescue and primary immunosuppression in transplanted children receiving tacrolimus. Transplantation 72:851–855, 2001

Singh N, Gayowski T, Wagener MM, et al: Depression in patients with cirrhosis: impact on outcome. Dig Dis Sci 42:1421–1427, 1997

Small S, Fukui M, Bramblett G, et al: Immunosuppression-induced leukoencephalopathy from tacrolimus. Ann Neurol 40:575–580, 1996

Snyder SL, Drooker M, Strain JJ: A survey estimate of academic liver transplant teams' selection practices for alcohol-dependent applicants. Psychosomatics 37:432–437, 1996

Starzl TE: The saga of liver replacement, with particular reference to the reciprocal influence of liver and kidney transplantation (1955–1967). J Am Coll Surg 195:587–610, 2002

Stevenson LW: Indications for listing and de-listing patients for cardiac transplantation (Chapter 233 [Cardiac Transplantation], reviews and editorials), in Harrison's Online. 2002. Available at: http://harrisons.accessmedicine.com. Accessed August 3, 2004.

Stilley CS, Miller DJ, Tarter RE: Measuring psychological distress in candidates of liver transplantation: a pilot study. J Clin Psychol 53:459–464, 1997

Stilley CS, Miller DJ, Gayowski T, et al: Psychological characteristics of candidates for liver transplantation: differences according to history of substance abuse and UNOS listing. United Network for Organ Sharing. J Clin Psychol 55:1287–1297, 1999

Stilley CS, Dew MA, Pilkonis P, et al: Personality characteristics among cardiothoracic transplant recipients. Gen Hosp Psychiatry 27:113–118, 2005

Stowe J, Kotz M: Addiction medicine in organ transplantation. Prog Transplant 11:50–57, 2001

Strouse TB, Fairbanks LA, Skotzko CE, et al: Fluoxetine and cyclosporine in organ transplantation: failure to detect significant drug interactions or adverse clinical events in depressed organ recipients. Psychosomatics 37:23–30, 1996

Strouse TB, el-Saden SM, Glaser NE, et al: Immunosuppressant neurotoxicity in liver transplant recipients: clinical challenges for the consultation-liaison psychiatrist. Psychosomatics 39:124–133, 1998

Stuber ML, Shemesh E, Seacord D, et al: Evaluating non-adherence to immunosuppressant medications in pediatric liver transplant recipients. Pediatr Transplant 12:284–288, 2008

Surman OS: Possible immunological effects of psychotropic medication. Psychosomatics 34:139–143, 1993

Surman OS: The ethics of partial-liver donation (comment). N Engl J Med 346:1038, 2002

Surman OS, Purtilo R: Reevaluation of organ transplantation criteria: allocation of scarce resources to borderline candidates. Psychosomatics 33:202–212, 1992

Taguchi T, Suita S: Segmental small-intestinal transplantation: a comparison of jejunal and ileal grafts. Surgery 131:S294–S300, 2002

Tan HP, Marcos A, Shapiro R (eds): Living Donor Transplantation. New York, Informa Healthcare, 2007a

Tan HP, Martin AE, Kilac A, et al: Donor outcomes (liver), in Living Donor Transplantation. Edited by Tan HP, Marcos A, Shapiro R. New York, Informa Healthcare, 2007b, pp 185–195

Tarter RE, Switala JA, Arria A, et al: Subclinical hepatic encephalopathy: comparison before and after orthotopic liver transplantation. Transplantation 50:632–637, 1990

Thoennissen NH, Schneider M, Allroggen A, et al: High level of cerebral microembolization in patients supported with the DeBakey left ventricular assist device. J Thorac Cardiovasc Surg 130:1159–1166, 2005

Thompson D, DiMartini A: Alternative routes of administration of psychiatric medications. Psychosomatics 40:185–192, 1999

Tringali RA, Trzepacz PT, DiMartini A, et al: Assessment and follow-up of alcohol-dependent liver transplantation patients: a clinical cohort. Gen Hosp Psychiatry 18 (suppl):70S–77S, 1996

Trotter JF, Talamantes M, McClure M, et al: Right hepatic lobe donation for living donor liver transplantation: impact on donor quality of life. Liver Transpl 7:485–493, 2001

Trotter JF, Hill-Callahan MM, Gillespie BW, et al: Severe psychiatric problems in right hepatic lobe donors for living donor liver transplantation. Transplantation 83:1506–1508, 2007

Trzepacz PT, DiMartini AF, Gupta B: Psychopharmacologic issues in transplantation, in The Transplant Patient. Edited by Trzepacz P, DiMartini A. Cambridge, UK, Cambridge University Press, 2000, pp 187–213

Twillman RK, Manetto C, Wellisch DK, et al: The Transplant Evaluation Rating Scale: a revision of the psychosocial levels system for evaluating organ transplant candidates. Psychosomatics 34:144–153, 1993

Umeshita K, Fujiwara K, Kiyosawa K, et al: Operative morbidity of living liver donors in Japan. Lancet 362:687–690, 2003

United Network of Organ Sharing (UNOS) Web site. Available at: http://www.optn.org. Accessed June 1, 2009.

U.S. Renal Data System: USRDS 2008 annual data report: atlas of chronic kidney disease and end-stage renal disease in the United States. Bethesda, MD, National Institutes of Health, National Institute of Diabetes and Digestive and Kidney Diseases, 2008. Available at: http://www.usrds.org/atlas_2008.htm. Accessed November 28, 2009.

Vaillant GE: The natural history of alcoholism and its relationship to liver transplantation. Liver Transpl Surg 3:304–310, 1997

Varney NR, Alexander B, MacIndoe JH: Reversible steroid dementia in patients without steroid psychosis. Am J Psychiatry 141:369–372, 1984

Venkataramanan R, Jain A, Warty VS, et al: Pharmacokinetics of FK 506 in transplant patients. Transplant Proc 23:2736–2740, 1991

Walter M, Papachristou C, Pascher A, et al: Impaired psychosocial outcome of donors after living donor liver transplantation: a qualitative case study. Clin Transplant 20:410–415, 2006

Watson CJ, Friend PJ, Jamieson NV, et al: Sirolimus: a potent new immunosuppressant for liver transplantation. Transplantation 67:505–509, 1999

Wein C, Koch H, Popp B, et al: Minimal hepatic encephalopathy impairs fitness to drive. Hepatology 39:739–745, 2004

Weinrieb RM: A matched comparison of medical/psychiatric complication and anesthesia/analgesia requirements in methadone maintained liver transplant patients. Poster presented at the Academy of Psychosomatic Medicine Annual Meeting, San Diego, CA, November 20, 2003

Weinrieb RM, Van Horn DH, McLellan AT, et al: Interpreting the significance of drinking by alcohol-dependent liver transplant patients: fostering candor is the key to recovery. Liver Transplant 6:769–776, 2000

Weinrieb RM, Van Horn DH, McLellan AT, et al: Alcoholism treatment after liver transplantation: lessons learned from a clinical trial that failed. Psychosomatics 42:111–115, 2001

Weinrieb RM, Barnett R, Lynch KG, et al: Psychiatric complications and anesthesia and analgesia requirements in methadone-maintained liver transplant recipients. Liver Transplant 10:97–106, 2004

Weitzner MA, Lehninger F, Sullivan D, et al: Borderline personality disorder and bone marrow transplantation: ethical considerations and review. Psychooncology 8:46–54, 1999

Wijdicks EF, Wiesner RH, Krom RA: Neurotoxicity in liver transplant recipients with cyclosporine immunosuppression. Neurology 45:1962–1964, 1995

Wijdicks EF, Eelco FM, Plevak DJ, et al: Causes and outcome of seizures in liver transplant recipients. Neurology 47:1523–1525, 1996

Wijdicks EF, Dahlke LJ, Wiesner RH: Oral cyclosporine decreases severity of neurotoxicity in liver transplant recipients. Neurology 52:1708–1710, 1999

Wilson JR, Conwit RA, Eidelman BH, et al: Sensorimotor neuropathy resembling CIDP in patients receiving FK506. Muscle Nerve 17:528–532, 1994

Wilson SE, de Groen PC, Aksamit AJ, et al: Cyclosporin A–induced reversible cortical blindness. J Clin Neuroophthalmol 8:215–220, 1988

Woodman CL, Geist LJ, Vance S, et al: Psychiatric disorders and survival after lung transplantation. Psychosomatics 40:293–297, 1999

Wright L, Pennington JJ, Abbey S, et al: Evaluation of a mentorship program for heart transplant patients. J Heart Lung Transplant 20:1030–1033, 2001

Yang RC, Thiessen-Philbrook H, Klarenbach S, et al: Insurability of living organ donors: a systematic review. Am J Transplant 7:1542–1551, 2007

Yates WR, Booth BM, Reed DA, et al: Descriptive and predictive validity of a high-risk alcoholism relapse model. J Stud Alcohol 54:645–651, 1993

Yates WR, LaBrecque DR, Pfab D: Personality disorder as a contraindication for liver transplantation in alcoholic cirrhosis. Psychosomatics 39:501–511, 1998

Zelikovsky N, Schast AP, Palmer JA, et al: Perceived barriers to adherence among adolescent renal transplant candidates. Pediatr Transplant 12:300–308, 2008

Zipfel S, Schneider A, Wild B, et al: Effect of depressive symptoms on survival after heart transplantation. Psychosom Med 64:740–747, 2002

Zitt N, Kollerits B, Neyer U, et al: Cigarette smoking and chronic allograft nephropathy. Nephrol Dial Transplant 22:3034–3039, 2007

CHAPTER 32

Neurology and Neurosurgery

Alan J. Carson, M.B.Ch.B., M.Phil., M.D., F.R.C.Psych.
Adam Zeman, M.A., D.M., F.R.C.P.
Jon Stone, M.B.Ch.B., Ph.D., F.R.C.P.
Michael C. Sharpe, M.A., M.D., F.R.C.P., F.R.C.Psych.

THE DIVIDE BETWEEN neurology and psychiatry is viewed by many as a historical artifact (Baker et al. 2002). Some psychiatrists have taken on primary responsibility for caring for brain injury, epilepsy, early-onset dementias, and sleep and movement disorders while retaining their more traditional role of diagnosing and treating "psychiatric" disorders in patients with neurological disease. Some neurologists have developed interests in cognitive and behavioral neurology and have focused on disorders traditionally considered to be psychiatric. New developments in neuroscience are bringing an understanding of the mechanisms of interaction between biological, psychological, and social aspects of illness, making this one of the most intellectually fascinating areas of work for a psychiatrist.

Psychiatrists working in a clinical neurosciences center are likely to be required to address four main categories of clinical problems:

1. Cognitive impairment—either as a primary presentation or as a secondary complication of a known condition such as multiple sclerosis
2. Neurological disease accompanied by emotional disturbance in excess of the clinical norm
3. Neurological symptoms that do not correspond to any recognized pattern of neurological disease
4. Postneurosurgery complications—usually involving behavioral, cognitive, or emotional disturbance

In this chapter, we concentrate on commonly encountered neurological conditions—stroke, Parkinson's disease, multiple sclerosis, amnestic syndromes, dementias with additional prominent neurological signs, epilepsy, headache, movement disorders, and conversion disorder—as well as on selected psychiatric aspects of neurosurgery. The principles of assessment applicable to these disorders are also relevant to other, rarer neurological conditions. Psychopharmacological and psychological treatments are not discussed in detail here because they are covered in other chapters. Although we refer to drug therapies, we wish to remind the reader that for many neuropsychiatric conditions, behavioral management and environmental manipulation are of equal importance.

Neuropsychiatric topics covered elsewhere in this book include the mental status examination (Chapter 1, "Psychiatric Assessment and Consultation"), delirium (Chapter 5, "Delirium"), dementia (Chapter 6, "Dementia"), conversion disorder (Chapter 12, "Somatization and Somatoform Disorders"), traumatic brain and spinal cord injuries (Chapter 35, "Physical Medicine and Rehabilitation"), pain syndromes (Chapter 36, "Pain"), and psychopharmacological interventions in neurological disease (Chapter 38, "Psychopharmacology").

Stroke

A cerebrovascular accident, or stroke, is a clinical syndrome characterized by rapidly developing clinical symptoms or signs of a focal (and sometimes global) disturbance of cerebral function of presumed vascular origin and of more than 24 hours' duration. One of two main pathological processes is responsible: cerebral infarction or hemorrhage. *Infarction* may result from thrombosis of vessels or emboli lodged within them. *Hemorrhage* can be either into brain tissue directly or into the subarachnoid space. Infarctions account for 85% of strokes and as a result of their lower immediate fatality rate are a much greater source of enduring disability than are hemorrhages, with approximately 75% survival at 1 year poststroke compared with 33% survival at 1 year after hemorrhage. Strokes are the third most common cause of death in the Western world. The Oxfordshire Community Stroke Project reported a population incidence of 2 per 1,000 for first-ever stroke (Bamford et al. 1988). Age is the major risk factor, although one-quarter of persons affected are younger than 65 years. Stroke occurs more commonly in men.

Psychiatrists are not usually involved in the diagnosis of acute stroke but occasionally are consulted when alterations in cognition, affect, or behavior dominate the clinical picture.

Clinical Features

The classical presentation of *middle cerebral artery* infarction is contralateral hemiparesis and sensory loss of a cortical type. These are often accompanied by hemianopsia if the optic radiation is affected. If the lesion is in the dominant hemisphere, then aphasia may be expected, whereas a lesion in the nondominant hemisphere may be accompanied by neglect, inattention, or perceptual disturbance.

Infarctions affecting the distribution of the *anterior cerebral artery* will lead to contralateral hemiparesis affecting the leg more severely than the arm. A grasp reflex and motor dysphasia may be present. Cognitive changes resembling a global dementia may occur, with incontinence. Residual personality changes (apathy and/or dysexecutive function) of a frontal type can also result.

Posterior cerebral artery infarction presents with a contralateral hemianopsia sometimes accompanied by visual hallucinations, visual agnosias, or spatial disorientation. Transient confusion may obscure the detection of hemianopsia. Vital memory structures are supplied from the posterior cerebral artery, and in some neurologically normal individuals both medial thalamic areas are supplied by a single penetrating artery. Dense amnestic symptoms occur if the hippocampus and other limbic structures are involved bilaterally. Diagnosis may be difficult, because early computed tomography (CT) scan findings are often negative; however, magnetic resonance imaging (MRI) will show the bilateral lesions.

Internal carotid artery occlusion can be entirely asymptomatic, but much depends on the collateral circulation. The clinical picture is often that of middle cerebral artery infarction. However, in some situations, cognitive and behavioral symptoms are predominant.

Vertebrobasilar strokes can be extremely diverse in their manifestations. Total occlusion of the basilar artery is usually rapidly fatal. Partial occlusions typically affect the brain stem, with a combination of uni- or bilateral pyramidal signs and ipsilateral cranial nerve palsies. One variant of brain stem stroke is the "locked in" syndrome, in which total paralysis is accompanied by full alertness and awareness. Occlusions of the rostral branches of the basilar artery can result in infarction of the midbrain, thalamus, and portions of the temporal and occipital lobes. An unusual consequence of basilar artery occlusion can be peduncular hallucinosis, in which patients have vivid, well-formed hallucinations that they recognize as unreal. One patient described seeing his wife growing a full and bushy black beard! States of bizarre disorientation can also occur and can be mistaken for confabulation or even deliberate playacting.

Cognitive Impairment and Delirium

Delirium affects 30%–40% of patients during the first week after a stroke, especially after a hemorrhagic stroke (Gustafson et al. 1993; Langhorne et al. 2000; Rahkonen et al. 2000). It is important to distinguish delirium from focal cognitive deficits affecting declarative memory. Some clinicians recommend the use of structured scales such as the Confusion Assessment Method or the Delirium Rating Scale (McManus et al. 2009b). Predictors of delirium include preexisting dementia, old age, impaired vision, impaired swallowing, and inability to raise both arms (McManus et al. 2009a; Sheng et al. 2006). The presence of delirium after stroke is associated with poorer prognosis, longer duration of hospitalization, increased mortality, increased risk of dementia, and institutionalization (Gustafson et al. 1991; Henon et al. 1999; Reitz et al. 2008).

Dementia following stroke is common, occurring in approximately one-quarter of patients at 3 months after stroke (Desmond et al. 2000; Tatimichi et al. 1994a, 1994b), and this effect is independent of prior cognitive function (Reitz et al. 2008). This figure rises significantly if focal impairments also are considered. *Vascular dementia* is an imprecise term referring to a heterogeneous group of dementing disorders caused by impairment of the brain's blood supply. These disorders fall into three principal categories: subcortical ischemic dementia, multi-infarct dementia, and dementia due to focal "strategic" infarction. Several sets of diagnostic criteria (e.g., the National Institute of Neurological Disorders and Stroke–Association Internationale pour la Recherche et l'Enseignement en Neurosciences [NINDS-AIREN] criteria) are available, with high specificity but low sensitivity for pathologically defined vascular dementia (Hachinski et al. 1974; Roman et al. 1993; Wiederkehr et al. 2008a, 2008b).

The common occurrence of relatively subtle cognitive decline, falling short of frank dementia, in the context of cerebrovascular disease has given rise to the broader concept of "vascular cognitive impairment." Subcortical ischemic dementia and multi-infarct dementia are described in more detail in Chapter 6 ("Dementia"). The term *strategic infarction* describes the occurrence of unexpectedly severe cognitive impairment following limited infarction, often in the absence of classic signs such as hemiplegia. Sites at which infarctions can have such an effect include the thalamus, especially the medial thalamus; the inferior genu of the internal capsule; the basal ganglia; the left angular gyrus (causing Gerstmann's syndrome of agraphia, acalculia, left-right disorientation, and finger agnosia); the basal forebrain; and the territory of the posterior cerebral arteries (Clark et al. 1994; Kumral et al. 1999; Rockwood et al. 1999; Tatimichi et al. 1992, 1995).

Behavioral Changes

The diverse behavioral changes following stroke are not unique to this condition and can therefore serve as a helpful model for understanding the clinical consequences of focal cerebral lesions of other causes (Bogousslavsky and Cummings 2000).

Aphasia

Global aphasia leads to the abolition of all linguistic faculties. Consequently, the physician must draw inferences about mental state from the patient's behavior and nonverbal communication. Some accounts associate Broca's aphasia with intense emotional frustration that may be secondary to problems in social interaction (Carota et al. 2000). Wernicke's aphasia is characterized by a lack of insight accompanied by irritability and rage, with recovered patients reporting that they believed the examiner was being deliberately incomprehensible (Lazar et al. 2000).

Anosognosia

Anosognosia refers to partial or complete unawareness of a deficit. It may coexist with depression (Starkstein et al. 1990), a finding that both implicates separate neural systems for different aspects of emotions (Damasio 1994) and suggests that depression after stroke cannot be explained solely as a psychological reaction to disability (Ramasubbu 1994). Anosognosia for hemiplegia is perhaps the most often described form of the condition, but anosognosia can occur with reference to any function and is commonly associated with visual and language dysfunction. Patients with anosognosia for hemiplegia have no spontaneous complaints and may indeed claim normal movements in the paralyzed limb. Behavioral correlates include attempting to walk normally despite the hemiplegia and paradoxical acceptance of a wheelchair while simultaneously maintaining that one has normal function. In extreme cases, ownership of the limb is denied—or, exceptionally, "extra" phantom limb sensations can occur. Anosognosia occurs more frequently with right-sided lesions, particularly those in the region of the middle cerebral artery (Breier et al. 1995; Jehkonen et al. 2006).

Affective Dysprosodia

Affective dysprosodia is impairment of the production and comprehension of those language components that communicate inner emotional states in speech. These components include stresses, pauses, cadence, accent, melody, and intonation. Affective dysprosodia is not associated with an actual deficit in the ability to experience emotions; rather, it is associated with a deficit in the ability to communicate or recognize emotions in the speech of others. Affective dysprosodia is particularly associated with right-hemispheric lesions. A depressed patient with dysprosodia will appear depressed and say that he or she is depressed, but the patient will not "sound" depressed. This is in contrast to a patient with anosognosia, who will both appear and sound depressed but may deny that he or she is depressed.

Apathy

Apathy is common after stroke, affecting up to 25% of patients, and appears to be distinct from depression (Brodaty et al. 2005). Patients with apathy show little spontaneous action or speech; their responses may be delayed, short, slow, or absent (Fisher 1995). Apathy is frequently associated with hypophonia, perseveration, grasp reflex, compulsive motor manipulations, cognitive impairment, and older age; it is also associated with poor functional outcomes (Hama et al. 2007). Apathy is usually a consequence of frontal or anterior temporal brain injury—in particular, lesions affecting the right fronto-subcortical pathways (Brodaty et al. 2005; Starkstein et al. 1993a).

Depression

Although depression following stroke is commonly defined according to DSM-IV-TR (American Psychiatric Association 2000) or ICD-10 (World Health Organization 1992) criteria (Starkstein and Robinson 1989), the imposition of these categorical diagnoses on patients who have suffered a stroke is problematic because it is often unclear which symptoms are attributable to the stroke and which are attributable to depression (Gainotti et al. 1997, 1999). Which definition is adopted has a substantive effect on prevalence rates of depressive illness after stroke (G. Andersen et al.

1994b; Herrmann et al. 1995; House et al. 2001; Morris et al. 1993a; Parikh et al. 1990; Pohjasvaara et al. 2001). Most studies suggest that poststroke depression is a common problem, affecting about one-quarter of stroke patients, although some high-quality studies have reported significantly lower prevalence rates (Brodaty et al. 2007). One solution to the dilemma of differential diagnosis is to focus on symptoms other than somatic ones, using scales specifically designed for that purpose, such as the Hospital Anxiety and Depression Scale and the Geriatric Depression Scale (Sivrioglu et al. 2009). Carota et al. (2005) persuasively argued that particular attention should be paid to crying and overt sadness. However, dismissing the somatic elements of depression may not be an adequate solution, given that the neurobehavioral consequences of cerebral lesions—such as aphasia, indifference, denial, cognitive impairment, and dissociation of subjective from displayed emotion—can obscure and complicate the diagnosis of depression. Most clinicians take a pragmatic approach, treating depression if the patient has symptoms suggestive of low mood or anhedonia accompanied by some somatic symptoms (e.g., insomnia, anorexia) as well as signs of lack of engagement with the environment (e.g., poor participation in physiotherapy).

Most epidemiological studies have suggested an association between depression and increased disability (G. Andersen et al. 1994b; Herrmann et al. 1995; Parikh et al. 1990; Pohjasvaara et al. 2001) and possibly mortality (House et al. 2001; Morris et al. 1993a). However, the direction of causality is unclear and is most probably circular. Some, but not all, pharmacological treatment studies have suggested that effective treatment of the depression leads to a reduction in overall disability (G. Andersen et al. 1994a; Lipsey et al. 1984).

There has been much speculation over the etiological mechanisms of depression after stroke, and emphasis has been placed on the site of the stroke lesion. One hypothesis put forward is that left frontal lesions are associated with an increased rate of depressive illness (Starkstein and Robinson 1989). There are, however, several limitations to this theory. First, it has been consistently found that patients with a premorbid history of depression are at higher risk of developing depression after stroke (G. Andersen et al. 1995). Second, it has proved impossible to clinically distinguish left frontal depression from depression associated with lesions in other brain regions (Gainotti et al. 1997). Finally, a meta-analysis reported that the available scientific literature did not support the left frontal hypothesis (Carson et al. 2000a).

It is generally recommended—but has not been conclusively demonstrated—that treatment for depression should be started early in order to maximize functional outcome. However, disappointingly few randomized controlled trials have tested this recommendation. Most studies suggest an improved outcome in mood with early treatment, but the effect on measures of functioning have been generally disappointing (G. Andersen et al. 1994a; Chemerinski et al. 2001; Gainotti et al. 2001; Hackett et al. 2008a, 2008b; Lipsey et al. 1984; Robinson et al. 2000; Wiart et al. 2000). Although both selective serotonin reuptake inhibitors (SSRIs) and tricyclic antidepressants (TCAs) have been reported to be effective, the SSRIs are probably preferable because they have fewer adverse effects, particularly for patients in whom cognitive or cardiac function is compromised. Nonetheless, this greater tolerability must be balanced against the finding that nortriptyline was more effective than fluoxetine in the only trial that compared these agents (Robinson et al. 2000). What is clear is that all stroke patients receiving antidepressants should be closely monitored for both treatment effectiveness and adverse drug effects. Whether due to lack of detection or concern about side effects, there is substantive evidence that depression after stroke tends to be undertreated (Paul et al. 2006). The adoption of a care management approach appears to confer significant advantages in the delivery of treatment (Williams et al. 2007). Psychological treatment—in particular, cognitive-behavioral therapy (CBT)—offers a potential solution for patients for whom pharmacotherapy is ineffective or contraindicated, but thus far, psychological approaches have received only limited support (Hackett et al. 2008b; Kneebone and Dunmore 2000; Lincoln and Flannagan 2003). Furthermore, it is likely that only a minority of patients with poststroke depression are suitable for such treatment (Lincoln et al. 1997).

A number of studies have examined the effectiveness of early interventions intended to prevent depression from developing after stroke. A 2008 Cochrane review found that antidepressant drugs were ineffective in preventing the development of depression (Hackett et al. 2008a)—although there have been dissenting voices (Chen et al. 2007)—but that there might be modest benefits to be gained from problem-solving therapy (Hackett et al. 2008a). However, a subsequent comparison of the antidepressant drug escitalopram and problem-solving therapy found the former to be more efficacious (Robinson et al. 2008); the trial itself and the relative effectiveness of treatments remains a controversial issue (J. Leo and Lacasse 2009; Robinson and Arndt 2009; Robinson and Penningworth 2009), and further studies are clearly required.

Anxiety

Anxiety disorders are common after stroke and probably share the same risk factors as depression (Astrom 1996). Estimates of prevalence have varied markedly, depending on whether the investigators subsumed anxiety symptoms within the construct of major depressive disorder. Thus, the reported prevalence of generalized anxiety disorder ranges from 4% to 28% (Astrom 1996). However, the percentage of patients experiencing anxiety symptoms appears to be 25%–30% (Burvill et al. 1995; De Wit et al. 2008). Female gender, a prior history of anxiety, and early symptoms of anxiety seem to be the main predictors (Morrison et al. 2005).

Stroke is a sudden and unpredictable life-threatening stressor and, not surprisingly, a highly aversive experience (McEwen 1996). Poststroke anxiety states may include posttraumatic stress symptoms, with compulsive and intrusive revisiting of the event, as well as health worries, with checking and reassurance seeking about the risk of recurrence (Lyndsay 1991). These worries can be associated with agoraphobia and the misinterpretation of somatic anxiety symptoms, especially headache and dizziness, as evidence of recurrence. Phobic states have a prevalence of 5%–10%, with an excess found in women (Burvill et al. 1995). Although there is a paucity of controlled-trial evidence, it is our experience that these symptoms respond to standard drug and behavioral therapies.

Emotional Lability

Emotionalism, or emotional lability, is an increase in laughing or crying that occurs with little or no warning. It is frequent in acute stroke but can also occur with delayed onset (Berthier et al. 1996; Cummings et al. 2006). The displayed emotions are not related to the patient's internal emotional state. Whether emotional lability is associated with depression is a moot point; both conditions can exist independently (House et al. 1989; Robinson et al. 1993). Others have suggested a link to executive dysfunction (Tang et al. 2009), although the experimental data show fairly weak correlations.

It has been suggested that the neurological basis is in serotonergic systems and that there is a specific response to SSRIs (G. Andersen et al. 1994a; Choi-Kwon et al. 2006). In practice, the evidence is contradictory, with reports of equivalent response to TCAs as well (House et al. 2004; Robinson et al. 1993). There is no consistently reported associated lesion location; pontine, subcortical, and frontal lesions have all been found (G. Andersen et al. 1994a; Derex et al. 1997; Morris et al. 1993b).

Catastrophic Reactions

Catastrophic reactions manifest as disruptive emotional behavior precipitated when a patient finds a task unsolvable (K. Goldstein 1939). The sudden, dramatic appearance of such marked self-directed and stereotypical anger or frustration can be startling for both staff and relatives. This symptom is often associated with aphasia, and it has been suggested that damage to language areas is a critical part of the etiology (Carota et al. 2001). Catastrophic reactions generally occur independently of depression in acute stroke; however, many patients who show early catastrophic reactions go on to develop depression (Starkstein et al. 1993b).

Psychosis

Psychosis—and, in particular, mania—has been observed following acute stroke. Its true incidence is unknown, although a rate of 1% has been reported (Starkstein et al. 1987). Psychotic symptoms have generally been associated with right-sided lesions (Cummings and Mendez 1984; Lampl et al. 2005), although we would suggest caution in accepting such claims. Old age and preexisting degenerative disease seem to increase the risk (Starkstein 1998) (see Chapter 10, "Psychosis, Mania, and Catatonia," for further details and treatment considerations). Reduplicative paramnesias can occur: one memorable patient believed he was being treated on a cruise liner; on looking out of the window and seeing hospital porters delivering goods, he surmised that the ship must be in "dry dock." Such paramnesias are usually short-lived, although a small number of chronic cases have been reported (Vighetto et al. 1980).

Obsessive-Compulsive Disorder

Obsessive-compulsive disorder (OCD) has been reported after cerebral infarctions, particularly those affecting the basal ganglia (Maraganore et al. 1991; Nighoghossian et al. 2006; Rodrigo et al. 1997).

Hyposexuality

Hyposexuality is a common complaint after stroke in both men and women (see also Chapter 16, "Sexual Dysfunction"). The symptoms generally are nonspecific, although health worries concerning body image and fear of recurrence may also be relevant. A relationship between reduced libido and emotionalism has also been proposed, suggesting a common serotonergic dysfunction (Kim and Choi-Kwon 2000).

Executive Function Impairment

Executive function, which includes decision making, judgment, and social cognition, is regulated by complex systems that are relatively resistant to damage after stroke (Carota et al. 2002; Zinn et al. 2007), although executive function is commonly impaired as part of a general dementia.

Inhibition Dyscontrol

Deficit of inhibition control occurs with impulsive behavior. The most striking examples of inhibition dyscontrol are grasp reflexes in patients with frontal lesions, but utilization behavior (a tendency to use objects present in the environment automatically), hyperphasia, and hypergraphia have all been described. Such behavior tends to improve during the first few months after stroke (Carota et al. 2002).

Loss of Empathy

Loss of empathy has been reported after bilateral orbitofrontal lesions (V.E. Stone et al. 1998). It has been suggested that this difficulty in understanding and adapting to the needs of others may underlie many of the personality changes associated with frontal lesions. These changes include lack of tact, inappropriate familiarity, loss of initiative and spontaneity, childish behavior, sexual disinhibition, and poverty of emotional expression (Carota et al. 2002).

Parkinson's Disease

Parkinson's disease (PD) is a degenerative condition traditionally characterized by motor features of tremor, rigidity, and bradykinesis. The nonmotor features are, however, numerous and include cognitive and psychiatric symptoms.

Incidence

Two incidence studies of PD, one in Minnesota (Bower et al. 1999) and one in Finland (Kupio et al. 1999), estimated 10.8 cases per 100,000 person-years and 17.2 per 100,000 population, respectively. Both studies found a slight excess in men and confirmed that incidence increases with age. The Finnish study also suggested that PD was more common in rural areas.

Etiology

The cause of PD remains unknown. Genetic forms of the disease have been described, but the implicated genes are not identified in most patients. Similarly, environmental causes have been suggested, but no single exposure has been consistently replicated, with the exception of cases associated with MPTP (1-methyl-4-phenyl-1,2,3,6-tetrahydropyridine) (Tanner and Aston 2000). Cigarette smoking is associated with decreased risk (Gorell et al. 1999).

Clinical Features

The core feature of PD is the triad of tremor, rigidity, and bradykinesia (Sethi 2002). Bradykinesia—usually of insidious onset and easily misdiagnosed as depression or boredom—is the most common first sign and ultimately is the most disabling symptom. Resting tremor is the most characteristic feature of PD, affecting more than 70% of patients. In the early stages of the disease, the tremor is described as "pill-rolling." The rigidity manifests as fixed abnormalities of posture and resistance to passive movement throughout the range of motion, often with a "cogwheel" sensation. Postural instability is a common additional feature, giving rise to an increasing liability to falls as the disorder progresses. Abnormal involuntary movements are a result both of the disease process and of dopaminergic therapy. Freezing of gait is particularly distressing to patients, but it is one of the most poorly understood features of PD, because such freezing may occur in response to visual cues (especially freezing during "off" periods), it can be misdiagnosed as willful behavior.

Nonmotor manifestations are common in PD and include autonomic (in particular, orthostatic hypotension and bladder and gastrointestinal dysfunction), sensory (pain), olfactory, sleep, cognitive, and other psychiatric symptoms.

Cognitive Features

Dementia with Lewy bodies (DLB), PD, and PD with dementia share common features, motor symptoms, and responses to treatment. The boundaries between these disorders are not distinct. Hallucinations and delusions occur in 57%–76% of DLB cases, in 29%–54% of cases of PD with dementia, and in 7%–14% of cases of PD without dementia (Aarsland et al. 2001). Delusions are often paranoid in type and mainly involve persecution and jealousy. Hallucinations usually occur in the presence of intact insight and frequently are visual and phenomenologically similar to those of Charles Bonnet syndrome (Diederich et al. 2000); these hallucinations are typically nonthreatening, worse at night, and often involve children and animals (Papapetropoulos et al. 2008).

In the early days of levodopa (L-dopa) treatment, adverse psychiatric reactions were reported in 10%–50% of patients (Goodwin 1971). Psychosis occurred in about 10% of patients initially, but this percentage rose to 60% after 6 years of treatment (R.D. Sweet et al. 1976). The addition of carbidopa to L-dopa made this adverse effect less common. More recent studies have suggested that dopaminomimetic medication is a significant risk factor for psychosis (Aarsland et al. 1999). Other studies have found correlations between psychotic symptoms and higher rates of cognitive dysfunction and depression (Ozer et al. 2007) but no association with dosage or length of exposure to dopaminomimetic medication (Giladi et al. 2000). The most likely etiology of psychosis in PD is a combination of cortical Parkinson's pathology and age-related loss of central cholinergic function. This is corroborated by the fact that psychotic symptoms in PD are often part of nondopaminomimetic medication–induced toxic (i.e., delirious) states and that psychosis was commonly reported in the pre-levodopa era (Wolters and Berendse 2001). Cognitive impairment and sleep disruption are predictive of the development of psychosis (Arnulf et al. 2000). Clinically, one should seek to distinguish dopaminomimetic medication-related psychosis from delirium of acute onset with disorientation, impaired attention, perceptive and cognitive disturbance, and alterations in the sleep-wake cycle. A true dopaminomimetic psychosis is a subacute, gradually progressive psychotic state unaccompanied by a primary deficit of attention. Delirium may be induced by drugs used in the treatment of PD, such as selegiline and anticholinergic medication.

Active treatment for dopaminomimetic psychosis is recommended only if symptoms begin to interfere with daily functioning. Dosage reduction of dopaminomimetic drugs is seldom effective, and antipsychotic drugs are often required (Wolters and Berendse 2001). The atypical antipsychotic drugs clozapine and quetiapine are preferred (Cummings 1999; Rabinstein and Shulman 2000), and high-potency typical antipsychotics should be avoided (see Chapter 10, "Psychosis, Mania, and Catatonia"). Early promising results suggesting a role for cholinesterase inhibitors in the treatment of dementia in PD have not been followed up with subsequent trials (McKeith et al. 2000; Ravina et al. 2005).

Emotional Symptoms

Depression is a common symptom in PD, with a prevalence of around 40%–50%. Timing of onset shows a bimodal distribution, with peaks during early and late stages of the disease (Cummings and Masterman 1999). Several large-scale studies have demonstrated that depression is one of the major determinants of quality of life in PD (Findlay 2002; Peto et al. 1995). The extent to which depression is caused by brain pathology as opposed to a psychological reaction to disability is unknown.

The diagnosis of depression in PD is difficult, because many depressive symptoms overlap with the core features of Parkinson's—motor retardation, attention deficit, sleep disturbance, hypophonia, impotence, weight loss, fatigue, preoccupation with health, and reduced facial expression. Therefore, anhedonia and sustained sadness are important diagnostic features, particularly if they are out of proportion to the severity of motor symptoms (D.J. Brooks and Doder 2001).

Mood changes can accompany the late-stage fluctuations in response to levodopa (known as "on-off" phenomena), and some patients fulfill criteria for major depressive disorder during the "off" phase but not during the "on" phase (Cantello et al. 1986; Menza et al. 1990). Bipolar mood changes reflecting the on-off phases have also been described (Keshavan et al. 1986). There is currently insufficient evidence to offer definitive recommendations for treatment of depression in PD (J. Andersen et al. 1980; Olanow et al. 2001; Rabey et al. 1996; Shabnam et al. 2003; Wermuth et al. 1998). Although SSRIs are popular, there have been case reports of exacerbation of motor symptoms with fluoxetine, citalopram, and paroxetine (Ceravolo et al. 2000; Chuinard and Sultan 1992; Jansen Steur 1993; R.J. Leo 1996; Tessei et al. 2000). In small-scale trials, TCAs have led to better motor outcomes than have SSRIs; however, TCAs with marked anticholinergic activity (e.g., amitriptyline) should be used with caution because of their potential adverse effects on cognition and autonomic function (Olanow et al. 2001). It may be that drugs such as mirtazapine will offer a compromise (Pact and Giduz 1999). It has been suggested that the non-ergot dopamine agonist pramipexole improves both mood and motivation in PD (Armin et al. 1997; Barone et al. 2006). Case report data suggest that both electroconvulsive therapy (ECT) and transcranial magnetic stimulation (TMS) can be used to treat depression in PD, although TMS is associated with short-lived adverse effects and seizures (Fregni et al. 2004; George et al. 1996; Olanow et al. 2001). The use of ECT in PD is reviewed in Chapter 40, "Electroconvulsive Therapy."

Anxiety phenomena are common in PD; they tend to occur later in the disease process than depression and are more closely associated with severity of motor symptoms (Witjas et al. 2002). In particular, marked anticipatory anxiety related to freezing of gait is common. Treatment with antidepressant drugs (Olanow et al. 2001) and CBT, particularly if delivered in conjunction with an active physiotherapy program, can be helpful. Occasionally, benzodiazepines may be required.

Medication-Related Impulse-Control Disorders

In recent years there has been increased recognition of complex behavioral problems associated with dopamine receptor stimulation in PD (Weintraub et al. 2006). These problems include pathological gambling, hypersexuality, punding (intense fascination with and repetitive handling, examining, sorting, and arranging of objects), compulsive shopping, and compulsive medication use. Sometimes described as "dopamine dysregulation syndrome" (Voon et al. 2007), these behaviors appear to affect up to 14% of patients with PD. Many patients are secretive about these behaviors and will not volunteer the symptoms unless specifically asked.

The etiology of these impulsive behaviors is believed to be linked to dopamine agonist use, although there is not a clear dose-related effect. It has been postulated that neuronal sensitization, particularly in mesolimbic dopaminergic tracts, to the intermittent administration of dopamine agonists leads to an increased behavioral response to similar levels of psychostimulation (Evans et al. 2006; Pessiglione et al. 2006). This process can be modified by a genetic predisposition to risk taking (there is a general association between PD and low risk-taking traits) and the environment. It is believed that younger age at onset, right-sided onset, and executive cognitive impairments can facilitate this.

Management involves transitioning patients from dopamine agonists to L-dopa and, if possible, reducing the total L-dopa dose. Several small trials have suggested some benefit for impulse-control disorders from SSRI antidepressants and antiandrogens (in hypersexuality). In one case series, subthalamic deep-brain stimulation resulted in improvement of pathological gambling in PD patients (Ardouin et al. 2006); however, a recent meta-analysis cautioned that a history of impulse-control disorders was a risk factor for postoperative suicide (Voon et al. 2007).

Sleep Disorders

Sleep disturbance is a very common symptom in PD. Rapid eye movement (REM) sleep behavior disorder, in which the sufferer acts out his or her dreams, may precede the onset of motor symptoms in PD by many years (Postuma et al. 2006). Daytime somnolence may also be a problem. There is increasing recognition that sudden somnolence can occur in PD, especially in relation to dopaminergic medication. Patients should therefore be warned about this possibility.

Multiple Sclerosis

Multiple sclerosis (MS) is a demyelinating disorder of the central nervous system (CNS) that causes some degree of cognitive impairment in almost half of cases and that can present with unexplained subcortical dementia. It can also be accompanied by affective disorders. The presence of high signal abnormalities on T2-weighted MRI and of oligoclonal bands of immunoglobulin in the cerebrospinal fluid (CSF) helps to confirm the diagnosis.

Demyelinating diseases are the most common nontraumatic cause of chronic neurological disability in young adults. Although a number of inflammatory demyelinating diseases can affect the CNS after vaccinations or systemic viral infection (collectively referred to as acute disseminated encephalomyelitis [ADEM]), MS is by far the most common of these. Other neuroinflammatory conditions include neurosarcoidosis and vasculitis (including cerebral lupus).

MS can occur at any age, but the median age at onset is 24 years, with a tendency for relapsing-remitting disease to present earlier than primary progressive MS. MS is more common in women. Epidemiological studies suggest that an exogenous or environmental factor, possibly viral infection, plays a part, although its nature remains unclear. The prevalence of the disorder rises with increasing distance from the equator which has given rise to theories that vitamin D deficiency may be a factor. Genetic factors appear to influence susceptibility. A family history in a first-degree relative increases the risk some 30- to 50-fold: the risk for siblings is usually estimated to be 3%–5%, with that for children slightly lower (Franklin and Nelson 2003).

Common neurological syndromes occurring at or close to the onset of MS include optic neuritis (unilateral visual impairment, usually painful), evolving sensory loss, and upper-motor-neuron or cerebellar disorders of the limbs and gait. These deficits typically develop and remit over the course of weeks and result from conduction block in regions of CNS inflammation. Transient worsening of function, lasting for minutes, can occur in partially demyelinated axons as a result of physiological changes (e.g., increase in body temperature). Positive symptoms, including Lhermitte's sign (electric shock–like sensations on flexing the neck) and trigeminal neuralgia, can also occur. Over time, the remissions and relapses of MS tend to give way to a progressive worsening of disability. A minority of patients present with a primary progressive form of the disease, with gradual worsening from onset without remissions (McDonald et al. 2001).

MS is characterized by multifocal areas of inflammatory demyelinating white matter lesions with glial scar formation and (as now recognized) axonal loss (Trapp et al. 1998). However, in recent years there has been emerging evidence of extensive gray matter and subpial lesions. These cortical lesions show distinct pathological features, with a notable lack of T cell and B cell infiltration, microglia activation, and astrogliosis. It has been suggested that this a neurodegenerative process that primarily affects cingulate, frontal, and temporal structures. It appears particularly relevant to the neuropsychiatric clinical features of MS. There is a general theoretical shift toward regarding MS as an inflammatory neurodegenerative condition (Stadelmann et al. 2008).

Patients with unsuspected MS may first present to psychiatrists with changes in cognitive function (Zarei et al. 2003), mood, or personality. More often, however, psychiatrists are involved in the treatment of established cases. MS demonstrates the interactive nature of many of the common symptoms of diffuse neurological disease, in particular the "vicious cycle" of mood symptoms, pain, and fatigue, necessitating intervention across the spectrum of complaints in order to improve outcome.

Cognitive Impairment

Cognitive impairment affects at least half of all patients with MS (W.W. Beatty et al. 1989; Heaton et al. 1985; Rao 1986; Rao et al. 1991). Impairment, when present, is generally a "subcortical dementia" with impaired attention and speed of processing as the hallmark signs. Executive function deficits are common. Deficits in working, semantic, and episodic memory are reported, but procedural and implicit memory functions are generally preserved. Cortical syndromes such as aphasia, apraxia, and agnosia are relatively rare. Neuropsychological tests such as the Paced Auditory Serial Addition Test (PASAT) appear most sensitive to changes (Hoffmann et al. 2007). At the bedside, tests of verbal fluency are of the most value. In general terms, processing speed is usually more impaired than accuracy (Henry and Beatty 2006). MRI studies show that cognitive impairment correlates with general atrophy; however, attempts to link specific cognitive deficits with particular gray or white matter lesions have so far yielded conflicting results (Rovaris et al. 2006). There is a paucity of well-designed studies on the effects of disease-modifying agents (e.g., beta interferon) on cognition and little evidence as to the utility of acetylcholinesterase inhibitors (Amato et al. 2006). There is slightly more robust evidence showing the utility of treating comorbid depression when present (Feinstein 2006).

Psychosis

A well-conducted population study has challenged the perceived orthodoxy that MS is not associated with an increased risk of psychosis (Patten et al. 2005b). The authors reported an increase in rate of psychosis to 2%–3%, with the highest prevalence, 4%, in 15- to 24-year-olds. In addition, the literature contains numerous case reports of well-described psychosis in MS.

Mood Disorders

Mood disorders are common in MS, with more than half of patients reporting depressive symptoms. Depression may be a direct physiologically mediated consequence of the disease, a psychological reaction to the illness, a complication of pharmacotherapy, or coincidental. Mania and emotional lability are also frequently reported (Joffe et al. 1987; Sadovnick et al. 1996) (see also Chapter 8, "Depression," and Chapter 10, "Psychosis, Mania, and Catatonia").

It is important to distinguish depression from the fatigue and pain that are commonly associated with MS (see subsections "Fatigue" and "Pain" below). As in stroke, there has been an attempt to separate out a "biological" depression from a "psychological reactive" depression (Patten and Metz 1997) and to link symptoms to the site of the brain lesions (Fassbender et al. 1998; Honer et al. 1987; Pujol et al. 1997). However, supporting evidence has been inconsistent and hampered by small study samples; for this reason, it appears to be more productive to consider depression in MS as multifactorial. There are few randomized controlled trials of antidepressant drug therapy in MS, but those available suggest modest efficacy for these agents (Feinstein 1997), similar to their efficacy for depression associated with neurological illness in general (Schiffer and Wineman 1990).

Interferon-beta therapy was reported to cause depression (and fatigue) in 40% of MS patients in an open-label trial (Neilley et al. 1996). However, depression is highly prevalent in untreated MS, and other studies have found no increase in depression following interferon-beta therapy (Patten and Metz 2001; Zephir et al. 2003). In one prospective study, the rate of depression actually fell with interferon-beta treatment (Feinstein et al. 2002). This discrepancy may lie in the fact that interferon-beta, particularly early in therapy, can cause symptoms that are mislabeled as depression (Patten et al. 2005a).

Fatigue

Fatigue is the most common single symptom in MS, affecting 80% of those with the disease (Fisk et al. 1994; Freal et al. 1984). It is generally a disabling and aversive experience and affects motivation as well as physical strength. It is important to differentiate fatigue from depression, adverse medication side effects, or pure physical exhaustion secondary to gait abnormalities, because management may differ (Multiple Sclerosis Council for Practice Guidelines 1998). The mechanism of fatigue is poorly understood and almost certainly multifactorial. A number of agents, including amantadine (Krupp et al. 1995; Pucci et al. 2007), 4-aminopyridine (Polman et al. 1994), 3,4-diaminopyridine (Sheean et al. 1997), and modafinil (Rammohan et al. 2002) and other stimulants, have been advocated, but results of studies with these drugs have been inconclusive. Some patients respond to SSRIs or bupropion, and CBT was found to be beneficial in one randomized controlled trial (van Kessel et al. 2008).

Pain

Pain, both acute and chronic, is a common and disabling complication of MS. One study found that one-quarter of MS patients in a large community-based sample had severe chronic pain (Ehde et al. 2003). Mechanisms may include dysesthesia, altered cognitive function, and other MS complications such as spasticity. Of the acute pain syndromes, trigeminal neuralgia is the most common and usually responds to carbamazepine (Thompson 1998). Widespread chronic pain is more frequent and harder to manage. There are small randomized controlled trials showing some benefit of lamotrigine (Breuer et al. 2007), levetiracetam (Rossi et al. 2009), and cannabinoids (Rog et al. 2005) for central pain syndromes in MS. Dysesthetic limb pain is particularly troublesome; treatment is usually with amitriptyline or gabapentin (Samkoff et al. 1997). Pain in the lumbar area, by contrast, usually tends to respond better to physiotherapy than to analgesia (Thompson 1998; see also Chapter 36, "Pain").

Amnestic Syndromes

The amnestic or amnesic syndrome is an abnormal mental state in which learning and memory are affected out of proportion to other cognitive functions in an otherwise alert and responsive patient (Victor et al. 1971). The most common cause of amnestic states is Wernicke-Korsakoff syndrome, which results from nutritional depletion, particularly thiamine deficiency. Other causes include carbon monoxide poisoning, herpes simplex encephalitis and other CNS infections, limbic encephalitis, hypoxic and other acquired brain injuries, stroke, deep midline cerebral tumors, and surgical resections, particularly for epilepsy. In the majority of cases, the pathology lies in midline or medial temporal structures, but there are also case reports of amnestic disorder following frontal lobe lesions.

Wernicke-Korsakoff Syndrome

Wernicke-Korsakoff syndrome results from thiamine depletion, and any cause of such depletion can lead to the syndrome—including, for example, hyperemesis gravidarum and gastric bypass surgery. However, the overwhelming majority of cases are associated with chronic alcohol abuse, which results in both decreased intake and decreased absorption of thiamine. A genetic defect for thiamine metabolism has been described in a small proportion of patients (Blass and Gibson 1977).

The syndrome presents acutely with Wernicke's encephalopathy, which is characterized by confusion, ataxia, nystagmus, and ophthalmoplegia. Peripheral neuropathy can also be present. Parenteral administration of high-dose B vitamins is required as *emergency* treatment if the chronic state of Korsakoff's syndrome is to be avoided. The majority of cases of Korsakoff's syndrome occur following Wernicke's encephalopathy.

On clinical examination, patients with Korsakoff's syndrome may perform well on standard tasks of attention and working memory (serial sevens and reverse digit span) (Kopelman 1985) but may struggle on more complex tasks involving shifting and dividing attention. A severe memory impairment involving both anterograde and retrograde deficits is present (Kopelman et al. 1999). The defective encoding of new information is the core component of this memory disorder (Meudell and Mayes 1982). In addition to a dense anterograde amnesia affecting declarative functions, there is inconsistent, poorly organized retrieval of retrograde memories with a temporal gradient (more impairment for relatively recent than for more remote memories). The retrograde amnesia is more pronounced in diencephalic amnestic syndromes such as Korsakoff's than in amnestic syndromes of hippocampal origin, in which retrograde amnesia is present but with a deficit measured in months rather than years (Kopelman et al. 1999). A limited degree of new learning may be possible, particularly if patients are given a strategy to follow. Confabulation commonly occurs, particularly early in the disorder. Procedural memory remains relatively intact (Schacter 1987).

Other cognitive impairments and behavioral changes may accompany the amnesia. Executive functions are commonly mildly affected, but this impairment may be secondary to chronic alcoholism rather than representing a specific deficit. Disorientation and apathy, often with lack of curiosity about the past, are common, yet such disengaged patients frequently demonstrate labile irritability.

The pathological process is neuronal loss, microhemorrhages, and gliosis in the paraventricular and periaqueductal gray matter (Victor et al. 1971). The mammillary bodies, mammillothalamic tract, and the anterior thalamus are the main structures affected (Mair et al. 1979; Mayes et al. 1988). There is often a degree of generalized cortical atrophy, more marked in the frontal lobes (Jacobson and Lishman 1990). The atrophy may, however, be nonspecific and secondary to alcohol abuse. MRI indicates specific atrophy in diencephalic structures (Colchester et al. 2001; Sullivan and Pfefferbaum 2009).

With vitamin replacement and abstinence from alcohol, the prognosis is fair: one-quarter of patients will recover, half will improve but with some persistent impairment, and one-quarter will show no change (Victor et al. 1971). High-dose B vitamins should be given to all patients acutely and probably continued, but it is unclear how long this therapy should be maintained.

Transient Amnestic Syndromes

Transient amnesia can occur in several contexts. Transient global amnesia (TGA) is a distinctive benign disorder affecting middle-aged or elderly persons, who become amnestic for recent events and unable to lay down new memories for a period of around 4 hours (Hodges and Ward 1989). Repetitive questioning by patients of their companions is a characteristic feature. Episodes can be provoked by physical or emotional stress and are usually isolated; the medium-term recurrence rate is 3% per year (Hodges 1991). There is good evidence that TGA results from reversible medial temporal lobe dysfunction, but the etiological mechanism is uncertain (Stillhard et al. 1990). Although temporal lobe epilepsy occasionally mimics TGA ("transient epileptic amnesia"), episodes are typically briefer (lasting less than an hour), recurrent (several per year), and tend to occur on waking (Butler et al. 2007; Zeman et al. 1998). Other causes of transient amnesia include transient cerebral ischemia (usually accompanied by other neurological symptoms and signs), migraine, drug ingestion, head injury, and dissociative disorders.

Dementias Accompanied by Neurological Signs

Dementia refers to a deterioration of intellectual faculties, such as memory, concentration, and judgment, that is sometimes accompanied by emotional disturbance and personality changes. An approach to management of dementing conditions (including Alzheimer's disease, vascular dementia, dementia with Lewy bodies, frontotemporal dementia, Huntington's disease, Parkinson's disease, and normal-pressure hydrocephalus, among others) is described in detail in Chapter 6, "Dementia." In this section, we concentrate on those disorders that are particularly likely to present with other neurological symptoms, often a movement disorder. Other causes of dementia are also discussed elsewhere in this volume: HIV (see Chapter 28, "HIV/AIDS"), other infections (see Chapter 27, "Infectious Diseases"), alcohol and other substance use (see Chapter 17, "Substance-Related Disorders"), toxic and metabolic conditions (see Chapter 22, "Endocrine and Metabolic Disorders," and Chapter 37, "Medical Toxicology"), rheumatological and inflammatory conditions (see Chapter 25, "Rheumatology"), and traumatic brain injury (see Chapter 35, "Physical Medicine and Rehabilitation").

Huntington's Disease

Huntington's disease (HD), also known as Huntington's chorea, was first described in Long Island in 1872 by George Huntington. This disorder is dominantly inherited and causes a combination of progressive motor, cognitive, psychiatric, and behavioral dysfunction.

Epidemiology

HD occurs at a prevalence of 5–7 per 100,000 population in the United States, with wide regional variations (Chua and Chiu 1994). The sexes are affected equally. Onset can be at any age but most commonly is in young or middle adulthood (Adams et al. 1988; Farrer and Conneally 1985). The disorder exhibits the phenomenon of *anticipation,* in which the age at onset tends to decrease over the generations, especially with paternal transmission (Brinkman et al. 1997) (see subsection "Pathology and Etiology" below).

Clinical Features

Chorea—involuntary, fidgety movements of the face and limbs—is the characteristic motor disorder. As the disease progresses, other extrapyramidal features can develop, including rigidity, dystonia, and bradykinesia, as well as dysphagia, dysarthria, and pyramidal signs (Harper 1991). Childhood-onset HD tends to be dominated by rigidity and myoclonus (the "Westphal variant"). Epilepsy can occur. Cognitive dysfunction goes hand in hand with the motor disorder. The dementia of HD is predominantly "subcortical," with impairment of attention, executive function, speed of processing, and memory (Zakzanis 1998). Psychiatric symptoms and behavioral changes are the norm (Mendez 1994; Zappacosta et al. 1996), with depression, apathy, and aggressiveness present in most cases (Burns et al. 1990; Levy et al. 1998) and psychosis, obsessional behavior, and suicide in a significant minority (Almqvist et al. 1999; Cummings and Cunningham 1992; Folstein et al. 1979). Obsessive behavior appears to be a trait marker in subjects who are gene carriers (see "Pathology and Etiology" below). Depression and irritability frequently precede the development of motor and cognitive symptoms. Psychosis, by contrast, rarely precedes the development of motor symptoms. Apathy tends to correlate positively with disease progression (Paulsen et al. 2005; Van Duijn et al. 2007). Progression to a state of immobility and dementia typically occurs over a period of 15–20 years (Feigin et al. 1995). Cognitive and behavioral changes may predate the clear-cut emergence of symptomatic HD (Kirkwood et al. 1999).

Pathology and Etiology

The key pathological processes of HD occur in the striatum, caudate, and putamen. The loss of small neurons in the striatum is accompanied by neuronal loss in the cerebral cortex, cerebral atrophy, ventricular dilatation, and, eventually, neuronal depletion throughout the basal ganglia (De la Monte et al. 1988; Vonsattel and DiFiglia 1998).

The underlying genetic abnormality in HD is expansion of a "base triplet repeat" of the *IT15* gene on chromosome 4, which codes for the *huntingtin* gene. The normal gene contains 10–35 CAG (cytosine-adenine-guanine) repeats; repeat lengths beyond 39 give rise to symptomatic HD over the course of a normal life span (Duyao et al. 1993). Repeat lengths between 36 and 39 can cause disease. Repeats in the 27–35 range appear to be unstable and liable to increase into the pathological range in the next generation. The tendency for pathologically expanded repeats to increase in length between generations, especially in paternal transmission, underlies the clinical phenomenon of *anticipation.* It has been suggested that the likelihood of psychopathology diminishes with increasing CAG repeat length (Vassos et al. 2008). The function of *huntingtin* remains uncertain.

Investigation and Differential Diagnosis

A number of disorders can cause the combination of chorea and cognitive change seen in HD, including other inherited disorders such as neuroacanthocytosis and dentato-rubro-pallido-luysian atrophy (DRPLA) and acquired disorders such as systemic lupus erythematosus. However, the diagnosis of HD can now be made with confidence by DNA analysis. Counseling by a clinical geneticist is mandatory before presymptomatic testing and should be considered in other circumstances as well (Codori et al. 1997).

Management

Chorea may require treatment, although patients often are not as concerned by it as their caregivers are. A range of agents have been suggested, of which tetrabenazine has the most supportive evidence (Mestre et al. 2009). However, given the cognitive and/or extrapyramidal side effects of the agents used to treat the chorea (neuroleptics, dopamine depleters [e.g., tetrabenazine], or benzodiazepines), this is often best avoided (Rosenblatt et al. 1999). Other psychiatric symptoms should be treated along standard lines (Leroi and Michalon 1998).

Wilson's Disease (Hepatolenticular Degeneration)

First described by Wilson in 1912, Wilson's disease is a very rare, autosomal recessive, progressive degenerative brain disease caused by a disorder of copper metabolism, producing personality change, cognitive decline, extrapyramidal signs, and cirrhosis of the liver.

Clinical Features

The onset of Wilson's disease most commonly occurs in childhood or adolescence but can occur as late as the fifth decade (Bearn 1957). Patients may present to psychiatrists with personality change, behavioral disturbance, depression, irritability, or dementia or to neurologists with a variety of extrapyramidal signs, including tremor, dysarthria and drooling, rigidity, bradykinesia, and dystonia (Walsh 1986; Walsh and Yelland 1992). Although commonly described, schizophreniform psychosis is in fact rare (Akil and Brewer 1995; Dening and Berrios 1989; Shanmugiah et al. 2008). Careful examination reveals these features and also, in virtually all symptomatic cases, the presence of *Kayser-Fleischer rings*—rings of greenish-brown copper pigment at the edge of the cornea (Wiebers et al. 1997). (In suspected cases, an ophthalmologist should be asked to look for this feature with a slit lamp.) The liver failure and the neuropsychiatric syndrome can occur together or independently.

Pathology and Etiology

The causative genetic mutation is in the copper-transporting P-type ATPase coded on chromosome 13 (Bull et al. 1993). The result is excessive copper deposition in the brain, cornea, liver, and kidneys and increased copper excretion in urine. The caudate and putamen are the brain regions most severely affected, but other parts of the basal ganglia and the cerebral cortex are also involved (Mochizuki et al. 1997; Starosta-Rubinstein et al. 1987).

Investigation and Differential Diagnosis

Ninety-five percent of patients with Wilson's disease have low serum levels of the copper-binding protein ceruloplasmin. Normal ceruloplasmin levels and an absence of Kayser-Fleischer rings render the diagnosis very unlikely in cases with neuropsychiatric features (Ferenci 1998). Uncertain cases may require measurement of urinary copper excretion and liver biopsy for measurement of copper content (Pfeil and Lynn 1999). DNA analysis is becoming increasingly available. The differential diagnosis varies with the type of presentation.

Management

Several copper-chelating agents (e.g., penicillamine, tetraethylene tetramine, zinc acetate) are available to treat patients with Wilson's disease, but the risk of significant side effects mandates care by a specialist (Pfeil and Lynn 1999).

Leukodystrophies

Leukodystrophies—recessively inherited or X-linked disorders of myelination—can be accompanied by neuropsychiatric syndromes, usually with associated neurological features. Metachromatic leukodystrophy, caused by a deficiency of the enzyme arylsulfatase A (Hyde et al. 1992), and adrenoleukodystrophy (see also Chapter 22, "Endocrine and Metabolic Disorders"), an X-linked disorder associated with abnormalities of very-long-chain fatty acids (James et al. 1984), are the most commonly encountered types.

Progressive Supranuclear Palsy

Progressive supranuclear palsy is characterized by supranuclear gaze palsy (an inability to direct eye movements voluntarily, especially vertical eye movements, in the presence of normal reflex eye movements); truncal rigidity, akinesia, postural instability, and early falls; bulbar features, with dysarthria and dysphagia; subcortical dementia; and alteration of mood (including pathological crying and laughing), personality, and behavior (De Bruin and Lees 1992). Neurofibrillary tangles, consisting of tau protein, are found in neurons of the basal ganglia and brain stem. Midbrain atrophy may be apparent on MRI.

Corticobasal Degeneration

Corticobasal degeneration typically manifests as a combination of limb apraxia, usually asymmetric at onset, alien limb phenomena, limb myoclonus, parkinsonism, and cognitive decline (Rinne et al. 1994). The neuropsychiatric features tend to be those of "frontal" disorders. Interestingly, unlike other parkinsonian syndromes, visual hallucinations appear to be rare (Geda et al. 2007). The pathology involves neuronal loss in both the basal ganglia and the frontal and parietal cortex, with intraneuronal accumulations of tau protein resembling those seen in progressive supranuclear palsy. MRI usually reveals frontoparietal atrophy.

Transmissible Spongiform Encephalopathies (Prion Dementias)

The transmissible spongiform encephalopathies are a group of rare dementias caused by an accumulation of abnormal prion protein within the brain (P. Brown 2001). Related illnesses occur in animals: indeed, one recently described disorder, variant Creutzfeldt-Jakob disease, is thought to result from infection of humans by consumption of beef products from cattle with bovine spongiform encephalopathy (BSE) (Will et al. 1996). The term *prion,* coined by Stanley Prusiner, stands for "proteinaceous infectious pathogen" (Prusiner 1994, 2001).

Epidemiology

All of the transmissible spongiform encephalopathies are rare. Sporadic Creutzfeldt-Jakob disease, the most common human transmissible spongiform encephalopathy, occurs with an annual incidence of one per million, usually affecting people between the ages of 55 and 70 years (P. Brown et al. 1987). At the time of this writing, variant Creutzfeldt-Jakob disease has been diagnosed in 168 individuals, almost all of them in the United Kingdom. Variant Creutzfeldt-Jakob disease more often develops in younger subjects than does sporadic Creutzfeldt-Jakob disease: most cases have occurred during the second through fourth decades of life (Will et al. 1996).

Clinical Features

Sporadic Creutzfeldt-Jakob disease typically causes a rapidly progressive dementia, with early changes in behavior, visual symptoms, and cerebellar signs. Within weeks to months, marked cognitive impairment develops, often progressing to mutism, with pyramidal, extrapyramidal, and cerebellar signs and myoclonus (P. Brown et al. 1994). The median duration of symptom onset to death is only 4 months, although in rare cases the disorder evolves over several years. Younger patients with sporadic Creutzfeldt-Jakob disease tend to have a more prolonged course and an early symptom profile closer to that of variant Creutzfeldt-Jakob (Boesenberg et al. 2005). Iatrogenic cases of Creutzfeldt-Jakob disease have occurred when CNS tissue from patients with sporadic Creutzfeldt-Jakob disease has unwittingly been transferred from patient to patient by surgical instruments or used in medical procedures as a source of growth hormone, gonadotropins, dura mater, or corneal grafts (P. Brown et al. 2000).

Variant Creutzfeldt-Jakob disease differs markedly from sporadic Creutzfeldt-Jakob disease (M.D. Spencer et al. 2002). The initial symptoms are usually psychiatric, most commonly anxiety or depression, and often of sufficient severity to lead to psychiatric referral. Limb pain or tingling is common early in the course of the illness. After some months, cognitive symptoms typically develop, causing difficulty at school or work, together with varied neurological features including pyramidal, extrapyramidal, and cerebellar signs and myoclonus. The disorder evolves more slowly than does sporadic Creutzfeldt-Jakob disease, with an average duration of 14 months from symptom onset to death.

Three other varieties of human transmissible spongiform encephalopathy have been described. *Kuru,* now extremely rare, causes a cerebellar syndrome with progression to dementia. It is confined to the Fore Indians of Papua New Guinea and was caused by cannibalism of CNS tissues from affected relatives (Gajdusek 1977). *Gerstmann-Straussler-Scheinker syndrome* is an autosomal-dominant prion dementia characterized primarily by cerebellar dysfunction and dementia with a protracted clinical course (Piccardo et al. 1998). *Fatal familial insomnia* is a very rare autosomal dominant prion disorder with severe insomnia and autonomic disturbance manifesting early in the course of the disease (Gambetti et al. 1995).

Pathology and Etiology

The light microscope reveals "spongiform change" in the brains of patients with transmissible spongiform encephalopathies; this change is associated with neuronal loss, gliosis, and deposition of "amyloid." Immunocytochemistry and direct biochemical analysis indicate that the amyloid is composed of a protease-resistant form of prion protein (PrP) (Prusiner 2001).

Investigation and Differential Diagnosis

In sporadic Creutzfeldt-Jakob disease, the electroencephalogram (EEG) shows 1- to 2-per-second triphasic waves in

80% of cases at some time during the course of the illness (Steinhoff et al. 1996). Detection of 14-3-3 protein in CSF has a sensitivity and specificity of approximately 90% for sporadic Creutzfeldt-Jakob disease (Hsich et al. 1996). Brain biopsy is usually diagnostic but is rarely performed. In variant Creutzfeldt-Jakob disease, the EEG and CSF examination are less useful, but characteristic MRI abnormalities (especially high signal in the pulvinar nucleus) are found in a substantial proportion of cases, with a reported sensitivity of 78% and a specificity of 100% (Zeidler et al. 2000). Tonsillar biopsy has also been used as a confirmatory test, because prion protein scrapie (PrPSc) is found in lymphoid tissue in variant Creutzfeldt-Jakob disease (Hill et al. 1999). In suspected cases of familial transmissible spongiform encephalopathy, sequencing of the *PrP* gene will identify the causative mutation.

Management

At present, there is no proven remedy for the disease.

Whipple's Disease

Whipple's disease is rare but important, because it is treatable. Infection with *Tropheryma whippelii* typically causes a multisystem disorder with prominent steatorrhea, weight loss, and abdominal pain (Fenollar et al. 2007; Fleming et al. 1988). CNS involvement is common, and neurological and psychiatric symptoms and signs occur in the absence of systemic features (A.P. Brown et al. 1990; Louis et al. 1996). Small-bowel biopsy, lymph node biopsy, brain MRI, and CSF examination, including polymerase chain reaction studies to identify the causative organism, can all be helpful in diagnosis (Louis et al. 1996). Antibiotic treatment can be effective.

Subacute Sclerosing Panencephalitis

Subacute sclerosing panencephalitis (SSPE) is a rare complication of childhood measles in which intraneuronal persistence of a defective form of the virus in the CNS results in a continuing immune response, with high levels of measles antibody in the CSF. Neurological signs, including myoclonus, accompany the dementia (Garg 2008; Lishman 1997; Risk et al. 1978). Average life expectancy from onset is 1–2 years.

Progressive Multifocal Leukoencephalopathy

Progressive multifocal leukoencephalopathy is caused by activation of JC papovavirus within the CNS in an immunocompromised patient. The resulting demyelination gives rise to pyramidal signs, visual impairment, and a subcortical dementia, usually with progression to death within months (Lishman 1997; Richardson 1961).

Limbic Encephalitis

Limbic encephalitis (LE) is an autoimmune-mediated inflammation centered on the limbic system. It can have a range of psychiatric and neurological presentations, including focal seizures, memory impairment, confusion, and alterations of mood, personality, and behavior (Schott 2006). LE may occur as a paraneoplastic phenomenon or (more often) as a primary autoimmune disease. The diagnosis is supported by MRI, which sometimes shows high signal change in the medial temporal lobes. The CSF often contains oligoclonal bands of immunoglobulin.

Paraneoplastic LE is most commonly caused by small-cell lung cancer, although breast, ovarian, renal, and testicular carcinoma and lymphoma can also be responsible. The tumor may be small and sometimes is initially undetectable by imaging. A range of antineuronal antibodies in serum or CSF may be found, most commonly "anti-Hu." Forty percent of cases are antibody-negative (Darnell and Prosser 2003).

Clues to the diagnosis of an autoimmune LE include hyponatremia and antibodies to voltage-gated potassium channels (Vincent et al. 2004). Some patients improve markedly with immunosuppressive treatment, with corresponding drops in antibody levels (see also Chapter 23, "Oncology").

Hashimoto's Encephalopathy

Hashimoto's encephalopathy, a severe encephalopathic illness manifesting in the presence of high serum antithyroid antibody concentrations, responds dramatically to steroids. Seizures, psychosis, confusion, stroke-like episodes, and raised CSF protein, often with normal MRI findings, are the common features. There is still controversy regarding whether thyroid autoantibodies are the cause of the illness or epiphenomena, leading to calls for the entity to be renamed steroid-responsive encephalopathy with autoimmune thyroiditis (SREAT) (Chong et al. 2003).

Amyotrophic Lateral Sclerosis (Motor Neurone Disease)

Amyotrophic lateral sclerosis (ALS) (known as *motor neurone disease* in Europe) is a neurodegenerative disorder, usually of unknown etiology, typically presenting in the seventh decade with progressive weakness either of limbs (limb onset) or of speech and swallowing (bulbar onset). Five percent to 10% of cases have a genetic basis. The diagnosis is made on the basis of progressive mixed upper and lower motor neuron signs in three limbs or in two limbs with bulbar symptoms (B.R. Brooks et al. 2000). Traditionally, ALS was thought of as one of the few neurodegenerative conditions without neuropsychiatric features. However, it is now clear that ALS has quite specific neuropsychiatric complications.

Around 5% of patients with sporadic ALS and 15% of those with familial ALS develop frontotemporal dementia. This may be a typical frontal syndrome (with impaired executive functions, apathy, and breakdown of social behavior) or a more specific focal dementia, especially primary progressive aphasia and semantic dementia. Because dementia often precedes the onset of motor symptoms, patients with frontotemporal dementia should be monitored for the development of ALS.

A large proportion of patients with ALS can be found to have subtle executive deficits on testing in the absence of symptoms (Abrahams et al. 2005). Emotional lability is also common in ALS, affecting up to 20% of patients (Palmieri et al. 2009).

CNS Tumors, Hydrocephalus, and Subdural Hematoma

CNS tumors, hydrocephalus, and subdural hematoma are discussed in the section "Neurosurgical Issues" later in this chapter.

Epilepsy

Epileptic seizures are transient cerebral dysfunctions resulting from an excessive and abnormal electrical discharge of neurons. The clinical manifestations are numerous. As a result, psychiatrists commonly encounter epilepsy, both when considering whether epilepsy is the primary cause of paroxysmal psychiatric symptoms and when treating its significant psychiatric complications.

Epidemiology

Problems with case definition and ascertainment complicate epidemiological estimates. However, incidence rates of 40–70 per 100,000 population in developed countries and 100–190 per 100,000 in developing countries are generally accepted. The prevalence of active epilepsy is around 7 per 1,000 population in the developed world (Bell and Sander 2001; Kotsopoulos et al. 2002; Sander and Shorvon 1996). Reasons for the higher incidence in developing nations are believed to include increased rates of birth trauma and head injury and lack of health services to manage them, and poor sanitation leading to high rates of CNS infection (e.g., cysticercosis; see Chapter 27, "Infectious Diseases"). Most studies show a bimodal distribution for age of incidence, with increased rates in persons younger than 10 years and older than 60 years. Epilepsy is more common in men and may be more common in black Africans (Sander and Shorvon 1996).

A specific etiological mechanism is identified in less than one-third of cases. These mechanisms include perinatal disorders, learning disabilities, cerebral palsy, head trauma, CNS infection, cerebrovascular disease, brain tumors, Alzheimer's disease, and substance misuse. In addition, many so-called idiopathic seizures are likely to have a genetic basis.

Estimates of seizure recurrence after a first event are widely varied and depend on the population being studied (Cockerell et al. 1997; Sander 1993). However, if seizures are going to recur, they usually do so within 6 months of the first event; the prognosis improves as the seizure-free period lengthens. In patients with established epilepsy, the prognosis is extremely variable. In some benign childhood epilepsies, anticonvulsant medication is unnecessary and remission the rule. In the majority of patients with epilepsy, remission occurs with treatment, and it may be possible to withdraw treatment in the long term. In some epilepsy syndromes, such as juvenile myoclonic epilepsy, treatment is effective but must be continued indefinitely. In around one-third of patients with epilepsy, anticonvulsants fail to provide adequate control of seizures. This is particularly likely in patients with aggressive pediatric epilepsy syndromes (e.g., infantile spasms, Lennox-Gastaut syndrome) or in patients whose epilepsy has a defined structural or congenital cause.

Clinical Features

Epilepsy constitutes a heterogeneous group of disorders with multiple causes, and its clinical features reflect this diversity. The key clinical distinction is between seizures with a focal and seizures with a generalized cerebral origin. The former are more likely to be associated with a detectable and potentially remediable cerebral lesion, whereas the latter are more likely to start in childhood or adolescence and to be familial. Despite the wide variety of possible seizure manifestations, an individual patient's seizures are usually stereotyped. Their clinical features result from a recurrent pattern of cortical hyperactivity during the ictal event followed by hypoactivity in the same area postictally.

Documentation of the clinical features of the seizure is the key to diagnosis. Because firsthand observation is seldom possible unless seizures are very frequent, the history of the episode, including an eyewitness account (or a home/mobile phone video), is of paramount importance.

Tonic-Clonic Seizures

Tonic-clonic seizures are the most dramatic manifestation of epilepsy and are characterized by motor activity and sudden loss of consciousness. In a typical seizure, a patient has no warning (with the possible exception of a couple of myoclonic jerks) of its onset. The seizure begins with sudden loss of consciousness and a tonic phase during which there are sustained muscle contractions lasting 10–20 seconds. This is followed by a clonic phase of repetitive muscle contractions that last approximately 30 seconds. A number of autonomic changes, including increase in blood pressure and pulse rate, apnea, mydriasis, incontinence, piloerection, cyanosis, and perspiration, may also occur. In the postictal period, the patient is drowsy and confused. Abnormal neurological signs are often elicited.

Partial Seizures

Partial seizures are categorized according to whether they are simple (without impairment in consciousness) or complex (with impairment of consciousness). This classification may be difficult to apply in practice, however.

Simple partial seizures. The clinical features of simple partial seizures depend on the brain region activated. Although the initial area is relatively localized, it is common for the abnormal activity to spread to adjacent areas, producing a progression of seizure pattern. If the activity originates in the motor cortex, there will be jerking movements in the contralateral body part. This can cause progressive jerking in contiguous regions (a phenomenon known as "Jacksonian march"). Activity in the supplementary motor cortex causes head turning with arm extension on the same side—the classic "fencer's posture."

Seizures originating in the *parietal lobe* can cause tingling or numbness in a bodily region or more complex sensory experiences such as a sense of absence on one side of the body, asomatognosia. Seizures in the inferior regions of the parietal lobe can cause severe vertigo and disorientation in space. Dominant-hemisphere parietal lobe seizures can cause language disturbance.

Seizures of the *occipital lobe* are associated with visual symptoms, which are usually elementary (e.g., simple flashing lights). However, if the seizure occurs at the border with the temporal lobe, more complex experiences can occur, including micropsia, macropsia, and metamorphosia, as well as visual hallucinations of previously experienced imagery.

Seizures affecting the *temporal lobe* can be the most difficult to diagnose, but this lobe is also the most common site of onset, accounting for 80% of partial seizures. Symptoms may include auditory hallucinations, ranging from simple sounds to complex language. Olfactory hallucinations, usually involving unpleasant odors, follow discharge in the mesial temporal lobe. Seizures in the Sylvian fissure or operculum will cause gustatory sensations; ictal epigastric sensations such as nausea or emptiness generally have a temporal lobe origin. The well-known emotional and psychic phenomena of temporal lobe seizure activity can occur in simple seizures but are more common in complex partial seizures.

Complex partial seizures. In a complex partial seizure, the patient frequently experiences an aura at the onset of the seizure. The aura is a simple partial seizure lasting seconds to minutes. It should be distinguished from a prodrome, which is not an ictal event and which can last for hours or even days before a seizure. Prodromes usually consist of a sense of nervousness or irritability. The content of the aura will depend on the location of the abnormal discharge within the brain. Thus, it may contain motor, sensory, visceral, or psychic elements. These can include hallucinations; intense affective symptoms such as fear, depression, panic, or depersonalization; and cognitive symptoms such as aphasia. Distortions of memory can include dreamy states, flashbacks, and distortions of familiarity with events (déjà vu or jamais vu). Occasionally, rapid recollection of episodes from earlier life experiences occurs (panoramic vision). Rage is rare; when it does occur, it is characterized by lack of provocation and abrupt abatement. This phase is followed by impairment of consciousness and a seizure usually lasting 60–90 seconds, which may generalize into a tonic-clonic seizure. Automatisms may occur and can involve an extension of the patient's actions prior to seizure onset. Common facial automatisms include chewing or swallowing, lip smacking, and grimacing; automatisms in the extremities include fumbling with objects, walking, or trying to stand up. Postictal confusion is usually significant and typically lasts 10 minutes or longer.

Complex partial seizures of frontal lobe origin tend to begin and end abruptly, with minimal postictal confusion. They often occur in clusters. The attacks are usually bizarre, with motor automatisms such as bicycling or with sexual automatisms and vocalizations.

Absence Seizures

Absence seizures are well-defined clinical and EEG events. The essential feature is an abrupt, brief episode of decreased awareness that occurs without any warning, aura, or postictal symptoms. At the onset there is a disruption of activity.

A *simple* absence seizure is characterized by only an alteration in consciousness. The patient remains mobile, breathing is unaffected, and there is no cyanosis or pallor and no loss of postural tone or motor activity. The ending is abrupt, and the patient resumes previous activity immediately, often unaware that a seizure has taken place. An attack usually lasts around 15 seconds. A *complex* absence seizure involves additional symptoms such as loss or increase of postural tone, minor clonic movements of the face or extremities, minor automatisms, or autonomic symptoms such as pallor, flushing, tachycardia, piloerection, mydriasis, and urinary incontinence.

Violent Behavior

Epilepsy, in particular epilepsy involving the temporal lobe, may cause emotional symptoms and very occasionally can result in undirected violent behavior (Kotagal 1997). However, in the majority of cases of epilepsy-related violence, the behavior occurs in response to being restrained during a seizure. One should be very cautious in attributing other violent assaults to a seizure. Indeed, a recent systematic review concluded that overall, patients with epilepsy have a reduced risk for violence compared with control subjects (Fazel et al. 2009). This issue is discussed in more detail in Chapter 7, "Aggression and Violence," which includes criteria for determining whether a violent act resulted from an epileptic seizure.

Differential Diagnosis

Differentiating epilepsy from nonepileptic attack disorder (psychogenic epilepsy or pseudoseizures) and syncope can be difficult (Roberts 1998). Other paroxysmal disorders should also be considered; these include transient ischemic attacks, hypoglycemia, migraine, transient global amnesia, cataplexy, paroxysmal movement disorders, and paroxysmal symptoms in multiple sclerosis. Attacks during sleep can pose particular difficulties, as informant reports are less useful.

Nonepileptic Attack Disorder

Nonepileptic attack disorder (NEAD)—also known as "pseudoseizures," "dissociative seizures," and "psychogenic seizures"—is the most common alternative diagnosis, accounting for about 30% of patients presenting to clinics with suspected epilepsy (Reuber and Elger 2003), and with a reported community prevalence of 33 cases per 100,000 population (Benbadis and Allen 2000). The terminology is confusing, and it is unclear whether NEAD is a specific diagnosis or a collective term for a number of psychiatric diagnoses or symptoms that may cause seizure-like spells, including conversion, panic attacks, hyperventilation syndrome (see Chapter 19, "Lung Disease"), posttraumatic stress disorder (PTSD), and catatonia. We personally favor the view that NEAD is often a variant of panic disorder with prominent dissociation (L.H. Goldstein and Mellers 2006). Although rates of psychiatric comorbidity are higher in patients with NEAD than in those with epilepsy, NEAD patients are paradoxically more likely to have an external locus of control in regard to health and to deny that psychological factors might contribute to their illness (J. Stone et al. 2004). Some patients have both epilepsy and nonepileptic attacks, but probably only about 10% of individuals with NEAD fall into this category (Benbadis et al. 2001; Reuber et al. 2002). Many of these patients are learning disabled and at increased risk of both epilepsy and psychiatric disorders.

The diagnosis of NEAD can often be made on the basis of a careful history and examination. Clinical clues include the presence of prior somatoform disorders; atypical varieties of seizure, especially the occurrence of frequent and prolonged seizures in the face of normal intellectual function and normal interictal EEG; a preponderance of seizures in public places, especially in clinics and hospitals; and behavior during an apparent generalized seizure that suggests preservation of awareness (e.g., resistance to attempted eye opening, persistent aversion of gaze from the examiner). Compared with patients with epilepsy, those with recent-onset NEAD are more likely to think that psychological factors are less important than somatic ones and have a greater tendency to deny nonhealth life stresses (J. Stone et al. 2004). Eye closure during the spell has been considered to be a reliable indicator that a spell is not epileptic (Chung et al. 2006), although this belief has been challenged (Syed et al. 2008). Previous childhood sexual abuse is common but not universal among those with the diagnosis (Binzer et al. 2004). When doubt remains after careful clinical assessment and standard investigations, the gold standard for diagnosis is observation of attacks during videotelemetry. A normal EEG during or immediately following an apparent generalized seizure also provides strong evidence for NEAD. However, surface EEG may be normal during focal seizures.

The diagnosis of NEAD is regarded as distinct from deliberate falsification of attacks (i.e., malingering or factitious disorder). The majority of patients will be cooperative with investigation and diagnosis, even when they know in advance that the purpose is to confirm NEAD and refute epilepsy (McGonigal et al. 2002).

Syncope

Syncope, usually due to temporary interruption of the blood supply to the brain, is often accompanied by myoclonic jerks that are frequently regarded as epileptic by lay and medical onlookers (Lempert et al. 1994). The occurrence of more complex movements, eye deviation, eyelid flicker, or vocalizations can confuse the diagnosis further, as can aura symptoms, which are recalled by the majority of subjects and which include epigastric, vertiginous, visual, and somatosensory experiences (Benke et al. 1997).

Sleep Disorders

Sleep disorders—including sleepwalking, night terrors, and confusional arousals, all of which occur during slow-wave sleep; REM sleep behavior disorder; and a variety of other parasomnias, including bruxism, rhythmic movement disorder, and periodic limb movements—must all be distinguished from epilepsy (see Chapter 15, "Sleep Disorders").

Investigation of Seizures

Epilepsy is above all a clinical diagnosis, and the use and interpretation of tests should reflect this. Routine blood tests should include a complete blood count and routine chemistries, including serum calcium and magnesium. An electrocardiogram (ECG) should always be performed. An EEG is helpful in confirming the diagnosis and in clarifying the type of epilepsy (i.e., generalized versus focal, a distinction particularly relevant for children and adolescents). However, the EEG is insensitive: a single interictal EEG will detect clearly epileptiform abnormalities in only about 30% of patients with epilepsy. Therefore, a normal EEG does not exclude epilepsy, just as minor nonspecific abnormalities do not confirm it. Serial recordings, including sleep-deprived recordings, increase the diagnostic yield to around 80% (Chabolla and Cascino 1997). EEG can be supplemented with video recording to allow examination of the correlation between the clinical symptoms and the EEG abnormalities (videotelemetry). Twenty-four-hour ambulatory monitoring is sometimes helpful.

Some form of neuroimaging should be performed in all patients with epilepsy, unless EEG has clearly demonstrated a syndrome of primary generalized epilepsy in a young patient. CT is adequate to exclude tumors and major structural abnormalities and has the benefit of ease of access in most developed countries; however, CT may miss subtle pathologies. MRI is undoubtedly the imaging modality of choice, capable of detecting pathological abnormalities in up to 90% of patients with intractable epilepsy, including mesial temporal sclerosis (S.S. Spencer 1994). It can, however, be difficult to access in some countries.

Prolactin will rise after a generalized seizure but not, as a rule, after a nonepileptic attack. However, interpretation of the test requires knowledge of the basal prolactin and concurrent drug treatment (e.g., antipsychotics). Partial seizures and syncope can also elevate prolactin (Oribe et al. 1996; Pohlmann-Eden et al. 1997).

Additional cardiac investigations that may be helpful in selected cases include 24-hour ambulatory ECG to identify cardiac dysrhythmias; echocardiography, to identify structural cardiac abnormalities; and tilt-table testing, to help confirm orthostatic syncope.

Psychiatric Complications

Record-linkage studies (Bredkjaer et al. 1998; Jalava and Sillanpaa 1996) have reported an increase in psychotic symptoms, particularly schizophreniform and paranoid psychoses, in men but not women with epilepsy. Studies have also shown a fourfold increase in overall rates of psychiatric disorder in both men and woman with epilepsy compared with individuals in the general population but not compared with patients with other medical diagnoses.

Psychosis

Psychotic symptoms may be categorized as transient postictal psychosis and chronic interictal psychosis. Patients with transient postictal psychosis often present with manic grandiosity with religious and mystical features (Kanemoto et al. 1996b). A number of small studies have suggested that such patients are more likely than other epilepsy patients to have psychic auras, bilateral interictal spikes, and nocturnal secondarily generalized seizures (Devinsky et al. 1995). In general, psychotic episodes do not start immediately after a seizure, but instead occur after a lucid interval of 2–72 hours. In one study, patients with chronic interictal psychosis had a higher frequency of perceptual delusions and auditory hallucinations than did patients with postictal psychoses (Kanemoto et al. 1996a).

Transient psychosis was reported in 1% of patients following temporal lobotomy for epilepsy. Men with right-sided foci who were not seizure free after surgery appeared to be at particular risk for this symptom (Manchanda et al. 1993). There may be an increased risk of postictal psychoses in patients with temporal lobe epilepsy and hippocampal sclerosis (in comparison with those with temporal lobe epilepsy and no sclerosis) (Kanemoto et al. 1996b). How mesial temporal sclerosis relates to psychosis is unclear.

The work of Landolt in the 1950s drew attention to the occurrence of psychosis in some patients in whom epileptiform EEG abnormalities were normalized by treatment ("forced normalization") (Krishnamoorthy and Trimble 1999; Landolt 1958). The concept remains controversial.

Psychosis is also a potential side effect of anticonvulsants, most frequently associated with levetiracetam and topiramate, but also with phenytoin, valproate, lamotrigine, zonisamide, pregabalin, and vigabatrin (Mula et al. 2003). This effect occurs more commonly in patients with a history of psychiatric illness.

Cognitive Disorders

Cognitive disorders are commonly associated with epilepsy (Hermann and Seidenberg 2007). Mild, generalized cognitive deficits, especially in memory, can be detected within months of onset; in children, academic records suggest that these deficits may predate onset (Oostrom et al. 2003). Quantitative volumetric MRI studies suggest associations with temporal lobe abnormalities (Bonilha et al. 2004; Lawson et al. 2002; Woermann et al. 1999). The impairment can be progressive but is not inevitably so, and patients can be reassured that they will not progress to dementia. Poor seizure control and cumulative effects of medication appear to be risk factors for deterioration. The direct impairments can be compounded by the indirect effects of epilepsy on scholastic achievement.

Depressive and Anxiety Disorders

It is well established that epilepsy is a significant risk factor for depressive illness (Jalava and Sillanpaa 1996; Kanner and Balabanov 2002; Stefansson et al. 1998). Depression arising from learned helplessness may occur in patients with epilepsy as a consequence of repeatedly experiencing unpredictable and unavoidable seizures (Weigartz et al. 1999). The stress of having to live with a stigmatized chronic illness may also be relevant. Finally, the antiepileptic drugs used in the treatment of epilepsy can themselves be a cause of depression. The relationship between depression and epilepsy is bidirectional (i.e., each is a risk factor for the other). Depression is an independent risk factor for unprovoked seizures (Hesdorffer et al. 2000). This effect seems to be particularly marked for partial seizures. However, recent data from three population-based studies have also shown that depression is associated with a four- to sevenfold increased risk for developing epilepsy (Kanner 2006). This bidirectional relationship does not imply causality but rather suggests common pathogenic mechanisms shared by both conditions, including abnormal CNS monoamine activity; atrophy of temporal and frontal lobe structures; decreased 5-HT_{1A} binding in mesial structures, raphe nuclei, thalamus, and cingulate; and disruption of the hypothalamic-pituitary-adrenal axis (Kanner 2006). Depressive symptoms not only affect onset of epilepsy but also are associated with poorer response to treatment and reduced quality of life.

Depressive disorders can be typical of their DSM-IV-TR mood disorder description (Jones et al. 2005), can be characterized by their relationship to the ictal event, or can present as "interictal dysphoric disorder" (Kanner et al. 2000). The latter concept was used originally by Kraepelin and then Bleuler to describe a pleomorphic pattern of symptoms consisting of prominent irritability intermixed with euphoria, anxiety, anergia, insomnia, and pain. Interictal dysphoric disorder is said to have a chronic relapsing remitting course but to respond well to antidepressants. Similarly, anxiety in epilepsy may have a complex etiology (M.A. Goldstein and Harden 2000). Anticipatory anxiety related to having a seizure without warning can lead to agoraphobic-like symptoms and behavior.

Treatment of depressive and anxiety disorders in epilepsy is generally the same as that of anxiety and depression in the medically ill (Hermann et al. 2000; see also Chapter 8, "Depression," and Chapter 11, "Anxiety Disorders"). Increased seizure risks associated with specific psychiatric drugs are reviewed in Chapter 38, "Psychopharmacology." Care needs to be taken not to exacerbate the epilepsy, given that TCAs, but not SSRIs, can lower the seizure threshold (Alper 2007). However, this effect is often exaggerated, and, in general, undertreatment has caused far more problems than overtreatment. Similarly, the risk of seizures with bupropion has been overstated in many sources; a systematic review concluded that the risk was lower than that associated with TCAs (Ruffmann et al. 2006).

Treatment

The basic principles of epilepsy treatment are as follows:

1. Use a single drug whenever possible. The Standard And New Antiepileptic Drugs (SANAD) trial has provided additional data on the relative merits of commonly used drugs, with lamotrigine suggested as first-line treatment for focal seizures and sodium valproate for generalized seizures (Marson et al. 2007).
2. Increase the dose slowly until either the seizures are controlled or toxicity occurs.
3. If a single drug does not control seizures without toxicity, then switch initially to another drug used alone.
4. Drug-level monitoring is generally unnecessary except in the case of phenytoin and carbamazepine and is sometimes misleading: some patients do well with drug levels below or above the "therapeutic range."
5. Consider using two drugs only when monotherapy is unsuccessful.
6. Be aware that the metabolism of drugs may be different in the young, the elderly, pregnant women, and patients with chronic disease, particularly chronic hepatic and renal disease, and be on the lookout for drug interactions.

Approximately 20%–30% of patients do not achieve seizure control with drug therapy. In carefully selected cases, surgery can be dramatically effective. Most surgical series report seizure freedom in the range of 50%–85%. The criteria for selection generally include the presence of a focal lesion on neuroimaging, evidence from videotelemetry that the lesion is the source of the habitual seizures, and neuropsychological evidence that resection of the lesion should not cause major cognitive deficits. Psychological factors are also often relevant to the decision to perform surgery (see section "Neurosurgical Issues" later in this chapter).

Vagal nerve stimulation has been shown to reduce seizure frequency in some patients with refractory epilepsy (Privitera et al. 2007), but it probably is no more effective than the addition of the newer anticonvulsants to established therapy.

Tic Disorders

Tics are habitual spasmodic muscular movements or contractions, usually of the face or extremities that are associated with a variety of disorders.

Gilles de la Tourette's syndrome (GTS) is characterized by a combination of multiple waxing and waning motor and vocal tics. These vary from simple twitches and grunts to complex stereotypies. Premonitory sensory sensations in body parts that "need to tic" are a common feature and complicate the picture, because their temporary suppressibility lends them a voluntary component. Other features are echolalia and coprolalia, particularly in severe cases. GTS is strongly associated with OCD but many claim that it is qualitatively different from pure OCD, with greater concern with symmetry, aggressive thoughts, forced touching, and fear of harming oneself in OCD-GTS compared with a more frequent focus on hygiene and cleanliness in pure OCD. Depressive symptoms are common (Cavanna et al. 2009). The prevalence of GTS is about 5 per 10,000 population, with a male:female ratio of 4:1. A debate exists as to whether OCD in itself constitutes a specific psychopathological entity comorbid with GTS or whether diverse pathological disorders—including attention-deficit/hyperactivity disorder (ADHD), eating disorders, anxiety, and substance misuse—should also be considered part of the phenotype. This issue clearly has implications for genetic studies, which have suggested a strong hereditary component in the disorder. Similarly, the neurobiology of GTS remains elusive, with evidence supporting dysfunctions in dopaminergic basal ganglia circuitry receiving the most attention. Structural imaging findings in GTS are usually normal; functional imaging data are contradictory.

A syndrome known as pediatric autoimmune neuropsychiatric disorders associated with streptococcal infection (PANDAS) has been proposed (Swedo et al. 1998), consisting of OCD accompanied by tics with abrupt onset or exacerbation associated with beta-hemolytic streptococcal infection (see Chapter 27, "Infectious Diseases") and the presence of anti–basal ganglia antibodies (ABGA). Studies finding ABGA in PANDAS, Sydenham's chorea, and GTS have excited interest in this area (Martino et al. 2007). However, there is continuing controversy regarding the status of PANDAS, with some studies suggesting that streptococcal infection is just one of many agents that can exacerbate tics (Shulman 2009).

Management of GTS is multidisciplinary, with clear need to address the educational, social, and family consequences of the disorder. Dopamine antagonists remain the mainstay of pharmacological management. Haloperidol has been the most widely used antipsychotic, but many authors advocate use of atypical antipsychotics on the basis of fewer extrapyramidal side effects. Of the newer antipsychotics, risperidone has attracted interest and sulpiride, (not available in the United States) is potentially useful (Scahill et al. 2003). Pimozide was shown to be superior to haloperidol in one of the few randomized controlled trials conducted, but potential cardiac side effects generally limit its use (Pringsheim et al. 2009). Tetrabenazine, a presynaptic monoamine depleter with postsynaptic blockade, has shown considerable efficacy in case series studies (Jankovic and Beach 1997), without a risk of dystonia or tardive dyskinesia but with a high risk of depression. Clonidine is used widely in the United States, but in the United Kingdom its use is generally restricted to patients with comorbid ADHD symptoms (Leckman et al. 1991). Deep brain stimulation is an emerging treatment for severe GTS, although it carries the usual risks of functional neurosurgery and as yet has not been proven in a sham-controlled trial (Servello et al. 2008). Behavioral treatments including habit reversal have also shown promise (Wilhelm et al. 2003). In establishing treatment priorities, one should bear in mind that the associated OCD and ADHD symptoms probably cause more functional and educational disability than the tics themselves. For many patients, tics are only a problem because of the attitudes of others.

Dystonias

The dystonias are a group of disorders characterized by involuntary twisting and repetitive movements and abnormal postures. The traditional clinical categorization is based on age at onset, distribution of symptoms, and site. Early-onset dystonia often starts in one limb, tends to generalize, and frequently has a genetic origin. By contrast, adult-onset dystonias usually spare the lower limbs, frequently involve the cervical or cranial muscles, and have a tendency to remain focal. They appear sporadic in most cases. Dystonias tend to improve with relaxation, hypnosis, and sleep. With the exception of cervical dystonia, pain is uncommon. Erroneous attribution of dystonia to a psychogenic cause was common because of the fluctuating nature of the symptoms, their often dramatic appearance, the ability of patients to use "tricks" to suppress them, and their association with task-specific symptoms (e.g., writer's cramp) (Eldridge et al. 1969). Dystonic movements may, however, be seen as the presentation of a conversion disorder. Psychogenic dystonia typically presents with a fixed posture, usually a clenched fist or inverted plantar-flexed foot (Schrag et al. 2004).

Generalized dystonia is associated with an expanding range of largely autosomal dominant genetic mutations (Geyer and Bressman 2006). The most common generalized dystonia is *primary torsion dystonia,* caused by a mutation in the *DYT1* gene. This usually begins in childhood in one limb and then generalizes to other body parts.

Focal dystonia is the most prevalent form. It starts in adulthood and usually remains localized (e.g., as an isolated torticollis [focal cervical dystonia], writer's cramp, blepharospasm, and musician's dystonia). The majority of cases are sporadic, although some family pedigree studies have shown an increased risk of focal dystonias in other family members.

Dopa-responsive dystonia is characterized by childhood onset, diurnal fluctuation of symptoms, and a dramatic response to L-dopa therapy. It may be confused with spastic paraparesis, leading to diagnostic delay. It generally has autosomal dominant inheritance associated with a mutation in the *DYT5* gene, although recessive forms associated with mutations in the tyrosine hydroxylase gene have been described (Clot et al. 2009).

It is important to remember the role of exposure to medications (e.g., antipsychotics, antiemetics) in the development of both acute and tardive dystonias (R.A. Sweet et al. 1995).

Medical treatment involves botulinum injections, oral drugs, and potentially neurosurgery. Botulinum therapy (both type A and type B) is more effective than placebo for focal dystonias such as cervical dystonia or writer's cramp (Kruisdijk et al. 2007; Snaith and Wade 2008). In generalized dystonia, a trial of L-dopa should be considered in all early-onset cases, given the possibility of dopa-responsive dystonia. Thereafter, oral drug treatment can be tried, although effects are usually disappointing. High-dose anticholinergics such as benzhexol can be of some effect. Occasionally, combination treatment with baclofen, tetrabenazine, and a dopamine antagonist can be considered. Surgical treatment can involve selective peripheral denervation or deep brain stimulation (Kupsch et al. 2006). Comorbid psychiatric disorders are commonly associated with dystonias, particularly OCD, panic disorder, and depression, and they should be actively treated in their own right.

Headache

Acute Headache

Headache of abrupt onset that is very severe and prolonged can be due to *subarachnoid hemorrhage,* usually from a ruptured aneurysm, or to migraine, meningitis, or other cranial infection such as otitis media or sinusitis. The diagnosis of subarachnoid hemorrhage is suggested by the rapidity of onset ("thunderclap" headache, at its worst within 1 minute or so) and associated loss of consciousness, photophobia, vomiting, and neck stiffness. A headache with these features requires immediate neurological referral for assessment with CT scan (which reveals subarachnoid blood in the majority of cases) and lumbar puncture, when CT is negative, to examine for xanthochromia (which is reliably present from 12 hours after subarachnoid hemorrhage) (Al-Shahi et al. 2006). Psychiatrists are predominantly involved in the management of the associated brain injury following subarachnoid hemorrhage. (For a further discussion of these management principles, see the section "Stroke" earlier in this chapter and Chapter 35, "Physical Medicine and Rehabilitation.")

Migraine can mimic subarachnoid hemorrhage. The diagnosis is usually suggested by a history of more typical intermittent headaches with evolving prodromal visual (or other focal neurological) disturbance and a hemicranial throbbing headache, worse on exercise, with photophobia and nausea or vomiting. *Meningitis* is suggested by a severe headache, usually worsening over hours, with photophobia, nausea, and neck stiffness in association with fever and other features of infection. There are many other causes of acute headache, such as spontaneous intracranial hypotension and venous sinus thrombosis.

Chronic Headache

Headache is an almost universal experience (see also Chapter 36 "Pain"). The exhaustive International Headache Society classification of headaches is available free online (http://ihs-classification.org/en/). *Migraine with aura* (previously classical migraine) has the features described above. In migraine without aura (previously common migraine), there is a throbbing hemicranial in the absence of focal neurological symptoms such as visual disturbance. *Tension-type headache* is familiar to most of us as a global headache, usually of mild to moderate severity, sometimes with a "bandlike" or pressing quality. It often worsens as the day goes on or following stress and has few associated symptoms. *Chronic tension-type headache,* defined as more than 15 headache days per month, is just one cause of chronic daily headache (CDH). Most patients with CDH have underlying migraine, which is frequently made worse by *analgesic overuse headache.* Prolonged exposure to any analgesic (not just opiates or ergotamine) can lead to overuse headache; analgesic withdrawal often results in improvement, although this must be done with careful explanation to the patient (Weatherall 2007). Thus, it is important in CDH to assess how much of the problem is migraine versus tension-type headache versus analgesic overuse headache.

A large literature has shown a close, probably bidirectional, association between CDH and psychiatric comorbidity, especially depression and anxiety (Hamelsky and Lipton 2006). The presence of psychiatric comorbidity is associated with poorer outcome. CDH is indicative of the need for more sophistication in our approach to understanding the complex interactions between brain biology, psychological processes, and behavioral responses. Treatment of comorbid mood disorders with antidepressants and CBT can be helpful (Kroenke and Swindle 2000).

Patients with chronic migraine headaches have often been described as having a "typical" personality characterized by conscientiousness, perfectionism, ambitiousness, rigidity, tenseness, and resentfulness; however, controlled studies have not consistently supported this profile. Specific personality traits in migraine appear more likely to be a consequence rather than a cause of suffering from recurrent headaches (Pompili et al. 2009). A community-based survey found more neuroticism and 2.5 times more psychological distress in migraine sufferers than in matched control subjects, but there was no relationship between headache frequency and the severity of psychological distress or personality abnormality (Brandt et al. 1990; Breslau et al. 2003).

Cervicogenic headache is strictly defined by the International Headache Society as headache arising from clearly defined pathology such as tumors, fractures, infections, and rheumatoid arthritis. Cervical spondylosis is a normal feature of aging and cannot be deemed a cause of cervicogenic headache. *Temporal arteritis* is a disorder of older people (it is very rare in persons younger than 55 years) that causes scalp pain and tenderness, jaw claudication, malaise, and an elevated erythrocyte sedimentation rate (usually >50 mm/hour). Treatment with corticosteroids should be started immediately and arrangements made for confirmatory temporal artery biopsy. *Raised intracranial pressure* typically causes a headache that is worse on lying down (and can be relieved by standing), disturbing sleep and present in the mornings. The pressure eventually causes nausea and vomiting and, if brain stem compression occurs, a progressive reduction of consciousness. The raised pressure can result from space-occupying lesions (e.g., tumors, subdural hematomas), hydrocephalus, or idiopathic intracranial hypertension. The typical features of raised intracranial pressure (i.e., headache, ataxia, drowsiness, confusion, coma) are not always present. If they are, or if headache is associated with papilledema or focal neurological signs, a CT scan should be obtained urgently. *Low CSF volume headache* is an increasingly well-recognized syndrome with features inverse to those of the headache of raised intracranial pressure: the headache comes on after getting up and is relieved by lying down. This type of headache is often iatrogenic (e.g., following lumbar puncture), but it can also occur as a result of spontaneous CSF leaks.

Certain "headaches" are felt mainly in the face. *Cluster headache,* a rare type of headache that is more common in young men, gives rise to severe retro-orbital pain occurring in bursts lasting an hour or so, that recur over a period of days to weeks (the "cluster"). The headache often wakes the sufferer in the middle of the night and usually makes him or her extremely restless (in contrast to migraine, which sends sufferers to their beds) (Matharu and Silver 2008). *Trigeminal neuralgia* causes stabs of lancinating pain in one of the three divisions of the trigeminal nerve (Graff-Radford 2000). *Atypical facial pain* is a diagnosis of exclusion, the facial equivalent of chronic daily headache.

Somatoform and Conversion Disorders in Neurology

Somatic symptoms unexplained by neurological disease are commonly encountered in neurological practice and may be diagnosed as somatoform disorders. Other names include medically unexplained symptoms, psychogenic disorders, and functional disorders. DSM-IV and its text revision DSM-IV-TR use the term *somatoform disorders,* although patients may prefer the term *functional disorders* (J. Stone et al. 2002).

Conversion disorder is regarded as a subgroup of somatoform disorders. The term is reserved to describe patients with motor and/or sensory symptoms or blackouts that suggest a neurological or other general medical condition but in whom no such condition is found by appropriate examination and investigation. DSM-IV-TR also requires that the psychological factors be judged to be associated with the symptoms because their initiation or exacerbation is *preceded by* conflicts or other stressors. This requirement is controversial, as its theoretical basis is unconfirmed. Furthermore, because psychological factors are common in all neurological presentations, the requirement is nonspecific and likely to be unreliable. Common conversion symptoms include paralysis, weakness, seizures, anesthesia, aphonia, blindness, amnesia, and stupor. Conversion disorder is also discussed in Chapter 12, "Somatization and Somatoform Disorders." (The epidemiology and clinical features of nonepileptic attacks were discussed earlier in this chapter under "Epilepsy.")

Epidemiology

Neurological symptoms in the absence of neurological disease or disproportionate to disease are observed in approximately one-third of patients attending neurological clinics (Carson et al. 2000b). Conversion weakness and paralysis have an incidence of at least 5 per 100,000 (Binzer and Kullgren 1998), a rate similar to that of multiple sclerosis. In less than half of patients do the symptoms remit spontaneously (Carson et al. 2003; Sharpe et al. 2010). Early expectation of nonrecovery, nonattribution of symptoms to psychological factors, and receipt of health-related benefits at the time of the initial consultation predict poorer outcome (Sharpe et al. 2010).

Clinical Features

A careful history is essential to diagnosis, first concentrating on the somatic symptoms, and only then exploring psychological and social factors. In considering the diagnosis, particular attention should be paid to the presence of multiple somatic symptoms (multiple symptoms make a somatoform disorder more likely), depression or anxiety (particularly panic), and a history of previous functional symptoms or of multiple surgical operations in the absence of organic pathology (Barsky and Borus 1999). Childhood abuse and neglect, personality factors, recent stressful life events, secondary gain (financial or otherwise), and strong beliefs about the causation may all be relevant to management, but these factors occur in all kinds of disease, and their presence does not allow one to infer a diagnosis of conversion disorder (J. Stone et al. 2005a).

At onset, patients with conversion weakness will often describe symptoms suggestive of depersonalization or derealization at the time of onset. These symptoms may be associated with a panic attack, physical trauma (often minor), or unexpected physiological events (e.g., postmicturition syncope, sleep paralysis) (J. Stone et al. 2009a).

The neurological examination has a crucial role in diagnosis of conversion disorder. Because of the difficulties in relying on features in the history, the diagnosis must usually be made in the presence of positive physical signs of internal inconsistency or marked incongruity with recognized neurological disorder. Helpful signs include Hoover's sign (Ziv et al. 1998), collapsing ("giveaway") weakness, and co-contraction (Knutsson and Martensson 1985), although none of these should be interpreted in isolation, as there may be false positives. A conversion tremor typically demonstrates variable frequency, marked attenuation with distraction, and entrainment (where the frequency entrains to a contralateral limb voluntarily making a 3- to 4-Hz movement). *Fixed dystonia* is a term used to describe the sustained posture of a limb, usually a clenched hand or a plantar-flexed inverted foot (Hallett et al. 2005; Schrag et al. 2004). Further evidence that an abnormality represents a conversion symptom must come from improvement after hypnosis, sedation, or placebo. There are many tests of visual conversion symptoms (S. Beatty 1999). The finding of a tubular visual field deficit at the bedside or of spiral fields on perimetry testing is suggestive. All of these signs should be demonstrated to patients in a collaborative, rather than confrontational, manner (J. Stone et al. 2005b).

Pathology and Etiology

The etiology of conversion disorder remains unknown, and there is value in remaining neutral about the relative contributions of biological, psychological, and social factors. In particular, one should be aware that although Freudian theory portrays conversion disorder as a mechanism for dealing with unconscious conflict and traumatic experience, this model can only be applied to some patients. Functional imaging studies (J. Stone et al. 2007; Vuilleumier et al. 2001) and neurophysiological investigations (Espay et al. 2006) have yielded intriguing results. The psychological and social risk factors for conversion disorder are similar to those for other somatoform disorders, as described in Chapter 12, "Somatization and Somatoform Disorders."

Investigation and Differential Diagnosis

Further imaging or neurophysiological testing may be required, depending on the symptoms present, but ultimately the diagnosis should be made at the bedside, not on the basis of normal test results. Diagnostic error has been a cause for concern for psychiatrists, although a systematic review of 27 studies found that the error rate since 1970 has been on average 4%. This is equivalent to the diagnostic error rates for most neurological and psychiatric conditions (Carson et al. 2003; J. Stone et al. 2005c, 2009b). Misdiagnosis may be more common in the presence of known psychiatric comorbidity, in patients with gait and movement disorders, and in patients who have not seen a neurologist. Although clinicians tend to worry about missing "organic" disease and therefore are often very conservative in making a diagnosis of conversion disorder, available evidence suggests that the reverse problem, misdiagnosing conversion disorder as "organic" disease, is more common, leading to iatrogenic complications of unneeded treatment and invalidism (Fink 1992; Nimnuan et al. 2000).

Management

The basis of treatment is an explicit acceptance of the reality of the symptoms and a nonstigmatizing, positive explanation of the diagnosis that emphasizes the potential reversibility of the problem. Explanation about how the diagnosis has been made and why this indicates the absence of neurological disease is likely to be more successful than simple reassurance alone (J. Stone et al. 2005b). Dismissing the symptoms as "nothing wrong" risks antagonizing or humiliating the patient and is rarely a good basis for collaborative management. Neurologists and psychiatrists need to work closely together for effective management of these patients. Neurologists who make the diagnosis need to be consistent in their explanations with the psychiatrists to whom they refer patients. Psychiatrists, for their own part, need to understand the positive basis on which the diagnosis has been made—first, to reduce their own uncertainty about the diagnosis, and second, so that they can explain this rationale to the patient. Only after the patient and doctor are reasonably satisfied that the diagnosis is correct can further treatment continue. In our own experience, conceptualizing the symptoms as functional symptoms—a problem with the functioning of the nervous system, in distinction to a structural disorder—works both theoretically and practically with patients (Sharpe and Carson 2000). The alternative approach of attempting to persuade patients that their symptoms are psychogenic or a manifestation of somatization is a more difficult route.

There is evidence for moderate effectiveness of antidepressant drugs, particularly TCAs, in other somatic symptom syndromes, with an odds ratio for improvement of 3.4 compared with placebo, regardless of the presence of depression (O'Malley et al. 1999), but unfortunately there are no studies of antidepressants in conversion disorder. A critical review of controlled trials evaluating the efficacy of CBT in patients with somatic symptom syndromes found that CBT-treated patients improved more than control subjects in 71% of the studies (Kroenke and Swindle 2000). Although studies of other treatment approaches are promising (Reuber et al. 2007; Ruddy and House 2005), there is little randomized evidence. Patients with physical disabilities need physical treatments like physiotherapy. There may be a role for hypnosis or therapeutic sedation in some conversion syndromes, especially those involving fixed dystonia (see Chapter 12, "Somatization and Somatoform Disorders," for further discussion of management).

Neurosurgical Issues

Many of the psychiatric issues arising in neurosurgical settings are described in other chapters in this book. Of particular relevance are Chapter 5, "Delirium"; Chapter 35, "Physical Medicine and Rehabilitation" (which discusses brain injury); and Chapter 36, "Pain." High doses of corticosteroids are used by neurosurgeons to reduce elevated intracranial pressure; the psychiatric adverse effects of corticosteroids are reviewed in Chapter 25, "Rheumatology." Mood disorders are frequent after neurosurgery, and their assessment should be guided by the discussion in the earlier sections of this chapter, particularly the section on stroke.

Central Nervous System Tumors

Psychiatric aspects of cancer are reviewed in Chapter 23, "Oncology." Psychiatrists generally become involved in neuro-oncology cases after tumor diagnosis, when the clinical issues are adjustment, mood disorder, or cognitive impairment. Patients with primary and metastatic CNS tumors typically present with headache, focal neurological signs, or seizures, but these tumors can also cause cognitive impairment, and occasionally their presentation mimics a dementing illness (Lishman 1997). Some brain tumors initially manifest with predominantly psychiatric symptoms, including depression, panic attacks, psychosis, disordered eating, and personality change. CT scanning should reveal their presence, although diffusely infiltrating tumors are sometimes missed in the early stages.

Hydrocephalus

Hydrocephalus is caused by dilatation of the ventricles within the brain resulting from elevation of CSF pressure. Hydrocephalus is termed *communicating* when the blockage to CSF flow is outside the ventricular system, *noncommunicating* when the blockage is within the ventricles. In "compensated" hydrocephalus, the clinical signs and CSF dynamics stabilize at an elevated level of CSF pressure. Normal-pressure hydrocephalus (NPH) describes ventricle enlargement with normal CSF pressure, possibly as the result of persistent elevation or intermittent surges of high pressure.

Clinical Features

Hydrocephalus can cause a wide range of psychiatric symptoms and signs. These include enlargement of the head (if present in infancy), depression, headache, sudden death due to "hydrocephalic attacks" with acute elevation of intracranial pressure, progressive visual failure, gait disturbance (often "gait apraxia"), incontinence, and subcortical cognitive impairment progressing to dementia. NPH in older individuals is classically associated with the triad of gait apraxia, incontinence, and cognitive decline. However, this triad is not specific for NPH and may occur in vascular dementia or other degenerative diseases.

Diagnosis

In younger persons, the radiological signs of hydrocephalus are usually clear-cut on CT scanning. This may also be the case in some elderly patients, but in other older patients apparent hydrocephalus is often due to ex vacuo atrophy of the subcortical white matter. The presence of easily visible cortical sulci should alert the clinician to this possibility. When enlargement of the ventricles raises a suspicion of communicating hydrocephalus in an older person, determination of whether the scan appearance is relevant to the clinical problem requires specialized studies—usually either serial lumbar punctures with observation of the clinical effects or neurosurgical studies of CSF pressure. However, there is no one test that can confirm a diagnosis of NPH or predict response to shunting, which means that appropriate investigations for NPH are controversial (Shprecher et al. 2008). Ultimately, only the insertion of a shunt can reliably determine whether a patient will benefit from shunting.

Management

Shunting of hydrocephalus—diversion of CSF from a CSF space to the venous system or peritoneum—can be beneficial in the long term (Pujari et al. 2008). However, the procedure is prone to complications—including subdural hematoma and shunt infection—in nearly half of patients (Hebb and Cusimano 2001) and thus should not be undertaken lightly.

Subdural Hematoma

Subdural hematoma is caused by accumulations of blood and blood products in the space between the fibrous dura mater and the more delicate arachnoid membrane that encloses the brain. Acute subdural hematomas accumulate rapidly following head injury; chronic hematomas can often (although not always) be traced back to a head injury.

Clinical Features

Acute subdural hematomas are, by definition, diagnosed close to the time of trauma, as a result of symptoms present at the time—headache, depressed level of consciousness, focal neurological signs—or seen on CT scan. Chronic subdural hematomas give rise to more gradually evolving symptoms and signs. Although they also can cause headache, depressed consciousness, and focal signs, chronic subdural hematomas sometimes result in predominantly cognitive features, including confusion and dementia, which can be reversed with surgery (Ishikawa et al. 2002). Marked variability of the mental state, and sometimes also of the neurological features, is often a clue to the diagnosis. Seizures can occur. Both acute and chronic subdural hematomas are especially common in alcoholic individuals, who frequently do not recall having experienced head trauma (Selecki 1965).

Pathology

The variability of the clinical features is explained by the tendency of the size of a chronic subdural hematoma to wax and wane as a result of alternating phases of bleeding and of breakdown of the contents of the hematoma (McIntosh et al. 1996). Subdural hematomas exert their effects both by local compression and irritation of adjacent cortical tissue and by global "brain shift" (with the risk of brain herniation and secondary brain stem compression).

Investigation and Differential Diagnosis

Subdural hematomas can generally be diagnosed on CT scanning. They are occasionally of the same density ("isodense") as adjacent brain tissue and therefore easily missed, especially if bilateral (Davenport et al. 1994). It is important to recognize that a small subdural hematoma can be an incidental finding; for example, cerebral atrophy occurring in the course of a dementing illness predisposes to subdural hematoma as vulnerable bridging veins are stretched between the dura and the arachnoid. In these circumstances, treatment of the subdural hematoma is unlikely to be helpful.

Management

Management requires liaison with a neurosurgical team. Small subdural hematomas often resorb spontaneously. If a subdural hematoma is considered to be relevant to a patient's problems and drainage is required, several surgical approaches are available. Reaccumulation is more likely for bilateral subdural hematomas and for subdural hematomas in patients receiving antiplatelet therapy (Torihashi et al. 2008).

Subarachnoid Hemorrhage

Severe, prolonged headache of abrupt onset can be due to a subarachnoid hemorrhage, usually arising from a ruptured berry aneurysm. A diagnosis of subarachnoid hemorrhage is suggested by the rapidity of onset ("thunderclap" headache, at its worst within a minute or so) and associated loss of consciousness, photophobia, vomiting, and neck stiffness (Al-Shahi et al. 2006). Psychiatrists are rarely involved in the diagnosis of subarachnoid hemorrhage but are frequently asked to evaluate patients in the postacute phase, as for stroke. In the first 21 days after a subarachnoid hemorrhage, one-third of patients may develop a fluctuating clinical course due to cerebral vasospasm. CT perfusion is a promising technique to monitor this condition (Wintermark et al. 2006). Symptoms and signs vary according to the territory affected, but variable akinetic mutism is particularly common in patients with vasospasm after an anterior cerebral artery aneurysmal hemorrhage.

Fitness for Surgery

Psychiatrists may be requested to assess patients for fitness for neurosurgery. Such requests occur most commonly for patients with epilepsy and with Parkinson's disease. A general assessment of capacity (see Chapter 2, "Legal Issues") and consideration of specific issues relevant to the operation in question are required, necessitating special attention when the operation is considered investigational.

Epilepsy Surgery

A psychiatric opinion should be sought prior to surgery if there are significant associated behavioral or social problems. Such problems include anticipated noncompliance with medication, severe personality disturbance, psychosis, severe mood disorder, unrealistic expectations of surgery, and an absence of social support. The presence of mental retardation is not an absolute contraindication to surgery but can complicate postsurgical care (Sperling 1994). The most commonly performed procedures are temporal lobectomy and amygdalohippocampectomy. Other procedures include extratemporal cortical resections, hemispherectomy, and white matter transections, including corpus callosotomy (Engel 1993). Approximately two-thirds of patients will become seizure free after surgery. Mortality is extremely low, and the rate of neurological complications has dropped significantly over the past few years, with hemiparesis now being exceptionally rare (S. Spencer 2008). Reported rates of complications after temporal lobectomies range from 0.4% to 4%, including partial hemianopsia, aphasia, and cranial nerve palsies (S. Spencer 2008). Cognitive changes—in particular, a decline in verbal memory—are reported in about one-third of patients (S. Spencer 2008). The likelihood of a new mood disorder is most closely related to preexisting mental state and whether the patient becomes seizure free (S. Spencer 2008). De novo development of psychosis is recognized, but the risk factors for its development are not (S. Spencer 2008). It is noteworthy that poor psychological outcomes occasionally accompany good postoperative seizure control, and some patients need considerable psychological help in adjusting to life without seizures (Vickrey et al. 1993).

Parkinson's Disease Surgery

Neurosurgery for Parkinson's disease is an evolving field. A number of different surgical interventions have been suggested (Olanow 2002), most of which can cause psychiatric complications (e.g., corticobulbar syndromes and psychic akinesia after bilateral pallidotomy) (de Bie et al. 2002; Merello et al. 2001). Subthalamic nucleus deep brain stimulation (STN DBS) appears the most promising technique (Deuschl et al. 2006). STN DBS is an effective treatment for motor symptoms in advanced Parkinson's disease; however, neurobehavioral side effects are relatively common and include executive impairments, delirium, depression, mania, hallucinations, and impulse-control disorders (Meagher et al. 2008). However, there is little evidence of any consistent effect of STN DBS in causing neuropsychiatric disturbance, although numerous study biases in terms of disease progression, medication effects, and control group selection may be influencing reporting. At the time of writing, it does seem likely that STN DBS is associated with significant neuropsychiatric complications, but how common they are is far less certain.

Conclusion

The practice of psychiatry in a neurological or neurosurgical setting is both challenging and rewarding. One of the challenges is the often complex task of determining the relationship between comorbid neurological and psychiatric symptoms. In this chapter we have outlined general principles of assessment and management in relation to the more commonly encountered conditions. These same principles apply to the more rarely encountered problems. Working closely with colleagues who share an interest in disorders of the brain can be very rewarding, and new developments in neuroscience are providing a greater understanding of the mechanisms by which biological, psychological, and social factors interact to cause both neurological and psychiatric illness. Consequently, the interface between these specialties is rapidly becoming one of the most intellectually fascinating areas of work for the specialist in psychosomatic medicine.

References

Aarsland D, Larsen JP, Cummins JL, et al: Prevalence and clinical correlates of psychotic symptoms in Parkinson disease: a community-based study. Arch Neurol 56:595–601, 1999

Aarsland D, Ballard C, Larsen JP, et al: A comparative study of psychiatric symptoms in dementia with Lewy bodies and Parkinson's disease with and without dementia. Int J Geriatr Psychiatry 16:528–536, 2001

Abrahams S, Goldstein LH, Leigh PN: Cognitive change in amyotrophic lateral sclerosis: a prospective study. Neurology 64:1222–1226, 2005

Adams P, Falek A, Arnold J: Huntington's disease in Georgia: age at onset. Am J Hum Genet 43:695–704, 1988

Akil M, Brewer GJ: Psychiatric and behavioral abnormalities in Wilson's disease. Adv Neurol 65:171–178, 1995

Almqvist EW, Bloch M, Brinkman R, et al: A worldwide assessment of the frequency of suicide, suicide attempts and psychiatric hospitalizations following predictive testing of Huntington disease. Am J Hum Genet 64:1293–1304, 1999

Alper K: Seizure incidence in psychopharmacological clinical trials: an analysis of Food and Drug Administration (FDA) summary basis of approval reports. Biol Psychiatry 62:345–354, 2007

Al-Shahi R, White PM, Davenport RJ, et al: Subarachnoid haemorrhage. BMJ 333:235–240, 2006

Amato MP, Portaccio E, Zipoli V: Are there protective treatments for cognitive decline in MS? J Neurol Sci 245:183–186, 2006

American Psychiatric Association: Diagnostic and Statistical Manual of Mental Disorders, 4th Edition, Text Revision. Washington, DC, American Psychiatric Association, 2000

Andersen G, Vestergaard K, Lauritzen L: Effective treatment of post-stroke depression with the selective reuptake inhibitor citalopram. Stroke 25:1099–1104, 1994a

Andersen G, Vestergaard K, Riis J, et al: Incidence of post-stroke depression during the first year in a large unselected stroke population determined using a valid standardized rating scale. Acta Psychiatr Scand 90:190–195, 1994b

Andersen G, Vestergaard K, Ingemann-Nielsen M, et al: Risk factors for post-stoke depression. Acta Psychiatr Scand 92:193–198, 1995

Andersen J, Aabro E, Gulmann N, et al: Anti-depressive treatment in Parkinson's disease. A controlled trial of the effect of nortriptyline in patients with Parkinson's disease treated with L-dopa. Acta Neurol Scand 62:210–219, 1980

Ardouin C, Voon V, Worbe Y, et al: Pathological gambling in Parkinson's disease improves on chronic subthalamic nucleus stimulation. Mov Disord 21:1941–1946, 2006

Armin S, Andreas H, Hermann W, et al: Pramipexole, a dopamine agonist, in major depression: antidepressant effects and tolerability in an open-label study with multiple doses. Clin Neuropharmacol 20:S36–S45, 1997

Arnulf I, Bonnet AM, Damier P, et al: Hallucinations, REM sleep and Parkinson's disease: a medical hypothesis. Neurology 55:281–288, 2000

Astrom M: Generalized anxiety disorder in stroke patients: a 3-year longitudinal study. Stroke 27:270–275, 1996

Baker MG, Kale R, Menken M: The wall between neurology and psychiatry: advances in neuroscience indicate it's time to tear it down. BMJ 324:1468–1469, 2002

Bamford J, Sandercock P, Dennis M, et al: A prospective study of acute cerebrovascular disease in the community: the Oxfordshire Community Stroke Project 1981–86, I: methodology, demography and incident cases of first-ever stroke. J Neurol Neurosurg Psychiatry 51:1373–1380, 1988

Barone P, Scarzella L, Marconi R, et al: Pramipexole versus sertraline in the treatment of depression in Parkinson's disease: a national multicenter parallel-group randomized study. J Neurol 253:601–607, 2006

Barsky AJ, Borus JF: Functional somatic syndromes. Ann Intern Med 130:910–921, 1999

Bearn AG: Wilson's disease: an unborn error of metabolism with multiple manifestations. Am J Med 22:747–757, 1957

Beatty S: Non-organic visual loss. Postgrad Med J 75:201–207, 1999

Beatty WW, Goodkin DE, Monson N, et al: Cognitive disturbances in patients with relapsing-remitting multiple sclerosis. Arch Neurol 46:1113–1119, 1989

Bell GS, Sander JW: The epidemiology of epilepsy: the size of the problem. Seizure 10:306–314, 2001

Benbadis SR, Allen HW: An estimate of the prevalence of psychogenic non-epileptic seizures. Seizure 9:280–281, 2000

Benbadis SR, Agrawal V, Tatum WO: How many patients with psychogenic non-epileptic seizures also have epilepsy? Neurology 57:915–917, 2001

Benke TH, Hockleitner M, Bauer G: Aura phenomena during syncope. Eur Neurol 37:28–32, 1997

Berthier ML, Kulisevsky J, Gironell A, et al: Poststroke bipolar affective disorder: clinical subtypes, concurrent movement disorders, and anatomical correlates. J Neuropsychiatry Clin Neurosci 8:160–170, 1996

Binzer M, Kullgren G: Motor conversion disorder: a prospective 2–5 year follow-up study. Psychosomatics 39:519–527, 1998

Binzer M, Stone J, Sharpe M: Recent onset pseudoseizures: clues to etiology. Seizure 13:146–155, 2004

Blass JP, Gibson GE: Abnormality of a thiamine-requiring enzyme in patients with Wernicke-Korsakoff syndrome. N Engl J Med 297:1367–1370, 1977

Boesenberg C, Schulz-Schaeffer WJ, Meissner B, et al: Clinical course in young patients with sporadic Creutzfeldt-Jakob disease. Ann Neurol 58:533–543, 2005

Bogousslavsky J, Cummings JL: Behavior and Mood Disorders in Focal Brain Lesions. New York, Cambridge University Press, 2000

Bonilha L, Rorden C, Castellano G, et al: Voxel based morphometry reveals gray matter network atrophy in refractory medial temporal lobe epilepsy. Arch Neurol 61:1379–1384, 2004

Bower JH, Maraganore DM, McDonnell SK, et al: Incidence and distribution of parkinsonism in Olmsted County, Minnesota, 1976–1990. Neurology 52:1214–1220, 1999

Brandt J, Celentano D, Stewart W, et al: Personality and emotional disorder in a community sample of migraine headache patients. Cephalagia 19:566–574, 1990

Bredkjaer SR, Mortensen PB, Parnas J: Epilepsy and non-organic non-affective psychosis: National Epidemiological Study. Br J Psychiatry 172:235–238, 1998

Breier JI, Adair JC, Gold M, et al: Dissociation of anosognosia for hemiplegia and aphasia during left-hemisphere anaesthesia. Neurology 45:65–67, 1995

Breslau N, Lipton RB, Stewart WF, et al: Comorbidity of migraine and depression: investigating potential etiology and prognosis. Neurology 60:1308–1312, 2003

Breuer B, Pappagallo M, Knotkova H, et al: A randomized, double-blind, placebo-controlled, two-period, crossover, pilot trial of lamotrigine in patients with central pain due to multiple sclerosis. Clin Ther 29:2022–2030, 2007

Brinkman RR, Mezei MM, Theilmann J, et al: The likelihood of being affected with Huntington's disease by a particular age, for a specific CAG size. Am J Hum Genet 60:1202–1210, 1997

Brodaty H, Sachdev PS, Withall A, et al: Frequency and clinical, neuropsychological and neuroimaging correlates of apathy following stroke—the Sydney Stroke Study. Psychol Med 35:1707–1716, 2005

Brodaty H, Withall A, Altendorf A, et al: Rates of depression at 3 and 15 months poststroke and their relationship with cognitive decline: the Sydney Stroke Study. Am J Geriatr Psychiatry 15:477–486, 2007

Brooks BR, Miller RG, Swash M, et al: El Escorial revisited: revised criteria for the diagnosis of amyotrophic lateral sclerosis. Amyotroph Lateral Scler Other Motor Neuron Disord 1:293–299, 2000

Brooks DJ, Doder M: Depression in Parkinson's disease. Curr Opin Neurol 14:465–470, 2001

Brown AP, Lane JC, Murayama S, et al: Whipple's disease presenting with isolated neurological symptoms: case report. J Neurosurg 73:623–627, 1990

Brown P: Transmissible spongiform encephalopathies, in Early-Onset Dementia: A Multidisciplinary Approach. Edited by Hodges JR. Oxford, UK, Oxford University Press, 2001, pp 367–384

Brown P, Cathala F, Raubertas RF, et al: The epidemiology of Creutzfeldt-Jakob disease: conclusion of a 15-year investigation in France and review of the world literature. Neurology 37:895–904, 1987

Brown P, Gibbs CJ Jr, Rodgers-Johnson P, et al: Human spongiform encephalopathy: the National Institutes of Health series of 300 cases of experimentally transmitted disease. Ann Neurol 35:513–529, 1994

Brown P, Preece M, Brandel J-P, et al: Iatrogenic Creutzfeldt-Jakob disease at the millennium. Neurology 55:1075–1081, 2000

Bull PC, Thomas GR, Rommens JM, et al: Wilson's disease gene is a putative copper transporting P-type ATPase similar to the Menkes gene. Nat Genet 5:327–337, 1993

Burns A, Folstein S, Brandt J, et al: Clinical assessment of irritability, aggression and apathy in Huntington and Alzheimer disease. J Nerv Ment Dis 178:20–26, 1990

Burvill PW, Johnson GA, Jamrozik KD, et al: Anxiety disorders after stroke: results from the Perth Community Stroke Study. Br J Psychiatry 166:328–332, 1995

Butler CR, Graham KS, Hodges JR, et al: The syndrome of transient epileptic amnesia. Ann Neurol 61:587–598, 2007

Cantello R, Gilli M, Ricco A, et al: Mood changes associated with "end of dose deterioration" in Parkinson's disease: a controlled study. J Neurol Neurosurg Psychiatry 49:1182–1190, 1986

Carota A, Nicola A, Aybek S, et al: Aphasia-related emotional behaviors in acute stroke. Neurology 54:A244, 2000

Carota A, Rossetti OA, Karapanayiotides T, et al: Catastrophic reaction in acute stroke: a reflex behavior in aphasic patients. Neurology 57:1902–1906, 2001

Carota A, Staub F, Bogousslavsky J: Emotions, behaviors and mood changes in stroke. Curr Opin Neurol 15:57–59, 2002

Carota A, Berney A, Aybek S, et al: A prospective study of predictors of poststroke depression. Neurology 64:428–433, 2005

Carson AJ, Machale S, Allen K, et al: Depression after stroke and lesion location: a systematic review. Lancet 356:122–126, 2000a

Carson AJ, Ringbauer B, Stone J, et al: Do medically unexplained symptoms matter? A study of 300 consecutive new referrals to neurology outpatient clinics. J Neurol Neurosurg Psychiatry 68:207–210, 2000b

Carson AJ, Postmas K, Stone J, et al: The outcome of neurology outpatients with medically unexplained symptoms: a prospective cohort study. J Neurol Neurosurg Psychiatry 74:897–900, 2003

Cavanna AE, Servo S, Monaco F, et al: The behavioral spectrum of Gilles de la Tourette syndrome. J Neuropsychiatry Clin Neurosci 21:13–23, 2009

Ceravolo R, Nuti A, Piccini A, et al: Paroxetine in Parkinson's disease: effects on motor and depressive symptoms. Neurology 55:1216–1218, 2000

Chabolla DR, Cascino GD: Interpretation of extracranial EEG, in The Treatment of Epilepsy: Principles and Practice, 2nd Edition. Edited by Wylie E. Baltimore, MD, Williams & Wilkins, 1997, pp 264–279

Chemerinski E, Robinson RG, Kosier JT: Improved recovery in activities of daily living associated with remission of PSD. Stroke 32:113–117, 2001

Chen Y, Patel NC, Guo JJ, et al: Antidepressant prophylaxis for poststroke depression: a meta-analysis. Int Clin Psychopharmacol 22:159–166, 2007

Choi-Kwon S, Han SW, Kwon SU, et al: Fluoxetine treatment in poststroke depression, emotional incontinence, and anger proneness: a double-blind, placebo-controlled study. Stroke 37:156–161, 2006

Chong JY, Rowland LP, Utiger RD: Hashimoto encephalopathy: syndrome or myth? Arch Neurol 60:164–171, 2003

Chua P, Chiu E: Huntington's disease, in Dementia. Edited by Burns A, Levy R. London, Chapman & Hall, 1994, pp 827–844

Chuinard G, Sultan S: A case of Parkinson's disease exacerbated by fluoxetine. Hum Psychopharmacol 7:63–66, 1992

Chung SS, Gerber P, Kirlin KA: Ictal eye closure is a reliable indicator for psychogenic nonepileptic seizures. Neurology 66:1730–1731, 2006

Clark S, Assal G, Bogousslavsky J, et al: Pure amnesia after unilateral left polar thalamic infarct: tomographic and sequential neuropsychological and metabolic (PET) correlations. J Neurol Neurosurg Psychiatry 57:27–34, 1994

Clot F, Grabli D, Cazeneuve C, et al: Exhaustive analysis of BH4 and dopamine biosynthesis genes in patients with Dopa-responsive dystonia. Brain 132:1753–1763, 2009

Cockerell OC, Johnson AL, Sander JW, et al: Prognosis of epilepsy: a review and further analysis of the first nine years of the British National General Practice Study of Epilepsy, a prospective population-based study. Epilepsy 38:31–46, 1997

Codori A-M, Slavney PR, Young C, et al: Predictors of psychological adjustment to genetic testing for Huntington's disease. Health Psychol 16:36–50, 1997

Colchester A, Kingsley D, Lasserson D, et al: Structural MRI volumetric analysis in patients with organic amnesia, I: methods and comparative findings across diagnostic groups. J Neurol Neurosurg Psychiatry 71:13–22, 2001

Cummings JL: Managing psychosis in patients with Parkinson's disease. N Engl J Med 340:801–803, 1999

Cummings JL, Cunningham K: Obsessive-compulsive disorder in Huntington's disease. Biol Psychiatry 31:263–270, 1992

Cummings JL, Masterman DL: Depression in patients with Parkinson's disease. Int J Geriatr Psychiatry 14:711–718, 1999

Cummings JL, Mendez MF: Secondary mania with focal cerebrovascular lesions. Am J Psychiatry 141:1084–1087, 1984

Cummings JL, Arciniegas DB, Brooks BR, et al: Defining and diagnosing involuntary emotional expression disorder. CNS Spectr 11:1–7, 2006

Damasio AR: Emotion, Reason and the Human Brain. New York, GP Putnam & Sons, 1994

Darnell RB, Posner JB: Paraneoplastic syndromes involving the nervous system. N Engl J Med 349:1543–1554, 2003

Davenport RJ, Statham PFX, Warlow CP: Detection of bilateral isodense subdural haematomas. BMJ 309:792–794, 1994

de Bie R, de Haan RJ, Schuurman PR, et al: Morbidity and mortality following pallidotomy in Parkinson's disease: a systematic review. Neurology 58:1008–1012, 2002

De Bruin VMS, Lees AJ: The clinical features of 67 patients with clinically definite Steele-Richardson-Olszeweski syndrome. Behav Neurol 5:229–232, 1992

De la Monte SM, Vonsattel JP, Richardson EP: Morphometric demonstration of atrophic changes in the cerebral cortex, white matter and neostriatum in Huntington's disease. J Neuropathol Exp Neurol 47:516–525, 1988

De Wit L, Putman K, Baert I, et al: Anxiety and depression in the first six months after stroke. A longitudinal multicenter study. Disabil Rehabil 30:1858–1866, 2008

Dening TR, Berrios GE: Wilson's disease: psychiatric symptoms in 195 cases. Arch Gen Psychiatry 46:1126–1134, 1989

Derex L, Ostrowsky K, Nighoghossian N, et al: Severe pathological crying after left anterior choroidal artery infarct: reversibility with paroxetine treatment. Stroke 28:1464–1469, 1997

Desmond DW, Moroney JT, Paik MC, et al: Frequency and clinical determinants of dementia after ischemic stroke. Neurology 54:1124–1131, 2000

Deuschl G, Schade-Brittinger C, Krack P, et al: A randomized trial of deep-brain stimulation for Parkinson's disease. N Engl J Med 355:896–908, 2006

Devinsky O, Abramson H, Alper K, et al: Postictal psychosis: a case control series of 20 patients and 150 controls. Epilepsy Res 20:247–253, 1995

Diederich NJ, Pieri V, Goetz CG: Visual hallucinations in Parkinson and Charles Bonnet syndrome patients: a phenomenological and pathogenetic comparison. Fortschr Neurol Psychiatr 68:129–136, 2000

Duyao M, Ambrose C, Myers R, et al: Trinucleotide repeat length: instability and age of onset of Huntington's disease. Nat Genet 4:387–392, 1993

Ehde DM, Gibbons LE, Chwastiak L, et al: Chronic pain in a large community sample of persons with multiple sclerosis. Mult Scler 9:605–611, 2003

Eldridge R, Riklan M, Cooper IS: The limited role of psychotherapy in torsion dystonia: experience with 44 cases. JAMA 210:705–708, 1969

Engel JJ: Update on surgical treatment of the epilepsies: summary of the Second International Palm Desert Conference on the Surgical Treatment of Epilepsies, 1992. Neurology 43:1612–1617, 1993

Espay AJ, Morgante F, Purzner J, et al: Cortical and spinal abnormalities in psychogenic dystonia. Ann Neurol 59:825–824, 2006

Evans AH, Pavese N, Lawrence AD, et al: Compulsive drug use linked to sensitized ventral striatal dopamine transmission. Ann Neurol 59:852–858, 2006

Farrer LA, Conneally PM: A genetic model for age at onset in Huntington's disease. Am J Hum Genet 37:350–357, 1985

Fassbender K, Schmidt R, Mossner R, et al: Mood disorders and dysfunction of the hypothalamic-pituitary-adrenal axis in multiple sclerosis: association with cerebral inflammation. Arch Neurol 55:66–72, 1998

Fazel S, Philipson J, Gardiner L, et al: Neurological disorders and violence: a systematic review and meta-analysis with a focus on epilepsy and traumatic brain injury. J Neurol 256:1591–1602, 2009

Feigin A, Kieburtz K, Bordwell K, et al: Functional decline in Huntington's disease. Mov Disord 10:211–214, 1995

Feinstein A: Multiple sclerosis, depression and suicide: clinicians should pay more attention to psychology. BMJ 315:691–692, 1997

Feinstein A: Mood disorders in multiple sclerosis and the effects on cognition. J Neurol Sci 245:63–66, 2006

Feinstein A, O'Connor P, Feinstein K: Multiple sclerosis, interferon beta-1b and depression: a prospective investigation. J Neurol 249:815–820, 2002

Fenollar F, Puéchal X, Raoult D: Whipple's disease. N Engl J Med 356:55–66, 2007

Ferenci P: Wilson's disease. Clin Liver Dis 2:31–49, 1998

Findlay LJ (for Global Parkinson's Disease Survey Steering Committee): Factors impacting on quality of life in Parkinson's disease: results from an international survey. Mov Disord 17:60–67, 2002

Fink P: Surgery and medical treatment in persistent somatizing patients. J Psychosom Res 36:439–447, 1992

Fisher CM: Abulia, in Stroke Syndromes. Edited by Bogousslavsky J, Caplan L. Cambridge, UK, Cambridge University Press, 1995, pp 182–187

Fisk JD, Pontefract A, Ritvo PG, et al: The impact of fatigue on patients with multiple sclerosis. Can J Neurol Sci 21:9–14, 1994

Fleming JL, Wiesner RH, Shorter RG: Whipple's disease: clinical, biochemical and histopathological features and assessment of treatment in 29 patients. Mayo Clin Proc 63:539–551, 1988

Folstein SE, Folstein MF, McHugh PR: Psychiatric syndromes in Huntington's disease. Adv Neurol 23:281–290, 1979

Franklin GM, Nelson MPH: Environmental risk factors in multiple sclerosis. Neurology 61:1032–1034, 2003

Freal JE, Kraft GH, Coryell JK: Symptomatic fatigue in multiple sclerosis. Arch Phys Med Rehabil 65:135–138, 1984

Fregni F, Santos CM, Myczkowski ML, et al: Repetitive transcranial magnetic stimulation is as effective as fluoxetine in the treatment of depression in patients with Parkinson's disease. J Neurol Neurosurg Psychiatry 75:1171–1174, 2004

Gainotti G, Azzoni A, Razzano C, et al: The Post-Stoke Depression Scale: a test specifically devised to investigate affective disorders of stroke patients. J Clin Exp Neuropsychol 19:340–356, 1997

Gainotti G, Azzoni A, Marra C: Frequency, phenomenology and anatomical-clinical correlates of major post-stroke depression. Br J Psychiatry 175:163–167, 1999

Gainotti G, Antonucci G, Marra C, et al: The relation between post-stroke depression, antidepressant, therapy and rehabilitation outcome. J Neurol Neurosurg Psychiatry 71:258–261, 2001

Gajdusek DC: Unconventional viruses and the origin and disappearance of kuru. Science 197:943–960, 1977

Gambetti P, Parchi P, Peterson RB, et al: Fatal familial insomnia and familial Creutzfeldt-Jakob disease: clinical, pathological, and molecular genetic features. Brain Pathol 5:43–51, 1995

Garg RK: Subacute sclerosing panencephalitis. J Neurol 255:1861–1871, 2008

Geda YE, Boeve BF, Negash S, et al: Neuropsychiatric features in 36 pathologically confirmed cases of corticobasal degeneration. J Neuropsychiatry Clin Neurosci 19:77–80, 2007

George MS, Wassermann EM, Post RM: Transcranial magnetic stimulation: a neuropsychiatric tool for the 21st century. J Neuropsychiatry Clin Neurosci 8:373–382, 1996

Geyer HL, Bressman SB: The diagnosis of dystonia. Lancet Neurol 5:780–790, 2006

Giladi N, Treves TA, Paleacu D, et al: Risk factors for dementia, depression and psychosis in long standing Parkinson's disease. J Neurol Transm 107:59–71, 2000

Goldstein K: The Organism: A Holistic Approach to Biology Derived From Pathological Data in Man. New York, American Books, 1939

Goldstein LH, Mellers JDC: Ictal symptoms of anxiety, avoidance behavior, and dissociation in patients with dissociative seizures. J Neurol Neurosurg Psychiatry 77:616–621, 2006

Goldstein MA, Harden CL: Epilepsy and anxiety. Epilepsy Behav 1:228–234, 2000

Goodwin FK: Behavioral effects of L-dopa in man. Semin Psychiatry 3:477–492, 1971

Gorell JM, Rybicki BA, Johnson CC, et al: Smoking and Parkinson's disease: a dose-response relationship. Neurology 52:115–119, 1999

Graff-Radford SB: Facial pain. Curr Opin Neurol 13:291–296, 2000

Gustafson Y, Olsson T, Erikkson S, et al: Acute confusional states (delirium) in stroke patients. Cerebrovasc Dis 1:257–264, 1991

Gustafson Y, Olsson T, Asplund K, et al: Acute confusional state (delirium) soon after stroke is associated with hypercortisolism. Cerebrovasc Dis 3:33–38, 1993

Hachinski VC, Lassen NA, Marshall J: Multi-infarct dementia: a cause of mental deterioration in the elderly. Lancet 2(7874): 207–210, 1974

Hackett ML, Anderson CS, House A, et al: Interventions for preventing depression after stroke. Cochrane Database Syst Rev (3):CD003689, 2008a

Hackett ML, Anderson CS, House A, et al: Interventions for treating depression after stroke. Cochrane Database Syst Rev (4):CD003437, 2008b

Hallett M, Lang AE, Fahn S, et al (eds): Psychogenic Movement Disorders: Neurology and Neuropsychiatry (Neurology Reference Series, American Neurological Association). Philadelphia, PA, Lippincott Williams & Wilkins, 2005

Hama S, Yamashita H, Shigenobu M, et al: Depression or apathy and functional recovery after stroke. Int J Geriatr Psychiatry 22:1046–1051, 2007

Hamelsky SW, Lipton RB: Psychiatric comorbidity of migraine. Headache 46:1327–1333, 2006

Harper PS: Huntington's Disease. London, WB Saunders, 1991

Heaton RK, Nelson LM, Thompson DS, et al: Neuropsychological findings in relapsing-remitting and chronic progressive multiple sclerosis. J Consult Clin Psychol 53:103–110, 1985

Hebb AO, Cusimano MD: Idiopathic normal pressure hydrocephalus: a systematic review of diagnosis and outcome. Neurosurgery 49:1166–1186, 2001

Henon H, Lebert F, Durieu I, et al: Confusional state in stroke: relation to pre-existing dementia, patient characteristics and outcome. Stroke 30:773–779, 1999

Henry JD, Beatty WW: Verbal fluency deficits in multiple sclerosis. Neuropsychologia 44:1166–1174, 2006

Hermann B, Seidenberg M: Epilepsy and cognition. Epilepsy Curr 7:1–6, 2007

Hermann BP, Seidenburg M, Bell B: Psychiatric comorbidity in chronic epilepsy: identification, consequences and treatment of major depression. Epilepsia 41:S31–S41, 2000

Herrmann M, Bartels C, Schumacher M, et al: Poststroke depression: is there a pathoanatomic correlate for depression in the postacute stage of stroke? Stroke 26:850–856, 1995

Hesdorffer DC, Hauser WA, Annegers JF, et al: Major depression is a risk factor for seizures in older adults. Ann Neurol 47:246–249, 2000

Hill AF, Butterworth RJ, Joiner S, et al: Investigation of variant Creutzfeldt-Jakob disease and other human prion diseases with tonsil biopsy samples. Lancet 353:183–189, 1999

Hodges JR: Transient Amnesia: Clinical and Neuropsychological Aspects. London, WB Saunders, 1991

Hodges JR, Ward CD: Observations during transient global amnesia: a behavioral and neuropsychological study of five cases. Brain 112:595–620, 1989

Hoffmann S, Tittgemeyer M, Yves von Cramon D: Cognitive impairment in multiple sclerosis. Curr Opin Neurol 20:275–280, 2007

Honer WG, Hurwitz T, Li DKB, et al: Temporal lobe involvement in multiple sclerosis patients with psychiatric disorders. Arch Neurol 44:187–190, 1987

House A, Dennis M, Molyneux A, et al: Emotionalism after stroke. BMJ 298:991–994, 1989

House A, Knapp P, Bamford J, et al: Mortality at 12 and 24 months after stroke may be associated with depressive symptoms at 1 month. Stroke 32:696–701, 2001

House A, Hackett ML, Anderson CS, et al: Pharmaceutical interventions for emotionalism after stroke. Cochrane Database Syst Rev (2):CD003690, 2004

Hsich G, Kenney K, Gibbs CJ Jr, et al: The 14-3-3 brain protein in cerebrospinal fluid as a marker for spongiform encephalopathies. N Engl J Med 335:924–930, 1996

Hyde TM, Ziegler JC, Weinberger DR: Psychiatric disturbances in metachromatic leukodystrophy: insights into the neurobiology of psychosis. Arch Neurol 49:401–406, 1992

Ishikawa E, Yanaka K, Sugimoto K, et al: Reversible dementia in patients with chronic subdural hematomas. J Neurosurg 96:680–683, 2002

Jacobson RR, Lishman WA: Cortical and diencephalic lesions in Korsakoff's syndrome: a clinical and CT scan study. Psychol Med 20:63–75, 1990

Jalava M, Sillanpaa M: Concurrent illnesses in adults with childhood-onset epilepsy: a population based 35-year follow up study. Epilepsia 37:1155–1163, 1996

James AC, Kaplan P, Lees A, et al: Schizophreniform psychosis and adrenomyeloneuropathy. J R Soc Med 77:882–884, 1984

Jankovic J, Beach J: Long-term effects of tetrabenazine in hyperkinetic movement disorders. Neurology 48:358–362, 1997

Jansen Steur ENH: Increase in Parkinson disability after fluoxetine medication. Neurology 43:211–213, 1993

Jehkonen M, Laihosalo M, Kettunen J: Anosognosia after stroke: assessment, occurrence, subtypes and impact on functional outcome reviewed. Acta Neurol Scand 114:293–306, 2006

Joffe RT, Lippert GP, Gray TA, et al: Mood disorders and multiple sclerosis. Arch Neurol 44:376–378, 1987

Jones JE, Hermann BP, Berry JJ, et al: Clinical assessment of Axis I psychiatric co-morbidity in chronic epilepsy: a multi-center investigation. J Neuropsychiatry Clin Neurosci 17:172–179, 2005

Kanemoto K, Kawasaki J, Kawai I: Postictal psychosis: a comparison with acute interictal and chronic psychoses. Epilepsia 37:551–556, 1996a

Kanemoto K, Takeuchi J, Kawasaki J, et al: Characteristics of temporal lobe epilepsy with mesial temporal sclerosis, with special reference to psychotic episodes. Neurology 47:1199–1203, 1996b

Kanner AM: Depression and epilepsy: a new perspective on two closely related disorders. Epilepsy Curr 6:141–146, 2006

Kanner AM, Balabanov A: Depression and epilepsy: how closely related are they? Neurology 58:S27–S39, 2002

Kanner AM, Kozak AM, Frey M: The use of sertraline in patients with epilepsy: is it safe? Epilepsy Behav 1:100–105, 2000

Keshavan MS, David AS, Narayanen HS, et al: "On-off" phenomena and manic-depressive mood shifts: case report. J Clin Psychiatry 47:93–94, 1986

Kim JS, Choi-Kwon S: Poststroke depression and emotional incontinence: correlation with lesion location. Neurology 54:1805–1810, 2000

Kirkwood SC, Siemers E, Stout JC, et al: Longitudinal cognitive and motor changes among presymptomatic Huntington disease gene carriers. Arch Neurol 56:563–568, 1999

Kneebone II, Dunmore E: Psychological management of poststroke depression. Br J Clin Psychol 39:53–65, 2000

Knutsson E, Martensson A: Isokinetic measurements of muscle strength in hysterical paresis. Electroencephalogr Clin Neurophysiol 61:370–374, 1985

Kopelman MD: Rates of forgetting in Alzheimer-type dementia and Korsakoff's syndrome. Neuropsychologia 23:623–638, 1985

Kopelman MD, Stanhope N, Kingsley DEP: Retrograde amnesia in patients with diencephalic temporal lobe or frontal lesions. Neuropsychologia 37:939–958, 1999

Kotagal P: Complex partial seizures with automatisms, in The Treatment of Epilepsy: Principles and Practice, 2nd Edition. Edited by Wylie E. Baltimore, MD, Williams & Wilkins, 1997, pp 385–400

Kotsopoulos IA, Merode T, Kessels FG, et al: Systematic review and meta-analysis of incidence studies of epilepsy and unprovoked seizures. Epilepsia 43:1402–1409, 2002

Krishnamoorthy ES, Trimble MR: Forced normalization: clinical and therapeutic relevance. Epilepsia 40:S57–S64, 1999

Kroenke K, Swindle R: Cognitive behavioral therapy for somatization and symptom syndromes: a critical review of controlled clinical trials. Psychother Psychosom 69:205–215, 2000

Kruisdijk JJ, Koelman JH, Ongerboer de V, et al: Botulinum toxin for writer's cramp: a randomised, placebo-controlled trial and 1-year follow-up. J Neurol Neurosurg Psychiatry 78:264–270, 2007

Krupp LB, Coyle PK, Doscher C, et al: Fatigue therapy in multiple sclerosis: results of a double-blind, randomized, parallel trial of amantadine, pemoline and placebo. Neurology 45:1956–1961, 1995

Kumral E, Evyapan D, Balkir K: Acute caudate vascular lesions. Stroke 30:100–108, 1999

Kupio AM, Marttila RJ, Helenius H, et al: Changing epidemiology of Parkinson's disease in southwestern Finland. Neurology 52:302–308, 1999

Kupsch A, Benecke R, Muller J, et al: Pallidal deep-brain stimulation in primary generalized or segmental dystonia. N Engl J Med 355:1978–1990, 2006

Lampl Y, Lorberboym M, Gilad R, et al: Auditory hallucinations in acute stroke. Behav Neurol 16:211–216, 2005

Landolt H: Serial electroencephalographic investigations during psychotic episodes in epileptic patients and during schizophrenic attacks, in Lectures on Epilepsy. Edited by Lorenz de Haas AM. Amsterdam, Elsevier, 1958, pp 256–284

Langhorne P, Stott DJ, Robertson L, et al: Medical complications after stroke: a multicenter study. Stroke 31:1223–1229, 2000

Lawson JA, Cook MJ, Vogrin S, et al: Clinical, EEG and quantitative MRI differences in pediatric frontal and temporal lobe epilepsy. Neurology 58:723–729, 2002

Lazar RM, Marshall RS, Prell GD, et al: The experience of Wernicke's aphasia. Neurology 55:1222–1224, 2000

Leckman JF, Hardin MT, Riddle MA, et al: Clonidine treatment of Gilles de la Tourette's syndrome. Arch Gen Psychiatry 48:324–328, 1991

Lempert T, Bauer M, Schmidt D: Syncope: a video metric analysis of 56 episodes of transient cerebral hypoxia. Ann Neurol 36:233–237, 1994

Leo J, Lacasse J: Clinical trials of therapy versus medication: even in a tie, medication wins (letter). BMJ: www.bmj.com/cgi/eletters/338/feb05_1/b463 (2009)

Leo RJ: Movement disorders associated with the serotonin selective reuptake inhibitors. J Clin Psychol 57:449–454, 1996

Leroi I, Michalon M: Treatment of the psychiatric manifestations of Huntington's disease: a review of the literature. Can J Psychiatry 43:933–940, 1998

Levy ML, Cummings JL, Fairbanks LA, et al: Apathy is not depression. J Neuropsychiatry Clin Neurosci 10:314–319, 1998

Lincoln NB, Flannagan T: Cognitive behavioral psychotherapy for depression after stroke: a randomised controlled trial. Stroke 34:111–115, 2003

Lincoln NB, Flannagan T, Sutcliff L, et al: Evaluation of cognitive behavioral treatment for depression after stroke: a pilot study. Clin Rehabil 11:114–122, 1997

Lipsey JR, Robinson RG, Pearlson GD, et al: Nortriptyline treatment of post-stroke depression: a double blind study. Lancet 1(8372):297–300, 1984

Lishman WA: Organic Psychiatry: The Psychological Consequences of Cerebral Disorder, 3rd Edition. Oxford, UK, Blackwell Science, 1997

Louis ED, Lynch T, Kaufmann P, et al: Diagnostic guidelines in central nervous system Whipple's disease. Ann Neurol 40:561–568, 1996

Lyndsay J: Phobic disorders in the elderly. Br J Psychiatry 159:531–541, 1991

Mair WGP, Warrington EK, Weiskrantz L: Memory disorder in Korsakoff's psychosis: a neuropathological and neuropsychological investigation of two cases. Brain 102:749–783, 1979

Manchanda R, Miller H, McLachlan RS: Postictal psychosis after right temporal lobectomy. J Neurol Neurosurg Psychiatry 56:277–279, 1993

Maraganore DM, Lees AJ, Marsden CD: Complex stereotypies after right putaminal infarction: a case report. Mov Disord 6:358–361, 1991

Marson AG, Al-Kharushi AM, Alwaidh M, et al: The SANAD study of effectiveness of carbamazepine, gabapentin, lamotrigine, oxcarbazepine, or topiramate for treatment of partial epilepsy: an unblinded randomised controlled trial. Lancet 369:1000–1015, 2007

Martino D, Church A, Giovannoni G: Are antibasal ganglia antibodies important, and clinically useful? Practical Neurology 7:32–41, 2007

Matharu M, Silver N: Cluster headache. Clin Evid (Online) pii:1212, 2008

Mayes AR, Meudell PR, Mann D, et al: Location of lesions in Korsakoff's syndrome: neuropsychological and neuropathological data on two patients. Cortex 24:367–388, 1988

McDonald WI, Compston A, Edan G, et al: Recommended diagnostic criteria for multiple sclerosis guidelines from the International Panel on the Diagnosis of Multiple Sclerosis. Ann Neurol 50:121–127, 2001

McEwen B: Stressful experience, brain and emotions: developmental genetic and hormonal influences, in The Cognitive Neurosciences. Edited by Gazzaniga MS. Cambridge, MA, MIT Press, 1996, pp 1117–1135

McGonigal A, Oto M, Russell AJ, et al: Outpatient video EEG recording in the diagnosis of non-epileptic seizures: a randomised controlled trial of simple suggestion techniques. J Neurol Neurosurg Psychiatry 72:549–551, 2002

McIntosh TK, Smith DH, Meaney DF, et al: Neuropathological sequelae of traumatic brain injury: relationship to neurochemical and biomechanical mechanisms. Lab Invest 74:315–342, 1996

McKeith IG, Grace JB, Walker Z, et al: Rivastigmine in the treatment of dementia with Lewy bodies: preliminary findings from an open trial. Int J Geriatr Psychiatry 15:387–392, 2000

McManus J, Pathansali R, Hassan H, et al: The course of delirium in acute stroke. Age Ageing 38:385–389, 2009a

McManus J, Pathansali R, Hassan H, et al: The evaluation of delirium post-stroke. Int J Geriatr Psychiatry 24:1251–1256, 2009b

Meagher LJ, Ilchef R, Silberstein, et al: Psychiatric morbidity in patients with Parkinson's disease following bilateral subthalamic deep brain stimulation: a literature review. Acta Neuropsychiatrica 20:182–192, 2008

Mendez MF: Huntington's disease: update and review of neuropsychiatric aspects. Int J Psychiatry Med 24:189–208, 1994

Menza MA, Sage J, Marshall E, et al: Mood changes and "on-off" phenomena in Parkinson's disease. Mov Disord 5:148–151, 1990

Merello M, Starkstein S, Nouzeilles M, et al: Bilateral pallidotomy for treatment of Parkinson's disease induced corticobulbar syndrome and psychic akinesia avoidable by globus pallidus lesion combined with contralateral stimulation. J Neurol Neurosurg Psychiatry 71:611–614, 2001

Mestre T, Ferreira J, Coelho MM, et al: Therapeutic interventions for symptomatic treatment in Huntington's disease. Cochrane Database Syst Rev (3):CD006456, 2009

Meudell P, Mayes AR: Normal and abnormal forgetting: some comments on the human amnesic syndrome, in Normality and Pathology in Cognitive Functions. Edited by Willis AW. London, Academic Press, 1982, pp 203–238

Mochizuki H, Kamakura K, Mazaki T, et al: Atypical MRI features of Wilson's disease: high signal in globus pallidus on T1 weighted images. Neuroradiology 39:171–174, 1997

Morris PL, Robinson RG, Andrzejewski P, et al: Association of depression with 10-year poststroke mortality. Am J Psychiatry 150:124–129, 1993a

Morris PL, Robinson RG, Raphael B: Emotional lability after stroke. Aust N Z J Psychiatry 27:601–605, 1993b

Morrison V, Pollard B, Johnston M, et al: Anxiety and depression 3 years following stroke: demographic, clinical, and psychological predictors. J Psychosom Res 59:209–213, 2005

Mula M, Trimble MR, Yuen A, et al: Psychiatric adverse events during levetiracetam therapy. Neurology 61:704–706, 2003

Multiple Sclerosis Council for Practice Guidelines: Fatigue and Multiple Sclerosis: Evidence-Based Management Strategies for Fatigue in Multiple Sclerosis. Washington, DC, Paralyzed Veterans of America, 1998

Neilley LK, Goodin DS, Goodkin DE, et al: Side effect profile of interferon beta-1b in multiple sclerosis: results of an open label trial. Neurology 46:552–554, 1996

Nighoghossian N, Zeng L, Derex L, et al: Warning compulsive behavior preceding acute ischemic stroke. Eur Neurol 56:39–40, 2006

Nimnuan C, Hotopf M, Wessely S: Medically unexplained symptoms: how often and why are they missed? Q J Med 93:21–28, 2000

Olanow CW, Watts RL, Koller WC: An algorithm (decision tree) for the management of Parkinson's disease: treatment guidelines. Neurology 56:S1–S88, 2001

Olanow CW: Surgical therapy for Parkinson's disease. Eur J Neurol 9:31–39, 2002

O'Malley PG, Jackson JL, Santoro J, et al: Antidepressant therapy for unexplained symptoms and symptom syndromes. J Fam Pract 48:980–990, 1999

Oostrom KJ, Smeets-Schouten A, Kruitwagen CL, et al: Not only a matter of epilepsy: early problems of cognition and behavior in children with "epilepsy only"—a prospective, longitudinal, controlled study starting at diagnosis. Pediatrics 112: 1338–1344, 2003

Oribe E, Amini R, Nissenbaum E, et al: Serum prolactin concentrations are elevated after syncope. Neurology 47:60–62, 1996

Ozer F, Meral H, Hanoglu L, et al: Cognitive impairment patterns in Parkinson's disease with visual hallucinations. J Clin Neurosci 14:742–746, 2007

Pact V, Giduz T: Mirtazapine treats resting tremor, essential tremor, and levodopa-induced dyskinesias. Neurology 53:1154, 1999

Palmieri A, Abrahams S, Sorarù G, et al: Emotional lability in MND: relationship to cognition and psychopathology and impact on caregivers. J Neurol Sci 278:16–20, 2009

Papapetropoulos S, Katzen H, Schrag A, et al: A questionnaire-based (UM-PDHQ) study of hallucinations in Parkinson's disease. BMC Neurol 20:8–21, 2008

Parikh RM, Robinson RG, Lipsey JR, et al: The impact of poststroke depression on recovery in activities of daily living over a 2-year follow-up. Arch Neurol 47:785–789, 1990

Patten SB, Metz LM: Depression in multiple sclerosis. Psychother Psychosom 66:286–292, 1997

Patten SB, Metz LM: Interferon beta-1 and depression in relapsing-remitting multiple sclerosis: an analysis of depression data from the PRISMS clinical trial. Mult Scler 7:243–248, 2001

Patten SB, Francis G, Metz LM, et al: The relationship between depression and interferon beta-1a therapy in patients with multiple sclerosis. Mult Scler 11:175–181, 2005a

Patten SB, Svenson LW, Metz LM: Psychotic disorders in MS: population based evidence of an association. Neurology 65:1123–1125, 2005b

Paul SL, Dewey HM, Sturm JW, et al: Prevalence of depression and use of antidepressant medication at 5 years poststroke in the North East Melbourne Stroke Incidence Study. Stroke 37:2854–2855, 2006

Paulsen JS, Nehl C, Hoth KF, et al: Depression and stages of Huntington's disease. J Neuropsychiatry Clin Neurosci 17:496–502, 2005

Pessiglione M, Seymour B, Flandin G, et al: Dopamine-dependent prediction errors underpin reward-seeking behavior in humans. Nature 31:1042–1045, 2006

Peto V, Jenkinson C, Fitzpatrick R, et al: The development and validation of a short measure of functioning and well being for individuals with Parkinson's disease. Qual Life Res 4:241–248, 1995

Pfeil SA, Lynn JD: Wilson's disease: copper unfettered. J Clin Gastroenterol 29:22–31, 1999

Piccardo P, Dlouhy SR, Lievens PJM: Phenotypic variability of Gerstmann-Straussler-Scheinker disease is associated with prion protein heterogeneity. J Neuropathol Exp Neurol 57: 979–988, 1998

Pohjasvaara T, Vataja R, Leppavuori A, et al: Depression is an independent predictor of poor long-term functional outcome poststroke. Eur J Neurol 8:315–319, 2001

Pohlmann-Eden B, Stefanou A, Wellhausser H: Serum prolactin in syncope. Neurology 48:1477–1478, 1997

Polman CH, Bertelsmann EW, Van Loenen AC, et al: 4-Aminopyridine in the treatment of patients with multiple sclerosis: long-term efficacy and safety. Arch Neurol 51:292–296, 1994

Pompili M, Di Cosimo D, Innamorati M, et al: Psychiatric comorbidity in patients with chronic daily headache and migraine: a selective overview including personality traits and suicide risk. J Headache Pain 10:283–290, 2009

Postuma RB, Lang AE, Massicotte-Marquez J, et al: Potential early markers of Parkinson disease in idiopathic REM sleep behavior disorder. Neurology 66:845–851, 2006

Pringsheim T, Marras C: Pimozide for tics in Tourette's syndrome. Cochrane Database Syst Rev (2):CD006996, 2009

Privitera MD, Welty TE, Ficker DM, et al: Vagus nerve stimulation for partial seizures. Cochrane Database Syst Rev (3):CD002896, 2007

Prusiner SB: Prion disease of humans and animals. J R Coll Phys Lond 28:1–30, 1994

Prusiner SB: Neurodegenerative disorders and prions. N Engl J Med 344:1516–1526, 2001

Pucci E, Brañas Tato P, D'Amico R, et al: Amantadine for fatigue in multiple sclerosis. Cochrane Database Syst Rev (1): CD002818, 2007

Pujari S, Kharkar S, Metellus P, et al: Normal pressure hydrocephalus: long-term outcome after shunt surgery. J Neurol Neurosurg Psychiatry 79:1282–1286, 2008

Pujol J, Bello J, Deus J, et al: Lesions in the left arcuate fasciculus region and depressive symptoms in multiple sclerosis. Neurology 49:1105–1110, 1997

Rabey J, Orlov E, Korczyn A: Comparison of fluvoxamine versus amitriptyline for treatment of depression in Parkinson's disease. Neurology (Abstract) 46:A374, 1996

Rabinstein AA, Shulman LM: Management of behavioral and psychiatric problems in Parkinson's disease. Parkinsonism Relat Disord 7:41–50, 2000

Rahkonen T, Makela H, Paanila S, et al: Delirium in elderly people without severe predisposing disorders: etiology and 1-year prognosis after discharge. Int Psychogeriatr 12:473–481, 2000

Ramasubbu R: Denial of illness and depression in stroke (letter). Stroke 25:226–227, 1994

Rammohan KW, Rosenburgh JH, Lynn DJ, et al: Efficacy and safety of modafinil (Provigil) for the treatment of fatigue in multiple sclerosis: a two center phase 2 study. J Neurol Neurosurg Psychiatry 72:179–183, 2002

Rao SM: Neuropsychology of multiple sclerosis. J Clin Exp Neuropsychol 8:503–542, 1986

Rao SM, Leo GJ, Bernardin L, et al: Cognitive dysfunction in multiple sclerosis, I: frequency, patterns and prediction. Neurology 41:685–691, 1991

Ravina B, Putt M, Siderowf A, et al: Donepezil for dementia in Parkinson's disease: a randomised, double blind, placebo controlled, crossover study. J Neurol Neurosurg Psychiatry 76:934–939, 2005

Reitz C, Bos MJ, Hofman A, et al: Prestroke cognitive performance, incident stroke, and risk of dementia: the Rotterdam Study. Stroke 39:36–41, 2008

Reuber M, Elger C: Psychogenic nonepileptic seizures: review and update. Epilepsy Behav 4:205–216, 2003

Reuber M, Fernandez G, Bauer J, et al: Diagnostic delay in psychogenic non-epileptic seizures. Neurology 58:493–495, 2002

Reuber M, Burness C, Howlett S, et al: Tailored psychotherapy for patients with functional neurological symptoms: a pilot study. J Psychosom Res 63:625–632, 2007

Richardson EP: Progressive multifocal leukoencephalopathy. N Engl J Med 265:815–823, 1961

Rinne JO, Lee MS, Thompson PD, et al: Corticobasal degeneration. A clinical study of 36 cases. Brain 117:1183–1196, 1994

Risk WS, Haddad FS, Chemali P: Substantial spontaneous long-term improvement in subacute sclerosing panencephalitis: six cases from the Middle East and a review of the literature. Arch Neurol 35:494–502, 1978

Roberts R: Differential diagnosis of sleep disorders, non-epileptic attacks and epileptic seizures. Curr Opin Neurol 11:135–139, 1998

Robinson RG, Arndt S: Incomplete financial disclosure in a study of escitalopram and problem solving therapy for prevention of poststroke depression. JAMA 301:1023–1024, 2009

Robinson RG, Penningworth PW: Re "Clinical trials of medication versus therapy: even in a tie, medication wins" (letter). BMJ www.bmj.com/cgi/eletters/338/feb05_1/b463 (2009)

Robinson RG, Parikh RM, Lipsey JR, et al: Pathological laughing and crying following stroke: validation of a measurement scale and a double-blind treatment study. Am J Psychiatry 150:286–293, 1993

Robinson RG, Schultz SK, Castillo C, et al: Nortriptyline versus fluoxetine in the treatment of depression and in short-term recovery after stroke: a placebo-controlled, double-blind investigation. Am J Psychiatry 157:351–359, 2000

Robinson RG, Jorge RE, Moser DJ, et al: Escitalopram and problem-solving therapy for prevention of poststroke depression: a randomized controlled trial. JAMA 299:2391–2400, 2008

Rockwood K, Bowler J, Erkinjuntti T, et al: Subtypes of vascular dementia. Alzheimer Dis Assoc Disord 13 (suppl 3):S59–S65, 1999

Rodrigo EP, Adair JC, Roberts BB, et al: Obsessive-compulsive disorder following bilateral globus pallidus infarction. Biol Psychiatry 42:410–412, 1997

Rog DJ, Nurmikko TJ, Friede T, et al: Randomized, controlled trial of cannabis-based medicine in central pain in multiple sclerosis. Neurology 65:812–819, 2005

Roman GC, Tatimichi TK, Erkinjuntti T: Vascular dementia: diagnostic criteria for research studies. Report of the NINDS-AIREN International Workshop. Neurology 43:250–260, 1993

Rosenblatt A, Ranen NG, Nance MA, et al: A Physician's Guide to the Management of Huntington's Disease, 2nd Edition. New York, Huntington's Disease Society of America, 1999

Rossi S, Mataluni G, Codecà C, et al: Effects of levetiracetam on chronic pain in multiple sclerosis: results of a pilot, randomized, placebo-controlled study. Eur J Neurol 16:360–366, 2009

Rovaris M, Comi G, Filippi M: MRI markers of destructive pathology in multiple sclerosis–related cognitive dysfunction. J Neurol Sci 245:111–116, 2006

Ruddy R, House A: Psychosocial interventions for conversion disorder. Cochrane Database Syst Rev (4):CD005331, 2005

Ruffmann C, Bogliun G, Beghi E: Epileptogenic drugs: a systematic review. Expert Rev Neurother 6:575–589, 2006

Sadovnick AD, Remick RA, Allen J, et al: Depression and multiple sclerosis. Neurology 46:628–632, 1996

Samkoff LM, Daras M, Tuchman AJ, et al: Amelioration of refractory dysesthetic limb pain in multiple sclerosis by gabapentin. Neurology 49:304–305, 1997

Sander JW: Some aspects of prognosis in the epilepsies: a review. Epilepsia 34:1007–1016, 1993

Sander JW, Shorvon SD: Epidemiology of the epilepsies. J Neurol Neurosurg Psychiatry 61:433–443, 1996

Scahill L, Leckman JF, Schultz RT, et al: A placebo-controlled trial of risperidone in Tourette syndrome. Neurology 60:1130–1135, 2003

Schacter DL: Implicit memory: history and current status. J Exp Psychol Learn Mem Cogn 13:501–518, 1987

Schiffer RB, Wineman NM: Antidepressant pharmacotherapy of depression associated with multiple sclerosis. Am J Psychiatry 147:1493–1497, 1990

Schott JM: Limbic encephalitis: a clinician's guide. Practical Neurology 6:143–153, 2006

Schrag A Trimble M, Quinn N, et al: The syndrome of fixed dystonia: an evaluation of 103 patients. Brain 127:2360–2372, 2004

Selecki BR: Intracranial space-occupying lesions among patients admitted to mental hospitals. Med J Aust 1:383–390, 1965

Servello D, Porta M, Sassi M, et al: Deep brain stimulation in 18 patients with severe Gilles de la Tourette syndrome refractory to treatment: the surgery and stimulation. J Neurol Neurosurg Psychiatry 79:136–142, 2008

Sethi KD: Clinical aspects of Parkinson disease. Curr Opin Neurol 15:457–460, 2002

Shabnam G, Chung TH, Deane K, et al: Therapies for depression in Parkinson's disease. Cochrane Database Syst Rev (2): CD003465, 2003

Shanmugiah A, Sinha S, Taly AB, et al: Psychiatric manifestations in Wilson's disease: a cross-sectional analysis. J Neuropsychiatry Clin Neurosci 20:81–85, 2008

Sharpe M, Carson A: Unexplained somatic symptoms, functional syndromes and somatization: do we need a paradigm shift? Ann Intern Med 134:926–930, 2000

Sharpe M, Stone J, Hibberd C, et al: Neurology out-patients with symptoms unexplained by disease: illness beliefs and financial benefits predict 1-year outcome. Psychol Med 40:689–698, 2010

Sheean GL, Murray NM, Rothwell JC, et al: An electrophysiological study of the mechanism of fatigue in multiple sclerosis. Brain 120:299–315, 1997

Sheng AZ, Shen Q, Cordato D, et al: Delirium within three days of stroke in a cohort of elderly patients. J Am Geriatr Soc 54:1192–1198, 2006

Shprecher D, Schwalb J, Kurlan R: Normal pressure hydrocephalus: diagnosis and treatment. Curr Neurol Neurosci Rep 8:371–376, 2008

Shulman ST: Pediatric autoimmune neuropsychiatric disorders associated with streptococci (PANDAS): update. Curr Opin Pediatr 21:127–130, 2009

Sivrioglu EY, Sivrioglu K, Ertan T, et al: Reliability and validity of the Geriatric Depression Scale in detection of poststroke minor depression. J Clin Exp Neuropsychol 3:1–8, 2009

Snaith A, Wade D: Dystonia. Clin Evid (Online) pii:1211, 2008

Spencer MD, Knight RSG, Will RG: First hundred cases of variant Creutzfeldt-Jakob disease: retrospective case note review of early psychiatric and neurological features. BMJ 324:1479–1482, 2002

Spencer SS: The relative contributions of MRI, SPECT and PET imaging in epilepsy. Epilepsia 35:S72–S89, 1994

Spencer S: Outcomes of epilepsy surgery in adults and children. Lancet Neurol 7:525–537, 2008

Sperling MR: Who should consider epilepsy surgery? Medical failure in the treatment of epilepsy, in The Surgical Management of Epilepsy. Edited by Wyler AR, Herman BR. Boston, MA, Butterworth-Heinemann, 1994, pp 26–31

Stadelmann C, Albert M, Wegner C, et al: Cortical pathology in multiple sclerosis. Curr Opin Neurol 21:229–234, 2008

Starkstein SE: Mood disorders after stroke, in Cerebrovascular Disease. Edited by Grinsberg M, Bogousslavsky J. Oxford, UK, Blackwell Science, 1998, pp 131–138

Starkstein SE, Robinson RG: Affective disorders and cerebral vascular disease. Br J Psychiatry 154:170–182, 1989

Starkstein SE, Pearlson GD, Boston J, et al: Mania after brain injury: a controlled study of causative factors. Arch Neurol 44:1069–1073, 1987

Starkstein SE, Berthier MI, Fedoroff P, et al: Anosognosia and major depression in 2 patients with cerebrovascular lesions. Neurology 40:1380–1382, 1990

Starkstein SE, Fedoroff JP, Price TR, et al: Apathy following cerebrovascular lesions. Stroke 24:1625–1630, 1993a

Starkstein SE, Fedoroff JP, Price TR, et al: Catastrophic reaction after cerebrovascular lesions: frequency, correlates, and validation of a scale. J Neuropsychiatry Clin Neurosci 5:189–194, 1993b

Starosta-Rubinstein S, Young AB, Kluin K, et al: Clinical assessment of 31 patients with Wilson's disease: correlations with structural changes on magnetic reasoning imaging. Arch Neurol 44:365–370, 1987

Stefansson SB, Olafsson E, Hauser WA: Psychiatric morbidity in epilepsy: a case controlled study of adults receiving disability benefits. J Neurol Neurosurg Psychiatry 64:238–241, 1998

Steinhoff BJ, Racker S, Herrendorf G, et al: Accuracy and reliability of periodic sharp wave complexes in Creutzfeldt-Jakob disease. Arch Neurol 53:162–166, 1996

Stillhard G, Landis T, Schiess R, et al: Bitemporal hypoperfusion in transient global amnesia: 99m-Tc-HM-PAO SPECT and neuropsychological findings during and after an attack. J Neurol Neurosurg Psychiatry 53:339–342, 1990

Stone J, Zeman A, Sharpe M: Physical signs: functional weakness and sensory disturbance. J Neurol Neurosurg Psychiatry 73:241–245, 2002

Stone J, Binzer M, Sharpe M: Illness beliefs and locus of control: a comparison of patients with pseudoseizures and epilepsy. J Psychosom Res 57:541–547, 2004

Stone J, Carson A, Sharpe M: Functional symptoms and signs in neurology: assessment and diagnosis. J Neurol Neurosurg Psychiatry 76:i2–i12, 2005a

Stone J, Carson A, Sharpe M: Functional symptoms and signs in neurology: management. J Neurol Neurosurg Psychiatry 76:i13–i21, 2005b

Stone J, Smyth R, Carson A, et al: Systematic review of misdiagnosis of conversion symptoms and "hysteria." BMJ 331:989–991, 2005c

Stone J, Zeman A, Simonotto E, et al: FMRI in patients with motor conversion symptoms and controls with simulated weakness. Psychosom Med 69:961–969, 2007

Stone J, Carson A, Aditya S, et al: The role of physical trauma in precipitating motor conversion disorder—a systematic and narrative review. J Psychosom Res 66:383–390, 2009a

Stone J, Carson A, Duncan R, et al: Symptoms "unexplained by organic disease" in 1,144 new neurology out-patients: how often does the diagnosis change at follow-up? Brain 132(pt 10):2878–2888, 2009b

Stone VE, Baron-Cohen S, Knight RT: Frontal lobe contributions to theory of mind. J Cogn Neurosci 10:640–656, 1998

Sullivan EV, Pfefferbaum A: Neuroimaging of the Wernicke-Korsakoff syndrome. Alcohol Alcohol 44:155–165, 2009

Swedo SE, Leonard HL, Garvey M, et al: Pediatric autoimmune neuropsychiatric disorders associated with streptococcal infections: clinical description of the first 50 cases. Am J Psychiatry 155:264–271, 1998

Sweet RA, Mulsant BH, Gupta B, et al: Duration of neuroleptic treatment and prevalence of tardive dyskinesia in late life. Arch Gen Psychiatry 52:478–486, 1995

Sweet RD, McDowell FH, Feigenson JS, et al: Mental symptoms in Parkinson's disease during chronic treatment with levodopa. Neurology 26:305–310, 1976

Syed TU, Arozullah AM, Suciu GP, et al: Do observer and self-reports of ictal eye closure predict psychogenic nonepileptic seizures? Epilepsia 49:898–904, 2008

Tang WK, Chen Y, Lam WW, et al: Emotional incontinence and executive function in ischemic stroke: a case-controlled study. J Int Neuropsychol Soc 15:62–68, 2009

Tanner CM, Aston DA: Epidemiology of Parkinson's disease and akinetic syndromes. Curr Opin Neurol 13:427–430, 2000

Tatimichi TK, Desmond DW, Prohovnik I, et al: Confusion and memory loss from capsular genu infarction: a thalamocortical disconnection syndrome? Neurology 42:1966–1979, 1992

Tatimichi TK, Desmon DW, Stern Y, et al: Cognitive impairment after stroke: frequency, patterns and relationship to functional abilities. J Neurol Neurosurg Psychiatry 57:202–207, 1994a

Tatimichi TK, Paik M, Begiella E, et al: Risk of dementia after stroke in a hospitalised cohort: results of a longitudinal study. Neurology 44:1885–1891, 1994b

Tatimichi TK, Desmond DW, Prohovnik I: Strategic infarcts in vascular dementia: a clinical and brain imaging experience. Arzneimittelforschung 54:371–385, 1995

Tessei S, Antonin A, Canesi M, et al: Tolerability of paroxetine in Parkinson's disease: a prospective study. Mov Disord 15:986–989, 2000

Thompson AJ: Symptomatic treatment in multiple sclerosis. Curr Opin Neurol 11:305–309, 1998

Torihashi K, Sadamasa N, Yoshida K, et al: Independent predictors for recurrence of chronic subdural hematoma: a review of 343 consecutive surgical cases. Neurosurgery 63:1125–1129, 2008

Trapp BD, Peterson J, Ranshohoff RM, et al: Axonal transection in the lesions of multiple sclerosis. N Engl J Med 338:278–285, 1998

Van Duijn E, Kingma EM, van der Mast M: Psychopathology in verified Huntington's disease gene carriers. J Neuropsychiatry Clin Neurosci 19:441–448, 2007

van Kessel K, Moss-Morris R, Willoughby E, et al: A randomized controlled trial of cognitive behavior therapy for multiple sclerosis fatigue. Psychosom Med 70:205–213, 2008

Vassos E, Panas M, Kladi A, et al: Effect of CAG repeat length on psychiatric disorders in Huntington's disease. J Psychiatr Res 42:544–549, 2008

Vickrey BG, Hays RD, Hermann BP, et al: Outcomes with respect to quality of life, in Surgical Treatment of Epilepsies, 2nd Edition. New York, Raven, 1993, pp 623–635

Victor M, Adams RD, Collins GH: The Wernicke-Korsakoff Syndrome. Philadelphia, PA, FA Davis, 1971

Vighetto A, Aimard G, Confavreux C, et al: Anatomo-clinical study of a case of topographic confabulation (or delusion) [in French]. Cortex 16:501–507, 1980

Vincent A, Buckley C, Schott JM, et al: Potassium channel antibody-associated encephalopathy: a potentially immunotherapy-responsive form of limbic encephalitis. Brain 127:701–712, 2004

Vonsattel JPG, DiFiglia M: Huntington disease. J Neuropathol Exp Neurol 57:369–384, 1998

Voon V, Potenza MN, Thomsen T: Medication-related impulse control disorders and repetitive behaviors in Parkinson's disease. Curr Opin Neurol 20:484–492, 2007

Vuilleumier P, Chicherio C, Assal F, et al: Functional neuroanatomical correlates of hysterical sensorimotor loss. Brain 124:1077–1090, 2001

Walsh JM: Wilson's disease, in Handbook of Clinical Neurology. Edited by Vinken PJ, Bruyn GW, Klawans HL. New York, Elsevier, 1986, pp 223–238

Walsh JM, Yealland M: Wilson's disease: the problem of delayed diagnosis. J Neurol Neurosurg Psychiatry 55:692–696, 1992

Weatherall MW: Chronic daily headache. Pract Neurol 7:212–221, 2007

Weigartz P, Seidenberg M, Woodard A, et al: Comorbid psychiatric disorder in chronic epilepsy: recognition and etiology of depression. Neurology 53:S3–S8, 1999

Weintraub D, Siderowf AD, Potenza MN, et al: Association of dopamine agonist use with impulse control disorders in Parkinson's disease. Arch Neurol 63:969–973, 2006

Wermuth L, Sorensen PS, Timm S, et al: Depression in idiopathic Parkinson's disease treated with citalopram. A placebo-controlled trial. Nord J Psychiatry 52:163–169, 1998

Wiart L, Petit H, Joseph PA, et al: Fluoxetine in early post-stroke depression: a double-blind placebo-controlled study. Stroke 31:1829–1832, 2000

Wiebers DO, Hollenhorst RW, Goldstein NP: The ophthalmologic manifestations of Wilson's disease. Mayo Clin Proc 52:409–416, 1997

Wiederkehr S, Simard M, Fortin C, et al: Comparability of the clinical diagnostic criteria for vascular dementia: a critical review: part I. J Neuropsychiatry Clin Neurosci 20:150–161, 2008a

Wiederkehr S, Simard M, Fortin C, et al: Validity of the clinical diagnostic criteria for vascular dementia: a critical review: part II. J Neuropsychiatry Clin Neurosci 20:162–177, 2008b

Wilhelm S, Deckersbach T, Coffey BJ, et al: Habit reversal versus supportive psychotherapy for Tourette's disorder: a randomized controlled trial. Am J Psychiatry 160:1175–1177, 2003

Will RG, Ironside JW, Zeidler M, et al: A new variant of Creutzfeldt-Jakob disease in the UK. Lancet 347:921–925, 1996

Williams LS, Kroenke K, Bakas T, et al: Care management of post-stroke depression: a randomized, controlled trial. Stroke 38:998–1003, 2007

Wintermark M, Ko NU, Smith WS, et al: Vasospasm after subarachnoid hemorrhage: utility of perfusion CT and CT angiography on diagnosis and management. Am J Neuroradiol 27:26–34, 2006

Witjas T, Kaphan E, Azulay JP, et al: Nonmotor fluctuations in Parkinson's disease: frequent and disabling. Neurology 59:408–413, 2002

Woermann FG, Free SL, Koepp MJ, et al: Voxel-by-voxel comparison of automatically segmented cerebral gray matter—a rater-independent comparison of structural MRI in patients with epilepsy. Neuroimage 10:373–384, 1999

Wolters ECH, Berendse HW: Management of psychosis in Parkinson's disease. Curr Opin Neurol 14:499–504, 2001

World Health Organization: The ICD-10 Classification of Mental and Behavioural Disorders: Clinical Descriptions and Diagnostic Guidelines. Geneva, World Health Organization, 1992

Zakzanis KK: The subcortical dementia of Huntington's disease. J Clin Exp Neuropsychol 20:565–578, 1998

Zappacosta B, Monza D, Meoni C, et al: Psychiatric symptoms do not correlate with cognitive decline, motor symptoms or

CAG repeat length in Huntington's disease. Arch Neurol 53:493–497, 1996

Zarei M, Chandran S, Compston A, et al: Cognitive presentation of multiple sclerosis: evidence for a cortical variant. J Neurol Neurosurg Psychiatry 74:872–877, 2003

Zeidler M, Sellar RJ, Collie DA, et al: The pulvinar sign on magnetic resonance imaging in variant CJD. Lancet 355:1412–1418, 2000

Zeman AZ, Boniface SJ, Hodges JR: Transient epileptic amnesia: a description of the clinical and neuropsychological features in 10 cases and a review of the literature. J Neurol Neurosurg Psychiatry 64:435–443, 1998

Zephir H, De Seze J, Stojkovic T, et al: Multiple sclerosis and depression: influence of interferon beta therapy. Mult Scler 9:284–288, 2003

Zinn S, Bosworth HB, Hoenig HM, et al: Executive function deficits in acute stroke. Arch Phys Med Rehabil 88:173–180, 2007

Ziv I, Djaldetti R, Zoldan Y, et al: Diagnosis of "nonorganic" limb paresis by a novel objective motor assessment: the quantitative Hoover's test. J Neurol 245:797–802, 1998

CHAPTER

33

Obstetrics and Gynecology

Donna E. Stewart, M.D., F.R.C.P.C.
Simone N. Vigod, M.D., F.R.C.P.C.
Nada Logan Stotland, M.D., M.P.H.

UNDERSTANDING OF WOMEN'S mental health is incomplete without consideration of the social context of their lives and reproductive factors across the life span. Traditionally, medical research has not taken sex differences into account when explaining behavior and illness nor when investigating treatment. However, the care of female patients requires an understanding not only of the biological substrates of reproduction and the nature of obstetric and gynecological diseases and treatments but also of the psychological considerations and social contexts at each stage of the reproductive life cycle. The interface between psychiatry and obstetrics and gynecology presents an important opportunity to understand the interaction between the two fields. Psychiatrists have a role in enhancing the care delivered by obstetricians and gynecologists, particularly as these specialists usually receive little training in mental health.

This chapter reviews a variety of topics relevant to reproductive psychiatry from a biological, psychological, and social perspective: gender identity, fertility, contraception, sterilization, hysterectomy, abortion (both spontaneous and induced), chronic pelvic pain, premenstrual mood disturbance, psychiatric disorders during pregnancy and postpartum, menopause, and urinary incontinence. Eating disorders are covered in Chapter 14, and cancers in women are discussed in Chapter 23.

It is important to note that some of the phenomena described in this chapter vary by culture and sexual orientation. Most research findings are derived from presumably heterosexual women in North America and Europe. Lesbian women, an often-neglected minority group, may be reluctant to seek health care because they fear or have experienced disapprobation and misunderstanding and may therefore suffer adverse health outcomes. Psychiatrists can help gynecologists and other primary care physicians to phrase questions about sexual orientation and activity in nonjudgmental terms. When possible, this chapter highlights some important considerations for treatment of women in often-overlooked minority groups, including immigrants and refugees. Unfortunately, it is beyond the scope of this chapter to address global variations in presentations and care.

Gender Identity

The first question about a newborn (or fetus) is whether it is a boy or girl, a determination made on the basis of the external genitalia. Ambiguous genitalia cause consternation; physicians and parents must decide whether to live with the ambiguity or assign the child to one gender or the other. Some believe that gender assignment should be made and carried out as early as possible so that the child can grow up with a clear gender, and others think that the child should be left as born and allowed to make a personal gender assignment when of age. Reproductive organs are the first defining feature of each human being, and gender remains a core aspect of identity throughout life. Sex hormones influence not only physical development and a host of physiological functions but also brain structure and activity. Environmental factors influence developing anatomy and ongoing physiology. A lifelong active interplay occurs among genetics, anatomy, physiology, social influences, and individual psychology.

The term *sex* refers to narrowly defined biological characteristics. The term *gender* includes social roles and an individual's sense of femininity or masculinity. Some evidence indicates that girls are aware of their sexual organs and identity as early as toddlerhood. As puberty approaches in females, the sense of gender identity is powerfully reinforced and reshaped by society and by physical changes: the development of breasts and pubic hair and the onset of menstruation. In some cultures, girls are told at menarche that they are now women. With menarche comes fertility and the possibility that sexual activity will lead to pregnancy. Although girls can be sexually abused at any age, the possibility of rape is more overt after puberty, and vulnerability to attack becomes part of gender identity. The possibility of pregnancy can be at once a worry and a wish. A young woman may feel that she is not truly a woman until she has had heterosexual intercourse or until she has borne a child. Girls who feel sexual attraction for other girls face a crisis in gender identity because society increasingly expects them to date, form relationships, and engage in sexual activity with males. Medical problems that interfere with any of these functions threaten core gender identity.

Infertility

A common definition of infertility is 12 months of appropriately timed unprotected intercourse that does not result in conception. However, a shorter time (6 months) is often used in women older than 35 years because the nature of fertility at this age makes it desirable to initiate diagnosis and treatment as soon as possible. The World Health Organization has reported that between 8% and 12% of couples, or approximately 50–80 million people worldwide, experience some type of fertility problem during their reproductive lives (World Health Organization Programme of Maternal and Child Health and Family Planning Unit 1991). A more recent study found an overall prevalence of infertility of 9% across countries (Boivin et al. 2007). In the United States, it has been estimated that 7.4% of married couples, or 2.1 million married women of childbearing age, have a fertility problem (Chandra et al. 2005). Although the popular impression is that the prevalence of infertility has risen over the past few decades, the rate of infertility has remained relatively stable since 1965 (Keye 1999). Rather, the use and availability of medical services, as well as willingness to disclose and public awareness of infertility treatment options, have increased (Burns and Covington 1999; Keye 1999).

As much as 40% of the time, infertility may be attributable to multiple causes (i.e., a combination of multiple male and female factors), and up to 10% of the time, the etiology remains completely unexplained. Historically, infertility that could not be explained on an organic basis was thought to be "psychogenic," related to ambivalence about becoming a parent, unconscious repudiation of femininity and motherhood, unconscious fears and conflict about sex, and wishes to remain dependent. However, these themes were based on psychoanalytic case reports and have been shown to be present in women with no trouble conceiving (Apfel and Keylor 2002). Thus, the focus of research on the relationship between mental health and fertility has shifted toward exploration of the biological, psychological, and social factors that mediate psychiatric illness or psychological distress in couples with infertility. This research suggests that the relationship between fertility and mental health is complex. Practitioners must take into account the stresses of infertility itself, with the associated investigations and treatment, as well as how psychiatric morbidity may influence fertility and the outcomes of fertility treatments (Williams et al. 2007).

Scope of Psychiatric Illness Affecting Couples With Infertility

Infertility is experienced as stressful, with 50% of women and 15% of men undergoing infertility diagnosis or treatment ranking it the most stressful event of their lives (Freeman et al. 1985). Although some studies show that women with infertility are distressed but do not meet criteria for a major psychiatric disorder, some studies reveal rates of major depressive disorder in infertile women that reach 50%, with anxiety disorders reaching 40% (Chen et al. 2004; Lukse and Vacc 1999; Ramezanzadeh et al. 2004). In a survey of 980 members of an infertility support group, 1 in 5 women reported suicidal feelings (despite the fact that approximately 50% had conceived by the time of the survey) (Kerr et al. 1999). Also, there are sex differences in the scope of psychiatric illness, with men reporting more symptoms of anxiety and depression than men in the general population (but far less than their female counterparts) (Volgsten et al. 2008). Although there is evidence to suggest that women become more depressed with every failed cycle of assisted reproductive technology treatment, successful conception may reduce depression scores (Verhaak et al. 2005, 2007).

Factors Mediating Psychiatric Illness in Couples With Infertility

Biological factors related to infertility that may impact mental health include the cause and duration of infertility, as well as the effects of fertility treatment. There is evidence that the difference in psychological profile between fertile and infertile couples increases with time. Ramezanzadeh et al. (2004) found scores on the Beck Depression Inventory increasing up to 9 years of infertility and that there is more distress when the cause is unexplained. Interestingly, men show greater distress and guilt when the infertility is attributable to male-factor etiology, but women are equally distressed regardless of the cause (Volgsten et al. 2010). Although the reasons for this sex difference have not been investigated, this may be a reflection of the association of fertility with virility, the social expectation on women for conception and delivery of a baby, and the pervasive shame associated with infertility.

Fertility treatments themselves may have adverse effects on mental health. Interventions can be time-consuming, embarrassing, and invasive. The psychological effects, particularly mood alterations, of fertility-enhancing drugs are underappreciated. Careful attention should be paid to the potential contribution of recent changes in drug regimens to recent-onset psychiatric symptoms such as depression, anxiety, mania, and psychosis (Choi et al. 2005). Progesterone is often used for luteal phase abnormalities of the endometrium and can cause depression, insomnia, and somnolence. Clomiphene induces follicle-stimulating hormone (FSH) and has been associated with anxiety, insomnia, and psychosis (related to ongoing treatment or upon discontinuation of treatment) (Burns 2007).

Both intrauterine insemination (IUI) and in vitro fertilization (IVF) are associated with multiple gestations, which often cause maternal and fetal problems. Maternal complications include significant increases in cardiac morbidity, hematological morbidity, amniotic fluid embolus, pre-eclampsia, obstetric intervention, hysterectomy, and blood transfusion (Walker et al. 2004). Preterm birth is very common in multiple gestations and may be associated with cerebral palsy and other long-term infant sequelae that may cause psychological stress to the whole family (Walker et al. 2004).

Psychological factors play an important role. Becoming a parent is a lifelong fantasy and is experienced as a developmental need for many women. Women experience anger, a sense of loss of control, and reduced self-esteem. Self-blame increases risk of depressive illness (Morrow et al. 1995). Guilt may manifest with respect to being the cause of the infertility (e.g., older age because of choice to establish a career, prior sexually transmitted infection) or from upsetting spouses and disappointing families. Important social factors include gender roles, marital expectations, and familial and societal attitudes (Dyer et al. 2004; Matsubayashi et al. 2004).

Effect of Psychiatric Illness on Fertility

The current understanding is that psychiatric illness may impact fertility directly through mechanisms related to chronic stress, altered immune responses, and hormonal changes, as well as indirectly through changes in behavior such as smoking, alcohol, poor nutrition, and lack of exercise. Eating disorders (anorexia nervosa, bulimia nervosa, obesity) are all associated with infertility. Restrictive or purging eating behaviors are often undisclosed and result in subfecundity and poor pregnancy outcomes (Stewart and Robinson 2001a). It is also important to consider the impact of psychotropic medications on fertility. For example, selective serotonin reuptake inhibitors (SSRIs) have been shown to be associated with a small but increased risk of early miscarriage, valproic acid is associated with polycystic ovarian syndrome (see Chapter 22, "Endocrine and Metabolic Disorders"), and many antipsychotic medications are associated with anovulation due to hyperprolactinemia (Joffe 2007).

Psychosocial Assessment in Infertility Patients

Although it is not common practice to refer all couples with infertility for a mental health assessment, the grueling nature of infertility diagnosis and treatment is becoming more widely appreciated. Normally intimate and private behaviors are asked about, subjected to strict timing, and brought into the clinical arena. Careful inquiry should be made regarding any psychiatric side effects of fertility-enhancing drugs, particularly alterations in mood.

Some have suggested that current levels of distress and coping strategies should be assessed in couples before initiating infertility treatment to provide the opportunity to learn and practice new adaptive behaviors that could enhance their ability to cope with infertility and the associated medical investigations and procedures. Counseling is sometimes recommended in couples considering donor eggs or sperm or surrogacy. The goal of mental health evaluation is to identify and treat any comorbid psychiatric disorders, to prepare the couple for infertility treatments, to raise emotional and ethical treatment issues that the couple may not have considered, and to offer support and coping strategies. Individual and group interventions are often helpful in providing mutual support, information, and coping techniques (Wischmann 2008).

Contraception

Contraceptive information and care are widely available in the Western world. Nevertheless, half of the pregnancies in North America each year are unintended, and one-third of births in the United States are classified as unwanted or mistimed. Contraceptive choices and use are affected by knowledge and misinformation, by women's comfort with their own sexuality and genitalia, by the preferences of sexual partners, by social custom, and by access to physicians for hormonal methods. Many women are ill-informed about contraception (Picardo et al. 2003).

Psychodynamics and psychiatric conditions can interfere with a woman's use of a contraceptive technique. Pregnancy may be sought, consciously or unconsciously, as a proof of fertility and womanhood. Contraception, because it requires planning, requires acknowledgment of future sexual activity. For example, because of views about sex outside of marriage or cultural sanctions, some unmarried women may only engage in sexual intercourse when "swept away" by a romantic situation (and are thus unprepared to prevent pregnancy). Some women may feel uncomfortable about touching their own genitalia, as some contraceptive methods require. Many women have limited knowledge about their own anatomy, are too anxious to absorb the information in a hurried office or clinic visit, and are too embarrassed to ask for information to be repeated (Sanders et al. 2003). In a review of 16 studies that examined reasons for unprotected intercourse in adult women, Ayoola et al. (2007) found that reasons for unprotected intercourse included perceived inconvenience; unexpected/unplanned sex; ambivalence about pregnancy; problems using, acquiring, or storing the method; lack of knowledge or misinformation (e.g., low perceived risk of getting pregnant, lack of understanding of how to use/acquire method, belief that contraception reduces pleasure or makes sex unnatural); and unwanted side effects from oral contraception. Other problems included access to contraception (e.g., problems getting appointment, cost, preferred method not available), lack of continuity in care providers, and lack of privacy at contraceptive clinics. Alcohol abuse, particularly binge drinking (the rates of which are rising in young women), may also be a contributing factor.

Unplanned pregnancy is by no means always the result of the factors described above. Contraceptive methods do fail. Forced or unwanted sex is also a reason for unprotected intercourse, and gender and relationship power differentials play a major role in the use of contraception. Some women are sexually assaulted, bullied, or cajoled into unprotected sexual intercourse (Rickert et al. 2002). Ayoola et al. (2007) found that interpersonal reasons for unprotected sex were often partner-related (partner did not want to use contraception, fear of negative reaction from partner) or attributable to the influence of social custom. In a U.S study of women at risk for sexually transmitted infections, a male partner's unwillingness to use condoms increased the odds of intercourse without barrier contraception by 4.1 (95% confidence interval [CI]=2.3 to 6.9) (Peipert et al. 2007). In a large sample of New Zealand women, those who experienced interpersonal violence were more likely to have a partner who had either refused to use condoms or tried to prevent the woman from using contraception (Fanslow et al. 2008). Despite these facts, it is women who are often blamed, both in societal and in medical contexts, for becoming pregnant at the wrong time or with the wrong partner. The resultant sense of shame and powerlessness can contribute to psychiatric symptoms and, paradoxically, can leave them more vulnerable to future unplanned pregnancies.

New Developments in Contraception

Newer developments in contraception have important psychosocial implications. For example, emergency contraception consists of higher doses of oral contraceptives taken after unprotected intercourse. Although most effective the earlier it is taken, it can be effective in preventing pregnancy within 3 days, and possibly up to 5 days, after unprotected intercourse. Emergency contraception can be obtained at family planning clinics, hospital emergency departments, or pharmacies. A recent study of women's preferences about obtaining emergency contraception found that women were more likely to use services perceived as sympathetic, nonjudgmental, and protective of privacy (Seston et al. 2007). Women who are young, especially those who are poor or from certain cultural groups, may be uninformed, embarrassed, unaware of their level of risk for pregnancy, worried about side effects of emergency contraception, and concerned about negative responses from others (Shoveller et al. 2007). In England, Australia, Canada, and some other countries, emergency contraception is available without a prescription. The U.S. Food and Drug Administration (FDA) recently notified the manufacturer of the emergency hormonal contraceptive pill Plan B (a 0.75 mg norgestrel) that it may market Plan B without a prescription to women 17 years or older (U.S. Food and Drug Administration 2009). A Cochrane Database systematic review of advance provision of emergency contraception found that it did not lead to increased rates of sexually transmitted infections (odds ratio [OR]=0.99; 95% CI=0.73 to 1.34), increased frequency of unprotected intercourse, or changes in contraceptive methods (Polis et al. 2007).

Another important consideration with respect to newer developments in contraception involves the use of hormonal contraceptives on a continuous rather than intermittent basis (e.g., hormonal implants, transdermal contraceptive patches, daily contraceptive pills). These methods have been developed to reduce the likelihood of contraceptive failure due to inconsistent use of the oral contraceptive pill or barrier contraceptive methods. They can also be used to treat dysmenorrhea and menorrhagia. However, continuous hormonal contraception does cause amenorrhea. This may have psychosocial implications for women who hold beliefs about menstruation as necessary for cleansing and confirmation of femininity (Glasier et al. 2003). Hormonal implants may also cause a decrease in bone density that is reversible when the implant is removed.

Management

Inquiries about sexual behavior and protection from unwanted consequences should be part of every medical, including psychiatric, history and treatment. Patients may be so accustomed to their birth control pills or injections that they fail to report them when asked what medications they are taking. Clinicians must ask about these contraceptives specifically in order to assess not only the adequacy of the contraceptive method but also the potential for drug-drug interactions. The major pathway of metabolism for both the estrogen and progesterone components of hormonal contraception is through the liver by cytochrome P450 (CYP) 3A4 (Oesterheld et al. 2008). Medications that induce CYP3A4, thus reducing the efficacy of hormonal contraception, include phenobarbital, oxcarbazepine, carbamazepine, topiramate (at dosages >200 mg/day), modafinil, and St. John's wort. Oral contraceptives can also inhibit the oxidation of various psychiatric medications via CYP1A2, 2B6, 2C19, and 3A4. Importantly, this can result in increased levels of benzodiazepines and tricyclic antidepressants (TCAs). Levels of valproate and lamotrigine can also be increased by oral contraceptives (likely via inhibition of glucuronidation).

In summary, access to care and adequate information about contraception is essential for all patients. Certain groups, such as women with severe and persistent psychiatric illness, adolescents, and recent immigrants, may have increased vulnerability to some of the factors cited above and have been shown to use contraceptive methods suboptimally (Gelberg et al. 2002; Magalhaes et al. 2009; Whitaker and Gilliam 2008). Atypical antipsychotic medications do not impair fertility as much as older antipsychotics and may result in unwanted pregnancies in women being treated for psychotic illnesses. Therefore, attention to contraceptive knowledge and use in these groups is of great importance.

Sterilization

Sterilization is the most commonly used method of contraception in the world for women ages 15–49 years who are married or in ongoing heterosexual relationships, with the highest rates in less developed countries (United Nations 2007). It is intended to be a permanent solution to unwanted fertility, although some tubal ligations are reversible. A psychiatrist may be asked to consult when a young nulliparous woman, or a patient with a mental illness, desires to be sterilized. Assessment of capacity to consent to treatment and to give informed consent is essential, highlighted by state laws enacted in the wake of past involuntary sterilization of individuals with mental illness. It may be appropriate for guardians to consent to sterilization procedures for severely cognitively impaired or developmentally delayed adult women who are unable to cope with the hygienic aspects of menstruation, are victimized by male predators, become pregnant, and are entirely unable to cope with the stresses of birth and parenting. However, mental illnesses cannot be equated with incapacity to make treatment decisions. Women may have psychotic symptoms, or a history of them, that interfere with capacity, but they also may make well-informed decisions not to have children, or more children, precisely because they recognize that their illness would interfere with their parenting. When there is uncertainty, a longitudinal assessment is appropriate. For example, the psychiatrist may ask the patient to return in a few months. If she is mature, not acutely psychotic, and persistent in her desire for sterilization, she may be as appropriate a candidate for the procedure as a woman without diagnosed psychiatric illness.

The occurrence of postsurgical regret ranges from 5% to 20%. A systematic review of 19 studies found that age was a significant risk factor for postsurgical regret, with women who were sterilized when younger than age 30 more than twice as likely to experience regret as women older than 30 years (Curtis et al. 2006). Other risk factors include marital conflict over the procedure and subsequent changes in marital partnerships (Jamieson et al. 2002). Death of a child has been associated with poststerilization regret, and a survey of women in India identified having few or no male children as a risk factor for regret (Machado et al. 2005; Malhotra et al. 2007). Sexual satisfaction does not appear to be affected (Peterson 2008). The provision of clear information about the nature, effectiveness, risks, and benefits of the procedure is a crucial factor in patient satisfaction.

Hysterectomy

Hysterectomy is the surgical removal of the uterus. It is one of the most common surgical procedures performed on North American women, with rates of approximately 5.3 per 1,000 women-years in the United States (Wu et al. 2007) (see also the "Pelvic Surgery" section in Chapter 30, "Surgery"). In North America, hysterectomy rates are between two and five times higher than in European countries, but small area rate variations are widespread in most countries. These variations appear to depend on women's socioeconomic class, race/ethnicity, education level, religion, physician practice, reimbursement schedules, and availability of new technologies (Stewart et al. 2002).

Hysterectomy may be total or subtotal (where the cervix is left intact) and also may be combined with removal of the fallopian tubes and ovaries (bilateral salpingo-oophorectomy [BSO]). Although vaginal hysterectomy is associated with lower mortality and shorter length of stay, abdominal hysterectomy remains the most common hysterectomy procedure. A small proportion of hysterectomies are performed to treat malignancies or catastrophic hemorrhage, but the vast majority are elective procedures performed primarily to improve quality of life in women with abnormal uterine bleeding, fibroids, uterine prolapse, chronic pelvic pain, or endometriosis. The mean age of women undergoing hysterectomy is the mid-40s, or an average of 6–7 years before the mean age of natural menopause, when some of these problems (abnormal uterine bleeding, fibroids) spontaneously resolve. However, hysterectomy is the treatment of choice for certain gynecological conditions. The predicted advantage must be carefully weighed against the risks of surgery and other treatment alternatives, such as hormonal therapy and endometrial ablation (Lefebvre et al. 2002).

Information Needs and Decision-Making Preferences

Well-informed women who have been involved in decision making about hysterectomy have the best outcomes (Stewart et al. 2002). Various studies and expert panels have concluded that women and their family physicians should be provided with an adequate level of knowledge to make a fully informed decision as to whether hysterectomy, less invasive procedures, medical management, or watchful waiting is the best option (Stewart et al. 2002; Uskul et al. 2003; Vigod and Stewart 2002). Similarly, the options for retention or removal of the cervix and ovaries and route of hysterectomy (vaginal vs. abdominal) should be discussed.

Women's decision making regarding discretionary hysterectomy (i.e., not for treatment of malignancy) is influenced by their age, socioeconomic status, education, desire for fertility, sexual orientation, ethnicity, and severity of their symptoms. The influence of family, friends, and partners as well as health care professionals also plays a major role (Graham et al. 2008). Women who require hysterectomy for the treatment of malignancies are understandably focused more on the cancer, its overall treatment, and its prognosis.

Variations With Ethnic, Socioeconomic, and Sexual Diversity

Several articles have explored ethnic differences and indications for hysterectomy (Bower et al. 2009; Farquhar and Steiner 2002; Lewis et al. 2000). African American women undergo hysterectomy at a younger age for most diagnostic categories, including leiomyomas, genital prolapse, and endometriosis. They are also more likely to have an abdominal hysterectomy, extended hospital stays, and higher in-hospital mortality (Lewis et al. 2000). Data from the Coronary Artery Risk Development in Young Adults (CARDIA) study in the United States were used to examine differences in hysterectomy rates between black and white women (N = 1,863). Black women demonstrated greater odds of hysterectomy compared with white women even after adjustment for age, educational attainment, perceived barriers to accessing medical care, body mass index, polycystic ovarian syndrome, tubal ligation, depressive symptoms, age at menarche, and geographic location (OR=3.70; 95% CI=2.44 to 5.61) (Bower et al. 2009). Qualitative analyses with Hispanic, African American, and lesbian women (Groff et al. 2000) have explored their capacity to acquire a second opinion about hysterectomy and available alternatives that may be limited by education, ethnicity, economics, and access.

Psychological and Sexual Outcomes

A literature review of psychological and sexual outcomes after hysterectomy located more than 100 studies (Flory et al. 2005). The methodological quality of many of the studies was poor, but the authors concluded that while psychosexual and psychosocial effects are minimal overall, a subgroup of women (10%–20%) do report sexual dysfunction, depressive symptoms, and/or impaired body image.

Risk factors for poor outcome appear to be related to preoperative pain, sexual dysfunction, and psychiatric morbidity. Outcome does not appear to depend on the method of surgical removal of the uterus or the type of hysterectomy that was performed (Flory et al. 2006). Hartmann et al. (2004) reported that women with preoperative pain and depression had less improvement after hysterectomy than women without pain and depression preoperatively. A prospective study of 68 women in Taiwan evaluated the risk of major depressive disorder in women who underwent hysterectomy for nonmalignant conditions. The authors found that although overall psychological symptoms improved postsurgery, risk factors for postoperative major depressive disorder were prior emotional problems, poorer body image, and poorer sexual functioning as well as higher stress 1 month postsurgery (Yen et al. 2008). Women with substantiated diagnoses and clear indications for hysterectomy have better physical and psychological outcomes than do women with less defined symptoms and indicators such as chronic pelvic pain.

Role of the Psychiatrist

There may be a role for psychiatrists in assessing mood, anxiety, understanding, and feelings about sexuality and fertility in vulnerable women undergoing hysterectomy. For the informed, psychologically healthy woman who has failed to respond to other treatment options and who has a significantly impaired quality of life because of a specific gynecological condition, hysterectomy may offer an improved quality of life. However, for women with premorbid depression, anxiety, or personality disorders, especially if accompanied by ambivalence about sexuality, fertility, or the procedure, hysterectomy may fail to ameliorate, or may even exacerbate, preexisting symptoms. It is important to consider that women undergoing hysterectomy with BSO have to confront the onset of sudden surgical menopause if estrogen therapy is not begun shortly after surgery. Even women whose ovaries were not removed may experience sudden menopause due to impaired blood supply to the ovaries. This sudden hormonal change may result in vasomotor symptoms, sleep loss, and depression, especially in vulnerable women with a history of depression associated with reproductive events (Stewart and Boydell 1993). Therefore, psychiatrists should ascertain the hormonal status of women with sudden mood changes following hysterectomy and consider short-term hormonal treatment as well as antidepressants. Psychiatrists who assess women undergoing hysterectomy should evaluate their understanding of the procedure, attitudes toward fertility and sexuality, and experience and expectations of surgery, as well as psychiatric history. The appropriate treatment, whether psychotherapy, hormones, or psychotropics, will, as always, depend on the individual woman.

Abortion

Spontaneous Abortion

Abortion can be spontaneous (miscarriage) or induced (usually just termed *abortion*). Approximately 15%–20% of recognized pregnancies end in spontaneous abortion, with the majority occurring in the first trimester of pregnancy. Spontaneous abortion generally evokes feelings of failure and loss. A woman's body has failed to perform one of its basic functions; she has failed to produce a child for her partner and parents; she has expelled her own potential child; and she may have conceived an embryo with genetic anomalies (Friedman and Gath 1989). Decades ago, miscarriage was sometimes attributed to the woman's unconscious rejection of motherhood, but this theory has never been validated by empirical research. Spontaneous abortion, like a stillbirth or neonatal death, may precipitate pathological grief, postpartum depression, or posttraumatic stress (Brier 2008; Engelhard et al. 2003). Although the psychological sequelae of miscarriage will be to some extent dependent on individual psychodynamic factors, psychiatric history, and prior experiences with loss, there are elements unique to spontaneous abortion that may play a role. Contrary to the traditional conceptualization of loss, a miscarriage often involves grief about anticipated outcomes. Women report that the failure of society in general and of friends and family to acknowledge their loss is painful and complicates the grieving process. People often say, "There must have been something wrong with the baby," "This is God's way of correcting mistakes," or "You can just get pregnant again." There are no ceremonies to mark the occasion. Friends and co-workers tend to avoid the subject and to expect the woman to recover within days or weeks, but grief may last for months. Gestational age and the degree to which a woman perceives the fetus as "real" have been shown to be associated with the nature and intensity of grief. The perception of the reality of the pregnancy increases when women have seen the fetus via ultrasonography or when they can feel fetal movement (both more likely with increased gestational age). It is important to note that although women are at higher risk of psychological reactions following miscarriage than men, their male partners can and do experience psychological sequelae, sometimes expressed as overinvolvement with work or sports.

Health care providers may have difficulty addressing the emotional effect of spontaneous abortion. They feel helpless to prevent it, and it is generally not associated with serious medical or obstetric complications. Psychiatrists can help them to understand and tolerate how their patients are feeling and to appreciate the benefits of simply allowing patients to express those feelings. Health care providers should be aware that emotional recovery, depending on the circumstances, can take months, and they need to know when and how to make the diagnosis of pathological grief. It is often helpful for them to meet with the patient some weeks after the event to go over the medical findings, if any; the prognosis; and the state of the woman's recovery.

The loss of pregnancy through miscarriage or stillbirth is associated with an increase in anxiety during a subsequent pregnancy (Bergner et al. 2008). Preliminary data suggest that fears related to pregnancy may have a negative impact on pregnancy and delivery outcomes (Fertl et al. 2009). Although patients are frequently counseled to wait 6 months or a year after such a loss, they often conceive as soon as possible, especially if they feel that the fertility clock is ticking. The obstetrician must be prepared to offer them enhanced support. There is evidence to suggest that medical counseling, either alone or combined with psychological counseling, can reduce a woman's distress with respect to grief, self-blame, and worry (Nikcevic et al. 2007).

Induced Abortion

Psychiatric Sequelae

Approximately 1.22 million abortions are performed every year in the United States; at least one in four women in the United States will have an abortion in their lifetime (Ventura et al. 2008). Psychiatrists are seldom consulted about abortion and abortion decisions, and no evidence shows that formal mental health consultation is routinely necessary. The psychiatric ramifications of abortion are a matter of some debate, but the findings are clear once methodological confounds are taken into account. Unbiased reviews of the literature indicate that self-limited feelings of guilt and sadness are common after abortion, although the predominant reaction is one of relief, and new episodes of psychiatric illness are rare (Charles et al. 2008). Although there may be initial increases in distress and anxiety around the time of abortion, adverse effects on self-esteem in the long term are not seen (Bradshaw et al. 2003). In fact, studies have shown that women's quality of life improves in the period from before to after an early abortion (Garg et al. 2001; Westhoff et al. 2003). The best outcomes prevail when women are able to make autonomous, supported choices about their pregnancies. When women seek, but are denied, abortion, the resulting children have significantly poorer outcomes than their siblings or matched control subjects (Kubicka et al. 2002).

Antiabortion groups and writers claim that abortion is associated with a higher risk of serious psychiatric disorders and suicide than is childbirth (Pro-Life Action Ministries, undated; Reardon et al. 2003; Thorp et al. 2003). These publications fail to address the circumstances of and reasons for abortion. Sometimes they confound common self-limited feelings of loss and guilt with diagnosable depression. Women often have abortions because they have been abandoned by the men who impregnated them, because those men threaten to leave if they continue the pregnancy, because the pregnancy is the result of rape or incest, because they are poor and overburdened with other responsibilities, or because they do not have the resources—educational, financial, emotional, or social—to provide adequate parenting. They may simply not want to be a parent. Preexisting serious psychiatric illness makes some women more vulnerable to unwanted pregnancy and less able to parent.

Risk Factors

Not surprisingly, coercion, lack of social support, poverty, rape, incest, and preexisting psychiatric illness are associated with increased risk for psychological difficulties following, but not causally related to, abortion. Women who belong to religious faiths opposed to abortion choose abortion as often as or more often than those who do not. Efforts have been made to reach out to this population, both to enlist them in antiabortion advocacy and to offer them spiritual support (Gay and Lynxwiler 1999; Jeal and West 2003; Ventura et al. 2000). Demonstrators or fear of terrorism at an abortion facility may exacerbate stress, and the attitudes and behaviors of medical personnel during the abortion procedure have a significant influence on patients' experience (Slade et al. 2001).

The delay of abortion into the second trimester, or later, is most often secondary to denial of pregnancy, difficulties with access, or diagnosis of a serious fetal defect, each of which increases the risk for negative postabortion reactions. The discovery of a fetal defect in a wanted pregnancy or the need to abort because of serious illness in the mother arouses the same sense of failure and loss as a miscarriage, with the added concern that one is carrying a genetic anomaly or is physically unable to bear a child. Consultation may be sought when a woman or family cannot decide, or manifests overwhelming anxiety, when making an abortion decision under these circumstances (Zlotogora 2002). Continuing a pregnancy and relinquishing the child for adoption pose a psychological burden as well (Cushman et al. 1993). There does not appear to be a difference in psychological outcome based on the type of abortion that a woman undergoes (i.e., medical or surgical abortion), although many women prefer the privacy of medical abortion (Ashok et al. 2005).

Minors and Abortion

The effect of abortion on minors, and their ability to make decisions about abortion, is another area of controversy. The vast majority of pregnant minors choose to involve their parents in the abortion decision. No evidence shows that those who think it is not safe or wise to inform their parents derive benefit from being forced to do so. Term pregnancy and delivery pose greater medical and psychological risks for adolescents than does abortion. Arguments that minors are too immature to elect abortion overlook the fact that these same minors, if their pregnancies are not terminated, will soon be mothers with responsibility for infants. In Zabin's classic study of inner-city girls who obtained pregnancy tests at a school clinic, girls who had abortions had better outcomes compared with those who carried their pregnancies to term and even compared with those whose pregnancy test results were negative. This does not imply that the abortion improved these teens' mental health; rather, it may indicate that the inability to confirm whether one is pregnant is associated with other psychosocial problems. Marriage of the pregnant teenager to the father of the baby does not improve outcome and may even worsen it (Zabin et al. 1989).

Chronic Pelvic Pain

Chronic pelvic pain is nonmenstrual pelvic pain of 6 or more months' duration that is severe enough to cause functional disability or require medical or surgical treatment (Howard 2003). It is a relatively common and significant disorder of women, with an estimated prevalence of 3.8% in adult women, similar to that of asthma or back pain (Zondervan et al. 1999). Chronic pelvic pain is one of the most common gynecological complaints and accounts for 2%–10% of outpatient gynecological referrals, although most women are managed by their primary care practitioners (Howard 2003). Chronic pelvic pain may lead to disability and suffering, with loss of employment, marital discord and divorce, and overall decline in quality of life (Howard 2003).

Etiology of Chronic Pelvic Pain

Despite the severity and frequency of chronic pelvic pain, its etiology is often difficult to discern. Disorders of the reproductive, gastrointestinal, urological, musculoskeletal, and neurological systems may be associated with chronic pelvic pain. In many cases, however, the pain is related to a combination of physical and psychological factors, such as endometriosis, adhesions, urological problems, irritable bowel syndrome, myofascial pain, depression, anxiety, somatization, and past abusive experiences (Dalpiaz et al. 2008). Endometriosis and pelvic adhesive disease are responsible for most cases of chronic pelvic pain with organic findings, but a significant number of patients have no obvious etiology for their pain at the time of laparoscopy (Gelbaya and El-Halwagy 2001). As with other chronic syndromes, especially those with ambiguous etiology, the biopsychosocial model offers the best way of integrating physical causes of pain with psychological and social factors. One model, the gate-control theory of pain, proposes that peripheral nociceptive signals can be modified by neurotransmitters, such as serotonin and endorphins, that control mood states, and accordingly, the gateway to chronic pain can be opened by a combination of depression and direct tissue irritation. Because interacting psychological and physical factors are likely to be present early in the course of pain, attempts to separate chronic pain into a simple cause-effect relation are usually unrewarding. An alternative theory, the diathesis-stress model, proposes that some patients are at increased risk for chronic pain because of preexisting acquired vulnerability. This might explain why a disproportionate number of patients with chronic pelvic pain report histories of physical and sexual abuse (Gelbaya and El-Halwagy 2001). Recent work on gene-environment interactions may also offer a promising model to explore chronic pelvic pain.

Psychological Factors Associated With Chronic Pelvic Pain

The relation of chronic pelvic pain to psychological state or personality style has received great attention. In general, the concept of psychogenic pain (emotional pain displaced onto the body) has been superseded. Cognitive-behavioral and psychophysiological theories have moved increasingly toward supporting more complex, multicausal views of chronic pelvic pain. Chronic pelvic pain is likely to be the outcome of several somatic, social, and psychological influences acting together in varying degrees. A systematic review evaluating the literature on factors predisposing women to chronic or recurrent pelvic pain (Latthe et al. 2006) identified psychological variables that appear to be consistently associated with chronic pelvic pain. Both cyclic (i.e., dysmenorrhea) and noncyclic pelvic pain are associated with anxiety, depression, and history of physical and sexual assault. Although very few of these studies were designed in a way to separate psychological predictors of chronic pelvic pain from psychological sequelae, it is clear that chronic pelvic pain is a long-standing condition and women with it are at greater risk of low self-esteem, depression or anxiety, low marital satisfaction and sexual dysfunction, and somatic symptoms (Weijenborg et al. 2007).

Management of Chronic Pelvic Pain

It is well recognized that a multidisciplinary, multifocal approach to chronic pelvic pain, individualized for each woman, is essential (Dalpiaz et al. 2008; Gunter 2003). Recent research suggests that many women become dissatisfied with the care they receive and refrain from seeking help, despite ongoing symptoms (Dalpiaz et al. 2008). This highlights the importance of attention to the therapeutic relationship. Goals of management include improving function, restoring quality of life, and maintaining even small gains in treatment. First-line management includes a combination of physical therapy, nonnarcotic pain management, and psychological support as indicated. Focused psychotherapy may be useful to address issues such as pain management, current conflicts, past sexual and physical abuse, current domestic violence, substance abuse problems, and sexual and marital dysfunction. Phases of treatment include education, skills acquisition, behavior modification, and maintenance. Special techniques may increase the patient's coping ability and sense of control; such techniques include muscle relaxation, deep breathing and imagery, and cognitive-behavioral techniques to identify and address maladaptive thoughts. Because patients with chronic pelvic pain frequently limit their activity to avoid possible pain, activity programs can be initiated to decrease disability behaviors. Additional interventions might include medical therapies (oral analgesics, antidepressants, drugs for dysmotility disorders, management of musculoskeletal pain, ovarian cycle suppression, and antibiotics), biofeedback, and surgical procedures. Unfortunately, the most recent Cochrane Database systematic review on the management of chronic pelvic pain identified only nine methodologically adequate studies (Stones and Mountfield 2000). Current evidence does not support SSRIs as beneficial in chronic pelvic pain (Cheong and William Stones 2006), but the role of serotonin-norepinephrine reuptake inhibitors (SNRIs) has not been fully explored.

Endometriosis

Endometriosis is defined as the presence of hormonally responsive endometrial tissue outside the uterine cavity. The precise pathogenesis is not clearly established but likely involves retrograde menstruation with seeding of endometrial glands in the dependent part of the pelvis and in or on the ovary, posterior cul-de-sac, broad ligament, uterosacral ligament, rectosigmoidal colon, bladder, and distal ureter. It has been proposed that retrograde menstruation occurs to some degree in all women, but that only those who are unable to clear the menstrual debris because of immune dysfunction will go on to develop endometriosis (Cramer and Missmer 2002). Family history is a risk factor for endometriosis, and current efforts are being made to investigate genetic factors. The mean age of women at diagnosis of endometriosis ranges from 25 to 30 years. This condition is often asymptomatic but is also found in association with dysmenorrhea, dyspareunia, infertility, chronic pelvic or back pain, and rectal discomfort. The pain from the disorder is often cyclic, although it can be constant. The gold standard for diagnosis and staging of endometriosis is laparoscopy; however, the intensity of pain and discomfort does not correlate well with the severity of the disease at laparoscopy (Lu and Ory 1995).

Management

Endometriosis can be treated by watchful waiting, medical or surgical management, or a combination of the latter two options. Current medical regimens to treat this condition with gonadotropin-releasing hormone (GnRH) agonists and other drugs attempt to create states of pseudopregnancy, pseudomenopause, or chronic anovulation. Nonsteroidal anti-inflammatory medication is widely used, but there is little evidence to suggest that it is helpful (Allen et al. 2009). Surgical treatments vary from conservative removal and destruction of endometrial implants by excision, electrocautery, or laser to total abdominal hysterectomy with BSO. Implants have been shown to recur in up to 28% of patients within 18 months and 40% after 9 years of follow-up. However, there is some evidence that perioperative medical management with GnRH agonists may improve outcomes and increase time to recurrence of symptoms (Yeung et al. 2009). Although surgical conservative treatment is widely used to enhance fertility, its efficacy for endometriosis-associated infertility has not yet been shown. Immunomodulators are being studied on the basis that the peritoneal immune system appears to be impaired in women with endometriosis. Preliminary evidence supports enhancement of fertility when surgery is combined with medical management with immune modulators (Creus et al. 2008).

Role of the Psychiatrist

Because endometriosis is often chronic, and its contribution to chronic pelvic pain is sometimes uncertain, psychiatric opinion may be sought. Women with endometriosis experience a range of problems for which they may not be adequately supported. In fact, some women report that their worst experience is their encounter with health professionals and the way in which their symptoms are trivialized and dismissed (Cox et al. 2003). Depression occurs commonly in cases where endometriosis is accompanied by chronic pain, dyspareunia, or infertility. In addition, GnRH agonists are often used to treat endometriosis, and depressive symptoms may be associated with this treatment. SSRI antidepressants appear to be significantly helpful in the treatment of mood symptoms during the course of GnRH agonists (Warnock et al. 2000). Psychotherapy and antidepressants also may be helpful in addressing other psychological issues and symptoms in women with endometriosis.

Vulvodynia

Vulvodynia is chronic burning, stinging, or pain in the vulva in the absence of objective clinical or laboratory findings. Vulvodynia is divided into two classes: 1) vulvar vestibulitis, which is restricted burning and pain in the vestibular region that is solicited by touch, and 2) dysesthetic vulvodynia, which is burning or pain not limited to the vestibule, which may occur without touch or pressure. A population-based National Institutes of Health study found that approximately 16% of women reported lower genital tract discomfort persisting for 3 months or longer (Edwards 2003), although a more recent national health survey estimated much lower rates for vulvodynia with a current prevalence of 3.8% for chronic vulvar pain for at least 6 months (Arnold et al. 2007). Variability in disease definition may account for these discordant findings.

The etiology of vulvodynia is unknown, and previously suspected agents such as subclinical yeast infections and human papillomavirus have largely been discounted. Many women with vulvodynia also have comorbid disorders, such as interstitial cystitis, headaches, fibromyalgia, and irritable bowel syndrome, as well as clinical depression.

Psychiatrists may be asked to assess the role of psychosexual factors and depression in women with vulvodynia. One recent study of 80 women being treated for vulvodynia reported that more than 50% of the sample showed anxiety and more than 50% had a depressive disorder (Tribo et al. 2008). A review of the literature in social science databases concluded that distress in women with vulvodynia is related to the woman's sense of sexual identity and impacted by social influences related to expectations of femininity (Cantin-Drouin et al. 2008). This formulation may be helpful in treating women with this disorder. Also, given the efficacy recently shown by dual-action antidepressants (SNRIs) in treating depression and chronic painful conditions, these antidepressants may be a promising treatment for vulvodynia. Although open trials with TCAs and SSRIs, lamotrigine, and gabapentin have shown some promise, no randomized controlled trials with these medications have been published to date (C.S. Brown et al. 2008; G. Harris et al. 2007; Meltzer-Brody et al. 2009; Reed et al. 2006).

Pregnancy

The entire range of psychiatric disorders occurs during pregnancy, and some conditions are unique to pregnancy. Treatment of these disorders is discussed later in this chapter.

Epidemiology of Psychiatric Disorders Occurring During Pregnancy

Depression

The incidence of depression during pregnancy is approximately the same as that for matched populations who are not pregnant. Data from face-to-face interviews in the 2001–2002 National Epidemiological Survey on Alcohol and Related Conditions (NESARC) in the United States found no difference in the 12-month prevalence of major depressive disorder between women with and without pregnancies in the preceding year (8.4% and 8.1%, respectively) (Vesga-Lopez et al. 2008). The signs and symptoms of depression must be carefully distinguished from the sleep, appetite, and energy changes often characteristic of pregnancy and from the signs and symptoms of thyroid dysfunction, anemia, or other diseases of pregnancy. Discontinuation of maintenance medication for women who have had recurrent depressions carries a high risk of relapse. In a prospective observational study of 201 women with a history of major depression, 43% experienced a relapse during pregnancy. Women who discontinued medication had a greater risk of relapse (68% vs. 26%) and more frequent relapses than women who continued antidepressant treatment in pregnancy (L.S. Cohen et al. 2006a).

Bipolar Disorder

There is a growing literature on bipolar disorder during pregnancy indicating that a substantial proportion of women with preexisting bipolar disorder may relapse. In a recent prospective study of 81 women with bipolar disorder, the overall risk of relapse in pregnancy was 71%. Women who discontinued medication had a twofold increased risk of relapse, had an earlier time to relapse, and spent more time being ill. Abrupt discontinuation led to earlier recurrence than gradual discontinuation (Viguera et al. 2007b). Serious episodes of mania pose a threat to the pregnancy, necessitating especially careful risk-benefit analysis with regard to psychotropic medication.

Anxiety Disorders

There has been increased attention to the course and impact of anxiety disorders in pregnancy. Maternal symptoms of anxiety during pregnancy may be associated with adverse fetal and developmental outcomes (O'Connor et al. 2002). The course of anxiety disorders during pregnancy may vary with the nature of the anxiety disorder. For example, panic disorder may remit, recur, or remain unchanged during pregnancy. There is little evidence that pregnancy is a high-risk time for new onset of panic disorder. Although an underlying medical etiology is uncommon, new-onset panic symptoms should be investigated because of the consequences of missing a medical etiology (e.g., hyperthyroidism) or medication side effect. Patients with panic disorder who wish to discontinue medication should be tapered off gradually and treated with cognitive-behavioral therapy. More than 10% of female patients with panic disorder report that their first episode occurred postpartum.

Obsessive-compulsive disorder (OCD) may worsen pre- and postpartum, and withdrawal of medication is very likely to result in recurrence. A systematic review of anxiety disorders in the peripartum period revealed five studies indicating that as many as 40% of childbearing OCD outpatients have onset during pregnancy (Ross et al. 2006). Patients with moderate to severe symptoms may require maintenance medication during pregnancy; patients with milder cases can be treated with cognitive-behavioral therapy.

Results from the NESARC survey do not suggest that pregnancy confers increased risk of posttraumatic stress disorder (PTSD) or generalized anxiety disorder (Vesga-Lopez et al. 2008), although PTSD in some women following traumatic deliveries has been reported (Ayers et al. 2008).

Psychotic Disorders

Since almost all women with psychotic disorders have been deinstitutionalized, and most newer antipsychotics do not impair fertility, their rate of fertility approximates that of the general population. Pregnancy does not ameliorate, and may exacerbate, psychotic symptoms (Davies et al. 1995). There is some evidence that women with schizophrenia have more obstetric complications such as bleeding in pregnancy and placental abnormalities (Jablensky et al. 2005). Psychotic episodes during pregnancy may be characterized by delusions that the fetus is evil or dangerous, leading the pregnant woman to stab herself in the abdomen or engage in other self-destructive behaviors. Alternatively, psychotic denial of pregnancy can lead to poor antenatal care and/or impair a woman's ability to recognize and react appropriately to the signs and symptoms of labor. Psychoeducation is essential in this population. Antipsychotic medication is a foundation of treatment, although electroconvulsive therapy (ECT) for acute affective psychotic episodes can be effective and is relatively safe for the fetus (Anderson and Reti 2009). Special consideration must be given to the use of restraints for agitated pregnant patients to avoid compression of the vena cava (Solari et al. 2009).

Prenatal assessment and treatment can mitigate wrenching custody disputes after the infant is born. Serious psychiatric illness, if treated, is not always incompatible with successful mothering. The psychiatrist and obstetrician, working together with the patient, family, and social agencies, can plan and make provision for the infant's needs. Psychiatrists may be called on to assist in the assessment of competency to parent an infant. When it is clear that the mother will not be able to care for the child, such as when her other children have been taken into state custody for their protection, the psychiatrist can help her come to terms with the painful separation that will occur.

Alcohol and Substance Abuse

Alcohol and substance abuse arouse heightened concern in a pregnant patient. Standing by while a woman's behavior puts her fetus at risk is a painful situation for prenatal care professionals. The most serious and well-documented result of alcohol abuse during pregnancy is fetal alcohol syndrome. A pregnant woman who drinks the equivalent of 10 beers per day has a one-third risk of delivering a child who has fetal alcohol syndrome and a similar risk of delivering a child who is developmentally delayed but does not have the full syndrome. The perinatal mortality in these circumstances is 17% (Greenfield and Sugarman 2001). More recent studies have not substantiated early fears of an epidemic of "crack babies." It appears that most or all of the negative cognitive and behavioral findings in these children are a result of the environment in which they grow up rather than intrauterine exposure to cocaine (Chiriboga 1998). However, misinformation and rage at pregnant women who abuse substances have led to instances in which women have been imprisoned, either for the protection of the fetus or as punishment for harm to the fetus. Many or most pregnant women who abuse drugs or alcohol will accept treatment if it is practical (e.g., providing child care) and humane. Evidence indicates that the threat of coercion and punishment leads women to avoid seeking prenatal care altogether, obviating any opportunity to treat them and improve the fetus's intrauterine environment (see also Chapter 17, "Substance-Related Disorders," and Chapter 2, "Legal Issues").

Goals for the treatment of substance-using pregnant women involve motivational enhancement and harm reduction. Clinicians should offer appropriate treatment for the substance use disorder (e.g., methadone maintenance for opioid dependence) and treat comorbid medical or psychiatric disorders. The safety of patient behaviors should be monitored throughout pregnancy and the postpartum period, and child and family services should be involved for risk reduction and facilitation of competent parenting behaviors as needed. The therapeutic relationship is of utmost importance and should be nonjudgmental. Continued motivation enhancement, behavioral skills training, and a multidisciplinary long-term treatment plan will be important, particularly for women returning to environments where they are at high risk of relapse.

Personality Disorders

Women with severe personality disorders may present with risky behaviors that raise concerns about fetal safety. It may also be challenging for prenatal providers to manage some of the interpersonal conflicts in which some of these patients excel. Psychiatrists may be helpful in assessing risk, explaining useful de-escalation strategies, emphasizing consistency in management, and providing ongoing support to staff and the patient.

Situational Anxiety

Some pregnant patients are referred for psychiatric consultation for evaluation of what seems to the primary care clinician to be an inordinate level of anxiety. A careful history often shows that the patient either has been frightened by the experiences of a close family member or has had a traumatic obstetric or general medical care experience herself (Saisto and Halmesmaki 2003). The degree of pain a woman experiences in labor is related to many factors, including her expectations of pain (Chang et al. 2002). When the source of the anxiety is identified, it can be addressed by reviewing the past experience and making plans to avoid the frightening aspects of care in the coming delivery, providing prenatal education about delivery, or using relaxation techniques or hypnosis. Domestic violence is another cause of prenatal anxiety. The World Health Organization (WHO) recently published its findings from a large multinational study of women and abuse. In 15 different countries, the prevalence of reported physical violence in pregnancy ranged from 1% to 28%. Between one-quarter and one-half of these women experienced direct trauma to the abdomen during pregnancy, and more than 90% of the assailants were the biological father of the fetus (Ellsberg et al. 2008).

Issues Unique to Pregnancy

Denial of Pregnancy

Some women go into full-term labor without having recognized, or their families having recognized, that they are pregnant. Many such patients are not psychotic, but some are women with schizophrenia who are delusional in denying pregnancy (Miller 1990). Older patients may report that they thought pregnancy was impossible at their age and therefore attributed their amenorrhea to menopause and the sensations of fetal movement to digestive problems. Younger patients in this situation are typically passive daughters isolated in very strict families without much knowledge about reproduction. Their preconscious or unconscious fears of the consequences of pregnancy are so terrifying that they keep its signs and symptoms out of awareness (Spielvogel and Hohener 1995). They wear loose-fitting clothing and go about their usual activities. These cases generally come to psychiatric attention only when the new mother kills the infant after birth. Therefore, these young women end up in the penal—rather than the mental health care—system, and there has been relatively little opportunity to work with them and their families to learn more about the dynamics of these situations. One epidemiological study in Germany reported an incidence of up to 1 case of pregnancy denial per 475 births (Wessel et al. 2002). Later, the authors attempted to characterize risk factors for denial of pregnancy in this group, but they concluded that the group was quite varied and were unable to define a "typology" of women at risk. Only 3 out of 65 women had a diagnosis of schizophrenia (Wessel et al. 2007).

Pseudocyesis

At the other end of the spectrum from the patient who does not realize she is pregnant is the patient who is convinced she is pregnant when she is not. This condition, referred to as *pseudocyesis,* is a fascinating example of psychobiological interplay. The patient ceases to have menstrual periods. Her abdomen grows, and her cervix may show signs of pregnancy. Some patients with the delusion that they are pregnant are psychotic, but that is not the case in classical pseudocyesis. Patients with pseudocyesis are a heterogeneous group, and they have no other signs or symptoms of frank psychiatric disorder (Rosch et al. 2002). They declare an expected date of delivery and move the date forward when delivery does not ensue. Their conviction may or may not be swayed by ultrasonographic evidence or physical examination. For unknown reasons, the incidence of this condition is decreasing. Frequent antecedents are pregnancy loss, infertility, isolation, naivety, and a belief that childbearing is a woman's crucial role. These individuals have no interest in psychiatric care, and little is known about how the condition eventually resolves (Whelan and Stewart 1990). It may be important to differentiate pseudocyesis from menstrual irregularity and lactation secondary to hyperprolactinemia in women taking antipsychotic medication. Case reports indicate that the symptoms of hyperprolactinemia may contribute to delusional beliefs about pregnancy in women with schizophrenia (Ahuja et al. 2008).

Hyperemesis

Pernicious vomiting in pregnancy was once thought to be the result of unconscious rejection of the pregnancy. Hyperemesis, which can result in dehydration and electrolyte imbalance and may require hospitalization and intravenous treatment, certainly could induce ambivalence about a pregnancy in a woman who had been very pleased at the prospect of becoming a mother, but no scientific evidence indicates that ambivalence induces the vomiting (O'Brien and Newton 1991). Hyperemesis is no longer considered a psychiatric disorder. Mental health intervention can, however, help the patient and family cope until the condition resolves (Deuchar 1995). In a survey of 808 women with hyperemesis, 83% reported negative psychosocial consequences, including socioeconomic stress (e.g., job loss), attitude changes like fear regarding future pregnancies, and psychiatric symptoms like feelings of depression and anxiety, which for some continued postpartum (Poursharif et al. 2008). There are several case reports of severe hyperemesis gravidarum resulting in Wernicke-Korsakoff encephalopathy. Treatment is usually with standard antiemetics, but mirtazapine may be helpful in treatment-resistant cases (Guclu et al. 2005).

Identification of Psychiatric Illness

Although routine screening for psychiatric illness in all patients is not supported by evidence, psychiatrists may advise obstetricians that an identification of psychiatric illness and appropriate referral and treatment during routine antenatal care will likely decrease the frequency and intensity of noncompliance with antenatal care and of psychiatric emergencies during pregnancy and labor. Patients who might not otherwise recognize that they are in labor, as well as their families, can receive special education so that infants are not delivered into the toilet or in some other less-than-ideal environment. Prenatal education can prepare them for labor and delivery so that they can best cooperate and communicate with medical staff when the time comes.

Postpartum Psychiatric Issues

Perinatal Death

Stillbirth and neonatal death provoke much the same reactions as do losses earlier in pregnancy (as discussed earlier in this chapter), with the added stresses of full-term labor and delivery and the probability that many practical provisions for the expected infant have been made. Clinical practice in dealing with the bereaved and disappointed parents has varied over time. It is probably best to offer parents the opportunity to see or not to see the stillborn infant and to allow them to decide. Many bereaved parents report that their grief is exacerbated by the failure of friends and relatives to acknowledge the loss. For some, naming the baby and having a funeral service, with or without a burial, are helpful rituals. A religious leader of the parents' choice also can help them reconcile their rage at God for depriving them of their child with their need to derive support from their faith.

When the cause of fetal or neonatal death is not clear, an autopsy or other tests may be performed. The results will not be immediately available. The obstetrician, pathologist, geneticist, and psychiatrist may want to meet with the parents some weeks later to convey the results, answer questions, observe the grieving process, and determine whether additional supports are necessary. Stillbirth increases the risk of posttraumatic stress, anxiety, and depression in a subsequent pregnancy, for both men and women (Turton et al. 2006). One study found these sequelae generally resolve within 1 year after the birth of a subsequent healthy child (Turton et al. 2001). Premature birth or the stress of complicated, or even normal, labor can precipitate posttraumatic stress symptoms as well, especially in women with preexisting psychiatric symptoms (particularly anxiety in late pregnancy) and poor social supports (Soderquist et al. 2009; Zaers et al. 2008).

Postpartum Psychiatric Disorders

"Baby Blues"

Within days after birth, 50%–80% of women experience significantly heightened emotional lability. After a few days, the symptoms abate. The phenomenon has been reported in a wide variety of cultures and is not related to demographic variables (Sakumoto et al. 2002). Although the patient may be moved to tears from time to time, none of the other signs or symptoms of depression are present, nor do they develop as an exacerbation of this condition. Some mothers also experience periods of joy or euphoria. This self-limited state may be caused by prolactin or other hormones. If these symptoms are excessive, an alternative diagnosis such as depression or psychosis should be considered. An interesting hypothesis is that "baby blues" may be related to the effects of oxytocin and other hormones involved in the initiation of mother–infant attachment and maternal behavior (Miller and Rukstalis 1999). Clinicians should offer reassurance. This is especially important because media reports of postpartum depression leading to the murder of children have frightened so many families. About 25% of women with baby blues will not improve within 10 days and will progress to postpartum depression.

Postpartum Depression

Postpartum depression occurs in up to 10%–15% of mothers in North America. Some cases of postpartum depression are simply continuations of antepartum depression. Symptoms can begin anytime from days to months after birth but generally later than "baby blues" and range from 4 weeks to 12 months postpartum. The diagnostic process can be complicated by the similarity of symptoms of the aftermath of delivery and the stresses of caring for a newborn and the signs and symptoms of depression. New mothers are often tired, sleepless, distracted, and preoccupied with infant care rather than the enjoyment of previous pursuits. Their meal schedules and sleep are disrupted. It is useful to ask whether the mother can sleep when the baby sleeps.

Risk factors include previous depression, especially postpartum depression; complications of birth; and poor social supports. Newly immigrant women, who often have poor social supports, are at higher risk (Stewart et al. 2008). There appears to be some cross-cultural variation in the incidence of postpartum depression; this may be related to contrasting patterns of antepartum and postpartum care and social support. In many cultures, the newly delivered woman is traditionally provided with rest, warmth, and enriched nutrition (Kaewsarn et al. 2003). In North America, medical attention decreases drastically after an infant is delivered; few medical and social resources are available to the new family. Some evidence shows that postpartum calls and visits from health care professionals decrease the incidence of postpartum depression (Chabrol et al. 2002). Endocrine factors also play a major role; some women are particularly vulnerable to rapid changes in hormone levels at any time across the life span, and some authors have proposed that there is a reproductive "subtype" of depression (Payne et al. 2009). Estradiol and progesterone are strongly implicated (Bloch et al. 2003). Women with thyroid autoantibodies have an increased risk for postpartum depression, but thyroxine administration does not appear to reduce that risk (B. Harris et al. 2002; Oretti et al. 2003).

Anxiety accompanies pre- and postpartum depression in up to 50% of cases (Ross et al. 2003). In an Australian study of 408 primigravidas, the inclusion of panic disorder and acute adjustment disorder with anxiety doubled the cases of postpartum psychiatric illness identified. Antecedent anxiety disorders were a more important risk factor for postpartum depression than was antecedent depression (Matthey et al. 2003a).

The thought content of a woman with postpartum depression centers on mothering (e.g., ruminating that she is not a good mother and that her infant is suffering as a result). Sometimes the woman becomes obsessed with thoughts of harm coming to the infant and vividly imagines his or her injury or death. These ruminations are found both in women with OCD and in those with other psychiatric illnesses (e.g., major depressive disorder). There are no reports of women harming their infants solely as a result of obsessional thinking. Most women realize that these thoughts are unreasonable and go to great lengths to avoid harming their infants. However, obsessions must be differentiated from postpartum psychosis, where women are out of touch with reality and are not aware that their thoughts are unreasonable. Reassurance of eventual recovery is crucial to patient care. One of the fears of women with postpartum depression, and their families, is that the depression is the first sign of a condition that will result in self-harm or infanticide. Relatives may be tempted to take over care of the infant of a depressed mother to allow her to rest and recuperate. This can be counterproductive, exacerbating her sense of failure and deprivation. It is preferable for them to help the mother with household tasks, allow her to care for the infant, and reinforce her sense of maternal adequacy.

Although obstetricians have become more aware of and responsive to postpartum depression as a result of the notorious cases in the media and educational initiatives by a variety of professional and advocacy organizations, they may not be in the optimal position to identify it. Women are discharged from the hospital within a day or two after delivery, with a rather cursory office follow-up visit 4–6 weeks later. Obstetric clinicians should be encouraged to increase their contacts with and availability to new mothers. A simple query about depressed mood is often successful in identifying cases (Wisner et al. 2002b). After the birth, the specialist women see most is the pediatrician. There have been attempts, with mixed success, to convince pediatricians to be vigilant for maternal postpartum depression. Several validated scales are available for screening: the Edinburgh Postnatal Depression Scale (Matthey et al. 2003b) is the best known. The efficacy and effectiveness of screening for PPD are controversial (especially if good systems are not available for referral and treatment). Researchers in Hong Kong determined that screening should be delayed for several days after delivery in order to be accurate (Lee et al. 2003), although earlier assessment has been found accurate in North America (Dennis 2003). Screening in an inner-city population in New York uncovered far more cases than were anticipated (Morris-Rush et al. 2003).

Postpartum Psychosis

Postpartum psychosis is characterized by extreme agitation, delirium, confusion, sleeplessness, and hallucinations and/or delusions. Onset can be sudden and usually occurs between days 3 and 14 postpartum, with 90% of episodes occurring within 4 weeks of delivery (Harlow et al. 2007). The overall incidence of postpartum psychosis is estimated at 0.1%–0.2% and appears to have been stable for more than a century and among cultures. A Swedish population-based study found that 40% of women who were hospitalized for psychosis or bipolar disorder during pregnancy were rehospitalized in the postpartum period (Harlow et al. 2007). Only a fraction of these women will go on to attempt suicide or infanticide, but the risk and the stakes are high enough to warrant considering postpartum psychosis as a medical emergency and hospitalizing the patient, at least for a period of observation. Women who have schizophrenic episodes may have more difficulty parenting their children after recovery from the acute episode than do women with other kinds of postpartum psychosis (Riordan et al. 1999).

Many experts believe that most episodes of postpartum psychosis are bipolar disorder (Attia et al. 1999; Chaudron and Pies 2003). The risk of postpartum relapse of bipolar disorder is 30%–50%; these relapses can be acute and severe. If pregnant women with bipolar disorder discontinue medication, there should be a plan for immediate medication resumption at delivery to lower the risk of recurrence (L.S. Cohen et al. 1995).

Trials and media coverage of cases of infanticide disclose major misunderstandings about the state and motivation of the perpetrators. Most often, the mother in these cases has command hallucinations or delusions and/or is suicidal and does not wish to leave the child behind but wants to be reunited with him or her in Heaven. Appleby et al. (1998) reported that the risk of suicide in the first postnatal year is "increased 70-fold" in women hospitalized for a postpartum psychiatric disorder. In some countries, there has been a very proactive stance toward the identification and treatment of women who are at particularly high risk of developing severe mental illness postpartum. For example, in England, the National Institute for Clinical Excellence (NICE) has issued guidelines that all health authorities in England are meant to implement (Department of Health 2007).

Custody

Psychiatric illness in and of itself does not rule out the possibility of adequate mothering. For general evaluation, and for the legal and medical records, when the question of custody arises, it is useful to perform a regular mental status examination. What are most important, however, are the parenting knowledge, attitudes, and behaviors of the newly delivered patient. Has she been able to arrange adequate accommodations for herself and the infant? How does she plan to feed the infant? Does she know approximately how often a newborn must be fed and its diaper changed? Does she have delusions about the infant?

Observation of mother-infant interaction is key. It is very difficult to predict how a person will behave with an infant in the absence of the infant. The postpartum staff should allow the mother as much observed time with the infant as possible and note how the mother responds to the infant's cries and other needs, whether she can feed the infant and change his or her diapers, and how she relates to the infant overall. New mothers without psychiatric disorders can be tired and overwhelmed; expectations should be realistic.

Custody decisions can be life-or-death decisions. Removing a child from his or her mother, unless a well-disposed and capable relative can take over his or her care, exposes the child to the possibility of a lifetime in transient foster care situations. Allowing a severely ill mother to retain custody exposes the child to possible abuse and neglect. Interactions with child protective services can be problematic. Depending on current resources and recent scandals, child protective services may take a child into custody without giving the mother a chance to show her ability to parent, or they may refuse to intervene with a dangerously psychotic mother because the infant has not yet been harmed. Often, the most appropriate approach, when available, is the provision of home help and/or visiting nurse services, which provide both support and further opportunities for observation of the parenting and the condition of the infant. Having a mental illness does not diminish, and may exacerbate, the grief and rage of a mother whose child is taken away.

Legal aspects of maternal competency are discussed in Chapter 2, "Legal Issues."

Psychotropic Drugs, Psychotherapy, and Electroconvulsive Therapy in Pregnancy and Lactation

No perfect solution exists for treating mental illness during pregnancy and lactation, and a risk-benefit decision must be made in the face of imprecise data. Three types of adverse fetal effects may occur when psychotropics are taken during pregnancy. Teratogenic effects may be incurred from first-trimester exposure, neonatal toxicity and withdrawal syndromes are related to third-trimester exposure, and behavioral or developmental effects may manifest later in childhood (Marcus et al. 2001; Wisner et al. 2002a).

How depression should be treated during pregnancy is a subject that receives continued scrutiny from the media and challenges both providers and patients. Untreated depression during pregnancy or postpartum is associated with increased morbidity in the mother and her offspring. Potential complications in pregnancy and at delivery include increased risk of poor prenatal care, substance use in pregnancy, preterm birth, and low birth weight (Oberlander et al. 2006; Steer et al. 1992; Suri et al. 2007; Yonkers et al. 2009). Women with depression in pregnancy are at high risk for postpartum depression and for impaired mother-infant interactions that have been associated with poor developmental and emotional outcomes in the offspring (Deave et al. 2008; DiPietro et al. 2006; Punamaki et al. 2006). Unfortunately, evidence indicates that depression is seriously undertreated during pregnancy, with less than 20% of women who experience depression during pregnancy and the postpartum seeking treatment (Marcus 2009).

Although psychotherapy is indicated as acute therapy for mild to moderate depression, it may not be adequate if a woman has severe depression. Also, even in mild to moderate depression, psychotherapy may not improve depression for several weeks to months, leaving the mother and fetus (or even infant) exposed to the effects of untreated depression during that time. Antidepressant medication is an effective treatment of antenatal depression (Dennis and Stewart 2004). However, concerns remain among patients and prescribing physicians about the safety of antidepressant exposure for the fetus/neonate. Previous meta-analyses of data examining potential relationships between antidepressant exposure and neonatal/fetal outcomes have been largely reassuring (Addis et al. 2000; Einarson and Einarson 2005). More recently, however, there has been renewal of the controversy regarding the safety of antidepressant use during pregnancy. Paroxetine has been shown in some, but not all, studies to be associated with heart defects.

Two large prospective databases on antidepressant use in pregnancy were recently published. The Danish database of 493,113 children born between 1996 and 2003 included 1,370 mothers who had had two or more prescriptions of an SSRI filled during the period 28 days before through 112 days after the beginning of gestation (Pedersen et al. 2009). After researchers controlled for maternal age, mental status, and smoking, antidepressant use showed no association with overall fetal major malformations. However, an increase in cardiac septal defects was observed (OR=1.99; 95% CI=1.13 to 3.53). Both sertraline and citalopram were associated with an increase in septal defects, and exposure to more than one type of SSRI was associated with the greatest increase in septal defects (OR=4.7; 95% CI=1.74 to 12.7). The absolute increase in risk for fetal septal defects was low (0.9% for exposure to one SSRI; 2.1% for exposure to more than one SSRI).

The Swedish Medical Birth Registry included 14,821 women who used antidepressant medication in pregnancy from 1995 to 2007 (Reis and Källén 2010). There was an excess of births before gestational week 37 and various pregnancy complications in women using antidepressants. The odds ratios were higher for hypoglycemia, respiratory distress, lower Apgar scores, and jaundice in babies exposed to antidepressants in utero. Atrial septal and ventricular septal defects were more frequent in infants exposed in utero to TCAs (OR=1.84; 95% CI=1.13 to 2.97) and paroxetine (OR=1.66; 95% CI=1.09 to 2.83). Paroxetine use was also associated with fetal hypospadias (OR=2.45; 95% CI=1.12 to 4.64). Although the investigators controlled for maternal age, smoking, and some other drug use, it was not possible to dissociate outcomes from the effects of depression, other comorbidities or exposure, or ascertainment bias.

Reports of small increases in fetal cardiovascular defects have been inconsistently reported for several other antidepressant drugs, leading to questions about possible drug class effects. Short-term adverse neonatal effects and neonatal pulmonary hypertension associated with late third-trimester exposure to SSRIs have been reported (Chambers et al. 2006; Koren and Boucher 2009). In all cases, the small absolute risks associated with antidepressant use in pregnancy must be weighed against the risk of not treating depression.

Hence, the decision about whether to take antidepressant medication in pregnancy is not straightforward. None of the treatment alternatives comes without risk of undesirable outcomes, and there is ongoing scientific uncertainty about risks and benefits of treatment. An added layer of complexity is that a woman is making this decision not only for her own health but also for the health and development of her unborn child. Wisner et al. (2000) presented a clinical decision-making model to aid both clinician and patient in making an optimal clinical decision about treatment for depression in pregnancy. The model guides physicians through the concepts of a diagnostic formulation and presentation of treatment options, including the risks of both untreated depression and antidepressant treatment in pregnancy. The model then guides physicians to help each patient make decisions about treatment based on the patient's values, perceptions of risk, and capacity to consent to treatment. Consideration should also be given to whether a woman has adequate support to make this complex decision.

Classification of Drugs

Current FDA risk assignments of drugs in pregnancy range from A (no risk) through B, C, D, and X (contraindicated). This classification is primarily based on concerns about teratogenicity and neonatal toxicity, because few or no data exist for later child behavior or development. The FDA classification lags behind current data and experience. At present, bupropion, clozapine, and buspirone have a B designation (absence of human risk) with a caveat of limited data. Most SSRI antidepressants, some TCAs (including desipramine), newer antidepressants (such as mirtazapine, nefazodone, and venlafaxine), clonazepam, and most conventional and atypical antipsychotics have received a C designation (human risk should not be eliminated because of inadequate human clinical trials and no or some risk in animals). Lithium, carbamazepine, sodium valproate, most TCAs, and some benzodiazepines (other than clonazepam) have received a D designation, indicating evidence of fetal risk without an absolute contraindication during pregnancy. As a result of concerns about the use of paroxetine (an SSRI) in pregnancy, it has been reclassified as a category "D" medication by the FDA (U.S Food and Drug Administration 2006). Because the FDA is currently revising its method of classifying drug risk in pregnancy, physicians should consult the most recent classification as well as other new literature.

Use of Psychotropic Medication

General principles of using psychotropic medication should guide management of the pregnant women. However, there are additional considerations. Changes in drug metabolism and extracellular fluid volume during pregnancy may require dosage adjustment for several drugs. For example, approximately twice the usual dose of lithium carbonate is required in the second and third trimesters to achieve therapeutic serum levels (Stewart and Robinson 2001b). (See also Chapter 38, "Psychopharmacology," for a discussion of pharmacotherapy during pregnancy.) A long-standing debate has existed, with contradictory data from several studies, on whether diazepam in pregnancy is associated with cleft lip or cleft palate. Some benzodiazepines, such as triazolam, temazepam, and flurazepam, have received an X designation, indicating complete contraindication in pregnancy (Marcus et al. 2001). A consensus statement by the American Psychiatric Association and American College of Obstetrics and Gynecology on the use of antidepressants in pregnancy gives current scientific findings and guidance (Yonkers et al. 2009). Insufficient data are available to ensure safety for most novel antipsychotics; however, high-potency antipsychotics, such as haloperidol, appear to be relatively safer in pregnancy (Einarson and Boscovic 2009).

Early reports warned of congenital heart disease in infants exposed in utero to lithium carbonate, but subsequent analyses have shown these risks to be only slightly greater than those in the general population (Altshuler et al. 1996). Other mood stabilizers such as carbamazepine and valproic acid are associated with greater teratogenicity than lithium (Stewart and Robinson 2001b). A recent study of antiepileptic drugs found that fetal exposure to valproate (although not carbamazepine or lamotrigine) was related to poorer cognitive development at age 3 years in children of mothers with epilepsy (Meador et al. 2009). For women with unstable bipolar disorder, it is reasonable to continue lithium throughout pregnancy while carefully monitoring serum levels. Divided doses may be safer than once-daily dosing. An ultrasound during the first trimester may be used to identify possible congenital cardiac malformations. Dosage should be reduced after delivery to avoid lithium toxicity in the early postpartum period.

Breast-Feeding and Psychotropic Drugs

The use of psychotropic drugs by breast-feeding women remains controversial. The amount of drug present in breast milk is small but extremely variable over time, even in the same woman. No controlled studies of the effects of psychotropic medication during breast-feeding exist, but several reviews provide further guidance (L.S. Cohen 2007; Yonkers et al. 2004). In general, it appears relatively safe for depressed women to take antidepressants and typical antipsychotics while breast-feeding full-term and healthy babies. Fewer data are available for premature infants or newer antidepressants and atypical antipsychotics. However, a systematic review of the literature on antipsychotics in breast-feeding advises that clozapine is not recommended due to risk of blood abnormalities and that olanzapine may increase the risk of extrapyramidal side effects in the infant (Gentile 2008). Useful reviews of mood stabilizers during lactation include Yonkers et al. (2004) and L.S. Cohen (2007). Lithium has been considered to be contraindicated while breast-feeding due to concerns about neonatal toxicity from passage of lithium into the breast milk (Stewart and Robinson 2001b). However, some experts are revisiting the postpartum use of lithium, given its unparalleled clinical efficacy for certain women who wish to breast-feed. A study measuring lithium levels in 10 breast-fed infants of mothers who were taking lithium found that breast milk levels were low and well tolerated. There were no adverse effects on the infants, but these results should be interpreted with caution (Viguera et al. 2007a). If lithium is used during lactation, both the infant's lithium levels and complete blood count should be monitored.

No adverse effects from the use of carbamazepine, valproate, or lamotrigine have been reported. However, serum concentrations of lamotrigine were 30% of maternal levels in one study, and Yonkers et al. (2004) recommend that such infants be monitored for rash if lamotrigine is used. Decisions about the care of women with a history of bipolar illness must be made on a case-by-case basis given the high risk of recurrence of bipolar disorder in the postpartum period (Viguera et al. 2007b).

Because new information on the use of drugs during pregnancy and lactation is frequently published, the reader is advised to consult the most recent reference in making risk-benefit decisions. The clinician must be cognizant that untreated mental illness in pregnancy and postpartum also has risks to the woman and the developing fetus and newborn child. Decisions should be made in consultation with the woman (and partner, if appropriate) and other health care providers (such as obstetricians and pediatricians), and discussions should be carefully documented in the patient's chart.

Psychotherapy in Pregnancy and Postpartum

Spinelli and Endicott (2003) and O'Hara et al. (2000) found interpersonal psychotherapy to be effective in the treatment of depressed pregnant and postpartum women, respectively. However, a 2007 Cochrane review concluded that there are still insufficient data to make generalized recommendations about the use of psychotherapy in pregnancy (Dennis et al. 2007). Because many women refuse to take medication while pregnant or breast-feeding, psychotherapy is often a viable alternative. However, its efficacy for severe depression is unproven.

Electroconvulsive Therapy

ECT is generally regarded as a safe and effective treatment for severe depression, affective psychosis, and catatonia in pregnancy and the puerperium. ECT is underused and should be considered in emergency situations in which the safety of the mother, fetus, or child is jeopardized; to avoid first-trimester exposure to teratogenic drugs; and in patients who are refractory to psychotropics or who have previously had successful treatment with ECT (Stewart and Robinson 2001b). ECT for acute affective psychotic episodes can be effective and is relatively safe for the fetus (Anderson and Reti 2009; see also Chapter 40, "Electroconvulsive Therapy"). Newer physical treatments for depression, such as vagal nerve stimulation, deep brain stimulation, and transcranial magnetic stimulation, have not been adequately studied in pregnant women.

Premenstrual Psychiatric Symptoms: Premenstrual Syndrome and Premenstrual Dysphoric Disorder

Background

The study of premenstrual symptoms poses unique methodological challenges. Most women in North America, if asked, report premenstrual mood, behavior, and somatic changes. There is a strong cultural belief that the menstrual cycle is associated with such negative changes. However, it is also clear that both women and men attribute unpleasant or problematic feelings and behaviors to the menstrual cycle regardless of whether they are related. The majority of women presenting for care of premenstrual symptoms, when assessed with prospective ratings and careful diagnostic interviews, have symptoms completely unrelated to their menstrual cycles. Nevertheless, premenstrual syndrome (PMS) and premenstrual dysphoric disorder (PMDD) remain popular attributions and diagnoses among women themselves, their families, and physicians. More commonly, women may experience premenstrual worsening of mood and anxiety disorders.

Etiology

Many attempts have been made, over decades, to identify circulating levels of reproductive hormones to account for mood symptoms occurring in concert with reproductive events and cycles. The reality is probably more complex than linear effects of hormone levels on mood. It would seem that some women are particularly sensitive not to specific levels but rather to changes in the levels of reproductive hormones. It has been reported for some time that women who report premenstrual symptoms are more likely to experience postpartum depression and may be predisposed to perimenopausal mood symptoms as well (Payne et al. 2007). Lending biological support to this hypothesis, Huo et al. (2007) reported that the risk of PMDD is associated with genetic variation in the estrogen receptor alpha gene, possibly representing abnormal estrogen signaling during the luteal phase of the menstrual cycle. This may lead to PMDD symptoms via estrogen's effects on serotonin, norepinephrine, gamma-aminobutyric acid (GABA), allopregnanolone, and various endorphins. Further corroborating evidence for treating PMDD as a distinct disorder involves emerging functional neuroimaging findings that women with PMDD may selectively respond to negative stimuli only during the premenstrual phase of their cycle (Protopopescu et al. 2008).

Diagnosis

Currently, premenstrual psychiatric symptoms are conceptualized and treated as part of the mood disorder spectrum. Experts, and the framers of DSM, have attempted to distinguish normative mood variations from symptoms worthy of medical attention by publishing research criteria for PMDD. For many years, the study of premenstrual psychiatric symptoms was complicated by the lack of a specific and uniform definition. More than 100 physical, emotional, and cognitive signs and symptoms have been attributed to PMS (Janowsky et al. 2002). PMDD is listed in DSM-IV-TR as an example of a depressive disorder not otherwise specified (NOS) and is described as follows:

> In most menstrual cycles during the past year, five (or more) of the following symptoms (e.g., markedly depressed mood, marked anxiety, marked affective lability, decreased interest in activities) were present for most of the time during the last week of the luteal phase, began to remit within a few days after the onset of the follicular phase, and were absent in the week postmenses. The disturbance markedly interferes with work or school or with usual social activities and relationships with others. (American Psychiatric Association 2000, p. 774)

According to DSM-IV TR, approximately 75% of women report mild premenstrual mood changes, and 20%–50% report at least moderate changes. Only 3%–5% of women report severe premenstrual mood symptoms rated prospectively over a 2-month period, fulfilling the proposed DSM IV-TR criteria for PMDD (American Psychiatric Association 2000). Given the tendency to retrospectively overattribute symptoms to the menstrual cycle, prospective daily ratings and careful evaluation for other psychiatric disorders are essential (Landen and Eriksson 2003; Lane and Francis 2003).

Irritability has been conceptualized as a common premenstrual symptom. Born et al. (2008) have validated a 14-item self-report and 5-item observer-rated rating scale for irritability. This scale covers the core elements of irritability—annoyance, anger, tension, hostile behavior, and sensitivity. Specific assessment of irritability may have relevance to both the impact of menstrual cycle–related mood disorders and their management. This may be of particular importance for women who do not meet criteria for DSM-IV mood and anxiety disorders but who present with guilt and shame related to their premenstrual irritability. The possibility of cyclical changes in symptoms and/or treatment response in all diagnostic categories should be considered in all menstruating women or at least in those whose diagnoses or treatment responses are puzzling or unsatisfactory (Lande and Karamchandani 2002).

Psychosocial Effects

Another controversial aspect of PMDD is the severity or effect of the symptoms. The DSM definition specifies a significant negative effect on life function. It has been difficult to specify the distinction between PMS and PMDD in this regard (Smith et al. 2003). Preexisting beliefs about work effect may color the findings in studies that use self-reports (Steiner et al. 2003). A large study of randomly selected members of a health maintenance organization found that women with PMDD reported decreased work productivity as compared with women with milder premenstrual symptoms, but the women with PMDD also reported lower productivity than the others in the follicular phase after the onset of menses, when their PMDD symptoms, according to the definition, should have been absent. This study did not produce significant evidence that premenstrual symptoms, regardless of their level of severity, caused women to stay in bed, reduce their hours at work, or decrease their activities at home or school (Chawla et al. 2002).

Management

No specific empirically supported treatments for PMS are available, but several approaches have proved helpful for both the symptoms and the patients' general health. These include taking vitamins (especially B vitamins), reducing or eliminating caffeine and nicotine, exercising, and using stress reduction techniques. Many women with premenstrual symptoms attempt complementary or alternative approaches (Domoney et al. 2003). In one study, cognitive-behavioral therapy was found to be equally effective as fluoxetine; fluoxetine produced more rapid results, and cognitive-behavioral therapy produced more lasting results (Hunter et al. 2002). Calcium carbonate also has produced promising results in one study (Thys-Jacobs et al. 1998).

Like other disorders in the mood spectrum, PMDD is well treated with SSRIs (Steiner et al. 2006). As of this writing, fluoxetine, sertraline, and paroxetine have received FDA indications for PMDD. For reasons still poorly understood, although SSRIs generally require 2–4 weeks for therapeutic effectiveness in depression, they are reported to be effective for PMDD when used only in the premenstrual phase (Halbreich et al. 2002). Perhaps because of the lack of continued administration, there is no discontinuation syndrome when they are used in this manner. A recent Cochrane Database meta-analysis confirmed effectiveness of either luteal-phase or continuous dosing of the SSRIs fluoxetine, paroxetine, sertraline, fluvoxamine, and citalopram and the highly serotonergic TCA clomipramine (J. Brown et al. 2009). Evidence does indicate that symptoms recur rapidly when luteal-phase treatment is discontinued (Pearlstein et al. 2003).

Exogenous hormones have not been traditionally effective for the treatment of PMDD. However, on the basis of randomized controlled trial evidence, the FDA has recently approved a combination of ethinyl estradiol and drospirenone for the treatment of PMDD (see Pearlstein and Steiner 2008 for summaries of these studies). It is thought that the antiandrogen and antimineralocorticoid properties of drospirenone account for the efficacy of this product (as compared to traditional oral contraceptive pills). This indication has been limited to women who desire to take an oral contraceptive to prevent pregnancy, likely because the potential for adverse effects (e.g., deep vein thrombosis, pulmonary embolism) exceeds that of the SSRIs.

Perimenopause and Menopause

The average age at menopause in North American and European women is 51 years, although the entire period of transition may extend over several years. By definition, menopause is said to have occurred after 12 months of amenorrhea, and perimenopause is that period of time leading up to menopause but before 12 consecutive months of amenorrhea. A National Institutes of Health Stages of Reproductive Aging Workshop recommended dividing perimenopause into early and late stages (Soules et al. 2001). During the perimenopause, the ovarian follicles gradually decline with age, estradiol and inhibin production by the ovary decreases, and FSH and luteinizing hormone levels rise (through loss of feedback inhibition). These changes are orchestrated through the hypothalamic-pituitary-ovarian axis, and cyclic variability often occurs throughout the transitional period. The perimenopause may be asymptomatic, but 70%–90% of women will experience some vasomotor symptoms consisting of hot flashes and night sweats. In addition, some women will experience palpitations, dizziness, fatigue, headaches, insomnia, joint pains, and paresthesias. Women also may complain of lack of concentration and loss of memory during the transitional period, but because men also complain of these symptoms, distinguishing them from normal aging is difficult. For a review incorporating the findings of the U.S. Women's Health Initiative (WHI) study with respect to the pathophysiology and management of vasomotor and vaginal symptoms during the menopausal transition, see Grady (2006).

The association of psychiatric symptoms with the perimenopause has traditionally been controversial. However, in a U.S. longitudinal prospective cohort study of premenopausal women with no lifetime diagnosis of major depressive disorder (MDD), women entering perimenopause had 1.8 times increased odds of developing depression compared to women who remained premenopausal (after adjustment for age and history of negative life events) (L.S. Cohen et al. 2006b). A 10-year follow-up of a population-based cohort of premenopausal women without depression or hot flashes at baseline found that 40% reported both symptoms during the study interval and that depressed mood was more likely to precede hot flashes (relative risk=2.1, 95% CI=1.5 to 2.9) (Freeman et al. 2009). Whether psychiatric symptoms are caused by hormonal changes, sociocultural factors, or psychological factors remains uncertain. Biological factors include estrogen shifts, whereas sociocultural theories focus on the importance of role changes in parenting, marriage, sex, and work. In addition, attitudes toward aging and female roles vary by culture. A consistent finding is that women with lower socioeconomic class and education report more perimenopausal symptoms. Psychological theories focus on stress during the perimenopausal years as a result of diminished personal and family health, socioeconomic status, family and work changes, other losses, retirement, illness, and death (Avis 2003). In addition, one study has shown that a lifetime history of major depression may be associated with an early decline in ovarian function and earlier menopause (Harlow et al. 2003). Women seeking treatment for physical symptoms in menopause clinics report a high prevalence of depression, irritability, mood lability, anxiety, lack of concentration, short-term memory loss, and decreased libido (Stewart and Boydell 1993). Other investigators have shown that prior depression is a risk factor for depression at perimenopause and that poor physical health, social circumstances, divorce, widowhood, and interpersonal stress are closely correlated with depression in menopausal women (Hunter 1990; Kaufert et al. 1992; Stewart and Boydell 1993). Women with bipolar disorder may be at increased risk for perimenopausal depression, although not necessarily mania (Marsh et al. 2008).

The incidence of depression in women mirrors estrogen shifts across the life cycle, at puberty, premenopause, postpartum, and perimenopause (Stahl 2001). This has led to studies to determine whether estrogen therapy in perimenopause can alleviate symptoms of clinical depression. Two small randomized controlled trials found that estradiol was a well-tolerated and effective treatment for perimenopausal depression (Schmidt et al. 2000; Soares et al. 2001), but this finding has not been replicated to date.

Although estrogen appears to have a salutary effect on depression in some perimenopausal women, in contrast, progesterone and progestins are known to cause dizziness, drowsiness, and sedation in many women and may be associated with negative moods (Bjorn et al. 2000). Progestins are primarily used in women with an intact uterus to prevent an increase in endometrial cancer caused by unopposed estrogen therapy.

Studies also have been conducted on the role of estrogen as an augmentation agent with antidepressants. In a pilot study, 17 women who had a partial response to antidepressants received augmentation with 0.625 mg conjugated estrogen or placebo in a double-blind design. Women receiving estrogen augmentation had significantly greater reductions in Hamilton Depression Rating Scale scores than women who received placebo (Morgan et al. 2005). Further studies of estrogen and selective estrogen receptor modulators as psychotropic augmentation agents are needed.

Moreover, the role of estrogen in psychiatric disorders is not limited to depression. Work by Kulkarni et al. (2001), Seeman (2002), and others has shown a worsening in preexisting schizophrenic illness and other psychoses associated with decreases in estradiol during perimenopause and beyond. Interestingly, some patients appear to respond to estrogen to augment antipsychotic drugs.

Of concern, however, are results from the WHI study indicating that estrogen-progesterone therapy is associated with an increased risk of breast cancer, cardiovascular disease (Writing Group for the Women's Health Initiative Investigators 2002), cognitive dysfunction, and dementia (Rapp et al. 2003; Shumaker et al. 2003). The estrogen-only arm of the WHI was also prematurely terminated in 2004 when estrogen monotherapy was found to be associated with increased rates of stroke, dementia, and mild cognitive impairment (but not breast cancer) (Women's Health Initiative Steering Committee 2004).

Emerging evidence may affect current use, but at present, estrogen is useful to control severe vasomotor symptoms and vaginal dryness, with current FDA guidelines recommending the smallest dosage for the shortest time possible. Systematic reviews and meta-analyses of nonhormonal therapies for menopausal hot flashes concluded that there is evidence for SSRIs, SNRIs, clonidine, and gabapentin, although the efficacy of these treatments is less than that of estrogen. Results were mixed with respect to the efficacy of isoflavone extracts (Toulis et al. 2009).

In conclusion, the many estrogen effects on brain function are complex. The role of estrogen in treating mood, cognition, and psychosis, and as a psychotropic augmentation agent, requires further adequately powered randomized controlled trials. Personal, social, and physical factors always should be considered in assessing the individual woman, and psychotherapy may be helpful in navigating the many transitions at midlife.

Urinary Incontinence

Urinary incontinence, the involuntary loss of urine, affects up to 23% of adults (Roe et al. 1999), with a prevalence in women that is twice that in men (Melville et al. 2002).

Urinary incontinence affects the physical, psychological, social, and economic well-being of individuals and their families and imposes a considerable economic burden on health and social services. Despite increasingly available and effective treatments for urinary incontinence, many women do not seek help. A Canadian population-based survey found that only 32% of women with urinary incontinence sought help from a physician, while 40% reported a significant impact of urinary incontinence on their quality of life (Vigod and Stewart 2007). Many people are reluctant to seek help because they are embarrassed or ashamed or believe that this problem is a part of normal aging

Etiology and Classification

The etiology of urinary incontinence is multifactorial and may be caused by impairment of the lower urinary tract or the nervous system or by various external factors. There are several subtypes of incontinence, but the most common are 1) stress incontinence (the involuntary loss of urine due to an increase in intra-abdominal pressure, such as coughing, laughing, or exercise); 2) urge incontinence (the involuntary loss of urine preceded by a strong urge to void whether or not the bladder is full); and 3) mixed incontinence (Melville et al. 2002).

Psychosocial Effects

Urinary incontinence may affect quality of life, sexual function, and mood. Studies have found that incontinence has a major negative effect on quality of life (Melville et al. 2002). A population-based cross-sectional study of nearly 6,000 American women between the ages of 50 and 69 years found that 16% reported mild, moderate, or severe incontinence. After adjustment for medical morbidity, functional status, and demographic variables, women with severe and mild to moderate incontinence were 80% and 40%, respectively, more likely to have depression than were continent women (Nygaard et al. 2003).

These findings were confirmed in a Canadian population-based cross-sectional study of 69,003 women, which found that the 12-month prevalence of major depression was 15.5% in women with urinary incontinence, compared to 9.9% in women without urinary incontinence. In this study, women with comorbid depression and urinary incontinence reported substantially worse quality of life than women with either condition alone (Vigod and Stewart 2006). In another population-based study, the severity of urinary incontinence was related to the risk of depressive illness (Melville et al. 2005).

A systematic review of the literature on sexual function in women with urinary incontinence (Shaw 2002) found that most studies were of poor quality. They concluded that further research in which standard definitions and measures of sexual impairment are used is needed to establish reliable information and prevalence estimates. The Female Sexual Function Index (FSFI) has been used for this purpose in more recent studies. Although results are not always consistent, urinary incontinence appears to negatively affect all domains of sexual function, including desire, arousal, and orgasm (Aslan et al. 2005; B.L. Cohen et al. 2008; Salonia et al. 2004).

Role of the Psychiatrist

Given the high prevalence of incontinence, particularly in middle-aged and older women, and women's frequent reluctance to disclose their symptoms, psychiatrists may wish to tactfully ask about urinary problems, as well as comorbid psychiatric conditions and adjustment problems.

TCAs and duloxetine (a dual-action SNRI) are useful treatments for stress urinary incontinence, particularly in women who have concurrent depression (Mariappan et al. 2007). However, although duloxetine is approved in Europe for urinary incontinence, it has not been approved in North America for this indication. Other treatments that have been used for urinary incontinence include behavioral training (with or without biofeedback), pelvic floor exercises, other drug therapies, intrapelvic devices such as pessaries, and surgical procedures (Rogers 2008).

Psychosomatic Obstetrics/ Gynecology and Men

A woman's significant other may be female or male, but published studies of relationships' effects on obstetric and gynecological events have been performed on heterosexual couples. Virtually every study of the psychosocial aspects of an obstetric and gynecological event or treatment indicates that the attitude of the male partner is a (or the) major determinant of outcome. Women turn to their significant others for reaffirmation of their worthiness if infertile, for reaffirmation of their femininity after hysterectomy, and for help deciding whether to take psychotropic medications while pregnant and whether to breast-feed or bottle-feed. Failure to achieve consensus on such decisions can cause serious long-term repercussions, as when a child is born with problems after (although not necessarily because of) the use of psychotropic medication during the mother's pregnancy, and the child's father blames the mother.

Fathers, brothers, sons, male partners, and husbands can be deeply affected by the obstetric and gynecological experiences of the women they care about, but they often feel uncomfortable, ignored, and excluded when their female loved ones are receiving care (Abboud and Liamputtong 2003; Buist et al. 2003). As mentioned in the section on infertility, men and women may manifest their feelings differently. Women are more likely to show emotion and to want to talk to friends and relatives. Men are more likely to keep their emotions to themselves and to withdraw into work or other activities. Women can mistake this behavior for a failure to care. Men can feel that their presence only makes their loved ones cry. Sometimes, one of the most useful interventions a psychiatric consultant can perform is to facilitate communication within the family.

Conclusion

Obstetricians and gynecologists are busy practitioners, challenged to deal with both specialized technological developments and primary care and burdened by the likelihood of lawsuits. Despite the intense emotional aspects of much of their clinical work, obstetricians and gynecologists have relatively little training or time for psychiatric problems. The scope of psychosomatic medicine in the area of obstetrics and gynecology includes psychopathological aspects of normal reproductive events, psychiatric aspects of obstetric and gynecological diseases and treatments, and psychiatric conditions specific to women's reproductive health. Gender-based medicine, which intersects psychosomatic obstetrics and gynecology at many points, is an exciting and promising area of research and clinical practice. Myriad opportunities exist for providing practical assistance to obstetricians and gynecologists and the women who are their patients, for educating fellow psychiatrists about developments in obstetrics and gynecology, and for conducting basic and clinical research.

References

Abboud LN, Liamputtong P: Pregnancy loss: what it means to women who miscarry and their partners. Soc Work Health Care 36:37–62, 2003

Addis A, Koren G: Safety of fluoxetine during the first trimester of pregnancy: a meta-analytical review of epidemiological studies. Psychol Med 30:89–94, 2000

Ahuja N, Moorhead S, Lloyd AJ, et al: Antipsychotic-induced hyperprolactinemia and delusion of pregnancy. Psychosomatics 49:163–167, 2008

Allen C, Hopewell S, Prentice A, et al: Nonsteroidal anti-inflammatory drugs for pain in women with endometriosis. Cochrane Database Syst Rev (2):CD004753, 2009

Altshuler L, Cohen L, Szuba M, et al: Pharmacologic management of psychiatric illness during pregnancy: dilemmas and guidelines. Am J Psychiatry 153:592–606, 1996

American Psychiatric Association: Diagnostic and Statistical Manual of Mental Disorders, 4th Edition, Text Revision. Washington, DC, American Psychiatric Association, 2000

Anderson EL, Reti IM: ECT in pregnancy: a review of the literature from 1941 to 2007. Psychosom Med 71:235–242, 2009

Apfel RJ, Keylor RG: Psychoanalysis and infertility. myths and realities. Int J Psychoanal 83:85–104, 2002

Appleby L, Mortensen PB, Faragher EB: Suicide and other causes of mortality after post-partum psychiatric admission. Br J Psychiatry 173:209–211, 1998

Arnold LD, Bachmann GA, Rosen R, et al: Assessment of vulvodynia symptoms in a sample of US women: a prevalence survey with a nested case control study. Am J Obstet Gynecol 196:128.e1–128.e6, 2007

Ashok PW, Hamoda H, Flett GM, et al: Psychological sequelae of medical and surgical abortion at 10–13 weeks gestation. Acta Obstet Gynecol Scand 84:761–766, 2005

Aslan G, Koseoglu H, Sadik O, et al: Sexual function in women with urinary incontinence. Int J Impot Res 17:248–251, 2005

Attia A, Downey J, Oberman M: Postpartum psychoses, in Postpartum Mood Disorders. Edited by Miller L. Washington, DC, American Psychiatric Press, 1999, pp 99–117

Avis NE: Depression during the menopausal transition. Psychol Women Q 27:91–100, 2003

Ayers S, Joseph S, McKenzie-McHarg K, et al: Post-traumatic stress disorder following childbirth: current issues and recommendations for future research. J Psychosom Obstet Gynaecol 29:240–250, 2008

Ayoola AB, Nettleman M, Brewer J: Reasons for unprotected intercourse in adult women. J Womens Health 16:302–310, 2007

Bergner A, Beyer R, Klapp BF, et al: Pregnancy after early pregnancy loss: a prospective study of anxiety, depressive symptomatology and coping. J Psychosom Obstet Gynaecol 29:105–113, 2008

Bjorn I, Bixo M, Nojd K, et al: Negative mood changes during hormone replacement therapy: a comparison between two progestogens. Am J Obstet Gynecol 183:1419–1426, 2000

Bloch M, Daly RC, Rubinow DR: Endocrine factors in the etiology of postpartum depression. Compr Psychiatry 44:234–246, 2003

Boivin J, Bunting L, Collins JA, et al: International estimates of infertility prevalence and treatment-seeking: potential need and demand for infertility medical care. Hum Reprod 22:1506–1512, 2007

Born L, Koren G, Lin E, et al: A new, female-specific irritability rating scale. J Psychiatry Neurosci 33:344–354, 2008

Bower JK, Schreiner PJ, Sternfeld B, et al: Black-white differences in hysterectomy prevalence: the CARDIA study. Am J Public Health 99:300–307, 2009

Bradshaw Z, Slade P: The effects of induced abortion on emotional experiences and relationships: a critical review of the literature. Clin Psychol Rev 23:929–958, 2003

Brier N: Grief following miscarriage: a comprehensive review of the literature. J Womens Health 17:451–464, 2008

Brown CS, Franks AS, Wan J, et al: Citalopram in the treatment of women with chronic pelvic pain: an open-label trial. J Reprod Med 53:191–195, 2008

Brown J, O'Brien PM, Marjoribanks J, et al: Selective serotonin reuptake inhibitors for premenstrual syndrome. Cochrane Database Syst Rev (2):CD001396, 2009

Buist A, Morse CA, Durkin S: Men's adjustment to fatherhood: implications for obstetric health care. J Obstet Gynecol Neonatal Nurs 32:172–180, 2003

Burns LH: Psychiatric aspects of infertility and infertility treatments. Psychiatr Clin North Am 30:689–716, 2007

Burns L, Covington S: Psychology of infertility, in Infertility Counseling. Edited by Burns LH, Covington SN. Pearl River, NY, Parthenon, 1999, pp 3–25

Cantin-Drouin M, Damant D, Turcotte D: Review of the literature on the psychoemotional reality of women with vulvodynia: difficulties met and strategies developed. Pain Res Manag 13:255–263, 2008

Chabrol H, Teissedre F, Saint-Jean M, et al: Prevention and treatment of post-partum depression: a controlled randomized study of women at risk. Psychol Med 32:1039–1047, 2002

Chambers CD, Hernandez-Diaz S, Van Marter LJ, et al: Selective serotonin-reuptake inhibitors and risk of persistent pulmonary hypertension of the newborn. N Engl J Med 354:579–587, 2006

Chandra A, Martinez GM, Mosher WD, et al: Fertility, family planning, and reproductive health of US women: data from the 2002 national survey of family growth. Vital Health Stat 23(25):1–160, 2005

Chang MY, Chen SH, Chen CH: Factors related to perceived labor pain in primiparas. Kaohsiung J Med Sci 18:604–609, 2002

Charles VE, Polis CB, Sridhara SK, et al: Abortion and long-term mental health outcomes: a systematic review of the evidence. Contraception 78:436–450, 2008

Chaudron LH, Pies RW: The relationship between postpartum psychosis and bipolar disorder: a review. J Clin Psychiatry 64:1284–1292, 2003

Chawla A, Swindle R, Long S, et al: Premenstrual dysphoric disorder: is there an economic burden of illness? Med Care 40:1101–1112, 2002

Chen TH, Chang SP, Tsai CF, et al: Prevalence of depressive and anxiety disorders in an assisted reproductive technique clinic. Hum Reprod 19:2313–2318, 2004

Cheong Y, William Stones R: Chronic pelvic pain: aetiology and therapy. Best Pract Res Clin Obstet Gynaecol 20:695–711, 2006

Chiriboga CA: Neurological correlates of fetal cocaine exposure. Ann N Y Acad Sci 846:109–125, 1998

Choi SH, Shapiro H, Robinson GE, et al: Psychological side effects of clomiphene citrate and human menopausal gonadotrophin. J Psychosom Obstet Gynaecol 26:93–100, 2005

Cohen BL, Barboglio P, Gousse A: The impact of lower urinary tract symptoms and urinary incontinence on female sexual dysfunction using a validated instrument. J Sex Med 5:1418–1423, 2008

Cohen LS: Treatment of bipolar disorder during pregnancy. J Clin Psychiatry 68 (suppl 9):4–9, 2007

Cohen LS, Sichel DA, Robertson LM, et al: Postpartum prophylaxis for women with bipolar disorder. Am J Psychiatry 152:1641–1645, 1995

Cohen LS, Altshuler LL, Harlow BL, et al: Relapse of major depression during pregnancy in women who maintain or discontinue antidepressant treatment. JAMA 295:499–507, 2006a

Cohen LS, Soares CN, Vitonis AF, et al: Risk for new onset of depression during the menopausal transition: the Harvard Study of Moods and Cycles. Arch Gen Psychiatry 63:385–390, 2006b

Cox H, Henderson L, Andersen N, et al: Focus group study of endometriosis: struggle, loss and the medical merry-go-round. Int J Nurs Pract 9:2–9, 2003

Cramer DW, Missmer SA: The epidemiology of endometriosis. Ann N Y Acad Sci 955:11–22; discussion 34–36, 396–406, 2002

Creus M, Fabregues F, Carmona F, et al: Combined laparoscopic surgery and pentoxifylline therapy for treatment of endometriosis-associated infertility: a preliminary trial. Hum Reprod 23:1910–1916, 2008

Curtis KM, Mohllajee AP, Peterson HB: Regret following female sterilization at a young age: a systematic review. Contraception 73:205–210, 2006

Cushman LF, Kalmuss K, Namerow PB: Placing an infant for adoption: the experience of young birth mothers. Soc Work 38:264–272, 1993

Dalpiaz O, Kerschbaumer A, Mitterberger M, et al: Chronic pelvic pain in women: still a challenge. BJU Int 102:1061–1065, 2008

Davies A, McIvor RJ, Kumar C: Impact of childbirth on a series of schizophrenic mothers: a comment on the possible influence of oestrogen on schizophrenia. Schizophr Res 16:25–31, 1995

Deave T, Heron J, Evans J, et al: The impact of maternal depression in pregnancy on early child development. BJOG 115:1043–1051, 2008

Dennis CL: The effect of peer support on postpartum depression: a pilot randomized controlled trial. Can J Psychiatry 48:115–124, 2003

Dennis CL, Stewart DE: Treatment of postpartum depression, part 1: a critical review of biological interventions. J Clin Psychiatry 65:1242–1251, 2004

Dennis CL, Ross LE, Grigoriadis S: Psychosocial and psychological interventions for treating antenatal depression. Cochrane Database Syst Rev (3):CD006309, 2007

Department of Health: Antenatal and postnatal mental health: clinical management and service guidance (NICE clinical guideline 45). London, National Institute for Health and Clinical Excellence, February 2007

Deuchar N: Nausea and vomiting in pregnancy: a review of the problem with particular regard to psychological and social aspects. Br J Obstet Gynecol 102:6–8, 1995

DiPietro JA, Novak MF, Costigan KA, et al: Maternal psychological distress during pregnancy in relation to child development at age two. Child Dev 77:573–587, 2006

Domoney CL, Vashisht A, Studd JW: Use of complementary therapies by women attending a specialist premenstrual syndrome clinic. Gynecol Endocrinol 17:13–18, 2003

Dyer SJ, Abrahams N, Mokoena NE, et al: "You are a man because you have children": experiences, reproductive health knowledge and treatment-seeking behaviour among men suffering from couple infertility in South Africa. Hum Reprod 19:960–967, 2004

Edwards L: New concepts in vulvodynia. Am J Obstet Gynecol 189:S24–S30, 2003

Einarson A, Boskovic R: Use and safety of antipsychotic drugs during pregnancy. J Psychiatr Pract 15:183–192, 2009

Einarson TR, Einarson A: Newer antidepressants in pregnancy and rates of major malformations: a meta-analysis of prospective comparative studies. Pharmacoepidemiol Drug Saf 14:823–827, 2005

Ellsberg M, Jansen HA, Heise L, et al: Intimate partner violence and women's physical and mental health in the WHO multi-country study on women's health and domestic violence: an observational study. Lancet 371:1165–1172, 2008

Engelhard IM, van den Hout MA, Kindt M, et al: Peritraumatic dissociation and posttraumatic stress after pregnancy loss: a prospective study. Behav Res Ther 41:67–78, 2003

Fanslow J, Whitehead A, Silva M, et al: Contraceptive use and associations with intimate partner violence among a population-based sample of New Zealand women. Aust N Z J Obstet Gynaecol 48:83–89, 2008

Farquhar CM, Steiner CA: Hysterectomy rates in the United States: 1990–1997. Obstet Gynecol 99:229–234, 2002

Fertl KI, Bergner A, Beyer R, et al: Levels and effects of different forms of anxiety during pregnancy after a prior miscarriage. Eur J Obstet Gynecol Reprod Biol 142:23–29, 2009

Flory N, Bissonnette F, Binik YM: Psychosocial effects of hysterectomy: literature review. J Psychosom Res 59:117–129, 2005

Flory N, Bissonnette F, Amsel RT, et al: The psychosocial outcomes of total and subtotal hysterectomy: a randomized controlled trial. J Sex Med 3:483–491, 2006

Freeman EW, Boxer AS, Rickels K, et al: Psychological evaluation and support in a program of in vitro fertilization and embryo transfer. Fertil Steril 43:48–53, 1985

Freeman EW, Sammel MD, Lin H: Temporal associations of hot flashes and depression in the transition to menopause. Menopause 16:728–734, 2009

Friedman T, Gath D: The psychiatric consequences of spontaneous abortion. Br J Psychiatry 155:810–813, 1989

Garg M, Singh M, Mansour D: Peri-abortion contraceptive care: can we reduce the incidence of repeat abortions? J Fam Plann Reprod Health Care 27:77–80, 2001

Gay D, Lynxwiler J: The impact of religiosity on race variations in abortion attitudes. Sociol Spectr 19:359–377, 1999

Gelbaya T, El-Halwagy E: Focus on primary care: chronic pelvic pain in women. Obstet Gynecol Surv 56:757–764, 2001

Gelberg L, Leake B, Lu MC, et al: Chronically homeless women's perceived deterrents to contraception. Perspect Sex Reprod Health 34:278–285, 2002

Gentile S: Infant safety with antipsychotic therapy in breast-feeding: a systematic review. J Clin Psychiatry 69:666–673, 2008

Glasier AF, Smith KB, van der Spuy ZM, et al: Amenorrhea associated with contraception—an international study on acceptability. Contraception 67:1–8, 2003

Grady D: Clinical practice. Management of menopausal symptoms. N Engl J Med 355:2338–2347, 2006

Graham M, James EL, Keleher H: Predictors of hysterectomy as a treatment for menstrual symptoms. Womens Health Issues 18:319–327, 2008

Greenfield SF, Sugarman DE: Treatment and consequences of alcohol abuse and dependence during pregnancy, in Management of Psychiatric Disorders During Pregnancy. Edited by Yonkers KA, Little B. London, Edward Arnold, 2001, pp 213–227

Groff JY, Mullen PD, Byrd T, et al: Decision making beliefs, and attitudes toward hysterectomy: a focus group study with medically underserved women in Texas. J Womens Health Gend Based Med 9 (suppl):S39–S50, 2000

Guclu S, Gol M, Dogan E, et al: Mirtazapine use in resistant hyperemesis gravidarum: report of three cases and review of the literature. Arch Gynecol Obstet 272:298–300, 2005

Gunter J: Chronic pelvic pain: an integrated approach to diagnosis and treatment. Obstet Gynecol Surv 58:615–623, 2003

Halbreich U, Bergeron R, Yonkers KA, et al: Efficacy of intermittent, luteal phase sertraline treatment of premenstrual dysphoric disorder. Obstet Gynecol 100:1219–1229, 2002

Harlow BL, Wise LA, Otto MW, et al: Depression and its influence on reproductive endocrine and menstrual cycle markers associated with perimenopause: the Harvard Study of Moods and Cycles. Arch Gen Psychiatry 60:29–36, 2003

Harlow BL, Vitonis AF, Sparen P, et al: Incidence of hospitalization for postpartum psychotic and bipolar episodes in women with and without prior prepregnancy or prenatal psychiatric hospitalizations. Arch Gen Psychiatry 64:42–48, 2007

Harris B, Oretti R, Lazarus J, et al: Randomised trial of thyroxine to prevent postnatal depression in thyroid-antibody-positive women. Br J Psychiatry 180:327–330, 2002

Harris G, Horowitz B, Borgida A: Evaluation of gabapentin in the treatment of generalized vulvodynia, unprovoked. J Reprod Med 52:103–106, 2007

Hartmann KE, Ma C, Lamvu GM, et al: Quality of life and sexual function after hysterectomy in women with preoperative pain and depression. Obstet Gynecol 104:701–709, 2004

Howard F: Chronic pelvic pain. Obstet Gynecol 101:594–611, 2003

Hunter MS: Somatic experience of the menopause: a prospective study. Psychosom Med 52:357–367, 1990

Hunter MS, Ussher JM, Browne SJ, et al: A randomized comparison of psychological (cognitive behavior therapy), medical fluoxetine and combined treatment for women with premenstrual dysphoric disorder. J Psychosom Obstet Gynaecol 23:193–199, 2002

Huo L, Straub RE, Roca C, et al: Risk for premenstrual dysphoric disorder is associated with genetic variation in ESR1, the estrogen receptor alpha gene. Biol Psychiatry 62:925–933, 2007

Jablensky AV, Morgan V, Zubrick SR, et al: Pregnancy, delivery, and neonatal complications in a population cohort of women with schizophrenia and major affective disorders. Am J Psychiatry 162:79–91, 2005

Jamieson DJ, Kaufman SC, Costello C, et al: A comparison of women's regret after vasectomy versus tubal sterilization. U.S. Collaborative Review of Sterilization Working Group. Obstet Gynecol 99:1073–1079, 2002

Janowsky DS, Rausch JL, Davis JM: Historical studies of premenstrual tension up to 30 years ago: implications for future research. Curr Psychiatry Rep 4:411–418, 2002

Jeal RR, West LA: Rolling away the stone: post-abortion women in the Christian community. J Pastoral Care Counsel 57:53–64, 2003

Joffe H: Reproductive biology and psychotropic treatments in premenopausal women with bipolar disorder. J Clin Psychiatry 68 (suppl 9):10–15, 2007

Kaewsarn P, Moyle W, Creedy D: Traditional postpartum practices among Thai women. J Adv Nurs 41:358–366, 2003

Kaufert PA, Gilbert P, Tate R: The Manitoba Project: a re-examination of the link between menopause and depression. Maturitas 14:143–155, 1992

Kerr J, Brown C, Balen AH: The experiences of couples who have had infertility treatment in the United Kingdom: results of a survey performed in 1997. Hum Reprod 14:934–938, 1999

Keye W: Medical aspects of infertility for the counselor, in Infertility Counseling. Edited by Burns LH, Covington SN. Pearl River, NY, Parthenon, 1999, pp 27–46

Koren G, Boucher N: Adverse effects in neonates exposed to SSRIs and SNRI in late gestation—Motherisk update 2008. Can J Clin Pharmacol 16:e66–e67, 2009

Kubicka L, Roth Z, Dytrych Z, et al: The mental health of adults born of unwanted pregnancies, their siblings, and matched controls: a 35 year follow-up study from Prague, Czech Republic. J Nerv Ment Dis 190:653–662, 2002

Kulkarni J, Riedel A, de Castella AR, et al: Estrogen: a potential treatment for schizophrenia. Schizophr Res 48:137–144, 2001

Lande RG, Karamchandani V: Chronic mental illness and the menstrual cycle. J Am Osteopath Assoc 102:655–659, 2002

Landen M, Eriksson E: How does premenstrual dysphoric disorder relate to depression and anxiety disorders? Depress Anxiety 17:122–129, 2003

Lane T, Francis A: Premenstrual symptomatology, locus of control, anxiety and depression in women with normal menstrual cycles. Arch Women Ment Health 6:127–138, 2003

Latthe P, Mignini L, Gray R, et al: Factors predisposing women to chronic pelvic pain: systematic review. BMJ 332:749–755, 2006

Lee DT, Yip AS, Chan SS, et al: Postdelivery screening for postpartum depression. Psychosom Med 65:357–361, 2003

Lefebvre G, Allaire C, Jeffrey J, et al: SOGC clinical guidelines: hysterectomy. J Obstet Gynaecol Can 24:37–61, 2002

Lewis CL, Groff JY, Herman CJ, et al: Overview of women's decision making regarding elective hysterectomy, oophorectomy, and hormone replacement therapy. J Womens Health Gend Based Med 9:S5–S14, 2000

Lu PY, Ory SJ: Endometriosis: current management. Mayo Clin Proc 70:453–463, 1995

Lukse M, Vacc N: Grief, depression and coping in women undergoing fertility treatments. Obstet Gynecol 93:245–251, 1999

Machado KM, Ludermir AB, da Costa AM: Changes in family structure and regret following tubal sterilization. Cad Saude Publica 21:1768–1777, 2005

Magalhaes PV, Kapczinski F, Kauer-Sant'Anna M: Use of contraceptive methods among women treated for bipolar disorder. Arch Womens Ment Health 12:183–185, 2009

Malhotra N, Chanana C, Garg P: Post-sterilization regrets in Indian women. Indian J Med Sci 61:186–191, 2007

Marcus SM: Depression during pregnancy: rates, risks and consequences—Motherisk update 2008. Can J Clin Pharmacol 16:e15–e22, 2009

Marcus S, Barry K, Flynn H, et al: Treatment guidelines for depression in pregnancy. Int J Obstet Gynecol 71:61–70, 2001

Mariappan P, Alhasso A, Ballantyne Z, et al: Duloxetine, a serotonin and noradrenaline reuptake inhibitor (SNRI) for the treatment of stress urinary incontinence: a systematic review. Eur Urol 51:67–74, 2007

Marsh WK, Templeton A, Ketter TA, et al: Increased frequency of depressive episodes during the menopausal transition in women with bipolar disorder: preliminary report. J Psychiatr Res 42:247–251, 2008

Matsubayashi H, Hosaka T, Izumi S, et al: Increased depression and anxiety in infertile Japanese women resulting from lack of husband's support and feelings of stress. Gen Hosp Psychiatry 26:398–404, 2004

Matthey S, Barnett B, Howie P, et al: Diagnosing postpartum depression in mothers and fathers: whatever happened to anxiety? J Affect Disord 74:139–147, 2003a

Matthey S, Barnett B, White T: The Edinburgh Postnatal Depression Scale. Br J Psychiatry 182:368–370, 2003b

Meador KJ, Baker GA, Browning N, et al: Cognitive function at 3 years of age after fetal exposure to antiepileptic drugs. N Engl J Med 360:1597–1605, 2009

Meltzer-Brody SE, Zolnoun D, Steege JF, et al: Open-label trial of lamotrigine focusing on efficacy in vulvodynia. J Reprod Med 54:171–178, 2009

Melville J, Walker E, Katon W, et al: Prevalence of comorbid psychiatric illness and its impact on symptom perception, quality of life and functional status in women with urinary incontinence Am J Obstet Gynecol 187:80–87, 2002

Melville JL, Delaney K, Newton K, et al: Incontinence severity and major depression in incontinent women. Obstet Gynecol 106:585–592, 2005

Miller LJ: Psychotic denial of pregnancy: phenomenology and clinical management. Hosp Community Psychiatry 41:1233–1237, 1990

Miller LJ, Rukstalis M: Beyond the "blues": hypotheses about postpartum reactivity, in Postpartum Mood Disorders. Edited by Miller LJ. Washington, DC, American Psychiatric Press, 1999, pp 3–19

Morgan ML, Cook IA, Rapkin AJ, et al: Estrogen augmentation of antidepressants in perimenopausal depression: a pilot study. J Clin Psychiatry 66:774–780, 2005

Morris-Rush JK, Freda MC, Bernstein PS: Screening for postpartum depression in an inner-city population. Am J Obstet Gynecol 188:1217–1219, 2003

Morrow KA, Thoreson RW, Penney LL: Predictors of psychological distress among infertility clinic patients. J Consult Clin Psychol 63:163–167, 1995

Nikcevic AV, Kuczmierczyk AR, Nicolaides KH: The influence of medical and psychological interventions on women's distress after miscarriage. J Psychosom Res 63:283–290, 2007

Nygaard I, Turvey C, Burns T, et al: Urinary incontinence and depression in middle-aged United States women. Obstet Gynecol 101:149–156, 2003

Oberlander TF, Warburton W, Misri S, et al: Neonatal outcomes after prenatal exposure to selective serotonin reuptake inhibitor antidepressants and maternal depression using population-based linked health data. Arch Gen Psychiatry 63:898–906, 2006

O'Brien B, Newton N: Psyche versus soma: historical evolution of beliefs about nausea and vomiting during pregnancy. J Psychosom Obstet Gynaecol 12:91–120, 1991

O'Connor TG, Heron J, Glover V, et al: Antenatal anxiety predicts child behavioral/emotional problems independently of postnatal depression. J Am Acad Child Adolesc Psychiatry 41:1470–1477, 2002

Oesterheld JR, Cozza K, Sandson NB: Oral contraceptives. Psychosomatics 49:168–175, 2008

O'Hara MW, Stuart S, Gorman LL, et al: Efficacy of interpersonal psychotherapy for postpartum depression. Arch Gen Psychiatry 57:1039–1045, 2000

Oretti RG, Harris B, Lazarus JH, et al: Is there an association between life events, postnatal depression and thyroid dysfunction in thyroid antibody positive women? Int J Soc Psychiatry 49:70–76, 2003

Payne JL, Roy PS, Murphy-Eberenz K, et al: Reproductive cycle-associated mood symptoms in women with major depression and bipolar disorder. J Affect Disord 99:221–229, 2007

Payne JL, Palmer JT, Joffe H: A reproductive subtype of depression: conceptualizing models and moving toward etiology. Harv Rev Psychiatry 17:72–86, 2009

Pearlstein T, Joliat MJ, Brown EB, et al: Recurrence of symptoms of premenstrual dysphoric disorder after the cessation of luteal-phase fluoxetine treatment. Am J Obstet Gynecol 188:887–895, 2003

Pearlstein T, Steiner M: Premenstrual dysphoric disorder: burden of illness and treatment update. J Psychiatry Neurosci 33:291–301, 2008

Peipert JF, Lapane KL, Allsworth JE, et al: Women at risk for sexually transmitted diseases: correlates of intercourse without barrier contraception. Am J Obstet Gynecol 197:474.e1–474.e8, 2007

Peterson HB: Sterilization. Obstet Gynecol 111:189–203, 2008

Pedersen LH, Henriksen TB, Vestergaard M, et al: Selective serotonin reuptake inhibitors in pregnancy and congenital malformations: population based cohort study. BMJ 339:b3569, 2009 {doi: 10.1136/bmj.b3569}

Picardo CM, Nichols M, Edelman A, et al: Women's knowledge and sources of information on the risks and benefits of oral contraception. J Am Med Womens Assoc 58:112–116, 2003

Polis CB, Schaffer K, Blanchard K, et al: Advance provision of emergency contraception for pregnancy prevention. Cochrane Database Syst Rev (2):CD005497, 2007

Poursharif B, Korst LM, Fejzo MS, et al: The psychosocial burden of hyperemesis gravidarum. J Perinatol 28:176–181, 2008

Pro-Life Action Ministries: What They Won't Tell You at the Abortion Clinic (flyer). St. Paul, MN, Pro-Life Action Ministries, undated

Protopopescu X, Tuescher O, Pan H, et al: Toward a functional neuroanatomy of premenstrual dysphoric disorder. J Affect Disord 108:87–94, 2008

Punamaki RL, Repokari L, Vilska S, et al: Maternal mental health and medical predictors of infant developmental and health problems from pregnancy to one year: does former infertility matter? Infant Behav Dev 29:230–242, 2006

Ramezanzadeh F, Aghssa MM, Abedinia N, et al: A survey of relationship between anxiety, depression and duration of infertility. BMC Womens Health 4:9, 2004

Rapp SR, Espeland MA, Shumaker SA, et al: Effect of estrogen plus progestin on global cognitive function in postmenopausal women. The Women's Health Initiative Memory Study: a randomized controlled trial. JAMA 289:2663–2672, 2003

Reardon DC, Cougle JR, Rue VM, et al: Psychiatric admissions of low-income women following abortion and childbirth. CMAJ 168:1253–1256, 2003

Reed BD, Caron AM, Gorenflo DW, et al: Treatment of vulvodynia with tricyclic antidepressants: efficacy and associated factors. J Low Genit Tract Dis 10:245–251, 2006

Reis M, Källén B: Delivery outcome after maternal use of antidepressant drugs in pregnancy: an update using Swedish data. Psychol Med 5:1–11, 2010

Rickert VI, Wiemann CM, Harrykissoon SD, et al: The relationship among demographics, reproductive characteristics, and intimate partner violence. Am J Obstet Gynecol 187:1002–1007, 2002

Riordan D, Appleby L, Faragher B: Mother-infant interaction in post-partum women with schizophrenia and affective disorders. J Psychol Med 29:991–995, 1999

Roe B, Doll H, Wilson K: Help seeking behaviour and health and social services utilization by people suffering from urinary incontinence. Int J Nurs Stud 36:245–253, 1999

Rogers RG: Urinary stress incontinence in women. N Engl J Med 358:1029–1036, 2008

Rosch DS, Sajatovic M, Sivec H: Behavioral characteristics in delusional pregnancy: a matched control group study. Int J Psychiatry Med 32:295–303, 2002

Ross LE, Gilbert Evans SE, Sellers EM, et al: Measurement issues in postpartum depression, part 1: anxiety as a feature of postpartum depression. Arch Womens Ment Health 6:51–57, 2003

Ross LE, McLean LM: Anxiety disorders during pregnancy and the postpartum period: a systematic review. J Clin Psychiatry 67:1285–1298, 2006

Saisto T, Halmesmaki E: Fear of childbirth: a neglected dilemma. Acta Obstet Gynecol Scand 82:201–208, 2003

Sakumoto K, Masamoto H, Kanazawa K: Post-partum maternity "blues" as a reflection of newborn nursing care in Japan. Int J Gynaecol Obstet 78:25–30, 2002

Salonia A, Zanni G, Nappi RE, et al: Sexual dysfunction is common in women with lower urinary tract symptoms and urinary incontinence: results of a cross-sectional study. Eur Urol 45:642–648; discussion 648, 2004

Sanders SA, Graham CA, Yarber WL, et al: Condom use errors and problems among young women who put condoms on their male partners. J Am Med Womens Assoc 58:95–98, 2003

Schmidt P, Nieman L, Danaceau M, et al: Estrogen replacement in perimenopause-related depression: a preliminary report. Am J Obstet Gynecol 183:414–420, 2000

Seeman MV: Does menopause intensify symptoms in schizophrenia? in Psychiatric Illness in Women: Emerging Treatments and Research. Edited by Lewis-Hall F, Williams TS, Panetta J, et al. Washington, DC, American Psychiatric Publishing, 2002, pp 239–248

Seston EM, Elliott RA, Noyce PR, et al: Women's preferences for the provision of emergency hormonal contraception services. Pharm World Sci 29:183–189, 2007

Shaw C: A systematic review of the literature on the prevalence of sexual impairment in women with urinary incontinence and the prevalence of urinary leakage during sexual activity. Eur Urol 42:432–440, 2002

Shoveller J, Chabot C, Soon JA, et al: Identifying barriers to emergency contraception use among young women from various sociocultural groups in British Columbia, Canada. Perspect Sex Reprod Health 39:13–20, 2007

Shumaker SA, Legault C, Rapp SR, et al: Estrogen plus progestin and the incidence of dementia and mild cognitive impairment in postmenopausal women. The Women's Health Initiative Memory Study: a randomized controlled trial. JAMA 289:2651–2662, 2003

Slade P, Heke S, Fletcher J, et al: Termination of pregnancy: patients' perceptions of care. J Fam Plann Reprod Health Care 27:72–77, 2001

Smith MJ, Schmidt PJ, Rubinow DR: Operationalizing DSM-IV criteria for PMDD: selecting symptomatic and asymptomatic cycles for research. J Psychiatr Res 37:75–83, 2003

Soares CN, Almeida OP, Joffe H, et al: Efficacy of estradiol for the treatment of depressive disorders in perimenopausal women: a double-blind, randomized, placebo-controlled trial. Arch Gen Psychiatry 58:529–534, 2001

Soderquist J, Wijma B, Thorbert G, et al: Risk factors in pregnancy for post-traumatic stress and depression after childbirth. BJOG 116:672–680, 2009

Solari H, Dickson KE, Miller L: Understanding and treating women with schizophrenia during pregnancy and postpartum—Motherisk update 2008. Can J Clin Pharmacol 16:e23–e32, 2009

Soules MR, Sherman S, Parrott L, et al: Executive summary: Stages of Reproductive Aging Workshop (STRAW). Menopause 8:402–407, 2001

Spielvogel AM, Hohener HC: Denial of pregnancy: a review and case reports. Birth 22:220–226, 1995

Spinelli MG, Endicott J: Controlled clinical trial of interpersonal psychotherapy versus parenting education program for depressed pregnant women. Am J Psychiatry 160:555–562, 2003

Stahl SM: Effects of estrogen on the central nervous system. J Clin Psychiatry 62:317–318, 2001

Steer RA, Scholl TO, Hediger ML, et al: Self-reported depression and negative pregnancy outcomes. J Clin Epidemiol 45:1093–1099, 1992

Steiner M, Brown E, Trzepacz P, et al: Fluoxetine improves functional work capacity in women with premenstrual dysphoric disorder. Arch Womens Ment Health 6:71–77, 2003

Steiner M, Pearlstein T, Cohen LS, et al: Expert guidelines for the treatment of severe PMS, PMDD, and comorbidities: the role of SSRIs. J Womens Health 15:57–69, 2006

Stewart DE, Boydell KM: Psychologic distress during menopause: associations across the reproductive life cycle. Int J Psychiatry Med 23:157–162, 1993

Stewart DE, Robinson G: Eating disorders and reproduction, in Psychological Aspects of Women's Health Care: The Interface Between Psychiatry and Obstetrics and Gynecology, 2nd Edition. Edited by Stotland N, Stewart D. Washington, DC, American Psychiatric Press, 2001a, pp 441–456

Stewart DE, Robinson G: Psychotropic drugs and electroconvulsive therapy during pregnancy and lactation, in Psychological Aspects of Women's Health Care: The Interface Between Psychiatry and Obstetrics and Gynecology, 2nd Edition. Edited by Stotland N, Stewart D. Washington, DC, American Psychiatric Press, 2001b, pp 67–93

Stewart DE, Leyland NA, Shime J, et al: Achieving Best Practices in the Use of Hysterectomy: Report of Ontario's Expert Panel on Best Practices in the Use of Hysterectomy. Ontario, Canada, Ontario Women's Health Council, 2002

Stewart DE, Gagnon A, Saucier JF, et al: Postpartum depression symptoms in newcomers. Can J Psychiatry 53:121–124, 2008

Stones RW, Mountfield J: Interventions for treating chronic pelvic pain in women. Cochrane Database Syst Rev (4): CD000387, 2000

Suri R, Altshuler L, Hellemann G, et al: Effects of antenatal depression and antidepressant treatment on gestational age at birth and risk of preterm birth. Am J Psychiatry 164:1206–1213, 2007

Thorp JM Jr, Hartmann KE, Shadigian E: Long-term physical and psychological health consequences of induced abortion: review of the evidence. Obstet Gynecol Surv 58:67–79, 2003

Thys-Jacobs S, Starkey P, Bernstein D, et al: Calcium carbonate and the premenstrual syndrome: effects on premenstrual and menstrual symptoms. Premenstrual Syndrome Study Group. Am J Obstet Gynecol 179:444–452, 1998

Toulis KA, Tzellos T, Kouvelas D, et al: Gabapentin for the treatment of hot flashes in women with natural or tamoxifen-induced menopause: a systematic review and meta-analysis. Clin Ther 31:221–235, 2009

Tribo MJ, Andion O, Ros S, et al: Clinical characteristics and psychopathological profile of patients with vulvodynia: an observational and descriptive study. Dermatology 216:24–30, 2008

Turton P, Hughes P, Evans CD, et al: Incidence, correlates and predictors of post-traumatic stress disorder in the pregnancy after stillbirth. Br J Psychiatry 178:556–560, 2001

Turton P, Badenhorst W, Hughes P, et al: Psychological impact of stillbirth on fathers in the subsequent pregnancy and puerperium. Br J Psychiatry 188:165–172, 2006

United Nations: World Contraceptive Use 2007. New York, Population Division, Department of Economic and Social Affairs, Population Division, United Nations November 2007. Available at: http://www.un.org/esa/population/publications/contraceptive2007/contraceptive_2007_table.pdf. Accessed May 17, 2009.

U.S. Food and Drug Administration: Drug Safety Oversight Board Update. Drug Information Association (DIA) Annual Meeting, Philadelphia, PA, June 21, 2006. Available at: http://www.fda.gov/downloads/AboutFDA/CentersOffices/CDER/ucm118835.pdf. Accessed October 28, 2009.

U.S. Food and Drug Administration: Plan B (0.75mg levonorgestrel) and Plan B One-Step (1.5 mg levonorgestrel) Tablets Information. July 13, 2009. Available at: http://www.fda.gov/Drugs/DrugSafety/PostmarketDrugSafetyInformationforPatientsandProviders/UCM109775. Accessed October 28, 2009.

Uskul AK, Ahmad F, Leyland NA, et al: Women's hysterectomy experiences and decision-making. Women Health 38:53–67, 2003

Ventura SJ, Mosher WD, Curtin SC, et al: Trends in pregnancies and pregnancy rates by outcome: estimates for the United States 1976–96. Vital Health Stat 21:1–47, 2000

Ventura SJ, Abma JC, Mosher WD, et al: Estimated pregnancy rates by outcome for the United States, 1990–2004. Natl Vital Stat Rep 56:1–25, 28, 2008

Verhaak CM, Smeenk JM, van Minnen A, et al: A longitudinal, prospective study on emotional adjustment before, during and after consecutive fertility treatment cycles. Hum Reprod 20:2253–2260, 2005

Verhaak CM, Smeenk JM, Evers AW, et al: Women's emotional adjustment to IVF: a systematic review of 25 years of research. Hum Reprod Update 13:27–36, 2007

Vesga-Lopez O, Blanco C, Keyes K, et al: Psychiatric disorders in pregnant and postpartum women in the United States. Arch Gen Psychiatry 65:805–815, 2008

Vigod SN, Stewart DE: The management of abnormal uterine bleeding by northern, rural and isolated primary care physicians, part II: what do we need? BMC Womens Health 2:11, 2002

Vigod SN, Stewart DE: Major depression in female urinary incontinence. Psychosomatics 47:147–151, 2006

Vigod SN, Stewart DE: Treatment patterns in Canadian women with urinary incontinence: a need to improve case identification. J Womens Health 16:707–712, 2007

Viguera AC, Newport DJ, Ritchie J, et al: Lithium in breast milk and nursing infants: clinical implications. Am J Psychiatry 164:342–345, 2007a

Viguera AC, Whitfield T, Baldessarini RJ, et al: Risk of recurrence in women with bipolar disorder during pregnancy: prospective study of mood stabilizer discontinuation. Am J Psychiatry 164:1817–1824; quiz 1923, 2007b

Volgsten H, Skoog Svanberg A, Ekselius L, et al: Prevalence of psychiatric disorders in infertile women and men undergoing in vitro fertilization treatment. Hum Reprod 23:2056–2063, 2008

Volgsten H, Skoog Svanberg A, Ekselius L, et al: Risk factors for psychiatric disorders in infertile women and men undergoing in vitro fertilization treatment. Fertil Steril 93:1088–1096, 2010

Walker MC, Murphy KE, Pan S, et al: Adverse maternal outcomes in multifetal pregnancies. BJOG 111:1294–1296, 2004

Warnock JK, Bundren JC, Morris DW: Depressive mood symptoms associated with ovarian suppression. Fertil Steril 74:984–986, 2000

Weijenborg PT, Greeven A, Dekker FW, et al: Clinical course of chronic pelvic pain in women. Pain 132 (suppl 1):S117–S123, 2007

Wessel J, Endrikat J, Buscher U: Frequency of denial of pregnancy: results and epidemiological significance of a 1-year prospective study in Berlin. Acta Obstet Gynecol Scand 81:1021–1027, 2002

Wessel J, Gauruder-Burmester A, Gerlinger C: Denial of pregnancy—characteristics of women at risk. Acta Obstet Gynecol Scand 86:542–546, 2007

Westhoff C, Picardo L, Morrow E: Quality of life following early medical or surgical abortion. Contraception 67:41–47, 2003

Whelan CI, Stewart DE: Pseudocyesis: a review and report of six cases. Int J Psychiatry Med 20:97–108, 1990

Whitaker AK, Gilliam M: Contraceptive care for adolescents. Clin Obstet Gynecol 51:268–280, 2008

Williams KE, Marsh WK, Rasgon NL: Mood disorders and fertility in women: a critical review of the literature and implications for future research. Hum Reprod Update 13:607–616, 2007

Wischmann T: Implications of psychosocial support in infertility—a critical appraisal. J Psychosom Obstet Gynaecol 29:83–90, 2008

Wisner KL, Zarin DA, Holmboe ES, et al: Risk-benefit decision making for treatment of depression during pregnancy. Am J Psychiatry 157:1933–1940, 2000

Wisner K, Gelenberg A, Leonard H, et al: Pharmacologic treatment of depression during pregnancy. JAMA 282:1264–1269, 2002a

Wisner KL, Parry BL, Piontek CM: Postpartum depression. N Engl J Med 347:194–199, 2002b

Women's Health Initiative Steering Committee: Effects of conjugated equine estrogen in postmenopausal women with hysterectomy: the Women's Health Initiative randomized controlled trial. JAMA 291:1701–1712, 2004

World Health Organization Programme of Maternal and Child Health and Family Planning Unit: Infertility: a tabulation of available data on prevalence of primary and secondary infertility (WHO/MCM/91.9). 1991. Available at: http://www.

who.int/reproductive-health/publications/Abstracts/infertility.html. Accessed October 28, 2009.

Writing Group for the Women's Health Initiative Investigators: Risks and benefits of estrogen plus progestin in healthy postmenopausal women: principal results from the Women's Health Initiative randomized controlled trial. JAMA 288:321–333, 2002

Wu JM, Wechter ME, Geller EJ, et al: Hysterectomy rates in the United Sates, 2003. Obstet Gynecol 110:1091–1095, 2007

Yen JY, Chen YH, Long CY, et al: Risk factors for major depressive disorder and the psychological impact of hysterectomy: a prospective investigation. Psychosomatics 49:137–142, 2008

Yeung PP Jr, Shwayder J, Pasic RP: Laparoscopic management of endometriosis: comprehensive review of best evidence. J Minim Invasive Gynecol 16:269–281, 2009

Yonkers KA, Wisner KL, Stowe Z, et al: Management of bipolar disorder during pregnancy and the postpartum period. Am J Psychiatry 161:608–620, 2004

Yonkers KA, Wisner KL, Stewart DE, et al: The management of depression during pregnancy: a report from the American Psychiatric Association and the American College of Obstetricians and Gynecologists. Gen Hosp Psychiatry 31:403–413, 2009

Zabin LS, Hirsch MB, Emerson MR: When urban adolescents choose abortion: effects on education, psychological status, and subsequent pregnancy. Fam Plann Perspect 21:248–255, 1989

Zaers S, Waschke M, Ehlert U: Depressive symptoms and symptoms of post-traumatic stress disorder in women after childbirth. J Psychosom Obstet Gynaecol 29:61–71, 2008

Zlotogora J: Parental decisions to abort or continue a pregnancy with an abnormal finding after an invasive prenatal test. Prenat Diagn 22:1102–1106, 2002

Zondervan K, Yudkin P, Vessey M, et al: Patterns of diagnosis and referral in women consulting for chronic pelvic pain in UK primary care. Br J Obstet Gynecol 106:1149–1155, 1999

CHAPTER 34

Pediatrics

Brenda Bursch, Ph.D.

Margaret Stuber, M.D.

IN THIS CHAPTER, WE PROVIDE a brief overview of the major issues in psychiatric or psychological consultation to pediatrics. (For pediatric topics discussed elsewhere in this book, see Chapter 13, "Deception Syndromes: Factitious Disorders and Malingering"; Chapter 14, "Eating Disorders"; Chapter 29, "Dermatology"; and Chapter 30, "Surgery.") Many of the issues addressed in pediatrics are similar to those seen with adults. However, because the relative importance of development and of the family is sufficiently different in pediatrics as opposed to working with adults, these issues should be considered at the start of any evaluation, and they infuse every intervention and recommendation.

General Principles in Evaluation and Management

Children's Developmental Understanding of Illness and Their Bodies

Children's conceptions of their bodies vary widely and are obviously influenced by experiences with illness. However, in general, children appear to follow a developmental path of understanding their bodies that roughly corresponds to Piaget's stages of cognitive development. *Sensorimotor children* (birth to approximately 2 years) are largely preverbal and do not have the capacity to create narratives to explain their experiences. Their perception of their bodies and of illness is therefore primarily built on sensory experiences and does not involve any formal reasoning. *Preoperational children* (approximately 2–7 years) also understand through perception, but they are able to use words and some very basic concepts of cause and effect. They tend to be most aware of parts of the body that they can directly sense, such as bones and heart (which they can feel) and blood (which they have seen come out of their bodies). However, they do not have a clear sense of cause and effect and are therefore inclined to see events that are temporally related as causally related. They also have no real sense of organs but conceptualize blood and food as going into or coming out of their bodies as though the body were itself the container. This leads to many humorous but confusing assumptions and misunderstandings. *Concrete operational children* (approximately 7–11 years) are able to apply logic to their perceptions in a more integrative manner. However, the logic is quite literal or concrete and allows for only one cause for an effect. They tend to be eager to learn factual information about the body and illness at this age but will have difficulty with any concepts that require abstract reasoning. *Formal operational children* (≥11 years) are able to use a level of abstract reasoning that allows discussion of systems rather than simple organs and can incorporate multiple causation of illness. It should not be assumed, however, that all adolescents approach the understanding of illness and their bodies at this level of cognition. In fact, most adults function at this level of thought only in areas of their own expertise, if at all.

As with all areas of cognition, education and experience make a difference. Children who have a medical problem (or who have a friend or family member with a medical history) may know more about the body and its function than do other children. However, children also will often be able to repeat what has been said to them without any real understanding of what it means. It is always important to assess children's level of understanding by asking them to explain in their own words or give their own version of why something is happening. This can alert you and the treating team to misunderstandings or fears that could influence adherence to the treatment plan.

Family Systems

No pediatric patient can be considered in isolation from his or her family. Parents are the legal decision makers for the child and thus are involved in all aspects of his or her care. Parents are also the ones to whom children look to understand the world. It is partially from their reactions to the illness and the treatment that the child determines how dangerous this is and how to respond (McLeod et al. 2007). Thus, parental fear, helplessness, anger, or withdrawal is important to address.

Psychiatric Issues

Psychological Responses to Illness

Overview

Psychological distress in response to serious pediatric illness has been a focus of many disease-specific and noncategorical studies over the years. Often symptoms of depression, anxiety, and behavior problems are grouped together. For example, a review of empirical studies of pediatric heart transplant recipients found that 20%–24% of these children experienced significant problems of psychological distress (Todaro et al. 2000). A study of children with epilepsy that used the State-Trait Anxiety Inventory and the Children's Depression Inventory (Oguz et al. 2002) found that the epileptic children reported significantly more depressed and anxious symptoms than did a control group. Even in children undergoing a surgical procedure as minor as a tonsillectomy, 17% of 89 children followed up prospectively had temporary symptoms consistent with a depressive episode (Papakostas et al. 2003). In some cases, the effects can be longer lasting, as was found in a study of 5,736 childhood cancer survivors, studied as young adults, who reported significantly more symptoms of depression than did their control siblings (Zebrack et al. 2002).

An area of increasing clinical focus is illness- or treatment-related trauma symptoms. For example, Kean et al. (2006) found that adolescents with asthma, especially those who have experienced a life-threatening event, as well as their parents, have high levels of posttraumatic stress symptoms (20% and 29% meeting posttraumatic stress disorder [PTSD] criteria, respectively). Rennick et al. (2002, 2004) found that children who were younger, were more severely ill, and experienced more invasive procedures had significantly more medical fears, a lower sense of health control, and chronic posttraumatic stress symptoms for 6 months after hospital discharge; they also found that exposure to high numbers of invasive procedures was the most important predictor of posttraumatic stress symptoms at 6 weeks after hospital discharge. The symptoms assessed in many of these cases would not necessarily meet criteria for a DSM diagnosis. However, these symptoms do appear to be associated with decrease in function. For example, the type of depression that is seen in association with chronic pain of various etiologies has been found to be strongly associated with functional disability (Kashikar-Zuck et al. 2001).

Social support appears to be a key element in psychological adjustment to illness. Social support was found to correlate negatively with problem behavior in adolescents with human immunodeficiency virus (HIV) over a period of 3 years (Battles and Wiener 2002). In a study of 160 pediatric rheumatology patients, children with higher classmate support had lower levels of depression (von Weiss et al. 2002). Depressed parents of chronically ill children have been found to have depressed children (Williamson et al. 2002). Social support has medical implications as well. For example, families that are less caring or are in more conflict are associated with poorer metabolic control of children with juvenile-onset diabetes (Schiffrin 2001). Studies have shown that serious pediatric illness or treatment may also lead to chronic and acute symptoms of emotional distress in the parents, which may interfere with their ability to provide support for the children. This has been found with pediatric cancer patients (Kazak et al. 1997) and pediatric transplant recipients (Young et al. 2003).

In some cases, psychological distress and behavior problems can be directly caused by physical manifestations of the illness or the treatment. For example, mood disorders and anxiety are relatively common manifestations of involvement of the central nervous system (CNS) in pediatric systemic lupus erythematosus (Sibbitt et al. 2002). Depression, anxiety, aggression, and school problems are observed as side effects of tacrolimus, given to prevent rejection of a transplanted kidney (Kemper et al. 2003). Use of steroids for inflammatory conditions, such as rheumatoid arthritis, can have significant effect on mood (Klein-Gitelman and Pachman 1998). Treatment of behavioral distress, depression, or anxiety in juvenile-onset diabetes mellitus must always consider the agitation that is symptomatic of hypoglycemia or the confusion associated with hyperglycemia (Goodnick et al. 1995).

Screening and Prevention

Because psychological adjustment problems appear to be relatively common, it is recommended that children who are chronically ill, acutely ill, or injured be screened by pediatricians or other professionals for depression, anxiety, and behavioral disturbance (Borowsky et al. 2003). Preventive programs are indicated for some pediatric inpatient services in which anxiety and depression are common. For example, in chronic painful treatment situations, such as pediatric burns, in which significant emotional distress is the norm, anxiety treatment programs are best built in along with pain management programs (Sheridan et al. 1997; Stoddard and Saxe 2001). Some evidence indicates that this may help prevent development of PTSD (see Saxe et al. 1998; Stoddard and Saxe 2001). In treatments with high mortality, such as bone marrow transplantation, in which different phases of treatment appear to have varying levels of depression or anxiety associated with them (Robb and Ebberts 2003), consistent psychosocial support should be available from the start. Kazak et al. (2006) have proposed a model for assessing and treating pediatric medical traumatic stress.

Treatment Considerations

Treatment studies targeting the psychiatric symptoms of medically ill children are rare. Consequently, treatment for anxiety that persists after normal adjustment and comfort issues are addressed is similar to that provided in general psychiatric practice: cognitive-behavioral therapy (In-Albon and Schneider 2007; Kendall 1994; Ollendick and King 1998; Walkup et al. 2008) and the use of selective serotonin reuptake inhibitors (SSRIs) (Research Unit on Pediatric Psychopharmacology Anxiety Study Group 2001; Walkup et al. 2008). Individual behavioral techniques, such as exposure and systematic desensitization, can be effective for patients with simple phobias such as needle phobia or food aversion. More extensive cognitive-behavioral treatment packages that address anxiety across many dimensions (including somatic, cognitive, and behavior problems) are indicated for children with more complex anxiety disorders (Piacentini and Bergman 2001). Treatment with a combination of cognitive-behavioral therapy and an SSRI has been shown to be more effective than a single strategy approach (Walkup et al. 2008).

Because hospitalized and chronically ill children often experience many of the symptoms seen in depression, making a decision as to whether a pediatric patient should receive treatment for depression can be difficult. A depressed or irritable mood, diminished interest or pleasure in activities, significant weight loss or change in appetite, insomnia or hypersomnia, psychomotor agitation or retardation, and fatigue or loss of energy may be secondary to the medical condition or to prolonged separation from friends and family. Although medication may be indicated, often supportive and cognitive-behavioral interventions can lead to significant improvements for such symptoms (Rey and Birmaher 2009). Less common, and more concerning, are feelings of worthlessness or inappropriate guilt, diminished ability to think or concentrate, or thoughts of suicide (Goldston et al. 1994). A careful assessment is necessary and should include suicidal fantasies or actions, concepts of what the child thinks would happen if suicide were attempted or achieved, previous experiences with suicidal behavior, circumstances at the time of the suicidal behavior, motivations for suicide, concepts and experiences of death, family situations, and environmental situations (Pfeffer 1986). Adolescents with suicidal intent and plan, family history of suicide, a comorbid psychiatric disorder, intractable pain, persistent insomnia, lack of social support, inadequate coping skills, a recent improvement in depressive symptoms, or impulsivity are at particular risk for suicide. Antidepressant medication should be started carefully in such cases. For some adolescents, the idea of suicide is an important source of control in the face of an unknown and uncontrollable illness course. Addressing a lack of perceived control, isolation, and distressing physical symptoms should be a high priority.

Pediatricians are often familiar with the use of stimulants and some antidepressants in their practice (Efron et al. 2003), but literature is limited on the use of these medications in medically ill children. The strongest research effort in child psychiatry on effective medication treatments for depression and anxiety has been with SSRIs. In multicenter trials, both fluvoxamine and sertraline have been shown to be superior to placebo in treating separation anxiety disorder, social anxiety disorder, or generalized anxiety disorder in children and adolescents (Research Unit on Pediatric Psychopharmacology Anxiety Study Group 2001; Walkup et al. 2008). Additionally, fluoxetine has been found to be effective for childhood obsessive-compulsive disorder (Liebowitz et al. 2002) and depression (Bridge et al. 2007). Antidepressants have been shown to increase the short-term risk of suicidal thinking and behavior in children and adolescents, requiring one to balance this potential risk with clinical indication (Bridge et al. 2007; Hammad et al. 2006; Mosholder and Willy 2006). When youths start taking an antidepressant, they should be closely monitored by clinicians and family members for clinical worsening, suicidal ideation, or unusual behavior changes (Birmaher et al. 2007). Meta-analysis has concluded that both fluoxetine and citalopram offer the most favorable risk-benefit profiles for the treatment of depression in children (Wallace et al. 2006). Strong evidence does not exist to support the use of tricyclic antidepressants (TCAs) or benzodiazepines as a first-line treatment for child anxiety disorders (Riddle et al. 1999). Despite a lack of supporting data, low doses of benzodiazepines are frequently prescribed by pediatricians for acute anxiety or agitation in the hospital because they can have a more immediate effect than SSRIs. Therefore, it is important to note that some anxious children have agitated reactions to benzodiazepines. Psychiatric consultants can offer alternatives, including antipsychotics, when immediate response is necessary.

Adherence

The term *adherence* is generally used to describe the extent to which a patient's health behavior is consistent with medical recommendations. Defined as such, adherence would include not only the taking of medications and attendance at clinical appointments but also diet, exercise, and other lifestyle issues such as smoking and use of sunscreen (Lemanek et al. 2001). Adherence is measured according to blood levels, pill counts, and self-report, all of which are problematic (Du Pasquier-Fediaevsky and Tubiana-Rufi 1999; Shemesh et al. 2004). With such a wide definition and different assessment strategies, the estimates vary as to the number of pediatric patients who adhere to medical regimens for chronic conditions (Rapoff 1999; Steele and Grauer 2003). Despite these problems, there is general agreement that nonadherence with medication regimens is a serious problem in pediatric patients with both acute and chronic conditions, resulting in significant clinical morbidity (Bauman et al. 2002; DiMatteo et al. 2002; Phipps and DeCuir-Whalley 1990; Serrano-Ikkos et al. 1998).

Many variables have been cited as potential predictors of nonadherence. Older age of the child and male sex are correlated with increased nonadherence, as is longer time receiving treatment, child self-responsibility for medication, and lack of appropriate family support in most studies across a variety of illnesses (Griffin and Elkin 2001; Kahana et al. 2008b; Lurie et al. 2000; Rapoff et al. 2002; Strunk et al. 2002). The patient's health beliefs about barriers to care, severity of the illness, and susceptibility to problems have been found to be related to nonadherence in some studies (Soliday and Hoeksel 2000), whereas other studies have found that parental health beliefs did not predict adherence (Steele et al. 2001). Some investigations have suggested that cultural beliefs may be equally or more important (Snodgrass et al. 2001; Tucker et al. 2002). Although lack of knowledge would seem to be an important predictor, this has proven more difficult to measure than might be expected (Ho et al. 2003; McQuaid et al. 2003). Although one study found that mild anxiety was associated with better adherence (Strunk et al. 2002), others suggested that psychological distress was associated with nonadherence (Kahana et al. 2008b; Simoni et al. 1997).

Interventions to increase adherence have fallen under the general categories of educational (written and verbal instructions), organizational (simplification of regimens, improved access, increased supervision), and behavioral (reminders, incentives, and self-monitoring). A recent meta-analysis of 12 intervention studies to increase medication adherence in pediatric otitis media and streptococcal pharyngitis found that multiple-strategy interventions appear to be more effective than single-strategy approaches, and education alone was not sufficient (Wu and Roberts 2008). Likewise, a meta-analysis of 70 psychological intervention studies for chronically ill youths (including children with asthma: 32 studies; diabetes: 16 studies; cystic fibrosis: 10 studies; juvenile rheumatoid arthritis: 2 studies; obesity: 2 studies; and 1 study each for hemodialysis, hemophilia, HIV, inflammatory bowel disease, phenylketonuria, seizure disorders, sickle cell disease, and tuberculosis) found medium effect sizes for behavioral and multiple-strategy interventions and a small effect size for education alone (Kahana et al. 2008a). Consistent with the larger health behavior literature, education appears to be necessary for adherence but is not always sufficient. One study found that treating liver transplant recipients for PTSD improved adherence to medication (Shemesh et al. 2000).

Death, Dying, and Bereavement

One of the most difficult issues for anyone to cope with is the death of a child (Field et al. 2003). Because of the tremendous advances in medicine over the past 20 years and the seeming unfairness of death in childhood, pediatricians and families often resist making the transition from an emphasis on cure to a focus on comfort care. The psychiatric consultant is often called when disagreement occurs within the team or between the team and the child and/or family about whether this point has been reached or about how this transition is to be approached. Sometimes these differences are the result of cultural or philosophical differences. Physicians who believe that life is to be pursued at all costs may have trouble understanding the feelings of nurses who feel that the child is being needlessly subjected to painful interventions. Families who are deeply religious and remain hopeful for a miracle may lead the medical team to request a psychiatric consult to address the family's "denial." Family members who wish to protect the child may feel that it is best to withhold information about disease prognosis or other potentially upsetting information. A dying child or adolescent might wish to be sedated to feel comfortable, whereas the family may want him or her to remain alert, or vice versa. The psychiatric consultant can serve as the interpreter and facilitate these often highly emotionally charged discussions to allow the individuals to understand one another well enough to plan together for the care of the child.

Although depression, withdrawal, and anxiety may be expected, a variety of emotional responses may be seen in terminally ill children and should be anticipated in conversations with parents. Children and adolescents may manifest their confusion and loss by negative, oppositional, aggressive, or emotional acting out, as well as with apathy and withdrawal from family and friends. They may frighten the medical staff or family as they talk about death or carry on conversations with someone who has died or with God. They may seem to know when they are going to die or "take a trip." What may initially appear to be confusion or delirium may actually be an attempt to communicate through a metaphor (Callanan and Kelley 1992). The approach of the consultant should be to allow such conversations to occur and to support the staff and parents to tolerate these attempts of the child to cope with the process of dying. Play therapy or art therapy may be particularly helpful for younger children and for older children who prefer these modalities. In some cases, children will choose to specifically address unfinished business, such as saying good-bye, making amends, being absolved of perceived transgressions, planning their memorial service, or deciding who gets particular belongings (Gyulay 1989). One study of parents of children who died of cancer found that parents rated medical care of their child higher when physicians clearly told them what to expect at the end of life, communicated in a sensitive and caring manner, and appropriately communicated with the child (Mack et al. 2005). Another study found that parents of children who died of severe malignant disease were more likely to have regrets if they had not discussed death with their child (almost a third of the parents interviewed), with no parents who discussed it having regrets about those discussions (Kreicbergs et al. 2004).

Environmental interventions can relieve many physical discomforts. Interventions to improve communication and understanding can relieve many emotional discomforts and fears. If such interventions are not sufficient to resolve distressing symptoms, medications should be considered. It is important to recognize that children and parents vary in their preferences for sedation or symptoms. It is important to understand these preferences when choosing medications. For a more thorough review of emotional and physical symptom management, see the chapter by Stuber and Bursch (2009) and the book by Behrman et al. (2004). For a more thorough review on the topic of talking to children about death, refer to the article by Stuber and Mesrkhani (2001).

Finally, consultants should be aware of community hospice services and be able to advocate for this approach to optimizing quality of life when indicated. Careful preparation and support are necessary if a family is to take a child home for the dying process. Parents typically need emotional and technical support as well as respite. Siblings will need age-appropriate information and emotional support. While it is often best for the child to be allowed to die at home, some families do not feel they can cope well with this plan. It is also important to consider that many palliative-care treatment approaches can be used for symptom management well before a transition to hospice care is indicated or decided.

Psychiatric Disorders

Delirium

Pediatric delirium (see Chapter 5, "Delirium") has received little research attention (Turkel et al. 2003) and is less often diagnosed in pediatrics than on the adult units (Manos and Wu 1997), especially among the younger pediatric patients (Schieveld et al. 2007). Critically ill children can develop delirium, with a hyperactive, hypoactive, mixed, or veiled presentation (Karnik et al. 2007; Schieveld et al. 2007). As in adults, it sometimes may present with what is interpreted to be psychotic symptoms (Webster and Holroyd 2000). The consultation request also may be put in terms of a request for an assessment of unexplained lethargy, depression, or confusion.

In adults, delirium has been found to be the strongest predictor of length of stay in the hospital, after studies have controlled for severity of illness, age, gender, race, and medication (Ely et al. 2001). A recent evaluation of the widely used Delirium Rating Scale found that it does appear to be applicable to children, with scores comparable to those of adults. However, the score or diagnosis of delirium in a child may not have the same implications that it has in adults. The scores for children, unlike those for adults, did not predict length of hospital stay or mortality (Turkel et al. 2003). Similarly, the Glasgow Coma Scale appears to be less effective in predicting prognosis for children than for adults (Lieh-Lai et al. 1992).

Common causes of delirium include infections, metabolic disturbances, and toxicity of medications. These can often be determined with a careful chart review. Other potentially severe or life-threatening causes of confusion include stroke (Kothare et al. 1998), confusional migraine (Shaabat 1996), neuropsychiatric symptoms of systemic lupus erythematosus (Turkel et al. 2001), or inflammatory encephalopathy (Vasconcellos et al. 1999). Less common causes of acute confusional state in children would be multiple sclerosis (Gadoth 2003) or thiamine deficiency (Hahn et al. 1998). Magnetic resonance imaging (MRI) and single photon emission computed tomography have been found to be useful in differentiation of inflammatory encephalopathy (Hahn et al. 1998) and systemic lupus erythematosus (Turkel et al. 2001), respectively.

Even after correction or treatment of the underlying etiology, the symptoms of delirium can last 1–2 weeks (Manos and Wu 1997). Therefore, symptomatic treatment is essential. Support and orienting cues can be very helpful in reducing the fear and confusion. These include the presence of familiar objects, photographs, and people who can reassure and orient the child, as well as age-appropriate clocks, calendars, or signs. Education can help the parents understand what is happening, reduce their distress, and help them to provide support for the child rather than irritation or fear.

Given the current lack of association between pediatric delirium and adverse outcomes, pharmacological intervention is indicated only if the child is distressed by the delirium or is becoming dangerous because of his or her lack of cooperation with care. Because the research into pharmacological approaches to pediatric delirium is almost nonexistent, the general guidelines are pragmatic and are based on the adult literature and the pediatric anesthesia literature. Treatment with haloperidol or risperidone is effective (Schieveld et al. 2007). Preliminary research suggests that there may be benefit from the use of risperidone for pediatric patients with hypoactive or mixed delirium and haloperidol for patients with hyperactive delirium (Karnik et al. 2007). Avoiding or weaning off benzodiazepines, which appear to compound the confusion with sedation (Breitbart et al. 1996), often should be recommended.

Factitious Disorders

Illness Falsification

The difference between factitious disorder and malingering relates to the primary motivation for the behavior. *Factitious disorder* is defined as the intentional production or feigning (falsification) of physical or psychological signs or symptoms to assume the sick role. *Malingering* is the intentional falsification of physical or psychological signs or symptoms to achieve external gain or to avoid unwanted responsibilities or outcomes.

Little research has been conducted on the topic of illness falsification in children and adolescents. More is known about illness falsification in adults and in child victims of adults (see Chapter 13, "Deception Syndromes: Factitious Disorders and Malingering"). The literature suggests that adult factitious disorder may have origins in childhood for some individuals (Libow 2002) and that some children and adolescents who falsify illness in themselves may have had earlier experiences as a victim of illness falsification or as a recipient of caregiver reinforcement for illness falsification. The child victim experience, including feelings of powerlessness, chronic lack of control, and disappointment in the medical care system, is a possible dynamic in the future development of illness falsification.

Libow (2000) conducted the only literature review to date for cases of child and adolescent patients who falsified illness. She identified 42 published cases in which patients had a mean age of 13.9 (range: 8–18 years). Most patients were female (71%), with the gender imbalance greater among older children. Patients engaged in false symptom reporting and induction, including active injections, bruising, and ingestions. The most commonly falsified or induced conditions were fevers, ketoacidosis, purpura, and infections. The average duration of the falsifications before detection was about 16 months. Many admitted to their deceptions when confronted, and some had positive outcomes at follow-up. The children were described as bland, depressed, and fascinated with health care.

Child Victims of Illness Falsification

Illness falsification can include exaggeration, fabrication, simulation, and induction. *Exaggeration* is embellishment of a true symptom or problem. *Fabrications* are false statements made by the abuser about the victim's medical history or symptoms. *Simulation* can include the alteration of records, medical test procedures, or symptoms to incorrectly suggest a problem. *Induction* is directly causing a problem or worsening a preexisting problem. Child victims of illness falsification (called *Munchausen syndrome by proxy* when the abuser's behavior is due to factitious disorder not otherwise specified [NOS]) experience significant psychological problems during childhood, including feelings of helplessness, self-doubt, and poor self-esteem; self-destructive ideation; eating disorders; behavioral growth problems; nightmares; and school concentration problems (Bools et al. 1993; Libow 1995; Porter et al. 1994). Adult survivors describe emotional difficulties, including suicidal feelings, anxiety, depression, low self-esteem, intense rage reactions, and PTSD symptoms (Libow 1995).

Ayoub (2002) presented longitudinal data on a sample of 40 children found by courts to be victims of illness falsification. The findings indicated that child victims frequently develop serious psychiatric symptoms that vary depending on the child's developmental age, the length and intensity of the child's exposure, and the current degree of protection and support. She found that PTSD and oppositional disorders are significant sequelae, as are patterns of reality distortion, poor self-esteem, and attachment difficulties. Although these children can superficially appear socially skilled and well adjusted, they often struggle with basic relationships. Lying is common, as is manipulative illness behavior and sadistic behavior toward other children. Many remain trauma-reactive and experience cyclical anger, depression, and oppositionality. Children who fared best were separated from their biological parents and remained in a single protected placement or had an abuser who admitted to the abuse and worked over a period of years toward reunification (Ayoub 2002).

Feeding Disorders

Food Refusal, Selectivity, and Phobias

Feeding problems and eating disturbances in toddlers and young school-age children (see also Chapter 14, "Eating Disorders") occur in 25%–40% of the population (Mayes et al. 1993). Most are transient and can be easily addressed with parent training, education about nutrition or normal child development, child–caregiver interaction advice, and suggestions for food preparation and presentation. However, severe eating disturbances requiring more aggressive treatment occur in 3%–10% of young children and are most common in children with other physical or developmental problems (Ahearn et al. 2001; Kerwin 1999). These children are at risk for aspiration, malnutrition, invasive medical procedures, hospitalizations, limitations in normal functioning and development, liver failure, and death.

Some physical factors that can impair normal eating include anatomical abnormalities, sensory perceptual impairments, oral motor dysfunction, and chronic medical problems (such as reflux, short-gut syndrome, inflammatory bowel disease, hepatic or pancreatic disease, or cancer). Other contributing factors can include the pairing of eating with an aversive experience (posttraumatic feeding disorders), inadvertent caregiver reinforcement of progressively more selective food choices, or a lack of normal early feeding experiences.

Munk and Repp (1994) developed methods for assessing feeding problems in individuals with cognitive and physical disabilities that allow categorization of individual feeding patterns based on responses to repeated presentations of food. Complete food refusal or food selectivity can occur with or without an associated phobia and can be assessed by observing for fear and anxiety behaviors on food presentation (Kerwin 1999).

Food aversion and oral motor dysfunction can be treated by a skilled mental health clinician, speech pathologist, or occupational therapist. Effective behavioral interventions include contingency management with positive reinforcement for appropriate feeding and ignoring or guiding inappropriate responses. Desensitization techniques can be effectively used to address phobias or altered sensory processing. Although no research has directly examined the use of psychotropic medication in treating food refusal, selectivity, or phobias, it may be valuable to consider for use with children with associated anxiety disorders.

Failure to Thrive

Children whose current weight or rate of weight gain is significantly below that of other children of similar age and sex are diagnosed by pediatricians with failure to thrive (FTT). It is helpful to think of FTT as a presenting symptom with varied and potentially multiple causes (Wren and Tarbell 1998). Parents might have a poor understanding of feeding techniques or might improperly prepare formula, or the mother may have an inadequate supply of breast milk. Biological contributors to FTT include defects in food assimilation, excessive loss of ingested calories, increased energy requirements, and prenatal insults; environmental contributors include economic or emotional deprivation.

Research examining the role of the child–parent attachment indicates that feeding problems and growth deficiencies can occur within the context of organized and secure attachments; however, insecure attachment relationships may intensify feeding problems and lead to more severe malnutrition (Chatoor et al. 1998). In one study of FTT children (who had no identifiable biological contributors), 80% of the mothers reported that they had a history of being victims of physical abuse (Weston et al. 1993).

Classic teaching has been that etiology can be determined by the child's ability to gain weight in the hospital, with a psychosocial etiology presumed if the child gains weight under these conditions. However, it is important to note that conclusions about likely FTT contributors cannot always be made on the basis of the child's ability to gain weight in the hospital. For example, some FTT children who have an inadequate caregiver will still lose weight in the hospital simply because they are separated from the caregiver. Former FTT children have been found to be smaller, less cognitively able, and more behaviorally disturbed than those children without a history of FTT, especially if their mothers are poorly educated (Drewett et al. 1999; Dykman et al. 2001).

The goal of treatment is to provide the medical, psychiatric, social, and environmental resources needed to promote satisfactory growth. Psychosocial treatment interventions need to be targeted at the likely contributors. Children with feeding skills deficits or maladaptive behavior related to food are likely to benefit from behavioral interventions. Primary caregivers with a history of abuse or with current psychopathology might require specific psychiatric assessment and treatment. Interventions targeting the child–parent relationship, sometimes including in-home intervention, might be effective for selected families (Black et al. 1995; Steward 2001). Interventions targeting the social-economic burdens of the family can be critical. In some cases of inadequate parenting, foster care is required while the parent receives needed parent training and psychiatric care. In such cases, the return to home should be closely monitored and based on the parents' demonstrated ability and resources to care adequately for their child.

Pica

Pica is defined as eating nonnutritious substances on a regular basis over a period of at least 1 month (Wren and Tarbell 1998). It is most frequently found in children with mental retardation or a pervasive developmental disorder. Pica also has a high prevalence in children with sickle cell disease, with preliminary studies suggesting that more than 30% are affected (Bond et al. 1994; Ivascu et al. 2001). Mouthing and occasional eating of nonnutritious substances are considered normal in children younger than 3 years. Young children with pica are most likely to eat sand, bugs, paint, plaster, paper, or other items within reach. Adolescents are more likely to eat clay, soil, paper, or similar substances. Pica can be a conditioned behavior, an indication of distress or environmental neglect, or evidence of a vitamin or mineral deficiency. One study (Singhi et al. 1981) in children with iron deficiency anemia (50 with pica and 50 without pica, individually matched for age, sex, socioeconomic class, and degree of anemia) found that stress factors significantly associated with pica included maternal deprivation, caregiver other than the mother, parental separation, parental neglect, joint family, child beating, and too little parent–child interaction (mother or father). Medical assessment includes screening for ingestion of toxic substances and evaluation for possible nutritional deficits. An evaluation and treatment plan to reduce psychosocial stress are also clearly important. Behavioral interventions have been shown to be effective in targeting the pica behavior, including food-versus-nonfood discrimination training, response interruption and positive practice overcorrection, habit reversal, and brief-duration physical restraint (Fisher et al. 1994; Johnson et al. 1994; Paniagua et al. 1986; Winton and Singh 1983; Woods et al. 1996). Psychiatric medications are not generally used to treat pica unless it is comorbid with another psychiatric disorder.

Rumination

Rumination syndrome is the effortless regurgitation into the mouth of recently ingested food followed by rechewing and reswallowing or expulsion (Clouse et al. 1999; Malcolm et al. 1997). Associated behavioral signs can include aversive posturing or gaze avoidance (C. Berkowitz 1999). Rumination can be conditioned after an illness, a sign of general distress, or a form of self-stimulation or self-soothing that appears to be associated with pleasure. It is most commonly seen in infants and the developmentally disabled but also occurs in children and adolescents with normal intelligence (O'Brien et al. 1995; Soykan et al. 1997).

Patients with rumination syndrome can be misdiagnosed as having bulimia nervosa, gastroesophageal reflux disease, or upper gastrointestinal motility disorders (such as gastroparesis or chronic intestinal pseudo-obstruction). They might undergo extensive, costly, and invasive medical testing before diagnosis. Complications can include weight loss, fatal malnutrition, dental erosions, halitosis, dehydration, school absenteeism, hospitalizations, and iatrogenic problems from the extensive diagnostic testing (O'Brien et al. 1995).

Rumination syndrome is a clinical diagnosis based on symptoms and the absence of structural disease. However, the Rome II diagnostic groups (defining diagnostic criteria for functional gastrointestinal disorders) include only "infant rumination syndrome," and criteria for older children have not been defined (Rasquin-Weber et al. 1999). Evaluation for gastroesophageal reflux disease is warranted if the rumination is accompanied by apnea, reactive airway disease, hematemesis, or food refusal.

In cases of rumination because of environmental neglect, the primary caregiver–child relationship and possible psychiatric disturbance in the primary caregiver should be evaluated and addressed. Operant behavioral methods can be used for conditioned rumination. Postmeal chewing gum has been used successfully to treat rumination in adolescents (Weakley et al. 1997). Habit reversal using diaphragmatic breathing as the competing response also can be effective in older children and adolescents (Chial et al. 2003; Kerwin 1999; Wagaman et al. 1998). Rumination in the presence of other psychosocial problems or psychiatric disorders in the child or primary caregiver may require additional therapeutic interventions. Later experiences of stress, loss, or isolation can trigger a relapse, requiring the reinstitution of the previously effective intervention (C. Berkowitz 1999).

Autism Spectrum Disorders

Given the prevalence of and comorbidities associated with autistic spectrum disorders, along with the additional coping challenges faced by children with autistic spectrum disorders, one would expect to regularly encounter pediatric inpatients with autistic spectrum disorders or autistic spectrum disorder traits. Autistic spectrum disorders such as autism or Asperger's disorder are neurodevelopmental disorders characterized by impairment in communication (verbal and/or nonverbal) and social interactions. Autistic spectrum disorders occur in all racial, ethnic, and socioeconomic groups but are four times more likely to occur in males than in females. In 2006, the Centers for Disease Control and Prevention (CDC) reported that among 8-year-old children in the United States, about 1 in 110 has an autistic spectrum disorder (Centers for Disease Control and Prevention 2009). Autistic spectrum disorders occur more often than expected among those who have fragile X syndrome, tuberous sclerosis, congenital rubella syndrome, and untreated phenylketonuria, as well as among those who were prenatally exposed to thalidomide.

A study published by the CDC in 2003 found that 62% of the children with an autistic spectrum disorder had at least one additional disability (most commonly, mental retardation) or epilepsy (Centers for Disease Control and Prevention 2007). Associated features of autistic spectrum disorders place affected individuals at higher risk for injuries, functional somatic disorders, and other medical problems. Associated features include hyperactivity, short attention span, impulsivity, aggressiveness, self-injury, temper tantrums, perseverative interests, unusual sensory responses, abnormal eating and/or sleeping habits, and seemingly unusual emotional reactions. Common medical presentations might, therefore, include seizures, weight loss or gain, nausea, vomiting, constipation, diarrhea (due to unusual eating habits, abnormal sensory signaling, or underlying gastrointestinal problems), injuries (due to self-injurious behavior, sensory signaling problems, physical altercations, lack of fear, inattentiveness, or clumsiness), pain or other sensory abnormalities, and addictions. Additional reasons for psychiatric consultation might include requests for evaluation and recommendations regarding difficulty coping with hospitalization or illness, nonadherence, capacity to refuse treatment, or pretransplant evaluations.

Individuals with autistic spectrum disorders may have great difficulty identifying and then explaining a symptom or telling the physician what they think is wrong with them. This sometimes requires the clinician to rely more heavily on objective data for diagnosis and monitoring (Smith 2009). Some individuals with autistic spectrum disorders cannot readily identify faces of individuals, potentially making it quite difficult to remember the various medical staff members providing care. Questions asked by clinicians can be difficult to answer if one is interpreting questions literally, if part of the question is implied nonverbally, or if questions are not precise enough (Smith 2007).

If patients have not yet received a diagnosis, it can be extremely helpful to children with autistic spectrum disorders and their parents to learn of their diagnosis and to be educated about the children's specific strengths, weaknesses, and needs. Hospitalized children with autistic spectrum disorders often benefit from being carefully prepared for procedures and daily routines, giving them time to adjust to unexpected changes, minimizing the number of staff involved with their care, and carefully managing distressing sensory stimuli. Extra effort may be required to communicate with a child with an autistic spectrum disorder and to learn how a specific child senses pain or other symptoms. Resources are now being developed for use by parents and medical staff to assist children with autistic spectrum disorders in the medical setting (e.g., see Hudson 2006).

Chronic Somatic Symptoms

Children and adolescents often report persistent physical concerns that are not clearly accounted for by identifiable medical illness (Campo and Fritsch 1994; Garber et al. 1991). In fact, the most common reason for a pediatric psychiatry consultation is for evaluation of unexplained physical symptoms (Simonds 1977; S.J. Tsai et al. 1995). Somatoform disorders can be considered the severe end of a continuum that includes functional somatic symptoms in the middle and minor transient symptoms at the other end (Fritz et al. 1997). Examples of symptoms and disorders on this continuum include atypical migraines, cyclic vomiting, chronic nausea, dizziness, fibromyalgia, chronic fatigue, functional abdominal pain, irritable bowel syndrome, myofascial pain, palpitations, conversion paralysis, and nonepileptic seizures (Heruti et al. 2002; Krilov et al. 1998; Li and Balint 2000; Plioplys et al. 2007; Schanberg et al. 1998; Volkmar et al. 1984). Disabling somatic symptoms can occur in the presence or absence of an identifiable etiology and in the presence or absence of other medical or psychiatric disorders.

Traditionally, disability and symptoms in excess of what would be expected given the amount of tissue pathology have been considered psychogenic. In such circumstances, children and families are sometimes informed by well-meaning clinicians that the symptoms have no physiological basis, with the intended or unintended suggestion that the children are fabricating the symptoms. It is sometimes misleading and confusing to families to dichotomize symptoms as organic or nonorganic because all symptoms are associated with neurosensory changes and influenced by psychosocial factors. Maintaining the organic versus nonorganic dichotomy can lead to unnecessary tests and treatments or to an unhelpful lack of empathy. Consequently, it is helpful to remember, and to communicate to families, that experiences of somatic symptoms are the result of an integration of biological processes, psychological and developmental factors, and social context (Bennett 1999; Li and Balint 2000; Mailis-Gagnon et al. 2003; Peyron et al. 2000; Terre and Ghiselli 1997; Zeltzer et al. 1997).

Psychiatric assessment is geared toward identifying psychiatric symptoms, behavioral reinforcements, and psychosocial stressors that could be exacerbating the symptoms. Common comorbid findings include anxiety disorders, alexithymia, depression, unsuspected learning disorders (in high-achieving children), developmental or communication disorders, social problems, physical or emotional trauma, family illness, and family distress (Bursch and Zeltzer 2002; Campo et al. 1999, 2002; Egger et al. 1998; Fritz et al. 1997; Garber et al. 1990; Hodges et al. 1985a, 1985b; Hyman et al. 2002; Lester et al. 2003; Livingston 1993; Livingston et al. 1995; Schanberg et al. 1998; Stuart and Noyes 1999; Zuckerman et al. 1987).

The family and treatment team often worry about missing a life-threatening problem or a diagnosis that could be remedied within a traditional biomedical model. This fear is particularly strong when the patient has significant distress about the symptoms. The treatment team must believe that a reasonable evaluation has been completed so that they can clearly communicate to the family that no further evaluation is indicated to understand and treat the problem. A rehabilitation approach can improve independent and normal functioning, enhance coping and self-efficacy, and serve to prevent secondary disabilities (Bursch 2010; Campo and Fritz 2001; Heruti et al. 2002). Functioning, rather than symptoms, should be tracked to determine whether progress is being made. As functioning, coping skills, and self-efficacy improve, symptoms and the distress related to the symptoms often remit.

Specific treatment plans target the biological, psychological, and social factors that are exacerbating or maintaining the symptoms and disability. Treatment techniques designed to target underlying sensory signaling mechanisms and specific symptoms can include cognitive-behavioral strategies (e.g., psychotherapy, hypnosis, biofeedback, or meditation), behavioral techniques, family interventions, physical interventions (e.g., massage, yoga, acupuncture, transcutaneous electrical nerve stimulation [TENS], physical therapy, heat and cold therapies, occupational therapy), sleep hygiene, and pharmacological interventions (Bursch 2008; Eccleston et al. 2009; Fritz et al. 1997; Minuchin et al. 1978; Sanders et al. 1989, 1994). In general, interventions that promote active coping are preferred over those that require passive dependency.

Most of the currently used pharmacological strategies are extrapolated from adult trials without evidence of efficacy in children. Classes of medications to consider include TCAs or anticonvulsants for neuropathic pain or irritable bowel syndrome; SSRIs for symptoms of functional abdominal pain, anxiety, or depression; muscle relaxants for myofascial pain; and low-dose antipsychotics (especially those with low potency) for acute anxiety, multiple somatic symptoms with significant distress, and chronic nausea (Bursch 2006; Campo et al. 2004; Garcia-Campayo and Sanz-Carillo 2002; J.E. Muller et al. 2008; T. Muller et al. 2004; Noyes et al. 1998; Saarto and Wiffen 2007; Volz et al. 2000, 2002; Wiffen et al. 2005a, 2005b). Benzodiazepines sometimes elicit paradoxical reactions in those children who are hypervigilant to their bodies and concerned about losing control. Blocks, trigger point injections, epidurals, and other invasive assessments and treatments that further stimulate the CNS can sometimes exacerbate the problem. Evidence-based treatments should be used whenever available.

Specific Medical Disorders

Oncology

In 2007, approximately 10,400 children in the United States younger than 15 years received a diagnosis of cancer (American Cancer Society 2007). Although cancer is the disease most frequently causing death among U.S. children ages 1–14 years, it is rare. Leukemias and brain or CNS cancers are the two most common cancer types among these children. Because of improved treatment approaches, survival rates have improved dramatically since 1975. However, many children do experience both short- and longer-term treatment side effects.

Psychological Short-Term Effects

Pediatric cancers present several challenges to patients and their families. Despite the numerous stressors, pediatric oncology patients report relatively few depressive symptoms during the time of active treatment. Children with cancer report fewer symptoms of depression than do healthy schoolchildren or children with asthma, and self-esteem concerns and somatic symptoms do not differentiate between depressed and nondepressed children with cancer (Gizynski and Shapiro 1990; Worchel et al. 1988). In fact, pediatric cancer patients report so few symptoms that clinical researchers have hypothesized that these children use an avoidant coping style to deal with their emotional response to cancer (Phipps and Srivastava 1997, 1999) or that their emotional response is shaped by traumatic avoidance (Erickson and Steiner 2000). Interventions that address the contextual issues that are precipitating distress are generally sufficient for the depressive symptoms seen during active treatment (Kazak et al. 2002).

Interventions for Invasive Procedures

One area of intervention that has been extensively researched is preparation for the many invasive procedures children experience during cancer treatment. Cognitive-behavioral techniques, including imagery, relaxation, distraction, modeling, desensitization, and positive reinforcement, are well established as effective (Powers 1999; Uman et al. 2008). This is consistent with the literature that suggests that depressive attributional style and avoidance coping are major predictors of anxiety and depression in pediatric oncology patients (Frank et al. 1997). Although all children have some distress with painful procedures, some appear to be more sensitive to pain and have differential responses to psychological interventions for procedural distress (Chen et al. 2000). In cases of children with severe distress, integration of pharmacological interventions has proven useful (Jay et al. 1991; Kazak et al. 1998). Topical anesthetic cream has been used with some success to alleviate the pain of venipuncture or the topical pain of other invasive procedures with pediatric oncology patients (Robieux et al. 1990). In comparisons of conscious sedation and general anesthesia for lumbar punctures, the outcomes were similar, and the conscious sedation was generally preferred and less expensive. However, for some children, the procedure could only be performed under general anesthesia because they were too distressed to cooperate (Ljungman et al. 2001). For conscious sedation, the amnestic effect of midazolam, as well as the ability to administer it nasally, rectally, or orally, has made it popular with anesthesiologists and intensivists. In a double-blind study, midazolam was shown to significantly reduce children's procedural anxiety, discomfort, and pain (Ljungman et al. 2000). For brief general anesthesia, a combination of midazolam and ketamine has been found effective (Parker et al. 1997). Interventions designed to enhance communication with youths with cancer have been developed but not rigorously assessed. Preliminary evidence suggests that some youths with cancer may benefit from informational interventions, support related to procedures, and interventions to facilitate reintegration into school and social activities (Ranmal et al. 2008).

Psychological Late Effects

With increasing survival of childhood cancer patients, the long-term effect of cancer has become a major focus of psycho-oncology research over the past 20 years. Here again, depression does not seem to be a problem (Zebrack et al. 2002). However, a rapidly growing area is investigations of PTSD. A study of 309 childhood cancer survivors (ages 8–20), an average of almost 6 years after cancer treatment, found similar rates of PTSD symptoms in the cancer and comparison groups (219 healthy children) (Kazak et al. 1997). However, in a study of 78 young adult (ages 18–37) survivors of childhood cancer, approximately 20% of the young adult survivors reported symptoms meeting diagnostic criteria for PTSD (Hobbie et al. 2000). Furthermore, PTSD in the young adults appeared predictive of adverse consequences. The young adult survivors who met criteria for PTSD were less likely to be married (none, compared with 23% of the non-PTSD group) and reported more psychological distress and poorer quality of life across all domains. The greatest differences reported were in social functioning, emotional well-being, and role limitations caused by emotional health and pain. Survivors without PTSD did not differ from population norms (Meeske and Stuber 2001). These findings indicate a need to prevent and intervene with children during the time of acute treatment, to prevent long-term consequences in much the same way that medical treatments are being adapted in light of the late effects of radiation and chemotherapy. Meta-analysis of survivors of childhood acute lymphoblastic leukemia treated solely with chemotherapy (no radiation) has identified neurocognitive sequelae, including deficits in intelligence and academic achievement, processing speed, verbal memory, executive functioning, and fine motor skills (Peterson et al. 2008). Visual-motor skills and visual memory appear to remain intact (Peterson et al. 2008).

Effect on Parents

Parents report significant distress and conflict both during and after their children's cancer treatment (Best et al. 2002; Pai et al. 2007). Although they do not appear to affect child outcomes, psychological interventions have been shown to decrease distress and improve adjustment among parents of youths with cancer (Pai et al. 2006). Specific problem-solving therapy has been found to be effective in helping mothers deal with the stresses of a child's treatment (Sahler et al. 2002), as have brief stress reduction techniques (Streisand et al. 2001). Rates of PTSD in parents of children off treatment appear comparable to those in adult cancer survivors (Manne et al. 1998). In a large study of pediatric cancer survivors' parents, 3% of the survivors' mothers reported severe, and 18.2% reported moderate, symptoms of PTSD, whereas 7% of the survivors' fathers reported severe, and 28.3% reported moderate, PTSD symptoms (Kazak et al. 1997).

Cystic Fibrosis

Cystic fibrosis (CF) affects approximately 30,000 children and adults in the United States and is the most common hereditary disease in white children. A defective gene causes the body to produce a thick, sticky mucus that clogs the lungs and leads to life-threatening lung infections. These secretions also obstruct the pancreas, preventing digestive enzymes from reaching the intestines. CF occurs in approximately 1 of every 3,200 live Caucasian births, with about 1,000 new cases diagnosed each year. More than 80% of patients are diagnosed by the age of 3 years; however, almost 10% are diagnosed at age 18 years or older. The median age of survival is 33.4 years, and nearly 40% of those with CF are adults.

People with CF have a variety of symptoms that vary from person to person but include very salty-tasting skin; persistent coughing; wheezing or shortness of breath; an excessive appetite but poor weight gain; and greasy, bulky stools. Malnutrition can lead to poor growth, delayed puberty, impaired respiratory function, reduced exercise tolerance, and increased risk of infection. CF patients with end-stage pulmonary disease show marked nutritional failure. Evidence shows that improving nutritional status may halt the decline in pulmonary function (Dalzell et al.

1992). Progressive respiratory failure is the most common cause of death.

The treatment of CF depends on the stage of the disease and the organs involved. Clearing mucus from the lungs is part of the daily CF treatment regimen; this entails vigorous clapping on the back and chest to dislodge the mucus from the lungs. Strict adherence to this important treatment has been measured to be only about 40% (Passero et al. 1981). Other types of treatments include antibiotics to treat lung infections and mucus-thinning drugs. A high-energy diet (a high-fat diet with significant amounts of carbohydrate and protein) aiming at 120% of the recommended daily intake for age has been linked to superior nutritional status. However, research has found that dietary adherence is poor, with up to 84% of CF children not reaching dietary goals. Both adherence and health status in children with CF are partially predicted by parental psychosocial variables, including knowledge specific to CF (Anthony et al. 1999; Patterson et al. 1993). More and more individuals with CF have received gene therapy or a lung, liver, and/or bowel transplant.

Many people with CF lead remarkably normal lives and maintain hope with the possibilities of gene therapy and organ transplantation in case of severe deterioration. Although early research suggested that eating disorders may be more prevalent in those with CF, recent work has suggested that this is not true. Similarly, rates of other psychiatric disorders among those with CF do not appear to be greater than the prevalence reported in the general population (Kashani et al. 1988a; Raymond et al. 2000). One study of health values in adolescents with CF found that they are willing to trade very little of their life expectancy or take more than a small risk of death to obtain perfect health (Yi et al. 2003). Although little research has been done on this topic, there are no apparent contraindications to standard assessment and treatment approaches for psychiatric disorders in those with CF. Currently, no clear evidence exists regarding the best psychological interventions to help those with CF and their families manage the disease (Glasscoe and Quittner 2008). Some data suggest that family interventions can be successfully used to improve maternal mental health and treatment adherence among those at high risk (Goldbeck and Babka 2001; Ireys et al. 2001).

Asthma

Asthma is the most common serious pediatric chronic illness, frequently responsible for missed school days and hospitalizations (American Lung Association 2010). Both prevalence and morbidity are rising, despite better pharmacological treatments. Comorbid psychiatric problems and increased levels of stress are cited as possible factors for the increases (Wamboldt and Gavin 1998). Comorbid psychiatric disorders may reduce asthma treatment compliance, impair daily functioning, or have a direct effect on autonomic reactions and pulmonary function (Norrish et al. 1977). The literature contains some contradictory findings about the prevalence and type of comorbid psychiatric problems, but it appears that internalizing disorders are more common and that more than one-third of asthmatic children have anxiety disorders. Additionally, those with moderate to severe asthma appear to be at a higher risk for anxiety disorders than those with mild disease. Kean et al. (2006) found that adolescents who have experienced a life-threatening asthma event, and their parents, have high levels of posttraumatic stress symptoms, with 20% and 29% meeting DSM criteria for PTSD, respectively. Although depression has been less consistently identified as a comorbid psychiatric disorder among pediatric asthma patients, the literature suggests that depression, along with other psychosocial problems, may be a risk factor for death in children with asthma. Consequently, the presence of depression in a child with uncontrolled or severe asthma requires serious attention (Bussing et al. 1996; Butz and Alexander 1993; Graham et al. 1967; Kashani et al. 1988b; MacLean et al. 1988; McNichol et al. 1973; Mrazek et al. 1985; Steinhausen et al. 1983; Strunk et al. 1985; Vila et al. 1999).

Twin studies suggest that there may be a genetic relation between atopic disorders and internalizing disorders (Wamboldt et al. 1998). One possible explanation is that panic anxiety acts as an asphyxia alarm system that is triggered by central chemoreceptors monitoring partial pressure of carbon dioxide in the blood ($PaCO_2$). Children with a genetic vulnerability for panic disorder who also have periodic increased $PaCO_2$ from asthma exacerbations thus may have panic anxiety triggered by their asthma attacks. Left undiagnosed and untreated, this anxiety can develop into panic disorder. Indeed, recent prospective epidemiological studies indicate that the primary risk factor for development of panic disorder in young adulthood is history of asthma as a child (Goodwin et al. 2003). Other reasons for increased comorbidity include the fact that most asthma medications (e.g., steroids and beta-agonists) are known to cause symptoms that appear psychiatric in nature. An inflammatory allergic response may release cytokines and other mediators that cause fatigue, trouble concentrating, and irritability that could also be interpreted as depression. The physiological response accompanying strong emotions can trigger wheezing in some patients. Recent research indicates not only that stress can lead to increased asthma exacerbations but also that those children with atopic illnesses have a reduced cortisol response to stress (Wamboldt et al. 2003). Stressors thus may have a direct effect on increased inflammation, leading to asthma symptoms or an increase in upper respiratory infections, which also exacerbate asthma. Depression and anxiety may indirectly influence asthma because distressed asthmatic patients tend to misperceive anxiety symptoms as asthma symptoms, often leading to unnecessary medication use.

Clinicians seeing children with asthma should assess for 1) psychosocial disruption and psychiatric symptoms, especially symptoms of anxiety and depression (including medical trauma); 2) the likelihood of nonadherence; 3) the ability to perceive symptoms; and 4) the presence of vocal cord dysfunction (see following subsection). Asthma can increase family burden, and having depressed primary caregivers increases the risk of poorer treatment adherence. New electronic monitoring of adherence with inhaled medications helps determine how much nonadherence is undermining outcome. Having patients guess their peak flow or rate their symptoms before spirometry or after a methacholine challenge is one way to assess whether these patients are accurate perceivers. Patients who have difficulty with symptom perception (either under- or overperceiving symptoms) can be trained to use objective assessment methods, such as peak flow meters. Asthma education has been found to be associated with decreases in hospitalizations and emergency department visits, with interactive learning opportunities and more educational sessions leading to a greater effect (Coffman et al. 2008).

Pharmacological and psychological treatments with efficacy to treat anxiety and depression in children are largely applicable to those with asthma. Focused family therapy to improve asthma management skills has been shown to be effective and efficient (Godding et al. 1997; Gustafsson et al. 1986; Lask and Matthew 1979; Panton and Barley 2000). Although some concern has been raised about the concurrent use of TCAs with medicines used in treating asthma, they appear to be safe, and the anticholinergic effects can sometimes be helpful (Wamboldt et al. 1997). Beta-receptor agonists are often used to treat asthma, which makes beta-blockers potentially dangerous. There is no contraindication to use of antipsychotics, and they may be particularly indicated for steroid-induced psychosis. Lithium increases theophylline clearance, requiring that levels of both drugs be monitored (Wamboldt and Gavin 1998). Some children with asthma have difficulty tolerating stimulants. Bupropion has shown efficacy in the treatment of attention-deficit/hyperactivity disorder in young patients in controlled trials (Barrickman et al. 1995; Conners et al. 1996) and does not interact with asthma medications.

Vocal Cord Dysfunction

Vocal cord dysfunction can mimic asthma and commonly occurs comorbidly with asthma. It is a condition of involuntary paradoxical adduction of the vocal cords during the inspiratory phase of the respiratory cycle (Wamboldt and Gavin 1998). It is often associated with anxiety or chronic stress; however, sexual abuse in this population is not as prevalent as previously believed (Brugman et al. 1994; Gavin et al. 1998). Patients with vocal cord dysfunction frequently present with stridulous breathing, experience tightness in their throats, and feel short of breath. It can be quite anxiety provoking that their symptoms are unrelieved by asthma medications. Clinicians can assess for vocal cord dysfunction by asking patients where they feel short of breath and if they have throat tightness. A flow volume loop can be helpful in showing vocal cord dysfunction, especially on the inspiratory part of the loop. Definitive diagnosis of vocal cord dysfunction is made by visualization of adducted cords during an acute episode via laryngoscopy. Provocation of symptoms during laryngoscopy has been achieved with methacholine, histamine, or exercise challenges. The primary treatment for vocal cord dysfunction is speech therapy or hypnotherapy geared toward increasing awareness and control of breathing and throat muscles (Wamboldt and Gavin 1998).

Childhood Obesity

Genetic factors may account for as much as 70% of the variability in human body weight (Allison et al. 1996; Stunkard et al. 1990). Nevertheless, there has been a disturbing increase during the past 20 years in the prevalence of obesity in children and adolescents in the United States. Children and adolescents are considered obese if they have a body mass index (BMI) of greater than or equal to the 95th percentile for age and sex, and they are considered overweight if their BMI is between the 85th and the 95th percentile (Dietz and Bellizzi 1999). Data from the third National Health and Nutrition Examination Survey, conducted from 1988 to 1994, indicated that approximately 11% of U.S. children were obese. An analysis of 1999–2002 data estimated childhood obesity prevalence at 16% (Hedley et al. 2004). These findings can be compared with the 5% obesity reported in a similar study conducted between 1976 and 1980 (Troiano et al. 1995). This dramatic increase in obesity has been attributed to the proliferation of inexpensive, calorie-rich foods that are quickly and readily available in the United States and the increased number of hours children spend in sedentary activities, such as watching television and playing computer games (Ebbeling et al. 2002). Similar increases in childhood obesity have been documented in Europe and Asia (Chinn and Rona 2001; Chunming 2000) and in developing societies (de Onis and Blossner 2000).

The effect of obesity is both immediate and long-lasting. Children and adolescents with a BMI at or above the 95th percentile for age and sex have been found to have significantly reduced health-related quality of life compared with healthy children and adolescents. In a study of 106 children, ages 5–18 years, the obese subjects were more than five times more likely to have significant impairment of physical functioning and almost six times as likely to have impaired psychosocial health. These findings are similar to those for children with cancer (Schwimmer et al. 2003). A survey of approximately 10,000 women, ages 16–24 years, found that obese adolescents were less likely to complete college than were nonoverweight adolescents with similar educational backgrounds. The obese young adults were much less likely to marry than were nonobese young adults, after the investigators controlled for IQ and parents' education or income level. Those obese women who did marry were more often married to men in a lower socioeconomic class (Gortmaker et al. 1993; Stunkard and Sabal 1995).

The immediate health consequences of childhood obesity are serious and include slipped capital femoral epiphysis, pseudotumor cerebri, asthma, sleep apnea, gallstones, insulin resistance, early puberty, dyslipidemia, and hypertension (for review, see Morgan et al. 2002). Although obese children are likely to become obese adults (Guo et al. 1994), the long-term health risks also include increased likelihood of atherosclerotic cardiovascular disease, gout, and colorectal cancer in men and arthritis and menstrual abnormalities in women, even after adult body mass is taken into account (Mossberg 1989; Must et al. 1999).

Importantly, research has found that with no treatment, the average overweight child can be expected to continue to gain weight over time (Wilfley et al. 2007). A meta-analysis of 61 trials determined that short-term medications, including sibutramine and orlistat, are effective in reducing BMI among overweight children and adolescents (McGovern et al. 2008). Interventions focused on physical activity have a moderate treatment effect on body fat but not BMI (McGovern et al. 2008). Short-term changes in weight status have been detected with combined lifestyle interventions, with preliminary evidence for a longer-term effect (McGovern et al. 2008; Wilfley et al. 2007). Some evidence suggests that behavioral interventions are more effective than cognitive interventions and that there is benefit in increasing the behavioral intervention "dose" and in including parents in the intervention (Gilles et al. 2008).

Among interventions designed to *prevent* pediatric obesity, small effects were detected on target behaviors but not related to BMI (Kamath et al. 2008). Lengthier interventions and interventions with postintervention outcome measurement fared better (Kamath et al. 2008).

Bariatric surgery is viewed as "a last resort option for severely obese adolescents" (Strauss et al. 2001, p. 503). Nevertheless, the bariatric surgery rate among adolescents (per 100,000 population) in the United States increased from 0.7 in 2000 to 2.3 in 2003 (W.S. Tsai et al. 2007). Meta-analysis of surgical interventions for adolescents identified sustained and clinically significant BMI reductions for both laparoscopic adjustable gastric banding (LAGB) and Roux-en-Y gastric bypass (RYGB), the two most commonly used surgical procedures. In LAGB surgery, a silicone band is placed around the upper portion of the stomach, creating a small pouch where food empties from the esophagus to the upper stomach. RYGB surgery also restricts intake through the creation of a small gastric pouch but includes bypass of the proximal small intestine to reduce food absorption. Complications were reported for both procedures, with more severe complications among the RYGB group (Brolin 2002; Treadwell et al. 2008). Given the likelihood of adolescents to be nonadherent with diet and other instructions, the potential interference with growth, the challenges of obtaining true informed consent from adolescents, and the lack of information on long-term consequences of these procedures, surgical interventions should be reserved for those who have not responded to more conventional interventions and have significant complications of their obesity (Treadwell et al. 2008; Yanovski 2001) (see also Chapter 30, "Surgery").

Sickle Cell Anemia

The sickle cell gene for hemoglobin S is the most common inherited blood condition in the United States, with an estimated 72,000 people affected. Symptoms do not usually appear until late in the first year of life and may include fever; swelling of the hands and feet; pain in the chest, abdomen, limbs, and joints; nosebleeds; and frequent upper respiratory infections. Pain is the most common complaint after infancy, as are the added problems of anemia, fatigue, irritability, and jaundice. Children and adolescents may experience delayed puberty, severe joint pain, progressive anemia, leg sores, gum disease, long-term damage to major organs, stroke, and acute chest syndrome. A compromised spleen can cause increased susceptibility to infections. Current treatments for sickle cell disease are prolonging and improving quality of life. Although most people with sickle cell anemia were not previously expected to survive childhood, most now live into adulthood with about half living beyond 50 years (Platt et al. 1994). Representing an important advance in treatment, preliminary data support the efficacy of hydroxyurea in adolescents to decrease severe painful episodes, hospitalizations, number of blood transfusio4ns, and episodes of acute chest syndrome (Brawley et al. 2008).

Sickle cell crises are acute pain episodes that are usually followed by periods of remission and a relatively normal life. Some patients have few crises, others need to be frequently hospitalized, and some have clusters of severe attacks with long intermittent remissions. Crises become less frequent with age for some. The risk for a crisis is increased by anything that boosts the body's oxygen requirement (including illness, physical stress, or being at high altitudes). The first day of the crisis is usually the worst, with sharp, intense, and throbbing pain in the arms, legs, and back. Shortness of breath, bone pain, and abdominal pain are also common. The liver can become enlarged, causing pain, nausea, low-grade fever, and jaundice. Males may experience priapism. Acute chest syndrome can be life threatening.

Stroke is a common cause of death for sickle cell patients older than 3 years (Kinney et al. 1999; Ohene-Frempong 1991; Ohene-Frempong et al. 1998). Although transfusions may be preventive, 8%–11% of those affected experience strokes. One study comparing sickle cell children with and without a history of stroke found relative deficits on measures of attention and executive functioning. Rodgers et al. (1984) provided positron emission tomography evidence of altered frontal lobe metabolism. Another study examined social information processing, social skills, and adjustment difficulties in children with sickle cell disease and learning and behavior problems, with or without CNS pathology on MRI. Children with CNS pathology had more errors on tasks of facial and vocal emotional decoding than did the control children (Boni et al. 2001). Some cognitive rehabilitation intervention development progress has been made to address cognitive deficits among children with sickle cell disease who have had a stroke (King et al. 2008).

Although children and adolescents with sickle cell disease do not appear to have a greater risk for psychiatric disorders than those in the same-race outpatient clinic control group, children attending outpatient medical clinics are at a higher risk for mental disorders than are nonmedical populations (Cepeda et al. 1997; Yang et al. 1994). Most well-designed studies report a prevalence rate of 25%–30% for psychiatric disorders among pediatric sickle cell patients, with internalizing disorders being most prevalent (Cepeda et al. 1997), similar to other pediatric outpatients (Costello and Shugart 1992; Costello et al. 1988). Psychosocial factors have accounted for more variability than biomedical ones in both depressive symptoms and anxiety, with social assertion, self-esteem, use of social support, and family factors accounting for a significant amount of the variability in adaptation (Burlew et al. 2000; Telfair 1994). Two studies suggest that pica (not often assessed) has a relatively high prevalence (up to 30%) in children with sickle cell disease (Bond et al. 1994; Ivascu et al. 2001).

Psychiatric assessment should look for 1) psychosocial disruption or psychiatric symptoms, especially related to pica, anxiety, and depression; 2) school or social problems that could reflect subtle neurocognitive problems; and 3) chronic pain problems. Pharmacological and psychological treatments with efficacy to treat psychiatric disorders in children are applicable to those with sickle cell anemia. Problems with academic or social functioning might be assessed via neurocognitive testing and addressed within the school system with an Individualized Educational Program (IEP). Pain in sickle cell patients is most commonly medically managed pharmacologically with nonsteroidal anti-inflammatory drugs (NSAIDs), opioids, and adjuvant medications (American Pain Society 1999). Chronic and acute pediatric pain also can be reduced with behavioral, psychological, or physical interventions (American Pain Society 1999). Behavioral interventions might include relaxation, deep breathing, biofeedback, behavioral modification, or exercise. Psychological interventions might include cognitive therapies, hypnotherapy, imagery, distraction, or social support. Physical interventions might include hydration, heat, massage, hydrotherapy, ultrasound, acupuncture, TENS, or physical therapy. Successful treatment of anxiety symptoms can reduce pain and pain-related distress. Although there are no contraindications for the use of psychotropic medications with this population, phenothiazines, TCAs, monoamine oxidase inhibitors, and other CNS depressants may potentiate adverse effects of opioids. It is important to note, however, that these agents also may serve to augment pain control efforts successfully and should be considered if needed. (See also Chapter 24, "Hematology.")

Renal Disease

Each year 20,000 children are born with kidney abnormalities, and 4,500 children require dialysis for renal failure. Hemodialysis (at a center or at home) and peritoneal dialysis are used in children. The basic principles of treatment of end-stage renal disease (ESRD) are similar in adults and children (see Chapter 21, "Renal Disease"). However, attention to dialysis adequacy, control of osteodystrophy, nutrition, and correction of anemia are crucial because these factors can influence growth, cognitive development, and school performance (Warady et al. 1999).

Pediatric patients with chronic renal failure have more problems in psychiatric adjustment than do healthy children, with a trend toward more psychological difficulties in those with higher illness severity (Garralda et al. 1988). However, even less severely physically ill children appear to have increased difficulties in school adjustment and feelings of loneliness (Garralda et al. 1988). Separation anxiety disorder in particular may be a relatively common disorder (up to 65.4%) among children receiving continuous ambulatory peritoneal dialysis (Fukunishi and Kudo 1995). This may be due to the forced dependence on parents for daily renal care. The burden for families caring for children with ESRD can be significant, especially when it involves dialysis. Disruption of family life, marital strain, and a tendency for more mental health problems in the parents also appear to be related to the severity of the child's renal illness and its associated care burdens (Reynolds et al. 1988). Children with ESRD (with or without transplant) have been shown to have lower-than-expected IQs and achievement scores. Lower achievement test scores were predicted by younger age at the time of renal disease diagnosis, increased time on dialysis, and caregiver's lower achievement (Brouhard et al. 2000; Fennell et al. 1984; Qvist et al. 2002). Overall, former pediatric ESRD adults appear to have a long-term favorable adjustment, with lower self-esteem related to early onset of the disease and to educational and social dysfunction (Morton et al. 1994).

According to the latest statistics (April 26, 2010) from the United Network for Organ Sharing (UNOS), 804 children were waiting for a kidney transplant in the United States, including 2 younger than 1 year, 150 in the 1- to 5-year-old age group, 142 in the 6- to 10-year-old group, and 508 in the 11- to 17-year-old group. Most transplanted kidneys come from cadavers. However, family members or unrelated individuals who are a good match may be able to donate one of their kidneys and live healthy lives with the kidney that remains. Pediatric kidney transplantation is associated with improved physical health, emotional health, and family functioning; however, poor peer relationships, school maladjustment, and other adjustment problems (as well as adherence problems) can remain after transplant (Fukunishi and Kudo 1995; Reynolds et al. 1991). Living with a transplant is a lifelong process requiring daily medications and monitoring for rejection. Medication nonadherence rates for pediatric renal transplant patients can be as high as 64% (Ettenger et al. 1991). Adverse consequences of nonadherence include medical complications and hospitalizations, higher health care costs and family stress, and increased risks for loss of the organ (Arbus et al. 1993; Bittar et al. 1992; Fukunishi and Honda 1995; Salvatierra et al. 1997; Swanson et al. 1992).

Those conducting mental health evaluations of children with renal disease should consider the effect of possible cognitive deficits, adaptation difficulties, and family strain on social and academic functioning, as well as adherence. The level of family stress and distress, as with all pediatric patients, is essential to evaluate and address as part of a larger treatment approach. Recommendations related to the use of psychotropic medication must be extrapolated from adult studies (see Chapter 21, "Renal Disease") because these data are not available for children.

Diabetes

Juvenile-onset diabetes mellitus affects 1.7 of every 1,000 school-age children in the United States (Centers for Disease Control and Prevention 2010). Type 1 diabetes mellitus is caused by autoimmune destruction of insulin-producing pancreatic beta cells and must be treated with exogenous insulin. Type 2 diabetes mellitus is the result of resistance to insulin rather than deficiency, can often be treated with diet or hypoglycemic agents, and is generally later in onset than type 1. There are genetic predispositions to both type 1 and type 2 diabetes mellitus (Drash 1993). Obesity and atypical antipsychotic medications appear to contribute to the development of type 2. Both can contribute to mortality and may cause significant morbidity, including retinopathy, nephropathy, peripheral neuropathy, and cardiovascular disease. Injected insulin also may precipitate potentially life-threatening episodes of hypoglycemia (DCCT Research Group 1993, 1994). A meta-analysis conducted by Gaudieri et al. (2008) with 1,393 children with type 1 diabetes and 751 control children determined that type 1 diabetes was associated with slightly lower overall cognitive abilities across a range of domains. Overall, learning and memory were similar for both groups. However, increased impairment was evident among those with early-onset disease. Verbal and visual learning and memory skills, along with attention and executive functioning skills, were more impaired among children with early-onset diabetes compared with those with late-onset diabetes.

The complexity of the management of type 1 diabetes mellitus leads to frequent problems with adherence to medical instructions. Patients on Humalog (or regular) and NPH (neutral protamine Hagedorn) regimens must inject themselves with insulin and test their blood glucose levels at least three times a day to maintain "tight" control, decreasing the incidence or delaying the onset of complications. Patients on Lantus must take an injection every day and another every time they eat more than 15 grams of carbohydrates (e.g., an apple). Even with an insulin pump, blood glucose must be tested at least four times a day. Diet and exercise must be regulated because both have significant effect on the need for exogenous insulin.

The physiological changes of puberty can lead to increased insulin resistance. In addition, the importance of peer acceptance and the withdrawal of parental supervision with the normal developmental focus on identity and autonomy lead to significant adherence problems during adolescence (Hauser et al. 1990). Poor control of diabetes has been repeatedly confirmed with HbA_{1c} (glycosylated hemoglobin), which allows one to get an estimate of glycemic control over the past 3 months. The medical consequences of such poor control were documented in a study of 78 adolescents with type 1 diabetes, ages 11–18 years, followed up for 8 years. Their mean HbA_{1c} peaked in late adolescence. Serious diabetic complications were seen in 38% of the females and 25% of the males (Bryden et al. 2001).

Psychiatric comorbidity in diabetic individuals is also a major issue for psychiatric consultants to pediatrics. Some moodiness and feelings of isolation and of loss or grief, as well as mild anxiety about the future, are to be expected as normal responses to diabetes. However, assessment for possible intervention is indicated if patients have aggression, school absences, hopelessness, or nonadherence to the insulin regimen (Jacobson 1996). In a study of 92 pediatric patients, ages 8–13 years, followed up over 9 years, 42% developed at least one psychiatric disorder, and 26% developed two or more disorders. Of these, the most common were depression in 26% and anxiety in 20%, with various behavior disorders in 16%. Children who were at higher risk for developing psychiatric comorbidity were those in the first year after diagnosis and those with preexisting anxiety or mothers with psychopathology (Kovacs et al. 1997). Eating disorders are also relatively common. A study of 91 adolescent girls, ages 12–18 years, followed up for 5 years found highly or moderately disordered eating in 29% at baseline and in 33% at follow-up (Rydall et al. 1997).

Treatment of comorbid psychiatric disorders with medications requires careful monitoring because most antidepressant, mood stabilizer, and atypical antipsychotic medications may stimulate appetite or affect glucose tolerance, inducing hypoglycemia or hyperglycemia. Beta-blockers should be avoided because they mask the early warning signs of hypoglycemia, eliminating the window of opportunity for patients to address the problem themselves before requiring the assistance of others (Goodnick et al. 1995).

Effective behavioral interventions for children with diabetes and their parents include identifying readiness for change and improving self-efficacy, the belief that one can maintain behavior change despite regular challenges (Anderson et al. 1996, 1999). In 110 young adults (ages 18–35 years) with type 1 diabetes mellitus, self-efficacy was more predictive of self-care and metabolic control than was self-esteem. After factoring in previous adherence, self-efficacy continues to be predictive of self-care and HbA_{1c} (Johnston-Brooks et al. 2002). A growing area of research is the application of motivational interviewing to improve health self-management among adolescents with diabetes mellitus (Berg-Smith et al. 1999; Dunn et al. 2001; Williams et al. 1998).

Cardiac Disease

Congenital Heart Defects and Disease

Congenital heart defects and disease include patent ductus arteriosus, atrial septal defects, and ventricular septal defects. About 40,000 children are born with a heart defect each year, and most can benefit from surgery. It appears that heart defects are multidetermined by factors that include genetics as well as exposure during pregnancy by the mother to certain viruses (such as rubella or German measles) or drugs (such as alcohol, anticonvulsants, or lithium). Acquired heart diseases that develop during childhood include Kawasaki disease, rheumatic fever, and infective endocarditis.

Van Horn et al. (2001) studied concerns expressed by mothers of children with congenital heart disease during hospitalization and again 2–4 weeks after discharge. During hospitalization, mothers were most concerned about medical prognosis. Mothers' concerns, anxiety, and depressed mood decreased after discharge. At follow-up, mothers' perceptions of medical severity were related to distress about psychosocial issues. Overall, it appears that children with heart disease psychiatrically resemble a healthy population without elevations in anxiety, depression, or behavior problems (Connolly et al. 2002; DeMaso et al. 2000; Visconti et al. 2002). However, similar to the case in healthy or other chronically ill children, demographic and socioeconomic factors, medical severity, and family distress appear to be related to symptoms of depression, anxiety, behavior problems, and cognitive effects (Alden et al. 1998; Karsdorp et al. 2007; Visconti et al. 2002; Yildiz et al. 2001). A meta-analysis by Karsdorp et al. (2007) found that older youths with congenital heart disease had a slightly increased risk of externalizing behavior problems and a greater increased risk of internalizing symptoms than did younger children with congenital heart disease. Additionally, they found that youths with severe congenital heart disease had lower cognitive functioning, across age groups, when compared with youths with mild disease. DeMaso et al. (2000) studied pediatric patients with recurrent cardiac arrhythmias who underwent radiofrequency catheter ablation of ectopic myocardial foci. Although these patients resembled a psychiatrically healthy population before the procedure, they experienced reductions in their "fear of their heart problem" and increases in "the things that they enjoy" after the ablation (DeMaso et al. 2000, p. 134). Those who experienced a curative ablation had better functioning than did those who did not experience improvement.

Heart Transplant Recipients

Serrano-Ikkos et al. (1999) compared the psychosocial outcome of pediatric heart and heart-lung transplant recipients with that of children and adolescents who underwent conventional cardiac surgery. Preoperatively, rates of psychiatric disorders (including anxiety and phobic states, depression, and adjustment reaction) were relatively the same in all groups (26%–28.5%). The prevalence of psychiatric disorder was unchanged after transplant in the transplant groups but decreased in the conventional cardiac surgery group. DeMaso et al. (1995) similarly found that most of the pediatric heart transplant patients studied (78.3%) had good psychological functioning after their heart transplantation. It was further noted that patients with psychological difficulties before and after transplantation had more hospitalizations after transplantation. Finally, Uzark et al. (1992) found that pediatric heart transplant recipients did not differ from peers on measures of self-concept and anxiety but showed less social competence and more behavior problems than a normative population. Behavior problems were frequently suggestive of depression and related to greater family stress and diminished family resources for managing stress. Relaxation and imagery techniques have been used successfully for routine endomyocardial biopsies after heart transplantation (Bullock and Shaddy 1993). A review of the literature related to cognition found that children and adolescents generally function normally on measures of cognitive functioning posttransplant, but a complicated transplant course (caused by infections or rejections) may increase risk for cognitive difficulties (Todaro et al. 2000). Serrano-Ikkos et al. (1998) found medication adherence to be relatively high, with 91% adherence confirmed by cyclosporine levels; however, adherence to medical diary keeping was lower, at about 70%. Variables associated with poor adherence to medication were heart-lung as opposed to heart transplantation, one-parent or blended families, and family adjustment.

Chest Pain

Chest pain as a presenting symptom in a previously healthy child is not as ominous a symptom as in an adult because it is rarely a sign of underlying cardiac disease (Driscoll et al. 1976; Tunaoglu et al. 1995). Idiopathic chest pain is the most common diagnosis made, followed by functional pain (associated with anxiety) and musculoskeletal pain (Selbst 1985). Laboratory tests are not typically helpful in establishing the etiology of chest pain. This topic is more fully discussed in the subsection "Chronic Somatic Symptoms" earlier in this chapter.

Psychotropic Medications

The American Heart Association (Gutgesell et al. 1999) has published recommendations for the use of psychotropic medications in children. Briefly, this document concludes that stimulants cause increases in heart rate and blood pressure that are typically considered clinically insignificant. (Although very rare incidences of sudden death have been reported since these guidelines were published, in 2006 the U.S. Food and Drug Administration Pediatric Psychopharmacology Advisory Panel concluded that there is no increased risk for sudden death in healthy patients taking stimulants for attention-deficit/hyperactivity disorder.) TCA treatment in pediatric patients is associated with cardiovascular changes that are likely of minor clinical significance (Wilens et al. 1996). The electrocardiographic effects of TCA administration include an increase in heart rate (by 20%–25%), PR interval (by 5%–10%), QRS duration (by 7%–25%), and QT interval (by 3%–10%). Malignant arrhythmias have not been documented except for the ventricular fibrillation observed in one pediatric patient with a family history of sudden death. To date, deaths in children taking TCAs have not been conclusively linked to the medication and have not been reported to be more frequent than expected in the population base. SSRIs have minimal cardiovascular effects. Clonidine has been associated with two deaths (in patients who also received methylphenidate), but the mechanism for these deaths is unknown and may have been sudden cessation of treatment. Adverse effects have occurred when the P450 system was inhibited, leading to elevated levels of medications that prolong the QT interval and produce ventricular tachycardia. Most notable have been deaths related to nonsedating histamine-blocking agents, now off the market. Other medications that inhibit or are metabolized by the cytochrome P450 system include antidepressants, calcium channel blockers, histamine blockers, gastrointestinal motility agents, and steroids. Antiarrhythmic drugs of class IA and class III prolong the QT interval, and therefore use of psychotropic medications with these drugs is not recommended. In addition to their effect on cardiac conduction, antipsychotic medications have a negative inotropic effect, reducing cardiac output and lowering blood pressure (Fayek et al. 2001).

American Heart Association recommendations include taking a careful history, obtaining an electrocardiogram (ECG) at baseline before TCA or phenothiazine therapy is begun (primarily to detect unsuspected instances of long-QT syndrome) and another when steady state is achieved, careful monitoring of all prescribed medications along with heart rate and blood pressure, and avoiding use of psychotropic medications with medications that are metabolized by or inhibit the P450 enzyme system (Gutgesell et al. 1999). The clinician should obtain a history of syncope, near syncope, or palpitations; family history of deafness (which can be associated with a congenital long-QT syndrome), sudden unexpected cardiac death, syncope, or tachydysrhythmias; and a medication history to document all medications that may have direct or indirect effects on the cytochrome P450 system or ECG intervals. Some cardiologists argue that ECG screening in children with no symptoms of cardiovascular disease is less efficient and helpful than simply asking about patient and family history of syncope or sudden death. However, no data are available to clearly settle this question. The American Academy of Child and Adolescent Psychiatry does not specifically address this issue in its policy statement related to prescribing. Nevertheless, the recommendation to conduct ECG screens was recently reiterated (Francis 2002; Labellarte et al. 2003).

Fetal Alcohol Syndrome and Alcohol-Related Neurological Disorder

Prenatal alcohol exposure represents one of the leading preventable causes of congenital neurological impairment, affecting as many as 1 in 100 children born in the United States yearly (May and Gossage 2001), with severe lifelong consequences for affected individuals. Fetal alcohol syndrome (FAS) is defined by a characteristic pattern of facial anomalies, growth retardation, and CNS dysfunction in one or more of the following areas: decreased cranial size at birth, structural brain abnormalities, and neurological hard or soft signs (Stratton et al. 1996). However, alcohol exposure to the fetus can result in neurocognitive changes even when none of the characteristic facial anomalies are present (Streissguth and O'Malley 2000).

The facial characteristics most frequently described in individuals with FAS include short palpebral fissures and abnormalities in the premaxillary zone, including a thin upper lip and flattened philtrum (Astley and Clarren 2001; Stratton et al. 1996). Neurocognitive changes include structural changes in the brain (Roebuck et al. 1998); verbal learning and memory problems; attention deficits; problems in executive functioning characterized by difficulties in planning, organizing, and sequencing behavior; and problems in abstract and practical reasoning and concept formation (Adnams et al. 2001; McGee et al. 2008), complex nonverbal problem solving (Goodman et al. 1999), flexible thinking (Schonfeld et al. 2001), and behavioral inhibition (Mattson et al. 1999). These changes appear to last into adulthood (Streissguth and O'Malley 2000). Children with FAS have been found to have lower levels of adaptive functioning related to social interaction and communication, personal living skills, and community living skills (Jirikowic et al. 2008). They also rated higher on maladaptive behavior scales (Jirikowic et al. 2008) and had motor delays (Kalberg et al. 2006). Secondary disabilities include high levels of psychiatric illness, school failure, social problems, alcohol and other drug abuse, impulsivity, history of trauma or abuse, delinquency, and trouble with the law, placing them at higher risk for suicidality (Baldwin 2007). No safe level of prenatal alcohol consumption has been established, making abstinence the best policy for those who are hoping to conceive. Because many women are often not aware of when they conceived and may continue to drink alcohol at least until pregnancy recognition, preconception counseling is suggested for all women of childbearing age who consume alcohol.

References

Adnams CM, Kodituwakku PW, Hay A, et al: Patterns of cognitive-motor development in children with fetal alcohol syndrome from a community in South Africa. Alcohol Clin Exp Res 25:557–562, 2001

Ahearn WH, Castine T, Nault K, et al: An assessment of food acceptance in children with autism or pervasive developmental disorder-not otherwise specified. J Autism Dev Disord 31:505–511, 2001

Alden B, Gilljam T, Gillberg C: Long-term psychological outcome of children after surgery for transposition of the great arteries. Acta Paediatr 87:405–410, 1998

Allison DB, Kaprio J, Korkeil M, et al: The heritability of body mass index among an international sample of monozygotic twins reared apart. Int J Obes Relat Metab Disord 20:501–506, 1996

American Cancer Society: Cancer Facts & Figures 2007. Atlanta, GA, American Cancer Society, 2007. Available at: http://www.cancer.org/downloads/STT/CAFF2007PWSecured.pdf. Accessed June 24, 2009.

American Lung Association: Asthma. Washington, DC, American Lung Association, 2010. Available at: http://www.lungusa.org/lung-disease/asthma. Accessed April 28, 2010.

American Pain Society: Guideline for the Management of Acute and Chronic Pain in Sickle-Cell Disease. Glenview, IL, American Pain Society, 1999

Anderson B, Ho J, Brackett J, et al: Parental involvement in diabetes management tasks: relationships to blood glucose monitoring adherence and metabolic control in young adolescents with insulin-dependent diabetes mellitus. J Pediatr 130:257–265, 1996

Anderson BJ, Bracett J, Ho J, et al: An office-based intervention to maintain parent-adolescent teamwork in diabetes management: impact on parent involvement, family conflict, and subsequent glycemic control. Diabetes Care 22:713–721, 1999

Anthony H, Paxton S, Bines J, et al: Psychosocial predictors of adherence to nutritional recommendations and growth outcomes in children with cystic fibrosis. J Psychosom Res 47:623–634, 1999

Arbus GS, Sullivan EK, Tejani A: Hospitalization in children during the first year after kidney transplantation. Kidney Int Suppl 43:83–86, 1993

Astley SJ, Clarren SK: Measuring the facial phenotype of individuals with prenatal alcohol exposure: correlations with brain dysfunction. Alcohol Alcohol 36:147–159, 2001

Ayoub CC: Munchausen by Proxy: Child Placement and Emotional Health. The 14th International Congress for the Prevention of Child Abuse and Neglect, Denver, CO, 2002

Baldwin MR: Fetal alcohol spectrum disorders and suicidality in a healthcare setting. Int J Circumpolar Health 66 (suppl 1): 54–60, 2007

Barrickman LL, Perry PJ, Allen AJ, et al: Bupropion versus methylphenidate in the treatment of attention-deficit hyperactivity disorder. J Am Acad Child Adolesc Psychiatry 34:649–657, 1995

Battles HB, Wiener LS: From adolescence through young adulthood: psychosocial adjustment associated with long-term survival of HIV. J Adolesc Health 30:161–168, 2002

Bauman LJ, Wright E, Leickly FE, et al: Relationship of adherence to pediatric asthma morbidity among inner-city children. Pediatrics 110(1 pt 1):e6, 2002

Behrman RE, Kliegman RM, Jenson HB (eds): Nelson Textbook of Pediatrics, 17th Edition. Philadelphia, PA, WB Saunders, 2004

Bennett RM: Emerging concepts in the neurobiology of chronic pain: evidence of abnormal sensory processing in fibromyalgia. Mayo Clin Proc 74:385–398, 1999

Berg-Smith SM, Stevens VJ, Brown KM, et al: A brief motivational intervention to improve dietary adherence in adolescents. Health Educ Res 14:339–410, 1999

Berkowitz C: Nonorganic failure to thrive and infant rumination syndrome, in Pediatric Functional Bowel Disorders. Edited by Hyman P. New York, Academy of Professional Information Services, 1999, pp 4.1–4.9

Best M, Streisand R, Catania L, et al: Parental distress during pediatric leukemia and parental posttraumatic stress symptoms after treatment ends. J Pediatr Psychol 26:299–307, 2002

Birmaher B, Brent D, AACAP Work Group on Quality Issues: Practice Parameter for the Assessment and Treatment of Children and Adolescents With Depressive Disorders. Washington, DC, American Academy of Child and Adolescent Psychiatry, 2007

Bittar AE, Keitel E, Garcia CD, et al: Patient noncompliance as a cause of late renal graft failure. Transplant Proc 24:2720–2721, 1992

Black MM, Dubowitz H, Hutcheson J, et al: A randomized clinical trial of home intervention for children with failure to thrive. Pediatrics 95:807–814, 1995

Bond S, Conner-Warren R, Sarnaik SA: Prevalence of pica in children with sickle cell disease. Paper presented at the 19th annual meeting of the National Sickle Cell Disease Program, New York, March 25, 1994

Boni LC, Brown RT, Davis PC, et al: Social information processing and magnetic resonance imaging in children with sickle cell disease. J Pediatr Psychol 26:309–319, 2001

Bools CN, Neale BA, Meadow SR: Follow up of victims of fabricated illness (Munchausen syndrome by proxy). Arch Dis Child 69:625–630, 1993

Borowsky IW, Mozayeny S, Ireland M: Brief psychosocial screening at health supervision and acute care visits. Pediatrics 112 (1 pt 1):129–133, 2003

Brawley OW, Cornelius LJ, Edwards LR, et al: National Institutes of Health Consensus Development Conference statement: hydroxyurea treatment for sickle cell disease. Ann Intern Med 148:932–938, 2008

Breitbart W, Marotta R, Platt MM, et al: A double-blind trial of haloperidol, chlorpromazine, and lorazepam in the treatment of delirium in hospitalized AIDS patients. Am J Psychiatry 153:231–237, 1996

Bridge JA, Iyengar S, Salary CB, et al: Clinical response and risk for reported suicidal ideation and suicide attempts in pediatric antidepressant treatment: a meta-analysis of randomized controlled trials. JAMA 297:1683–1696, 2007

Brolin RE: Bariatric surgery and long-term control of morbid obesity. JAMA 288:2793–2796, 2002

Brouhard BH, Donaldson LA, Lawry KW, et al: Cognitive functioning in children on dialysis and post-transplantation. Pediatr Transplant 4:261–267, 2000

Brugman SM, Howell JH, Mahler JL, et al: The spectrum of pediatric vocal cord dysfunction. Am Rev Respir Dis 149:A353, 1994

Bryden KS, Peveler RC, Stein A, et al: Clinical and psychological course of diabetes from adolescence to young adulthood. Diabetes Care 24:1536–1540, 2001

Bullock EA, Shaddy RE: Relaxation and imagery techniques without sedation during right ventricular endomyocardial biopsy in pediatric heart transplant patients. J Heart Lung Transplant 12(1 pt 1):59–62, 1993

Burlew K, Telfair J, Colangelo L, et al: Factors that influence adolescent adaptation to sickle cell disease. J Pediatr Psychol 25:287–299, 2000

Bursch B: Somatization disorders, in Comprehensive Handbook of Personality and Psychopathology, Vol III: Child Psychopathology. Edited by Hersen M, Thomas JC (Ammerman RT, volume editor). New York, Wiley, 2006, pp 403–421

Bursch B: Psychological/cognitive behavioral treatments for childhood functional abdominal pain and irritable bowel syndrome J Pediatr Gastroenterol Nutr 47:706–707, 2008

Bursch B: Pediatric pain, in Textbook of Pediatric Psychosomatic Medicine: Edited by Shaw RJ, DeMaso DR. Washington, DC, American Psychiatric Publishing, 2010, pp 141–154

Bursch B, Zeltzer LK: Autism spectrum disorders presenting as chronic pain syndromes: case presentations and discussion. Journal of Developmental and Learning Disorders 6:41–48, 2002

Bussing R, Burket RC, Kelleher ET: Prevalence of anxiety disorders in a clinic-based sample of pediatric asthma patients. Psychosomatics 37:108–115, 1996

Butz AM, Alexander C: Anxiety in children with asthma. J Asthma 30:199–209, 1993

Callanan M, Kelley P: Final Gifts: Understanding the Special Awareness, Needs, and Communications of the Dying. New York, Bantam, 1992

Campo JV, Fritsch SL: Somatization in children and adolescents. J Am Acad Child Adolesc Psychiatry 33:1223–1235, 1994

Campo JV, Fritz G: A management model for pediatric somatization. Psychosomatics 42:467–476, 2001

Campo JV, Jansen-McWilliams L, Comer DM, et al: Somatization in pediatric primary care: association with psychopathology, functional impairment and use of services. J Am Acad Child Adolesc Psychiatry 38:1093–1101, 1999

Campo JV, Comer DM, Jansen-McWilliams L, et al: Recurrent pain, emotional distress, and health service use in childhood. J Pediatr 141:76–83, 2002

Campo JV, Perel, J, Lucas A, et al: Citalopram treatment of pediatric recurrent abdominal pain and comorbid internalizing disorders: an exploratory study. J Am Acad Child Adolesc Psychiatry 43:1234–1242, 2004

Centers for Disease Control and Prevention: Prevalence of autism spectrum disorders—Autism and Developmental Disabilities Monitoring Network, 14 sites, United States, 2002. Autism and Developmental Disabilities Monitoring Network Surveillance Year 2002 Principal Investigators. MMWR Surveill Summ 56(SS01):12–28, 2007

Centers for Disease Control and Prevention: Prevalence of autism spectrum disorders—Autism and Developmental Disabilities Monitoring Network, United States, 2006. Autism and Developmental Disabilities Monitoring Network Surveillance Year 2006 Principal Investigators. MMWR Surveill Summ 58(SS10):1–20, 2009

Centers for Disease Control and Prevention: Diabetes Public Health Resource. Children and Diabetes—More Information. 2010. Available at: http://www.cdc.gov/diabetes/projects/cda2.htm. Accessed April 28, 2010.

Cepeda ML, Yang YM, Price CC, et al: Mental disorders in children and adolescents with sickle cell disease. South Med J 90:284–287, 1997

Chatoor I, Ganiban J, Colin V, et al: Attachment and feeding problems: a reexamination of nonorganic failure to thrive and attachment insecurity. J Am Acad Child Adolesc Psychiatry 37:1217–1224, 1998

Chen E, Craske MG, Katz ER, et al: Pain-sensitive temperament: does it predict procedural distress and response to psychological treatment among children with cancer? J Pediatr Psychol 25:269–278, 2000

Chial HJ, Camilleri M, Williams DE, et al: Rumination syndrome in children and adolescents: diagnosis, treatment, and prognosis. Pediatrics 111:158–162, 2003

Chinn S, Rona RJ: Prevalence and trends in overweight and obesity in three cross-sectional studies of British children, 1974–1994. BMJ 322:24–26, 2001

Chunming C: Fat intake and nutritional status in children in China. Am J Clin Nutr 72:1368S–1372S, 2000

Clouse RE, Richter JE, Heading RC, et al: Functional esophageal disorders. Gut 45 (suppl 2):II31–II36, 1999

Coffman JM, Cabana MD, Halpin HA, et al: Effects of asthma education on children's use of acute care services: a meta-analysis. Pediatrics 121:575–586, 2008

Conners CK, Casat CD, Gualtieri CT, et al: Bupropion hydrochloride in attention deficit disorder with hyperactivity. J Am Acad Child Adolesc Psychiatry 35:1314–1321, 1996

Connolly D, Rutkowski M, Auslender M, et al: Measuring health-related quality of life in children with heart disease. Appl Nurs Res 15:74–80, 2002

Costello EJ, Shugart MA: Above and below the threshold: severity of psychiatric symptoms and functional impairment in a pediatric sample. Pediatrics 90:359–368, 1992

Costello EJ, Costello AJ, Edelbrock C, et al: Psychiatric disorders in pediatric primary care: prevalence and risk factors. Arch Gen Psychiatry 45:1107–1116, 1988

Dalzell AM, Shepherd RW, Dean B, et al: Nutritional rehabilitation in cystic fibrosis: a 5 year follow-up study. J Pediatr Gastroenterol Nutr 15:141–145, 1992

DCCT Research Group: The effects of intensive treatment of diabetes on the development and progression of long-term complications in insulin-dependent diabetes mellitus. N Engl J Med 329:977–986, 1993

DCCT Research Group: Effects of intensive diabetes treatment on the development and progression of long-term complications in adolescents with insulin-dependent diabetes mellitus: Diabetes Control and Complications Trial. J Pediatr 125:177–188, 1994

de Onis M, Blossner M: Prevalence and trends of overweight among preschool children in developing countries. Am J Clin Nutr 72:1032–1039, 2000

DeMaso DR, Twente AW, Spratt EG, et al: Impact of psychologic functioning, medical severity, and family functioning in pediatric heart transplantation. J Heart Lung Transplant 14(6 pt 1):1102–1108, 1995

DeMaso DR, Spratt EG, Vaughan BL, et al: Psychological functioning in children and adolescents undergoing radiofrequency catheter ablation. Psychosomatics 41:134–139, 2000

Dietz WH, Bellizzi MC: Introduction: the use of body mass index to assess obesity in children. Am J Clin Nutr 70:123S–125S, 1999

DiMatteo MR, Giordani PJ, Lepper HS, et al: Patient adherence and medical treatment outcomes: a meta-analysis. Med Care 40:794–811, 2002

Drash AL: The child, the adolescent, and the diabetes control and complications trial. Diabetes Care 16:1515–1516, 1993

Drewett RF, Corbett SS, Wright CM: Cognitive and educational attainments at school age of children who failed to thrive in infancy: a population-based study. J Child Psychol Psychiatry 40:551–561, 1999

Driscoll DJ, Glicklich LB, Gallen WJ: Chest pain in children: a prospective study. Pediatrics 57:648–651, 1976

Du Pasquier-Fediaevsky L, Tubiana-Rufi N: Discordance between physician and adolescent assessments of adherence to treatment: influence of HbA1c level. The PEDIAB Collaborative Group. Diabetes Care 22:1445–1449, 1999

Dunn C, Deroo L, Rivara F: The use of brief interventions adapted from motivational interviewing across behavioral domains: a systemic review. Addiction 96:1725–1742, 2001

Dykman RA, Casey PH, Ackerman PT, et al: Behavioral and cognitive status in school-aged children with a history of failure to thrive during early childhood. Clin Pediatr (Phila) 40:63–70, 2001

Ebbeling CA, Pawlak DB, Ludwig DS: Childhood obesity: public-health crisis, common sense cure. Lancet 360:473–482, 2002

Eccleston C, Palermo TM, Williams AC, et al: Psychological therapies for the management of chronic and recurrent pain in children and adolescents (review). Cochrane Database Syst Rev (2):CD003968, 2009

Efron D, Hiscock H, Sewell JR, et al: Prescribing of psychotropic medications for children by Australian pediatricians and child psychiatrists. Pediatrics 111:372–375, 2003

Egger HL, Angold A, Costello EJ: Headaches and psychopathology in children and adolescents. J Am Acad Child Adolesc Psychiatry 37:951–958, 1998

Ely EW, Gautam S, Margolin R, et al: The impact of delirium in the intensive care unit on hospital length of stay. Intensive Care Med 27:1892–1900, 2001

Erickson SJ, Steiner H: Trauma spectrum adaptation: somatic symptoms in long-term pediatric cancer survivors. Psychosomatics 41:339–346, 2000

Ettenger RB, Rosenthal JT, Marik JL, et al: Improved cadaveric renal transplant outcome in children. Pediatr Nephrol 5:137–142, 1991

Fayek M, Kingsbury SJ, Zada J, et al: Psychopharmacology: cardiac effects of antipsychotic medications. Psychiatr Serv 52:607–609, 2001

Fennell RS 3rd, Rasbury WC, Fennell EB, et al: Effects of kidney transplantation on cognitive performance in a pediatric population. Pediatrics 74:273–278, 1984

Field MJ, Institute of Medicine, Behrman RE: When Children Die: Improving Palliative and End-of-Life Care for Children and Their Families. Washington, DC, National Academies Press, 2003

Fisher WW, Piazza CC, Bowman LG, et al: A preliminary evaluation of empirically derived consequences for the treatment of pica. J Appl Behav Anal 27:447–457, 1994

Francis PD: Effects of psychotropic medications on the pediatric electrocardiogram and recommendations for monitoring. Curr Opin Pediatr 14:224–230, 2002

Frank NC, Blount RL, Brown RT: Attributions, coping, and adjustment in children with cancer. J Pediatr Psychol 22:563–576, 1997

Fritz GK, Fritsch S, Hagino O: Somatoform disorders in children and adolescents: a review of the past 10 years. J Am Acad Child Adolesc Psychiatry 36:1329–1338, 1997

Fukunishi I, Honda M: School adjustment of children with end-stage renal disease. Pediatr Nephrol 9:553–557, 1995

Fukunishi I, Kudo H: Psychiatric problems of pediatric end-stage renal failure. Gen Hosp Psychiatry 17:32–36, 1995

Gadoth N: Multiple sclerosis in children. Brain Dev 25:229–232, 2003

Garber J, Zeman J, Walker L: Recurrent abdominal pain in children: psychiatric diagnoses and parental psychopathology. J Am Acad Child Adolesc Psychiatry 29:648–656, 1990

Garber J, Walker LS, Zeman J: Somatization symptoms in a community sample of children and adolescents: further validation of the children's somatization inventory. J Consult Clin Psychol 3:588–595, 1991

Garcia-Campayo J, Sanz-Carillo C: Topiramate as a treatment for pain in multisomatoform disorder patients: an open trial. Gen Hosp Psychiatry 24:417–421, 2002

Garralda ME, Jameson RA, Reynolds JM, et al: Psychiatric adjustment in children with chronic renal failure. J Child Psychol Psychiatry 29:79–90, 1988

Gaudieri PA, Chen R, Greer TF, et al: Cognitive function in children with type 1 diabetes: a meta-analysis. Diabetes Care 31:1892–1897, 2008

Gavin LA, Wamboldt M, Brugman S, et al: Psychological and family characteristics of adolescents with vocal cord dysfunction. J Asthma 35:409–417, 1998

Gilles A, Cassano M, Shepherd EJ, et al: Comparing active pediatric obesity treatments using meta-analysis. J Clin Child Adolesc Psychol 37:886–892, 2008

Gizynski M, Shapiro V: Depression and childhood illness. Child Adolesc Social Work J 7:179–197, 1990

Glasscoe CA, Quittner AL: Psychological interventions for people with cystic fibrosis and their families. Cochrane Database Syst Rev (3):CD003148, 2008

Godding V, Kruth M, Jamart J: Joint consultation for high-risk asthmatic children and their families, with pediatrician and child psychiatrist as co-therapists: model and evaluation. Fam Process 36:265–280, 1997

Goldbeck L, Babka C: Development and evaluation of a multifamily psychoeducational program for cystic fibrosis. Patient Educ Couns 44:187–192, 2001

Goldston DB, Kovacs M, Ho VY, et al: Suicidal ideation and suicide attempts among youth with insulin-dependent diabetes mellitus. J Am Acad Child Adolesc Psychiatry 33:240, 1994

Goodman AM, Mattson SN, Lang AR, et al: Concept formation and problem solving in children with heavy prenatal alcohol exposure. Alcohol Clin Exp Res 23 (suppl 5):32A, 1999

Goodnick PJ, Henry JH, Buki VM: Treatment of depression in patients with diabetes mellitus. J Clin Psychiatry 56:128–136, 1995

Goodwin RD, Pine DS, Hoven CW: Asthma and panic attacks among youth in the community. J Asthma 40:139–145, 2003

Gortmaker SL, Must A, Perrin JM, et al: Social and economic consequences of overweight in adolescence and young adulthood. N Engl J Med 329:1008–1012, 1993

Graham PJ, Rutter ML, Pless IB: Childhood asthma: a psychosomatic disorder? Some epidemiological considerations. Br J Prev Soc Med 2:78–85, 1967

Griffin KJ, Elkin TD: Non-adherence in pediatric transplantation: a review of the existing literature. Pediatr Transplant 5:246–249, 2001

Guo SS, Roche AF, Chumlea WC, et al: The predictive value of childhood body mass index values for overweight at age 35 years. Am J Clin Nutr 59:810–819, 1994

Gustafsson PA, Kjellman NI, Cederblad M: Family therapy in the treatment of severe childhood asthma. J Psychosom Res 30:369–374, 1986

Gutgesell H, Atkins D, Barst R, et al: AHA Scientific Statement: cardiovascular monitoring of children and adolescents receiving psychotropic drugs. J Am Acad Child Adolesc Psychiatry 38:1047–1050, 1999

Gyulay JE: Home care for the dying child. Issues Compr Pediatr Nurs 12:33–69, 1989

Hahn JS, Berquist W, Alcorn DM, et al: Wernicke encephalopathy and beriberi during total parenteral nutrition attributable to multivitamin infusion shortage. Pediatrics 101:E10, 1998

Hammad TA, Laughren T, Racoosin J: Suicidality in pediatric patients treated with antidepressant drugs. Arch Gen Psychiatry 63:332–339, 2006

Hauser ST, Jacobson AM, Lavori P, et al: Adherence among children and adolescents with insulin-dependent diabetes mellitus over a four-year longitudinal follow-up, II: immediate and long-term linkages with the family milieu. J Pediatr Psychol 15:527–542, 1990

Hedley AA, Ogden CL, Johnson CL, et al: Prevalence of overweight and obesity among US children, adolescents, and adults, 1999–2002. JAMA 291:2847–2850, 2004

Heruti RJ, Levy A, Adunski A, et al: Conversion motor paralysis disorder: overview and rehabilitation model. Spinal Cord 40:327–334, 2002

Ho J, Bender BG, Gavin LA, et al: Relations among asthma knowledge, treatment adherence, and outcome. J Allergy Clin Immunol 111:498–502, 2003

Hobbie WL, Stuber M, Meeske K, et al: Symptoms of posttraumatic stress in young adult survivors of childhood cancer. J Clin Oncol 18:4060–4066, 2000

Hodges K, Kline JJ, Barbero G, et al: Depressive symptoms in children with recurrent abdominal pain and in their families. J Pediatr 107:622–626, 1985a

Hodges K, Kline JJ, Barbero G, et al: Anxiety in children with recurrent abdominal pain and their parents. Psychosomatics 26:859, 862–866, 1985b

Hudson J: Prescription for Success: Supporting Children With Autism Spectrum Disorders in the Medical Environment. Shawnee Mission, KS, Autism Asperger Publishing, 2006

Hyman PE, Bursch B, Lopez E, et al: Visceral pain-associated disability syndrome: a descriptive analysis. J Pediatr Gastroenterol Nutr 35:663–668, 2002

In-Albon T, Schneider S: Psychotherapy of childhood anxiety disorders: a meta-analysis. Psychother Psychosom 76:15–24, 2007

Ireys HT, Chernoff R, DeVet KA, et al: Maternal outcomes of a randomized controlled trial of a community-based support program for families of children with chronic illnesses. Arch Pediatr Adolesc Med 155:771–777, 2001

Ivascu NS, Sarnaik S, McCrae J, et al: Characterization of pica prevalence among patients with sickle cell disease. Arch Pediatr Adolesc Med 155:1243–1247, 2001

Jacobson AM: The psychological care of patients with insulin-dependent diabetes mellitus. N Engl J Med 334:1249–1253, 1996

Jay SM, Elliott CH, Woody PD, et al: An investigation of cognitive-behavioral therapy combined with oral Valium for children undergoing painful medical procedures. Health Psychol 10:317–322, 1991

Jirikowic T, Kartin D, Olson HC: Children with fetal alcohol spectrum disorders: a descriptive profile of adaptive function. Can J Occup Ther 75:238–248, 2008

Johnson CR, Hunt FM, Siebert MJ: Discrimination training in the treatment of pica and food scavenging. Behav Modif 18:214–229, 1994

Johnston-Brooks CH, Lewis MA, Garg S: Self-efficacy impacts self-care and HbA1c in young adults with type 1 diabetes. Psychosom Med 64:43–51, 2002

Kahana SY, Drotar D, Frazier TW: Meta-analysis of psychological interventions to promote adherence to treatment in pediatric chronic health conditions. J Pediatr Psychol 33:590–611, 2008a

Kahana SY, Frazier TW, Drotar D: Preliminary quantitative investigation of predictors of treatment non-adherence in pediatric transplantation: a brief report. Pediatr Transplant 12:656–660, 2008b

Kalberg WO, Provost B, Tollison SJ, et al: Comparison of motor delays in young children with fetal alcohol syndrome to those with prenatal alcohol exposure and with no prenatal alcohol exposure. Alcohol Clin Exp Res 30:2037–2045, 2006

Kamath CC, Vickers KS, Ehrlich A, et al: Clinical review: behavioral interventions to prevent childhood obesity: a systematic review and meta-analyses of randomized trials. J Clin Endocrinol Metab 93:4606–4615, 2008

Karnik NS, Joshi SV, Paterno C, et al: Subtypes of pediatric delirium: a treatment algorithm. Psychosomatics 48:253–257, 2007

Karsdorp PA, Everaerd W, Kindt M, et al: Psychological and cognitive functioning in children and adolescents with congenital heart disease: a meta-analysis. J Pediatr Psychol 32:527–541, 2007

Kashani JH, Barbero GJ, Wilfley DE, et al: Psychological concomitants of cystic fibrosis in children and adolescents. Adolescence 23:873–880, 1988a

Kashani JH, König P, Shepperd JA, et al: Psychopathology and self-concept in asthmatic children. J Pediatr Psychol 13:509–520, 1988b

Kashikar-Zuck S, Goldschneider KR, Powers SW, et al: Depression and functional disability in chronic pediatric pain. Clin J Pain 17:341–349, 2001

Kazak AE, Barakat LP, Meeske K, et al: Posttraumatic stress symptoms, family functioning, and social support in survivors of childhood leukemia and their mothers and fathers. J Consult Clin Psychol 65:120–129, 1997

Kazak AE, Penati B, Brophy P, et al: Pharmacological and psychological interventions for procedural pain. Pediatrics 102:59–66, 1998

Kazak AE, Simms S, Rourke M: Family systems practice in pediatric psychology. J Pediatr Psychol 27:133–143, 2002

Kazak AE, Kassam-Adams N, Schneider S, et al: An integrative model of pediatric medical traumatic stress. J Pediatr Psychol 31:343–355, 2006

Kean EM, Kelsay K, Wamboldt F, et al: Posttraumatic stress in adolescents with asthma and their parents. J Am Acad Child Adolesc Psychiatry 45:78–86, 2006

Kemper MJ, Sparta G, Laube GF, et al: Neuropsychologic side effects of tacrolimus in pediatric renal transplantation. Clin Transplant 17:130–134, 2003

Kendall P: Treating anxiety disorders in children: results of a randomized clinical trial. J Consult Clin Psychol 62:100–110, 1994

Kerwin ME: Empirically supported treatments in pediatric psychology: severe feeding problems. J Pediatr Psychol 24:193–214, 1999

King AA, DeBaun MR, White DA: Need for cognitive rehabilitation for children with sickle cell disease and strokes. Expert Rev Neurother 8:291–296, 2008

Kinney TR, Sleeper LA, Wang WC, et al: Silent cerebral infarcts in sickle cell anemia: a risk factor analysis. Pediatrics 103:640–645, 1999

Klein-Gitelman MS, Pachman LM: Intravenous corticosteroids: adverse reactions are more variable than expected in children. J Rheumatol 25:1995–2002, 1998

Kothare SV, Ebb DH, Rosenberger PB, et al: Acute confusion and mutism as a presentation of thalamic strokes secondary to deep cerebral venous thrombosis. J Child Neurol 13:300–303, 1998

Kovacs M, Goldston D, Obrosky DS, et al: Psychiatric disorders in youth with IDDM: rates and risk factors. Diabetes Care 20:36–44, 1997

Kreicbergs U, Valdimarsdottir U, Onelov E, et al: Talking about death with children who have severe malignant disease. N Engl J Med 351:1175–1186, 2004

Krilov LR, Fisher M, Friedman SB, et al: Course and outcome of chronic fatigue in children and adolescents. Pediatrics 102 (2 pt 1):360–366, 1998

Labellarte MJ, Crosson JE, Riddle MA: The relevance of prolonged QTc measurement to pediatric psychopharmacology. J Am Acad Child Adolesc Psychiatry 42:642–650, 2003

Lask B, Matthew D: Childhood asthma: a controlled trial of family psychotherapy. Arch Dis Child 54:116–119, 1979

Lemanek KL, Kamps J, Chung MB: Empirical supported treatments in pediatric psychology: regimen adherence. J Pediatr Psychol 26:253–275, 2001

Lester P, Stein JA, Bursch B: Developmental predictors of somatic symptoms in adolescents of parents with HIV: a 12-month follow-up. J Dev Behav Pediatr 24:242–250, 2003

Li B, Balint JP: Cyclic vomiting syndrome: the evolution of understanding of a brain-gut disorder. Adv Pediatr 47:117–160, 2000

Libow JA: Munchausen by proxy victims in adulthood: a first look. Child Abuse Negl 19:1131–1142, 1995

Libow JA: Child and adolescent illness falsification. Pediatrics 105:336–342, 2000

Libow JA: Beyond collusion: active illness falsification. Child Abuse Negl 26:525–536, 2002

Liebowitz MR, Turner SM, Piacentini J, et al: Fluoxetine in children and adolescents with OCD: a placebo-controlled trial. J Am Acad Child Adolesc Psychiatry 41:1431–1438, 2002

Lieh-Lai MW, Theodorou AA, Sarnaik AP, et al: Limitations of the Glasgow Coma Scale in predicting outcome in children with traumatic brain injury. J Pediatr 120(2 pt 1):195–199, 1992

Livingston R: Children of people with somatization disorder. J Am Acad Child Adolesc Psychiatry 32:536–544, 1993

Livingston R, Witt A, Smith GR: Families who somatize. J Dev Behav Pediatr 16:42–46, 1995

Ljungman G, Kreuger A, Andreasson S, et al: Midazolam nasal spray reduces procedural anxiety in children. Pediatrics 105 (1 pt 1):73–78, 2000

Ljungman G, Gordh T, Sorensen S, et al: Lumbar puncture in pediatric oncology: conscious sedation vs. general anesthesia. Med Pediatr Oncol 36:372–379, 2001

Lurie S, Shemesh E, Sheiner PA, et al: Non-adherence in pediatric liver transplant recipients—an assessment of risk factors and natural history. Pediatr Transplant 4:200–206, 2000

Mack JW, Hilden JM, Watterson J, et al: Parent and physician perspectives on quality of care at the end of life in children with cancer. J Clin Oncol 23:9155–9161, 2005

MacLean W Jr, Perrin J, Gortmarkers S, et al: Psychological adjustment of children with asthma: effects of illness severity and recent stressful life events. J Pediatr Psychol 17:159–171, 1988

Mailis-Gagnon A, Giannoylis I, Downar J, et al: Altered central somatosensory processing in chronic pain patients with "hysterical" anesthesia. Neurology 60:1501–1507, 2003

Malcolm A, Thumshirn MB, Camilleri M, et al: Rumination syndrome. Mayo Clin Proc 72:646–652, 1997

Manne SL, Du Hamel K, Gallelli K, et al: Posttraumatic stress disorder among mothers of pediatric cancer survivors: diagnosis, comorbidity, and utility of the PTSD checklist as a screening instrument. J Pediatr Psychol 23:357–366, 1998

Manos PJ, Wu R: The duration of delirium in medical and postoperative patients referred for psychiatric consultation. Ann Clin Psychiatry 9:219–226, 1997

Mattson SN, Goodman AM, Caine C, et al: Executive functioning in children with heavy prenatal alcohol exposure. Alcohol Clin Exp Res 23:1808–1815, 1999

May PA, Gossage JP: Estimating the prevalence of fetal alcohol syndrome. Alcohol Health Res World 25:159–167, 2001

Mayes L, Volkmar F, Hooks M, et al: Differentiating pervasive developmental disorder not otherwise specified from autism and language disorders. J Autism Dev Disord 23:79–90, 1993

McGee CL, Schonfeld AM, Roebuck-Spencer TM, et al: Children with heavy prenatal alcohol exposure demonstrate deficits on multiple measures of concept formation. Alcohol Clin Exp Res 32:1388–1397, 2008

McGovern L, Johnson JN, Paulo R, et al: Clinical review: treatment of pediatric obesity: a systematic review and meta-analysis of randomized trials. J Clin Endocrinol Metab 93:4600–4605, 2008

McLeod BD, Wood JJ, Weisz JR: Examining the association between parenting and childhood anxiety: a meta-analysis. Clin Psychol Rev 27:155–172, 2007

McNichol K, Williams H, Allan J, et al: Spectrum of asthma in children, III: psychological and social components. BMJ 4:16–20, 1973

McQuaid EL, Kopel SJ, Klein RB, et al: Medication adherence in pediatric asthma: reasoning, responsibility, and behavior. J Pediatr Psychol 28:323–333, 2003

Meeske K, Stuber ML: PTSD, quality of life and psychological outcome in young adult survivors of pediatric cancer. Oncol Nurs Forum 28:481–489, 2001

Minuchin S, Rosman B, Baker L: Psychosomatic Families. Boston, MA, Harvard University Press, 1978

Morgan CM, Tanofsky-Kraff M, Wilfley DE, et al: Childhood obesity. Child Adolesc Psychiatr Clin N Am 11:257–278, 2002

Morton MJ, Reynolds JM, Garralda ME, et al: Psychiatric adjustment in end-stage renal disease: a follow up study of former paediatric patients. J Psychosom Res 38:293–303, 1994

Mosholder AD, Willy M: Suicidal adverse events in pediatric randomized, controlled clinical trials of antidepressant drugs are associated with active drug treatment: a meta-analysis. J Child Adolesc Psychopharmacol 16:25–32, 2006

Mossberg HO: Forty year follow-up of overweight children. Lancet 2(8661):491–493, 1989

Mrazek DA, Anderson IS, Strunk RC: Disturbed emotional development of severely asthmatic preschool children. J Child Psychol Psychiatry 4:81–94, 1985

Muller JE, Wentzel I, Koen L, et al: Escitalopram in the treatment of multisomatoform disorder: a double-blind, placebo-controlled trial. Int Clin Psychopharmacol 23:43–48, 2008

Muller T, Mannel M, Murck H, et al: Treatment of somatoform disorders with St. John's wort: a randomized, double-blind and placebo-controlled trial. Psychosom Med 66:538–547, 2004

Munk DD, Repp AC: Behavioral assessment of feeding problems of individuals with severe disabilities. J Appl Behav Anal 27:241–250, 1994

Must A, Spandano J, Coakley EH, et al: The disease burden associated with overweight and obesity. JAMA 282:1523–1529, 1999

Norrish M, Tooley M, Godfry S: Clinical, physiological, and psychological study of asthmatic children attending a hospital clinic. Arch Dis Child 52:912–917, 1977

Noyes R, Happel RL, Muller BA, et al: Fluvoxamine for somatoform disorders: an open trial. Gen Hosp Psychiatry 20:339–344, 1998

O'Brien MD, Bruce BK, Camilleri M: The rumination syndrome: clinical features rather than manometric diagnosis. Gastroenterology 108:1024–1029, 1995

Oguz A, Kurul S, Dirik E: Relationship of epilepsy-related factors to anxiety and depression scores in epileptic children. J Child Neurol 17:37–40, 2002

Ohene-Frempong K: Stroke in sickle cell disease: demographic, clinical, and therapeutic considerations. Semin Hematol 28:213–219, 1991

Ohene-Frempong K, Weiner SJ, Sleeper LA, et al: Cerebrovascular accidents in sickle cell disease: rates and risk factors. Blood 91:288–294, 1998

Ollendick TH, King NJ: Empirically supported treatments for children with phobic and anxiety disorders: current status. J Clin Child Psychol 27:156–167, 1998

Pai AL, Drotar D, Zebracki K, et al: A meta-analysis of the effects of psychological interventions in pediatric oncology on outcomes of psychological distress and adjustment. J Pediatr Psychol 31:978–988, 2006

Pai AL, Greenley RN, Lewandowski A, et al: A meta-analytic review of the influence of pediatric cancer on parent and family functioning. J Fam Psychol 21:407–415, 2007

Paniagua FA, Braverman C, Capriotti RM: Use of a treatment package in the management of a profoundly mentally retarded girl's pica and self-stimulation. Am J Ment Defic 90:550–557, 1986

Panton J, Barley EA: Family therapy for asthma in children. Cochrane Database Syst Rev (2):CD000089, 2000

Papakostas K, Moraitis D, Lancaster J, et al: Depressive symptoms in children after tonsillectomy. Int J Pediatr Otorhinolaryngol 67:127–132, 2003

Parker RI, Mahan RA, Giugliano D, et al: Efficacy and safety of intravenous midazolam and ketamine as sedation for therapeutic and diagnostic procedures in children. Pediatrics 99:427–431, 1997

Passero MA, Remor B, Solomon J: Patient-reported compliance with cystic fibrosis therapy. Clin Pediatr 20:264–268, 1981

Patterson JM, Budd J, Goetz D, et al: Family correlates of a 10-year pulmonary health trend in cystic fibrosis. Pediatrics 91:383–389, 1993

Peterson CC, Johnson CE, Ramirez LY, et al: A meta-analysis of the neuropsychological sequelae of chemotherapy-only treatment for pediatric acute lymphoblastic leukemia. Pediatr Blood Cancer 51:99–104, 2008

Peyron R, Laurent B, Garcia-Larrea L: Functional imaging of brain responses to pain: a review and meta-analysis 2000. Neurophysiol Clin 30:263–288, 2000

Pfeffer CR: Suicide prevention: current efficacy and future promise. Ann N Y Acad Sci 487:341–350, 1986

Phipps S, DeCuir-Whalley S: Adherence issues in pediatric bone marrow transplantation. J Pediatr Psychol 15:459–475, 1990

Phipps S, Srivastava DK: Repressive adaptation in children with cancer. Health Psychol 16:521–528, 1997

Phipps S, Srivastava DK: Approaches to the measurement of depressive symptomatology in children with cancer: attempting to circumvent the effects of defensiveness. J Dev Behav Pediatr 20:150–156, 1999

Piacentini J, Bergman RL: Developmental issues in cognitive therapy for childhood anxiety disorders. Journal of Cognitive Psychotherapy 15:165–182, 2001

Platt OS, Brambilla DJ, Rosse WF, et al: Mortality in sickle cell disease: life expectancy and risk factors for early death. N Engl J Med 330:1639–1644, 1994

Plioplys S, Asato M, Bursch B, et al: Multidisciplinary management of pediatric nonepileptic seizures. J Am Acad Child Adolesc Psychiatry 46:1491–1495, 2007

Porter GE, Heitsch GM, Miller MD: Munchausen syndrome by proxy: unusual manifestations and disturbing sequelae. Child Abuse Negl 18:789–794, 1994

Powers SW: Empirically supported treatments in pediatric psychology: procedure-related pain. J Pediatr Psychol 24:131–145, 1999

Qvist E, Pihko H, Fagerudd P, et al: Neurodevelopmental outcome in high-risk patients after renal transplantation in early childhood. Pediatr Transplant 6:53–62, 2002

Ranmal R, Prictor M, Scott JT: Interventions for improving communication with children and adolescents about their cancer. Cochrane Database Syst Rev (4):CD002969, 2008

Rapoff MA: Adherence to Pediatric Medical Regimens. New York, Kluwer/Plenum, 1999

Rapoff MA, Belmont J, Lindsley C, et al: Prevention of nonadherence to nonsteroidal anti-inflammatory medications for newly diagnosed patients with juvenile rheumatoid arthritis. Health Psychol 21:620–623, 2002

Rasquin-Weber A, Hyman PE, Cucchiara S, et al: Childhood functional gastrointestinal disorders. Gut 45 (suppl 2):II60–II68, 1999

Raymond NC, Chang PN, Crow SJ, et al: Eating disorders in patients with cystic fibrosis. J Adolesc 23:359–363, 2000

Rennick JE, Johnston CC, Dougherty G, et al: Children's psychological responses after critical illness and exposure to invasive technology. J Dev Behav Pediatr 23:133–144, 2002

Rennick JE, Morin I, Kim D, et al: Identifying children at high risk for psychological sequelae after pediatric intensive care unit hospitalization. Pediatr Crit Care Med 5:358–363, 2004

Research Unit on Pediatric Psychopharmacology Anxiety Study Group: Fluvoxamine for the treatment of anxiety disorders in children and adolescents. N Engl J Med 344:1279–1285, 2001

Rey JM, Birmaher B: Treating Child and Adolescent Depression. Philadelphia, PA, Lippincott Williams & Wilkins, 2009

Reynolds JM, Garralda ME, Jameson RA, et al: How parents and families cope with chronic renal failure. Arch Dis Child 63:821–826, 1988

Reynolds JM, Garralda ME, Postlethwaite RJ, et al: Changes in psychosocial adjustment after renal transplantation. Arch Dis Child 66:508–513, 1991

Riddle MA, Bernstein GA, Cook EH, et al: Anxiolytics, adrenergic agents, and naltrexone. J Am Acad Child Adolesc Psychiatry 38:546–556, 1999

Robb SL, Ebberts AG: Songwriting and digital video production interventions for pediatric patients undergoing bone marrow transplantation, part I: an analysis of depression and anxiety levels according to phase of treatment. J Pediatr Oncol Nurs 20:2–15, 2003

Robieux IC, Kumar R, Rhadakrishnan S, et al: The feasibility of using EMLA (eutectic mixture of local anaesthetics) cream in pediatric outpatient clinics. Can J Hosp Pharm 43:235–236, xxxii, 1990

Rodgers GP, Clark CM, Kessler RM: Regional alterations in brain metabolism in neurologically normal sickle cell patients. JAMA 256:1692–1700, 1984

Roebuck RM, Mattson SN, Riley EP: Behavioral and psychosocial profiles of alcohol-exposed children. Alcohol Clin Exp Res 22:339–344, 1998

Rydall AC, Rodin GM, Olmsted MP, et al: Disordered eating behavior and microvascular complications in young women with insulin-dependent diabetes mellitus. N Engl J Med 336:1849–1854, 1997

Saarto T, Wiffen PJ: Antidepressants for neuropathic pain. Cochrane Database Syst Rev (4):CD005454, 2007

Sahler OJ, Varni JW, Fairclough DL, et al: Problem-solving skills training for mothers of children with newly diagnosed cancer: a randomized trial. J Dev Behav Pediatr 23:77–86, 2002

Salvatierra O, Alfrey E, Tanne DC, et al: Superior outcomes in pediatric renal transplantation. Arch Surg 132:842–847, 1997

Sanders MR, Rebyetz M, Morrison M, et al: Cognitive-behavioral treatment of recurrent nonspecific abdominal pain in children: an analysis of generalization, maintenance and side effects. J Consult Clin Psychol 57:294–300, 1989

Sanders MR, Shepherd RW, Cleghorn G, et al: The treatment of recurrent abdominal pain in children: a controlled comparison of cognitive-behavioral family intervention and standard pediatric care. J Consult Clin Psychol 62:306–314, 1994

Saxe GN, Stoddard FJ, Sheridan RL: PTSD in children with burns: a longitudinal study. J Burn Care Rehabil 19(1 pt 2):S206, 1998

Schanberg LE, Keefe FJ, Lefebvre JC, et al: Social context of pain in children with juvenile primary fibromyalgia syndrome: parental pain history and family environment. Clin J Pain 14:107–115, 1998

Schieveld JN, Leroy PL, van Os J, et al: Pediatric delirium in critical illness: phenomenology, clinical correlates and treatment response in 40 cases in the pediatric intensive care unit. Intensive Care Med 33:1033–1040, 2007

Schiffrin A: Psychosocial issues in pediatric diabetes. Curr Diab Rep 1:33–40, 2001

Schonfeld A, Mattson SN, Lang A, et al: Verbal and nonverbal fluency in children with heavy prenatal alcohol exposure. J Stud Alcohol 62:239–246, 2001

Schwimmer JB, Burwinkle TM, Varni JW: Health-related quality of life of severely obese children and adolescents. JAMA 289:1813–1819, 2003

Selbst SM: Chest pain in children. Pediatrics 75:1068–1070, 1985

Serrano-Ikkos E, Lask B, Whitehead B, et al: Incomplete adherence after pediatric heart and heart-lung transplantation. J Heart Lung Transplant 17:1177–1183, 1998

Serrano-Ikkos E, Lask B, Whitehead B, et al: Heart or heart-lung transplantation: psychosocial outcome. Pediatr Transplant 3:301–308, 1999

Shaabat A: Confusional migraine in childhood. Pediatr Neurol 15:23–25, 1996

Shemesh E, Lurie S, Stuber ML, et al: A pilot study of posttraumatic stress and nonadherence in pediatric liver transplant recipients. Pediatrics 105:E29, 2000

Shemesh E, Shneider BL, Savitzky JK, et al: Medication adherence in pediatric and adolescent liver transplant recipients. Pediatrics 113:825–832, 2004

Sheridan RL, Hinson M, Nackel A, et al: Development of a pediatric burn pain and anxiety management program. J Burn Care Rehabil 18:455–459, 1997

Sibbitt WL Jr, Brandt JR, Johnson CR, et al: The incidence and prevalence of neuropsychiatric syndromes in pediatric onset systemic lupus erythematosus. J Rheumatol 29:1536–1542, 2002

Simonds JF: Psychiatric consultations for 112 pediatric inpatients. South Med J 70:980–984, 1977

Simoni JM, Asarnow JR, Munford PR, et al: Psychological distress and treatment adherence among children on dialysis. Pediatr Nephrol 11:604–606, 1997

Singhi S, Singhi P, Adwani GB: Role of psychosocial stress in the cause of pica. Clin Pediatr (Phila) 20:783–785, 1981

Smith J: NTs are weird: an autistic's view of the world. 2007. Available at: http://thiswayoflife.org/blog/?p=143. Accessed May 13, 2009.

Smith J: Unexpected difficulties. 2009. Available at: http://thiswayoflife.org/unexpected.html. Accessed May 13, 2009.

Snodgrass SR, Vedanarayanan VV, Parker CC, et al: Pediatric patients with undetectable anticonvulsant blood levels: comparison with compliant patients. J Child Neurol 16:164–168, 2001

Soliday E, Hoeksel R: Health beliefs and pediatric emergency department after-care adherence. Ann Behav Med 22:299–306, 2000

Soykan I, Chen J, Kendall BJ, et al: The rumination syndrome: clinical and manometric profile, therapy, and long-term outcome. Dig Dis Sci 42:1866–1872, 1997

Steele RG, Grauer D: Adherence to antiretroviral therapy for pediatric HIV infection: review of the literature and recommendations for research. Clin Child Fam Psychol Rev 6:17–30, 2003

Steele RG, Anderson B, Rindel B, et al: Adherence to antiretroviral therapy among HIV-positive children: examination of the role of caregiver health beliefs. AIDS Care 13:617–630, 2001

Steinhausen HC, Schindler HP, Stephan H: Comparative psychiatric studies on children and adolescents suffering from cystic fibrosis and bronchial asthma. Child Psychiatry Hum Dev 14:117–130, 1983

Steward DK: Behavioral characteristics of infants with nonorganic failure to thrive during a play interaction. MCN Am J Matern Child Nurs 26:79–85, 2001

Stoddard FJ, Saxe G: Ten-year research review of physical injuries. J Am Acad Child Adolesc Psychiatry 40:1128–1145, 2001

Stratton K, Howe C, Battaglia F (eds): Fetal Alcohol Syndrome: Diagnosis, Prevention, and Treatment. Washington, DC, National Academy Press, 1996

Strauss RS, Bradley LJ, Brolin RE: Gastric bypass surgery in adolescents with morbid obesity. J Pediatr 138:499–504, 2001

Streisand R, Braniecki S, Tercyak KP, et al: Childhood illness-related parenting stress: the pediatric inventory for parents. J Pediatr Psychol 26:155–162, 2001

Streissguth AP, O'Malley K: Neuropsychiatric implications and long-term consequences of fetal alcohol spectrum disorders. Semin Clin Neuropsychiatry 5:177–190, 2000

Strunk RC, Mrazek DA, Wolfson Fuhrmann GS, et al: Psychologic and psychological characteristics associated with death due to asthma in childhood: a case-controlled study. JAMA 254:1193–1198, 1985

Strunk RC, Bender B, Young DA, et al: Predictors of protocol adherence in a pediatric asthma clinical trial. J Allergy Clin Immunol 110:596–602, 2002

Stuart S, Noyes R: Attachment and interpersonal communication in somatization. Psychosomatics 40:34–43, 1999

Stuber ML, Bursch B: Psychiatric care of the terminally ill child, in Handbook of Psychiatry in Palliative Medicine, 2nd Edition. Edited by Chochinov HM, Breitbart W. New York, Oxford University Press, 2009, pp 519–530

Stuber ML, Mesrkhani VH: "What do we tell the children?": understanding childhood grief. West J Med 174:187–191, 2001

Stunkard A, Sabal J: Psychosocial consequences of obesity, in Eating Disorders and Obesity. Edited by Brownell KD, Fairburn CG. New York, Guilford, 1995, pp 417–421

Stunkard AJ, Harris JR, Pederson NL, et al: The body-mass index of twins who have been reared apart. N Engl J Med 322:1483–1487, 1990

Swanson M, Hall D, Bartas S, et al: Economic impact of noncompliance in kidney transplant recipients. Transplant Proc 24:2723–2724, 1992

Telfair J: Factors in the long term adjustment of children and adolescents with sickle cell disease: conceptualizations and review of the literature. J Health Soc Policy 5:69–96, 1994

Terre L, Ghiselli W: A developmental perspective on family risk factors in somatization. J Psychosom Res 42:197–208, 1997

Todaro JF, Fennell EB, Sears SF, et al: Review: cognitive and psychological outcomes in pediatric heart transplantation. J Pediatr Psychol 25:567–576, 2000

Treadwell JR, Sun F, Schoelles K: Systematic review and meta-analysis of bariatric surgery for pediatric obesity. Ann Surg 248:763–776, 2008

Troiano RP, Flegal KM, Kuczmarski RJ, et al: Overweight prevalence and trends for children and adolescents: the National Health and Nutrition Examination Surveys, 1963 to 1991. Arch Pediatr Adolesc Med 149:1085–1091, 1995

Tsai SJ, Lee YC, Chang K, et al: Psychiatric consultations in pediatric inpatients. Zhonghua Min Guo Xiao Er Ke Yi Xue Hui Za Zhi 36:411–414, 1995

Tsai WS, Inge TH, Burd RS: Bariatric surgery in adolescents: recent national trends in use and in-hospital outcome. Arch Pediatr Adolesc Med 161:217–221, 2007

Tucker CM, Fennell RS, Pedersen T, et al: Associations with medication adherence among ethnically different pediatric patients with renal transplants. Pediatr Nephrol 17:251–256, 2002

Tunaoglu FS, Olgunturk R, Akcabay S, et al: Chest pain in children referred to a cardiology clinic. Pediatr Cardiol 16:69–72, 1995

Turkel SB, Miller JH, Reiff A: Case series: neuropsychiatric symptoms with pediatric systemic lupus erythematosus. J Am Acad Child Adolesc Psychiatry 40:482–485, 2001

Turkel SB, Braslow K, Tavare CJ, et al: The Delirium Rating Scale in children and adolescents. Psychosomatics 44:126–129, 2003

Uman LS, Chambers CT, McGrath PJ, et al: Psychological interventions for needle-related procedural pain and distress in children and adolescents. J Pediatr Psychol 33:842–854, 2008

United Network for Organ Sharing (UNOS): Organ by Age. Current U.S. Waiting List. Based on OPTN data as of April 16, 2010. Available at: http://optn.transplant.hrsa.gov/data/. Accessed April 26, 2010.

U.S. Food and Drug Administration: Sudden death with drugs used to treat ADHD. February 28, 2006. Available at: www.fda.gov/OHRMS/DOCKETS/AC/06/briefing/2006-4210b_07_01_safetyreview.pdf. Accessed June 28, 2009.

Uzark KC, Sauer SN, Lawrence KS, et al: The psychosocial impact of pediatric heart transplantation. J Heart Lung Transplant 11:1160, 1992

Van Horn M, DeMaso DR, Gonzalez-Heydrich J, et al: Illness-related concerns of mothers of children with congenital heart disease. J Am Acad Child Adolesc Psychiatry 40:847–854, 2001

Vasconcellos E, Pina-Garza JE, Fakhoury T, et al: Pediatric manifestations of Hashimoto's encephalopathy. Pediatr Neurol 20:394–398, 1999

Vila G, Nollet-Clemencon C, Vera M, et al: Prevalence of DSM-IV disorders in children and adolescents with asthma versus diabetes. Can J Psychiatry 44:562–569, 1999

Visconti KJ, Saudino KJ, Rappaport LA, et al: Influence of parental stress and social support on the behavioral adjustment of children with transposition of the great arteries. J Dev Behav Pediatr 23:314–321, 2002

Volkmar FR, Poll J, Lewis M: Conversion reactions in childhood and adolescence. J Am Acad Child Adolesc Psychiatry 23:424–430, 1984

Volz HP, Möller HJ, Reimann I, et al: Opipramol for the treatment of somatoform disorders: results from a placebo-controlled trial. Eur Neuropsychopharmacol 10:211–217, 2000

Volz HP, Murck, H, Kasper S, et al: St John's wort extract (LI 160) in somatoform disorders: results of a placebo-controlled trial. Psychopharmacology 164:294–300, 2002

von Weiss RT, Rapoff MA, Varni JW, et al: Daily hassles and social support as predictors of adjustment in children with pediatric rheumatic disease. J Pediatr Psychol 27:155–165, 2002

Wagaman JR, Williams DE, Camilleri M: Behavioral intervention for the treatment of rumination. J Pediatr Gastroenterol Nutr 27:596–598, 1998

Walkup JT, Albano AM, Piacentini J, et al: Cognitive behavioral therapy, sertraline, or a combination in childhood anxiety. N Engl J Med 359:2753–2766, 2008

Wallace AE, Neily J, Weeks WB, et al: A cumulative meta-analysis of selective serotonin reuptake inhibitors in pediatric depression: did unpublished studies influence the efficacy/safety debate? J Child Adolesc Psychopharmacol 16:37–58, 2006

Wamboldt MZ, Gavin L: Pulmonary disorders, in Handbook of Pediatric Psychology and Psychiatry, Vol I: Disease, Injury and Illness. Edited by Ammerman R, Campo J. Needham Heights, MA, Allyn & Bacon, 1998, pp 266–297

Wamboldt MZ, Yancey AG Jr, Roesler TA: Cardiovascular effects of tricyclic antidepressants in childhood asthma: a case series and review. J Child Adolesc Psychopharmacol 7:45–64, 1997

Wamboldt MZ, Schmitz S, Mrazek D: Genetic association between atopy and behavioral symptoms in middle childhood. J Child Psychol Psychiatry 39:1007–1016, 1998

Wamboldt MZ, Laudenslager M, Wamboldt FS, et al: Adolescents with atopic disorders have an attenuated cortisol response to laboratory stress. J Allergy Clin Immunol 111:509–514, 2003

Warady BA, Alexander SR, Watkins S, et al: Optimal care of the pediatric end-stage renal disease patient on dialysis. Am J Kidney Dis 33:567–583, 1999

Weakley MM, Petti TA, Karwisch G: Case study: chewing gum treatment of rumination in an adolescent with an eating disorder. J Am Acad Child Adolesc Psychiatry 36:1124–1127, 1997

Webster R, Holroyd S: Prevalence of psychotic symptoms in delirium. Psychosomatics 41:519–522, 2000

Weston JA, Colloton M, Halsey S, et al: A legacy of violence in nonorganic failure to thrive. Child Abuse Negl 17:709–714, 1993

Wiffen PJ, McQuay HJ, Edwards JE, et al: Gabapentin for acute and chronic pain. Cochrane Database Syst Rev (3): CD005452, 2005a

Wiffen PJ, McQuay HJ, Moore RA: Carbamazepine for acute and chronic pain. Cochrane Database Syst Rev (3):CD005451, 2005b

Wilens TE, Biederman J, Baldessarini RJ, et al: Cardiovascular effects of therapeutic doses of tricyclic antidepressants in children and adolescents. J Am Acad Child Adolesc Psychiatry 35:1491–1501, 1996

Wilfley DE, Tibbs TL, Van Buren DJ, et al: Lifestyle interventions in the treatment of childhood overweight: a meta-analytic review of randomized controlled trials. Health Psychol 26:521–532, 2007

Williams GC, Freedman ZR, Deci EL: Supporting autonomy to motivate patients with diabetes for glucose control. Diabetes Care 21:1644–1651, 1998

Williamson GM, Walters AS, Shaffer DR: Caregiver models of self and others, coping, and depression: predictors of depression in children with chronic pain. Health Psychol 21:405–410, 2002

Winton AS, Singh NN: Suppression of pica using brief-duration physical restraint. J Ment Defic Res 27(pt 2):93–103, 1983

Woods DW, Miltenberger RG, Lumley VA: A simplified habit reversal treatment for pica-related chewing. J Behav Ther Exp Psychiatry 27:257–262, 1996

Worchel FF, Nolan BF, Wilson VL, et al: Assessment of depression in children with cancer. J Pediatr Psychol 13:101–112, 1988

Wren F, Tarbell S: Feeding and growth disorders, in Handbook of Pediatric Psychology and Psychiatry, Vol I: Disease, Injury and Illness. Edited by Ammerman R, Campo J. Needham Heights, MA, Allyn & Bacon, 1998, pp 133–165

Wu YP, Roberts MC: A meta-analysis of interventions to increase adherence to medication regimens for pediatric otitis media and streptococcal pharyngitis. J Pediatr Psychol 33:789–796, 2008

Yang YM, Cepeda M, Price C, et al: Depression in children and adolescents with sickle-cell disease. Arch Pediatr Adolesc Med 148:457–460, 1994

Yanovski JA: Intensive therapies for pediatric obesity. Pediatr Clin North Am 48:1041–1053, 2001

Yi MS, Britto MT, Wilmott RW, et al: Health values of adolescents with cystic fibrosis. J Pediatr 142:133–140, 2003

Yildiz S, Savaser S, Tatlioglu GS: Evaluation of internal behaviors of children with congenital heart disease. J Pediatr Nurs 16:449–452, 2001

Young GS, Mintzer LL, Seacord D, et al: Symptoms of posttraumatic stress disorder in parents of transplant recipients: incidence, severity, and related factors. Pediatrics 111 (6 pt 1): e725–e731, 2003

Zebrack B, Zeltzer L, Whitton J, et al: Psychological outcomes in long-term survivors of childhood leukemia, Hodgkin's disease, and non-Hodgkin's lymphoma: a report from the childhood cancer survivors study. Pediatrics 110:42–52, 2002

Zeltzer LK, Bursch B, Walco GA: Pain responsiveness and chronic pain: a psychobiological perspective. J Dev Behav Pediatr 18:413–422, 1997

Zuckerman B, Stevenson J, Bailey V: Stomachaches and headaches in a community sample of preschool children. Pediatrics 79:677–682, 1987

CHAPTER

35

Physical Medicine and Rehabilitation

Jesse R. Fann, M.D., M.P.H.

Richard Kennedy, M.D.

Charles H. Bombardier, Ph.D.

PHYSICAL MEDICINE AND rehabilitation, or *rehabilitation medicine,* is concerned with helping people reach the fullest physical, psychological, social, vocational, and educational potential consistent with their physiological or anatomical impairment, environmental limitations, and desires and life plans (DeLisa et al. 1998). The patients encountered in the rehabilitation setting are highly diverse, and their problems include those listed in Table 35–1. As can be seen, the medical and surgical issues range from acute to chronic and can involve nearly any organ system. Rehabilitation can take place in outpatient, inpatient, and extended-care programs and includes both prevention and treatment of disorders. Striving for maximum independence is central to the goal of maximizing quality of life.

Rehabilitation is generally a multi- or interdisciplinary effort. Rehabilitation medicine physicians (physiatrists) usually lead the team of other specialized professionals, including physical therapists, occupational therapists, speech pathologists, clinical and neuropsychologists, vocational rehabilitation counselors, recreation therapists, social workers, and nurses. Rehabilitation programs often have a dedicated psychologist on staff whose job is to conduct psychological and neuropsychological assessments; provide counseling to patients and families; oversee behavioral programs; and generally assist staff in the management of cognitive, behavioral, affective, and social aspects of rehabilitation.

Psychiatrists have an increasing role in the care of patients in the rehabilitation setting. As advances in medical care have increased survival in many medical and traumatic conditions that previously were fatal—the so-called epidemic of survival—opportunities and challenges have emerged that did not previously exist in the rehabilitation of thousands of individuals each year. Data from the 2007 National Health Interview Survey suggest that 12% of the U.S. population has a limitation in usual activities because of one or more chronic health conditions (Adams et al. 2008). For the first time, *Healthy People 2010: Understanding and Improving Health* (U.S. Department of Health and Human Services 2001), the national agenda for improving the health of Americans, included a chapter on "Disability and Secondary Conditions," acknowledging that disability is a critical risk factor for many other health-related conditions.

The World Health Organization has shifted its framework for classifying functioning, health, and health-related states from an emphasis on "consequences of disease" found in the previous *International Classification of Impairments, Disabilities and Handicaps* (World Health Organi-

Work on this chapter was funded by grants from the National Institutes of Health (R21HD053736) and the National Institute on Disability and Rehabilitation Research (H133G070016, H133N060033).

TABLE 35–1. Problems treated in rehabilitation medicine

Stroke
Traumatic brain injury
Multiple sclerosis
Spinal cord injury
Degenerative movement disorders
Cancer
Human immunodeficiency virus and acquired immunodeficiency syndrome
Cardiac disease
Respiratory dysfunction
Chronic pain
Spinal and muscle pain
Osteoporosis
Rheumatological disorders
Peripheral vascular disease
Peripheral neuropathy and myopathy
Motor neuron diseases
Burn injury
Organ transplantation
Sports injuries
Occupational disorders
Cumulative trauma disorders
Total hip and knee replacements
Hand trauma and disorders
Visual impairment
Hearing impairment
Vestibular disorders

zation 1980) to an emphasis on "components of health" in the current *International Classification of Functioning, Disability and Health* (ICF; World Health Organization 2001). The ICF conceptually differentiates health and health-related components of the disabling process at the levels of 1) *body structures* (anatomical parts of the body, such as organs, limbs, and their components) and *functions* (physiological functions of body systems, including psychological functions) and 2) *activities* (execution of a task or an action by an individual) and *participation* (involvement in a life situation). The ICF defines *impairments* as problems in body function or structure, such as a significant deviation or loss, and focuses on *activity limitations* rather than disabilities and *participation limitations* rather than handicaps. A further change has been the inclusion of a section on *environmental factors* as part of the classification, with the recognition of the important role of environment in either facilitating functioning or creating barriers for people with disabilities. Environmental factors interact with a health condition to restore functioning or create a disability, depending on whether the environmental factor is a facilitator or barrier. Figure 35–1 illustrates the interactive and dynamic dimensions of this model. The ICF puts the burden of all diseases and health conditions, including mental illness, on an equal footing. Psychosocial factors can cause impairment and limit activities and participation in many ways, thus affording opportunities for multifaceted psychosocial interventions in the rehabilitation setting.

In this chapter, we focus on the psychiatric issues encountered in the treatment of traumatic brain injury (TBI) and spinal cord injury (SCI), two common and highly complex rehabilitation problems with aspects that may require psychiatric intervention. Although many of the other disorders encountered in the rehabilitation setting are covered in other chapters of this text, many of the principles discussed in this chapter also apply to them.

Traumatic Brain Injury

Epidemiology

TBI is a significant problem from both an individual and a public health perspective. An estimated 1.7 million Americans sustain TBI each year; of these, approximately 275,000 are hospitalized and survive, 1.365 million are treated and released from an emergency department, and 52,000 die (Faul et al. 2010). These figures likely underestimate the incidence of TBI as a result of underreporting of milder injuries. According to data from hospitalized individuals, at least 5.3 million persons in the United States, or about 2% of the population, live with disabilities resulting from TBI (Thurman et al. 1999). Although about 75% of TBIs are mild in severity, many of these individuals experience long-term somatic and psychiatric problems that may lead to disability (Brown et al. 1994; Guerrero et al. 2000). TBI is often referred to as the *invisible epidemic* because TBI-related disabilities are not readily visible to the general public.

With improved medical care, TBI mortality and hospitalizations have declined 20% and 50%, respectively, since 1980 (Thurman et al. 1999), leading to more long-term morbidity and disability. Decreases in TBI mortality also have been seen in military injuries because of advances in body armor (Okie 2005). The peak incidence of TBI is in 0- to 4-year-old and 15- to 19-year-old persons (mostly from falls and motor vehicle accidents, respectively), with a secondary peak among those 65 years and older (mostly from falls).

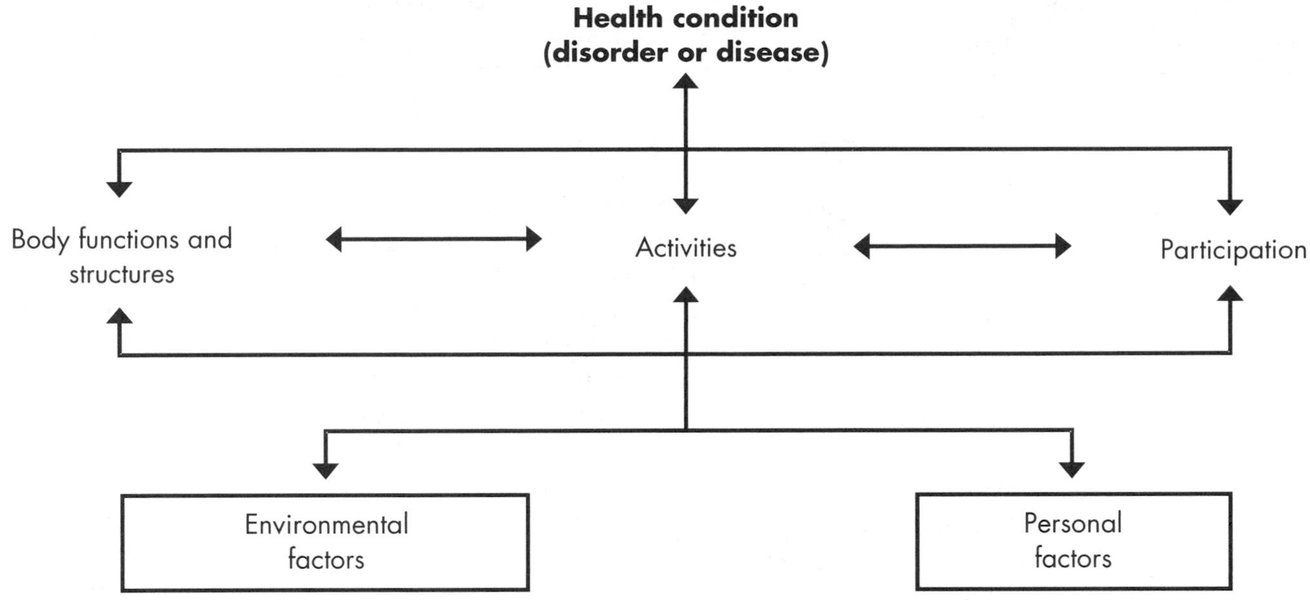

FIGURE 35–1. Interactions between components of health as defined in the *International Classification of Functioning, Disability and Health.*

Source. Reprinted from World Health Organization: *International Classification of Functioning, Disability and Health: ICF.* Geneva, Switzerland, World Health Organization, 2001. Used with permission.

Early studies differentiated between military and civilian injuries, with injuries to military personnel outside of combat zones more closely resembling the latter than the former. TBI sustained during combat was noted to be predominantly posterior injuries to the occipital and parietal lobes, whereas civilian TBI was noted to be predominantly anterior injuries to the frontal and temporal lobes. The incidence of penetrating TBI among military groups also was higher than that among civilian groups. These findings have not held up in recent conflicts. Blast injuries are now the predominant cause of injury among personnel in combat zones (Warden et al. 2006), which present with a more diffuse form of TBI (Ritenour and Baskin 2008) that some experts categorize as being distinct from both penetrating and nonpenetrating injuries in civilians (Arciniegas and McAllister 2008). However, penetrating injuries are still more common in military than in civilian settings (Galarneau et al. 2008). The demographics of those injured in current military operations are thought to reflect the overall demographics of those deployed, with most of those injured younger than 30 years (Hoge et al. 2008; Vasterling et al. 2006).

Because TBI affects a predominantly younger population, the effects of disability are much greater than for illnesses occurring later in life. Approximately one in four adults with TBI is unable to return to work 1 year after injury (Centers for Disease Control and Prevention 1999), and approximately 43% of the individuals hospitalized for TBI have long-term disability (Selassie et al. 2008). In the United States in 2000, direct and indirect costs of TBI totaled an estimated $60 billion (Finkelstein et al. 2006). Figures show that the total acute care and rehabilitation costs of TBI are $9–$10 billion per year (National Institutes of Health Consensus Development Panel on Rehabilitation of Persons With Traumatic Brain Injury 1999), and about $13.5 billion is necessary for continuing care of those who experienced TBI in previous years (J.F. Kraus and McArthur 1999). About 65% of TBI-related costs are accrued among survivors. Statistics from 1985 estimate that TBI-related work loss and disability cost approximately $20.6 billion (Max et al. 1991); this figure would be much higher today because of the rapid increase in the number of individuals with TBI surviving their injury but requiring supportive care (J.F. Kraus and McArthur 1999). Similar results have been reported among the military for recent conflicts, with the estimated total cost of $600–$900 million in the first year after diagnosis of TBI (Tanielian and Jaycox 2008). Long-term disability has primarily been attributed to psychiatric disorders and to behavior problems such as irritability (Sander et al. 1997; Whelan-Goodinson et al. 2008). Finally, self-reported TBI appears to be more frequent among psychiatric inpatients compared with the general population, with rates of approximately 66% in studies examining the issue (Burg et al. 1996, 2000). Thus, many psychiatrists will be involved in some level in the care of individuals with TBI.

Severity Classification

Original severity classifications for TBI focused on the Glasgow Coma Scale (GCS) (Jennett and Bond 1975) because of its widespread use. A TBI with a low postresuscitation GCS score of 3–8 is considered severe, 9–12 is moderate, and 13–15 is mild. However, although the GCS is useful for predicting mortality after TBI, it has less utility in predicting level of disability and neurobehavioral outcome, particularly at the upper end of the scale. It is recognized that individuals with GCS scores of 13–15 are quite heterogeneous in terms of levels of impairment and outcome (Dikmen et al. 2001; Saatman et al. 2008; Williams et al. 1990). Durations of coma and of posttraumatic amnesia are also used to describe TBI severity. These variables are difficult to determine in the civilian and combat setting, making TBI ascertainment and severity classification problematic.

The American Congress of Rehabilitation Medicine has put forth a definition of mild TBI that is widely used, requiring at least one of the following: 1) loss of consciousness (LOC) of 30 minutes or less, with an initial GCS score of 13–15; 2) posttraumatic amnesia of 24 hours or less; 3) presence of any alteration of mental state at the time of the injury (e.g., feeling dazed, disoriented, or confused); or 4) a focal neurological deficit (Kay et al. 1993). Patients with a GCS score of 13–15 who have imaging evidence of intracranial pathology have outcomes more similar to those of moderate TBI and are often classified as "complicated mild" injuries (see Williams et al. 1990).

Functional Pathophysiology

There has been considerable progress in understanding the pathophysiological mechanisms of TBI in recent years. The physical forces in TBI initiate mechanical and chemical changes that lead to neurological dysfunction. These are divided into *primary damage,* which occurs at the moment of injury, and *secondary damage,* which is initiated at injury but evolves over time. The latter is subdivided into direct injury, occurring within the neuron itself, and indirect injury, occurring outside the neuron but affecting its function.

Primary damage consists of injuries such as skull fractures, brain contusions and lacerations, and intracranial hemorrhage (McIntosh et al. 1996). Because these occur at the time of injury, the key treatment is prevention. Diffuse axonal injury is the predominant mechanism of injury in most cases of TBI (Meythaler et al. 2001), with shearing forces resulting in temporary or permanent disruption of axonal function. Diffuse axonal injury can evolve over a period of 24–72 hours after injury (Povlishock et al. 1983), making it potentially responsive to pharmacological intervention; however, no currently used therapeutic modality is known to influence its progression (Doppenberg and Bullock 1997).

Direct secondary injury occurs via neurochemical changes evolving over time after the mechanical disruption of neuronal pathways (McIntosh et al. 1996). The acute phase of this process has been well described, with a global increase in cerebral metabolism after injury (Bergsneider et al. 2001; Yoshino et al. 1991). This is accompanied by a period of excessive activity of neurotransmitters, including acetylcholine, glutamate, dopamine, norepinephrine, and various growth factors (Hayes et al. 1992; McIntosh et al. 1996). This may lead to abnormal activation of receptors, causing changes in intracellular signaling that lead to long-lasting modifications of cell function (Hamm et al. 2000). In addition, excessive transmitter activity may have direct neurotoxic effects, leading to apoptosis and permanent dysfunction. A key event in the early phase of injury is excessive influx of calcium (Gennarelli and Graham 1998), which may lead to gene activation, triggering preprogrammed cell death and enzyme activation, leading to damage to the cellular cytoskeleton and free radical generation.

The neurochemical changes in the subacute phase of TBI have been less intensively investigated, but current evidence indicates that this phase is associated with a dramatic reversal of acute processes. Cerebral metabolism and function of many neurotransmitters, including glutamate, acetylcholine, dopamine, and norepinephrine, become depressed (Hamm et al. 2000; Hayes and Dixon 1994); given the prominence of these neurotransmitters in psychiatric disorders, these alterations would potentially account for cognitive and neurobehavioral deficits in TBI. Research in animal models of TBI has successfully identified pharmacotherapies to reduce behavioral and histological complications (Marklund et al. 2006). However, clinical investigations of such agents have been disappointing (Wang et al. 2006). Interventions explored include anticholinergics, cholinomimetics, anti-inflammatory agents, calcium channel blockers, free radical scavengers, glutamate antagonists, and hypothermia (Beauchamp et al. 2008; Kokiko and Hamm 2007).

Psychiatric Disorders in Traumatic Brain Injury

Although useful data have been collected regarding the epidemiology of psychiatric disorders after TBI, the numbers of studies and subjects for each disorder remain small. Other limitations of many studies include selection bias (examining only hospitalized subjects or those referred for psychiatric evaluation), varying assessment periods, use of unstructured psychiatric interviews, and limited assessment of premorbid psychiatric history (Van Reekum et al. 2000). Such factors lead to wide variation in the estimates of incidence and prevalence of psychiatric disorders after TBI. Other complex disturbances seen after TBI are not adequately captured by current diagnostic systems such as DSM-IV-TR (American Psychiatric Association 2000). Some symptoms, such as fatigue or impulsivity, may cause significant impairment but may not fit into a specific diagnosis. Also, individuals with TBI may lack insight into, and not report, their deficits. Psychiatrists may give greater weight to the reports of family and treating clinicians for this reason. However, family ratings may be influenced by other factors, including caregiver personality characteristics (McKinlay and Brooks 1984). Similarly, the clinician's emotional response to the patient may interfere with accurate assessment of deficits (Heilbronner et al. 1989). In addition to these general concerns, there may be differences in the presentation and phenomenology of specific disorders in the context of TBI.

The development of psychiatric disorders involves a complex interplay between premorbid biological and psychological factors, postinjury biological changes, and psychosocial and environmental factors. The role of many risk factors has yet to be well elucidated, and many are specific to a given disorder. A review by Rao and Lyketsos (2002) compiled risk factors for the development of psychiatric sequelae in general (Table 35–2). These are divided into highly significant risk factors (sufficient evidence exists for their role in psychiatric disorders) and less significant risk factors (evidence is still controversial). In a large unselected primary care population, Fann et al. (2004) found psychiatric history to be a highly significant risk factor for psychiatric illness in the 3 years following TBI. Their data suggested that moderate to severe TBI may be associated with higher initial risk for psychiatric problems, whereas mild TBI and prior psychiatric illness may increase the risk for more persistent psychiatric problems. The authors hypothesized that psychiatric symptoms that arise immediately after TBI may be etiologically related to the neurophysiological effects of the injury, consistent with the early relation between TBI severity and psychiatric risk, whereas other factors, such as psychological vulnerability, self-awareness of deficits, social influences, and secondary gain, may play roles over time, particularly in individuals with prior psychiatric illness and prior injury.

The role of TBI in the etiology of psychiatric disorders after TBI may have significant implications for prognosis and treatment, as well as medicolegal ramifications (Van Reekum et al. 2001). Although several psychiatric disorders are common after TBI, establishing a causal link between these remains difficult. Both Van Reekum et al. (2000, 2001) and Rogers and Read (2007) noted that some evidence for causality exists, in that studies (particularly in experimental animals) have shown that TBI disrupts neuronal systems involved in mood and behavior. However, other lines of evidence are inconclusive. The following suggestive findings point to other possible associations: 1) the psychiatric disorder increases the risk for TBI (Fann et al. 2002); 2) the risk for both TBI and the psychiatric disorder is due to a common third factor, such as substance abuse; and 3) a postinjury condition, such as pain or change in family status, contributes to the psychiatric disorder. Evidence for a biological gradient, in which more severe injuries are associated with higher risk for psychiatric disorders, is mixed. There is also a lack of specificity: TBI has been postulated to cause a variety of psychiatric disorders and conditions rather than a single specific syndrome. Assigning TBI as the definitive cause of psychiatric disturbances in most instances is not possible under current evidence.

TABLE 35–2. Risk factors for psychiatric illness after traumatic brain injury

Highly significant risk factors
Preinjury psychiatric history
Preinjury social impairments
Increased age
Alcohol abuse
Arteriosclerosis
Less significant risk factors
More severe injury
Poor neuropsychological functioning
Marital discord
Financial instability
Poor interpersonal relationships
Low preinjury level of education
Compensation claims
Female gender
Short time since injury
Lesion location (especially left prefrontal)

Source. Adapted from Rao and Lyketsos 2002.

Depression

Several studies have used structured interviews to examine rates of depression. Fann et al. (1995) used the National Institute of Mental Health Diagnostic Interview Schedule (DIS) to assess 50 consecutive outpatients presenting to a rehabilitation clinic for evaluation of TBI. Of these, 26% received the diagnosis of major depression, and another 28% had had major depression with onset after injury that had since resolved. Hibbard et al. (1998) administered the Structured Clinical Interview for DSM-IV (SCID) to 100 patients with TBI who were randomly selected from a larger quality-of-life study. Depression was found in 61%, with the onset of depression after injury in 48%. Deb et al.

(1999) examined 164 outpatients previously admitted to the emergency department with a diagnosis of TBI. Assessment based on the Schedules for Clinical Assessment in Neuropsychiatry (SCAN) indicated that the rate of depression was 18%. Ashman et al. (2004) administered the SCID to 188 outpatients 3 months to 4 years after injury as part of a longitudinal follow-up of TBI. Major depression was present in 20% of patients before injury and in 24%–35% of patients during the first year of follow-up. Levin et al. (2005) prospectively followed up 239 consecutive subjects admitted with a diagnosis of mild TBI; of the 129 returning for follow-up at 3 months, 11.6% met criteria for major depression according to the SCID. Among the estimated 20% of Iraq and Afghanistan veterans who sustain a TBI, 7.3% report both TBI and posttraumatic stress disorder (PTSD) or depression, and 5% report all three conditions (Tanielian and Jaycox 2008). Among army soldiers with mild TBI with and without LOC, 23% and 8%, respectively, had major depression, compared with 7% with other injuries and 3% with no injuries (Hoge et al. 2008). Bryant et al. (2010) reported on 1,084 randomly selected admissions to four Australian trauma centers. Using the Mini International Neuropsychiatric Interview (MINI; Sheehan et al. 1998), 16% of patients were diagnosed with major depression at 12 months, with 11.6% being new onset after TBI. Bombardier et al. (2010) examined 559 consecutive admissions to a single trauma center with complicated mild to severe TBI. Assessments with the nine-item Patient Health Questionnaire (PHQ-9; Kroenke et al. 2001) at 1- to 2-month intervals identified 53.1% of patients with major depression during the 12-month follow-up period. Point prevalence ranged between 31% at 1 month and 21% at 6 months. Fann et al. (2005) found that the PHQ-9 was highly correlated with the SCID diagnosis of depression and other measures of depressive symptoms. Use of the criteria of at least five PHQ-9 symptoms being present for at least several days over the past 2 weeks, with at least one symptom being depressed mood or anhedonia, showed excellent operating characteristics with a sensitivity of 93% and a specificity of 89% for major depression.

In a systematic examination of depression after TBI, Federoff et al. (1992) examined 66 consecutive trauma center admissions with the Present State Examination (PSE), a forerunner of the SCAN. Approximately 1 month after injury, 26% had symptoms that met criteria for major depression. Jorge et al. (1993a, 1993b) carried out follow-up examinations on this cohort. At 3 months after injury, 12 of 54 patients (22%) had major depression; at 6 months, 10 of 43 (23%) had major depression; and at 12 months, 8 of 43 (19%) had major depression. Although the prevalence of depression remained fairly stable, some individuals had resolution of depression during the course of the year, whereas others had onset of depression. Of the 41 patients without depression seen for follow-up, 11 (27%) developed depression during the study: 4 (10%) at 3 months, 4 (10%) at 6 months, and 3 (7%) at 12 months. Jorge et al. (2004) subsequently replicated these results in another cohort of 91 consecutive hospital admissions for TBI, showing 33% of the patients developing major depression during the first year after injury: 17% at initial evaluation, 10% at 3 months, and 6% at 6 months. Dikmen et al. (2004) followed up 283 consecutive hospital admissions with complicated mild to severe TBI with the Center for Epidemiological Studies Depression (CES-D) Scale. At 1 month postinjury, 46% of the subjects had at least mild depression. The rates declined to 35% at 6 months and remained stable at approximately 30% at 1 and 3–5 years postinjury.

Kreutzer et al. (2001) examined the scores of 722 outpatient referrals for neuropsychological evaluation with the Neurobehavioral Functioning Inventory (NFI), which assesses a wide range of functions after TBI. By mapping 37 of the NFI items to DSM-IV-TR (American Psychiatric Association 2000) diagnostic criteria, the authors reported that the prevalence of depression was 42%. A subsequent study (Seel et al. 2003) that used the same methodology in 666 patients at 17 TBI Model Systems centers found a rate of 27%. These studies had large sample sizes, but it remains unclear how the authors' mapping of NFI items corresponds with the diagnosis of depression on the basis of DSM-IV criteria in a clinical interview.

In their cohort, Jorge et al. (1993b) noted no difference between depressed and nondepressed patients with respect to demographic variables, type or severity of TBI, family history of psychiatric disorder, or degree of physical or cognitive impairment. Those with depression were significantly more likely to have a premorbid history of psychiatric disorders, including substance abuse. Subjects with depression had significantly poorer social functioning prior to injury, and poor social functioning was the strongest and most consistent correlate of depression on follow-up. Findings from their later cohort were generally consistent with these observations, except that individuals with depression were not more likely than individuals without depression to have a history of substance abuse (Jorge et al. 2004). In their original study (Federoff et al. 1992), depression at 1 month was strongly associated with lesions in the left dorsolateral frontal and/or left basal ganglia regions on computed tomography (CT) scanning. Right parieto-occipital lesions were associated with depression to a lesser extent. Pure cortical lesions were associated with a decreased probability of depression. However, no relation was found between lesion location and depression in subsequent follow-ups (Jorge et al. 1993a). In their later study (Jorge et al. 2004), major depression was associated with reduced volume in the left prefrontal cortex at 3-month follow-up. Replication is needed to confirm these correlations.

Fann et al. (2004) found that patients with mild TBI had a higher risk for mood disorders (including depressive and anxiety disorders) than did patients with moderate to severe TBI (e.g., relative risk = 2.7 vs. 1.0 in the first 6 months following TBI) among 939 health maintenance organization enrollees with TBI. This finding is consistent with other reports that more severe TBI is not necessarily associated with a higher risk of depression (Fann et al. 1995; Hibbard et al. 1998). Dikmen et al. (2004) also found no relation between injury severity and risk for major depression but did find that less education, an unstable preinjury work history, and alcohol abuse increased the risk. Levin et al. (2005) noted that increasing age, presence of CT abnormalities, and higher CES-D scores at 1 week were strong predictors of major depression at 3 months. Finally, Bombardier et al. (2010) identified presence of major depression at the time of injury, history of major depression prior to injury, older age, and lifetime history of alcohol dependence as risk factors for major depression after TBI. Half of patients with MDD in the year following TBI were depressed within the first 3 months. These findings suggest that early evaluation for depressive symptoms can be helpful in identifying patients at risk for subsequent depression and that preventive measures may be useful in select subgroups of patients with mild TBI.

Early studies of major depression showed high rates of vegetative symptoms among individuals with TBI that exceeded the reported rate of depression in these patients. These symptoms included psychomotor slowing, reported at 67%–74% (Cavallo et al. 1992; McKinlay et al. 1981); difficulty concentrating, 38%–88% (Cavallo et al. 1992; Oddy et al. 1978b); fatigue, 33%–71% (Cavallo et al. 1992; Oddy et al. 1978b); insomnia, 27%–56% (Fichtenberg et al. 2001); and decreased interest, 21%–55% (Oddy et al. 1978b; Thomsen 1984). Although these investigations did not include a structured psychiatric assessment, the findings raised concern about the validity of using physical symptoms in the diagnosis of depression after TBI. The "inclusive," "etiological," "substitutive," and "exclusive" approaches used in the medically ill have similar advantages and disadvantages in the TBI population. Although no studies have compared these approaches per se in TBI, Jorge et al. (1993a) did use a similar methodology to explore this issue. They found that TBI patients who reported depressed mood had higher rates of both physical and psychological symptoms of depression (as assessed with the PSE) than did those without depressed mood. The group with depressed mood also endorsed more DSM-III-R (American Psychiatric Association 1987) symptoms of major depression than did those without depressed mood. The symptoms of suicidal ideation, inappropriate guilt, anergia, psychomotor agitation, and weight loss or poor appetite occurred with significantly greater frequency in the depressed group. Studies from patients with other forms of brain injury are similarly encouraging for the use of DSM diagnostic criteria. Paradiso et al. (1997) examined patients with acute stroke; the frequency of major depression was 18% by the inclusive strategy and 22% by the substitutive strategy. Dikmen et al. (2004) found that depressed affect and lack of positive affect, as well as somatic symptoms, contributed to elevated scores on the CES-D among subjects with major depression. R.E. Kennedy et al. (2005) compared the NFI depression subscale scores of subjects with and without a diagnosis of major depression according to the SCID. The highest between-group differences were not restricted to vegetative symptoms but included psychological symptoms such as loss of pleasure, being uncomfortable around others, feelings of hopelessness, and lack of confidence. Thus, it appears that the diagnosis of major depression can be accurately made with DSM criteria in brain-injured patients.

The course of major depression is the best described of disorders that develop after TBI. Jorge et al. (1993b) found that the mean duration of depression was 4.7 months. Subjects with anxious depression had a significantly longer duration of symptoms than did those with depression and no anxiety (7.5 months vs. 1.5 months). In their follow-up study, 33% of the patients met criteria for major depression during the year after injury. In half of these patients, the depression developed acutely; in the other half, the depression was of delayed onset. The mean duration of depression was 4.7 months for those who received antidepressants and 5.8 months for those who did not. Bombardier et al. (2010) found that among patients depressed within the first 3 months of injury, the median duration of depression was 4 months, with 27% depressed for only 1 month and 36% depressed for 6 months or more. Collectively, these data show that the onset of depression is not immediately linked to the occurrence of TBI in a significant number of individuals and that the duration of depression varies widely.

Mania

The prevalence of bipolar disorder after TBI is difficult to determine because most reports have been single cases or small case series. Varney et al. (1987) noted that 5% of their sample met the criteria for manic episodes, although it is unclear how many of these cases of mania predated the injury. A prevalence of 2% was reported by Hibbard et al. (1998), with all occurring after TBI; and Jorge et al. (1993c) reported that 9% of their subjects met the criteria for mania at some point during the year after injury. In contrast, none of the subjects developed bipolar disorder in the study by Fann et al. (1995). Thus, although TBI may increase the risk for developing bipolar disorder, it still appears to be a relatively rare consequence of injury.

Phenomenologically, all forms of bipolar disorder, including bipolar I, bipolar II, and rapid-cycling variants, have been reported (McAllister 1992). The largest study addressing this topic suggested that patients are more likely to present with irritable than with euphoric mood (Shukla et al. 1987). Shukla et al. (1987) observed that mania after TBI was associated with posttraumatic seizures but not with family history of bipolar disorder. Jorge et al. (1993c) noted that mania after TBI was significantly related to basopolar temporal lesions but was not associated with type or severity of TBI, degree of physical or intellectual impairment, family or personal history of psychiatric illness, or posttraumatic epilepsy. They also reported on the course of mania occurring in their subjects. Of the six cases of subjects developing mania after TBI, five occurred within 3 months after injury and one within 6 months after injury. The duration of the manic episode was only 2 months, but elevated or expansive mood persisted for a mean of 5.7 months. These limited data suggest that episodes of bipolar disorder may occur soon after TBI. Its duration is relatively brief, although patients may have subsyndromal disturbances present after mania resolves.

Anxiety

A continuing topic of interest and controversy has been the development of acute stress disorder and PTSD after TBI. Early opinion was that PTSD could not develop after TBI; investigators argued that LOC or posttraumatic amnesia would prevent patients from having reexperiencing and avoidance because memories were not encoded (Harvey et al. 2003). This hypothesis was supported by the studies of Mayou et al. (1993), Sbordone and Liter (1995), and Warden et al. (1997), each noting that none of their sample who had LOC during injury went on to develop PTSD. However, the first two studies relied on clinical interviews to determine PTSD, and the last used a modified version of the PSE, which assessed only two of the five criterion B (reexperiencing) symptoms. Thus, some experts have raised legitimate concerns that these studies did not adequately assess for PTSD.

Studies with more detailed, structured assessments of PTSD have yielded different results. Hibbard et al. (1998) noted that 19% of their subjects had symptoms that met criteria for PTSD. Mayou et al. (2000) examined consecutive admissions to an emergency department with the PTSD Symptom Scale, another structured interview providing DSM-IV diagnosis. Ten of the 21 subjects (48%) with definite LOC met the criteria for PTSD at 3 months, compared with 9 of 39 (23%) with probable LOC and 179 of 796 (22%) without LOC. At 1-year follow-up, the rates of PTSD were 33%, 14%, and 17%, respectively. Levin et al. (2001) interviewed a sample of 69 patients with mild to moderate TBI drawn from admissions to a major trauma center. Of the patients, 12% received diagnoses of PTSD at 3 months according to the SCID, which was identical to the rate in general trauma control subjects. Ashman et al. (2004) found that 10% of their subjects met criteria for PTSD prior to injury, with 18%–30% meeting criteria during the first year of follow-up. Bombardier et al. (2006) prospectively examined 125 consecutive hospital admissions with complicated mild to severe TBI over 6 months with the PTSD Checklist–Civilian version (PCL-C). Only 5.6% of the subjects met full DSM-IV criteria for PTSD. The highest rates of PTSD symptoms (11.3%) were observed in the first month after injury, with a gradual attenuation of symptoms in the remaining months. This suggests that other studies that use referral samples may overestimate the prevalence of PTSD. Among military personnel, Hoge et al. (2008) found that 44% of those with mild TBI who reported LOC met criteria for PTSD, compared with 27% of those who reported mild TBI with altered mental status but no LOC, 16% of those with injuries other than TBI, and 9% of those with no injury.

Harvey and Bryant (1998) reported on 79 consecutive hospital admissions with mild TBI. According to the Acute Stress Disorder Interview, a structured clinical interview based on DSM-IV symptoms of acute stress disorder, 14% fulfilled diagnostic criteria. Of these subjects, 71 participated in follow-up at 6 months (Bryant and Harvey 1998), undergoing assessment with the PTSD module of the Composite International Diagnostic Interview, and 50 in follow-up at 2 years (Harvey and Bryant 2000). Rates of PTSD were 25% at 6 months and 22% at 2 years. Bryant et al. (2000) also examined 96 subjects drawn from admissions to a brain injury rehabilitation unit with severe TBI. Approximately 27% of the subjects met criteria for PTSD on the basis of the PTSD Interview; however, again, subjects were not consecutive admissions, and these data cannot be used to estimate overall prevalence of PTSD after TBI. In the largest study to date, Broomhall et al. (2009) used the Clinician-Administered PTSD Scale to examine 1,116 subjects consecutively admitted to the hospital with mild TBI. Approximately 4.6% of the subjects met criteria for acute stress disorder, again indicating that the rates of noncombat PTSD may be artificially inflated with referral samples or nonconsecutive admissions. Bryant et al. (2010) reported that 9.7% of their 1,084 patients had PTSD at 12 months, with 7% of these cases being new onset. Several of these studies also examined risk factors for, and the phenomenology of, PTSD. Bryant and Harvey (1998) noted that 82% of the mild TBI patients who met criteria for acute stress disorder went on to develop PTSD, whereas only 11% of those without acute stress disorder eventually developed PTSD. It is not entirely clear whether memory of the traumatic event is necessary for the development of PTSD. In some cases, those who are "amnestic" for the event will actually have "islands" of traumatic memories that are involved in PTSD. In other cases, patients who do not recall their injury may develop PTSD around traumatic experiences involved in hospitalization, which they do recall. However, patients with mild TBI initially may have low rates of posttraumatic symptoms such as intrusive memories, but these may increase over time to meet criteria for PTSD (Bryant and Harvey 1999). Among those with severe TBI, Bryant et al. (2000) noted that the overwhelming majority of patients with PTSD did not have nightmares or intrusive memories but met reexperiencing criteria on the basis of marked psychological distress in response to reminders of the trauma. This area clearly warrants further investigation to determine the appropriateness of a PTSD diagnosis for such individuals.

It seems rather certain that those who do have memories of traumatic events are at increased risk for developing PTSD and should be monitored accordingly (Hiott and Labbate 2002). This is supported by the study of Gil et al. (2005), which prospectively examined 120 subjects with mild TBI for the development of PTSD. Memory of the traumatic event significantly increased the risk of developing PTSD; 23% of the subjects with memory of the traumatic event received a diagnosis of PTSD at 6 months postinjury, compared with only 6% of those without such memory. The differing rates of diagnosis were largely explained by differences in reexperiencing symptoms between subjects with and without memory of the traumatic event. Such findings are particularly important in light of research suggesting that PTSD occurring after TBI may be less likely to remit spontaneously, with more than 80% of the patients meeting criteria for acute stress disorder having PTSD on reassessment 2 years later (Harvey and Bryant 2000).

Bombardier et al. (2006) noted that being assaulted, feeling terrified or helpless at the time of the injury, and having stimulant (cocaine or amphetamine) intoxication increased the risk for developing PTSD. Lower levels of education also were associated with increased risk for PTSD, although it is unclear if this association would remain after the study controlled for other factors. Gil et al. (2005) found that acute posttraumatic symptoms, presence of depressive or anxiety disorders, and history of psychiatric illness increased the risk for PTSD. Among military personnel, Schneiderman et al. (2008) found that mild TBI approximately doubled the risk of PTSD among recently returned service members. In contrast, a recent review (Institute of Medicine 2008) found only limited or suggestive evidence of a link between mild TBI and PTSD among Gulf War veterans; the reasons for these discrepant findings are unclear but may relate to differing mechanisms of injury. Finally, Vanderploeg et al. (2009) noted that subsequent mild TBI was associated with a significantly increased risk for persistence of PTSD symptoms among Vietnam War–era veterans compared with those who did not experience TBI.

Overall, the evidence indicates that PTSD is a common occurrence after TBI; however, the precise incidence is less certain, particularly for more severe injuries with posttraumatic amnesia. Individuals with acute stress disorder and other psychiatric disorders appear particularly vulnerable to the development of PTSD and should be monitored accordingly.

Other anxiety disorders also may be fairly common, although the number of investigations into this topic remains quite small. Fann et al. (1995) found that 24% of subjects met the criteria for generalized anxiety disorder (GAD) and 4% had panic disorder after TBI. In the follow-up study by Jorge et al. (1993b), 23 (76.7%) of the patients with major depression also met criteria for comorbid anxiety disorder, compared with 9 (20.4%) of the patients without major depression. Bombardier et al. (2010) reported that patients with TBI who were depressed were 9 times more likely to have a panic or other anxiety disorder compared with those who were not depressed. Hibbard et al. (1998) reported rates of 14% for obsessive-compulsive disorder (OCD), 11% for panic disorder, 7% for phobias, and 8% for GAD after injury. Deb et al. (1999) noted that 9% of their subjects had panic disorder, 3% had GAD, 2% had OCD, and 1% had phobias. Ashman et al. (2004) found that 16% of their subjects met criteria for other anxiety disorders besides PTSD prior to injury, with 19%–27% having other anxiety disorders during the first year of follow-up. Finally, Bryant et al. (2010) reported rates of 11.1% for GAD, 9.7% for agoraphobia, 6.9% for social phobia, 5.9% for panic disorder, and 3.5% for OCD at 12 months postinjury. The paucity of studies precludes any firm statements about risk factors for the development of anxiety disorders other than PTSD.

Psychosis

Relatively few studies have examined psychosis after TBI. Davison and Bagley (1969) reviewed eight studies before 1960, which showed that between 0.7% and 9.8% of the patients with TBI had a schizophrenia-like psychosis (although diagnosis was not based on structured criteria). In a different approach, Wilcox and Nasrallah (1987) performed a retrospective review of 659 hospital admissions and found a significantly higher rate of prior head trauma in patients with schizophrenia compared with control subjects admitted for depression, mania, or general surgery. However, this study would not allow causal inferences to be made. Malaspina et al. (2001) examined 1,830 individuals who were first-degree relatives of patients with schizophrenia or bipolar disorder. Compared with other first-degree relatives, those individuals with a history of TBI were significantly more likely to develop schizophrenia. This suggested a synergistic relation between schizophrenia and TBI, in which familial factors among schizophrenic patients and their relatives increased the risk of TBI, and TBI further increased the risk of schizophrenia in those with genetic vulnerability.

Only a few studies have examined other forms of psychosis. Violon and DeMol (1987) performed a retrospective review of 530 patients with TBI admitted to a neurosurgical unit, noting that 3% had delusions during follow-up. Koponen et al. (2002) noted that three patients (5%) in their sample met criteria for delusional disorder, and one (2%) met criteria for psychotic disorder not otherwise specified. Fann et al. (2004) also found a higher rate of psychotic disorders among patients with TBI, compared with matched non-TBI control subjects, especially in those with moderate to severe TBI and with prior psychiatric illness.

Risk factors and phenomenology are similarly understudied. Sachdev et al. (2001) compared symptoms of 45 patients with TBI and psychosis with symptoms of 45 patients with TBI but no psychosis. They noted that auditory hallucinations and paranoid delusions were more common than negative symptoms. Fujii and Ahmed (2002) reviewed descriptions of psychosis after TBI in 69 patients from 39 publications, with particular emphasis on studies that used neuroimaging or neurophysiological measures. Delusions, most commonly persecutory, were much more common than hallucinations, and hallucinations were more likely to be observed in delayed-onset psychosis. Negative symptoms seen in schizophrenia were relatively uncommon.

In their review, Davison and Bagley (1969) identified several risk factors for psychosis, including left hemisphere and temporal lobe lesions, closed head injury, and increasing severity of TBI. Others have noted that more extensive brain injury, greater cognitive impairment, male gender, and having TBI in childhood were associated with psychosis (Fujii and Ahmed 2002; Sachdev et al. 2001).

Electroencephalogram abnormalities (especially in the temporal lobe) were common, and the rates of seizure disorders among individuals with psychosis after TBI were much higher than estimates for the rates of seizures after TBI in general (Fujii and Ahmed 2002). Neuroimaging lesions (predominantly in the frontal and temporal lobes) were also frequent. Finally, the severity and duration of psychosis occurring after TBI may be less than those of idiopathic psychotic disorders, with only about one-third of patients with psychosis after TBI having a chronic course similar to schizophrenia in the studies examining this issue (Hillbom 1960; Violon and DeMol 1987). The onset of psychotic symptoms is typically gradual and delayed, often occurring more than a year after injury (Fann et al. 2004; Fujii and Ahmed 2002; Sachdev et al. 2001).

Anger, Aggression, and Agitation

Many patients with TBI have difficulty modulating emotional reactions and controlling impulses (Rao and Lyketsos 2002), often described in the TBI literature as *posttraumatic agitation* (Sandel and Mysiw 1996). However, as noted by Yudofsky et al. (1997), *agitation* is a poorly defined term encompassing behaviors ranging from "constant unwarranted requests" to assaultiveness. Although measures such as the Agitated Behavior Scale (ABS; Corrigan 1989) have been well validated for TBI, they are rarely used in clinical practice (Fugate et al. 1997). Similarly, the Overt Aggression Scale (OAS; Yudofsky et al. 1986) was developed to provide objective measurement of the severity of aggression and, to a lesser extent, agitation. Other authors have expanded the OAS to make it more applicable to the rehabilitation setting by including a greater number of choices for antecedents and outcomes (Overt Aggression Scale–Modified for Neurorehabilitation–Extended [OAS-MNR-E]; Giles and Mohr 2007). Brooke et al. (1992b) used the OAS to measure agitation in 100 patients with severe TBI. Only 11% of the patients had agitation; an additional 35% were classified as "restless" but not severely enough to be labeled "agitated." Bogner and Corrigan (1995) examined 100 consecutive patients admitted to an inpatient TBI unit. Of these, 42% had agitation (as measured by the ABS) during at least one shift. Episodes of anger or aggression are also common (Auerbach 1989). In their validation study of the OAS-MNR-E, Giles and Mohr (2007) noted 158 episodes of aggression in 34 subjects over a 6-week study period.

Although aggression may be a symptom of many disorders, several features are characteristic of aggression after TBI (Yudofsky et al. 1990). Such behavior is typically *nonreflective,* occurring without any premeditation or planning, and *nonpurposeful,* achieving no particular goals for the individual. It is also *reactive,* triggered by a stimulus, but often a stimulus that would not normally provoke a strong reaction. Aggression after TBI is *periodic,* occurring at intervals with relatively calm behavior in between, and *explosive,* occurring without a prodromal buildup. Finally, it is *egodystonic,* creating a great deal of distress for the patient.

The lack of precise definitions of agitation and aggression in the literature makes identification of risk factors difficult, although some have been reported. Agitation is more likely to occur with frontotemporal injuries (Van der Naalt et al. 1999). Disorientation, comorbid medical illness, and use of anticonvulsant medications are also associated with agitation (Galski et al. 1994). Risk of aggression is increased with a premorbid history of impulsive aggression (Greve et al. 2001), impaired executive-attention function (Wood and Liossi 2006), arrest (Kreutzer et al. 1995), substance abuse (Dunlop et al. 1991), or depression (Jorge et al. 2004). For these risk factors, it is often difficult to ascertain whether the aggression is a direct result of TBI, premorbid character pathology, or both (Kim 2002).

Little is known about the course of agitation or aggression after TBI. However, in their review of the literature, Silver and Yudofsky (1994a) noted that 31%–71% of the individuals had these behaviors in long-term follow-up ranging from 1 to 15 years. Similarly, Baguley et al. (2006) noted that approximately 25% of inpatient rehabilitation patients with TBI showed aggression on the OAS at 6, 24, and 60 months postinjury. Greater depressive symptomatology and younger age at injury were the most significant predictors of later aggression. These authors also reported that 70% of the inpatient rehabilitation patients with TBI had agitation at discharge and at 6 and 24 months postdischarge in a retrospective chart review (Nott et al. 2006). Increased agitation was found to be associated with longer duration of posttraumatic amnesia, increased length of stay, and greater cognitive impairment. Thus, it appears that agitation and aggression may be chronic problems not confined to the early stage of recovery. This would be expected for such behaviors that predate the injury; it is currently unclear whether agitation and aggression directly resulting from TBI follow this chronic course.

Substance Use Disorders

Substance abuse and dependence are of great concern in the TBI population, at the time of injury and afterward. Substance use disorders not only are highly prevalent and often the underlying cause of injury but also adversely affect outcomes, including agitation, length of coma, risk of reinjury, return to work, and ability to reintegrate into the community (Bombardier and Turner 2009; Corrigan and Cole 2008). Alcohol intoxication at the time of injury may influence initial injury severity; however, preinjury alcohol abuse and problems do not necessarily predict poorer postacute cognitive functioning (Turner et al. 2006). Preinjury history of alcohol and substance abuse among individuals with TBI may not differ significantly from that of demographically similar control groups (Ponsford et al. 2007), although this requires further investigation. Literature reviews have shown that in higher-quality studies, 44%–66% of the patients with TBI had a history of significant alcohol-related problems before injury and that 31%–51% were intoxicated at the time of injury (Bombardier and Turner 2009; Ponsford et al. 2007; Vickery et al. 2008). Those with a history of significant alcohol-related problems before injury are 11 times more likely to have alcohol problems after injury compared with those without alcohol problems before injury (Bombardier et al. 2003). Studies that used informal interviews and screening measures found that 21%–37% reported a history of illicit drug use (Bombardier et al. 2002; Kolakowsky-Hayner et al. 1999; Kreutzer et al. 1991, 1996; Ruff et al. 1990). In one study, 37.7% had a positive toxicology screen at the time of injury for one or more illicit drugs (marijuana 23.7%, cocaine 13.2%, amphetamine 8.8%; Bombardier et al. 2002). Bryant et al. (2010), using structured interviews to diagnose substance abuse, found that 9.9% of patients met criteria at 12 months, with 2.5% having onset after TBI. Substance abuse declines after TBI but remains significant. Longitudinal data indicate that, depending on the criteria used, rates of remission from alcohol problems range from 31% to 56% during the first year after injury (Bombardier et al. 2003). However, the initial decrease in alcohol use may subsequently increase with additional time since injury (Ponsford et al. 2007). Data on postacute heavy drinking and alcohol problems are relatively consistent in that 22%–29% of patients were moderate to heavy drinkers (Bombardier et al. 2002; Kreutzer et al. 1996) or met the criteria for substance abuse or dependence (Hibbard et al. 1998). However, some studies reported much lower rates of substance abuse or dependence—8% by Fann et al. (1995), 4% by Deb et al. (1999), and 10%–14% by Ashman et al. (2004). Research in which less formal measures were used has shown that 14%–43% of individuals reported significant alcohol or drug use after their injury (Kolakowsky-Hayner et al. 2002; Kreutzer et al. 1990, 1991). Timing of assessment and sensitivity of screening measures, as well as whether patients were unselected or from referral populations, may play critical roles in explaining some of these variations. Risk factors for postinjury substance abuse include male gender, history of legal problems related to substance abuse, substance abuse problems among family or friends, postinjury diagnosis of depression, younger age, and less severe injuries (Horner et al. 2005; Jorge et al. 2005; Ponsford et al. 2007; Taylor et al. 2003).

Brain injury rehabilitation may represent a window of opportunity for intervening in substance abuse disorders (Bombardier et al. 1997). More than 75% of TBI patients considered to be "at-risk" drinkers indicated that they were intending to reduce or were contemplating reductions in their alcohol use during inpatient rehabilitation (Bombardier et al. 2002). Of these patients, 17%–20% reported wanting to enter treatment or try Alcoholics Anonymous, and about 70% wanted to try changing on their own. A simple typology based on lifetime history of alcohol-related consequences combined with recent alcohol consumption and toxicology results can be used to recommend tailored interventions: 1) TBI-specific education and advice, 2) brief motivational interventions, 3) relapse prevention training, or 4) referral to comprehensive substance abuse treatment (Turner et al. 2003). Referral to outside substance abuse treatment programs may be most helpful when staff members at available programs are comfortable with the cognitive and physical disabilities associated with TBI. Small financial incentives can facilitate substance abuse treatment attendance and completion in people with TBI (Corrigan and Bogner 2007). If such specialized programs are not available, efforts can be made to integrate evidence-based substance abuse interventions within rehabilitation programs (Bombardier and Turner 2009; Taylor et al. 2003).

Cognitive Impairment

Much effort has been devoted to characterizing the cognitive deficits that occur after TBI. Some have suggested that deficits can be divided into four time periods (Rao and Lyketsos 2000). The first is the period of LOC that results from the injury. After emerging from unconsciousness, many individuals enter a phase consisting of multiple cognitive and behavioral deficits, which some have described as posttraumatic delirium (Kwentus et al. 1985; Trzepacz 1994). The third period is a rapid recovery of cognitive function, which plateaus over time. This leads to the fourth period of permanent cognitive deficits. TBI is associated with deficits in multiple domains, including impaired memory, language deficits, reduced attention and concentration, slowed information processing, and executive dysfunction (Capruso and Levin 1996).

Although TBI is associated with an acute decrement in cognitive function that typically improves over time, recovery is very individualized, and no universally applicable description of the recovery process exists. Rao and Lyketsos (2000) offered the following general timeline: the first two periods of recovery will last from a few days to a month, the third period will last 6–12 months, and the fourth period will last 12–24 months. Such guidelines are more characteristic of moderate to severe injuries. By definition, individuals with mild TBI will have LOC of less than 30 minutes, with many having none at all (Kay et al. 1993). It is also estimated that about 95% of patients with mild TBI will recover to baseline status within 3–6 months and not enter the fourth phase of permanent deficits (Binder et al. 1997). Even among individuals with moderate to severe TBI, some recovery of cognitive function may occur 2 years or more after injury, although the gains are typically small (Millis et al. 2001). A few patients may experience decline late in the course of recovery, perhaps caused by depression (Millis et al. 2001). Thus, these time frames must be considered general approximations only.

Descriptions of the period of recovery from TBI vary in the rehabilitation literature. One classical term is *posttraumatic amnesia,* which occurs "from injury until recovery of full consciousness and the return of ongoing memory" (Grant and Alves 1987). This would include the first two periods described earlier and potentially extend into the third. However, characterization of the deficits after TBI as purely amnestic is an oversimplification because multiple cognitive deficits occur (D.I. Katz 1992). Stuss et al. (1999) advocated discarding *posttraumatic amnesia* for the concept of *posttraumatic confusion,* although this has not gained widespread use in the TBI literature. Another common term for the period of recovery after TBI is *posttraumatic agitation,* characterized by "excesses of behavior that include some combination of aggression, akathisia, disinhibition, and/or emotional lability" (Sandel and Mysiw 1996, p. 619). This would correspond closely to the second period described earlier.

Unfortunately, the terminology used in the rehabilitation literature does not correspond exactly to DSM-IV-TR psychiatric diagnoses. Most definitions of posttraumatic amnesia would be consistent with a period of delirium followed by an amnestic phase (Trzepacz and Kennedy 2005). The term *posttraumatic confusion* more closely resembles the diagnosis of delirium yet still omits features such as mood and perceptual disturbances. *Posttraumatic agitation* is defined by some experts as a subtype of delirium (Sandel and Mysiw 1996), yet others have noted that agitation may resolve while the confusional state persists (Van der Naalt et al. 1999). Thompson et al. (2001) examined this issue in detail by concurrently rating inpatients with TBI on the Delirium Rating Scale (Trzepacz et al. 1988), a standardized measure for delirium; the Galveston Orientation and Amnesia Test (GOAT; Levin et al. 1979), a measure of posttraumatic amnesia; and the ABS (Corrigan 1989), a measure of posttraumatic agitation. Of those with a diagnosis of delirium, 22.5% had normal scores on the ABS, and 7.5% had normal scores on the GOAT. Among those without delirium, 7.5% had abnormal scores on the ABS, and 27.5% had abnormal scores on the GOAT. A combination of GOAT and ABS scores classified the delirium diagnosis with 77.5% accuracy. Thus, although the terms *delirium, posttraumatic amnesia,* and *posttraumatic agitation* describe conditions that share many common features, they are not synonymous.

The long-term diffuse cognitive deficits seen after TBI would be categorized as dementia due to head trauma or cognitive disorder not otherwise specified under DSM-IV-TR. This would include the fourth period described earlier and potentially the third period when the recovery process is slow. Rehabilitation experts have expressed concern with use of the term *dementia* in the TBI population (Leon-Carrion 2002). The impairments seen after TBI, unlike those seen in most dementias, tend to be either static or improving over time. Experts also have expressed concern that application of DSM criteria would lead to diagnoses of dementia in the vast majority of individuals with moderate and severe TBI, with potential legal and social ramifications. Clearly, these implications should be further studied and addressed, but the DSM framework provides a useful standardized approach to diagnosis in this population that might otherwise be lacking.

Preliminary studies suggest that delirium after TBI shows phenomenological similarities to other types of delirium (Sherer et al. 2003b), with both hypo- and hyperactive subtypes noted in other patient populations. The hyperactive subtype appears more common and is associated with agitation and high frequency of hallucinations or delusions. Several risk factors for delirium in the medical-surgical population would likely apply to individuals with TBI (Trzepacz and Kennedy 2005), who are at increased risk for several medical illnesses (Kalisky et al. 1985; Shavelle et al. 2001). Risk factors for prolonged posttraumatic amnesia include older age, low initial GCS score, nonreactive pupils, longer coma duration, higher number of lesions detected by neuroimaging, and use of phenytoin (Ellenberg et al. 1996; J.T. Wilson et al. 1994). These would likely be risk factors for delirium as well. Unfortunately, patients who are traditionally considered to have a higher risk for delirium—especially alcoholic patients, elderly patients, those with psychiatric and neurological histories, and those with prior brain injury—are nearly always excluded from posttraumatic amnesia studies (Trzepacz and Kennedy 2005). Finally, more recent studies have highlighted the prognostic significance of delirium after TBI, which is an important predictor of length of rehabilitation stay (Sherer et al. 2005) and later employability and productivity (Nakase-Richardson et al. 2007; Sherer et al. 2008).

For dementia, severity of injury is consistently associated with the degree and duration of cognitive impairments. The extent of impairment is also influenced by premorbid intellectual abilities and the time after injury at which the patient is assessed (Dikmen et al. 1995). As with other dementias, the cognitive domains affected will vary from patient to patient (Kreutzer et al. 1993). Patients with TBI also may be at increased risk for developing dementia from other causes, such as Alzheimer's disease (Amaducci et al. 1986; Graves et al. 1990).

Postconcussive Syndrome

The diagnosis of postconcussive syndrome has been a source of wide controversy. It is important to differentiate postconcussive *symptoms* from postconcussive *syndrome*. The symptoms of postconcussive syndrome are nonspecific and include disturbances such as headache, dizziness, irritability, fatigue, and insomnia. Indeed, several studies have documented high base rates of postconcussive symptoms among subjects without TBI, often at rates similar to those in individuals with mild TBI (Boake et al. 2005; Caveness 1966; Gouvier et al. 1988; McLean et al. 1983; Meares et al. 2008; Tuohimaa 1978). There is disagreement as to the number and types of symptoms required for postconcussive syndrome. Most experts concur that the diagnosis of postconcussive syndrome requires the presence of multiple concurrent symptoms (Brown et al. 1994; Mittenberg and Strauman 2000), although disagreement may remain over which specific symptoms are required. Standardized diagnostic criteria for postconcussive syndrome have been developed; DSM-IV-TR lists provisional criteria for postconcussional disorder (Table 35–3), indicating that the diagnosis may still undergo refinement. The most widely published criteria are those in ICD-10 (World Health Organization 1992), listed in Table 35–4. Differences between the two sets of criteria do exist, but the implications have not been well studied. Boake et al. (2005) found the ICD-10 criteria to be much more inclusive than the DSM-IV criteria, with 64% of individuals hospitalized for mild to moderate TBI meeting criteria for postconcussive syndrome at 3 months using the former but only 11% with the latter. Unfortunately, few studies have used either of these criteria sets (Mittenberg and Strauman 2000). The adoption of such standard definitions will be a necessary step in advancing the study and treatment of postconcussive syndrome.

Because postconcussive symptoms are not specific to TBI, it is important to consider their differential diagnosis. Alexander (1995) and Mittenberg and Strauman (2000) noted that postconcussive syndrome has significant overlap with psychiatric disorders. Both major depression and postconcussive syndrome have symptoms of depressed mood, irritability, sleep disturbance, fatigue, and difficulty with concentration. However, unlike major depression, postconcussive syndrome does not include symptoms of changes in appetite, psychomotor changes, or suicidal ideation. Stein and McAllister (2009) specifically described the overlap between PTSD and postconcussive syndrome. PTSD and postconcussive syndrome have common symptoms of anxious mood, difficulty sleeping, irritability, poor concentration, and difficulty recalling the injury. Postconcussive syndrome is not associated with persistent reexperiencing of the event or with numbing of responsiveness, and PTSD is not associated with the headaches, dizziness, and general memory disturbance that characterize postconcussive syndrome. Symptoms such as head-

TABLE 35–3. DSM-IV-TR research criteria for postconcussional disorder

A. A history of head trauma that has caused significant cerebral concussion.

Note: The manifestations of concussion include loss of consciousness, posttraumatic amnesia, and, less commonly, posttraumatic onset of seizures. The specific method of defining this criterion needs to be established by further research.

B. Evidence from neuropsychological testing or quantified cognitive assessment of difficulty in attention (concentrating, shifting focus of attention, performing simultaneous cognitive tasks) or memory (learning or recalling information).

C. Three (or more) of the following occur shortly after the trauma and last at least 3 months:

(1) becoming fatigued easily
(2) disordered sleep
(3) headache
(4) vertigo or dizziness
(5) irritability or aggression on little or no provocation
(6) anxiety, depression, or affective lability
(7) changes in personality (e.g., social or sexual inappropriateness)
(8) apathy or lack of spontaneity

D. The symptoms in Criteria B and C have their onset following head trauma or else represent a substantial worsening of preexisting symptoms.

E. The disturbance causes significant impairment in social or occupational functioning and represents a significant decline from a previous level of functioning. In school-age children, the impairment may be manifested by a significant worsening in school or academic performance dating from the trauma.

F. The symptoms do not meet criteria for dementia due to head trauma and are not better accounted for by another mental disorder (e.g., amnestic disorder due to head trauma, personality change due to head trauma).

Source. Reprinted from American Psychiatric Association: *Diagnostic and Statistical Manual of Mental Disorders,* 4th Edition, Text Revision. Washington, DC, American Psychiatric Association, 2000, pp. 761–762. Used with permission.

TABLE 35–4. ICD-10 criteria for postconcussive syndrome

A. History of head trauma with loss of consciousness precedes symptom onset by maximum of 4 weeks.

B. Three or more symptom categories

1. Headache, dizziness, malaise, fatigue, noise intolerance
2. Irritability, depression, anxiety, emotional lability
3. Subjective concentration, memory, or intellectual difficulties without neuropsychological evidence of marked impairment
4. Insomnia
5. Reduced alcohol tolerance
6. Preoccupation with above symptoms and fear of brain damage with hypochondriacal concern and adoption of sick role

Source. Reprinted from World Health Organization: *International Statistical Classification of Diseases and Related Health Problems,* 10th Edition. Geneva, Switzerland, World Health Organization, 1992. Used with permission.

ache, fatigue, dizziness, blurred vision, memory disturbance, and hypochondriacal preoccupation with health may be part of postconcussive syndrome or of a somatoform disorder. Postconcussive syndrome is not associated with the gastrointestinal symptoms often seen in somatization disorder, and it is also not associated with marked motor or sensory deficits or nonepileptic seizures often seen in conversion disorder. Patients with chronic pain also may have symptoms of headaches, fatigue, poor sleep, poor concentration, depressed mood, and dizziness that overlap with postconcussive syndrome. Thus, the presence of psychiatric disorders may lead to high rates of reporting of postconcussive symptoms, regardless of TBI history (Fox et al. 1995; Suhr and Gunstad 2002; Trahan et al. 2001). Careful history taking and diagnosis are needed to avoid mislabeling these patients as having postconcussive syndrome. The clinician also must keep in mind that individuals may have both postconcussive syndrome and a psychiatric disorder, which may blur the boundaries between the two.

Studies have examined risk factors and time course for the development of postconcussive syndrome. However, failure to use standardized diagnostic criteria for postconcussive syndrome in most studies makes generalization difficult. Most studies of postconcussive syndrome have focused on individuals with mild TBI, although postconcussive syndrome can occur with more severe injuries as well. The symptoms of postconcussive syndrome are extremely common after mild TBI, with 80%–100% of patients experiencing one or more symptoms in the immediate postinjury period (Levin et al. 1987a). Several studies have shown that such symptoms resolve completely within 3 months in most patients (Alves et al. 1986; R.W. Evans 1996; Leininger et al. 1990). However, other prospective studies have shown that 20%–66% of patients have persistent symptoms at 3 months (Englander et al. 1992) and that 1%–50% have persistent symptoms at 1 year (Middleboe et al. 1992; Rutherford et al. 1979). Alves et al. (1993) followed up the resolution of these symptoms in 587 consecutive adult hospital admissions with mild TBI, with assessments at baseline and at 3, 6, and 12 months. Approximately two-thirds of the patients had symptoms of postconcussive syndrome at discharge, with progressive decline in prevalence during recovery. At 3 months, 40%–60% experienced such symptoms; at 6 months, 25%–45%; and at 12 months, 10%–40%. Most of these subjects reported only one or two postconcussive symptoms and would not qualify for a diagnosis of postconcussive syndrome under DSM or ICD. Subjects with multiple symptoms consistent with a diagnosis of postconcussive syndrome were rare—between 1.9% and 5.8% of those studied. For this and many other studies, the lack of an appropriate control group makes it difficult to determine how many of these symptoms could be attributed to the TBI itself.

Because the symptoms of postconcussive syndrome are nonspecific, some have questioned whether it constitutes a true disorder or syndrome (King 1997, 2003). There also is a long-standing debate as to whether postconcussive syndrome constitutes a neurological or a psychiatric syndrome (King 2003; Mittenberg et al. 1996). Currently, the acute syndrome is thought to be related to neurological factors, whereas chronic symptoms are more likely to persist because of psychological factors (Larrabee 1997; Mittenberg and Strauman 2000). Complaints of poor sleep, difficulty concentrating, and memory disturbances that arise shortly after TBI may be caused by direct neuronal injury (Alexander 1997). Dizziness may be due to central or peripheral vestibular injury, and pain complaints may be due to musculoskeletal or scalp injury (Alexander 1997). It is not known how these putative neurological injuries, which should resolve quickly, transition into chronic postconcussive syndrome. Symptom expectations, in which patients fear that their symptoms will not resolve, may play a role (King 2003; Mittenberg and Strauman 2000; Mittenberg et al. 1996). However, the precise role of psychological factors in persistent postconcussive syndrome is far from clear (Dikmen et al. 1989). Thus, the risk factors for postconcussive syndrome are a mixture of biological and psychological.

The more commonly reported risk factors are female gender (Bazarian et al. 1999; McCauley et al. 2001; McClelland et al. 1994; Meares et al. 2008), older age (Alexander 1997; McCauley et al. 2001), history of TBI (McCauley et al. 2001; Schneiderman et al. 2008), psychosocial stress (Fenton et al. 1993; Moss et al. 1994), and poor social support (Fenton et al. 1993; McCauley et al. 2001). Dikmen et al. (2010) also found that preinjury history of alcohol abuse and psychiatric history were associated with greater endorsement of posttraumatic symptoms. Low socioeconomic status and ongoing litigation also increase risk (Alexander 1997; Binder and Rohling 1996; McCauley et al. 2001). However, for the latter, it should be noted that few individuals involved in litigation have improvement in postconcussive syndrome after settlement (King 2003). Self-reported rates of specific postconcussive symptoms (anxiety, noise sensitivity, and difficulty concentrating) also have been associated with increased risk of long-term postconcussive syndrome (Dischinger et al. 2009). Finally, in examining postconcussive symptoms among individuals without TBI, Gouvier et al. (1992; Santa Maria et al. 2001) noted that females had higher rates of symptom reporting, and rates of reporting increased with levels of psychosocial stress.

A significant association is seen between depression and postconcussive symptoms, including those postconcussive symptoms that do not overlap with depression (Fann et al. 1995; King 2003), and severity of depressive symptoms predicts risk for postconcussive syndrome (McCauley et al. 2001; Meares et al. 2008). McCauley et al. (2001) used portions of the SCID to identify major depression and PTSD as significant moderators of postconcussive syndrome. It appears that psychiatric disorders, particularly depression, may significantly amplify the presentation of postconcussive symptoms. Meares et al. (2008) had similar findings with the Mini International Neuropsychiatric Interview and the ICD-10 criteria for postconcussive syndrome, with major depression, PTSD, and other anxiety disorders increasing the risk for postconcussive symptoms within 2 weeks of injury. They also noted that increasing levels of pain raised the risk for postconcussive syndrome. Schneiderman et al. (2008) found PTSD to be a significant predictor of postconcussive symptoms among combat veterans with mild TBI, even after overlapping symptoms of PTSD and postconcussive syndrome were eliminated. Hoge et al. (2008), in their study of recently returned soldiers, found that the association of mild TBI with postconcussive symptoms was no longer significant after they controlled for major depression and PTSD, suggesting that elevated rates of postconcussive symptoms after mild TBI in this population were mediated to a large degree by the latter two diagnoses. In contrast, Vanderploeg et al. (2009) noted that mild TBI and PTSD had independent contributions to postconcussive symptoms among Vietnam War–era veterans. In the latter study, mild TBI occurred several years after the development of PTSD, whereas in the former, the traumatic event and mild TBI occurred in the same period, so the results cannot be directly compared.

Although the vast majority of the persons with mild TBI experience good recovery (Binder et al. 1997), Ruff (1999) identified a "miserable minority" of 10%–20% of mild TBI patients with poor outcome, and Malec (1999) noted that 20%–40% of mild TBI patients have residual long-term symptoms or disability. In many cases, such individuals complain of symptoms of postconcussive syndrome, indicating that ongoing postconcussive syndrome may be an important source of disability. Studies of such patients also have found significant deficits on a variety of neuropsychological tests (Bohnen et al. 1992; Guilmette and Rasile 1995; Leininger et al. 1990), although it remains unclear how these difficulties develop during the course of postconcussive syndrome. The severity of postconcussive symptoms is consistently correlated with severity of impairment in information-processing speed, but correlations with other cognitive domains (such as verbal and visuospatial abilities) are equivocal (King 2003). In particular, Larrabee (1999) commented on two of these studies, which consisted of patients experiencing postconcussive symptoms after TBI involving LOC of less than 30 minutes. The effects on neuropsychological testing observed in these patients were equivalent to the effects observed in other studies in patients who had undergone 1–4 weeks of coma (Dikmen et al. 1995). These data suggest that individuals with persistent postconcussive syndrome differ in significant respects from most individuals with TBI, although the reasons for these differences remain unexplained. Investigators also have found that high rates of postconcussive symptoms were better predictors of neuropsychological test performance than was actual history of mild TBI (Hanna-Pladdy et al. 1997; Pinkston et al. 2000). These results cast further doubt on the contention that the cognitive impairment in persistent postconcussive syndrome is due to TBI.

Sleep Disorders

Sleep disturbances are a common component of many neuropsychiatric disorders occurring after TBI, including delirium, major depression, bipolar disorder, anxiety disorders, and postconcussive syndrome. TBI also may have significant effects on sleep architecture that are independent of these illnesses by altering the levels of several neurotransmitters involved in the regulation of sleep. The prevalence of sleep disturbance after TBI is high, with estimates ranging from 30% to 70% (Ouellet et al. 2004). Although insomnia is a frequent focus in the literature, other forms of sleep disturbances, such as fatigue and daytime sleepiness, have been reported. Reports also have found increased rates of obstructive sleep apnea, periodic limb movements, and narcolepsy among individuals after TBI compared with control populations (Castriotta et al. 2007; Lai and Castriotta 1999; Verma et al. 2007; J.B. Webster et al. 2001). In at least some cases, evidence suggested that the sleep disorder predated the TBI, raising the possibility that the sleep disorder increased the risk for TBI rather than vice versa. Orff et al. (2009) provided a comprehensive review of the literature concerning sleep and TBI. They noted several deficiencies in existing studies, including poor descriptions of comorbid physical and psychological conditions that may contribute to sleep disturbances, inadequate information about TBI severity and injury location, and few long-term studies. More recent studies also indicate that sleep disturbance, particularly insomnia, is more likely with mild TBI than with more severe injuries, although the reasons for this difference are unknown.

Psychological Aspects

In addition to the defined DSM-IV-TR psychiatric disorders, TBI is associated with psychological challenges that may not fit into specific diagnostic categories. Four areas of importance are the neurological injury and resultant cognitive deficits, the psychological meaning of deficits and their effect on the patient, the psychological factors that exist independently of TBI, and the broader social context (Lewis 1991).

Deficits due to neurological impairment may have a direct effect on psychological functioning. Impaired self-awareness is common after TBI, with 76%–97% of TBI patients showing some degree of impairment (Sherer et al. 1998c, 2003a). Many individuals with TBI also have deficits in awareness of their behavioral limitations (Prigatano and Altman 1990), which may be one of their most troubling problems (Ben-Yishay et al. 1985; Prigatano and Fordyce 1986). Awareness of cognitive and emotional changes tends to be worse than awareness of physical dysfunction (Sherer et al. 1998c). There is little agreement on the most appropriate way to measure lack of awareness (Sherer et al. 1998b, 2003a). Comparisons of patient reports with those of family members (D.J. Fordyce and Roueche 1986; Hendryx 1989; McKinlay and Brooks 1984; Prigatano 1996; Prigatano and Altman 1990; Prigatano et al. 1990; Walker et al. 1987) or rehabilitation providers (D.J. Fordyce and Roueche 1986; Gasquione 1992; Gasquione and Gibbons 1994; Heilbronner et al. 1989; Ranseen et al. 1990) may be biased by respondent characteristics. Comparing patient reports with neuropsychological test results can eliminate much of this subjectivity but may not allow the consultant to gauge the accuracy of patient self-reports of real-world functioning (Allen and Ruff 1990; Anderson and Tranel 1989; Heaton and Pendleton 1981). The method of questioning is also important because studies have shown that patients are much less likely to report deficits when asked general questions rather than specific ones (Gasquione 1992; Sherer et al. 1998b).

Impaired awareness has both neurological and psychological dimensions. At one extreme is anosognosia, wherein the person has no awareness of neurological impairments

(Prigatano 1999). At the other extreme is "defensive denial," which represents the person's attempt to cope with overwhelming anxiety associated with neurological impairment by minimizing the implications. Apparent impaired awareness also can be the result of moderate to severe memory impairment that prevents the person from consolidating and acting on new information about his or her condition. The neuroanatomical underpinnings of impaired self-awareness are not well documented, but hypoarousal associated with subcortical damage and various types of cortical damage is thought to contribute (Prigatano 1999). Few studies have attempted to separate neurological from psychological causes of decreased awareness (Boake et al. 1995; McGlynn and Schacter 1989). Phenomenologically, decreased awareness might appear the same regardless of cause but has significant treatment implications. Interventions designed to address denial and other forms of decreased awareness resulting from psychological causes may be ineffective when the decreased awareness is due to neurological dysfunction that cannot be reversed.

Finally, most studies of awareness have focused on individuals who overestimate their abilities compared with the reports of others. However, some patients underestimate their abilities; the deficits that these individuals have in awareness have not been well studied (Prigatano and Altman 1990). Although more than a half-dozen instruments have been developed for measurement of awareness in the TBI population, there has been little work on the psychometric properties or factor structures of these instruments (Seel et al. 1997; Sherer et al. 1998b). Research in this area is ongoing, and the most systematically studied scales are the Patient Competency Rating Scale (Prigatano and Fordyce 1986) and the Awareness Questionnaire (Sherer et al. 1998a). Other measures are also being developed and validated. Nimmo-Smith et al. (2005) specifically investigated a bedside examination of anosognosia for hemiplegic deficits with questions related to bilateral arm and leg use to find maximum discrimination between groups that did and did not overestimate their physical abilities. Murrey et al. (2005) reported that the Mayo-Portland Adaptability Inventory had good discrimination between patients with severe TBI having frontal lobe damage and anosognosia and patients with mild TBI having no demonstrable frontal lobe damage. Both the total score and four of the subscale scores (Communications, Emotions, Independent Living Skills, and Relationship) differed between groups, whereas no differences were noted on the Mobility subscale, indicating that the scale was useful for measuring specific deficits of awareness. The available literature suggests that deficits in awareness are common immediately after TBI, with gradual improvement over time (C. Evans et al. 2003).

The patient's psychological state and the perceived meaning of physical and cognitive deficits may be strongly linked. Patients with depression or anxiety appear to perceive their injury and associated cognitive problems as more severe (Fann et al. 1995, 2000). Many patients with TBI experience grief in reaction to their disability and loss of their "former self." For many years, rehabilitation researchers have relied on bereavement concepts to explain the adjustment-to-disability process (Stewart and Shields 1985; Vargo 1978). However, long-held assumptions about the symptoms and process of normal bereavement have not withstood empirical testing (Marwit 1996; Stroebe et al. 2001; Wortman and Silver 1989). For example, the 2-month time limit placed on a "normal" grieving process in DSM-IV has been called into question (Parkes and Weiss 1983; Wortman and Silver 1989). Also, contrary to the belief that a person must make a "show" of grief, some support exists for the benefits of focusing on positive emotions (Bonanno and Kaltman 1999). Finally, advances in the understanding of grief following loss of a loved one, with few exceptions (Niemeier et al. 2004), have not yet been applied to the emotional experience of individuals with functional and cognitive losses due to illness or injury.

Psychological defenses and adaptations used by the individual prior to TBI are also important. In many cases, patients will continue to use previously learned defenses. However, in some instances, coping mechanisms used before the injury may no longer be available because of the degree of neurocognitive impairment; this can cause considerable distress for the patient. Evidence indicates that many behavioral traits are exacerbated by TBI rather than developing de novo after injury (Prigatano 1991). Such alterations would be diagnosed as personality change due to TBI in DSM-IV-TR.

Finally, as with many other chronic illnesses, TBI has a significant effect on family and social functioning. Individuals with TBI may be unable to return to their former roles as breadwinner, parent, or spouse, placing significant demands on other members of the family system (Kay and Cavallo 1994). In general, neurobehavioral disturbances are the most important source of stress for the family, but this effect can be mediated by good social support (Ergh et al. 2002; Groom et al. 1998). Family members are at significantly increased risk for psychiatric disorders, particularly anxiety and depression, and for increased substance use (Hall et al. 1994; Kreutzer et al. 1994; Livingston et al. 1985). Caregivers may experience problems such as unemployment or financial loss, placing additional stresses on the patient and family (Hall et al. 1994). Sexual dysfunction after TBI places further stress on intimate relationships (Hibbard et al. 2000a), and partners may be uncomfortable with the dual role of caregiver (parentlike) and sexual partner (spouse) (Gosling and Oddy 1999). Rates of separation and divorce are also elevated for individuals with TBI (G. Webster et al. 1999).

Spinal Cord Injury

Epidemiology

SCI results from trauma to the spinal cord and may cause changes in motor, sensory, or autonomic functioning. SCI is an uncommon but often catastrophic injury with an annual incidence of 30–40 per million and a point prevalence of 183,000–230,000 in the United States (Go et al. 1995). However, a recent unpublished report commissioned by the Christopher Reeve Foundation suggests that the prevalence of SCI may be as high as 1,275,000 (www.christopherreeve.org). Those who sustain SCIs are predominantly males (80%), young (half are ages 16–30), and Caucasian (89%). At the time that they are injured, those sustaining SCI are less likely to be married, twice as likely to be divorced, and slightly less educated than the general population. The most common causes of SCI are motor vehicle crashes (44.5%), falls (18.1%), violence (16.6%), and sports activities (12.7%).

Early survival and overall life expectancy rates for persons with SCI have improved dramatically over the past 30 years. However, life expectancy with SCI remains below that of the general population, especially among those who are ventilator dependent (DeVivo et al. 1999). Leading causes of death are heart disease (19%); external causes such as accidents, suicide, and violence (18%); respiratory illness, especially pneumonia (18%); and septicemia (10%) (DeVivo et al. 1999). Death from suicide is approximately five times more common among people with SCI than in the general population (59.2 per 100,000) and represents about 9% of deaths. Most suicides occur within 5 years of injury (Charlifue and Gerhart 1991).

Severity Classification

Tetraplegia (or quadriplegia) denotes SCI that affects all four limbs, whereas *paraplegia* denotes injuries that affect only the lower extremities. SCI usually is described in terms of the level and the completeness of injury. The level of injury refers to the most caudal segment with normal motor or sensory function. Neurological level of injury may vary on the right and the left side, and segments also may be partially innervated. More than half of all injuries (54%) result in tetraplegia, whereas 46% are classified as resulting in paraplegia. The midcervical region is the most common site of injury. Injury severity is most commonly described according to the American Spinal Injury Association (ASIA) Impairment Scale (Table 35–5). Approximately half of all injuries are considered ASIA-A or "complete." Of those admitted with an ASIA-A SCI, only about 2% are expected to improve to the point of having functional motor recovery below the level of their injury. In contrast, those admitted with an ASIA-B injury have about a 35% chance of regaining functional motor abilities below the level of their lesion. Those admitted with an ASIA-C injury have a 71% chance of regaining functional motor ability below the level of their injury (Marino et al. 1999).

TABLE 35–5. American Spinal Injury Association (ASIA) Impairment Scale

A. **Complete**—No sensory or motor function is preserved in the sacral segments S4/5.

B. **Sensory Incomplete**—Sensory but no motor function is preserved below the neurological level and includes the sacral segments S4/5.

C. **Motor Incomplete**—Motor function is preserved below the neurological level, and more than half of the key muscles below the neurological level have muscle grade less than 3 (active movement against gravity). There must be some sparing of sensory and/or motor function in the sacral segments S4/5.

D. **Motor Incomplete**—Motor function is preserved below the neurological level, and at least half of the key muscles below the neurological level have a muscle grade greater than or equal to 3. There must be some sparing of sensory and/or motor function in the sacral segments S4/5.

E. **Normal**—Sensory and motor functions are normal. Patient may have abnormalities of reflex examination.

Source. Reprinted from American Spinal Injury Association: *International Standards for Neurological and Functional Classification of Spinal Cord Injury.* Chicago, IL, American Spinal Injury Association, 1996. Used with permission.

Acute Management and Management of Secondary Complications

Emergency management of SCI involves immobilizing the spine as well as ensuring an open airway, breathing, and circulation. In many settings, standard practice is to administer a large intravenous bolus of methylprednisolone within 8 hours of injury to minimize secondary injury due to swelling within the spinal canal. Unstable spine fractures may require surgical decompression and stabilization. Various orthoses are used to maintain external spinal stabilization after surgery, typically for 3 months.

Key aspects of postsurgical care include respiratory management and prevention of pneumonia, management of orthostatic hypotension associated with blood pooling in the lower extremities, and prevention of deep venous thrombosis and pulmonary embolus from venous stasis and hypercoagulability. Neurogenic bladder and bowel management begins with indwelling or intermittent catheterization and establishment of a regular bowel regimen. After injury, heterotopic ossification, the deposition of new bone in and around joints, may cause loss of range of motion. Spinal reflexes are initially depressed during the period of "spinal shock" but then become hyperactive during the first 6 months after injury. Daily range of motion and static muscle stretch are used to reduce spasticity and prevent contractures, along with medication such as baclofen, diazepam, and clonidine. Pain is a common problem; 25% complain of severe pain, and 44% report that pain interferes with daily activities (Staas et al. 1998). SCI-related pain classification remains controversial, but important dimensions include whether the pain is above, at, or below the lesion level and whether the pain is judged to be nociceptive or neuropathic (Bryce et al. 2007). Concurrent TBI is present in about 60% of patients with SCI, although 57% of brain injuries are mild (Macciocchi et al. 2008). Of the patients with recent SCI, 10%–60% may have cognitive impairment (Davidoff et al. 1992). Cognitive deficits may be attributable to a variety of factors, including preinjury learning disabilities, substance abuse, and traumatic or hypoxic brain injury sustained at the time of SCI. Behavior problems such as noncompliance, anger, and agitation may be attributable to premorbid traits or undetected brain injury. A severe complication for people with midthoracic or higher spinal cord injuries is autonomic dysreflexia. Autonomic dysreflexia is often triggered by a noxious stimulus below the level of lesion that leads to sympathetic discharge uninhibited by descending neural control. Immediate steps must be taken to control hypertension and to identify and reverse the triggering stimulus. The most common secondary medical complication during the first year postinjury is pressure ulcers (McKinley et al. 1999).

Acute Rehabilitation

Patients are usually transferred to specialized rehabilitation programs once they are medically stable and can participate in therapies for at least 3 hours per day. Inpatient rehabilitation typically focuses on education, physical training, strengthening, and basic skill building needed to return to maximal functional independence for living in the community. Individuals with paraplegia are usually expected to be able to function and live independently once their rehabilitation is complete (Consortium for Spinal Cord Medicine 1999). Those with low cervical lesions (C7–8) should be independent in most functional tasks. Depending on their neurological level, people with higher cervical lesions require different degrees of assistance for activities of daily living, such as managing bowel and bladder, bathing, dressing, eating, and transferring to and from a wheelchair. Whatever his or her level of injury, the person with SCI is expected to be independent in guiding others to care for him or her in areas the person cannot perform on his or her own.

Adjustment to Spinal Cord Injury

Following discharge from acute rehabilitation, 91% of the people with SCI are discharged to a home environment (Eastwood et al. 1999). Estimates of employment rates after SCI have varied from 13% to 69%. One study found that, overall, 27% were employed, with 14% employed within 1 year and 35% employed within 10 years postinjury (Krause et al. 1999). Subjective well-being and quality of life are somewhat controversial, especially with regard to patients with high tetraplegia. The controversy relates to the tendency of health care workers to overestimate depressed mood and underestimate potential quality of life in survivors of SCI (Caplan 1983; Gerhart et al. 1994; Trieschmann 1988). In sharp contrast with what health care workers predict, more than 90% of the people living in the community with high tetraplegia, including those with ventilator dependence, report that they are "glad to be alive" (Gerhart et al. 1994). Nevertheless, people with SCI tend to report lower subjective quality of life compared with nondisabled persons (Barker et al. 2009). It is somewhat surprising that quality of life is generally unrelated to level of injury or injury severity, weakly related to physical impairment, and more strongly related to one's ability to carry out day-to-day tasks and participate in school, work, or other community activities (Barker et al. 2009; Mortenson et al. 2010). These studies suggest that quality of life is related to several modifiable risk factors such as pain, subjective health competence, mood, social participation, and environmental barriers.

Common biased expectations among rehabilitation staff and their misapplication of stage models have interfered with appropriate understanding and intervention to promote psychological adjustment to SCI (Elliott and Frank 1996; Trieschmann 1988). In numerous studies, rehabilitation staff, primarily nurses and therapists, have been found to overestimate depressed mood regularly in SCI patients (Trieschmann 1988). Rehabilitation staff also tend to view signs of depression as a normal, even necessary, stage of grief. An SCI patient wrote that the most depressing part of his rehabilitation program was that staff expected him to be depressed, an expectation dubbed "the requirement of mourning" (Trieschmann 1988). Empirical data contradict popular conceptualizations of grief. Most people who sustain significant losses (including SCI) do not become depressed and do not go through traditional "stages of grief" (Bonanno et al. 2002; Wortman and

Silver 1989). Rather, resilience is the modal response to loss (Bonanno et al. 2002), and acceptance of loss begins early and is more prominent than any other emotional response (Maciejewski et al. 2007). In a study that used the Beck Depression Inventory to measure depressive symptoms weekly during inpatient rehabilitation, about 60% of the SCI patients never scored in the depressed range, 20% endorsed significant depressive symptoms only once, and 20% reported significant depressive symptoms at multiple time points and required treatment with antidepressants (Judd et al. 1989). Viewing persisting depression as a normal or even healing part of the grief process may interfere with appropriate recognition and treatment of major depression. Conversely, staff may judge the absence of depression to be pathological, a sign of denial or poor adjustment and an indication that the staff should confront the patient more forcefully with the implications of his or her impairments.

In the absence of empirically supported approaches to manage grief and poor adjustment, the consultant is advised to "do no harm" by eschewing confrontational approaches that may only damage relatively healthy defenses or increase patient resistance. We recommend tolerance of adjustment patterns that are not interfering with rehabilitation. We also attempt to educate staff and family members about countertherapeutic myths of coping with loss, such as the belief that it is necessary to "work through" the loss, that patients should reach a state of "acceptance," and that the absence of grief is pathological (Wortman and Silver 1989).

Psychiatric Disorders in Spinal Cord Injury

Depression

Major depressive disorder is probably the most common psychiatric disorder after SCI (Banerjea et al. 2009; Fullerton et al. 1981; Migliorini et al. 2008). According to studies that used DSM criteria, the prevalence of major depression ranged from 9.8% to 37.5%, with most estimates falling between 15% and 23% (Bombardier et al. 2004). Some studies suggest that depression may be more common soon after injury but may remit after several months (Kishi et al. 1994, 1995). In unselected cases, mood tends to improve over the first year after injury (Richards 1986). However, other studies suggest that a subgroup of about 30% of patients develop significant depressive and anxiety symptoms soon after injury and remain highly depressed and anxious through at least 2 years after injury (Craig et al. 1994).

Depression is a significant and disabling problem for persons with SCI. Depression is associated with longer lengths of hospital stay and fewer functional improvements (Malec and Neimeyer 1983) as well as less functional independence and mobility at discharge (Umlauf and Frank 1983). Depression is associated with the occurrence of pressure sores and urinary tract infections (Herrick et al. 1994), poorer self-appraised health (Bombardier et al. 2004), less leisure activity (Elliott and Shewchuck 1995), poorer community mobility and social integration, and fewer meaningful social pursuits (Fuhrer et al. 1993; MacDonald et al. 1987). Persons with SCI and significant depression spend more days in bed and fewer days outside the home, require greater use of paid personal care, and incur greater medical expenses (Tate et al. 1994). Symptoms consistent with depression, such as documented expressions of despondency, hopelessness, shame, and apathy, are the variables most predictive of suicide 1–9 years after SCI (Charlifue and Gerhart 1991). Probable major depression predicts all-cause mortality after SCI (Krause et al. 2008).

Anxiety

Relatively few studies have examined PTSD or other anxiety disorders in this population. Rates of current PTSD range from 14% to 22% in patients with SCI (P. Kennedy and Evans 2001; Radnitz et al. 1998). Rates of PTSD appear to vary as a function of level of injury, with lower rates found among those with tetraplegia (2%) compared with those with paraplegia (22%; Radnitz et al. 1998). This variability has been attributed to diminished experience of psychophysiological arousal, which may occur in higher-level injuries (P. Kennedy and Duff 2001). Current PTSD appears to be no more prevalent in persons with SCI than in other trauma survivors. People with SCI who are war theater veterans, have prior exposure to violence, or have limited social support may be at higher risk for PTSD (P. Kennedy and Duff 2001). Elevated levels of general anxiety also have been found in people with SCI (Craig et al. 1994; P. Kennedy and Rogers 2000), particularly in a subgroup of patients with chronic comorbid depression. Anxiety and depression are associated with lower quality of life (Budh and Österåker 2007).

PTSD symptoms are also common in families of persons with SCI. Boyer et al. (1998) found that 25% of pediatric SCI survivors reported significant current PTSD symptoms, but 41% of mothers and 36% of fathers also endorsed significant PTSD symptoms on self-report measures.

Substance Use Disorders

High rates of alcohol and drug abuse problems are found among trauma patients generally and SCI patients specifically (Bombardier and Turner 2009). Preinjury alcohol problems are common (35%–49%; Bombardier and Rimmele 1998; Heinemann et al. 1988). Rates of alcohol intoxication at the time of injury range from 36% to 40% (Heinemann et al. 1988; Kiwerski and Krasuski 1992). After SCI, substance abuse appears to decline but remains somewhat higher than in the general population and, importantly, may be more harmful because of its association with poorer health maintenance behaviors (Krause 1992), including pressure ulcers (Tate et al. 2004). Acute SCI rehabilitation is a potential "teachable moment" for patients with a history of alcohol abuse or dependence to initiate changes in their drinking behavior (Bombardier and Rimmele 1998). Most do not have severe dependence and, depending on the person's history, may benefit from advice, brief motivational interventions, relapse prevention skills, or referral to specialist treatment (Turner et al. 2003).

Sexual Dysfunction

SCI affects erectile functioning, ejaculation, and emission in males and lubrication in females as a function of level (upper motor neuron vs. lower motor neuron) and completeness of injury (Table 35–6). Approximately 70% of men with SCI recover some degree of erectile function (Sipski and Alexander 1997). Reflex erection ability is dependent on the parasympathetic reflex arc in the sacral segments (S2 to S4) and can be brought on by direct stimulation of the penis or other erogenous areas. Psychogenic erection is dependent on the integrity of the hypogastric plexus, which includes both the T11–L2 segments and the sacral plexus, and can be elicited by sexual thoughts or feelings (Sipski and Alexander 1997).

Laboratory research confirms that women with complete upper motor lesions affecting the sacral segments are likely to have vaginal lubrication from reflexive but not psychogenic mechanisms (Sipski et al. 1995). Women with incomplete upper motor lesions affecting the sacral segments retain the capacity for reflex lubrication but will have psychogenic lubrication only if they have intact pinprick sensation in the T11–L2 dermatomes. Women with incomplete lower motor lesions affecting the sacral segments are expected to achieve psychogenic lubrication in 25% of cases and no reflex lubrication.

By contrast, achieving orgasm is less well studied but appears to be relatively independent of level and completeness of injury. Among males with SCI, 38%–47% report achieving orgasm, which may be experienced as similar to or different from preinjury experiences. In a laboratory study, about 50% of the women with SCI reported experiencing orgasm, with longer stimulation, greater sexual knowledge, and higher sexual drive associated with higher rates of orgasm (Sipski et al. 1995). Sexual desire, activity, and pleasure tend to decrease after SCI for both women and men, but most remain interested in sexual activity. Erogenous zones and preferences for type of sexual activity may change.

Numerous treatments are available for sexual dysfunction related to SCI (Consortium for Spinal Cord Medicine 2010; see also Chapter 16, "Sexual Dysfunction"). First-line treatment for erectile dysfunction is with sildenafil and other phosphodiesterase type 5 (PDE-5) inhibitors (Lombardi et al. 2009). Large increases in successful intercourse rates can be achieved with the use of PDE-5 inhibitors. Ejaculation and orgasm rates also improve. All PDE-5 inhibitors appear safe with the caveat that most studies have been short term. Second-line treatments include vacuum erection devices, pharmacological penile injections, and penile implants. Ejaculatory dysfunction and related infertility are treated with vibratory or electroejaculation procedures in conjunction with intrauterine insemination, in vitro fertilization, or intracytoplasmic sperm injection, depending on sperm quality and motility (Amador et al. 2000). Decreased lubrication in females can be managed by water-based lubricants. Regarding sexual enjoyment, patients can benefit from many standard counseling strategies adapted for people with SCI, such as enhancing communication skills, teaching sensate focus exercises, addressing performance anxiety, and generally dispelling common counterproductive beliefs about sexual relationships (Consortium for Spinal Cord Medicine 2010; Zilbergeld 1978). It is important to broach the subjects of sexuality and fertility while the person is undergoing acute rehabilitation, but studies indicate that during this time many patients rate other rehabilitation concerns as more important and may prefer to discuss sexual concerns in more detail after the acute rehabilitation phase (Hanson and Franklin 1976).

TABLE 35–6. Male sexual functioning by level and type of lesion

<table>
<tr><th>Male sexual functioning</th><th>Psychogenic erection (%)</th><th>Reflex erection (%)</th><th>Anterograde ejaculation (%)</th></tr>
<tr><td>Upper motor neuron—complete</td><td>0</td><td>70–93</td><td>4</td></tr>
<tr><td>Upper motor neuron—incomplete</td><td>19</td><td>80</td><td>32</td></tr>
<tr><td>Lower motor neuron—complete</td><td>26–50</td><td>0</td><td>18</td></tr>
<tr><td>Lower motor neuron—incomplete</td><td colspan="2">67–95</td><td>70</td></tr>
</table>

Source. Adapted from Sipski and Alexander 1997.

The PLISSIT sexual counseling model is a useful framework when offering sexually related counseling to patients in a rehabilitation setting (Consortium for Spinal Cord Medicine 2010). First, one asks for **P**ermission to discuss sexuality during acute rehabilitation with all patients. If permitted, the clinician should provide **L**imited **I**nformation, generally educational in nature, about sexual functioning. The clinician should give **S**pecific **S**uggestions about how to manage sexuality or fertility problems and refer the patient to a sexual counseling specialist for **I**ntensive **T**herapy when indicated.

Personality and Psychological Testing

Personality assessment among persons with SCI has received justifiable criticism. Critics allege that clinicians are guilty of a negative bias, of overreliance on measures designed only to detect pathology, and of attribution of behavior patterns only to intrapsychic and not to situational or environmental factors (Elliott and Umlauf 1995). Measures such as the Minnesota Multiphasic Personality Inventory and the Hopkins Symptom Checklist–90 should be interpreted cautiously and with the aid of norms correcting for disability-related factors (Barncord and Wanlass 2000). Nonpathological measures such as the NEO Personality Inventory (NEO-PI), the 16 Personality Factor Questionnaire (16PFQ), and the Meyers-Briggs Type Indicator may be more appropriate tests of personality functioning in this population (Elliott and Shewchuck 1995). Yet evidence indicates that certain premorbid personality characteristics are more prominent among individuals with SCI than in the uninjured population. Nearly two-thirds of the patients with SCI have personality characteristics suggesting a strong physical orientation, difficulty expressing emotion, a preference for working with things rather than people, and a dislike of intellectual or academic interests (Rohe and Krause 1998). Neuropsychological evaluation that documents areas of cognitive impairment and strength can be critical in guiding treatment and vocational rehabilitation, especially because comorbid TBI can be expected in most cases, particularly those with cervical SCI (Macciocchi et al. 2008).

Treatment of Psychiatric Disorders in Traumatic Brain Injury and Spinal Cord Injury

General Principles

A patient's specific physical (e.g., spasticity) and cognitive (e.g., defects in executive functions) impairments must be considered in designing a treatment plan for psychiatric disorders in the rehabilitation setting. A detailed understanding of the patient's physical and psychological stage in rehabilitation and functional goals will help in choosing the most appropriate psychopharmacological or psychotherapeutic treatment modality. Consulting with other members of the multidisciplinary rehabilitation team will provide clues as to the patient's motivation and treatment limitations. Knowledge of the patient's current functional, social, and vocational status is required to tailor the psychiatric treatment to specific practical needs and limitations. For example, initial treatment with an activating antidepressant in a fatigued, cognitively impaired, depressed TBI patient who is not participating optimally in physical therapy may be more appropriate than attempting to engage the patient in cognitive-behavioral therapy (CBT).

Once rapport has been established, it is helpful to discuss the events that led up to the patient's impairment (e.g., the circumstances of the car crash that led to the TBI, the stroke that led to the left-sided hemiparesis) to explore the psychodynamic significance of these events. For example, patients will often blame themselves for their predicament, with such self-attribution leading to guilt and depression. In contrast, patients may not associate their psychiatric symptoms with their physical impairment, which may affect readiness for psychotherapy.

Interviewing the patient's family, friends, and caregivers can provide critical information about the patient's past and present mental state. How patients handled prior losses and health problems can provide clues as to how resilient they will be during rehabilitation. Moreover, patients may report different symptoms from those observed by those close to them. For example, a patient often focuses on physical and cognitive deficits, whereas family members may consider the patient's emotional changes as more disabling (Hendryx 1989; Oddy et al. 1978a; Sherer et al. 1998b). Patients often report significantly less frequent symptoms of depression, aggression, and memory and attention problems on self-ratings compared with ratings by their significant others (Hart et al. 2003). Close communication with family and other caregivers and acquaintances can provide critical longitudinal information about the progress of psychiatric treatment.

Because SCI may result in marked weight loss, alterations in appetite and sleep, and reduced energy and activity, diagnosing depression can be complicated. However, vegetative symptoms should not be dismissed, because altered psychomotor activity, appetite change, and sleep disturbance are predictive of major depression (Clay et al. 1995). Core symptoms of depression in people with physical disabilities such as arthritis and SCI are worthlessness or self-blame, depressed mood, and suicidal ideation (Frank et al. 1992). The patient's own experience and interpretation of the vegetative symptoms can aid the diagnostic process (Elliott and Frank 1996).

As discussed earlier with TBI and SCI, the phenomenological presentation of psychiatric symptoms in rehabilitation patients may differ from symptoms that arise de novo or in other medical settings. Although psychopathology based on DSM-IV-TR criteria should be thoroughly explored, psychiatric symptoms that do not meet DSM diagnostic criteria but that still lead to significant functional impairment are common in the rehabilitation setting (e.g., the depressed TBI patient who has four depressive symptoms but shows apathy that affects his or her level of functioning, or the severely anxious SCI patient with few autonomic symptoms). These syndromes, or symptom clusters, still may warrant close monitoring and treatment to maximize functioning. Therefore, in addition to monitoring and documenting psychiatric signs and symptoms, functional status (e.g., activities of daily living, progress in physical and occupational therapy, role functioning) should be monitored closely as an indicator of overall progress. Consistent with the rehabilitation process's basic tenet of working toward realistic and measurable goals, psychiatric intervention should begin with defining treatment end points according to measurable outcomes. Examples of useful measures include the PHQ (Spitzer et al. 1999) for depression and anxiety, the Brief Symptom Inventory for general distress (Meachen et al. 2008), the Neurobehavioral Rating Scale (Levin et al. 1987b) for behavior and cognition, and the Rivermead Post Concussion Symptoms Questionnaire (King et al. 1995) or the OAS (Giles and Mohr 2007; Yudofsky et al. 1986) for severe agitation. Improved participation in rehabilitation therapies, which may be the outcome of most concern to the referring physician, can be monitored easily with the Pittsburgh Rehabilitation Participation Scale (Lenze et al. 2004).

Realistic expectations, including the possibility of incomplete remission of symptoms, must be conveyed at the outset so that the patient, who is already frustrated with the often slow and arduous rehabilitation process, does not become even more hopeless or overwhelmed if some symptoms persist (Roy-Byrne and Fann 1997). A survey of 16,403 community-dwelling elderly and disabled Medicare beneficiaries found that persons with disabilities reported poor communication and lack of thorough care as negative aspects of their care (Iezzoni et al. 2003). Because patients may have strong preexisting preferences for specific treatment approaches (Fann et al. 2009b), adequate time must be spent on providing education about evidence-based approaches. Collaboration with rehabilitation psychologists and counselors can provide significant depth of assessment and breadth of intervention. Attending rehabilitation team meetings is often a valuable and efficient way of communicating and coordinating needs and treatment. Because the patient is likely already feeling overwhelmed about his or her situation, framing the psychiatric consultation and intervention as another modality similar to, for example, occupational or speech therapy that can help him or her achieve the rehabilitation goals during a period of intense stress and adaptation can quickly put the patient at ease. Often, appropriately applied treatments may not have been given ample time to work. This problem may be exacerbated by imposed pressures on rehabilitation centers to work within predetermined payment structures and lengths of stay on the basis of medical diagnoses (Carter et al. 2000).

Treatment of psychiatric problems in the rehabilitation setting typically warrants a combination of pharmacological and psychosocial interventions. Because treatments for most chronic diseases are covered in other chapters, the following treatment recommendations focus on TBI and SCI.

Psychopharmacology

Several common physiological changes in SCI (Table 35-7), often more pronounced in tetraplegia than in paraplegia, can have an effect on the pharmacokinetics and tolerability of many psychotropic medications. The goals and potential side effects of pharmacotherapy should be explained thoroughly to the patient and caregivers because unanticipated symptoms caused by medications may be viewed as a sign that the underlying condition is worsening. For example, urinary retention from an anticholinergic psychotropic drug may signal to the patient with SCI that the spinal lesion is progressing. Medications that can cause weight gain, constipation, dry mouth, orthostatic hypotension, or sexual dysfunction also may exacerbate already present pathophysiology. Medications that are sedating are of particular concern in TBI and SCI because they may impair mobility and cognition, increase risk for pressure sores, and interfere

TABLE 35-7. Common physiological changes associated with spinal cord injury

Increased body fat and glucose intolerance
Decreased gastrointestinal motility
Reduced cardiac output
Anemia
Orthostatic hypotension
Bradyarrhythmia
Decreased blood flow to skeletal muscle
Venous thrombosis
Osteoporosis

with rehabilitation. Sedation is a frequent problem because many patients with TBI and SCI are taking multiple central nervous system (CNS) depressants, such as anticonvulsants, muscle relaxants, and opioid analgesics (for discussion of interactions between neurological and psychiatric drugs, see Chapter 38, "Psychopharmacology").

Because patients with TBI or SCI are often more susceptible to sedative, extrapyramidal, anticholinergic, epileptogenic, and spasticity effects (Fann 2002), psychotropic dosages should be started at lower-than-standard levels and be titrated slowly. Despite this need for caution, some patients still may ultimately need full standard doses (Silver and Yudofsky 1994b).

Neuropsychiatric polypharmacy is common in TBI patients and should be critically examined. When multiple psychotropics are needed, they should be initiated one at a time, when possible, to accurately determine the therapeutic and adverse effects of each medication. This practice may become difficult to follow if patients' behavior endangers them or staff or significantly impairs rehabilitation, but it usually will prove beneficial in the long term.

Because few randomized, placebo-controlled studies have tested pharmacotherapy for psychiatric conditions in TBI and SCI populations, many of the following recommendations are based on case series and expert consensus (Warden et al. 2006) or are extrapolated from other neurological populations. Heterogeneous study populations, including those varying in time elapsed since injury, confound the interpretation of study results. When TBI or SCI occurs in the context of a preexisting psychiatric illness, it is logical to continue a previously effective medication regimen, but previously absent side effects may emerge that require changes in dosages and/or drugs. Electroconvulsive therapy for refractory depression (Crow et al. 1996; Martino et al. 2008), mania (Clark and Davison 1987), and prolonged posttraumatic delirium and agitation (Kant et al. 1995) may be considered. However, efforts should be made to lessen cognitive dysfunction in TBI patients (e.g., by using high-dose unilateral electrode placement or twice-weekly treatment frequency), and caution should be exercised in treating patients with SCI who may have unstable spinal columns. Preliminary studies of low-intensity magnetic field exposure (Baker-Price and Persinger 2003), biofeedback with electroencephalogram recording and photic feedback (Schoenberger et al. 2001), acupuncture (Donnellan 2006), and music therapy (Guetin et al. 2009) for improving mood after TBI have been reported and require further study.

Depression, Apathy, and Fatigue

The literature on the efficacy of pharmacological treatment of depression after TBI is limited to small studies varying widely in design, diagnostic and outcome assessment, severity of brain injury, and time after injury (see systematic review on treatment of depression after TBI by Fann et al. 2009a).

Because of a favorable side-effect profile, a selective serotonin reuptake inhibitor (SSRI) usually is the first-line antidepressant for patients with TBI. Ashman et al. (2009) randomly assigned 52 depressed patients at an average of 17.7 years postinjury to sertraline or placebo. Although no statistically significant group differences in response rates or decreases in Hamilton Rating Scale for Depression scores were found over 10 weeks, 59% of the sertraline group responded compared with only 32% of the placebo group. A single-blind, placebo run-in study of sertraline in 15 patients with mild TBI (Fann et al. 2000) and an open study of citalopram in 54 patients with mild to moderate TBI (Rapoport et al. 2008) suggested that SSRIs are efficacious and well tolerated in TBI populations. The study by Fann et al. (2000) found that 67% had remission of their major depression after 8 weeks of sertraline and that treatment also was associated with improvements in postconcussive symptoms, neuropsychological functioning, functional status, and self-ratings of injury severity and distress. The areas of cognitive functioning that improved included short-term memory, mental flexibility, cognitive efficiency, and psychomotor speed. In a 4-week study of depressed patients, H. Lee et al. (2005) found both sertraline and methylphenidate to be superior to placebo in decreasing depression scores. Perino et al. (2001) assessed 20 depressed post-TBI patients before and after administration of citalopram and carbamazepine and found that depression, anxiety, inappropriate and labile affect, and somatic overconcern improved significantly. SSRIs should be started at about half of their usual starting dose and titrated slowly. SSRI-induced akathisia sometimes can be mistaken for TBI-related agitation (Hensley and Reeve 2001). Escitalopram, citalopram, and sertraline all have low potential for significant drug–drug interactions. For patients at high risk for noncompliance (e.g., because of cognitive impairment), fluoxetine should be considered because of its lower risk for withdrawal symptoms.

No clinical trials of antidepressants in persons with SCI are available to help guide pharmacotherapy. The Paralyzed Veterans of America and their partners in the Consortium for Spinal Cord Medicine (1998) have published a clinical practice guideline on depression following SCI for primary care physicians, extrapolated from research conducted in the general population or among other disability groups. Combining an antidepressant and psychotherapy may be effective for major depression (Kemp et al. 2004). Although SSRIs are likely efficacious in patients with SCI, the risk for spasticity may be increased (Stolp-Smith and Wainberg 1999). Similarly, there may be an increased risk of spasticity and autonomic dysreflexia with tricyclic antidepressants (TCAs) in patients with SCI (Cardenas et al. 2002; Fullerton et al. 1981). Although not yet studied for depression after SCI, venlafaxine may improve voiding in SCI patients with urinary retention (Inghilleri et al. 2005).

The literature on the tolerability and safety of TCAs and monoamine oxidase inhibitors (MAOIs) after TBI is more inconsistent (Dinan and Mobayed 1992; Saran 1985; Wroblewski et al. 1996). Because of the potentially problematic adverse effects of TCAs and MAOIs (e.g., sedation, hypotension, and anticholinergic effects) in patients with CNS impairment and their narrow therapeutic index (which can lead to inadvertent overdose in patients with cognitive impairment), these medications should be used with extreme caution in TBI patients. Autonomic dysfunction in patients with SCI makes them more vulnerable to TCA-related anticholinergic and orthostatic side effects. If a TCA is chosen, nortriptyline or desipramine may cause the fewest side effects.

Although not yet systematically studied, dual-action serotonin–norepinephrine reuptake inhibitors (SNRIs) such as venlafaxine and duloxetine are likely safe and effective in patients with TBI. The one open study (N= 10) that examined a dual-action SNRI (milnacipran) for minor or major depression after mild to moderate TBI also suggested that it may be efficacious (66.7% responded, 44.4% remitted) and well tolerated (Kanetani et al. 2003). Mirtazapine, nefazodone, and trazodone may prove to be too sedating for some patients, particularly if they have cognitive impairment or gait instability, but if insomnia is a major problem, these drugs may be helpful. Venlafaxine and mirtazapine have low drug–drug interaction potential. Moclobemide, a reversible inhibitor of monoamine oxidase A, showed efficacy in an open subgroup analysis of 26 depressed patients with TBI (Newburn et al. 1999).

Some data suggest that antidepressants, especially TCAs and bupropion, are associated with an increased risk of seizures (Davidson 1989), a particular concern following severe TBI (Wroblewski et al. 1990); however, if the drugs are titrated cautiously, most patients will not experience increased seizures, particularly if they are taking an anticonvulsant (Ojemann et al. 1987).

The symptoms of apathy and fatigue, often associated with CNS impairment, can occur concomitantly with or independently of depression and are often mistaken for primary depression (Marin 1991). For apathy and fatigue, medications that augment dopaminergic activity appear to be the most useful (Marin et al. 1995). Methylphenidate and dextroamphetamine are generally safe at standard dosages (e.g., methylphenidate 10–30 mg/day in divided doses) (Alban et al. 2004) and have been used successfully to enhance participation in rehabilitation (C.T. Gualtieri and Evans 1988). Methylphenidate and dextroamphetamine also have been shown in case series and double-blind studies to be effective in improving some aspects of mood, mental speed, attention, and behavior, although improvement was not always sustained long term (Bleiberg et al. 1993; C.T. Gualtieri and Evans 1988; Kaelin et al. 1996; Mooney and Haas 1993; Plenger et al. 1996; Speech et al. 1993; Whyte et al. 1997, 2004). Dextroamphetamine may exacerbate dystonia and dyskinesia in some cases. Therapeutic use of these oral psychostimulants in the medically ill rarely leads to abuse in patients without a personal or family history of substance abuse (Masand and Tesar 1996), but substance abuse is overrepresented in the TBI and SCI populations.

Modafinil has been efficacious in treating fatigue in patients with multiple sclerosis (Rammahan et al. 2000; Terzoudi et al. 2000; Zifko et al. 2002) and excessive daytime sleepiness in patients with TBI (Teitelman 2001). Bupropion (Marin et al. 1995) and dopamine agonists such as amantadine (Green et al. 2004; M.F. Kraus et al. 2005; Sawyer et al. 2008), bromocriptine (McDowell et al. 1998; Powell et al. 1996), and levodopa/carbidopa (Lal et al. 1988) have been used for apathy states, fatigue, and cognitive impairment. Bupropion's stimulating properties may be of particular benefit in the fatigued or apathetic depressed patient. Stimulants and dopamine agonists can increase the risk for delirium and psychosis and thus should be used with caution in more vulnerable patients. Amantadine has been associated with an increased risk of seizures (T. Gualtieri et al. 1989), but methylphenidate, dextroamphetamine, and bromocriptine do not appear to lower seizure threshold at typical doses.

There is great interest in pharmacological agents that could improve not only arousal and attention following TBI but also memory; however, data are lacking. Preliminary evidence indicates that the acetylcholinesterase inhibitor donepezil may improve memory and global functioning (Khateb et al. 2005; Whelan et al. 2000; Zhang et al. 2004), but no large randomized controlled trials of cholinesterase inhibitors have been done in patients with TBI.

Another secondary benefit of some antidepressants in TBI and SCI patients is their analgesic properties (Onghena and Van Houdenhove 1992) (see also Chapter 36, "Pain"). TCAs have been shown to be effective for the treatment of chronic nonmalignant pain, including neuropathic pain (McQuay et al. 1996). Amitriptyline improves SCI-related neuropathic pain in the context of comorbid depressive symptomatology (Rintala et al. 2007). SSRIs have not been shown to be effective in neuropathic pain (Jung et al. 1997). Venlafaxine and duloxetine may be effective in treating a variety of pain syndromes, including neuropathic pain (Diamond 1995; Lang et al. 1996; Schreiber et al. 1999).

Mania

For mania following TBI, the mood stabilizers lithium carbonate (Oyewumi and Lapierre 1981; Stewart and Nemsath 1988), valproic acid (Pope et al. 1988), and carbamazepine (Stewart and Nemsath 1988) all have been used successfully. Successful use of the antipsychotics haloperidol, thioridazine, chlorpromazine, olanzapine, and quetiapine, often in combination with another mood-stabilizing agent, also has been documented in case reports (Daniels and Felde 2008; Oster et al. 2007). Electroconvulsive therapy (Clark and Davison 1987) can be used as a second-line modality. Dikmen et al. (2000) have shown that valproic acid is well tolerated after TBI, but lithium and carbamazepine have been associated with neurocognitive adverse effects (Hornstein and Seliger 1989; Schiff et al. 1982). Lithium has a narrow therapeutic window and also can lower the seizure threshold; thus, caution is required when lithium is used in TBI patients whose cognitive impairment may lead to poor adherence or inadvertent overdosage. Although serum blood levels of valproic acid and carbamazepine help in monitoring adherence and absorption, dosing should be guided primarily by therapeutic response and side effects. Possible roles for other anticonvulsants in secondary mania are reviewed in Chapter 10, "Psychosis, Mania, and Catatonia." Carbamazepine, gabapentin, pregabalin, and clonazepam also can be effective for the treatment of neuropathic pain.

Anxiety

Benzodiazepines are the treatment of choice for acute anxiety in TBI, but they should be used initially at lower doses because of their propensity to exacerbate or cause cognitive impairment and oversedation. The high prevalence of substance abuse in patients with TBI and SCI adds to the risk of benzodiazepine use and may preclude their use in some patients. Although few studies exist in TBI patients, antidepressants also appear to be effective for anxiety, particularly in the context of depression. SSRIs also have been found to be effective in decreasing mood lability after brain injury (Nahas et al. 1998; Sloan et al. 1992), although this effect may take as long as their antidepressant effects. In a case report, venlafaxine, 150 mg/day, successfully treated compulsions after TBI (Khouzam and Donnelly 1998). Valproic acid, gabapentin, and pregabalin may be of benefit, especially in patients with concomitant mood lability or seizures (Pande et al. 1999, 2000). Buspirone is another option for generalized anxiety symptoms; however, it has been associated, albeit rarely, with seizures and movement disorders (Levitt et al. 1993).

Sleep Disorders

Treatment of sleep problems in patients with TBI and SCI ideally should be based on diagnosis of a specific sleep disorder. Sleep apnea is fairly common in TBI (Castriotta and Lai 2001; Masel et al. 2001) and SCI (Burns et al. 2000), and nocturnal periodic leg movements are frequent in SCI (Dickel et al. 1994). Fichtenberg et al. (2000) found that insomnia often appeared to be associated with depression in post-acute TBI patients. No specific data exist on treating insomnia or other sleep disorders in TBI or SCI, but trazodone is widely used in these patients for middle or late insomnia, and hypnotics are used in as many as 20% of TBI patients (Worthington and Melia 2006). Trazodone-associated orthostatic hypotension may be particularly problematic in the rehabilitation setting, however. Antihistamines such as diphenhydramine should be avoided because of their anticholinergic properties (see Chapter 15, "Sleep Disorders," for general diagnosis and treatment of sleep disorders).

Anger, Aggression, and Agitation

Anger, aggression, and agitation are common following TBI and can occur in isolation or as part of delirium or other psychiatric disorders (see Chapter 7, "Aggression and Violence," for a full review of agitation and aggression in the medically ill). The published literature regarding their treatment is often not diagnostically specific and consists largely of case reports, case series, and reviews (e.g., Fleminger et al. 2006; Krieger et al. 2003; Levy et al. 2005; Maryniak et al. 2001).

Treatment can be divided into acute treatment, in which the goal is timely management of behavior to prevent injury to self or others, and chronic treatment, in which the goal is long-term management and prevention (Silver et al. 2002). Many agents take from 2 to 8 weeks to gain full effectiveness. It is important to keep in mind that medications that worsen cognition or sedation can actually worsen confusion and may, therefore, worsen agitation during the confusional state of posttraumatic amnesia after TBI. Because the effects of medications on the patient with TBI can be unpredictable and because their side effects actually may potentiate the behavior problem (e.g., akathisia from antipsychotics), systematically eliminating certain medications, including those that were initially prescribed to treat the behavioral dyscontrol, can prove beneficial. A rationale for such an approach is the clinical observation that some patients have a natural course of recovery and that some medication efficacy may decrease over time.

A survey published in 1997 (Fugate et al. 1997) showed that physiatrist experts in TBI most often treated agitation with carbamazepine, TCAs, trazodone, amantadine, and beta-blockers. Psychiatrists appear more likely than physiatrists to use atypical antipsychotics (Burnett et al. 1999) and SSRIs.

The atypical antipsychotics afford the clinician many more options in the acute setting than were available a decade ago (Battaglia et al. 2003; Currier and Simpson 2001; Lesem et al. 2001). The efficacy of the atypical antipsychotics in treating acute aggression and agitation in TBI patients is still emerging (Scott et al. 2009), and evidence is mounting to support their efficacy in treating other agitated states associated with neurological syndromes (M.A. Lee et al. 2001; Meehan et al. 2002). The typical antipsychotics given orally or intramuscularly also may be useful in the acute setting (Stanislav and Childs 2000), but the elevated risks of extrapyramidal and anticholinergic effects in TBI patients must be considered. Studies in animals have suggested that haloperidol and other antipsychotics may impede neuronal and cognitive recovery (Hoffman et al. 2008; M.S. Wilson et al. 2003), but this finding has not been supported in humans with TBI.

Antipsychotic use for chronic agitation ideally should be reserved for situations when aggression occurs in the context of psychotic symptoms. Risperidone (Cohen et al. 1998; De Deyn et al. 1999; I.R. Katz et al. 1999; McDougle et al. 1998) and olanzapine (Street et al. 2000) show promise in neuropsychiatric patients, although efficacy data in TBI patients for these and the other atypical antipsychotics such as quetiapine (Kim and Bijlani 2006) are sparse. Clozapine use in TBI patients is limited by its seizure risk, although it has been found to be effective for chronic aggression (J.E. Kraus and Sheitman 2005; Michals et al. 1993).

The benzodiazepines offer rapid sedation that may be useful in the acute setting; however, they also have a high potential for neurocognitive effects, such as mental slowing, amnesia, disinhibition, and impaired balance, in patients with TBI. As a result, low doses of a short-acting agent, such as lorazepam, 1–2 mg orally or parenterally, should be used initially and titrated as needed. If agitation is frequent, a longer-acting agent, such as clonazepam, 0.5–1.0 mg two or three times a day, may be used for short durations. The combination of haloperidol and low-dose lorazepam (e.g., 0.5–1.0 mg) may offer a synergistic calming effect for some acutely agitated patients.

Serotonergic antidepressants, such as the SSRIs, trazodone, and amitriptyline, have been used to treat agitation and aggression in TBI populations (Mysiw et al. 1988; Rowland et al. 1992). In 8-week nonrandomized trials with sertraline, Fann et al. (2000) showed that improved depression was associated with improved anger and aggression scores in patients with mild TBI, whereas Kant et al. (1998) found improved aggression independent of depression scores. One rationale for the use of antidepressants is the observation that serotonin and norepinephrine levels are reduced in the cerebrospinal fluid of agitated patients with brain injury (van Workeom et al. 1977). SSRIs are also effective in treating emotional incontinence, such as pathological crying or laughter (Muller et al. 1999; Nahas et al. 1998; Sloan et al. 1992).

Buspirone also has shown some efficacy for agitation in TBI and other neurological patients (C.T. Gualtieri 1991; Silver and Yudofsky 1994a; Stanislav et al. 1994) and can be particularly useful when anxiety also is present. Although one 6-week placebo-controlled trial found that methylphenidate significantly reduced anger an average of 27 months after severe TBI (Mooney and Haas 1993), stimulants should be used with caution in the agitated TBI patient because of the risks of exacerbating agitation and psychosis and of abuse.

Among the anticonvulsants, carbamazepine (Azouvi et al. 1999; Chatham-Showalter 1996) and valproic acid (Chatham-Showalter and Kimmel 2000; Lindenmayer and Kotsaftis 2000; Wroblewski et al. 1997) have been studied the most for treatment of behavioral dyscontrol in TBI populations. Although evidence of seizures or epileptiform activity on electroencephalogram is a strong indication for anticonvulsant use in the agitated patient, these agents also have shown efficacy in those without electroencephalographic abnormalities. Oxcarbazepine, gabapentin, lamotrigine, and topiramate also may be efficacious, although data are more limited. Some TBI patients may experience paradoxical agitation with gabapentin (Childers and Holland 1997). Lamotrigine was found to decrease aggressive and agitated behavior in one patient with severe TBI (Pachet et al. 2003), but it could possibly exacerbate aggression, as is seen in some mentally retarded patients with epilepsy (Beran and Gibson 1998; Ettinger et al. 1998). Cognitive functioning may worsen with topiramate in some cases (Martin et al. 1999; Tatum et al. 2001). Topiramate also has been found to attenuate binge-eating behavior in some patients (Dolberg et al. 2005). Some patients may need to achieve serum levels of anticonvulsants that exceed therapeutic levels used for seizure prophylaxis to ensure adequate behavioral control. Lithium is also an effective mood stabilizer and has antiaggressive properties in TBI patients, according to case reports; however, its narrow therapeutic window and high potential for neurotoxicity limit its routine use, particularly in those with significant cognitive impairment or history of seizures.

When anger, aggression, or agitation occurs without signs of other psychiatric syndromes, beta-blockers such as propranolol, pindolol, metoprolol, and nadolol should be considered. Placebo-controlled studies have shown their efficacy in treating agitation in TBI patients (Brooke et al. 1992a; Greendyke and Kanter 1996; Greendyke et al. 1996). A Cochrane review (Fleminger et al. 2006) concluded that among the drugs used to treat agitation and aggression in

TBI, beta-blockers have the best evidence for efficacy. Dosages of propranolol in the range of 160–320 mg/day have been effective. Bradycardia and hypotension are potential side effects; contraindications include asthma, chronic obstructive pulmonary disease, type 1 diabetes mellitus, congestive heart failure, persistent angina, significant peripheral vascular disease, and hyperthyroidism. Pindolol is less likely to cause bradycardia.

Psychosis

Because of the increased susceptibility of patients with TBI to experience anticholinergic and extrapyramidal side effects and of patients with SCI to experience problematic anticholinergic sequelae, the newer-generation atypical antipsychotics are the drugs of first choice for psychotic symptoms that emerge after TBI or SCI (Burnett et al. 1999) (see also earlier discussion of antipsychotics for agitation in the "Anger, Aggression, and Agitation" subsection and Chapter 10, "Psychosis, Mania, and Catatonia"). Case reports suggest that olanzapine, 5–20 mg/day, alone and with valproic acid may be helpful and safe for treating post-TBI psychosis (Butler 2000; Umansky and Geller 2000). Despite the relative tolerability of newer-generation antipsychotics, tardive dyskinesia has been reported with aripiprazole after TBI (Zaidi and Faruqui 2008). Clozapine carries a risk of seizures and should be used with extreme caution in TBI patients, particularly when compliance is in question. Augmenting risperidone with the anticholinesterase inhibitor galantamine was effective in decreasing both negative and positive psychotic symptoms following a severe TBI (Bennouna et al. 2005).

Cognitive Impairment

Little evidence is available to guide pharmacological treatments to enhance cognitive recovery following TBI; most data are derived from theoretical or animal models or case reports. Medications targeting the dopaminergic, cholinergic, and noradrenergic neurotransmitter systems have been tried (McElligott et al. 2003). Dopaminergic agents include levodopa/carbidopa, bromocriptine, amantadine, pergolide, the newer dopamine agonists (ropinirole, pramipexole), catecholamine-*O*-methyltransferase (COMT) inhibitors (entacapone, tolcapone), and the monoamine oxidase–B (MAO-B) inhibitor selegiline (McDowell et al. 1998; Meythaler et al. 2002; Zafonte et al. 2001). The SSRI sertraline, which has some dopaminergic activity, may have a cognition-enhancing effect in addition to its antidepressant effect (Fann et al. 2001), although larger controlled studies are needed to confirm this finding and to determine whether sertraline's effect on cognition is independent of its effect on depression. Medications that enhance cholinergic activity include cholinergic precursors such as lecithin and acetylcholinesterase inhibitors such as physostigmine (Cardenas et al. 1994), donepezil (Khateb et al. 2005; Whelan et al. 2000; Zhang et al. 2004), and galantamine (Bennouna et al. 2005). The noradrenergic agents most commonly used to enhance cognition, perhaps by improving arousal, attention, and awareness, are the psychostimulants methylphenidate (H. Lee et al. 2005; Whyte et al. 2004) and dextroamphetamine, which also have dopaminergic effects. Modafinil also may show some benefit. The opioid antagonist naltrexone helped improve TBI-associated memory impairment in a case series (Tennant and Wild 1987). Although evidence-based guidelines support post-TBI use of methylphenidate and donepezil for deficits of attention and speed of processing, donepezil for memory deficits, and bromocriptine for deficits in executive functioning (Warden et al. 2006), these agents require further study to better delineate appropriate indications, dosages, and treatment durations.

Psychological Treatment

Traumatic Brain Injury

A widely accepted model of psychological effects of TBI distinguishes among symptoms that are reactions to the effects of TBI (e.g., depression, anxiety, irritability, anger, hopelessness, helplessness, social withdrawal, distrust, and phobias), symptoms that are neurologically based (e.g., affective lability, impulsivity, agitation, paranoia, unawareness), and symptoms that reflect long-standing personality traits (e.g., obsessiveness, antisocial behavior, work attitude, social connectedness, dependence, entitlement) (Prigatano 1986). Although the genesis of symptoms can be multifactorial, it is useful to consider the potential contributions of all three factors to observed problem behaviors. Prigatano (1986) argued that reactive problems may be most amenable to psychotherapeutic interventions, whereas neurologically mediated symptoms may require multimodal interventions that also target underlying cognitive impairment. Characterological problems may require making coordinated changes in important environmental contingencies and working with families or caregivers.

Although psychotherapy is considered an important aspect of brain injury rehabilitation (National Institutes of Health Consensus Development Panel 1999), there are few controlled studies of psychotherapeutic interventions in persons with TBI and little guidance on the indications for psychotherapeutic interventions. A systematic review of the literature on psychotherapeutic and rehabilitation interventions for depression after TBI (Fann et al. 2009a) suggests that cognitive-behavioral approaches, particularly holistic treatment programs for TBI that include activity scheduling and increasing positive interaction with the environment, may improve mood along with functional outcomes and productivity. Other treatment components such as problem-solving and goal-setting training that are commonly used in multidisciplinary programs for TBI, including two reviewed here (Powell et al. 2002; Svendsen et al. 2004), also may be important. A telephone-based psychoeducational and problem-solving program aimed at improving functioning after TBI also shows promise in improving depressive symptoms while overcoming barriers to treatment (Bombardier et al. 2009). Empirically supported psychotherapies have been adapted for use in brain-injured individuals (e.g., modified CBT for anxiety [Bryant et al. 2003; Hibbard et al. 2000b; Tiersky et al. 2005], depression [Hibbard et al. 1992], and insomnia [Ouellet and Morin 2004]). Psychological interventions are more likely to require involvement of family members or caregivers to help cue follow-through and generalization to real-world situations. Psychotherapy has been used with selected patients to foster insight in comprehensive post acute neurorehabilitation programs (Prigatano and Ben-Yishay 1999). Insight-focused psychotherapy often begins with providing the patient with a simple model to explain what has happened. These explanations and coping strategies must be rehearsed repeatedly until they are automatic. Group therapy may be used to foster more insight through feedback from peers.

When insight and self-management approaches are not feasible, applied behavioral analysis can be used to manage a wide variety of brain injury–related behavioral deficits or excesses, such as emotional lability, anger management, compulsions, and impulsivity. Mainly case studies have shown the efficacy of contingency management for enhancing appropriate social behavior, improving participation in rehabilitation, and increasing independent functioning (Horton and Howe 1981). In some cases, such as anger management, both self-control and environmental control strategies can be combined to achieve better outcomes (Uomoto and Brockway 1992).

Therapy for impaired awareness is in its infancy but has included several different strategies. Mildly impaired patients may benefit from information about the effects of brain injury coupled with test data and observations about the specific ways they have been affected, including limited awareness. Basic cognitive compensatory strategies should be used to help patients attend to, understand, and recall this information. Family, friends, or caregivers should be included in these educational processes. With more severe or persistent problems, treatment may include more comprehensive, coordinated, and real-time feedback about impairments, such as via videotaping. Experiential learning paradigms can be used in which the person is asked to predict how well he or she will perform on a given test and is reinforced for successively improving the accuracy of his or her predictions. Failure experiences may be permitted, although staff should minimize the potential for shame or humiliation that may occur with failures. Improvements may be made in safety behaviors without corresponding changes in verbal awareness, so at times it may be therapeutic to ignore verbal denial and work strictly on the level of behavior. With intractable unawareness, it may be essential to enlist relatives and friends to create a protective environment by ensuring 24-hour supervision, removing access to cars or other dangerous equipment, contacting employers, and providing a written letter signed by the physician that lists all the behavioral restrictions to support caregivers when the restrictions are challenged. When adaptive denial is present, staff may benefit from information about how the denial helps the person psychologically. Staff may be inclined to confront the denial, not realizing the value of defensive denial in managing anxiety and maintaining a sense of self-efficacy.

Cognitive rehabilitation. The science of cognitive rehabilitation has grown tremendously in the past 15 years to the point that evidence-based guidelines have been derived from significant efficacy and effectiveness trials (Cicerone et al. 2000, 2005). Empirically validated approaches are available for remediation of visuoperceptual deficits, language deficits, and impaired pragmatic communication and for memory compensation in patients with mild memory impairment (Cicerone et al. 2000). Some evidence suggests that attention training, including computer-based training modules, is effective (Park and Ingles 2001). Effective strategies are available to train patients to improve visual scanning, reading comprehension, language formation, and problem solving (Cicerone et al. 2000). Optional rehabilitation strategies that may be effective include the use of memory books for persons with moderate to severe impairment, verbal self-instructional training, and self-questioning and self-monitoring to address deficits in executive functioning. Isolated use of computer-based training procedures is not recommended for any form of impairment (Cicerone et al. 2000).

Controlled trials of comprehensive rehabilitation programs are rare for postacute rehabilitation and absent for acute rehabilitation, primarily because of cost and ethical issues associated with withholding usual care. In a recent randomized controlled trial, Cicerone et al. (2008) showed the superiority of a holistic rehabilitation program compared with a standard multidisciplinary rehabilitation program. The holistic program emphasized the integration of cognitive, interpersonal, and functional interventions within a therapeutic environment and produced greater improvements in community integration and self-efficacy for the management of TBI-related symptoms than did standard neurorehabilitation. The data suggested that greater effectiveness of the holistic program may be attributable to interventions directed at self-regulation of cognitive and emotional processes, including metacognitive processes of self-appraisal, prediction, self-monitoring, and self-evaluation. A current synthesis of the available evidence on comprehensive rehabilitation concluded that the greatest benefits accrue to those patients who receive individualized and integrated treatment oriented toward both cognitive and interpersonal areas of function (Cicerone et al. 2000).

Spinal Cord Injury

Three types of problems may require psychological interventions in the context of SCI: 1) primary psychiatric disorders, 2) problems with adjustment to disability, and 3) problems with adherence to medical and rehabilitation therapies. With the caveat that there may be significant time constraints on implementing psychotherapy during a relatively short rehabilitation stay, abbreviated forms of standard empirically supported psychotherapies can be used in many cases if cognition is intact. Additionally, if a rehabilitation psychologist is on staff, responsibilities for therapeutic interventions can be negotiated between the psychiatrist and the psychologist.

For depression and anxiety disorders, brief CBT is often indicated in conjunction with initiating pharmacotherapy. Rehabilitation activities should afford the patient numerous opportunities to practice CBT skills, such as identification of irrational thoughts and positive reframing within a supportive context. The consultant also can work within the rehabilitation team to accomplish additional therapy goals by proxy. For example, the recreation therapist can carry out graded exposure to being in a motor vehicle for a patient with acute PTSD-related anxiety and avoidance of cars.

Cognitive-behavioral interventions have been adapted for, and studied to a limited degree in, the SCI population. Craig et al. (1997) used a group-based skills-oriented approach for teaching relaxation, cognitive restructuring, social skills, assertiveness, pleasant activity scheduling, and ways to begin sexual adjustment. Subjects with high levels of depressed mood before treatment were significantly less depressed than were historical control subjects 1 year after treatment. At 2-year follow-up, subjects who had received CBT had fewer hospital readmissions, used fewer drugs, and reported higher levels of adjustment compared with subjects in the control group (Craig et al. 1999). P. Kennedy et al. (2003) tested a "coping effectiveness training" approach that involves teaching cognitive appraisal and coping skills in small groups. Compared with matched historical control subjects, the treated subjects reported reduced depression and anxiety, although improvements were unrelated to changes in coping skills.

Group-based interventions provide unique opportunities to capitalize on the positive coping abilities modeled by participants with better adjustment. Therefore, group-based coping skills training is recommended for people with significant anxiety or depressive symptoms after SCI as an adjunct to or in lieu of individual psychotherapy.

Poor adjustment to disability and management of grief are also common reasons for referrals. As noted earlier, potentially harmful myths exist about the nature and course of grief. Empirically supported approaches to manage grief are lacking (Bonanno et al. 2002), especially with regard to loss of physical function as in SCI. Nevertheless, current conceptualizations of the grieving process may be instructive. Stroebe and Shut (1999) described a dual process model of grief in which aggrieved individuals alternate between confronting and avoiding loss and restoration-related stressors. This model normalizes the transient denial shown by people with SCI and emphasizes that oscillation between confronting and seeking respite from loss experiences is an aspect of adaptive coping. Maciejewski et al. (2007) found that acceptance, not disbelief, is the first most dominant normal grief indicator; that acceptance increases steadily over time; and that by 6 months postloss, disbelief, yearning, anger, and depression have all peaked. Their data suggested that grief indicators that have not begun to subside after 6 months may merit specialized treatment. Finally, effective treatment of more chronic grief requires integration of strategies from interpersonal therapy and exposure therapy (Shear et al. 2001).

Applying these findings to adjustment to SCI suggests that clinicians should resist the temptation to confront patients with their prognosis when they, for example, insist that they are going to walk again. Such denial may simply reflect the loss-avoidance phase of the dual process model and the understandable hope or wish for neurological recovery. Overly direct confrontation may interfere with normal oscillations and damage adaptive defenses. Confrontation also may increase resistance and risk eliciting excessive distress. Tolerance of verbal denial and other adjustment patterns is recommended as long as they do not interfere with rehabilitation progress for more than a day or so. For these patients, staff education about the dual process model may be the main intervention. In the uncommon instance when verbal denial is accompanied by behavioral denial (e.g., refusing to learn adaptive strategies such as wheelchair use and self-catheterization) or persistently interferes with rehabilitation progress, more exposure-based interventions may be needed. In such cases, the psychiatrist may recommend that patients review information about the nature and extent of their injury (including radiographic evidence), prognosis for recovery, and current SCI research with the attending physician, possibly with the consultant present.

Given the action-oriented behavioral style of many patients with SCI (Rohe and Krause 1998), we believe that much adjustment is behaviorally mediated; that is, rather than verbally processing losses associated with SCI, patients accommodate to their impairments largely through physical and occupational therapy wherein they repeatedly experience their abilities and limitations through activities. To the extent that therapists can set attainable incremental goals and maximize the patients' sense of mastery, positive adjustment can be facilitated. Therapies also can be organized to help patients resume participation in their most meaningful, rewarding, and pleasant life activities. Prospective descriptive studies of bereavement (Bonanno et al. 2002) and the incipient empirical use of combined interpersonal therapy and exposure therapy for "traumatic grief" (Shear et al. 2001) may lead to more valid approaches to treating adjustment to loss in SCI.

Nonadherence to treatment, and the associated conflicts with staff, often triggers psychiatric consultation. Causes of nonadherence are varied and include depression, amotivational states due to concomitant TBI, antisocial personality traits, ongoing substance abuse, and unrealistic staff expectations. Adherence is a function of the interaction among somatic, psychological, and environmental variables (Trieschmann 1988). Environmental factors may be particularly salient in cases of nonadherence. Once primary psychiatric disorders are ruled out, the consultant should examine how adherence to prescribed therapies may not be as rewarding for the patient as it should be, perhaps because of pain, withdrawal of social contact, or relinquishing a sense of control. In some cases, nonadherence may inadvertently be rewarded by engaging staff in negative social interactions, asserting independence, or avoiding unwanted responsibilities. One example is patients with dependent traits not improving toward independence because staff attention and expressions of support are contingent on dependent behavior. Behavioral principles such as rewarding successive approximations, ignoring disability-inappropriate behaviors, initiating behavioral activation, using quota systems, and explicitly linking progress in rehabilitation to desired outcomes (such as earlier discharge) may improve adherence to treatment (W.E. Fordyce 1976).

Conclusion

As society's attitudes toward disability continue to evolve and researchers work toward better understanding the potent effects of psychosocial factors in disability, psychiatrists will have an increasing role in the rehabilitation setting. To achieve comprehensive evaluation and treatment of TBI and SCI, psychiatrists must appreciate and address the multiple complex facets of these conditions, from the acute neurological injury and its attendant psychological trauma through the chronic neurological, medical, psychiatric, and social sequelae of the injury. The multidisciplinary rehabilitation setting affords an environment in which psychiatrists can use their pharmacological and psychotherapeutic skills in psychosomatic medicine to maximize the long-term functional potential of their patients.

References

Adams PF, Barnes PM, Vickerie JL: Summary health statistics for the U.S. population: National Health Interview Survey, 2007. Vital Health Stat 10 (238):1–104, 2008

Alban JP, Hopson MM, Ly V, et al: Effect of methylphenidate on vital signs and adverse effects in adults with traumatic brain injury. Am J Phys Med Rehabil 83:131–137, 2004

Alexander MP: Mild traumatic brain injury: pathophysiology, natural history, and clinical management. Neurology 45:1253–1260, 1995

Alexander MP: Mild traumatic brain injury: a review of physiogenesis and psychogenesis. Semin Clin Neuropsychiatry 2:177–187, 1997

Allen CC, Ruff RM: Self-rating versus neuropsychological performance of moderate versus severe head-injured patients. Brain Inj 4:7–17, 1990

Alves WM, Colohan ART, O'Leary TJ, et al: Understanding posttraumatic symptoms after minor head injury. J Head Trauma Rehabil 1:1–12, 1986

Alves W, Macciocchi SN, Barth JT. Postconcussive symptoms after uncomplicated mild head injury. J Head Trauma Rehabil 8:48–59, 1993

Amador M, Lynne C, Brackett N: A Guide and Resource Directory to Male Fertility Following Spinal Cord Injury/Dysfunction: Miami Project to Cure Paralysis. Miami, FL, University of Miami, 2000

Amaducci LA, Fratiglioni L, Rocca WA, et al: Risk factors for clinically diagnosed Alzheimer's disease: a case-control study of an Italian population. Neurology 36:922–931, 1986

American Psychiatric Association: Diagnostic and Statistical Manual of Mental Disorders, 3rd Edition, Revised. Washington, DC, American Psychiatric Association, 1987

American Psychiatric Association: Diagnostic and Statistical Manual of Mental Disorders, 4th Edition. Washington, DC, American Psychiatric Association, 1994

American Psychiatric Association: Diagnostic and Statistical Manual of Mental Disorders, 4th Edition, Text Revision. Washington, DC, American Psychiatric Association, 2000

Anderson SW, Tranel D: Awareness of disease states following cerebral infarction, dementia, and head trauma: standardized assessment. Clin Neuropsychol 3:327–339, 1989

Arciniegas DB, McAllister TW: Neurobehavioral management of traumatic brain injury in the critical care setting. Crit Care Clin 24:737–765, 2008

Ashman TA, Spielman LA, Hibbard MR, et al: Psychiatric challenges in the first 6 years after traumatic brain injury: cross-sequential analyses of Axis I disorders. Arch Phys Med Rehabil 85 (4 suppl 2):S36–S42, 2004

Ashman TA, Cantor JB, Gordon WA, et al: A randomized controlled trial of sertraline for the treatment of depression in persons with traumatic brain injury. Arch Phys Med Rehabil 90:733–740, 2009

Auerbach SH: The pathophysiology of traumatic brain injury. Phys Med Rehabil 3:1–11, 1989

Azouvi P, Jokic C, Attal N, et al: Carbamazepine in agitation and aggressive behaviour following severe closed-head injury: results of an open trial. Brain Inj 13:797–804, 1999

Baguley IJ, Cooper J, Felmingham K: Aggressive behavior following traumatic brain injury: how common is common? J Head Trauma Rehabil 21:45–56, 2006

Baker-Price L, Persinger MA: Intermittent burst-firing weak (1 microtesla) magnetic fields reduce psychometric depression in patients who sustained closed head injuries: a replication and electroencephalographic validation. Percept Mot Skills 96:965–974, 2003

Banerjea R, Findley PA, Smith B, et al: Co-occurring medical and mental illness and substance use disorders among veteran clinic users with spinal cord injury patients with complexities. Spinal Cord 47:789–795, 2009

Barker RN, Kendall MD, Amsters DI, et al: The relationship between quality of life and disability across the lifespan for people with spinal cord injury. Spinal Cord 47:149–155, 2009

Barncord SW, Wanlass RL: A correction procedure for the Minnesota Multiphasic Personality Inventory–2 for persons with spinal cord injury. Arch Phys Med Rehabil 81:1185–1190, 2000

Battaglia J, Lindborg SR, Alaka K, et al: Calming versus sedative effects of intramuscular olanzapine in agitated patients. Am J Emerg Med 21:192–198, 2003

Bazarian JJ, Wong T, Harris M, et al: Epidemiology and predictors of post-concussive syndrome after minor head injury in an emergency population. Brain Inj 13:173–189, 1999

Beauchamp K, Mutlak H, Smith WR, et al: Pharmacology of traumatic brain injury: where is the "golden bullet"? Mol Med 14:731–740, 2008

Ben-Yishay Y, Rattok J, Piasetsky EB, et al: Neuropsychologic rehabilitation: quest for a holistic approach. Semin Neurol 5:252–259, 1985

Bennouna M, Green VB, Defranoux L: Adjuvant galantamine to risperidone improves negative and cognitive symptoms in a patient presenting with schizophrenic like psychosis after traumatic brain injury. J Clin Psychopharmacol 25:505–507, 2005

Beran RG, Gibson RJ: Aggressive behavior in intellectually challenged patients with epilepsy treated with lamotrigine. Epilepsia 39:280–282, 1998

Bergsneider M, Hovda DA, McArthur DL, et al: Metabolic recovery following human traumatic brain injury based on FDG-PET: time course and relationship to neurological disability. J Head Trauma Rehabil 16:135–148, 2001

Binder LM, Rohling ML: Money matters: meta-analytic review of the effects of financial incentives on recovery after closed head injury. Am J Psychiatry 153:7–10, 1996

Binder LM, Rohling ML, Larrabee GJ: A review of mild head trauma, part I: meta-analytic review of neuropsychological studies. J Clin Exp Neuropsychol 19:421–431, 1997

Bleiberg J, Garmoe W, Cederquist J, et al: Effects of dexedrine on performance consistency following brain injury: a double-blind placebo crossover case study. Neuropsychiatry Neuropsychol Behav Neurol 6:245–248, 1993

Boake C, Freeland JC, Ringholz GM, et al: Awareness of memory loss after severe closed-head injury. Brain Inj 9:273–283, 1995

Boake C, McCauley SR, Levin HS, et al: Diagnostic criteria for postconcussional syndrome after mild to moderate traumatic brain injury. J Neuropsychiatry Clin Neurosci 17:350–356, 2005

Bogner J, Corrigan JD: Epidemiology of agitation following brain injury. NeuroRehabilitation 5:293–297, 1995

Bohnen N, Jolles J, Twijnstra A: Neuropsychological deficits in patients with persistent symptoms six months after mild head injury. Neurosurgery 30:692–696, 1992

Bombardier CH, Rimmele C: Alcohol use and readiness to change after spinal cord injury. Arch Phys Med Rehabil 79:1110–1115, 1998

Bombardier CH, Turner AT: Alcohol and other drug use in traumatic disability, in The Handbook of Rehabilitation Psychology. Edited by Frank R, Rosenthal M, Caplan B. Washington, DC, American Psychological Association, 2009, pp 241–258

Bombardier CH, Kilmer J, Ehde D: Screening for alcoholism among persons with recent traumatic brain injury. Rehabil Psychol 42:259–271, 1997

Bombardier CH, Rimmele C, Zintel H: The magnitude and correlates of alcohol and drug use before traumatic brain injury. Arch Phys Med Rehabil 83:1765–1773, 2002

Bombardier CH, Temkin N, Machamer J, et al: The natural history of drinking and alcohol-related problems after traumatic brain injury. Arch Phys Med Rehabil 84:185–191, 2003

Bombardier CH, Richards JS, Krause JS, et al: Symptoms of major depression in people with spinal cord injury: implication for screening. Arch Phys Med Rehabil 85:1749–1756, 2004

Bombardier CH, Fann JR, Temkin N, et al: Posttraumatic stress disorder symptoms during the first six months after traumatic brain injury. J Neuropsychiatry Clin Neurosci 18:501–508, 2006

Bombardier CH, Bell KR, Temkin NR, et al: The efficacy of telephone counseling as a treatment for depressive symptoms during the first year following traumatic brain injury. J Head Trauma Rehabil 24:230–238, 2009

Bombardier CH, Fann JR, Temkin NR, et al: Rates of major depressive disorder and clinical outcomes following traumatic brain injury. JAMA 303:1938–1945, 2010

Bonanno G, Kaltman S: Toward an integrative perspective on bereavement. Psychol Bull 125:760–776, 1999

Bonanno GA, Wortman CB, Lehman DR, et al: Resilience to loss and chronic grief: a prospective study from preloss to 18-months postloss. J Pers Soc Psychol 83:1150–1164, 2002

Boyer B, Tollen L, Kafkalas C: A pilot study of posttraumatic stress disorder in children and adolescents with spinal cord injury. SCI Psychosocial Process 11:75–81, 1998

Brooke MM, Questad KA, Patterson PR, et al: Agitation and restlessness after closed head injury: a prospective study of 100 consecutive admissions. Arch Phys Med Rehabil 73:320–323, 1992a

Brooke MM, Patterson DR, Questad KA, et al: The treatment of agitation during initial hospitalization after traumatic brain injury. Arch Phys Med Rehabil 73:917–921, 1992b

Broomhall LG, Clark CR, McFarlane AC, et al: Early stage assessment and course of acute stress disorder after mild traumatic brain injury. J Nerv Ment Dis 197:178–181, 2009

Brown SJ, Fann JR, Grant I: Postconcussional disorder: time to acknowledge a common source of neurobehavioral morbidity. J Neuropsychiatry Clin Neurosci 6:15–22, 1994

Bryant RA, Harvey AG: Relationship between acute stress disorder and posttraumatic stress disorder following mild traumatic brain injury. Am J Psychiatry 155:625–629, 1998

Bryant RA, Harvey AG: The influence of traumatic brain injury on acute stress disorder and posttraumatic stress disorder following motor vehicle accidents. Brain Inj 13:15–22, 1999

Bryant RA, Marosszeky JE, Crooks J, et al: Posttraumatic stress disorder following severe traumatic brain injury. Am J Psychiatry 157:629–631, 2000

Bryant RA, Moulds MM, Guthrie R, et al. Treating acute stress disorder following mild traumatic brain injury. Am J Psychiatry 160:585–587, 2003

Bryant RA, O'Donnell ML, Creamer M, et al: The psychiatric sequelae of traumatic injury. Am J Psychiatry 167:312–320, 2010

Bryce TN, Budh CN, Cardenas DD, et al: Pain after spinal cord injury: an evidence-based review for clinical practice and research: report of the National Institute on Disability and Rehabilitation Research Spinal Cord Injury Measures meeting. J Spinal Cord Med 30:421–440, 2007

Budh CN, Osteråker AL: Life satisfaction in individuals with a spinal cord injury and pain. Clin Rehabil 21:89–96, 2007

Burg JS, McGuire LM, Burright RG, et al: Prevalence of head injury in an inpatient psychiatric population. J Clin Psychol Med Settings 3:243–251, 1996

Burg JS, Williams R, Burright RG, et al: Psychiatric treatment outcome following traumatic brain injury. Brain Inj 14:513–533, 2000

Burnett DM, Kennedy RE, Cifu DX, et al: Using atypical neuroleptic drugs to treat agitation in patients with a brain injury: a review. NeuroRehabilitation 13:165–172, 1999

Burns SP, Little JW, Hussey JD, et al: Sleep apnea syndrome in chronic spinal cord injury: associated factors and treatment. Arch Phys Med Rehabil 81:1334–1339, 2000

Butler PV: Diurnal variation in Cotard's syndrome (copresent with Capgras delusion) following traumatic brain injury. Aust N Z J Psychiatry 34:684–687, 2000

Caplan B: Staff and patient perception of patient mood. Rehabil Psychol 28:67–77, 1983

Capruso DX, Levin HS: Neurobehavioral outcome of head trauma, in Neurology and Trauma. Edited by Evans RW. Philadelphia, PA, WB Saunders, 1996, pp 201–221

Cardenas DD, McLean A, Farrell-Robers L, et al: Oral physostigmine and impaired memory in adults with brain injury. Brain Inj 8:579–587, 1994

Cardenas DD, Warms CA, Turner JA, et al: Efficacy of amitriptyline for relief of pain in spinal cord injury: results of a randomized clinical trial. Pain 96:365–373, 2002

Carter GM, Relles DA, Wynn BO, et al: Interim Report on an Inpatient Rehabilitation Facility Prospective Payment System. Rand Corp, DRU-2309-HCFA [Health Care Financing Administration], July 2000. Available at: http://www.rand.org/pubs/drafts/DRU2309/index.html. Accessed May 14, 2010.

Castriotta RJ, Lai JM: Sleep disorders associated with traumatic brain injury. Arch Phys Med Rehabil 82:1403–1406, 2001

Castriotta RJ, Wilde MC, Lai JM, et al: Prevalence and consequences of sleep disorders in traumatic brain injury. J Clin Sleep Med 3:349–356, 2007

Cavallo MM, Kay T, Ezrachi O: Problems and changes after traumatic brain injury: differing perceptions within and between families. Brain Inj 6:327–335, 1992

Caveness WF: Posttraumatic sequelae, in Head Injury Conference Proceedings. Edited by Caveness WF, Walker A. Philadelphia, PA, JB Lippincott, 1966, pp 209–219

Centers for Disease Control and Prevention, National Center for Injury Prevention and Control: Traumatic Brain Injury in the United States: A Report to Congress. Atlanta, GA, Centers for Disease Control and Prevention, 1999

Charlifue SW, Gerhart KA: Behavioral and demographic predictors of suicide after traumatic spinal cord injury. Arch Phys Med Rehabil 72:488–492, 1991

Chatham-Showalter PE: Carbamazepine for combativeness in acute traumatic brain injury. J Neuropsychiatry Clin Neurosci 8:96–99, 1996

Chatham-Showalter PE, Kimmel DN: Agitated symptom response to divalproex following acute brain injury. J Neuropsychiatry Clin Neurosci 12:395–397, 2000

Childers MK, Holland D: Psychomotor agitation following gabapentin use in brain injury. Brain Inj 11:537–540, 1997

Cicerone K, Dahlberg C, Kalmar K: Evidence-based cognitive rehabilitation: recommendations for clinical practice. Arch Phys Med Rehabil 81:1596–1615, 2000

Cicerone KD, Dahlberg C, Malec JF, et al: Evidence-based cognitive rehabilitation: updated review of the literature from 1998 through 2002. Arch Phys Med Rehabil 86:1681–1692, 2005

Cicerone KD, Mott T, Azulay J, et al: A randomized controlled trial of holistic neuropsychologic rehabilitation after traumatic brain injury. Arch Phys Med Rehabil 89:2239–2249, 2008

Clark AF, Davison K: Mania following head injury: a report of two cases and a review of the literature. Br J Psychiatry 150:841–844, 1987

Clay DL, Hagglund KJ, Frank RG, et al: Enhancing the accuracy of depression diagnosis in patients with spinal cord injury using Bayesian analysis. Rehabil Psychol 40:171–180, 1995

Cohen SA, Ihrig K, Lott RS, et al: Risperidone for aggression and self-injurious behavior in adults with mental retardation. J Autism Dev Disord 28:229–233, 1998

Consortium for Spinal Cord Medicine: Depression Following Spinal Cord Injury: A Clinical Practice Guideline for Primary Care Physicians. Washington, DC, Paralyzed Veterans of America, 1998. Available at: http://www.pva.org/site/PageServer?pagename=pubs_main#CPG. Accessed May 14, 2010.

Consortium for Spinal Cord Medicine: Outcomes Following Spinal Cord Injury: A Clinical Practice Guideline for Health Care Professionals. Washington, DC, Paralyzed Veterans of America, 1999. Available at: http://www.pva.org/site/PageServer?pagename=pubs_main#CPG. Accessed May 14, 2010.

Consortium for Spinal Cord Medicine: Sexuality and Reproductive Health in Adults with Spinal Cord Injury: A Clinical Practice Guideline for Health Care-Professionals. Washington, DC, Paralyzed Veterans of America, 2010. Available at: http://www.pva.org/site/PageServer?pagename=pubs_main#CPG. Accessed May 14, 2010.

Corrigan JD: Development of a scale for assessment of agitation following traumatic brain injury. J Clin Exp Neuropsychol 11:261–277, 1989

Corrigan JD, Bogner J: Interventions to promote retention in substance abuse treatment. Brain Inj 21:343–356, 2007

Corrigan JD, Cole TB: Substance use disorders and clinical management of traumatic brain injury and posttraumatic stress disorder. JAMA 300:720–721, 2008

Craig AR, Hancock KM, Dickson HG: A longitudinal investigation into anxiety and depression in the first 2 years following a spinal cord injury. Paraplegia 32:675–679, 1994

Craig AR, Hancock K, Dickson H, et al: Long-term psychological outcomes in spinal cord injured persons: results of a controlled trial using cognitive behavior therapy. Arch Phys Med Rehabil 78:33–38, 1997

Craig A, Hancock K, Dickson H: Improving the long-term adjustment of spinal cord injured persons. Spinal Cord 37:345–350, 1999

Crow S, Meller W, Christensen G, et al: Use of ECT after brain injury. Convuls Ther 12:113–116, 1996

Currier GW, Simpson GM: Risperidone liquid concentrate and oral lorazepam versus intramuscular haloperidol and intramuscular lorazepam for treatment of psychotic agitation. J Clin Psychiatry 62:153–157, 2001

Daniels JP, Felde A: Quetiapine treatment for mania secondary to brain injury in 2 patients. J Clin Psychiatry 69:497–498, 2008

Davidoff GN, Roth EJ, Richards JS: Cognitive deficits in spinal cord injury: epidemiology and outcome. Arch Phys Med Rehabil 73:275–284, 1992

Davidson J: Seizures and bupropion: a review. J Clin Psychiatry 50:256–261, 1989

Davison K, Bagley CR: Schizophrenia-like psychosis associated with organic disorders of the central nervous system. Br J Psychiatry 114:113–184, 1969

De Deyn PP, Rabheru K, Rasmussen A, et al: A randomized trial of risperidone, placebo, and haloperidol for behavioral symptoms of dementia. Neurology 53:946–955, 1999

Deb S, Lyons I, Koutzoukis C, et al: Rate of psychiatric illness 1 year after traumatic brain injury. Am J Psychiatry 156:374–378, 1999

DeLisa JA, Currie DM, Martin GM: Rehabilitation medicine: past, present, and future, in Rehabilitation Medicine: Principles and Practice, 3rd Edition. Philadelphia, PA, Lippincott Williams & Wilkins, 1998, pp 3–32

DeVivo MJ, Krause JS, Lammertse DP: Recent trends in mortality and causes of death among persons with spinal cord injury. Arch Phys Med Rehabil 80:1411–1419, 1999

Diamond S: Efficacy and safety profile of venlafaxine in chronic headache. Headache Quarterly 6:212–214, 1995

Dickel MJ, Renfrow SD, Moore PT, et al: Rapid eye movement sleep periodic leg movements in patients with spinal cord injury. Sleep 17:733–738, 1994

Dikmen SS, Temkin N, Armsden G: Neuropsychological recovery: relationship to psychosocial functioning and postconcussional complaints, in Mild Head Injury. Edited by Levin HS, Eisenberg HM, Benton AL. New York, Oxford University Press, 1989, pp 229–241

Dikmen S, Machamer JE, Winn HR, et al: Neuropsychological outcome at 1-year post head injury. Neuropsychology 9:80–90, 1995

Dikmen SS, Machamer JE, Winn HR, et al: Neuropsychological effects of valproate in traumatic brain injury: a randomized trial. Neurology 54:895–902, 2000

Dikmen S, Machamer J, Temkin N: Mild head injury: facts and artifacts. J Clin Exp Neuropsychol 23:729–738, 2001

Dikmen SS, Bombardier CH, Machamer JE, et al: Natural history of depression in traumatic brain injury. Arch Phys Med Rehabil 85:1457–1464, 2004

Dikmen S, Machamer J, Fann JR, et al: Rates of symptom reporting after traumatic brain injury. J Int Neuropsychol Soc 16:401–411, 2010

Dinan TG, Mobayed M: Treatment resistance of depression after head injury: a preliminary study of amitriptyline response. Acta Psychiatr Scand 85:292–294, 1992

Dischinger PC, Ryb GE, Kufera JA, et al: Early predictors of postconcussive syndrome in a population of trauma patients with mild traumatic brain injury. J Trauma 66:289–296, 2009

Dolberg OT, Barkai G, Gross Y, et al: Differential effects of topiramate in patients with traumatic brain injury and obesity: a case series. Psychopharmacology 179:838–845, 2005

Donnellan CP: Acupuncture for central pain affecting the ribcage following traumatic brain injury and rib fractures—a case report. Acupunct Med 24:129–133, 2006

Doppenberg EMR, Bullock R: Clinical neuro-protection trials in severe traumatic brain injury: lessons from previous studies. J Neurotrauma 14:71–80, 1997

Dunlop TW, Udvarhelyi GB, Stedem AFA, et al: Comparison of patients with and without emotional/behavioral deterioration during the first year after traumatic brain injury. J Neuropsychiatry Clin Neurosci 3:150–156, 1991

Eastwood EA, Hagglund KJ, Ragnarsson KT, et al: Medical rehabilitation length of stay and outcomes for persons with traumatic spinal cord injury: 1990–1997. Arch Phys Med Rehabil 80:1457–1463, 1999

Ellenberg JH, Levin HS, Saydjari C: Posttraumatic amnesia as a predictor of outcome after severe closed head injury. Arch Neurol 53:782–791, 1996

Elliott TR, Frank RG: Depression following spinal cord injury. Arch Phys Med Rehabil 77:816–823, 1996

Elliott T, Shewchuck R: Social support and leisure activities following severe physical disability: testing the mediating effects of depression. Basic Appl Soc Psychol 16:471–587, 1995

Elliott T, Umlauf R: Measurement of personality and psychopathology in acquired disability, in Psychological Assessment in Medical Rehabilitation Settings. Edited by Cushman L, Scherer M. Washington, DC, American Psychological Association, 1995, pp 325–358

Englander J, Hall K, Simpson T, et al: Mild traumatic brain injury in an insured population: subjective complaints and return to employment. Brain Inj 6:161–166, 1992

Ergh TC, Rapport LJ, Coleman RD, et al: Predictors of caregiver and family functioning following traumatic brain injury: social support moderates caregiver distress. J Head Trauma Rehabil 17:155–174, 2002

Ettinger AB, Weisbrot DM, Saracco J, et al: Positive and negative psychotropic effects of lamotrigine in patients with epilepsy and mental retardation. Epilepsia 39:874–877, 1998

Evans C, Sherer M, Nakase Thompson R, et al: Early impaired self-awareness, depression, and subjective well-being following TBI. J Int Neuropsychol Soc 9:253–254, 2003

Evans RW: The postconcussion syndrome and the sequelae of mild head injury, in Neurology and Trauma. Edited by Evans RW. Philadelphia, PA, WB Saunders, 1996, pp 91–116

Fann JR: Neurological effects of psychopharmacological agents. Semin Clin Neuropsychiatry 7:196–206, 2002

Fann JR, Katon WJ, Uomoto JM, et al: Psychiatric disorders and functional disability in outpatients with traumatic brain injuries. Am J Psychiatry 152:1493–1499, 1995

Fann JR, Uomoto JM, Katon WJ: Sertraline in the treatment of major depression following mild traumatic brain injury. J Neuropsychiatry Clin Neurosci 12:226–232, 2000

Fann JR, Uomoto JM, Katon WJ: Cognitive improvement with treatment of depression following mild traumatic brain injury. Psychosomatics 42:48–54, 2001

Fann JR, Leonetti A, Jaffe K, et al: Psychiatric illness and subsequent traumatic brain injury: a case-control study. J Neurol Neurosurg Psychiatry 72:615–620, 2002

Fann JR, Burington B, Leonetti A, et al: Psychiatric illness following traumatic brain injury in an adult health maintenance organization population. Arch Gen Psychiatry 61:53–61, 2004

Fann JR, Bombardier CH, Dikmen S, et al: Validity of the Patient Health Questionnaire-9 in assessing depression following traumatic brain injury. J Head Trauma Rehabil 20:501–511, 2005

Fann JR, Hart T, Schomer KG: Treatment for depression after traumatic brain injury: a systematic review. J Neurotrauma 26:2383–2402, 2009a

Fann JR, Jones AL, Dikmen SS, et al: Depression treatment preferences after traumatic brain injury. J Head Trauma Rehabil 24:272–278, 2009b

Faul M, Xu L, Wald MM, Coronado VG: Traumatic Brain Injury in the United States: Emergency Department Visits, Hospitalizations and Deaths 2002–2006. Atlanta, GA, Centers for Disease Control and Prevention, National Center for Injury Prevention and Control, 2010

Federoff JP, Starkstein SE, Forrester AW, et al: Depression in patients with acute traumatic brain injury. Am J Psychiatry 149:918–923, 1992

Fenton G, McClelland R, Montgomery A, et al: The postconcussional syndrome: social antecedents and psychological sequelae. Br J Psychiatry 162:493–497, 1993

Fichtenberg NL, Millis SR, Mann NR, et al: Factors associated with insomnia among post-acute traumatic brain injury survivors. Brain Inj 14:659–667, 2000

Fichtenberg NL, Putnam SH, Mann NR, et al: Insomnia screening in postacute traumatic brain injury: utility and validity of the Pittsburgh Sleep Quality Index. Am J Phys Med Rehabil 80:339–345, 2001

Finkelstein E, Corso P, Miller T, et al: The Incidence and Economic Burden of Injuries in the United States. New York, Oxford University Press, 2006

Fleminger S, Greenwood RJ, Oliver DL: Pharmacological management for agitation and aggression in people with acquired brain injury. Cochrane Database Syst Rev (4):CD003299, 2006

Fordyce DJ, Roueche JR: Changes in perspectives of disability among patients, staff, and relatives during rehabilitation of brain injury. Rehabil Psychol 31:217–229, 1986

Fordyce WE: Behavioral Methods for Chronic Pain and Illness. St. Louis, MO, Mosby Year Book, 1976

Fox DD, Lees-Haley PR, Earnest K, et al: Post-concussive symptoms: base rates and etiology in psychiatric patients. Clin Neuropsychol 9:89–92, 1995

Frank RG, Chaney JM, Clay DL, et al: Dysphoria: a major symptom factor in persons with disability or chronic illness. Psychiatry Res 43:231–241, 1992

Fugate LP, Spacek LA, Kresty LA, et al: Measurement and treatment of agitation following traumatic brain injury, II: a survey of the Brain Injury Special Interest Group of the American Academy of Physical Medicine and Rehabilitation. Arch Phys Med Rehabil 78:924–928, 1997

Fuhrer M, Rintala D, Hart K, et al: Depressive symptomatology in persons with spinal cord injury who reside in the community. Arch Phys Med Rehabil 74:255–260, 1993

Fujii D, Ahmed I: Characteristics of psychotic disorder due to traumatic brain injury: an analysis of case studies in the literature. J Neuropsychiatry Clin Neurosci 14:130–140, 2002

Fullerton D, Harvey R, Klein M, et al: Psychiatric disorders in patients with spinal cord injury. Arch Gen Psychiatry 32:369–371, 1981

Galarneau MR, Woodruff SI, Dye JL, et al: Traumatic brain injury during Operation Iraqi Freedom: findings from the United States Navy-Marine Corps Combat Trauma Registry. J Neurosurg 108:950–957, 2008

Galski T, Palasz J, Bruno RL, et al: Predicting physical and verbal aggression on a brain trauma unit. Arch Phys Med Rehabil 75:380–383, 1994

Gasquione PG: Affective state and awareness of sensory and cognitive effects after closed head injury. Neuropsychology 4:187–196, 1992

Gasquione PG, Gibbons TA: Lack of awareness of impairment in institutionalized, severely and chronically disabled survivors of traumatic brain injury: a preliminary investigation. J Head Trauma Rehabil 9:16–24, 1994

Gennarelli TA, Graham DI: Neuropathology of the head injuries. Semin Clin Neuropsychiatry 3:160–175, 1998

Gerhart KA, Koziol-McLain J, Lowenstein SR, et al: Quality of life following spinal cord injury: knowledge and attitudes of emergency care providers. Ann Emerg Med 23:807–812, 1994

Gil S, Caspi Y, Ben-Ari IZ, et al: Does memory of a traumatic event increase the risk of posttraumatic stress disorder in patients with traumatic brain injury? A prospective study. Am J Psychiatry 162:963–969, 2005

Giles GM, Mohr JD: Overview and interrater reliability of an incident-based rating scale for aggressive behavior following traumatic brain injury: the Overt Aggression Scale, Modified for Neurorehabilitation-Extended (OAS-MNR-E). Brain Inj 21:505–511, 2007

Go BK, DeVivo MJ, Richards JS: The epidemiology of spinal cord injury, in Spinal Cord Injury: Clinical Outcomes From the Model Systems. Edited by Stover S, DeLisa JA, Whiteneck GG. Gaithersburg, MD, Aspen, 1995, pp 21–55

Gosling J, Oddy M: Rearranged marriages: marital relationships after head injury. Brain Inj 13:785–796, 1999

Gouvier WD, Uddo-Crane M, Brown LM: Base rates of postconcussional symptoms. Arch Clin Neuropsychol 3:273–278, 1988

Gouvier WD, Cubic B, Jones G, et al: Postconcussion symptoms and daily stress in normal and head-injured college populations. Arch Clin Neuropsychol 7:193–211, 1992

Grant I, Alves W: Psychiatric and psychosocial disturbances in head injury, in Neurobehavioral Recovery From Head Injury. Edited by Levin HS, Grafman J, Eisenberg HM. New York, Oxford University Press, 1987, pp 234–235

Graves AB, White E, Koepsell TD, et al: The association between head trauma and Alzheimer's disease. Am J Epidemiol 131:491–501, 1990

Green LB, Hornyak JE, Hurvitz EA: Amantadine in pediatric patients with traumatic brain injury: a retrospective, case-controlled study. Am J Phys Med Rehabil 83:893–897, 2004

Greendyke RM, Kanter DR: Therapeutic effects of pindolol on behavioral disturbances associated with organic brain disease: a double-blind study. J Clin Psychiatry 47:423–426, 1996

Greendyke RM, Kanter DR, Schuster DB, et al: Propranolol treatment of assaultive patients with organic brain disease: a double-blind, crossover, placebo-controlled study. J Nerv Ment Dis 174:290–294, 1996

Greve KW, Sherwin E, Stanford MW, et al: Personality and neurocognitive correlates of impulsive aggression in long-term survivors of severe traumatic brain injury. Brain Inj 15:255–262, 2001

Groom KN, Shaw TG, O'Connor ME, et al: Neurobehavioral symptoms and family functioning in traumatically brain-injured adults. Arch Clin Neuropsychol 13:695–711, 1998

Gualtieri CT: Buspirone for the behavior problems of patients with organic brain disorders. J Clin Psychopharmacol 11:280–281, 1991

Gualtieri CT, Evans RW: Stimulant treatment for the neurobehavioural sequelae of traumatic brain injury. Brain Inj 2:273–290, 1988

Gualtieri T, Chandler M, Coons TB, et al: Amantadine: a new clinical profile for traumatic brain injury. Clin Neuropharmacol 12:258–270, 1989

Guerrero J, Thurman DJ, Sniezek JE: Emergency department visits associated with traumatic brain injury: United States, 1995–1996. Brain Inj 14:181–186, 2000

Guetin S, Soua B, Voiriot G, et al: The effect of music therapy on mood and anxiety-depression: an observational study in institutionalized patients with traumatic brain injury. Ann Phys Rehabil Med 52:30–40, 2009

Guilmette TJ, Rasile D: Sensitivity, specificity, and diagnostic accuracy of three verbal memory measures in the assessment of mild brain injury. Neuropsychology 9:338–344, 1995

Hall KM, Karzmark P, Stevens M, et al: Family stressors in traumatic brain injury: a two-year follow-up. Arch Phys Med Rehabil 75:876–884, 1994

Hamm RJ, Temple MD, Buck DL, et al: Cognitive recovery from traumatic brain injury: results of post-traumatic experimental interventions, in Neuroplasticity and Reorganization of Function After Brain Injury. Edited by Levin HS, Grafman J. New York, Oxford University Press, 2000, pp 49–67

Hanna-Pladdy B, Gouvier WD, Berry ZM: Postconcussional symptoms as predictors of neuropsychological deficits (abstract). Arch Clin Neuropsychol 12:329–330, 1997

Hanson R, Franklin M: Sexual loss in relation to other functional losses for spinal cord injured males. Arch Phys Med Rehabil 57:291–303, 1976

Hart T, Whyte J, Polansky M, et al: Concordance of patient and family report of neurobehavioral symptoms at 1 year after traumatic brain injury. Arch Phys Med Rehabil 84:204–213, 2003

Harvey AG, Bryant RA: Acute stress disorder following mild traumatic brain injury. J Nerv Ment Dis 186:333–337, 1998

Harvey AG, Bryant RA: A two-year prospective evaluation of the relationship between acute stress disorder and posttraumatic stress disorder following mild traumatic brain injury. Am J Psychiatry 157:626–628, 2000

Harvey AG, Brewin CR, Jones C, et al: Coexistence of posttraumatic stress disorder and traumatic brain injury: towards a resolution of the paradox. J Int Neuropsychol Soc 9:663–676, 2003

Hayes RL, Dixon CE: Neurochemical changes in mild head injury. Semin Neurol 14:25–31, 1994

Hayes RL, Jenkins LW, Lyeth BG: Neurotransmitter-mediated mechanisms of traumatic brain injury: acetylcholine and excitatory amino acids. J Neurotrauma 9 (suppl 1):173–187, 1992

Heaton RK, Pendleton MG: Use of neuropsychological test to predict adult patients' everyday functioning. J Consult Clin Psychol 49:807–821, 1981

Heilbronner RL, Roueche JR, Everson SA, et al: Comparing patient perspectives of disability and treatment effects with quality of participation in a post-acute brain injury rehabilitation programme. Brain Inj 3:387–389, 1989

Heinemann A, Keen M, Donohue R, et al: Alcohol use in persons with recent spinal cord injuries. Arch Phys Med Rehabil 69:619–624, 1988

Hendryx PM: Psychosocial changes perceived by closed-head-injured adults and their families. Arch Phys Med Rehabil 70:526–530, 1989

Hensley PL, Reeve A: A case of antidepressant-induced akathisia in a patient with traumatic brain injury. J Head Trauma Rehabil 16:302–305, 2001

Herrick S, Elliott T, Crow F: Social support and the prediction of health complications among persons with SCI. Rehabil Psychol 39:231–250, 1994

Hibbard MR, Grober SE, Stein PN, et al: Poststroke depression, in Comprehensive Casebook of Cognitive Therapy. Edited by Freeman A, Dattilio F. New York, Guilford, 1992, pp 303–310

Hibbard MR, Uysal S, Kepler K, et al: Axis I psychopathology in individuals with traumatic brain injury. J Head Trauma Rehabil 13:24–39, 1998

Hibbard MR, Gordon WA, Flanagan S, et al: Sexual dysfunction after traumatic brain injury. NeuroRehabilitation 15:107–120, 2000a

Hibbard MR, Gordon WA, Kothera LM: Traumatic brain injury, in Cognitive-Behavioral Strategies in Crisis Intervention, 2nd Edition. Edited by Dattilio F, Freeman A. New York, Guilford, 2000b, pp 219–242

Hillbom E: After-effects of brain-injuries: research on the symptoms causing invalidism of persons in Finland having sustained brain-injuries during the wars of 1939–1940 and 1941–1944. Acta Psychiatr Scand 35 (suppl 142):1–95, 1960

Hiott DW, Labbate L: Anxiety disorders associated with traumatic brain injuries. NeuroRehabilitation 17:345–355, 2002

Hoffman AN, Cheng JP, Zafonte RD, et al: Administration of haloperidol and risperidone after neurobehavioral testing hinders the recovery of traumatic brain injury-induced deficits. Life Sci 83:602–607, 2008

Hoge CW, McGurk D, Thomas JL, et al: Mild traumatic brain injury in U.S. soldiers returning from Iraq. N Engl J Med 358:453–463, 2008

Horner MD, Ferguson PL, Selassie AW, et al: Patterns of alcohol use 1 year after traumatic brain injury: a population-based, epidemiological study. J Int Neuropsychol Soc 11:322–330, 2005

Hornstein A, Seliger G: Cognitive side effects of lithium in closed head injury (letter). J Neuropsychiatry Clin Neurosci 1:446–447, 1989

Horton A, Howe N: Behavioral treatment of the traumatically brain injured: a case study. Percept Mot Skills 53:349–350, 1981

Iezzoni LI, Davis RB, Soukup J, et al: Quality dimensions that most concern people with physical and sensory disabilities. Arch Intern Med 163:2085–2092, 2003

Inghilleri M, Conte A, Frasca V, et al: Venlafaxine and bladder function. Clin Neuropharmacol 28:270–273, 2005

Institute of Medicine: Gulf War and Health, Vol 7: Long-Term Consequences of Traumatic Brain Injury. Washington, DC, National Academies Press, 2008

Jennett B, Bond M: Assessment of outcome after severe brain damage. Lancet 1:480–484, 1975

Jorge RE, Robinson RG, Arndt S: Are there symptoms that are specific for depressed mood in patients with traumatic brain injury? J Nerv Ment Dis 181:91–99, 1993a

Jorge RE, Robinson RG, Starkstein SE, et al: Depression and anxiety following traumatic brain injury. J Neuropsychiatry Clin Neurosci 5:369–374, 1993b

Jorge RE, Robinson RG, Starkstein SE, et al: Secondary mania following traumatic brain injury. Am J Psychiatry 150:916–921, 1993c

Jorge RE, Robinson RG, Moser D, et al: Major depression following traumatic brain injury. Arch Gen Psychiatry 61:42–50, 2004

Jorge RE, Starkstein SE, Arndt S, et al: Alcohol misuse and mood disorders following traumatic brain injury. Arch Gen Psychiatry 62:742–749, 2005

Judd FK, Stone J, Webber JE, et al: Depression following spinal cord injury: a prospective in-patient study. Br J Psychiatry 154:668–671, 1989

Jung AC, Staiger T, Sullivan M: The efficacy of selective serotonin reuptake inhibitors for the management of chronic pain. J Gen Intern Med 12:384–389, 1997

Kaelin DL, Cifu DX, Matthies B: Methylphenidate effect on attention deficit in the acutely brain-injured adult. Arch Phys Med Rehabil 77:6–9, 1996

Kalisky Z, Morrison DP, Meyers CA, et al: Medical problems encountered during rehabilitation of patients with head injury. Arch Phys Med Rehabil 66:25–29, 1985

Kanetani K, Kimura M, Endo S: Therapeutic effects of milnacipran (serotonin noradrenalin reuptake inhibitor) on depression following mild and moderate traumatic brain injury. J Nippon Med Sch 70:313–320, 2003

Kant R, Bogyi AM, Carosella NW, et al: ECT as a therapeutic option in severe brain injury. Convuls Ther 11:45–50, 1995

Kant R, Smith-Seemiller L, Zeiler D: Treatment of aggression and irritability after head injury. Brain Inj 12:661–666, 1998

Katz DI: Neuropathology and neurobehavioral recovery from closed head injury. J Head Trauma Rehabil 7:1–15, 1992

Katz IR, Jeste DV, Mintzer JE, et al: Comparison of risperidone and placebo for psychosis and behavioral disturbances associated with dementia: a randomized, double-blind trial. J Clin Psychiatry 60:107–115, 1999

Kay T, Cavallo MM: The family system: impact, assessment and intervention, in Neuropsychiatry of Traumatic Brain Injury. Edited by Hales RE. Washington, DC, American Psychiatric Press, 1994, pp 533–568

Kay T, Harrington DE, Adams R, et al: Definition of mild traumatic brain injury. Mild Traumatic Brain Injury Committee of the Head Injury Interdisciplinary Special Interest Group of the American Congress of Rehabilitation Medicine. J Head Trauma Rehabil 8:86–87, 1993

Kemp BJ, Kahan JS, Krause JS, et al: Treatment of major depression in individuals with spinal cord injury. J Spinal Cord Med 27:22–28, 2004

Kennedy P, Duff J: Post traumatic stress disorder and spinal cord injuries. Spinal Cord 39:1–10, 2001

Kennedy P, Evans MJ: Evaluation of post traumatic distress in the first 6 months following SCI. Spinal Cord 39:381–386, 2001

Kennedy P, Rogers BA: Anxiety and depression after spinal cord injury: a longitudinal analysis. Arch Phys Med Rehabil 81:932–937, 2000

Kennedy P, Duff J, Evans M, et al: Coping effectiveness training reduces depression and anxiety following traumatic spinal cord injuries. Br J Clin Psychol 42(pt 1):41–52, 2003

Kennedy RE, Livingston L, Riddick A, et al: Evaluation of the Neurobehavioral Functioning Inventory as a depression screening tool after traumatic brain injury. J Head Trauma Rehabil 20:512–526, 2005

Khateb A, Ammann J, Annoni JM, et al: Cognitive-enhancing effects of donepezil in traumatic brain injury. Eur Neurol 54:39–45, 2005

Khouzam HR, Donnelly NJ: Remission of traumatic brain injury-induced compulsions during venlafaxine treatment. Gen Hosp Psychiatry 20:62–63, 1998

Kim E: Agitation, aggression, and disinhibition syndromes after traumatic brain injury. NeuroRehabilitation 17:297–310, 2002

Kim E, Bijlani M: A pilot study of quetiapine treatment of aggression due to traumatic brain injury. J Neuropsychiatry Clin Neurosci 18:547–549, 2006

King N: Mild head injury: neuropathology, sequelae, measurement and recovery. Br J Clin Psychol 36:161–184, 1997

King NS: Post-concussion syndrome: clarity amid the controversy? Br J Psychiatry 183:276–278, 2003

King NS, Crawford S, Wenden FJ, et al: The Rivermead Post Concussion Symptoms Questionnaire: a measure of symptoms commonly experienced after head injury and its reliability. J Neurol 242:587–592, 1995

Kishi Y, Robinson RG, Forrester AW: Prospective longitudinal study of depression following spinal cord injury. J Neuropsychiatry Clin Neurosci 6:237–244, 1994

Kishi Y, Robinson RG, Forrester AW: Comparison between acute and delayed onset major depression after spinal cord injury. J Nerv Ment Dis 183:286–292, 1995

Kiwerski JE, Krasuski M: Influence of alcohol intake on the course and consequences of spinal cord injury. Int J Rehabil Res 15:240–245, 1992

Kokiko ON, Hamm RJ: A review of pharmacological treatments used in experimental models of traumatic brain injury. Brain Inj 21:259–274, 2007

Kolakowsky-Hayner SA, Gourley EV III, Kreutzer JS, et al: Pre-injury substance abuse among persons with brain injury and persons with spinal cord injury. Brain Inj 13:571–581, 1999

Kolakowsky-Hayner SA, Gourley EV III, Kreutzer JS, et al: Post-injury substance abuse among persons with brain injury and persons with spinal cord injury. Brain Inj 16:583–592, 2002

Koponen S, Taiminen T, Portin R, et al: Axis I and II psychiatric disorders after traumatic brain injury: a 30-year follow-up study. Am J Psychiatry 159:1315–1321, 2002

Kraus JE, Sheitman BB: Clozapine reduces violent behavior in heterogeneous diagnostic groups. J Neuropsychiatry Clin Neurosci 17:36–44, 2005

Kraus JF, McArthur DL: Incidence and prevalence of, and costs associated with, traumatic brain injury, in Rehabilitation of the Adult and Child With Traumatic Brain Injury, 3rd Edition. Edited by Rosenthal M, Kreutzer JS, Griffith ER, et al. Philadelphia, PA, FA Davis, 1999, pp 3–18

Kraus MF, Smith GS, Butters M, et al: Effects of the dopaminergic agent and NMDA receptor antagonist amantadine on cognitive function, cerebral glucose metabolism and D2 receptor availability in chronic traumatic brain injury: a study using positron emission tomography (PET). Brain Inj 19:471–479, 2005

Krause J: Delivery of substance abuse services during spinal cord injury rehabilitation. NeuroRehabilitation 2:45–51, 1992

Krause JS, Kewman D, DeVivo MJ, et al: Employment after spinal cord injury: an analysis of cases from the Model Spinal Cord Injury Systems. Arch Phys Med Rehabil 80:1492–1500, 1999

Krause JS, Carter RE, Pickelsimer EE, et al: A prospective study of health and risk of mortality after spinal cord injury. Arch Phys Med Rehabil 89:1482–1491, 2008

Kreutzer JS, Doherty KR, Harris JA, et al: Alcohol use among persons with traumatic brain injury. J Head Trauma Rehabil 5:9–20, 1990

Kreutzer JS, Wehman PH, Harris JA, et al: Substance abuse and crime patterns among persons with traumatic brain injury referred for supported employment. Brain Inj 5:177–187, 1991

Kreutzer JS, Gordon WA, Rosenthal M, et al: Neuropsychological characteristics of patients with brain injury: preliminary findings from a multicenter investigation. J Head Trauma Rehabil 8:47–59, 1993

Kreutzer JS, Gervasio AH, Camplair PS: Primary caregivers' psychological status and family functioning after traumatic brain injury. Brain Inj 8:197–210, 1994

Kreutzer JS, Marwitz JH, Witol AD: Interrelationship between crime, substance abuse, and aggressive behaviours among persons with traumatic brain injury. Brain Inj 9:757–768, 1995

Kreutzer JS, Witol AD, Marwitz JH: Alcohol and drug use among young persons with traumatic brain injury. J Learn Disabil 29:643–651, 1996

Kreutzer JS, Seel RT, Gourley E: The prevalence and symptom rates of depression after traumatic brain injury: a comprehensive examination. Brain Inj 15:563–576, 2001

Krieger D, Hansen K, McDermott C, et al: Loxapine versus olanzapine in the treatment of delirium following traumatic brain injury. NeuroRehabilitation 18:205–208, 2003

Kroenke K, Spitzer RL, Williams JB: The PHQ-9: validity of a brief depression severity measure. J Gen Intern Med 16:606–613, 2001

Kwentus JA, Hart RP, Peck ET, et al: Psychiatric complications of closed head trauma. Psychosomatics 26:8–17, 1985

Lai J, Castriotta R: Sleep disorders associated with traumatic brain injury. Sleep 22(suppl):314, 1999

Lal S, Merbitz CP, Grip JC: Modification of function in head-injured patients with Sinemet. Brain Inj 2:225–233, 1988

Lang E, Hord AH, Denson D: Venlafaxine hydrochloride (Effexor) relieves thermal hyperalgesia in rats with an experimental mononeuropathy. Pain 68:151–155, 1996

Larrabee GJ: Neuropsychological outcome, post concussion symptoms and forensic considerations in mild closed head injury. Semin Clin Neuropsychiatry 2:196–206, 1997

Larrabee GJ: Current controversies in mild head injury, in The Evaluation and Treatment of Mild Traumatic Brain Injury. Edited by Varney NR, Roberts RJ. Mahwah, NJ, Lawrence Erlbaum Associates, 1999, pp 327–346

Lee H, Kim SW, Kim JM, et al: Comparing effects of methylphenidate, sertraline and placebo on neuropsychiatric sequelae in patients with traumatic brain injury. Hum Psychopharmacol Clin Exp 20:97–104, 2005

Lee MA, Leng MEF, Tierman EJJ: Risperidone: a useful adjunct for behavioural disturbance in primary cerebral tumours. Palliative Med 15:255–256, 2001

Leininger BE, Gramling SE, Farrell AD, et al: Neuropsychological deficits in symptomatic minor head injury patients after concussion and mild concussion. J Neurol Neurosurg Psychiatry 53:293–296, 1990

Lenze EJ, Munin MC, Quear T, et al: The Pittsburgh Rehabilitation Participation Scale: reliability and validity of a clinician-rated measure of participation in acute rehabilitation. Arch Phys Med Rehabil 85:380–384, 2004

Leon-Carrion J: Dementia due to head trauma: an obscure name for a clear neurocognitive syndrome. NeuroRehabilitation 17:115–122, 2002

Lesem MD, Zajecka JM, Swift RH, et al: Intramuscular ziprasidone, 2 mg versus 10 mg, in the short-term management of agitated psychotic patients. J Clin Psychiatry 62:12–18, 2001

Levin HS, O'Donnell VM, Grossman RG: The Galveston Orientation and Amnesia Test: a practical scale to assess cognition after head injury. J Nerv Ment Dis 167:675–684, 1979

Levin HS, Mattis S, Ruff RM, et al: Neurobehavioral outcome following minor head injury: a three-center study. J Neurosurg 66:234–243, 1987a

Levin HS, High WM, Goethe KE, et al: The Neurobehavioral Rating Scale: assessment of the behavioral sequelae of head injury by the clinician. J Neurol Neurosurg Psychiatry 50:183–193, 1987b

Levin HS, Brown SA, Song JX, et al: Depression and posttraumatic stress disorder at three months after mild to moderate traumatic brain injury. J Clin Exp Neuropsychol 23:754–769, 2001

Levin HS, McCauley SR, Josic CP, et al: Predicting depression following mild traumatic brain injury. Arch Gen Psychiatry 62:523–528, 2005

Levitt P, Henry W, McHale D: Persistent movement disorder induced by buspirone. Mov Disord 8:331–334, 1993

Levy M, Berson A, Cook T, et al: Treatment of agitation following traumatic brain injury: a review of the literature. NeuroRehabilitation 20:279–306, 2005

Lewis L: A framework for developing a psychotherapy treatment plan with brain-injured patients. J Head Trauma Rehabil 6:22–29, 1991

Lindenmayer JP, Kotsaftis A: Use of sodium valproate in violent and aggressive behaviors: a critical review. J Clin Psychiatry 61:123–128, 2000

Livingston MG, Brooks DN, Bond MR: Patient outcome in the year following severe head injury and relatives' psychiatric and social functioning. J Neurol Neurosurg Psychiatry 48:876–881, 1985

Lombardi G, Macchiarella A, Cecconi F, et al: Ten years of phosphodiesterase type 5 inhibitors in spinal cord injured patients. J Sex Med 6:1248–1258, 2009

Macciocchi S, Seel RT, Thompson N, et al: Spinal cord injury and co-occurring traumatic brain injury: assessment and incidence. Arch Phys Med Rehabil 89:1350–1357, 2008

MacDonald M, Nielson W, Cameron M: Depression and activity patterns of spinal cord injured persons living in the community. Arch Phys Med Rehabil 68:339–343, 1987

Maciejewski P, Zhang B, Block S, et al: An empirical examination of the stage theory of grief. JAMA 297:716–723, 2007

Malaspina D, Goetz RR, Friedman JH, et al: Traumatic brain injury and schizophrenia in members of schizophrenia and bipolar disorder pedigrees. Am J Psychiatry 158:440–446, 2001

Malec JF: Mild traumatic brain injury: scope of the problem, in The Evaluation and Treatment of Mild Traumatic Brain Injury. Edited by Varney NR, Roberts RJ. Mahwah, NJ, Lawrence Erlbaum Associates, 1999, pp 15–38

Malec J, Neimeyer R: Psychologic prediction of duration of inpatient spinal cord injury rehabilitation performance of self care. Arch Phys Med Rehabil 64:359–363, 1983

Marin RS: Apathy: a neuropsychiatric syndrome. J Neuropsychiatry Clin Neurosci 3:243–254, 1991

Marin RS, Fogel BS, Hawkins J, et al: Apathy: a treatable syndrome. J Neuropsychiatry Clin Neurosci 7:23–30, 1995

Marino RJ, Ditunno JF Jr, Donovan WH, et al: Neurologic recovery after traumatic spinal cord injury: data from the Model Spinal Cord Injury Systems. Arch Phys Med Rehabil 80:1391–1396, 1999

Marklund N, Bakshi A, Castelbuono DJ, et al: Evaluation of pharmacological treatment strategies in traumatic brain injury. Curr Pharm Des 12:1645–1680, 2006

Martin R, Kuzniecky R, Ho S, et al: Cognitive effects of topiramate, gabapentin, and lamotrigine in healthy young adults. Neurology 52:321–327, 1999

Martino C, Krysko M, Petrides G, et al: Cognitive tolerability of electroconvulsive therapy in a patient with a history of traumatic brain injury. J ECT 24:92–95, 2008

Marwit SJ: Reliability of diagnosing complicated grief: a preliminary investigation. J Consult Clin Psychol 64:563–568, 1996

Maryniak O, Manchanda R, Velani A: Methotrimeprazine in the treatment of agitation in acquired brain injury patients. Brain Inj 15:167–174, 2001

Masand PS, Tesar GE: Use of stimulants in the medically ill. Psychiatr Clin North Am 19:515–547, 1996

Masel BE, Scheibel RS, Kimbark T, et al: Excessive daytime sleepiness in adults with brain injuries. Arch Phys Med Rehabil 82:1526–1532, 2001

Max W, MacKenzie EJ, Rice DP: Head injuries: costs and consequences. J Head Trauma Rehabil 6:76–91, 1991

Mayou R, Bryant B, Duthie R: Psychiatric consequences of road traffic accidents. BMJ 307:647–651, 1993

Mayou R, Black J, Bryant B: Unconsciousness, amnesia and psychiatric symptoms following road traffic accident injury. Br J Psychiatry 177:540–545, 2000

McAllister TW: Neuropsychiatric sequelae of head injuries. Psychiatr Clin North Am 15:395–413, 1992

McCauley SR, Boake C, Levin HS, et al: Postconcussional disorder following mild to moderate traumatic brain injury: anxiety, depression, and social support as risk factors and comorbidities. J Clin Exp Neuropsychol 23:792–808, 2001

McClelland RJ, Fenton GW, Rutherford W: The post-concussional syndrome revisited. J R Soc Med 87:508–510, 1994

McDougle CJ, Holmes JP, Carlson DC, et al: A double-blind, placebo-controlled study of risperidone in adults with autistic disorder and other pervasive developmental disorders. Arch Gen Psychiatry 55:633–641, 1998

McDowell S, Whyte J, D'Esposito M: Differential effect of a dopaminergic agonist on prefrontal function in traumatic brain injury patients. Brain 121:1155–1164, 1998

McElligott JM, Greenwald BD, Watanabe TK: Congenital and acquired brain injury, 4: new frontiers: neuroimaging, neuroprotective agents, cognitive-enhancing agents, new technology, and complementary medicine. Arch Phys Med Rehabil 84 (suppl 1):18–22, 2003

McGlynn SM, Schacter DL: Unawareness of deficits in neuropsychological syndromes. J Clin Exp Neuropsychol 11:143–205, 1989

McIntosh TK, Smith DH, Meaney DF, et al: Neuropathological sequelae of traumatic brain injury: relationship to neurochemical and biomechanical mechanisms. Lab Invest 74:315–342, 1996

McKinlay WW, Brooks DN: Methodological problems in assessing psychosocial recovery following severe head injury. J Clin Neuropsychol 6:87–99, 1984

McKinlay WW, Brooks DN, Bond MR, et al: The short-term outcome of severe blunt head injury as reported by relatives of the injured persons. J Neurol Neurosurg Psychiatry 44:527–533, 1981

McKinley WO, Seel RT, Hardman JT: Nontraumatic spinal cord injury: incidence, epidemiology, and functional outcome. Arch Phys Med Rehabil 80:619–623, 1999

McLean A Jr, Temkin NR, Dikmen S, et al: The behavioral sequelae of head injury. J Clin Neuropsychol 5:361–376, 1983

McQuay HJ, Tramer M, Nye BA, et al: A systematic review of antidepressants in neuropathic pain. Pain 68:217–227, 1996

Meachen SJ, Hanks RA, Millis SR, et al: The reliability and validity of the Brief Symptom Inventory-18 in persons with traumatic brain injury. Arch Phys Med Rehabil 89:958–965, 2008

Meares S, Shores EA, Taylor AJ, et al: Mild traumatic brain injury does not predict acute postconcussion syndrome. J Neurol Neurosurg Psychiatry 79:300–306, 2008

Meehan KM, Wang H, David SR, et al: Comparison of rapidly acting intramuscular olanzapine, lorazepam, and placebo: a double-blind, randomized study in acutely agitated patients with dementia. Neuropsychopharmacology 26:494–504, 2002

Meythaler JM, Peduzzi JD, Eleftheriou E, et al: Current concepts: diffuse axonal injury-associated traumatic brain injury. Arch Phys Med Rehabil 82:1461–1471, 2001

Meythaler JM, Brunner RC, Johnson A, et al: Amantadine to improve neurorecovery in traumatic brain injury-associated diffuse axonal injury: a pilot double-blind randomized trial. J Head Trauma Rehabil 17:300–313, 2002

Michals ML, Crismon ML, Robers S, et al: Clozapine response and adverse effects in nine brain-injured patients. J Clin Psychopharmacol 13:198–203, 1993

Middleboe T, Anderson HS, Birket-Smith M, et al: Minor head injury: impact on general health after one year. Acta Neurol Scand 85:5–9, 1992

Migliorini C, Tonge B, Taleporos G: Spinal cord injury and mental health. Aust N Z J Psychiatry 42:309–314, 2008

Millis SR, Rosenthal M, Novack TA, et al: Long-term neuropsychological outcome after traumatic brain injury. J Head Trauma Rehabil 16:343–355, 2001

Mittenberg W, Strauman S: Diagnosis of mild head injury and the postconcussion syndrome. J Head Trauma Rehabil 15:783–791, 2000

Mittenberg W, Tremont G, Zielinski RE, et al: Cognitive-behavioral prevention of postconcussion syndrome. Arch Clin Neuropsychol 11:139–145, 1996

Mooney GF, Haas LJ: Effect of methylphenidate on brain injury-related anger. Arch Phys Med Rehabil 74:153–160, 1993

Mortenson WB, Noreau L, Miller WC: The relationship between and predictors of quality of life after spinal cord injury at 3 and 15 months after discharge. Spinal Cord 48:73–79, 2010

Moss NE, Crawford S, Wade DT: Postconcussion symptoms: is stress a mediating factor? Clin Rehabil 8:149–156, 1994

Muller U, Murai T, Bauer-Wittmund T, et al: Paroxetine versus citalopram treatment of pathological crying after brain injury. Brain Inj 13:805–811, 1999

Murrey GJ, Hale FM, Williams JD: Assessment of anosognosia in persons with frontal lobe damage: clinical utility of the Mayo-Portland Adaptability Inventory (MPAI). Brain Inj 19:599–603, 2005

Mysiw WJ, Jackson RD, Corrigan JD: Amitriptyline for post-traumatic agitation. Am J Phys Med Rehabil 67:29–33, 1988

Nahas Z, Arlinghaus KA, Kotrla KJ, et al: Rapid response of emotional incontinence to selective serotonin reuptake inhibitors. J Neuropsychiatry Clin Neurosci 10:453–455, 1998

Nakase-Richardson R, Yablon SA, Sherer M: Prospective comparison of acute confusion severity with duration of post-traumatic amnesia in predicting employment outcome after traumatic brain injury. J Neurol Neurosurg Psychiatry 78:872–876, 2007

National Institutes of Health Consensus Development Panel on Rehabilitation of Persons With Traumatic Brain Injury: Rehabilitation of persons with traumatic brain injury. JAMA 282:974–983, 1999

Newburn G, Edwards R, Thomas H, et al: Moclobemide in the treatment of major depressive disorder (DSM-3) following traumatic brain injury. Brain Inj 13:637–642, 1999

Niemeier J, Kennedy R, McKinley W, et al: The Loss Inventory: preliminary reliability and validity data for a new measure of emotional and cognitive responses to disability. Disabil Rehabil 26:614–623, 2004

Nimmo-Smith I, Marcel AJ, Tegnér R: A diagnostic test of unawareness of bilateral motor task abilities in anosognosia for hemiplegia. J Neurol Neurosurg Psychiatry 76:1167–1169, 2005

Nott MT, Chapparo C, Baguley IJ: Agitation following traumatic brain injury: an Australian sample. Brain Inj 20:1175–1182, 2006

Oddy M, Humphrey M, Uttley D: Stresses upon the relatives of head-injured patients. Br J Psychiatry 133:507–513, 1978a

Oddy M, Humphrey M, Uttley D: Subjective impairment and social recovery after closed head injury. J Neurol Neurosurg Psychiatry 41:611–616, 1978b

Ojemann LM, Baugh-Bookman C, Dudley DL: Effect of psychotropic medications on seizure control in patients with epilepsy. Neurology 37:1525–1527, 1987

Okie S: Traumatic brain injury in the war zone. N Engl J Med 352:2043–2047, 2005

Onghena P, Van Houdenhove B: Antidepressant-induced analgesia in chronic non-malignant pain: a meta-analysis of 39 placebo-controlled studies. Pain 49:205–219, 1992

Orff HJ, Ayalon L, Drummond SPA: Traumatic brain injury and sleep disturbance: a review of current research. J Head Trauma Rehabil 24:155–165, 2009

Oster TJ, Anderson CA, Filley CM, et al: Quetiapine for mania due to traumatic brain injury. CNS Spectr 12:764–769, 2007

Ouellet MC, Morin CM: Cognitive behavioral therapy for insomnia associated with traumatic brain injury: a single-case study. Arch Phys Med Rehabil 85:1298–1302, 2004

Ouellet MC, Savard J, Morin CM: Insomnia following traumatic brain injury: a review. Neurorehabil Neural Repair 18:187–198, 2004

Oyewumi LK, Lapierre YD: Efficacy of lithium in treating mood disorder occurring after brain stem injury. Am J Psychiatry 138:110–112, 1981

Pachet A, Friesen S, Winkelaar D, et al: Beneficial behavioural effects of lamotrigine in traumatic brain injury. Brain Inj 17:715–722, 2003

Pande AC, Davidson JR, Jefferson JW, et al: Treatment of social phobia with gabapentin: a placebo-controlled study. J Clin Psychopharmacol 19:341–348, 1999

Pande AC, Pollack MH, Crockatt J, et al: Placebo-controlled study of gabapentin treatment of panic disorder. J Clin Psychopharmacol 20:467–471, 2000

Paradiso S, Ohkubo T, Robinson RG: Vegetative and psychological symptoms associated with depressed mood over the first two years after stroke. Int J Psychiatry Med 27:137–157, 1997

Park NW, Ingles JL: Effectiveness of attention rehabilitation after an acquired brain injury: a meta-analysis. Neuropsychology 15:199–210, 2001

Parkes CM, Weiss RS: Recovery From Bereavement. New York, Basic Books, 1983

Perino C, Rago R, Cicolini A, et al: Mood and behavioural disorders following traumatic brain injury: clinical evaluation and pharmacological management. Brain Inj 15:139–148, 2001

Pinkston JB, Gouvier WD, Santa Maria MP: Mild head injury: differentiation of long-term differences on testing. Brain Cogn 44:74–78, 2000

Plenger PM, Dixon CE, Castillo RM, et al: Subacute methylphenidate treatment for moderate to moderately severe traumatic brain injury: a preliminary double-blind placebo-controlled study. Arch Phys Med Rehabil 77:536–540, 1996

Ponsford J, Whelan-Goodinson R, Bahar-Fuchs A: Alcohol and drug use following traumatic brain injury: a prospective study. Brain Inj 21:1385–1392, 2007

Pope HG Jr, McElroy SL, Satlin A, et al: Head injury, bipolar disorder, and response to valproate. Compr Psychiatry 29:34–38, 1988

Povlishock JT, Becker DP, Cheng CL, et al: Axonal change in minor head injury. J Neuropathol Exp Neurol 42:225–242, 1983

Powell JH, al-Adawi S, Morgan J, et al: Motivational deficits after brain injury: effects of bromocriptine in 11 patients. J Neurol Neurosurg Psychiatry 60:416–421, 1996

Powell J, Heslin J, Greenwood R: Community based rehabilitation after severe traumatic brain injury: a randomised controlled trial. J Neurol Neurosurg Psychiatry 72:193, 2002

Prigatano GP: Personality and psychosocial consequences of brain injury, in Neuropsychological Rehabilitation After Brain Injury. Edited by Prigatano GP, Fordyce DJ, Zeiner HK, et al. Baltimore, MD, Johns Hopkins University Press, 1986, pp 29–50

Prigatano GP: Disordered mind, wounded soul: the emerging role of psychotherapy in rehabilitation after brain injury. J Head Trauma Rehabil 6:1–10, 1991

Prigatano GP: Behavioral limitations TBI patients tend to underestimate: a replication and extension to patients with lateralized cerebral dysfunction. Clin Neuropsychol 10:191–201, 1996

Prigatano GP: Principles of Neuropsychological Rehabilitation. New York, Oxford University Press, 1999

Prigatano GP, Altman IM: Impaired awareness of behavioral limitations after traumatic brain injury. Arch Phys Med Rehabil 71:1058–1064, 1990

Prigatano GP, Ben-Yishay Y: Psychotherapy and psychotherapeutic interventions in brain injury rehabilitation, in Rehabilitation of the Adult and Child With Traumatic Brain Injury. Edited by Rosenthal M, Griffith ER, Kreutzer JS, et al. Philadelphia, PA, FA Davis, 1999, pp 271–283

Prigatano GP, Fordyce DJ: Cognitive dysfunction and psychosocial adjustment after brain injury, in Neuropsychological Rehabilitation After Brain Injury. Edited by Prigatano GP, Fordyce DJ, Zeiner HK, et al. Baltimore, MD, Johns Hopkins University Press, 1986, pp 1–17

Prigatano GP, Altman IM, O'Brien KP: Behavioral limitations that brain injured patients tend to underestimate. Clin Neuropsychol 4:163–176, 1990

Radnitz CL, Hsu L, Tirch DD, et al: A comparison of posttraumatic stress disorder in veterans with and without spinal cord injury. J Abnorm Psychol 107:676–680, 1998

Rammahan KW, Rosenberg JH, Pollak CP, et al: Modafinil: efficacy for the treatment of fatigue in patients with multiple sclerosis (abstract). Neurology 54 (suppl 3):24, 2000

Ranseen JD, Bohaska LA, Schmidt FA: An investigation of anosognosia following traumatic head injury. Int J Clin Neuropsychol 12:29–36, 1990

Rao V, Lyketsos C: Neuropsychiatric sequelae of traumatic brain injury. Psychosomatics 41:95–103, 2000

Rao V, Lyketsos CG: Psychiatric aspects of traumatic brain injury. Psychiatr Clin North Am 25:43–69, 2002

Rapoport MJ, Chan F, Lanctot K, et al: An open-label study of citalopram for major depression following traumatic brain injury. J Psychopharmacol 22:860–864, 2008

Richards JS: Psychologic adjustment to spinal cord injury during first postdischarge year. Arch Phys Med Rehabil 67:362–365, 1986

Rintala DH, Holmes SA, Courtade D, et al: Comparison of the effectiveness of amitriptyline and gabapentin on chronic neuropathic pain in persons with spinal cord injury. Arch Phys Med Rehabil 88:1547–1560, 2007

Ritenour AE, Baskin TW: Primary blast injury: update on diagnosis and treatment. Crit Care 36:S311–317, 2008

Rogers JM, Read CA: Psychiatric comorbidity following traumatic brain injury. Brain Inj 21:1321–1333, 2007

Rohe DE, Krause JS: Stability of interests after severe physical disability: an 11-year longitudinal study. J Vocat Behav 52:45–58, 1998

Rowland T, Mysiw WJ, Bogner J, et al: Trazodone for post traumatic agitation (abstract). Arch Phys Med Rehabil 73:963, 1992

Roy-Byrne P, Fann JR: Psychopharmacologic treatment for patients with neuropsychiatric disorders, in The American Psychiatric Press Textbook of Neuropsychiatry, 3rd Edition. Edited by Yudofsky SC, Hales RE. Washington, DC, American Psychiatric Press, 1997, pp 943–981

Ruff RM: Discipline-specific approach versus individual care, in The Evaluation and Treatment of Mild Traumatic Brain Injury. Edited by Varney NR, Roberts RJ. Mahwah, NJ, Lawrence Erlbaum Associates, 1999, pp 99–114

Ruff RM, Marshall LF, Klauber MR, et al: Alcohol abuse and neurological outcome of the severely head injured. J Head Trauma Rehabil 5:21–31, 1990

Rutherford WH, Merrett JD, McDonald JR: Symptoms at one year following concussion from minor head injuries. Injury 10:225–230, 1979

Saatman KE, Duhaime AC, Bullock R, et al: Classification of traumatic brain injury for targeted therapies. J Neurotrauma. 25:719–738, 2008

Sachdev P, Smith JS, Cathcart S: Schizophrenia-like psychosis following traumatic brain injury: a chart-based descriptive and case-control study. Psychol Med 31:231–239, 2001

Sandel ME, Mysiw WJ: The agitated brain injured patient, part 1: definitions, differential diagnosis, and assessment. Arch Phys Med Rehabil 77:617–623, 1996

Sander AM, Kreutzer JS, Fernandez CC: Neurobehavioral functioning, substance abuse, and employment after brain injury: implications for vocational rehabilitation. J Head Trauma Rehabil 12:28–41, 1997

Santa Maria MP, Pinkston JB, Miller SR, et al: Stability of postconcussion symptomatology differs between high and low responders and by gender but not by mild head injury status. Arch Clin Neuropsychol 16:133–140, 2001

Saran AS: Depression after minor closed head injury: role of dexamethasone suppression test and antidepressants. J Clin Psychiatry 46:335–338, 1985

Sawyer E, Mauro LS, Ohlinger MJ: Amantadine enhancement of arousal and cognition after traumatic brain injury. Ann Pharmacother 42:247–252, 2008

Sbordone RJ, Liter JC: Mild traumatic brain injury does not produce post-traumatic stress disorder. Brain Inj 9:405–412, 1995

Schiff HB, Sabin TD, Geller A, et al: Lithium in aggressive behavior. Am J Psychiatry 139:1346–1348, 1982

Schneiderman AI, Braver ER, Kang HK: Understanding sequelae of injury mechanisms and mild traumatic brain injury incurred during the conflicts in Iraq and Afghanistan: persistent postconcussive symptoms and posttraumatic stress disorder. Am J Epidemiol 167:1446–1452, 2008

Schoenberger NE, Shiflett SC, Esty ML, et al: Flexyx neurotherapy system in the treatment of traumatic brain injury: an initial evaluation. J Head Trauma Rehabil 16:260–274, 2001

Schreiber S, Backer MM, Pick CG: The antinociceptive effect of venlafaxine in mice is mediated through opioid and adrenergic mechanisms. Neurosci Lett 273:85–88, 1999

Scott LK, Green R, McCarthy PJ, et al: Agitation and/or aggression after traumatic brain injury in a pediatric population treated with ziprasidone: clinical article. J Neurosurg Pediatr 3:484–487, 2009

Seel RT, Kreutzer JS, Sander AM: Concordance of patients' and family members' ratings of neurobehavioral functioning after traumatic brain injury. Arch Phys Med Rehabil 78:1254–1259, 1997

Seel RT, Kreutzer JS, Rosenthal M, et al: Depression after traumatic brain injury: a National Institute on Disability and Rehabilitation Research Model Systems multicenter investigation. Arch Phys Med Rehabil 84:177–184, 2003

Selassie AW, Zaloshnja E, Langlois JA, et al: Incidence of long-term disability following traumatic brain injury hospitalization, United States, 2003. J Head Trauma Rehabil 23:123–131, 2008

Shavelle RM, Strauss D, Whyte J, et al: Long-term causes of death after traumatic brain injury. Am J Phys Med Rehabil 80:510–516, 2001

Shear MK, Frank E, Foa E, et al: Traumatic grief treatment: a pilot study. Am J Psychiatry 158:1506–1508, 2001

Sheehan DV, Lecrubier Y, Sheehan KH, et al: The Mini-International Neuropsychiatric Interview (M.I.N.I.): the development and validation of a structured diagnostic psychiatric interview for DSM-IV and ICD-10. J Clin Psychiatry Suppl 20:22–33, 1998

Sherer M, Bergloff P, Boake C, et al: The Awareness Questionnaire: factor structure and internal consistency. Brain Inj 12:63–68, 1998a

Sherer M, Boake C, Levin E, et al: Characteristics of impaired awareness after traumatic brain injury. J Int Neuropsychol Soc 4:380–387, 1998b

Sherer M, Bergloff P, Levin E, et al: Impaired awareness and employment outcome after traumatic brain injury. J Head Trauma Rehabil 13:52–61, 1998c

Sherer M, Hart T, Nick TG, et al: Early impaired self-awareness after traumatic brain injury. Arch Phys Med Rehabil 84:168–176, 2003a

Sherer M, Nakase Thompson R, Nick T, et al: Patterns of neurobehavioral deficits in TBI patients at rehabilitation admission (abstract). J Int Neuropsychol Soc 9:251–252, 2003b

Sherer M, Nakase-Thompson R, Yablon SA, et al: Multidimensional assessment of acute confusion after traumatic brain injury. Arch Phys Med Rehabil 86:896–904, 2005

Sherer M, Yablon SA, Nakase-Richardson R, et al: Effect of severity of post-traumatic confusion and its constituent symptoms on outcome after traumatic brain injury. Arch Phys Med Rehabil 89:42–47, 2008

Shukla S, Cook BL, Mukherjee S, et al: Mania following head trauma. Am J Psychiatry 144:93–96, 1987

Silver JM, Yudofsky SC: Aggressive disorders, in Neuropsychiatry of Traumatic Brain Injury. Edited by Silver JM, Yudofsky SC, Hales RE. Washington, DC, American Psychiatric Press, 1994a, pp 313–353

Silver JM, Yudofsky SC: Psychopharmacology, in Neuropsychiatry of Traumatic Brain Injury. Edited by Silver JM, Yudofsky SC, Hales RE. Washington, DC, American Psychiatric Press, 1994b, pp 631–670

Silver JM, Hales RE, Yudofsky SC: Neuropsychiatric aspects of traumatic brain injury, in The American Psychiatric Publishing Textbook of Neuropsychiatry and Clinical Neurosciences, 4th Edition. Edited by Yudofsky SC, Hales RE. Washington, DC, American Psychiatric Publishing, 2002, pp 625–672

Sipski M, Alexander C: Sexual Function in People With Disabilities and Chronic Illness. Gaithersburg, MD, Aspen Publishers, 1997

Sipski ML, Alexander CJ, Rosen RC: Orgasm in women with spinal cord injuries: a laboratory-based assessment. Arch Phys Med Rehabil 76:1097–1102, 1995

Sloan RL, Brown KW, Pentland B: Fluoxetine as a treatment for emotional lability after brain injury. Brain Inj 6:315–319, 1992

Speech TJ, Rao SM, Osmon DC, et al: A double-blind controlled study of methylphenidate treatment in closed head injury. Brain Inj 7:333–338, 1993

Spitzer RL, Kroenke K, Williams JB: Validation and utility of a self-report version of PRIME-MD: the PHQ primary care study. Primary Care Evaluation of Mental Disorders. Patient Health Questionnaire. JAMA 282:1737–1744, 1999

Staas W, Formal C, Freedman M, et al: Spinal cord injury and spinal cord injury medicine, in Rehabilitation Medicine: Principles and Practice. Edited by DeLisa J, Gans BM. Philadelphia, PA, Lippincott-Raven Publishers, 1998, pp 1259–1291

Stanislav SW, Childs A: Evaluating the usage of droperidol in acutely agitated persons with brain injury. Brain Inj 14:261–265, 2000

Stanislav SW, Fabre T, Crismon ML, et al: Buspirone's efficacy in organic-induced aggression. J Clin Psychopharmacol 14:126–130, 1994

Stein MB, McAllister TW: Exploring the convergence of posttraumatic stress disorder and mild traumatic brain injury. Am J Psychiatry 166:768–776, 2009

Stewart JT, Nemsath RH: Bipolar illness following traumatic brain injury: treatment with lithium and carbamazepine. J Clin Psychiatry 49:74–75, 1988

Stewart T, Shields CR: Grief in chronic illness: assessment and management. Arch Phys Med Rehabil 66:447–450, 1985

Stolp-Smith K, Wainberg K: Antidepressant exacerbation of spasticity. Arch Phys Med Rehabil 80:339–342, 1999

Street JS, Clark WS, Gannon KS, et al: Olanzapine treatment of psychotic and behavioral symptoms in patients with Alzheimer disease in nursing care facilities: a double-blind, randomized, placebo-controlled trial. The HGEU Study Group. Arch Gen Psychiatry 57:968–976, 2000

Stroebe M, Shut H: The dual process model of coping with bereavement: rationale and description. Death Studies 23:197–224, 1999

Stroebe MS, Hansson RO, Stroebe W, et al: Handbook of Bereavement Research. Washington, DC, American Psychological Association, 2001

Stuss DT, Binns MA, Carruth FG, et al: The acute period of recovery from traumatic brain injury: posttraumatic amnesia or posttraumatic confusional state? J Neurosurg 90:635–643, 1999

Suhr JA, Gunstad J: Postconcussive symptom report: the relative influence of head injury and depression. J Clin Exp Neuropsychol 24:981–993, 2002

Svendsen HA, Teasdale TW, Pinner M: Subjective experience in patients with brain injury and their close relatives before and after a rehabilitation programme. Neuropsychol Rehabil 14:495–515, 2004

Tanielian T, Jaycox LH (eds): Invisible Wounds of War: Psychological and Cognitive Injuries, Their Consequences, and Services to Assist Recovery. Santa Monica, CA, RAND Center for Military Health Policy Research, 2008

Tate DG, Stiers W, Daugherty J, et al: The effects of insurance benefits coverage on functional and psychosocial outcomes after spinal cord injury. Arch Phys Med Rehabil 75:407–414, 1994

Tate DG, Forchheimer MB, Krause JS, et al: Patterns of alcohol and substance use and abuse in persons with spinal cord injury: risk factors and correlates. Arch Phys Med Rehabil 85:1837–1847, 2004

Tatum WO, French JA, Faught E, et al: Postmarketing experience with topiramate and cognition. Epilepsia 42:1134–1140, 2001

Taylor LA, Kreutzer JS, Demm SR, et al: Traumatic brain injury and substance abuse: a review and analysis of the literature. Neuropsychol Rehabil 13:165–188, 2003

Teitelman E: Off-label uses of modafinil (letter). Am J Psychiatry 158:8, 2001

Tennant FS, Wild J: Naltrexone treatment for postconcussional syndrome. Am J Psychiatry 144:813–814, 1987

Terzoudi M, Gavrielidou P, Heilakos G, et al: Fatigue in multiple sclerosis: evaluation of a new pharmacological approach (abstract). Neurology 54 (suppl 3):A61–A62, 2000

Thompson RN, Sherer M, Yablon SA, et al: Confusion following TBI: inspection of indices of delirium and amnesia. J Int Neuropsychol Soc 7:177, 2001

Thomsen IV: Late outcome of very severe blunt head trauma: a 10–15 year second follow-up. J Neurol Neurosurg Psychiatry 47:260–268, 1984

Thurman DJ, Alverson C, Dunn KA, et al: Traumatic brain injury in the United States: a public health perspective. J Head Trauma Rehabil 14:602–615, 1999

Tiersky LA, Anselmi V, Johnston MV, et al: A trial of neuropsychological rehabilitation in mild-spectrum traumatic brain injury. Arch Phys Med Rehabil 86:1565–1574, 2005

Trahan DE, Ross CE, Trahan SL: Relationships among postconcussional-type symptoms, depression, and anxiety in neurologically normal young adults and victims of mild brain injury. Arch Clin Neuropsychol 16:435–445, 2001

Trieschmann RB: Spinal Cord Injuries: Psychological, Social and Vocational Rehabilitation. New York, Demos Publication, 1988

Trzepacz PT: Delirium, in Neuropsychiatry of Traumatic Brain Injury. Edited by Silver JM, Yudofsky SC, Hales RE. Washington, DC, American Psychiatric Press, 1994, pp 189–218

Trzepacz PT, Kennedy RE: Delirium and posttraumatic amnesia, in Textbook of Traumatic Brain Injury. Edited by Silver JM, McAllister TW, Yudofsky SC. Washington, DC, American Psychiatric Publishing, 2005, pp 175–200

Trzepacz PT, Baker RW, Greenhouse J: A symptom rating scale for delirium. Psychiatry Res 23:89–97, 1988

Tuohimaa P: Vestibular disturbances after acute mild head injury. Acta Otolaryngol Suppl 359:3–67, 1978

Turner AP, Bombardier CH, Rimmele CT: A typology of alcohol use patterns among persons with recent traumatic brain injury or spinal cord injury: implications for treatment matching. Arch Phys Med Rehabil 84:358–364, 2003

Turner AP, Kivlahan DR, Rimmele CT, et al: Does preinjury alcohol use or blood alcohol level influence cognitive functioning after traumatic brain injury? Rehabil Psychol 51:78–86, 2006

Umansky R, Geller V: Olanzapine treatment in an organic hallucinosis patient. Int J Neuropsychopharmacol 3:81–82, 2000

Umlauf R, Frank RG: A cluster-analytic description of patient subgroups in the rehabilitation setting. Rehabil Psychol 28:157–167, 1983

Uomoto J, Brockway J: Anger management training for brain injured patients and their family members. Arch Phys Med Rehabil 73:674–679, 1992

U.S. Department of Health and Human Services: Healthy People 2010: Understanding and Improving Health. Washington, DC, U.S. Department of Health and Human Services, 2001

Van der Naalt J, Van Zomeren AH, Sluiter WJ, et al: Acute behavioral disturbances related to imaging studies and outcome in mild-to-moderate head injury. Brain Inj 14:781–788, 1999

Van Reekum R, Cohen T, Wong J: Can traumatic brain injury cause psychiatric disorders? J Neuropsychiatry Clin Neurosci 12:316–327, 2000

Van Reekum R, Streiner DL, Conn DK: Applying Bradford Hill's criteria for causation to neuropsychiatry: challenges and opportunities. J Neuropsychiatry Clin Neurosci 13:318–325, 2001

van Workeom TC, Teelken AW, Minderhous JM: Difference in neurotransmitter metabolism in frontotemporal-lobe contusion and diffuse cerebral contusion. Lancet 1:812–813, 1977

Vanderploeg RV, Belanger HG, Curtiss G: Mild traumatic brain injury and posttraumatic stress disorder and their associations with health symptoms. Arch Phys Med Rehabil 90:1084–1093, 2009

Vargo JW: Some psychological effects of physical disability. Am J Occup Ther 32:31–34, 1978

Varney NR, Martzke JS, Roberts RJ: Major depression in patients with closed head injuries. Neuropsychology 1:7–9, 1987

Vasterling JJ, Proctor SP, Amoroso P, et al: Neuropsychological outcomes of army personnel following deployment to the Iraq war. JAMA 296:519–529, 2006

Verma A, Anand V, Verma NP: Sleep disorders in chronic traumatic brain injury. J Clin Sleep Med 3:357–362, 2007

Vickery CD, Sherer M, Nick TG, et al: Relationships among premorbid alcohol use, acute intoxication, and early functional status after traumatic brain injury. Arch Phys Med Rehabil 89:48–55, 2008

Violon A, DeMol J: Psychological sequelae after head trauma in adults. Acta Neurochir (Wien) 85:96–102, 1987

Walker DE, Blankenship V, Ditty JA, et al: Prediction of recovery for closed-head-injured adults: an evaluation of the MMPI, the Adaptive Behavior Scale, and a "Quality of Life" Rating Scale. J Clin Psychol 43:699–707, 1987

Wang KK, Larner SF, Robinson G, et al: Neuroprotection targets after traumatic brain injury. Curr Opin Neurol 19:514–519, 2006

Warden DL, Labbate LA, Salazar AM, et al: Posttraumatic stress disorder in patients with traumatic brain injury and amnesia for the event? J Neuropsychiatry Clin Neurosci 9:18–22, 1997

Warden DL, Gordon B, McAllister TW, et al: Neurobehavioral Guidelines Working Group. Guidelines for the pharmacologic treatment of neurobehavioral sequelae of traumatic brain injury. J Neurotrauma 23:1468–1501, 2006

Webster G, Daisley A, King N: Relationship and family breakdown following acquired brain injury: the role of the rehabilitation team. Brain Inj 13:593–603, 1999

Webster JB, Bell KR, Hussey JD, et al: Sleep apnea in adults with traumatic brain injury: a preliminary investigation. Arch Phys Med Rehabil 82:316–321, 2001

Whelan FJ, Walker MS, Schultz SK: Donepezil in the treatment of cognitive dysfunction associated with traumatic brain injury. Ann Clin Psychiatry 12:131–135, 2000

Whelan-Goodinson R, Ponsford J, Schonberger M: Association between psychiatric state and outcome following traumatic brain injury. J Rehabil Med 40:850–857, 2008

Whyte J, Hart T, Schuster K, et al: Effects of methylphenidate on attentional function after traumatic brain injury: a randomized placebo-controlled trial. Am J Phys Med Rehabil 76:440–450, 1997

Whyte J, Hart T, Vaccaro M, et al: Effects of methylphenidate on attention deficits after traumatic brain injury: a multidimensional, randomized, controlled trial. Am J Phys Med Rehabil 83:401–420, 2004

Wilcox JH, Nasrallah HA: Childhood head trauma and psychosis. Psychiatry Res 21:303–306, 1987

Williams DH, Levin HS, Eisenberg HM: Mild head injury classification. Neurosurgery 27:422–428, 1990

Wilson JT, Teasdale GM, Hadley DM, et al: Posttraumatic amnesia: still a valuable yardstick. J Neurol Neurosurg Psychiatry 57:198–201, 1994

Wilson MS, Gibson CJ, Hamm RJ: Haloperidol, but not olanzapine, impairs cognitive performance after traumatic brain injury in rats. Am J Phys Med Rehabil 82:871–879, 2003

Wood RL, Liossi C: Neuropsychological and neurobehavioral correlates of aggression following traumatic brain injury. J Neuropsychiatry Clin Neurosci 18:333–341, 2006

World Health Organization: International Classification of Impairments, Disabilities and Handicaps: ICIDH. Geneva, Switzerland, World Health Organization, 1980

World Health Organization: International Statistical Classification of Diseases and Related Health Problems, 10th Revision. Geneva, Switzerland, World Health Organization, 1992

World Health Organization: International Classification of Functioning, Disability and Health: ICF. Geneva, Switzerland, World Health Organization, 2001

Worthington AD, Melia Y: Rehabilitation is compromised by arousal and sleep disorders: results of a survey of rehabilitation centres. Brain Inj 20:327–332, 2006

Wortman CB, Silver RC: The myths of coping with loss. J Consult Clin Psychol 57:349–357, 1989

Wroblewski BA, McColgan K, Smith K, et al: The incidence of seizures during tricyclic antidepressant drug treatment in a brain-injured population. J Clin Psychopharmacol 10:124–128, 1990

Wroblewski BA, Joseph AB, Cornblatt RR: Antidepressant pharmacotherapy and the treatment of depression in patients with severe traumatic brain injury: a controlled, prospective study. J Clin Psychiatry 57:582–587, 1996

Wroblewski BA, Joseph AB, Kupfer J, et al: Effectiveness of valproic acid on destructive and aggressive behaviors in patients with acquired brain injury. Brain Inj 11:37–47, 1997

Yoshino A, Hovda DA, Kawamata T, et al: Dynamic changes in local cerebral glucose utilization following cerebral concussion in rats: evidence of hyper- and subsequent hypometabolic state. Brain Res 561:106–119, 1991

Yudofsky SC, Silver JM, Jackson W, et al: The Overt Aggression Scale for the objective rating of verbal and physical aggression. Am J Psychiatry 143:35–39, 1986

Yudofsky SC, Silver JM, Hales RE: Pharmacological management of aggression in the elderly. J Clin Psychiatry 51:22–28, 1990

Yudofsky SC, Kopecky HJ, Kunik M, et al: The Overt Agitation Severity Scale for the objective rating of agitation. J Neuropsychiatry Clin Neurosci 9:541–548, 1997

Zafonte RD, Lexell J, Cullen N: Possible applications for dopaminergic agents following traumatic brain injury: part 2. J Head Trauma Rehabil 16:112–116, 2001

Zaidi SH, Faruqui RA: Aripiprazole is associated with early onset of tardive dyskinesia like presentation in a patient with ABI and psychosis. Brain Inj 22:99–102, 2008

Zhang L, Plotkin RC, Wang G, et al: Cholinergic augmentation with donepezil enhances recovery in short-term memory and sustained attention after traumatic brain injury. Arch Phys Med Rehabil 85:1050–1055, 2004

Zifko UA, Rupp M, Schwarz S, et al: Modafinil in treatment of fatigue in multiple sclerosis: results of an open-label study. J Neurol 249:983–987, 2002

Zilbergeld B: Male Sexuality. New York, Bantam Books, 1978

CHAPTER

36

Pain

Michael R. Clark, M.D., M.P.H., M.B.A.

IN THIS CHAPTER, I FIRST review definitions, assessment, and epidemiology of pain. I then discuss selected specific acute and chronic pain syndromes, followed by the major psychiatric comorbidities of chronic pain, including somatization, substance use, depression, anxiety, and other emotional states. Finally, treatments are reviewed, including medications, psychological therapies, and interdisciplinary programs. Some pain topics are covered elsewhere in this book, including arthritis (see Chapter 25, "Rheumatology"), fibromyalgia (see Chapter 26, "Chronic Fatigue and Fibromyalgia Syndromes"), postoperative pain (see Chapter 30, "Surgery"), headache (see Chapter 32, "Neurology and Neurosurgery"), pelvic pain and vulvodynia (see Chapter 33, "Obstetrics and Gynecology"), spinal cord injury (SCI; see Chapter 35, "Physical Medicine and Rehabilitation"), and palliative care (see Chapter 41, "Palliative Care").

Definition and Assessment

Pain is a complex experience that integrates affective, cognitive, and behavioral factors with an extensive neurobiology. Pain has been defined by the International Association for the Study of Pain as "an unpleasant sensory and emotional experience associated with actual or potential tissue damage, or described in terms of such damage" (Merskey 2007, p. 13). Many terms are used to describe different types of painful experiences (Table 36–1). Pain is the most common reason a patient presents to a physician for evaluation. This physician is rarely a psychiatrist. If the patient has chronic pain, pain persisting on a daily basis for a month beyond what would be considered the usual time for healing of underlying pathology, then many specialists may be involved in the care of the patient (Bonica 1990).

Pain is a subjective experience and difficult to assess, especially in patients with terminal illnesses, cognitive impairments, and other chronic degenerative diseases of the brain (Nikolaus 1997). Pain rating scales attempt to measure the severity and intensity of pain. Many factors can influence these ratings, including disease states, mental disorders, distress, personality traits, and meaningful interpretations based on personal beliefs. In a comparison study of several pain rating scales, such as a vertically oriented visual analog scale (VAS), a verbal descriptor scale (VDS), a pain thermometer, and a numeric rating scale, the VDS was rated as the preferred, easiest, and best assessment tool for rating pain by the elderly (Herr and Mobily 1993). The Geriatric Pain Measure short form is a 12-item self-administered questionnaire targeted at community-dwelling elderly people to improve assessment of pain intensity, pain with ambulation, and disengagement because of pain (Clough-Gorr et al. 2008).

Epidemiology

The U.S. Center for Health Statistics conducted an 8-year follow-up survey and found that 32.8% of the general population experienced chronic pain symptoms (Magni et al. 1993). Health status surveys in six European countries found pain to be a significant problem in 28.5% of the general population (König et al. 2009). In Israel, 46% reported at least one chronic pain complaint, and more than a third of individuals reported severe pain with impaired life activities (Neville et al. 2008). A World Health Organization (WHO) study of more than 25,000 primary care patients in 14 countries found that 22% of patients had pain that was present for most of the time for at least 6 months (Gureje et al. 1998). In people age 65 years or older, musculoskeletal

TABLE 36–1. Definitions relating to pain sensations

Allodynia	Pain from a stimulus that does not normally provoke pain
Deafferentation pain	Pain resulting from loss of sensory input into the central nervous system
Dysesthesia	Unpleasant, abnormal sensation that can be spontaneous or evoked
Hyperalgesia	Increased response to a stimulus that is normally painful
Hyperesthesia	Increased sensitivity to stimulation that excludes the special senses
Hyperpathia	Pain characterized by an increased reaction to a stimulus, especially a repetitive stimulus, and an increased threshold
Hypoesthesia	Diminished sensitivity to stimulation that excludes the special senses
Nociception	Detection of tissue damage by transducers in skin and deeper structures and the central propagation of this information via A delta and C fibers in the peripheral nerves
Paresthesia	Abnormal sensation, spontaneous or evoked, that is not unpleasant
Sensitization	Lowered threshold and prolonged/enhanced response to stimulation

Source. Adapted from Merskey et al. 1986.

pain is associated with three times the likelihood of significant difficulty performing three or more physical activities (Scudds and Robertson 1998). In a community sample of individuals older than 70, chronic pain was present in 52%, and obesity was associated with a two- to fourfold increase in risk of having chronic pain (McCarthy et al. 2009). In persons older than 75, more than two-thirds reported pain, almost half reported pain in multiple sites, and a third rated pain as severe in at least one location (Brattberg et al. 1996).

Acute Pain

The Joint Commission on Accreditation of Healthcare Organizations has implemented pain management standards for all patient encounters (Phillips 2000). In the Veterans Affairs medical centers, pain intensity is defined and tracked as the "fifth vital sign." Acute pain is usually the result of trauma from a surgery, an injury, or an exacerbation of chronic disease, especially musculoskeletal conditions. Treatment is focused on controlling inflammation, preventing tissue destruction, and repairing injury, with more emphasis placed on pain relief to facilitate reaching these goals.

The approach to acute pain management usually will be successful with straightforward strategies such as relaxation, immobilization, analgesic medications (aspirin, acetaminophen, nonsteroidal anti-inflammatory drugs [NSAIDs], opioids), massage, and transcutaneous electrical nerve stimulation (Institute for Clinical Systems Improvement [ICSI] 2008). The absence of signs consistent with acute pain, such as elevated heart rate, blood pressure, and diaphoresis, does not rule out the presence of pain. Acute pain management initiated as early as possible and focused on preventing occurrence and reemergence of pain may allow for lower total doses of analgesics. Analgesics, especially opioids, should be prescribed only for pain relief. Although analgesia may produce many benefits, other symptoms commonly coinciding with acute pain such as insomnia or anxiety should be managed separately from pain. Sleep deprivation and anxiety may intensify the sensation of pain and increase requests for more medication. Reducing anxiety and insomnia often reduces analgesic requirements.

In acute pain management, psychiatric consultation is requested when a patient requires more analgesia than expected or has a history of substance abuse. Patients with an active or recent history of opioid addiction and those receiving methadone maintenance therapy have increased tolerance to opioids and may require up to 50% higher doses of short-acting opioids being used for acute pain management. Although it is important to monitor opioid use carefully in these patients, adequate treatment of acute pain is a priority. Inadequate dosing is significantly more common than abuse or diversion in these patients.

Psychiatric Comorbidity

Pain Disorder and Somatization

When a somatic cause for pain cannot be identified, many clinicians begin to seek psychological causes. Pain "caused" by emotional factors was first classified in DSM-II (American Psychiatric Association 1968) under psychophysiological disorders, and DSM-III (American Psychiatric Association 1980) introduced psychogenic pain disorder.

The lifetime prevalence of somatoform pain disorder (DSM-III-R; American Psychiatric Association 1987) in the general population was 34%, and the 6-month prevalence was 17%. The addition of the DSM-IV (American Psychiatric Association 1994) requirement of "significant distress or psychosocial impairment due to somatoform pain" reduced the lifetime prevalence of pain disorder to 12% and the 6-month prevalence to 5%, with a female-to-male ratio of 2:1 (Grabe et al. 2003).

Pain is the chief complaint, but the experience of pain is augmented by psychological factors. Injured workers with somatoform pain disorder compared with those workers without this disorder had more sites of pain with spread of pain beyond the area of original injury, more opioid and benzodiazepine use, and greater involvement with compensation and litigation (Streltzer et al. 2000). Pain disorder is often equated with "psychogenic" pain with no "real" cause. However, neuroimaging studies show significant decreases in gray matter density in prefrontal, cingulate, and insular cortex that modulate the subjective experience of pain (Valet et al. 2009). Unfortunately, the either/or concept of psychological and physical dualism remains inherent in this diagnosis instead of appreciating how these domains interrelate with each other.

Multiple pain complaints are typical in somatization disorder, but somatization disorder is very uncommon in patients with chronic pain. More common in patients with multiple unexplained painful symptoms are subsyndromal forms of somatization disorder, such as multisomatoform disorder, which affects 4%–18% of primary care patients and is associated with high rates of health care use and persistent somatic complaints (Jackson and Kroenke 2008). These patients are more likely to have catastrophic thinking, believe the cause of their pain to be a mysterious medical disease, have feelings of losing control, and think that physicians believe their pain is imaginary. Patients with chronic pain and medically unexplained symptoms also are at risk for iatrogenic consequences of excessive diagnostic tests, inappropriate medications, and unnecessary surgery. Increased psychiatric morbidity is associated with levels of unexplained medical symptoms far below the number required for the diagnosis of somatization disorder. Overlap between somatoform disorders and depressive or anxiety disorders is common. Patients with somatization experience significant functional disability and role impairment independent of psychiatric and medical comorbidity (Harris et al. 2009). The concept of somatization is more likely a dimensional process based on somatic distress and care-eliciting behavior with varying degrees of severity and persistence across the entire population rather than a set of categorical disorders affecting only a small subset of people (Noyes et al. 2008).

Substance Abuse and Dependence

The prevalence of substance dependence or addiction in patients with chronic pain is estimated to range from 3% to 19% (Dersh et al. 2002; McWilliams et al. 2003). The essential criteria for a substance use disorder in patients with chronic pain include the loss of control in the use of the medication, excessive preoccupation with the medication despite adequate analgesia, and adverse consequences associated with its use. The Researched Abuse, Diversion and Addiction-Related Surveillance System (RADARS) reported that prescription opioid abuse has significantly increased (Cicero et al. 2007). Americans represent less than 5% of the world's population but consume 80% of the global opioid supply, including 99% of the hydrocodone produced (Manchikanti and Singh 2008).

Aberrant medication-taking behaviors can be mistaken for addiction. Persistent pain can lead to an increased focus on taking opioid medications, with the patient taking measures to ensure an adequate medication supply. Patients understandably fear the reemergence of pain and withdrawal symptoms if they run out of medication. Medication-seeking behavior may be the result of an anxious patient trying to maintain a previous level of pain control or improve on a partial but inadequate response to analgesics. These actions may represent pseudoaddiction that results from therapeutic dependence and current or potential undertreatment but not addiction (Kirsh et al. 2002). The distinction between pseudoaddiction and true addiction is based on whether these behaviors abate with adequate analgesic therapy and functioning improves or whether these behaviors persist in the context of deteriorating function.

Several patterns of nonadherence to or misuse of prescribed medications occur when patients have concerns about medications (McCracken et al. 2006). The taking of *more* medication than prescribed was associated with patients' concerns about addiction, tolerance, withdrawal, excessive scrutiny of medication use by others, and a greater perceived need for medication. These factors are likely risk factors for developing an addiction to prescribed medications. During the first 5 years after the onset of a chronic pain problem, patients are at increased risk for developing new drug use problems and disorders. The risk was highest among those with a history of drug use disorder or psychiatric comorbidity. Not infrequently, a history of substance abuse emerges only after the current misuse of medications has been identified, thus requiring physicians to monitor treatment closely. Aberrant medication-taking behaviors occur in approximately 50% of the patients with chronic pain receiving chronic opioid analgesic therapy, with even higher rates in patients with a history of substance abuse (Passik et al. 2006). The Pain Assessment and Documentation Tool is an effective means to standardize follow-up care and decrease the risk of poor outcome with opioid therapy (Passik et al. 2005). These studies suggest that aberrant medication-taking behavior is a manifestation of addiction or diversion in only 10% of patients.

The process of relapse back to substance abuse in these patients is not well understood and probably involves multiple factors. A cycle of pain followed by relief after taking medications is an excellent example of operant reinforcement of their future use (Fordyce et al. 1973). For patients with chronic pain who develop new substance use disorders, the problem most commonly involved the medications prescribed by their physicians (Long et al. 1988). In a recent comprehensive review, a calculated rate of abuse or addiction in patients with chronic pain was only 3.27% (Fishbain et al. 2008a). In the subgroup of patients with chronic pain who had no history of substance abuse, this rate declined to 0.19%. However, as expected, rates for aberrant medication-taking behaviors and abnormal urine toxicology results were significantly higher, reinforcing the need for risk screening and monitoring. Risk prediction instruments such as the Screener and Opioid Assessment for Patients With Pain (SOAPP), Opioid Risk Tool (ORT), and Current Opioid Misuse Measure (COMM) offer valuable guidance but have significant limitations (Chou et al. 2009). Strategies to optimize outcome and minimize abuse require careful analysis of the behavior of both patients and physicians (Passik and Kirsh 2008).

From the opposite perspective, patients with substance use disorders have increased rates of chronic pain and are at the greatest risk for stigmatization and undertreatment. Opioid-dependent patients with chronic pain have even higher rates of drug use than do those without chronic pain (Peles et al. 2005; Rosenblum et al. 2003). Surprisingly, 84% of the patients with chronic pain who abused prescription opioids and entered a drug abuse treatment facility reported that they had legitimately received a prescription from a physician for the treatment of pain (Passik et al. 2006). However, 91% had purchased prescription opioids through illegitimate sources, and 80% had altered the delivery system of the prescription drug, which suggests that they had progressed to more severe forms of addiction. For example, patients with substance abuse and back pain were less likely to complete a substance abuse treatment program compared with those without pain, although the other factors associated with poor outcome were difficult to define (Stack et al. 2000). Integrating care for chronic pain with innovative stepped-care models of substance abuse treatment would likely improve outcomes by tailoring the intensity of treatment to an individual patient's needs (Clark et al. 2008).

Depression and Affective Distress

The relation between pain and depression is intimate and bidirectional. Physical symptoms are common in patients with major depression. Approximately 60% of patients with depression report pain symptoms at diagnosis. In the WHO's data from 14 countries on 5 continents, 69% (range: 45%–95%) of patients with depression presented with only somatic symptoms, of which pain complaints were most common (Simon et al. 1999). A survey of almost 19,000 Europeans found a fourfold increase in the prevalence of chronic painful conditions in subjects with major depression (Ohayon and Schatzberg 2003). A depressive disorder doubles the risk of developing chronic musculoskeletal pain, headache, and chest pain up to 13 years later (Larson et al. 2004). In patients with early inflammatory arthritis, baseline symptoms of depression predicted future pain better than did initial ratings of pain and disease activity (Schieir et al. 2009).

Individuals with chronic physical complaints have higher rates of lifetime major depression. The prevalence of major depression in patients with chronic low back pain (LBP) is more than three times the rate in the general population (Sullivan et al. 1992). Among patients presenting to chronic pain clinics, one-third to more than one-half meet criteria for current major depression (Dersh et al. 2002). Depression in patients with chronic pain is associated with greater pain intensity, more pain persistence, application for early retirement, and greater interference from pain, including more pain behaviors observed by others (Hasenbring et al. 1994). Depression is a better predictor of disability than are pain intensity and duration. Primary care patients with musculoskeletal pain complicated by depression are significantly more likely than nondepressed patients with musculoskeletal pain to use medications daily, including sedative-hypnotics, and in combinations (Mäntyselkä et al. 2002). In a study of more than 15,000 employees who filed health claims, the cost of managing chronic conditions such as back problems was almost doubled when they had comorbid depression (Druss et al. 2000). In older adults with chronic pain, depression may be characterized by the absence of self-blame and significantly influenced by cognitive-behavioral variables such as catastrophizing and maladaptive coping styles (Lopez-Lopez et al. 2008).

Patients with chronic pain syndromes, such as migraine, chronic abdominal pain, and orthopedic pain syndromes, have increased rates of suicidal ideation, suicide attempts, and suicide completion (Magni et al. 1998). Patients with chronic pain completed suicide at two to three times the rate in the general population (Fishbain et al. 1991). The decrease in self-efficacy experienced by patients with chronic pain is highly associated with depressive symptoms that result in feelings of hopelessness (Rahman et al. 2008). Although other psychosocial variables play a role, depression is the most consistent and strongest predictor of suicidal ideation and behaviors in patients with chronic pain (Braden and Sullivan 2008). Pain is even more likely to be an independent risk factor for suicide in patients with head or multiple types of pain (Ilgen et al. 2008).

Depression with comorbid pain can be more resistant to treatment (Kroenke et al. 2009). Depression should be treated aggressively and not simply "understood" as an expected outcome of suffering with chronic pain. Pain often subsides with improvement in depressive symptoms. In patients older than 60 years with arthritis, antidepressants and/or problem-solving-oriented psychotherapy not only reduced depressive symptoms but also improved pain, functional status, and quality of life (Lin et al. 2003). In addition to having greater efficacy for the treatment of neuropathic pain, serotonin-norepinephrine reuptake inhibitors (SNRIs) and tricyclic antidepressants (TCAs) are associated with faster rates of improvement in depressive symptoms and lower rates of relapse of major depressive disorder compared with selective serotonin reuptake inhibitors (SSRIs) (Rosenzweig-Lipson et al. 2007). These findings may be explained by the fact that the neurobiology of pain and depression overlap (Bair et al. 2003).

Anxiety, Fear, Catastrophizing, and Anger

Almost 50% of patients with chronic pain report anxiety symptoms, and up to 30% of patients have an anxiety disorder such as generalized anxiety disorder, panic disorder, agoraphobia, and posttraumatic stress disorder (PTSD) (Dersh et al. 2002; McWilliams et al. 2003). One prospective study of 1,007 young adults found that a baseline history of migraine was significantly associated with an increased risk (odds ratio [OR] = 12.8) of first-incidence panic disorder (Breslau and Davis 1993). In patients with noncardiac chest pain, the presence of panic disorder significantly worsened health-related quality of life (Dammen et al. 2008).

PTSD is increasingly recognized as a comorbid condition with significant consequences for patients with medical illnesses, especially chronic pain disorders (Liebschutz et al. 2007). More than half of fibromyalgia patients reported clinically relevant PTSD-like symptoms that were significantly associated with greater levels of pain, emotional distress, interference, and disability (Sherman et al. 2000). Compared with accident-related factors, PTSD symptoms and other psychological factors were the strongest predictors of the development of chronic pain in people who had severe accidents 3 years earlier (Jenewein et al. 2009).

Conversely, anxiety symptoms and disorders are associated with high levels of somatic preoccupation and physical symptoms. Pain intensity in rheumatoid arthritis patients was significantly influenced by the presence of anxiety and depression, even after disease activity had been controlled for (Smedstad et al. 1995). Almost two-thirds of patients with panic disorder reported at least one current pain symptom (Schmidt et al. 2002). Pain was related to higher levels of anxiety symptoms, panic frequency, and cognitive features of anxiety. Pain severity, pain-related disability, and health-related quality of life were significantly worse in patients with chronic musculoskeletal pain and comorbid anxiety or depression (Bair et al. 2008).

Fear of pain, movement, reinjury, and other negative consequences that result in the avoidance of activities promote the transition to and sustaining of chronic pain and its associated disabilities (Greenberg and Burns 2003). Patients with chronic LBP who restricted their activities developed physiological changes (muscle atrophy, weight gain) and functional deterioration attributed to deconditioning (Verbunt et al. 2003). This process is reinforced by low self-efficacy, catastrophic interpretations, and increased expectations of failure regarding attempts to engage in rehabilitation. The fear-avoidance model of musculoskeletal pain incorporates components such as pain severity, pain catastrophizing, attention to pain, pain-related fear, escape or avoidance behavior, disability, disuse, and vulnerabilities to explain the transition from acute to chronic LBP (Leeuw et al. 2007).

Fear-avoidance beliefs were one of the most significant predictors of failure to return to work in patients with chronic LBP (Waddell et al. 1993). Operant conditioning reinforces disability if the avoidance provides any short-term benefits, such as reducing anticipatory anxiety or relieving the patient of unwanted responsibilities. In patients with chronic LBP, improvements in disability following physical therapy were associated with decreases in pain, psychological distress, and fear-avoidance beliefs but not specific physical deficits (Mannion et al. 2001). Decreasing work-specific fears was a more important outcome than addressing general fears of physical activity in predicting improved physical capability for work (Vowles and Gross 2003).

Catastrophic thinking about pain has been attributed to the amplification of threatening information, and it interferes with patients' ability to remain involved with productive activities (Crombez et al. 1998). Catastrophizing intensifies the experience of pain and increases emotional distress and self-perceived disability (Sullivan et al. 2001). This multidimensional construct includes elements of cognitive rumination, symptom magnification, feelings of helplessness, and expectations of pessimism (Edwards et al. 2006). Early treatment catastrophizing and feelings of helplessness in patients attending a 4-week multidisciplinary pain program predicted late-treatment outcomes (Burns et al. 2003). Pain-related cognitions such as catastrophizing and fear-avoidance beliefs predict poor coping and adjustment to chronic pain better than do objective factors such as disease status, physical impairment, or occupational descriptions (Hasenbring et al. 2001). High levels of catastrophizing and fear of injury prospectively predicted disability due to new-onset LBP 6 months later (Picavet et al. 2002). Catastrophizing has been shown to be a predictor of suicidal ideation independent of depressive symptoms and pain severity (Edwards et al. 2006).

Chronic Pain Conditions

Postherpetic Neuralgia

Postherpetic neuralgia (PHN) is defined as pain persisting or recurring at the site of shingles at least 3 months after the onset of the acute varicella zoster viral rash. PHN occurs in about 10% of patients with acute herpes zoster. More than half of patients older than 65 years with shingles develop PHN, and it is more likely to occur in patients with cancer, diabetes mellitus, and immunosuppression. Other risk factors include longer duration of prodromal symptoms, greater acute pain and rash severity, sensory impairment, and psychological distress (Volpi et al. 2008). Most cases gradually improve over time, with only about 25% of patients with PHN experiencing pain at 1 year after diagnosis. Approximately 15% of referrals to pain clinics are for the treatment of PHN.

Although degeneration and destruction of motor and sensory fibers of the mixed dorsal root ganglion characterize acute varicella zoster, other neurological damage may include inflammation of the spinal cord, myelin disruption, axonal damage, and decreases in the number of nerve endings from the affected skin. Studies have suggested the role of both peripheral and central mechanisms resulting from the loss of large caliber neurons and subsequent central sensitization or adrenergic receptor activation and alterations in C-fiber activity (Truini et al. 2008). Early treatment of varicella zoster with low-dose amitriptyline reduced the prevalence of pain at 6 months by 50% (Johnson 1997). TCAs, SNRIs, anticonvulsants, and opioids are the most common effective treatments for PHN and may have potential for its prevention (Attal et al. 2006; Saarto and Wiffen 2007; Zin et al. 2008). Topical lidocaine recently has been approved by the U.S. Food and Drug Administration for treatment of PHN. A live attenuated varicella vaccine decreased the incidence of herpes zoster and PHN as well as the burden of illness in adults older than 60 years (Harpaz et al. 2008; Johnson et al. 2008).

Peripheral Neuropathy Pain

The most common cause of painful peripheral neuropathy is diabetes mellitus (Veves et al. 2008; Zochodne 2008). Approximately 25% of patients with diabetes mellitus will experience painful diabetic neuropathy, and longer duration of illness and poor glycemic control increase this risk (Tavakoli and Malik 2008). If C-fiber input is preserved but large-fiber input is lost, dysesthesias and pain are the predominant sensory experiences. The pain of a peripheral neuropathy can range from a constant burning to a pain that is episodic, paroxysmal, and lancinating in quality (Mendell and Sahenk 2003). These phenomena are primarily the result of axonal degeneration and segmental demyelination (Tomlinson and Gardiner 2008). Sites of ectopic impulse generation can be found at any point along the peripheral nerve, including the dorsal root ganglion, regardless of where the nerve is actually damaged. Other changes can alter the magnitude and frequency of impulse generation, such as sensitivity to mechanical or neurochemical stimuli. The paroxysms of pain that result from stimulation of hyperexcitable damaged neurons and subsequent recruitment of nearby undamaged sensory afferents may be explained by several forms of nonsynaptic (ephaptic) and prolonged (afterdischarge) impulse transmission. Voltage-dependent sodium channels contribute to hyperexcitability, and central sensitization amplifies and sustains neuronal activity by a variety of mechanisms such as reduced inhibition of dorsal horn cells, *N*-methyl-D-aspartate (NMDA) receptor activation, and excessive glutamate release (Carozzi et al. 2008). Pharmacological treatments are almost identical to those used in the treatment of PHN (Jain 2008; T.S. Jensen and Finnerup 2007).

Parkinson's Disease

Most patients with Parkinson's disease have pain, which is more common in women (Beiske et al. 2009). The pain is typically described as cramping and aching, located in the lower back and extremities, but not associated with muscle contraction or spasm. All forms of chronic pain are represented, including musculoskeletal, neuropathic (radicular, central), and dystonic (Schestatsky et al. 2007). These pains often decrease when the patient is given levodopa, which suggests a central origin. The loss of dopaminergic input could explain how pain is produced. Dopamine is now consistently implicated as having a role in the endogenous pain modulation system (Potvin et al. 2009; Wood 2008). In a review of French health system data, 82% of patients with Parkinson's disease were prescribed analgesics (Brefel-Courbon et al. 2009). Although patients with Parkinson's disease were more commonly prescribed chronic analgesics such as opioids and adjuvant medications when compared with the general population and diabetic patients, only a minority of patients continued taking these medications. In an open-label trial of duloxetine in patients with Parkinson's disease, their pain improved significantly (Djaldetti et al. 2007). Subthalamic deep brain stimulation may offer relief to patients with symptoms refractory to other therapies (Kim et al. 2008).

Central Poststroke Pain and Spinal Cord Injury

Pain associated with lesions of the central nervous system is common after stroke (8%) or spinal cord trauma (60%–70%) (Finnerup 2008; Ullrich 2007). Symptoms of SCI pain or central poststroke pain are often poorly localized, vary over time, and include allodynia (>50% of central poststroke pain patients), hyperalgesia, dysesthesias, lancinating pain, and muscle and visceral pain regardless of sensory deficits. Pain is described as burning, aching, lacerating, or pricking. Radiographic lesions are present in the thalamus, although other sites are often involved such as the spinothalamic tracts, especially in SCI (Hari et al. 2009). Excitatory amino acids are likely involved in the development of central sensitization associated with this syndrome, and the onset of pain can occur more than a month after the stroke, suggesting multiple processes (Hains and Waxman 2007; Hulsebosch et al. 2009).

As a result, central poststroke pain is difficult to treat, and conventional analgesics and opioids have been shown to be ineffective. Randomized clinical trials have reported efficacy for amitriptyline and for drugs that reduce neuronal hyperexcitability, including lidocaine (intravenous), mexiletine, lamotrigine, fluvoxamine, and gabapentin, but not carbamazepine, phenytoin, or topiramate (Frese et al. 2006). Fluvoxamine significantly improved pain ratings but only in patients within 1 year after stroke (Shimodozono et al. 2002). In contrast, patients with SCI experience reductions in continuous and evoked pain with ketamine and opioids, suggesting different mechanisms in different central pain states (Eide et al. 1995). Morphine may be effective against allodynia but not other components of central pain syndromes (Nicholson 2004). Intravenous lidocaine has been efficacious, but the need for intravenous administration and its adverse effects limit its use. Recent reviews support the efficacy of amitriptyline, gabapentin, and pregabalin for the neuropathic pain associated with SCI (Baastrup and Finnerup 2008; Tzellos et al. 2008).

Migraine and Chronic Daily Headache

The International Headache Society has published guidelines for the classification of headache. The peak incidence of migraine occurs between the third and sixth decade of life and then decreases with age (Silberstein et al. 2007). Over the life span, 18% of women and 6% of men will experience migraine headaches (Lipton et al. 2007). Theories of pathogenesis include the trigeminovascular system and plasma protein extravasation, antagonism of serotonin receptors, modulation of central aminergic control mechanisms, membrane-stabilizing effects through action at voltage-sensitive calcium channels, and increased levels of substance P (Goadsby et al. 2009). Common migraine is a unilateral pulsatile headache, which may be associated with other symptoms such as nausea, vomiting, photophobia, and phonophobia. The classic form of migraine adds visual prodromal symptoms such as scintillating scotomata. Complicated migraine includes focal neurological signs such as cranial nerve palsies and is often described by the name of the primary deficit (e.g., hemiplegic, vestibular, or basilar migraine).

Placebo-controlled clinical trials support use of NSAIDs and triptans for acute treatment of migraine attacks, with propranolol, metoprolol, flunarizine, valproate, and topiramate recommended as the best prophylactic agents (Evers et al. 2006; Mulleners and Chronicle 2008). In general, calcium channel blockers, beta-blockers, antidepressants, and anticonvulsants are the treatments of choice for more refractory migraine (Evers et al. 2006; Silberstein 2008). Behavioral treatments such as cognitive-behavioral psychotherapy and biofeedback or relaxation training are effective therapies (Holroyd and Drew 2006). A group-based multidisciplinary treatment for migraine consisting of stress management, supervised exercise, dietary education, and massage therapy significantly improved various pain characteristics, functional status, quality of life, depression, and pain-related disability (Lemstra et al. 2002).

Headache is the most common pain condition reported by the U.S. workforce as the reason for lost productivity (Stewart et al. 2003). Chronic daily headache affects about 5% of the population and is composed of constant (transformed) migraine, medication-overuse headache, chronic tension-type headaches, new-onset daily persistent headache, and hemicrania continua (Dodick 2006). Individuals with chronic daily headache are more likely to overuse analgesics, leading to rebound headache; to have psychiatric comorbidity such as depression and anxiety; to report functional disability; and to experience stress-related headache exacerbations (Fernández-de-las-Peñas and Schoenen 2009). Patients with transformed migraine have poor quality of life and the worst Short Form 36 (SF-36) Health Survey profile when compared with patients with episodic migraine or chronic tension-type headaches (Wang et al. 2001).

Chronic tension-type headaches typically manifest as daily pain that is difficult to manage and unresponsive to many treatments. Placebo-controlled clinical trials are few but support the use of amitriptyline, gabapentin, tizanidine, mirtazapine, topiramate, memantine, and botulinum toxin type A (Dodick 2006). Various medications have been recommended and include serotonin agonists, serotonin antagonists, and alpha$_2$-adrenergic agonists. Olanzapine decreased headache severity and frequency in patients with refractory headaches who failed treatment with at least four preventive medications (Silberstein et al. 2002). Topiramate decreased migraine frequency and severity, number of headache days, and use of abortive medications in patients with both episodic and transformed migraine (Mathew et al. 2002). TCAs coupled with stress management therapy significantly reduced headache activity, analgesic medication use, and headache-related disability (Holroyd et al. 2001). Combined medication and cognitive-behavioral psychotherapy is more effective than either treatment alone (Lake 2001; Lipchik and Nash 2002).

Fibromyalgia

Fibromyalgia is a chronic pain syndrome characterized by widespread musculoskeletal pain in all four limbs and trunk, stiffness, and exaggerated tenderness. These symptoms are usually accompanied by poor sleep, cognitive difficulties, depression, and fatigue. Fibromyalgia is diagnosed in 3.4% of women and 0.5% of men and is clustered in families (Arnold et al. 2004). Current research suggests that fibromyalgia may be a syndrome of dysfunctional central pain processing influenced by a variety of processes, including infection, physical trauma, psychological traits, and psychopathology (Abeles et al. 2007). Guidelines for fibromyalgia treatment have been recently released and recommend multidisciplinary treatment regimens (Carville et al. 2008; Hauser et al. 2009). Placebo-controlled trials suggest pain reduction with cyclobenzaprine, milnacipran, gabapentin, pregabalin, duloxetine, and tramadol (Crofford 2008; Mease et al. 2009). Fibromyalgia is discussed in detail in Chapter 26, "Chronic Fatigue and Fibromyalgia Syndromes."

Phantom Limb Pain

Pain in a body part that has been removed occurs in 50%–80% of amputees within a year of the amputation (Schley et al. 2008). *Phantom limb pain,* considered to be neuropathic and described as stabbing, throbbing, burning, or cramping, is more intense in the distal portion of the phantom limb (Flor 2002). Any area of the body can manifest phantom pain, with phantom breast syndrome common after mastectomy (Bjorkman et al. 2008; Spyropoulou et al. 2008). Although TCAs, gabapentin, and carbamazepine are considered first-line treatments for phantom pain, no controlled trials support their use. Newer antidepressants and anticonvulsants with generally fewer side effects may result in greater effectiveness if patients can tolerate higher doses. However, morphine, calcitonin, and ketamine have been shown to reduce phantom pain in controlled studies. Morphine, but not mexiletine, decreased postamputation pain lasting more than 6 months (Wu et al. 2008). Controlled trials have discredited anecdotal reports of the effectiveness of neural blockade (Manchikanti and Singh 2004).

Complex Regional Pain Syndrome

Complex regional pain syndrome (CRPS; formerly reflex sympathetic dystrophy and causalgia) is an array of painful conditions characterized by ongoing spontaneous burning pain that is precipitated by a specific noxious trauma or cause of immobilization and often is associated with hyperalgesia or allodynia to cutaneous stimuli (Hsu 2009; Sharma et al. 2009). Pain is regional but is not limited to a single peripheral nerve or dermatome. Edema, blood flow abnormalities, or sudomotor dysfunction is often evident in the pain region—usually an extremity (Albazaz et al. 2008). These changes may be a result of neurogenic inflammation and neuropeptides such as calcitonin gene–related peptide, cytokines, substance P, and nerve growth factors (Birklein and Schmelz 2008). Motor changes such as weakness, tremor, dystonia, and limitations in movement are common (Harden et al. 2007). Sympathetically maintained pain is present in most, but not all, cases and may result from coupling of sympathetic and sensory neurons or adrenoreceptor supersensitivity in nociceptive fibers (Gibbs et al. 2008). Patients with sympathetically maintained pain often report hyperalgesia to cold stimuli and report temporary relief with sympathetic blockade (Pontell 2008).

Patients with CRPS often have mood (46%), anxiety (27%), and substance abuse disorders (14%), generally considered to be a consequence of chronic pain rather than its cause, when coupled with maladaptive personality traits and coping styles (Bruehl and Chung 2006).

Pharmacotherapy for CRPS has limited success, and few randomized controlled studies are available to guide treatment selection (Mackey and Feinberg 2007; Rowbotham 2006). Symptoms often improve with NSAIDs or corticosteroids in the acute, or inflammatory, stage of the disease. Evidence suggests efficacy for gabapentin, pregabalin, carbamazepine, TCAs, and opioids. Randomized controlled trials of calcitonin and bisphosphonates in CRPS found reduced pain and improved joint mobility. Clinical trials of local anesthetic sympathetic blockade, once considered the gold standard therapy for CRPS, have proven inconclusive (Sharma et al. 2006). Other therapies include early intervention with reactivating physical therapies, electrical stimulation, and possibly even surgical sympathectomy (Pontell 2008).

Orofacial Pain

Trigeminal neuralgia (tic douloureux) is a chronic pain syndrome with severe, paroxysmal, recurrent, lancinating pain in the distribution of cranial nerve V that is unilateral and most commonly involves the mandibular division (Obermann and Katsarava 2009; Prasad and Galetta 2009). Sensory or motor deficits are not usually present. Episodes of pain can be spontaneous or evoked by nonpainful stimuli to trigger zones, activities such as talking or chewing, or environmental conditions. Between episodes, patients are typically pain free.

Less common syndromes involving the intermedius branch of the facial nerve or the glossopharyngeal nerve present with pain that can involve the ear, posterior pharynx, tongue, or larynx (Zakrzewska 2002). Other related conditions include cluster headache, which occurs predominantly in men with an onset before age 25 and presents with pain that is episodic, unilaterally surrounds the eye, is described as excruciating, lasts minutes to hours, and is associated with autonomic symptoms. Short-lasting, unilateral neuralgia-form pain with conjunctival injection and tearing (SUNCT) syndrome is a rare condition that more commonly affects older men. Tolosa-Hunt syndrome presents with pain in the ocular area accompanied by ipsilateral paresis of oculomotor nerves and the first branch of the trigeminal nerve that is associated with compromise of ophthalmic venous circulation and improves with steroids. The residual category of atypical facial pain includes atypical odontalgia and is more commonly associated with psychopathology or other psychological factors that amplify the patient's pain, distress, disability, and risk for suicide (List et al. 2007).

Most patients with classic trigeminal neuralgia show evidence of trigeminal nerve root compression by blood vessels (85%), mass lesions, or other diseases (multiple sclerosis, herpes zoster, PHN) that cause demyelination and hyperactivity of the trigeminal nucleus (Joffroy et al. 2001; Love and Coakham 2001). Uncontrolled pain with frequent or severe prolonged attacks increases the risk of insomnia, weight loss, social withdrawal, anxiety, and depression, including suicide.

Pharmacological treatment includes anticonvulsants, antidepressants, baclofen, mexiletine, lidocaine, and opioids (Cheshire 2002; Fisher et al. 2002; Sindrup and Jensen 2002). Placebo-controlled trials identify carbamazepine (number needed to treat of 1.8) as first-line treatment. Trials also support the use of oxcarbazepine and lamotrigine. Evidence is insufficient to recommend clonazepam, gabapentin, phenytoin, tizanidine, topical capsaicin, or valproate (Cruccu et al. 2008). Given the pathophysiological similarities to PHN and painful peripheral neuropathies, other medications such as the TCAs and SNRIs would be appropriate pharmacological treatments to consider. When pharmacological treatments fail, a variety of surgical procedures such as microvascular decompression via suboccipital craniectomy, percutaneous gangliolysis, and stereotactic radiosurgery may be undertaken (Gronseth et al. 2008; Miller et al. 2009).

Temporomandibular disorder (TMD) is a general term referring to complaints that involve the temporomandibular joint, muscles of mastication, and other orofacial musculoskeletal structures. Pain most commonly arises from the muscles of mastication and is precipitated by jaw function such as opening the mouth or chewing. Associated symptoms include feelings of muscle fatigue, weakness, and tightness as well as changes in bite (malocclusion) or the ability to open or close the jaw. In contrast to the vague, diffuse pain of myalgia, temporomandibular joint dysfunction causes sharp, sudden, and intense pain with joint movement that is often localized to the preauricular area. Joint sounds such as clicking, popping, and crepitation are common. Patients may experience limitations in jaw movements such as catching sensations or actual locking of the jaw. Joint problems are classified as relating to the condyle-disk complex, structural incompatibility of the articular surfaces, and inflammatory joint disorders.

Psychological distress is common in patients with TMD. Patients with pain of muscular origin are usually more distressed and depressed, with greater levels of disability, than are those with temporomandibular joint pain. These factors are responsive to behavioral treatment (Auerbach et al. 2001). Longitudinal data suggest that negative affect in patients with orofacial pain is more likely than pain to cause poor sleep quality (Riley et al. 2001).

Burning mouth syndrome (BMS) is characterized as pain in oral and pharyngeal cavities, especially the tongue, often associated with dryness and taste alterations. Most cases are idiopathic, but BMS may coincide with a plethora of conditions, such as bruxism, poorly fitting dentures, oral candidiasis, xerostomia, malnutrition, food allergies and contact dermatitis, gastroesophageal reflux disease, diabetes mellitus, hypothyroidism, neoplasia, and menopause, as well as psychiatric disorders such as depression, anxiety, and somatization (Drage and Rogers 2003; Grushka et al. 2002). The condition mainly affects middle-aged and postmenopausal women, and the oral mucosa is usually normal. Psychological factors such as severe life events have been associated with the condition.

Potential underlying etiologies, such as depression or anxiety, nutritional deficiencies (iron, folate, B_{12}, and other B vitamins), maladaptive oral habits, and iatrogenic causes such as medications, should be identified and treated (Pinto et al. 2003). Treatment with TCAs or anticonvulsants has brought pain relief in some patients with BMS.

Other treatments include benzodiazepines, topical analgesics, soft desensitizing oral appliances, serotonin reuptake inhibitors, vitamin and hormonal supplements, and habit awareness counseling (Maina et al. 2002; Pinto et al. 2003).

Low Back Pain

LBP is one of the most common physical symptoms and the most expensive condition when lost productivity and health care costs are included (Deyo et al. 2009). Psychological factors, including distress, depressed mood, and somatization, which predict the transition from acute to chronic LBP, are highly correlated with LBP. In one prospective cohort study of 1,246 patients with acute LBP who sought treatment, about 8% had chronic, continuous symptoms for 3 months, and fewer than 5% had unremitting pain for 22 months (Carey et al. 2000). Two-thirds of patients with chronic LBP at 3 months had functional disability at 22 months. The most powerful predictor of chronicity was poor functional status 4 weeks after seeking treatment. In a study of secondary gain, both economic and social rewards were associated with higher levels of disability and depression in patients with chronic nonmalignant back pain (Ciccone et al. 1999). Anxiety, depression, and occupational mental stress predicted lower rates of return to work in patients undergoing lumbar surgeries (DeBerard et al. 2001; Schade et al. 1999; Trief et al. 2000).

The presence of a depressive disorder has been shown to increase the risk of developing chronic musculoskeletal pain. In a 15-year prospective study of workers in an industrial setting, initial depression symptom scores were predictive of LBP and a positive clinical back examination in men but not women (Leino and Magni 1993). In a community-based sample, depression was associated with a nearly fourfold increase in the likelihood of seeking a consultation for a new complaint of back pain lasting longer than 3 months at follow-up (Waxman et al. 1998). In a 13-year follow-up study that examined the longitudinal relation between LBP and depressive disorder by using lifetime reports of symptoms and that excluded other forms of affective distress such as demoralization, grief, and adjustment disorders, depressive disorder was a significant risk factor for incident LBP (Larson et al. 2004). One study concluded that as much as 16% of LBP in the general population may be attributable to psychological distress (Croft et al. 1996). In contrast, these findings do not undermine the fact that chronic, disabling occupational spinal disorders result in high levels of psychopathology that affect outcomes and benefit from treatment (Dersh et al. 2007).

The treatment of chronic LBP has been pursued with multiple modalities alone and in combination (Deyo and Weinstein 2001). Patients with chronic LBP exemplify the complexity of chronic pain treatment. Their symptoms usually represent numerous diagnoses that require multimodal treatment plans. Although treatments often produce symptom reductions, conflicting evidence exists about their ability to improve functional status, particularly with respect to returning to work (Staiger et al. 2003). Even conservative interventions such as education, exercise, massage, and transcutaneous electrical stimulation produce inconsistent results (Furlan et al. 2002; Pengel et al. 2002). A study of physiotherapy for chronic LBP showed that physiotherapist-led pain management classes offered a cost-effective alternative to outpatient physiotherapy and spinal stabilization classes, with greater reductions in health care use and similar improvements in pain, quality of life, and time off from work (Critchley et al. 2007). Studies of behavior therapies support their effectiveness in comparison with wait-list or no-treatment control conditions, but the efficacy data are less convincing when compared with usual treatment for chronic LBP (van Tulder et al. 2001). Evidence indicates that surgery may be effective for a carefully selected group of patients with chronic LBP (Fritzell et al. 2001). Interdisciplinary rehabilitation programs usually offer the best outcomes for reducing pain and pain-related disability but are the most expensive approach, and high-quality randomized controlled trials are still needed to document long-term efficacy (Huge et al. 2006). Combined therapy with antidepressants and self-management education was effective in the treatment of patients with both depression and musculoskeletal pain (Kroenke et al. 2009). One review found efficacy for intensive multidisciplinary rehabilitation emphasizing functional restoration, but less intensive interventions were ineffective (Guzman et al. 2007). The patient's perception of disability is a critical factor that must be addressed for treatment to succeed.

Pharmacological Treatment

Numerous medications are used in the treatment of chronic pain, especially neuropathic pain, which affects 2%–3% of the world's population (Moulin et al. 2007). The pharmacological targets are mechanisms of peripheral and central nervous system sensitization such as sodium and calcium channel upregulation, spinal hyperexcitability, descending modulation, and aberrant sympathetic–somatic nervous system interactions. Antidepressants and anticonvulsants are the best studied and recommended as first-line therapies (Dworkin et al. 2007). Unfortunately, these medications remain underused and underdosed. In one study of patients with neuropathic pain, 73% complained of inadequate pain control, but 72% had never received anticonvulsants, 60% had never received TCAs, 41% had never received opioids, and 25% had never received any of the above (Gilron et al. 2002). No medication algorithm can provide a simple, straightforward approach to the complexities encountered during the treatment of chronic pain.

Opioids

Opioids reduce the sensory and affective components of pain by interacting with mu, delta, and kappa opioid receptors located in both the peripheral and the central nervous systems of pain transmission and modulation. Controversy surrounds the long-term use of opioids for chronic nonmalignant pain (Noble et al. 2008). Studies generally last less than 18 months and are complicated by high rates of discontinuation because of adverse events or insufficient pain relief. Opioids should be slowly tapered to avoid withdrawal and completely discontinued if the risks (side effects, toxicities, aberrant drug-related behaviors) outweigh the objective benefits (analgesia, functional improvements).

Guidelines have been established for the use of opioids in chronic pain (American Academy of Pain Medicine and American Pain Society 2008). The U.S. Food and Drug Administration is now discussing risk evaluation and mitigation strategies to standardize the use of opioids and minimize their liabilities. Appropriate patients are those with moderate or severe pain persisting for more than 3 months and adversely affecting functioning or quality of life. Before initiating opioid therapy, additional factors such as the patient's specific pain syndrome, response to other therapies, and potential for aberrant drug-related behaviors (misuse, abuse, addiction, diversion) should be considered (Ballantyne and LaForge 2007). A patient's suitability for chronic opioid therapy can be assessed with standardized questionnaires such as the Opioid Risk Tool (ORT); the Diagnosis, Intractability, Risk, Efficacy (DIRE); and the Screener and Opioid Assessment for Patients in Pain (SOAPP). Treatment outcomes, including analgesia, activities of daily living, adverse events, and potential aberrant drug-related behaviors, can be assessed more easily with the Pain Assessment and Documentation Tool (PADT; Passik et al. 2004). The Current Opioid Misuse Measure (COMM) evaluates patients who are taking opioids for concurrent signs or symptoms of intoxication, emotional volatility, poor response to medications, addiction, inappropriate health care use patterns, and problematic medication behaviors. These scales can be downloaded from the Pain Treatment Topics Web site (www.pain-topics.org/opioid_rx/risk.php#AssessTools).

Clinically available opioids include naturally occurring compounds (morphine and codeine), semisynthetic derivatives (hydromorphone, oxymorphone, hydrocodone, oxycodone, dihydrocodeine, and buprenorphine), and synthetic opioid analgesics (meperidine, fentanyl, methadone, tramadol, pentazocine, and propoxyphene). *Morphine,* because of its hydrophilicity, has poor oral bioavailability (22%–48%) and delayed central nervous system absorption and onset of action. This delay prolongs the analgesic effect of morphine relative to its plasma half-life, which decreases the potential for accumulation and toxicity with repeated dosing. Morphine is a more effective epidural spinal analgesic than oxycodone. *Oxycodone* is an opiate analgesic with higher oral bioavailability (>60%), a faster onset of action, and more predictable plasma levels compared with morphine. Oxycodone, in comparison to morphine, has similar analgesic efficacy but releases less histamine and causes fewer hallucinations (Riley et al. 2008). *Hydrocodone* is similar to oxycodone, with rapid oral absorption and onset of analgesia. Hydrocodone is metabolized by *N*-demethylation to hydromorphone, which has properties similar to those of morphine, except for lower rates of side effects. *Fentanyl* is highly lipophilic with affinity for neuronal tissues, which allows for transdermal or transmucosal delivery. The duration of action of transdermal preparations is up to 72 hours, but interindividual variability is considerable.

Methadone warrants special consideration in the treatment of chronic pain because of its stigma, low cost, high bioavailability, rapid onset of action, slow hepatic clearance, multiple receptor affinities, lack of neurotoxic metabolites, and incomplete cross-tolerance with other opioids. Methadone has significantly greater risk of overdose because of the longer time needed for adaptation with oral use and greater variation in plasma half-life (15–120 hours) (Sandoval et al. 2005). Methadone is unique among opioids in its risk for increasing the QTc interval and causing torsade de pointes (Andrews et al. 2009). Extensive tissue distribution and prolonged half-life prevent withdrawal symptoms with once-daily dosing. However, elimination is biphasic, and the more rapid elimination phase equates with analgesia that is limited to approximately 6 hours. Repeated dosing, with accumulation in tissue, may increase the duration of analgesia to 8–12 hours. In one of the longer follow-up studies, methadone was shown to be effective for decreasing chronic pain in a study of 100 patients over a mean treatment duration of 11 months (Peng et al. 2008b).

The most common side effect of chronic opioid therapy is decreased gastrointestinal motility, causing constipation, vomiting, and abdominal pain. Oral opioids differ in their propensity to cause these symptoms. Transdermal opioids (fentanyl, buprenorphine) have fewer gastrointestinal side effects than do oral opioids (Tassinari et al. 2008). Long-term opiate administration may result in analgesic tolerance or opioid-induced hyperalgesia (Mitra 2008). When tolerance develops, coadministration of other analgesics, opioid rotation to a more potent agonist, or intermittent cessation of certain agents may restore analgesic effect (Dumas and Pollack 2008; Vorobeychik et al. 2008). Opioid rotation from either morphine or hydromorphone may be beneficial because 3-glucuronide metabolites can accumulate within the cerebrospinal fluid and produce neuroexcitatory effects such as allodynia, myoclonus, delirium, and seizures (Smith 2000). Rotation to mixed agonist–antagonist opiates (buprenorphine, pentazocine) may precipitate withdrawal symptoms in patients receiving chronic opioid therapy. The concomitant use of opioids with monoamine oxidase inhibitors (MAOIs), dextromethorphan, and meperidine should be avoided.

Antidepressants

The neurobiology of pain suggests that all antidepressants would be effective for treatment of chronic pain, but the analgesic properties of these medications remain underappreciated (McCleane 2008). The TCAs and SNRIs, in particular, are effective treatments for many chronic pain syndromes, including diabetic neuropathy, PHN, central pain, poststroke pain, tension-type headache, migraine, and orofacial pain but not nonspecific LBP (Saarto and Wiffen 2007; Verdu et al. 2008). The analgesic effect of antidepressants is thought to be independent of their antidepressant effect and is primarily mediated by the blockade of reuptake of norepinephrine and serotonin, increasing their levels, and enhancing the activation of descending inhibitory neurons in the dorsal horn of the spinal cord (McCleane 2008; Mico et al. 2006). However, antidepressants may produce antinociceptive effects through a variety of pharmacological mechanisms, including modulation by monoamines; interactions with opioid systems; inhibition of ion channel activity; and antagonism by NMDA, histamine, and cholinergic receptors (Dick et al. 2007).

Tricyclic Antidepressants

Meta-analyses of randomized controlled trials concluded that TCAs are the most effective agents for neuropathic pain and effective for headache syndromes. A recent meta-analysis of fibromyalgia treatment trials found positive but diminishing effect when comparing classes of antidepressants: TCAs > MAOIs > SSRIs = SNRIs (Hauser et al. 2009). TCAs have been shown to effectively treat central poststroke pain, PHN, many painful polyneuropathies, and postmastectomy pain syndrome but not SCI pain, phantom limb pain, or painful HIV neuropathy. TCA agents are equally effective for pain, but secondary amine TCAs (e.g., nortriptyline) are better tolerated than are tertiary agents (e.g., amitriptyline) (Dworkin et al. 2007). Antidepressants generally produce analgesia at lower doses and with earlier onset of action than expected for the treatment of depression (Rojas-Corrales et al. 2003). However, lack of analgesic effects may be a result of inadequate dosing and necessitates optimal titration and confirmation with serum level monitoring. Chronic pain of PHN and diabetic peripheral neuropathy has been treated successfully with TCAs at average doses of 100–250 mg/day (Max 1994). In contrast, a U.S. health insurance claims database found that the average dose of TCAs for the treatment of neuropathic pain in patients age 65 and older was only 23 mg (Berger et al. 2006). Patients in a multidisciplinary pain center study were prescribed the equivalent of 50 mg or less of amitriptyline, suggesting unrealized potential for additional pain relief. Cost-effectiveness research strongly supports the use of TCAs (Cepeda and Farrar 2006).

Serotonin–Norepinephrine Reuptake Inhibitors

Duloxetine, venlafaxine, desvenlafaxine, and milnacipran inhibit the presynaptic reuptake of serotonin, norepinephrine, and, to a lesser extent, dopamine with fewer side effects and less toxicity than TCAs. Duloxetine more potently blocks serotonin and norepinephrine transporters than does venlafaxine (Berrocoso and Mico 2008). Milnacipran has antihyperalgesic effects mediated by monoamine and opioid systems. Clinical trials show efficacy for treatment of fibromyalgia (Clauw et al. 2008; Mease et al. 2009). SNRIs produce better analgesic efficacy compared with SSRIs, even in combination with selective noradrenergic reuptake inhibitors (Jones et al. 2006).

In placebo-controlled trials, venlafaxine significantly reduced neuropathic pain following breast cancer treatment (Tasmuth et al. 2002). Venlafaxine significantly prevents migraine and decreases allodynia and hyperalgesia in both neuropathic pain and atypical facial pain (Bulut et al. 2004; Ozyalcin et al. 2005; Yucel et al. 2005). Response improved with higher doses attributable to increased reuptake inhibition of norepinephrine. In a study of painful diabetic neuropathy, 150–225 mg/day of venlafaxine produced a greater percentage reduction in pain than did 75 mg/day (50% vs. 32%) (Rowbotham et al. 2004). Duloxetine possesses analgesic efficacy in both preclinical models and clinical populations such as patients with fibromyalgia and painful diabetic neuropathy (Arnold et al. 2005; Wernicke et al. 2006). Guidelines for the treatment of neuropathic pain recommend duloxetine as an effective treatment (Argoff et al. 2006). The efficacy of duloxetine in painful diabetic neuropathy was greater in patients with more severe pain but was not related to the severity of diabetes or neuropathy (Ziegler et al. 2007). Patients with depression and painful somatic symptoms experience relief when taking duloxetine, but the analgesic effects were independent of antidepressant actions (Perahia et al. 2006).

Selective Serotonin Reuptake Inhibitors

In clinical trials, the efficacy of SSRIs in chronic pain syndromes has been inconsistent, especially in the treatment of neuropathic pain (Finnerup et al. 2005). A Cochrane review found SSRIs no more efficacious than placebo for migraine and less efficacious than TCAs for tension-type headache (Moja et al. 2005). However, fluoxetine improved outcome measures in women with fibromyalgia and was comparable to amitriptyline in significantly reducing rheumatoid arthritis pain (Arnold et al. 2002). Citalopram improved abdominal pain in irritable bowel syndrome independent of effects on anxiety and depression (Tack et al. 2006). Patients with DSM-IV-TR pain disorder experienced significant analgesic effects, independent of changes in depression, with citalopram but not with the noradrenergic reuptake inhibitor reboxetine (Aragona et al. 2005). Paroxetine and citalopram, but not fluoxetine, decreased the pain of diabetic peripheral neuropathy in controlled studies (Goodnick 2001). Also, in a comparison study of gabapentin, paroxetine, and citalopram for painful diabetic peripheral neuropathy, patients reported better satisfaction, compliance, and mood with SSRIs with similar efficacy for pain (Giannopoulos et al. 2007). Overall, SSRIs are not recommended as a first-line therapy for chronic pain but are a recommended alternative to TCAs or SNRIs, with a favorable risk-benefit profile.

Novel Antidepressants

Few controlled trials have examined the efficacy of novel antidepressants in pain syndromes, but their pharmacology suggests antinociceptive properties. Mirtazapine decreased the duration and intensity of treatment-refractory chronic tension-type headache in a controlled trial (Bendtsen and Jensen 2004). In a controlled trial of patients with neuropathic pain, bupropion sustained-release decreased pain intensity and interference of pain with quality of life (Semenchuk et al. 2001). Although several reports suggested efficacy for trazodone in chronic pain, controlled studies did not support its use in chronic LBP (Goodkin et al. 1990).

Anticonvulsants

Anticonvulsants inhibit excessive neuronal activity by blocking voltage-gated sodium channels, modulating calcium channels, inhibiting excitatory amino acid neurotransmission, or enhancing gamma-amino acid–mediated inhibitory neurotransmission (Stefan and Feuerstein 2007). Anticonvulsants are effective for trigeminal neuralgia, diabetic neuropathy, PHN, and migraine recurrence. The number needed to treat ranges from approximately 2 to 4 for anticonvulsants, with better compliance when compared with TCAs because of fewer adverse effects (Finnerup et al. 2005).

First-Generation Anticonvulsants

Phenytoin was first reported as a successful treatment for trigeminal neuralgia in 1942 (Bergouignan 1942). Carbamazepine is the most widely studied anticonvulsant effective for neuropathic pain (Tanelian and Victory 1995). Valproic acid is most commonly used in the prophylaxis of migraine but is also effective for neuropathic pain. Valproate was an effective prophylactic treatment in more than two-thirds of patients with migraine and almost 75% of those with cluster headache (Gallagher et al. 2002). Improvement occurred in multiple domains of headache severity, use of other medications for acute treatment of headache, the patient's opinion of treatment, and ratings of depression and anxiety (Kaniecki 1997; Klapper 1997; Rothrock 1997).

Second-Generation Anticonvulsants

Pregabalin and gabapentin decrease the influx of calcium and modulate the release of neurotransmitters such as substance P and glutamate (Han et al. 2007; Taylor et al. 2007). They also activate the descending noradrenergic inhibitory system of nociception (Tanabe et al. 2008). Pregabalin and gabapentin are effective for the treatment of painful diabetic neuropathy, PHN, fibromyalgia, post-amputation phantom limb pain, and central neuropathic pain associated with SCI (Arezzo et al. 2008; Richter et al. 2005; Sandercock et al. 2009; Tassone et al. 2007). Patients with chronic pain were more likely to respond to gabapentin if they experienced allodynia. Pregabalin was more cost-effective than gabapentin for the treatment of painful diabetic neuropathy and PHN (Tarride et al. 2006). In patients with PHN, flexible titration strategies resulted in fewer discontinuations, higher final dose, and slightly better pain relief compared with fixed-dose schedules (Stacey et al. 2008).

Lamotrigine has multiple pharmacological actions and produced positive results for pain associated with HIV-related neuropathy and central poststroke pain but was disappointing for other neuropathic pains in a meta-analysis of controlled trials (Wiffen and Rees 2007). Doses greater than 300 mg/day with serum levels lower than 15 mg/L were more effective for the treatment of painful diabetic neuropathy (Jose et al. 2007; Vinik et al. 2007). Topiramate offers the advantages of minimal hepatic metabolism and unchanged renal excretion, few drug interactions, a long half-life, and the unusual side effect of weight loss. Topiramate was effective for migraine prophylaxis and decreased pain from chronic LBP, lumbar radiculopathy, and painful diabetic neuropathy (Keskinbora and Aydinli 2008; Muehlbacher et al. 2006; Silberstein et al. 2006; Van Passel et al. 2006).

Next-Generation Anticonvulsants

Oxcarbazepine is a carbamazepine derivative with an improved safety and tolerability profile. Oxcarbazepine for refractory PHN decreased pain with rapid onset of action and improvements in function and quality of life (Nasreddine and Beydoun 2007). A randomized, placebo-controlled trial in painful diabetic neuropathy found that about 35% of the patients taking oxcarbazepine experienced greater than 50% improvement in their pain (Grosskopf et al. 2006). Tiagabine, vigabatrin, retigabine, levetiracetam, and zonisamide are new anticonvulsants with a spectrum of pharmacological actions and antinociceptive effects in animal models, but few clinical studies exist to support their use as a first-line therapy for chronic pain (Cutrer 2001; Marson et al. 1997). Variable adverse drug reactions from these agents can cause significant cognitive impairment. Tiagabine reduced pain by comparable amounts to gabapentin but resulted in significantly greater improvements in sleep quality (Todorov et al. 2005). Despite multiple mechanisms of action, zonisamide showed mixed results for the treatment of neuropathic pain (Kothare et al. 2008). Riluzole (sodium channel blocker), retigabine (potassium channel opener), ethosuximide (T-type calcium channel blocker), and levetiracetam attenuated nociceptive responses in animals (Munro et al. 2007).

Combinations of anticonvulsants with complementary mechanisms of action may increase effectiveness and decrease adverse effects of treatment. Patients with multiple sclerosis or trigeminal neuralgia who had responded to but had to discontinue treatment with carbamazepine or lamotrigine at therapeutic doses because of intolerable side effects were given gabapentin as an augmentation agent (Solaro et al. 2000). Gabapentin was successfully titrated to pain relief, with no new side effects up to a maximum dose of 1,200 mg/day, at which time either carbamazepine or lamotrigine was tapered until its side effects were no longer present without loss of analgesia. When anticonvulsants were combined with tramadol, synergistic effects were found for inhibiting allodynia and blocking nociception (Codd et al. 2008). Carbamazepine and oxcarbazepine combined with clonidine produced a synergistic antihyperalgesic effect on inflammatory pain (Vuckovic et al. 2006).

Benzodiazepines

Benzodiazepines are commonly prescribed for insomnia, anxiety, and spasticity. In patients with chronic pain, no studies found any significant benefit for these target symptoms (Taricco et al. 2000). Benzodiazepines decreased pain in only a limited number of chronic pain conditions, such as trigeminal neuralgia, tension headache, and TMD (Dellemijn and Fields 1994). Clonazepam may provide long-term relief of the episodic lancinating variety of phantom limb pain (Bartusch et al. 1996). Benzodiazepines cause sedation and cognitive impairment, especially in the elderly and other neurologically vulnerable populations (Buffett-Jerrott and Stewart 2002). In patients with chronic pain, the use of benzodiazepines, but not opioids, was associated with decreased activity levels, higher rates of health care visits, increased domestic instability, depression, and more disability days (Ciccone et al. 2000). Combining benzodiazepines with opioids may be countertherapeutic and potentially dangerous. Benzodiazepines may exacerbate pain and interfere with opioid analgesia (Sawynok 1987). Studies of methadone-related mortality found high rates of benzodiazepine use, with the cause of death being attributed to a combination of drug effects, especially in patients with chronic pain (Darke et al. 2010; McCowan et al. 2009).

Antipsychotics

Atypical antipsychotics offer a broader therapeutic spectrum, lower rates of extrapyramidal side effects, and the potential for augmentation of antidepressants and mood stabilizers. These benefits have been offset by concerns about weight gain, new-onset diabetes, hyperlipidemias, and cardiac arrhythmias. Antipsychotics have been tried in diabetic neuropathy, PHN, headache, facial pain, pain associated with AIDS and cancer, and musculoskeletal pain, with increasing evidence to support their effectiveness (Fishbain et al. 2004). A meta-analysis of 11 controlled trials concluded that some antipsychotics have analgesic efficacy in headache (haloperidol) and trigeminal neuralgia (pimozide) (Seidel et al. 2008).

Recent trials have focused on fibromyalgia because evidence suggests that dopaminergic D_2 receptor hypersensitivity and decreased release of dopamine from the basal ganglia occur in response to pain (Wood et al. 2007). An open-label study of the addition of quetiapine to patients' existing but ineffective fibromyalgia treatment regimens did not report decreased pain but did produce significant functional improvements on the Fibromyalgia Impact Questionnaire and quality-of-life measures (Hidalgo et al. 2007). Studies of ziprasidone and olanzapine showed beneficial effects but low response rates and poor tolerability (Calandre et al. 2007; Rico-Villademoros et al. 2005). Results are difficult to interpret because of comorbid depressive, anxiety, and sleep disorders in patients with fibromyalgia that might respond to treatment with antipsychotics.

Local Anesthetics

Topical lidocaine has been approved for the treatment of PHN and does not produce significant serum levels (Argoff 2000). It is ineffective against HIV neuropathy pain (Estanislao et al. 2004). Oral mexiletine is an effective treatment for neuropathic pain in painful diabetic neuropathy, peripheral nerve injury, and alcoholic neuropathy; mixed results are reported for phantom limb, and mexiletine is ineffective for cancer-related pain (Wu et al. 2008). Mexiletine decreased not only reports of pain but also the accompanying paresthesias and dysesthesias. Analgesic effects did not correlate with mexiletine serum levels.

Calcium Channel Blockers

Verapamil is the most commonly prescribed calcium channel blocker for chronic pain and has proven effective in the treatment of migraine and cluster headaches (Lewis and Solomon 1996). Ziconotide, a neuron-specific calcium channel blocker, has been approved for the intrathecal treatment of refractory pain of cancer or AIDS. It has potent analgesic, antihyperesthetic, and antiallodynic activity as well as synergistic analgesic effects with morphine without producing tolerance (Christo and Mazloomdoost 2008).

Psychological Treatments

Cognitive-Behavioral Models

Psychological treatment for chronic pain was pioneered by Fordyce, who used an operant conditioning behavioral model (Fordyce et al. 1973). The behavioral approach is based on an understanding of pain occurring in a social context. The behaviors of the patient with chronic pain not only reinforce the behaviors of others, including physicians, but also are reinforced by others. Pain behaviors such as grimacing, guarding, and taking pain medication are indicators of perceived pain severity and functional disability (Turk and Matyas 1992). In a study of medical practice patterns, only observed pain behaviors were predictive of whether opioid medications were prescribed to patients with chronic pain (Turk and Okifuji 1997). Other aspects of the patient's presentation to a health care practitioner, such as reports of functional disability, distress, pain severity, objective physical pathology, duration of pain, and demographic variables, were not predictive. If pain behaviors are reinforced, the behavioral model assumes pain and disability will persist. In treatment, healthy behaviors are targeted for reinforcement to replace extinguished pain behaviors.

Many psychological interventions have been effective in the reduction of pain and its associated distress (Molton et al. 2007). The cognitive-behavioral model of chronic pain assumes individual beliefs, attitudes, and expectations affect emotional and behavioral reactions to life experiences. Pain and the resultant pain behaviors are influenced by biomedical, psychological, and socioenvironmental variables. If patients believe pain, depression, and disability are inevitable and uncontrollable, then they will likely experience more negative affective responses, increased pain, and even more impaired physical and psychosocial functioning. The components of cognitive-behavioral therapy (CBT), such as relaxation, guided imagery, biofeedback, meditation, hypnosis, motivational interviewing, external reinforcement, cognitive restructuring, and coping self-statement training, interrupt this cycle of disability. Patients are taught to become active participants in the management of their pain by using methods that minimize distressing thoughts and feelings. The goals of CBT, regardless of techniques used, focus the patient on self-control and self-management to increase activity, independence, and resourcefulness (Turk et al. 2008). Outcome studies of CBT in patients with a variety of chronic pain syndromes have shown significant improvements in pain intensity, pain behaviors, distress, depression, and coping (Eccleston et al. 2009; Turk et al. 2008). The benefits of CBT have been found to continue up to 6 months after the completion of active treatment sessions.

Beliefs

The success of CBT in chronic pain treatment has led to focused attention on many elements of the chronic pain experience, including concepts such as *psychological resilience* and *illness adaptation* (Karoly and Ruehlman 2006). *Adjustment* is defined as the ability to carry out normal physical and psychosocial activities. Three dimensions of adjustment have been defined: social functioning, morale, and somatic health (Lazarus and Folkman 1984). Examples of these domains include pain intensity, medication use, depression, anxiety, employment, health care use, and functional ability.

Beliefs are conceptualized as the thoughts of an individual about his or her personal pain problem (Morley and Wilkinson 1995). Psychosocial dysfunction has been correlated with receiving overly solicitous responses from family, believing emotions are related to pain, and attributing the inability to function to pain (M.P. Jensen et al. 1994b). In contrast, although physical disability was correlated with beliefs about pain interfering with function, patients also endorsed the belief that pain signifies injury, and, therefore, activity should be avoided. A change in perceived control over pain was the most significant predictor of beneficial effects of cognitive-behavioral therapies for chronic TMD pain (Turner et al. 2007).

Cognitive variables derived from social learning theory associated with chronic pain include self-efficacy, outcome expectancies, and locus of control (Solberg et al. 2009). A self-efficacy expectancy is a belief about one's ability to perform a specific behavior, whereas an outcome expectancy is a belief about the consequences of performing a behavior. Individuals are considered more likely to engage in coping efforts they believe are within their capabilities and will result in a positive outcome. Patients with a variety of chronic pain syndromes who score higher on measures of self-efficacy or have an internal locus of control report lower levels of pain, higher pain thresholds, increased exercise performance, and more positive coping efforts. Interestingly, physician expectations of pain relief were significant predictors of patient pain relief ratings, which supports the important role of other persons in an individual's chronic pain experience.

Acceptance of chronic pain is a two-factor construct (Activity Engagement, Pain Willingness) associated with multiple domains of the experience of chronic pain. Acceptance of pain was found to be associated with reports of lower pain intensity, less pain-related anxiety and avoidance, less depression, less physical and psychosocial disability, more daily uptime, and better work status (McCracken 1998). Acceptance has been found to mediate the effects of catastrophizing on depression, avoidance, and functioning in patients with chronic pain (Vowles et al. 2008). One's acceptance of chronic pain predicts his or her adjustment to the illness and is independent of catastrophizing, coping skills, and pain-related beliefs and cognitions (Esteve et al. 2007; Vowles et al. 2007).

Coping

Coping is "a person's cognitive and behavioral efforts to manage the internal and external demands of the person–environment transaction that is appraised as taxing or exceeding the person's resources" (Folkman et al. 1986, p. 571). Coping strategies, whether active versus passive or adaptive versus maladaptive, generally support the cognitive-behavioral model of chronic pain (M.P. Jensen 2009). Higher levels of disability were found in persons who remain passive or use maladaptive coping strategies of catastrophizing, ignoring or reinterpreting pain sensations, diverting attention from pain, and praying or hoping for relief. In a 6-month follow-up study of patients completing an inpatient pain program, improvement was associated with decreases in the use of passive coping strategies and changing beliefs about pain being an incurable illness (M.P. Jensen et al. 1994a).

The effectiveness of particular coping strategies with improved adjustment to chronic pain is dependent on many aspects of a patient's experience with illness. For example, reinterpreting pain sensations as not being signs of ongoing injury typically has been formulated as useful for reducing the effects of experimentally induced pain. However, in a study of amputees with phantom limb pain, this coping strategy was not associated with reduced pain levels but instead with greater psychosocial dysfunction (Hill et al. 1995). Attempting to reinterpret pain sensations may not always be an appropriate technique for individuals with persistent pain because it requires greater amounts of time spent focusing on pain and disability. This may prevent patients from engaging in social activities and healthy behaviors. Catastrophic thinking about pain involves the amplification of threatening information and interference with the attentional focus needed to facilitate patients remaining involved with productive instead of pain-related activities (Crombez et al. 1998). In one study, high levels of catastrophizing combined with lower levels of active pain coping predicted higher levels of depressive symptoms and disability (Buenaver et al. 2008). The use of adaptive coping skills decreased pain and disability when patients perceived an increase in the effectiveness of their new skills and reduced their use of maladaptive coping strategies such as catastrophic thinking.

Placebo Response

Placebo effects and patient responses to them are complex phenomena but similar to those of active treatments (Kleinman et al. 1994; Turner et al. 1994). The literature supporting the placebo effect has been criticized as flawed, misinterpreted, and overrated (Kienle and Kienle 1997). Placebo analgesia is a biologically measurable phenomenon (Greene et al. 2009). In a clinical setting, it is difficult to separate "true" improvements from placebo responses to treatment and other factors such as regression to the mean and the natural history of the condition. Multiple patient and practitioner characteristics such as expectancy, conditioning, and learning affect the placebo response, and most are almost impossible to control (Ploghaus et al. 2003; Price et al. 1999). Evidence supports a role for the endogenous opioid and sympathetic nervous systems in placebo-induced analgesia that can be reversed with opioid antagonists (Pollo et al. 2003; ter Riet et al. 1998).

Historically, on the basis of Beecher's original article, placebo interventions were a part of paternalistic medicine's treatment armamentarium (Kaptchuk 1998). In the era of randomized controlled trials, placebos may be used if the cooperation of informed patients is secured. The magnitude of placebo analgesic effects was found to be significantly higher in studies that specifically investigated placebo analgesic mechanisms compared with those controlled trials that simply used a placebo for comparison (Vase et al. 2002). Several important strategies can be used to decrease excessive placebo responses in clinical trials (Dworkin et al. 2005). However, controversy exists about the evidence of clinically important effects to justify the use of placebo interventions (Hrobjartsson and Gotzsche 2003). Use of placebo to determine whether the patient's pain is "real" or to "cure" a psychogenic condition by replacing an analgesic with a "neutral" substance is dishonest, misleading, and counterproductive. A positive placebo response neither proves that the patient's pain is psychogenic nor shows that the patient would not benefit from an active treatment. Such an intervention also can result in loss of the patient's trust and render future treatment less effective.

Interdisciplinary Rehabilitation

Patients with chronic pain have dramatic reductions in physical, psychological, and social well-being with lower-rated health-related quality of life than do those with almost all other medical conditions (O'Connor 2009). A study of sequential trials of different treatment modalities found that the success of nerve blocks was diminished when used later in the treatment sequence. These results suggest that early failures of a single-modality treatment for chronic pain can have devastating consequences for future treatment attempts (Davies et al. 1997). In another study of more than 3,000 patients with low back or neuropathic pain, wide variations in medical practice decreased significantly after the practitioners received information that updated them about treatment modalities being used in the clinic and other available options (Davies et al. 1996). Education programs led by laypeople have produced short-term gains in self-efficacy, cognitive symptom management, and frequency of exercise (Foster et al. 2007). Collaborative care initiatives incorporating pain specialist assistance to primary care practitioners significantly improved pain-related outcomes (Dobscha et al. 2009).

Self-management programs for elderly people with chronic pain show significant reductions in pain intensity and disability (Morrison et al. 2009; Reid et al. 2008). Evidence-based practice guidelines emphasize interdisciplinary rehabilitation, integrated treatment, and well-delineated patient selection criteria (Sanders et al. 2005). The interdisciplinary pain rehabilitation program provides a full range of treatments for the most difficult pain syndromes within a framework of collaborative ongoing communication among team members, patients, and other interested parties (Stanos and Houle 2006). Unfortunately, the type of practitioners and scope of practice of "multidisciplinary" pain clinics vary considerably (Peng et al. 2008a). A recent survey in North Carolina found that only 7% of these clinics met the criteria of having a medical physician, registered nurse, physical therapist, and mental health specialist (Castel et al. 2009).

Substantial evidence indicates that interdisciplinary pain rehabilitation programs improve patient functioning in several areas for patients with various chronic pain syndromes, even the severely disabled (Angst et al. 2006; Lake et al. 2009; McCracken et al. 2007; van Wilgen et al. 2009). In a seminal review, a meta-analysis of 65 studies evaluated the efficacy of treatments in patients who attended multidisciplinary pain clinics (Flor et al. 1992). Although the study had limitations, it concluded that multidisciplinary pain clinics are efficacious. Combination treatments were superior to unimodal treatments or no treatment, treatment effects were maintained over a period of up to 7 years, and improvements were found not only on subjective but also on objective measures of effectiveness such as return to work and decreased health care use. Current smoking status has been associated with poorer treatment outcome from multidisciplinary treatment, suggesting that these patients should receive targeted or more intensive treatments (Fishbain et al. 2008b). More recent analyses of interdisciplinary programs that use comprehensive assessments, severity-adapted or stepped-care treatments, and rehabilitation goals report significant reductions in pain along with functional and quality-of-life improvements (Kainz et al. 2006; Marnitz et al. 2008).

The goal of treating chronic pain is to end disability and return people to work or other productive activities. Multidisciplinary interventions do show efficacy in returning patients to work (Norlund et al. 2009). In a long-term follow-up study, only half of the patients remained unemployed after treatment in an inpatient pain management program (Maruta et al. 1998). In a 30-month follow-up study of patients with chronic pain receiving multidisciplinary treatment, employment status was predicted by the patient's desire to return to work, the perception of a job's dangerousness, and the patient's education level (Fishbain et al. 1997). Patients not intending to return to work were more likely to complain of their job's excessive physical demands and reported more job dissatisfaction and feelings of disability. *Individualized subjective quality of life* is defined as the appraisal of quality of life based on personal values, desired goal attainment, and life priorities (Moliner et al. 2007). Poorer individualized subjective quality of life was not predicted by work status but by higher levels of distress, pain intensity, and perceived disability.

Conclusion

Chronic pain is a significant public health problem and frustrating to everyone affected by it, especially the patients who feel that health care has failed them. Psychiatrists as medical specialists should take an active role in the care of these patients because pharmacological and psychological treatments are now recognized as effective in the management of chronic pain. Recent advances in the treatment of chronic pain include the diagnosis and treatment of psychiatric comorbidity, the application of psychiatric treatments to chronic pain, and the development of interdisciplinary efforts to provide comprehensive health care to the patient with disabling and refractory chronic pain syndromes. Specifically, the psychiatrist provides the expertise of examining mental life and behavior as well as understanding the individual person and the systems in which he or she interacts. Finally, psychiatrists can facilitate the integration of the delivery of medical care with other health care professionals and medical specialists.

References

Abeles AM, Pillinger MH, Solitar BM, et al: Narrative review: the pathophysiology of fibromyalgia. Ann Intern Med 146:726–734, 2007

Albazaz R, Wong YT, Homer-Vanniasinkam S: Complex regional pain syndrome: a review. Ann Vasc Surg 22:297–306, 2008

American Academy of Pain Medicine and American Pain Society: The use of opioids for the treatment of chronic pain. 2008. Available at: www.ampainsoc.org/advocacy/opioids.htm. Accessed December 16, 2008.

American Psychiatric Association: Diagnostic and Statistical Manual of Mental Disorders, 2nd Edition. Washington, DC, American Psychiatric Association, 1968

American Psychiatric Association: Diagnostic and Statistical Manual of Mental Disorders, 3rd Edition. Washington, DC, American Psychiatric Association, 1980

American Psychiatric Association: Diagnostic and Statistical Manual of Mental Disorders, 3rd Edition, Revised. Washington, DC, American Psychiatric Association, 1987

American Psychiatric Association: Diagnostic and Statistical Manual of Mental Disorders, 4th Edition. Washington, DC, American Psychiatric Association, 1994

Andrews CM, Krantz MJ, Wedam EF, et al: Methadone-induced mortality in the treatment of chronic pain: role of QT prolongation. Cardiol J 16:210–217, 2009

Angst F, Brioschi R, Main CJ, et al: Interdisciplinary rehabilitation in fibromyalgia and chronic back pain: a prospective outcome study. J Pain 7:807–815, 2006

Aragona M, Bancheri L, Perinelli D, et al: Randomized double-blind comparison of serotonergic (citalopram) versus noradrenergic (reboxetine) reuptake inhibitors in outpatients with somatoform, DSM-IV-TR pain disorder. Eur J Pain 9:33–38, 2005

Arezzo JC, Rosenstock J, Lamoreaux L, et al: Efficacy and safety of pregabalin 600 mg/d for treating painful diabetic peripheral neuropathy: a double-blind placebo-controlled trial. BMC Neurol 8:33, 2008

Argoff CE: New analgesics for neuropathic pain: the lidocaine patch. Clin J Pain 16:S62–S66, 2000

Argoff CE, Backonja MM, Belgrade MJ, et al: Consensus guidelines: treatment planning and options. Diabetic peripheral neuropathic pain [published erratum appears in Mayo Clin Proc 81:854, 2006]. Mayo Clin Proc 81 (4 suppl):S12–S25, 2006

Arnold LM, Hess EV, Hudson JI, et al: A randomized, placebo-controlled, double-blind, flexible-dose study of fluoxetine in the treatment of women with fibromyalgia. Am J Med 112:191–197, 2002

Arnold LM, Hudson JI, Hess EV, et al: Family study of fibromyalgia. Arthritis Rheum 50:944–952, 2004

Arnold LM, Rosen A, Pritchett YL, et al: A randomized, double-blind, placebo-controlled trial of duloxetine in the treatment of women with fibromyalgia with or without major depressive disorder. Pain 119:5–15, 2005

Attal N, Cruccu G, Haanpaa M, et al: EFNS guidelines on pharmacological treatment of neuropathic pain. Eur J Neurol 13:1153–1169, 2006

Auerbach SM, Laskin DM, Frantsve LM, et al: Depression, pain, exposure to stressful life events, and long-term outcomes in temporomandibular disorder patients. J Oral Maxillofac Surg 59:628–633, 2001

Baastrup C, Finnerup NB: Pharmacological management of neuropathic pain following spinal cord injury. CNS Drugs 22:455–475, 2008

Bair MJ, Robinson RL, Katon W, et al: Depression and pain comorbidity: a literature review. Arch Intern Med 163:2433–2445, 2003

Bair MJ, Wu J, Damush TM, et al: Association of depression and anxiety alone and in combination with chronic musculoskeletal pain in primary care patients. Psychosom Med 70:890–897, 2008

Ballantyne JC, LaForge KS: Opioid dependence and addiction during opioid treatment of chronic pain. Pain 129:235–255, 2007

Bartusch SL, Sanders BJ, D'Alessio JG, et al: Clonazepam for the treatment of lancinating phantom limb pain. Clin J Pain 12:59–62, 1996

Beiske AG, Loge JH, Ronningen A, et al: Pain in Parkinson's disease: prevalence and characteristics. Pain 141:173–177, 2009

Bendtsen L, Jensen R: Mirtazapine is effective in the prophylactic treatment of chronic tension-type headache. Neurology 62:1706–1711, 2004

Berger A, Dukes EM, Edelsberg J, et al: Use of tricyclic antidepressants in older patients with painful neuropathies. Eur J Clin Pharmacol 62:757–764, 2006

Bergouignan M: Cures heureuses de nevralgies faciaales essentielles par le diphenyl-hydantoinate de soude. Rev Laryngol Otol Rhinol 63:34–41, 1942

Berrocoso E, Mico JA: Role of serotonin 5-HT1A receptors in the antidepressant-like effect and the antinociceptive effect of venlafaxine in mice. Int J Neuropsychopharmacol 14:1–11, 2008

Birklein F, Schmelz M: Neuropeptides, neurogenic inflammation and complex regional pain syndrome (CRPS). Neurosci Lett 437:199–202, 2008

Bjorkman B, Arner S, Hyden LC: Phantom breast and other syndromes after mastectomy: eight breast cancer patients describe their experiences over time: a 2-year follow-up study. J Pain 9:1018–1025, 2008

Bonica JJ: Definitions and taxonomy of pain, in The Management of Pain. Edited by Bonica JJ. Philadelphia, PA, Lea & Febiger, 1990, pp 18–27

Braden JB, Sullivan MD: Suicidal thoughts and behavior among adults with self-reported pain conditions in the National Comorbidity Survey Replication. J Pain 9:1106–1115, 2008

Brattberg G, Parker MG, Thorslund M: The prevalence of pain among the oldest old in Sweden. Pain 67:29–34, 1996

Brefel-Courbon C, Grolleau S, Thalamas C, et al: Comparison of chronic analgesic drugs prevalence in Parkinson's disease, other chronic diseases and the general population. Pain 141:14–18, 2009

Breslau N, Davis GC: Migraine, physical health and psychiatric disorder: a prospective epidemiologic study in young adults. J Psychiatr Res 27:211–221, 1993

Bruehl S, Chung OY: Psychological and behavioral aspects of complex regional pain syndrome management. Clin J Pain 22:430–437, 2006

Buenaver LF, Edwards RR, Smith MT, et al: Catastrophizing and pain-coping in young adults: associations with depressive symptoms and headache pain. J Pain 9:311–319, 2008

Buffett-Jerrott SE, Stewart SH: Cognitive and sedative effects of benzodiazepine use. Curr Pharm Des 8:45–58, 2002

Bulut S, Berilgen MS, Baran A, et al: Venlafaxine versus amitriptyline in the prophylactic treatment of migraine: randomized, double-blind, crossover study. Clin Neurol Neurosurg 107:44–48, 2004

Burns JW, Kubilus A, Bruehl S, et al: Do changes in cognitive factors influence outcome following multidisciplinary treatment for chronic pain? A cross-lagged panel analysis. J Consult Clin Psychol 71:81–91, 2003

Calandre EP, Hidalgo J, Rico-Villademoros F: Use of ziprasidone in patients with fibromyalgia: a case series. Rheumatol Int 27:473–476, 2007

Carey TS, Garrett JM, Jackman AM: Beyond the good prognosis: examination of an inception cohort of patients with chronic low back pain. Spine 25:115–120, 2000

Carozzi V, Marmiroli P, Cavaletti G: Focus on the role of glutamate in the pathology of the peripheral nervous system. CNS Neurol Disord Drug Targets 7:348–360, 2008

Carville SF, Arendt-Nielsen S, Bliddal H, et al: EULAR evidence-based recommendations for the management of fibromyalgia syndrome. Ann Rheum Dis 67:536–541, 2008

Castel LD, Freburger JK, Holmes GM, et al: Spine and pain clinics serving North Carolina patients with back and neck pain: what do they do, and are they multidisciplinary? Spine 34:615–622, 2009

Cepeda MS, Farrar JT: Economic evaluation of oral treatments for neuropathic pain. J Pain 7:119–128, 2006

Cheshire WP: Defining the role for gabapentin in the treatment of trigeminal neuralgia: a retrospective study. J Pain 3:137–142, 2002

Chou R, Fanciullo GJ, Fine PG, et al: Opioids for chronic noncancer pain: prediction and identification of aberrant drug-related behaviors: a review of the evidence for an American Pain Society and American Academy of Pain Medicine clinical practice guideline. J Pain 10:131–146, 2009

Christo PJ, Mazloomdoost D: Interventional pain treatments for cancer pain. Ann N Y Acad Sci 1138:299–328, 2008

Ciccone DS, Just N, Bandilla EB: A comparison of economic and social reward in patients with chronic nonmalignant back pain. Psychosom Med 61:552–563, 1999

Ciccone DS, Just N, Bandilla EB, et al: Psychological correlates of opioid use in patients with chronic nonmalignant pain: a preliminary test of the downhill spiral hypothesis. J Pain Symptom Manage 20:180–192, 2000

Cicero TJ, Dart RC, Inciardi JA, et al: The development of a comprehensive risk-management program for prescription opioid analgesics: researched abuse, diversion and addiction-related surveillance (RADARS). Pain Med 8:157–170, 2007

Clark MR, Stoller KB, Brooner RK: Assessment and management of chronic pain in individuals seeking treatment for opioid dependence disorder. Can J Psychiatry 53:496–508, 2008

Clauw DJ, Mease P, Palmer RH, et al: Milnacipran for the treatment of fibromyalgia in adults: a 15-week, multicenter, randomized, double-blind, placebo-controlled, multiple-dose clinical trial. Clin Ther 30:1988–2004, 2008

Clough-Gorr KM, Blozik E, Gillmann G, et al: The self-administered 24-item geriatric pain measure (GPM-24-SA): psychometric properties in three European populations of community-dwelling older adults. Pain Med 9:695–709, 2008

Codd EE, Martinez RP, Molino L, et al: Tramadol and several anticonvulsants synergize in attenuating nerve injury-induced allodynia. Pain 134:254–262, 2008

Critchley DJ, Ratcliffe J, Noonan S, et al: Effectiveness and cost-effectiveness of three types of physiotherapy used to reduce chronic low back pain disability: a pragmatic randomized trial with economic evaluation. Spine 32:1474–1481, 2007

Crofford LJ: Pain management in fibromyalgia. Curr Opin Rheumatol 20:246–250, 2008

Croft PR, Papageorgiou AC, Ferry S, et al: Psychological distress and low back pain: evidence from a prospective study in the general population. Spine 20:2731–2737, 1996

Crombez G, Eccleston C, Baeyens F, et al: When somatic information threatens, catastrophic thinking enhances attentional interference. Pain 75:187–198, 1998

Cruccu G, Gronseth G, Alksne J, et al: AAN-EFNS guidelines on trigeminal neuralgia management. Eur J Neurol 15:1013–1028, 2008

Cutrer FM: Antiepileptic drugs: how they work in headache. Headache 41:S3–10, 2001

Dammen T, Ekeberg O, Arnesen H, et al: Health-related quality of life in non-cardiac chest pain patients with and without panic disorder. Int J Psychiatry Med 38:271–286, 2008

Darke S, Duflou J, Torok M: The comparative toxicology and major organ pathology of fatal methadone and heroin toxicity cases. Drug Alcohol Depend 106:1–6, 2010

Davies HT, Crombie IK, Macrae WA, et al: Audit in pain clinics: changing the management of low-back and nerve-damage pain. Anaesthesia 51:641–646, 1996

Davies HT, Crombie IK, Brown JH, et al: Diminishing returns or appropriate treatment strategy? An analysis of short-term outcomes after pain clinic treatment. Pain 70:203–208, 1997

DeBerard MS, Masters KS, Colledge AL, et al: Outcomes of posterolateral lumbar fusion in Utah patients receiving workers' compensation: a retrospective cohort study. Spine 26:738–746, 2001

Dellemijn PL, Fields HL: Do benzodiazepines have a role in chronic pain management? Pain 57:137–152, 1994

Dersh J, Polatin PB, Gatchel RJ: Chronic pain and psychopathology: research findings and theoretical considerations. Psychosom Med 64:773–786, 2002

Dersh J, Mayer T, Theodore BR, et al: Do psychiatric disorders first appear preinjury or postinjury in chronic disabling occupational spinal disorders? Spine 32:1045–1051, 2007

Deyo RA, Weinstein JN: Low back pain. N Engl J Med 344:363–370, 2001

Deyo RA, Mirza SK, Turner JA, et al: Overtreating chronic back pain: time to back off? J Am Board Fam Med 22:62–68, 2009

Dick IE, Brochu RM, Purohit Y, et al: Sodium channel blockade may contribute to the analgesic efficacy of antidepressants. J Pain 8:315–324, 2007

Djaldetti R, Yust-Katx S, Kolianov V, et al: The effect of duloxetine on primary pain symptoms in Parkinson disease. Clin Neuropharmacol 30:201–205, 2007

Dobscha SK, Corson K, Perrin NA, et al: Collaborative care for chronic pain in primary care: a cluster randomized trial. JAMA 301:1242–1252, 2009

Dodick DW: Clinical practice: chronic daily headache. N Engl J Med 354:158–165, 2006

Drage LA, Rogers RS 3rd: Burning mouth syndrome. Dermatol Clin 21:135–145, 2003

Druss BG, Rosenheck RA, Sledge WH: Health and disability costs of depressive illness in a major U.S. corporation. Am J Psychiatry 157:1274–1278, 2000

Dumas EO, Pollack GM: Opioid tolerance development: a pharmacokinetic/pharmacodynamic perspective. AAPS J 10:537–551, 2008

Dworkin RH, Katz J, Gitlin MJ: Placebo response in clinical trials of depression and its implications for research on chronic neuropathic pain. Neurology 65 (12 suppl 4):S7–S19, 2005

Dworkin RH, O'Connor AB, Backonja M, et al: Pharmacologic management of neuropathic pain: evidence-based recommendations. Pain 132:237–251, 2007

Eccleston C, Williams AC, Morley S: Psychological therapies for the management of chronic pain (excluding headache) in adults. Cochrane Database Syst Rev (2):CD007407, 2009

Edwards RR, Smith MT, Kudel I, et al: Pain-related catastrophizing as a risk factor for suicidal ideation in chronic pain. Pain 126:272–279, 2006

Eide PK, Stubhaug A, Stenehjem AE: Central dysesthesia pain after traumatic spinal cord injury is dependent on N-methyl-D-aspartate receptor activation. Neurosurgery 37:1080–1087, 1995

Estanislao L, Carter K, McArthur J, et al: A randomized controlled trial of 5% lidocaine gel for HIV-associated distal symmetric polyneuropathy. J Acquir Immune Defic Syndr 37:1584–1586, 2004

Esteve R, Ramirez-Maestre C, Lopez-Marinez AE: Adjustment to chronic pain: the role of pain acceptance, coping strategies, and pain-related cognitions. Ann Behav Med 33:179–188, 2007

Evers S, Afra J, Frese A, et al: EFNS guideline on the drug treatment of migraine—a report of an EFNS task force. Eur J Neurol 13:560–572, 2006

Fernández-de-las-Peñas C, Schoenen J: Chronic tension-type headache: what is new? Curr Opin Neurol 22:254–261, 2009

Finnerup NB: A review of central neuropathic pain states. Curr Opin Anaesthesiol 21:586–589, 2008

Finnerup NB, Otto M, McQuay HJ, et al: Algorithm for neuropathic pain treatment: an evidence based proposal. Pain 118:289–305, 2005

Fishbain DA, Goldberg M, Rosomoff RS, et al: Completed suicide in chronic pain. Clin J Pain 7:29–36, 1991

Fishbain DA, Cutler RB, Rosomoff HL, et al: Impact of chronic pain patients' job perception variables on actual return to work. Clin J Pain 13:197–206, 1997

Fishbain DA, Cutler RB, Lewis J, et al: Do the second-generation "atypical neuroleptics" have analgesic properties? A structured evidence-based review. Pain Med 5:359–365, 2004

Fishbain DA, Cole B, Lewis J, et al: What percentage of chronic nonmalignant pain patients exposed to chronic opioid analgesic therapy develop abuse/addiction and/or aberrant drug-related behaviors? A structured evidence-based review. Pain Med 9:444–459, 2008a

Fishbain DA, Lewis JE, Cutler R, et al: Does smoking status affect multidisciplinary pain facility treatment outcome? Pain Med 9:1081–1090, 2008b

Fisher A, Zakrzewska JM, Patsalos PN: Trigeminal neuralgia: current treatments and future developments. Expert Opin Emerg Drugs 8:123–143, 2002

Flor H: Phantom-limb pain: characteristics, causes, and treatment. Lancet Neurol 1:182–189, 2002

Flor H, Fydrich T, Turk DC: Efficacy of multidisciplinary pain treatment centers: a meta-analytic review. Pain 49:221–230, 1992

Folkman S, Lazarus RS, Gruen RJ, et al: Appraisal, coping, health status, and psychological symptoms. J Per Soc Psychol 50:571–579, 1986

Fordyce WE, Fowler RS Jr, Lehmann JF, et al: Operant conditioning in the treatment of chronic pain. Arch Phys Med Rehabil 54:399–408, 1973

Foster G, Taylor SJ, Eldridge SE, et al: Self-management education programmes by lay leaders for people with chronic conditions. Cochrane Database Syst Rev (4):CD005108, 2007

Frese A, Husstedt IW, Ringelstein EB, et al: Pharmacologic treatment of central post-stroke pain. Clin J Pain 22:252–260, 2006

Fritzell P, Hagg O, Wessberg P, et al: 2001 Volvo Award Winner in Clinical Studies: Lumbar fusion versus nonsurgical treatment for chronic low back pain: a multicenter randomized controlled trial from the Swedish Lumbar Spine Study Group. Spine 26:2521–2532, 2001

Furlan AD, Brosseau L, Imamura M, et al: Massage for low-back pain: a systematic review within the framework of the Cochrane Collaboration Back Review Group. Spine 27:1896–1910, 2002

Gallagher RM, Mueller LL, Freitag FG: Divalproex sodium in the treatment of migraine and cluster headache. J Am Osteopath Assoc 102:92–94, 2002

Giannopoulos S, Kosmidou M, Sarmas I, et al: Patient compliance with SSRIs and gabapentin in painful diabetic neuropathy. Clin J Pain 23:267–269, 2007

Gibbs GF, Drummond PD, Finch PM, et al: Unravelling the pathophysiology of complex regional pain syndrome: focus on sympathetically maintained pain. Clin Exp Pharmacol Physiol 35:717–724, 2008

Gilron I, Bailey J, Weaver DF, et al: Patients' attitudes and prior treatments in neuropathic pain: a pilot study. Pain Res Manag 7:199–203, 2002

Goadsby PJ, Charbit AR, Andreou AP, et al: Neurobiology of migraine. Neuroscience 161:327–341, 2009

Goodkin K, Gullion C, Agras WS: A randomized, double-blind, placebo-controlled trial of trazodone hydrochloride in chronic low back pain syndrome. J Clin Psychopharmacol 10:269–278, 1990

Goodnick PJ: Use of antidepressants in treatment of comorbid diabetes mellitus and depression as well as in diabetic neuropathy. Ann Clin Psychiatry 13:31–41, 2001

Grabe HJ, Meyer C, Hapke U, et al: Somatoform pain disorder in the general population. Psychother Psychosom 72:88–94, 2003

Greenberg J, Burns JW: Pain anxiety among chronic pain patients: specific phobia or manifestation of anxiety sensitivity? Behav Res Ther 41:223–240, 2003

Greene CS, Goddard G, Macaluso GM, et al: Topical review: placebo responses and therapeutic responses: how are they related? J Orofac Pain 23:93–107, 2009

Gronseth G, Cruccu G, Alksne J, et al: Practice parameter: the diagnostic evaluation and treatment of trigeminal neuralgia (an evidence-based review): report of the Quality Standards Subcommittee of the American Academy of Neurology and the European Federation of Neurological Societies. Neurology 71:1183–1190, 2008

Grosskopf J, Mazzola J, Wan Y, et al: A randomized, placebo-controlled study of oxcarbazepine in painful diabetic neuropathy. Acta Neurol Scand 114:177–180, 2006

Grushka M, Epstein JB, Gorsky M: Burning mouth syndrome. Am Fam Physician 65:615–620, 622, 2002

Gureje O, Von Korff M, Simon GE, et al: Persistent pain and well-being: a World Health Organization study in primary care. JAMA 280:147–151, 1998

Guzman J, Esmail R, Karjalainen K, et al: Multidisciplinary bio-psycho-social rehabilitation for chronic low-back pain. Cochrane Database Syst Rev (2):CD000963, 2007

Hains BC, Waxman SG: Sodium channel expression and the molecular pathophysiology of pain after SCI. Prog Brain Res 161:195–203, 2007

Han DW, Kweon TD, Lee JS, et al: Antiallodynic effect of pregabalin in rat models of sympathetically maintained and sympathetic independent neuropathic pain. Yonsei Med J 48:41–47, 2007

Harden RN, Bruehl S, Stanton-Hicks M, et al: Proposed new diagnostic criteria for complex regional pain syndrome. Pain Med 8:326–331, 2007

Hari AR, Wydenkeller S, Dokladal P, et al: Enhanced recovery of human spinothalamic function is associated with central neuropathic pain after SCI. Exp Neurol 216:428–430, 2009

Harpaz R, Ortega-Sanchez IR, Seward JF; Advisory Committee on Immunization Practices (ACIP) Centers for Disease Control and Prevention (CDC): Prevention of herpes zoster: recommendations of the Advisory Committee on Immunization Practices (ACIP) [published erratum appears on MMWR Recomm Rep 57:779, 2008]. MMWR Recomm Rep 57(RR-5):1–30, 2008

Harris AM, Orav EJ, Bates DW, et al: Somatization increases disability independent of comorbidity. J Gen Intern Med 24:155–161, 2009

Hasenbring M, Marienfeld G, Kuhlendahl D, et al: Risk factors of chronicity in lumbar disc patients: a prospective investigation of biologic, psychologic, and social predictors of therapy outcome. Spine 19:2759–2765, 1994

Hasenbring M, Hallner D, Klasen B: Psychological mechanisms in the transition from acute to chronic pain: over- or underrated? [in German]. Schmerz 15:442–447, 2001

Hauser W, Bernardy K, Uceyler N, et al: Treatment of fibromyalgia syndrome with antidepressants: a meta-analysis. JAMA 301:198–209, 2009

Herr KA, Mobily PR: Comparison of selected pain assessment tools for use with the elderly. Appl Nurs Res 6:39–46, 1993

Hidalgo J, Rico-Villademoros F, Calandre EP: An open-label study of quetiapine in the treatment of fibromyalgia. Prog Neuropsychopharmacol Biol Psychiatry 31:71–77, 2007

Hill A, Niven CA, Knussen C: The role of coping in adjustment to phantom limb pain. Pain 62:79–86, 1995

Holroyd KA, Drew JB: Behavioral approaches to the treatment of migraine. Semin Neurol 26:199–207, 2006

Holroyd KA, O'Donnell FJ, Stensland M, et al: Management of chronic tension-type headache with tricyclic antidepressant medication, stress management therapy, and their combination: a randomized controlled trial. JAMA 285:2208–2215, 2001

Hrobjartsson A, Gotzsche PC: Placebo treatment versus no treatment. Cochrane Database Syst Rev (1):CD003974, 2003

Hsu ES: Practical management of complex regional pain syndrome. Am J Ther 16:147–154, 2009

Huge V, Schloderer U, Steinberger M, et al: Impact of a functional restoration program on pain and health-related quality of life in patients with chronic low back pain. Pain Med 7:501–508, 2006

Hulsebosch CE, Hains BC, Crown ED, et al: Mechanisms of chronic central neuropathic pain after spinal cord injury. Brain Res Rev 60:202–213, 2009

Ilgen MA, Zivin K, McCammon RJ, et al: Pain and suicidal thoughts, plans and attempts in the United States. Gen Hosp Psychiatry 30:521–527, 2008

Institute for Clinical Systems Improvement (ICSI): Health Care Guideline: Assessment and Management of Acute Pain, 6th Edition. March 2008. Available at: http://www.icsi.org/pain_acute/pain__acute__assessment_and_management_of__3.html. Accessed June 7, 2010.

Jackson JL, Kroenke K: Prevalence, impact, and prognosis of multisomatoform disorder in primary care: a 5-year follow-up study. Psychosom Med 70:430–434, 2008

Jain KK: Current challenges and future prospects in management of neuropathic pain. Expert Rev Neurother 8:1743–1756, 2008

Jenewein J, Moergeli H, Wittmann L, et al: Development of chronic pain following severe accidental injury: results of a 3-year follow-up study. J Psychosom Res 66:119–126, 2009

Jensen MP: Research on coping with chronic pain: the importance of active avoidance of inappropriate conclusions. Pain 147:3–4, 2009

Jensen MP, Turner JA, Romano JM: Correlates of improvement in multidisciplinary treatment of chronic pain. J Consult Clin Psychol 62:172–179, 1994a

Jensen MP, Turner JA, Romano JM, et al: Relationship of pain-specific beliefs to chronic pain adjustment. Pain 57:301–309, 1994b

Jensen TS, Finnerup NB: Management of neuropathic pain. Curr Opin Support Palliat Care 1:126–131, 2007

Joffroy A, Levivier M, Massager N: Trigeminal neuralgia: pathophysiology and treatment. Acta Neurol Belg 101:20–25, 2001

Johnson RW: Herpes zoster and postherpetic neuralgia: optimal treatment. Drugs Aging 10:80–94, 1997

Johnson RW, Wasner G, Saddier P, et al: Herpes zoster and postherpetic neuralgia: optimizing management in the elderly patient. Drugs Aging 25:991–1006, 2008

Jones CK, Eastwood BJ, Need AB, et al: Analgesic effects of serotonergic, noradrenergic or dual reuptake inhibitors in the carrageenan test in rats: evidence for synergism between serotonergic and noradrenergic reuptake inhibition. Neuropharmacology 51:1172–1180, 2006

Jose VM, Bhansali A, Hota D, et al: Randomized double-blind study comparing the efficacy and safety of lamotrigine and amitriptyline in painful diabetic neuropathy. Diabet Med 24:377–383, 2007

Kainz B, Gulich M, Engel EM, et al: Comparison of three outpatient therapy forms for treatment of chronic low back pain—findings of a multicentre, cluster randomized study. Rehabilitation 45:65–77, 2006

Kaniecki RG: A comparison of divalproex with propranolol and placebo for the prophylaxis of migraine without aura. Arch Neurol 54:1141–1145, 1997

Kaptchuk TJ: Powerful placebo: the dark side of the randomized controlled trial. Lancet 351:1722–1725, 1998

Karoly P, Ruehlman LS: Psychological "resilience" and its correlates in chronic pain: findings from a national community sample. Pain 123:90–97, 2006

Keskinbora K, Aydinli I: A double-blind randomized controlled trial of topiramate and damitriptyline either alone or in combination for the prevention of migraine. Clin Neurol Neurosurg 110:979–984, 2008

Kienle GS, Kienle H: The powerful placebo effect: fact or fiction? J Clin Epidemiol 50:1311–1318, 1997

Kim HJ, Paek SH, Kim JY, et al: Chronic subthalamic deep brain stimulation improves pain in Parkinson disease. J Neurol 255:1889–1894, 2008

Kirsh KL, Whitcomb LA, Donaghy K, et al: Abuse and addiction issues in medically ill patients with pain: attempts at clarification of terms and empirical study. Clin J Pain 18:S52–S60, 2002

Klapper J: Divalproex sodium in migraine prophylaxis: a dose-controlled study. Cephalalgia 17:103–108, 1997

Kleinman I, Brown P, Librach L: Placebo pain medication: ethical and practical considerations. Arch Fam Med 3:453–457, 1994

König HH, Bernert S, Angermeyer MC, et al: Comparison of population health status in six European countries: results of a representative survey using the EQ-5D questionnaire. Med Care 47:255–261, 2009

Kothare SV, Kaleyias J: Zonisamide: review of pharmacology, clinical efficacy, tolerability, and safety. Expert Opin Drug Metab Toxicol 4:493–506, 2008

Kroenke K, Bair MJ, Damush TM, et al: Optimized antidepressant therapy and pain self-management in primary care patients with depression and musculoskeletal pain: a randomized controlled trial. JAMA 301:2099–2110, 2009

Lake AE 3rd: Behavioral and nonpharmacologic treatments of headache. Med Clin North Am 85:1055–1075, 2001

Lake AE 3rd, Saper JR, Hamel RL: Comprehensive inpatient treatment of refractory chronic daily headache. Headache 49:555–562, 2009

Larson SL, Clark MR, Eaton WW: Depressive disorder as a long-term antecedent risk factor for incident back pain: a thirteen year followup study from the Baltimore Epidemiological Catchment Area Sample. Psychol Med 34:1–9, 2004

Lazarus RA, Folkman S: Stress, Appraisal, and Coping. New York, Springer, 1984

Leeuw M, Goossens ME, Linton SJ, et al: The fear-avoidance model of musculoskeletal pain: current state of scientific evidence. J Behav Med 30:77–94, 2007

Leino P, Magni G: Depressive and distress symptoms as predictors of low back pain, neck-shoulder pain, and other musculoskeletal morbidity: a 10 year follow-up of metal industry employees. Pain 53:89–94, 1993

Lemstra M, Stewart B, Olszynski WP: Effectiveness of multidisciplinary intervention in the treatment of migraine: a randomized clinical trial. Headache 42:845–854, 2002

Lewis TA, Solomon GD: Advances in cluster headache management. Cleve Clin J Med 63:237–244, 1996

Liebschutz J, Saitz R, Brower V, et al: PTSD in urban primary care: high prevalence and low physician recognition. J Gen Intern Med 22:719–726, 2007

Lin EH, Katon W, Von Korff M, et al: Effect of improving depression care on pain and functional outcomes among older adults with arthritis: a randomized controlled trial. JAMA 290:2428–2429, 2003

Lipchik GL, Nash JM: Cognitive-behavioral issues in the treatment and management of chronic daily headache. Curr Pain Headache Rep 6:473–479, 2002

Lipton RB, Bigal ME, Diamond M, et al: Migraine prevalence, disease burden, and the need for preventive therapy. Neurology 68:343–349, 2007

List T, Leijon G, Helkimo M, et al: Clinical findings and psychological factors in patients with atypical odontalgia: a case-control study. J Orofac Pain 21:89–98, 2007

Long DM, Filtzer DL, BenDebba M, et al: Clinical features of the failed-back syndrome. J Neurosurg 69:61–71, 1988

Lopez-Lopez A, Montorio I, Izal M, et al: The role of psychological variables in explaining depression in older people with chronic pain. Aging Ment Health 12:735–745, 2008

Love S, Coakham HB: Trigeminal neuralgia: pathology and pathogenesis. Brain 124:2347–2360, 2001

Mackey S, Feinberg S: Pharmacologic therapies for complex regional pain syndrome. 11:38–43, 2007

Magni G, Marchetti M, Moreschi C, et al: Chronic musculoskeletal pain and depressive symptoms in the National Health and Nutrition Examination, I: epidemiologic follow-up study. Pain 53:163–168, 1993

Magni G, Rigatti-Luchini S, Fracca F, et al: Suicidality in chronic abdominal pain: an analysis of the Hispanic Health and Nutrition Examination Survey (HHANES). Pain 76:137–144, 1998

Maina G, Vitalucci A, Gandolfo S, et al: Comparative efficacy of SSRIs and amisulpride in burning mouth syndrome: a single-blind study. J Clin Psychiatry 63:38–43, 2002

Manchikanti L, Singh V: Managing phantom pain. Pain Physician 7:365–375, 2004

Manchikanti L, Singh A: Therapeutic opioids: a ten-year perspective on the complexities and complications of the escalating use, abuse, and nonmedical use of opioids. Pain Physician 11 (2 suppl):S63–S88, 2008

Mannion AF, Junge A, Taimela S, et al: Active therapy for chronic low back pain, part 3: factors influencing self-rated disability and its change following therapy. Spine (Phila Pa 1976) 26:920–929, 2001

Mäntyselkä P, Ahonen R, Viinamäki H, et al: Drug use by patients visiting primary care physicians due to nonacute musculoskeletal pain. Eur J Pharm Sci 17:210–206, 2002

Marnitz U, Weh L, Muller G, et al: Multimodal integrated assessment and treatment of patients with back pain: pain related results and ability to work. Schmerz 22:415–423, 2008

Marson AG, Kadir ZA, Hutton JL, et al: The new antiepileptic drugs: a systematic review of their efficacy and tolerability. Epilepsia 38:859–880, 1997

Maruta T, Malinchoc M, Offord KP, et al: Status of patients with chronic pain 13 years after treatment in a pain management center. Pain 74:199–204, 1998

Mathew NT, Kailasam J, Meadors L: Prophylaxis of migraine, transformed migraine, and cluster headache with topiramate. Headache 42:796–803, 2002

Max MB: Treatment of post-herpetic neuralgia: antidepressants. Ann Neurol 35:850–853, 1994

McCarthy LH, Bigal ME, Katz M, et al: Chronic pain and obesity in elderly people: results from the Einstein aging study. J Am Geriatr Soc 57:115–119, 2009

McCleane G: Antidepressants as analgesics. CNS Drugs 22:139–156, 2008

McCowan C, Kidd B, Fahey T: Factors associated with mortality in Scottish patients receiving methadone in primary care: retrospective cohort study. BMJ 338:b2225, 2009

McCracken LM: Learning to live with the pain: acceptance of pain predicts adjustment in persons with chronic pain. Pain 74:21–27, 1998

McCracken LM, Hoskins J, Eccleston C: Concerns about medication and medication use in chronic pain. J Pain 7:726–734, 2006

McCracken LM, MacKichan F, Eccleston C: Contextual cognitive-behavioral therapy for severely disabled chronic pain sufferers: effectiveness and clinically significant change. Eur J Pain 11:314–322, 2007

McWilliams LA, Cox BJ, Enns MW: Mood and anxiety disorders associated with chronic pain: an examination in a nationally representative sample. Pain 106:127–133, 2003

Mease PJ, Clauw DJ, Gendreau RM, et al: The efficacy and safety of milnacipran for treatment of fibromyalgia: a randomized, double-blind, placebo-controlled trial. J Rheumatol 36:398–409, 2009

Mendell JR, Sahenk Z: Clinical practice: painful sensory neuropathy. N Engl J Med 348:1243–1255, 2003

Merskey H: The taxonomy of pain. Med Clin North Am 91:13–20, vii, 2007

Merskey H, Lindblom U, Mumford JM, et al: Pain terms: a current list with definitions and notes on usage. Pain Suppl 3:S215–S221, 1986

Mico JA, Ardid D, Berrocoso E, et al: Antidepressants and pain. Trends Pharmacol Sci 27:348–354, 2006

Miller JP, Magill ST, Acar F, et al: Predictors of long-term success after microvascular decompression for trigeminal neuralgia. J Neurosurg 110:620–626, 2009

Mitra S: Opioid-induced hyperalgesia: pathophysiology and clinical implications. J Opioid Manag 4:123–130, 2008

Moja PL, Cusi C, Sterzi RR, et al: Selective serotonin re-uptake inhibitors (SSRIs) for preventing migraine and tension-type headaches. Cochrane Database Syst Rev (3):CD002919, 2005

Moliner CE, Durand MJ, Desrosiers J, et al: Subjective quality of life according to work status following interdisciplinary work rehabilitation consequent to musculoskeletal disability. J Occup Rehabil 17:667–682, 2007

Molton IR, Graham C, Stoelb BL, et al: Current psychological approaches to the management of chronic pain. Curr Opin Anaesthesiol 20:485–489, 2007

Morley S, Wilkinson L: The Pain Beliefs and Perception Inventory: a British replication. Pain 61:427–433, 1995

Morrison RS, Flanagan S, Fischberg D, et al: A novel interdisciplinary analgesic program reduces pain and improves function in older adults after orthopedic surgery. J Am Geriatr Soc 57:1–10, 2009

Moulin DE, Clark AJ, Gilron I, et al: Pharmacological management of chronic neuropathic pain—consensus statement and guidelines from the Canadian Pain Society. Pain Res Manag 12:13–21, 2007

Muehlbacher M, Nickel MK, Kettler C, et al: Topiramate in treatment of patients with chronic low back pain: a randomized, double-blind, placebo-controlled study. Clin J Pain 22:526–531, 2006

Mulleners WM, Chronicle EP: Anticonvulsants in migraine prophylaxis: a Cochrane review. Cephalalgia 28:585–597, 2008

Munro G, Erichsen HK, Mirza NR: Pharmacological comparison of anticonvulsant drugs in animal models of persistent pain and anxiety. Neuropharmacology 53:609–618, 2007

Nasreddine W, Beydoun A: Oxcarbazepine in neuropathic pain. Expert Opin Investig Drugs 16:1615–1625, 2007

Neville A, Peleg R, Singer Y, et al: Chronic pain: a population-based study. Isr Med Assoc J 10:676–680, 2008

Nicholson BD: Evaluation and treatment of central pain syndromes. Neurology 62:S30–S36, 2004

Nikolaus T: Assessment of chronic pain in elderly patients. Ther Umsch 54:340–344, 1997

Noble M, Tregear SJ, Treadwell JR, et al: Long-term opioid therapy for chronic noncancer pain: a systematic review and meta-analysis of efficacy and safety. J Pain Symptom Manage 35:214–228, 2008

Norlund A, Ropponen A, Alexanderson K: Multidisciplinary interventions: review of studies of return to work after rehabilitation for low back pain. J Rehabil Med 41:115–121, 2009

Noyes R Jr, Stuart SP, Watson DB: A reconceptualization of the somatoform disorders. Psychosomatics 49:14–22, 2008

Obermann M, Katsarava Z: Update on trigeminal neuralgia. Expert Rev Neurother 9:323–329, 2009

O'Connor AB: Neuropathic pain: quality-of-life impact, costs and cost effectiveness of therapy. Pharmacoeconomics 27:95–112, 2009

Ohayon MM, Schatzberg AF: Using chronic pain to predict depressive morbidity in the general population. Arch Gen Psychiatry 60:39–47, 2003

Ozyalcin SN, Falu GK, Kiziltan E, et al: The efficacy and safety of venlafaxine in the prophylaxis of migraine. Headache 45:144–152, 2005

Pain Treatment Topics: Opioid Risk Management. Glenview, IL, SBL Ltd, 2010. Available at: http://www.pain-topics.org/opioid_rx/risk.php#AssessTools. Accessed June 7, 2010.

Passik SD, Kirsh KL: The interface between pain and drug abuse and the evolution of strategies to optimize pain management while minimizing drug abuse. Exp Clin Psychopharmacol 16:400–404, 2008

Passik SD, Kirsh KL, Whitcomb L, et al: A new tool to assess and document pain outcomes in chronic pain patients receiving opioid therapy. Clin Ther 26:552–561, 2004

Passik SD, Kirsh KL, Whitcomb L, et al: Monitoring outcomes during long term opioid therapy for noncancer pain: results with Pain Assessment and Documentation Tool. J Opioid Manag 1:257–266, 2005

Passik SD, Kirsh KL, Donaghy KB, et al: Pain and aberrant drug-related behaviors in medically ill patients with and without histories of substance abuse. Clin J Pain 22:173–181, 2006

Peles E, Schreiber S, Gordon J, et al: Significantly higher methadone dose for methadone maintenance treatment (MMT) patients with chronic pain. Pain 113:340–346, 2005

Peng P, Stinson JN, Choiniere M, et al: Role of health care professionals in multidisciplinary pain treatment facilities in Canada. Pain Res Manag 13:484–488, 2008a

Peng P, Tumber P, Stafford M, et al: Experience of methadone therapy in 100 consecutive chronic pain patients in a multidisciplinary pain center. Pain Med 9:786–794, 2008b

Pengel HM, Maher CG, Refshauge KM: Systematic review of conservative interventions for subacute low back pain. Clin Rehabil 16:811–820, 2002

Perahia DG, Pritchett YL, Desaiah D, et al: Efficacy of duloxetine in painful symptoms: an analgesic or antidepressant effect? Int Clin Psychopharmacol 21:311–317, 2006

Phillips DM: JCAHO pain management standards are unveiled. Joint Commission on Accreditation of Healthcare Organizations. JAMA 284:428–429, 2000

Picavet HS, Vlaeyen JW, Schouten JS: Pain catastrophizing and kinesiophobia: predictors of chronic low back pain. Am J Epidemiol 156:1028–1034, 2002

Pinto A, Sollecito TP, DeRossi SS: Burning mouth syndrome: a retrospective analysis of clinical characteristics and treatment outcomes. N Y State Dent J 69:18–24, 2003

Ploghaus A, Becerra L, Borras C, et al: Neural circuitry underlying pain modulation: expectation, hypnosis, placebo. Trends Cogn Sci 7:197–200, 2003

Pollo A, Vighetti S, Rainero I, et al: Placebo analgesia and the heart. Pain 102:125–133, 2003

Pontell D: A clinical approach to complex regional pain syndrome. Clin Podiatr Med Surg 25:361–380, 2008

Potvin S, Grignon S, Marchand S: Human evidence of a supraspinal modulating role of dopamine on pain perception. Synapse 63:390–402, 2009

Prasad S, Galetta S: Trigeminal neuralgia: historical notes and current concepts. Neurologist 15:87–94, 2009

Price DD, Milling LS, Kirsch I, et al: An analysis of factors that contribute to the magnitude of placebo analgesia in an experimental paradigm. Pain 83:147–156, 1999

Rahman A, Reed E, Underwood M, et al: Factors affecting self-efficacy and pain intensity in patients with chronic musculoskeletal pain seen in a specialist rheumatology pain clinic. Rheumatology (Oxford) 47:1803–1808, 2008

Reid MC, Papaleontiou M, Ong A, et al: Self-management strategies to reduce pain and improve function among older adults in community settings: a review of the evidence. Pain Med 9:409–424, 2008

Richter RW, Pertenoy R, Sharma U, et al: Relief of painful diabetic peripheral neuropathy with pregabalin: a randomized, placebo-controlled trial. J Pain 6:253–260, 2005

Rico-Villademoros F, Hidalgo J, Dominguez I, et al: Atypical antipsychotics in the treatment of fibromyalgia: a case series with olanzapine. Prog Neuropsychopharmacol Biol Psychiatry 29:161–164, 2005

Riley JL 3rd, Benson MB, Gremillion HA, et al: Sleep disturbance in orofacial pain patients: pain-related or emotional distress? Cranio 19:106–113, 2001

Riley J, Eisenberg E, Muller-Schwefe G, et al: Oxycodone: a review of its use in the management of pain. Curr Med Res Opin 24:175–192, 2008

Rojas-Corrales MO, Casas J, Moreno-Brea MR, et al: Antinociceptive effects of tricyclic antidepressants and their noradrenergic metabolites. Eur Neuropsychopharmacol 13:355–363, 2003

Rosenblum A, Joseph H, Fong C, et al: Prevalence and characteristics of chronic pain among chemically dependent patients in methadone maintenance and residential treatment facilities. JAMA 289:2370–2378, 2003

Rosenzweig-Lipson S, Beyer CE, Hughes ZA, et al: Differentiating antidepressants of the future: efficacy and safety. Pharmacol Ther 113:134–153, 2007

Rothrock JF: Clinical studies of valproate for migraine prophylaxis. Cephalalgia 17:81–83, 1997

Rowbotham MC: Pharmacologic management of complex regional pain syndrome. Clin J Pain 22:425–429, 2006

Rowbotham MC, Goli V, Kunz NR, et al: Venlafaxine extended release in the treatment of painful neuropathy: a double-blind, placebo-controlled study. Pain 110:697–706, 2004

Saarto T, Wiffen PJ: Antidepressants for neuropathic pain. Cochrane Database Syst Rev (4):CD005454, 2007

Sandercock D, Cramer M, Wu J, et al: Gabapentin extended release for the treatment of painful diabetic peripheral neuropathy: efficacy and tolerability in a double-blind, randomized, controlled clinical trial. Diabetes Care 32:e20, 2009

Sanders SH, Harden RN, Vicente PJ: Evidence-based clinical practice guidelines for interdisciplinary rehabilitation of chronic nonmalignant pain syndrome patients. Pain Pract 5:303–315, 2005

Sandoval JA, Furlan AD, Mailis-Gagnon A: Oral methadone for chronic noncancer pain: a systematic literature review of reasons for administration, prescription patterns, effectiveness, and side effects. Clin J Pain 21:503–512, 2005

Sawynok J: GABAergic mechanisms of analgesia: an update. Pharmacol Biochem Behav 26:463–474, 1987

Schade V, Semmer N, Main CJ, et al: The impact of clinical, morphological, psychosocial and work-related factors on the outcome of lumbar diskectomy. Pain 80:239–249, 1999

Schestatsky P, Jumru H, Valls-Sole J, et al: Neurophysiologic study of central pain in patients with Parkinson disease. Neurology 69:2162–2169, 2007

Schieir O, Thombs BD, Hudson M, et al: Symptoms of depression predict the trajectory of pain among patients with early inflammatory arthritis: a path analysis approach to assessing change. J Rheumatol 36:231–239, 2009

Schley MT, Wilms P, Toepfner S, et al: Painful and nonpainful phantom and stump sensations in acute traumatic amputees. J Trauma 65:858–864, 2008

Schmidt NB, Santiago HT, Trakowski JH, et al: Pain in patients with panic disorder: relation to symptoms, cognitive characteristics and treatment outcome. Pain Res Manag 7:134–141, 2002

Scudds RJ, McD Robertson J: Empirical evidence of the association between the presence of musculoskeletal pain and physical disability in community-dwelling senior citizens. Pain 75:229–235, 1998

Seidel S, Aigner M, Ossege M, et al: Antipsychotics for acute and chronic pain in adults. Cochrane Database Syst Rev (4): CD004844, 2008

Semenchuk MR, Sherman S, Davis B: Double-blind, randomized trial of bupropion SR for the treatment of neuropathic pain. Neurology 57:1583–1588, 2001

Sharma A, Williams K, Raja SN: Advances in treatment of complex regional pain syndrome: recent insights on a perplexing disease. Curr Opin Anaesthesiol 19:566–572, 2006

Sharma A, Agarwal S, Broatch J, et al: A web-based cross-sectional epidemiological survey of complex regional pain syndrome. Reg Anesth Pain Med 34:110–115, 2009

Sherman JJ, Turk DC, Okifuji A: Prevalence and impact of posttraumatic stress disorder-like symptoms on patients with fibromyalgia syndrome. Clin J Pain 16:127–134, 2000

Shimodozono M, Kawhira K, Kamishita T, et al: Reduction of central poststroke pain with the selective serotonin reuptake inhibitor fluvoxamine. Int J Neurosci 112:1173–1181, 2002

Silberstein SD: Treatment recommendations for migraine. Nat Clin Pract Neurol 4:482–489, 2008

Silberstein SD, Peres MF, Hopkins MM, et al: Olanzapine in the treatment of refractory migraine and chronic daily headache. Headache 42:515–518, 2002

Silberstein SD, Hulihan J, Karim MR, et al: Efficacy and tolerability of topiramate 200 mg/d in the prevention of migraine with/without aura in adults: a randomized, placebo controlled, double-blind, 12-week pilot study. Clin Ther 28:1002–1011, 2006

Silberstein S, Loder E, Diamond S, et al: Probable migraine in the United States: results of the American Migraine Prevalence and Prevention (AMPP) study. Cephalalgia 27:220–234, 2007

Simon GE, VonKorff M, Piccinelli M, et al: An international study of the relation between somatic symptoms and depression. N Engl J Med 341:1329–1335, 1999

Sindrup SH, Jensen TS: Pharmacotherapy of trigeminal neuralgia. Clin J Pain 18:22–27, 2002

Smedstad LM, Vaglum P, Kvien TK, et al: The relationship between self-reported pain and sociodemographic variables, anxiety, and depressive symptoms in rheumatoid arthritis. J Rheumatol 22:514–520, 1995

Smith MT: Neuroexcitatory effects of morphine and hydromorphone: evidence implicating the 3-glucuronide metabolites. Clin Exp Pharmacol 27:524–528, 2000

Solaro C, Messmer UM, Uccelli A, et al: Low-dose gabapentin combined with either lamotrigine or carbamazepine can be useful therapies for trigeminal neuralgia in multiple sclerosis. Eur Neurol 44:45–48, 2000

Solberg Nes L, Roach AR, Segerstrom SC: Executive functions, self-regulation, and chronic pain: a review. Ann Behav Med 37:173–183, 2009

Spyropoulou AC, Papageorgiou C, Markopoulos C, et al: Depressive symptomatology correlated with phantom breast syndrome in mastectomized women. Eur Arch Psychiatry Clin Neurosci 258:165–170, 2008

Stacey BR, Barrett JA, Whalen E, et al: Pregabalin for postherpetic neuralgia: placebo-controlled trial of fixed and flexible dosing regimens on allodynia and time to onset of pain relief. J Pain 9:1006–1017, 2008

Stack K, Cortina J, Samples C, et al: Race, age, and back pain as factors in completion of residential substance abuse treatment by veterans. Psychiatr Serv 51:1157–1161, 2000

Staiger TO, Gaster B, Sullivan MD, et al: Systematic review of antidepressants in the treatment of chronic low back pain. Spine 28:2540–2545, 2003

Stanos S, Houle TT: Multidisciplinary and interdisciplinary management of chronic pain. Phys Med Rehabil Clin N Am 17:435–450, 2006

Stefan H, Feuerstein TJ: Novel anticonvulsant drugs. Pharmacol Ther 113:165–183, 2007

Stewart WF, Ricci JA, Chee E, et al: Lost productive time and cost due to common pain conditions in the US workforce. JAMA 290:2443–2454, 2003

Streltzer J, Eliashof BA, Kline AE, et al: Chronic pain disorder following physical injury. Psychosomatics 41:227–234, 2000

Sullivan MJ, Reesor K, Mikail S, et al: The treatment of depression in chronic low back pain: review and recommendations. Pain 50:5–13, 1992

Sullivan MJ, Thorn B, Haythornthwaite JA, et al: Theoretical perspectives on the relation between catastrophizing and pain. Clin J Pain 17:52–64, 2001

Tack J, Broekaert D, Fischler B, et al: A controlled crossover study of the selective serotonin reuptake inhibitor citalopram in irritable bowel syndrome. Gut 55:1095–1103, 2006

Tanabe M, Takasu K, Takeuchi Y, et al: Pain relief by gabapentin and pregabalin via supraspinal mechanisms after peripheral nerve injury. J Neurosci Res 86:3258–3264, 2008

Tanelian DL, Victory RA: Sodium channel-blocking agents: their use in neuropathic pain conditions. Pain Forum 4:75–80, 1995

Taricco M, Adone R, Pagliacci C, et al: Pharmacological interventions for spasticity following spinal cord injury. Cochrane Database Syst Rev (2):CD001131, 2000

Tarride JE, Gordon A, Vera-Llonch M, et al: Cost-effectiveness of pregabalin for the management of neuropathic pain associated with diabetic peripheral neuropathy and postherpetic neuralgia: a Canadian perspective. Clin Ther 28:1922–1934, 2006

Tasmuth T, Hartel B, Kalso E: Venlafaxine in neuropathic pain following treatment of breast cancer. Eur J Pain 6:17–24, 2002

Tassinari D, Sartori S, Tamburini E, et al: Adverse effects of transdermal opiates treating moderate-severe cancer pain in comparison to long-acting morphine: a meta-analysis and systematic review of the literature. J Palliat Med 11:492–501, 2008

Tassone DM, Boyce E, Guyer J, et al: Pregabalin: a novel gamma-aminobutyric acid analogue in the treatment of neuropathic pain, partial-onset seizures, and anxiety disorders. Clin Ther 29:26–48, 2007

Tavakoli M, Malik RA: Management of painful diabetic neuropathy. Expert Opin Pharmacother 9:2969–2978, 2008

Taylor CP, Angelotti T, Fauman E: Pharmacology and mechanism of action of pregabalin: the calcium channel alpha2-delta subunit as a target for antiepileptic drug discovery. Epilepsy Res 73:137–150, 2007

ter Riet G, de Craen AJ, de Boer A, et al: Is placebo analgesia mediated by endogenous opioids? A systematic review. Pain 76:273–275, 1998

Todorov AA, Kolchev CB, Todorov AB: Tiagabine and gabapentin for the management of chronic pain. Clin J Pain 21:358–361, 2005

Tomlinson DR, Gardiner NJ: Diabetic neuropathies: components of etiology. J Peripher Nerv Syst 13:112–121, 2008

Trief PM, Grant W, Fredrickson B: A prospective study of psychological predictors of lumbar surgery outcome. Spine 25:2616–2621, 2000

Truini A, Galeotti F, Haanpaa M, et al: Pathophysiology of pain in postherpetic neuralgia: a clinical and neurophysiological study. Pain 140:405–410, 2008

Turk DC, Matyas TA: Pain-related behaviors: communication of pain. Am Pain Soc J 1:109–111, 1992

Turk DC, Okifuji A: What features affect physicians' decisions to prescribe opioids for chronic noncancer pain patients? Clin J Pain 13:330–336, 1997

Turk DC, Swanson KS, Tunks ER: Psychological approaches in the treatment of chronic pain patients—when pills, scalpels, and needles are not enough. Can J Psychiatry 53:213–223, 2008

Turner JA, Deyo RA, Loeser JD, et al: The importance of placebo effects in pain treatment and research. JAMA 271:1609–1614, 1994

Turner JA, Holtzman S, Mancl L: Mediators, moderators, and predictors of therapeutic change in cognitive-behavioral therapy for chronic pain. Pain 127:197–198, 2007

Tzellos TG, Papazisis G, Amaniti E, et al: Efficacy of pregabalin and gabapentin for neuropathic pain in spinal-cord injury: an evidence-based evaluation of the literature. Eur J Clin Pharmacol 64:851–858, 2008

Ullrich PM: Pain following spinal cord injury. Phys Med Rehabil Clin N Am 18:217–233, 2007

Valet M, Gundel H, Sprenger T, et al: Patients with pain disorder show gray-matter loss in pain-processing structures: a voxel-based morphometric study. Psychosom Med 71:49–56, 2009

Van Passel L, Arif H, Hirsch LJ: Topiramate for the treatment of epilepsy and other nervous system disorders. Expert Rev Neurother 6:19–31, 2006

van Tulder MW, Ostelo R, Vlaeyen JW, et al: Behavioral treatment for chronic low back pain: a systematic review within the framework of the Cochrane Back Review Group. Spine 26:270–281, 2001

Van Wilgen CP, Dijkstra PU, Versteegen GJ, et al: Chronic pain and severe disuse syndrome: long-term outcome of an inpatient multidisciplinary cognitive behavioural programme. J Rehabil Med 41:122–128, 2009

Vase L, Riley JL 3rd, Price DD: A comparison of placebo effects in clinical analgesic trials versus studies of placebo analgesia. Pain 99:443–452, 2002

Verbunt JA, Seelen HA, Vlaeyen JW, et al: Disuse and deconditioning in chronic low back pain: concepts and hypotheses on contributing mechanisms. Eur J Pain 7:9–21, 2003

Verdu B, Decosterd I, Buclin T, et al: Antidepressants for the treatment of chronic pain. Drugs 68:2611–2632, 2008

Veves A, Backonja M, Malik RA: Painful diabetic neuropathy: epidemiology, natural history, early diagnosis, and treatment options. Pain Med 9:660–674, 2008

Vinik AI, Tuchman M, Safirstein B, et al: Lamotrigine for treatment of pain associated with diabetic neuropathy: results of two randomized, double-blind, placebo-controlled studies. Pain 128:169–179, 2007

Volpi A, Gatti A, Pica F, et al: Clinical and psychosocial correlates of post-herpetic neuralgia. J Med Virol 80:1646–1652, 2008

Vorobeychik Y, Chen L, Bush MC, et al: Improved opioid analgesic effect following opioid dose reduction. Pain Med 9:724–727, 2008

Vowles KE, Gross RT: Work-related beliefs about injury and physical capability for work in individuals with chronic pain. Pain 101:291–298, 2003

Vowles KE, McCracken LM, Eccleston C: Processes of change in treatment for chronic pain: the contributions of pain, acceptance, and catastrophizing. Eur J Pain 11:779–787, 2007

Vowles KE, McCracken LM, Eccleston C: Patient functioning and catastrophizing in chronic pain: the mediating effects of acceptance. Health Psychol 27 (2 suppl):S136–S143, 2008

Vuckovic SM, Tomic MA, Stepanovic-Petrovic RM, et al: The effects of alpha2-adrenoceptor agents on anti-hyperalgesic effects of carbamazepine and oxcarbazepine in a rat model of inflammatory pain. Pain 125:10–19, 2006

Waddell G, Newton M, Henderson I, et al: A fear-avoidance beliefs questionnaire (FABQ) and the role of fear-avoidance beliefs in chronic low back pain and disability. Pain 52:157–168, 1993

Wang SJ, Fuh JL, Lu SR, et al: Quality of life differs among headache diagnoses: analysis of SF-36 survey in 901 headache patients. Pain 89:285–292, 2001

Waxman R, Tennant A, Helliwell P: Community survey of factors associated with consultation for low back pain. BMJ 317:1564–1567, 1998

Wernicke JF, Pritchett YL, D'Souza DN, et al: A randomized controlled trial of duloxetine in diabetic peripheral neuropathic pain. Neurology 67:1411–1420, 2006

Wiffen PJ, Rees J: Lamotrigine for acute and chronic pain. Cochrane Database Syst Rev (2):CD006044, 2007

Wood PB: Role of central dopamine in pain and analgesia. Expert Rev Neurother 8:781–797, 2008

Wood PB, Schweinhardt P, Jaeger E, et al: Fibromyalgia patients show an abnormal dopamine response to pain. Eur J Neurosci 25:3576–3582, 2007

Wu CL, Agarwal S, Tella PK, et al: Morphine versus mexiletine for treatment of postamputation pain: a randomized, placebo-controlled, crossover trial. Anesthesiology 109:289–296, 2008

Yucel A, Ozyalcin S, Koknel TG, et al: The effect of venlafaxine on ongoing and experimentally induced pain in neuropathic pain patients: a double blind, placebo controlled study. Eur J Pain 9:407–416, 2005

Zakrzewska JM: Diagnosis and differential diagnosis of trigeminal neuralgia. Clin J Pain 18:14–21, 2002

Ziegler D, Pritchett YL, Wang F, et al: Impact of disease characteristics on the efficacy of duloxetine in diabetic peripheral neuropathic pain. Diabetes Care 30:664–669, 2007

Zin CS, Nissen LM, Smith MT, et al: An update on the pharmacological management of post-herpetic neuralgia and painful diabetic neuropathy. CNS Drugs 22:417–442, 2008

Zochodne DW: Diabetic polyneuropathy: an update. Curr Opin Neurol 21:527–533, 2008

CHAPTER

37

Medical Toxicology

J. J. Rasimas, M.D., Ph.D.

TOXICOLOGY IS THE CLINICAL SPECIALTY dedicated to caring for illnesses induced by exposure to exogenous compounds. At the intersection of psychiatry and toxicology are several types of conditions, including deliberate overdoses, surreptitious ingestions, accidental poisonings, environmental or occupational exposures to toxins causing neuropsychiatric symptoms, delirium, adverse drug reactions and interactions, and illnesses that represent feared or imagined toxic exposures. Formal toxicology education in the training of psychiatrists is rare (Ingels et al. 2003). This chapter focuses on the presentation, evaluation, and treatment of toxicology patients with particular relevance to psychiatric practice.

As observed by Paracelsus, the first scientist of toxicology, any substance can be a medicine or a poison, depending upon the dose (Deichmann et al. 1986). With very few exceptions, minimal exposures rarely produce progressive or persistent deficits. The level of medical acuity in toxic exposures can vary widely. The effects of toxins may be delayed after exposure, abruptly appearing and progressing. This means that a diagnosis of poisoning may not be obvious upon initial presentation, and seemingly stable patients may suddenly deteriorate and succumb to seizures, arrhythmias, or refractory hypotension (Donovan et al. 2005). Therefore, psychiatrists need to know enough toxicology to make their own assessments, rather than always relying upon another physician's determination that a patient is "medically clear."

Since the brain is the organ most commonly affected by acute poisoning, any patient whose behavior, level of consciousness, or cognition is acutely disturbed should prompt concerns about toxicity (Flomenbaum et al. 2006; Maldonado 2008). Barriers to recognition of a toxic exposure include lack of awareness, deception by patients after intentional ingestion, physicians' failure to consider iatrogenic toxicity, and manifestations of the toxic exposure itself. The most important diagnostic factor in uncovering a toxic etiology is the clinician's consideration of its possibility.

Toxicology in Psychiatric Practice

The psychosomatic medicine physician is likely to encounter three categories of patients with possible toxic exposures, requiring different approaches:

1. The acutely presenting toxic patient, most often with a purposeful ingestion (the suicidal patient)
2. The neurobehaviorally disturbed hospital patient, sometimes with a mental illness history, whose symptoms may be toxically mediated
3. The subacutely or chronically afflicted outpatient about whom there is a question of toxin exposure versus somatoform illness

Nearly 20% of Americans who die by their own hand accomplish suicide by ingesting toxic substances (Miniño et al. 2007). If an individual remains acutely suicidal after an overdose, the medical setting must be a secure environment with close observation. A patient whose intentional ingestion does not result in a substantial change in mental status and/or level of consciousness may be at high risk due to ongoing self-injurious urges from unmodulated psychiatric distress. Repeat deliberate self-poisoning is quite common after an index medical encounter has ended; 4.5% of overdose patients present to the hospital again within a month, 10% within 6 months, and 14% within 1 year (Carter et al. 1999). In addition, prospective longitudinal research suggests that mortality rates specific to suicide in those with an episode of deliberate self-poisoning are over 10% within 10 years (Nordentoft et al. 1993). General principles in the psychiatric management of the suicidal patient in medical settings are discussed in Chapter 9, "Suicidality."

A number of studies have highlighted the unreliability of patients' reports regarding the identities and amounts of what they ingest in overdose, although stated times of ingestion are typically more accurate and can help to guide management (Pohjola-Sintonen et al. 2000). Cognitive disorders can introduce additional complications, increasing the risk for medication errors that may lead to self-poisoning (irrespective of intent) and interfering with communication of a reliable history to inform toxicological care. The subjective data in any case must therefore always be considered in light of the vital signs, objective physical findings, and laboratory results, all of which more accurately tell the tale of pharmacological misadventure. A short period of observation for a minimally symptomatic patient may be sufficient, but some substances—including extended-release, anticholinergic, and opioid medications—can produce delayed and/or prolonged toxicity.

Physical Examination

Clues evident on physical examination can be particularly helpful in identifying possible overdose or toxin exposure. The most common early presentations of drug toxicity involve gastrointestinal tract symptoms and central/autonomic nervous system effects. Withdrawal states manifest in these physiological systems as well—opioids with a clear-thinking, self-limited though uncomfortable syndrome and alcohol or sedatives with potentially life-threatening hemodynamic changes and delirium. Nystagmus is a nonspecific physical finding, but its new onset strongly suggests a toxic process. Although much attention is paid to examination of the pupils, size and reactivity are highly variable, except in opioid toxicity when they are almost always miotic. Cutaneous abnormalities may suggest specific toxins or indicate intravenous drug use. Unusual odors of the patient's breath, skin, clothing, vomitus, or nasogastric aspirate may also provide useful diagnostic clues (Table 37–1) (Goldfrank et al. 1992). The absence of such odors, however, should not be taken as evidence that suspected agents are not present.

Laboratory Testing

Patients in whom purposeful ingestion is suspected or known will frequently have specific testing for acetaminophen and salicylate levels, because these are readily available, potentially lethal, frequently coingested drugs with nonspecific clinical presentations, and test results can be obtained rapidly to guide management (Hepler et al. 1986). Many other serum levels can be ordered, but intervention is typically required well before the results of quantitative testing become available (Boehnert and Lovejoy 1985).

Abnormalities in conventional laboratory tests such as electrolytes, renal functions, and blood gas analysis can point to specific ingestions. Metabolic acidosis with an increased anion gap suggests the ingestion of methanol, ethylene glycol, paraldehyde, toluene, iron, isoniazid, nonsteroidal anti-inflammatory drugs (NSAIDs), or salicylates. The latter often produces a mixed acid–base picture, with

TABLE 37–1. Selected odors from toxic exposures

Characteristic odor	Possible intoxicant
Bitter almonds/sweaty locker room	Cyanide
Burned rope	Cannabis, opium
Carrots	Water hemlock (cicutoxin)
Fruity	Ethanol, acetone, isopropyl alcohol, paraldehyde, nitrites, chlorinated hydrocarbons (e.g., chloroform)
Garlic	Arsenic, dimethyl sulfoxide (DMSO), organophosphates, white phosphorus, selenium, thallium
Glue	Toluene, organic solvents
Mothballs	Paradichlorobenzene, naphthalene, camphor
Acrid/pearlike	Chloral hydrate, paraldehyde
Violets	Turpentine (metabolites in the urine)
Rotten eggs	Disulfiram, hydrogen sulfide, sulfa drugs, stibine
Shoe polish	Nitrobenzene
Wintergreen	Methyl salicylate

coexisting respiratory alkalosis, as well. An elevated measured serum osmolarity compared with a calculated osmolarity (i.e., osmolar gap) indicates the presence of low-molecular-weight osmotically active compounds, such as ethylene glycol, methanol, and isopropanol. Hypoglycemia is common in patients poisoned with these toxic alcohols and by isoniazid, acetaminophen, salicylates, propranolol, valproic acid, and sulfonylureas. Serum aminotransferase levels are useful, since they will be elevated in most cases of hepatotoxicity caused by medications; and liver function is crucial in the metabolism of so many compounds. Rhabdomyolysis, indicated by elevated serum creatine phosphokinase and myoglobinuria, may be due to prolonged immobility after any overdose with central nervous system (CNS) depressive effects, but it is also caused directly by compounds that produce muscle rigidity and/or seizures (e.g., strychnine, antipsychotics, antidepressants, lithium, stimulants).

Decreased oxygen saturation of hemoglobin with a normal or increased arterial oxygen partial pressure is found in patients with carbon monoxide poisoning or in methemoglobinemia, which can be caused by metoclopramide, phenacetin, nitroglycerin, topical anesthetics, and some antimicrobials like dapsone. Noncardiogenic pulmonary edema on a chest radiograph suggests opioid or salicylate toxicity. Some drugs are radiopaque (e.g., heavy metals, phenothiazines, potassium, calcium, chlorinated hydrocarbons) and can occasionally be visualized within the gastrointestinal tract on roentgenography, but abdominal X rays are rarely helpful in the evaluation of a poisoned patient except to monitor the decontamination of metals or body packets (Craig 2001).

Toxicological Testing

In some cases, a detailed history, physical examination, and targeted laboratory studies still leave the specifics of a poisoning concealed. Toxicology testing may be helpful in confirming the clinical diagnosis. However, identifying all available toxins with a high degree of specificity and sensitivity is impossible due to limitations of time and expense. Instead, drug screening is sometimes performed. Standard urine drug screening is conducted using immunoassay techniques, offering the advantage of rapid turnaround time with detection of some commonly used and abused compounds. Urine screening utility is limited by relatively high false-negative and false-positive rates.

Comprehensive toxicology screening detects a wide range of analgesics, narcotics, psychotropics, and various other drugs, also by immunoassay, but takes time to complete. Available tests vary between and among institutions. The best chance to detect an unknown toxin is usually via assay of the urine where drugs are excreted in concentrated form; testing concurrently drawn blood can be useful for quantitation to correlate drug levels with the clinical picture. It is important to note that negative results of comprehensive testing do not rule out a toxic state, because even many commonly ingested agents cannot be assayed and because the gathering of bodily fluids may be mistimed. Even true-positive tests can be misleading, since drugs found on screening may not be those responsible for the patient's symptoms (Donovan et al. 2005; Montague et al. 2001). Substances with a large volume of distribution and/or high fat solubility can be detected in urine for a long time after the last dose, but the clinical presentation may not be the result of those compounds. The history and physical examination (including an account of all available and administered medications before and during hospitalization) are therefore far more important in the acute management of drug toxicity than is a comprehensive drug screen (Pohjola-Sintonen et al. 2000). Toxicology screening may in fact be more useful in the outpatient setting when chronic exposure is suspected and symptoms are less severe, rather than in the acute hospital where the demand for intervention does not allow time for assay (Rainey 2006).

Principles of Acute Exposure Management

The three main goals in the acute phase of toxicological treatment are preventing further drug absorption, providing antidotal therapy, and hastening the elimination of an absorbed poison. Sometimes, toxic effects on patients' behavior can interfere with these goals. Rapid sedation with benzodiazepines can protect against injury, prevent seizures, and allow vital medical interventions to proceed. Antipsychotics are effective as well (Battaglia 2005), but their potential for more adverse effects or interactions with unknown ingestants (e.g., precipitation of seizures, induction of arrhythmias) requires caution in their use (Martel et al. 2005; Olson 2007). If information is available to confirm the specifics of the poisoning and if comorbid conditions and/or toxicities do not preclude its safe use, direct antidote therapy should be instituted immediately. A list of antidotes for selected known exposures is provided in Table 37-2. Guidance from a medical toxicologist or poison control is needed regarding these therapies, since their use is not required in all cases, and some carry risk of adverse effects. Poison control centers and medical toxicologists can provide specific recommendations, especially for more esoteric or unfamiliar poisons and for management of multidrug ingestions with complex clinical courses.

Except for specific lifesaving antidotes against certain toxins, many poisoned patients require only recognition

TABLE 37–2. Emergency antidotes for selected ingestions

Toxin	Antidote
Acetaminophen	*N*-acetylcysteine (NAC)
Anticholinergics	Physostigmine
Benzodiazepines and nonbenzodiazepine hypnotics	Flumazenil
Beta-adrenergic blockers	Glucagon
Calcium channel blockers	Calcium, insulin + glucose
Cyanide, hydrogen sulfide	Sodium thiosulfate, hydroxocobalamin
Digitalis glycosides	Digoxin immune fab
Ethylene glycol, methanol	Fomepizole (preferred over ethanol)
Iron	Deferoxamine
Lead	Dimercaprol (BAL), calcium disodium versanate ($CaNa_2EDTA$), succimer (DMSA)
Opioids, $alpha_2$ agonists	Naloxone, nalmefene
Organophosphates and carbamates	Atropine, pralidoxime
Sulfonylureas	Octreotide
Valproic acid	L-Carnitine

Note. BAL=British anti-Lewisite (2,3-dimercaptopropanol); DMSA=dimercaptosuccinic acid; EDTA=ethylenediaminetetraacetic acid.

and removal of the offending agent with supportive therapy. A standard historical home remedy was gastric emptying by induction of emesis with ipecac. However, ipecac can sensitize the myocardium to arrhythmogenic effects of other ingested substances and also perpetuate bulimic behavior, so it is no longer recommended (American Academy of Pediatrics 2003). Inducing emesis does not improve toxin retrieval significantly when used in the emergency department and may delay the effective use of more beneficial treatments such as activated charcoal and specific antidotes (Kulig et al. 1985).

Activated charcoal minimizes the gastrointestinal absorption of many toxins by adsorptive binding, producing better toxin recovery and fewer complications than emesis or gastric lavage. Therefore, it should be considered as the primary means of decontamination in most overdoses (Albertson et al. 1989). It is not recommended for ingestions of agents that do not adsorb to charcoal, including ions, solvents, alcohols, and most metals (Table 37–3).

TABLE 37–3. Toxins poorly adsorbed by activated charcoal

Ethanol, methanol, isopropanol, ethylene glycol
Acids
Alkalis
Hydrocarbons
Lithium
Iron
Heavy metals
Cyanide
Borates
Bromides

Activated charcoal may be beneficial if given early after an ingestion (most effective within an hour) or for drugs that have delayed absorption, including aspirin, anticholinergics, opioids, sustained-release medications, or drug packets in "body stuffers." For patients who present hours after ingestion, charcoal is usually ineffective. Furthermore, charcoal aspiration can occur, causing bronchospasm and pneumonitis (Givens et al. 1992). Its use should therefore be limited to conscious patients with an intact gag reflex, unless airway protection is insured via intubation before nasogastric administration in obtunded patients (Chyka et al. 2005). Activated charcoal in multiple doses enhances the serum clearance of certain medications

(Table 37–4), taking advantage of enterohepatic recirculation and adsorption of drugs across the gastrointestinal mucosa (Howland 2006).

Gastric decontamination does not generally improve outcomes in overdose patients, even though it is frequently performed (Bond 2002). Whole-bowel irrigation with a polyethylene glycol solution may be useful in certain cases of massive, recent ingestion of medications with sustained release and delayed absorption, such as some calcium channel antagonists and enteric-coated aspirin. It can aid in the clearance of other toxins, like lead or lithium, which are not well adsorbed by activated charcoal. Whole-bowel irrigation has also been used to aid in the evacuation of large pill fragments and drug packets from "body packers" (Tenenbein 1997).

Gastric lavage with the aim of removing unabsorbed compounds is rarely indicated and should be considered only when a patient is seen less than an hour after ingesting a highly toxic substance (e.g., calcium channel blocker, tricyclic antidepressant [TCA]) and/or one that delays gastric emptying (e.g., opioid, anticholinergic) or forms concretions (Vale and Kulig 2004). It is contraindicated in alkali ingestions because of the increased risk for esophageal perforation. Some studies have shown an increase in adverse outcomes with the use of gastric lavage, including aspiration pneumonitis and prolonged intensive care (Merigian et al. 1990). Given the uncertain benefits of gastric lavage, patients who are otherwise asymptomatic should not be sedated and intubated for the sole purpose of performing this procedure (Vale and Kulig 2004). In general, decontamination procedures should only be used when an ingestion is recent and potentially life-threatening and when such procedures can be performed without undue risk.

For enhancing the elimination of an absorbed poison, the available procedures that have the greatest value are manipulation of urine pH, dialysis, and hemoperfusion. These methods, too, should be used only when the danger of the persisting poison likely exceeds that of removing it and when the method is known to be effective for that toxin.

For alteration of urinary pH to be effective in hastening elimination, the toxin must be excreted primarily by the kidneys. Diuresis does little to clear compounds that are highly protein-bound, highly lipid-soluble, or hepatically excreted. Alkalinization of the urine enhances excretion of weak acid compounds ($3.0<pK<7.2$), aspirin and phenobarbital being the most commonly overdosed drugs in this category. Elevation of urine pH is accomplished by adding sodium bicarbonate to intravenous fluids. In theory, weak bases ($7.2<pK<9.8$) like phencyclidine and amphetamine can be eliminated more rapidly in acidified urine, but this course is almost never recommended. Acidosis (metabolic or respiratory) frequently accompanies severe overdoses, and therefore treatment with acidifying compounds risks worsening the clinical course (Olson 2007), especially in patients with underlying kidney or liver disease (Fortenberry and Mariscalco 2006).

TABLE 37–4. Toxins with enhanced elimination by multiple-dose activated charcoal

Valproic acid and other anticonvulsants (phenobarbital, carbamazepine, phenytoin)
Salicylates
Theophylline, aminophylline
Digoxin, digitoxin
Cyclosporine
Quinine
Tricyclic antidepressants
Phenothiazines

In the setting of impaired renal function or overwhelming intoxication, hemodialysis or hemoperfusion may effectively remove drugs that are poorly protein-bound, are highly water-soluble, and have a low volume of distribution (Table 37–5). Lithium ions and small molecules such as methanol, ethylene glycol, salicylates, and phenobarbital rapidly diffuse across synthetic membranes and are therefore removed effectively by hemodialysis. Hypotension, hemolysis, hypoxemia, and arrhythmias can result from the procedure.

Hemoperfusion has been shown to be a very effective method of extracting some drugs, including barbiturates, TCAs, theophylline, and aspirin. The facilities and skills necessary for hemoperfusion are essentially the same as those needed to perform hemodialysis. Complications include hypotension, thrombocytopenia, hypothermia, and hypocalcemia (Cutler et al. 1987); these risks often outweigh therapeutic benefits of the procedure.

TABLE 37–5. Selected toxins with enhanced elimination by extracorporeal techniques

Ethanol, isopropanol, methanol, ethylene glycol
Lithium
Salicylates
Theophylline
Acetaminophen
Chloral hydrate
Some anticonvulsants (phenobarbital, carbamazepine, valproic acid, phenytoin)

Overdoses and Toxic Exposures

What follows is a survey of common overdoses and exposures not primarily involving psychotropic compounds; the reader is referred to Chapters 38 ("Psychopharmacology") and 17 ("Substance-Related Disorders") and to the "Toxidromes" section later in this chapter for information regarding psychotropic medication and illicit drug toxicities.

Acetaminophen

Acetaminophen is the pharmaceutical most frequently involved in overdose, both readily available and potentially lethal. Of the 2,054 reported deaths resulting from pharmaceutical substances in 2003, 327 (16%) were attributed to acetaminophen either singly or in combination with other agents (Watson et al. 2004). Over half of the cases of toxicity are reported in patients under 20 years of age, but very few deaths occur in children. Accidental poisoning is more common in young children and in the elderly, whereas almost all adolescents and adults with acute acetaminophen toxicity have intentionally harmed themselves. An acute overdose of as little as 15 g can cause toxicity in adults, and a single ingestion of 200 mg/kg can bring serious harm to children. The analgesic is regularly sold in amounts far in excess of these thresholds. In 1998, the United Kingdom took measures to limit its nonprescription availability, and since the requirement for limited sale of acetaminophen (there, paracetamol) in small blister packs, severity of overdoses and liver transplant rates secondary to overdose have fallen (Hawkins et al. 2007).

Hepatotoxicity is the primary concern and the target for medical intervention. Following oral ingestion, approximately 94% of the drug is metabolized to the glucuronide or sulfate conjugate, and about 2% is excreted unchanged in the urine. Neither the parent drug, nor the conjugated forms are hepatotoxic. The remaining 4%, however, is metabolized primarily through cytochrome P450 (CYP) 2E1 and, to some extent, CYP3A4, to form a toxic metabolite, *N*-acetyl-*p*-benzoquinone imine (NAPQI). After therapeutic dosing, any NAPQI formed is conjugated with normal hepatic stores of glutathione (GSH) to produce the nontoxic mercapturic acid, which is excreted in the urine. In the setting of a significant overdose, CYP2E1 metabolizes more acetaminophen, large amounts of NAPQI are formed, and the pool of GSH is rapidly depleted. Direct effects of excess NAPQI and liver failure can impact the function of other organ systems including kidneys, pancreas, and CNS.

Clinically, patients present with diaphoresis, nausea, vomiting, and malaise within 24 hours of acute ingestion. Despite evolving liver injury as reflected by elevations in hepatocellular enzymes and prolongation of prothrombin time, there can be a window of time when patients look and feel better. If they present for care at this stage, and clinicians fail to consider acetaminophen overdose because of the patient's benign appearance, the consequences can be fatal. Coagulation status declines and transaminase levels can exceed 10,000 IU/L before metabolic acidosis, jaundice, and encephalopathy herald fulminant hepatic failure.

Hence, it is vital to quickly identify patients with significant acetaminophen overdose and institute the antidote *N*-acetylcysteine (NAC) without delay. NAC repletes GSH stores to detoxify NAPQI and works as an antioxidant to prevent evolving toxicity until nondamaging metabolic pathways clear the parent drug. The need for treatment after a single overdose can be calculated based on a timed plasma acetaminophen level drawn at least 4 hours after ingestion (Rumack and Matthew 1975).

NAC can be administered either orally/intragastrically or intravenously. No studies have demonstrated the superiority of one particular route, but the intravenous route is more tolerable since the oral agent is highly distasteful and emetogenic (Perry and Shannon 1998). Furthermore, nearly 50% of patients have repetitive vomiting after a serious acetaminophen ingestion, so the intravenous route is certainly preferred to ensure delivery. For a patient who has ingested a potentially toxic amount of acetaminophen and in whom an acetaminophen level cannot be obtained within 8 hours after the ingestion, a loading dose of NAC should be administered immediately (Heard 2008). The same is true for cases of repeat or chronic overdosing. If the acetaminophen level then returns in the nontoxic range and transaminases are normal, the antidote is stopped. Even after 24 hours from the time of ingestion, late administration of NAC has been shown to be of some benefit and should not be withheld if there is evidence of hepatic injury (Tucker 1998). A pregnant woman should be administered a loading dose of NAC as soon as possible, regardless of the time since overdose, because potential exists for fetal toxicity after maternal overdose, and fetal demise has been correlated with treatment delay.

Poor prognostic factors generally relate to propensity of a given individual to produce more of the toxic acetaminophen metabolite or to be less able to withstand its oxidative effects. Advanced age, states of malnutrition (e.g., anorexia nervosa), and active liver disease predispose patients to greater toxicity. Obesity is correlated with higher levels of CYP2E1 activity. Chronic alcohol use also induces CYP2E1 and depletes GSH stores, thus increasing the possibility of a poorer outcome. Alcohol coingestion at the time of overdose, however, can be slightly protective, since ethanol competes with acetaminophen for CYP2E1, thus decreasing production of the toxic NAPQI.

Once NAC treatment is complete, if the patient is asymptomatic and transaminase levels and liver function tests return to normal, the patient can be discharged to the appropriate psychiatric disposition.

Salicylates

Toxicity from aspirin and other salicylates (found in literally hundreds of medicinal agents) is also a significant source of morbidity and mortality. Child-resistant packaging has decreased the incidence of aspirin ingestion in children, but intentional overdoses of this ubiquitous analgesic still result in adolescent and adult deaths. The diagnosis of salicylism is often delayed because its symptoms of fever, vomiting, and tachypnea may be attributed to the disease process for which the salicylate is used therapeutically.

Aspirin is absorbed rapidly from the upper small intestine under normal circumstances. In the setting of overdose, absorption is slowed, and salicylate serum concentrations can increase for more than 24 hours after ingestion. At therapeutic doses, most salicylate is bound to plasma proteins, but in overdose, the amount of non-protein-bound drug increases, which increases the potential for significant toxicity. Conditions that deplete albumin and other proteins (e.g., anorexia nervosa) predispose patients to a disproportionate risk of toxicity at a given plasma concentration (Alván et al. 1981). Salicylates are eliminated primarily through the kidneys via both glomerular filtration and tubular secretion.

The toxic pathophysiology of salicylism is complex. Acute overdose, particularly in children, produces nausea and vomiting, which can cause metabolic alkalosis. Metabolic acidosis subsequently results from several systemic effects of salicylates. Salicylates also produce hyperventilation secondary to direct stimulation of the CNS respiratory center leading to respiratory alkalosis; unexplained hyperpnea should raise suspicion for aspirin overdose and not merely be attributed to anxiety. The classic acid-base presentation is a mixed one of anion-gap metabolic acidosis with a slight alkalemia driven by respiratory alkalosis (Gabow et al. 1978). Severe dehydration, electrolyte disturbances, and significant glycemic shifts can occur with salicylate toxicity, as well.

The usual symptoms of acute toxicity include tinnitus, nausea, vomiting, dehydration, hyperpnea, hyperpyrexia, acute tubular necrosis, and oliguria, with progression to delirium, seizures, and coma. Other less common findings include bleeding, hemolysis, pulmonary edema, bronchospasm, and anaphylaxis. Reversible ototoxicity is directly related to unbound serum salicylate concentration. The onset of symptoms usually occurs within 1–2 hours of an acute ingestion, but may be delayed 4–6 hours due to sustained-release preparations, pylorospasm, or formation of gastric concretions.

There is no direct antidote for salicylates, so management is aimed at preventing further absorption and increasing elimination, including activated charcoal and fluid resuscitation with sodium bicarbonate solutions to promote alkaline diuresis (Proudfoot et al. 2004). Plasma salicylate levels should be drawn every 2 to 4 hours until they are clearly decreasing. In severe cases, hemodialysis should be considered. Most salicylate-poisoned patients survive with minimal sequelae (Stolbach et al. 2008).

Nonsteroidal Anti-Inflammatory Drugs

Although much less toxic than salicylates, other NSAIDs are even more widely used in nonprescription products and therefore more frequently encountered in recent cases of suicidal ingestion. Ibuprofen, naproxen, and ketoprofen exert both therapeutic and toxic effects through competitive, reversible inhibition of type I cyclooxygenase. Enzymatic selectivity with the type II cyclooxygenase inhibitors (celecoxib, meloxicam, rofecoxib, and valdecoxib) is lost at extremely high doses, so these agents can produce a similar toxic presentation in massive overdose.

After an acute ingestion, gastrointestinal distress in the form of epigastric pain, nausea, and vomiting is virtually always present, and its absence makes toxicity unlikely (Hall et al. 1988). Metabolic acidosis with an elevated anion gap is common. In very large overdoses, confusion and depressed level of consciousness with progression to seizures, coma, and death can result (Halpern et al. 1993). Activated charcoal effectively binds NSAIDs. In addition to supportive measures, aggressive intravenous fluid therapy is indicated to more rapidly eliminate the drug, resolve acidosis, and protect the kidneys from acute damage. Unless complications develop from CNS depression, most patients poisoned with NSAIDs survive without long-term consequences.

Carbon Monoxide

Carbon monoxide (CO) is a toxic gas that is essentially undetectable by human sensory modalities. Sources of exposure include automobile exhaust, smoke from fires, fuel stoves, and, to a lesser extent, cigarette smoke. Purposeful exposure to exhaust fumes or burning charcoal is a particularly lethal suicide method from which only a fraction of attempters are rescued. In fact, carbon monoxide is the leading cause of poisoning morbidity and mortality in the United States, with most events being the result of intentional acts involving car exhaust (Mott et al. 2002). The toxin binds to hemoglobin with 250 times greater affinity than oxygen, thereby markedly reducing tissue oxygen delivery. Most patients experience nausea, headache, and dizziness. Psychosis, depression, mutism, amnesia, and delirium have all been reported as presenting symptoms. Syncope and coma follow more severe exposures. Cardiovascular toxicity progresses from dyspnea and angina to hypotension, myocardial infarction, and potentially lethal arrhythmia.

When a patient is thwarted in the midst of a suicide attempt, CO poisoning may be obvious. With a mild presentation in the absence of such a history, diagnosis can be challenging. Very few patients actually display classic cherry-red skin; most appear "shocky" and gray. Routine blood gas analysis and pulse oximetry fail to identify poisoning despite profound systemic hypoxia. Serum carboxyhemoglobin concentration is diagnostic and helps to guide therapy; it should be assayed without delay in any overdose patient found in a vehicle. Treatment with 100% oxygen is critically important, as it helps to address hypoxia and enhance elimination of the toxic gas. Hyperbaric oxygenation further speeds elimination of CO and may produce better outcomes in more severely poisoned patients. Persistently altered mental status with poor visuospatial functioning and signs of ataxia and apraxia are the most important indicators of the need for hyperbaric treatment (Weaver 2009). The potential for in utero toxicity due to avid binding interactions between CO and fetal hemoglobin lowers the threshold for more aggressive oxygen therapy in pregnant patients.

Survivors of severe CO poisoning are likely to have residual deficits from hypoxic injury to the CNS. Neuroimaging can reveal cerebral atrophy, periventricular white matter changes, and low-density lesions in the basal ganglia (J.S. Brown 2002). Neuropsychiatric sequelae may be present in up to one-half of patients and range from mild memory and concentration deficits to mood and personality changes, parkinsonism, and dense encephalopathy (Asian et al. 2004; Ku et al. 2006; S.P. Lam et al. 2004). Patients have similar complaints after chronic exposure to low levels of carbon monoxide (Myers et al. 1998), but no studies have demonstrated objective neuropsychiatric effects in the absence of a severe, acute episode of poisoning.

Toxic Alcohols

A handful of liquids that are more acutely dangerous than ethanol are occasionally consumed as substitutes by severe alcoholics. Sometimes children are drawn to their attractive colors and/or sweet tastes. More frequently, however, these agents are ingested with suicidal intent. Ethylene glycol is the primary ingredient in antifreeze. Propylene glycol is also found in antifreeze and as a diluent in parenteral formulations of lorazepam, diazepam, esmolol, and other medications, making continuous infusions a potential source of toxicity (Zar et al. 2007). Windshield washer fluid and fuel additives contain methanol. Isopropanol is found in rubbing alcohol. Like ethanol, all of these compounds are rapidly absorbed after oral ingestion, and their metabolism depends upon alcohol dehydrogenase. It is the body's enzymatic handling of ethylene glycol, propylene glycol, and methanol that creates much of their toxicity.

The toxic alcohols produce an initial clinical presentation that is similar to ethanol, with slurred speech, ataxia, and CNS depression that can progress to stupor and coma in severe overdose. Because rapid breakdown by alcohol dehydrogenase produces organic acids from both methanol (formic acid) and ethylene glycol (glycolic and oxalic acids), metabolic acidosis with an elevated anion gap is a key finding. Isopropanol is metabolized to acetone, so the result of this ingestion is CNS depression and ketosis (along with the characteristic fruity breath odor) without significant acidosis. The parent compounds and some of their breakdown products are also osmotically active, so an osmolar gap is present. Acidosis and the direct toxic effects of the alcohols and their metabolites lead to end-organ damage with potentially lethal consequences, including nephrotoxicity with ethylene glycol, and blindness with methanol. Methanol also can cause necrotic damage to the putamen, the result being an irreversible movement disorder with symptoms similar to parkinsonism (Sefidbakht et al. 2007).

In addition to supportive care, the mainstay of toxic alcohol treatment is to inhibit metabolism while enhancing elimination. For years, the acute intervention was administration of ethanol to metabolically compete for alcohol dehydrogenase and slow the formation of toxic species from ethylene glycol and methanol. (Inhibiting metabolism of isopropanol only prolongs CNS effects without providing systemic protection from toxicity and is therefore not appropriate therapy in a rubbing alcohol overdose.) Continuous titrated infusion of ethanol to maintain serum concentrations between 100 and 150 mg/dL was the therapeutic goal (Barceloux et al. 1999, 2002). More recently, a synthetic inhibitor of alcohol dehydrogenase has become available. Fomepizole has a much higher affinity for the enzyme than does ethanol and, although more expensive, is preferred. It does not compound CNS depression induced by the original ingestion and also avoids other ethanol toxicities such as hepatitis and pancreatitis (Brent et al. 1999, 2001). Elimination of the toxic alcohols can then be effectively enhanced by hemodialysis if necessary. If any delay to advanced hospital treatment is anticipated, oral doses of ethanol can be temporizing and potentially lifesaving (Jacobsen and McMartin 1997). Supplementation with pyridoxine and thiamine after ethylene glycol ingestion, and folic or folinic acid after methanol ingestion, can also reduce production of toxic metabolites and support recovery.

Hydrocarbons and Inhalants

Like the toxic alcohols, hydrocarbons are found in commonly available products, most of them polishes, solvents, lubricants, and fuels. They are typically ingested orally in error by children and with suicidal intent by adults, but fatal outcomes are rare. Several hydrocarbons are abused as inhalants; sniffing, huffing, and bagging these agents are all intended to produce a euphoric high. Psychiatric consequences of intentional or unintentional inhalation of hydrocarbons include mood disorders (e.g., affective lability, irritability, depression, mania), psychosis, insomnia, amnesia, confusion, and bizarre/violent behavior. While purposeful solvent abuse was not documented until 1951, the history of accidental exposure with serious consequences is much older. In the nineteenth-century rubber industry, carbon disulfide toxicity induced mood and psychotic symptoms that resulted in suicides of factory workers (Hartman 1988). Neuropsychiatric impairment is a serious problem with other agents such as trichloroethylene, methyl chloride, toluene, ethylene oxide, propane, acetone, and nitrous oxide. However, the magnitude and duration of solvent exposure necessary to cause psychiatric problems remains controversial, as does the potential duration of CNS symptoms following cessation of use. Inhalant abusers have high rates of comorbid psychiatric disorders (Wu and Howard 2007). Many will show brain abnormalities on computed tomography (CT) or magnetic resonance imaging (MRI), including diffuse white matter changes, cerebral and cerebellar atrophy, callosal thinning, and damage to the basal ganglia (J.S. Brown 2002). After chronic abuse of sufficient dose and duration, such changes are frequently irreversible (Schaumberg 2000). Psychometric testing may delineate functional correlates for the anatomic pathology and help to guide rehabilitation (Filley et al. 1988). Neuropathies can also develop with chronic use and persist long after discontinuation. Large acute exposures may lead to ataxia, cranial nerve palsies, delirium, seizures, and coma. "Sudden sniffing death" can result from cardiac dysrhythmias, usually involving inhalation of fluorinated hydrocarbons (Kulig and Rumack 1981). The primary danger with oral ingestion of hydrocarbons and other solvents is aspiration, leading to chemical pneumonitis. Pneumonitis and associated respiratory compromise can occur merely with huffing, even when the solvent is not aspirated in liquid form.

The management of acute hydrocarbon ingestion is primarily symptomatic. Gastric emptying procedures should be avoided, as they increase the risk of aspiration. Activated charcoal is ineffective in hydrocarbon ingestion, and there are no specific antidotes. Care of patients with chronic toxicity involves rehabilitative therapies, chemical dependency intervention, targeted psychopharmacology, and neuropsychiatric reassessment.

Pesticides

Agents used to kill animal, plant, and fungal pests have the potential to cause significant acute and chronic toxicity in humans. They represent a variety of chemical classes with diverse mechanisms of action. In the United States exposures rarely cause death, but intentional ingestions of more toxic mixtures in Africa and the Indian subcontinent result in thousands of completed suicides every year (Gunnell et al. 2007). In the West, environmental toxicity causing more subtle, chronic somatic and neuropsychiatric manifestations is the major public health issue. Additionally, the use of some of these compounds in times of war has produced questions about whether they may have an etiological role in unexplained symptoms found in veterans (J.S. Brown 2007; see also "Gulf War Syndrome" later in this chapter). The following subsections focus on selected pesticides most relevant to psychiatrists.

Strychnine

Strychnine is an alkaloid botanical derivative that was once marketed for therapeutic uses, but is now commercially available only as a laboratory reagent and in products used to kill small mammals and birds. It is, however, a fairly common adulterant in illicit drugs such as heroin, ecstasy, and cocaine (O'Callaghan et al. 1982). Strychnine is occasionally employed with suicidal or homicidal intent. It has been found in some Chinese and Cambodian herbal medicines designed to treat rheumatism and gastrointestinal illness (Chan 2002; Katz et al. 1996). Strychnine toxicity causes rapid, widespread peripheral manifestations of neural excitation including nystagmus, hyperreflexia, and severe generalized painful skeletal muscle contraction, often resulting in hyperthermia, rhabdomyolysis, renal failure, tonic respiratory paralysis, and death.

The myoclonus, *risus sardonicus,* and opisthotonic posturing of strychnine toxicity may be mistaken for seizures. The differential diagnosis also includes tetanus, serotonin syndrome, neuroleptic malignant syndrome, stimulant toxicity, and drug-induced dystonia. Patients have both metabolic and respiratory acidosis, as well as myoglobinuria and elevated levels of creatine phosphokinase and serum aminotransferases. Activated charcoal can be useful early after an oral ingestion. Benzodiazepines and, in severe cases, nondepolarizing paralytics such as pancuronium are most effective for muscular hyperactivity (Smith 1990). Patients who survive strychnine poisoning do not generally have long-term physical sequelae, but posttraumatic stress disorder may be very common in light of the harrowing conscious experience of painful physical symptoms.

Insecticides

There are a number of insecticides that produce toxicity in man. Although resolution of even severe, acute exposure to many insecticides is expected to proceed without sequelae, chronic exposure is a well-documented source of morbidity that may be misattributed or remain medically unexplained. Case reports of low-level exposures suggest a range of chronic problems, including memory loss, peripheral neuropathy, and nonspecific dermatological findings (Roldan-Tapia et al. 2006).

Organophosphates are not only used to eliminate pests, but some (sarin, tabun, and soman) have also been used in chemical warfare. In rural areas of Taiwan, China, and India, purposeful ingestion of organophosphates leads to many deaths every year (Wei and Chua 2008). Accidental exposure on the farm or in the garden, particularly in children, is also a significant source of toxicity. Medication errors or overdoses with carbamates (e.g., pyridostigmine, neostigmine) pose a similar danger. These substances all exert their effects through inhibition of acetylcholinesterase, resulting in characteristic manifestations of excess cholinergic activity (discussed in the "Toxidromes" section later in this chapter). Organophosphates, as a rule, more readily cross the blood-brain barrier than do carbamates (Gallo and Lawryk 1991) and are likely to produce seizures with progression to coma. Organophosphates are also more deadly if there is any delay in treatment, because their binding to the enzyme is irreversible and produces more severe, longer-lasting cholinergic toxicity (Gallo and Lawryk 1991).

Treatment first involves careful decontamination of skin and clothing to prevent further exposure to the patient (and health care providers), followed by specific antidotes. Atropine counteracts the effects of excessive vagal stimulation; multiple doses are usually necessary. Pralidoxime reactivates cholinesterase by dislodging the toxin from the active site (Wong et al. 2000). Patients who do recover from acute poisoning often suffer no sequelae, although delirium, mood changes, anxiety, and self-limited parkinsonian movements have been described, and some psychiatric symptoms can last for months after the event (Gallo and Lawryk 1991; Gershon and Shaw 1961; Merrill and Mihm 1982; Rosenstock et al. 1990).

Chronic organophosphate toxicity usually arises from work-related exposure. Symptoms include blurred vision with miosis, nausea, diarrhea, diaphoresis, weakness, and other neurological complaints (Clark 2006). Pyramidal tract signs are sometimes found (Bhatt et al. 1999; Müller-Vahl et al. 1999); data are mixed on the association between organophosphate exposure and the development of frank parkinsonism (L.S. Engel et al. 2001; Stephenson 2000; Taylor et al. 1999). Peripheral neuropathy and CNS effects, including memory complaints, mood changes, and irritable or otherwise abnormal behavior have also been reported secondary to chronic organophosphate exposure (Jamal 1997). Red blood cell cholinesterase testing is a sensitive assay that can reveal the diagnosis (Gallo and Lawryk 1991).

Other insecticides have been implicated in toxic syndromes with relatively low levels of exposure. Organic chlorines (e.g., dichlorodiphenyltrichloroethane [DDT]) all lower the seizure threshold (Ecobichon and Joy 1994). Some related compounds such as the antihelminthic lindane may adversely affect cognition and behavior, particularly in children for whom this low-cost scabies treatment is most frequently prescribed. Chronic occupational exposure to chlordecone, a highly lipophilic insecticide, can cause diffuse tremors, ataxia, an exaggerated startle reflex, opsoclonus, weakness, weight loss, and metabolic liver injury (Faroon et al. 1995). Intentional overdose of *N,N*-diethyl-3-methylbenzamide (DEET), found commonly in commercial bug sprays, may cause seizures. Encephalopathy and seizures have been reported in young children with excessive skin exposure to DEET (Briassoulis et al. 2001).

Radiation

Ionizing radiation sources include nuclear weapons and reactors, natural elements (e.g., radon), and consumer products, as well as diagnostic and therapeutic isotopes. Ionizing radiation preferentially harms cells with high turnover rates, including those of the skin, immune system, pulmonary epithelium, and gastrointestinal tract. In the CNS, damage and necrosis can produce neurological dysfunction and mental status changes, although the mere stress from perceived or actual exposure to ionizing radiation can also result in psychiatric impairment. Symptoms of toxicity include depression, sleep disturbance, fatigue, memory problems, poor concentration, and, rarely, psychosis (J.S. Brown 2007). Cranial irradiation, while often necessary for cancer survival increases the risk of neuropsychiatric abnormalities, particularly in children (V.A. Anderson et al. 2004; Cole and Kamen 2006). However, not all cranial irradiation causes dysfunction, and in some cases, improvement in cognition results, depending on the location and type of tumor, and the specifics of treatment (P.D. Brown et al. 2003; L.C. Lam et al. 2003; Torres et al. 2003). Ionizing radiation is a developmental teratogen, so high-level exposure to fetuses can cause mental retardation.

The question of whether low levels of ionizing radiation cause neurocognitive dysfunction has been confounded by the frequently high levels of comorbid stress and unrelated illness and injury in those who are suspected to suffer exposure. Gulf War veterans with bodily retained fragments of depleted uranium from exploded ammunition have demonstrated subtle changes in neurological status (McDiarmid et al. 2000, 2002), although objective neurological signs are rare. Studies of Hiroshima survivors did not correlate radiation exposure with dementia (Yamada et al. 1999, 2002, 2003). One nested case-control study of female nuclear weapons workers did find a small but significant increased risk of dementia-related death associated with total lifetime radiation exposure (Sibley et al. 2003). Most long-term studies of radiation survivors conclude that survivors are at high risk for mood and anxiety disorders, particularly the latter due to lasting worries about health consequences of the exposure (Honda et al. 2002; Kawano et al. 2006; Yamada and Izumi 2002). Posttraumatic responses to the mere threat of irradiation after an accident or attack are significant, and psychiatric symptoms are commonly reported even when little or no energy has been released (J.S. Brown 2002). "Radiophobia" refers to the substantial burden of psychological and functional somatic syndromes that appear after radiation exposure, which are forms of stress response not due to the radiation itself (Dawson and Madsen 1995; Pastel 2002; Pastel and Mulvaney 2001). It typically accompanies fears about cancer and other illnesses being caused by various exposures from nuclear power plants to natural sources to diagnostic radiography.

Non-ionizing radiation does not have the toxic potential outlined above, because the low energy of electromagnetic frequencies (e.g., radar, microwaves, television signals, mobile telephone transmission) is not sufficient to induce atomic reactive change. Nevertheless, there are patients with syndromic symptoms similar to those reported in idiopathic environmental intolerance (see "Psychosomatic Medicine and Blame-X Syndromes" section later in this chapter) who are "sensitive" to radiation in the electromagnetic range and who demonstrate some perceptual differences relative to study control subjects (Landgrebe et al. 2008). A clear causal relationship between exposure and symptoms is lacking (Feychting et al. 2005; Rubin et al. 2005), but patients may be helped with psychological interventions such as cognitive-behavioral therapy (Hillert et al. 1998; Rubin et al. 2006).

Metals

Despite advances in preventing exposures, metal poisonings continue to cause serious illness, with frequent neuropsychiatric symptoms. The neurotoxic metals of greatest importance to psychosomatic practice are lead, arsenic, thallium, manganese, selenium, and mercury. Toxicity can occur from acute ingestion, but most cases are the result of chronic exposures with insidious development of vague physical symptoms and psychiatric manifestations. A general workup for neuropsychiatric symptoms suspected to be the result of metal toxicity includes a careful neurological and mental status examination, complete blood count, and screening assays of serum and urine for metals. Neuropsychological testing can help to delineate cognitive impairment and guide rehabilitation. Specific details about each element follow.

Lead

The syndrome resulting from lead poisoning was classically referred to as *plumbism*. Although acute symptomatic lead poisoning and plumbic encephalopathy are rare since the removal of this metal from house paints and gasoline, lead toxicity remains a major problem, particularly in pediatrics, where it is still underdiagnosed. The fact that the major source of lead for children is old paint places inner-city residents at increased risk simply from the high metal content of dust in their homes (Chiodo et al. 2004; Reyes et al. 2006). Lead paint has a sweet flavor, and consumption of a single 1 g flake can exceed the permissible weekly intake for any individual (especially a small child) by orders of magnitude. Some imported toys and low-cost jewelry may be decorated with lead-based paints as well (Weidenhamer and Clement 2007).

Adult lead poisoning results from occupational or environmental exposures to lead-based products (H.A. Anderson and Islam 2006). Removing lead from gasoline has markedly reduced airborne emissions, and blood lead concentrations have correspondingly declined. But hobbies such as stained glass and ceramics may introduce lead into household air and dust. Some cosmetics traditionally used by Hindu and Muslim populations have extremely high concentrations of lead. Some Mexican folk remedies, such as azarcon and greta, used for gastrointestinal disorders, contain large amounts of lead as well.

Lead interferes with normal development and function of the CNS. Elevated serum levels are associated with lower IQ, poor concentration, sleep problems, and mood dysregulation (Bellinger et al. 1987). With acute, progressive poisoning, headache, vomiting, clumsiness, staggering, and drowsiness may presage the onset of encephalopathy, which may progress to convulsions, stupor, and coma (Wiley et al. 1995). Other systemic signs and symptoms can help to distinguish milder, chronic plumbism in differential diagnosis. Gastrointestinal effects include crampy pain, anorexia, weight loss, nausea, and constipation. Lead also causes anemia, peripheral motor neuropathy, nephropathy, and adverse reproductive outcomes. The metal has a long half-life in neuronal tissue and is stored for an extremely long time in bone. Because the majority of total body lead is found in bone, and late-life demineralization allows the metal back into systemic circulation, early exposure has been proposed as a risk factor for Alzheimer's dementia (Shcherbatykh and Carpenter 2007). Conditions such as massive traumatic fracture, hyperthyroidism, and pregnancy can also remobilize lead, with the potential for toxicity to emerge in an adult or in a developing fetus.

An elevated whole-blood lead level is the most useful indicator of exposure. The threshold for acceptable lead levels was originally set at 60 µg/dL, but evidence of attributable risk with lesser exposures has led to steady reductions to the current 10 µg/dL level. Over 2% of children in the United States under 6 years of age have blood lead levels greater than 10 µg/dL (Woolf et al. 2007). And even in the absence of other physical symptoms, there is good evidence for toxic neuronal injury below 10 µg/dL in the form of cognitive and behavioral impairment (Chiodo et al. 2004; Shannon 2003). Deficits in speech and language, attention, and classroom behavior also have been reported in relation to low-level lead exposure. A follow-up of lead-exposed but apparently asymptomatic subjects into young adulthood found that the high-lead group had a sevenfold increase in high school graduation failure and a sixfold increase in reading disabilities (Needleman et al. 1990). Behavioral dyscontrol and antisocial features are also found more commonly in lead-exposed cohorts in a dose–response relationship.

The cornerstone of lead toxicity treatment is identifying the source of lead and terminating exposure. In an acute ingestion (e.g., lead paint chips), activated charcoal is frequently used but may do little to adsorb the metal. Whole-bowel irrigation should be strongly considered. It is also important to consider removing lead-containing buckshot, shrapnel, or bullets from firearm trauma patients to prevent plumbism from delayed absorption.

The three major chelating agents for lead toxicity are ethylenediaminetetraacetic acid (EDTA), dimercaptosuccinic acid (DMSA, or succimer), and 2,3 dimercaptopropanol (British anti-Lewisite, or BAL). Encephalopathic patients should be treated with BAL and EDTA (Goyer et al. 1995). Less severely affected or asymptomatic patients can be treated with the oral chelator DMSA. It is unlikely that patients with a serum level lower than 10 µg/dL will benefit from chelation therapy of any kind; the mainstay of treatment in these cases is to minimize further exposure. Neuropsychiatric impairments may resolve slowly and incompletely, with a resulting need for rehabilitation, symptomatic psychopharmacology, and psychosocial and educational accommodations (Needleman 2006).

Arsenic

Arsenic is found in commercial, industrial, and pharmaceutical products, and a range of different exposures results in toxicity. Poisoning has been reported from unintentional, suicidal, homicidal, occupational, environmental, and iatrogenic means (Hunt et al. 1999). Contaminated water, soil, and food are the primary sources of exposure for most people. Arsenic is also found in herbicides, fungicides, and pesticides. Arsenic trioxide is used to treat acute promyelocytic leukemia. Asian natural remedy preparations sometimes contain significant levels of arsenic (Saper et al. 2008). Inorganic arsenic is odorless and tasteless and well absorbed by a variety of routes.

Acute oral poisoning produces nausea, vomiting, and severe diarrhea within minutes to hours (Schoolmeester and White 1980). Hypotension, tachyarrhythmias, and shock often follow. Delirium typically manifests early, but can be delayed in onset by days. Peripheral neuropathy with severe dysesthesias and dermatological changes emerge within weeks of ingestion.

Low-level exposure to arsenic over time produces a different picture (Yoshida et al. 2004). Fatigue, anemia, leukopenia, skin hypopigmentation, and hyperkeratosis are common. Peripheral vascular insufficiency, including Raynaud's phenomenon, is observed. Patients suffer from noncirrhotic portal hypertension with elevated transaminases. Memory loss, cerebellar dysfunction, and mild cortical impairment are seen in adults with chronic exposure. Anxiety, irritability, and personality changes have also been reported (J.S. Brown 2007). Children show signs of mental retardation.

Diagnosis should be confirmed by 24-hour urine collection, given that single-specimen urinary excretion and serum levels of arsenic are highly variable. In a case where arsenism is suspected but urinary assays are negative, hair or nail testing can reveal the diagnosis. Acutely poisoned patients should receive chelation therapy with dimercaprol (BAL) as soon as possible (Muckter et al. 1997). Chronically intoxicated patients should not begin chelation therapy until confirmatory testing results are received, and the drug of choice is oral succimer (Muckter et al. 1997).

Thallium

Poisoning with thallium is much less common in recent years, since removal of depilatory and rodenticide compounds from the market has drastically reduced its availability. It still occurs, however, from accidental exposures as well as homicide and suicide attempts (Rusyniak et al. 2002). Thallium is used in the manufacture of some jewelry. It may be ingested in herbal preparations and adulterated illicit drugs like heroin and cocaine (Insley et al. 1986; Questel et al. 1996; Schaumberg and Berger 1992). Occupational exposures are rare. Delirium, seizures, and respiratory failure mark the mortal trajectory after acute ingestion.

Chronic thallium toxicity should be suspected in patients when neuropsychiatric complaints (e.g., depression, irritability, paranoia, memory loss, confusion) are accompanied by alopecia, nail dystrophy, painful neuropathy and gastrointestinal disturbances (Bank 1980). Chorea and ophthalmoplegia are sometimes observed. CNS pathology includes cerebral and brain stem edema. Psychiatric symptoms may persist long after resolution of other toxic sequelae (Rusyniak et al. 2002).

Multiple-dose activated charcoal, potassium supplementation, and Prussian blue can be helpful to enhance elimination and prevent end-organ toxicity (Thompson and Callen 2004). In chronic toxicity, removal of the source of exposure is the most crucial intervention, although there may be a role for potassium and Prussian blue therapy.

Manganese

Manganese intoxication is usually the result of chronic occupational exposure in miners, metalworkers, and welders who inhale the metal. The earliest descriptions of poisoning in Chilean manganese miners in the early twentieth century outlined symptoms of uncontrollable affective expression with agitation and psychosis, and a similar syndrome is still recognized (Bouchard et al. 2006; Bowler et al. 2007). "Manganese madness" was the term used to describe the initial psychiatric syndrome of compulsive behavior, emotional lability, and hallucinations. Memory and concentration deficits are common. There is also a manganese based fungicide that is suspected as a cause of chronic neuropsychiatric toxicity. Parkinsonism and other movement disorders are frequently comorbid but usually do not manifest until psychiatric problems have been present for some time. In these cases, brain MRI often identifies manganese deposition, especially in the basal ganglia (Bowler et al. 2006). Serum and urine assays can be performed, but results do not correlate with symptoms in chronic toxicity. Treatment for acute inhalation is supportive, and therapy of chronic neuropsychiatric sequelae is frequently ineffective after manganese has damaged the brain (Bouchard et al. 2006).

Selenium

Selenium is an essential trace element that causes toxicity from exposure to industrial compounds or dietary supplements. Fatalities are usually the result of purposeful ingestion of selenous acid or selenium salts (Pentel et al. 1985). The acid (found most commonly in gun bluing solutions) causes corrosive injury to the upper gastrointestinal tract, vomiting, diarrhea, hypotension, myopathy, renal impairment, respiratory failure, and progressive CNS depression (Köppel et al. 1986). Chronic selenosis results in fatigue, brittle hair and nails, and a variety of dermatological changes. Accumulation of selenium also causes hyperreflexia, paresthesias, irritability, depression, and anxiety (Holness et al. 1989).

Assays for whole-blood and erythrocyte concentrations of selenium are more reliable for confirming toxicity than serum levels (Barceloux 1999). Activated charcoal may be useful in acute ingestions, but no other treatments apart from supportive care have established efficacy. Reversing chronic selenosis depends primarily upon identifying and removing the source of ongoing exposure. The antioxidants ascorbic acid and NAC may have some value in acute or chronic toxicity.

Mercury

Mercury is found in pharmaceuticals, folk medicines, laboratory and agricultural chemicals, industrial devices, and substituted alkyl compounds that accumulate in the bodies of large carnivorous fish. Toxicity from the metallic form of mercury is mediated through inhalational exposure, whereas organic mercury and its salts cause poisoning via ingestion.

Acute inhalation can cause severe chemical pneumonitis. Acute ingestion of mercury salts produces hemorrhagic gastroenteritis. It is more chronic exposure that gives rise to neuropsychiatric symptoms. Chronic inhalation can lead to a singular combination of personality changes with shyness and withdrawal alternating with explosive, flushed-face irritability. This syndrome is known as *erethism*. Volatile mercury was once used to prepare fur for hats; erethism is the condition referenced when labeling someone "mad as a hatter" (J.S. Brown 2002). Anxiety, mania, memory loss, and poor concentration have been reported with elemental mercury poisoning. Patients can also develop tremors and choreiform movements (Sue 2006).

The CNS is the primary site of toxicity with ingestion of organic mercury, as well. Symptoms usually differ from those caused by inorganic mercury and include paresthesias, dysarthria, ataxia, and loss of vision and hearing (Winship 1986). Organic mercury compounds are also teratogenic, manifest as mental retardation and neurological impairment that mimics cerebral palsy. As a result, pregnant and nursing women are advised to limit their intake of predatory fish (Mozaffarian and Rimm 2006).

Much attention has been given to the possibility that autism is caused by ethylmercury thiosalicylate (Thimerosal), a preservative used in childhood vaccines. Rigorous epidemiological studies have found no evidence to support a link between mercury in vaccines and autism (Andrews et al. 2004; Heron et al. 2004; Parker et al. 2004; Smeeth et al. 2004). Randomized controlled trials of chelation therapy for autism were halted in late 2008 due to safety concerns (Mitka 2008). See also Chapter 27, "Infectious Diseases."

Laboratory testing for mercury toxicity is complicated and is best undertaken with a combination of both whole-blood and urine assays (Rosenman et al. 1986). Acute toxicity management is focused on supportive care. Early activated charcoal and gastric decontamination are recommended, except with oral ingestion of liquid mercury, since it passes through unabsorbed in patients without preexisting gastrointestinal abnormalities. Succimer will chelate metallic mercury well. Salts are best bound by dimercaprol, but this chelator should not be used in other states of mercurism, because it can transport more of the toxic metal to the brain. Organic mercury poisoning, with its high risk of CNS pathology, may be treated with succimer plus either NAC or *N*-acetyl-*d*,L-penicillamine, but data are limited regarding effectiveness in reversing neuropsychiatric sequelae (Clarkson et al. 1981). There is no evidence to suggest that the small amount of mercury in dental amalgam produces systemic toxicity that warrants filling extraction or chelation therapy (Y.K. Fung and Molvar 1992).

Over-the-Counter Remedies

Medicines available without a prescription are commonly used in supratherapeutic doses (both mistakenly and purposely) and are also ingested with suicidal intent. Cough and cold preparations are too often administered by parents and other child care providers to induce sedation, even in the absence of allergic or infectious symptoms, occasionally with lethal consequences for young children (Dart et al. 2009). In addition to analgesics (discussed above) some products contain a number of different potentially toxic compounds in combinations that can complicate diagnosis and treatment.

Dextromethorphan

Dextromethorphan is ubiquitous in cough and cold products. This antitussive is a synthetic analog of codeine that is frequently abused by teenagers (Baker and Borys 2002). Its potency in cough suppression is roughly equivalent to that of codeine, but it has very weak opioid activity, even in overdose. The drug primarily inhibits serotonin reuptake mechanisms and, to a lesser degree, glutamate receptors. These neurotransmitter alterations mediate both its desirable and harmful effects. At low levels of intoxication, euphoria and hallucinosis can occur along with dizziness, ataxia, nystagmus, and akathisia. Serotonin syndrome is common in large overdose and in cases of coingestion with other serotonergic agents. More severe poisoning causes seizures and CNS depression with progression to respiratory failure and coma. The drug is bound well by activated charcoal in the recent wake of an acute ingestion. Naloxone has been reported to improve mental status in some symptomatic cases (Schneider et al. 1991), but benzodiazepines and supportive care (i.e., to treat serotonin syndrome and its sequelae) are the cornerstone of management (Chyka et al. 2007).

Decongestants and Related Drugs

Some sympathomimetic drugs are used to induce local and peripheral vasoconstriction, thereby acting as nasal decongestants. They can be found alone or in combination preparations for use in managing symptoms of upper respiratory infection and environmental allergies. Pseudoephedrine and phenylephrine are the most commonly used, both of which are alpha-adrenergic agonists with the former carrying some beta-stimulatory activity, as well (Johnson and Hricik 1993). Ephedrine also has more nonspecific adrenergic effects and is found in herbal preparations used recreationally, to enhance energy, or as adjuncts to fitness regimens (Nelson and Perrone 2000). The U.S. Food and Drug Administration (2004) declared ephedrine-containing dietary supplements illegal in 2004, but they remain readily available on the Internet. Hypertension is the main toxic effect of acute concern with all of these agents, particularly in large overdose. However, they have psychiatric effects as well, including anxiety, irritability, euphoria, and insomnia—the presentation of acute and/or chronic abuse can resemble mania and lasts considerably longer than the physical effects on hemodynamics (Dalton 1990; Lake et al. 1983). After an acute ingestion, aggressive blood pressure control and intensive monitoring are essential, with readiness to manage seizures, intracranial hemorrhage, and arrhythmias. Direct vasodilators such as phentolamine or nitroprusside are the preferred agents; as with acute cocaine intoxication, beta-blockers are to be avoided. Survival of the acute phase of toxicity from these short-acting compounds without an adverse vascular event generally leads to full recovery.

Antihistamines

Histamine receptor antagonists are used for the treatment of allergies, motion sickness, and short-term insomnia. This discussion is confined to histamine 1 (H_1) receptor blockers, since the H_2 blockers are relatively harmless, even in massive overdose (Illingworth and Jarvie 1979; Krenzelok et al. 1987). Accidental supratherapeutic ingestions occur (frequently in children), but toxicity from H_1 blockers is most commonly encountered either in elderly patients with delirium or in suicidal patients after intentional overdose with the most widely available and potentially toxic agent in the class, diphenhydramine. Doxylamine and hydroxyzine are also problematic in overdose. Newer H_1 blockers are more selective for peripheral H_1 receptors and correspondingly less toxic (Nolen 1997).

Acute intoxication presents as anticholinergic poisoning due to direct activity of these compounds on muscarinic receptors and the overlap of histaminergic and cholinergic neurotransmission pathways. Patients often have classic symptoms of flushed dry skin, fever, tachycardia, impaired consciousness, hallucinations, and abnormal movements. Given that H_1 receptor activity is important in memory, attention, concentration, executive function, and regulation of the sleep-wake cycle, it is no surprise that antihistamines precipitate delirium. Slowing of gastrointestinal motility may prolong absorption and the duration of toxicity. Seizures and rhabdomyolysis occur in serious overdose. Massive diphenhydramine ingestion can produce cardiac conduction disturbances and precipitate lethal arrhythmias secondary to sodium channel blockade (similar to TCA toxicity). Activated charcoal is recommended in patients with intact airway protection. Cardiotoxicity, as with TCAs, requires alkalinization of the serum using bicarbonate-containing intravenous fluids. The cholinesterase inhibitor physostigmine is an effective antidote for anticholinergic symptoms (Burns et al. 2000). In more severe poisonings, multiple doses of this short-acting remedy may be required; its use is discussed in more detail in the following section.

Toxidromes

Certain constellations of signs and symptoms, commonly called toxidromes, may suggest poisoning by a specific class of compounds (Table 37–6). The findings represent direct physiological manifestations of the pharmacology of the agents in question, thus providing objective clinical data about the status of the patient and what has been ingested. Recognition of such patterns can be very helpful, but clinical pictures are not always so obvious. It is important to seek historical information regarding all the potential medications and substances to which a patient may have access and attend well to the details of the presentation and evolving course, because polydrug overdoses may result in overlapping and confusing mixed syndromes that require careful management. Nevertheless, recognizing the dominant features of particular classes of pharmacological toxicities can be a vital diagnostic and therapeutic starting point in psychosomatic consultation.

Anticholinergics

The anticholinergic syndrome occurs frequently because many common medications and other xenobiotics have anticholinergic properties. It is a particularly prevalent problem in the elderly medically ill who, on average, take more medications and are more sensitive to their adverse effects. Polypharmacy is a major concern, as a number of commonly used drugs not typically classified as anticholinergics (e.g., antipsychotics, muscle relaxants, antihypertensives) do possess some anticholinergic activity (Tune 2000). Anticholinergic toxicity in the CNS causes delirium, frequently with mumbling speech and carphology or floccillation—aimless "picking movements" of the fingers. Vivid visual hallucinosis and undressing behavior are not uncommon. Peripheral anticholinergic syndrome signs include tachycardia, dry mouth, flushed skin, temperature elevation, mydriasis, ileus, and urinary retention. The duration and severity of CNS manifestations typically exceed peripheral effects (Tune 2001).

Most patients recover with removal of offending agents and supportive therapy, but delirium may last for over 24 hours after an acute overdose of anticholinergics—considerably longer if medications that add to the problem continue to be administered. Physostigmine is a useful intravenous antidote that can rapidly resolve delirium. It has a short half-life, and repeated 2-mg doses may be needed in severe anticholinergic toxicity. Primarily on the basis of two case reports of asystole, its use has been curtailed in the setting of a possible TCA overdose or in patients with prolonged QRS or QTc intervals (Pentel and Peterson 1980). However, extensive subsequent clinical experience has documented its safety and utility in anticholinergic states induced by medications that can affect cardiac conduction (Burns et al. 2000; Schneir et al. 2003). Relative contraindications to the use of physostigmine include reactive airway disease, parkinsonism, and atrioventricular blockade. Side effects of excessive physostigmine dosing include nausea, vomiting, diarrhea, bronchospasm, bradycardia, and seizures.

Cholinergics

The cholinergic syndrome is uncommon but is important to recognize because lifesaving treatment is available. Cholinergic toxicity produces a "wet" patient (profuse sweating, sialorrhea, lacrimation, vomiting, diarrhea, urinary incontinence) as opposed to the anticholinergic syndrome, which causes the patient to be "dry." The CNS (e.g., seizures, coma) and skeletal muscles (e.g., weakness, fasciculations) can also be involved. Cholinergic excess is most frequently caused by accidental organophosphate or carbamate pesticide exposure, which may occur through unsuspected dermal contamination (Hodgson and Parkinson 1985). Such agents and cholinesterase inhibitors used therapeutically for dementia can be employed in suicide attempts, as well. Cholinergic effects are also the cause of toxicity from "nerve gases" like sarin and from clitocybe and inocybe mushrooms. Recognition of the syndrome should prompt the use of atropine and, in cases of severe toxicity, the cholinesterase regenerator pralidoxime (Eddleston et al. 2002). Some phosphate-based insecticides

TABLE 37–6. Toxidromes: prominent clinical findings

Drug class	Examples	Clinical signs	Antidote
Anticholinergics	Atropine, antihistamines, scopolamine, antispasmodics, TCAs, phenothiazines, antiparkinsonian agents, jimsonweed	Agitation, hallucinations, picking movements, tachycardia, mydriasis, dry membranes, hyperthermia, decreased bowel sounds, urinary retention, flushed/dry skin	Physostigmine
Cholinergics	Organophosphates, carbamate insecticides, cholinesterase inhibitors	Hypersalivation, lacrimation, incontinence, gastrointestinal cramping, emesis, bradycardia, diaphoresis, miosis, pulmonary edema, weakness, paralysis, fasciculations	Atropine, pralidoxime
Opioids	Oxycodone, hydrocodone, hydromorphone, fentanyl, morphine, propoxyphene, codeine, methadone, heroin	CNS and respiratory depression, miosis, bradycardia, hypotension, hypothermia, pulmonary edema, hyporeflexia	Naloxone, nalmefene
Sedative-hypnotics	Benzodiazepines, zolpidem, zaleplon, eszopiclone, barbiturates, ethanol, chloral hydrate, ethchlorvynol, meprobamate	CNS depression, hyporeflexia, slow respirations, hypotension, hypothermia, bradycardia	Flumazenil (for some)
Sympathomimetics	Psychostimulants, amphetamines, pseudoephedrine, phenylephrine, ephedrine, cocaine	Hypertension, tachycardia, arrhythmias, agitation, paranoia, hallucinations, mydriasis, nausea, vomiting, abdominal pain, piloerection	Benzodiazepines
Neuroleptics	Typical and atypical antipsychotics, phenothiazine antiemetics	Hypotension, oculogyric crisis, trismus, dystonia, ataxia, parkinsonism, anticholinergic manifestations (some)	Physostigmine (for some)
Serotonergics	SSRIs, SNRIs, TCAs, MAOIs, buspirone, tramadol, dextromethorphan, antiemetics, triptans, sibutramine	Akathisia, tremor, agitation, hyperthermia, hypertension, diaphoresis, hyperreflexia, clonus, lower extremity muscular hypertonicity, diarrhea	Benzodiazepines, cyproheptadine?

Note. CNS = central nervous system; MAOIs = monoamine oxidase inhibitors; SNRIs = serotonin–norepinephrine reuptake inhibitors; SSRIs = selective serotonin reuptake inhibitors; TCAs = tricyclic antidepressants.

are very long acting due to their fat solubility and therefore may require prolonged pralidoxime treatment.

Opioids

Toxicity from opioids progresses from analgesia to anesthetic CNS depression, coma, and death. Respiratory depression is particularly pronounced with opioid overdose, and the tidal volume or respiratory rate can be diminished before decreases in blood pressure or pulse occur. Miosis is also characteristic and, in pure opioid toxicity, a fairly reliable finding (Sporer 1999). The diagnosis of opioid overdose is often confirmed by the use of naloxone or nalmefene in adequate doses that reverse the toxidrome (Hoffman and Goldfrank 1995). Naloxone has an elimination half-life of about 1 hour, whereas that of nalmefene is over 10 hours, thus making the latter antidote potentially useful in the case of opioid toxicity from a long-acting drug (e.g., methadone) (Glass et al. 1994). In most patients, naloxone is the preferred agent, since a shorter-acting antidote allows for more careful titration of toxidrome reversal without precipitation of withdrawal. A dose of 0.4 mg is adequate; higher doses merely increase the likelihood of agitated withdrawal without added benefit to neurological or respiratory status—unless the antidote is being employed to reverse imidazoline (e.g., clonidine, guanfacine, tizanidine) toxicity, where doses of 2 mg or more may be useful (Seger 2002). Conversely, in known chronic users of opioids, unless apnea is present and not yet addressed with adequate assisted ventilation, starting with 0.2 mg doses of naloxone and carefully repeating as needed is reasonable to avoid dangerously agitated withdrawal. Ongoing monitoring after antidote administration is vital, since cardiopulmonary symptoms are not reversed as durably as CNS depression, and life-threatening symptoms can recur.

Sedative-Hypnotics

Sedative-hypnotic agents can produce neurological depression similar to opioids, and are frequently coingested (or, unfortunately, coadministered in the hospital) to the point of toxicity. "Pure" gamma-aminobutyric acid (GABA)–ergic toxidromes can sometimes be distinguished on the basis of history, relatively preserved pulmonary function, and the absence of constricted pupils (see Table 37–6). When taken in sufficient dosage, sedative-hypnotics cause general anesthesia with a complete loss of awareness and reflex activity, and ultimately, deterioration in cardiopulmonary function. Reversal of this syndrome can be accomplished with the benzodiazepine antagonist flumazenil. In addition to toxicity from benzodiazepines and nonbenzodiazepine hypnotics (e.g., zolpidem, zaleplon, eszopiclone), this antidote has also shown some efficacy in overdoses of the centrally acting skeletal muscle relaxants baclofen, carisoprodol, and metaxalone (Kim 2007). It should not, however, be used without caution in a mixed overdose that may include agents that are proarrhythmic or proconvulsant, since GABA activity is protective against drug-induced arrhythmias and seizures (Seger 2004). As long as doses are kept low (0.5 mg) and delivered over at least 30 seconds into a flowing intravenous line, side effects due to flumazenil (including benzodiazepine withdrawal) are generally mild, although patients can emerge from sedation in a state of anxiety (Ngo et al. 2007). Flumazenil is short acting, so multiple doses may be necessary, and continued neurological and cardiopulmonary monitoring is vital.

Sympathomimetics

The sympathomimetic syndrome is usually seen after acute or chronic abuse of cocaine, amphetamines, or decongestants, the latter of which have been previously discussed. The clinical picture overlaps with serotonin syndrome, as these compounds have multiple catecholamine effects. Signs include agitation, tachycardia, hypertension, mydriasis, and piloerection. In contrast to anticholinergic poisoning, the skin is typically not dry, but the two toxidromes can be difficult to distinguish on clinical examination. Mild toxicity rarely leads to cardiac complications, but large overdoses of sympathomimetic agents can produce arrhythmias, cardiovascular compromise, and shock. Patients may be psychotic, with intricate and paranoid delusions (Berman et al. 2009). Seizures are common, and the postictal state can contribute further to alterations in mental status. No specific antidotes exist, but benzodiazepines are the cornerstone of treatment because they attenuate catecholamine release, reduce hypertension, prevent seizures, and provide helpful sedation. Beta-blockers are contraindicated because they would leave alpha-adrenergic stimulation unopposed; thus, direct vasodilators such as hydralazine, nitroprusside, or phentolamine are preferred for treatment of severe hypertension that does not respond to benzodiazepines. Failure of confusion and agitation to resolve with physostigmine can help to distinguish this toxidrome and serotonin syndrome from anticholinergic delirium. Psychiatric sequelae from sympathomimetic toxicity can linger long after physical symptoms have resolved and may require antipsychotic medication (Berman et al. 2009).

Antipsychotics

Toxidromes involving psychotropic compounds that block dopaminergic transmission are discussed in depth in Chapter 38, "Psychopharmacology." While antidopaminergic effects may dominate adverse reactions with therapeutic use, many antipsychotic medications are highly anticholinergic in overdose, making physostigmine a potentially useful antidote. Neuroleptic malignant syndrome is an idiopathic reaction that results in severe muscle rigidity, hyperthermia, autonomic instability, and altered mental status; it requires discontinuation of antipsychotic medication and aggressive symptom-focused medical interventions. The varied and complex pharmacological effects of neuroleptics make supportive care after removal of the offending agent key to management in any case of toxicity.

Serotonergics

Serotonergic agents (sometimes in suicidal monoingestion or unintentional combined polypharmacy, but even more frequently with concomitant use of cocaine) can produce serotonin syndrome, characterized by neuromuscular symptoms, hyperthermia, and altered mental status. Classic signs of lower extremity muscle rigidity, hyperreflexia, and especially clonus, along with increased gastrointestinal motility and diaphoresis help to distinguish this potentially lethal toxidrome from anticholinergic poisoning (see Table 37–6). In addition to differences in precipitating medications, neuroleptic malignant syndrome does not cause gastrointestinal symptoms and typically results in more generalized and severe muscle rigidity without hyperreflexia (Boyer and Shannon 2005; Caroff 2003). Serotonin toxicity demands removal of the offending agents and supportive care with fluids and cooling measures; benzodiazepines are the mainstay of pharmacological treatment. The oral antihistamine cyproheptadine has some antiserotinergic activity and has often been prescribed, but it has not been demonstrated to improve outcomes. It may reduce symptoms but can only be administered orally, so severely afflicted patients are unable to benefit from its use and instead require large doses of parenteral benzodiazepines. Serotonin syndrome is discussed further in Chapter 38, "Psychopharmacology."

Gulf War Syndrome

Gulf War syndrome refers to the medically unexplained somatic symptoms of thousands of military and civilian personnel who served in conflicts in the Persian Gulf. Over 10% of returning troops have reported a variable host of symptoms, including rashes, gastrointestinal upset, fatigue, muscle aches, paresthesias, headaches, memory impairment, concentration difficulties, irritability, and insomnia (Cohn et al. 2008). These presentations, however, do not constitute a toxidrome, for with the majority of the symptoms being subjective, nonspecific, and referable to multiple organ systems requiring multiple pharmacological mechanisms, the likelihood of a toxic etiology is quite low (Iversen et al. 2007; Kang et al. 2009).

In order to protect troops from insect pests and chemical warfare, they received preemptive repellants and antidotes in therapeutic doses. Vaccinations against botulism and anthrax were also provided. The question has been raised of whether the combination of these agents may have precipitated Gulf War syndrome. Although combinations of DEET, pyridostigmine, and the pyrethroid permethrin have shown synergistic neurotoxicity in very-high-dose animal models, low-level exposure to these and other agents is unlikely to account for soldiers' myriad symptoms through toxicological mechanisms (Abou-Donia et al. 1996; McCain et al. 1997). Similarities between the troops' presentations following the latest conflict and those returning from previous wars lead some experts to conclude that Gulf War syndrome represents a complex reaction of psyche and soma to the many severe traumas of armed conflict (Holland 2006). Subtle CNS effects of insecticides and/or as-yet-unidentified toxins (e.g., combustion products, warfare agents) may contribute, in part, to the complex symptoms in some patients. Treatment, however, is not best accomplished using a disease model that anticipates identification of a specific etiological agent. Since toxicological mechanisms neither explain the disability nor suggest interventions to address it, a population-based approach to anticipatory management coupled with multidisciplinary biopsychosocial attention to individual patient needs is advised (C.C. Engel et al. 2006; Mahoney 2001).

Psychosomatic Medicine and Blame-X Syndromes

In some cases, not only does the history fail to reveal a specific toxic exposure, but also the examination and laboratory testing do not suggest that a xenobiotic is responsible for the patient's suffering. Similar to the Gulf War syndrome, there is a growing number of conditions in which a constellation of complaints are attributed to an exposure with lack of corresponding objective toxicological data. Some involve a single suspected exposure, while others involve concern about repeated or continuous dosing from the environment. Many times, specific agents have been investigated but failed to meet causality standards, and in other instances, a toxic etiology seems plausible but no compounds have yet been identified. Although it is clear that psychiatric factors play a major role for many such patients, it is important to remember that the history of medicine is filled with illnesses viewed as psychogenic until treatable physiological causes were elucidated.

A helpful framework for conceptualizing the emergence and evolution of these syndromes in the modern world has been laid out by Dr. Alvan Feinstein. He refers to functional somatic presentations with external attributions as the Blame-X syndrome (Feinstein 2001). Availability of almost limitless diagnostic (including toxicological) testing contributes to medicalization of distress. On the basis of mere statistical probability, some abnormal results are bound to arise, even if they have nothing to do with a patient's complaints. There is then a tendency to abandon the demand for pathophysiological correlation of symptoms and objective findings. As a result, early suspicion and a corresponding desire for answers prompts the appellation of new diseases before etiologies have been rigorously established. Such Blame-X rendering of diagnoses can stand in the way of patients' functional recovery and also impede ongoing critical research that could properly elucidate underlying causes (Feinstein 2001). Three of these related syndromes involving toxicological issues are discussed below.

In all of these Blame-X syndromes involving medically unexplained symptoms, there is a broad psychiatric differential diagnostic spectrum, including somatoform, posttraumatic stress, obsessive-compulsive, psychotic, and factitious disorders, as well as hypochondriasis, abnormal illness behavior, and malingering. The longitudinal course of symptoms that are initially unexplained is variable, depending upon a host of factors including their nature and severity as well as the demographics of the population in which they arise (Carson et al. 2003; Crimlisk et al. 1998). It is true that long-term complaints, especially those that wax and wane or worsen with time, are very unlikely to be toxicological in origin unless some ongoing exposure can be documented (Leikin et al. 2004). In some cases, a medical etiology is uncovered for initially unexplained symptoms, but even if it is not, diagnosis of a psychological cause by exclusion alone is not appropriate (see discussion of medically unexplained symptoms in Chapter 12, "Somatization and Somatoform Disorders").

Medication Sensitivity

Some patients have an extensive list of medication intolerances. The term *medication sensitivity* is not being used here to label a new syndrome, but merely to describe a characteristic of patients commonly encountered in psychosomatic practice. It is distinguished from multiple chemical sensitivity, a condition synonymous with idiopathic environmental intolerance (discussed next), particularly with reference to those who are sensitive to odors and airborne substances. Some patients have concerns about both therapeutics and environmental xenobiotics, so medication sensitivity is used here to describe a phenomenon that defines patients whose adverse experiences are attributed specifically to medications. Patients with extensive medication sensitivity may blame current symptoms on a relatively benign medication given in the recent or remote past, but they lack objective physical or pathological findings. As a group these patients, indeed, display an attributional cognitive style similarly seen in idiopathic environmental intolerance (Waddell 1993).

The majority of drug allergy entries in most charts are not indicative of true allergic reactions, but are instead presumed medication toxicities. Most patients who seem to respond poorly to a number of drugs do not have elevated allergic sensitivity to antigenic challenge (Mitchell et al. 2000). Medication rechallenge studies, especially double-blinded trials, which would help to document a starting point for further toxicological study of these patients, are also lacking (Waddell 1993). Some of these drug reactions are "nocebo" responses—adverse effects that would occur even with placebo due to the patient's anticipatory anxiety and pessimistic expectation that a drug will produce unpleasant or harmful side effects (Amanzio et al. 2009). Although little research has been performed to better understand patients with extensive nonallergic medication intolerance, clinical experience indicates a high rate of psychiatric comorbidity (Black 2000). Advising other providers as to the potential for intolerance of rather than relief from new prescriptions can be an important consultative intervention in such cases.

Idiopathic Environmental Intolerance

Some patients report a constellation of symptoms that they ascribe to the toxic effects of one or more components of the external environment. They are distinguished here from the previous category of individuals in that most do not identify a medication as the precipitant, and many cite ongoing exposures to various agents as the driving force for chronic impairment. Idiopathic environmental intolerance has also been labeled multiple chemical sensitivity, environmental somatization syndrome, environmental allergy syndrome, and, in earlier terms, total allergy syndrome or twentieth-century disease (the latter name emphasizing the suspected role of ecological threats from the modern industrialized world). Characteristics of the syndrome include 1) acquisition after environmental exposure that may have produced minimal (or no) objective evidence of health effects, 2) waxing and waning of symptoms that may vary in response to stimuli and are referable to multiple organs and systems, and 3) lack of evidence of organ damage or abnormal test results to account for symptoms (F. Fung 2004a).

Suspected toxins include construction materials, fabrics, food additives, drinking water, fumes, and agrochemicals. Symptoms are as varied as the causes, and they may include shortness of breath, palpitations, headaches, fatigue, insomnia, cough, nausea, diarrhea, constipation, paresthesias, muscle twitching, skeletal pain, bloating, and diaphoresis. Controlled studies reveal no evidence of toxic exposures or positive allergy testing that might explain the symptoms (Mitchell et al. 2000). "Clinical ecologists" have advanced the hypothesis that low-level exposure to multiple environmental compounds that are generally deemed nontoxic can, in susceptible individuals, precipitate multisystem disease (Stewart and Raskin 1985). Their treatments have included homeopathic remedies and rotary diets. Patients often use air and water purifiers and make moves or take holidays to avoid exposures. Hygienic factors should be considered but rarely contribute to an effective treatment plan unless an epidemic of exposure—and therefore, perhaps, a bona fide toxin—is suspected (Göthe et al. 1995). Relief of symptoms from all these remedies is usually minimal, although outcome studies are lacking.

Sufferers of idiopathic environmental intolerance are more commonly female and have a high rate of psychiatric comorbidity. In one series from a university-based consultation psychiatry service, every patient had at least one DSM diagnosis of mood, anxiety, psychotic, or personality disorder (Stewart and Raskin 1985). Malingering is also not uncommon. Patients share features with those suffering from somatoform disorders to such a great extent that formal research has failed to distinguish the two groups (Bailer et al. 2005; Bornschein et al. 2002). In outpatient toxicology clinic studies, lack of objective physical findings in patients presenting with concerns about a single toxin correlate with negative chemical assay results and high degrees of maladaptive projection and somatization (Leikin et al. 2004; Zilker 2002). Unfortunately, these individuals typically resist psychiatric intervention or any suggestion of psychogenic etiology (Göthe et al. 1995). Initial treatment of idiopathic environmental intolerance should be directed toward minimizing external attributions and emphasizing functionality through behavioral and cognitive therapies (Staudenmayer 2000). Management of comorbid psychiatric illness is indicated and can provide a starting point for longer-term mental health intervention in this group that otherwise tends to flee from psychotherapeutic interventions.

Sick Building Syndrome

Concerns about symptoms attributable to a particular indoor environment, usually the workplace, characterize the sick building syndrome. Patients frequently complain of lethargy, blocked nasal airways, dry throat, mucosal irritation, and headaches. Some feel chest tightness and dyspnea. Suspected toxins include insulation and other construction materials, residues from office products, and inadequately ventilated airborne contaminants, including fungal spores. In cases where toxic precipitants are identified, susceptible individuals have elevated histamine release that appears to correlate with respiratory symptoms (Meggs 1994). Although direct evidence of infectious disease or toxic exposure in individual patients is typically lacking, there are some studies supporting the possible role of mold species in buildings where prevalence rates are high (Burge 2004; Cooley et al. 1998), but other studies have been inconclusive (Straus et al. 2003). Some patients present with complaints of neuropsychiatric impairment claimed secondary to brain damage from mold exposure, but medical workups do not correlate any neural pathology. Malingering on neuropsychological testing of litigious individuals in this group is not uncommon (Stone et al. 2006).

Psychosocial factors related to workplace stress and job satisfaction do also correlate with somatic symptoms but in limited controlled studies do not account for patient differences attributable to factors about the buildings themselves (Skov et al. 1989). The prevalence of sick building syndrome is higher in women who have desk jobs involving computer work and who perform a substantial amount of photocopying. Toxins in these specific environments, however, have not been identified, and variable symptoms are found in similar workspaces. Infectious agents have been considered, but treatment studies with antibiotics and antifungals have yet to yield benefit (Straus et al. 2003). When an underlying disease such as bronchitis, asthma, or hypersensitivity pneumonitis is discovered, targeted treatment can be effective. Staying away from the building in question does resolve many, but not all cases of this illness (F. Fung 2004b). Supportive mental health treatment to aid with management of associated stress and comorbid conditions is the only currently relevant psychiatric intervention in sick building syndrome.

Conclusion

A thorough history (often gathered from several sources) and astute physical examination are key to toxicological diagnosis. Medication toxicities are a frequent and commonly misdiagnosed problem in hospitalized patients. Many psychiatric patients misuse drugs with a variety of motivations and corresponding outcomes. Exposures to other poisons may be intentional or accidental, obvious or hidden, at home, in the workplace, or even in the hospital. The CNS toxicity of many agents should include them in the differential diagnosis of unexplained acute or chronic neuropsychiatric symptoms. Removal of ongoing exposure and institution of selected treatments are required. In patients with functional impairment and attributed toxic reactions who have no demonstrable underlying toxic pathology, psychotherapeutic interventions beginning with a supportive stance and an eye toward other etiological factors help to facilitate well-being and recovery.

References

Abou-Donia M, Wilmarth K, Jensen K, et al: Neurotoxicity resulting from coexposure to pyridostigmine bromide, DEET, and permethrin: implications of Gulf War chemical exposures. J Toxicol Environ Health 48:35–56, 1996

Albertson TE, Derlet RW, Foulke GE, et al: Superiority of activated charcoal alone compared with ipecac and activated charcoal in the treatment of acute toxic ingestions. Ann Emerg Med 18:56–59, 1989

Alván G, Bergman U, Gustafsson LL: High unbound fraction of salicylate in plasma during intoxication. Br J Clin Pharmacol 11:625–626, 1981

Amanzio M, Corazzini LL, Vase L, et al: A systematic review of adverse events in placebo groups of anti-migraine clinical trials. Pain 146:261–269, 2009

American Academy of Pediatrics: Poison treatment in the home. American Academy of Pediatrics Committee on Injury, Violence, and Poison Prevention. Pediatrics 112:1182–1185, 2003

Anderson HA, Islam KM: Trends in occupational and adult lead exposure in Wisconsin 1988–2005. WMJ 105:21–25, 2006

Anderson VA, Godber T, Smibert E, et al: Impairments of attention following treatment with cranial irradiation and chemotherapy in children. J Clin Exp Neuropsychol 26:684–697, 2004

Andrews N, Miller E, Grant A, et al: Thimerosal exposure in infants and developmental disorders: a retrospective cohort study in the United Kingdom does not support a causal association. Pediatrics 114:584–591, 2004

Asian S, Karcioglu O, Bilge F, et al: Post-interval syndrome after carbon monoxide poisoning. Vet Hum Toxicol 46:183–185, 2004

Bailer J, Witthöft M, Paul C, et al: Evidence for overlap between idiopathic environmental intolerance and somatoform disorders. Psychosom Med 67:921–919, 2005

Baker SD, Borys DJ: A possible trend suggesting increased abuse from Coricidin exposures reported to the Texas Poison Network: comparing 1998 to 1999. Vet Hum Toxicol 44:169–171, 2002

Bank WJ: Thallium, in Experimental and Clinical Neurotoxicology. Edited by Spencer PS, Schaumberg HH. Baltimore, MD, Williams & Wilkins, 1980, pp 570–577

Barceloux DG: Selenium. J Toxicol Clin Toxicol 37:145–172, 1999

Barceloux DG, Krenzelok EP, Olson K, et al: American Academy of Clinical Toxicology practice guidelines on the treatment of ethylene glycol poisoning. J Toxicol Clin Toxicol 37:537–560, 1999

Barceloux DG, Bond GR, Krenzelok EP, et al: American Academy of Clinical Toxicology practice guidelines on the treatment of methanol poisoning. J Toxicol Clin Toxicol 40:415–446, 2002

Battaglia J: Pharmacological management of acute agitation. Drugs 65:1207–1222, 2005

Bellinger D, Leviton A, Waternaux C, et al: Longitudinal analyses of prenatal and postnatal lead exposure and early cognitive development. N Engl J Med 316:1037, 1987

Berman SM, Kuczenski R, McCracken JT, et al: Potential adverse effects of amphetamine treatment on brain and behavior: a review. Mol Psychiatry 14:123–142, 2009

Bhatt MH, Elias MA, Mankodi AK: Acute and reversible parkinsonism due to organophosphate pesticide intoxication: five cases. Neurology 52:1467–1471, 1999

Black DW: The relationship of mental disorders and idiopathic environmental intolerance. Occup Med 15:557–570, 2000

Boehnert MT, Lovejoy FH Jr: Value of the QRS duration versus the serum drug level in predicting seizures and ventricular arrhythmias after an acute overdose of tricyclic antidepressants. N Engl J Med 313:474–479, 1985

Bond GR: The role of activated charcoal and gastric emptying in gastrointestinal decontamination: a state-of-the-art review. Ann Emerg Med 39:273–286, 2002

Bornschein S, Hausteiner C, Zilker T, et al: Psychiatric and somatic disorders and multiple chemical sensitivity (MCS) in 264 "environmental patients." Psychol Med 32:1387–1394, 2002

Bouchard M, Mergler D, Baldwin M, et al: Neuropsychiatric symptoms and past manganese exposure in a ferro-alloy plant. Neurotoxicology 28:290–297, 2006

Bowler RM, Koller W, Schulz PE: Parkinsonism due to manganism in a welder: neurological and neuropsychological sequelae. Neurotoxicology 27:327–332, 2006

Bowler RM, Roels HA, Nakagawa S, et al: Dose-effect relationships between manganese exposure and neurological, neuropsychological and pulmonary function in confined space bridge welders. Occup Environ Med 64:167–177, 2007

Boyer EW, Shannon M: The serotonin syndrome. N Engl J Med 352:1112–1120, 2005

Brent J, McMartin K, Phillips S, et al: Fomepizole for the treatment of ethylene glycol poisoning. N Engl J Med 340:832–838, 1999

Brent J, McMartin K, Phillips S, et al: Fomepizole for the treatment of methanol poisoning. N Engl J Med 344:424–429, 2001

Briassoulis G, Narlioglou M, Hatzis T: Toxic encephalopathy associated with use of DEET insect repellents: a case analysis of its toxicity in children. Hum Exp Toxicol 20:8–14, 2001

Brown JS: Environmental and Chemical Toxins and Psychiatric Illness. Washington, DC, American Psychiatric Publishing, 2002

Brown JS: Psychiatric issues in toxic exposures. Psychiatr Clin North Am 30:837–854, 2007

Brown PD, Buckner JC, O'Fallon JR, et al: Effects of radiotherapy on cognitive function in patients with low-grade glioma measured by the Folstein mini-mental state examination. J Clin Oncol 21:2519–2524, 2003

Burge PS: Sick building syndrome. Occup Environ Med 61:185–190, 2004

Burns MJ, Linden CH, Graudins A, et al: A comparison of physostigmine and benzodiazepines for the treatment of anticholinergic poisoning. Ann Emerg Med 35:374–381, 2000

Caroff SN: Neuroleptic malignant syndrome, in Neuroleptic Malignant Syndrome and Related Conditions, 2nd Edition. Edited by Mann SC, Caroff SN, Keck PE, et al. Washington, DC, American Psychiatric Publishing, 2003, pp 1–44

Carson AJ, Best S, Postma K, et al: The outcome of neurology outpatients with medically unexplained symptoms: a prospective cohort study. J Neurol Neurosurg Psychiatry 74:897–900, 2003

Carter GL, Whyte IM, Ball K, et al: Repetition of deliberate self-poisoning in an Australian hospital-treated population. Med J Aust 170:307–311, 1999

Chan TY: Herbal medicine causing likely strychnine poisoning. Hum Exp Toxicol 21:467–468, 2002

Chiodo LM, Jacobson SW, Jacobson JL: Neurodevelopmental effects of postnatal lead exposure at very low levels. Neurotoxicol Teratol 26:359–371, 2004

Chyka PA, Seger D, Krenzelok EP, et al: Position paper: Single-dose activated charcoal. Clin Toxicol (Phila) 43:61–87, 2005

Chyka PA, Erdman AR, Manoguerra AS, et al: Dextromethorphan poisoning: an evidence-based consensus guideline for out-of-hospital management. Clin Toxicol (Phila) 45:662–677, 2007

Clark RF: Insecticides: organic phosphorous compounds and carbamates, in Goldfrank's Toxicologic Emergencies, 8th Edition. Edited by Flomenbaum NE, Goldfrank LR, Hoffman RS, et al. New York, McGraw-Hill, 2006, pp 1497–1512

Clarkson TW, Magos L, Cox C, et al: Tests of efficacy of antidotes for removal of methylmercury in human poisoning during the Iraq outbreak. J Pharmacol Exp Ther 218:74–83, 1981

Cohn S, Dyson C, Wessely S: Early accounts of Gulf War illness and the construction of narratives in UK service personnel. Soc Sci Med 67:1641–1649, 2008

Cole PD, Kamen BA: Delayed neurotoxicity associated with therapy for children with acute lymphoblastic leukemia. Ment Retard Dev Disabil Res Rev 12:174–183, 2006

Cooley JD, Wong WC, Jumper CA, et al: Correlation between the prevalence of certain fungi and sick building syndrome. Occup Environ Med 55:579–584, 1998

Craig SA: Radiology, in Clinical Toxicology. Edited by Ford M, Delaney K, Ling L, et al. Philadelphia, PA, WB Saunders, 2001, pp 61–72

Crimlisk HL, Bhatia K, Cope H, et al: Slater revisited: 6 year follow up study of patients with medically unexplained motor symptoms. BMJ 316:582–586, 1998

Cutler RE, Forland SC, Hammond PG, et al: Extracorporeal removal of drugs and poisons by hemodialysis and hemoperfusion. Annu Rev Pharmacol Toxicol 27:169–191, 1987

Dalton R: Mixed bipolar disorder precipitated by pseudoephedrine hydrochloride. South Med J 83:64–65, 1990

Dart RC, Paul IM, Bond GR, et al: Pediatric fatalities associated with over the counter (nonprescription) cough and cold medications. Ann Emerg Med 53:411–417, 2009

Dawson SE, Madsen GE: American Indian uranium millworkers: a study of the perceived effects of occupational exposure. J Health Soc Policy 7:19–31, 1995

Deichmann WB, Henschler D, Holmsted B, et al: What is there that is not poison? A study of the Third Defense by Paracelsus. Arch Toxicol 58:207–213, 1986

Donovan JW, Burkhart KK, Brent J: General management of the critically poisoned patient, in Critical Care Toxicology: Diagnosis and Management of the Critically Poisoned Patient. Edited by Brent J, Wallace KL, Burkhart KK, et al. Philadelphia, PA, Elsevier Mosby, 2005, pp 1–11

Ecobichon DJ, Joy RM: Pesticides and Neurological Diseases, 2nd Edition. Boca Raton, FL, CRC Press, 1994

Eddleston M, Szinicz L, Eyer P, et al: Oximes in acute organophosphorus pesticide poisoning: a systematic review of clinical trials. QJM 95:275–283, 2002

Engel CC, Hyams KC, Scott K: Managing future Gulf War Syndromes: international lessons and new models of care. Philos Trans R Soc Lond B Biol Sci 361:707–720, 2006

Engel LS, Checkoway H, Keifer MC, et al: Parkinsonism and occupational exposure to pesticides. Occup Environ Med 58:582–589, 2001

Faroon O, Kueberuwa S, Smith L, et al: ATSDR evaluation of health effects of chemicals, II: mirex and chlordecone: health effects, toxicokinetics, human exposure, and environmental fate. Toxicol Ind Health 11:1–203, 1995

Feinstein AR: The Blame-X syndrome: problems and lessons in nosology, spectrum, and etiology. J Clin Epidemiol 54:433–439, 2001

Feychting M, Ahlbom A, Kheifets L: EMF and health. Ann Rev Pub Health 26:165–189, 2005

Filley CM, Franklin GM, Keaton RK, et al: White matter dementia: clinical disorders and implications. Neuropsychiatry Neuropsychol Behav Neurol 1:239–254, 1988

Flomenbaum NE, Goldfrank LR, Hoffman RS, et al: Principles of managing the poisoned or overdosed patient, in Goldfrank's Toxicologic Emergencies, 8th Edition. Edited by Flomenbaum NE, Goldfrank LR, Hoffman RS, et al. New York, McGraw-Hill, 2006, pp 42–50

Fortenberry JD, Mariscalco MM: General principles of poisoning management, in Oski's Pediatrics: Principles and Practice, 4th Edition. Edited by McMillan JA, Feigin RD, DeAngelis CD, et al. New York, Lippincott Williams & Wilkins, 2006, pp 747–753

Fung F: Multiple chemical sensitivity and idiopathic environmental intolerance, in Medical Toxicology, 3rd Edition. Edited by Dart RC, Caravate EM, McGuigan MA, et al. Philadelphia, PA, Lippincott Williams & Wilkins, 2004a, pp 98–101

Fung F: Sick building syndrome, in Medical Toxicology, 3rd Edition. Edited by Dart RC, Caravate EM, McGuigan MA, et al. Philadelphia, PA, Lippincott Williams & Wilkins, 2004b, pp 131–135

Fung YK, Molvar MP: Toxicity of mercury from dental environment and from amalgam restorations. J Toxicol Clin Toxicol 30:49–61, 1992

Gabow PA, Anderson RJ, Potts DE, et al: Acid-base disturbances in the salicylate-intoxicated adult. Arch Intern Med 138:1481–1484, 1978

Gallo MA, Lawryk NJ: Organic phosphorous pesticides, in Handbook of Pesticide Toxicology. Edited by Hayes WJ, Laws ER. San Diego, CA, Academic Press, 1991, pp 917–1090

Gershon S, Shaw FH: Psychiatric sequelae of chronic exposure to organophosphorus insecticides. Lancet 1:1371–1374, 1961

Givens T, Holloway M, Wason S: Pulmonary aspiration of activated charcoal: a complication of its misuse in overdose management. Pediatr Emerg Care 8:137–140, 1992

Glass PS, Jhaveri RM, Smith LR: Comparison of potency and duration of action of nalmefene and naloxone. Anesth Analg 78:536–541, 1994

Goldfrank L, Weisman R, Flomenbaum N: Teaching the recognition of odors. Ann Emerg Med 11:684–686, 1982

Göthe CJ, Molin C, Nilsson CG: The environmental somatization syndrome. Psychosomatics 36:1–11, 1995

Goyer RA, Cherian MG, Jones MM, et al: Role of chelating agents for prevention, intervention, and treatment of exposures to toxic metals. Environ Health Perspect 103:1048–1052, 1995

Gunnell D, Eddleston M, Phillips MR, et al: The global distribution of fatal pesticide self-poisoning: systematic review. BMC Public Health 7:357, 2007

Hall AH, Smolinske SC, Kulig KW, et al: Ibuprofen overdose—a prospective study. West J Med 148:653–656, 1988

Halpern SM, Fitzpatrick R, Volans GN: Ibuprofen toxicity. A review of adverse reactions and overdose. Adverse Drug React Toxicol Rev 12:107–128, 1993

Hartman DE: Neuropsychological Toxicology: Identification and Assessment of Human Neurotoxic Syndromes. New York, Pergamon, 1988

Hawkins LC, Edwards JN, Dargan PI: Impact of restricting paracetamol pack sizes on paracetamol poisoning in the United Kingdom: a review of the literature. Drug Saf 30:465–479, 2007

Heard KJ: Acetylcysteine for acetaminophen poisoning. N Engl J Med 359:285–292, 2008

Hepler BR, Sutheimer CA, Sunshine I: Role of the toxicology laboratory in the treatment of acute poisoning. Med Toxicol 1:61–75, 1986

Heron J, Golding J, ALSPAC Study Team: Thimerosal exposure in infants and developmental disorders: a prospective cohort study in the United Kingdom does not support a causal association. Pediatrics 114:577–583, 2004

Hillert L, Kolmodin-Hedman B, Dölling BF, et al: Cognitive behavioural therapy for patients with electric sensitivity—a multidisciplinary approach in a controlled study. Psychother Psychosom 67:302–310, 1998

Hodgson MJ, Parkinson DK: Diagnosis of organophosphate intoxication. N Engl J Med 313:329, 1985

Hoffman RS, Goldfrank LR: The poisoned patient with altered consciousness. Controversies in the use of a "coma cocktail." JAMA 274:562–569, 1995

Holland MG: Insecticides: organic chlorines, pyrethrins/pyrethroids, and DEET, in Goldfrank's Toxicologic Emergencies, 8th Edition. Edited by Flomenbaum NE, Goldfrank LR, Hoffman RS, et al. New York, McGraw-Hill, 2006, pp 1523–1535

Holness DL, Taraschuk IG, Nethercott JR: Health status of copper refinery workers with specific reference to selenium exposure. Arch Environ Health 44:291–297, 1989

Honda S, Shibata Y, Mine M, et al: Mental health conditions among atomic bomb survivors in Nagasaki. Psychiatry Clin Neurosci 56:575–583, 2002

Howland MA: Activated charcoal, in Goldfrank's Toxicologic Emergencies, 8th Edition. Edited by Flomenbaum NE, Goldfrank LR, Hoffman RS, et al. New York, McGraw-Hill, 2006, pp 128–134

Hunt E, Hader SL, Files D, et al: Arsenic poisoning seen at Duke Hospital, 1965–1998. N C Med J 60:70–74, 1999

Illingworth RN, Jarvie DR: Absence of toxicity in cimetidine overdosage. Br Med J 1:453–454, 1979

Ingels M, Marks D, Clark RF: A survey of medical toxicology training in psychiatry residency programs. Acad Psychiatry 27:50–53, 2003

Insley BM, Grufferman S, Ayliffe HE: Thallium poisoning in cocaine abusers. Am J Emerg Med 4:545–548, 1986

Iversen A, Chalder T, Wessely S: Gulf War illness: lessons from medically unexplained symptoms. Clin Psychol Rev 27:842–854, 2007

Jacobsen D, McMartin KE: Antidotes for methanol and ethylene glycol poisoning. J Toxicol Clin Toxicol 35:127–143, 1997

Jamal GA: Neurological syndromes of organophosphorus compounds. Adverse Drug React Toxicol Rev 16:133–170, 1997

Johnson DA, Hricik JG: The pharmacology of alpha-adrenergic decongestants. Pharmacotherapy 13:110S-115S, 1993

Kang HK, Li B, Mahan CM, et al: Health of US veterans of the 1991 Gulf War: a follow-up survey in 10 years. J Occup Environ Med 51:401–410, 2009

Katz J, Prescott K, Woolf AD: Strychnine poisoning from a Cambodian traditional remedy. Am J Emerg Med 14:475–477, 1996

Kawano N, Hirabayashi K, Matsuo M, et al: Human suffering effects of nuclear tests at Semipalatinsk, Kazakhstan: established on the basis of questionnaire surveys. J Radiat Res 47:A209–A217, 2006

Kim S: Skeletal muscle relaxants, in Poisoning and Drug Overdose, 5th Edition. Edited by Olson KR, Anderson IB, Benowitz NL, et al. New York, McGraw-Hill, 2007, pp 341–343

Köppel C, Baudisch H, Beyer KH, et al: Fatal poisoning with selenium dioxide. J Toxicol Clin Toxicol 24:21–35, 1986

Krenzelok EP, Litovitz T, Lippold KP, et al: Cimetidine toxicity: an assessment of 881 cases. Ann Emerg Med 16:1217–1221, 1987

Ku BD, Shin HY, Kim EJ, et al: Secondary mania in a patient with delayed anoxic encephalopathy after carbon monoxide intoxication. J Clin Neurosci 13:860–862, 2006

Kulig K, Rumack B: Hydrocarbon ingestion. Curr Top Emerg Med 3:1–5, 1981

Kulig K, Bar-Or D, Cantrill SV, et al: Management of acutely poisoned patients without gastric emptying. Ann Emerg Med 14:562–567, 1985

Lake CR, Tenglin R, Chernow B, et al: Psychomotor stimulant-induced mania in a genetically predisposed patient: a review of the literature and report of a case. J Clin Psychopharmacol 3:97–100, 1983

Lam LC, Leung SF, Chan YL: Progress of memory function after radiation therapy in patients with nasopharyngeal carcinoma. J Neuropsychiatry Clin Neurosci 15:90–97, 2003

Lam SP, Fong SY, Kwok A, et al: Delayed neuropsychiatric impairment after carbon monoxide poisoning from burning charcoal. Hong Kong Med J 10:428–431, 2004

Landgrebe M, Frick U, Hauser S, et al: Cognitive and neurobiological alterations in electromagnetic hypersensitive patients: results of a case-control study. Psychol Med 38:1781–1791, 2008

Leikin JB, Mycyk MB, Bryant S, et al: Characteristics of patients with no underlying toxicologic syndrome evaluated in a toxicology clinic. J Toxicol Clin Toxicol 42:643–648, 2004

Mahoney DB: A normative construction of Gulf War syndrome. Perspect Biol Med 44:575–583, 2001

Maldonado JR: Delirium in the acute care setting: characteristics, diagnosis and treatment. Crit Care Clin 24:657–722, 2008

Martel M, Sterzinger A, Miner J, et al: Management of acute undifferentiated agitation in the emergency department: a randomized double-blind trial of droperidol, ziprasidone, and midazolam. Acad Emerg Med 12:1167–1172, 2005

McCain WC, Lee R, Johnson MS, et al: Acute oral toxicity study of pyridostigmine bromide, permethrin, DEET in the laboratory rat. J Toxicol Environ Health 50:113–124, 1997

McDiarmid MA, Keogh JP, Hooper FJ, et al: Health effects of depleted uranium on exposed Gulf War veterans. Environ Res 82:168–180, 2000

McDiarmid MA, Hooper FJ, Squibb K, et al: Health effects and biological monitoring results of Gulf War veterans exposed to depleted uranium. Mil Med 167:123–124, 2002

Meggs WJ: RADS and RUDS—the toxic induction of asthma and rhinitis. J Toxicol Clin Toxicol 32:487–501, 1994

Merigian KS, Woodard M, Hedges JR, et al: Prospective evaluation of gastric emptying in the self-poisoned patient. Am J Emerg Med 8:479–483, 1990

Merrill DG, Mihm FG: Prolonged toxicity of organophosphate poisoning. Crit Care Med 10:550–551, 1982

Miniño AM, Heron MP, Murphy SL, et al: Deaths: final data for 2004. Natl Vital Stat Rep 55:1–119, 2007

Mitchell CS, Donnay A, Hoover DR, et al: Immunologic parameters of multiple chemical sensitivity. Occup Med 15:647–665, 2000

Mitka M: Chelation therapy trials halted. JAMA 300:2236, 2008

Montague RE, Grace RF, Lewis JH, et al: Urine drug screens in overdose patients do not contribute to immediate clinical management. Ther Drug Monit 23:47–50, 2001

Mott JA, Wolfe MI, Alverson CJ, et al: National vehicle emissions policies and practices and declining US carbon monoxide-related mortality. JAMA 288:988–995, 2002

Mozaffarian D, Rimm EB: Fish intake, contaminants, and human health: evaluating the risks and benefits. JAMA 296:1885–1899, 2006

Muckter H, Liebl B, Reichl FX, et al: Are we ready to replace dimercaprol (BAL) as an arsenic antidote? Hum Exp Toxicol 16:460–465, 1997

Müller-Vahl KR, Kolbe H, Dengler R: Transient severe parkinsonism after acute organophosphate poisoning. J Neurol Neurosurg Psychiatry 66:253–254, 1999

Myers RA, DeFazio A, Kelly MP: Chronic carbon monoxide exposure: a clinical syndrome detected by neuropsychological tests. J Clin Psychol 54:555–567, 1998

Needleman HL: Lead poisoning, in Oski's Pediatrics: Principles and Practice, 4th Edition. Edited by McMillan JA, Feigin RD, DeAngelis CD, et al. New York, Lippincott Williams & Wilkins, 2006, pp 767–772

Needleman HL, Schell A, Bellinger D, et al: The long-term effects of exposure to low doses of lead in childhood: an 11-year follow-up report. N Engl J Med 322:83, 1990

Nelson L, Perrone J: Herbal and alternative medicine. Emerg Med Clin North Am 18:709–722, 2000

Ngo AS, Anthony CR, Samuel M, et al: Should a benzodiazepine antagonist be used in unconscious patients presenting to the emergency department? Resuscitation 74:27–37, 2007

Nolen TM: Sedative effects of antihistamines: safety, performance, learning, and quality of life. Clin Ther 19:39–55, 1997

Nordentoft M, Breum L, Munck LK, et al: High mortality by natural and unnatural causes: a 10 year follow up study of patients admitted to a poisoning treatment centre after suicide attempts. BMJ 306:1637–1641, 1993

O'Callaghan WG, Joyce N, Counihan HE, et al: Unusual strychnine poisoning and its treatment: report of eight cases. Br Med J (Clin Res Ed) 285:478, 1982

Olson KR: Emergency evaluation and treatment, in Poisoning and Drug Overdose, 5th Edition. Edited by Olson KR, Anderson IB, Benowitz NL, et al. New York, McGraw-Hill, 2007, pp 1–57

Parker SK, Schwartz B, Todd J, et al: Thimerosal-containing vaccines and autistic spectrum disorder: a critical review of published original data. Pediatrics 114:793–804, 2004

Pastel RH: Radiophobia: long-term psychological consequences of Chernobyl. Mil Med 167:134–136, 2002

Pastel RH, Mulvaney J: Fear of radiation in US military medical personnel. Mil Med 166:80–82, 2001

Pentel P, Peterson CD: Asystole complicating physostigmine treatment of tricyclic antidepressant overdose. Ann Emerg Med 9:588–590, 1980

Pentel P, Fletcher D, Jentzen J: Fatal acute selenium toxicity. J Forensic Sci 30:556–562, 1985

Perry HE, Shannon MW: Efficacy of oral versus intravenous N-acetylcysteine in acetaminophen overdose: results of an open-label, clinical trial. J Pediatr 132:149–152, 1998

Pohjola-Sintonen S, Kivistö KT, Vuori E, et al: Identification of drugs ingested in acute poisoning: correlation of patient history with drug analyses. Ther Drug Monit 22:749–752, 2000

Proudfoot AT, Krenzelok EP, Vale JA: Position paper on urine alkalinization. J Toxicol Clin Toxicol 42:1–26, 2004

Questel F, Dugarin J, Dally S: Thallium-contaminated heroin. Ann Intern Med 124:616, 1996

Rainey PM: Laboratory principles, in Goldfrank's Toxicologic Emergencies, 8th Edition. Edited by Flomenbaum NE, Goldfrank LR, Hoffman RS, et al. New York, McGraw-Hill, 2006, pp 88–108

Reyes NL, Wong LY, MacRoy PM, et al: Identifying housing that poisons: a critical step in eliminating childhood lead poisoning. J Public Health Pract 12:563–569, 2006

Roldan-Tapia L, Nieto-Escamez FA, del Aguila EM, et al: Neuropsychological sequelae from acute poisoning and long-term exposure to carbamate and organophosphate pesticides. Neurotoxicol Teratol 28:694–703, 2006

Rosenman KD, Valciukas JA, Glickman L, et al: Sensitive indicators of inorganic mercury toxicity. Arch Environ Health 41:208–215, 1986

Rosenstock L, Daniell W, Barnhart S, et al: Chronic neuropsychological sequelae of occupational exposure to organophosphate insecticides. Am J Ind Med 18:321–325, 1990

Rubin GJ, Das Munshi MJ, Wessely S: Electromagnetic hypersensitivity: a systematic review of provocation studies. Psychosom Med 67:224–232, 2005

Rubin GJ, Das Munshi MJ, Wessely S: A systematic review of treatments for electromagnetic hypersensitivity. Psychother Psychosom 75:12–18, 2006

Rumack BH, Matthew H: Acetaminophen poisoning and toxicity. Pediatrics 55:871–876, 1975

Rusyniak DE, Furbee RB, Kirk MA: Thallium and arsenic poisoning in a small Midwestern town. Ann Emerg Med 39:307–311, 2002

Saper RB, Phillips RS, Sehgal A, et al: Lead, mercury, and arsenic in US- and Indian-manufactured Ayurvedic medicines sold via the Internet. JAMA 300:915–923, 2008

Schaumberg HH: Toluene, in Experimental and Clinical Neurotoxicology, 2nd Edition. Edited by Spencer PS, Schaumberg HH. New York, Oxford University Press, 2000, pp 1183–1189

Schaumberg HH, Berger A: Alopecia and sensory polyneuropathy from thallium in a Chinese herbal medication. JAMA 268:3430–3431, 1992

Schneider SM, Michelson EA, Boucek CD, et al: Dextromethorphan poisoning reversed by naloxone. Am J Emerg Med 9:237–238, 1991

Schneir AB, Offerman SR, Ly BT, et al: Complications of diagnostic physostigmine administration to emergency department patients. Ann Emerg Med 42:14–19, 2003

Schoolmeester WL, White DR: Arsenic poisoning. South Med J 73:198–208, 1980

Sefidbakht S, Rasekhi AR, Kamali K, et al: Methanol poisoning: acute MR and CT findings in nine patients. Neuroradiology 49:427–435, 2007

Seger DL: Clonidine toxicity revisited. J Toxicol Clin Toxicol 40:145–155, 2002

Seger DL: Flumazenil—treatment or toxin. J Toxicol Clin Toxicol 42:209–216, 2004

Shannon M: Lead levels in children: how low must they go? Child Health Alert 21:1–2, 2003

Shcherbatykh I, Carpenter DO: The role of metals in the etiology of Alzheimer's disease. J Alzheimers Dis 11:191–205, 2007

Sibley RF, Moscato BS, Wilkinson GS, et al: Nested case-control study of external ionizing radiation dose and mortality from dementia within a pooled cohort of female nuclear weapons workers. Am J Ind Med 44:351–358, 2003

Skov P, Valbjørn O, Pedersen BV: Influence of personal characteristics, job-related factors and psychosocial factors on the sick building syndrome. Danish Indoor Climate Study Group. Scand J Work Environ Health 15:286–295, 1989

Smeeth L, Cook C, Fombonne E, et al: MMR vaccination and pervasive developmental disorders: a case-control study. Lancet 364:963–969, 2004

Smith BA: Strychnine poisoning. J Emerg Med 8:321–325, 1990

Sporer KA: Acute heroin overdose. Ann Intern Med 130:584–590, 1999

Staudenmayer H: Psychological treatment of psychogenic idiopathic environmental intolerance. Occup Med 15:627–646, 2000

Stephenson J: Exposure to home pesticides linked to Parkinson disease. JAMA 283:3055–3056, 2000

Stewart DE, Raskin J: Psychiatric assessment of patients with "20th-century disease" ("total allergy syndrome"). CMAJ 133:1001–1006, 1985

Stolbach AI, Hoffman RS, Nelson LS: Mechanical ventilation was associated with acidemia in a case series of salicylate-poisoned patients. Acad Emerg Med 15:866–869, 2008

Stone DC, Boone KB, Back-Madruga C, et al: Has the rolling uterus finally gathered moss? Somatization and malingering of cognitive deficit in six cases of "toxic mold" exposure. Clin Neuropsychol 20:766–785, 2006

Straus DC, Cooley JD, Wong WC, et al: Studies on the role of fungi in Sick Building Syndrome. Arch Environ Health 58:475–478, 2003

Sue Y: Mercury, in Goldfrank's Toxicologic Emergencies, 8th Edition. Edited by Flomenbaum NE, Goldfrank LR, Hoffman RS, et al. New York, McGraw-Hill, 2006, pp 1334–1344

Taylor CA, Saint-Hilaire MH, Cupples LA, et al: Environmental, medical, and family history risk factors for Parkinson's disease: a New England-based case control study. Am J Med Genet 88:742–749, 1999

Tenenbein M: Position statement: whole bowel irrigation. American Academy of Clinical Toxicology; European Association of Poisons Centres and Clinical Toxicologists. J Toxicol Clin Toxicol 35:753–762, 1997

Thompson DF, Callen ED: Soluble or insoluble Prussian blue for radiocesium or thallium poisoning? Ann Pharmacother 38:1509–1514, 2004

Torres IJ, Mundt AJ, Sweeney PJ, et al: A longitudinal neuropsychological study of partial brain radiation in adults with brain tumors. Neurology 60:1113–1118, 2003

Tucker JR: Late-presenting acute acetaminophen toxicity and the role of N-acetylcysteine. Pediatr Emerg Care 14:424–426, 1998

Tune LE: Serum anticholinergic activity levels and delirium in the elderly. Semin Clin Neuropsychiatry 5:149–153, 2000

Tune LE: Anticholinergic effects of medication in elderly patients. J Clin Psychiatry 62 (suppl 21):11–14, 2001

U.S. Food and Drug Administration, HHS: Final rule declaring dietary supplements containing ephedrine alkaloids adulterated because they present an unreasonable risk. Final rule. Fed Regist 69:6787–6854, 2004

Vale JA, Kulig K: Position paper: gastric lavage. J Toxicol Clin Toxicol 42:933–943, 2004

Waddell WJ: The science of toxicology and its relevance to MCS. Regul Toxicol Pharmacol 18:13–22, 1993

Watson WA, Litovitz TL, Klein-Scwhartz W, et al: 2003 annual report of the American Association of Poison Control Centers Toxic Exposure Surveillance System. Am J Emerg Med 22:335, 2004

Weaver LK: Clinical practice. Carbon monoxide poisoning. N Engl J Med 360:1217–1225, 2009

Wei KC, Chua HC: Suicide in Asia. Int Rev Psychiatry 20:434–440, 2008

Weidenhamer JD, Clement ML: Widespread lead contamination of imported low-cost jewelry in the US. Chemosphere 67:961–965, 2007

Wiley J, Henretig F, Foster R: Status epilepticus and severe neurologic impairment from lead encephalopathy. J Toxicol Clin Toxicol 33:529–530, 1995

Winship KA: Organic mercury compounds and their toxicity. Adverse Drug React Acute Poisoning Rev 5:141–180, 1986

Wong L, Radic Z, Brüggemann RJ, et al: Mechanism of oxime reactivation of acetylcholinesterase analyzed by chirality and mutagenesis. Biochemistry 39:5750–5757, 2000

Woolf AD, Goldman R, Bellinger DC: Update on the clinical management of childhood lead poisoning. Pediatr Clin North Am 54:271–294, 2007

Wu LT, Howard MO: Psychiatric disorders in inhalant users: results from the National Epidemiologic Survey on Alcohol and Related Conditions. Drug Alcohol Depend 88:146–155, 2007

Yamada M, Izumi S: Psychiatric sequelae in atomic bomb survivors in Hiroshima and Nagasaki two decades after the explosion. Soc Psychiatry Psychiatr Epidemiol 37:409–415, 2002

Yamada M, Sasaki H, Mimori Y, et al: Prevalence and risks of dementia in the Japanese population: RERF's adult health study Hiroshima subjects. J Am Geriatr Soc 47:189–195, 1999

Yamada M, Sasaki H, Kasagi F, et al: Study of cognitive function among the Adult Health Study (AHS) population in Hiroshima and Nagasaki. Radiat Res 158:236–240, 2002

Yamada M, Kasagi F, Sasaki H, et al: Association between dementia and midlife risk factors: the Radiation Effects Research Foundation Adult Health Study. J Am Geriatr Soc 51:410–414, 2003

Yoshida T, Yamauchi H, Fan SG: Chronic health effects in people exposed to arsenic via the drinking water: dose-response relationships in review. Toxicol Appl Pharmacol 198:243–252, 2004

Zar T, Yusufzai I, Sullivan A, et al: Acute kidney injury, hyperosmolality and metabolic acidosis associated with lorazepam. Nat Clin Pract Nephrol 3:515–520, 2007

Zilker T: Assessment of risks from environmental exposure: practical implications in clinical toxicology. J Toxicol Clin Toxicol 40:296–297, 2002

PART IV

Treatment

CHAPTER

38

Psychopharmacology

James A. Owen, Ph.D.

PSYCHOPHARMACOLOGICAL interventions are an essential part of the management of the medically ill; at least 35% of psychiatric consultations include recommendations for medication (Bronheim et al. 1998). Appropriate use of psychopharmacology in the medically ill requires careful consideration of the underlying medical illness, potential alterations to pharmacokinetics, drug–drug interactions, and contraindications. This chapter reviews basic psychopharmacological concepts, including pharmacokinetics and pharmacodynamics in the medically ill, side effects, toxicity, drug interactions, and alternative routes of administration for each psychotropic drug class, as well as safety in pregnancy and lactation. Important considerations are critically examined for the use of psychotropic drugs in patients with major organ disorders. The use of complementary medicines, including herbal medicines and nonherbal dietary supplements, is also briefly reviewed.

Pharmacokinetics in the Medically Ill

Pharmacokinetics describes what the body does to the drug. It characterizes the rate and extent of drug absorption, distribution, metabolism, and excretion. These pharmacokinetic processes determine the rate of drug delivery to, and its concentration at, its sites of action. *Pharmacodynamics* describes the effects of a drug on the body. Pharmacodynamic processes determine the relationship between drug concentration and response for both therapeutic and adverse effects.

Absorption

Absorption of a drug is influenced by the characteristics of the absorption site and the physiochemical properties of a drug. Specific site properties that may affect absorption include surface area, ambient pH, mucosal integrity and function, and local blood flow. Orally administered drugs absorbed through the gastrointestinal tract may be extensively altered by "first-pass" hepatic metabolism before entering the systemic circulation. Sublingual, intranasal, topical, and intramuscular administration of drugs minimizes this first-pass effect, and rectal administration may reduce the first-pass effect by 50%. Drug formulation, drug interactions, gastric motility, and the characteristics of the absorptive surface all influence the *rate* of absorption, a key factor when rapid onset is desired. The *extent* of drug absorption, however, is more important with chronic administration. The *bioavailability* of a drug describes the rate and extent to which the drug ingredient is absorbed from the drug product and available for drug action. Intravenous drug delivery has 100% bioavailability.

Distribution

Systemic drug distribution is influenced by serum pH, blood flow, protein binding, lipid solubility, and the degree of ionization. Most drugs bind to proteins, either albumin or alpha$_1$ acid glycoprotein (AAGP), to a greater or lesser extent. Disease may alter the concentrations of serum proteins as well as binding affinities. For example, albumin binding is decreased in pregnancy and in a number of illnesses (e.g., cirrhosis, bacterial pneumonia, acute pancreatitis, renal failure, surgery, and trauma). In contrast, some disease states, such as hypothyroidism, may increase protein binding. AAGP concentrations may increase in Crohn's disease, myocardial infarction, stress, surgery, and trauma.

Typically, acidic drugs (e.g., valproate, barbiturates) bind mostly to albumin, and more basic drugs (e.g., phenothiazines, tricyclic antidepressants [TCAs], amphetamines, most benzodiazepines) bind to globulins. In general, only free (unbound to plasma proteins) drug is pharmacologically active. Decreases in protein binding increase the availability of the "free" drug for pharmacological action, metabolism, and excretion. Providing metabolic and excretory processes are unchanged by disease, any changes to protein binding of a drug are compensated by an increase in drug elimination (metabolism and excretion) resulting in little change of steady-state plasma concentrations of pharmacologically active free drug. However, although free drug levels may remain unchanged, changes in protein binding will reduce plasma levels of total drug (free + bound fractions). While of no consequence therapeutically, therapeutic drug monitoring procedures that measure total drug levels could mislead the clinician by suggesting lower, possibly subtherapeutic, levels and might prompt a dosage increase with possible toxic effects. For this reason, during pregnancy or in patients with uremia, chronic hepatic disease, hypoalbuminemia, or a protein-binding drug interaction, the use of therapeutic drug monitoring for dosage adjustment requires caution; clinical response to the drug (e.g., international normalized ratio [INR] for warfarin), rather than laboratory-determined drug levels, should guide dosage. Where therapeutic drug monitoring is employed, methods selective for unbound drug should be used, if available, for phenytoin, valproate, tacrolimus, cyclosporine, amitriptyline, haloperidol, and possibly carbamazepine (Dasgupta 2007).

Most diseases that affect protein binding also affect metabolism and excretion. In this case, disease-induced changes in free drug availability may have clinically significant consequences, especially for drugs with a low therapeutic index.

Volume of distribution is a function of a drug's lipid solubility and plasma- and tissue-binding properties. Most psychotropic drugs are lipophilic but are also extensively bound to plasma proteins. Volume of distribution is unpredictably altered by disease and is not useful in guiding dosage adjustments for medically ill patients.

Metabolism (or Biotransformation) and Elimination

Biotransformation occurs throughout the body, with the greatest activity in the liver and gut wall. Most psychotropic drugs are eliminated by hepatic metabolism and renal excretion. Two phases of hepatic metabolism enable drug excretion by increasing its water solubility. Phase I metabolism consists of oxidation (i.e., cytochrome P450 monooxygenase system), reduction, or hydrolysis, which prepares medications for excretion or further metabolism by phase II pathways. The monoamine oxidases (MAOs) are also considered part of phase I processes. Phase II metabolism consists of many conjugation pathways, the most common being glucuronidation, acetylation, and sulfation. The hepatic clearance of drugs may be limited by either the rate of delivery (i.e., hepatic blood flow) of the drug to the hepatic metabolizing enzymes or the intrinsic capacity of the enzymes to metabolize the substrate. Clinically significant decreases in hepatic blood flow occur only in severe cirrhosis, and when possible, parenteral administration of drugs is preferred because this route bypasses first-pass metabolism. Hepatic disease may preferentially affect anatomic regions of the liver, thereby altering specific metabolic processes. For example, oxidative metabolic reactions are more concentrated in the pericentral regions affected by acute viral hepatitis or alcoholic liver disease. Disease affecting the periportal regions, such as chronic hepatitis (in the absence of cirrhosis), may spare some hepatic oxidative function. In addition, acute and chronic liver diseases generally spare glucuronide conjugation reactions. Metabolic reactions altering the intrinsic capacity of the enzymes through inhibition and induction are discussed in the next section ("Drug–Drug Interactions").

The kidney's primary pharmacokinetic role is drug elimination. However, renal disease may affect absorption, distribution, and metabolism of drugs. Creatinine clearance is a more useful indicator of renal function than serum creatinine. Specific drugs and their use in renal failure are covered later in this chapter. In general, despite the complexity of pharmacokinetic changes in renal failure, most psychotropics, other than lithium, gabapentin, pregabalin, topiramate, memantine, paliperidone, paroxetine, desvenlafaxine, and venlafaxine, do not require drastic dosage adjustment.

Disease processes, particularly those involving the gastrointestinal tract, liver, heart, and kidneys, can alter absorption, distribution, metabolism, and elimination. Table 38–1 summarizes how disease in these organ systems may alter the pharmacokinetics of psychotropic medications.

Drug–Drug Interactions

Drug–drug interactions are pharmacodynamic or pharmacokinetic in nature. Pharmacodynamic interactions involve alterations in the pharmacological response to a drug, which may be additive, synergistic, or antagonistic. These interactions may occur directly, by altering drug binding to the receptor site, or indirectly through other mechanisms. Pharmacokinetic interactions include altered absorption, distribution, metabolism, or excretion and often change the drug concentration in tissues.

Pharmacokinetic interactions are understood in terms of the actions of an interacting drug (a metabolic inhibitor or inducer) on a substrate drug. A *substrate* is an agent or a

TABLE 38–1. Pharmacokinetics in the medically ill

Pharmacokinetic parameter	Potential factors	Clinical significance
Liver disease		
Absorption	Gastric acidity Gastric and intestinal motility Small intestine surface area (e.g., short gut) Enteric blood flow Reduced hepatic blood flow Portosystemic shunting	Minimize gastrointestinal side effects of psychotropics Liquid formulations may be better or more quickly absorbed than solid drug formulations Motility, secretory, and enteric blood flow changes in gastrointestinal disease usually do not require dosage change Consider parenteral administration
Distribution	Alterations in liver blood flow Changes in plasma proteins Albumin may fall AAGP may rise Decreases in binding affinities Fluid shifts (e.g., ascites)	Reduce dose Serum levels of drugs (bound + free) may be misleading
Metabolism and excretion	Reduced hepatic blood flow Reduced intrinsic capacity of the enzymes	Clinically significant reductions only occur in severe cirrhosis
Renal disease		
Absorption	Ammonia buffering may raise gastric pH	Rarely clinically significant changes in pharmacokinetics Major exceptions—lithium and gabapentin
Distribution	Altered body water volume Reduced protein binding	Exact prediction of pharmacokinetic changes in the context of renal disease is impractical clinically Monitor drug levels more frequently but interpretation of blood levels difficult Serum levels of drugs (bound + free) may be misleading
Metabolism and excretion	Reduced renal blood flow Glomerular function	Creatinine clearance is a useful indicator of renal function to guide dose adjustments Serum creatinine may be confounded by some diseases that affect creatinine metabolism Dialysis alters pharmacokinetics
Cardiac disease		
Absorption	Decreased perfusion of drug absorption sites Intestinal wall edema may reduce absorption Changes in autonomic activity may affect GI motility and cause vasoconstriction	Congestive heart failure may decrease absorption of drugs through the gastrointestinal tract Intramuscular drug absorption may be decreased by vasoconstriction
Distribution	Changes in plasma proteins AAGP may rise Albumin may fall Volume of distribution is reduced Regional blood flow redistributions	Acute doses should be reduced by approximately 50% Intravenous infusions should be given at a slower rate to avoid toxicity
Metabolism and excretion	Reduced renal and hepatic blood flow	A 50% reduction of dosage for chronic drug administration should be considered

Note. AAGP=alpha$_1$ acid glycoprotein; GI=gastrointestinal.

drug that is metabolized by an enzyme. An *inducer* is an agent or drug that increases the activity of the metabolic enzyme, allowing for an increased rate of metabolism. Induction may decrease the amount of circulating parent drug and increase the number and amount of metabolites produced. The clinical effect may be a loss or decrease in therapeutic efficacy or an increase in toxicity from metabolites. An *inhibitor* has the opposite effect, decreasing or blocking enzyme activity needed for the metabolism of other drugs. An enzyme inhibitor increases the concentration of any drug dependent on that enzyme for biotransformation, thereby prolonging the pharmacological effect or increasing toxicity.

The hepatic cytochrome P450 (CYP) enzyme system catalyzes most phase I reactions and is involved in most metabolic drug interactions. Three CYP enzyme families are important in humans: CYP1, CYP2, and CYP3. The families are divided into subfamilies identified by a capital letter (e.g., CYP3A), and the subfamilies further divided into isozymes based on the homology between subfamily proteins. CYP enzymes for drug metabolism are CYP1A2, 2C9, 2C19, 2D6, and 3A4. Because some of these enzymes exist in a polymorphic form, a small percentage of the population has one or more CYP enzymes with significantly altered activity. These individuals are identified as either poor or extensive metabolizers for that specific isozyme.

Phase II reactions are conjugation reactions in which the drug is coupled to water-soluble molecules to enhance its excretion. The most abundant phase II enzymes belong to the superfamily of uridine glucuronosyltransferases (UGTs). The UGT superfamily of enzymes is classified by a system similar to that for CYP enzymes. There are two clinically significant UGT subfamilies: 1A and 2B. As with the CYP system, there can be substrates, inhibitors, and inducers of UGT enzymes. For example, the benzodiazepines primarily metabolized by conjugation (oxazepam, lorazepam, and temazepam) are glucuronidated by UGT2B7. A number of nonsteroidal anti-inflammatory drugs (NSAIDs) are competitive inhibitors of UGT2B7. Phenobarbital, rifampin, and oral contraceptive drugs appear to be inducers of UGT2B7. The role of UGTs in clinical pharmacology is being increasingly recognized.

A third system involved in drug elimination is P-glycoprotein (P-gp). P-gp is an efflux transporter present in the gut, liver and biliary systems, gonads, kidneys, brain, and other organs. P-gps protect the body from harmful substances by transporting certain hydrophobic compounds out of the brain and other organs and into the gut, urine, and bile. The distribution and elimination of many clinically important therapeutic substances are altered by P-gps. For example, P-gps in the gut limit absorption of certain compounds and significantly influence oral bioavailability and "first-pass" effects. P-gps in the blood-brain barrier contribute to the functional integrity of the barrier.

As with the CYP and UGT enzyme systems, there are substrates, inhibitors, and inducers of the P-gp transporters. Administration of a P-gp inhibitor will increase oral bioavailability and central nervous system (CNS) access of a substrate drug, with opposite effects for an inducer. For example, loperamide (an over-the-counter antidiarrheal) is a P-gp substrate normally transported out of the brain and therefore without central opiate effects. When coadministered with quinidine (a P-gp inhibitor), loperamide brain concentrations increase and signs of respiratory depression can occur (Sadeque et al. 2000). Many factors can alter P-gp function and influence P-gp–based interactions; these include genetic differences, gender, herbal supplements, foods, and hormones (Cozza et al. 2003). As with UGTs, the role and interactions of P-gps in clinical pharmacology is being increasingly recognized.

General Principles

Prescribing in a polypharmacy environment, usually the norm in medically ill patients, requires vigilance regarding the many potential drug–drug interactions. To commit to memory all potential drug–drug interactions associated with psychotropic medications is practically impossible as these interactions are constantly changing with our knowledge and the development of new medications. Knowing a drug's metabolic pathways and the metabolic inhibitory or inductive effects of the coadministered drug enables a rough prediction of potential interactions. However, it should be remembered that drug concentration changes do not necessarily translate into clinically meaningful interactions. Cozza et al. (2003) advised that physicians prescribing in a polypharmacy environment should, whenever possible, avoid medications that significantly inhibit or induce CYP enzymes and prefer those eliminated by multiple pathways and with a wide safety margin.

Identification of Potential Pharmacokinetic Interactions

Most pharmacokinetic drug–drug interactions involve the effects of an interacting drug on the CYP-mediated metabolism of a substrate drug. The interacting drug may be either an inhibitor or an inducer of the critical CYP isozymes involved in the substrate drug's metabolism. However, not all combinations of interacting drug with substrate will result in clinically significant drug–drug interactions. For these interactions to be clinically relevant, the substrate must have certain characteristics. A *critical substrate* drug is a drug with a narrow therapeutic index and one primary CYP isozyme mediating its elimination. For example, nifedipine, like all calcium channel blockers, is primarily metabolized by the CYP3A4 isozyme. The addition of a drug that is a potent CYP3A4 inhibitor, such as fluoxetine, will inhibit nifedipine's metabolism. Without a compensatory reduction in nifedipine dose, nifedipine levels will rise and toxicity may result. On the other hand, the addition of an inhibitor or inducer that interacts with a CYP isozyme other than CYP3A4 will have no significant effect on nifedipine levels. Table 38–2 lists those drugs that are critical substrates and significant inhibitors and inducers of CYP isozymes, MAO, UGT, and P-gp.

Metabolic drug interactions are most likely to occur in three situations:

1. The addition of an interacting drug to a medication regime containing a substrate drug at steady-state levels may dramatically alter substrate drug concentration. If the interacting drug is an inhibitor, substrate drug concentrations will rise as its elimination is reduced and toxicity may result. Conversely, addition of an enzyme inducer will increase elimination of the substrate, thereby lowering its concentration and therapeutic effect.
2. A much overlooked interaction involves the withdrawal of an interacting drug from an established drug regimen containing a critical substrate drug. Previously, the substrate drug dosage will have been titrated in the presence of the interacting drug to optimize therapeutic effect and minimize adverse effects. Withdrawal of an enzyme inhibitor will allow metabolism to return (increase) to normal levels. This increased substrate drug metabolism will result in lower levels and decreased therapeutic effect. In contrast, removal of an enzyme inducer will increase substrate drug levels and may lead to drug toxicity as metabolism of the substrate decreases to a normal rate.
3. The addition of a critical substrate drug to a drug regimen containing an interacting drug can result in a clinically significant interaction if the substrate is dosed according to established guidelines. Dosing guidelines do not account for the presence of a metabolic inhibitor or inducer and thus may lead to substrate concentrations that are, respectively, toxic or subtherapeutic.

Metabolic drug interactions can be minimized by avoiding drugs that are known critical substrates or potent inhibitors or inducers. Unfortunately, this is not always possible. However, by identifying medications that are critical substrates or potent inhibitors or inducers, making appropriate dosage adjustments, and monitoring drug levels (where possible), the adverse effects of these metabolic interactions will be reduced.

Drug interactions that affect renal drug elimination are clinically significant only if the parent drug or its active metabolite undergoes appreciable renal elimination. Changes in urine pH can modify the elimination of those compounds whose ratio of ionized/un-ionized forms is dramatically altered across the physiological range of urine pH (4.6 to 8.2) (i.e., the compound has a pKa within this pH range). Common drugs that alkalinize urine include antacids and carbonic anhydrase inhibitor diuretics. Un-ionized forms of drugs undergo greater glomerular resorption, whereas ionized drug forms are resorbed less and so have greater urinary excretion. For a basic drug such as amphetamine, alkalinization of urine increases the un-ionized fraction, enhancing resorption and so prolonging activity. Other basic psychotropic drugs, such as amitriptyline, imipramine, meperidine, methadone (Nilsson et al. 1982), memantine, and flecainide, may be similarly affected (Cadwallader 1983; Freudenthaler et al. 1998).

Side Effects and Toxicity of Major Psychotropic Drug Classes

Antidepressants

Antidepressant drugs are used to treat affective, anxiety, eating, and some somatoform disorders as well as insomnia, enuresis, incontinence, headaches, and chronic pain.

Selective Serotonin Reuptake Inhibitors and Novel/Mixed-Action Agents

Adverse effects of selective serotonin reuptake inhibitors (SSRIs) and novel/mixed-action agents are common, but they are usually mild, dose related, and abate over time. However, serotonergic agents, especially when used in combination, can induce the potentially fatal serotonin syndrome (see "Serotonin Syndrome" subsection later in this section).

Common short-term side effects with SSRIs and serotonin–norepinephrine reuptake inhibitors (SNRIs) include nausea, vomiting, anxiety, headache, sedation, tremors, and anorexia. Common long-term side effects include sexual dysfunction, dry mouth, sweating, impaired sleep, and potential weight gain. Trazodone and nefazodone do not disrupt sexual function or sleep. Trazodone causes sedation in 20%–50% of patients and is often used for its sedating properties. It also rarely causes priapism. Trazodone and nefazodone can cause orthostatic hypotension, and nefazodone can cause hepatotoxicity.

Frequent duloxetine side effects are nausea, dry mouth, fatigue, dizziness, constipation, somnolence, decreased appetite, and increased sweating (Eli Lilly 2010c). Mirtazapine is associated with a high incidence of sedation, increased

TABLE 38–2. Drugs with clinically significant pharmacokinetic interactions

	Cytochrome P450 (CYP) isozyme						
Drug	**1A2**	**2C[a]**	**2D6**	**3A4**	**MAO-A**	**UGT**	**P-gp**
ACE inhibitors							
captopril							X
Antianginals							
ranolazine			X	S			S, X
Antiarrhythmics							
amiodarone	X	S, X	X	S, X			X
disopyramide				S			
flecainide			S				
lidocaine	S, X			S			X
mexiletine	X, S		S				
propafenone	X		S, X	S		S	X
quinidine			X	S			S, X
Anticoagulants/antiplatelet agents							
ticlopidine		X		S			
R-warfarin	S	S		S			
S-warfarin		S					
Anticonvulsants							
carbamazepine	I	I		S, I		S, I	
ethosuximide				S, I			
felbamate							S
lamotrigine						S	S
phenytoin	I	S, I		I		I	S
tiagabine		S	S	S			
valproate		I				S, X	
Antidepressants							
amitriptyline	S	S	S	S			S, X
bupropion			X	S			
clomipramine	S	S	S, X	S			
desipramine			S, X				X
desvenlafaxine						S	
doxepin			S				
duloxetine	S		S, X				
fluoxetine	X	X	S, X	S, X			
fluvoxamine	S, X	X		X			S
gepirone				S			
imipramine	S	S	S	S			X
maprotiline			S				X
mirtazapine			S	S			
moclobemide		S	X		X		
nefazodone				S, X			
nortriptyline			S				S

TABLE 38–2. Drugs with clinically significant pharmacokinetic interactions *(continued)*

	Cytochrome P450 (CYP) isozyme						
Drug	**1A2**	**2C[a]**	**2D6**	**3A4**	**MAO-A**	**UGT**	**P-gp**
paroxetine			S, X				S, X
phenelzine					X		
sertraline							X
tranylcypromine		X			X		
trazodone			S	S			I
trimipramine			S				
venlafaxine			S	S			S
Antidiarrheal agents							
loperamide							S
Antiemetics							
ondansetron							S
Antihyponatremics							
conivaptan				S, X			X
Antihyperlipidemics							
atorvastatin				S			X
fenofibrate							X
fluvastatin		X		S			
gemfibrozil		X					
lovastatin		X		S			S, X
pravastatin				S			
simvastatin		X		S			X
Antimicrobials							
chloramphenicol		X					
ciprofloxacin	X			X			S
clarithromycin	X			S, X			X
co-trimoxazole		X					
enoxacin	X						S
erythromycin	X			S, X			S, X
fluconazole		X		X			
grepafloxacin							S
griseofulvin	I						
isoniazid	X			I	X		
itraconazole				S, X			S, X
ketoconazole	X			S, X			X
levofloxacin	X						
linezolid					X		
metronidazole				X			
miconazole		S, X		S, X			
nafcillin				S, I			
norfloxacin	X			X			
ofloxacin	X						X

TABLE 38–2. Drugs with clinically significant pharmacokinetic interactions *(continued)*

	Cytochrome P450 (CYP) isozyme						
Drug	**1A2**	**2C[a]**	**2D6**	**3A4**	**MAO-A**	**UGT**	**P-gp**
Antimicrobials *(continued)*							
posaconazole				X		S	S
rifabutin				I			
rifampin (rifampicin)	I	I		S, I		I	S, I
roxithromycin				X			
sulfaphenazole		X					
sulfonamides		X					
troleandomycin	X			S, X			
valinomycin							S
Antimigraine agents							
eletriptan				S			S
ergotamine				S			
frovatriptan	S						
rizatriptan					S		
sumatriptan					S		
zolmitriptan	S				S		
Antineoplastic agents							
dactinomycin							S, X
dasatinib				S, X			
docetaxel				S			S
doxorubicin							S, X
etoposide				S			S
gefitinib				S			
ifosfamide				S			
imatinib			X	S, X			S
irinotecan				S		S	S
lapatinib				S, X			S, X
methotrexate							S
nilotinib		X	X	S, X		X	S, X
paclitaxel		S		S			S
procarbazine					X		
sorafenib		X		S		S, X	
sunitinib				S			
tamoxifen			S	S			S, X
tegafur (ftorafur)	S, I			I			
teniposide				S			S
topotecan							S
vinblastine				S			S, X
vincristine				S			S
vinorelbine				S			S

TABLE 38–2. Drugs with clinically significant pharmacokinetic interactions *(continued)*

Drug	Cytochrome P450 (CYP) isozyme						
	1A2	2C[a]	2D6	3A4	MAO-A	UGT	P-gp
Antiparkinsonian agents							
rasagiline	S						
selegiline					X		
Antipsychotics							
aripiprazole			S	S			
asenapine	S					S	
chlorpromazine	S		S				X
clozapine	S		S	S			
fluphenazine			S				
haloperidol	S		S, X				X
iloperidone			S	S			
olanzapine	S		S			S	S
perphenazine			S				
pimozide				S			X
quetiapine				S			S
risperidone			S				S
thioridazine	S	S	S				
trifluoperazine							X
ziprasidone				S			
Antiretroviral agents							
amprenavir				S			S, I
atazanavir		X		S, X		X	X
darunavir				S, X			
delavirdine		X		S, X			
efavirenz		X		S, X			
indinavir				S, X			S
lopinavir				S			S
maraviroc				S			S
nelfinavir				S, X			S, X
nevirapine				S, I			
raltegravir						S	
ritonavir	I	X	X	S, X			S, X
saquinavir				S, X			S, X
tipranavir/ritonavir			X	S, X			S, I
zidovudine						S	
Anxiolytics/sedative-hypnotics							
alprazolam				S			
bromazepam				S			
buspirone				S			
clonazepam				S			
diazepam		S		S			

TABLE 38–2. Drugs with clinically significant pharmacokinetic interactions *(continued)*

	Cytochrome P450 (CYP) isozyme						
Drug	**1A2**	**2C[a]**	**2D6**	**3A4**	**MAO-A**	**UGT**	**P-gp**
Anxiolytics/sedative-hypnotics *(continued)*							
hexobarbital		S					
lorazepam						S	
midazolam				S			X
oxazepam						S	
phenobarbital	I	I		I			
ramelteon	S			S			
temazepam						S	
triazolam				S			
Beta-blockers							
alprenolol			S				
bisoprolol			S				
bufuralol			S				
labetalol			S				
metoprolol			S				
pindolol			S				
propranolol	S	S	S				X
talinolol							S, X
timolol		S	S				
Bronchodilators							
theophylline	S			S			
Calcium channel blockers							
amlodipine				S			
diltiazem				S, X			S, X
felodipine				S			X
isradipine				S			
nicardipine				S			X
nifedipine				S			
nimodipine				S			
nisoldipine				S			
verapamil	S			S			S, X
Cardiac glycosides							
digoxin							S
Cognitive enhancers							
tacrine	S						
Gastrointestinal motility modifier							
domperidone							S
Gout therapy							
colchicine							S, X
probenecid						X	
sulfinpyrazone		X					

TABLE 38–2. Drugs with clinically significant pharmacokinetic interactions *(continued)*

	Cytochrome P450 (CYP) isozyme						
Drug	**1A2**	**2C[a]**	**2D6**	**3A4**	**MAO-A**	**UGT**	**P-gp**
Histamine H_2 antagonists							
cimetidine	X	X	X	X			S
ranitidine						X	S
Immunosuppressive agents							
cyclosporine				S, X			S, X
sirolimus				S			
tacrolimus							S
Muscle relaxants							
cyclobenzaprine	S		S	S			
Nonsteroidal anti-inflammatory drugs and analgesic agents							
acetaminophen						S	
diclofenac		X					X
flurbiprofen		X					X
naproxen							X
phenylbutazone		S, X					
Opiate analgesics							
alfentanil				S			
codeine			S	S		S	
fentanyl				S			X
hydrocodone			S				
meperidine			S				
methadone			S	S			X
morphine						S	S
oxycodone			S				
tramadol			S				
Oral hypoglycemics							
chlorpropamide		S					
glimepiride		S					
glipizide		S					
glyburide		S					
nateglinide		S					
pioglitazone		S					
rosiglitazone		S		S			
tolbutamide		S, X					
Proton pump inhibitors							
esomeprazole							X
lansoprazole	I	S					S, X
omeprazole	I	S, X		S			S, X
pantoprazole							S, X

TABLE 38–2. Drugs with clinically significant pharmacokinetic interactions *(continued)*

	Cytochrome P450 (CYP) isozyme						
Drug	**1A2**	**2C[a]**	**2D6**	**3A4**	**MAO-A**	**UGT**	**P-gp**
Psychostimulants							
armodafinil	I	X		S, I			
atomoxetine			S, X				
modafinil	I	X		S, I			
Steroids							
aldosterone							S
cortisol				S			S
dexamethasone				I			S, I
estradiol				S			S
estrogen				S			
ethinylestradiol				S, X			
hydrocortisone							S, X
prednisolone				S			S
prednisone				S			S
progesterone				S			X
testosterone				S			
triamcinolone							S
Foods and herbal medicines							
caffeine	S			S			
cannabinoids		S		S, X			
cruciferous vegetables[b]	I						
grapefruit juice				X			X
smoking (tobacco, etc.)	I				S		
St. John's wort				I			I
Tyramine-containing foods, including banana peel, beer (all tap, "self-brew," and nonalcoholic), broad bean pods (not beans), fava beans, aged cheese (tyramine content increases with age), sauerkraut, sausage (fermented or dry), soy sauce and soy condiments, and concentrated yeast extract (Marmite)					S		

Note. Pharmacokinetic drug interactions: S, substrate; X, inhibitor; I, inducer. Only drugs with significant interactions are listed. This list is a general consensus of drugs with significant potential to interact metabolically as substrate, inhibitor, or inducer. Minor differences in pharmacokinetic interactions between this listing and individual reports may be expected because of experimental design, genetic differences, incomplete data, etc. ACE=angiotensin-converting enzyme; MAO-A=monoamine oxidase type A; P-gp=P-glycoprotein efflux transporter; UGT=uridine 5′-diphosphate glucuronosyltransferase.

[a]Combined properties on 2C8/9/10 and 2C19 CYP isozymes.

[b]Cruciferous vegetables include cabbage, cauliflower, broccoli, brussels sprouts, kale, etc.

Source. Compiled in part from. Armstrong and Cozza 2002; Balayssac et al. 2005; Bezchlibnyk-Butler et al. 2007; Bristol-Myers Squibb 2010; Cozza et al. 2003; DeVane and Nemeroff 2002; Eli Lilly 2010a; Gardner et al. 1996; Gillman 2005; Guedon-Moreau et al. 2003; Kiang et al. 2005; Michalets 1998; Pal and Mitra 2006; USPDI Editorial Board 2007.

appetite, and weight gain (Thompson 1999). Common adverse effects of bupropion include agitation, insomnia, anxiety, dry mouth, constipation, postural hypotension, and tachycardia. Nausea and vomiting are much less common with bupropion than with SSRIs (Vanderkooy et al. 2002). Patients treated with reboxetine (used only in Europe) often report dry mouth, insomnia, constipation, sweating, and hypotension (Andreoli et al. 2002). Milnacipran, an SNRI approved for depression in Europe and Japan and approved by the U.S. Food and Drug Administration (FDA) for fibromyalgia, is associated with constipation, flushing, sweating, vomiting, palpitations, increased heart rate and hypertension, and dry mouth (Cypress Bioscience 2010), similar to the other SNRIs.

Central nervous system. An association between SSRI use and increased suicidal ideation was proposed by Teicher et al. in 1990 on the basis of case reports. However, an early review of controlled antidepressant trial reports by the FDA suggested no difference in suicide risk between antidepressant- and placebo-treated depressed patients or between SSRIs and other antidepressants (Khan et al. 2003). In contrast, Fergusson et al. (2005), following a review of 345 controlled trials, suggested that SSRIs have a suicide attempt rate similar to that of TCAs and more than double the rate of placebo. Supporting these findings, a later FDA meta-analysis of 23 placebo-controlled pediatric clinical trials for nine modern antidepressants in 4,582 patients identified a twofold increased risk for suicide for all drugs examined (Hammad et al. 2006). In May 2007, the FDA concluded that all antidepressants increase the risk of suicidal thinking and behavior in young adults (age ≤24 years) during initial treatment and required manufacturers to include in their labeling a warning statement that recommends close observation of young adult and pediatric patients treated with these agents for worsening depression or the emergence of suicidality.

Bupropion causes a dose-related lowering of the seizure threshold and may precipitate seizures in susceptible patients receiving dosages above 450 mg/day. The incidence of seizure rises with increasing dosage, from 0.1% at 100–300 mg/day, through 0.4% at 300–450 mg/day, to 2.3% at dosages over 600 mg/day (McEvoy 2008). The seizure risk reported for other antidepressants ranges from 0.04% for mirtazapine to 0.5% for clomipramine (Harden and Goldstein 2002; Rosenstein et al. 1993). Given that the annual incidence of first unprovoked seizure is 0.06% in the general population, seizure risk for patients taking most antidepressants is not elevated. However, it is clear that certain antidepressants, including bupropion, clomipramine, maprotiline, and venlafaxine, are associated with a greater seizure risk than are other antidepressants (Harden and Goldstein 2002; Whyte et al. 2003), but this is rarely significant except at toxic doses.

Potential side effects of SSRIs include SSRI-induced extrapyramidal symptoms (EPS), likely resulting from serotonergic antagonism of dopaminergic pathways in the CNS. Akathisia, dystonia, parkinsonism, and tardive dyskinesia–like states have been reported, with akathisia being the most common effect and tardive dyskinesia–like states being the least common. Certain patients appear to be at increased risk, such as the elderly, patients with Parkinson's disease, and patients concurrently treated with dopamine antagonists (Leo 1996).

Serotonin syndrome. Serotonin syndrome is an uncommon but potentially life-threatening complication of treatment with serotonergic agents. Overall, there is considerable heterogeneity in the reported clinical features of serotonin syndrome (Table 38–3), reflecting the variation in the degree of severity of the syndrome. The incidence of the syndrome is unknown, in part because many physicians are unaware of the syndrome as a clinical diagnosis (Mackay et al. 1999) and because uniform diagnostic criteria are lacking. Virtually all medications that potentiate serotonergic neurotransmission in the CNS have been reported in association with serotonin syndrome. The antidepressant combinations most commonly implicated have been monoamine oxidase inhibitors (MAOIs; reversible and irreversible) and TCAs, MAOIs and SSRIs, and MAOIs and venlafaxine. Table 38–4 lists other serotonergic drugs.

Currently there is no formal consensus regarding diagnostic criteria for serotonin syndrome. The first operationalized criteria were proposed by Sternbach (1991) but were found to have low specificity. The Hunter Serotonin Toxicity Criteria have subsequently gained acceptance as a simple set of highly sensitive and specific decision rules; these criteria are listed in Table 38–5 (Dunkley et al. 2003). Laboratory findings have not been commonly reported in cases of serotonin syndrome, but some reports have noted leukocytosis, rhabdomyolysis with elevated creatine phosphokinase (CPK), serum hepatic transaminase elevations, electrolyte abnormalities (hyponatremia, hypomagnesemia, hypercalcemia), and disseminated intravascular coagulopathy. The differential diagnosis includes CNS infection (e.g., encephalitis, meningitis), delirium tremens, poisoning with anticholinergic or adrenergic agents, neuroleptic malignant syndrome (NMS), and malignant hyperthermia. Differentiating serotonin syndrome from NMS can be very difficult in patients receiving both serotonergic and antipsychotic medications (see "Neuroleptic Malignant Syndrome" subsection under "Antipsychotics" later in this chapter).

TABLE 38–3. Clinical features of serotonin syndrome

Category	Clinical features
Mental status and behavioral	Delirium, confusion, agitation, anxiety, irritability, euphoria, dysphoria, restlessness
Neurological and motor	Ataxia/incoordination, tremor, muscle rigidity, myoclonus, hyperreflexia, clonus, seizures, trismus, teeth chattering
Gastrointestinal	Nausea, vomiting, diarrhea, incontinence
Autonomic nervous system	Hypertension, hypotension, tachycardia, diaphoresis, shivering, sialorrhea, mydriasis, tachypnea, pupillary dilation
Thermoregulation	Hyperthermia

Source. Compiled in part from Keck and Arnold 2000.

Serotonin syndrome is often self-limited and usually resolves quickly after discontinuation of serotonergic agents. Management includes the following basic principles: 1) discontinue all serotonergic agents, 2) provide necessary supportive care, 3) anticipate potential complications, 4) consider administering antiserotonergic agents, and 5) reassess the need for psychopharmacological therapy before reinstituting drug therapy (Keck and Arnold 2000). Some patients will require admission to an intensive care unit, but most will show some improvement within 24 hours with supportive care alone. There are no specific antidotes available for the treatment of serotonin syndrome. The antihistamine cyproheptadine is the most consistently effective serotonin antagonist reported. The recommended adult dose is 4–8 mg and may be repeated every 1–4 hours up to a maximum daily dose of 32 mg. There is limited information on drug rechallenge in patients who have developed serotonin syndrome. General guidelines include reevaluating the necessity for drug therapy, considering a switch to a nonserotonergic medication, using single-drug therapy when serotonergic medications are required, and considering an extended (6-week) serotonin "drug-free" period before restarting a serotonergic agent (Mills 1997).

Autonomic and cardiovascular. The SSRIs and the novel/mixed-action antidepressants have a much safer cardiovascular profile than the TCAs and MAOIs. In general, the SSRIs have little effect on blood pressure or cardiac conduction (Glassman et al. 2002). Fluoxetine has been reported to rarely cause mild bradycardia in elderly patients with preexisting cardiac arrhythmias (Upward et al. 1988), and this may occur with other SSRIs as well (Roose and Miyazaki 2005).

TABLE 38–4. Drugs that potentiate serotonin in the central nervous system

Mechanism	Drug
Enhance serotonin synthesis	L-Tryptophan
Increase serotonin release	Cocaine
	Amphetamine
	Sibutramine
	Dextromethorphan, meperidine, fentanyl
	MDMA (Ecstasy)
	Lithium
Stimulate serotonin receptors	Buspirone
	Triptans
	Ergot alkaloids
	Trazodone, nefazodone
Inhibit serotonin catabolism	Antidepressant MAOIs
	Moclobemide
	Selegiline
	Linezolid
	Isoniazid
	Procarbazine
Inhibit serotonin reuptake	SSRIs
	Mirtazapine
	Trazodone, nefazodone
	Venlafaxine, desvenlafaxine, duloxetine, milnacipran
	TCAs
	Dextromethorphan, meperidine (pethidine)
	Tramadol

Note. MAOIs = monoamine oxidase inhibitors; MDMA = 3, 4-methylenedioxymethamphetamine; SSRIs = selective serotonin reuptake inhibitors; TCAs = tricyclic antidepressants.

The novel/mixed-action agents venlafaxine, desvenlafaxine, duloxetine, bupropion, nefazodone, mirtazapine, and reboxetine have little effect on cardiac conduction but may affect blood pressure or heart rate (Khawaja and Feinstein 2003; Pfizer 2010b). Venlafaxine exhibits dose-related increases in heart rate (mean increase of 4 beats/minute over placebo) and blood pressure. Placebo-controlled clinical trials of venlafaxine observed an average diastolic pressure increase of 7 mm Hg at dosages of more than 300 mg/day and clinically significant diastolic pressure increases (≥15 mm Hg) in 5.5% of patients taking the drug at dosages of more than 200 mg/day (Feighner 1995). Similar effects would be expected for desvenlafaxine. Duloxetine appears to be without clinically significant effects on heart rate, blood pres-

TABLE 38–5. Diagnostic criteria for serotonin syndrome

Use of a serotonergic agent

Plus any of the following symptoms:

Spontaneous clonus

Inducible clonus plus either agitation or diaphoresis

Tremor plus hyperreflexia

Muscle rigidity plus elevated body temperature plus either ocular clonus or inducible clonus

Exclude:

Infection, metabolic, endocrine, or toxic causes

Neuroleptic malignant syndrome

Delirium tremens

Malignant hyperthermia

Source. Compiled from Boyer and Shannon 2005; Dunkley et al. 2003; Prator 2006.

sure, or QT interval (Wernicke et al. 2007b). Bupropion is reported to cause hypertension without affecting heart rate in some patients. In patients using transdermal nicotine, bupropion is associated with a 6.1% incidence of hypertension (Khawaja and Feinstein 2003). Reboxetine has also been associated with an increase in heart rate of 8–11 beats/minute (Fleishaker et al. 2001) but without any significant effect on electrocardiography (Andreoli et al. 2002). Trazodone lacks significant effects on cardiac conduction but in rare cases was reported to cause ventricular ectopy and ventricular tachycardia. The most frequent cardiovascular adverse effect of trazodone is postural hypotension, which may be associated with syncope. Nefazodone is structurally related to trazodone but has a lower incidence of postural hypotension (3%). Mirtazapine does not have significant effects on cardiac conduction, but because of its moderate alpha$_1$-antagonist activity, it has a 7% incidence of orthostatic hypotension (Khawaja and Feinstein 2003). Hypotension is observed in 10% of patients receiving reboxetine.

Gastrointestinal. Nausea is the most common adverse effect associated with the serotonergic antidepressants. Nausea is most likely to occur in patients receiving fluvoxamine (36%), venlafaxine (37%), and duloxetine at a starting dose of 60 mg/day (35%–40%) (Detke et al. 2002a, 2002b). Other serotonergic antidepressants have a lower incidence (20%–26%) of nausea, but these incidences are still much higher than those seen with placebo (9.3%–11.8%) (Nelson 1997; Repchinsky 2009). Diarrhea was more prevalent with sertraline than with other SSRIs (Meijer et al. 2002).

Although most adverse gastrointestinal effects of serotonergic antidepressants are dose related and generally decrease with continued treatment, sometimes severe side effects require antidepressant discontinuation. Potential severe hepatotoxicity with nefazodone has led to its removal from the market in a number of countries, and it should not be used in patients with preexisting liver disease (D.E. Stewart 2002). Duloxetine-related hepatotoxicity in 1.1% of patients has prompted product monograph warnings (Eli Lilly 2010c); however, a review of duloxetine hepatic safety suggested no increase in hepatotoxicity compared with other conventional antidepressants (McIntyre et al. 2008). Pancreatitis has also rarely been reported with mirtazapine (Hussain and Burke 2008).

Hematological. SSRIs are associated with a slightly increased risk of bleeding disorders, including gastrointestinal bleeding. This effect is discussed in the "Psychotropic Drug Use in the Medically Ill" section later in this chapter.

Weight gain/loss. Weight gain is a relatively common problem during both acute and long-term treatment with antidepressants. TCAs and the MAOI phenelzine are more likely to cause weight gain than other antidepressants, with the exception of mirtazapine. Mirtazapine was associated with weight gain (defined as ≥7% weight increase during treatment) in 26% of patients followed by SSRIs and venlafaxine (16%–19%). Bupropion and nefazodone rarely cause weight gain (12%) (Papakostas 2007). Duloxetine may cause less weight gain than SSRIs (Dunner et al. 2008).

Sexual dysfunction. Refer to Chapter 16, "Sexual Dysfunction," for a discussion of the sexual side effects of psychotropic medications.

Drug interactions. Many SSRIs and novel/mixed-action antidepressants are potent inhibitors of CYP isozymes and may significantly increase the blood levels, and the potential for toxic effects, of other coadministered narrow-therapeutic-index medications metabolized by these enzymes. See Table 38–2 for a listing of critical narrow-therapeutic-index drug substrates for these enzymes.

The use of multiple serotonergic drugs can induce serotonin syndrome (see "Serotonin Syndrome" subsection earlier in the chapter).

Serotonin discontinuation syndrome. Abrupt discontinuation of SSRIs or SNRIs, especially those with short half-lives (e.g., fluvoxamine, paroxetine, venlafaxine), may give rise to a discontinuation syndrome characterized by a wide variety of symptoms, including psychiatric, neurological, and flulike symptoms (nausea, vomiting, sweats); sleep disturbances; and headache (Haddad 1998), usually resolving within 3 weeks. Antidepressants, like all psychoactive medications, should be gradually withdrawn. Discontinuation symptoms can cause misdiagnosis and inappropriate treatment, particularly in a patient with an active medical illness, as well as erode future compliance.

Tricyclic Antidepressants

TCAs are now viewed as second-line treatments for depression because their adverse-effect profile is less benign than that of SSRIs and novel/mixed-action agents. Death from TCA-induced cardiac conduction abnormalities was not uncommon in overdose.

Many adverse effects of TCAs are due not to their effects on serotonin (5-HT) or norepinephrine reuptake inhibition but rather to secondary pharmacological activities. TCAs are antagonists at histamine H_1, adrenergic $alpha_1$, and muscarinic receptors and have Type 1A antiarrhythmic (quinidine-like) effects from their blockade of voltage-dependent Na^+ channels. Adverse effects of TCAs include sedation, anticholinergic effects (dry mouth, dry eyes, constipation, urinary retention, decreased sweating, confusion, memory impairment, tachycardia, blurred vision), and postural hypotension. Tolerance to these effects usually develops over time. TCAs at or just above therapeutic plasma levels frequently prolong PR, QRS, and QTc intervals but rarely to a clinically significant degree in patients without preexisting cardiac disease or conduction defects (Glassman 1984). TCAs can cause heart block, arrhythmias, palpitations, tachycardia, syncope, and heart failure and should be used with caution in patients with preexisting cardiovascular disease or at risk of suicide. Following the discovery that class I antiarrhythmic drugs can increase mortality in patients with ischemic heart disease, it is prudent to assume that TCAs may carry the same risk in these patients (Cardiac Arrhythmia Suppression Trial [CAST] Investigators 1989; Roose and Miyazaki 2005).

Drug interactions. The combination of TCAs and other drugs with sedating, hypotensive, antiarrhythmic, or seizure threshold-lowering properties may lead to additive toxicity.

Concomitant use of TCAs and drugs with anticholinergic properties may cause an anticholinergic crisis characterized by delirium, hyperthermia (especially in hot environments), tachycardia, and paralytic ileus.

Coadministration of TCAs with MAOIs and other drugs with MAOI activity may precipitate serotonin syndrome or hyperpyretic crisis (hyperpyrexia, sweating, confusion, myoclonus, seizures, hypertension, and tachycardia), either of which may be fatal. The combination of serotonergic effects from cotherapy with some TCAs and SSRIs may precipitate serotonin syndrome (see "Serotonin Syndrome" subsection earlier in this chapter).

TCAs are narrow-therapeutic-index drugs, each metabolized predominantly by either CYP2D6 or CYP3A4. Inhibitors of these enzymes can cause TCA toxicity by dramatically increasing TCA serum levels. Many agents, including several SSRIs and novel/mixed-action antidepressants, are potent inhibitors of these CYP isozymes (see Table 38-2). Plasma levels of TCAs should be monitored if they are coadministered with such inhibitors.

Toxicity/overdose. TCA overdose carries a risk of death from cardiac conduction abnormalities that result in malignant ventricular arrhythmias. Initial symptoms of overdose involve CNS stimulation, in part due to anticholinergic effects, and include hyperpyrexia, delirium, hypertension, hallucinations, seizure, agitation, hyperreflexia, and parkinsonian symptoms. The initial stimulation phase is typically followed by CNS depression with drowsiness, areflexia, hypothermia, respiratory depression, severe hypotension, and coma. Risk of cardiotoxicity is high if the QRS interval is 100 msec or more (Boehnert and Lovejoy 1985) or if the total TCA plasma concentration is greater than 1,000 ng/mL; concentrations greater than 2,500 ng/mL are often fatal (Foulke and Albertson 1987).

Treatment for overdose includes removal of any unabsorbed medication from the stomach (gastric lavage and then activated charcoal to reduce absorption), followed by supportive therapy and close monitoring (see Chapter 37, "Medical Toxicology"). Cardiac conduction abnormalities, arrhythmias, and hypotension may be treated with administration of intravenous sodium bicarbonate to produce a serum pH of 7.4–7.5. Life-threatening anticholinergic effects may be managed with physostigmine. Because of their large volumes of distribution and extensive protein binding, TCAs are not removed by dialysis.

Abrupt discontinuation of TCAs may give rise to a discontinuation syndrome characterized by dizziness, lethargy, headache, nightmares, and symptoms of anticholinergic rebound, including gastrointestinal upset, nausea, vomiting, diarrhea, excessive salivation, sweating, anxiety, restlessness, piloerection, and delirium (Dilsaver and Greden 1984). This syndrome can be avoided by gradual withdrawal.

Monoamine Oxidase Inhibitors

MAOIs, with the possible exception of moclobemide (not available in the United States), are seen as third-line antidepressants because of their significant drug interactions and the dietary restrictions that accompany their use (Howland 2006). Moclobemide, a short-half-life reversible inhibitor of monoamine oxidase type A (MAO-A), is less susceptible to dietary interactions provided that it is taken after meals. Common adverse effects of MAOIs include orthostatic hypotension, dizziness, headache, sedation, insomnia or hypersomnia, tremor, and hyperreflexia. Interactions between MAOIs and direct- or indirect-acting sympathomimetics or dopaminergic agonists may cause a hypertensive crisis. MAOIs may trigger serotonin syndrome when combined with other medications (see "Serotonin Syndrome" subsection earlier in chapter). Moclobemide shares the potential to cause hypertensive crises and serotonin syndrome with the irreversible agents. MAOIs may greatly potentiate the hypotensive effects of antihypertensive agents, including diuretics.

Selegiline, a semiselective monoamine oxidase type B (MAO-B) inhibitor used to treat Parkinson's disease, and now as a transdermal patch indicated for depression, may also contribute to serotonin syndrome. At oral dosages greater than 10 mg/day, and with patch strengths greater than 6 mg, selegiline also inhibits MAO-A and thus shares many of the adverse effects and drug–food interactions, including hypertensive crisis, of the antidepressant MAOIs.

Toxicity/overdose. Symptoms of MAOI overdose are an extension of the normal adverse-effect profile. Treatment for overdose includes removal of any unabsorbed medication from the stomach and supportive measures.

Treatment for hypertensive crisis involves discontinuing the MAOI and slowly administering intravenous phentolamine (typical adult dose: 5 mg). ***Beta-blockers should never be used;*** beta-blockade allows unrestrained alpha-adrenergic stimulation, which further exacerbates the hypertension.

Mood Stabilizers/Anticonvulsants

Mood stabilizers are used in the medically ill to treat primary and secondary mood disorders as well as for symptoms such as headache and chronic pain.

Many, but not all, anticonvulsants appear to have mood-stabilizing properties. Valproate, carbamazepine, and oxcarbazepine are the most commonly used anticonvulsant mood stabilizers. Controlled studies do not support the use of gabapentin as a mood stabilizer (Evins 2003).

Lithium

Most patients using lithium experience some side effects, both acute (gastrointestinal distress and tremor) and long term (polyuria and polydipsia, hypothyroidism, weight gain, impaired cognition, sedation, impaired coordination, edema, acne, and hair loss), most of which are mild and dose related (Freeman and Freeman 2006; Peet and Pratt 1993). Adverse effects of lithium can be minimized by reducing the dose or decreasing the rate of absorption from the gut by administering the drug either in divided doses with meals or in a slow-release dosage form.

Central nervous system. Headache, fatigue, hand tremor, and mild cognitive impairment are reported by up to 50% of patients beginning lithium treatment. Hand tremor is usually a benign, fine, rapid, intention tremor that resolves over time or can be managed by dose reduction or low-dose beta-blockers. The tremor does not respond to antiparkinsonian drugs. Muscle weakness, fatigue, and ataxia are also common initial adverse effects that usually resolve (McEvoy 2008). Mild cognitive impairment may be experienced during the first 6–8 months of treatment; although rarely progressive, this impairment is the most common reason for noncompliance (Gitlin et al. 1989). Compliance may be improved by patient education and use of the lowest effective dose (Berk and Berk 2003).

Autonomic and cardiovascular. Lithium causes benign reversible repolarization electrocardiographic changes in 20%–30% of patients (Mitchell and Mackenzie 1982), including T wave depression and inversion. Other cardiovascular effects of lithium include decreased heart rate, prolonged QT interval, and arrhythmias (Burggraf 1997; van Noord et al. 2009).

Renal. Lithium reduces renal response to antidiuretic hormone, resulting in polyuria and/or polydipsia initially in 30%–50% of patients and persisting in 10%–25%. Stopping lithium usually reverses this nephrogenic diabetes insipidus (McEvoy 2008). Apart from dry mouth, patients do not generally exhibit signs of dehydration. Management of polyuria may include changing to a single daily bedtime dose of lithium, decreasing dosage, and/or administering amiloride, considered the treatment of choice, or thiazide diuretics. If thiazide diuretics are added, lithium dosage should be reduced by 50% to compensate for thiazide-induced reduction of lithium excretion (Jefferson et al. 1987). Use of amiloride does not require a reduction in lithium dosage (Bendz and Aurell 1999). Edema has been reported in patients with a high sodium intake (>170 mEq/day), responsive to reduction in sodium intake or spironolactone (Stancer and Kivi 1971).

Both functional and morphological changes of the kidneys have been reported in lithium-poisoned patients. Chronic use of lithium may result in altered kidney morphology—including interstitial fibrosis, tubular atrophy, urinary casts, and, occasionally, glomerular sclerosis—in 10%–20% of patients (Bendz et al. 1996). These changes are not generally associated with impaired renal function. Although long-term lithium treatment is the only well-established factor associated with lithium-induced nephropathy, other factors such as age, previous episodes of lithium toxicity, and the presence of comorbid disorders may also contribute. Lithium dose is not strongly related to nephrotoxic effects (Freeman and Freeman 2006). The progression of lithium nephrotoxicity to end-stage renal disease is rare (0.2% to 0.7%) and requires lithium use for several decades (Presne et al. 2003). Lithium is so efficacious in bipolar disorder that the risk of renal dysfunction during chronic use is considered acceptable with yearly monitoring of renal function.

Endocrine and metabolic. The prevalence of overt hypothyroidism has been reported to be as high as 8%–19% for patients taking lithium, compared with a prevalence of 0.5%–1.8% in the general population. Subclinical hypothyroidism has been reported in up to 23% of patients receiving lithium therapy, compared with rates of up to 10.4% in the general population. Elevated thyroid-stimulating hormone is present in approximately 30% of patients taking lithium for 6 months or more, and progression to overt hypothyroidism (elevated thyroid-stimulating hormone and low free T_4) may occur in as many as 5%–10% of patients per year (Kleiner et al. 1999) with greater risk in thyroid antibody-positive individuals (Bocchetta et al. 2007). Thyroid function should be assessed before lithium is started and periodically during therapy. Hypothyroidism can be treated with L-thyroxine and is not a contraindication to continuing lithium (Bauer and Whybrow 1990; see also Chapter 22, "Endocrine and Metabolic Disorders").

Lithium-induced weight gain (>8% of baseline body weight) (Chengappa et al. 2002) is the second most common reason cited by patients for lithium noncompliance (Gitlin et al. 1989). Weight gain is a consequence of increased caloric intake in part due to consumption of high-calorie fluids in response to increased thirst (McEvoy 2008).

Dermatological. Dermatological adverse effects include dry skin, hair loss, and acne. Lithium-induced acne occurs in more than 30% of patients (Chan et al. 2000). These effects usually respond to standard treatment and rarely require lithium discontinuation. Alopecia and exacerbation of psoriasis occur less frequently. Lithium-induced psoriasis has been shown to respond to inositol supplements (Allan et al. 2004; see also Chapter 29, "Dermatology").

Drug interactions. Lithium is almost entirely renally excreted, and most lithium filtered by the glomeruli is reabsorbed with sodium in the proximal tubule. Serum lithium levels are increased by thiazide diuretics, NSAIDs, angiotensin-converting enzyme inhibitors, sodium depletion, dehydration (Dunner 2003), and possibly verapamil (Wright and Jarrett 1991) and angiotensin receptor antagonists (Su et al. 2007). Acutely, loop diuretics increase lithium excretion, but with chronic use, compensatory changes leave lithium levels not greatly changed. Carbonic anhydrase inhibitors and osmotic diuretics reduce lithium levels. Potassium-sparing diuretics may increase lithium excretion (Owen and Levenson 2010). The effect of the direct renin inhibitor aliskiren on lithium excretion is presently unknown. (See Thomsen and Schou [1999] for a review of lithium drug interactions.)

Lithium may potentiate the neurological adverse effects of other drugs, for example, EPS and tremor (Dunner 2000). Several case reports suggest that lithium in combination with other serotonin-enhancing drugs may precipitate serotonin syndrome (Adan-Manes et al. 2006; Schweitzer and Tuckwell 1998).

Toxicity/overdose. Toxicity increases markedly as serum lithium levels exceed 1.5 mEq/L, and serum levels greater than 2.0 mEq/L are dangerous. However, some patients experience toxicity at "therapeutic" levels. Initial symptoms of toxicity include marked tremor, nausea, diarrhea, blurred vision, vertigo, confusion, and increased deep tendon reflexes, progressing to seizures, coma, cardiac arrhythmia, and possibly permanent neurological impairment as lithium levels increase.

Treatment for lithium toxicity includes gastric lavage or emesis followed by supportive measures. These measures include volume resuscitation with isotonic or one-half isotonic sodium chloride solution to enhance renal elimination of lithium in individuals with mild to moderate toxicity or hemodialysis for patients with severe toxicity and/or lithium levels of 3.5 mEq/L or higher (Jaeger et al. 1993; Menghini and Albright 2000).

Anticonvulsants

Central nervous system. The anticonvulsants valproate, carbamazepine, gabapentin, lamotrigine, oxcarbazepine, topiramate, tiagabine, zonisamide, and levetiracetam share a similar profile of CNS adverse effects. Sedation, ataxia, dizziness, muscle weakness, fatigue, and vision disturbances such as nystagmus and diplopia are common and often resolve with time, dosage reduction, or discontinuation. Studies of oxcarbazepine in epilepsy suggest a lower rate of most adverse effects than carbamazepine (Schmidt and Elger 2004). Patients with a previous psychiatric history were more likely to experience psychiatric adverse effects with levetiracetam, including affective disorder (1%), psychosis (3%), and aggression (2%) (Mula et al. 2003). Psychotic symptoms are an infrequent adverse effect with topiramate (Crawford 1998). Cognitive impairment is a common complication of anticonvulsant use. Among anticonvulsants used in psychiatry, the ranking of cognitive profile is (best to worst) gabapentin, valproate, lamotrigine, carbamazepine, levetiracetam > zonisamide, phenytoin, oxcarbazepine >> topiramate (Arif et al. 2009).

The incidence of adverse effects increases with anticonvulsant multitherapy.

Gastrointestinal. Symptoms of gastrointestinal distress, including nausea, vomiting, dyspepsia, diarrhea, and anorexia, are the most frequent adverse effects experienced with most anticonvulsants. These effects are often dose related and transient and can be minimized by giving the drug in divided doses, with meals, or with slow titration. Gastrointestinal effects appear less often with divalproex sodium than with valproate or sodium valproate. There are fewer gastrointestinal complaints with oxcarbazepine than with carbamazepine. Transient elevations in liver enzymes occur commonly with anticonvulsants (Bjornsson 2008). Significant changes in hepatic function are usually reversible with dosage reduction or discontinuation. However, fatal hepatotoxicity has been reported with valproate and carbamazepine. The risk of hepatic failure may be increased by combination therapy and comorbid hepatic disorders (Konig et al. 1999). Several anticonvulsants, including valproate, carbamazepine, and lamotrigine, are infrequently associated with drug-induced pancreatitis. (For further discussion, see "Gastrointestinal Disorders," below.)

Hematological. Carbamazepine is frequently associated with transient leukopenia and rarely may cause aplastic anemia. Carbamazepine should be discontinued in patients with white blood cell (WBC) counts less than 3.0×10^9/L or neutrophil counts less than 1.0×10^9/L, and patients must be educated to report early signs of anemia, infection, or bleeding (Sobotka et al. 1990).

Mild, asymptomatic leukopenia and thrombocytopenia have been observed with valproate and are generally reversible with dosage reduction or discontinuation. More severe cases of thrombocytopenia and agranulocytosis have also been reported (Finsterer et al. 2001; Tohen et al. 1995).

Renal. Carbamazepine and oxcarbazepine frequently cause the syndrome of inappropriate antidiuretic hormone secretion (SIADH), leading to hyponatremia and water intoxication. Hyponatremia is twice as likely with oxcarbazepine (29.9% of patients) than with carbamazepine (14.4%) (Dong et al. 2005), and more common in the elderly (van Amelsvoort et al. 1994). (For further discussion of SIADH, see the "Antipsychotics" section later in this chapter.)

Endocrine and metabolic. Weight gain is a common factor in noncompliance (Mendlewicz et al. 1999). Weight gain is especially a problem with valproate, with an average weight gain of >8% of baseline body weight (Chengappa et al. 2002). Gabapentin causes a 1% weight gain (Wang et al. 2002). Although carbamazepine is also reported to cause weight gain, the incidence is less than with valproate (Corman et al. 1997). Lamotrigine has little effect on weight (Biton et al. 2001), whereas topiramate causes a weight loss of about 0.7% of body weight (Chengappa et al. 2002).

Topiramate inhibits carbonic anhydrase and can cause hyperchloremic, non-anion gap metabolic acidosis; in adult clinical trials, persistent reductions in serum bicarbonate occurred in 32% of patients, and levels were markedly low (<17 mEq/L) in up to 7%, depending on dose. The incidence of a persistent reduction in serum bicarbonate is greater in pediatric patients (Ortho-NcNeil 2010). Valproate can cause asymptomatic hyperammonemia and hyperammonemic encephalopathy.

Polycystic ovarian syndrome is 3.8-fold more prevalent in women with epilepsy than in the general population. This increase has been variously attributed to either epilepsy (Joffe et al. 2001) or anticonvulsant medications, especially valproate. Valproate appears to present a reduced risk when used as a mood stabilizer (Bilo and Meo 2008; see Chapter 22, "Endocrine and Metabolic Disorders").

Immune system. Benign skin rashes occur in 5%–20% of patients receiving anticonvulsants, including valproate, carbamazepine, and lamotrigine. However, serious and potentially fatal immune reactions to anticonvulsants are not uncommon. Anticonvulsant hypersensitivity syndrome has been observed in up to 1% of patients, with initial signs of rash, fever, malaise, and pharyngitis progressing to internal organ involvement. Severe and often fatal hypersensitivity cutaneous reactions in 0.01% to 0.1% of new anticonvulsant users include Stevens-Johnson syndrome and toxic epidermal necrolysis (Mockenhaupt et al. 2005). Mortality occurs in about 5%–10% of patients with Stevens-Johnson syndrome and in up to 45% of those with toxic epidermal necrolysis. In comparison with general medical patients, the risk of developing Stevens-Johnson syndrome or toxic epidermal necrolysis during the first 2 months of anticonvulsant therapy is increased by 120-fold for carbamazepine, 25-fold for lamotrigine, and 24-fold for valproate (Rzany et al. 1999). Clinical trials suggest that 25% of patients with hypersensitivity reactions to carbamazepine will also cross-react to oxcarbazepine (USPDI Editorial Board 2007). The presence of an anticonvulsant-induced rash should prompt drug discontinuation (Hebert and Ralston 2001).

Drug interactions. Significant CYP isoenzyme induction occurs with carbamazepine (CYP1A2, CYP2C, and CYP 3A4), oxcarbazepine (CYP3A4), and valproate (CYP2C) (see Table 38–2). Because valproate is highly bound to plasma proteins, it can significantly displace other highly protein-bound drugs. Valproate can also compete for hepatic glucuronidation and so inhibit the elimination of drugs primarily using this route of metabolism, such as lamotrigine and morphine.

Toxicity/overdose. Symptoms of anticonvulsant overdose are often an extension of the normal adverse effects, including stupor, conduction disturbances, and hypotension. Treatment for overdose includes gastric lavage or emesis followed by supportive therapy. Hemodialysis is an effective means of enhancing drug elimination for valproate, gabapentin, pregabalin, topiramate, and levetiracetam.

Antipsychotics

Antipsychotic drugs are used in the medically ill to treat nearly all forms of psychosis, including psychosis secondary to general medical conditions, delirium, and dementia, and less frequently for nonspecific sedation and as analgesic adjuvants.

Central Nervous System

Acute extrapyramidal symptoms. Acute EPS—akathisia, akinesia, and dystonia—occur in as many as 50%–75% of patients who take typical antipsychotics (Collaborative Working Group on Clinical Trial Evaluations 1998). High-potency typical antipsychotics are associated with higher rates of EPS than are low-potency agents. Among the currently available atypical antipsychotics, the hierarchy of EPS risk (greater to lesser) is ziprasidone > aripiprazole > risperidone = paliperidone (estimated) > asenapine (estimated) > iloperidone (estimated) > olanzapine > quetiapine > clozapine (Citrome 2009; Gao et al. 2008; Tandon 2002; Weber and McCormack 2009).

Most akathisia and acute dystonic reactions in the medically ill are caused by phenothiazine antiemetics or metoclopramide, especially at high intravenous doses. When agitated medically ill patients are being treated with haloperidol, it can be very difficult to distinguish akathisia from the original target symptoms. It is also important to exclude other causes of restlessness that may mimic akathisia in medically ill patients, such as hypoglycemia, hypoxia, drug withdrawal, pain, electrolyte disturbances, iron deficiency, and restless legs syndrome. Severe dystonic reactions (e.g., opisthotonus) may be misdiagnosed in the medically ill as status epilepticus.

Chronic extrapyramidal symptoms. Parkinsonian signs and tardive dyskinesia may result from chronic use of antipsychotics, phenothiazine antiemetics, or metoclopramide. Bradykinesia may easily be missed in the elderly or disabled medical patients. Tardive dyskinesias may be difficult to distinguish from other dyskinesias in elderly patients (e.g., "senile dyskinesias," ill-fitting dentures).

Seizures. Most antipsychotics lower seizure threshold and increase seizure risk. Various reports suggest a dose-dependent seizure risk with phenothiazines of 0.3%–1.2% compared with a rate of first unprovoked seizure in the general population of about 0.1%. Most of the early case reports were of seizures with chlorpromazine. Although there are no controlled comparative studies to allow an accurate assessment of relative seizure risk, it appears that high-potency typical antipsychotics and risperidone (and likely paliperidone) have the lowest rate of seizures, followed by quetiapine, then olanzapine and low-potency typical antipsychotics with an intermediate risk, and finally clozapine with the highest risk (1% at 300 mg/day, increasing to 4.4% at >600 mg/day) (Alldredge 1999; Alper et al. 2007; Devinsky et al. 1991).

Sedation. Sedation is the most common single side effect, especially with the low-potency typical antipsychotics. Among the atypical antipsychotics, the hierarchy of potential for sedation (greater to lesser) is quetiapine > ziprasidone = clozapine > olanzapine > asenapine (estimated) = iloperidone (estimated) > risperidone = paliperidone (estimated) > aripiprazole (Citrome 2009; Leucht et al. 2009; Weber and McCormack 2009). Sedation is most prominent in the early stages of therapy, with some degree of tolerance developing over time.

Thermoregulation. Antipsychotics may interfere with temperature regulation, especially low-potency typical and anticholinergic atypical agents. Medically ill patients, especially elderly ones, are at particular risk because of other anticholinergic drugs and comorbidities impairing thermoregulation (e.g., congestive heart failure, cerebrovascular disease). Depending on environmental exposure, either hyperthermia (heatstroke) or hypothermia may result (S.C. Mann et al. 2003).

Neuroleptic malignant syndrome. NMS is a rare, potentially fatal, idiosyncratic reaction to antipsychotics. NMS (or a similar syndrome) is also reported among patients with extrapyramidal disorders such as Wilson's disease, striatonigral degeneration, and Parkinson's disease who have received antipsychotics or dopamine-depleting agents or who have had dopamine agonists abruptly withdrawn (Friedman et al. 1985; Gibb 1988; Gibb and Griffith 1986; Kontaxakis et al. 1988). However, NMS is not specific to any neuropsychiatric diagnosis and has been reported in non-psychiatrically ill individuals who were treated with other dopamine antagonists such as metoclopramide and prochlorperazine (Nonino and Campomori 1999; Pesola and Quinto 1996). Estimates of the incidence of NMS, once thought to be as high as 3%, are now suggested from more recent data to be 0.01%–0.02% (Stubner et al. 2004). Mortality ranges from 11% to 38% (Jahan et al. 1992). Malnutrition, dehydration, and iron deficiency all appear to increase risk for NMS.

NMS generally develops over a 1- to 3-day period and lasts for 5–10 days after a nondepot antipsychotic is discontinued. Mortality is high, often quoted at 20%–30% but probably lower now because of earlier recognition of the syndrome. The main clinical features of NMS include hyperthermia (>37°C), generalized muscle rigidity, mental status changes and autonomic instability (Table 38–6). Hyperthermia is greater than 38°C in the majority of cases and can exceed 40°C, which predisposes the patient to severe complications, including irreversible CNS and other organ damage. Muscle rigidity is often heterogeneous and can be "lead-pipe" or cogwheeling, but may be absent. Autonomic dysfunction in NMS may include hypertension, orthostatic hypotension, labile blood pressure, tachycardia, tachypnea, sialorrhea, diaphoresis, skin pallor, and urinary incontinence. Neurological dysfunction may consist of tremor, myoclonus, focal dystonias, dysphagia, dysarthria, opisthotonus, oculogyric crisis, and dyskinesias. Altered level of consciousness may range from decreased awareness to coma. CPK levels are elevated in NMS secondary to muscle necrosis from rigidity, hyperthermia, and ischemia. Elevated CPK levels are not proof of NMS, because they may result from agitation, use of physical restraints, and intramuscular injections. Extreme elevation of CPK (>100,000 U/L) constitutes rhabdomyolysis, which may be a consequence of NMS and/or other causes in the medically ill (e.g., sepsis, shock, alcohol). Serial CPK levels decline with the resolution of NMS. Leukocytosis with or without a left shift is common. Complications may include respiratory or renal failure, pulmonary embolus, electrolyte disturbances, and coagulopathy (Caroff and Mann 1993; Pelonero et al. 1998) as well as neuropsychiatric sequelae (Adityanjee et al. 2005).

The differential diagnosis of NMS is large (Table 38–7). Although the vast majority of patients receiving antipsychotics who develop fever and rigidity will be found to have other conditions, the possibility of NMS should be considered because of the importance of promptly withholding antipsychotics. Diagnosis may be guided by the use of an NMS rating scale (Sachdev 2005).

The main interventions in NMS are early diagnosis, rapid cessation of the antipsychotic treatment, and intensive supportive care. Lithium, antipsychotics, and all other dopamine-blocking agents (including antiemetics, metoclopramide, and droperidol) should be discontinued. No specific therapy (e.g., benzodiazepines, dantrolene, or bromocriptine) has been proven superior to other measures (reviewed by Strawn et al. 2007). Meta-analyses of dantrolene therapy of NMS have demonstrated results which vary from a beneficial effect (Rosenberg and Green 1989) to a higher overall mortality or slower clinical recovery (Reulbach et al. 2007). Most cases of NMS require initial treatment in a medical intensive care unit and should be transferred back to a psychiatric service only after the patient is medically stable. Among patients who recover from NMS, there may be a 30% risk of recurrent episodes following subsequent antipsychotic rechallenge, but the majority of patients who require antipsychotic therapy can be cautiously re-treated at least two weeks after resolution of NMS. Additional information is available from the Neuroleptic Malignant Syndrome Information Service (www.nmsis.org).

TABLE 38–6. Diagnostic criteria for neuroleptic malignant syndrome

Use of dopamine-blocking agents

Antipsychotics
Antiemetics
Droperidol
Metoclopramide

Muscle rigidity

Generalized or localized (tongue, facial muscles)
Elevated creatine phosphokinase

Pyrexia

Mild pyrexia to >42°C

Altered level of consciousness

Mild confusion to coma

Autonomic dysfunction

Hypertension, orthostatic hypotension, labile blood pressure, tachycardia, tachypnea, sialorrhea, diaphoresis, skin pallor, and urinary incontinence

Autonomic and cardiovascular. Autonomic side effects result from cholinergic and alpha$_1$-adrenergic blockade, seen more frequently with low-potency typical antipsychotics. Among the atypical agents, the hierarchy for producing hypotension (from greatest risk to least risk) is clozapine > quetiapine > iloperidone (estimated) > risperidone = paliperidone (estimated) > olanzapine = ziprasidone = aripiprazole (estimated) (Tandon 2002; Vanda 2010). Clozapine and quetiapine have been reported to cause tachycardia in 25% and 7% of cases, respectively. Tachycardia occurs in 5% of patients receiving risperidone or olanzapine, and in 2% of ziprasidone patients (Drici and Priori 2007).

QTc prolongation and torsade de pointes. A number of antipsychotics may be associated with QTc interval prolongation and risk for torsade de pointes. Sertindole was never

TABLE 38–7. Differential diagnosis of neuroleptic malignant syndrome

Differential diagnosis	Distinguishing clinical features
Serotonin syndrome	Occurs with combinations of drugs that increase serotonin transmission. Rapid onset over 24 hours; altered mental state, hyperreflexia, spontaneous or inducible clonus, autonomic instability; nausea, vomiting, diarrhea are common. Muscle rigidity present only in very severe form.
Malignant hyperthermia	Occurs after general anesthesia; familial
Lethal catatonia	Similar symptoms but occurs independent of antipsychotic exposure
Heatstroke	Pyrexia, agitation, and confusion. Skin is hot and dry and muscles are flaccid; prior neuroleptic exposure may increase risk for heatstroke
Severe EPS or Parkinson's disease	No fever, leukocytosis, or autonomic changes
Central nervous system infection	Seizures more likely; abnormal CSF
Allergic drug reaction	Rash, urticaria, wheezing, eosinophilia
Toxic encephalopathy, lithium toxicity	No fever; low CPK
Anticholinergic delirium	Dry skin, flaccid muscles, and low CPK
Systemic infection plus severe EPS	May appear identical to neuroleptic malignant syndrome

Note. CPK = creatine phosphokinase; CSF = cerebrospinal fluid; EPS = extrapyramidal symptoms.
Source. Compiled from Haddad and Dursun 2008; Pelonero et al. 1998.

marketed in the United States for this reason, but it is available in Europe with a restrictive label. Ziprasidone, thioridazine, and droperidol carry a black-box warning regarding dose-related QTc prolongation and risk for sudden death. Mean QTc interval prolongation (greatest to least) for antipsychotics is: thioridazine (36 msec) > ziprasidone (21 msec) > quetiapine (15 msec) > paliperidone (12 msec) = risperidone (10 msec) = asenapine (estimated) = iloperidone (9 msec) > olanzapine (6 msec) > haloperidol (5 msec) > aripiprazole (<1 msec) (Citrome 2009; Janssen 2010; Otsuka 2002; Pfizer 2010a; Weber and McCormack 2009). Almost 30% of patients taking thioridazine had a change in QTc of 60 msec, followed by 21% for ziprasidone, 11% for quetiapine, and 4% each for risperidone, olanzapine, and haloperidol. A few subjects receiving thioridazine (10%) or ziprasidone (3%) had a QTc prolongation of 75 msec or greater. Case reports have also associated droperidol and pimozide with QTc prolongation. Controlled trials confirm QTc prolongation with droperidol (Carroll et al. 2002).

Other cardiac side effects. Potentially fatal myocarditis, cardiomyopathy, and heart failure have been reported with clozapine. Estimated rates of clozapine-associated myocarditis range from 1 in 10,000 to 1 in 500. Eighty-five percent of these cases develop during the first 2 months of therapy and may be accompanied by eosinophilia. Clozapine-associated cardiomyopathy has most often occurred in patients younger than 50 years, with dilated cardiomyopathy accounting for two-thirds of the cases and one-third of the deaths. Withdrawal of the drug might result in improvement of the cardiomyopathy (Wooltorton 2002). Myocarditis and cardiomyopathy have also been reported in association with chlorpromazine, fluphenazine, risperidone, haloperidol, and quetiapine (Bush and Burgess 2008), but a causal link has not been demonstrated (Coulter et al. 2001).

Endocrine and Metabolic

For a fuller discussion of the endocrine and metabolic effects of antipsychotic drugs, the reader is referred to Chapter 22, "Endocrine and Metabolic Disorders."

Glucose tolerance. Pharmacoepidemiological studies and case reports reveal an association between the use of various atypical antipsychotics and hyperglycemia, new-onset type 2 diabetes, and occasionally ketoacidosis. These effects are not fully understood and are not solely explained by weight gain; schizophrenia is itself a risk factor for type 2 diabetes regardless of treatment. A large retrospective study suggests the risk of new-onset diabetes is greatest with clozapine and declines through olanzapine, quetiapine, and risperidone (E.A. Miller et al. 2005). Other surveys suggest little difference in risk between olanzapine, quetiapine, and risperidone (Lambert et al. 2006). A U.S. consensus statement concluded that hyperglycemia is associated with all marketed atypical antipsychotics but is less with aripiprazole and ziprasidone (American Diabetes

Association et al. 2004). To date, however, the only report of hyperglycemia associated with ziprasidone has been in the context of possible NMS with rhabdomyolysis and pancreatitis (Yang and McNeely 2002). Diabetic ketoacidosis has been reported in association with all atypical antipsychotics, including aripiprazole, except for ziprasidone and paliperidone.

Lipids. Phenothiazines, but not butyrophenones were long ago noted to elevate serum levels of cholesterol and triglycerides. Among atypical antipsychotics, risk of hyperlipidemia is highest with clozapine, olanzapine, and quetiapine, and lowest with risperidone, ziprasidone and aripiprazole (Meyer and Koro 2004). Serum triglycerides usually peak in the first year of therapy.

Hyperprolactinemia. Hyperprolactinemia is relatively common, especially with high-potency typical antipsychotics, risperidone, and paliperidone, and can result in amenorrhea or irregular menses, galactorrhea, gynecomastia, sexual dysfunction, and osteoporosis. Risperidone and paliperidone (Melkersson 2006) often elevate prolactin levels; clozapine, quetiapine, olanzapine, and ziprasidone are regarded as prolactin-sparing; aripiprazole decreases prolactin levels (Haddad and Sharma 2007).

Weight gain. All currently marketed antipsychotics (with the possible exception of ziprasidone and aripiprazole) are associated with weight gain, which may increase health risks (e.g., hypertension, atherosclerosis, type 2 diabetes, cardiovascular disease, and stroke), stigmatization, noncompliance, impairment in quality of life, and social withdrawal. The relative propensity to cause weight gain among the atypical antipsychotics (from greatest to least) is clozapine > olanzapine >> quetiapine > risperidone = paliperidone (estimated) > iloperidone (estimated) > asenapine (estimated) >> aripiprazole > ziprasidone (Citrome 2009; Haddad 2005; Weber and McCormack 2009). Current consensus guidelines for monitoring patients receiving atypical antipsychotics, including monitoring forms and risk criteria, are available from the Center for Quality Assessment and Improvement in Mental Health (www.cqaimh.org/pdf/tool_metabolic.pdf).

Syndrome of inappropriate antidiuretic hormone secretion. SIADH can occur with typical as well as atypical antipsychotics (and some antidepressants and anticonvulsants). SIADH is characterized by a reduced ability to excrete water, resulting in extracellular dilution and hyponatremia. SIADH is distinguished from polydipsia (water intoxication) by urine osmolality, with relatively high urine osmolality in SIADH versus very low urine osmolality in polydipsia. Common symptoms include weakness, lethargy, headache, anorexia, and weight gain and may progress to confusion, convulsions, coma, and death.

Hematological. Hematological side effects of antipsychotics include agranulocytosis, aplastic anemia, neutropenia, eosinophilia, and thrombocytopenia (reviewed in Flanagan and Dunk 2008). Transient leukopenia and leukocytosis are not uncommon in the first few weeks of therapy and are usually not clinically significant. Agranulocytosis is the most common serious hematological side effect with clozapine, low-potency typical antipsychotics (<0.1%) and olanzapine. Clozapine-associated agranulocytosis occurs in about 0.5%–2.0% of patients, with highest risk in the first 6 months. Clozapine use is through a controlled distribution system dependent on routine assessment of WBC count and absolute neutrophil count (ANC). A WBC count less than 2,000/mm^3 or an ANC less than 1,000/mm^3 is an indication for immediate cessation of clozapine.

Hepatic. Liver function abnormalities during antipsychotic therapy have long been reported but seldom require drug discontinuation. Mild to moderate elevations in liver aminotransferases and alkaline phosphatase usually occur early in treatment and are unlikely to result in hepatic impairment. Cholestatic jaundice is an idiosyncratic reaction that occurs rarely with phenothiazines.

Allergic, dermatological, and ophthalmological. Dermatological adverse reactions include early allergic rashes, photosensitivity, and skin hyperpigmentation, especially with chlorpromazine. Pigmentary retinopathy occurred in patients taking more than 800 mg/day of thioridazine. Acute angle closure glaucoma may occur in patients with a physiologically narrow anterior chamber angle who take anticholinergic medications.

Sexual. Antipsychotics may cause sexual dysfunction, in some cases related to their causing hyperprolactinemia (see also Chapter 22, "Endocrine and Metabolic Disorders," and Chapter 16, "Sexual Dysfunction").

Toxicity/overdose. Generally, antipsychotic overdose is associated with low morbidity and mortality. Most patients who have taken an antipsychotic overdose remain asymptomatic or develop mild sedation within 1–2 hours, but particular antipsychotics can cause serious cardiac effects (e.g., QTc prolongation from ziprasidone or thioridazine) or neurotoxicity (e.g., clozapine-induced seizures), especially in medically vulnerable patients.

Drug interactions. Most antipsychotic drugs have sedating, hypotensive, anticholinergic, antiarrhythmic, and seizure threshold–lowering properties. Predictable drug interactions may occur when combining antipsychotics with other drugs also possessing these characteristics. For example, antipsychotics may strongly potentiate the sedative effects of other CNS depressants, and anticholinergic antipsychotics will have additive adverse effects with other anticholinergic drugs. Antipsychotics may greatly enhance the hypotensive effects of antihypertensive agents. Low-potency antipsychotics and ziprasidone should be avoided in patients receiving other drugs with type 1A antiarrhythmic (quinidine-like) properties.

Many antipsychotics, including aripiprazole, clozapine, olanzapine, risperidone, and asenapine, are prone to pharmacokinetic drug interactions because of the limited number of CYP isozymes involved in their metabolism (see Table 38–2).

Anxiolytics and Sedative-Hypnotics

Benzodiazepines have long been considered the cornerstone of pharmacotherapy for anxiety and insomnia. Alternatives include buspirone for anxiety and the nonbenzodiazepine hypnotics eszopiclone, zopiclone, zolpidem, zaleplon, and ramelteon (a melatonin receptor agonist). These newer agents appear to have less tolerance and abuse potential and fewer adverse effects than benzodiazepines. Chloral hydrate has been used as a sedative-hypnotic since 1869, but because dependence occurs rapidly and withdrawal can be fatal, its use has greatly declined. Chloral hydrate is no longer FDA-approved for use in the United States.

Benzodiazepines

Benzodiazepines commonly cause dose-related CNS adverse effects but rarely affect organ systems other than the respiratory system, although in cirrhosis they may precipitate hepatic encephalopathy.

Central nervous system. Acute adverse CNS effects, including sedation, fatigue and weakness, ataxia, slurred speech, confusion, and memory impairment, are common, especially in older individuals and the medically ill. When used for the treatment of insomnia, long-half-life benzodiazepines are more likely to cause daytime sedation and cognitive impairment than short-half-life drugs. The elderly and patients with brain injury are also susceptible to benzodiazepine-induced behavioral disinhibition resulting in excitement, aggression, and paradoxical rage (Mancuso et al. 2004).

Physical tolerance often develops with chronic use of benzodiazepines, and some therapeutic effects (not anxiolysis) and adverse effects (sedation and psychomotor impairment) may diminish (O'Brien 2005). Studies suggest little or no long-term cognitive deterioration following chronic benzodiazepine use in the elderly (Bierman et al. 2007; McAndrews et al. 2003).

Respiratory. Benzodiazepines decrease the central respiratory response to hypoxia. Benzodiazepines differ in their ability to cause respiratory depression (Cohn 1983; Guilleminault 1990), with long-acting agents such as flurazepam (Dolly and Block 1982; Mendelson et al. 1981) and nitrazepam (Model 1973; Sanger and Zivkovic 1992) having the most pronounced effects. These drugs can cause apnea when used alone or in combination with other CNS depressants, most commonly alcohol (Guilleminault 1990; Mendelson et al. 1981). The respiratory depressant effects of benzodiazepines may become clinically significant in individuals with preexisting respiratory disorders, such as chronic obstructive pulmonary disease (COPD) (Clarke and Lyons 1977; Model 1973) or sleep apnea (Mendelson et al. 1981), or in those with seizure disorders (which also can cause respiratory depression).

The incidence of respiratory depression associated with benzodiazepine treatment of seizure disorder ranges from 10.6% for lorazepam in adults (Alldredge et al. 2001) to 14% in children treated mainly with lorazepam (W.A. Stewart et al. 2002) and 9%–20% for children treated with diazepam (Appleton et al. 1995; Norris et al. 1999). Benzodiazepines should be used with caution in patients with compromised respiratory function or seizure disorders. Use in patients with obstructive sleep apnea is potentially fatal (Dolly and Block 1982; see also Chapter 15, "Sleep Disorders").

Drug interactions. Additive CNS depressant effects, including respiratory depression, result from the combination of benzodiazepines and other CNS depressants, including alcohol.

Many benzodiazepines, including alprazolam, bromazepam, clonazepam, diazepam, midazolam, and triazolam, undergo hepatic and intestinal metabolism mediated by CYP3A4. Significant inhibitors of CYP3A4 may reduce the elimination of these benzodiazepines, whereas CYP3A4 inducers can increase their hepatic metabolism (see Table 38–2). Oxazepam, lorazepam, and temazepam are eliminated primarily by conjugation and renal excretion and thus may be less problematic in patients with hepatic impairment.

Toxicity/overdose. Benzodiazepines have a wide margin of safety; death from overdose is rare unless part of a polydrug overdose. Overdose may result in sedation, ataxia, slurred speech, confusion, seizures, respiratory depression, and coma. Treatment includes removal of any unabsorbed drug from the stomach (gastric lavage or emesis) followed by supportive therapy. The benzodiazepine antagonist flumazenil can also be used but may cause seizures.

Sudden discontinuation of benzodiazepines may result in severe withdrawal symptoms, including anxiety, agitation, dysphoria, anorexia, insomnia, sweating, vomiting, diarrhea, abdominal cramps, ataxia, psychosis, and seizures. The intensity of withdrawal symptoms is greater with higher doses, prolonged treatment, abrupt discontinuation, and short-half-life benzodiazepines. Patients should be gradually withdrawn from benzodiazepines; this is especially crucial for those with a history of seizure disorder. Withdrawal from short-half-life agents can be facilitated by switching to a long-half-life agent before tapering.

Nonbenzodiazepine Sedatives (Eszopiclone, Zopiclone, Zolpidem, Zaleplon, and Ramelteon)

Eszopiclone, zopiclone, zolpidem, and zaleplon are very well tolerated short-half-life hypnotics with very few dose-related adverse effects. Adverse effects of eszopiclone and zopiclone include bitter taste, dry mouth, difficulty arising in the morning, sleepiness, nausea, and nightmares (Allain et al. 1991; Najib 2006). Clinical trials of zaleplon report adverse effects comparable to those seen with placebo (Hedner et al. 2000). Zolpidem's adverse effects include CNS (dizziness, drowsiness, and headache) and gastrointestinal (nausea) effects (Krystal et al. 2008). Tolerance to the hypnotic effects of these agents occurs less frequently than with benzodiazepines, and they may be useful for treatment of rebound insomnia associated with benzodiazepine withdrawal (Pat-Horenczyk et al. 1998). Mild withdrawal symptoms have been reported in a small number of patients after discontinuation of zolpidem (Elie et al. 1999) and zopiclone (Bianchi and Musch 1990). These agents have less abuse potential than benzodiazepines (Wagner and Wagner 2000).

Ramelteon, a melatonin agonist FDA approved for insomnia, demonstrated efficacy for insomnia, with no next-morning residual effects, an adverse-effect profile similar to that of placebo, and no withdrawal symptoms upon discontinuation in a 6-month controlled clinical trial (Mayer et al. 2009).

Reports of complex sleep behaviors (e.g., sleep driving, sleep cooking, sleep eating, sleep conversations, sleep sex) in individuals taking these nonbenzodiazepine sedatives has prompted the FDA to require new safety warnings in product information. Although such reports are rare, the majority have been associated with zolpidem (Dolder and Nelson 2008).

Respiratory. Unlike benzodiazepines, typical doses of zolpidem, zopiclone, eszopiclone, and ramelteon have no significant effect on respiratory drive and central control of breathing in healthy subjects or patients with mild to moderate COPD (Girault et al. 1996; Kryger et al. 2007; Muir et al. 1990; Rosenberg et al. 2007). However, at high doses, zolpidem has been reported to cause respiratory depression (Cirignotta et al. 1988). A preliminary trial of zaleplon suggested an absence of significant respiratory effects (George 2000). Ramelteon did not worsen sleep apnea when administered to subjects with mild to moderate obstructive sleep apnea (Kryger et al. 2007).

Drug interactions. Ramelteon is oxidatively metabolized primarily by CYP1A2, with a much lesser contribution by CYP3A4. Fluvoxamine, a potent CYP1A2 inhibitor, has been reported to increase blood levels of ramelteon by 70-fold and area under the curve (AUC) by 190-fold (Takeda 2010). Ramelteon should not be used in combination with CYP1A2 inhibitors (e.g., fluvoxamine) or CYP1A2 inducers (e.g., rifampicin; see Table 38–2 for a listing). Coadministration with strong CYP3A4 inhibitors (e.g., conazole antifungals, macrolide antibiotics, grapefruit juice) should also be avoided.

Toxicity/overdose. Fatal overdose of zolpidem is rare. A review of zolpidem (n = 5,842) and zaleplon (n = 467) overdoses identified 2 deaths with zolpidem and no fatalities with zaleplon (Forrester 2006). In a survey of 344 cases of intentional acute zolpidem overdose, death occurred in 6% of the cases but could not be directly linked to zolpidem because of multiple drug involvement (Garnier et al. 1994). Symptoms of intentional overdose of zolpidem and zaleplon are similar and include drowsiness, slurred speech, ataxia, vomiting, and coma. Treatment is generally limited to supportive measures and/or gastric lavage. Symptoms of toxicity rapidly subside in most cases (Garnier et al. 1994).

Fatal overdose with zopiclone has been reported but, as with zolpidem, appears rare (Boniface and Russell 1996; Bramness et al. 2001).

Buspirone

Buspirone is a well-tolerated anxiolytic with no apparent effects on cognitive function or seizure threshold. Buspirone has little or no potential for physiological or psychological tolerance and so has no abuse liability or withdrawal syndrome on discontinuation. Dizziness, drowsiness, nervousness, nausea, and headache are the most frequent adverse affects and occur in about 5%–10% of patients. Adverse effects appear to be dose and age-related and diminish with continued therapy. Unlike benzodiazepines, buspirone does not potentiate the effects of alcohol (Seppala et al. 1982) or suppress respiration (Garner et al. 1989). Buspirone does not exhibit cross-tolerance with benzodiazepines and so cannot be used to manage benzodiazepine withdrawal. Buspirone stimulates prolactin secretion in a dose-related manner, but the clinical significance of this effect is uncertain. Menstrual irregularities and galactorrhea have occasionally been reported, but their relation to buspirone is unclear.

Drug interactions. Case reports suggest that buspirone may very rarely precipitate serotonin syndrome when used in combination with St. John's wort (Dannawi 2002) or SSRIs (G.H. Manos 2000). Buspirone should not be combined with drugs possessing MAOI activity (see Table 38-2 for list).

Buspirone undergoes hepatic and intestinal metabolism mediated by CYP3A4, so interactions are similar to those described earlier for benzodiazepines. Oral absorption of buspirone is greatly limited (~4%) by intestinal P-gp. Coadministration with drugs which inhibit P-gp (e.g., macrolide antibiotics; see Table 38-2) can increase buspirone bioavailability manyfold (5 to 10 times) and possibly cause symptoms of overdose.

Toxicity/overdose. No fatalities have been reported from buspirone overdose. Overdose symptoms include nausea, vomiting, drowsiness, miosis, and gastric distention. Treatment includes removal of any unabsorbed drug from the stomach (gastric lavage or emesis), followed by supportive therapy.

Psychostimulants

Psychostimulants are used in the treatment of attention-deficit/hyperactivity disorder (ADHD), narcolepsy, depression, apathy, and analgesia augmentation in the medically ill. The well-established psychostimulant medications include methylphenidate, dexmethylphenidate, and amphetamines (a mixture of amphetamine salts; dextroamphetamine). Pemoline has been withdrawn in many regions due to potentially fatal hepatotoxicity.

Newer compounds include atomoxetine (a specific norepinephrine reuptake inhibitor) and lisdexamfetamine, an amphetamine prodrug, for ADHD (Gibson et al. 2006) and modafinil and armodafinil for excessive sleepiness due to narcolepsy, shift work sleep disorder and obstructive sleep apnea. Modafinil and armodafinil have demonstrated efficacy for excessive daytime sleepiness accompanying obstructive sleep apnea (Black and Hirshkowitz 2005; Roth et al. 2008). Modafinil improves fatigue and cognition accompanying multiple sclerosis (Lange et al. 2009).

Methylphenidate, Dexmethylphenidate, and Amphetamines

Common adverse effects include CNS (insomnia, headache, nervousness, and social withdrawal) and gastrointestinal (stomachache and anorexia) symptoms. Adverse effects are generally mild and diminish with continued treatment, adjustment of dose, or dose timing. Lisdexamfetamine has a longer duration of action than dexamphetamine but otherwise has similar therapeutic and adverse effects (Cowles 2009).

Although psychostimulants may suppress appetite, this does not tend to occur with the low doses used in medically ill patients (Masand et al. 1991). In healthy adults, methylphenidate (≤30 mg) and dextroamphetamine (≤15 mg) did not significantly alter heart rate or blood pressure (Martin et al. 1971). However, psychostimulants can cause elevated heart rate and blood pressure, palpitations, hypertension, hypotension, and cardiac arrhythmias when taken at doses higher than those routinely used in the medically ill. In a review of side effects associated with methylphenidate therapy in children with ADHD, methylphenidate increased heart rate by 3-10 beats/minute and blood pressure by 3.3-8.0 mm Hg systolic and 1.5-14.0 mm Hg diastolic (Rapport and Moffitt 2002). Dexmethylphenidate and methylphenidate have similar therapeutic and adverse effects.

Drug interactions. Psychostimulants may interact with sympathomimetics and MAOIs (including selegiline), resulting in headache, arrhythmias, hypertensive crisis, and hyperpyrexia. Psychostimulants should not be administered with MAOIs or within 14 days of their discontinuation. Despite the paucity of empirical evidence regarding TCA-stimulant metabolic interactions, warning statements are included in many drug manuals. One review of the effects of stimulants on the pharmacokinetics of desipramine in children found no statistically or clinically significant interaction regardless of age, gender, or type of stimulant (L.G. Cohen et al. 1999). Several reports suggest that methylphenidate may interact pharmacodynamically with TCAs to cause increased anxiety, irritability, agitation, and aggression. Symptoms subsided on drug discontinuation (Grob and Coyle 1986; Gwirtsman et al. 1994; Markowitz and Patrick 2001).

Higher doses of psychostimulants may also reduce the therapeutic effectiveness of antihypertensive medications. When psychostimulants are used concurrently with beta-blockers, the excessive alpha-adrenergic activity may cause hypertension, reflex bradycardia, and possible heart block.

Toxicity/overdose. Symptoms of overdose include cardiovascular (flushing, palpitations, hypertension, arrhythmias, and tachycardia), CNS (delirium, euphoria, hyperreflexia, and psychosis), and autonomic (hyperpyrexia and sweating) effects. Treatment is primarily supportive. Any unabsorbed drug should be removed from the stomach (gastric lavage or emesis). A short-acting sedative may be needed in patients with severe intoxication.

Modafinil, Armodafinil, and Atomoxetine

Modafinil, armodafinil (the active R-enantiomer of modafinil), and atomoxetine have adverse-effect profiles different from those of other psychostimulants and do not have their same abuse potential. Modafinil's adverse effects include delayed sleep onset, nausea, and rhinitis (U.S. Modafinil in Narcolepsy Multicenter Study Group 2000). Palpitations, tachycardia, hypertension, excitation, and aggression have also been infrequently observed. Modafinil has been associated in rare cases with chest pain, palpitations, dyspnea, and transient ischemic T wave changes in association with mitral valve prolapse or left ventricular hypertrophy. Modafinil does not cause appetite reduction (Rugino and Copley 2001). Serious skin rash and possible Stevens-Johnson syndrome have been observed in modafinil trials and may occur with armodafinil (Cephalon 2010). Modafinil and armodafinil have similar therapeutic and adverse effects.

Atomoxetine side effects reported in clinical trials included insomnia, nausea, dry mouth, constipation, dizziness, decreased appetite, urinary hesitancy, sexual dysfunction, and palpitations (Adler et al. 2009; Eli Lilly 2010a).

Elimination of atomoxetine, modafinil, and armodafinil is reduced in patients with hepatic impairment. Atomoxetine dose should be reduced by 50% in patients with moderate hepatic impairment and by 75% in those with severe hepatic impairment (Eli Lilly 2010a). In patients with severe hepatic impairment, modafinil and armodafinil dose should be reduced by 50% (McEvoy 2008). Blood levels of modafinil acid, a modafinil metabolite, increase ninefold in patients with severe renal insufficiency, but its effects are unknown.

Drug interactions. Atomoxetine is a potent inhibitor of CYP2D6 and is primarily eliminated through metabolism by CYP2D6 (see Table 38–2). Atomoxetine may increase the toxicity of other coadministered narrow-therapeutic-index medications primarily metabolized by CYP2D6.

Modafinil and armodafinil are moderate inducers of CYP3A4 and moderate inhibitors of CYP2C19 (Darwish et al. 2008). Drug interaction data for modafinil and armodafinil are limited. Clinical studies suggest that significant metabolic drug interactions are most likely with compounds, such as ethinylestradiol and triazolam, that undergo significant gastrointestinal CYP3A4-mediated first-pass metabolism (Robertson and Hellriegel 2003; Robertson et al. 2002). Modafinil–clozapine interactions have been the subject of two case reports, one showing an increase in clozapine level (Dequardo 2002) and the other showing a decrease in clozapine's therapeutic effect (Narendran et al. 2002).

Like other psychostimulants, atomoxetine, modafinil, and armodafinil should not be administered to patients receiving MAOIs or within 14 days of MAOI withdrawal.

Cognitive Enhancers

The currently approved treatments for dementia of the Alzheimer's type are cholinesterase inhibitors, including tacrine, donepezil, rivastigmine, and galantamine, and the *N*-methyl-D-aspartate (NMDA) receptor antagonist memantine.

Cholinesterase Inhibitors

Tacrine is now rarely prescribed because of frequent reversible hepatotoxicity (Watkins et al. 1994). Other mainstream cholinesterase inhibitors are well tolerated; most of their adverse effects are mild, dose-related, and gastrointestinal in nature (nausea, vomiting, and diarrhea), as expected from procholinergic agents. Gastrointestinal side effects can be minimized by slow dose titration and administration with food. Adequate hydration reduces nausea. Procholinergic properties increase vagotonic and bronchoconstrictor effects. These agents should be used with caution in patients with cardiac conduction abnormalities or a history of asthma or obstructive pulmonary disease.

Agent-specific side effects include muscle cramps and insomnia with donepezil and anorexia with rivastigmine and galantamine.

Overdose. Overdose of cholinesterase inhibitors can cause a potentially fatal cholinergic crisis, with bradycardia, hypotension, muscle weakness, nausea, vomiting, respiratory depression, sialorrhea, diaphoresis, and seizures. Treatment is with atropine (1–2 mg intravenously, repeat as required) and supportive care.

Drug interactions. Donepezil and galantamine are metabolized by CYP2D6 and CYP3A4 isozymes but are not associated with any clinically important CYP-mediated pharmacokinetic interactions (reviewed in Jann et al. 2002). Rivastigmine is metabolized primarily by esterase-mediated hydrolysis and has been shown not to interact with CYP isozymes in vitro (Grossberg 2002).

Cholinesterase inhibitors do, however, have the potential to exacerbate the effects of other cholinesterase inhibitors (e.g., physostigmine) or cholinomimetic agents (e.g., bethanechol). Cholinesterase inhibitors prolong the duration of action of the depolarizing neuromuscular blocking agent succinylcholine (suxamethonium) by inhibiting metabolism of succinylcholine by plasma cholinesterase and increasing acetylcholine-mediated neuromuscular depolarization (Crowe and Collins 2003). In contrast, the cholinesterase inhibitor-mediated increase in acetylcholine levels antagonizes the actions of nondepolarizing neuromuscular blockers (e.g., atracurium, mivacurium) (Baruah et al. 2008). Cholinesterase inhibitors should be discontinued several weeks before surgery (Russell 2009).

Many prescription and nonprescription drugs possess anticholinergic activity that may impair cognitive function. In addition to those drug classes commonly recognized as having anticholinergic effects, such as antiparkinsonian agents, antispasmodics, TCAs, low-potency antipsychotics, and antihistamines, many individual drugs from unrelated drug classes also have these effects. Drugs with anticholinergic properties may decrease the effect of cognitive enhancers. In a study of long-term care residents, 21% of those receiving acetylcholinesterase inhibitors were receiving concurrent medications with anticholinergic activity (J.L. Mann et al. 2003). The use of anticholinergic agents in a patient with compromised cognitive function should be minimized. A partial listing of drugs with significant CNS anticholinergic effects is presented in Table 38–8. Conversely, cholinesterase inhibitors may have a countertherapeutic effect in those patients receiving anticholinergic medication for medical conditions.

NMDA Receptor Antagonists

Memantine has been shown in a meta-analysis of controlled long-term trials in patients with Alzheimer's disease to be well tolerated, with an adverse-effect profile similar to that of placebo (Farlow et al. 2008). Memantine has no effect on respiration and is generally benign in patients with cardiovascular disease, although it may rarely cause bradycardia (Gallini et al. 2008). Memantine is primarily renally eliminated and requires reduced dosage in patients with moderate renal impairment.

Drug interactions. Memantine has no significant interactions with other drugs.

Alternative Routes of Administration

Psychotropic medications are usually delivered orally, but this may not represent the best administration route or even be possible for many patients. Oral administration of medications may be difficult in the medically compromised including: patients with severe nausea or vomiting, dysphagia, severe malabsorption; unconscious or uncooperative patients; and patients unable to take medications by mouth. Alternative nonoral routes of administration include intravenous, intramuscular, subcutaneous, sublingual/buccal, rectal, topical or transdermal, and intranasal.

The potential advantages of nonoral administration of psychotropics include guaranteed compliance, providing options for those patients who cannot take oral medications, and potential pharmacokinetic advantages such as greater bioavailability, bypassing first-pass hepatic metabolism, and potential reduction in toxic metabolites or adverse effects. Intravenous delivery can be controlled from very rapid to slow infusion with 100% bioavailability and rapid drug distribution. Intramuscular administration provides fast absorption, avoidance of first-pass metabolism and ensured compliance, but bioavailability is often less than 100% because of drug retention or metabolism by local tissues. Sublingual/buccal routes have rapid absorption and good bioavailability for small lipid-soluble drugs. Drugs absorbed sublingually avoid first-pass metabolism and may have fewer gastrointestinal adverse effects. Significant sublingual/buccal absorption of oral liquids or oral disintegrating tablets cannot be assumed and must be evaluated on a drug-by-drug basis. Rectal absorption is often incomplete and erratic, but in comparison with oral administration, first-pass metabolism is reduced by about 50% (reviewed by van Hoogdalem et al. 1991a, 1991b). Transdermal drug delivery bypasses the gut, avoids first-pass metabolism, reduces gastrointestinal adverse effects, and is unaffected by food intake. Continuous drug delivery from a transdermal patch reduces the peak to trough fluctuation of drug levels produced by oral dosing and provides near-constant plasma drug levels, even for short-half-life drugs, over longer dosing intervals. The intranasal route has been suggested as the best alternative to parenteral injections for rapid systemic drug delivery. However, there are no approved intranasal formulations of psychotropic medications.

Many formulations discussed are commercially available, although not necessarily in the United States or Canada. The Lundbeck Institute provides an international database of approved psychotropic formulations (www.psychotropics.dk) that may help to locate their sources. Customized formulations are reported for a few agents. Caution is indicated when using a medication for which adequate studies of safety and efficacy regarding parenteral administration are lacking.

Antidepressants

Few antidepressants are available for parenteral administration. Intravenous clomipramine, amitriptyline, imipramine, maprotiline, doxepin, viloxazine, trazodone, and citalopram have been studied or widely used, mainly in Europe. None are currently available in the United States or Canada. Intravenous mirtazapine (15 mg/day) was found to be well tolerated and effective in two small uncontrolled trials in moderately to severely depressed inpatients (Kon-

TABLE 38–8. Common drugs with significant anticholinergic effects

Antidepressants		**Antiparkinsonian agents**		**Antispasmodics**	
Tertiary amine TCAs	+++	Amantadine	++	Atropine	+++
Secondary amine TCAs	++	Benztropine	+++	Clidinium	+++
Citalopram	+	Biperiden	+++	Dicyclomine	+++
Escitalopram	+	Entacapone	+	Flavoxate	++
Fluoxetine	+	Ethopropazine	+++	Glycopyrrolate	++
Mirtazapine	+	Orphenadrine	+++	Homatropine	+++
Paroxetine	++	Pramipexole	+	Hyoscine	+++
Trazodone	+	Procyclidine	+++	Hyoscyamine	+++
		Selegiline	+	Methscopolamine	+++
Antidiarrheals		Trihexyphenidyl	+++	Oxybutynin	+++
Loperamide	++			Propantheline	++
		Antipsychotics		Scopolamine	+++
Antiemetics		Chlorpromazine	++	Tolterodine	++
Metoclopramide	+	Clozapine	+++		
Perphenazine	+++	Haloperidol	+	**Mood stabilizers**	
Promethazine	+++	Olanzapine	++	Lithium	+
		Quetiapine	+		
Antihistamines		Risperidone	+	**Skeletal muscle relaxants**	
Brompheniramine	+++	Thioridazine	+++	Baclofen	++
Chlorpheniramine	++	Ziprasidone	+	Carisoprodol	+++
Cyproheptadine	++			Chlorzoxazone	+++
Dimenhydrinate	+++	**Anxiolytics and sedative-hypnotics**		Cyclobenzaprine	+++
Diphenhydramine	+++	Temazepam	+	Metaxalone	+++
Hydroxyzine	+++			Methocarbamol	+++
Meclizine	+++	**H_2 antagonists**		Tizanidine	+++
		Cimetidine	++		
		Ranitidine	+		

Note. Risk of anticholinergic adverse effects at therapeutic doses: +++, high; ++, medium; +, low. Risk is increased in the elderly and with multiple agents with anticholinergic activity.
Source. Compiled from Bezchlibnyk-Butler et al. 2007; Cancelli et al. 2009; Chew et al. 2008; McEvoy 2008; Repchinsky 2009; Rudolph et al. 2008.

stantinidis et al. 2002; Muhlbacher et al. 2006). Citalopram is the only SSRI available for parenteral administration. To date, open and double-blind randomized, controlled clinical trials have shown citalopram infusion followed by oral citalopram (Kasper and Muller-Spahn 2002) or escitalopram (Schmitt et al. 2006) to be effective and well tolerated for severe depression. However, the safety and efficacy of intravenous antidepressants in the medically ill is uncertain because studies to date have been performed only in medically healthy patients.

No antidepressants are currently marketed in a rectal preparation including enema, foam, semisolid suppository, or gelatin capsules. However, several antidepressants, including trazodone, amitriptyline, imipramine, and clomipramine, have been compounded as rectal suppositories with anecdotal reports of success in depression (Koelle and Dimsdale 1998; Mirassou 1998). Therapeutic serum levels of doxepin were produced in 3 of 4 cancer patients following rectal insertion of oral capsules (Storey and Trumble 1992). The rectal bioavailability of fluoxetine oral capsules, administered rectally, was only 15% of oral administration but was reasonably well tolerated in 7 healthy subjects (Teter et al. 2005). With an appropriate dosage adjustment, rectal administration of antidepressants may be feasible in patients who cannot take oral medications. Serum drug levels (if available) and clinical response should guide dosage.

The MAOI selegiline, available in a transdermal patch, is the only nonoral antidepressant formulation approved in the United States. The antidepressant dose of oral selegiline requires dietary tyramine restriction because of clinically significant inhibition of intestinal MAO-A. By avoiding intestinal exposure to selegiline, transdermal administration reduces intestinal MAO-A inhibition and the need for dietary tyramine restrictions at doses of 6 mg/day or less, as well as circumventing first-pass metabolism to provide higher plasma levels and reduced metabolite formation. Short-term (8-week; Feiger et al. 2006) and long-term (52-week; Amsterdam and Bodkin 2006) placebo-controlled, double-blind clinical trials have demonstrated antidepressant efficacy, with adverse effects similar to those of placebo, except for application-site reactions and insomnia. An oral disintegrating tablet of selegiline, designed for buccal absorption, has been approved in the United States for Parkinson's disease (Valeant 2010). There are no reports of its use for the treatment of depression.

Transdermal amitriptyline was reported to be well absorbed and effective in a case report (Scott et al. 1999) but showed no significant systemic absorption in a small open trial (Lynch et al. 2005). This variability may be due to use of different transdermal formulations.

Sublingual administration of fluoxetine oral solution produced therapeutic plasma levels of fluoxetine plus norfluoxetine and improved depressive symptoms in two medically compromised patients with depression (Pakyurek and Pasol 1999).

Mirtazapine is available in an oral disintegrating tablet for gut absorption, but the extent of sublingual/buccal absorption from this formulation is unknown.

Anxiolytics and Sedative-Hypnotics

Internationally, many benzodiazepines are available in intravenous, intramuscular, rectal, sublingual, and intranasal preparations. Injectable forms of diazepam, lorazepam, and midazolam and diazepam rectal gel are marketed in the United States and Canada. Sublingual lorazepam is available in Canada. Intravenous benzodiazepines are commonly used to treat status epilepticus or to calm severely agitated patients. Compared with diazepam, lorazepam pharmacokinetics after intravenous administration are more predictable. Because intravenous lorazepam redistributes more slowly from the CNS to peripheral tissues than diazepam or midazolam, it has a longer duration of effect after a single dose. Midazolam is a short-acting, water-soluble benzodiazepine frequently used in preoperative sedation, induction and maintenance of anesthesia, anxiolysis, and the treatment of status epilepticus. Midazolam's onset of action following intravenous administration is usually within 1–5 minutes, and the action lasts usually less than 2 hours. Intravenous flunitrazepam (Rohypnol), available in Europe and Japan, has been used for severe insomnia (Matsuo and Morita 2007) and for the treatment and the prevention of alcohol withdrawal (Pycha et al. 1993). Intravenous benzodiazepine administration should always occur in a setting where there is ready access to personnel and equipment necessary for respiratory resuscitation.

Injectable forms of lorazepam, midazolam, and diazepam are available for intramuscular delivery. For behavioral emergencies, lorazepam is the preferred agent because it is readily absorbed and has no active metabolites. Midazolam is also rapidly absorbed after intramuscular administration, with an onset of action between 5 and 15 minutes. Intermittent or sustained continuous subcutaneous infusion of injectable midazolam is reported for management of delirium, especially in a palliative care setting (Bottomley and Hanks 1990). Intramuscular diazepam is not recommended because of its erratic absorption (Rey et al. 1999).

Sublingual benzodiazepines are often used to control anxiety in patients undergoing dental procedures. Only lorazepam in Canada and temazepam in Europe (Russell et al. 1988) are marketed in a sublingual form, although several benzodiazepines, including alprazolam, triazolam, prazepam, midazolam, clonazepam, diazepam, flunitrazepam, and lormetazepam have been administered sublingually using commercial nonsublingual formulations (such as oral tablets) or custom preparations. Pharmacokinetic studies comparing sublingual administration of oral tablets against intramuscular administration suggest slightly slower sublingual drug absorption but similar bioavailability.

Rectal administration of benzodiazepines is useful for the acute management of seizures in children. Diazepam is available as a rectal gel for use when other routes are not readily available. A pharmacokinetic study of a parenteral solution of lorazepam administered rectally to healthy adults describes average bioavailability of 80% but with considerable variation in the rate and extent of absorption (Graves et al. 1987). Other benzodiazepines, such as clonazepam, triazolam, and midazolam, have also been administered rectally. Although rectal benzodiazepine absorption is rapid, it is not always reliable because rectal bioavailability is highly variable and the onset of action is delayed (Rey et al. 1999). Since lorazepam may be given intravenously, intramuscularly, or sublingually, there is little need for rectal administration of benzodiazepines in adults.

Other routes of administration for benzodiazepines include intrathecal and nasal midazolam. Intrathecal midazolam has been used principally for adjunctive pain management and has been found to be safe and effective in a variety of settings (Duncan et al. 2007). While no benzodiazepines are available in intranasal formulations, intranasal formulations of midazolam and lorazepam sprays have been reported to be effective with rapid absorption and high bioavailability (Bjorkman et al. 1997; Wermeling et al. 2006).

Two sublingual formulations of zolpidem, a nonbenzodiazepine hypnotic, have recently been approved in the United States: a sublingual tablet and an oral spray. In a clinical study, the sublingual tablet produced significantly earlier sleep initiation than the oral preparation (Staner et al. 2010). The sublingual spray has been demonstrated to provide more rapid systemic absorption of zolpidem than the oral formulation (NovaDel 2010).

Antipsychotics

The atypical antipsychotics aripiprazole, olanzapine, and ziprasidone and many typical agents are available as short-acting intramuscular preparations. Haloperidol has been given intravenously and subcutaneously. Long-acting intramuscular depot formulations for risperidone, olanzapine, paliperidone, haloperidol, and fluphenazine are available in the United States. In Canada, long-acting depot formulations of risperidone, fluphenazine, haloperidol, flupenthixol, pipotiazine, and zuclopenthixol are approved. Olanzapine is the only atypical antipsychotic available in oral, short-acting intramuscular and depot intramuscular formulations.

Intravenous agents are usually reserved for acute agitation in which a rapid onset of effect is desirable. Droperidol is FDA approved for use as an intravenous anesthetic adjunct (but not for psychiatric conditions) but has been used for rapid tranquilization in the medical/surgical setting. Droperidol causes dose-dependent prolongation of the QTc interval and has been withdrawn from the United Kingdom and received a black-box warning in North America. Although haloperidol is not approved by the FDA for intravenous use, it is often administered intravenously in medical inpatient settings, especially for delirium, aggression, or mania. The FDA recommends electrocardiogram monitoring for QT prolongation and arrhythmia if haloperidol is administered intravenously. High doses of haloperidol, up to 1,000 mg daily, in patients with severe delirium have been reported to have minimal effects on heart rate, respiratory rate, blood pressure, and pulmonary artery pressure, with minimal EPS (Levenson 1995; Stern 1985).

Intramuscular antipsychotic formulations can be categorized on the basis of their pharmacokinetic features: short-acting preparations and long-acting depot preparations. Long-acting antipsychotics are typically used as antipsychotic maintenance treatment to ensure adherence and to eliminate bioavailability problems. Short-acting antipsychotics are usually used in acute management of delirium, psychosis, mania, or aggression (see Chapter 5, "Delirium"; Chapter 7, "Aggression and Violence"; and Chapter 10, "Psychosis, Catatonia, and Mania," for further discussion). Haloperidol is the most common (and least costly) intramuscularly administered antipsychotic in medical settings. However, acute parenteral administration of high-potency antipsychotics such as haloperidol is associated with more dystonia and other EPS. In patients with existing extrapyramidal disorders, an intramuscular antipsychotic other than haloperidol would be preferred. Parenteral administration of low-potency agents may cause more hypotension and lowered seizure threshold.

Intramuscular forms of atypical antipsychotics are less likely to cause acute dystonia and akathisia than haloperidol (Currier and Medori 2006; Zimbroff 2008), but there has been much less experience using them in the medically ill, and they are considerably more expensive. Haloperidol, but none of the atypical antipsychotics, can be mixed with a benzodiazepine in the same syringe. Ziprasidone and aripiprazole can be administered in conjunction with an intramuscular benzodiazepine, but concurrent intramuscular olanzapine with a parenteral benzodiazepine is not recommended because of excessive sedation and cardiorespiratory depression (Eli Lilly 2010b). Ziprasidone (oral or intramuscular) is contraindicated in patients with a known history of QT prolongation (including congenital long QT syndrome) or cardiac arrhythmias, with recent acute myocardial infarction, or with uncompensated heart failure, and caution should be used when coadministering ziprasidone with other drugs that prolong the QT interval (Pfizer 2010a). Intramuscular ziprasidone has not been systematically studied in patients with significant hepatic or renal impairment. Intramuscular olanzapine is recommended for the management of agitation in patients with schizophrenia, bipolar mania, or dementia. At this time, there are no data on intramuscular ziprasidone or olanzapine in the management of agitation in medically ill patients without an underlying psychiatric condition, so caution is advised.

Asenapine, recently FDA approved, is the only antipsychotic available in a sublingual preparation; it is not available in other delivery forms at this time. Oral disintegrating tablets, designed to deliver drug for intestinal absorption, are available for most atypical agents. Sublingual absorption of olanzapine oral disintegrating tablet has been studied in healthy volunteers (Markowitz et al. 2006). Sublingual administration resulted in a similar extent and rate of drug absorption compared with regular administration of the oral disintegrating tablet and faster absorption than the standard oral tablet. Sublingual/buccal absorption of oral disintegrating tablets for other antipsychotics has not been reported.

Subcutaneous administration of haloperidol and methotrimeprazine (available in Canada and Europe) and fluphenazine (Health Canada–approved for subcutaneous administration) can be used to manage terminal restlessness and for nausea/vomiting in palliative care patients. Loxapine has also been used subcutaneously in the palliative care setting. Most other phenothiazines are too irritating for subcutaneous injection.

Psychostimulants

Transdermal methylphenidate was approved for children in 2006 in the United States. The patch is worn for 9 hours but provides therapeutic effect through 12 hours. Several patch doses are available and the duration of effect can be modified by early removal of the patch (M.J. Manos et al. 2007). In children with ADHD, the adverse-effect profile is similar to that of a placebo patch (McGough et al. 2006). A placebo-controlled comparison of transdermal methylphenidate and the osmotic-release oral capsule in children revealed similar treatment efficacy for the active formulations but a higher incidence of tics and anorexia for transdermal methylphenidate (Findling et al. 2008). No clinical trials of transdermal methylphenidate in adults with serious medical illness have been published.

Although no other nonoral forms of psychostimulants are available, custom preparations are described. Dextroamphetamine has been administered intravenously to human subjects in research but not clinically (C.L. Ernst and Goldberg 2002). There is one published case report of 5-mg dextroamphetamine suppositories compounded by a pharmacy for treating depressed mood in a woman with gastrointestinal obstruction (Holmes et al. 1994).

Mood Stabilizers/Anticonvulsants

Mood stabilizers that have been administered intravenously include lithium carbonate and valproate. Because lithium is not metabolized, parenteral administration has fewer potential pharmacokinetic advantages than for other psychotropics. Parenteral lithium has rarely been used in the treatment of psychiatric disorders but has been used as a possible treatment in thyroid storm. Lithium was administered intraperitoneally in patients on continuous ambulatory peritoneal dialysis (Flynn et al. 1987). Lithium carbonate is not approved by the FDA for parenteral use, and there is not enough clinical experience or data to recommend its use by nonenteral routes.

Valproate has been available in parenteral form (Depacon) in Europe for more than 18 years and was approved by the FDA in the United States in 1997 (it was discontinued in Canada in 2004). Valproate is the only mood stabilizer, apart from several atypical antipsychotics, with an approved parenteral formulation where case reports exist for its use in psychiatric conditions (Norton 2001; Norton and Quarles 2000; Regenold and Prasad 2001). The intravenous solution, prepared in dextrose, saline, or lactated Ringer's solution, should not be infused at more than 20 mg/minute, with the dosage reduced in the elderly and in those with organic brain syndromes. The infusion does not require cardiac monitoring and causes no significant risk of orthostatic hypotension (Norton 2001). There are no randomized controlled trials documenting its safety and efficacy for psychiatric disorders.

Several studies report that rectal administration of carbamazepine, lamotrigine, and topiramate provides acceptable bioavailability and tolerability. Carbamazepine has been rectally administered as a solution (Neuvonen and Tokola 1987) and as a crushed tablet in a gelatin capsule (Storey and Trumble 1992), attaining therapeutic blood levels in some, but not all, patients. Rectal preparations of lamotrigine and topiramate have been prepared from oral formulations. Compared with oral dosing, rectal lamotrigine had reduced bioavailability (approximately 50%) leading to lower drug levels and slower absorption (Birnbaum et al. 2001), while blood levels were identical after rectal topiramate (Conway et al. 2003). Provided relative bioavailability is considered, rectal administration of an aqueous suspension of these tablets may be acceptable. Rectal absorption of other anticonvulsants including oxcarbazepine, gabapentin, felbamate, and phenytoin is not reliable (Clemens et al. 2007). Oxcarbazepine is available as an oral suspension, but its rectal administration achieved only 10% of the oral bioavailability for the parent drug or active metabolite (Clemens et al. 2007). Thus, rectal delivery is not an appropriate route for oxcarbazepine.

Cholinesterase Inhibitors

Rivastigmine, as a transdermal patch, is the only cognitive enhancer available in a nonoral formulation. The rivastigmine patch is dosed daily and provides less fluctuating plasma levels than the twice-daily oral capsules or solution. The patch provides greater bioavailability but with slower absorption, which reduces peak drug levels by 20%. This more consistent drug exposure might improve efficacy, but this remains to be investigated. The incidence of nausea and vomiting declined from 33% with the oral form to 20% with the patch (Lefevre et al. 2008).

Complementary Medicines

Surveys suggest that approximately 20% of U.S. adults have used herbal medicines and nonherbal dietary supplements within the past year (Barnes et al. 2004), often without disclosing their use. Many people assume that complementary medicines are "naturally" safe, and they combine complementary and conventional therapies, believing that the combination will be more effective (Eisenberg et al. 2001). This raises concerns about the appropriate therapeutic use, contraindications, adverse effects, and drug interactions of herbal and nonherbal drugs. Patients with chronic disease may be especially vulnerable to adverse effects from herbal medicines because of compromised organ function and polypharmacy with conventional agents.

Recently, the FDA Office of Nutritional Products, Labeling, and Dietary Supplements (www.cfsan.fda.gov/~dms/supplmnt.html) and Health Canada, Office of Natural Health Products (www.hc-sc.gc.ca/dhp-mps/prodnatur), have moved to provide a regulatory framework to encourage good manufacturing practice and adverse-effect reporting for natural health products (Bent 2008; Morrow 2008). However, the FDA does not require efficacy or safety data for products marketed as dietary supplements.

The lack of government oversight and regulation has complicated attempts to assess the safety of herbal medicines. Manufacturers are not required to standardize the concentration of active ingredients or even to identify them (Chandler 2000; De Smet 2002). Herbal preparations may contain several plant species used under a single name (Chandler 2000) and may be adulterated with unlisted pharmacological agents, pesticides, and heavy metals, including cadmium, lead, mercury, or arsenic (Crone and Wise 1998; Saper et al. 2008). Drugs such as anti-inflammatory agents, steroids, diuretics, antihistamines, sildenafil-like compounds, and benzodiazepines may be intentionally added to the herbal product for therapeutic effect (G.M. Miller and Stripp 2007; Wooltorton 2003).

Contraindications, major adverse effects, and significant drug interactions for those herbal medicines and nonherbal dietary supplements commonly used for neuropsychiatric symptoms are summarized in the following subsections, derived from available reviews (Ang-Lee et al. 2001; Bent and Ko 2004; Brazier and Levine 2003; Chandler 2000; De Smet 2002; C.L. Ernst and Goldberg 2002; E. Ernst 2003; Gardiner et al. 2008; Gurley et al. 2008; Hu et al. 2005; Mahady et al. 2008; Tracy and Kingston 2007).

Selected Herbal Medicines

Black Cohosh

Purported use. Menopausal symptoms

Pharmacological effects and drug interactions. Black cohosh binds to estrogen receptors and lowers levels of luteinizing hormone. It is contraindicated in pregnancy and lactation and should be avoided by women with estrogen-dependent tumors. Hepatotoxicity has prompted the FDA to require a cautionary notice on black cohosh products.

Feverfew

Purported use. Migraine prophylaxis, anti-inflammatory

Pharmacological effects and drug interactions. Used as an abortifacient in animals, feverfew is contraindicated in pregnancy in humans. It inhibits platelet activation factor and may prolong bleeding time. Risk is increased with drugs known to increase bleeding times, such as anticoagulants, NSAIDs, SSRIs, and platelet inhibitors. Allergic reactions are common. Withdrawal syndrome (anxiety, fatigue, joint ache) may occur on sudden discontinuation.

Ginkgo Biloba

Purported use. Ginkgo biloba improves peripheral and CNS blood flow and has been used for ischemia associated with peripheral artery disease and vascular dementia.

Pharmacological effects and drug interactions. Ginkgo biloba inhibits platelet activation factor and prolongs bleeding time. It carries an increased risk for bleeding disorders when used with drugs known to increase bleeding times (anticoagulants, NSAIDs, SSRIs, platelet inhibitors). Intracerebral and intraocular hemorrhages have been reported, and it may cause palpitations. Seizures have been reported in children, and efficacy of anticonvulsants may be reduced. The ginkgo biloba fruit, including the seeds, is poisonous and very allergenic. Ingestion of the fruit has resulted in loss of consciousness, seizures, and death, with a mortality rate of 27%. Ingestion of fruit also causes contact dermatitis of mucous membranes. Ginkgo biloba should be discontinued at least 2 days before surgery.

Ginseng

Purported use. Ginseng is promoted as a physical, mental, and sexual tonic, immunostimulant, and mood enhancer.

Pharmacological effects and drug interactions. Ginseng possesses estrogenic activity; it is contraindicated in patients with estrogen receptor–positive breast cancer. It may cause estrogen-related bleeding disorders (vaginal bleeding) and breast nodules. Sympathomimetic activity may cause tachycardia, hypertension, nervousness, agitation, mania, and headache. It also has hypoglycemic and antiplatelet aggregation properties. Ginseng may reduce the effects of loop diuretics (furosemide), antihypertensives, anxiolytics, antidepressants, mood stabilizers, and antiestrogens. It inhibits platelet activation factor and prolongs bleeding time. Ginseng increases the risk of bleeding disorders with drugs known to increase bleeding times (anticoagulants, NSAIDs, SSRIs, platelet inhibitors). Risk is increased in patients with diabetes, hypertension, anxiety disorders, and bipolar disorder or those using estrogen therapy, antiestrogen therapy, or anticoagulants. Long-term use may result in "ginseng abuse syndrome" with symptoms including hypertension, nervousness, insomnia, skin eruptions, diarrhea, and tremor. A withdrawal syndrome (hypotension, weakness, tremor) may occur upon discontinuation. Ginseng should be discontinued at least 7 days before surgery.

Kava Kava

Purported use. Anxiolytic, sedative

Pharmacological effects and drug interactions. Kava kava exerts effects on several neurotransmitter systems, including gamma-aminobutyric acid (GABA), norepinephrine, and dopamine, and should not be used with antipsychotics and drugs used to treat Parkinson's disease. It potentiates the effects of CNS depressants, such as barbiturates, benzodiazepines, and alcohol. Dermopathy is common with heavy use. Antithrombotic action may prolong bleeding time. Risk is increased with drugs known to increase bleeding times. Kava kava is also hallucinogenic. Sale of kava has been banned in many jurisdictions because of several incidents of fatal hepatotoxicity. Kavalactones, the proposed active constituents of kava, inhibit major CYP enzymes and may cause interactions with concurrent medications. Kava kava should be discontinued at least 24 hours before surgery.

Ma Huang (Ephedra)

Purported use. Weight loss, stimulant

Pharmacological effects and drug interactions. Ma huang is an indirect sympathomimetic; it contains ephedrine and pseudoephedrine, which cause release of epinephrine and norepinephrine. Excessive sympathetic stimulation can lead to dizziness, headache, decreased appetite, gastrointestinal distress, irregular heartbeat, tachycardia, hypertension, insomnia, flushing, seizures, stroke, and death. Drug interactions include increased risk of cardiac arrhythmia with cardiac glycosides and antiarrhythmics; reduced effects of antihypertensives, beta-blockers, sedative-hypnotics, and anesthetics; hypertensive crisis with MAOIs; and increased stimulant effects with theophylline and caffeine. Several ephedra-related deaths have occurred. The FDA banned the sale of ephedra in 2004.

St. John's Wort

Purported use. Antidepressant for mild to moderate depression, sedative

Pharmacological effects and drug interactions. St. John's wort increases serotonin and norepinephrine activity, which may cause sinus tachycardia and gastrointestinal distress and may exacerbate bipolar disorder, causing mania. Photosensitizing properties may cause sun-induced skin rash, neuropathy, and possibly increased incidence of cataracts, and may exacerbate photosensitivity due to tetracycline, piroxicam, and phenothiazines. St. John's wort induces CYP3A4 and has the potential to interact with medications metabolized by this enzyme to lower drug levels and decrease therapeutic effect (see Table 38–2). It induces P-gp drug efflux systems, reducing bioavailability and systemic exposure to several drugs, including digoxin, cyclosporine, and TCAs. St. John's wort may induce serotonin syndrome in combination with other serotonergic drugs. It should be discontinued at least 5 days before surgery.

Valerian

Purported use. Sedative, short-term treatment of insomnia, anxiolytic

Pharmacological effects and drug interactions. Tolerance to valerian may develop and lead to withdrawal effects with abrupt discontinuation following prolonged use. Withdrawal effects are similar to benzodiazepine withdrawal and can be managed with benzodiazepines. Valerian potentiates the sedative effects of CNS depressants.

Yohimbe, Yohimbine

Purported use. Aphrodisiac, stimulant

Pharmacological effects and drug interactions. Yohimbine, an $alpha_2$ antagonist, has indirect sympathomimetic activity. Adverse effects include insomnia, anxiety, panic attacks, hallucinations, hypertension, tachycardia, nausea, and vomiting. It should be avoided in patients with hypertension, sleep disorders, anxiety disorders, and psychosis. Yohimbine exacerbates the CNS and autonomic effects of stimulants and TCAs. It should be discontinued at least 2 days before surgery.

Selected Nonherbal Supplements

DHEA (Dehydroepiandrosterone)

Purported use. Depression, postmenopausal osteoporosis, systemic lupus erythematosus, erectile dysfunction, multiple sclerosis, dementia

Pharmacological effects and drug interactions. DHEA is an endogenous anabolic steroid that may undergo conversion in vivo to testosterone or androstenedione followed by conversion to estriol, estrone, and estradiol. DHEA may cause weight gain, voice change, hirsutism, and menstrual irregularities in females and gynecomastia and prostatic hypertrophy in males. DHEA is contraindicated in patients who have liver dysfunction, prostate cancer, or hormone-dependent diseases such as estrogen-dependent breast cancer. DHEA may inhibit CYP3A4.

Gamma-Hydroxybutyrate (GHB or Sodium Oxybate), Gamma-Butyrolactone, and 1,4-Butanediol

Purported use. Narcolepsy, recreational fast-acting hypnotic

Pharmacological effects and drug interactions. GHB is a partial agonist at $GABA_B$ receptors with fast-onset hypnotic action. Gamma-butyrolactone and 1,4-butanediol are metabolized to GHB in vivo. Adverse effects include nystagmus, ataxia, apnea, sedation, dizziness, and respiratory depression. Coma, bradycardia, and death can result. Psychiatric side effects of GHB include hallucinations, delusions, agitation, confusion, and euphoria. A withdrawal syndrome (consisting of anxiety, insomnia, tremor, muscle cramps) has been observed. GHB is approved in the United States and Canada for narcolepsy under a controlled prescription program, but it is a banned drug in many other jurisdictions. Its precursors, gamma-butyrolactone and 1,4-butanediol, are industrial solvents and are available as street drugs (see also Chapter 17, "Substance-Related Disorders").

S-Adenosyl-L-Methionine (SAMe)

Purported use. Depression, osteoarthritis, chronic liver disease

Pharmacological effects and drug interactions. SAMe is the principal endogenous methyl donor for methylation reactions. Adverse effects include nausea, vomiting, and diarrhea. SAMe may increase anxiety and restlessness in patients with depression and mania and hypomania in patients with bipolar disorder. Serotonin syndrome has been reported. Risk is increased in patients with bipolar disorder, patients with movement disorders, or patients taking serotonergic drugs.

Psychotropic Drug Use in the Medically Ill

Psychosomatic medicine specialists routinely prescribe and advise other physicians regarding the use of psychotropic medications in patients with multiple complex medical problems. This gives rise to many issues regarding changes in pharmacokinetics and pharmacodynamics as previously outlined in this chapter. This section outlines clinical recommendations for the use of psychotropic medications in specific medical/surgical populations.

Gastrointestinal Disorders

Hepatic Disease

Psychopharmacological concerns in patients with liver disease largely center on pharmacokinetic changes brought about by the disease (discussed earlier in this chapter). Acute hepatitis usually does not require dose alteration of psychotropics, but chronic hepatitis may require dosage adjustment depending on the severity of liver dysfunction. In patients with cirrhosis, drug dose will require significant modification. The severity of liver disease can be approximated using the Child-Pugh scoring system (see Chapter 20, "Gastrointestinal Disorders"). All plasma proteins are synthesized in the liver, so protein binding is altered in liver disease. The main clinical effect of chronically decreased protein binding is on the interpretation of blood levels (see discussion in the "Distribution" subsection under "Pharmacokinetics in the Medically Ill" at the beginning of this chapter). When prescribing hepatically metabolized psychotropic drugs to patients with impaired hepatic function, it is prudent to reduce the initial dose and titrate more slowly, to carefully monitor for clinical response and side effects, and to choose drugs with a wide therapeutic index. Table 38–9 lists recommendations regarding dosing of psychotropics in patients with hepatic disease.

Antidepressants. Most antidepressants undergo extensive phase I hepatic oxidative metabolism and should be dosed according to the recommendations described. Anticholinergic TCAs may exacerbate hepatic encephalopathy in susceptible individuals via intestinal stasis and central anticholinergic effects. The use of newer antidepressants in patients with hepatic disease has received very little study. Citalopram, paroxetine, sertraline, and fluoxetine have all been used safely in patients with hepatitis C, usually in the context of interferon-alpha treatment (Hauser et al. 2002; Kraus et al. 2008; Raison et al. 2007; Sammut et al. 2002; Schramm et al. 2000).

Hepatotoxicity is a known rare side effect of many antidepressants, but nefazodone has a higher reported inci-

TABLE 38–9. Selected psychotropic drugs in hepatic insufficiency (HI)

Antidepressants	
MAOIs	Potentially hepatotoxic. No dosing guidelines.
SSRIs	Extensively metabolized. Decreased clearance and prolonged half-life. Initial dose should be reduced 50% and subsequent increments at longer intervals than usual. Target doses are typically substantially lower than usual.
TCAs	Extensively metabolized. Potentially serious hepatic effects. No dosing guidelines.
Bupropion	Extensively metabolized; decreased clearance. In even mild cirrhosis, use at reduced dose and/or frequency. In severe cirrhosis, dose should not exceed 75 mg daily for conventional tablets, or 100 mg daily or 150 mg every other day for sustained-release formulations.
Desvenlafaxine	Primarily metabolized by conjugation. No adjustment in starting dose necessary in HI. Dosage should not exceed 100 mg/day in severe HI.
Duloxetine	Extensively metabolized; reduced metabolism and elimination. Do not use in patients with any HI.
Mirtazapine	Extensively metabolized; decreased clearance. No dosing guidelines.
Nefazodone	May cause hepatic failure. Avoid use in patients with active liver disease.
Selegiline	Extensively metabolized; caution in HI. No dosing guidelines.
Trazodone	Extensively metabolized. No dosing guidelines.
Venlafaxine	Decreased clearance of venlafaxine and its active metabolite *O*-desmethylvenlafaxine. Dosage should be reduced by 50% in mild to moderate HI per manufacturer.
Atypical antipsychotics	
Asenapine	No dosage adjustment required in mild to moderate HI. Not recommended in patients with severe HI per manufacturer.
Aripiprazole	Extensively metabolized. No dosage adjustment required in mild to severe HI per manufacturer.
Clozapine	Extensively metabolized. Clozapine should be discontinued in patients with marked transaminase elevations or jaundice. No dosing guidelines.
Iloperidone	Extensively metabolized. Pharmacokinetics in mild or moderate HI are unknown. Not recommended in patients with HI per manufacturer.
Olanzapine	Extensively metabolized. Periodic assessment of transaminases is recommended. No dosage adjustment needed per manufacturer.
Paliperidone	Primarily renally excreted. No dosage adjustment required in mild to moderate HI. No dosing guidelines in severe HI.
Quetiapine	Extensively metabolized; clearance decreased 30%. Start at 25 mg/day; increase by 25–50 mg daily.
Risperidone	Extensively metabolized; free fraction increased 35%. Starting dosage and dose increments not to exceed 0.5 mg bid. Increases over 1.5 mg bid should be made at intervals of ≥1 week.
Ziprasidone	Extensively metabolized; increased half-life and serum level in mild to moderate HI. In spite of this, manufacturer recommends no dosage adjustment.
Conventional antipsychotics	
Haloperidol et al.	All metabolized in the liver. No specific dosing recommendations. Phenothiazines (e.g., thioridazine, trifluoperazine) should be avoided. If nonphenothiazines are used, dosage should be reduced and titration should proceed more slowly than usual.
Anxiolytic and sedative-hypnotic drugs	
Alprazolam	Decreased metabolism and increased half-life. Dosage should be reduced by 50%. Avoid use in patients with cirrhosis.
Buspirone	Extensively metabolized; half-life may be prolonged. Reduce dose and frequency in mild to moderate cirrhosis. Do not use in patients with severe impairment.
Chlordiazepoxide, clonazepam, diazepam, flurazepam, triazolam	Extensively metabolized; reduced clearance and prolonged half-life. Avoid use if possible.

TABLE 38–9. Selected psychotropic drugs in hepatic insufficiency (HI) *(continued)*

Lorazepam, oxazepam, temazepam	Metabolized by conjugation; clearance not affected. No dosage adjustment needed. Lorazepam is the preferred choice.
Ramelteon	Extensively metabolized. Exposure to ramelteon increased 4-fold in mild HI and 10-fold in moderate HI. Use with caution in patients with moderate HI. Not recommended in severe HI.
Zaleplon, zolpidem	Metabolized in the liver. Reduced clearance. Usual ceiling dose is 5 mg. Not recommended in severe HI.
Eszopiclone, zopiclone	Metabolized in liver. No dosage adjustment for mild to moderate HI. Reduce dose by 50% in severe HI.
Mood stabilizers/anticonvulsants	
Carbamazepine	Extensively metabolized. Perform baseline liver function tests and periodic evaluations during therapy. Discontinue for active liver disease or aggravation of liver dysfunction. No dosing guidelines.
Oxcarbazepine	Manufacturer states that no dosage adjustment is needed in mild to moderate HI.
Gabapentin	Renally excreted; not appreciably metabolized. No dosage adjustment needed.
Lamotrigine	Initial, escalation, and maintenance dosages should be reduced by 50% in moderate HI (Child-Pugh B) and by 75% in severe HI (Child-Pugh C).
Lithium	Renally excreted; not metabolized. Dosage adjustment depends on fluid status.
Pregabalin	Renally excreted; not appreciably metabolized. No dosage adjustment recommended.
Topiramate	Reduced clearance. No dosing guidelines.
Valproate	Extensively metabolized; reduced clearance and increased half-life. Reduce dosage, monitor liver function tests frequently, especially in first 6 months of therapy. Avoid in patients with substantial hepatic dysfunction. Use with caution in patients with prior history of hepatic disease.
Cholinesterase inhibitors and memantine	
Donepezil	Mildly reduced clearance in cirrhosis. No specific recommendations for dose adjustment.
Galantamine	Use with caution in mild to moderate HI. Dose should not exceed 16 mg daily in moderate HI (Child-Pugh 7–9). Use not recommended in severe HI (Child-Pugh 10–15).
Rivastigmine	Clearance reduced 60%–65% in mild to moderate HI, but dose adjustment may not be necessary.
Memantine	Primarily renally eliminated. No dosage adjustment expected in HI per manufacturer.
Central nervous system stimulants	
Atomoxetine	Extensively metabolized; reduce initial and target dose by 50% in moderate HI and 75% in severe HI as per manufacturer.
Methylphenidate	Unclear association with hepatotoxicity, particularly when coadministered with other adrenergic drugs. No dosing guidelines.
Armodafinil, modafinil	Decreased clearance. Reduce dose by 50% in severe HI.

Note. MAOI = monoamine oxidase inhibitor; SSRI = selective serotonin reuptake inhibitor; TCA = tricyclic antidepressant.
Source. Compiled from Crone et al. 2006; Jacobson 2002; Monti and Pandi-Perumal 2007; and manufacturer's product information.

dence than other current antidepressants and thus should be avoided in patients with preexisting hepatic disease (Carvajal Garcia-Pando et al. 2002; D.E. Stewart 2002). As a general guideline, minor elevations in transaminases are common and usually benign. Elevation of aspartate transaminase (AST) or alanine transaminase (ALT) levels of two to three times baseline or two times normal is significant, and any elevation of alkaline phosphatase (ALP) or bilirubin may be significant.

Antipsychotics. Although very little has been written about the use of antipsychotics in individuals with liver failure, haloperidol remains the most commonly chosen antipsychotic agent for patients with hepatic disease. Chlorpromazine should be avoided because of its greater risk for hepatotoxicity. Low-potency typical antipsychotic medications, which are more anticholinergic than high-potency typical agents, may precipitate hepatic encephalopathy in patients with cirrhosis (as previously described for TCAs). Hepatotoxicity from atypical antipsychotics is rare, and agents in this class remain viable alternatives. All antipsychotics except paliperidone and aripiprazole require dosage reduction in patients with hepatic insufficiency.

Anxiolytics and sedative-hypnotics. Most benzodiazepines are metabolized by phase I processes, and liver disease affects phase I processes significantly more than phase II processes. For this reason, the preferred benzodiazepines for any patient with liver disease are lorazepam, oxazepam, and temazepam because they are metabolized by phase II conjugation. All benzodiazepines should be avoided in patients at risk for developing hepatic encephalopathy because they may precipitate its onset. When their use cannot be avoided (e.g., alcohol withdrawal in a patient with cirrhosis), lorazepam, oxazepam, and temazepam are preferred, with vigilant monitoring of changes in mental status.

Mood stabilizers/anticonvulsants. Because of the risk of hepatotoxicity, carbamazepine and valproate are relatively contraindicated in patients with preexisting liver disease. If either of these agents is used, reduce dose and monitor liver function regularly, especially during the first 6 months of therapy. Gabapentin is renally excreted and does not require dosage adjustment in patients with hepatic disease. Lithium, although renally excreted, may require dosage adjustment and close monitoring secondary to fluctuating fluid balance in patients with liver disease accompanied by ascites (secondary hyperaldosteronism). Lithium pharmacokinetics is also influenced by diuretics for treatment of ascites (see discussion of lithium drug interactions, above). Oxcarbazepine's manufacturer states that no disease adjustment is needed for patients with mild to moderate hepatic insufficiency. Lamotrigine dose should be reduced according to the severity of hepatic impairment. There are no current dosing recommendations for topiramate.

Cholinesterase inhibitors and memantine. Donepezil clearance may be reduced in cirrhosis, but there are no specific dosing recommendations for hepatic insufficiency. Galantamine should be used with caution in patients with mild to moderate hepatic insufficiency, and its dose should not exceed 16 mg daily in patients with a Child-Pugh Score of 7–9 (see Chapter 20, "Gastrointestinal Disorders"). Rivastigmine clearance may be reduced by 60%–65% in patients with mild to moderate hepatic insufficiency, and dosing should be guided by monitoring efficacy and tolerability. Memantine is mainly renally eliminated and requires no dosage reduction in hepatic insufficiency.

Psychostimulants. There are no specific dosing recommendations for methylphenidate. Modafinil and armodafinil clearance is reduced in hepatic insufficiency, and its dosage should be reduced by 50% in patients with severe hepatic insufficiency. For atomoxetine, initial and target doses should be reduced by 50% and 75% of the normal dose for patients with moderate and severe hepatic impairment, respectively (Eli Lilly 2010a).

Gastrointestinal Bleeding

Antidepressants. SSRIs have hemorrhagic potential by interfering with serotonin-induced platelet aggregation through depletion of platelet serotonin stores. The absolute effects are modest and about equal to low-dose ibuprofen. Cohort studies confirm an increased risk of upper gastrointestinal bleeding (3.6-fold), especially with concurrent NSAID or acetylsalicylic acid (ASA; aspirin) use (12-fold) (Dalton et al. 2003; Turner et al. 2007). Concurrent use of SSRIs and warfarin increased the risk of clinically relevant nongastrointestinal bleeding in patients receiving warfarin (3.5-fold) (Wallerstedt et al. 2009). Risk also increases in the presence of medical conditions, such as thrombocytopenia or clotting disorders, which predispose to prolonged bleeding time (see Chapter 24, "Hematology," for a more complete discussion).

Cholinesterase inhibitors. Increased cholinergic activity is expected to increase gastric acid secretion, thereby increasing risk of peptic ulcers. Therefore, caution is warranted when using cholinesterase inhibitors in patients who are at increased risk of developing ulcers or who are receiving NSAIDs.

Drug-Induced Pancreatitis

Several psychotropic agents are infrequently associated with drug-induced pancreatitis. Risk may be elevated in patients with AIDS/HIV, cancer, Crohn's disease, cystic fibrosis, or alcohol abuse or those on multiple medications. Symptoms usually resolve with prompt discontinuation of medication. Among psychotropics, valproate is most frequently associated with acute pancreatitis with an incidence of 0.0025%. Although transient asymptomatic hyperamylasemia occurs in 20% of adult valproate patients, it is unrelated to risk of pancreatitis (Gerstner et al. 2007). Anticonvulsant drug–induced pancreatitis is also infrequently reported with carbamazepine, lamotrigine, topiramate, levetiracetam, and vigabatrin (Zaccara et al. 2007). Antipsychotic-induced pancreatitis, usually occurring within 6 months of starting therapy, has been reported with clozapine and olanzapine, and less often with risperidone and haloperidol (Koller et al. 2003). Mirtazapine, and less frequently bupropion, venlafaxine, and SSRIs may also cause antidepressant-induced pancreatitis (Hussain and Burke 2008; Spigset et al. 2003).

Following recovery from drug-induced pancreatitis, the offending drug should not be re-instated; use of a drug from a different class is preferred (Dhir et al. 2007).

Other Gastrointestinal Disorders

Many diseases can cause malabsorption. Depending on the type of malabsorption syndrome and the mechanism involved, varied effects on pharmacokinetics may be observed. In general, however, orally administered drugs may be poorly absorbed in the presence of malabsorption syndromes. In patients with delayed gastric emptying (due to diabetes mellitus, atrophic gastritis, gastric cancer, pyloric stenosis, pancreatitis, gastric ulcer, or drug effects), absorption rate may be slowed resulting in a delay in the onset of the medication's therapeutic effect. The effects of gastric dysfunction on drug absorption, including reduced gastric acidity and reduced gastric emptying, are complex (see Gubbins and Bertch 1991; Parsons 1977). For non-enteric-coated preparations, increased gastric emptying is likely to increase the rate of drug absorption, and conversely, delayed gastric emptying will slow the rate of drug absorption. However, because of the large intestinal surface area, overall absorption is not likely to change significantly. Similarly, for most drugs, reduced gastric acidity is unlikely to significantly affect the extent of absorption. For enteric-coated preparations, however, reduced gastric acidity increases the rate of drug absorption because dissolution of the preparation will occur in the stomach. The rate and extent of absorption of drugs, such as clorazepate, that require gastric acid–induced hydrolysis for conversion to the active form (desmethyldiazepam in the case of clorazepate) are impaired by agents, and presumably disease states, that reduce gastric acidity (Greenblatt et al. 1978; Parsons 1977). Anticholinergic drugs should be avoided in patients with gastroparesis, constipation, or ulcerative colitis. SSRIs may be undesirable in patients with increased gastric motility or diarrhea. When conditions or disease states may significantly alter oral drug absorption, an alternate route of drug administration should be considered (see "Alternative Routes of Administration" subsection earlier in this chapter).

Renal Disease

Although most psychotropic drugs do not depend on the kidney for excretion, renal failure may alter drug pharmacokinetics including changes in absorption, distribution, and protein binding (discussed earlier in this chapter). Despite the complexity of pharmacokinetic changes in renal failure, most psychotropics, other than lithium, gabapentin, pregabalin, memantine, paliperidone, paroxetine, desvenlafaxine, topiramate, and venlafaxine, do not require drastic dosage adjustment. However, many problems associated with use of psychotropics in patients with end-stage renal disease (ESRD) are related to comorbid illnesses rather than to the renal failure per se. Specific dosing guidelines based on creatinine clearance are not available for most psychotropics, but many clinicians use the rule of "two-thirds"—that is, for patients with renal insufficiency, use two-thirds of the dose (except for drugs listed above) used for patients with normal renal function.

Because most psychotropics are lipophilic compounds with large volumes of distribution, they are not dialyzable. Only lithium, gabapentin, pregabalin, valproate, topiramate, and levetiracetam are removed by dialysis. Significant fluid shifts occur during and several hours after each hemodialysis treatment, making dialysis patients more prone to orthostasis. Hence, drugs that frequently cause orthostatic hypotension should ideally be avoided.

Table 38–10 provides recommendations for dosing psychotropics in patients with renal disease.

Antidepressants

Virtually all antidepressants may be used in patients with renal failure, although the greatest experience is with the TCAs. However, patients with ESRD tend to be more sensitive to the side effects of TCAs, including sedation, anticholinergic toxicity, and orthostatic hypotension. Hydroxylated metabolites have been shown to be markedly elevated in patients with ESRD and may be responsible for some TCA side effects. Nortriptyline is considered the preferred TCA because its blood levels correlate well with clinical effect, and the "therapeutic window" is the same in renal failure patients as in physically healthy patients. Limited data are available on the use of newer antidepressants in patients with renal failure. Some evidence suggests that dosage adjustments may not be needed for citalopram and fluoxetine in those with ESRD. However, the half-life of venlafaxine is prolonged in renal insufficiency; its clearance is reduced by over 50% in patients undergoing dialysis. Desvenlafaxine undergoes significant renal elimination requiring dosage reduction in moderate and severe renal impairment. Paroxetine clearance is also reduced in renal insufficiency. Because most antidepressants are metabolized by the liver and excreted by the kidney, initial dosage reduction of all antidepressants is reasonable as a way to reduce the possibility that potentially active metabolites will accumulate.

Antipsychotics

All antipsychotics may be used in patients with renal failure, however, paliperidone clearance is significantly decreased in all degrees of renal impairment requiring a reduction in initial and target dose. Difficulties arise from the complications of renal failure and dialysis or from the chronic disease causing renal failure (e.g., diabetes). For example, patients with ESRD who also have diabetic autonomic neuropathy will be at higher risk for drug side ef-

TABLE 38–10. Psychotropic drugs in renal insufficiency (RI)[a]

Antidepressants	
MAOIs	May accumulate in RI.
TCAs	Water-soluble active metabolites may accumulate. No recommended dosage adjustments.
Most SSRIs	Mild to moderate RI: no dosage adjustment needed. Severe RI: may need to reduce dosage or lengthen dosing interval.
Paroxetine	Mild RI: no dosage adjustment needed. Moderate RI: 50%–75% of usual dose. Severe RI: initial dosage of 10 mg/day; increase as needed by 10 mg at weekly intervals to a maximum dosage of 40 mg/day. Controlled-release formulation: initial dose of 12.5 mg/day; increase if needed by 12.5 mg at weekly intervals to a maximum of 50 mg/day.
Bupropion	Water-soluble active metabolites may accumulate. Reduce initial dosage.
Desvenlafaxine	Approximately 45% of desvenlafaxine is excreted unchanged in urine. No dosage adjustment is required in mild RI. Dosage should not exceed 50 mg/day in moderate RI, or 50 mg every other day in severe RI, per manufacturer.
Duloxetine	Mild RI: population CPK analyses suggest no significant effect on apparent clearance. No data regarding use in moderate to severe RI. Not recommended for patients with end-stage renal disease.
Mirtazapine	Moderate RI: clearance decreased by 30%. Severe RI: clearance decreased by 50%.
Nefazodone	No dosage adjustment needed.
Trazodone	Mild RI: use with caution. No data regarding use in moderate to severe RI.
Selegiline	Active metabolite (methamphetamine) renally eliminated. Use with caution in renal impairment. No dosing guidelines.
Venlafaxine	Mild to moderate RI: 75% of usual dose. Severe RI: 50% of usual dose. Hemodialysis patients should have dosage reduced by 50% and receive dose after dialysis session.
Atypical antipsychotics	
Asenapine, aripiprazole, clozapine, olanzapine, quetiapine	No dosage adjustment needed.
Iloperidone	Dosage adjustment not needed in mild to moderate RI, per manufacturer. No recommendations for dosing in severe RI.
Paliperidone	Clearance decreased in RI. For mild impairment, start at 3 mg/day. increasing to a maximum of 6 mg/day. For moderate to severe impairment start at 1.5 mg/day, increasing to 3 mg/day, as tolerated.
Risperidone	Clearance decreased in RI. Initiate therapy at 0.25–0.5 mg bid. Increase beyond 1.5 mg should be made at intervals of at least 7 days.
Ziprasidone	No recommendations made regarding dosage adjustment.
Conventional antipsychotics	
Haloperidol et al.	No dosage adjustment needed.
Anxiolytics and sedative-hypnotics	
Most benzodiazepines	No dosage adjustment needed.
Chlordiazepoxide	Severe RI: 50% of usual dose.
Buspirone	Use in severe RI not recommended.
Ramelteon	No dosage adjustment needed.
Zaleplon	Mild to moderate RI: no dosage adjustment needed. Severe RI not adequately studied.
Zolpidem	Dosage adjustment may not be needed in RI.
Eszopiclone, zopiclone	No dosage adjustment needed.

TABLE 38–10. Psychotropic drugs in renal insufficiency (RI)[a] *(continued)*

Mood stabilizers/anticonvulsants	
Carbamazepine	Severe RI: 75% of usual dose.
Gabapentin	Cl_{cr} >60 mL/min: 1,200 mg/day (400 mg tid). Cl_{cr} 30–60 mL/min: 600 mg/day (300 mg bid). Cl_{cr} 15–30 mL/min: 300 mg/day. Cl_{cr} <15 mL/min: 150 mg/day (300 mg every other day). Hemodialysis: 300–400 mg loading dose to patients who have never received gabapentin, then 200–300 mg after each dialysis session.
Lamotrigine	Reduced dose may be effective in significant RI.
Lithium	Moderate RI: 50%–75% of usual dose. Hemodialysis: supplemental dose of 300 mg once after each dialysis session.
Oxcarbazepine	Initiate therapy at 300 mg/day (50% of usual starting dose).
Pregabalin	Cl_{cr} 30–60 mL/min: 50% of usual dosage. Cl_{cr} 15–30 mL/min: 25% of usual dosage. Cl_{cr} <15 mL/min: 12.5% of usual dosage. Hemodialysis: supplemental dose may be needed after every 4-hour dialysis. See manufacturer's recommendations.
Topiramate	Mild RI: 100% of usual dosage. Moderate RI: 50% of usual dosage. Severe RI: 25% of usual dosage. Supplemental dose may be needed after hemodialysis.
Valproate	No dosage adjustment needed in RI, but valproate level measurements are misleading.
Cholinesterase inhibitors and memantine	
Donepezil	Limited data suggest no dosage adjustment needed.
Galantamine	Moderate RI: maximum dose 16 mg/day. Severe RI: use not recommended.
Rivastigmine	Dosage adjustment not recommended.
Memantine	Extensive renal elimination. No dosage reduction needed in mild to moderate RI. Reduce dose to 5 mg bid in severe RI.
Central nervous system stimulants	
Atomoxetine	No dosage adjustment needed.
Methylphenidate	No dosage adjustment needed.
Armodafinil, modafinil	No dosage adjustment needed.
Antiparkinsonian agents	
Amantadine	Cl_{cr} 80 mL/min: 100 mg twice daily. Cl_{cr} 60 mL/min: alternating daily doses of 100 mg once daily and 100 mg twice daily. Cl_{cr} 40 mL/min: 100 mg/day. Cl_{cr} 30 mL/min: 200 mg twice weekly. Cl_{cr} 20 mL/min: 100 mg three times weekly. Cl_{cr} 10 mL/min: alternating weekly doses of 100 mg once weekly and 200 mg once weekly. Hemodialysis: 200 mg once weekly.
Pramipexole	90% renal elimination: clearance of pramipexole is 75% lower in severe RI (Cl_{cr} 20 mL/min) and 60% lower in patients with moderate RI (Cl_{cr} 40 mL/min) compared with healthy volunteers. Interval between titration steps should be increased to 14 days in restless legs syndrome (RLS) patients with severe or moderate RI (Cl_{cr} 20–60 mL/min).

Note. Cl_{cr} = creatinine clearance; CPK = creatine phosphokinase; MAOIs = monoamine oxidase inhibitors; SSRIs = selective serotonin reuptake inhibitors; TCAs = tricyclic antidepressants.

[a]Mild RI is >50 mL/min; moderate RI is 10–50 mL/min; severe RI is <10 mL/min.

Source. Compiled from L.M. Cohen et al. 2004; Crone et al. 2006; Jacobson 2002; Periclou et al. 2006; and manufacturer's product information.

fects, including postural hypotension and bladder, gastrointestinal, and sexual dysfunction.

Anxiolytics and Sedative-Hypnotics

Virtually all sedative-hypnotics can be used in patients with renal failure with the exception of barbiturates. Barbiturates should be avoided because they may increase osteomalacia and because of excessive sedation. Preferred benzodiazepines include those with inactive metabolites such as lorazepam and oxazepam. Even so, the half-lives of lorazepam and oxazepam may almost quadruple in patients with ESRD, and dosage reduction is required. Other benzodiazepines with inactive metabolites include clonazepam and temazepam, but less is known about changes in their half-lives in ESRD.

Mood Stabilizers/Anticonvulsants

Lithium is almost entirely excreted by the kidneys. It is contraindicated in patients with acute renal failure, but not in those with chronic renal failure. For patients with stable partial renal insufficiency, dose conservatively and monitor renal function frequently. For patients on dialysis, lithium is completely dialyzed and may be given as a single oral dose (300–600 mg) following hemodialysis treatment. Lithium levels should not be checked until at least 2–3 hours after dialysis, because re-equilibration from tissue stores occurs in the immediate postdialytic period. For patients on peritoneal dialysis, lithium can be given in the dialysate. Dosage adjustment recommendations based on creatinine clearance are available for gabapentin, lithium, pregabalin, topiramate, and carbamazepine (Jacobson 2002).

Cholinesterase Inhibitors and Memantine

It appears, from the limited data available, that dosage adjustment of donepezil is not required. As in patients without renal disease, rivastigmine dose should be titrated according to efficacy and individual tolerability. Galantamine should be used cautiously in patients with moderate renal insufficiency; according to the manufacturer, its use in patients with severe renal insufficiency is not recommended. Memantine undergoes extensive renal elimination requiring a dosage reduction in severe renal insufficiency.

Psychostimulants

No specific dosing recommendations are currently available for psychostimulants.

Cardiovascular Disease

Potential adverse cardiovascular effects of psychotropics include orthostatic hypotension, conduction disturbances, and arrhythmias (see also Chapter 18, "Heart Disease"). Orthostatic hypotension can be a serious problem for many debilitated patients, aggravated by dehydration, with increased morbidity resulting in patients with poor tissue perfusion and leading to injuries due to falls (fractures, subdural hematomas).

Antidepressants

The safety of antidepressant drugs in patients with cardiac disease is extensively reviewed by Alvarez and Pickworth (2003) and Taylor (2008). In summary, patients most at risk for developing cardiac side effects include those with unstable coronary artery disease (especially recent myocardial infarction), conduction abnormalities, orthostatic hypotension, and congestive heart failure (Taylor 2008). Although there are more studies of TCAs than of other antidepressants in cardiac patients, the SSRIs have been studied in the largest number of patients.

Tricyclic antidepressants. The TCAs have been shown to be relatively safe for short-term treatment of patients with stable ischemic heart disease, previous myocardial infarction, and congestive heart failure. Long-term safety has not been studied. In healthy individuals, the cardiovascular complications from TCAs administered at therapeutic levels are largely limited to orthostatic hypotension (Glassman 1984). In patients with heart disease, the cardiovascular risks become clinically significant. TCAs are more likely to cause orthostatic hypotension in patients with impairment in left ventricular function but are relatively safe to use in most patients with congestive heart failure. Caution is required if the patient has symptomatic orthostatic hypotension or markedly reduced cardiac ejection fraction. Nortriptyline is considered the safest TCA in patients with congestive heart failure because it is least likely to cause orthostasis (Roose et al. 1981) and has little to no effect on cardiac ejection fraction (Giardina et al. 1985; Roose et al. 1986).

All TCAs have quinidine-like Type 1A antiarrhythmic properties that delay cardiac conduction and increase heart rate. In healthy individuals, this is usually not clinically significant. Patients with existing conduction delays (e.g., bundle branch block) may have clinically relevant deleterious effects on conduction time. In patients with bundle branch block (especially those with second-degree heart block), dissociative (third-degree) atrioventricular heart block may develop. Some calcium channel blockers (diltiazem and verapamil, but not nifedipine) may also slow atrioventricular conduction, making their combination with TCAs more dangerous.

The quinidine-like effect of TCAs prolongs the QTc interval, which may lead to the potentially fatal arrhythmia torsade de pointes. Patients at particular risk include those with preexisting familial long QTc syndrome or who develop undue QTc prolongation during treatment with TCAs (or other QTc-prolonging drugs including antipsychotics and antimicrobials). An electrocardiogram is indicated for patients treated with TCAs who have a family history of sudden death or syncope or a personal history of angina, syncope, myocardial infarction, congestive heart failure, arrhythmias, hypokalemia, hypomagnesemia, or other significant cardiac risk factors (Vieweg 2002). TCAs are not recommended in patients with existing conduction disturbances, however, if necessary, a cardiology consultation should be sought prior to the use of TCAs in these patients.

Wolff-Parkinson-White syndrome, or atrioventricular nodal reentrant tachycardia, affects approximately 0.15%–0.2% of the general population. Of these individuals, 60%–70% have no other evidence of heart disease. In some, more serious and potentially life-threatening abnormal rhythms may develop. The most common of these is atrial fibrillation. Quinidine-like drugs given to patients with atrial flutter-fibrillation may lead to ventricular tachycardia or fibrillation. All patients with Wolff-Parkinson-White syndrome should be evaluated by a cardiologist prior to considering TCA treatment.

Newer antidepressants. SSRIs are currently considered the safest antidepressants in patients with cardiac disease. Cardiovascular effects of SSRIs include modest slowing of heart rate, minimal effects on blood pressure (rare hypotension) or conduction, and no effects on ventricular function (Taylor 2008; Vieweg et al. 2006). Venlafaxine, desvenlafaxine, and duloxetine may increase supine diastolic blood pressure through their noradrenergic effects. Although trazodone is considered safe, it causes orthostatic hypotension not infrequently and, rarely, premature ventricular contractions and ventricular tachycardia (Winkler et al. 2006). Bupropion may elevate blood pressure, but other cardiovascular effects are generally rare. Bupropion has been used safely in patients with conduction disease and left ventricular dysfunction (Roose et al. 1991). Mirtazapine has been studied in patients with post–myocardial infarction depressive disorder and found to have no significant cardiac effects (Honig et al. 2007).

Antipsychotics

Antipsychotics causing orthostatic hypotension, including low-potency antipsychotics, clozapine, and quetiapine, should be avoided in patients with congestive heart failure. Because olanzapine and high-potency typical antipsychotics such as haloperidol cause orthostasis far less frequently, they can usually be used safely even during acute unstable cardiac disease.

Patients with preexisting intraventricular conduction delays are at increased risk of heart block when given antipsychotics with quinidine-like properties such as thioridazine. Although the cardiovascular risks with antipsychotics may vary, pimozide, thioridazine, mesoridazine, droperidol, sertindole, ziprasidone, and quetiapine carry the highest risk for prolonging the QTc interval and causing torsade de pointes. Other atypical antipsychotics and haloperidol appear to demonstrate the least risk for prolonging the QTc interval. Although haloperidol has caused QTc prolongation and torsade de pointes, especially when parenterally administered at a high dosage (>100 mg/day), it is generally accepted to be minimally cardiotoxic. It is prudent to obtain an electrocardiogram for any patient at increased cardiac risk when prescribed an antipsychotic drug, and especially for those drugs associated with a significantly increased risk of QTc prolongation (ziprasidone, quetiapine, droperidol, mesoridazine, thioridazine, pimozide, high-dose intravenous haloperidol).

Anxiolytics and Sedative-Hypnotics

Generally, benzodiazepines are free of cardiovascular effects. Their safety has been documented even in the immediate post–myocardial infarction period (Risch et al. 1982). However, rapid intravenous administration may cause hypotension. Buspirone is essentially free of cardiovascular effects. Zolpidem has been reported to be without effect on systolic blood pressure or heart rate in healthy human volunteers (McCann et al. 1993). To date, there are no reports of the cardiovascular effects of zopiclone, eszopiclone, zaleplon, or ramelteon.

Mood Stabilizers/Anticonvulsants

The cardiac effects of lithium at nontoxic levels are generally insignificant; there may be nonspecific electrocardiographic changes, which are usually benign. Lithium uncommonly causes sinus node dysfunction or first-degree atrioventricular block (Dasgupta and Jefferson 1990) and QTc prolongation (van Noord et al. 2009) and should be used cautiously in patients at risk. For patients with congestive heart failure, reduced doses are required secondary to decreased lithium clearance. However, lithium is difficult to use in these patients because of salt restriction and coadministration of diuretics, angiotensin-converting enzyme inhibitors, and angiotensin receptor blockers. Valproate is safe to use in patients with cardiovascular disease. Carbamazepine is more cardiotoxic and has been associated with the development of atrioventricular conduction disturbances (Chong et al. 2001). Before carbamazepine is prescribed, a baseline electrocardiogram should be obtained in patients at risk, and alternative therapy should be considered if there is evidence of heart block or atrioventricular conduction delay. Lamotrigine has been associated with clinically insignificant prolongation of the PR interval. Caution is warranted with other mood stabilizers because they have not been systematically studied in patients with cardiac disease.

Cholinesterase Inhibitors and Memantine

Cholinesterase inhibitors may have vagotonic effects on the heart (e.g., bradycardia). This effect may be of particular concern in patients with "sick sinus syndrome" or other supraventricular conduction abnormalities. Cholinesterase inhibitors should be avoided in patients with most cardiac conduction abnormalities and those with unexplained syncopal episodes. Memantine is generally benign in patients with cardiovascular disease, but it may rarely cause bradycardia (Gallini et al. 2008).

Psychostimulants

Methylphenidate and dextroamphetamine in low doses have no significant cardiovascular effects, including no effect on blood pressure or heart rate. While safe use has been described in many cardiac patients, including those with congestive heart failure, coronary artery disease, arrhythmias, and hypertension (Masand and Tesar 1996), use of these stimulants in patients with structural cardiac abnormalities, cardiomyopathy, coronary artery disease or serious rhythm abnormalities is contraindicated according to FDA-approved product monographs.

There are no studies of the cardiovascular effects of modafinil, armodafinil, or atomoxetine in cardiac patients. Modafinil increased blood pressure more than placebo in obstructive sleep apnea patients subjected to mental and physical stress (Heitmann et al. 1999). In noncardiac patients, cardiovascular adverse effects of atomoxetine are restricted to small increases in heart rate and blood pressure with no prolongation of the QT interval (Wernicke et al. 2003).

Because stimulants can increase heart rate and blood pressure, it would seem prudent to use caution when prescribing stimulants to patients with underlying medical conditions that might be compromised by increases in heart rate or blood pressure.

Central Nervous System Disease

Cerebrovascular Disease

The most common problems encountered when prescribing psychotropics to patients with cerebrovascular disease include lowered threshold for CNS side effects, orthostatic hypotension, and comorbid disorders (e.g., cardiac disease, diabetes).

Antidepressants. Poststroke depression is a common neuropsychiatric complication of stroke in up to one-half of patients (see also Chapter 8, "Depression," and Chapter 32, "Neurology and Neurosurgery"). Antidepressant prophylaxis of poststroke depression has been studied in several meta-analyses. Chen et al. (2007) suggested that SSRIs and TCAs are effective in reducing the incidence of poststroke depression by more than 50%, especially in patients with ischemic stroke. Many, but not all (Hackett et al. 2005), analyses support a beneficial prophylactic effect for antidepressants in poststroke depression. Treatment of existing poststroke depression has been most studied with nortriptyline, trazodone, fluoxetine, sertraline, citalopram, and escitalopram, with favorable therapeutic effects in those patients able to tolerate these medications. Mirtazapine, venlafaxine, and milnacipran are also reportedly of benefit (Tharwani et al. 2007). Evidence for the safety and efficacy of desvenlafaxine and duloxetine in poststroke patients is lacking.

Antipsychotics. Concerns of an increased risk of cerebrovascular events (stroke, transient ischemic attack), including fatalities, arose from analysis of four placebo-controlled trials of risperidone in elderly patients with dementia-related psychosis (Health Canada 2002). Further pharmacovigilance suggested an increased risk of cerebrovascular events with all atypical antipsychotics prompting Britain's Committee on Safety of Medicines in 2004 to recommend against use of atypical antipsychotics in dementia patients. In 2005, the FDA ordered a black-box warning for all atypical antipsychotics of an increased risk of death in elderly patients with dementia-related psychosis. Recent studies suggest that all antipsychotics (both typical and atypical agents) are associated with an increased risk of stroke in the elderly. A large cohort study identified risk of stroke as greater for elderly users of phenothiazines (5.8-fold), butyrophenones (3.6-fold), and atypical agents (2.5-fold) than for elderly nonusers (Sacchetti et al. 2008). An increase in stroke incidence was also observed in a within-person case series examining the risk of stroke while taking an antipsychotic drug. For elderly patients, the risk of stroke increased while taking antipsychotics 2.3-fold for atypical agents and 1.7-fold for typical agents. The presence of dementia approximately doubled the risk of stroke for each drug class (Douglas and Smeeth 2008). To date, identified risk factors that may predispose to cerebrovascular adverse events are limited to age greater than 80 years, antipsychotic use, and presence of dementia, although other factors—including sedation, concomitant use of benzodiazepines, and the presence of pulmonary conditions (e.g., pneumonia with or without aspiration)—have been suggested.

Psychostimulants. Psychostimulants offer an alternative in treating poststroke depression, but poststroke patients may be more sensitive to their side effects. Hence, psychostimulants should be initiated at a very low dose and gradually increased as necessary (Masand and Tesar 1996).

Seizures

Psychotropics that may lower seizure threshold at normal doses primarily pose a risk in patients with untreated (or undertreated) seizure disorder.

Antidepressants. Seizure disorder patients are frequently prescribed psychotropic medications, including antidepressants, because of high psychiatric comorbidity. Naturally, the use of antidepressants in these patients raises concerns over the possibility of increased seizure risk. Studies estimating seizure risk are difficult to interpret because of methodological limitations and confounding factors. TCAs consistently increase seizure risk a small amount. An analysis of FDA Phase II and Phase III clinical trials suggests that in comparison with placebo, SSRIs and SNRIs actually lower the incidence of seizure by more than 50% (Alper et al. 2007). Risk of seizures with the sustained-release (SR) formulation of bupropion (dosage of 450 mg/day) is comparable to that with SSRIs but is elevated at dosages greater than 450 mg/day. Bupropion immediate release (IR) has a greater risk of seizures than bupropion SR. The use of bupropion in patients with preexisting seizure disorder, or in patients who may be at higher risk for developing seizures (e.g., in bulimia), warrants caution, especially with the IR form.

Antipsychotics. Low-potency typical antipsychotics, especially at high dose (≥1,000 mg/day chlorpromazine), and clozapine have higher reported risk of seizures and should be avoided in patients with existing seizure disorders. Seizures have been reported with most antipsychotics; however, haloperidol and risperidone (and likely paliperidone) have the lowest rate of seizures, followed by quetiapine, then olanzapine and low-potency typical antipsychotics with an intermediate risk (Alldredge 1999; Alper et al. 2007). Generally, antipsychotic seizure risk increases with sedating effect.

Cholinesterase inhibitors and memantine. Cholinomimetics may reduce the seizure threshold, and seizures have been reported during clinical trials with all cholinesterase inhibitors. However, seizure activity may also be a manifestation of Alzheimer's disease. Donepezil has been reported to increase seizure frequency in patients with epilepsy (Fisher et al. 2001). The risk-benefit ratio of cholinesterase treatment for patients with seizures must be carefully evaluated. Memantine may lower seizure threshold but clinical trials do not suggest an increase in seizure risk (Forest 2010).

Psychostimulants. Many physicians believe that psychostimulants can lower seizure threshold, but evidence is lacking. One study of traumatic brain injury patients with posttraumatic seizures concluded that methylphenidate can be safely used even in those at high risk for seizures (Wroblewski et al. 1992). A small number of patients may experience an increase in seizure frequency when they are treated with psychostimulants. If seizure frequency rises, the drug should be discontinued. A review of pharmaceutical company databases suggests that atomoxetine does not increase the risk of seizures in ADHD (Wernicke et al. 2007a).

Migraine Headache

Antidepressants. Many patients with migraine headaches take triptans, which are potent 5-$HT_{1B/1D}$ receptor agonists. Antidepressants are also frequently prescribed for migraine prophylaxis or comorbid depression. Risk of serotonin syndrome with antidepressant and triptan coadministration is quite rare, with only a few cases reported (Gardner and Lynd 1998). Triptan use does not contraindicate the use of serotonergic antidepressants. The triptans vary widely in their potential for pharmacokinetic interactions (Dodick and Martin 2004). Some triptans, including sumatriptan, rizatriptan, and zolmitriptan, are metabolized by MAO and should not be used during MAOI therapy (including selegiline) or within 2 weeks of MAOI discontinuation (McEvoy 2008). Almotriptan, eletriptan, frovatriptan, and naratriptan are eliminated primarily through metabolism by CYP enzymes and/or renal elimination and thus can be more safely used in conjunction with MAOIs.

Parkinsonism

For additional discussion of use of medications in patients with Parkinson's disease, see Chapter 32, "Neurology and Neurosurgery."

Antidepressants. Double-blind studies of imipramine, nortriptyline, desipramine, and bupropion demonstrate antidepressant efficacy with no change in Parkinson's disease symptoms. The anticholinergic effects of TCAs may even be therapeutic for parkinsonism.

There is a theoretical concern that serotonergic antidepressants could worsen parkinsonism through serotonin-mediated inhibition of nigrostriatal dopamine release—this effect occurs rarely (Richard et al. 1999). In a retrospective analysis of patients with Parkinson's disease stabilized on L-dopa, initiation of an SSRI was no more likely to result in a change in antiparkinsonian medication dose than initiation of any other antidepressant class including TCAs, venlafaxine, bupropion, or mirtazapine (Arbouw et al. 2007). The clinical efficacy of antidepressants for Parkinson's disease depression has been studied in few controlled antidepressant drug trials. Placebo-controlled trials suggest nortriptyline, desipramine, and citalopram (Devos et al. 2008) but not paroxetine (Menza et al. 2009) or sertraline (Wermuth et al. 1998) to be superior to placebo for the treatment of Parkinson's-related depression. TCAs may be more efficacious but less tolerable than SSRIs for depression in Parkinson's disease.

Early reports suggest that mirtazapine may reduce tremor (Gordon et al. 2002; Pact and Giduz 1999). Selegiline, a highly selective MAO-B inhibitor at doses used in the treatment of Parkinson's disease, is another antidepressant option, but it loses selectivity at the oral doses required for antidepressant efficacy and so requires standard MAOI precautions.

Antipsychotics. The major concern regarding antipsychotic use in Parkinson's disease is the degree of dopamine D_2 receptor blockade—especially with high-potency typical antipsychotics—potentially aggravating the disease. Clozapine is the only atypical antipsychotic demonstrated in a number of controlled trials in patients with Parkinson's disease to be effective against psychosis without aggravating the disease (reviewed in Frieling et al. 2007), and it may even be beneficial in reducing tremor (Parkinson Study Group 1999). In two placebo-controlled trials, quetiapine was well tolerated but failed to demonstrate efficacy. Olanzapine was without therapeutic effect but increased EPS in four controlled trials.

To date, case reports and open-label studies suggest that aripiprazole and ziprasidone may be effective for psychosis in Parkinson's disease and well tolerated (Gomez-Esteban et al. 2005; Lopez-Meza et al. 2005; Schonfeldt-Lecuona and Connemann 2004), but controlled trials are needed to confirm these results.

Cholinesterase inhibitors. Cholinesterase inhibitors are currently the most promising alternative to antipsychotics for the treatment of psychosis in Parkinson's disease. Rivastigmine, in both an open-label study and a placebo-controlled trial involving 188 patients with Parkinson's disease and visual hallucinations, exhibited efficacy without increased EPS (Burn et al. 2006). Although case studies suggest an improvement in psychosis with donepezil, results from two controlled clinical trials are less encouraging; donepezil was not significantly better than placebo (Aarsland et al. 2002; Ravina et al. 2005).

Dementia With Lewy Bodies

Antipsychotics. Patients with dementia with Lewy bodies typically present with extreme sensitivity to EPS of antipsychotics—an important consideration when prescribing antipsychotics for the treatment of hallucinations, delusions, and/or agitation in patients with dementia. No randomized controlled trials of antipsychotics in patients with dementia with Lewy bodies exist. Overall, atypical antipsychotics are probably safer than typical antipsychotics but should be used at very low doses.

Cholinesterase inhibitors. Patients with Lewy body dementia (see Chapter 6, "Dementia") typically present with cognitive, behavioral, and psychiatric symptoms. Cholinesterase inhibitors are now considered by many to be first-line therapy for dementia with Lewy bodies. A review of open-label trials of donepezil and galantamine and a placebo-controlled trial of rivastigmine concluded that all three cholinesterase inhibitors significantly improve cognitive and psychiatric symptoms in patients with this condition (Bhasin et al. 2007). More recent case-control studies and open-label trials support these conclusions for galantamine (Edwards et al. 2007) and rivastigmine (Rozzini et al. 2007). A placebo-controlled trial of all three agents is necessary to identify the most efficacious and tolerable cholinesterase inhibitor for Lewy body dementia.

Endocrine Disease

Diabetes Mellitus

Antidepressants. Elevated catecholamine levels increase serum glucose levels while reducing both insulin release and insulin sensitivity. In contrast, increases in serotonergic function seem to increase sensitivity to insulin and reduce serum glucose. Thus, in this light, SSRIs may be preferred agents in patients with diabetes because of their minimal effects on glucose metabolism. However, in diabetic neuropathic pain, SNRIs are more effective at lower doses than SSRIs, perhaps because both catecholamines and serotonin have been implicated in pain pathways (Goodnick 2001). First-line pharmacological treatments for diabetic neuropathic pain include TCAs, SNRIs, and the anticonvulsants gabapentin and pregabalin (Zin et al. 2008), which appear to be of comparable efficacy (Chou et al. 2009; Quilici et al. 2009). Duloxetine, venlafaxine, desvenlafaxine, and milnacipran have fewer side effects than TCAs.

Antipsychotics. An assessment of relative risks of particular antipsychotics in diabetes should include the risks of weight gain, glucose intolerance, and hyperlipidemia. Where these factors are of concern it is generally agreed that clozapine and olanzapine should be avoided. Weight gain is minimal for ziprasidone and aripiprazole (Haddad 2005). Clozapine, olanzapine, quetiapine, and risperidone on rare occasions have precipitated diabetic ketoacidosis. Current consensus guidelines for monitoring patients receiving atypical antipsychotics, including monitoring forms and risk criteria, are available from the Center for Quality Assessment and Improvement in Mental Health (www.cqaimh.org/pdf/tool_metabolic.pdf).

Obesity

Antidepressants. Many patients receiving antidepressants experience weight gain. The proportion of patients who gained at least 7% of their body weight over 1 year of treatment was greatest for mirtazapine (26%), less for SSRIs (16%–19%) and similar to placebo for venlafaxine, duloxetine (at doses ≤60 mg/day), nefazodone, and bupropion (Papakostas 2008).

Antipsychotics. Almost all antipsychotics can cause weight gain, but they vary in their propensity to cause this effect. There is some controversy as to who is more likely to gain weight on antipsychotics—those at normal weight to begin with or those who are already obese. Nevertheless, in patients who are already obese, weight-neutral antipsychotics such as ziprasidone and aripiprazole are sensible as preferred agents.

Anticonvulsants. Many anticonvulsants are associated with significant weight changes with long-term treatment for epilepsy. Weight gain has been reported for gabapentin (57% of patients gain >5% baseline weight), pregabalin (11% of patients gain >7% baseline weight), valproate (average weight gain 3%–8% of baseline weight), and possibly carbamazepine. Lamotrigine, levetiracetam, and phenytoin are weight neutral. Felbamate, topiramate, and zonisamide are associated with weight loss (Ben-Menachem 2007; Biton et al. 2001; Privitera et al. 2003).

Lipids

Antidepressants. Several antidepressants, including mirtazapine, paroxetine, and sertraline, are reported to increase low-density lipoprotein cholesterol (LDL-C), especially in women (Le Melledo et al. 2004). Generally, lipid disruptions are most likely with antidepressants associated with weight gain (McIntyre et al. 2006).

Antipsychotics. Phenothiazines, clozapine, olanzapine, and quetiapine are known to elevate serum triglyceride levels and thus should be avoided in patients with hypertriglyceridemia or hypercholesterolemia.

Respiratory Disease

For additional discussion of use of medications in patients with respiratory disease, see Chapter 19, "Lung Disease."

Antidepressants

Antidepressants generally do not cause problems in patients with respiratory disease. However, MAOIs are problematic in asthmatic patients because of their potential to interact with epinephrine and other sympathomimetic medications. Use of antidepressants with anticholinergic properties is of theoretical benefit because of their mild bronchodilator effect. Cyclic antidepressants, SSRIs, and other newer antidepressants have little to no effect on respiratory function.

Anxiolytics and Sedative-Hypnotics

The respiratory depressant effects of all benzodiazepines are well established; most of these agents can significantly reduce the ventilatory response to hypoxia. This may precipitate respiratory failure in a patient with marginal respiratory reserve. Patients with moderate-to-severe COPD are at risk for carbon dioxide retention with long-acting benzodiazepines, even at relatively low doses. However, benzodiazepines should not automatically be rejected for use in patients with COPD. Anxiety can often reduce respiratory efficiency, and benzodiazepines may actually improve respiratory status in some patients, especially those with asthma or emphysema ("pink puffers") (Mitchell-Heggs et al. 1980). Patients with severe bronchitis ("blue bloaters") or severe restrictive lung disease are the most vulnerable to the adverse effects of benzodiazepines. Intermediate-acting agents (e.g., oxazepam, temazepam, lorazepam) have fewer respiratory depressant effects and are the benzodiazepines of first choice for anxiolysis in patients with COPD. For patients with severe COPD, baseline assessment of blood gases and pulmonary consultation may be necessary in deciding whether benzodiazepines are appropriate for use. Oximetry is likely adequate for ongoing monitoring of the patient's clinical status during benzodiazepine use unless the patient is a known CO_2 retainer, in which case blood gases are more appropriate. Benzodiazepines are currently contraindicated in individuals with sleep apnea.

Controlled trials with the short-acting nonbenzodiazepine hypnotics zopiclone, eszopiclone, zolpidem, and zaleplon suggest that they may be safely used in selected patients who have mild to moderate COPD without daytime hypercapnia (George 2000). Zopiclone and zolpidem have been found to have no significant effects on ventilatory drive or central control of breathing in patients with mild to moderate COPD (Girault et al. 1996; Ranlov and Nielsen 1987). Zopiclone has been studied in patients with upper airway resistance syndrome and has no adverse effects on sleep architecture, respiratory parameters during sleep, and daytime sleepiness (Lofaso et al. 1997). Ramelteon, a melatonin agonist, is a recently introduced hypnotic that reduces sleep latency. Ramelteon has been shown in controlled clinical trials to be safe in patients with mild to moderate COPD (Kryger et al. 2008) and moderate to severe COPD (Kryger et al. 2009) without effect on arterial oxygen saturation. Further study is needed to better define the risk–benefit ratio of hypnotics in patients with COPD.

Buspirone is potentially a safer anxiolytic in pulmonary patients because it does not depress respiration in patients with COPD (Argyropoulou et al. 1993). It also does not adversely affect sleep apnea (Mendelson et al. 1991). In the one open-label study of buspirone in subjects with severe lung disease, none of the subjects showed deterioration in respiratory function or increased carbon dioxide retention (Craven and Sutherland 1991). In patients with COPD, a double-blind study demonstrated no adverse effects on respiratory measures but also failed to show clinical benefit (Singh et al. 1993). Although buspirone does not adversely affect pulmonary function, its limitations are its potency and delayed therapeutic effect (Robinson and Levenson 2000).

Antipsychotics

Antipsychotics may be helpful in pulmonary patients who are incapacitated by extreme panic and dyspnea that mutually exacerbate each other. Most typical and atypical antipsychotics can be used in patients with chronic respiratory disease. Uncommon but serious concerns include the provocation of laryngeal dystonia and development of tardive dyskinesia affecting respiratory musculature. Low-potency typical antipsychotics may have some additional bronchodilatory effects because of their anticholinergic properties. Clozapine has been associated with respiratory arrest and depression as well as allergic asthma (Lieberman and Safferman 1992; Stoppe et al. 1992).

Cholinesterase Inhibitors and Memantine

Because acetylcholine is a potent mediator of bronchoconstriction, cholinesterase inhibitors should be used with caution in patients with a history of asthma or obstructive pulmonary disease. Memantine has no effect on respiration and can be used safely in patients with COPD.

Cancer

For additional discussion of use of medications in patients with cancer, see Chapter 23, "Oncology."

Antidepressants

Serotonin-enhancing antidepressants elevate prolactin levels, and hyperprolactinemia has been associated with increased risk of postmenopausal breast cancer. However, several recent large population-based case–control surveys reported no association between the risk of breast cancer and the use of antidepressants overall, or by antidepressant class or individual agent (Chien et al. 2006; Coogan et al. 2005; Fulton-Kehoe et al. 2006). Similar methodologies identified no evidence of increased risk of ovarian cancer with antidepressants in general or for SSRIs (Moorman et al. 2005). SSRI use did not increase the risk of prostate cancer (Tamim et al. 2008) and was related to a decreased risk of lung (Toh et al. 2007) and colorectal cancer (Xu et al. 2006).

Antipsychotics

Both increased and decreased rates of cancer in patients taking (mostly typical) antipsychotics have been reported in a number of epidemiological studies (Dalton et al. 2006; Hippisley-Cox et al. 2007; Mortensen 1987). No findings have been clearly replicated. Risperidone, and possibly its major metabolite paliperidone, may be associated with pituitary tumors according to a retrospective pharmacovigilance review of the U.S. FDA Adverse Event Reporting System database (Szarfman et al. 2006). Studies to date do not support withholding antipsychotics based on fear of increasing cancer risk. It would seem prudent to avoid risperidone and paliperidone in patients with present or past history of pituitary endocrine tumors.

Anxiolytics and Mood Stabilizers/Anticonvulsants

Benzodiazepines, and the mood stabilizers lithium, valproate, and lamotrigine are not associated with increased cancer risk. Carbamazepine carcinogenicity has not been studied in humans.

HIV/AIDS

See Chapter 28, "HIV/AIDS," and reviews by Repetto and Petitto (2008) and Robinson and Qaqish (2002) for further discussion of the use of psychotropics in patients with HIV/AIDS.

Psychotropic Drug Use During Pregnancy and Breast-Feeding

For additional discussion of the issues regarding medication use by pregnant or breast-feeding women, including consideration of the risks of withholding medication, see Chapter 33, "Obstetrics and Gynecology." Current information on drug use in pregnancy and breast-feeding is available through the Motherisk program (www.motherisk.org). Patient information handouts on medication use during pregnancy and breast-feeding can be obtained from the Organization of Teratology Information Specialists (www.otispregnacy.org).

Pregnancy

Fetal exposure to medications is common, especially during the first trimester. Because approximately 50%–65% of all pregnancies in the United States are unplanned (Koren et al. 1998; Rosenfeld and Everett 1996), the fetus may be exposed to a variety of drugs during the first trimester before the mother is aware of her pregnancy. Even during an established pregnancy, surveys estimate that 80% of women take prescription medications and 21%–33% are exposed to psychotropic drugs (Barki et al. 1998; Doering and Stewart 1978). For any woman of childbearing age, all drugs should be considered for their safety in pregnancy and breast-feeding. Risks for teratogenicity have been identified for lithium, carbamazepine, valproate, phenytoin, benzodiazepines, and paroxetine.

Fetal risks associated with drug use during pregnancy include teratogenicity, direct toxicity, perinatal effects, and possible long-term effects on behavior and development. Known and possible risks of pharmacotherapy, however, must be balanced against the risks to the fetus from withholding therapy. Exacerbation of the mother's psychiatric illness may endanger the fetus in utero through maternal self-harm, suicide, malnutrition, lack of proper prenatal care, or excessive exposure to risks through impulsivity, delusions, disorientation, or denial of the pregnancy. Treatments for psychotic and bipolar disorders in severely ill patients should not be discontinued during pregnancy because of the fetal risks associated with the high incidence of relapse (Viguera et al. 2007).

Physiological changes associated with pregnancy alter drug pharmacokinetics and complicate therapy. In general, drug levels decline during pregnancy because of increases in renal elimination, volume of distribution, and cardiac output (R.M. Ward 1995, 1996). Over the course of the pregnancy, lithium clearance doubles (Schou et al. 1973) and TCA elimination increases 1.6 times (Wisner et al. 1993).

Drug levels should be monitored during the pregnancy, and dosage should be adjusted to maintain a therapeutic response consistent with the lowest effective dose. However, with the decline in albumin levels during pregnancy, therapeutic drug monitoring results may be misleading unless methods selective for unbound drug are used (see discussion in the "Distribution" subsection under "Pharmacokinetics in the Medically Ill" at the beginning of this chapter). During the early postpartum period, these physiological changes reverse. As maternal drug elimination returns to normal, any dosage adjustment required during pregnancy should be gradually reversed.

At parturition, the delivery of maternal drug to the neonate is discontinued and neonatal withdrawal symptoms may appear. Neonatal benzodiazepine withdrawal symptoms include irritability, tremor, diarrhea, vomiting, hypertonicity, and high-pitched crying (Rementeria and Bhatt 1977). Symptoms of TCA withdrawal in neonates include irritability, abdominal cramps, insomnia, tachycardia, tachypnea, and cyanosis. SSRIs have also been associated with a neonatal withdrawal syndrome (irritability, constant crying, shivering, increased tonus, eating and sleeping difficulties, and convulsions) (Klinger and Merlob 2008). When possible, tapering and discontinuation of benzodiazepines and TCAs over a few weeks before delivery has been recommended to prevent neonatal withdrawal (L.J. Miller 1991, 1994), but this must be balanced against the risk of postpartum depression. Discontinued medications should be reinstated postpartum.

Neonates exposed to SSRIs and SNRIs late in the third trimester have developed complications requiring prolonged hospitalization, respiratory support, and tube feeding. Such complications can arise immediately upon delivery. Reported clinical findings have included respiratory distress, cyanosis, apnea, seizures, temperature instability, feeding difficulty, vomiting, hypoglycemia, hypotonia, hyperreflexia, tremor, jitteriness, irritability, and constant crying (Nordeng et al. 2001). These features are consistent with either a direct toxic effect of SSRIs and SNRIs or possibly a drug discontinuation syndrome. Before making the decision to treat a pregnant woman with an antidepressant during the third trimester, the physician should carefully consider the potential risks and benefits of treatment.

Breast-Feeding

During the postpartum period, women are at risk for the development of depression, mania, or psychosis. More than 60% of mothers breast-feed their infants (Llewellyn and Stowe 1998), and many will wish to do so while taking psychotropic medications. If informed that a medication is incompatible with breast-feeding, a mother may covertly breast-feed and discontinue her medication. Recurrence of the psychiatric disorder not only is dangerous for the mother but may place the infant at greater risk than that posed by breast-feeding while the mother is taking medication.

Unfortunately, case reports are the only source of information on adverse psychotropic effects during breast-feeding; there are no clinical trials of drug effects in breast-fed infants. With a few exceptions, psychotropic drugs seem to be relatively safe in breast-feeding (Menon 2008; Rubin et al. 2004).

Risks of Psychotropic Drug Use During Pregnancy and Breast-Feeding

The use of medications during pregnancy and breast-feeding, including the risks, benefits, and treatment alternatives, must be discussed with the patient. Failure to fully inform may result in the patient discontinuing treatment because of excessive fear of risk to the fetus or neonate.

Increasing evidence suggests that most psychotropic medications are safe in pregnancy and breast-feeding. However, there are concerns about the anticonvulsant mood stabilizers, lithium, low-potency antipsychotics, paroxetine, and benzodiazepines. Concerns about psychotropic drug use in pregnancy and breast-feeding are listed below (American Academy of Pediatrics Committee on Drugs 2000; C.L. Ernst and Goldberg 2002; Gentile 2008; Gjere 2001; Jain and Lacy 2005; Menon 2008; Rubin et al. 2004; R.K. Ward and Zamorski 2002).

Antipsychotics

Pregnancy. *Typical agents*—Not associated with any evidence of teratogenic, behavioral, emotional, or cognitive abnormalities.

Low-potency drugs—Can cause neonatal tachycardia, gastrointestinal dysfunction, sedation, and hypotension for a few days after birth. Best avoided so as to minimize anticholinergic, hypotensive, and antihistaminic effects.

High-potency drugs—Preferred despite the risk of fetal EPS. Incidence of fetal EPS (hyperactivity, hyperreflexia, abnormal movements, tremor, hand flapping, and crying that may persist for several months) is dose related.

Atypical agents—Limited evidence from cohort studies suggests no evidence of increased risk of malformations for olanzapine, risperidone, and quetiapine (McKenna et al. 2005). Antipsychotic use increases the risk of gestational diabetes (Reis and Kallen 2008).

Depot preparations—Avoid because of long duration of action.

Breast-feeding. Compatibility of antipsychotics with breast-feeding is unknown. Clozapine may be of concern because of possible agranulocytosis, sedation, and seizures (Iqbal et al. 2001). Sedating drugs such as chlorpromazine may produce drowsiness and lethargy in the infant. Monitor the neonate for antipsychotic side effects such as sedation, muscle rigidity, or tremor (Gentile 2008).

Antidepressants

Pregnancy. *TCAs*—Not associated with evidence of teratogenic effects. Avoid maprotiline because of increased maternal seizure risk. Neonatal TCA withdrawal symptoms include seizures, irritability, abdominal cramps, insomnia, tachycardia, tachypnea, and cyanosis. Desipramine is the recommended TCA because of low anticholinergic effects.

SSRIs/SNRIs—Paroxetine has been associated with a risk of cardiovascular birth defects by the FDA and Health Canada (U.S. Food and Drug Administration 2005), although this has been disputed (Einarson et al. 2008). Fluoxetine is not associated with teratogenic effects. Other SSRIs/SNRIs do not appear to be teratogenic from limited human data. Infants exposed to SSRIs in late pregnancy may have an increased risk for persistent pulmonary hypertension (Chambers et al. 2006).

Bupropion—Early reports from the GlaxoSmithKline bupropion pregnancy registry suggested an increase in cardiovascular malformations in infants exposed to bupropion during the first trimester. More recent analysis of data from this registry do not support a teratogenic effect for first-trimester exposure to bupropion (Cole et al. 2007).

MAOIs—Avoid because of hypotensive effects and potential for drug and food interactions.

Breast-feeding. Compatibility with breast-feeding is unknown. Sedating drugs such as doxepin, fluoxetine, and trazodone may cause neonatal lethargy. Limited case reports suggest that SSRIs are relatively safe. Data for SNRIs, mirtazapine and bupropion are too limited for recommendations.

Antiparkinsonian Agents

Pregnancy. *Anticholinergics*—Not recommended for the treatment of EPS during pregnancy. Associated with increased risk of congenital anomalies, complications of pregnancy, and neonatal adverse effects (Gjere 2001). Akathisia can be treated during pregnancy with propranolol or atenolol.

Breast-feeding. Anticholinergic drugs and amantadine are not classified.

Mood Stabilizers/Anticonvulsants

Pregnancy. *Lithium*—Teratogenic potential is less than earlier thought. First-trimester exposure associated with a 10-fold increase in Ebstein's anomaly, a rare (1 in 20,000) cardiovascular malformation. Cardiac ultrasonography at 16–18 weeks, neonatal electrocardiogram, and monitoring the infant for the first 10 days for lithium toxicity are recommended. Regular monitoring of serum lithium levels is required during pregnancy (every 4 weeks early in pregnancy; weekly in the latter half) (Jain and Lacy 2005; Menon 2008).

Carbamazepine and valproate—Associated with neural tube defects—carbamazepine (~1%) and valproate (~1% to

2%)—and fetal hydantoin syndrome (facial dysmorphism, cleft lip and palate, cardiac defects and digit hypoplasia). Valproate is relatively contraindicated during pregnancy. Screening for neural tube defects (amniocentesis and serum alpha-fetoprotein) before week 20 is advised. To minimize risk, all women of childbearing age should consume 0.4 mg folate daily. Women taking valproate or carbamazepine should supplement with 4 mg folate daily when planning to start pregnancy. Carbamazepine and valproate may cause transient vitamin K deficiency, resulting in neonatal clotting disorders. This risk can be minimized by supplementing with 20 mg oral vitamin K daily from week 36 to delivery, plus 1 mg intramuscularly to the newborn (Jain and Lacy 2005; Menon 2008).

Gabapentin, lamotrigine, topiramate—Insufficient human data for recommendation. There is evidence of fetal toxicity (gabapentin) and teratogenicity (topiramate) in animal studies. Lamotrigine decreases folate in rats; consider folate supplementation (see previous item).

Breast-feeding. Carbamazepine and valproate are compatible with breast-feeding; monitor for possible neonatal thrombocytopenia and hepatotoxicity. Avoid breast-feeding if patient is taking lithium. High levels of lithium are present in breast milk, and therapeutic serum levels are found in breast-fed infants (Chaudron and Jefferson 2000), with reports of neonatal electrocardiographic changes and hypotonia (C.L. Ernst and Goldberg 2002). Gabapentin is excreted into breast milk at near 100% of maternal levels; avoid breast-feeding if possible. For lamotrigine and topiramate, compatibility with breast-feeding is unknown. Lamotrigine may be of concern.

Anxiolytics and Sedative-Hypnotics

Pregnancy. *Benzodiazepines*—May be associated with a twofold increase in orofacial clefts. Neonatal benzodiazepine withdrawal (irritability, tremor, diarrhea, vomiting, hypertonicity, and high-pitched crying) may occur. "Floppy infant syndrome" is characterized by lethargy, hypothermia, respiratory depression, and feeding difficulties.

Other anxiolytics/sedatives—Insufficient data for recommendation.

Breast-feeding. Compatibility with breast-feeding is unknown. Sedating drugs may cause neonatal lethargy. Short half-life agents with no active metabolites (e.g., oxazepam or lorazepam) may be preferred. Buspirone, zaleplon, zopiclone, and eszopiclone achieve high concentrations in breast milk and are contraindicated in breast-feeding. Zolpidem is hydrophilic and compatible with breast-feeding.

General Guidelines for Psychotropic Drug Use in Pregnancy and Breast-Feeding

General guidelines for psychotropic drug use in pregnancy and breast-feeding (adapted from Fait et al. 2002; Newport et al. 2002; R.K. Ward and Zamorski 2002) include the following:

1. For any woman of childbearing age, carefully select all drugs for their safety in pregnancy and breast-feeding.
2. Remember that the benefit of any medication to the mother must outweigh the risk to the fetus.
3. Discuss with the mother the risks and benefits of using psychotropic medications while pregnant or breast-feeding.
4. Avoid all drugs during pregnancy and breast-feeding if possible, including over-the-counter and herbal medicines.
5. Use the lowest effective dose.
6. Prefer monotherapy to combination therapy.
7. Select established drugs with known effects in pregnancy and breast-feeding rather than agents with little supporting data.
8. Select medications for minimum teratogenic and behavioral toxicity.
9. Monitor clinical response and drug levels where possible during pregnancy. Adjust dosage as necessary to maintain therapeutic effect. At delivery, slowly return drug dose to prepregnancy levels.
10. Minimize drug exposure for the nursing infant by instructing the mother to take medication just after breast-feeding or before the infant is due for a long sleep (American Academy of Pediatrics 2001). SSRI levels peak in breast milk at 8–9 hours postdose. Infant exposure can be minimized if the milk during this period is "pumped and dumped" (Newport et al. 2002).
11. Consider electroconvulsive therapy for treatment of depression and especially for psychotic depression.

Conclusion

Rapid developments in medical care in general, and psychopharmacology in particular, challenge clinicians to remain current with new agents, new indications for established agents, and potential pharmacokinetic and pharmacodynamic interactions in a polypharmacy environment, which also includes over-the-counter and herbal preparations. In this chapter the many key considerations relevant to the use of psychopharmacological agents in complex medically ill patients and during pregnancy and lactation have been discussed. Detailed adverse effects, toxicities, drug interactions, and alternate administration routes for each major psychotherapeutic drug class have been described. Where possible, the use of Internet resources provides access to the most up-to-date information. Many of these Internet sources are cited in the References below, and their general use as a means of following developments in this area is encouraged.

References

Aarsland D, Laake K, Larsen JP, et al: Donepezil for cognitive impairment in Parkinson's disease: a randomised controlled study. J Neurol Neurosurg Psychiatry 72:708–712, 2002

Adan-Manes J, Novalbos J, Lopez-Rodriguez R, et al: Lithium and venlafaxine interaction: a case of serotonin syndrome. J Clin Pharm Ther 31:397–400, 2006

Adityanjee, Sajatovic M, Munshi KR: Neuropsychiatric sequelae of neuroleptic malignant syndrome. Clin Neuropharmacol 28:197–204, 2005

Adler LA, Spencer T, Brown TE, et al: Once-daily atomoxetine for adult attention-deficit/hyperactivity disorder: a 6-month, double-blind trial. J Clin Psychopharmacol 29:44–50, 2009

Allain H, Delahaye C, Le Coz F, et al: Postmarketing surveillance of zopiclone in insomnia: analysis of 20,513 cases. Sleep 14:408–413, 1991

Allan SJ, Kavanagh GM, Herd RM, et al: The effect of inositol supplements on the psoriasis of patients taking lithium: a randomized, placebo-controlled trial. Br J Dermatol 150:966–969, 2004

Alldredge BK: Seizure risk associated with psychotropic drugs: clinical and pharmacokinetic considerations. Neurology 53:S68–S75, 1999

Alldredge BK, Gelb AM, Isaacs SM, et al: A comparison of lorazepam, diazepam, and placebo for the treatment of out-of-hospital status epilepticus. N Engl J Med 345:631–637, 2001

Alper K, Schwartz KA, Kolts RL, et al: Seizure incidence in psychopharmacological clinical trials: an analysis of Food and Drug Administration (FDA) summary basis of approval reports. Biol Psychiatry 62:345–354, 2007

Alvarez W Jr, Pickworth KK: Safety of antidepressant drugs in the patient with cardiac disease: a review of the literature. Pharmacotherapy 23:754–771, 2003

American Academy of Pediatrics: Transfer of drugs and other chemicals into human milk. Pediatrics 108:776–789, 2001

American Academy of Pediatrics Committee on Drugs: Use of psychoactive medication during pregnancy and possible effects on the fetus and newborn. Committee on Drugs. American Academy of Pediatrics. Pediatrics 105:880–887, 2000

American Diabetes Association, American Psychiatric Association, American Association of Clinical Endocrinologists: Consensus development conference on antipsychotic drugs and obesity and diabetes. Diabetes Care 27:596–601, 2004

Amsterdam JD, Bodkin JA: Selegiline transdermal system in the prevention of relapse of major depressive disorder: a 52-week, double-blind, placebo-substitution, parallel-group clinical trial. J Clin Psychopharmacol 26:579–586, 2006

Andreoli V, Caillard V, Deo RS, et al: Reboxetine, a new noradrenaline selective antidepressant, is at least as effective as fluoxetine in the treatment of depression. J Clin Psychopharmacol 22:393–399, 2002

Ang-Lee MK, Moss J, Yuan C-S: Herbal medicines and perioperative care. JAMA 286:208–216, 2001

Appleton R, Sweeney A, Choonara I, et al: Lorazepam versus diazepam in the acute treatment of epileptic seizures and status epilepticus. Dev Med Child Neurol 37:682–688, 1995

Arbouw ME, Movig KL, Neef C, et al: Influence of initial use of serotonergic antidepressants on antiparkinsonian drug use in levodopa-using patients. Eur J Clin Pharmacol 63:181–187, 2007

Argyropoulou P, Patakas D, Koukou A, et al: Buspirone effect on breathlessness and exercise performance in patients with chronic obstructive pulmonary disease. Respiration 60:216–220, 1993

Arif H, Buchsbaum R, Weintraub D, et al: Patient-reported cognitive side effects of antiepileptic drugs: predictors and comparison of all commonly used antiepileptic drugs. Epilepsy Behav 14:202–209, 2009

Armstrong SC, Cozza KL: Triptans. Psychosomatics 43:502–504, 2002

Balayssac D, Authier N, Cayre A, et al: Does inhibition of P-glycoprotein lead to drug-drug interactions? Toxicol Lett 156:319–329, 2005

Barki ZHK, Kravitz HM, Berki TM: Psychotropic medications in pregnancy. Psychiatric Annals 28:486–500, 1998

Barnes PM, Powell-Griner E, McFann K, et al: Complementary and alternative medicine use among adults: United States, 2002. Adv Data (343):1–19, 2004. Available at: http://nccam.nih.gov/news/camstats/2002/report.pdf. Accessed May 14, 2010.

Baruah J, Easby J, Kessell G: Effects of acetylcholinesterase inhibitor therapy for Alzheimer's disease on neuromuscular block. Br J Anaesth 100:420, 2008

Bauer MS, Whybrow PC: Rapid cycling bipolar affective disorder, II: treatment of refractory rapid cycling with high-dose levothyroxine: a preliminary study. Arch Gen Psychiatry 47:435–440, 1990

Ben-Menachem E: Weight issues for people with epilepsy—a review. Epilepsia 48 (suppl 9):42–45, 2007

Bendz H, Aurell M: Drug-induced diabetes insipidus: incidence, prevention and management. Drug Saf 21:449–456, 1999

Bendz H, Sjodin I, Aurell M: Renal function on and off lithium in patients treated with lithium for 15 years or more. A controlled, prospective lithium-withdrawal study. Nephrol Dial Transplant 11:457–460, 1996

Bent S: Herbal medicine in the United States: review of efficacy, safety, and regulation: grand rounds at University of California, San Francisco Medical Center. J Gen Intern Med 23:854–859, 2008

Bent S, Ko R: Commonly used herbal medicines in the United States: a review. Am J Med 116:478–485, 2004

Berk M, Berk L: Mood stabilizers and treatment adherence in bipolar disorder: addressing adverse events. Ann Clin Psychiatry 15:217–224, 2003

Bezchlibnyk-Butler KZ, Jeffries JJ, Virani A: Clinical Handbook of Psychotropic Drugs, 17th Revised Edition. Ashland, OH: Hogrefe & Huber, 2007

Bhasin M, Rowan E, Edwards K, et al: Cholinesterase inhibitors in dementia with Lewy bodies: a comparative analysis. Int J Geriatr Psychiatry 22:890–895, 2007

Bianchi M, Musch B: Zopiclone discontinuation: review of 25 studies assessing withdrawal and rebound phenomena. Int Clin Psychopharmacol 5 (suppl 2):139–145, 1990

Bierman EJ, Comijs HC, Gundy CM, et al: The effect of chronic benzodiazepine use on cognitive functioning in older persons: good, bad or indifferent? Int J Geriatr Psychiatry 22:1194–1200, 2007

Bilo L, Meo R: Polycystic ovary syndrome in women using valproate: a review. Gynecol Endocrinol 24:562–570, 2008

Birnbaum AK, Kriel RL, Im Y, et al: Relative bioavailability of lamotrigine chewable dispersible tablets administered rectally. Pharmacotherapy 21:158–162, 2001

Biton V, Mirza W, Montouris G, et al: Weight change associated with valproate and lamotrigine monotherapy in patients with epilepsy. Neurology 56:172–177, 2001

Bjorkman S, Rigemar G, Idvall J: Pharmacokinetics of midazolam given as an intranasal spray to adult surgical patients. Br J Anaesth 79:575–580, 1997

Bjornsson E: Hepatotoxicity associated with antiepileptic drugs. Acta Neurol Scand 118:281–290, 2008

Black JE, Hirshkowitz M: Modafinil for treatment of residual excessive sleepiness in nasal continuous positive airway pressure-treated obstructive sleep apnea/hypopnea syndrome. Sleep 28:464–471, 2005

Bocchetta A, Cocco F, Velluzzi F, et al: Fifteen-year follow-up of thyroid function in lithium patients. J Endocrinol Invest 30:363–366, 2007

Boehnert MT, Lovejoy FH Jr: Value of the QRS duration versus the serum drug level in predicting seizures and ventricular arrhythmias after an acute overdose of tricyclic antidepressants. N Engl J Med 313:474–479, 1985

Boniface PJ, Russell SG: Two cases of fatal zopiclone overdose. J Anal Toxicol 20:131–133, 1996

Bottomley DM, Hanks GW: Subcutaneous midazolam infusion in palliative care. J Pain Symptom Manage 5:259–261, 1990

Boyer EW, Shannon M: The serotonin syndrome. N Engl J Med 352:1112–1120, 2005

Bramness JG, Arnestad M, Karinen R, et al: Fatal overdose of zopiclone in an elderly woman with bronchogenic carcinoma. J Forensic Sci 46:1247–1249, 2001

Brazier NC, Levine MA: Drug-herb interaction among commonly used conventional medicines: a compendium for health care professionals. Am J Ther 10:163–169, 2003

Bristol-Myers Squibb: Abilify (aripiprazole) home page. 2010. Available at: http://www.abilify.com. Accessed May 14, 2010.

Bronheim HE, Fulop G, Kunkel EJ, et al: The Academy of Psychosomatic Medicine practice guidelines for psychiatric consultation in the general medical setting. The Academy of Psychosomatic Medicine. Psychosomatics 39:S8–S30, 1998

Burggraf GW: Are psychotropic drugs at therapeutic levels a concern for cardiologists? Can J Cardiol 13:75–80, 1997

Burn D, Emre M, McKeith I, et al: Effects of rivastigmine in patients with and without visual hallucinations in dementia associated with Parkinson's disease. Mov Disord 21:1899–1907, 2006

Bush A, Burgess C: Fatal cardiomyopathy due to quetiapine. N Z Med J 121:U2909, 2008

Cadwallader DE: Biopharmaceutics and Drug Interactions. New York, Raven, 1983

Cancelli I, Beltrame M, Gigli GL, et al: Drugs with anticholinergic properties: cognitive and neuropsychiatric side-effects in elderly patients. Neurol Sci 30:87–92, 2009

Cardiac Arrhythmia Suppression Trial (CAST) Investigators: Preliminary report: effect of encainide and flecainide on mortality in a randomized trial of arrhythmia suppression after myocardial infarction. N Engl J Med 321:406–412, 1989

Caroff SN, Mann SC: Neuroleptic malignant syndrome. Med Clin North Am 77:185–202, 1993

Carroll DH, Shyam R, Scahill L: Cardiac conduction and antipsychotic medication: a primer on electrocardiograms. J Child Adolesc Psychiatr Nurs 15:170–177, 2002

Carvajal Garcia-Pando A, Garcia dP, Sanchez AS, et al: Hepatotoxicity associated with the new antidepressants. J Clin Psychiatry 63:135–137, 2002

Cephalon: Nuvigil (armodafinil) home page. 2010. Available at: http://www.nuvigil.com. Accessed May 14, 2010.

Chambers CD, Hernandez-Diaz S, Van Marter LJ, et al: Selective serotonin-reuptake inhibitors and risk of persistent pulmonary hypertension of the newborn. N Engl J Med 354:579–587, 2006

Chan HH, Wing Y, Su R, et al: A control study of the cutaneous side effects of chronic lithium therapy. J Affect Disord 57:107–113, 2000

Chandler F (ed): Herbs: Everyday Reference for Health Professionals. Ottawa, ON, Canadian Pharmacist Association and Canadian Medical Association, 2000

Chaudron LH, Jefferson JW: Mood stabilizers during breastfeeding: a review. J Clin Psychiatry 61:79–90, 2000

Chen Y, Patel NC, Guo JJ, et al: Antidepressant prophylaxis for poststroke depression: a meta-analysis. Int Clin Psychopharmacol 22:159–166, 2007

Chengappa KN, Chalasani L, Brar JS, et al: Changes in body weight and body mass index among psychiatric patients receiving lithium, valproate, or topiramate: an open-label, nonrandomized chart review. Clin Ther 24:1576–1584, 2002

Chew ML, Mulsant BH, Pollock BG, et al: Anticholinergic activity of 107 medications commonly used by older adults. J Am Geriatr Soc 56:1333–1341, 2008

Chien C, Li CI, Heckbert SR, et al: Antidepressant use and breast cancer risk. Breast Cancer Res Treat 95:131–140, 2006

Chong SA, Mythily S, Mahendran R: Cardiac effects of psychotropic drugs. Ann Acad Med Singapore 30:625–631, 2001

Chou R, Carson S, Chan BK: Gabapentin versus tricyclic antidepressants for diabetic neuropathy and post-herpetic neuralgia: discrepancies between direct and indirect meta-analyses of randomized controlled trials. J Gen Intern Med 24:178–188, 2009

Cirignotta F, Mondini S, Zucconi M, et al: Zolpidem-polysomnographic study of the effect of a new hypnotic drug in sleep apnea syndrome. Pharmacol Biochem Behav 29:807–809, 1988

Citrome L: Iloperidone for schizophrenia: a review of the efficacy and safety profile for this newly commercialised second-generation antipsychotic. Int J Clin Pract 63:1237–1248, 2009

Clarke RS, Lyons SM: Diazepam and flunitrazepam as induction agents for cardiac surgical operations. Acta Anaesthesiol Scand 21:282–292, 1977

Clemens PL, Cloyd JC, Kriel RL, et al: Relative bioavailability, metabolism and tolerability of rectally administered oxcarbazepine suspension. Clin Drug Investig 27:243–250, 2007

Cohen LG, Prince J, Biederman J, et al: Absence of effect of stimulants on the phamacokinetics of desipramine in children. Pharmacotherapy 19:746–752, 1999

Cohen LM, Tessier EG, Germain MJ, et al: Update on psychotropic medication use in renal disease. Psychosomatics 45:34–48, 2004

Cohn MA: Hypnotics and the control of breathing: a review. Br J Clin Pharmacol 16 (suppl 2):245S–250S, 1983

Cole JA, Modell JG, Haight BR, et al: Bupropion in pregnancy and the prevalence of congenital malformations. Pharmacoepidemiol Drug Saf 16:474–484, 2007

Collaborative Working Group on Clinical Trial Evaluations: Assessment of EPS and tardive dyskinesia in clinical trials. J Clin Psychiatry 59 (suppl 12):23–27, 1998

Conway JM, Birnbaum AK, Kriel RL, et al: Relative bioavailability of topiramate administered rectally. Epilepsy Res 54:91–96, 2003

Coogan PF, Palmer JR, Strom BL, et al: Use of selective serotonin reuptake inhibitors and the risk of breast cancer. Am J Epidemiol 162:835–838, 2005

Corman CL, Leung NM, Guberman AH: Weight gain in epileptic patients during treatment with valproic acid: a retrospective study. Can J Neurol Sci 24:240–244, 1997

Coulter DM, Bate A, Meyboom RH, et al: Antipsychotic drugs and heart muscle disorder in international pharmacovigilance: data mining study. BMJ 322:1207–1209, 2001

Cowles BJ: Lisdexamfetamine for treatment of attention-deficit/hyperactivity disorder. Ann Pharmacother 43:669–676, 2009

Cozza K, Armstrong S, Oesterheld J: Concise Guide to the Cytochrome P450 System: Drug Interaction Principles for Medical Practice. Washington, DC, American Psychiatric Publishing, 2003

Craven J, Sutherland A: Buspirone for anxiety disorders in patients with severe lung disease. Lancet 338:249, 1991

Crawford P: An audit of topiramate use in a general neurology clinic. Seizure 7:207–211, 1998

Crone C, Wise T: Use of herbal medicines among consultation-liaison populations. Psychosomatics 39:3–13, 1998

Crone CC, Gabriel GM, DiMartini A: An overview of psychiatric issues in liver disease for the consultation-liaison psychiatrist. Psychosomatics 47:188–205, 2006

Crowe S, Collins L: Suxamethonium and donepezil: a cause of prolonged paralysis. Anesthesiology 98:574–575, 2003

Currier GW, Medori R: Orally versus intramuscularly administered antipsychotic drugs in psychiatric emergencies. J Psychiatr Pract 12:30–40, 2006

Cypress Bioscience: Savella (milnacipran) home page. 2010. Available at: http://www.savella.com. Accessed May 14, 2010.

Dalton SO, Johansen C, Mellemkjaer L, et al: Use of selective serotonin reuptake inhibitors and risk of upper gastrointestinal tract bleeding: a population-based cohort study. Arch Intern Med 163:59–64, 2003

Dalton SO, Johansen C, Poulsen AH, et al: Cancer risk among users of neuroleptic medication: a population-based cohort study. Br J Cancer 95:934–939, 2006

Dannawi M: Possible serotonin syndrome after combination of buspirone and St John's wort. J Psychopharmacol 16:401, 2002

Darwish M, Kirby M, Robertson P Jr, et al: Interaction profile of armodafinil with medications metabolized by cytochrome P450 enzymes 1A2, 3A4 and 2C19 in healthy subjects. Clin Pharmacokinet 47:61–74, 2008

Dasgupta A: Usefulness of monitoring free (unbound) concentrations of therapeutic drugs in patient management. Clin Chim Acta 377:1–13, 2007

Dasgupta K, Jefferson JW: The use of lithium in the medically ill. Gen Hosp Psychiatry 12:83–97, 1990

De Smet PA: Herbal remedies. N Engl J Med 347:2046–2056, 2002

Dequardo JR: Modafinil-associated clozapine toxicity. Am J Psychiatry 159:1243–1244, 2002

Detke MJ, Lu Y, Goldstein DJ, et al: Duloxetine 60 mg once daily dosing versus placebo in the acute treatment of major depression. J Psychiatr Res 36:383–390, 2002a

Detke M, Lu Y, Goldstein DJ, et al: Duloxetine, 60 mg once daily, for major depressive disorder: a randomized double-blind placebo-controlled trial. J Clin Psychiatry 63:308–315, 2002b

DeVane CL, Nemeroff CB: 2002 Guide to psychotropic drug interactions. Primary Psychiatry 9:28–57, 2002

Devinsky O, Honigfeld G, Patin J: Clozapine-related seizures. Neurology 41:369–371, 1991

Devos D, Dujardin K, Poirot I, et al: Comparison of desipramine and citalopram treatments for depression in Parkinson's disease: a double-blind, randomized, placebo-controlled study. Mov Disord 23:850–857, 2008

Dhir R, Brown DK, Olden KW: Drug-induced pancreatitis: a practical review. Drugs Today (Barc) 43:499–507, 2007

Dilsaver SC, Greden JF: Antidepressant withdrawal phenomena. Biol Psychiatry 19:237–256, 1984

Dodick DW, Martin V: Triptans and CNS side-effects: pharmacokinetic and metabolic mechanisms. Cephalalgia 24:417–424, 2004

Doering PL, Stewart RB: The extent and character of drug consumption during pregnancy. JAMA 239:843–846, 1978

Dolder CR, Nelson MH: Hypnosedative-induced complex behaviours: incidence, mechanisms and management. CNS Drugs 22:1021–1036, 2008

Dolly FR, Block AJ: Effect of flurazepam on sleep-disordered breathing and nocturnal oxygen desaturation in asymptomatic subjects. Am J Med 73:239–243, 1982

Dong X, Leppik IE, White J, et al: Hyponatremia from oxcarbazepine and carbamazepine. Neurology 65:1976–1978, 2005

Douglas IJ, Smeeth L: Exposure to antipsychotics and risk of stroke: self controlled case series study. BMJ 337:a1227, 2008

Drici MD, Priori S: Cardiovascular risks of atypical antipsychotic drug treatment. Pharmacoepidemiol Drug Saf 16:882–890, 2007

Duncan MA, Savage J, Tucker AP: Prospective audit comparing intrathecal analgesia (incorporating midazolam) with epidural and intravenous analgesia after major open abdominal surgery. Anaesth Intensive Care 35:558–562, 2007

Dunkley EJ, Isbister GK, Sibbritt D, et al: The Hunter Serotonin Toxicity Criteria: simple and accurate diagnostic decision rules for serotonin toxicity. QJM 96:635–642, 2003

Dunner DL: Optimizing lithium treatment. J Clin Psychiatry 61 (suppl 9):76–81, 2000

Dunner DL: Drug interactions of lithium and other antimanic/mood-stabilizing medications. J Clin Psychiatry 64 (suppl 5):38–43, 2003

Dunner DL, Wilson M, Fava M, et al: Long-term tolerability and effectiveness of duloxetine in the treatment of major depressive disorder. Depress Anxiety 25:E1–E8, 2008

Edwards K, Royall D, Hershey L, et al: Efficacy and safety of galantamine in patients with dementia with Lewy bodies: a 24-week open-label study. Dement Geriatr Cogn Disord 23:401–405, 2007

Einarson A, Pistelli A, DeSantis M, et al: Evaluation of the risk of congenital cardiovascular defects associated with use of paroxetine during pregnancy. Am J Psychiatry 165:749–752, 2008

Eisenberg DM, Kessler RC, Van Rompay MI, et al: Perceptions about complementary therapies relative to conventional therapies among adults who use both: results from a national survey. Ann Intern Med 135:344–351, 2001

Eli Lilly: Strattera (atomoxetine) home page. 2010a. Available at: http://www.strattera.com. Accessed May 14, 2010.

Eli Lilly: Zyprexa (olanzapine) home page. 2010b. Available at: http://www.zyprexa.com. Accessed May 14, 2010.

Eli Lilly: Cymbalta (duloxetine) home page. 2010c. Available at: http://www.cymbalta.com. Accessed May 14, 2010.

Elie R, Ruther E, Farr I, et al: Sleep latency is shortened during 4 weeks of treatment with zaleplon, a novel nonbenzodiazepine hypnotic. Zaleplon Clinical Study Group. J Clin Psychiatry 60:536–544, 1999

Ernst CL, Goldberg JF: The reproductive safety profile of mood stabilizers, atypical antipsychotics, and broad-spectrum psychotropics. J Clin Psychiatry 63 (suppl 4):42–55, 2002

Ernst E: Complementary medicine. Curr Opin Rheumatol 15:151–155, 2003

Evins AE: Efficacy of newer anticonvulsant medications in bipolar spectrum mood disorders. J Clin Psychiatry 64 (suppl 8): 9–14, 2003

Fait ML, Wise MG, Jachna JS, et al: Psychopharmacology, in The American Psychiatric Publishing Textbook of Consultation-Liaison Psychiatry: Psychiatry in the Medically Ill, 2nd Edition. Edited by Wise MG, Rundell JR. Washington, DC, American Psychiatric Publishing, 2002, pp 939–987

Farlow MR, Graham SM, Alva G: Memantine for the treatment of Alzheimer's disease: tolerability and safety data from clinical trials. Drug Saf 31:577–585, 2008

Feiger AD, Rickels K, Rynn MA, et al: Selegiline transdermal system for the treatment of major depressive disorder: an 8-week, double-blind, placebo-controlled, flexible-dose titration trial. J Clin Psychiatry 67:1354–1361, 2006

Feighner JP: Cardiovascular safety in depressed patients: focus on venlafaxine. J Clin Psychiatry 56:574–579, 1995

Fergusson D, Doucette S, Glass KC, et al: Association between suicide attempts and selective serotonin reuptake inhibitors: systematic review of randomised controlled trials. BMJ 330:396, 2005

Findling RL, Bukstein OG, Melmed RD, et al: A randomized, double-blind, placebo-controlled, parallel-group study of methylphenidate transdermal system in pediatric patients with attention-deficit/hyperactivity disorder. J Clin Psychiatry 69:149–159, 2008

Finsterer J, Pelzl G, Hess B: Severe, isolated thrombocytopenia under polytherapy with carbamazepine and valproate. Psychiatry Clin Neurosci 55:423–426, 2001

Fisher RS, Bortz JJ, Blum DE, et al: A pilot study of donepezil for memory problems in epilepsy. Epilepsy Behav 2:330–334, 2001

Flanagan RJ, Dunk L: Haematological toxicity of drugs used in psychiatry. Hum Psychopharmacol 23 (suppl 1):27–41, 2008

Fleishaker JC, Francom SF, Herman BD, et al: Lack of effect of reboxetine on cardiac repolarization. Clin Pharmacol Ther 70:261–269, 2001

Flynn CT, Chandran PK, Taylor MJ, et al: Intraperitoneal lithium administration for bipolar affective disorder in a patient on continuous ambulatory peritoneal dialysis. Int J Artif Organs 10:105–107, 1987

Forest Pharmaceuticals Inc: Namenda (memantine) home page. 2010. Available at: http://www.namenda.com. Accessed May 14, 2010.

Forrester MB: Comparison of zolpidem and zaleplon exposures in Texas, 1998–2004. J Toxicol Environ Health A 69:1883–1892, 2006

Foulke GE, Albertson TE: QRS interval in tricyclic antidepressant overdosage: inaccuracy as a toxicity indicator in emergency settings. Ann Emerg Med 16:160–163, 1987

Freeman MP, Freeman SA: Lithium: clinical considerations in internal medicine. Am J Med 119:478–481, 2006

Freudenthaler S, Meineke I, Schreeb KH, et al: Influence of urine pH and urinary flow on the renal excretion of memantine. Br J Clin Pharmacol 46:541–546, 1998

Friedman JH, Feinberg SS, Feldman RG: A neuroleptic malignantlike syndrome due to levodopa therapy withdrawal. JAMA 254:2792–2795, 1985

Frieling H, Hillemacher T, Ziegenbein M, et al: Treating dopamimetic psychosis in Parkinson's disease: structured review and meta-analysis. Eur Neuropsychopharmacol 17:165–171, 2007

Fulton-Kehoe D, Rossing MA, Rutter C, et al: Use of antidepressant medications in relation to the incidence of breast cancer. Br J Cancer 94:1071–1078, 2006

Gallini A, Sommet A, Montastruc JL: Does memantine induce bradycardia? A study in the French PharmacoVigilance Database. Pharmacoepidemiol Drug Saf 17:877–881, 2008

Gao K, Kemp DE, Ganocy SJ, et al: Antipsychotic-induced extrapyramidal side effects in bipolar disorder and schizophrenia: a systematic review. J Clin Psychopharmacol 28:203–209, 2008

Gardiner P, Phillips R, Shaughnessy AF: Herbal and dietary supplement—drug interactions in patients with chronic illnesses. Am Fam Physician 77:73–78, 2008

Gardner DM, Lynd LD: Sumatriptan contraindications and the serotonin syndrome. Ann Pharmacother 32:33–38, 1998

Gardner DM, Shulman KI, Walker SE, et al: The making of a user friendly MAOI diet. J Clin Psychiatry 57:99–104, 1996

Garner SJ, Eldridge FL, Wagner PG, et al: Buspirone, an anxiolytic drug that stimulates respiration. Am Rev Respir Dis 139:946–950, 1989

Garnier R, Guerault E, Muzard D, et al: Acute zolpidem poisoning—analysis of 344 cases. J Toxicol Clin Toxicol 32:391–404, 1994

Gentile S: Infant safety with antipsychotic therapy in breast-feeding: a systematic review. J Clin Psychiatry 69:666–673, 2008

George CF: Perspectives on the management of insomnia in patients with chronic respiratory disorders. Sleep 23 (suppl 1): S31–S35, 2000

Gerstner T, Busing D, Bell N, et al: Valproic acid-induced pancreatitis: 16 new cases and a review of the literature. J Gastroenterol 42:39–48, 2007

Giardina EG, Johnson LL, Vita J, et al: Effect of imipramine and nortriptyline on left ventricular function and blood pressure in patients treated for arrhythmias. Am Heart J 109:992–998, 1985

Gibb WR: Neuroleptic malignant syndrome in striatonigral degeneration. Br J Psychiatry 153:254–255, 1988

Gibb WR, Griffith DN: Levodopa withdrawal syndrome identical to neuroleptic malignant syndrome. Postgrad Med J 62:59–60, 1986

Gibson AP, Bettinger TL, Patel NC, et al: Atomoxetine versus stimulants for treatment of attention deficit/hyperactivity disorder. Ann Pharmacother 40:1134–1142, 2006

Gillman PK: Monoamine oxidase inhibitors, opioid analgesics and serotonin toxicity. Br J Anaesth 95:434–441, 2005

Girault C, Muir JF, Mihaltan F, et al: Effects of repeated administration of zolpidem on sleep, diurnal and nocturnal respiratory function, vigilance, and physical performance in patients with COPD. Chest 110:1203–1211, 1996

Gitlin MJ, Cochran SD, Jamison KR: Maintenance lithium treatment: side effects and compliance. J Clin Psychiatry 50:127–131, 1989

Gjere NA: Psychopharmacology in pregnancy. J Perinat Neonatal Nurs 14:12–25, 2001

Glassman AH: Cardiovascular effects of tricyclic antidepressants. Annu Rev Med 35:503–511, 1984

Glassman AH, O'Connor CM, Califf RM, et al: Sertraline treatment of major depression in patients with acute MI or unstable angina. JAMA 288:701–709, 2002

Gomez-Esteban JC, Zarranz JJ, Velasco F, et al: Use of ziprasidone in parkinsonian patients with psychosis. Clin Neuropharmacol 28:111–114, 2005

Goodnick PJ: Use of antidepressants in treatment of comorbid diabetes mellitus and depression as well as in diabetic neuropathy. Ann Clin Psychiatry 13:31–41, 2001

Gordon PH, Pullman SL, Louis ED, et al: Mirtazapine in parkinsonian tremor. Parkinsonism Relat Disord 9:125–126, 2002

Graves NM, Kriel RL, Jones-Saete C: Bioavailability of rectally administered lorazepam. Clin Neuropharmacol 10:555–559, 1987

Greenblatt DJ, Allen MD, MacLaughlin DS, et al: Diazepam absorption: effect of antacids and food. Clin Pharmacol Ther 24:600–609, 1978

Grob CS, Coyle JT: Suspected adverse methylphenidate-imipramine interactions in children. J Dev Behav Pediatr 7:265–267, 1986

Grossberg GT: The ABC of Alzheimer's disease: behavioral symptoms and their treatment. Int Psychogeriatr 14 (suppl 1):27–49, 2002

Gubbins PO, Bertch KE: Drug absorption in gastrointestinal disease and surgery. Clinical pharmacokinetic and therapeutic implications. Clin Pharmacokinet 21:431–447, 1991

Guedon-Moreau L, Ducrocq D, Duc MF, et al: Absolute contraindications in relation to potential drug interactions in outpatient prescriptions: analysis of the first five million prescriptions in 1999. Eur J Clin Pharmacol 59:689–695, 2003

Guilleminault C: Benzodiazepines, breathing, and sleep. Am J Med 88:25S–28S, 1990

Gurley BJ, Swain A, Williams DK, et al: Gauging the clinical significance of P-glycoprotein-mediated herb-drug interactions: comparative effects of St. John's wort, Echinacea, clarithromycin, and rifampin on digoxin pharmacokinetics. Mol Nutr Food Res 52:772–779, 2008

Gwirtsman HE, Szuba MP, Toren L, et al: The antidepressant response to tricyclics in major depressives is accelerated with adjunctive use of methylphenidate. Psychopharmacol Bull 30:157–164, 1994

Hackett ML, Anderson CS, House AO: Management of depression after stroke: a systematic review of pharmacological therapies. Stroke 36:1098–1103, 2005

Haddad P: The SSRI discontinuation syndrome. J Psychopharmacol 12:305–313, 1998

Haddad P: Weight change with atypical antipsychotics in the treatment of schizophrenia. J Psychopharmacol 19:16–27, 2005

Haddad PM, Dursun SM: Neurological complications of psychiatric drugs: clinical features and management. Hum Psychopharmacol 23 (suppl 1):15–26, 2008

Haddad PM, Sharma SG: Adverse effects of atypical antipsychotics: differential risk and clinical implications. CNS Drugs 21:911–936, 2007

Hammad TA, Laughren T, Racoosin J: Suicidality in pediatric patients treated with antidepressant drugs. Arch Gen Psychiatry 63:332–339, 2006

Harden CL, Goldstein MA: Mood disorders in patients with epilepsy: epidemiology and management. CNS Drugs 16:291–302, 2002

Hauser P, Khosla J, Aurora H, et al: A prospective study of the incidence and open-label treatment of interferon-induced major depressive disorder in patients with hepatitis C. Mol Psychiatry 7:942–947, 2002

Health Canada: Important Drug Safety Information: RISPERDAL (risperidone) and Cerebrovascular Adverse Events in Placebo-Controlled Dementia Trials Janssen-Ortho Inc. October 11, 2002. Available at: http://www.hc-sc.gc.ca/dhp-mps/medeff/advisories-avis/prof/_2002/risperdal_hpc-cps-eng.php. Accessed May 14, 2010.

Hebert AA, Ralston JP: Cutaneous reactions to anticonvulsant medications. J Clin Psychiatry 62 (suppl 14):22–26, 2001

Hedner J, Yaeche R, Emilien G, et al: Zaleplon shortens subjective sleep latency and improves subjective sleep quality in elderly patients with insomnia. The Zaleplon Clinical Investigator Study Group. Int J Geriatr Psychiatry 15:704–712, 2000

Heitmann J, Cassel W, Grote L, et al: Does short-term treatment with modafinil affect blood pressure in patients with obstructive sleep apnea? Clin Pharmacol Ther 65:328–335, 1999

Hippisley-Cox J, Vinogradova Y, Coupland C, et al: Risk of malignancy in patients with schizophrenia or bipolar disorder: nested case-control study. Arch Gen Psychiatry 64:1368–1376, 2007

Holmes TF, Sabaawi M, Fragala MR: Psychostimulant suppository treatment for depression in the gravely ill. J Clin Psychiatry 55:265–266, 1994

Honig A, Kuyper AM, Schene AH, et al: Treatment of post-myocardial infarction depressive disorder: a randomized, placebo-controlled trial with mirtazapine. Psychosom Med 69:606–613, 2007

Howland RH: MAOI antidepressant drugs. J Psychosoc Nurs Ment Health Serv 44:9–12, 2006

Hu Z, Yang X, Ho PC, et al: Herb-drug interactions: a literature review. Drugs 65:1239–1282, 2005

Hussain A, Burke J: Mirtazapine associated with recurrent pancreatitis—a case report. J Psychopharmacol 22:336–337, 2008

Iqbal MM, Gundlapalli SP, Ryan WG, et al: Effects of antimanic mood-stabilizing drugs on fetuses, neonates, and nursing infants. South Med J 94:304–322, 2001

Jacobson S: Psychopharmacology: prescribing for patients with hepatic or renal dysfunction. Psychiatric Times 19:65–70, 2002

Jaeger A, Sauder P, Kopferschmitt J, et al: When should dialysis be performed in lithium poisoning? A kinetic study in 14 cases of lithium poisoning. J Toxicol Clin Toxicol 31:429–447, 1993

Jahan MS, Farooque AI, Wahid Z: Neuroleptic malignant syndrome. J Natl Med Assoc 84:966–970, 1992

Jain AE, Lacy T: Psychotropic drugs in pregnancy and lactation. J Psychiatr Pract 11:177–191, 2005

Jann MW, Shirley KL, Small GW: Clinical pharmacokinetics and pharmacodynamics of cholinesterase inhibitors. Clin Pharmacokinet 41:719–739, 2002

Janssen: Invega (paliperidone) home page. 2010. Available at: http://www.invega.com. Accessed May 14, 2010.

Jefferson JW, Greist JH, Ackerman DL, et al: Lithium Encyclopedia for Clinical Practice, 2nd Edition. Washington, DC, American Psychiatric Press, 1987

Joffe H, Taylor AE, Hall JE: Polycystic ovarian syndrome—relationship to epilepsy and antiepileptic drug therapy. J Clin Endocrinol Metab 86:2946–2949, 2001

Kasper S, Muller-Spahn F: Intravenous antidepressant treatment: focus on citalopram. Eur Arch Psychiatry Clin Neurosci 252:105–109, 2002

Keck PE Jr, Arnold LM: The serotonin syndrome. Psychiatric Annals 30:333–343, 2000

Khan A, Khan S, Kolts R, et al: Suicide rates in clinical trials of SSRIs, other antidepressants, and placebo: analysis of FDA reports. Am J Psychiatry 160:790–792, 2003

Khawaja IS, Feinstein RE: Cardiovascular effects of selective serotonin reuptake inhibitors and other novel antidepressants. Heart Dis 5:153–160, 2003

Kiang TK, Ensom MH, Chang TK: UDP-glucuronosyltransferases and clinical drug-drug interactions. Pharmacol Ther 106:97–132, 2005

Kleiner J, Altshuler L, Hendrick V, et al: Lithium-induced subclinical hypothyroidism: review of the literature and guidelines for treatment. J Clin Psychiatry 60:249–255, 1999

Klinger G, Merlob P: Selective serotonin reuptake inhibitor induced neonatal abstinence syndrome. Isr J Psychiatry Relat Sci 45:107–113, 2008

Koelle JS, Dimsdale JE: Antidepressants for the virtually eviscerated patient: options instead of oral dosing. Psychosom Med 60:723–725, 1998

Koller EA, Cross JT, Doraiswamy PM, et al: Pancreatitis associated with atypical antipsychotics: from the Food and Drug Administration's MedWatch surveillance system and published reports. Pharmacotherapy 23:1123–1130, 2003

Konig SA, Schenk M, Sick C, et al: Fatal liver failure associated with valproate therapy in a patient with Friedreich's disease: review of valproate hepatotoxicity in adults. Epilepsia 40:1036–1040, 1999

Konstantinidis A, Stastny J, Ptak-Butta J, et al: Intravenous mirtazapine in the treatment of depressed inpatients. Eur Neuropsychopharmacol 12:57–60, 2002

Kontaxakis V, Stefanis C, Markidis M, et al: Neuroleptic malignant syndrome in a patient with Wilson's disease. J Neurol Neurosurg Psychiatry 51:1001–1002, 1988

Koren G, Pastuszak A, Ito S: Drugs in pregnancy. N Engl J Med 338:1128–1137, 1998

Kraus MR, Schafer A, Schottker K, et al: Therapy of interferon-induced depression in chronic hepatitis C with citalopram: a randomised, double-blind, placebo-controlled study. Gut 57:531–536, 2008

Kryger M, Wang-Weigand S, Roth T: Safety of ramelteon in individuals with mild to moderate obstructive sleep apnea. Sleep Breath 11:159–164, 2007

Kryger M, Wang-Weigand S, Zhang J, et al: Effect of ramelteon, a selective MT(1)/MT(2)-receptor agonist, on respiration during sleep in mild to moderate COPD. Sleep Breath 12:243–250, 2008

Kryger M, Roth T, Wang-Weigand S, et al: The effects of ramelteon on respiration during sleep in subjects with moderate to severe chronic obstructive pulmonary disease. Sleep Breath 13:79–84, 2009

Krystal AD, Erman M, Zammit GK, et al: Long-term efficacy and safety of zolpidem extended-release 12.5 mg, administered 3 to 7 nights per week for 24 weeks, in patients with chronic primary insomnia: a 6-month, randomized, double-blind, placebo-controlled, parallel-group, multicenter study. Sleep 31:79–90, 2008

Lambert BL, Cunningham FE, Miller DR, et al: Diabetes risk associated with use of olanzapine, quetiapine, and risperidone in veterans health administration patients with schizophrenia. Am J Epidemiol 164:672–681, 2006

Lange R, Volkmer M, Heesen C, et al: Modafinil effects in multiple sclerosis patients with fatigue. J Neurol 256:645–650, 2009

Lefevre G, Pommier F, Sedek G, et al: Pharmacokinetics and bioavailability of the novel rivastigmine transdermal patch versus rivastigmine oral solution in healthy elderly subjects. J Clin Pharmacol 48:246–252, 2008

Le Melledo JM, Pilar Castillo AM, Newman S, et al: The effects of newer antidepressants on low-density lipoprotein cholesterol levels. J Clin Psychiatry 65:1017–1018, 2004

Leo RJ: Movement disorders associated with the serotonin selective reuptake inhibitors. J Clin Psychiatry 57:449–454, 1996

Leucht S, Corves C, Arbter D, et al: Second-generation versus first-generation antipsychotic drugs for schizophrenia: a meta-analysis. Lancet 373:31–41, 2009

Levenson JL: High-dose intravenous haloperidol for agitated delirium following lung transplantation. Psychosomatics 36:66–68, 1995

Lieberman JA, Safferman AZ: Clinical profile of clozapine: adverse reactions and agranulocytosis. Psychiatr Q 63:51–70, 1992

Llewellyn A, Stowe ZN: Psychotropic medications in lactation. J Clin Psychiatry 59 (suppl 2):41–52, 1998

Lofaso F, Goldenberg F, Thebault C, et al: Effect of zopiclone on sleep, night-time ventilation, and daytime vigilance in upper airway resistance syndrome. Eur Respir J 10:2573–2577, 1997

Lopez-Meza E, Ruiz-Chow A, Ramirez-Bermudez J: Aripiprazole in psychosis associated with Parkinson's disease. J Neuropsychiatry Clin Neurosci 17:421–422, 2005

Lynch ME, Clark AJ, Sawynok J, et al: Topical amitriptyline and ketamine in neuropathic pain syndromes: an open-label study. J Pain 6:644–649, 2005

Mackay FJ, Dunn NR, Mann RD: Antidepressants and the serotonin syndrome in general practice. Br J Gen Pract 49:871–874, 1999

Mahady GB, Low DT, Barrett ML, et al: United States Pharmacopoeia review of the black cohosh case reports of hepatotoxicity. Menopause 15:628–638, 2008

Mancuso CE, Tanzi MG, Gabay M: Paradoxical reactions to benzodiazepines: literature review and treatment options. Pharmacotherapy 24:1177–1185, 2004

Mann JL, Evans TS, Taylor RD, et al: The use of medications with known or potential anticholinergic activity in patients with dementia receiving cholinesterase inhibitors. Consult Pharm 18:1042–1049, 2003

Mann SC, Caroff SN, Keck PE Jr, et al: Neuroleptic Malignant Syndrome and Related Conditions, 2nd Edition. Washington, DC, American Psychiatric Publishing, 2003

Manos GH: Possible serotonin syndrome associated with buspirone added to fluoxetine. Ann Pharmacother 34:871–874, 2000

Manos MJ, Tom-Revzon C, Bukstein OG, et al: Changes and challenges: managing ADHD in a fast-paced world. J Manag Care Pharm 13:S2–S13, 2007

Markowitz JS, Patrick KS: Pharmacokinetic and pharmacodynamic drug interactions in the treatment of attention-deficit hyperactivity disorder. Clin Pharmacokinet 40:753–772, 2001

Markowitz JS, DeVane CL, Malcolm RJ, et al. Pharmacokinetics of olanzapine after single-dose oral administration of standard tablet versus normal and sublingual administration of an orally disintegrating tablet in normal volunteers. J Clin Pharmacol 46:164–171, 2006

Martin WR, Sloan JW, Sapira JD, et al: Physiologic, subjective, and behavioral effects of amphetamine, methamphetamine, ephedrine, phenmetrazine, and methylphenidate in man. Clin Pharmacol Ther 12:245–258, 1971

Masand PS, Tesar GE: Use of stimulants in the medically ill. Psychiatr Clin North Am 19:515–547, 1996

Masand P, Pickett P, Murray GB: Psychostimulants for secondary depression in medical illness. Psychosomatics 32:203–208, 1991

Matsuo N, Morita T: Efficacy, safety, and cost effectiveness of intravenous midazolam and flunitrazepam for primary insomnia in terminally ill patients with cancer: a retrospective multicenter audit study. J Palliat Med 10:1054–1062, 2007

Mayer G, Wang-Weigand S, Roth-Schechter B, et al: Efficacy and safety of 6-month nightly ramelteon administration in adults with chronic primary insomnia. Sleep 32:351–360, 2009

McAndrews MP, Weiss RT, Sandor P, et al: Cognitive effects of long-term benzodiazepine use in older adults. Hum Psychopharmacol 18:51–57, 2003

McCann CC, Quera-Salva MA, Boudet J, et al: Effect of zolpidem during sleep on ventilation and cardiovascular variables in normal subjects. Fundam Clin Pharmacol 7:305–310, 1993

McEvoy GE: American Hospital Formulary Service (AHFS) Drug Information 2008. Bethesda, MD, American Society of Health-System Pharmacists, 2008

McGough JJ, Wigal SB, Abikoff H, et al: A randomized, double-blind, placebo-controlled, laboratory classroom assessment of methylphenidate transdermal system in children with ADHD. J Atten Disord 9:476–485, 2006

McIntyre RS, Soczynska JK, Konarski JZ, et al: The effect of antidepressants on lipid homeostasis: a cardiac safety concern? Expert Opin Drug Saf 5:523–537, 2006

McIntyre RS, Panjwani ZD, Nguyen HT, et al: The hepatic safety profile of duloxetine: a review. Expert Opin Drug Metab Toxicol 4:281–285, 2008

McKenna K, Koren G, Tetelbaum M, et al: Pregnancy outcome of women using atypical antipsychotic drugs: a prospective comparative study. J Clin Psychiatry 66:444–449, 2005

Meijer WE, Heerdink ER, van Eijk JT, et al: Adverse events in users of sertraline: results from an observational study in psychiatric practice in The Netherlands. Pharmacoepidemiol Drug Saf 11:655–662, 2002

Melkersson KI: Prolactin elevation of the antipsychotic risperidone is predominantly related to its 9-hydroxy metabolite. Hum Psychopharmacol 21:529–532, 2006

Mendelson WB, Garnett D, Gillin JC: Flurazepam-induced sleep apnea syndrome in a patient with insomnia and mild sleep-related respiratory changes. J Nerv Ment Dis 169:261–264, 1981

Mendelson WB, Maczaj M, Holt J: Buspirone administration to sleep apnea patients. J Clin Psychopharmacol 11:71–72, 1991

Mendlewicz J, Souery D, Rivelli SK: Short-term and long-term treatment for bipolar patients: beyond the guidelines. J Affect Disord 55:79–85, 1999

Menghini VV, Albright RC Jr: Treatment of lithium intoxication with continuous venovenous hemodiafiltration. Am J Kidney Dis 36:E21, 2000

Menon SJ: Psychotropic medication during pregnancy and lactation. Arch Gynecol Obstet 277:1–13, 2008

Menza M, Dobkin RD, Marin H, et al: A controlled trial of antidepressants in patients with Parkinson disease and depression. Neurology 72:886–892, 2009

Meyer JM, Koro CE: The effects of antipsychotic therapy on serum lipids: a comprehensive review. Schizophr Res 70:1–17, 2004

Michalets E: Clinically significant cytochrome P-450 drug interactions. Pharmacotherapy 18:84–112, 1998

Miller EA, Leslie DL, Rosenheck RA: Incidence of new-onset diabetes mellitus among patients receiving atypical neuroleptics in the treatment of mental illness: evidence from a privately insured population. J Nerv Ment Dis 193:387–395, 2005

Miller GM, Stripp R: A study of western pharmaceuticals contained within samples of Chinese herbal/patent medicines collected from New York City's Chinatown. Leg Med (Tokyo) 9:258–264, 2007

Miller LJ: Clinical strategies for the use of psychotropic drugs during pregnancy. Psychiatr Med 9:275–298, 1991

Miller LJ: Psychiatric medication during pregnancy: Understanding and minimizing risks. Psychiatric Annals 24:69–75, 1994

Mills KC: Serotonin syndrome. A clinical update. Crit Care Clin 13:763–783, 1997

Mirassou MM: Rectal antidepressant medication in the treatment of depression. J Clin Psychiatry 59:29, 1998

Mitchell JE, Mackenzie TB: Cardiac effects of lithium therapy in man: a review. J Clin Psychiatry 43:47–51, 1982

Mitchell-Heggs P, Murphy K, Minty K, et al: Diazepam in the treatment of dyspnoea in the "Pink Puffer" syndrome. Q J Med 49:9–20, 1980

Mockenhaupt M, Messenheimer J, Tennis P, et al: Risk of Stevens-Johnson syndrome and toxic epidermal necrolysis in new users of antiepileptics. Neurology 64:1134–1138, 2005

Model DG: Nitrazepam induced respiratory depression in chronic obstructive lung disease. Br J Dis Chest 67:128–130, 1973

Monti JM, Pandi-Perumal S: Eszopiclone: its use in the treatment of insomnia. Neuropsychiatr Dis Treat 3:441–453, 2007

Moorman PG, Berchuck A, Calingaert B, et al: Antidepressant medication use [corrected] and risk of ovarian cancer. Obstet Gynecol 105:725–730, 2005

Morrow JD: Why the United States still needs improved dietary supplement regulation and oversight. Clin Pharmacol Ther 83:391–393, 2008

Mortensen PB: Neuroleptic treatment and other factors modifying cancer risk in schizophrenic patients. Acta Psychiatr Scand 75:585–590, 1987

Muhlbacher M, Konstantinidis A, Kasper S, et al: Intravenous mirtazapine is safe and effective in the treatment of depressed inpatients. Neuropsychobiology 53:83–87, 2006

Muir JF, DeFouilloy C, Broussier P, et al: Comparative study of the effects of zopiclone and placebo on respiratory function in patients with chronic obstructive respiratory insufficiency. Int Clin Psychopharmacol 5 (suppl 2):85–94, 1990

Mula M, Trimble MR, Yuen A, et al: Psychiatric adverse events during levetiracetam therapy. Neurology 61:704–706, 2003

Najib J: Eszopiclone, a nonbenzodiazepine sedative-hypnotic agent for the treatment of transient and chronic insomnia. Clin Ther 28:491–516, 2006

Narendran R, Young CM, Valenti AM, et al: Is psychosis exacerbated by modafinil? Arch Gen Psychiatry 59:292–293, 2002

Nelson JC: Safety and tolerability of the new antidepressants. J Clin Psychiatry 58 (suppl 6):26–31, 1997

Neuvonen PJ, Tokola O: Bioavailability of rectally administered carbamazepine mixture. Br J Clin Pharmacol 24:839–841, 1987

Newport DJ, Hostetter A, Arnold A, et al: The treatment of postpartum depression: minimizing infant exposures. J Clin Psychiatry 63 (suppl 7):31–44, 2002

Nilsson MI, Widerlov E, Meresaar U, et al: Effect of urinary pH on the disposition of methadone in man. Eur J Clin Pharmacol 22:337–342, 1982

Nonino F, Campomori A: Neuroleptic malignant syndrome associated with metoclopramide. Ann Pharmacother 33:644–645, 1999

Nordeng H, Lindemann R, Perminov KV, et al: Neonatal withdrawal syndrome after in utero exposure to selective serotonin reuptake inhibitors. Acta Paediatr 90:288–291, 2001

Norris E, Marzouk O, Nunn A, et al: Respiratory depression in children receiving diazepam for acute seizures: a prospective study. Dev Med Child Neurol 41:340–343, 1999

Norton J: The use of intravenous valproate in psychiatry. Can J Psychiatry 46:371–372, 2001

Norton JW, Quarles E: Intravenous valproate in neuropsychiatry. Pharmacotherapy 20:88–92, 2000

NovaDel: Zolpimist (zolpidem) information page. 2010. Available at: http://www.novadel.com/pipeline/zolpimist.htm. Accessed May 18, 2010.

O'Brien CP: Benzodiazepine use, abuse, and dependence. J Clin Psychiatry 66 (suppl 2):28–33, 2005

Ortho-NcNeil: Topamax (topiramate) home page. 2010. Available at: http://www.topamax.com. Accessed May 14, 2010.

Otsuka: Abilify (Aripiprazole) Tablets, Application No. 21-436, Drug Approval Package, Medical review(s). Food and Drug Administration Center for Drug Evaluation and Research, November 15, 2002. Available at: http://www.accessdata.fda.gov/drugsatfda_docs/nda/2002/21-436_Abilify_medr_P2.pdf. Accessed May 14, 2010.

Owen JA, Levenson JL: Renal and urological disorders, in Clinical Manual of Psychopharmacology in the Medically Ill. Edited by Ferrando SJ, Levenson JL, Owen JA. Arlington, VA, American Psychiatric Publishing, 2010, pp 149–180

Pact V, Giduz T: Mirtazapine treats resting tremor, essential tremor, and levodopa-induced dyskinesias. Neurology 53:1154, 1999

Pakyurek M, Pasol E: Sublingually administered fluoxetine for major depression in medically compromised patients. Am J Psychiatry 156:1833–1834, 1999

Pal D, Mitra AK: MDR- and CYP3A4-mediated drug-drug interactions. J Neuroimmune Pharmacol 1:323–339, 2006

Papakostas GI: Limitations of contemporary antidepressants: tolerability. J Clin Psychiatry 68 (suppl 10):11–17, 2007

Papakostas GI: Tolerability of modern antidepressants. J Clin Psychiatry 69 (suppl E1):8–13, 2008

Parkinson Study Group: Low-dose clozapine for the treatment of drug-induced psychosis in Parkinson's disease. N Engl J Med 340:757–763, 1999

Parsons RL: Drug absorption in gastrointestinal disease with particular reference to malabsorption syndromes. Clin Pharmacokinet 2:45–60, 1977

Pat-Horenczyk R, Hacohen D, Herer P, et al: The effects of substituting zopiclone in withdrawal from chronic use of benzodiazepine hypnotics. Psychopharmacology (Berl) 140:450–457, 1998

Peet M, Pratt JP: Lithium. Current status in psychiatric disorders. Drugs 46:7–17, 1993

Pelonero AL, Levenson JL, Pandurangi AK: Neuroleptic malignant syndrome: a review. Psychiatr Serv 49:1163–1172, 1998

Periclou A, Ventura D, Rao N, et al: Pharmacokinetic study of memantine in healthy and renally impaired subjects. Clin Pharmacol Ther 79:134–143, 2006

Pesola GR, Quinto C: Prochlorperazine-induced neuroleptic malignant syndrome. J Emerg Med 14:727–729, 1996

Pfizer: Geodon (ziprasidone) home page. 2010a. Available at: http://www.geodon.com. Accessed May 14, 2010.

Pfizer: Pristiq (desvenlafaxine) home page. 2010b. Available at: http://www.pristiq.com. Accessed May 14, 2010.

Prator BC: Serotonin syndrome. J Neurosci Nurs 38:102–105, 2006

Presne C, Fakhouri F, Noel LH, et al: Lithium-induced nephropathy: rate of progression and prognostic factors. Kidney Int 64:585–592, 2003

Privitera MD, Brodie MJ, Mattson RH, et al: Topiramate, carbamazepine and valproate monotherapy: double-blind comparison in newly diagnosed epilepsy. Acta Neurol Scand 107:165–175, 2003

Pycha R, Miller C, Barnas C, et al: Intravenous flunitrazepam in the treatment of alcohol withdrawal delirium. Alcohol Clin Exp Res 17:753–757, 1993

Quilici S, Chancellor J, Lothgren M, et al: Meta-analysis of duloxetine vs. pregabalin and gabapentin in the treatment of diabetic peripheral neuropathic pain. BMC Neurol 9:6, 2009

Raison CL, Woolwine BJ, Demetrashvili MF, et al: Paroxetine for prevention of depressive symptoms induced by interferon-alpha and ribavirin for hepatitis C. Aliment Pharmacol Ther 25:1163–1174, 2007

Ranlov PJ, Nielsen SP: Effect of zopiclone and diazepam on ventilatory response in normal human subjects. Sleep 10 (suppl 1): 40–47, 1987

Rapport MD, Moffitt C: Attention deficit/hyperactivity disorder and methylphenidate. A review of height/weight, cardiovascular, and somatic complaint side effects. Clin Psychol Rev 22:1107–1131, 2002

Ravina B, Putt M, Siderowf A, et al: Donepezil for dementia in Parkinson's disease: a randomised, double blind, placebo controlled, crossover study. J Neurol Neurosurg Psychiatry 76:934–939, 2005

Regenold WT, Prasad M: Uses of intravenous valproate in geriatric psychiatry. Am J Geriatr Psychiatry 9:306–308, 2001

Reis M, Kallen B: Maternal use of antipsychotics in early pregnancy and delivery outcome. J Clin Psychopharmacol 28:279–288, 2008

Rementeria JL, Bhatt K: Withdrawal symptoms in neonates from intrauterine exposure to diazepam. J Pediatr 90:123–126, 1977

Repchinsky CE: CPS 2009: Compendium of Pharmaceuticals and Specialties: The Canadian Drug Reference for Health Professionals. Ottawa, ON, Canadian Pharmacists Association, 2009

Repetto MJ, Petitto JM: Psychopharmacology in HIV-infected patients. Psychosom Med 70:585–592, 2008

Reulbach U, Dütsch C, Biermann T, et al: Managing an effective treatment for neuroleptic malignant syndrome. Crit Care 11:R4, 2007

Rey E, Treluyer JM, Pons G: Pharmacokinetic optimization of benzodiazepine therapy for acute seizures. Focus on delivery routes. Clin Pharmacokinet 36:409–424, 1999

Richard IH, Maughn A, Kurlan R: Do serotonin reuptake inhibitor antidepressants worsen Parkinson's disease? A retrospective case series. Mov Disord 14:155–157, 1999

Risch SC, Groom GP, Janowsky DS: The effects of psychotropic drugs on the cardiovascular system. J Clin Psychiatry 43:16–31, 1982

Robertson P Jr, Hellriegel ET: Clinical pharmacokinetic profile of modafinil. Clin Pharmacokinet 42:123–137, 2003

Robertson P Jr, Hellriegel ET, Arora S, et al: Effect of modafinil on the pharmacokinetics of ethinyl estradiol and triazolam in healthy volunteers. Clin Pharmacol Ther 71:46–56, 2002

Robinson MJ, Levenson JL: The use of psychotropics in the medically ill. Curr Psychiatry Rep 2:247–255, 2000

Robinson MJ, Qaqish RB: Practical psychopharmacology in HIV-1 and acquired immunodeficiency syndrome. Psychiatr Clin North Am 25:149–175, 2002

Roose SP, Miyazaki M: Pharmacologic treatment of depression in patients with heart disease. Psychosom Med 67 (suppl 1): S54–S57, 2005

Roose SP, Glassman AH, Siris SG, et al: Comparison of imipramine- and nortriptyline-induced orthostatic hypotension: a meaningful difference. J Clin Psychopharmacol 1:316–319, 1981

Roose SP, Glassman AH, Giardina EG, et al: Nortriptyline in depressed patients with left ventricular impairment. JAMA 256:3253–3257, 1986

Roose SP, Dalack GW, Glassman AH, et al: Cardiovascular effects of bupropion in depressed patients with heart disease. Am J Psychiatry 148:512–516, 1991

Rosenberg MR, Green M: Neuroleptic malignant syndrome. Review of response to therapy. Arch Intern Med 149:1927–1931, 1989

Rosenberg R, Roach JM, Scharf M, et al: A pilot study evaluating acute use of eszopiclone in patients with mild to moderate obstructive sleep apnea syndrome. Sleep Med 8:464–470, 2007

Rosenfeld JA, Everett KD: Factors related to planned and unplanned pregnancies. J Fam Pract 43:161–166, 1996

Rosenstein DL, Nelson JC, Jacobs SC: Seizures associated with antidepressants: a review. J Clin Psychiatry 54:289–299, 1993

Roth T, Rippon GA, Arora S: Armodafinil improves wakefulness and long-term episodic memory in nCPAP-adherent patients with excessive sleepiness associated with obstructive sleep apnea. Sleep Breath 12:53–62, 2008

Rozzini L, Chilovi BV, Bertoletti E, et al: Cognitive and psychopathologic response to rivastigmine in dementia with Lewy bodies compared to Alzheimer's disease: a case control study. Am J Alzheimers Dis Other Demen 22:42–47, 2007

Rubin ET, Lee A, Ito S: When breastfeeding mothers need CNS-acting drugs. Can J Clin Pharmacol 11:e257-e266, 2004

Rudolph JL, Salow MJ, Angelini MC, et al: The anticholinergic risk scale and anticholinergic adverse effects in older persons. Arch Intern Med 168:508–513, 2008

Rugino TA, Copley TC: Effects of modafinil in children with attention-deficit/hyperactivity disorder: an open-label study. J Am Acad Child Adolesc Psychiatry 40:230–235, 2001

Russell WJ: The impact of Alzheimer's disease medication on muscle relaxants. Anaesth Intensive Care 37:134–135, 2009

Russell WJ, Badcock NR, Frewin DB, et al: Pharmacokinetics of a new sublingual formulation of temazepam. Eur J Clin Pharmacol 35:437–439, 1988

Rzany B, Correia O, Kelly JP, et al: Risk of Stevens-Johnson syndrome and toxic epidermal necrolysis during first weeks of antiepileptic therapy: a case-control study. Study Group of the International Case Control Study on Severe Cutaneous Adverse Reactions. Lancet 353:2190–2194, 1999

Sacchetti E, Trifiro G, Caputi A, et al: Risk of stroke with typical and atypical anti-psychotics: a retrospective cohort study including unexposed subjects. J Psychopharmacol 22:39–46, 2008

Sachdev PS: A rating scale for neuroleptic malignant syndrome. Psychiatry Res 135:249–256, 2005

Sadeque AJ, Wandel C, He H, et al: Increased drug delivery to the brain by P-glycoprotein inhibition. Clin Pharmacol Ther 68:231–237, 2000

Sammut S, Bethus I, Goodall G, et al: Antidepressant reversal of interferon-alpha-induced anhedonia. Physiol Behav 75:765–772, 2002

Sanger DJ, Zivkovic B: Differential development of tolerance to the depressant effects of benzodiazepine and non-benzodiazepine agonists at the omega (BZ) modulatory sites of GABAA receptors. Neuropharmacology 31:693–700, 1992

Saper RB, Phillips RS, Sehgal A, et al: Lead, mercury, and arsenic in US- and Indian-manufactured Ayurvedic medicines sold via the Internet. JAMA 300:915–923, 2008

Schmidt D, Elger CE: What is the evidence that oxcarbazepine and carbamazepine are distinctly different antiepileptic drugs? Epilepsy Behav 5:627–635, 2004

Schmitt L, Tonnoir B, Arbus C: Safety and efficacy of oral escitalopram as continuation treatment of intravenous citalopram in patients with major depressive disorder. Neuropsychobiology 54:201–207, 2006

Schonfeldt-Lecuona C, Connemann BJ: Aripiprazole and Parkinson's disease psychosis. Am J Psychiatry 161:373–374, 2004

Schou M, Amdisen A, Steenstrup OR: Lithium and pregnancy, II: hazards to women given lithium during pregnancy and delivery. BMJ 2:137–138, 1973

Schramm TM, Lawford BR, Macdonald GA, et al: Sertraline treatment of interferon-alfa-induced depressive disorder. Med J Aust 173:359–361, 2000

Schweitzer I, Tuckwell V: Risk of adverse events with the use of augmentation therapy for the treatment of resistant depression. Drug Saf 19:455–464, 1998

Scott MA, Letrent KJ, Hager KL, et al: Use of transdermal amitriptyline gel in a patient with chronic pain and depression. Pharmacotherapy 19:236–239, 1999

Seppala T, Aranko K, Mattila MJ, et al: Effects of alcohol on buspirone and lorazepam actions. Clin Pharmacol Ther 32:201–207, 1982

Singh NP, Despars JA, Stansbury DW, et al: Effects of buspirone on anxiety levels and exercise tolerance in patients with chronic airflow obstruction and mild anxiety. Chest 103:800–804, 1993

Sobotka JL, Alexander B, Cook BL: A review of carbamazepine's hematologic reactions and monitoring recommendations. DICP 24:1214–1219, 1990

Spigset O, Hagg S, Bate A: Hepatic injury and pancreatitis during treatment with serotonin reuptake inhibitors: data from the

World Health Organization (WHO) database of adverse drug reactions. Int Clin Psychopharmacol 18:157–161, 2003

Stancer HC, Kivi R: Lithium carbonate and oedema. Lancet 2:985, 1971

Staner C, Joly F, Jacquot N, et al. Sublingual zolpidem in early onset of sleep compared to oral zolpidem: polysomnographic study in patients with primary insomnia. Curr Med Res Opin 26:1423–1431, 2010

Stern TA: The management of depression and anxiety following myocardial infarction. Mt Sinai J Med 52:623–633, 1985

Sternbach H: The serotonin syndrome. Am J Psychiatry 148:705–713, 1991

Stewart DE: Hepatic adverse reactions associated with nefazodone. Can J Psychiatry 47:375–377, 2002

Stewart WA, Harrison R, Dooley JM: Respiratory depression in the acute management of seizures. Arch Dis Child 87:225–226, 2002

Stoppe G, Muller P, Fuchs T, et al: Life-threatening allergic reaction to clozapine. Br J Psychiatry 161:259–261, 1992

Storey P, Trumble M: Rectal doxepin and carbamazepine therapy in patients with cancer. N Engl J Med 327:1318–1319, 1992

Strawn JR, Keck PE Jr, Caroff SN: Neuroleptic malignant syndrome. Am J Psychiatry 164:870–876, 2007

Stubner S, Rustenbeck E, Grohmann R, et al: Severe and uncommon involuntary movement disorders due to psychotropic drugs. Pharmacopsychiatry 37 (suppl 1):S54–S64, 2004

Su YP, Chang CJ, Hwang TJ: Lithium intoxication after valsartan treatment. Psychiatry Clin Neurosci 61:204, 2007

Szarfman A, Tonning JM, Levine JG, et al: Atypical antipsychotics and pituitary tumors: a pharmacovigilance study. Pharmacotherapy 26:748–758, 2006

Takeda: Rozerem (ramelteon) home page. 2010. Available at: http://www.rozerem.com. Accessed May 14, 2010.

Tamim HM, Mahmud S, Hanley JA, et al: Antidepressants and risk of prostate cancer: a nested case-control study. Prostate Cancer Prostatic Dis 11:53–60, 2008

Tandon R: Safety and tolerability: how do newer generation “atypical” antipsychotics compare? Psychiatr Q 73:297–311, 2002

Taylor D: Antidepressant drugs and cardiovascular pathology: a clinical overview of effectiveness and safety. Acta Psychiatr Scand 118:434–442, 2008

Teicher MH, Glod C, Cole JO: Emergence of intense suicidal preoccupation during fluoxetine treatment. Am J Psychiatry 147:207–210, 1990

Teter CJ, Phan KL, Cameron OG, et al: Relative rectal bioavailability of fluoxetine in normal volunteers. J Clin Psychopharmacol 25:74–78, 2005

Tharwani HM, Yerramsetty P, Mannelli P, et al: Recent advances in poststroke depression. Curr Psychiatry Rep 9:225–231, 2007

Thompson C: Mirtazapine versus selective serotonin reuptake inhibitors. J Clin Psychiatry 60 (suppl 17):18–22, 1999

Thomsen K, Schou M: Avoidance of lithium intoxication: advice based on knowledge about the renal lithium clearance under various circumstances. Pharmacopsychiatry 32:83–86, 1999

Toh S, Rodriguez LA, Hernandez-Diaz S: Use of antidepressants and risk of lung cancer. Cancer Causes Control 18:1055–1064, 2007

Tohen M, Castillo J, Baldessarini RJ, et al: Blood dyscrasias with carbamazepine and valproate: a pharmacoepidemiological study of 2,228 patients at risk. Am J Psychiatry 152:413–418, 1995

Tracy TS, Kingston RL (eds): Herbal Products, 2nd Edition. Totowa, NJ, Humana Press, 2007

Turner MS, May DB, Arthur RR, et al: Clinical impact of selective serotonin reuptake inhibitors therapy with bleeding risks. J Intern Med 261:205–213, 2007

Upward JW, Edwards JG, Goldie A, et al: Comparative effects of fluoxetine and amitriptyline on cardiac function. Br J Clin Pharmacol 26:399–402, 1988

U.S. Food and Drug Administration: FDA advising risk of birth defects with Paxil: agency requiring updated product labeling. Rockville, MD, Food and Drug Administration, December 8, 2005. Available at: http://www.fda.gov/NewsEvents/Newsroom/PressAnnouncements/2005/ucm108527.htm. Accessed May 14, 2010.

U.S. Modafinil in Narcolepsy Multicenter Study Group: Randomized trial of modafinil as a treatment for the excessive daytime somnolence of narcolepsy. Neurology 54:1166–1175, 2000

USPDI Editorial Board (eds): United States Pharmacopoeia Dispensing Information, Vol 1: Drug Information for the Health Care Professional, 27th Edition. Greenwood Village, CO, Thompson Micromedex, 2007

Valeant: Zelapar (selegiline oral disintegrating tablets) home page. 2010. Available at: http://www.zelapar.com. Accessed May 14, 2010.

van Amelsvoort T, Bakshi R, Devaux CB, et al: Hyponatremia associated with carbamazepine and oxcarbazepine therapy: a review. Epilepsia 35:181–188, 1994

van Hoogdalem E, De Boer AG, Breimer DD: Pharmacokinetics of rectal drug administration, part I: general considerations and clinical applications of centrally acting drugs. Clin Pharmacokinet 21:11–26, 1991a

van Hoogdalem EJ, De Boer AG, Breimer DD: Pharmacokinetics of rectal drug administration, part II: clinical applications of peripherally acting drugs, and conclusions. Clin Pharmacokinet 21:110–128, 1991b

van Noord C, Straus SM, Sturkenboom MC, et al: Psychotropic drugs associated with corrected QT interval prolongation. J Clin Psychopharmacol 29:9–15, 2009

Vanda: Fanapt (iloperidone) home page. 2010. Available at: http://www.fanapt.com. Accessed May 14, 2010.

Vanderkooy JD, Kennedy SH, Bagby RM: Antidepressant side effects in depression patients treated in a naturalistic setting: a study of bupropion, moclobemide, paroxetine, sertraline, and venlafaxine. Canadian Journal of Psychiatry—Revue Canadienne de Psychiatrie 47:174–180, 2002

Vieweg WV: Mechanisms and risks of electrocardiographic QT interval prolongation when using antipsychotic drugs. J Clin Psychiatry 63 (suppl 9):18–24, 2002

Vieweg WV, Julius DA, Fernandez A, et al: Treatment of depression in patients with coronary heart disease. Am J Med 119:567–573, 2006

Viguera AC, Whitfield T, Baldessarini RJ, et al: Risk of recurrence in women with bipolar disorder during pregnancy: prospective study of mood stabilizer discontinuation. Am J Psychiatry 164:1817–1824, 2007

Wagner J, Wagner ML: Non-benzodiazepines for the treatment of insomnia. Sleep Med Rev 4:551–581, 2000

Wallerstedt SM, Gleerup H, Sundstrom A, et al: Risk of clinically relevant bleeding in warfarin-treated patients—influence of SSRI treatment. Pharmacoepidemiol Drug Saf 18:412–416, 2009

Wang PW, Santosa C, Schumacher M, et al: Gabapentin augmentation therapy in bipolar depression. Bipolar Disord 4:296–301, 2002

Ward RK, Zamorski MA: Benefits and risks of psychiatric medications during pregnancy. Am Fam Physician 66:629–636, 2002

Ward RM: Pharmacological treatment of the fetus. Clinical pharmacokinetic considerations. Clin Pharmacokinet 28:343–350, 1995

Ward RM: Pharmacology of the maternal-placental-fetal-unit and fetal therapy. Progress in Pediatric Cardiology 5:79–89, 1996

Watkins PB, Zimmerman HJ, Knapp MJ, et al: Hepatotoxic effects of tacrine administration in patients with Alzheimer's disease. JAMA 271:992–998, 1994

Weber J, McCormack PL: Asenapine. CNS Drugs 23:781–792, 2009

Wermeling DP, Record KA, Kelly TH, et al: Pharmacokinetics and pharmacodynamics of a new intranasal midazolam formulation in healthy volunteers. Anesth Analg 103:344–349, Table of Contents, 2006

Wermuth L, Sørensen PS, Timm S, et al: Depression in idiopathic Parkinson's disease treated with citalopram: a placebo-controlled trial. Nord J Psychiatry 52:163–169, 1998

Wernicke JF, Faries D, Girod D, et al: Cardiovascular effects of atomoxetine in children, adolescents, and adults. Drug Saf 26:729–740, 2003

Wernicke JF, Holdridge KC, Jin L, et al: Seizure risk in patients with attention-deficit-hyperactivity disorder treated with atomoxetine. Dev Med Child Neurol 49:498–502, 2007a

Wernicke J, Lledo A, Raskin J, et al: An evaluation of the cardiovascular safety profile of duloxetine: findings from 42 placebo-controlled studies. Drug Saf 30:437–455, 2007b

Whyte IM, Dawson AH, Buckley NA: Relative toxicity of venlafaxine and selective serotonin reuptake inhibitors in overdose compared to tricyclic antidepressants. QJM 96:369–374, 2003

Winkler D, Ortner R, Pjrek E, et al: Trazodone-induced cardiac arrhythmias: a report of two cases. Hum Psychopharmacol 21:61–62, 2006

Wisner KL, Perel JM, Wheeler SB: Tricyclic dose requirements across pregnancy. Am J Psychiatry 150:1541–1542, 1993

Wooltorton E: Antipsychotic clozapine (Clozaril): myocarditis and cardiovascular toxicity. CMAJ 166:1185–1186, 2002

Wooltorton E: Hua Fo tablets tainted with sildenafil-like compound. J Can Med Assoc 166:1568, 2003

Wright BA, Jarrett DB: Lithium and calcium channel blockers: possible neurotoxicity. Biol Psychiatry 30:635–636, 1991

Wroblewski BA, Leary JM, Phelan AM, et al: Methylphenidate and seizure frequency in brain injured patients with seizure disorders. J Clin Psychiatry 53:86–89, 1992

Xu W, Tamim H, Shapiro S, et al: Use of antidepressants and risk of colorectal cancer: a nested case-control study. Lancet Oncol 7:301–308, 2006

Yang SH, McNeely MJ: Rhabdomyolysis, pancreatitis, and hyperglycemia with ziprasidone. Am J Psychiatry 159:1435, 2002

Zaccara G, Franciotta D, Perucca E: Idiosyncratic adverse reactions to antiepileptic drugs. Epilepsia 48:1223–1244, 2007

Zimbroff DL: Pharmacological control of acute agitation: focus on intramuscular preparations. CNS Drugs 22:199–212, 2008

Zin CS, Nissen LM, Smith MT, et al: An update on the pharmacological management of post-herpetic neuralgia and painful diabetic neuropathy. CNS Drugs 22:417–442, 2008

CHAPTER

39

Psychotherapy

Elspeth Guthrie, M.B., Ch.B., M.R.C.Psych., M.Sc., M.D.

> The heartbeat of therapy is a process of learning how to go on becoming a person together with others. That learning never ends.
>
> R.F. Hobson 1985, p. xii

THE TERM *PSYCHOTHERAPY* has a very broad meaning. At its heart, however, it implies the intent to help another person or persons through the medium of an interpersonal professional relationship. People usually seek or are referred for therapy because they are distressed or are struggling to cope with some major life problem or difficulty. Physical illness is scary, stressful, and at times unimaginably difficult to bear. What must it be like to be told that the tremor you have developed is the first sign of Parkinson's disease, or that the cough that will not go away has been confirmed as lung cancer?

This chapter focuses on the role of psychological treatments in physical illness and is divided into two parts. In the first part, psychological approaches to helping people cope with physical illness are discussed, and in the second part, evidence for the effectiveness of psychological treatments in physical illness is reviewed. In this textbook there are separate chapters on psychological treatments and pharmacotherapy. The two, however, are commonly used together to good effect, particularly in people with physical illness, and it is usually helpful when considering psychological treatment to also consider the potential benefits of pharmacological interventions. This will be discussed further in relation to collaborative and stepped-care models (see later in chapter).

Psychological Approaches to Helping People Cope With Physical Illness

Rationale for Psychological Therapies in Physical Illness

Many people find it difficult to cope or adapt to physical illness, but given time and the right environment, most manage this process without the need to seek professional help. Approximately 10% of medically ill patients require specific psychiatric treatment (Royal College of Physicians and Royal College of Psychiatrists 2003). Although certain forms of physical illness (e.g., terminal cancer) carry huge emotional burdens, people's individual perceptions of their illness have a powerful influence on how they cope with the illness and how emotionally stressful they find it. At a very basic human level, physical illness can be understood as a threat to the self (Cassell 1982), and it can "attack" the very heart of who we are as people and human beings. For example, physical illness can interfere with our ability to work, parent, make love, socialize, and take part in sports, music, and other creative activities. It can threaten our body image, our physical independence, and our ability to care for ourselves. It can undermine and destabilize us—and, of course, in its most extreme form, threaten our very existence.

Minute Particulars of the Patient's Story of Illness

Whatever the modality of therapy, the starting point for most therapies involving patients with physical illness is a detailed account of the person's own illness story. Most people "need" to tell their story, retell it and reshape it, and finally, hopefully, make peace with it. William Blake wrote, "He who would do good to another must do it in the Minute Particulars: General Good is the plea of the scoundrel, hypocrite and flatterer, for Art and Science cannot exist but in minutely organized particulars" (William Blake, *Jerusalem* III, 55:60–68).

It is through the exploration of the "minute particulars" of the person's illness that a real sharing and understanding of the person's suffering emerges. At its best, this process can foster a deep and positive therapeutic alliance with the client, which can provide a springboard for further work involving any therapeutic modality. In itself it can bring relief from suffering, an understanding of the self and of the experience of illness, and a sense of mastery and empowerment.

Necessary Adaptations

Participation in any form of meaningful psychotherapy requires an individual to be able to concentrate during the therapy and to recall and think about the therapy in between sessions. In structured therapies, there is an explicit expectation that homework will be carried out between sessions. However, physical illness may prevent some people from participating in psychological treatments because they are too physically unwell. It is hard to concentrate in therapy if one is nauseous or exhausted or is very short of breath. It may also be physically difficult for some people to attend psychotherapy sessions because of problems with mobility or transport. Sessions may have to be rescheduled or fitted around other medical commitments (e.g., investigations, renal dialysis). The duration of sessions may have to be modified or breaks in therapy accommodated because of relapses in the person's illness or participation in challenging treatment regimes.

It is often appropriate for the therapist to involve other members of the patient's family in the therapeutic process, particularly if they have a role as a care provider. It may also be important for the therapist to liaise with other members of the health care team and to spend time with the patient discussing relationships with nursing, medical, and other professional staff.

Therapists who work in medical settings need to have an understanding of the illnesses the patients they see are suffering from and the kinds of investigations and treatment that patients are likely to experience. This will involve spending time with other health professionals and patients on medical or surgical units or in the community setting.

Therapists vary in their competence, and more competent therapists produce better outcomes than less competent ones (Barber et al. 2006). There is some evidence for cognitive-behavioral therapy (CBT) that use of so-called concrete CBT techniques (e.g., establish the session agenda, set homework tasks, or help clients identify and modify negative automatic thoughts) is associated with good outcomes (DeRubeis and Feeley 1990). In relational therapies, better outcomes have been associated with therapists who can repair ruptures in the alliance (Bennett and Parry 2004).

In the medical setting, it may be particularly important that therapists have a high level of competence because of the complexity of patients' problems and the need for the adaptations described above, which are required when working with people who have both physical and mental illness.

Although there are many different types of psychological treatment, three main approaches will be described in this chapter: basic supportive techniques and problem solving, relational therapies, and cognitive-behavioral therapies.

Supportive and Problem-Solving Approaches

Health care professionals play a key role in helping people adjust to illness and may prevent the development of long-term distress by a sensitive and judicious approach. This should involve establishing a trusting relationship with the patient based on warmth and a genuine desire to help. Fear and uncertainty can be reduced by providing individuals with clear information. This may need to be repeated on several occasions, and it is important to convey the right amount of information so that individuals are not overwhelmed. The information should be presented in an authoritative but jargon-free manner. There should be a continual process of checking out what the person knows and doesn't know and what they want to know. The health professional should be guided by the person's responses and tailor the information accordingly. The health professional should be optimistic but realistic and avoid false reassurance.

There should be a collaborative approach to treatment so that patients themselves can make most of the decisions about their treatment. However, sometimes patients want doctors to play a more active, authoritative role in decision making, as was found in women attending clinics for breast cancer (Wright et al. 2004). This emphasizes the need to find out what different people want and tailor responses accordingly.

If possible, patients should be given emotional space to voice their fears and uncertainties about their illness or reflect on loss and explore ways of coping. This is rarely possible in busy hospital clinics or ward settings, but it should be an ideal to which all health professionals aspire. Any opportunity to foster beliefs in the controllability of the disease process will help the patient feel more empowered and less vulnerable. Involvement of patients' families in the treatment process is crucial, as illness affects the whole family and not just the individual with the illness.

Positive reassurance can be very helpful but must be based on and grow out of the physician's understanding of the patient's anxiety. The physician should explore any fears and not presume that he or she knows why the patient is asking without asking. Facile, nonspecific reassurance can undermine the therapeutic relationship, because the patient is likely to feel that the physician is out of touch with and not really interested in what he or she is actually feeling. Knowing, not presuming, the patient's specific fears leads the physician to appropriate therapeutic interventions.

The spiritual and cultural dimensions of peoples' lives are often overlooked by busy health professionals. Many religious organizations offer support and help for people at times of adversity, and other forms of cultural support may be available for certain groups of patients (e.g., gay men who are HIV positive).

Managing Uncertainty and Breaking Bad News

Physicians and other health professionals play a key role in providing patients and relatives with information. Often, information that is painful, difficult, and upsetting has to be conveyed. Common mistakes when giving bad news are to provide too little information about prognosis and to fail to explore people's concerns, fears, and associated feelings. Patients thus remain preoccupied with their fears and fail to take on board anything positive that the health professional has told them. Professionals also mistakenly think that once they have told a patient something, he or she will retain the information and will not need to be told again. However, people often need to be told something several times before they are able to assimilate the information.

People's responses to bad news are highly variable and unpredictable. There may be a whole range of emotions from extreme distress to utter blankness and denial. Two of the key principles of giving bad news well are 1) to tailor the information to what the patient wishes and is able and ready to hear and 2) to give enough time to the process. It is important to give the patient and his or her family members time to take in the information, without provoking denial or overwhelming distress. The physician should check out from the patient what he or she wants to know and in how much detail and tailor responses accordingly. A third principle is to acknowledge distress, to explore reasons for it, and to check that the patients would like to continue the discussion. Further guidelines on communicating risk and uncertainty and breaking bad news are provided in Chapter 2 of *The Psychological Care of Medical Patients: A Practical Guide*, 2nd Edition (Royal College of Physicians and Royal College of Psychiatrists 2003).

Illness Narratives

Writing about emotionally charged experiences in comparison with emotionally neutral topics appears to have a beneficial and cathartic effect (Pennebaker and Seagal 1999). Expressive writing has been shown to promote good health with beneficial outcomes on reported physical health, psychological well-being, physiological functioning, and general functioning (Smyth 1998).

Patients with chronic illness (either asthma or rheumatoid arthritis) also appear to benefit from being asked to write about an emotionally stressful experience (Stone et al. 2000). An interesting study involving women with early-stage breast cancer found that women who were rated low in avoidance found writing about "their deepest thoughts and feelings about breast cancer" to be very beneficial, and they reported significantly reduced physical symptoms over a 3-month follow-up period (Stanton et al. 2002). However, women who were rated high in avoidance gained greater benefit from writing about "positive thoughts and feelings about their experience of breast cancer." This suggests that although emotional writing may not be helpful for all people, it may be a simple and beneficial strategy for some people who are struggling to cope with physical illness. Emotional writing may be helpful because it enables people to express things that they cannot put into words (Bolton 2008).

Use of narratives has also been taken to a deeper level to help patients make sense of their depression in the context of physical illness (Viederman and Perry 1980). In this approach, the psychiatrist, after eliciting the patient's illness and life history, presents a statement that places the patient's physical illness in the context of his or her life trajectory and demonstrates the psychodynamic logic of the patient's depression (or other psychological response).

Counseling

There are many different forms of counseling, ranging from the imparting of information (educational counseling) to quite intensive psychotherapeutic interventions. One of the most common forms of therapeutic counseling is person-centered counseling. This is nondirective counseling in which emphasis is placed on the development of a personal relationship in which an individual can talk openly and freely about his or her problems. The counselor employs specific skills, such as warmth, empathy, and attentive listening. Counseling involves skilled use of nonspecific psychotherapeutic techniques.

Counseling is widely employed in health service settings to help people adjust better to illness. There are relatively few controlled evaluations of the benefits of counseling in relation to physical illness. An exception is in the field of cancer, where there have been several evaluations by different research groups of the effects of counseling (Christensen 1983; Maguire et al. 1980, 1983). A recent systematic review of psychosocial interventions for anxiety and depression in adult cancer patients concluded that interventions involving counseling can be currently recommended for improving patients' general functional ability or quality of life, degree of depression, and interpersonal relationships (Jacobsen and Jim 2008). However, the review noted the general poor methodological quality of many studies. Counseling has been shown to be helpful for improving the psychological status of persons with systemic lupus erythematosus (Maisiak et al. 1996).

Hypnosis

Hypnosis has been used as a treatment for medical conditions for more than 300 years. There is no consensus view as to what exactly hypnosis is, but it involves the induction of a state of mind in which a person's normal critical nature is bypassed, allowing for acceptance of suggestions. In hypnosis used for the treatment of medical conditions, suggestions are made to the patient, while he or she is hypnotized, about the patient's bodily state, which hopefully results in an improvement in function or a reduction in pain. The role of hypnosis in contemporary medicine has been reviewed by Stewart (2005). The best evidence for hypnotherapy in the field of liaison psychiatry comes from work in relation to irritable bowel syndrome (Whorwell et al. 1984). Hypnotherapy for irritable bowel syndrome is gut directed. The treatment involves the induction of a hypnotic trance using progressive relaxation and other induction procedures to deepen the hypnotic state. This is followed by suggestions, imagery, and other techniques appropriate to the individual, such as inducing warmth through the patient's hands on the abdomen, directed toward control and normalization of gut function, in addition to relevant ego-strengthening interventions. Patients are given one-to-one treatment over several weeks and also asked to practice skills on a daily basis using an autohypnosis tape. This kind of treatment can also be delivered in a group format.

Problem-Solving Therapy

Problem-solving therapy improves individuals' abilities to cope with stressful life difficulties. It has three main steps: 1) symptoms and problems are identified, and the two are linked together; 2) the problems are defined and clarified; and 3) strategies are developed in a collaborative fashion with the patient to help solve the problems in a systematic way. The overall intention is to break problems down into very small components which then become easier to tackle and solve. Problem solving has been employed in a pure form to treat depression or other problems in primary care. It is a relatively brief intervention, with one of the earliest studies involving six sessions and a total contact time of less than 4 hours (Hawton and Kirk 1989).

Problem-solving therapy has been used to help patients with cancer (Nezu et al. 2003) and has also been incorporated into more complex treatment interventions involving stepped-care models for treating depression or collaborative care models.

Self-Management Programs

Self-management programs or chronic care models are becoming increasingly popular for patients with chronic illness. They consist of a structured primary care–based framework aimed at improving the self-care and management of patients with chronic illnesses. Most include proactive involvement and support from care managers or case workers, with an emphasis on patient education, psychosocial support, and promotion of self-management strategies and skills. A meta-analysis of data from 112 studies involving interventions to improve self-care for chronic illness (e.g., asthma, diabetes, congestive heart failure, and depression) concluded that interventions that contain at least one element of a chronic care model improve clinical outcomes and quality of life for patients with chronic illness (Tsai et al. 2005).

Supportive–Expressive Therapies and Support Groups

A variety of different kinds of supportive therapy groups have been used in the psychosocial treatment for patients with cancer, and several randomized investigations have shown positive effects on psychosocial adjustment (Cain et al. 1986; Edmonds et al. 1999; Fawzy et al. 1990, 1993; Spiegel et al. 1981), trauma symptoms (Classen et al. 2009), physical status (Fawzy et al. 1990, 1993; Spiegel et al. 1981), and survival (Cunningham et al. 1998; Fawzy et al. 1993; Spiegel et al. 1989). The effects on survival are controversial and have not been replicated by other researchers (Goodwin et al. 2001), although the positive effects on emotional adjustment seem robust.

The group therapeutic approaches that have received most attention are those employing supportive–expressive group therapy, which is an unstructured but quite intensive and existentially based treatment (Spiegel and Glafkides 1983). The rationale for the existential orientation presumes that living with a terminal illness amplifies existential concerns of death, meaning, freedom, and isolation. Thus, one aim of the group intervention is to give patients an opportunity to discuss these concerns. The treatment strategy is to facilitate discussion of issues that are uppermost in patients' minds rather than imposing the topics to be discussed, although the group experience can be quite challenging and intensive.

The supportive-expressive group-based approach should not be confused with supportive-expressive therapy, which is a short-term psychodynamic treatment and is discussed under "Relational Therapies" below.

Relational Therapies

A broad group of therapies have in common a model of human development and the mind in which the nature and quality of human interpersonal relationships play a key role in the maintenance of "emotional homeostasis." Close interpersonal relationships can either be a source of stress or act as a buffer against adversity to provide emotional support and foster resilience. The earliest relationship, that between mother and infant or main caregiver and infant, is crucially important in shaping identity, cognitive function, and the ability to regulate and control feelings. As adults, the bonds that we form with others help us to maintain our sense of "self." If the bonds break down or become noxious, this may precipitate anxiety and depression. Relational therapies are based on the premise that feelings, thoughts, and relationships are intimately tied up with each other. How we feel and think about others affects how we behave toward them, and this, in turn, affects how we feel about ourselves.

A variety of different theories and models of development, including psychodynamic, attachment, and interpersonal, link together previous relationship experiences, current relationship experiences, and emotions and coping. Individuals with a history of childhood adversity have an increased likelihood of both emotional and physical problems as adults. People with certain kinds of insecure attachment styles find physical illness more difficult to manage than those with secure attachment and may default on medical appointments or find it more difficult to establish trusting relationships with health professionals (Ciechanowski et al. 2004).

Physical illness is a threat to the self, and nearly all aspects of being physically ill impact the interpersonal domain. At a very deep level, some people construe their illness as a personal attack on themselves, asking "Why me?" At other levels, physical illness can put an immense strain on families and their relationships. Severe or chronic physical illness often changes people and forces them to reappraise themselves and their relationships. Issues of loss—for example, fears of loss or dying, fears of becoming dependent and a burden on others, fears of having to cope alone—are extremely common in the physically ill and can be addressed by relational therapies (see also Chapter 4, "Psychological Responses to Illness").

Interpersonal Therapy

Interpersonal therapy (IPT) was developed at Yale University in the late 1960s as a time-limited treatment for depression (Klerman et al. 1984). The basic underlying assumption of the treatment approach is that there is a relationship between the onset and recurrence of a depressive episode and a person's social and interpersonal relationships at the time. The model was influenced by the work of Sullivan (1953) and Bowlby (1969).

There are three stages of development in IPT when it is used to treat depression. In the first phase, depression is diagnosed and explained to the patient so there is a clear understanding of the nature of the condition and its symptoms. An interpersonal inventory is compiled that lists all of the patient's relationships, and the main problem areas are identified. Problem areas are classified into four groups: grief, role transitions, role disputes, and interpersonal deficits.

During the intermediate sessions of therapy, the therapist and client work on a specific problem area. If this is grief, treatment includes facilitating the grieving process, helping the client accept difficult or painful feelings, and exploring ways of replacing lost relationships. If the problem is a role transition, treatment is focused on helping the client give up the old role, accepting feelings of loss about this, and acquiring skills and support in the new role the client has to take on (e.g., becoming a parent). If the problem area is a role dispute, the focus of the treatment is about gaining a better understanding of the nature of the dispute and exploring ways that it could be resolved. If the problem area is an interpersonal deficit or deficits, the focus of the treatment is to gain a better understanding of the nature of the deficit and any problems the client has with the way he or she interacts and communicates with people. Attempts are made to try to modify these problematic interactions using a variety of techniques, including role-play.

In the final part of the therapy, the therapist works to consolidate the client's gains and addresses the termination of therapy, with a focus on strategies that can prevent the depression from recurring.

IPT has a solid evidence base, with a recent systematic review concluding that it is an effective treatment for depression, superior to placebo and comparable to antidepressants (de Mello et al. 2005). IPT has been modified to treat depression in a variety of different settings with different populations (e.g., maintenance therapy for recurrent depression, bipolar disorder, eating disorders, anxiety disorders, borderline personality disorders, postpartum depression, and depression in developing countries) (Weissman 2006).

Several elements of IPT are highly relevant to the general medical setting and to patients who have emotional difficulties secondary to physical illness. In particular, grief (e.g., loss of a body part) and role transition (e.g., having to change from being an active and healthy person to someone who is confined to a wheelchair) are extremely common problem areas. IPT has been used to good effect to treat depression in HIV-positive patients (Markowitz et al. 1995), and it has also been adapted for the treatment of posttraumatic stress disorder, which is common in some medical settings. Two small studies of telephone IPT have been published (Badger et al. 2005; Donnelly et al. 2000), in which IPT was used to help alleviate emotional distress in cancer patients and their spouses.

IPT has also been adapted for use in hypochondriasis (Stuart and Noyes 2005). In this condition, the therapy has been adapted to focus on the interpersonal consequences of being preoccupied with physical illness.

Psychodynamic Interpersonal Therapy ("Conversational Model" Therapy)

This form of treatment has been developed by Hobson (1985), a psychiatrist and psychotherapist. Psychodynamic interpersonal therapy (PIT) combines elements of psychodynamic and interpersonal therapies. It places greater emphasis on the patient–therapist relationship as a tool for resolving interpersonal issues than does IPT, and there is less emphasis on the interpretation of transference than in psychodynamic therapies. One of the central tenets of PIT is the importance of human experience and an individual's sense of self within a personal relationship. Human existence is regarded as being essentially relational, and man is regarded as a "creature of the between." This applies even to people who live a solitary existence.

The emphasis in the therapy is on getting to know someone, rather than merely knowing *about* them. In the words of Hobson (1985), "In an unrepeatable moment, I hope to respond to my unique client by sharing in an ongoing act of creation, expressing and shaping immediate experience in the making and remaking of a verbal and nonverbal language of feeling. It is not only a matter of 'knowing about' someone but also, and mainly, of sharing a language of 'knowing'" (p. xiii). Hobson believed that the heart of psychotherapy is that of a personal relationship—a meeting between two people and a process of symbolic transformation of self and experience by means of a personal conversation.

The process of symbolic transformation is particularly valuable when using the PIT model with people who have both physical and psychological symptoms (Moorey and Guthrie 2003). The client and therapist begin by exploring the "minute particulars" of the client's physical symptom experience. The client is encouraged to explore and describe his or her physical symptoms in great depth, and the therapist assumes an attitude of intense listening, concern, and fascination. It is in the detail of the conversation that metaphors or feeling language emerges, as the client and therapist go deeper and deeper into the client's physical experience. Expressions such as "off balance," used to describe neurological symptoms, come to also represent psychological and emotional states of mind. The process is collaborative, gradual, and nonthreatening. The conversation gradually moves from being about physical symptoms to what Hobson (1985) described as a "feeling language." This process of symbolic transformation leads to a change in the experience of the self and a move toward a greater understanding of the connection between physical and psychological, followed by psychological and emotional change.

Key features of the model include 1) the assumption that the patient's problems arise from or are exacerbated by disturbances of significant personal relationships; 2) a tentative, encouraging, supportive approach from the therapist, who seeks to develop deeper understanding with the patient through negotiation, exploration of feelings, and use of metaphor; 3) the linkage of the patient's distress to specific interpersonal problems; and 4) the use of the therapeutic relationship to address problems and test out solutions in the "here and now." Emphasis is placed on identifying repeated patterns of behavior within relationships that result in conflict and emotional distress. Support and encouragement is provided to the patient to challenge difficult problem areas in relationships and to develop more adaptive ways of coping.

PIT has efficacy comparable to that of cognitive therapy for the treatment of depression (Shapiro et al. 1994) and has been adapted for use in medically unexplained symptoms. PIT has been evaluated in several large randomized controlled trials (RCTs) (Creed et al. 2003; Guthrie et al. 1991; J. Hamilton et al. 2000). It is cost effective, with the costs of therapy being recouped by reductions in health care use in the months posttherapy (Creed et al. 2003; Guthrie et al. 1999). It has also been used after self-harm and was found to result in a reduction in repetition in the subsequent 6 months following the index episode (Guthrie et al. 2001).

Cognitive-Behavioral Therapy

The central tenet of CBT is that emotions, behavior, and cognitions are all interlinked. According to the cognitive model, when a person shows distressing emotions such as anxiety or depression, these emotions are linked to particular beliefs, assumptions, or thoughts. It is assumed that persistent distress is linked to underlying maladaptive beliefs, which if modified results in a reduction in emotional distress.

In the general medical setting, the way a person thinks about his or her illness or bodily sensations is central to the cognitive model. If, for example, benign sensations are regarded by the person as being symptomatic of disease, several consequences ensue. First, the patient will become emotionally distressed, which may cause further bodily sensations. Second, the patient will pay increased attention to these symptoms and may worry about them more. Third, the types of behaviors the person employs to cope with the symptoms may exacerbate the symptoms rather than relieve them (e.g., rubbing one's chest if it is painful). Fourth, other people, including doctors, may respond to the patient in a way that intensifies, rather than reduces, the patient's concern with disease, attention to bodily sensations, and dysfunctional coping (Sharpe et al. 1992).

This model is applicable to patients with medically unexplained symptoms, but also to patients with medical disease (e.g., concerns about recurrence of a breast lump after previous diagnosis and treatment for breast cancer).

Sensky (2004) has described in detail how CBT has been adapted for use in people with physical illnesses. Crucial to the development of any treatment intervention is an understanding of the patient's model of his or her illness, and a useful model or framework for doing this has been developed by Moss-Morris et al. (2002) in relation to illness perception. This concept was originally developed by Leventhal et al. (1997). Within Leventhal's model, illness representations are considered to be multidimensional, comprising five main components: identity, perceived consequences, timeline, perceived cause, and control/cure (Table 39–1).

A key principle in cognitive therapy is that the patient, rather than the therapist, is the expert in understanding the patient's problems. A detailed understanding of the patient's illness perceptions often leads to identification of maladaptive beliefs and underlying fears or anxieties, which can then be addressed.

CBT is tailored to the individual patient's beliefs and behavior, although certain cognitions are likely to be associated with particular presenting symptoms. For example, it is common for patients who experience chest pain to fear that they are going to have a heart attack, and they will become very anxious every time chest pain is experienced.

If someone believes that his chest pain is indicative of a heart attack and repeatedly seeks reassurance every time chest pain is experienced, that reassurance is characteristically short-lived, and the behavior becomes counterproductive. The therapist can address this kind of behavior in the therapy session, particularly if the client develops pain or seeks reassurance from the therapist during the session itself. The therapist can ask the patient to keep a diary between sessions, quantifying at various times the extent of his worry and/or reassurance on a 0–10 scale. Having identified that the behavior is unhelpful and only increases anxiety and worry, patient and therapist can then collaborate to devise ways of managing the problem behavior and beliefs more effectively.

This is done by devising behavioral and/or cognitive experiments aiming to produce more favorable outcomes. Thus, in the above example, a behavioral experiment might be for the patient to delay seeking reassurance about his chest pain for progressively longer periods, to demonstrate that he is able to tolerate the anxiety involved. A cognitive task might be to prepare a statement (and perhaps even to write the statement down on a "cue card") regarding the unhelpful outcomes of reassurance seeking that the patient can remind himself about when he experiences the urge to seek reassurance. Each of these tasks might be rehearsed in the therapy session, so that the patient has some confidence that the possible benefits of carrying out the tasks between sessions outweigh the perceived risks.

In some cases, the entire focus of treatment can remain on the present and the recent past, particularly if the patient experiences symptoms in the "here and now" in the therapy session. However, beliefs that are maladaptive commonly have their origins in the more distant past, particularly during childhood, and when this occurs, it is an appropriate focus in therapy to make links between the present and the past.

TABLE 39–1. Leventhal and colleagues' five components of illness representations

Identity:	Label or name given to the condition and the symptoms that go with it.
Cause:	Ideas about the perceived cause of the condition (may or may not be based on biomedical evidence).
Timeline:	Predictive beliefs about how long the condition will last.
Consequences:	Individual beliefs about the consequences of the condition and how these affect people physically and socially.
Curability/controllability:	Beliefs about whether the condition can be cured or kept under control.

Source. Leventhal et al. 1997.

TABLE 39–2. Cognitive factors in the assessment of the physically ill

Illness model and illness perception: What is the patient's understanding of his/her illness, and how does this contribute to worry or distress, or to maladaptive behaviors and beliefs?

Personalized formulation of the patient's problem: How can the patient's physical symptoms, emotional response, behavior, and cognitions be linked together in an understandable and meaningful formulation?

Affective disturbance: Is the patient experiencing anxiety, fears, depression, or hopelessness?

Motivation: Prochaska's stages of change model (Prochaska et al. 1994):

Precontemplation—Is the patient avoiding thinking about the consequences of illness?
Contemplation—Is the patient beginning to face that changes have to be made to adapt to the impact of the illness?
Preparation—Is the patient taking steps necessary for action?
Action—Is the patient making the required changes?
Maintenance—Are the changes/adaptations being maintained?

Coping: What are the patient's emotion-focused and problem-focused ways of coping? Which of these are helpful? Which are not helpful?

Life transitions: How is the individual managing the impact of illness on his/her life, and what can be learned from the way he/she has managed previous life transitions?

Influence of others: How are the patient's relationships with doctors and other professionals, family, and friends influenced by the patient's beliefs about his/her illness? Conversely, how do the patient's illness beliefs influence his/her relationships with others?

Resilience: What are the patient's areas of vulnerability in regard to his/her responses to stress? What are his/her strengths?

Source. Adapted from Guthrie and Sensky 2008.

Other cognitive factors in the assessment of the physically ill have been described by Guthrie and Sensky (2008) and are summarized in Table 39–2.

CBT is a recognized treatment for many different psychiatric disorders (Butler et al. 2006). There is a substantial evidence base for CBT, both for the treatment of medically unexplained symptoms and for the treatment of depression in physical illness (Fekete et al. 2007). Both of these areas will be reviewed later in the chapter. Areas for development in the future include computer-delivered CBT (Kaltenthaler et al. 2006) and Internet-based CBT (Cuijpers et al. 2008).

Mindfulness-Based Stress Reduction Interventions

Mindfulness-based stress reduction (MBSR) is a well-defined systematic educational, patient-focused intervention with formal training in mindfulness meditation and its applications in everyday life, which includes managing physical and emotional pain. It was developed by Jon Kabat-Zinn and colleagues at the University of Massachusetts. MBSR has grown rapidly in the medical setting, and MBSR programs are now offered in health care settings around the world. A useful review of its practice in the medical setting has been written by Ott et al. (2006). MBSR programs generally consist of 7–10 weekly group sessions. Each session lasts 1 to 1.5 hours, and in addition there is one silent retreat. Classes include both an educational component and an experiential component. During the groups, participants are taught meditation fundamentals and practice sitting meditation, awareness of sensations, body scan and mindfulness movement, which they are expected to practice for 45 minutes on a daily basis. During the first class, participants receive an audiotape so they can practice at home for 45 minutes every day. Participants are also encouraged to bring informal mindfulness into day-to-day activities whenever the opportunity arises.

MBSR has been particularly developed in relation to helping patients cope with cancer. Patients with cancer often experience a loss of control and feelings of helplessness. MBSR is a useful skill that can be used by patients to help reduce and cope with stress, promote relaxation, and alleviate physical discomfort and emotional distress. Mindfulness helps patients to take a proactive stance by consciously directing their attention to present-moment experiences.

Bringing attention to the senses is generally unthreatening and easy to experience. Patients are also asked to focus on their breathing during sitting meditation. They may become aware that they are not breathing fully but rather are limiting inspiration to the upper part of the chest, losing the benefit of abdominal breathing. As patients continue to focus on breathing, the breath becomes a familiar focal point, and they are then able to move on and focus on other physical sensations. Even strong physical sensations such as pain can become less intense and less frightening using MBSR.

The body scan enables patients to develop a focused concentrated awareness of the body, moving attention methodically from the toes to the head. Patients become aware of subtle changes which are happening on a moment-to-moment basis, and unpleasant sensations become more tolerable. Mindfulness movement invites a compassionate, ongoing awareness of the body in motion (Ott et al. 2006).

Mindfulness-Based Cognitive Therapy

Mindfulness-based cognitive therapy (MBCT) has been adapted from mindfulness stress reduction program approaches as a treatment for depression (Segal et al. 2002). It includes simple breathing meditations and yoga stretches to help participants become more aware of the present moment, including getting in touch with moment-to-moment changes in the mind and the body. Participants attend eight weekly educational classes where they are taught and practice the techniques of mindfulness meditation, and also listen to tapes at home during the week. MBCT also includes basic education about depression and several exercises from cognitive therapy that show the links between thinking and feeling and how best participants can look after themselves when depression threatens to overwhelm them. These more structured exercises make MBCT different from mindfulness meditation as it is normally taught at retreat centers, but the approach is embedded within and seeks to remain true to the insight meditation tradition.

MBCT helps participants in the classes to see more clearly the patterns of the mind and to learn how to recognize when their mood is beginning to go down. Unlike formal CBT, which seeks to link negative thoughts and mood and then change negative thoughts to lift mood, MBCT encourages participants to "let go" of their thoughts and break the link between negative mood and the negative thinking. Participants develop the capacity to allow distressing mood, thoughts, and sensations to come and go, without having to battle with them. They find that they can stay in touch with the present moment without having to ruminate about the past or worry about the future.

MBCT is rapidly becoming established as a treatment for depression and as a treatment to prevent depression recurring in vulnerable individuals (Teasdale et al. 2000). MBCT reduces overgeneral autobiographical memory, which has been implicated as a potential mediator of self-harm, and MBCT is now being evaluated as a treatment to alleviate suicidal thinking in vulnerable people. Individuals with overgeneralized autobiographical memory present vague, nonspecific memories when asked about their past or ways in the past they have solved problems. Unlike individuals with more specific memory recall, they do not have a range of specific past experiences from which to draw to attempt to solve current difficulties or problems.

Mindfulness-based therapies have been used to treat a wide range of stress disorders, including chronic pain (Kabat-Zinn et al. 1987), fibromyalgia (Kaplan et al. 1993; Sephton et al. 2007), mood symptoms in cancer (Carlson et al. 2001, 2003; Smith et al. 2005), and depression (Teasdale et al. 2000). A recent systematic review of meditation techniques for medical illness identified 20 RCTs involving a total of 958 subjects (Arias et al. 2006). The reviewers concluded that the strongest evidence for the efficacy of meditative techniques was found for epilepsy, symptoms of premenstrual syndrome, and menopausal symptoms. Benefit was also demonstrated for mood and anxiety disorders, autoimmune illness, and emotional disturbance in neoplastic disease. Ott et al. (2006) identified nine studies in the field of cancer that had used mindfulness meditation, of which four were RCTs and the other five were one-group pretest–posttest design studies. The reviewers concluded that mindfulness interventions showed promising results in the field of cancer but that more RCTs were required before firm conclusions about efficacy could be established. Ledesma and Kumano (2009) recently published a meta-analysis of 10 MBSR studies in the field of cancer which included 4 RCTs and 6 non-RCTs. Three of the 4 RCTs in this latter study were included in the earlier review by Ott et al. (2006). Ledesma and Kumano (2009) computed an effect size (Cohen's d) for change in mental and physical health resulting from MBSR. The effect size for improvement in mental health was moderate ($d=0.48$), whereas the effect size for improvement in physical health was quite small ($d=0.18$).

Organization and Delivery of Psychological Treatments

Although psychological treatments can be offered as stand-alone treatments, they are increasingly delivered as part of a package of care or part of a stepped-care model. This is particularly so for the treatment of depression but applies to many other psychological conditions including medically unexplained symptoms and depression in the context of chronic physical illness.

The stepped-care model involves five different intensities of treatment that are offered to the patient or client according to the severity or complexity of his or her problems. Most patients start at the bottom of this model and progress to the next step only if their symptoms do not improve:

- Step 1 involves watchful waiting, as many patients who present with symptoms will find that their symptoms resolve spontaneously without requiring any help.

- Step 2 usually involves some form of guided self-help and may include computerized CBT, psychoeducation, or help from voluntary organizations. Exercise may also be recommended or even prescribed if such treatment is available from a relevant health service organization.
- Step 3 involves brief psychological therapy (e.g., CBT, counseling, interpersonal therapies) for 6–8 sessions. Antidepressants may be prescribed if there is a previous history of moderate to severe depression.
- Step 4 involves depression case management, and the patient may be assigned a case manager or key worker. Medication and more intensive psychological treatments may be offered, with care coordinated by the case manager working with the patient's primary care physician.
- Step 5 is for patients who have not responded to the previous 4 steps. Step 5 may involve crisis intervention services, inpatient treatment, or even more intensive multicomponent treatment packages.

Collaborative care models have five essential elements:

1. Collaborative definition of problems, in which patient-defined problems are identified alongside medical problems diagnosed by health care professionals
2. Focus on specific problems and use of problem-solving techniques
3. Creation of a range of self-management training and support services
4. Provision of active follow-up in which patients are contacted at regular intervals to monitor health status and check and reinforce progress in implementing the care plan
5. Assignment of a case manager who has responsibility for delivering the care plan

Sometimes stepped-care programs are incorporated into collaborative care interventions, as in the Pathways Study (Katon et al. 2004), which tested a complex intervention to treat depression in patients with diabetes. The intervention involved an initial choice of two treatments, either an antidepressant or problem-solving therapy, followed by a stepped-care algorithm in which patients received different types and intensities of treatment according to their observed outcomes. In comparison with usual care, patients who received the complex intervention improved significantly in relation to depression, but there was no impact on glycemic control.

Evidence Base for Psychological Treatments for Specific Conditions

Patients With Medically Unexplained Symptoms or Somatoform Disorders

There is a substantial evidence base for the efficacy and effectiveness of psychological treatments for people with medically unexplained symptoms or somatoform disorders. Most studies have involved patients with specific symptom-defined syndromes, such as chronic fatigue syndrome and irritable bowel syndrome. It remains unclear whether these conditions are discrete entities (W.T. Hamilton et al. 2009) or share a common underlying problem of bodily symptom distress (Fink et al. 2007). There is, however, substantial overlap among the conditions, and psychological approaches that are shown to be helpful for one condition are likely to benefit patients who present with a different symptom pattern but similar psychological concerns.

Psychosocial factors such as depression, anxiety, childhood adversity, stressful life events, and chronic difficulties are common in people who have medically unexplained symptoms that are persistent and severe and who seek treatment. Psychological morbidity is less prevalent in community subjects with medically unexplained symptoms who do not seek treatment. Most studies that have evaluated the efficacy or effectiveness of psychological interventions in patients with medically unexplained symptoms have been carried out on patients in secondary- or tertiary-care settings who have moderate to severe symptoms. There are far fewer primary care–based studies, and these tend to show less substantial treatment effects than studies conducted in secondary-care settings (Raine et al. 2002). A recent systematic review of the efficacy of treatment (pharmacological and nonpharmacological) for fibromyalgia concluded that there was little difference in treatment effects according to whether patients were treated in primary or secondary care (Garcia-Campayo et al. 2008).

Several systematic or critical reviews summarizing the effects of psychological treatment for medically unexplained symptoms or somatoform disorders have been published over the past 10–15 years as the evidence base has been growing. The majority of studies have focused on CBT interventions, although (as discussed earlier in this chapter) other relational therapies have been evaluated and shown to be of benefit in certain conditions, although there are far fewer "non-CBT" studies.

Tables 39–3 through 39–5 summarize the findings of reviews carried out on three common functional somatic syndromes: fibromyalgia, chronic fatigue syndrome, and irritable bowel syndrome. Most of the reviews comment on the variability of the psychological interventions studied

TABLE 39–3. Systematic reviews, critical reviews, and meta-analyses of trials of psychological treatment in fibromyalgia

Authors	Therapy	Type of review	Outcome
Rossy et al. 1999	Pharmacological and nonpharmacological treatment	Meta-analysis (4 studies)	Evidence for benefits for CBT and exercise.
Hadhazy et al. 2000	Mind–body therapies	Systematic review (13 studies)	Moderate evidence that mind–body therapies are more effective for some clinical outcomes than wait list, treatment as usual, or placebo.
Sim and Adams 2002	Nonpharmacological treatment	Systematic review (25 RCTs)	Strong evidence did not emerge for any single intervention. Preliminary support for aerobic exercise.
Van Koulil et al. 2007	CBT and exercise programs	Systematic review (30 studies)	Nonpsychological treatments such as CBT have a limited effect on pain, disability, and mood.
Garcia-Campayo et al. 2008	Pharmacological and nonpharmacological outpatient and inpatient treatments	Meta-analysis (33 RCTs)	Treating fibromyalgia in specialized care centers offers no clear advantages over outpatient treatment.
Häuser et al. 2009	Multicomponent treatments	Meta-analysis (9 RCTs)	Strong evidence that multicomponent treatment has beneficial short-term effects.

Note. CBT=cognitive-behavioral therapy; RCT=randomized controlled trial.

and the diverse population groups included in the RCTs and highlight a variety of methodological concerns, including small numbers and therefore a lack of power, lack of blinded assessments in some trials, and poor quality of randomization procedures. In general, methodological rigor has improved over time, with more recent studies showing evidence of improved methodological quality.

Fibromyalgia

Several different psychological approaches have been evaluated for patients with fibromyalgia, such as multicomponent treatment, CBT, exercise programs, relaxation therapy, and educational interventions. There appears to be evidence for modest effects for these treatments, with the best evidence for multicomponent treatment (at least one educational intervention plus one psychological therapy plus one exercise therapy) rather than specific individual treatments. Multicomponent treatment appears to have beneficial short-term effects on the key symptoms of fibromyalgia, including pain, low physical fitness, and depressive symptoms, but there is little evidence of long-term gain.

Chronic Fatigue Syndrome

There is better evidence for the benefits of CBT for chronic fatigue syndrome, with the most recent meta-analytic review (which included 13 studies) suggesting that CBT is "moderately efficacious" (Malouff et al. 2008). The reviewers also reported a substantial but nonsignificant association between the number of treatment hours and the effect size, which supports the dose–response literature for psychotherapy (i.e., clients tend to show sequential improvements per session, up to 10–16 sessions [Lambert and Ogles 2004]). Malouff et al. (2008) additionally carried out a comparison between treatments with and without cognitive elements and found no evidence that including cognitive components led to a greater effect. In fact, a trend occurred in favor of *not* including cognitive components. This supports the findings of an earlier review of studies employing a variety of different psychological treatment interventions, which reported evidence for the effectiveness of CBT and graded exercise programs (Whiting et al. 2001).

Irritable Bowel Syndrome

The most recent systematic review of treatment interventions for irritable bowel syndrome included the evaluation of the efficacy of antidepressants and psychological therapies (Ford et al. 2009). The reviewers concluded that both antidepressants and psychological therapies were effective in the treatment of irritable bowel syndrome and of comparable efficacy (number needed to treat [NNT]=4 for

TABLE 39–4. Systematic reviews, critical reviews, and meta-analyses of trials of psychological treatment in chronic fatigue syndrome (CFS)

Authors	Therapy	Type of review	Outcome
Whiting et al. 2001	Pharmacological and nonpharmacological	Systematic review (36 RCTs, 8 controlled trials)	Mixed results in terms of effectiveness. CBT and graded exercise showed promising results.
Looper and Kirmayer 2002	CBT	Critical review (4 studies)	Positive outcomes in most studies.
Rimes and Chalder 2005	Pharmacological and nonpharmacological	Systematic review	Most promising results were for CBT and graded exercise therapy.
Chambers et al. 2006	Pharmacological and nonpharmacological	Systematic review (70 studies)	Increase in size and quality of evidence base on interventions for CFS/ME. Promising results shown for some behavioral interventions in reducing symptoms of CFS/ME and improving physical functioning.
Malouff et al. 2008	CBT	Meta-analysis (13 RCTs)	Significant difference (Cohen's d=0.48) in posttreatment fatigue between CBT and control conditions.

Note. CBT=cognitive-behavioral therapy; ME=myalgic encephalomyelitis; RCT=randomized controlled trial.

both types of treatment), although there was less high-quality evidence for routine use of psychological therapies.

Seven studies included in the Ford et al. (2009) review involved CBT, with an estimated NNT of 3, although there was statistically significant heterogeneity between studies and evidence of funnel plot asymmetry. When some of the smaller studies were removed from the analysis, the beneficial effect of CBT on irritable bowel syndrome symptoms disappeared. There were two studies on hypnotherapy (NNT=2) and two studies on dynamic therapy (NNT=3.5). Multicomponent treatment was evaluated in three studies (NNT=4).

A previous systematic review of psychological treatments for irritable bowel syndrome by Lackner et al. (2004) identified 10 studies eligible for inclusion in a meta-analysis, involving a total of 185 patients, and reported a number needed to treat of 2. The more recent review by Ford et al. (2009), however, included data on almost 1,300 patients

TABLE 39–5. Systematic reviews, critical reviews, and meta-analyses of trials of psychological treatment in irritable bowel syndrome (IBS)

Authors	Therapy	Type of review	Outcome
Lackner et al. 2004	Psychological treatment	Systematic review and meta-analysis (17 RCTs)	Psychological treatments were effective for IBS (NNT=2).
Blanchard 2005	CBT	Critical review	Good evidence for efficacy of CBT interventions in the short term. Long-term outcome was rarely evaluated.
Wilson et al. 2006	Hypnotherapy	Systematic review (6 controlled/RCT, 12 uncontrolled)	Suggestive evidence of significant benefit.
Ford et al. 2009	Antidepressants and psychological therapies	Systematic review and meta-analysis (32 RCTs)	Antidepressants are effective in the treatment of IBS. There is less high-quality evidence for psychological therapies, although they may be of comparable efficacy. (NNT=4 for both interventions.)

Note. CBT=cognitive-behavioral therapy; NNT=number needed to treat; RCT=randomized controlled trial.

randomly assigned to some form of psychological intervention and employed much more rigorous methods. Ford and colleagues' more conservative estimate of number needed to treat (NNT=4) is probably a better indicator of likely treatment effects but still suggests that psychological treatments have a good evidence base for the treatment of irritable bowel syndrome.

Chronic Pain

Several systematic or meta-analytic reviews of psychological treatment or CBT for chronic pain have been published over the past 20 years. Each review has included different groups of pain patients (e.g., patients with headache and dental pain, with low back pain, with back pain and fibromyalgia). Table 39-6 summarizes the main conclusions from these reviews. Of particular interest, A. Williams and Morley (2009) recently updated an influential review of psychological treatments for persistent pain (excluding headache) that they first published in 1999 (Morley et al. 1999).

The original review identified 25 trials suitable for meta-analysis but commented that most trials were underpowered with small numbers, and some were overcomplex with multiple treatment and control groups (Morley et al. 1999). The authors concluded that CBT, when compared with wait-list control conditions, was associated with significant effect sizes on all domains of measurement (median effect size across domains=0.5). However, when CBT was compared with other treatments or control conditions across the same range of outcomes, the efficacy of CBT was of a smaller magnitude and limited to fewer outcome measures of pain and coping.

The updated review identified 50 studies suitable for data extraction. Treatments were classified as behavioral treatment (BT) or CBT. The authors found that pain improved with BT and CBT compared with treatment as usual at the assessment immediately posttreatment but not at the follow-up assessment (A. Williams and Morley 2009). Effect sizes were small to medium: 0.18 for CBT (22 studies, >1,200 patients) and 0.48 for BT (8 studies, 564 patients). The authors found no difference between BT or CBT when compared with other active treatment control conditions.

They found a small but positive effect on mood for CBT compared with both treatment as usual conditions and active control conditions, immediately posttreatment (16 trials, 1,001 patients, effect size=0.16) and at follow-up (17 trials, 873 patients, effect size=0.19). They concluded that CBT showed disappointingly small effects on pain and other primary treatment targets (A. Williams and Morley 2009).

The evidence for multidisciplinary interventions as opposed to single-modality treatments for chronic pain

TABLE 39–6. Systematic reviews, critical reviews, and meta-analyses of trials of psychological treatment in chronic pain

Authors	Therapy	Type of review	Outcome
Carroll and Seers 1998	Relaxation	Systematic review (9 RCTs)	Insufficient evidence to confirm that relaxation can reduce chronic pain.
Morley et al. 1999	CBT and BT	Systematic review and meta-analysis (25 RCTs)	Psychological treatments based on CBT are effective. Median effect size across domains was 0.5 for CBT vs. wait-list controls.
Raine et al. 2002	CBT	Systematic review (16 studies)	Sustained improvements in pain, depression, and disability.
Bailey 2002	Psychological treatment	Meta-analysis (146 interventions)	Psychological interventions showed small effects.
Hoffman et al. 2007	Psychosocial interventions	Meta-analysis (22 RCTs)	CBT and self-regulatory treatments were efficacious.
Scascighini et al. 2008	Multidisciplinary treatments	Systematic review (35 RCTs)	Strong evidence for multidisciplinary treatments vs. standard medical treatment for pain.
A. Williams and Morley 2009	Psychological treatments	Systematic review and meta-analysis (62 RCTs)	Effect sizes for pain were small to medium for CBT (0.18) and BT (0.48) vs. treatment as usual immediately posttreatment, although there was no difference at follow-up.

Note. BT=behavior therapy; CBT=cognitive-behavioral therapy; RCT=randomized controlled trial.

seems to be stronger. A minimum standard of multidisciplinary therapy would include the following: specific individual exercising, regular training in relaxation techniques, group therapy led by a clinical psychologist (1.5 hours per week), patient education sessions (once per week), physiotherapy treatments (two per week) for pacing strategies, medical training therapy, and neurophysiology information given by a trained physician (Scascighini et al. 2008).

A recent systematic review of multidisciplinary interventions for chronic pain identified 27 studies involving a total of 2,407 patients (Scascighini et al. 2008). Eighteen of the studies were performed in an outpatient setting, 4 in an inpatient setting, and 4 studies compared inpatient treatment with outpatient treatment. The duration of programs varied, ranging from 4 to 15 weeks for outpatient programs and from 3 to 8 weeks for inpatient programs. Based on available data, the median duration of all treatments was 45 hours. The quality of the trials varied, with many being judged to suffer from a lack of quality of design, execution, or reporting of main outcome variables. The reviewers did not perform a meta-analysis. Fifteen studies comparing multidisciplinary treatment (MDT) versus wait-list control or treatment as usual showed strong evidence (according to the reviewers) for the superiority of MDT. There was moderate evidence that comprehensive inpatient programs were more beneficial than outpatient treatment. There was no evidence that specific treatment variables, such as duration or specific program components, were influential in the success of the intervention.

Somatoform Disorders

There have been relatively few trials involving patients that meet strict criteria for somatoform disorders. Kroenke (2007) recently carried out a critical review of this area and included studies of interventions in somatization disorder, undifferentiated somatoform disorder, hypochondriasis, conversion disorder, pain disorder, and body dysmorphic disorder. Kroenke identified 34 RCTs involving 3,922 patients. He reported that a meta-analysis was not possible because of the small number of trials within each diagnostic category and the wide variability between studies in terms of study design, outcome measures, etc.

Two-thirds of the studies involved somatization disorder (n=4 studies) or lower-threshold variants such as abridged somatization disorder (n=9) and medically unexplained symptoms (n=10). CBT was effective in 11 out of 13 studies, as were antidepressants in a small number (4 out of 5) of studies. Trials involving other treatment modalities showed benefit in 8 out of 16 studies. The other treatments for somatization disorder and its variants were a psychiatric consultation letter to the patient's primary care physician with advice on how to better manage somatizing patients (n=4), training of primary care physicians to better manage somatizing patients (n=3), non-CBT therapy (n=2), a multicomponent nurse care management intervention (n=1), aerobic exercise (n=1), and writing disclosure (n=1). There were two studies of hypnosis and one of paradoxical intention for conversion disorder, and one study of explanatory therapy in hypochondriasis. The most consistent evidence among these other treatments was for a consultation letter to the primary care physician. Kroenke (2007) concluded that CBT is the best-established treatment for a variety of somatoform disorders.

Treatment of Depression in Physical Illness

There is a growing evidence base for the treatment of depression in physical illness using either psychological interventions alone or psychological interventions as part of a package of collaborative care.

Collaborative and Stepped Care

The United Kingdom's National Institute of Clinical Excellence (NICE) recently published a new guideline for the treatment of depression in chronic physical illness (National Institute for Health and Clinical Excellence 2009). In the NICE guideline, 17 trials involving service-led interventions for the treatment of depression in physical illness were identified which provided data on 4,994 participants. Fifteen of the studies assessed the efficacy of collaborative care versus either standard or enhanced standard care (Table 39–7).

There was considerable variation between the different collaborative care interventions, with the complexity of the intervention and treatment components differing among studies. In the stepped-care approaches, participants were given a choice between an antidepressant or a psychological intervention as first-line treatment.

The NICE guideline concluded that there was consistent evidence that collaborative care had small to medium benefits on a range of depression outcomes, including response and remission, when compared with any form of standard care (National Institute for Health and Clinical Excellence 2009). Few conclusions could be drawn regarding the efficacy of collaborative care on improving physical health outcomes. Trials differed in the kind of physical illness from which patients were suffering, and the reporting of physical health outcomes was sparse, with different papers reporting a diverse range of outcomes.

Cognitive-Behavioral Therapy

NICE identified seven trials of individual-based CBT for depression in chronic physical illness (Table 39–8). Following analysis, NICE reported that individual-based CBT had a moderate effect on depression at the end of treatment in

TABLE 39–7. Studies of collaborative care for the treatment of depression in chronic physical illness

Medical condition	Study
Diabetes	Katon et al. 2004; J.W. Williams et al. 2004
Asthma or diabetes	Landis et al. 2007
Cancer	Dwight-Johnson et al. 2005; Ell et al. 2008; Strong et al. 2008
Stroke	L.S. Williams et al. 2007
Arthritis	Lin et al. 2003
Hypertension	Bogner and de Vries 2008
General medical illness	Cole et al. 2006; Cullum et al. 2007; Ell et al. 2007; Fortney et al. 2007; Katzelnick et al. 2000; Oslin et al. 2003

Source. Adapted from National Institute for Health and Clinical Excellence 2009.

comparison with standard care (standardized mean difference [SMD] = –0.55; 95% confidence interval [CI] = –0.97 to –0.13) for people with minor to mild depression. There were no differences between individual-based cognitive and behavioral interventions and counseling for depression at the end of treatment (SMD = –0.13, 95% CI = –0.46 to 0.20).

NICE also reported on group-based CBT interventions and identified 11 studies (Table 39–9). Following analysis, group CBT was found to have a moderate effect on depression at the end of treatment in comparison with standard care (SMD = –0.54; 95% CI = –0.86 to –0.21) for people with mild to moderate depression (National Institute for Health and Clinical Excellence 2009). The quality of evidence was "moderate" for depression because a possible publication bias was identified. There was also high heterogeneity; a sensitivity analysis was performed removing an outlier, which had a large effect on depression at the end of treatment and reduced the effect of the intervention on depression from a moderate to a small effect at the end of treatment (SMD = –0.42; 95% CI = –0.63 to –0.21).

Non-CBT Psychological Therapies

There are relatively few studies of non-CBT treatment for depression in physical illness. Gellis et al. (2008) evaluated problem solving as a treatment for depression in older adults with a range of medical conditions living in a care home. Very positive results on depression following a 6-session intervention were reported.

There have been four trials of IPT. Two of the trials involved patients with HIV (Markowitz et al. 1995; Ransom et al. 2008), one trial involved patients with cardiovascular disease (Lesperance et al. 2007), and one trial involved older adults with general medical illness (Mossey et al. 1996). The results of the trials were mixed. Lesperance et al. (2007) did not find IPT to be superior to clinical management for the treatment of major depression in patients with cardiovascular disease. Ransom et al. (2008) found a small but statistically nonsignificant effect of IPT in comparison to standard care for patients with HIV, while Markowitz et al. (1995) found IPT to be superior to CBT

TABLE 39–8. Studies of individual-based cognitive-behavioral therapy for depression in chronic physical illness

Medical condition	Study
Multiple sclerosis	Mohr et al. 2001; Foley et al. 1987
Cancer	Savard et al. 2006
Celiac disease	Addolorato et al. 2004
HIV	Markowitz et al. 1995

Source. Adapted from National Institute for Health and Clinical Excellence 2009.

TABLE 39–9. Studies of group-based cognitive-behavioral interventions for depression in chronic physical illness

Medical condition	Study
HIV	Antoni et al. 2006; Chesney et al. 2003; Heckman and Carlson 2007; Kelly et al. 1993
Epilepsy	Davis et al. 1984
Cancer	Evans and Connis 1995; Penedo et al. 2008
Diabetes	Henry et al. 1997; Lustman et al. 1998
Multiple sclerosis	Larcombe and Wilson 1984

Source. Adapted from National Institute for Health and Clinical Excellence 2009.

for the treatment of depression in HIV and equivalent to counseling. No clear picture emerged for IPT, and further studies are required before its usefulness as a treatment for depression in medical illness can be fully evaluated.

There have been three trials that have included a counseling arm. One involved depressed patients with cancer (Manne et al. 2007), one involved patients with cardiovascular disease (Brown et al. 1993), and one involved patients with multiple sclerosis (Mohr et al. 2005). All three studies compared counseling with individual CBT, and one also compared counseling with a "standard care" control condition. There was no difference between counseling versus standard care, and there was no difference between counseling and CBT for depression over the three studies (SMD=0.06; 95% CI=-0.16 to 0.27).

Psychological Therapies for Patients With Cancer

Psychosocial care is increasingly being recognized as an essential component of the comprehensive care of the individual with cancer. A wide range of therapies have been evaluated for patients with cancer and include behavioral therapy, cognitive therapy, CBT, communication skills training, counseling, family therapy/counseling, guided imagery, mindfulness therapy, music therapy, problem-solving therapy, psychotherapy, stress management training, support groups, and supportive-expressive group therapy (Jacobsen and Jim 2008).

There have been many systematic reviews published over the past 20 years evaluating the evidence supporting psychosocial treatments for anxiety and depression in patients with cancer. Jacobsen and Jim (2008) recently carried out a "review of reviews" summarizing findings from 14 previous systematic reviews that had evaluated psychosocial interventions. The studies are shown in Table 39–10, which has been adapted from Jacobsen and Jim (2008).

Thirteen of the 14 studies reached conclusions about the efficacy of psychosocial interventions for depression in cancer patients. Nine out of the 13 reviews reached positive conclusions, with the best evidence for behavioral therapy and counseling/psychotherapy. One of the reviews (Uitterhoeve et al. 2004) specifically evaluated interventions for patients with advanced cancer. These reviewers identified 13 trials and reported that 12 trials evaluating behavior therapy found positive effects on one or more indicators of quality of life (e.g., depression).

Eight of the 14 publications identified offered conclusions about the efficacy of psychosocial interventions for anxiety in cancer patients, with 6 out of the 8 publications reaching positive conclusions.

Jacobsen and Jim (2008) reported that many of the reviews had identified areas of weakness in the evidence base which had important implications for clinical practice. First, few of the studies included men or members of ethnic and racial minority groups. Second, there were inconsistent findings across studies due to differences in type of disease, number and timing of outcome measures, and demographics of patients recruited to the studies. Third, many of the studies were rated as being of poor quality. Finally, relatively few of the studies included patients with clinically significant levels of anxiety and depression, and many people included in the trials may not have been depressed or anxious at all, or suffering from subthreshold symptoms.

TABLE 39–10. Systematic reviews and meta-analyses of psychosocial interventions for anxiety or depression in adults with cancer

Authors	Intervention	Main findings
Devine and Westlake 1995	Psychoeducational care	Positive results for anxiety (Cohen's d=0.56; 95% CI=0.42 to 0.70)
Lovejoy and Matteis 1997	CBT	Knowledge base for CBT for treatment of depression in cancer is in early stages
Bottomley 1998	Pharmacological and psychological	Positive results for depression with individual and groups
Sellick and Crooks 1999	Individual counseling	Magnitude of treatment effects for depression in the 10 studies reviewed were classified as large (5), moderate (2), low (2), and none (1)
Sheard and Maguire 1999	Psychosocial	Anxiety: Cohen's d=0.42 (95% CI=0.08 to 0.74); d=0.36 when based on criteria for developing a robust estimate
Luebbert et al. 2001	Relaxation training	Anxiety: Cohen's d=0.45 (95% CI=0.23 to 0.67) Depression: d=0.54 (95% CI=0.30 to 0.78)
Redd et al. 2001	Behavioral interventions for cancer treatment side effects	Four of 5 studies demonstrated beneficial effects on anxiety

TABLE 39–10. Systematic reviews and meta-analyses of psychosocial interventions for anxiety or depression in adults with cancer *(continued)*

Authors	Intervention	Main findings
Barsevick et al. 2002	Psychoeducational	Positive results for depression reported in 63% of studies reviewed
Newell et al. 2002	Psychosocial	Recommendations for depression were tentatively against 7 strategies, neither for nor against 6 strategies, and tentatively for 0 strategies
Uitterhoeve et al. 2004	Psychosocial	Six of 10 studies showed a significant effect for depression; 1 of 10 studies showed a significant effect for anxiety
Jacobsen et al. 2006	Psychosocial and pharmacological	Forty-one percent of analyses yielded significant results for depression favoring intervention condition; 36% yielded significant results for anxiety favoring intervention condition
Osborn et al. 2006	Psychosocial	Anxiety: Hedges' g=1.99 (95% CI=0.69 to 3.31) (CBT); g=–0.02 (95% CI=–0.36 to 0.31) (psychoeducation)
S. Williams and Dale 2006	Psychosocial and pharmacological	Three of 4 studies showed benefit of intervention in treating depression; 7 of 10 trials showed a benefit of CBT in reducing depression
Rodin et al. 2007	Psychological and pharmacological	Two of 4 studies showed a benefit of psychosocial intervention in reducing depressive symptoms

Note. CBT=cognitive-behavioral therapy; CI=confidence interval; RCT=randomized controlled trial.
Source. Adapted from Jacobsen and Jim 2008.

Conclusion

There is evidence that psychological therapies are beneficial for patients with physical and psychological problems. The best evidence is for CBT, but other therapies are also developing evidence bases. Psychological therapies are particularly helpful for patients with medically unexplained symptoms but have less impact on patients who present with chronic pain, unless the treatments are provided as part of a multicomponent package. Increasingly, psychological treatments are being delivered as components of either stepped-care or collaborative care models. Psychological therapies are often provided in conjunction with pharmacological treatments, particularly if there is poor initial response to psychological treatments alone.

In the coming decade there is likely to be a growth in studies evaluating the role of psychological therapies in chronic illness, particularly in view of the possibility that such treatments may result in reduced health care costs.

Access to appropriate psychological treatment for patients with physical and psychological health problems remains a serious problem in many countries. Improvement in access is unlikely to occur to a significant extent unless psychological therapies are better integrated into physical health care systems, which can be done via liaison psychiatry services or via primary care–based services.

References

Addolorato G, De Lorenzi L, Abenavoli L, et al: Psychological support counseling improves gluten-free diet compliance in celiac patients with affective disorders. Aliment Pharmacol Ther 20:777–782, 2004

Antoni MH, Carrico MS, Duran RE, et al: Randomized clinical trial of cognitive behavioral stress management on human immunodeficiency virus viral load in gay men treated with highly active antiretroviral therapy. Psychosom Med 68:143–151, 2006

Arias AJ, Steinberg K, Banga A, et al: Systematic review of the efficacy of meditation techniques as treatments for medical illness. J Altern Complement Med 12:817–832, 2006

Badger T, Segrin C, Meek P, et al: Telephone interpersonal counseling with women with breast cancer: symptom management and quality of life. Oncol Nurs Forum 32:273–279, 2005

Bailey GW: The psychological treatment of back pain: a meta-analysis. Dissertation Abstracts International, Section B: The Sciences and Engineering 63:515, 2002

Barber JP, Gallop R, Crits-Christoph P, et al: The role of therapist adherence, therapist competence, and alliance in predicting outcome of individual drug counseling: results from the National Institute Drug Abuse Collaborative Cocaine Treatment Study. Psychother Res 16:220–240, 2006

Barsevick AM, Sweeney C, Haney E, et al: A systematic qualitative analysis of psychoeducational interventions for depression in patients with cancer. Oncol Nurs Forum 29:73–84, 2002

Bennett D, Parry G: Maintaining the therapeutic alliance: resolving alliance-threatening interactions related to the transference, in Core Processes in Brief Psychodynamic Psychotherapy. Edited by Charman DP. Mahwah, NJ, Lawrence Erlbaum, 2004, pp 251–274

Blake W: Jerusalem Chapter III, Plate 55: verses 60–68, in The Complete Poetry and Prose of William Blake. Edited by Erdman DV. New York, Anchor Books, 1988, p 205

Blanchard EB: A critical review of cognitive, behavioral, and cognitive-behavioral therapies for irritable bowel syndrome. Journal of Cognitive Psychotherapy19:101–123, 2005

Bogner HR, de Vries HF: Integration of depression and hypertension treatment: a pilot, randomized controlled trial. Ann Fam Med 6:295–301, 2008

Bolton G: "Writing is a way of saying things I can't say"—therapeutic creative writing: a quantitative study. BMJ 34:40–46, 2008

Bottomley A: Depression in cancer patients: a literature review. Eur J Cancer Care 7:181–191, 1998

Bowlby J Attachment and Loss, Vol 1: Attachment. New York, Basic Books, 1969

Brown MA, Munford AM, Munford PR: Behavior therapy of psychological distress in patients after myocardial infarction or coronary bypass. J Cardiopulm Rehabil 13:201–210, 1993

Butler AC, Chapman JE, Forman EM, et al: The empirical status of cognitive-behavioral therapy: a review of meta-analyses. Clin Psychol Rev 26:17–31, 2006

Cain EN, Kohorn EI, Quinlan DM, et al: Psychosocial benefits of a cancer support group. Cancer 57:183–189, 1986

Carroll D, Seers K: Relaxation for the relief of chronic pain: a systematic review. J Adv Nurs 27:476–487, 1998

Carlson LE, Ursuliak Z, Goodey E, et al: The effects of a mindfulness meditation-based stress reduction program on mood and symptoms of stress in cancer outpatients: 6-month follow-up. Support Care Cancer 9:112–123, 2001

Carlson LE, Speca M, Patel KD, et al: Mindfulness-based stress reduction in relation to quality of life, mood, symptoms of stress, and immune parameters in breast and prostate cancer outpatients. Psychosom Med 65:571–581, 2003

Cassell EJ: The nature of suffering and the goals of medicine. N Engl J Med 306:639–645, 1982

Chambers D, Bagnall A, Hempel S, et al: Interventions for the treatment, management, and rehabilitation of patients with chronic fatigue syndrome/myalgic encephalomyelitis: an updated systematic review. J R Soc Med 99:506–520, 2006

Chesney MA, Chambers DB, Taylor JM, et al: Coping effectiveness training for men living with HIV: results from a randomized clinical trial testing a group-based intervention. Psychosom Med 65:1038–1046, 2003

Christensen DN: Postmastectomy couple counseling: an outcome study of a structured treatment protocol. J Sex Marital Ther 9:266–275, 1983

Ciechanowski P, Russo J, Katon W, et al: Influence of patient attachment style on self-care and outcomes in diabetes. Psychosom Med 66:720–728, 2004

Classen C, Butler LD, Koopman C, et al: Supportive-expressive group therapy and distress in patients with metastatic breast cancer. Arch Gen Psychiatry 58:494–501, 2009

Cole MG, McCusker J, Elie M, et al: Systematic detection and multidisciplinary care of depression in older medical inpatients: a randomized trial. CMAJ 174:38–44, 2006

Creed F, Fernandes L, Guthrie E, et al: The cost-effectiveness of psychotherapy and paroxetine for severe irritable bowel syndrome. Gastroenterology 124:303–317, 2003

Cuijpers P, van Straten A, Andersson G: Internet-administered cognitive behavior therapy for health problems: a systematic review. J Behav Med 31:169–177, 2008

Cullum S, Tucker S, Todd C, et al: Effectiveness of liaison psychiatric nursing in older medical inpatients with depression: a randomised controlled trial. Age Ageing 36:436–442, 2007

Cunningham AJ, Edmonds CVI, Jenkins GP, et al: A randomized controlled trial of the effects of group psychological therapy on survival in women with metastatic breast cancer. Psychooncology 7:508–517, 1998

Davis GR, Armstrong HE, Donovan DM, et al: Cognitive-behavioral treatment of depressed affect among epileptics: preliminary findings. J Clin Psychol 40:930–935, 1984

de Mello MF, de Jesus Mari J, Bacaltchuk J, et al: A systematic review of research findings on the efficacy of interpersonal therapy for depressive disorders. Eur Arch Psychiatry Clin Neurosci 255:75–82, 2005

DeRubeis RJ, Feeley M: Determinants of change in cognitive therapy for depression. Cogn Ther Res 14:469–482, 1990

Devine EC, Westlake SK: The effects of psychoeducational care provided to adults with cancer: meta-analysis of 116 studies. Oncol Nurs Forum 22:1369–1381, 1995

Donnelly JM, Kornblith AB, Fleishman S, et al: A pilot study of interpersonal psychotherapy by telephone with cancer patients and their partners. Psychooncology 9:44–56, 2000

Dwight-Johnson M, Ell K, Pey-Juian L: Can collaborative care address the needs of low-income Latinas with comorbid depression and cancer? Results from a randomized pilot study. Psychosomatics 46:224–232, 2005

Edmonds CV, Lockwood GA, Cunningham AJ: Psychological response to long-term group therapy: a randomized trial with metastatic breast cancer patients. Psychooncology 8:74–91, 1999

Ell K, Unützer D, Aranda M, et al: Managing depression in home health care: a randomized clinical trial. Home Health Care Serv Q 26:81–104, 2007

Ell K, Xie B, Quon B, et al: Randomized controlled trial of collaborative care management of depression among low-income patients with cancer. J Clin Oncol 26:4488–4496, 2008

Evans RL, Connis RT: Comparison of brief group therapies for depressed cancer patients receiving radiation treatment. Public Health Reports 110:306–311, 1995

Fawzy FI, Cousins N, Fawzy NW, et al: A structured psychiatric intervention for cancer patient, I: changes over time in method of coping and affective disturbance. Arch Gen Psychiatry 47:720–725, 1990

Fawzy FI, Fawzy NW, Hyun CS, et al: Malignant melanoma: effects of an early structured psychiatric intervention, coping, and affective state on recurrence and survival 6 years later. Arch Gen Psychiatry 50:681–689, 1993

Fekete EM, Antoni MH, Schneiderman N: Psychosocial and behavioral interventions for chronic medical conditions. Curr Opin Psychiatry 20:152–157, 2007

Fink P, Toft T, Hansen MS: Symptoms and syndromes of bodily distress: an exploratory study of 978 internal medical, neurological, and primary care patients. Psychosom Med 69:30–39, 2007

Foley FW, Bedell JR, LaRocca NG, et al: Efficacy of stress-inoculation training in coping with multiple sclerosis. J Consult Clin Psychol 55:919–922, 1987

Ford AC, Talley NJ, Schoenfeld PS, et al: Efficacy of antidepressants and psychological therapies in irritable bowel syndrome: systematic review and meta-analysis. Gut 58:367–378, 2009

Fortney JC, Pyne JM, Edlund MJ, et al: A randomized trial of telemedicine-based collaborative care for depression. Gen Intern Med 22:1086–1093, 2007

Garcia-Campayo J, Magdalena J, Magallón R, et al: A meta-analysis of the efficacy of fibromyalgia treatment according to level of care. Arthritis Res Ther 10:R81, 2008

Gellis ZD, McGinty J, Tierney L, et al: Randomized controlled trial of problem solving therapy for minor depression in home care. Research on Social Work Practice 18:596–606, 2008

Goodwin PJ, Leszcz M, Ennis M: The effect of group psychosocial support on survival in metastatic breast cancer. N Engl J Med 345:1719–1726, 2001

Guthrie E, Sensky T: The role of psychological treatments, in Handbook of Liaison Psychiatry. Edited by Lloyd GG, Guthrie E. Cambridge, UK, Cambridge University Press, 2008, pp 800–817

Guthrie E, Creed F, Dawson D: A controlled trial of psychological treatment for irritable bowel syndrome. Gastroenterology 100:450–457, 1991

Guthrie E, Moorey J, Margison F, et al: Cost-effectiveness of brief psychodynamic-interpersonal therapy in high utilizers of psychiatric services. Arch Gen Psychiatry 56:519–526, 1999

Guthrie E, Kapur N, Mackway-Jones K, et al: Randomised controlled trial of brief psychological intervention after deliberate self poisoning. BMJ 323:135–138, 2001

Hadhazy VA, Ezzo J, Creamer P, et al: Mind-body therapies for the treatment of fibromyalgia. A systematic review. J Rheumatol 27:2911–2918, 2000

Hamilton J, Guthrie E, Creed F, et al: Randomized controlled trial of psychotherapy in patients with chronic functional dyspepsia. Gastroenterology 119:661–669, 2000

Hamilton WT, Gallagher AM, Thomas JM, et al: Risk markers for both chronic fatigue and irritable bowel syndromes: a prospective case-control study in primary care. Psychol Med 39:1913–1921, 2009

Häuser W, Bernardy K, Arnold B, et al: Efficacy of multicomponent treatment in fibromyalgia syndrome: a meta-analysis of randomized controlled clinical trials. Arthritis Rheum 61:216–224, 2009

Hawton K, Kirk J: Problem-solving, in Cognitive Behaviour Therapy for Psychiatric Problems: A Practical Guide. Edited by Hawton K, Salkovskis P, Kirk J, et al. Oxford, UK, Oxford Medical Publications, 1989, pp 406–427

Heckman TG, Carlson B: A randomized clinical trial of two telephone-delivered mental health interventions for HIV infected persons in rural areas of the United States. AIDS Behav 11:5–14, 2007

Henry JL, Wilson PH, Bruce DG, et al: Cognitive-behavioural stress management for patients with non-insulin dependent diabetes mellitus. Psychology, Health and Medicine 2:109–118, 1997

Hobson RF: Forms of Feeling. London, Tavistock, 1985

Hoffman BM, Papas RK, Chatkoff DK, et al: Meta-analysis of psychological interventions for chronic low back pain. Health Psychol 26:1–9, 2007

Jacobsen PB, Jim HS: Psychosocial interventions for anxiety and depression in adult cancer patients: achievements and challenges. CA Cancer J Clin 58:214–230, 2008

Jacobsen PB, Donovan KA, Swaine ZN, et al: Management of anxiety and depression in adult cancer patients: toward an evidence-based approach, in Oncology: An Evidence-Based Approach. Edited by Chang AE, Ganz PA, Hayes DF, et al. New York, Springer, 2006, pp 1552–1579

Kabat-Zinn J, Lipworth L, Burney R, et al: Four-year follow-up of a meditation-based program for the self-regulation of chronic pain: treatment outcomes and compliance. The Clinical Journal of Pain 2(3):159–173, 1987

Kaltenthaler E, Brazier J, De Nigris E, et al: Computerised cognitive behaviour therapy for depression and anxiety update: a systematic review and economic evaluation. Health Technol Assess 10:iii, xi–xiv, 1–168, 2006

Kaplan KH, Goldenberg DL, Galvin-Nadeau M: The impact of a meditation-based stress reduction program on fibromyalgia. Gen Hosp Psychiatry 15:284–298, 1993

Katon WJ, Von Korff M, Lin EH, et al: The Pathways Study: a randomized trial of collaborative care in patients with diabetes and depression. Arch Gen Psychiatry 61:1042–1049, 2004

Katzelnick DJ, Simon GE, Pearson SD, et al: Randomized trial of depression management program in high utilizers of medical care. Arch Fam Med 9:345–351, 2000

Kelly JA, Murphy DA, Bahr GR, et al: Outcome of cognitive-behavioral and support group brief therapies for depressed, HIV-infected persons. Am J Psychiatry 150:1679–1686, 1993

Klerman G, Weissman M, Rounsaville B, et al: Interpersonal Psychotherapy of Depression. New York, Basic Books, 1984

Kroenke K: Efficacy of treatment for somatoform disorders: a review of randomized controlled trials. Psychosom Med 69:881–888, 2007

Lackner JM, Mesmer C, Morley S: Psychological treatments for irritable bowel syndrome: a systematic review and meta-analysis. J Consul Clin Psychol 72:1100–1113, 2004

Lambert MJ, Ogles BM: The efficacy and effectiveness of psychotherapy, in Bergin and Garfield's Handbook of Psychotherapy and Behavior Change, 5th Edition. Edited by Lambert MJ. New York, Wiley, 2004, pp 139–193

Landis SE, Bradley NG, Morrissey JP, et al: Generalist care managers for the treatment of depressed Medicaid patients in North Carolina: a pilot study. BMC Family Practice 8:7, 2007

Larcombe NA, Wilson PH: An evaluation of cognitive-behaviour therapy for depression in patients with multiple sclerosis. Br J Psychiatry 145:366–371, 1984

Ledesma D, Kumano H: Mindfulness-based stress reduction and cancer: a meta-analysis. Psychooncology 18:571–579, 2009

Lesperance F, Frasure-Smith N, Koszycki D, et al: Effects of citalopram and interpersonal psychotherapy on depression in patients with coronary artery disease. JAMA 297:367–379, 2007

Leventhal H, Benyamini Y, Brownlee S: Illness representations: theoretical foundations, in Perceptions of Health and Illness: Current Research and Applications. Edited by Petrie KJ, Weinman J. Amsterdam, The Netherlands, Harwood Academic Publishers, 1997, pp 19–45

Lin EHB, Katon W, Von Korff M, et al: Effect of improving depression care on pain and functional outcomes among older adults with arthritis: a randomized controlled trial. JAMA 290:2428–2429, 2003

Looper KJ, Kirmayer LJ: Behavioral medicine approaches to somatoform disorders. J Consult Clin Psychol 70:810–827, 2002

Lovejoy NC, Matteis M: Cognitive-behavioral interventions to manage depression in patients with cancer: research and theoretical initiatives. Cancer Nurs 20:155–167, 1997

Luebbert K, Dahme B, Hasenbring M: The effectiveness of relaxation training in reducing treatment-related symptoms and improving emotional adjustment in acute non-surgical cancer treatment: a meta-analytical review. Psychooncology 10:490–502, 2001

Lustman PJ, Griffith LS, Freedland KE, et al: Cognitive behavior therapy for depression in type 2 diabetes mellitus. Ann Intern Med 129:613–621, 1998

Maguire P, Tait A, Brooke M, et al: Effect of counselling on the psychiatric morbidity associated with mastectomy. BMJ 281:1454–1456, 1980

Maguire P, Tait A, Brooke M, et al: The effect of counselling on physical disability and social recovery after mastectomy. Clin Oncol 9:319–324, 1983

Maisiak R, Austin J, West S, et al: The effect of person-centered counseling on the psychological status of persons with systemic lupus erythematosus or rheumatoid arthritis: a randomized, controlled trial. Arthritis Care Res 9:60–66, 1996

Malouff JM, Thorsteinsson EB, Rooke SE, et al: Efficacy of cognitive behavioral therapy for chronic fatigue syndrome: a meta-analysis. Clin Psychol Rev 28:736–745, 2008

Manne SL, Rubin S, Edelson M, et al: Coping and communication-enhancing intervention versus supportive counseling for women diagnosed with gynecological cancers. J Consult Clin Psychol 75:615–628, 2007

Markowitz JC, Klerman GL, Clougherty KF, et al: Individual psychotherapies for depressed HIV-positive patients. Am J Psychiatry 152:1504–1509, 1995

Mohr DC, Boudewyn AC, Goodkin DE, et al: Comparative outcomes for individual cognitive-behavior therapy, supportive-expressive group psychotherapy, and sertraline for the treatment of depression in multiple sclerosis. J Consult Clin Psychol 69:942–949, 2001

Mohr DC, Burke H, Beckner V, et al: A preliminary report on a skills-based telephone-administered peer support programme for patients with multiple sclerosis. Mult Scler 11:222–226, 2005

Moorey J, Guthrie E: Persons and experience: essential aspects of psychodynamic interpersonal therapy. Psychodynamic Practice 9:547–564, 2003

Morley S, Eccleston C, Williams A: Systematic review and meta-analysis of randomized controlled trials of cognitive behaviour therapy and behaviour therapy for chronic pain in adults, excluding headache. Pain 80:1–13, 1999

Mossey JM, Knott KA, Higgins M, et al: Effectiveness of a psychosocial intervention, interpersonal counseling, for subdysthymic depression in medically ill elderly. J Gerontol A Biol Sci Med Sci 51:M172–M178, 1996

Moss-Morris R, Weinman J, Petrie KJ: The Revised Illness Perception Questionnaire (IPQ-R). Psychol Health 17:1–16, 2002

National Institute for Health and Clinical Excellence: Depression in Adults With a Chronic Physical Health Problem: Treatment and Management (CG91). London, National Institute for Health and Clinical Excellence, October 2009. Available at: http://guidance.nice.org.uk/CG91. Accessed February 5, 2010.

Newell SA, Sanson-Fisher RW, Savolainen NJ: Systematic review of psychological therapies for cancer patients: overview and recommendations for future research. J Natl Cancer Inst 94:558–584, 2002

Nezu AM, Nezu CM, Felgoise SH: Project Genesis: assessing the efficacy of problem-solving therapy for distressed adult cancer patients. J Consult Clin Psychol 71:1036–1048, 2003

Osborn RL, Demoncada AC, Feuerstein M: Psychosocial interventions for depression, anxiety, and quality of life in cancer survivors: meta-analyses. Int J Psych Med 36:13–34, 2006

Oslin DW, Sayers S, Ross J, et al: Disease management for depression and at-risk drinking via telephone in an older population of veterans. Psychosom Med 65:931–937, 2003

Ott MJ, Norris RL, Bauer-Wu SM: Mindfulness meditation for oncology patients: a discussion and critical review. Integr Cancer Ther 5:98–108, 2006

Penedo FJ, Molton I, Dahn JR, et al: A randomized clinical trial of group-based cognitive-behavioral stress management in localized prostate cancer. Ann Behav Med 31:261–270, 2008

Pennebaker JW, Seagal JD: Forming a story: the health benefits of narrative. J Clin Psychol 55:1243–1254, 1999

Prochaska JO, Norcross JC, DiClemente CC: Changing for Good: A Revolutionary Six-Stage Program for Overcoming Bad Habits and Moving Your Life Positively Forward. New York, William Morrow, 1994

Raine R, Haines A, Sensky T, et al: Systematic review of mental health interventions for patients with common somatic symptoms: can research evidence from secondary care be extrapolated to primary care? BMJ 325:1082–1085, 2002

Ransom D, Heckman TG, Anderson T, et al: Telephone-delivered, interpersonal psychotherapy for HIV-infected rural persons with depression: a pilot trial. Psychiatr Serv 59:871–877, 2008

Redd WH, Montgomery GH, DuHamel KN: Behavioral intervention for cancer treatment side effects. J Natl Cancer Inst 93:810–823, 2001

Rimes KA, Chalder T: Treatments for chronic fatigue syndrome. Occup Med 55:32–39, 2005

Rodin G, Lloyd N, Katz M, et al: The treatment of depression in cancer patients: a systematic review. Supportive Care Guidelines Group of Cancer Care Ontario Program in Evidence-Based Care. Support Care Cancer 15:123–136, 2007

Rossy LA, Buckelew SP, Dorr N, et al: A meta-analysis of fibromyalgia treatment interventions. Ann Behav Med 21:180–191, 1999

Royal College of Physicians and Royal College of Psychiatrists: The Psychological Care of Medical Patients: A Practical Guide, 2nd Edition. London, Royal College of Physicians, 2003. Available at: http://www.rcpsych.ac.uk/files/pdfversion/cr108.pdf. Accessed February 5, 2010.

Savard J, Simard S, Giguere I, et al: Randomized clinical trial on cognitive therapy for depression in women with metastatic breast cancer: psychological and immunological effects. Palliat Support Care 4:219–237, 2006

Scascighini L, Toma V, Dober-Spielmann S, et al: Multidisciplinary treatment for chronic pain: a systematic review of interventions and outcomes. Rheumatology 47:670–678, 2008

Segal Z, Teasdale J, Williams M: Mindfulness-Based Cognitive Therapy for Depression. New York, Guilford, 2002

Sellick SM, Crooks DL: Depression and cancer: an appraisal of the literature for prevalence, detection, and practice guideline development for psychological interventions. Psychooncology 8:315–333, 1999

Sensky T: Cognitive therapy with medical patients, in Cognitive-Behavior Therapy. Edited by Wright JH (Review of Psychiatry Series, Vol 23; Oldham JM and Riba MB, series eds). Washington, DC, American Psychiatric Publishing, 2004, pp 83–121

Sephton SE, Salmon P, Weissbecker I, et al: Mindfulness meditation alleviates depressive symptoms in women with fibromyalgia: results of a randomized clinical trial. Arthritis Rheum (Arthritis Care Res) 57:77–85, 2007

Shapiro DA, Barkham M, Rees A, et al: Effects of treatment duration and severity of depression on the effectiveness of cognitive-behavioral and psychodynamic-interpersonal psychotherapy. J Consult Clin Psychol 62:522–534, 1994

Sharpe M, Peveler R, Mayou R: The functional treatment of patients with functional somatic symptoms: a practical guide. J Psychosom Res 36:515–529, 1992

Sheard T, Maguire P: The effect of psychological interventions on anxiety and depression in cancer patients: results of two meta-analyses. Br J Cancer 80:1770–1780, 1999

Sim J, Adams N: Systematic review of randomized controlled trials of nonpharmacological interventions for fibromyalgia. Clin J Pain:18:324–336, 2002

Smith JE, Richardson J, Hoffman C, et al: Mindfulness-Based Stress Reduction as supportive therapy in cancer care: a systematic review. J Adv Nurse 52:315–327, 2005

Smyth JM: Written emotional expression: effect sizes, outcome types and moderating variables. J Consult Clin Psychol 66:174–184, 1998

Spiegel D, Glafkides MC: Effects of group confrontation with death and dying: Int J Group Psychother 33:433–447, 1983

Spiegel D, Bloom JR, Yalom I: Group support for patients with metastatic cancer: a randomized outcome study. Arch Gen Psychiatry 38:527–533, 1981

Spiegel D, Bloom JR, Kraemer HC, et al: Effect of psychosocial treatment on survival of patients with metastatic breast cancer. Lancet 2(8668):888–891, 1989

Stanton AL, Danoff-Burg S, Sworowski LA, et al: Randomized controlled trial of written emotional expression and benefit finding in breast cancer. J Clin Oncology 20:4160–4168, 2002

Stewart JH: Hypnosis in contemporary medicine. Mayo Clinic Proc 80:511–524, 2005

Stone AA, Smyth JM, Kaell A: Structured writing about stressful events: exploring potential psychological mediators of positive health events. Health Psychol 19:619–624, 2000

Strong V, Waters R, Hibberd C, et al: Management of depression for people with cancer (SMaRT oncology 1): a randomised trial. Lancet 372:40–48, 2008

Stuart S, Noyes R Jr: Treating hypochondriasis with interpersonal psychotherapy. Journal of Contemporary Psychotherapy 35:269–283, 2005

Sullivan HS: The Interpersonal Theory of Psychiatry. New York, WW Norton, 1953

Teasdale JD, Segal ZV, Williams JMG: Prevention of relapse/recurrence in major depression by mindfulness-based cognitive therapy. J Consult Clin Psychol 68:615–623, 2000

Tsai AC, Morton SC, Mangione CM, et al: A meta-analysis of interventions to improve care for chronic illnesses. Am J Manag Care 11:478–488, 2005

Uitterhoeve RJ, Vernooy M, Litjens M, et al: Psychosocial interventions for patients with advanced cancer—a systematic review of the literature. Br J Cancer 91:1050–1062, 2004

van Koulil S, Effting M, Kraaimaat FW, et al: Cognitive-behavioural therapies and exercise programmes for patients with fibromyalgia: state of the art and future directions. Ann Rheum Dis 66:571–581, 2007

Viederman M, Perry SW 3rd: Use of a psychodynamic life narrative in the treatment of depression in the physically ill. Gen Hosp Psychiatry 2:177–185, 1980

Weissman MW: A brief history of interpersonal psychotherapy. Psychiatric Annals 36:553–557, 2006

Whiting P, Bagnall A, Sowde A, et al: Interventions for the treatment and management of chronic fatigue syndrome: a systematic review. JAMA 286:1360–1401, 2001

Whorwell PJ, Prior A, Faragher EB: Controlled trial of hypnotherapy in the treatment of severe refractory irritable bowel syndrome. Lancet 2(8414):1232–1234, 1984

Williams A, Morley S: Systematic review and meta-analysis of psychological treatments for persistent pain in adults, excluding headache. Papers and Abstracts Presented at the 28th Annual Scientific Meeting of the American Pain Society. The Journal of Pain 10 (4, suppl):S62, 2009

Williams JW, Katon W, Lin E, et al: The effectiveness of depression care management on depression and diabetes related outcomes in older patients with both conditions. Ann Intern Med 140:1015–1024, 2004

Williams LS, Kroenke K, Bakas T, et al: Care management of poststroke depression. Stroke 38:998–1003, 2007

Williams S, Dale J: The effectiveness of treatment for depression/depressive symptoms in adults with cancer: a systematic review. Br J Cancer 94:372–390, 2006

Wilson S, Maddison T, Roberts L, et al: Systematic review: the effectiveness of hypnotherapy in the management of irritable bowel syndrome. Aliment Pharmacol Ther 24:769–780, 2006

Wright EB, Holcombe C, Salmon P: Doctors' communication of trust, care, and respect in breast cancer: qualitative study. BMJ 328:864, 2004

CHAPTER

40

Electroconvulsive Therapy

Keith G. Rasmussen, M.D.

ELECTROCONVULSIVE THERAPY (ECT) is a safe procedure with low mortality rates (Nuttall et al. 2004). Nonetheless, medical comorbidity in ECT patients is so common that the clinician should be familiar with strategies to prevent complications. Management of medically ill patients receiving ECT includes careful pretreatment assessment of medical comorbidity, proper treatment technique, vigilant assessment of the patients' medical status between treatments, and identification and management of treatment-emergent medical complications. Two overriding principles for the ECT clinician are ongoing vigilance and communication. Vigilance refers to the need for the ECT clinician to have a thorough awareness of all significant medical problems the prospective ECT patient has and the results and recommendations of medical tests and consultations. Because ECT fundamentally involves a team approach in patient care, the ECT clinician is the coordinator of the team and must ensure ongoing communication among the various caregivers. For example, if the pre-ECT workup detects cervical spine disease, then the ECT clinician must pass this information on to whoever manages the airway during the treatments. Thus, even though a psychiatrist probably will not determine specialized testing performed before treatments, deliver anesthesia, or manage the airway, the psychiatrist must ensure that the relevant parties are fully informed.

The basic questions covered in this chapter are 1) What are the risks with a particular medical condition during ECT? and 2) How can they be reduced? Ideally, large prospective case series would be available to inform us of morbidity and mortality risks, and controlled trials would inform us about preventive strategies, but both are lacking in this field. We do have case reports and relatively small case series as well as the clinical expertise of experienced ECT practitioners. In this chapter, I review, in an organ system–based format, the current state of knowledge of ECT risk reduction strategies. It is assumed that all prospective ECT patients will undergo a thorough medical history, review of systems, and physical examination. Laboratory studies, radiological examinations, cardiac testing, and specialty consultation (e.g., cardiology or neurology) are individualized and discussed in the relevant sections later in this chapter.

Cardiovascular Disorders

Cardiac Physiology of ECT

Over the past several decades, numerous carefully conducted studies have investigated the hemodynamic, electrocardiographic, and echocardiographic findings during and shortly after ECT treatments. In brief, a sharp rise in pulse and blood pressure occurs during the seizures but returns to baseline usually within a few minutes postictally (Rasmussen et al. 1999).

After the electrical stimulus, there is a vagally (i.e., parasympathetically) mediated short-lived bradycardia, occasionally with asystole of several seconds. If the electrical stimulus is strong enough to cause a seizure, this initial parasympathetic phase is rapidly replaced by a sympathetically mediated tachycardia and rise in blood pressure during the seizure. Myocardial workload and cardiac output increase significantly. These effects generally subside within a few minutes to an hour. In the immediate postictal phase, if no antimuscarinic premedication has been given, there is often transient bradycardia, followed again by a smaller increase in heart rate that typically reverts to prestimulus levels within a few minutes. A mild increase in heart rate may persist over the preanesthesia baseline depending on the half-life of the antimuscarinic premedication, if given.

Thus, from a hemodynamic standpoint, the factor that is most relevant to cardiac patients is the sympathetically mediated sharp increase in myocardial workload.

If the electrical stimulus is not of sufficient intensity to cause a seizure, then the initial parasympathetic effects will not be offset by the sympathetic phase. Thus, there have been rare reports of prolonged asystole requiring resuscitation, especially in patients who have not been given antimuscarinic premedication or who received beta-blockers. For this reason, the use of antimuscarinic premedication is encouraged in ECT. This is especially true at the first treatment session, when a stimulus dose titration is performed to determine seizure threshold and subconvulsive stimuli are likely. However, at subsequent treatment sessions, subconvulsive stimuli are much less likely. If a patient experienced uncomfortable urinary hesitancy with the first treatment when an antimuscarinic agent was administered, then it should be withheld at subsequent sessions.

As would be expected given this stress on the heart, it is not uncommon to see a variety of transient electrocardiogram (ECG) abnormal findings during this time, including ST segment depression and T wave changes (Rasmussen et al. 2004) as well as temporary echocardiographic abnormalities, mainly abnormal wall motion (McCully et al. 2003). The parameters that are monitored routinely include blood pressure and ECG, and any untoward measurements can be treated promptly by the anesthesiologist (e.g., with blood pressure medication or antiarrhythmics) to prevent serious complications. It is easy to appreciate that these physiological changes might predispose cardiac patients to higher-than-usual risks during ECT, but the literature does not permit confident precise conclusions about such risks. Pre-ECT consultation with a cardiologist or an anesthesiologist familiar with the cardiac physiology of ECT should be undertaken. No universally agreed-upon standards of pre-ECT cardiac testing have been developed, but such testing should be individualized according to the particular patient's cardiac status.

Congestive Heart Failure

Patients with congestive heart failure (CHF) are particularly sensitive to increased myocardial demand such as occurs in ECT. The key for maximum safety with such patients is to stabilize ventricular pump function optimally before proceeding with treatments. What is known about risks comes from a few small case series. Zielinski et al. (1993) reported on 40 ECT patients with a variety of cardiac diagnoses, 12 of whom had CHF. There were no deaths in this series. Of the patients with CHF, 2 had (unspecified) ischemic changes on electrocardiography, and 1 had dysrhythmias. Seven of the CHF patients had minor cardiac complications, consisting usually of transient dysrhythmias (atrial or ventricular). Finally, 2 of the CHF patients underwent ECT without cardiac complications. The authors found that in patients who did not receive initial pretreatment with antimuscarinic medication, bradycardia and brief periods of asystole were common and preventable with subsequent atropine.

Stern et al. (1997) described three patients with CHF who received ECT without any cardiac complications. The authors used nitroglycerin patch, sublingual nifedipine, and intravenous labetalol pre-ECT to lower the risk of decompensation of heart failure during the procedure. Goldberg and Badger (1993) treated two patients with CHF and implantable cardioverter defibrillators (ICDs). The first tolerated eight ECT treatments without consequence. The second, a 65-year-old man with dilated cardiomyopathy and pre-ECT ejection fraction of 20%, underwent four treatments. After recovery from the first and third treatments, he had respiratory difficulties and bouts of hypotension that responded to ephedrine. After the fourth treatment, he developed a wide complex tachycardia without palpable pulse and was resuscitated. No further ECT was administered, but he had a hypotensive episode 5 days later that ultimately led to his death from progressive heart failure several days thereafter.

Gerring and Shields (1982) provided detailed outcome data on four patients with CHF who were treated with ECT for depressive illness. A 60-year-old woman with mitral stenosis received ECT without complication. A 58-year-old woman, also with mitral stenosis in addition to CHF, experienced atrial fibrillation leading to severe decompensation of the CHF after the second treatment; on stabilization, she went on to receive another course of ECT without complication. A 71-year-old woman with a history of myocardial infarction (MI) in addition to CHF had a cardiopulmonary arrest 45 minutes after her fifth treatment and died. Finally, a 69-year-old woman showed transient ventricular and atrial dysrhythmias after several of her ECT treatments, which she otherwise tolerated well.

Petrides and Fink (1996), in a series of ECT patients with atrial fibrillation, reported that one 89-year-old woman with CHF converted to sinus rhythm after receiving a course of ECT. Also, a 76-year-old woman with CHF and atrial fibrillation received a course of seven ECT treatments, during which she fluctuated between atrial fibrillation and sinus rhythm. The CHF did not seem to worsen. In summary, most CHF patients have received ECT without worsening of ECT or other complications except transient arrhythmias in some, but there have been rare deaths.

CHF should optimally be treated and stabilized prior to ECT treatments. Once the patient is scheduled for ECT, cardiac medications should be administered in the morning before the treatment with a small amount of water, with enough time to ensure absorption. Practice guidelines caution against administration of diuretic agents the morning of ECT to avoid bladder rupture or incontinence during the seizure (American Psychiatric Association 2001). However, the author generally recommends administering patients' usual stable medications, including diuretics, to avoid any abrupt changes in their medical regimen. The full bladder problem can be managed simply by having the patient void just before the treatment or, if necessary, by making transient use of a urinary catheter.

Whether to use an antimuscarinic agent in the patient with CHF must be decided on a case-by-case basis. The potential for such medication to increase myocardial workload through added tachycardia and hypertension is established (Rasmussen et al. 1999). However, if a patient receives a subconvulsive electrical stimulus, especially if he or she is also receiving beta-blocking medication, the risk of unopposed parasympathetic stimulation and resultant prolonged asystole is real (Tang and Ungvari 2001).

The attending anesthesiologist may elect to use other cardioprotective agents when ECT is being administered to the patient with CHF. For example, a beta-blocker such as esmolol or labetalol may dampen the seizure-induced sympathetic stimulation. Other strategies include preload reduction (e.g., nitrates), peripheral vasodilators (e.g., hydralazine), and calcium channel blockade (e.g., verapamil or diltiazem).

Finally, intertreatment assessment in patients with CHF is especially important, as shown by the case report of a patient who died of congestive decompensation that began several days after the last ECT treatment (Goldberg and Badger 1993). Daily rounds should include not only assessment of mood and cognitive status but also inquiries about symptoms of CHF (e.g., shortness of breath, orthopnea) and physical examination for signs of CHF (e.g., gallops, jugular venous distension, peripheral edema, pulmonary crackles). Any new or worsening findings should prompt careful evaluation and, if necessary, halting of ECT (even if temporarily) to stabilize the patient. Patients with known CHF should be evaluated by an internist or a cardiologist prior to initiating treatment.

Coronary Artery Disease/ Post–Myocardial Infarction

Easing the rise in myocardial oxygen demand is the goal in care of patients with coronary artery disease (CAD) during ECT. In several case series (Gerring and Shields 1982; Magid et al. 2005; Petrides and Fink 1996; Rice et al. 1994; Zielinski et al. 1993), numerous patients with CAD—some with remote history of MI—underwent ECT without major complications. Unfortunately, patients with precisely defined severity of CAD were prospectively followed up for any effects of ECT in only a few reports. In an echocardiographic/sestamibi study by Ruwitch et al. (1994) in patients with known CAD, ECT did not cause any clinical complications (e.g., angina, MI, clinically significant ventricular dysfunction).

After the prospective ECT patient with CAD has had the appropriate pretreatment evaluation and stabilization, some measures may further reduce cardiac risk. Many studies have shown that pretreatment with a variety of antihypertensive agents (e.g., beta-blockers, calcium channel blockers, other vasodilators, nitrates) lowers the seizure-induced rise in heart rate or blood pressure (Abrams 2002, pp. 77–81). Whether this reliably translates into actual protection against cardiac complications is unknown. In fact, Castelli et al. (1995), O'Connor et al. (1996), and Zvara et al. (1997) found no evidence that use of beta-blockers during ECT reduced evidence of myocardial ischemia despite beneficial effects on blood pressure rises during the treatments. Thus, it remains uncertain whether beta-blocker pretreatment reduces morbidity associated with ECT. Given the well-documented salutary effects of such drugs in patients with ischemic heart disease, it seems reasonable to use them in selected cases before, during, or shortly after the treatment depending on the patient's hemodynamic status, after carefully weighing the risks and potential benefits of such treatment.

Dysrhythmias, Pacemakers, and Implantable Defibrillators

The most common dysrhythmia in ECT patients is atrial fibrillation. There are several reports of patients in atrial fibrillation who safely received ECT (Petrides and Fink 1996). Occasionally, such patients will convert to sinus rhythm during ECT or convert back to atrial fibrillation if already converted before ECT to sinus rhythm. Atrial fibrillation newly identified before ECT should be assessed by a cardiologist for optimal management, including the decision whether to choose rate control or cardioversion. Therapeutic anticoagulation should be maintained throughout the course of ECT if the patient is already anticoagulated. Close and meticulous monitoring of the patient's hemodynamic status, oxygenation, and electrocardiographic changes in response to treatment is critically important during ECT. Electrocardiographic rhythm should be inspected before each treatment. The patient without history of atrial fibrillation who develops this rhythm during ECT obviously should have a cardiac evaluation before treatment is resumed. In patients taking warfarin, therapeutic anticoagulation should be continued throughout ECT (Mehta et al. 2004).

Because cardiac patients are predisposed to a variety of atrial or ventricular dysrhythmias, it is important to ensure that electrolytes are normal. Electrolyte abnormalities and other metabolic perturbations (e.g., thyroid dysfunction) can be even more proarrhythmic, along with medications that may prolong the QT interval, including many psychotropics, which are often prescribed for ECT patients (Rasmussen et al. 2006a). Some intriguing recent data suggest that high QTc dispersion (i.e., inhomogeneity of the QTc interval on the 12-lead ECG) is common in ECT patients (Dodd et al. 2008) and may predispose to arrhythmias during ECT treatments (Rasmussen et al. 2007a).

A related issue concerns the prospective ECT patient with a cardiac pacemaker or an ICD. There have been numerous case reports of patients with pacemakers who have undergone successful and uncomplicated ECT (Dolenc et al. 2004), as well as a few reports of patients with ICDs (Dolenc et al. 2004; Lynch et al. 2008). Pre-ECT device assessment to ensure normal functioning is advisable. Some practitioners have used a magnet placed on the chest above the device to convert a demand mode pacemaker to fixed mode during ECT to avoid spurious discharge of the device, which theoretically could occur as the result of muscle electrical activity; however, no evidence supports this practice. ICDs should be turned off prior to each ECT treatment while the patient is on an electrocardiographic monitor, the latter being continued until the ICD is turned back on. All patients with ICDs or pacemakers that have been reprogrammed prior to ECT should have device assessment after the procedure.

Aneurysms

Several case reports cite safe use of ECT in patients with aortic aneurysms, some after surgical correction (Mueller et al. 2009; Porquez et al. 2003). Assuming that patients have no preexisting conditions or surgical complications, there is no specific reason to assume that patients who have had an aneurysm repair are at increased risk during ECT.

The chief concern in patients with aneurysms is the potential risk of rupture or leakage caused by the rapid rise in blood pressure during ECT. If a patient is known to have an aortic aneurysm, the size should be evaluated (e.g., by ultrasound) prior to ECT. Consultation with a vascular surgeon would be prudent to evaluate the stability of the aneurysm and strategies for risk reduction. Pretreatment with antihypertensives before ECT anesthesia can optimize control of blood pressure and reduce arterial wall stress. Labetalol is ideal for this purpose because it has both alpha and beta blockade and thus can reduce peripheral vascular resistance and attenuate the rise in blood pressure during and shortly after the seizure. Repetitive imaging may be necessary during the course of ECT treatments if there is any concern with respect to the stability of the aneurysm.

Hypertension

There are two overarching concerns regarding blood pressure and ECT. The first is how well controlled blood pressure should be before it is safe to proceed with ECT in hypertensive patients. Hypertension is the most common cardiovascular condition in patients receiving ECT. Presumably, with the rise in blood pressure during seizures, uncontrolled hypertension might predispose to complications such as MI or cerebral infarction. A recent review concluded by suggesting that patients with blood pressure measurements greater than 140/90 mm Hg should be treated until blood pressure is normal before proceeding with ECT (Tess and Smetana 2009), but such an arbitrary cutoff is problematic. Although it seems intuitively obvious that good control of blood pressure is ideal before ECT, undue delays while waiting for complete normalization seem unwarranted. Furthermore, gaining tight control of blood pressure is difficult in many hypertensive patients, especially those with severe psychopathology such as catatonia, psychosis, or melancholia. Insisting on "normal" blood pressure effectively eliminates ECT for some patients. The author has personally overseen ECT in many patients over the years who have had somewhat elevated blood pressure, none of whom have had a peri-ECT stroke or MI. If the anesthesiologist is concerned about a patient's blood pressure at the time of a treatment, intravenous beta blockade can effectively dampen the rise in pressure during the seizure. Furthermore, Albin et al. (2007) found that no sustained rise in blood pressure occurs in hypertensive patients during a course of ECT treatment. With the availability of short-acting antihypertensive agents (e.g., esmolol or labetalol), high blood pressure generally can be managed rapidly and effectively during the treatments. Data also indicate that labetalol does not predispose to orthostatic hypotension in the hours after ECT (Rasmussen et al. 2008c). Thus, although attempting to achieve good blood pressure control in hypertensive patients is obviously an excellent idea, the author recommends against strict limits that might lead to withholding ECT. The practitioner must weigh the urgency of ECT, the severity of the elevated pressure, and any comorbid cardiac condition (e.g., presence of known CHF) while taking reassurance from the knowledge that cardiac complications during ECT are extremely rare.

The second blood pressure concern in ECT is the management of spikes that occur during ECT treatments. As described earlier, there is no evidence that control of blood pressure spikes during ECT reduces complications. Given that the complication rate during ECT is so low, the sample size of a prospective controlled trial of antihypertensive administration at ECT sessions that would provide adequate statistical power to detect a meaningful difference would probably be prohibitively large. In the meantime, it seems reasonable to use an agent to dampen the rise in ECT-induced blood pressure in selected patients (e.g., those with very high baseline blood pressure or concomitant cardiac conditions). Some data indicate that beta-blockers may shorten seizure length in ECT (Howie et al. 1990; Van den Broek et al. 1999), whereas other studies have not found this effect (Dannon et al. 1998; Howie et al. 1992; McCall et al. 1991). In either case, no evidence indicates that beta-blockers reduce the efficacy of ECT, and no correlation is found between seizure length and ECT efficacy (Abrams 2002, p. 122). To underscore this point, the anesthetic agent propofol is known to reduce seizure length potently in ECT, but several controlled trials indicate that it does not reduce ECT efficacy (Abrams 2002, p. 156). Thus, not all experts would agree with the recent review advising caution in the use of beta-blockers in ECT (Tess and Smetana 2009). Concomitant use of an anticholinergic agent at the time of treatment, typically either glycopyrrolate or atropine, is recommended if beta-blockers are used to prevent prolonged asystole after the electrical stimulus.

Valvular Abnormalities

Patients with aortic stenosis are at risk for low cardiac output under conditions of increased myocardial workload. Numerous reports exist of safe use of ECT in patients with aortic stenosis without prior surgical correction (Mueller et al. 2007; Rasmussen 1997), although a case of hypotension in such a patient (Sutor et al. 2008) illustrates the fragile hemodynamic status of this population Aortic stenosis is common, especially in elderly patients, and may require special attention by the anesthesiologist during ECT treatments to balance the risk of hyper- or hypotension, both of which may be problematic (Mueller et al. 2007). If a patient has had mechanical valve replacement and has received appropriate anticoagulation, the risk of ECT treatment should not be significantly increased (assuming that no other cardiac dysfunction, such as impaired ventricular function or dysrhythmia, is present). However, if a patient has a valvular abnormality that has not been optimally treated or is newly identified, then cardiac consultation should be obtained.

Heart Transplant

Heart transplant patients are rarely encountered in ECT practice. Three cases of uncomplicated ECT in heart transplant recipients have been published (Kellner et al. 1991; Lee et al. 2001; Pargger et al. 1995). Obviously, one should undertake ECT in a cardiac transplant patient only in close consultation with the patient's cardiologist.

Neurological Disorders

Neurophysiology of ECT

In contrast to cardiac physiology and testing, no known neurodiagnostic tests specifically predict neurological risk with ECT, and neuroprotective strategies are unavailable. Thus, brain imaging and electroencephalogram are not routinely indicated to assess ECT risk. If there is some other reason to perform a neurodiagnostic procedure, such as a newly found focal neurological sign, then that should be done prior to ECT as part of the diagnostic evaluation. ECT causes a brief rise in intracranial pressure, which theoretically implies risk of brain stem herniation in patients who already have increased intracranial pressure. However, such patients rarely are considered for ECT.

Dementia

Dementia, of course, is a term encompassing heterogeneous conditions causing progressive cognitive impairment. In ECT practice, the typical scenario is the elderly patient with known neurodegenerative dementia such as Alzheimer's or Lewy body disease or, less frequently, frontotemporal dementia. There is no reason to believe that these conditions per se would increase risk of medical complications during ECT. It would not be surprising that such patients may have greater-than-average acute cognitive impairment with ECT, but is the trajectory of their dementia worsened by a series of electrically induced seizures? The definitive study would be to randomly assign patients with well-characterized dementia syndromes who have psychopathology that normally would indicate ECT treatment to ECT or other interventions and follow up carefully with longitudinal assessments of cognition. Such a study has never been done and is not likely to be. We have only a set of relatively small case series of heterogeneous dementia patients with depression or agitation who seemed to benefit from ECT and who, in the opinion of the authors, did not seem to experience undue cognitive impairment (Rasmussen et al. 2003; Sutor and Rasmussen 2008).

Prudent advice for the ECT practitioner treating patients with dementia is to use unilateral electrode placement and twice-weekly scheduling. If improvement seems to lag from what is expected, then more aggressive treatment (i.e., bitemporal electrode placement or thrice-weekly treatments) can be given. Dementia patients with either depression or agitation who are referred for ECT may improve, but if maintenance treatments are not administered, rapid relapse tends to occur. Furthermore, the frequency of maintenance treatments often needs to be no less than every other week or even weekly to maintain the gains of the index course. This often leads to ongoing worsening of cognition, a side effect that obviously needs to be weighed against improvements in mood and behavior.

Some authors have cautioned against prescribing cholinesterase inhibitors such as donepezil during ECT, which synergistically increase the effects of succinylcholine and similar neuromuscular blocking agents (Walker and Perks 2002). However, Rasmussen et al. (2003) found no problems in their case series of ECT patients who received donepezil. The ECT practitioner may wish to discontinue such medication before ECT, but the time required for several half-lives of the medication delays what may be urgently needed treatment. Whether initial evidence in patients without dementia of lesser cognitive effects with ECT while using donepezil (Prakash et al. 2006) extends to patients with dementia awaits controlled trials.

Parkinson's Disease

Several case reports and series indicate that ECT is effective for treating depression and even the motor manifestations in patients with Parkinson's disease (PD) (Rasmussen and Abrams 1991, 1992; Rasmussen et al. 2002). Common side effects of ECT in patients with PD include delirium and treatment-emergent dyskinesias (Douyon et al. 1989). The duration of ECT-related antiparkinsonian effects has been variable (Fall and Granerus 1999) and may be extended with maintenance ECT, although the benefits must be balanced against cognitive impairment (Pridmore and Pollard 1996). Acute confusional states and dyskinesias are common during ECT in PD and may be reduced with cautious lowering of dopamine agonist dosage. As for patients with dementia, the ECT clinician should consider twice-weekly treatment frequency and the use of right-unilateral electrode placement.

With the introduction of deep brain stimulation to the PD treatment landscape, one would expect to see an occasional such patient receive ECT. There are a few reports of uncomplicated use of ECT in patients with deep brain stimulators (Bailine et al. 2008; Chou et al. 2005; Moscarillo and Annunziata 2000). In all three of these patients, one of whom had essential tremor and the other two parkinsonism, the stimulator was turned off for the duration of the patients' courses of ECT. So far, damage to the pulse generator, overheating of the electrode tip, and dislocation of the electrode during the seizure have not been reported.

Cerebrovascular Disease

In several small case series, patients with poststroke depression improved with ECT without development of further neurological injury (Weintraub and Lippmann 2000). No randomized prospective comparisons of ECT and other antidepressant treatment modalities have been done, however. Prudent advice for the ECT practitioner is not to use ECT in patients with recent stroke if possible. However, occasionally such a patient is profoundly depressed with marked decrease in psychomotor effort, has low or no food intake, or is at high acute suicidal risk. In such cases, if ECT is judged to be necessary, risk reduction strategies include continuing anticoagulation if it already is indicated (i.e., it should not be started just for ECT) and paying close attention to blood pressure to avoid high spikes and potentially dangerous declines.

There is concern that intracerebral aneurysms may rupture during ECT because of the rapid increase in blood pressure during seizures. Several cases of safe use of ECT in such patients have been reported (Okamura et al. 2006; Sharma et al. 2005). Two cases of ECT-associated intracerebral hemorrhages have been reported (Rikher et al. 1997; Weisberg et al. 1991), both in patients without known pre-ECT cerebrovascular disease. Most investigators reporting on ECT in patients with known aneurysms used antihypertensive drugs to dampen the ECT-related increase in blood pressure.

Epilepsy

ECT has anticonvulsant activity, as indicated by a progressive increase in seizure threshold and decrease in seizure length during the course of treatments (Rasimas et al. 2007; Sackeim et al. 1983). In the pre-anticonvulsant era and sporadically in the modern era, ECT has been used successfully to treat intractable epilepsy (Regenold et al. 1998) and even status epilepticus (Lisanby et al. 2001). These effects are short-lived, however, and the use of ECT to treat epilepsy is largely only of historical interest.

There are two reports of status epilepticus following ECT in epileptic patients: one patient had been administered multiple monitored ECT (Maletzky 1981), a technique no longer recommended for routine use (American Psychiatric Association 2001); the other had previously unrecognized seizures and was not receiving anticonvulsant medication during ECT (Moss-Herjanic 1967). At present, no evidence indicates that spontaneous seizure frequency increases with ECT in epileptic patients. Furthermore, it does not appear that the incidence of chronic epilepsy is increased in nonepileptic patients who receive ECT (Blackwood et al. 1980). However, because epilepsy is fairly common in the general population, recurrent seizures do occasionally develop in patients receiving extended courses of maintenance ECT (Rasmussen and Lunde 2007).

A common clinical challenge is how to treat the epileptic patient whose psychiatric illness requires ECT. Several case reports, small case series, and one fairly large series suggested that such patients can be given ECT effectively without worsening spontaneous seizure frequency (Lunde et al. 2006; Sienaert and Puskens 2007). Before undertaking a course of ECT in a patient with epilepsy, consultation with the patient's neurologist is advised. Pretreatment brain imaging or electroencephalography is not needed unless such testing is indicated as part of the patient's neurological care.

The most common technical problem in ECT with epileptic patients is elicitation of therapeutic seizures in the face of concomitant treatment with anticonvulsant medications. Cautious lowering of the patient's anticonvulsant medication dosages might be needed but increases the risk of spontaneous seizures and should be undertaken with the aid of a neurologist (Lunde et al. 2006). At present, it is not known whether various anticonvulsant agents differentially affect seizure threshold and duration in ECT.

Intracranial Tumors

Some reports indicate safe use of ECT in patients with a variety of intracranial masses (Kohler and Burock 2001; Patkar et al. 2000; Perry et al. 2007; Rasmussen and Flemming 2006; Rasmussen et al. 2007c). Presence of any central nervous system tumor may lead to an increased risk for neurological complications caused by ECT. In the absence of focal neurological signs, brain edema, mass effect, or papilledema, the risks likely are relatively small. In the presence of such findings, ECT should be considered only when no other reasonable option exists and after consultation with a neurosurgeon or neurologist to discuss strategies to reduce the increase in intracranial pressure that accompanies seizures.

Other Neurological Disorders

ECT may be lifesaving in some cases of refractory neuroleptic-induced malignant catatonia, which includes neuroleptic malignant syndrome (American Psychiatric Association 2001). Additionally, there are reports of patients with protracted delirium after traumatic brain injury or other neurological illness who responded to ECT (Rasmussen et al. 2008b). A prudent summary statement on this issue would be that although ECT is not a primary treatment for delirium, it sometimes may be dramatically effective in cases in which, despite intense medical and neurological assessment and management, severe agitation, psychosis, or catatonic features persist.

Several cases have been reported of patients with multiple sclerosis receiving ECT for psychopathology (Rasmussen and Keegan 2007). Isolated case reports and small series also describe, with varying details on outcome, the safe use of ECT for psychopathology in patients with other diverse neurological conditions such as cerebral palsy (Rasmussen et al. 1993). Of course, these do not prove that ECT has the same risk profile as for patients without these conditions. A prudent approach in such patients is to be alert for signs of neurological worsening and especially for excessive cognitive side effects.

Other Medical Disorders

The heart and brain bear most of the physiological effects of ECT. Fortunately, most of the other organ systems are not substantially affected, nor do their diseases generally cause much concern for greater risk of complications during ECT. Some additional considerations are discussed below.

Pulmonary Conditions

Large case series attest to the safe use of ECT in patients with asthma (Mueller et al. 2006) and chronic obstructive pulmonary disease (Schak et al. 2008). Patients who are using inhalers should do so in the morning shortly before treatment. Theophylline has been associated with a risk of prolonged seizures and status epilepticus in ECT (Abrams 2002, pp. 170–171), and discontinuation before ECT if medically safe has been recommended (American Psychiatric Association 2001), although Rasmussen and Zorumski (1993) described seven patients with therapeutic theophylline levels during ECT, none of whom developed status epilepticus. If discontinuing theophylline is medically contraindicated, then the lowest therapeutic blood level should be maintained, and caffeine augmentation should be avoided.

Two cases of successful and safe use of ECT after a pulmonary embolus have been reported (Suzuki et al. 2008). Attention should focus on continuation of therapeutic anticoagulation during ECT in such patients.

Pregnancy

The most common adverse events in pregnant women during ECT are aspiration and those related to premature labor, uterine contractions, and vaginal bleeding, although ECT can be delivered safely during pregnancy (Bozkurt et al. 2007; Kasar et al. 2007). Measures to prevent aspiration pneumonitis include tracheal intubation and alkalinizing intragastric pH with a nonparticulate antacid. Pretreatment obstetrical assessment, preferably to include fetal ultrasound, can identify high-risk pregnancies. Noninvasive monitoring of fetal heart tones before and after the seizure can document that no fetal distress occurred. Finally, probably the most important aspect of safe ECT in pregnant women is ready availability of obstetrical intervention in case of untoward events (American Psychiatric Association 2001).

Diabetes Mellitus

Single ECT treatments cause a brief approximately 8%–10% rise in blood sugar immediately after treatment in both diabetic and nondiabetic patients (Rasmussen and Ryan 2005; Rasmussen et al. 2006b). However, very little change occurs in blood sugar control over a course of treatments (Netzel et al. 2002). Diabetic patients should have blood glucose levels monitored closely during the ECT course, including fingerstick checks before treatment. Typically, type 1 diabetic patients are administered half their morning insulin dose and are treated with ECT promptly. They are then fed breakfast and given the remaining half of their insulin dose. Alternatively, the whole dose can be withheld, ECT can be delivered promptly early in the morning, and then posttreatment breakfast and the insulin dose can be given.

Chronic Pain

Chronic pain syndromes are quite common in psychiatric patients. When the pain symptom is clearly secondary to a melancholic or psychotic depression, the ECT clinician can be optimistic about resolution of the pain symptoms along with other psychiatric symptoms. When a chronic pain patient seems to have developed secondary depression, results are more mixed with ECT (Rasmussen 2003; Rasmussen and Rummans 2002). Patients who are highly entrenched in a "pain lifestyle" are not likely to benefit from ECT. An intriguing finding is that phantom limb pain may abate with ECT even in the absence of apparent mood disturbance (Rasmussen and Rummans 2000).

Miscellaneous Considerations

Mild sodium abnormalities have not proven to be problematic for safe administration of ECT (Rasmussen et al. 2007b). Some anesthesiologists prefer to give an extra dose of steroid—so-called stress doses—prior to ECT in patients who are already taking such medication. However, in a large series (Rasmussen et al. 2008a), this was found to be unnecessary. Histamine-2 antagonists or antacids may decrease gastric acid secretion and the risk of aspiration pneumonitis in patients with gastroesophageal reflux disease, gastroparesis, or obesity (as well as pregnancy, as discussed earlier). Patients at severe risk for aspiration may require intubation. Urinary retention from antimuscarinic agents given during ECT is quite uncomfortable for patients and can predispose to urinary tract infections and even bladder rupture if not monitored. In those patients who do experience significant urinary retention after treatments, antimuscarinic agents can be avoided, recognizing that the vagal effect of the electrical stimulus is not blocked and prolonged asystole can occur. Patients with severe osteoporosis or recent fractures require careful titration of muscle relaxant dosing; the adequacy of paralysis can be tested with a peripheral nerve stimulator. Extra care should be exercised when ventilating the patient with unstable cervical spine disease to avoid spinal cord injury. With the brief increase in intraocular pressure lasting a few minutes after the seizures (Good et al. 2004), glaucoma patients should receive their medications in the mornings before treatment, an exception being anticholinesterase drugs, which may prolong the action of succinylcholine.

Conclusion

ECT represents a remarkably safe and effective treatment option for depressed, manic, or psychotic patients with concomitant medical illnesses. With proper attention to pretreatment medical evaluation, rational use of cardioprotective medications during the treatments, and ongoing monitoring of medical status in between treatments, virtually all patients requiring ECT can be safely treated.

References

Abrams R: Electroconvulsive Therapy, 4th Edition. New York, Oxford University Press, 2002

Albin SM, Stevens SR, Rasmussen KG: Blood pressure before and after electroconvulsive therapy in hypertensive and nonhypertensive patients. J ECT 23:9–10, 2007

American Psychiatric Association, Committee on Electroconvulsive Therapy: The Practice of Electroconvulsive Therapy, 2nd Edition. Washington, DC, American Psychiatric Association, 2001

Bailine S, Kremen N, Kohen I, et al: Bitemporal electroconvulsive therapy for depression in a Parkinson disease patient with a deep-brain stimulator. J ECT 24:171–172, 2008

Blackwood DHR, Cull RE, Freeman CPL, et al: A study of the incidence of epilepsy following ECT. J Neurol Neurosurg Psychiatry 43:1098–1102, 1980

Bozkurt A, Karlidere T, Isintas M, et al: Acute and maintenance electroconvulsive therapy for treatment of psychotic depression in a pregnant patient. J ECT 23:185–187, 2007

Castelli I, Steiner LA, Kaufman MA, et al: Comparative effects of esmolol and labetalol to attenuate hyperdynamic states after electroconvulsive therapy. Anesth Analg 80:557–561, 1995

Chou KL, Hurtig HI, Jaggi JL, et al: Electroconvulsive therapy for depression in a Parkinson's disease patient with bilateral subthalamic nucleus deep brain stimulators. Parkinsonism Relat Disord 11:403–406, 2005

Dannon PN, Iancu I, Hirschmann S, et al: Labetalol does not lengthen asystole during electroconvulsive therapy. J ECT 14:245–250, 1998

Dodd ML, Dolenc TJ, Karpyak VM, et al: QTc dispersion in patients referred for electroconvulsive therapy. J ECT 24:131–133, 2008

Dolenc TJ, Barnes RD, Hayes DL, et al: Electroconvulsive therapy in patients with pacemakers and ICDs. Pacing Clin Electrophysiol 27:1257–1263, 2004

Douyon R, Serby M, Klutchko B, et al: ECT and Parkinson's disease revisited: a "naturalistic" study. Am J Psychiatry 146:1451–1455, 1989

Fall P-A, Granerus A-K: Maintenance ECT in Parkinson's disease. J Neural Transm 106:737–741, 1999

Gerring JP, Shields HM: The identification and management of patients with a high risk for cardiac arrhythmias during modified ECT. J Clin Psychiatry 43:140–143, 1982

Goldberg RK, Badger JM: Major depressive disorder in patients with the implantable cardioverter defibrillator: two cases treated with ECT. Psychosomatics 34:273–277, 1993

Good MS, Dolenc TJ, Rasmussen KG: Electroconvulsive therapy in a patient with glaucoma. J ECT 20:48–49, 2004

Howie MB, Black HA, Zvara D, et al: Esmolol reduces autonomic hypersensitivity and length of seizures induced by electroconvulsive therapy. Anesth Analg 71:384–388, 1990

Howie MB, Hiestland DC, Zvara DA, et al: Defining the dose range for esmolol used in electroconvulsive therapy hemodynamic attenuation. Anesth Analg 75:805–810, 1992

Kasar M, Saatcioglu O, Kutlar T: Electroconvulsive therapy use in pregnancy. J ECT 23:183–184, 2007

Kellner CH, Monroe RR, Burns C, et al: Electroconvulsive therapy in a patient with a heart transplant (letter). N Engl J Med 325:663, 1991

Kohler CG, Burock M: ECT for psychotic depression associated with a brain tumor (letter). Am J Psychiatry 158:2089, 2001

Lee HB, Jayaram G, Teitelbaum ML: Electroconvulsive therapy for depression in a cardiac transplant patient. Psychosomatics 42:362–364, 2001

Lisanby SH, Bazil CW, Resor SR, et al: ECT in the treatment of status epilepticus. J ECT 17:210–215, 2001

Lunde ME, Lee EK, Rasmussen KG: Electroconvulsive therapy in patients with epilepsy. Epilepsy Behav 9:355–359, 2006

Lynch AM, Pandurangi A, Levenson JL: Electroconvulsive therapy in a candidate for heart transplant with an implantable cardioverter defibrillator and cardiac contractility modulator. Psychosomatics 49:341–344, 2008

Magid M, Lapid MI, Sampson SM, et al: Use of electroconvulsive therapy in a patient 10 days after myocardial infarction. J ECT 21:182–185, 2005

Maletzky BM: Multiple Monitored Electroconvulsive Therapy. Boca Raton, FL, CRR Press, 1981

McCall WV, Shelp FE, Weiner RD, et al: Effects of labetalol on hemodynamics and seizure duration during ECT. Convuls Ther 7:5–14, 1991

McCully RB, Karon BL, Rummans TA, et al: Frequency of left ventricular dysfunction after electroconvulsive therapy. Am J Cardiol 91:1147–1150, 2003

Mehta V, Mueller PS, Gonzalez-Arriaza HL, et al: Safety of electroconvulsive therapy in patients receiving long-term warfarin therapy. Mayo Clin Proc 79:1396–1401, 2004

Moscarillo FM, Annunziata CM: ECT in a patient with deep brain-stimulating electrode in place. J ECT 16:287–290, 2000

Moss-Herjanic B: Prolonged unconsciousness following electroconvulsive therapy. Am J Psychiatry 124:112–114, 1967

Mueller PS, Schak K, Barnes RD, et al: The safety of electroconvulsive therapy in patients with asthma. Neth J Med 64:417–421, 2006

Mueller PS, Barnes RD, Nishimura R, et al: ECT in patients with aortic stenosis. Mayo Clin Proc 82:1360–1363, 2007

Mueller PS, Albin SM, Barnes RD, et al: Safety of electroconvulsive therapy in patients with unrepaired abdominal aortic aneurysm: report of 8 patients. J ECT 25:165–169, 2009

Netzel PJ, Mueller PS, Rummans TA, et al: Safety, efficacy, and effects on glycemic control of electroconvulsive therapy in insulin-requiring type 2 diabetic patients. J ECT 18:16–21, 2002

Nuttall GA, Bowersox MR, Douglass SB, et al: Morbidity and mortality in the use of electroconvulsive therapy. J ECT 20:237–241, 2004

O'Connor CJ, Rothenberg DM, Soble JS, et al: The effect of esmolol pretreatment on the incidence of regional wall motion abnormalities during electroconvulsive therapy. Anesth Analg 82:143–147, 1996

Okamura T, Kudo K, Sata N, et al: Electroconvulsive therapy after coil embolization of cerebral aneurysm: a case report and literature review. J ECT 22:148–149, 2006

Pargger H, Kaufmann MA, Schouten R, et al: Hemodynamic responses to electroconvulsive therapy in a patient 5 years after cardiac transplantation. Anesthesiology 83:625–627, 1995

Patkar AA, Hill KP, Weinstein SP, et al: ECT in the presence of brain tumor and increased intracranial pressure: evaluation and reduction of risk. J ECT 16:189–197, 2000

Perry CL, Lindell EP, Rasmussen KG: ECT in patients with arachnoid cysts. J ECT 23:36–37, 2007

Petrides G, Fink M: Atrial fibrillation, anticoagulation, and electroconvulsive therapy. Convuls Ther 12:91–98, 1996

Porquez JN, Thompson TR, McDonald WM: Administration of ECT in a patient with inoperable abdominal aortic aneurysm: serial imaging of the aorta during maintenance. J ECT 19:118–120, 2003

Prakash J, Kotwal A, Prabhu HRA: Therapeutic and prophylactic utility of the memory-enhancing drug donepezil hydrochloride on cognition of patients undergoing electroconvulsive therapy: a randomized controlled trial. J ECT 22:163–168, 2006

Pridmore S, Pollard C: Electroconvulsive therapy in Parkinson's disease: 30 month follow up (letter). J Neurol Neurosurg Psychiatry 61:693, 1996

Rasimas JJ, Stevens SR, Rasmussen KG: Seizure length in ECT as a function of age, gender, and treatment number. J ECT 23:14–16, 2007

Rasmussen KG: Electroconvulsive therapy in patients with aortic stenosis. Convuls Ther 13:196–199, 1997

Rasmussen KG: The role of electroconvulsive therapy in chronic pain. Reviews in Analgesia 7:1–8, 2003

Rasmussen K, Abrams R: Treatment of Parkinson's disease with electroconvulsive therapy. Psychiatr Clin North Am 14:925–933, 1991

Rasmussen KG, Abrams R: The role of electroconvulsive therapy in Parkinson's disease, in Parkinson's Disease: Neurobehavioral Aspects. Edited by Huber S, Cummings J. New York, Oxford University Press, 1992, pp 255–270

Rasmussen KG, Flemming KD: Electroconvulsive therapy in patients with cavernous hemangiomas. J ECT 22:272–273, 2006

Rasmussen KG, Keegan BM: ECT in patients with multiple sclerosis. J ECT 23:179–180, 2007

Rasmussen KG, Lunde ME: Patients who develop epilepsy during extended treatment with electroconvulsive therapy. Seizure 16:266–270, 2007

Rasmussen KG, Rummans TA: Electroconvulsive therapy for phantom limb pain. Pain 85:297–299, 2000

Rasmussen KG, Rummans TA: Electroconvulsive therapy in the management of chronic pain. Curr Pain Headache Rep 6:17–22, 2002

Rasmussen KG, Ryan DA: The effect of electroconvulsive therapy treatments on blood sugar in nondiabetic patients. J ECT 21:232–234, 2005

Rasmussen KG, Zorumski CF: Electroconvulsive therapy in patients taking theophylline. J Clin Psychiatry 54:427–431, 1993

Rasmussen KG, Zorumski CF, Jarvis MR: ECT in patients with cerebral palsy. Convuls Ther 9:205–208, 1993

Rasmussen KG, Jarvis MR, Zorumski CF, et al: Low-dose atropine in electroconvulsive therapy. J ECT 15:213–221, 1999

Rasmussen KG, Rummans TA, Richardson JR: Electroconvulsive therapy in the medically ill. Psychiatr Clin North Am 25:177–194, 2002

Rasmussen KG, Russell JC, Kung S, et al: ECT in major depression with probable Lewy body dementia. J ECT 19:103–109, 2003

Rasmussen KG, Karpyak VM, Hammill SC: Lack of effect of ECT on Holter monitor recordings before and after treatment. J ECT 20:45–47, 2004

Rasmussen KG, Mueller M, Kellner CH, et al: Patterns of psychotropic medication use among severely depressed patients referred for ECT: data from the Consortium for Research in ECT. J ECT 22:116–123, 2006a

Rasmussen KG, Ryan DA, Mueller PS: Blood glucose before and after ECT treatments in type 2 diabetic patients. J ECT 22:124–126, 2006b

Rasmussen KG, Hooten WM, Dodd ML, et al: QTc dispersion on the baseline ECG predicts arrhythmias during electroconvulsive therapy. Acta Cardiol 62:345–347, 2007a

Rasmussen KG, Mohan A, Stevens SR: Serum sodium does not correlate with seizure length or seizure threshold in electroconvulsive therapy. J ECT 23:175–176, 2007b

Rasmussen KG, Perry CL, Sutor B, et al: ECT in patients with intracranial masses. J Neuropsychiatry Clin Neurosci 19:191–193, 2007c

Rasmussen KG, Albin SM, Mueller PS, et al: Electroconvulsive therapy in patients taking steroid medication: should supplemental doses be given on the days of treatment? J ECT 24:128–130, 2008a

Rasmussen KG, Hart DA, Lineberry TW, et al: ECT in patients with psychopathology secondary to acute neurologic illness. Psychosomatics 49:67–72, 2008b

Rasmussen KG, Leise AD, Stevens SR: Orthostatic hemodynamic changes after ECT treatments. J ECT 24:134–136, 2008c

Regenold WT, Weintraub D, Taller A: Electroconvulsive therapy for epilepsy and major depression. Am J Geriatr Psychiatry 6:180–183, 1998

Rice EH, Sombrotto LB, Markowitz JC, et al: Cardiovascular morbidity in high-risk patients during ECT. Am J Psychiatry 151:1637–1641, 1994

Rikher KV, Johnson R, Kamal M: Cortical blindness after electroconvulsive therapy. J Am Board Fam Pract 10:141–143, 1997

Ruwitch JF, Perez JE, Miller TR, et al: Myocardial ischemia induced by electroconvulsive therapy (abstract 2034). Circulation 90 (suppl 4, pt 2):I379, 1994

Sackeim HA, Decina P, Prohovnik I, et al: Anticonvulsant and antidepressant properties of electroconvulsive therapy: a proposed mechanism of action. Biol Psychiatry 18:1301–1310, 1983

Schak KM, Mueller PS, Barnes RD, et al: The safety of ECT in patients with chronic obstructive pulmonary disease. Psychosomatics 49:208–211, 2008

Sharma A, Ramaswamy S, Bhatia SC: Electroconvulsive therapy after repair of cerebral aneurysm. J ECT 21:180–181, 2005

Sienaert P, Puskens J: Anticonvulsants during electroconvulsive therapy: review and recommendations. J ECT 23:120–123, 2007

Stern L, Hirschmann S, Grunhaus L: ECT in patients with major depressive disorder and low cardiac output. Convuls Ther 13:68–73, 1997

Sutor B, Rasmussen KG: Electroconvulsive therapy for agitation in Alzheimer disease: a case series. J ECT 24:239–241, 2008

Sutor B, Mueller PS, Rasmussen KG: Bradycardia and hypotension in a patient with severe aortic stenosis receiving electroconvulsive therapy dose titration for treatment of depression. J ECT 24:281–282, 2008

Suzuki K, Takamatsu K, Takano T, et al: Safety of electroconvulsive therapy in psychiatric patients shortly after the occurrence of pulmonary embolism. J ECT 24:286–288, 2008

Tang W-K, Ungvari GS: Asystole during electroconvulsive therapy: a case report. Aust N Z J Psychiatry 35:382–385, 2001

Tess AV, Smetana GW: Medical evaluation of patients undergoing electroconvulsive therapy. N Engl J Med 360:1437–1444, 2009

Van den Broek WW, Leentjens AF, Mulder PG, et al: Low-dose esmolol bolus reduces seizure duration during electroconvulsive therapy: a double-blind, placebo-controlled study. Br J Anaesth 83:271–274, 1999

Walker C, Perks D: Do you know about donepezil and succinylcholine? (letter) Anaesthesia 57:1041, 2002

Weintraub D, Lippmann S: Electroconvulsive therapy in the acute poststroke period. J ECT 16:415–418, 2000

Weisberg LA, Elliott D, Mielke D: Intracerebral hemorrhage following electroconvulsive therapy (letter). Neurology 41:1849, 1991

Zielinski RJ, Roose SP, Devanand DP, et al: Cardiovascular complications of ECT in depressed patients with cardiac disease. Am J Psychiatry 150:904–909, 1993

Zvara DA, Brooker RF, McCall WV, et al: The effect of esmolol on ST-segment depression and arrhythmias after electroconvulsive therapy. Convuls Ther 13:165–174, 1997

CHAPTER 41

Palliative Care

William Breitbart, M.D.

Harvey Max Chochinov, M.D., Ph.D., F.R.C.P.C.

Yesne Alici, M.D.

ONE OF THE MOST CHALLENGING roles for the psychosomatic medicine psychiatrist is to help guide terminally ill patients physically, psychologically, and spiritually through the dying process. Patients with advanced cancer, AIDS, and other life-threatening medical illnesses are at increased risk for developing major psychiatric complications and have an enormous burden of both physical as well as psychological symptoms (Breitbart et al. 2004a). In fact, surveys suggest that psychological symptoms such as depression, anxiety, and hopelessness are as frequent, if not more so, than pain and other physical symptoms (Portenoy et al. 1994; Vogl et al. 1999). The psychiatrist, as a consultant to or member of a palliative care team, has a unique role and opportunity to offer competent and compassionate palliative care to those with life-threatening illness.

In 1999 the Academy of Psychosomatic Medicine published its position statement titled "Psychiatric Aspects of Excellent End-of-Life Care" (Shuster et al. 1999), which stressed the importance of psychiatric issues in palliative care and the need for competent psychiatric care to be an integral component of palliative care. Major textbooks provide comprehensive reviews of the interface of psychiatry and palliative medicine (Chochinov and Breitbart 2009; Lloyd-Williams 2008), and an international journal with that focus has been in existence since 2003 (Breitbart 2003).

The importance of the psychiatric, psychosocial, and spiritual aspects of palliative care has also been recognized in reports from the American Board of Internal Medicine (Subcommittee on Psychiatric Aspects of Life-Sustaining Technology 1996), the Institute of Medicine (Field and Cassel 1997; Foley and Helband 2001), the National Comprehensive Cancer Network (Levy et al. 2009), the U.S. Health Resources and Services Administration (O'Neill et al. 2003), and the National Consensus Project for Quality Palliative Care (2009). Several major national and international palliative care organizations also exist, and more than 10 national and international palliative care scientific journals have been published (Stjernsward and Clark 2004).

This chapter guides the psychosomatic medicine practitioner through the most salient aspects of effective psychiatric care of patients with advanced, life-threatening medical illnesses. In this chapter, we review basic concepts and definitions of palliative care and the experience of dying in the United States; the role of the psychiatrist in palliative care, including assessment and management of common psychiatric disorders in the terminally ill, with special attention to suicide and desire for hastened death. We describe the psychotherapies developed for use in palliative care settings and then discuss spirituality, cultural sensitivity, communication, grief and bereavement, and psychiatric contributions to the control of common physical symptoms.

Related topics are discussed elsewhere in this book, including advance directives and end-of-life decisions (see Chapter 3, "Ethical Issues," and Chapter 4, "Psychological Responses to Illness"), physician assisted suicide (see Chapter 9, "Suicidality"), terminal sedation (see Chapter 19, "Lung Disease"), dialysis discontinuation (see Chapter 21, "Renal Disease"), and pain management (see Chapter 36, "Pain").

Palliative Care

Historical Perspectives

The term *palliation* is derived from the Latin root word *palliare,* which means "to cloak" or "to conceal." *Pallium* also refers to the cloth that covers or cloaks burial caskets. These root words suggest that the dying patient, although not amenable to cure, can be "cloaked" or "embraced" in the comforting arms of the caregiver. What cannot be cured can always be comforted. The terms *palliative care* and *palliative medicine* are often used interchangeably. Palliative medicine refers to the medical discipline of palliative care, an approach to improve the quality of life of patients and their families facing life-threatening illness. The nature and focus of palliative care have evolved over the past century, expanding beyond just comfort for the dying to include palliative care and symptom control that begins with the onset of a life-threatening illness and proceeds past death to include bereavement interventions for family and others (Sepulveda et al. 2002).

Modern palliative care is an outgrowth of the hospice movement that began in the 1840s with Calvaires in Lyon, France, and progressed through 1900 and the establishment of the St. Joseph's Hospice in London, finally culminating with the progenitor of all modern hospices, St. Christopher's Hospice, established in 1967 by Cicely Saunders. By 1975, a large number of independent hospices had been developed in the United Kingdom, Canada, and Australia. The first hospice in the United States was established in 1974 in Connecticut. Soon after, the U.S. government established limited Medicare coverage for hospice benefits. This period also saw the establishment of the first "palliative care" program at Royal Victoria Hospital in Montreal, founded by Balfour Mount and his colleagues. This period of evolution from the traditional stand-alone, home-based hospice also saw the development of hospital-based pain and palliative care consultation services such as the pain service established in 1978 by Kathleen Foley at the Memorial Sloan-Kettering Cancer Center. Modern palliative care thus evolved from the hospice movement into a mixture of academic and nonacademic clinical care delivery systems that had components of home care and hospital-based services (Berger et al. 2006; Stjernsward and Clark 2004).

Definition of Palliative Care

The Palliative Care Foundation (1981) defined *palliative care* as "active compassionate care of the terminally ill at a time that their disease is no longer responsive to traditional treatment aimed at cure or prolongation of life, and when the control of symptoms is paramount" (p. 10). According to this definition, palliative care applies primarily at the end of life. In 1990, the World Health Organization defined *palliative care* as

> the active total care of patients whose disease is not responsive to curative treatment. Control of pain, of other symptoms, and of psychological, social and spiritual problems, is paramount. The goal of palliative care is achievement of the best quality of life for patients and their families. Many aspects of palliative care are also applicable earlier in the course of the illness in conjunction with anti-cancer treatment. (p. 2)

This definition was the first to suggest applicability even at stages of disease that precede the end of life (World Health Organization 1990).

In 1995, the Canadian Palliative Care Association published its definition of *palliative care:*

> Palliative care, as a philosophy of care, is the combination of active and compassionate therapies, intended to comfort and support individuals and families who are living with a life-threatening illness. During periods of illness and bereavement, palliative care strives to meet physical, psychological, social and spiritual expectations and needs, while remaining sensitive to personal, cultural and religious values, beliefs and practices. Palliative care may be combined with therapies aimed at reducing or curing illness or it may be the total focus of care. (p. 3)

This definition was perhaps the first to suggest that palliative care is not only applicable at all stages of life-threatening disease (intensifying once cure is no longer possible) but also that psychological, social, spiritual, and cultural issues are elements of palliative care as important as the control of pain and other physical symptoms.

The World Health Organization definition of palliative care has been revised and expanded through the years (Sepulveda et al. 2002; World Health Organization 2002). The most recent and comprehensive definition of palliative care as outlined by the World Health Organization (2002, 2009) provides a framework for palliative care in all settings. According to this definition, palliative care

- provides relief from pain and other distressing symptoms.
- affirms life and regards dying as a normal process.
- intends neither to hasten nor to postpone death.
- integrates psychological and spiritual aspects of patients care.
- offers a support system to help patients live as actively as possible until death.
- offers a support system to help families cope during the patient's illness and in their own bereavement.
- is interdisciplinary and uses a team approach including physicians, nurses, mental health professionals,

clergy, and volunteers to address the needs of patients and their families.
- will enhance quality of life and may also positively influence the course of illness.
- is applicable early in the course of illness, in conjunction with other therapies that are intended to prolong life, and includes those investigations needed to better understand and manage distressing complications.

Palliative Care Programs/Models of Care Delivery

Palliative care is not restricted to those who are dying or those who are enrolled in hospice programs, but rather can be applied cost-effectively to the control of symptoms and provision of support to those living with chronic life-threatening illnesses (Taylor et al. 2007). Palliative care has been successfully instituted for patients with AIDS and cancer as national policy in countries that are neither wealthy nor industrialized (Bruera et al. 2000).

Fully developed, model palliative care programs ideally include all of the following components: 1) a home care program (e.g., hospice program); 2) a hospital-based palliative care consultation service; 3) a day care program or ambulatory care clinic; 4) a palliative care inpatient unit (or dedicated palliative care beds in hospital); 5) a bereavement program; 6) training and research programs; and 7) Internet-based services. An updated U.S. national expert consensus process produced the Clinical Practice Guidelines for Quality Palliative Care, which notes the need for adaptation to specific care settings and training for all providers (National Consensus Project for Quality Palliative Care 2009).

It is estimated that there are currently more than 4,500 hospices and over 1,000 hospital-based pain and palliative care services in the United States, serving around 1.4 million patients (National Hospice and Palliative Care Organization 2008). The subspecialty of Hospice and Palliative Medicine has recently achieved recognition within the American Board of Medical Subspecialties (ABMS) and the Accreditation Council for Graduate Medical Education (ACGME), with the American Board of Psychiatry and Neurology one of the co-sponsoring boards. There are a total of 48 accredited hospice and palliative medicine fellowship programs in the United States (American Academy of Hospice and Palliative Medicine Web site 2009).

Death in America

To understand and treat psychiatric issues in the dying patient today, one must have an appreciation of why, when, where, and how Americans now die.

Where and How Do Americans Die?

Population surveys continue to show that the majority of people would prefer to be cared for and die at home (Higginson and Sen-Gupta 2000; Stajduhar et al. 2008). Despite these findings, most Americans die in institutions, surrounded by medical caregivers.

The SUPPORT clinical trial (Study to Understand Prognoses and Preferences for Outcomes and Risks of Treatments) (SUPPORT Principal Investigators 1995) and other studies have suggested that a technological imperative characterizes Western medical practice, including care of the dying. SUPPORT found substantial shortcomings in the care of seriously ill hospitalized patients—including poor communication between physicians and dying patients and implementation of overly aggressive treatment, often against patients' wishes. The findings of this study emphasized the need for greater skills and education in end-of-life issues as well as increased communication with and support of dying patients. Perhaps the most perturbing conclusion from this study was that in general, Americans were dying not good deaths but bad deaths, characterized by needless suffering and disregard for patients' or families' wishes or values.

The concept of death trajectories (Figure 41–1) has been used to describe the unique as well as relatively predictable patterns of approaching death (Field and Cassel 1997). Some people die suddenly and unexpectedly, as shown in Figure 41–1A (e.g., cardiac arrest). Among those with forewarning of death, many have a steady and relatively predictable decline, as shown in Figure 41–1B (e.g., advanced cancer). There is a third pattern (Figure 41–1C) of long periods of chronic illness punctuated by crises, any of which may result in death (e.g., AIDS, congestive heart failure, or chronic obstructive pulmonary disease). Each type of death trajectory brings with it a unique set of problems and illustrates the challenges of determining prognoses for patients with life-threatening illnesses.

What Is a "Good" Death?

A meaningful dying process is one throughout which the patient is physically, psychologically, spiritually, and emotionally supported by his or her family, friends, and caregivers. Weisman (1972) described four criteria for what he called an "appropriate death": 1) internal conflicts, such as fears about loss of control, should be reduced as much as possible; 2) the individual's personal sense of identity should be sustained; 3) critical relationships should be enhanced or at least maintained, and conflicts should be resolved, if possible; and 4) the person should be encouraged to set and attempt to reach meaningful goals, even though limited, such as attending a graduation, a wedding, or the

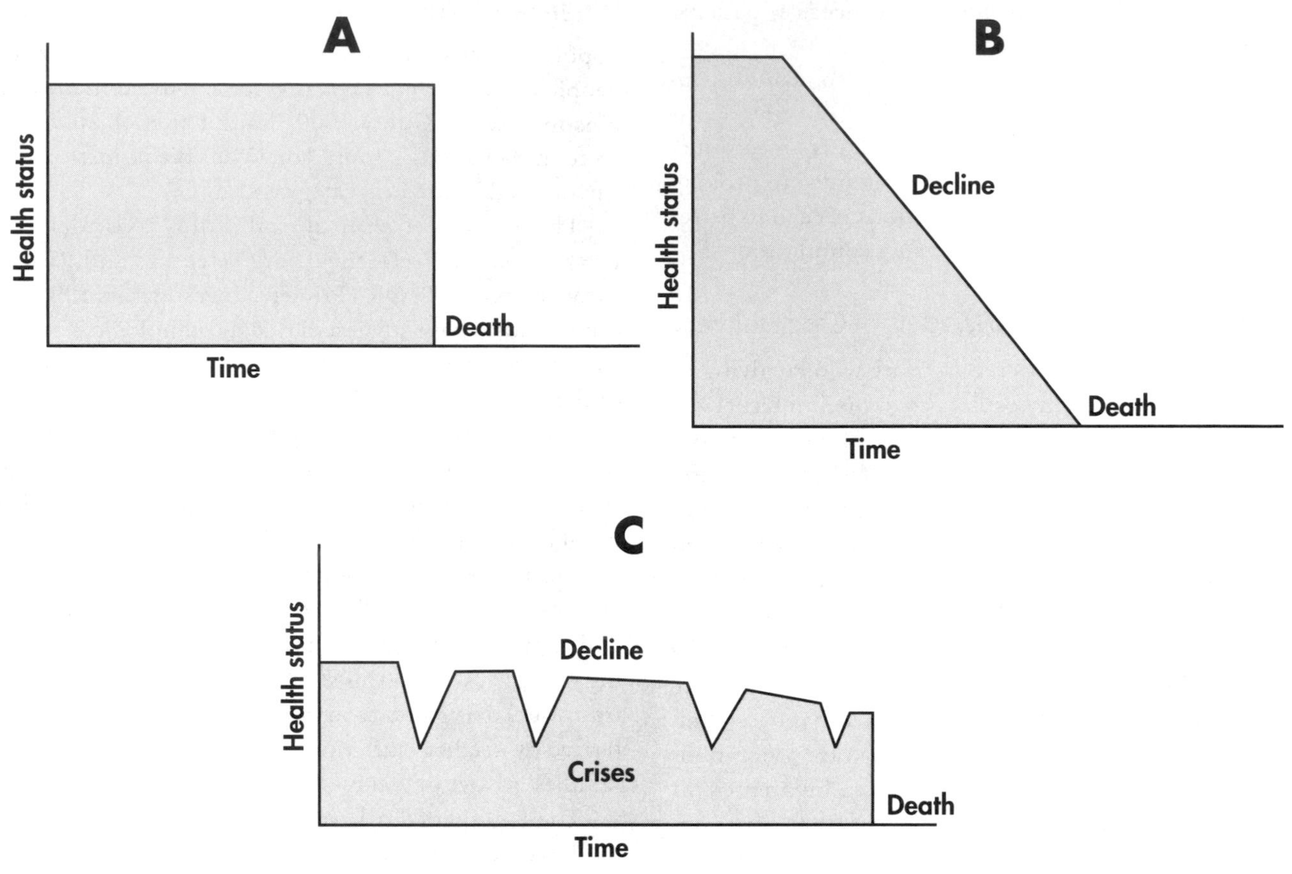

FIGURE 41–1. Prototypical death trajectories.

(A) Sudden death from an unexpected cause. (B) Steady decline from a progressive disease with a "terminal" phase. (C) Advanced illness marked by slow decline with periodic crises and "sudden" death.

birth of a child, as a way to provide a sense of continuity into the future. The World Health Organization (2002, 2009) outlined guidelines characterizing a "good" death as one that is 1) free from avoidable distress and suffering for patient, family, and caregivers; 2) in general accord with the patient's and family's wishes; and 3) reasonably consistent with clinical, cultural, and ethical standards. These guidelines and the aforementioned considerations for achieving a good death can serve as general principles for the psychosomatic medicine psychiatrist in caring for the dying.

What Is the Role of the Psychiatrist?

The traditional role of the psychiatrist is broadened in several ways in the care of the dying patient. The psychiatrist's primary role in the palliative care setting is the diagnosis and treatment of comorbid psychiatric disorders. Psychosomatic medicine psychiatrists can provide expert care and teaching about the management of depression, suicide, anxiety, delirium, fatigue, and pain in terminally ill patients (Breitbart and Holland 1993; Chochinov and Breitbart 2009). The role of the psychiatrist, in the care of the dying, extends beyond the management of psychiatric symptoms and syndromes into existential issues, family and caregiver support, bereavement, doctor–patient communication, and education and training. Psychiatrists can play an important role in the management of social, psychological, ethical, legal, and spiritual issues that complicate the care of dying patients. The psychiatrist can provide assistance in dealing with the existential crisis posed by a terminal diagnosis. Through discussions with the primary care physician, the patient and family may have begun to confront the reality that the disease is no longer curable or controllable. The psychiatrist can help the patient deal with the prognosis and explore treatment options, including palliative care.

The psychiatrist helps resolve conflicts among patient, family, and staff by opening lines of communication and helping families to deal with the strong emotions that surround the imminent death of a loved one. Conflicts with the physician and staff are common because the clinicians are also stressed; resolution of these conflicts is a critical intervention for the patient's physical and psychological well-being.

Psychotherapeutic interventions for patients and families who are experiencing anticipatory grief are also important. During the bereavement period, the family may turn to the psychiatrist who participated in the patient's care and who shares memories of the patient for continuing support.

The psychiatrist also has an ethical role in encouraging discussion of end-of-life decisions regarding treatment, withholding resuscitation, and life support. The capacity of the patient to make rational judgments and the proxy's ability to make an appropriate decision for the patient may require psychiatric evaluation. The decision to withdraw life support is highly emotional and may require psychiatric consultation (Subcommittee on Psychiatric Aspects of Life-Sustaining Technology 1996).The psychiatrist's role can include teaching the medical staff about the psychological issues involved in care of dying patients, including how to deliver bad news and discuss do-not-resuscitate (DNR) orders and other treatment preferences ideally with the patient or with family when the patient is unable to make such decisions (Levin et al. 2008; Misbin et al. 1993; Weissman 2004).

Psychiatric Disorders in the Palliative Care Setting

Patients with advanced disease, such as advanced cancer, are particularly vulnerable to psychiatric disorders and complications (Breitbart et al. 1995, 2004a; Miovic and Block 2007). Unfortunately, medical specialists frequently fail to recognize emotional distress and common psychiatric disorders in terminally ill patients (Breitbart and Alici 2008; Miovic and Block 2007). In this section we review psychiatric disorders frequently encountered in palliative care settings including anxiety disorders, depression, and delirium. The incidence, assessment, and treatment of specific psychiatric disorders in advanced diseases are discussed in earlier chapters in this volume—for example, cancer (Chapter 23, "Oncology"), heart failure (Chapter 18, "Heart Disease"), chronic obstructive pulmonary disease (Chapter 19, "Lung Disease"), end-stage renal disease (Chapter 21, "Renal Disease"), and AIDS (Chapter 28, "HIV/AIDS").

Anxiety Disorders

The terminally ill patient presents with a complex mixture of physical and psychological symptoms in the context of a frightening reality, making the identification of anxious symptoms requiring treatment challenging (see also Chapter 11, "Anxiety Disorders"). Patients with anxiety complain of tension or restlessness, or they exhibit jitteriness, autonomic hyperactivity, vigilance, insomnia, distractibility, shortness of breath, numbness, apprehension, worry, or rumination. Often the physical or somatic manifestations of anxiety overshadow the psychological or cognitive ones and are the symptoms that the patient most often presents (Holland 1989). The consultant must use these symptoms as a cue to inquire about the patient's psychological state, which is commonly one of fear, worry, or apprehension.

The assumption that a high level of anxiety is inevitably encountered during the terminal phase of illness is neither helpful nor accurate. In deciding whether to treat anxiety during the terminal phase of illness, the clinician should consider the patient's subjective level of distress as the primary impetus for the initiation of treatment. Other considerations include problematic patient behavior such as noncompliance due to anxiety, family and staff reactions to the patient's distress, and the balancing of the risks and benefits of treatment (Roth and Massie 2009).

Prevalence

Prevalence of anxiety disorders among terminally ill cancer and AIDS patients ranges from 15% to 28% (Kerrihard et al. 1999). Prevalence studies of anxiety, primarily in cancer populations, report a higher prevalence of mixed anxiety and depressive symptoms rather than anxiety alone (Roth and Massie 2009). Prevalence of anxiety increases with advancing disease and decline in the patient's physical status (Rabkin et al. 1997). Brandberg et al. (1995) reported that 28% of advanced melanoma patients were anxious compared with 15% of control subjects. In the Canadian National Palliative Care Survey, 24.4% of the patients receiving palliative care for cancer were found to have at least one DSM-IV (American Psychiatric Association 1994) anxiety or depressive disorder. The prevalence of anxiety disorders in that survey was 13.9%. Younger patients and those with a lower performance status, smaller social networks, and less participation in organized religious services were more likely to have a psychiatric disorder (Wilson et al. 2007a). It was also notable that palliative care patients with a DSM-IV anxiety and/or depressive disorder reported more severe distress from several physical symptoms, social concerns, and existential issues (Wilson et al. 2007a).

Assessment

As outlined in Table 41–1, anxiety can occur in terminally ill patients as an adjustment disorder, a disease- or treatment-related condition, or an exacerbation of a preexisting anxiety disorder (Kerrihard et al. 1999; Massie 1989). Adjustment disorder with anxiety is related to adjusting to the existential crisis and the uncertainty of the prognosis and the future (Holland 1989). When faced with terminal

TABLE 41–1. Anxiety in terminally ill patients

Types of anxiety	Causes
Adjustment disorder with anxiety	Awareness of terminal condition
	Fears and uncertainty about death
	Conflicts with family or staff
	Do-not-resuscitate order discussion
Disease- and treatment-related anxiety	Poor pain control
	Delirium (can be misdiagnosed as an anxiety disorder in medical settings)
	Related metabolic disturbances Hypoxia Hypoglycemia Electrolyte imbalance
	Sepsis
	Bleeding
	Pulmonary embolus
Substance-induced anxiety	Anxiety-producing drugs
	Corticosteroids
	Antipsychotics (akathisia)
	Antiemetics (akathisia) Methoclopramide Prochlorperazine, promethazine
	Bronchodilators
	Withdrawal Opioids Benzodiazepines Alcohol
Preexisting anxiety disorders General anxiety disorder Panic Phobias Posttraumatic stress disorder	Exacerbation of symptoms related to fears and distressing medical symptoms

illness, patients with preexisting anxiety disorders are at risk for reactivation of symptoms. Generalized anxiety disorder or panic disorder are apt to recur, especially in the presence of dyspnea or pain. Persons with phobias will have an especially difficult time if the disease or treatment confronts them with their fears (e.g., claustrophobia, fear of needles, fear of isolation). Posttraumatic stress disorder (PTSD) may be activated in dying patients as they relate their situation to some prior frightening experience, such as the Holocaust, a combat experience, or a cardiac arrest. Patients with PTSD may present with high levels of anxiety, insomnia, frequent panic attacks, comorbid depressive symptoms, and avoidance of medical settings that trigger traumatic memories (Miovic and Block 2007).

As noted in Table 41–1, symptoms of anxiety in the terminally ill patient may arise from a medical complication of the illness or treatment (Breitbart et al. 1995; Roth and Massie 2009). Hypoxia, sepsis, poorly controlled pain, medication side effects such as akathisia, and withdrawal states often present as anxiety (Miovic and Block 2007). In the dying patient, anxiety can represent impending cardiac or respiratory arrest, pulmonary embolism, sepsis, electrolyte imbalance, or dehydration (Strain et al. 1981). Delirium can present with anxiety and restlessness in palliative care settings. Disturbance in level of consciousness, impaired concentration, cognitive impairment, altered perception, and fluctuation of symptoms are important diagnostic indicators of delirium as opposed to a diagnosis of anxiety disorder (Roth and Massie 2009). During the terminal phase of illness, when patients become less alert, there is a tendency to minimize the use of sedating medications. It is important to consider the need to slowly taper benzodiazepines and opioids, which may have been sustained at high doses for extended relief of anxiety or pain, in order to prevent acute withdrawal states. Withdrawal states in terminally ill patients often manifest first as agitation or anxiety and become clinically evident days later than might be expected in younger, healthier patients due to impaired metabolism.

As disease progresses, patients' anxiety may include fears about the disease process, the clinical course, possible treatment outcomes, and death. In addition, anxiety may result from fear of increasing social stigma as the medical illness becomes more evident as well as from fear of the increasing financial consequences of treatment.

Despite the fact that anxiety in terminal illness commonly results from medical complications, it is important to consider psychological factors that may play a role, particularly in patients who are alert and not confused (Holland 1989; Roth and Massie 2009). Patients frequently fear the isolation and separation of death. Claustrophobic patients may fear the idea of being confined and buried in a coffin. These issues can be disconcerting to consultants, who may find themselves at a loss for words that are consoling to the patient.

Treatment

The most effective management of anxiety is multimodal and usually involves a combination of psychotherapy and pharmacological management. The treatment of anxiety in terminal illness has been extensively reviewed (Breitbart et al. 1995; Levin and Alici 2010; Roth and Massie 2009) and is similar in most respects to its treatment in the medically ill in general (see Chapter 11, "Anxiety Disorders," and Chapter 38, "Psychopharmacology"). In this subsection, we note selected aspects specific to the terminally ill.

Pharmacological treatment. For patients who feel persistently anxious, the first-line antianxiety drugs are the benzodiazepines. For patients with severely compromised hepatic function, the use of shorter-acting benzodiazepines such as lorazepam, oxazepam, or temazepam is preferred, since these drugs are metabolized by conjugation with glucuronic acid and have no active metabolites (Roth and Massie 2009). Dying patients can be administered diazepam rectally when no other route is available, with dosages equivalent to those used in oral regimens. Rectal diazepam (Twycross and Lack 1984) has been used widely in palliative care to control anxiety, restlessness, and agitation associated with the final days of life. Clonazepam is available in an orally disintegrating formulation for patients with swallowing difficulties. The American College of Clinical Care Medicine and the Society of Critical Care Medicine guidelines for the management of anxiety in critically ill adult patients recommend use of lorazepam for prolonged (i.e., more than 24 hours) treatment of anxiety in critically ill patients (Shapiro et al. 1995). See also "Alternative Routes of Administration" section in Chapter 38, "Psychopharmacology." These guidelines may prove useful in palliative care settings as well (Levin and Alici 2010). On the other hand, a Cochrane review of pharmacotherapy for anxiety in palliative care concluded that there was lack of high level evidence on the role of antianxiety medications in terminally ill patients (Jackson and Lipman 2004). The excessive use of benzodiazepines may result in mental status changes. In anxious patients with severely compromised pulmonary function, the use of benzodiazepines that suppress central respiratory mechanisms may be unsafe. Low doses of a neuroleptic or an antihistamine can be useful, but the anticholinergic effects of antihistamines make them problematic in the debilitated patient prone to develop delirium. Anxiety symptoms in patients with delirium are better treated with antipsychotics than with benzodiazepines (Breitbart et al. 1996); however, none of the antipsychotics have been systematically studied in the treatment of anxiety among patients receiving palliative care (Jackson and Lipman 2004; Levin and Alici 2010).

Sedating antidepressants such as trazodone or mirtazapine may help patients with persistent anxiety, insomnia, and anorexia. Selective serotonin reuptake inhibitors (SSRIs) are also effective in the management of anxiety disorders (Roth and Massie 2009). The utility of antidepressants and buspirone for anxiety disorders is often limited in the dying patient because they require weeks to achieve therapeutic effect.

Opioid drugs such as the narcotic analgesics are primarily indicated for the control of pain but are also effective in the relief of dyspnea and associated anxiety (Elia and Thomas 2008). Continuous intravenous infusions of morphine or other narcotic analgesics allow for careful titration and control of respiratory distress, anxiety, pain, and agitation (Portenoy et al. 1989). Occasionally one must maintain the patient in a state of unresponsiveness in order to maximize comfort. When respiratory distress is not a major problem, it is preferable to use the opioid drugs solely for analgesia and to add more specific anxiolytics to control concomitant anxiety.

Nonpharmacological treatment. Nonpharmacological interventions for anxiety and distress include supportive psychotherapy, behavioral interventions, and cognitive-behavioral therapy that are used alone or in combination (see discussion later in this chapter and in Chapter 11, "Anxiety Disorders," and Chapter 39, "Psychotherapy"). Brief supportive psychotherapy is often useful in dealing with both crises and existential issues confronted by the terminally ill

(Roth and Massie 2009). Supportive-expressive group therapy has been shown to reduce distress and subsyndromal symptoms of PTSD in women with advanced breast cancer (Classen et al. 2001). Inclusion of the family in psychotherapeutic interventions should be considered, particularly as the patient with advanced illness becomes increasingly debilitated and less able to interact.

Relaxation, guided imagery, and hypnosis may help reduce anxiety and thereby increase the patient's sense of control. Many patients with advanced illness are still appropriate candidates for the use of behavioral techniques despite physical debilitation. A feasibility study of a brief cognitive-behavioral intervention has been shown to reduce anxiety and depression symptoms in a small population of hospice patients (T. Anderson et al. 2008). However the utility of such interventions for a terminally ill patient is limited by the degree of mental clarity of the patient (Breitbart et al. 1995). In some cases, techniques can be modified so as to include even mildly cognitively impaired patients. This involves the therapist taking a more active role by orienting the patient, creating a safe and secure environment, and evoking a conditioned response to his or her voice or presence. A typical behavioral intervention for anxiety in a terminally ill patient would include a relaxation exercise combined with some distraction or imagery technique. The patient is first taught to relax using passive breathing accompanied by either passive or active muscle relaxation. When in a relaxed state, the patient is taught a pleasant, distracting imagery exercise. In a randomized study comparing a relaxation technique with alprazolam in the treatment of anxiety and distress in non-terminally ill cancer patients, both treatments were demonstrated to be quite effective for mild to moderate degrees of anxiety or distress. Alprazolam was more effective for greater levels of distress or anxiety and had more rapid onset of beneficial effect (Holland et al. 1987). Of course, relaxation techniques can be prescribed concurrently with anxiolytic medications in highly anxious terminal patients.

Depression

See also Chapter 8, "Depression," for additional information.

Epidemiology

Most studies on the prevalence of major depression in patients with advanced cancer in palliative care settings suggest that the prevalence of depression in patients with advanced disease ranges from 9% to 20% (Breitbart et al. 2000; Wilson et al. 2000, 2007a). The Canadian National Palliative Care Survey has shown a prevalence rate of 20.7% for any depressive disorder among patients (n=381) receiving palliative care (Wilson et al. 2007a). Family history of depression and history of previous depressive episodes further increase the patient's risk of developing a depressive episode (Miovic and Block 2007). Loss of meaning and low scores on measures of spiritual well-being have been associated with higher levels of depressive symptoms, suggesting that the relationship between existential distress and depression in terminal illness warrants further investigation (Nelson et al. 2002). Depression is associated with poor treatment compliance, reduced quality of life, poor survival, and desire for hastened death among terminally ill patients (Breitbart et al. 2000; Chochinov et al. 1995; Lloyd-Williams et al. 2009; Potash and Breitbart 2002; van der Lee et al. 2005). Many studies have also found a correlation between depression, pain, and functional status (Breitbart 1989b; Potash and Breitbart 2002; Wilson et al. 2007a). Younger age and poor social support have also been identified as risk factors for depression in the terminally ill (Potash and Breitbart 2002). Corticosteroids (Stiefel et al. 1989), chemotherapeutic agents (e.g., vincristine, vinblastine, asparaginase, intrathecal methotrexate, interferon, interleukin) (Adams et al. 1984; Denicoff et al. 1987; Holland et al. 1974; Young 1982), amphotericin (Weddington 1982), whole brain radiation (DeAngelis et al. 1989), central nervous system (CNS) metabolic-endocrine complications (Breitbart 1989a), and paraneoplastic syndromes (Patchell and Posner 1989; Posner 1988) can all cause depressive symptoms (Potash and Breitbart 2002). The phenomenological similarities between depression and "sickness behavior syndrome" have led researchers to consider the role of proinflammatory cytokines in the development of depressive syndromes among patients with advanced disease (Jacobson et al. 2008).

Assessment

Depressed mood and sadness can be appropriate responses as the terminally ill patient faces death. These emotions can be manifestations of anticipatory grief over the impending loss of one's life, health, loved ones, and autonomy (Block 2000). Despite this, major depression is common in the palliative care setting, where it has been underdiagnosed and undertreated. Minimization of depressive symptoms as "normal reactions" by clinicians and the difficulties of accurately diagnosing depression in the terminally ill both contribute to the underdiagnosis of depression, and undertreatment is due in part to the concern that severely medically ill patients will not be able to tolerate the side effects of antidepressants (Block 2000). However, recent evidence from the increasing prevalence of antidepressant utilization among cancer patients suggests that clinicians have become more vigilant in recognition and treatment of depression in the medically ill (Wilson et al. 2009). Strategies for accurately diagnosing depression in seriously medically ill patients are reviewed in Chapter 8, "Depression." A detailed description of their application in palliative care settings can be found in Wilson et al. 2009.

The diagnosis of a major depressive syndrome in a terminally ill patient, as in medically ill patients in general, often relies more on the psychological or cognitive symptoms of major depression than the neurovegetative symptoms. The strategy of relying on the psychological symptoms of depression for diagnostic specificity is itself not without problems. How is the clinician to interpret feelings of hopelessness in the dying patient when there is no hope for cure or recovery? Feelings of hopelessness, worthlessness, or suicidal ideation must be explored in detail. Although many dying patients lose hope for a cure, they are able to maintain hope for better symptom control. For many patients hope is contingent on the ability to find continued meaning in their day-to-day existence. Hopelessness that is pervasive and accompanied by a sense of despair or despondency is more likely to represent a symptom of a depressive disorder. Such patients often state that they feel they are burdening their families unfairly, causing them great pain and inconvenience. Those beliefs are less likely to represent a symptom of depression than if the patient feels that his or her life has never had any worth or that the illness is punishment for evil things he or she has done. Even mild and passive forms of suicidal ideation are very often indicative of significant degrees of depression in terminally ill patients (Breitbart 1987, 1990).

Several screening instruments have been studied for detection of depression in palliative care settings, a detailed description of these instruments can be found elsewhere (Wilson et al. 2009). Chochinov et al. (1997) studied brief screening instruments to measure depression in the terminally ill, including a single-item interview assessing depressed mood ("Have you been depressed most of the time for the past 2 weeks?"), a two-item interview assessing depressed mood and loss of interest in activities, a visual analogue scale for depressed mood, and the Beck Depression Inventory. Semistructured diagnostic interviews served as the standard against which the screening performance of the four brief screening methods was assessed. Most noteworthy, the single-item question correctly identified the diagnosis of every patient, substantially outperforming the questionnaire and visual analogue measures. The single-item depression question has been incorporated into routine clinical assessments in a variety of clinical settings to identify depression among medically ill patients (Wilson et al. 2009).

Treatment

Treatment of depression in the medically ill is reviewed in detail in Chapter 8, "Depression," Chapter 38, "Psychopharmacology," and Chapter 39 "Psychotherapy," and in this discussion we note specific aspects relevant to palliative care. A combination of pharmacotherapy, supportive psychotherapy, cognitive-behavioral therapy, and psychoeducation is the mainstay of treatment for depression in palliative care settings (Miovic and Block 2007; Wilson et al. 2000). It is important to treat the distressing physical symptoms (such as pain, dyspnea, nausea) concurrently while managing depression in patients with advanced disease (Potash and Breitbart 2002).

Pharmacological treatment. Antidepressant medications are the mainstay of pharmacological management for gravely ill patients meeting diagnostic criteria for major depression (Block 2000; Wilson et al. 2000) and have established efficacy (Wilson et al. 2000, 2009). Factors such as prognosis and the time frame for treatment may play an important role in determining the type of pharmacotherapy for depression in the terminally ill. A depressed patient with several months of life expectancy can afford to wait the 2–4 weeks it may take to respond to a standard antidepressant. For the terminally ill, antidepressants are usually initiated at approximately half the usual starting dose because of patients' sensitivity to adverse effects. A Cochrane review supported the use of antidepressants in this patient population but emphasized the methodological weaknesses in reviewed studies (Gill and Hatcher 2000). The depressed dying patient with less than 3 weeks to live may do best with a rapid-acting psychostimulant (Block 2000; Homsi et al. 2001; Tremblay and Breitbart 2001). Patients who are within hours to days of death and in distress are likely to benefit most from the use of sedatives or narcotic analgesic infusions.

Psychostimulants are particularly helpful in the treatment of depression in the terminally ill because they have a rapid onset of action and energizing effects and typically do not cause anorexia, weight loss, or insomnia at therapeutic doses (Candy et al. 2008; Pessin et al. 2008; Potash and Breitbart 2002). In fact, at low doses, stimulants may actually increase appetite (see also Chapter 8, "Depression," and Chapter 38, "Psychopharmacology"). Abuse is almost always an irrelevant concern in the terminally ill, and stimulants should not be withheld on the basis of a patient's previous history of substance abuse. Occasionally, treatment with an SSRI and a psychostimulant may be initiated concurrently so that depressed patients may receive the immediate benefits of the psychostimulant drug while waiting the necessary weeks for the SSRI to work. At that point the psychostimulant may be withdrawn. Methylphenidate and dextroamphetamine are usually initiated at low doses (2.5–5.0 mg in the morning and at noon). The benefits can be assessed during the first 1–2 days of treatment and the dose gradually titrated (usually to no greater than 30 mg/day total). An additional benefit of stimulants is that they have been shown to reduce sedation secondary to opioid analgesics and provide adjuvant analgesic effects (Bruera et al. 1987). A recent review of 19 controlled trials of methylphenidate in medically ill older adults and patients in palliative care has concluded that the use of low-dose methylphenidate is appropriate in the treatment of depression, fatigue, or apathy in this patient population with monitoring for response and adverse effects (Hardy 2009).

Nonpharmacological treatment. Depression in cancer patients with advanced disease is optimally managed with a combination of supportive psychotherapy, cognitive-behavioral techniques, psychoeducation, and antidepressant medications as discussed above (Miovic and Block 2007; Wilson et al. 2000). Psychotherapeutic interventions, in the form of either individual or group counseling, have been shown to effectively reduce psychological distress and depressive symptoms in advanced-stage cancer patients (Savard et al. 2006; Spiegel and Bloom 1983; Spiegel et al. 1981; Wilson et al. 2009). Cognitive-behavioral interventions such as relaxation and distraction with pleasant imagery also have been shown to decrease depressive symptoms in patients with mild to moderate levels of depression (Holland et al. 1987).

Supportive psychotherapy for the dying patient consists of active listening with supportive verbal interventions and the occasional interpretation (Peck et al. 1983). Despite the seriousness of the patient's plight, it is not necessary for the psychiatrist or psychologist to appear overly solemn or emotionally restrained. Often the psychotherapist is the only person among all of the patient's caregivers who is comfortable enough to converse lightheartedly and to allow the patient to talk about his or her life and experiences rather than focus solely on impending death. The dying patient who wishes to talk or ask questions about death should be encouraged to do so freely, with the therapist maintaining an interested, interactive stance.

Psychotherapies other than supportive psychotherapy have been described as potentially useful in the treatment of depressive symptoms and distress in palliative care patients. Chochinov and Breitbart (2009) extensively reviewed interpersonal, existential, life narrative, and group psychotherapies in palliative care. Several novel psychotherapies have been developed and are being tested in the treatment of depression, hopelessness, loss of meaning, and demoralization; these new modalities include meaning-centered psychotherapy (Breitbart 2002) and dignity-conserving care (Chochinov 2002), both of which are described later in this chapter.

Suicide and Desire for Hastened Death

Suicide, suicidal ideation, and desire for hastened death are all important and serious consequences of unrecognized and inadequately treated clinical depression (see also Chapter 9, "Suicidality"). Although clinical depression has been demonstrated to be a critically important factor in desire for hastened death (through suicide or other means), understanding more fully why some patients with a terminal illness wish or seek to hasten their death remains an important element in the practice of palliative care. Despite the continued legal prohibitions against assisted suicide in most of the United States, a substantial number of patients think about and discuss those alternatives with their physicians, family, and friends (Olden et al. 2009; Rosenfeld 2000).

Suicide

Factors associated with increased risk of suicide in patients with serious medical illnesses are reviewed in Chapter 9, "Suicidality," and elsewhere (Breitbart 1987; Olden et al. 2009).

Cancer patients commit suicide most frequently in the advanced stages of disease. With advancing disease the incidence of significant pain increases, and uncontrolled pain is a dramatically important risk factor for suicide.

Hopelessness is a key variable linking depression and suicide in the terminally ill. Chochinov et al. (1998) demonstrated that hopelessness was correlated more highly with suicidal ideation in terminally ill cancer patients than was level of depression. In Scandinavia, the highest incidence of suicide was found in cancer patients who were offered no further treatment and no further contact with the health care system (Bolund 1985; Louhivuori and Hakama 1979). Being left to face illness alone creates a sense of isolation and abandonment that is critical to the development of hopelessness.

The prevalence of delirium reaches as high as 85% during the terminal stages of illness (Massie et al. 1983). Although early work suggested that delirium was a protective factor in regard to suicide among cancer patients (Farberow et al. 1963), clinical experience has found confusional states to be a major contributing factor in impulsive suicide attempts, especially in the hospital setting (see Chapter 9, "Suicidality"). Delirium or any cognitive impairment often impairs one's ability to reason and increases risk of impulsive behavior (Olden et al. 2009). Pessin et al. (2003) reported that advanced AIDS patients with cognitive impairment were more likely to express a desire for hastened death than patients without cognitive impairment.

Loss of control and a sense of helplessness in the face of terminal illness are important factors in suicide vulnerability. *Control* refers to the helplessness induced by symptoms, deficits due to the illness or its treatments, and the excessive need on the part of some patients to be in control of all aspects of living or dying. Farberow et al. (1971) noted that patients who were accepting and adaptable were much less likely to commit suicide than those who exhibited a need to be in control of even the most minute details of their care. However, it is not uncommon for terminal illness to induce a great sense of helplessness even in those who are not typically controlling individuals, for example through loss of mobility, paraplegia, loss of bowel and bladder function, amputation, aphonia, sensory loss, and inability to eat or swallow. Most distressing to patients is the sense that they are losing control of their minds, especially when they are confused or sedated by medications. The risk of suicide is increased with such impairments, especially when accompanied by psychological distress and disturbed interpersonal relationships (Farberow et al. 1971).

Fatigue in the form of emotional, spiritual, financial, familial, communal, and other resource exhaustion increases risk of suicide in patients with terminal illness (Breitbart 1987). Increased survival in cancer, AIDS, chronic obstructive pulmonary disease, congestive heart failure, and other diseases is accompanied by increased numbers of hospitalizations, complications, and expenses. Symptom control thus becomes a prolonged process with frequent advances and setbacks. The dying process also can become extremely long and arduous for all concerned. It is not uncommon for both family members and health care providers to withdraw prematurely from the patient under these circumstances. A suicidal patient can thus feel even more isolated and abandoned. The presence of a strong support system for the patient that may act as an external control of suicidal behavior reduces risk of suicide significantly.

Suicidal Ideation

It is widely held that most terminally ill patients experience occasional thoughts of suicide as a means of escaping the threat of being overwhelmed by their illness ("If it gets too bad, I always have a way out") and will reveal this to a sensitive interviewer. However, some studies suggest that suicidal ideation is relatively infrequent and is limited to those who are significantly depressed (Achte and Vanhkouen 1971; Brown et al. 1986; Silberfarb et al. 1980). Among a cohort of cancer patients with pain, suicidal ideation was found in just 17% (Breitbart 1987). The actual prevalence of suicidal ideation may be higher, because patients may be less likely to disclose these thoughts to a research interviewer than in a well-established doctor–patient relationship.

Assessment and Management of the Suicidal Terminally Ill Patient

Assessment and management of suicidal ideation in the medically ill are discussed in Chapter 9, "Suicidality." Some physicians, nurses, and other caregivers fail to intervene for suicidal ideation in the terminally ill, either because they think it is rational ("I would feel that way too") or because they think that intervention is futile ("He's going to die anyway"). This is a serious error for several reasons. Suicide can be very traumatic to family and health caregivers, even in the terminally ill. Patients often reconsider and reject the idea of suicide after they have an opportunity to express underlying issues to an attentive physician, particularly fears of loss of control over aspects of their death. Suicidal ideation is often driven by unbearable symptoms that may not have been recognized and should become the focus of palliative care.

Psychiatric hospitalization can sometimes be helpful but is usually not desirable in the terminally ill patient. Thus, the medical hospital or home is the setting in which management most often takes place. Although it is appropriate to intervene when medical or psychiatric factors are clearly the driving force in a cancer patient's suicide, there are circumstances when usurping control from the patient and family with overly aggressive intervention may be contraindicated. This is most evident in those with advanced illness for whom comfort and symptom control are the primary concerns.

Ultimately, palliative care clinicians are not able to prevent all suicides in terminally ill patients for whom they provide care. Intervention should emphasize an aggressive attempt to prevent suicide that is driven by the desperation of physical and psychological symptoms, such as uncontrolled pain and unrecognized or untreated delirium or depression. Prolonged suffering caused by poorly controlled symptoms can lead to such desperation, and it is the appropriate role of the palliative care team to provide effective management of physical and psychological symptoms as an alternative to desire for death, suicide, or request for assisted suicide by patients. (Requests for assisted suicide are covered in Chapter 9, "Suicidality.")

Desire for Hastened Death

Desire for hastened death may be thought of as a unifying construct underlying requests for assisted suicide or euthanasia, as well as suicidal thoughts in general. Several studies have demonstrated that depression plays a significant role in the terminally ill patient's desire for hastened death (Olden et al. 2009; Rodin et al. 2007, 2009). Chochinov et al. (1995) found that 45% of terminally ill patients in a palliative care facility acknowledged at least a fleeting desire to die, but these episodes were mostly brief and did not reflect a sustained or committed desire to die. However, 9% reported an unequivocal desire for death to come soon and indicated that they held this desire consistently over time. Among this group, 59% received a diagnosis of depression, compared with a prevalence of 8% in patients who did not endorse a genuine, consistent desire for death. Patients with depression were approximately six to seven times more likely to have a desire for hastened death than patients without depression. Patients with a desire for death were also found to have significantly more pain and less social support than those patients without a desire for death.

Breitbart et al. (2000) studied the relationships among depression, hopelessness, and desire for death in terminally ill cancer patients. Seventeen percent of the patients were classified as having a high desire for death (Rosenfeld et al. 1999, 2000), and 16% met criteria for a current major depressive episode. Of the patients who met criteria for major depressive episode, 47% were classified as having a high desire for hastened death; only 12% of those without a desire for death met criteria for depression. Thus, patients with major depression were four times more likely to have a high desire for hastened death. In addition, Breitbart et al. (2000) found that both depression and hopelessness, characterized as a pessimistic cognitive style rather than an assessment of one's poor prognosis, appear to be synergistic determinants of desire for hastened death. No significant association with the presence or the intensity of pain was found. Conversely, Mystakidou et al. (2005) have found that the severity of pain and the interference with daily activities due to pain significantly predicted desire for hastened death.

Researchers have also explored the desire for hastened death among patients with a better prognosis to determine whether similar contributing factors played a role (Rodin et al. 2007; Rosenfeld et al. 2006). In a sample of metastatic cancer patients with an expected prognosis of 6 months or longer, 5% of patients had a high desire for hastened death, a relatively lower rate compared to the 17% rate among patients with less than 1 month of survival expectancy. The desire for hastened death significantly correlated with high levels of depression and hopelessness in all of the individuals in that sample (Rodin et al. 2007).

Desire for hastened death also appears to be a function of psychological distress and social factors such as social support, spiritual well-being, quality of life, and perception of oneself as a burden to others (Chochinov et al. 2005a; Hudson et al. 2006; Olden et al. 2009). Among dying patients, the "will to live," as measured with a visual analogue scale, was found to fluctuate rapidly over time and correlated with anxiety, depression, and shortness of breath as death approached (Chochinov et al. 1999).

In a Canadian study of terminally ill cancer patients, detailed interviews of the patients with desire for hastened death revealed the following seven themes underlying their wishes for death including the futility of existence due to functional limitations and the imminence of death, physical and emotional suffering, sense of being a burden to others, readiness for death, the wish for a compassionate death that minimized suffering, preserving their autonomy of choice in the timing of death, and the influence of witnessing the death of others (Wilson et al. 2007b).

Interventions for Despair at the End of Life

The response of a clinician to despair at the end of life as manifest by a patient's expression of desire for death or request for assisted suicide has important and obvious implications for all aspects of care and affects patients, family, and staff (Breitbart et al. 2004a). These issues must be addressed both rapidly and thoughtfully, offering the patient a nonjudgmental willingness to discuss the factors contributing to the kind of suffering and despondency that leads to such a desire for death. Such despair has been variably described as "spiritual" suffering, "demoralization," loss of "dignity," and "loss of meaning" (Breitbart 2002; Cherny 2004; Chochinov et al. 2002b, 2005a; Greenstein and Breitbart 2000; Kissane et al. 2001; Rousseau 2000).

Although most palliative care clinicians believe that aggressive management of physical and psychological distress (such as depression) will prevent desire for hastened death or requests for assisted suicide, few studies have been conducted to validate this (Olden et al. 2009). A recent study demonstrated that desire for hastened death can often be ameliorated through treatment of depression with antidepressants (Breitbart et al. 2010a). If the treatment of depression reduces the wish for hastened death, it may also result in increased desire for life-sustaining medical therapies (Ganzini et al. 1994). When it is practical to do so, in severely depressed patients—particularly those who are hopeless—decisions about withdrawal of treatment should be discouraged until after treatment of their depression.

Several psychosocial interventions—some using cognitive techniques to restructure beliefs underlying hopelessness or demoralization, and others focusing on enhancing patients' sense of meaning and dignity—have been proposed and studied in terminally ill patients with a desire for hastened death (Breitbart et al. 2010b; Chochinov 2002; Chochinov et al. 2005b; Griffith et al. 2005). Specific therapeutic approaches for despair at the end of life are described in detail in the section on "Psychotherapy Interventions in Palliative Care" later in the chapter.

Delirium

Delirium is discussed in detail in Chapter 5, "Delirium"; in this discussion we focus on aspects most relevant to palliative care. In the palliative care literature, delirium occurring in the last days of life is often referred to as "terminal delirium," "terminal restlessness," or "terminal agitation." Despite being the most common neuropsychiatric complication of advanced illness, delirium is often underdiagnosed and untreated in palliative care settings. Delirium is a harbinger of impending death among terminally ill patients, and also a significant source of distress for patients, families, and staff. Delirium can interfere dramatically with the recognition and control of other physical and psychological symptoms such as pain in later stages of illness. Palliative care clinicians should thus be familiar with the assessment and management of delirium, as well as the controversies regarding the goals of management in the terminally ill (Breitbart and Alici 2008; Breitbart et al. 2002a; Coyle et al. 1994).

Prevalence

Delirium is the most common and serious neuropsychiatric complication in patients with advanced illnesses such as cancer and AIDS, particularly in the last weeks of life, with prevalence rates ranging from 25% to 85% (Breitbart 2001; Breitbart et al. 1996; Bruera et al. 1992; Fainsinger et al. 1991; Levine et al. 1978; Massie et al. 1983; Murray 1987). Pereira et al. (1997) found the prevalence of cognitive impairment in cancer inpatients to be 44%, and just prior to death, the prevalence rose to 62%. Lawlor et al. (2000a) reported that whereas 42% of advanced cancer patients had delirium upon admission to their palliative care unit, terminal delirium occurred in 88% of patients before their deaths.

The Experience of Delirium for Patients, Families, and Staff

Delirium causes significant distress in patients, families, and staff (Breitbart et al. 2002a; Buss et al. 2007; Morita et al. 2004). In a study of terminally ill cancer patients, Breitbart et al. (2002a) found that 54% of patients recalled their delirium experience after recovery from delirium. Factors predicting delirium recall included the degree of short-term memory impairment, delirium severity, and the presence of perceptual disturbances (the more severe, the less likely recall). Patients, spouses or other caregivers, and nurses each rated distress related to the episode of delirium. The most significant factor predicting distress for patients was the presence of delusions. Patients with hypoactive delirium were just as distressed as patients with hyperactive delirium. Spouse distress was predicted by the patients' Karnofsky Performance Status (the lower the Karnofsky score, the worse the spouse distress), and nurse distress was predicted by delirium severity and perceptual disturbances.

Assessment and Reversibility of Delirium in the Terminally Ill

Delirium, in contrast with dementia, is classically conceptualized as a reversible process. Reversibility of delirium is often possible even in the patient with advanced illness, but it may not be reversible in the last 24–48 hours of life, with the outcome probably attributable to irreversible processes such as multiple organ failure occurring in the final hours of life.

Instruments available for diagnosing and monitoring severity of delirium are described in Chapter 5, "Delirium." Of those, the Memorial Delirium Assessment Scale (MDAS) and the Confusion Assessment Method have been validated in palliative care settings (Breitbart et al. 1997; Lawlor et al. 2000b; Ryan et al. 2009). The MDAS, validated in hospitalized patients with advanced cancer and AIDS, is a 10-item tool useful both for diagnostic screening and for assessing delirium severity among patients with advanced disease (Breitbart et al. 1997). Lawlor et al. (2000b) found that a cutoff score of 7 out of 30 yielded the highest sensitivity (98%) and specificity (76%) for a delirium diagnosis in advanced cancer patients in a palliative care unit. The Confusion Assessment Method (CAM), validated in palliative care settings with a sensitivity of 88% and a specificity of 100% when administered by well-trained clinicians, is a nine-item delirium diagnostic scale based on the DSM-III-R (American Psychiatric Association 1987) criteria for delirium (Inouye et al. 1990; Ryan et al. 2009).

The standard approach to managing delirium outlined in Chapter 5, "Delirium," remains relevant in the terminally ill, including a search for underlying causes, correction of those factors, and management of the symptoms of delirium (Breitbart 2001; Breitbart and Alici 2008; Breitbart et al. 2000). The ideal and often achievable outcome is a patient who is awake, alert, calm, cognitively intact, not psychotic, and communicating coherently with family and staff. In the terminally ill patient who develops delirium in the last days of life (terminal delirium), the management differs, presenting a number of dilemmas, and the desired clinical outcome may be significantly altered by the dying process.

Delirium can have multiple potential etiologies (Table 41–2). In patients with advanced cancer, for instance, delirium can be due to the direct effects of cancer on the CNS, indirect CNS effects of the disease or treatments (e.g., medications, electrolyte imbalance, failure of a vital organ, infection, vascular complications), and/or preexisting CNS disease (e.g., dementia) (Bruera et al. 1992; Lawlor et al. 2000a). Given the large numbers of drugs terminally ill pa-

TABLE 41–2. Causes of delirium in patients with advanced disease

Direct central nervous system (CNS) causes
Primary brain tumor
Metastatic spread to CNS
Seizures
CNS infection
Indirect causes
Hyperthermia
Organ failure
Uremia
Hepatic encephalopathy
Congestive heart failure
Pulmonary failure
Pulmonary edema
Pulmonary emboli
Electrolyte imbalance
Treatment side effects from
Chemotherapeutic agents
Corticosteroids
Radiation
Opioid analgesics
Anticholinergics
Antivirals
Infection
Sepsis
Opportunistic infections
Hematological abnormalities
Severe anemia
Disseminated intravascular coagulopathy (DIC) and other hypercoagulable states
Nutritional deficiencies
Paraneoplastic syndromes

tients require and the fragile state of their physiological functioning, even routinely ordered hypnotic agents may be enough to tip patients over into delirium. Narcotic analgesics, especially meperidine, are common causes of confusional states, particularly in the elderly and terminally ill.

In confronting delirium in the terminally ill or dying patient, a differential diagnosis should always be formulated as to the likely etiology. However, there is an ongoing debate as to the appropriate extent of diagnostic evaluation that should be pursued in a dying patient with a terminal delirium (Breitbart 2001). Most palliative care clinicians would undertake diagnostic studies only when a clinically suspected etiology can be identified easily, with minimal use of invasive procedures, and treated effectively with simple interventions that carry minimal burden or risk of causing further distress. Diagnostic workup in pursuit of an etiology for delirium may be limited by either practical constraints such as the setting (home, hospice) or the focus on patient comfort, so that unpleasant or painful diagnostics may be avoided. Most often, however, the etiology of terminal delirium is multifactorial or may not be determined. Bruera et al. (1992) reported that an etiology is discovered in less than 50% of terminally ill patients with delirium. When a distinct cause is found for delirium in the terminally ill, it may be irreversible or difficult to treat. Studies in patients with earlier stages of advanced cancer have demonstrated the potential utility of a thorough diagnostic assessment (Bruera et al. 1992; Coyle et al. 1994). When such diagnostic information is available, specific therapy may be able to reverse delirium. A prospective study of delirium in patients on a palliative care unit found that 68% of delirious cancer patients could be improved, despite a 30-day mortality of 31% (Lawlor et al. 2000a). The etiology of delirium was multifactorial in the great majority of cases in that study. Although delirium occurred in 88% of dying patients in the last week of life, delirium was reversible in approximately 50% of episodes. Causes of delirium that were most associated with reversibility included dehydration and psychoactive or opioid medications. Hypoxic and metabolic encephalopathies were less likely to be reversible in terminal delirium (Lawlor et al. 2000a). Another study found a cause in 43% of the patients evaluated, and of these, one-third of the episodes of cognitive failure improved (Bruera et al. 1992). Leonard et al. (2008) have reported a delirium reversibility rate of 27% among patients in a palliative care unit. A study of patients with advanced cancer admitted to hospice found an overall delirium reversibility rate of 20% with a 30-day mortality rate of 83%. Reversibility of delirium was highly dependent on the etiology. Delirium due to hypercalcemia or medications was likely to be reversible, whereas delirium due to infections, hepatic failure, hypoxia, disseminated intravascular coagulation, or dehydration was likely to be irreversible (Morita et al. 2001).

Even in terminal delirium, a diagnostic workup should include basic assessment of potentially reversible causes of delirium while minimizing any investigation that would be burdensome for the patient. A full physical examination should be conducted to assess for evidence of sepsis, fecal impaction, dehydration, or major organ failure. Medications that could contribute to delirium should be reviewed. Oximetry can rule out hypoxia; one set of blood draws can screen for metabolic disturbances (e.g., hypercalcemia) and hematological abnormalities (e.g., anemia, leukocytosis). Imaging studies of the brain and assessment of the cerebrospinal fluid may be appropriate in some instances if they have the potential to identify lesions amenable to palliative treatment (e.g., radiosensitive CNS metastases).

Interventions

Pharmacological

Pharmacotherapy of delirium is reviewed in detail in Chapter 5, "Delirium." A detailed review of the use of antipsychotic medications in the treatment of delirium is available elsewhere (Boettger and Breitbart 2005). While no medications have been approved by the U.S. Food and Drug Administration (FDA) for treatment of delirium, treatment with antipsychotics or sedatives is often required to control the symptoms of delirium in palliative care settings. Low doses of neuroleptic medication are usually sufficient in treating delirium in the terminally ill, but high doses have sometimes been required (Breitbart and Alici 2008). Haloperidol remains the drug of first choice and may be given orally or parenterally (Breitbart and Alici 2008; Breitbart et al. 1996). Delivery of haloperidol by the subcutaneous route is utilized by many palliative care practitioners (Bruera et al. 1992; Twycross and Lack 1983).

Many palliative care clinicians use low dose atypical antipsychotics in the management of delirium in terminally ill patients (Boettger and Breitbart 2005; Breitbart 2001; Breitbart and Alici 2008; Breitbart et al. 2002b). A Cochrane review comparing the efficacy and the adverse effects of haloperidol and atypical antipsychotics concluded that haloperidol, risperidone, and olanzapine were all effective in managing delirium, and that extrapyramidal adverse effects did not differ significantly between atypical antipsychotics and haloperidol (Lonergan et al. 2007).

Psychostimulants have been suggested in the treatment of hypoactive subtype of delirium, alone or in combination of antipsychotics (Keen and Brown 2004; Lawlor et al. 2000c). A prospective study (n=14) of methylphenidate use in advanced cancer patients with hypoactive delirium have shown improvement in cognitive functioning and psychomotor activities (Gagnon et al. 2005).

Although neuroleptic drugs are generally very beneficial in reducing agitation, anxiety, and confusion in delirium, this is not always possible in terminal delirium. A significant group (at least 10%–20%) of terminally ill patients experience delirium that can only be controlled by sedation to the point of a significantly decreased level of consciousness (Fainsinger et al. 2000; Lo and Rubenfeld 2005; Rietjens et al. 2008). The goal of treatment in those cases is quiet sedation only. Midazolam, given by subcutaneous or intravenous infusion in doses ranging from 30 to 100 mg per 24 hours, can be used to control agitated terminal delirium (Bottomley and Hanks 1990; de Sousa and Jepson 1988). Propofol, a short-acting anesthetic agent, is also used for this purpose, given in, for example, an intravenous loading dose of 20 mg followed by a continuous infusion with initial doses of 10–70 mg/hour titrated up to as high as 400 mg/hour in severely agitated patients (Mercadante et al. 1995; Moyle 1995). Propofol's level of sedation may be more easily controlled, with more rapid recovery upon decreasing the rate of infusion than with midazolam (Mercadante et al. 1995).

Nonpharmacological

In addition to seeking out and potentially correcting underlying causes for delirium, environmental and supportive interventions are important, as described in Chapter 5, "Delirium." In fact, in the dying patient, these may be the only steps taken. The presence of family, frequent reorientation, correction of hearing and visual impairment, reversal of dehydration, and a quiet well-lit room with familiar objects all are helpful in reducing the severity and impact of delirium in seriously ill patients. However, these interventions are less applicable in the last days of life, and there is little likelihood that they would prevent terminal delirium.

Controversies in the Management of Terminal Delirium

Several aspects of the use of neuroleptics and other pharmacological agents in the management of delirium in the dying patient remain controversial in some circles. Some view delirium as a natural part of the dying process that should not be altered and argue that pharmacological interventions are inappropriate in the dying patient. In particular, some who care for the dying view hallucinations and delusions in which dead relatives communicate with dying patients or welcome them to heaven as important elements in the transition from life to death. There are some patients who experience hallucinations during delirium that are pleasant and even comforting, and many clinicians question the appropriateness of intervening pharmacologically in such instances.

Another concern often raised is that these patients are so close to death that aggressive treatment is unnecessary. Parenteral neuroleptics or sedatives may be mistakenly avoided because of exaggerated fears that they might hasten death through hypotension or respiratory depression. There is the possibility that sedation may worsen confusion in delirium. Many clinicians are unnecessarily pessimistic about the possible results of neuroleptic treatment for delirium. They argue that since the underlying pathophysiological process (such as hepatic or renal failure) often continues unabated, no improvement can be expected in the patient's mental status.

Clinical experience in managing delirium in dying patients suggests that the use of neuroleptics in the management of agitation, paranoia, hallucinations, and altered sensorium is safe, effective, and often quite appropriate

(Breitbart 2001; Breitbart and Alici 2008). Management of delirium on a case-by-case basis seems wisest. The agitated, delirious dying patient should usually receive a trial of neuroleptics to help restore calm. A "wait and see" approach prior to using neuroleptics may be appropriate with some patients who have a lethargic, somnolent presentation of delirium or those who are having frankly pleasant or comforting hallucinations. Such an approach must be tempered by the knowledge that a lethargic delirium may very quickly and unexpectedly become an agitated delirium that can threaten the serenity and safety of the patient, family, and staff. An additional rationale for intervening pharmacologically with patients who have "hypoactive" delirium is evidence that neuroleptics are effective in controlling the symptoms of delirium in both the hyperactive and hypoactive subtypes of delirium (Breitbart et al. 1996).

Finally, a very challenging clinical problem is management of terminal delirium that is unresponsive to standard neuroleptics and for which symptoms can only be controlled by sedation to the point of significantly decreased consciousness. Before undertaking interventions such as midazolam or propofol infusions, in which the aim is a calm, comfortable, but sedated and unresponsive patient, the clinician should discuss with the family (and the patient if he or she has lucid moments) the concerns and wishes for the type of care that can best honor the patient's and family's values. Family members should be informed that the goal of sedation is to provide comfort and symptom control and not to hasten death. Terminal sedation intended to maximize the patient's comfort is not euthanasia. After the patient receives this degree of sedation, the family may experience a premature sense of loss, and they may feel their loved one is in some sort of limbo state, not yet dead but yet no longer alive in the vital sense. The distress and confusion that family members can experience during such a period can be ameliorated by including them in the decision making and emphasizing the shared goals of care. Sedation in such patients is not always complete or irreversible; some patients have periods of wakefulness despite sedation, and many clinicians will periodically lighten sedation to reassess the patient's condition.

Psychotherapy Interventions in Palliative Care

The potential benefits of psychotherapy for seriously medically ill patients are frequently underestimated by clinicians (Rodin 2009). This bias against psychotherapeutic interventions tends to be even more pronounced in patients who are months away from death. However, psychotherapeutic interventions have been demonstrated to be useful and effective for patients struggling with advanced life-threatening medical illness (Kissane et al. 2009). This section briefly describes different psychotherapeutic interventions and their relative applicability and efficacy for patients near the end of life. Psychotherapy in the medically ill is reviewed in detail in Chapter 39, "Psychotherapy."

Individual Psychotherapy

Traditional insight-oriented psychotherapy has had limited application among dying patients. Insight-oriented psychotherapy is based on the development of a trusting relationship between the psychotherapist and the patient and an exploration of various unconscious conflicts and issues. Resolution of conflicts, through a process involving interpretation, catharsis, and enhanced insight, requires time, energy, and commitment. This approach may be too demanding for most patients nearing death, but elements of psychodynamic therapy have an important role in all palliative psychotherapies. Cognitive-behavioral and interpersonal therapies have been widely studied in the medically ill (Kissane et al. 2009; Rodin 2009). In full extended form they too may not be practical in imminently dying patients, but there are important cognitive and interpersonal elements in the specific psychotherapies as described in the following sections.

Existential Therapies

Existential therapies explore ways in which suffering can be experienced from a more positive and meaningful perspective. *Logotherapy* is one approach with the primary tenet that one always has control over one's attitude or outlook, no matter the enormity of the adversity. The goal is to decrease patients' suffering and encourage them to live life to its fullest by engaging in activities that bring the greatest amount of meaning and purpose to their lives (Frankl 1959/1992). The focus is on goals to achieve, tasks to fulfill, and responsibilities toward others. Rather than covering up patients' distress, logotherapy acknowledges and fully explores patients' suffering (Spira 2000). Although logotherapy was not designed for patients who were imminently dying, Zuehlke and Watkins (1975) explored the use of logotherapy with six dying patients and reported them to have a greater sense of freedom to change their attitudes and to see themselves and their lives as meaningful and worthwhile.

Another form of existential therapy useful with dying patients is the *life narrative*. This treatment explores the meaning of the physical illness in the context of the patient's life trajectory. It is designed to create a new perspective of dealing with the illness, emphasize past strengths, increase self-esteem, and support effective past coping strategies. The therapist emphatically summarizes the patient's life history and response to the illness to convey a sense that the therapist understands the patient over time (Viederman 2000; Viederman and Perry 1980). Life narrative can bolster patients' psychological and physical well-being. One study by Pennebaker and Seagal (1999) demonstrated that when patients wrote about important personal experiences in an emotional way for 15 minutes over 3 days, improvements in mental and physical health occurred. Life narrative has traditionally been used for treating depressed patients whose depression is a response to physical illness. However, the written form of this approach can be too demanding for patients at the end stage of their illness.

A similar method of intervention is the *life review*, which provides patients with the opportunity to identify and reexamine past experiences and achievements to find meaning, resolve old conflicts and make amends, or resolve unfinished business (Byock 1996; Heiney 1995; Lichter et al. 1993). The process of life review can be achieved through written or taped autobiographies, by reminiscing, through storytelling about past experiences or discussion of the patient's career or life work, and by creating family trees (Lewis and Butler 1974). Examples of other life review activities include going on pilgrimages, artistic expression (e.g., creating a collage or drawings, writing poetry), and journal writing (Pickrel 1989). Life review has traditionally been used in the elderly as a means of conflict resolution and to facilitate a dignified acceptance of death (Butler 1963). For dying patients, their stories have a special meaning. In negotiating one's way through serious illness and its treatment, the telling of one's own story takes on a renewed urgency. This approach has not, however, been widely utilized in palliative care settings.

Group Psychotherapy

Group interventions may offer benefits less available in individual therapies, such as a sense of universality, sharing a common experience and identity, a feeling of helping oneself by helping others, hopefulness fostered by seeing how others have coped successfully, and a sense of belonging to a larger group (self-transcendence, meaning, common purpose). However, patients in advanced stages of terminal illness are often too sick to participate in group therapy.

Emerging Psychotherapeutic Interventions in the Terminally Ill

Spiritual Suffering

Palliative care practitioners have recognized the importance of spiritual suffering in their patients and have begun to design interventions to address it (Puchalski and Romer 2000; Rousseau 2000). Rousseau (2000) has developed an approach for the treatment of spiritual suffering that centers on facilitating religious expression while also controlling physical symptoms; providing a supportive presence; encouraging life review to assist in recognizing purpose, value, and meaning; exploring guilt, remorse, forgiveness, and reconciliation; reframing goals; and encouraging meditative practices. Although this approach blends basic principles common to many psychotherapies, it should be noted that Rousseau's intervention includes a heavy emphasis on facilitating religious expression and confession and thus, although very useful to many patients, is not applicable to all and is not an intervention that all clinicians feel comfortable providing.

Meaning-Centered Psychotherapy

Breitbart and colleagues (Breitbart 2002; Breitbart and Heller 2003; Greenstein and Breitbart 2000) have applied Viktor Frankl's (1955/1986, 1959/1992, 1963, 1969/1988, 1975/1997) concepts of meaning-based psychotherapy (logotherapy) to address spiritual suffering in dying patients. This "Meaning-Centered Group Psychotherapy" (Greenstein and Breitbart 2000) utilizes a mixture of didactics, discussion, and experiential exercises that focus on particular themes related to meaning and advanced cancer. It is designed to help patients with advanced cancer sustain or enhance a sense of meaning, peace, and purpose in their lives even as they approach the end of life. In a recent randomized controlled trial comparing meaning-centered group psychotherapy (MCGP) and supportive group psychotherapy among advanced cancer patients, Breitbart et al. (2010b) showed that the MCGP resulted in significant improvements in spiritual well-being and sense of meaning, with reductions in anxiety and desire for hastened death.

Demoralization

Kissane et al. (2001) described a syndrome of "demoralization" in the terminally ill that is distinct from depression and consists of a triad of hopelessness, loss of meaning, and existential distress expressed as a desire for death. It is associated with life-threatening medical illness, disability, bodily disfigurement, fear, loss of dignity, social isolation, and feelings of being a burden (Kissane et al. 2009). Because of the sense of impotence and hopelessness, those with the syndrome predictably progress to a desire to die or commit suicide. The authors (Kissane et al. 2001) formulated a treatment approach for demoralization syndrome that emphasizes a multidisciplinary, multimodal approach consisting of 1) ensuring continuity of care and active symptom management; 2) ensuring dignity in the dying process; 3) using various types of psychotherapy to help sustain a sense of meaning, limit cognitive distortions, and maintain family relationships (i.e., meaning-based, cognitive-behavioral, interpersonal, and family psychotherapy interventions); 4) using life review and narrative and attention to spiritual issues; and 5) administering pharmacotherapy for comorbid anxiety, depression, and delirium.

Dignity-Conserving Care

Ensuring dignity in the dying process is a critical goal of palliative care. Despite use of the term *dignity* in arguments for and against a patient's self-governance in matters pertaining to death, there is little empirical research on how this term has been used by patients who are nearing death. Chochinov et al. (2002a, 2002b) examined how dying patients understand and define *dignity* in order to develop a model of dignity in the terminally ill (Figure 41-2). A semistructured interview was designed to explore how patients cope with their illness and their perceptions of dignity. Three major categories emerged, which included illness-related concerns (concerns related to the illness itself that threaten or impinge on the patient's sense of dignity), dignity-conserving repertoire (internally held qualities or personal approaches that patients use to maintain their sense of dignity), and social dignity inventory (social concerns or relationship dynamics that enhance or detract from a patient's sense of dignity). These broad categories and their carefully defined themes and subthemes form the foundation for an emerging model of dignity among the dying (Chochinov et al. 2006). The concept of dignity and the notion of dignity-conserving care offer a way of understanding how patients face advancing terminal illness and present an approach that clinicians can use to explicitly target the maintenance of dignity as a therapeutic objective.

Accordingly, Chochinov (2002) has developed a short-term dignity-conserving care intervention for palliative care patients coined "dignity therapy," which incorporates various facets from this model most likely to bolster the dying patient's will to live, lessen their desire for death or overall level of distress, and improve their quality of life. The dignity model establishes the importance of generativity as a significant dignity theme. As such, the sessions are taped, transcribed, and edited, and the transcription is returned to the patient within 1-2 days. The creation of a tangible product that will live beyond the patient acknowledges the importance of generativity as a salient dignity issue. The immediacy of the returned transcript is intended to bolster the patient's sense of purpose, meaning, and worth while giving them the tangible experience that their thoughts and words continue to be valued. In most instances, these transcripts will be left for family or loved ones and form part of a personal legacy that the patient will have actively participated in creating and shaping.

Spirituality in Palliative Care

Addressing spirituality as an essential element of quality palliative care has been identified as a priority by medical professionals as well as by patients (Chochinov and Cann 2005; Dufault and Pulchalski 2006). Spirituality encompasses concepts of faith and/or meaning. Viewing spirituality as a construct composed of faith and meaning is reflected in the FACIT Spiritual Well-Being Scale (Brady et al. 1999; Peterman et al. 1996). This scale generates a total score as well as two subscale scores; one corresponding to "Faith" and a second corresponding to "Meaning/Peace." Other measures that are commonly used to gauge aspects of spirituality include the Daily Spiritual Experiences Scale (Underwood and Teresi 2002) and the Spiritual Beliefs Inventory (Baider et al. 2001).

Spirituality and Life-Threatening Medical Illness

There has been great interest in spirituality, faith, and religious beliefs and their impact on health outcomes and their role in palliative care. Sloan et al. (1999) concluded in their review of the literature that evidence of an association between religion and health was weak and inconsistent and that it was premature to promote faith and religion as adjunctive treatments. Researchers theorize that religious beliefs may help patients construct meaning from the suffering inherent in illness, which may in turn facilitate acceptance (Koenig et al. 1998). A number of studies have found that religion and spirituality generally play a positive role in patients' coping with illnesses such as cancer or HIV (Baider et al. 1999; Nelson et al. 2002; Peterman et al. 1996).

Several studies (Breitbart et al. 2000; McClain et al. 2003; Nelson et al. 2002; Whitford et al. 2008) have demonstrated a central role for spiritual well-being and meaning as a buffering agent against depression, hopelessness, and desire for hastened death among advanced cancer patients. Although spiritual well-being (per the FACIT Spiritual Well-Being Scale) has a generally positive influence on the incidence of depression, hopelessness, and desire for death, it is the score on the Meaning/Peace subscale that has the most significant effect.

Communication About Spiritual Issues

Several factors may inhibit effective communication with patients about spirituality in a palliative care setting (C.L. Clayton 2000; Ellis et al. 1999; Post et al. 2000; Sloan et al. 1999). Promoting religion, faith, or specific religious beliefs or rituals (e.g., prayer, belief in an afterlife) in an effort to deal with patients' spiritual concerns or suffering at the end of life has limited acceptance among health care pro-

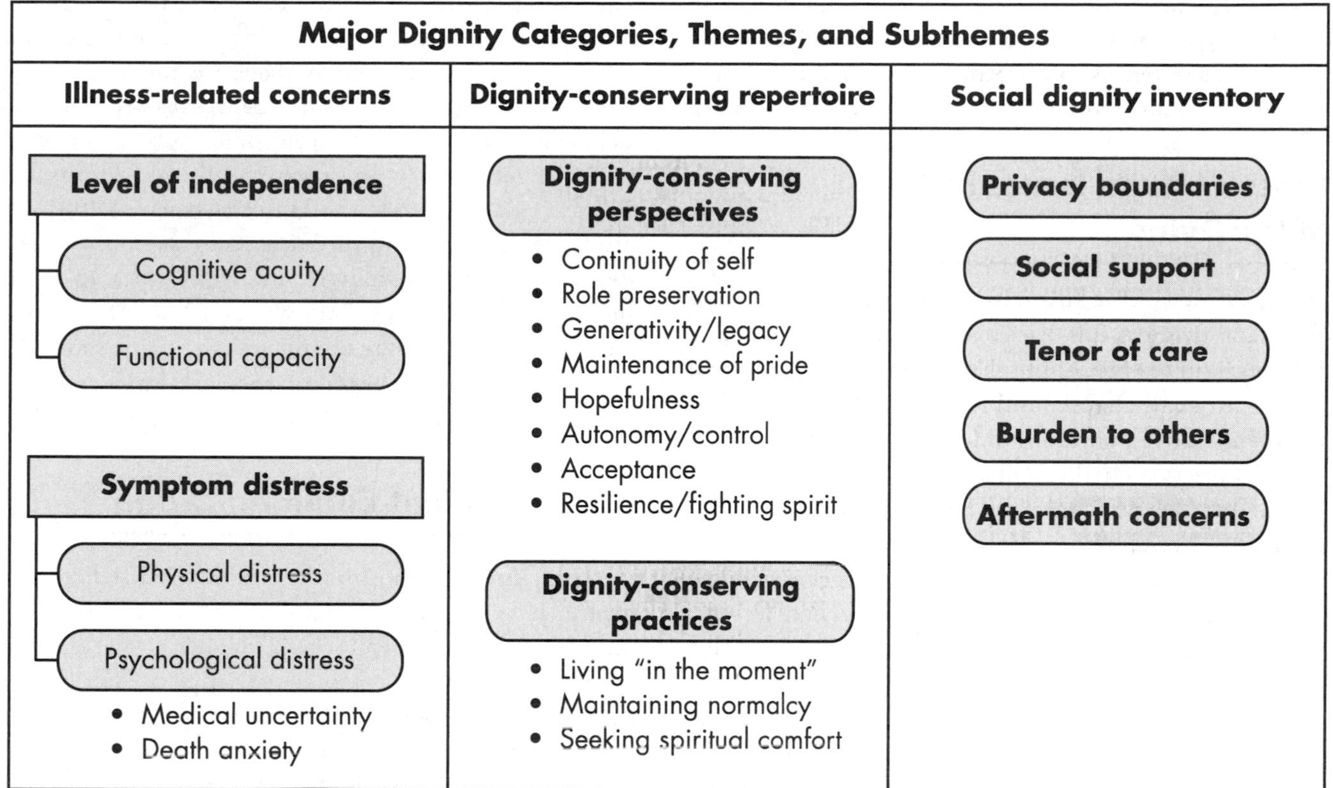

FIGURE 41–2. Model of dignity for the terminally ill.

viders and is not universally applicable to all patients. Maugans and Wadland (1991) suggested that there is often a great discrepancy between physicians and patients on such issues as belief in God, belief in an afterlife, regular prayer, and feeling close to God, with physicians endorsing such beliefs or practices less than half as often as patients (none greater than 40%).

Additional barriers include lack of time on the part of the provider, lack of training, fear of projecting one's own beliefs onto the patient, and concerns about patient autonomy (Ellis et al. 1999). Finally, providers may feel that these discussions are inappropriate because they are outside of their area of expertise or intrusive to the patient's privacy (Ellis et al. 1999; Post et al. 2000; Sloan et al. 1999). However, the majority of studies have demonstrated that patients welcome these discussions (J.M. Anderson et al. 1993; King and Bushwick 1994; Maugans 1996).

Communicating effectively with patients about spirituality requires comfort in several domains. These include 1) a basic knowledge of common spiritual concerns and sources of spiritual pain for patients; 2) the principles and beliefs of the major religions common to the patient populations one treats; 3) basic clinical communication skills, such as active and empathic listening, with an ability to identify and highlight spiritually relevant issues; and 4) the ability to remain present while patients struggle with spiritual issues in light of their mortality (Storey and Knight 2001). This final domain is often the most trying, especially for clinicians early in their career.

The American Academy of Hospice and Palliative Medicine offers the following guidelines for clinicians when communicating about spiritual issues (Doyle 1992; Hay 1996; Storey and Knight 2001). First, it is important to recognize that every patient is an individual and has a unique belief system that should be honored and respected. A patient's spiritual views may or may not incorporate religious beliefs, as *spirituality* is considered the more inclusive category. Therefore, initial discussions should focus on broad spiritual issues and then, when appropriate, on more specific religious beliefs. Caregivers should maintain appropriate boundaries and avoid discussions of their own religious beliefs because they are usually not relevant. Finally, fostering hope and integrating meaning into a patient's life is a more important aspect of providing spiritual healing than adherence to a particular belief system or religious affiliation. Methods for taking a spiritual history are reviewed elsewhere (Puchalski and Romer 2000). Formal assessment tools are also available (Kuhn 1988; Maugans 1996).

Psychosomatic medicine clinicians should be aware of the importance of spirituality and the value of pastoral care services not only for the patient but also for the family coping with a terminal illness. Referrals to chaplains are as important as referrals to any other specialist and an essential part of comprehensive care (Thiel and Robinson 1997).

Cross-Cultural Issues in Care of the Dying

Ethnicity and culture strongly influence attitudes toward death and dying. A full discussion of cultural and ethnic differences in the face of life-threatening illness is beyond the scope of this chapter and is described elsewhere, but some illustrative points should be noted (National Consensus Project for Quality Palliative Care 2009; Schim et al. 2006). Although fears of cancer and other debilitating diseases are universal (Butow et al. 1997), it appears that individuals from mainstream Western cultures generally use different coping strategies than those used in non-Western cultures (Barg and Gullatte 2001). Wide differences also exist within countries.

Blackhall et al. (1995) studied ethnic attitudes in the United States toward patient autonomy regarding disclosure of the diagnosis and prognosis of a terminal illness and toward end-of-life decision making. They found that different cultures have distinct opinions about how much information physicians should provide concerning diagnoses and prognoses. The investigators determined that African Americans (88%) and European Americans (87%) are significantly more likely than Mexican Americans (65%) or Korean Americans (47%) to believe that a patient should always be informed of a diagnosis of metastatic cancer. They also found that African Americans (63%) and European Americans (69%) are more likely than Korean Americans (35%) and Mexican Americans (48%) to believe a patient should be informed of a terminal prognosis and be actively involved in decisions concerning use of life-sustaining technology. They concluded that physicians should ask their patients whether they wish to be informed of their diagnoses and prognoses and to be involved in treatment decisions or prefer to let family members or caregivers handle such matters.

A similar study of Navajo Indian beliefs concerning autonomy in patient diagnosis and prognosis found that in the Navajo culture, physicians and patients must speak in only a positive way, avoiding any negative thought or speech (Carrese and Rhodes 1995). Because Navajos believe that language can "shape reality and control events," informing patients of a negative diagnosis or prognosis is considered disrespectful and physically and emotionally dangerous (Carrese and Rhodes 1995). As these two studies show, physicians must be careful to respect their patients' cultural beliefs in disclosing the diagnosis and prognosis of a terminal illness. Important differences between cultures include those that exist in the roles of religion (Musick et al. 1998a, 1998b), family, alternative healing traditions and folk healers (Canive and Castillo 1997; Chan et al. 2001), attitudes toward pain and suffering (Gordon 2002), beliefs about afterlife, and customs regarding the deceased's body and burial preparations (Parkes et al. 1997). At the same time, one should beware of cultural stereotypes and not assume that every member of a particular ethnic or cultural group holds identical shared values.

Doctor–Patient Communication

Doctor–patient communication is an essential component in caring for a dying patient (Baile and Beale 2001; Buckman 1993, 1998; Fallowfield 2004; Parker et al. 2001; Smith 2000). A study of cancer patients' predictions regarding outcome and the treatments they chose revealed that inadequate communication between cancer patients and their physicians resulted in overestimation of survival by patients and a resulting tendency to choose more aggressive treatment (Weeks et al. 1996).

In a study of oncologists' communication skills (Fallowfield et al. 1998), less than 35% reported having received any previous communication training, but most desired to learn better communication techniques. Psychosomatic medicine specialists can help improve communication skills in physicians and other health care professionals caring for dying patients. Intensive training programs in doctor–patient communication that use a variety of teaching methods, including role-playing, videotaped feedback, experiential exercises, and didactics, have been demonstrated to have both short-term as well as long-term efficacy in improving communication skills among physicians (Fallowfield 2004; Maguire 1999). Bylund et al. (2010) reported on the successful implementation of a curriculum for oncologists at Memorial Sloan-Kettering Cancer Center with improved communication skills following training.

One critical aspect of doctor–patient communication is how to break bad news. A useful six-step protocol for breaking bad news includes 1) getting the physical context right, 2) finding out how much the patient knows, 3) finding out how much the patient wants to know, 4) sharing information (aligning and educating), 5) responding to the patient's feelings, and 6) planning and following through (Baile and Beale 2001; Buckman 1998).

Bereavement

Bereavement care is an integral dimension of palliative care, particularly for the 20% of bereaved individuals who develop complicated grief, for which effective therapies are available (Kissane 2004). Normal grief is an inevitable dimension of humanity, an adaptive adjustment process, and one that, with support, can be approached with courage.

Although words such as *grief, mourning,* and *bereavement* are commonly used interchangeably, the following definitions may be helpful:

- *Bereavement* is the state of loss resulting from death (Parkes 1998).
- *Grief* is the emotional response associated with loss (Stroebe et al. 1993).
- *Mourning* is the process of adaptation, including the cultural and social rituals prescribed as accompaniments (Raphael 1983).
- *Anticipatory grief* precedes the death and results from the expectation of that event (Raphael 1983).
- *Complicated grief* represents a pathological outcome involving psychological, social, or physical morbidity (Rando 1983).
- *Disenfranchised grief* represents the hidden sorrow of the marginalized patient, for whom there is less social permission to express many dimensions of loss (Doka 2000).

Nature of Normal Grief

The expression of normal grief is evident through its emotional, cognitive, physical, and behavioral features (Parkes 1998). In Lindemann's (1944) classic study of people who lost a relative in Boston's Coconut Grove Nightclub fire, he identified key features of grief including somatic distress with numbness, preoccupation with sad memories of the deceased, guilt, anger, loss of regular patterns of conduct, and identification with the deceased.

Emotional distress occurs in waves with unavoidable crying and a range of associated affects including sadness, anger, despair, anxiety, and guilt. Cognitive processes become dominated by memories, reflected in storytelling, reminiscences, and conversations about the deceased. Physical responses include numbness, restlessness, tension, tremors, sleep disturbance, anorexia, weight loss, fatigue, and painful symptoms. Finally, behavioral aspects are variously reflected in social withdrawal, wandering, searching, and seeking company and consolation.

A number of physiological changes have been identified in grief in neuroendocrine functioning (Jacobs et al. 1997), immune indices (Esterling et al. 1996), and sleep efficiency (Hall et al. 1998).

Clinical Presentations of Grief

As the patient and family journey through palliative care, the clinical phases of grief progress from anticipatory grief through to the immediate news of the death, to the stages of acute grief, and potentially for some, to the complications of bereavement.

Anticipatory Grief

Anticipatory grief generally draws the supportive family closer. In contrast, for some families difficulties emerge as they express their anticipatory grief. Impaired coping is exhibited through protective avoidance, denial of the seriousness of the threat, anger, or withdrawal from involvement. Sometimes family dysfunction is glaring. More commonly, however, subthreshold or mild depressive or anxiety disorders develop gradually as individuals struggle to adapt to unwelcome changes. Although anticipatory grief was historically suggested to reduce postmortem grief (Parkes 1975), intense distress is now well recognized as a marker of risk for complicated grief. During this phase of anticipatory grief, families that are capable of effective communication should be encouraged to openly share their feelings as they go about the care of their dying family member or friend. Saying goodbye needs to be recognized as a process that evolves over time, with opportunities for reminiscence, celebration of the life and contribution of the dying person, expressions of gratitude, and completion of any unfinished business (Meares 1981). These tasks have the potential to generate creative and positive emotional aspects of what is otherwise a sad time for all.

Sometimes staff will have concerns about the emotional response of the bereaved. If there is uncertainty about its cultural appropriateness, consultation with an informed cultural intermediary may prove helpful.

Caution is needed in those settings where grief could be marginalized, well exemplified by ageism (see Doka 2000). If a death is normalized because it appears in step with the life cycle, family members may receive less support and reduced permission to express many aspects of their loss.

Acute Grief and Time Course of Bereavement

The sequence or stages through which the bereaved move over time are not rigidly demarcated but merge gradually one into the other (Parkes 1998; Raphael 1983). Starting with initial numbness and a sense of unreality, waves of distress begin to occur as bereaved individuals experience intense pining and yearning for their lost one. Memories of the deceased trigger these acute pangs of grief. Then, as the pain of separation grows, a phase of disorganization emerges as loneliness resulting from the loss sets in. Hofer (1984) described this phase aptly as a constant background disturbance of restlessness, inattention, sadness, and despair, with social withdrawal that can last for several months. Eventually a phase of reorganization and recovery develops as nostalgia replaces sadness, morale improves, and an altered worldview is constructed.

The time course of mourning is proportional to the strength of attachment to the lost person and also varies with cultural expression, there being no sharply defined end point to grief. Just as a mother's grief following sudden infant death syndrome usually lasts longer than grief following a neonatal death, so too with adult loss—the mourning that follows many years of marriage is generally longer than that in brief relationships. Some, including older widows and widowers, may continue to display their grief for several years (Zisook and Shuchter 1985). This may represent a continuing relationship with the deceased that, for some, is their choice and leads to a prolonged period of bereavement that may be quite appropriate and within the normal range of grief experience. The clinical task is then to differentiate those that remain within the spectrum of normality from those that cross the threshold of complicated grief.

Complicated Grief

Normal and abnormal responses to bereavement span a spectrum in which intensity of reaction, presence of a range of related grief behaviors, and time course determine the differentiation. Complicated grief has been conceptualized as a stress response syndrome that results from failure to integrate the loss, making it difficult to function in a world without the deceased, with avoidance a central feature (Shear et al. 2007). In complicated grief, yearning for the lost one is even more common than depressed mood (Maciejewski et al. 2007). Diagnostic criteria have been proposed for "complicated grief disorder" by Zhang et al. (2006) to be included in DSM-V. The proposed criteria capture the essential features of complicated grief including daily yearning for the deceased to a distressing or disruptive degree accompanied by any four of the following symptoms: difficulty accepting death, inability to trust others, anger about the death, feeling uneasy about moving on with one's life, feeling numb, feeling life is empty, feeling the future holds no meaning, and feeling agitated or on edge since the death.

Inhibited or Delayed Grief

Although avoidance may serve some as a temporary coping mechanism, its persistence is usually associated with relationship or other difficulties. Cultural and individual variation significantly influences grief expression; a placid external emotional response cannot be equated with internal avoidance. Empirical studies have generally identified avoidant forms of complicated grief in up to 5% of the bereaved—the grief may not always present clinically but may reappear in later years as an unresolved issue.

Chronic Grief

A common form of complicated grief, chronic grief is particularly associated with overly dependent relationships in which a sense of abandonment is avoided by perpetuation of the relationship through memorialization of the deceased and maintenance of continuing bonds. Social withdrawal and depression are common. A fantasy of reunion with the deceased can cause suicide to be an increasingly attractive option. Active treatment using antidepressants and cognitive-behavioral therapy to reality test the loss and promote socialization (via activity scheduling) is often appropriate for chronic grief (keeping in mind that not all persistent grief is pathological).

Traumatic Grief

When death has been unexpected or its nature in some way shocking—traumatic, violent, stigmatized, or perceived as undignified—its integration and acceptance may be interfered with by the arousal and increased distress that memories can trigger. Intensive recollections including flashbacks, nightmares, and recurrent intrusive memories cause hyperarousal, disbelief, insomnia, irritability, and disturbed concentration that distort normal grieving (Prigerson and Jacobs 2001). The shock of the death can precipitate mistrust, anger, detachment, and an unwillingness to accept its reality. These reactions at a subthreshold level are on a continuum with the full features of acute and posttraumatic stress disorders, but subthreshold states have been observed to persist for years and contribute substantial morbidity. Palliative care deaths involving profound breakdown of bodily surfaces, gross disfigurement due to head and neck cancers, or other changes eliciting fear, disgust, or mortification may generate traumatic memories in the bereaved. Schut et al. (1997) found that PTSD was often correlated with the perceived inadequacy of the goodbye and suggested that rituals to complete this be incorporated into related grief therapies. The researchers who initially proposed the term "traumatic grief" have suggested returning to the original term "complicated grief" in order to avoid confusion between traumatic grief and posttraumatic stress disorder (Zhang et al. 2006).

Psychiatric Disorders in Bereavement

Psychiatric disorders commonly complicating grief include clinical depression, anxiety disorders, alcohol abuse or other substance abuse, and psychotic disorders. When frank psychiatric disorders complicate bereavement, they are more likely to be recognized and treated than subthreshold states. Studies of the bereaved identify clusters of intense grief symptoms distinct from uncomplicated grief (Parkes and Weiss 1983; Prigerson et al. 1995a, 1995b). Their recognition calls for an experienced clinical judgment that does not normalize the distress as understandable.

Rates of major depression in the bereaved have varied between 16% and 50%, peaking during the first 2 months (P. Clayton 1990; Zisook and Shuchter 1991) and gradually decreasing to 15% across the next 2 years (Harlow et al. 1991; Zisook et al. 1994). The features of any major depressive episode following bereavement resemble major depression at other points of the life cycle (Kendler et al. 2008). There is a tendency toward chronicity, considerable social morbidity, and risk of inadequate treatment.

Anxiety disorders take the form of adjustment disorders, generalized anxiety disorder, acute and posttraumatic stress disorders, and phobias and occur in up to 30% of the bereaved (Jacobs 1993).

Individuals predisposed to alcohol or other substance use disorders are at higher risk for relapse during grief (Jacobs 1993), as are those with psychotic disorders. The latter should not be confused with the "normal" hallucinations that can occur in grief, typically limited to the voice, sight, and/or sense of presence of the deceased.

Risk factors that, when present, can aid recognition of those at greater risk of complicated grief are summarized in Table 41–3.

TABLE 41–3. Risk factors for complicated grief

Category	Range of circumstances
Nature of the death	Untimely within the life cycle (e.g., death of a child) Sudden and unexpected Traumatic/shocking Stigmatized
Strengths and vulnerabilities of the caregiver/bereaved	Past history of psychiatric disorder Personality and coping style Cumulative experience of losses
Nature of the relationship with the deceased	Overly dependent Ambivalent
Family and support network	Dysfunctional family Isolated Alienated

Grief Therapies

The most basic model is a supportive-expressive intervention in which the person is invited to share his or her feelings about the loss to a health professional who will listen and seek to understand the other's distress in a comforting manner. The key therapeutic aspects of this encounter are the sharing of distress and, through the relational understanding that is acknowledged, some shift in cognitive appraisal of the reality that has been forever altered. There are multiple possible formal interventions for bereaved people, but the first question is whether an intervention is actually warranted. For most, although bereavement is painful, personal resilience will ensure normal adaptation. There can therefore be no justification for routine intervention, because grief is not a disease. Early intervention should be considered for those at risk of maladaptive outcomes, and those who later develop complicated bereavement need active treatments.

The spectrum of interventions spans individual-, group-, and family-oriented therapies and encompasses all schools of psychotherapy as well as appropriately indicated pharmacotherapy. A typical intervention entails six to eight sessions over several months. In this sense, grief therapy is focused and time limited, but multimodal therapies are common (Kissane 2004). Table 41–4 lists commonly used forms of grief therapy (Kissane 2004).

Pharmacotherapy is widely used to support the bereaved, but prescribing should be judicious. Benzodiazepines allay anxiety and assist sleep, but excessive use may interfere with adaptive mourning. Antidepressants are indicated when bereavement is complicated by major depression or panic disorder (Pasternak et al. 1991; Zisook et al. 2001).

Palliation of Selected Physical Symptoms

Although the diagnosis and treatment of psychiatric disorders in the patient with advanced illness is important, pain and other distressing physical symptoms must also be aggressively treated to enhance the patient's quality of life. Some key points are noted in this discussion, but a comprehensive review of pharmacological and nonpharmacological interventions for common physical symptoms encountered in the terminally ill can be found in a curriculum published by the American Society of Clinical Oncology (2001) and in major palliative care texts (Chochinov and Breitbart 2009; Doyle et al. 2003; Portenoy et al. 2009).

Pain

The Agency for Health Care Policy and Research (Jacox et al. 1994) published a practice guideline for management of cancer pain in the early 1990s, with more recent guidelines from the National Comprehensive Cancer Network (NCCN Adult Cancer Pain Panel Members 2008). Breitbart et al. (2004b) provided an up-to-date detailed discussion of the

TABLE 41–4. Models of grief therapy

Model	Potential focus for application	Clinical issues when indicated
Supportive–expressive therapy (guided grief work, crisis intervention)	Individual and/or group	Avoidance of emotional expression Inhibited or delayed grief Isolated and needing support Established psychiatric disorders including depression
Interpersonal or psychodynamic therapy	Individual and/or group	Relational issues dominate Role transition difficulties
Cognitive-behavioral therapy	Individual and/or group	Chronic grief with "stuck" behaviors Traumatic grief Posttraumatic stress disorder
Family-focused grief therapy	Family	Family either at risk or clearly dysfunctional in its relating Adolescents or children at risk
Combined pharmacotherapies with any of the psychotherapeutic models	Individual	Depressive disorders Anxiety disorders Sleep disorders

use of behavioral, psychotherapeutic, and psychopharmacological interventions for pain control in palliative care (see also Chapter 36, "Pain"). After adequate medical treatment, mild to moderate levels of residual pain can be effectively managed with behavioral techniques that are quite similar to those used for anxiety, phobias, and anticipatory nausea and vomiting. Relaxation techniques, imagery, hypnosis, biofeedback, and multicomponent cognitive-behavioral interventions have been used to provide comfort and minimize pain in adults, children, and adolescents.

Anorexia and Weight Loss

While physiological changes associated with terminal illness account for most of the anorexia and cachexia in the terminally ill, with additional contributions from adverse effects of treatments, psychological and psychiatric factors, including anxiety, depression, and conditioned food aversions, may also play a role (Lesko 1989). The treatment of anorexia and weight loss begins with the identification and correction of reversible causes (e.g., opioid-induced nausea, stomatitis from chemotherapy, or thrush) (NCCN Palliative Care Panel Members 2009). Progestational drugs (medroxyprogesterone or megestrol acetate) or corticosteroids are often tried for nonspecific cachexia (NCCN Palliative Care Panel Members 2009). Appetite-stimulating antidepressants (e.g., tricyclic antidepressants [TCAs], trazodone, mirtazapine) should be considered when the cause is major depression, but depression should never be diagnosed solely on the basis of unexplained anorexia and weight loss. Treatment of conditioned nausea and vomiting is discussed later.

Asthenia/Fatigue

Asthenia and fatigue are extremely common in patients with advanced cancer, AIDS, and organ failure as a result of deconditioning, catabolism, malnutrition, infection, profound anemia, metabolic abnormalities, or adverse effects of treatment, but a reversible cause often cannot be identified. As with unexplained weight loss in advanced disease, there is a tendency to overdiagnose depression in the terminally ill patient with extreme fatigue.

The literature in support of the pharmacotherapy of fatigue in cancer patients is limited, but practice guidelines are available (Mock et al. 2000; NCCN Cancer-Related Fatigue Panel Members 2008). Antidepressants have been recommended to treat the underlying depression when present (NCCN Cancer-Related Fatigue Panel Members 2008). Identifiable causes should be specifically treated when possible, for example, erythropoietin for anemia. Some patients respond to corticosteroids, but the benefits tend to be fleeting and prolonged use can cause proximal myopathy. Psychostimulants have been used in the treatment of asthenia with good results, however further research is needed (Breitbart et al. 2001; NCCN Cancer-Related Fatigue Panel Members 2008; see also Chapter 28, "HIV/AIDS"). Low doses of stimulants do not appear to cause appetite suppression or weight loss and may actually improve energy and appetite in fatigued terminally ill patients.

Nausea and Vomiting

Common causes of nausea and vomiting in advanced cancer patients include radiation, medications, toxins, metabolic derangements, obstruction of the gastrointestinal tract, and chemotherapy (NCCN Antiemesis Panel Members 2009). Conditioned by the experience of profound nausea and vomiting secondary to highly emetic chemotherapy agents, some patients report being nauseated in anticipation of treatment. Anticipatory nausea and vomiting used to be very frequent but has become less so with current antiemetic therapy.

Antiemetic drugs are the mainstay of managing chemotherapy-induced nausea and vomiting in patients with advanced disease. Several antiemetics (e.g., metoclopramide, prochlorperazine, promethazine) have dopamine-blocking properties and so can cause the same extrapyramidal side effects as neuroleptics, with acute akathisia and dystonia common. Extrapyramidal side effects are not a problem with newer antiemetics like ondansetron. Rapid-onset, short-acting benzodiazepines are also helpful in controlling anticipatory nausea and vomiting once they have developed (Greenberg et al. 1987). Behavioral control of anticipatory nausea and vomiting was shown to be highly effective (Barnes 1988) but has largely been replaced by antiemetic drugs.

Conclusion

The psychosomatic medicine practitioner can play an important role in the care of patients with advanced, life-threatening medical illnesses. Palliative care for terminally ill patients must include not only control of pain and physical symptoms but also assessment and management of psychiatric and psychosocial complications. The psychosomatic medicine practitioner working in the palliative care setting must be knowledgeable in the assessment and management of major psychiatric complications, such as anxiety, depression, and delirium, and also must be adept in dealing with issues of existential despair and spiritual suffering. Cultural issues, communication issues, ethical issues, and issues of bereavement are all areas requiring attention and awareness. As part of an interdisciplinary team, the psychosomatic medicine practitioner can play an important role in the provision of comprehensive palliative care.

References

Achte KA, Vanhkouen ML: Cancer and the psyche. Omega 2:46–56, 1971

Adams F, Quesada JR, Gutterman JU: Neuropsychiatric manifestations of human leukocyte interferon therapy in patients with cancer. JAMA 252:938–941, 1984

American Academy of Hospice and Palliative Medicine: American ABMS Certification. 2009. Available at: http://www.aahpm.org/certification/abms.html. Accessed May 24, 2009.

American Psychiatric Association: Diagnostic and Statistical Manual of Mental Disorders, 3rd Edition, Revised. Washington, DC, American Psychiatric Association, 1987

American Psychiatric Association: Diagnostic and Statistical Manual of Mental Disorders, 4th Edition. Washington, DC, American Psychiatric Association, 1994

American Society of Clinical Oncology: Optimizing Cancer Cure: The Importance of Symptom Management. Alexandria, VA, American Society of Clinical Oncology Publishing, 2001

Anderson JM, Anderson LJ, Felsenthal G: Pastoral needs for support within an inpatient rehabilitation unit. Arch Phys Med Rehabil 74:574–578, 1993

Anderson T, Watson M, Davidson R: The use of cognitive behavioural therapy techniques for anxiety and depression in hospice patients: a feasibility study. Palliat Med 22:814–821, 2008

Baider L, Russak SM, Perry S, et al: The role of religious and spiritual beliefs in coping with malignant melanoma: an Israeli sample. Psychooncology 8:27–35, 1999

Baider L, Holland JC, Russak SM, et al: The System of Belief Inventory-15 (SBI-15). Psychooncology 10:534–540, 2001

Baile W, Beale E: Giving bad news to cancer patients: matching process and content. J Clin Oncol 19:2575–2577, 2001

Barg FK, Gullatte MM: Cancer support groups: meeting the needs of African Americans with cancer. Semin Oncol Nurs 17:171–178, 2001

Barnes M: Nausea and vomiting in the patient with advanced cancer. J Pain Symptom Manage 3:81–85, 1988

Berger AM, Shuster JL, Von Roenn JH (eds): Principles and Practice of Palliative Care and Supportive Oncology, 3rd Edition. Philadelphia, PA, Lippincott, Williams & Wilkins, 2006

Blackhall LJ, Murphy ST, Frank G, et al: Ethnicity and attitudes toward patient autonomy. JAMA 274:820–825, 1995

Block SD: Assessing and managing depression in the terminally ill patient. Ann Intern Med 132:209–218, 2000

Boettger S, Breitbart W: Atypical antipsychotics in the management of delirium: a review of the empirical literature. Palliat Support Care 3:227–237, 2005

Bolund C: Suicide and cancer, II: medical and care factors in suicide by cancer patients in Sweden. Journal of Psychosocial Oncology 3:17–30, 1985

Bottomley DM, Hanks GW: Subcutaneous midazolam infusion in palliative care. J Pain Symptom Manage 5:259–261, 1990

Brady MJ, Peterman AH, Fitchett G, et al: A case for including spirituality in quality of life measurement in oncology. Psychooncology 8:417–428, 1999

Brandberg Y, Mansson-Brahme E, Ringborg U, et al: Psychological reactions in patients with malignant melanoma. Eur J Cancer 31A:157–162, 1995

Breitbart W: Suicide in cancer patients. Oncology (Huntingt) 1:49–55, 1987

Breitbart W: Endocrine-related psychiatric disorders, in Handbook of Psychooncology: Psychological Care of the Patient With Cancer. Edited by Holland JC, Rowland JH. New York, Oxford University Press, 1989a, pp 356–368

Breitbart W: Psychiatric management of cancer pain. Cancer 63:2336–2342, 1989b

Breitbart W: Cancer pain and suicide, in Advances in Pain Research and Therapy, Vol 16. Edited by Foley K, Bonica JJ, Ventafridda V, et al. New York, Raven, 1990, pp 399–412

Breitbart W: Diagnosis and management of delirium in the terminally ill, in Topics in Palliative Care, Vol 5. Edited by Bruera E, Portenoy R. New York, Oxford University Press, 2001, pp 303–321

Breitbart W: Spirituality and meaning in supportive care: spirituality- and meaning-centered group psychotherapy interventions in advanced cancer. Support Care Cancer 10:272–280, 2002

Breitbart W: Palliative and Supportive Care: introducing a new international journal; the "care" journal of palliative medicine. Palliat Support Care 1:1–2, 2003

Breitbart W, Alici Y: Agitation and delirium at the end of life: "We couldn't manage him." JAMA 300:2898–2910, 2008

Breitbart W, Heller KS: Reframing hope: meaning-centered care for patients near the end of life. J Palliat Med 6:979–988, 2003

Breitbart W, Holland JC (eds): Psychiatric Aspects of Symptom Management in Cancer Patients. Washington, DC, American Psychiatric Press, 1993

Breitbart W, Bruera E, Chochinov H, et al: Neuropsychiatric syndromes and psychological symptoms in patients with advanced cancer. J Pain Symptom Manage 10:131–141, 1995

Breitbart W, Marotta R, Platt MM, et al: A double-blind comparison trial of haloperidol, chlorpromazine, and lorazepam in the treatment of delirium in hospitalized AIDS patients. Am J Psychiatry 153:231–237, 1996

Breitbart W, Rosenfeld B, Roth A, et al: The Memorial Delirium Assessment Scale. J Pain Symptom Manage 13:128–137, 1997

Breitbart W, Rosenfeld B, Pessin H, et al: Depression, hopelessness, and desire for death in terminally ill patients with cancer. JAMA 284:2907–2911, 2000

Breitbart W, Rosenfeld B, Kaim M, et al: A randomized, double-blind, placebo-controlled trial of psychostimulants for the treatment of fatigue in ambulatory patients with human immunodeficiency virus disease. Arch Intern Med 161:411–420, 2001

Breitbart W, Gibson C, Tremblay A: The delirium experience: delirium recall and delirium-related distress in hospitalized patients with cancer, their spouses/caregivers, and their nurses. Psychosomatics 43:183–194, 2002a

Breitbart W, Tremblay A, Gibson C: An open trial of olanzapine for the treatment of delirium in hospitalized cancer patients. Psychosomatics 43:175–182, 2002b

Breitbart W, Chochinov H, Passik S: Psychiatric symptoms in palliative medicine, in Oxford Textbook of Palliative Medicine, 3rd Edition. Edited by Doyle D, Hanks G, Cherny N, et al. New York, Oxford University Press, 2004a, pp 746–771

Breitbart W, Payne D, Passik S: Psychological and psychiatric interventions in pain control, in Oxford Textbook of Palliative Medicine, 3rd Edition. Edited by Doyle D, Hanks G, Cherny N, et al. New York, Oxford University Press, 2004b, pp 424–438

Breitbart W, Rosenfeld B, Gibson C, et al: Impact of treatment for depression on desire for hastened death in patients with advanced AIDS. Psychosomatics 51:98–105, 2010a

Breitbart W, Rosenfeld B, Gibson C, et al: Meaning-centered group psychotherapy for patients with advanced cancer: a pilot randomized controlled trial. Psychooncology 19:21–28, 2010b

Brown JH, Henteleff P, Barakat S, et al: Is it normal for terminally ill patients to desire death? Am J Psychiatry 143:208–211, 1986

Bruera E, Chadwick S, Brenneis C, et al: Methylphenidate associated with narcotics for the treatment of cancer pain. Cancer Treat Rep 71:67–70, 1987

Bruera E, Miller L, McCallion J, et al: Cognitive failure in patients with terminal cancer: a prospective study. J Pain Symptom Manage 7:192–195, 1992

Bruera E, Neumann CM, Gagnon B, et al: The impact of a regional palliative care program on the cost of palliative care delivery. J Palliat Med 3:181–186, 2000

Buckman R: How to Break Bad News: A Guide for Healthcare Professionals. London, Macmillan Medical, 1993

Buckman R: Communication in palliative care: a practical guide, in Oxford Textbook of Palliative Medicine, 2nd Edition. Edited by Doyle D, Hanks GWC, MacDonald N. New York, Oxford University Press, 1998, pp 141–156

Buss MK, Vanderwerker LC, Inouye SK, et al: Associations between caregiver-perceived delirium in patients with cancer and generalized anxiety in their caregivers. J Palliat Med 10:1083–1092, 2007

Butler RN: The life review: an interpretation of reminiscence in the aged. Psychiatry 26:65–75, 1963

Butow P, Tattersall M, Goldstein D: Communication with cancer patients in culturally diverse societies. Ann N Y Acad Sci 809:317–329, 1997

Bylund CL, Brown R, Gueguen JA, et al: The implementation and assessment of a comprehensive communication skills training curriculum for oncologists. Psychooncology 19:583–593, 2010

Byock IR: The nature of suffering and the nature of opportunity at the end of life. Clin Geriatr Med 12:237–252, 1996

Canadian Palliative Care Association: Palliative Care: Towards a Consensus in Standardized Principles of Practice. Ottawa, ON, Canadian Palliative Care Association, 1995

Candy M, Jones L, Williams R, et al: Psychostimulants for depression. Cochrane Database Syst Rev 16(2):CD006722, 2008

Canive JM, Castillo D: Hispanic veterans diagnosed with PTSD: assessment and treatment issues. NCP Clinical Quarterly 7(1), Winter 1997

Carrese J, Rhodes L: Western bioethics on the Navajo reservation. JAMA 274:826–829, 1995

Chan C, Ho P, Chow E: A body-mind-spirit model in health: an Eastern approach. Soc Work Health Care 34:261–282, 2001

Cherny N: The problem of suffering, in Oxford Textbook of Palliative Medicine, 3rd Edition. Edited by Doyle D, Hanks G, Cherny N, et al. New York, Oxford University Press, 2004, pp 7–13

Chochinov HM: Dignity-conserving care—a new model for palliative care: helping the patient feel valued. JAMA 287:2253–2260, 2002

Chochinov HM, Breitbart W (eds): Handbook of Psychiatry in Palliative Medicine. New York, Oxford University Press, 2009

Chochinov HM, Cann BJ: Interventions to enhance the spiritual aspects of dying. J Palliat Med 8 (suppl 1):103–115, 2005

Chochinov HM, Wilson KG, Enns M, et al: Desire for death in the terminally ill. Am J Psychiatry 152:1185–1191, 1995

Chochinov H, Wilson K, Enns M, et al: "Are You Depressed?" screening for depression in the terminally ill. Am J Psychiatry 154:674–676, 1997

Chochinov H, Wilson K, Enns M, et al: Depression, hopelessness, and suicidal ideation in the terminally ill. Psychosomatics 39:366–370, 1998

Chochinov HM, Tataryn D, Clinch JJ, et al: Will to live in the terminally ill. Lancet 354:816–819, 1999

Chochinov HM, Hack T, Hassard T, et al: Dignity in the terminally ill: a cross-sectional, cohort study. Lancet 360:2026–2030, 2002a

Chochinov HM, Hack T, McClement S, et al: Dignity in the terminally ill: an empirical model. Soc Sci Med 54:433–443, 2002b

Chochinov HM, Hack T, Hassard T, et al: Understanding the will to live in patients nearing death. Psychosomatics 46:7–10, 2005a

Chochinov HM, Hack T, Hassard T, et al: Dignity therapy: a novel psychotherapeutic intervention for patients near the end of life. J Clin Oncol 23:5520–5525, 2005b

Chochinov HM, Krisjanson LJ, Hack TF, et al: Dignity in the terminally ill: revisited. J Palliat Med 9:666–672, 2006

Classen C, Butler LD, Koopman C, et al: Supportive-expressive group therapy and distress in patients with metastatic breast cancer: a randomized clinical intervention trial. Arch Gen Psychiatry 58:494–501, 2001

Clayton CL: Barriers, boundaries, and blessings: ethical issues in physicians' spiritual involvement with patients. Medical Humanities Report 21:234–256, 2000

Clayton P: Bereavement and depression. J Clin Psychiatry 51:34–38, 1990

Coyle N, Breitbart W, Weaver S, et al: Delirium as a contributing factor to "crescendo" pain: three case reports. J Pain Symptom Manage 9:44–47, 1994

DeAngelis LM, Delattre J, Posner JB: Radiation-induced dementia in patients cured of brain metastases. Neurology 39:789–796, 1989

Denicoff KD, Rubinow DR, Papa MZ, et al: The neuropsychiatric effects of treatment with interleukin-2 and lymphokine activated killer cells. Ann Intern Med 107:293–300, 1987

de Sousa E, Jepson BA: Midazolam in terminal care (letter). Lancet 1(8575–6):67–68, 1988

Doka K: Disenfranchised grief, in Disenfranchised Grief: Recognizing Hidden Sorrow. Edited by Doka K. Lexington, MA, Lexington Books, 2000, pp 3–11

Doyle D: Have we looked beyond the physical and psychosocial? J Pain Symptom Manage 7:302–311, 1992

Doyle D, Hanks GWC, Cherny N, et al (eds): Oxford Textbook of Palliative Medicine, 3rd Edition. New York, Oxford University Press, 2003

Dufault K, Pulchalski C: Hospital-based spirituality initiative: integration of spiritual care into daily care. J Palliat Care 22:192–193, 2006

Elia G, Thomas J: The symptomatic relief of dyspnea. Curr Oncol Rep 10:319–325, 2008

Ellis M, Vinson D, Ewigman B: Addressing spiritual concerns of patients: family physicians' attitudes and practices. J Fam Pract 48:105–109, 1999

Esterling B, Kiecolt-Glaser J, Glaser R: Psychosocial modulation of cytokine-induced natural killer cell activity in older adults. Psychosomatics 38:529–534, 1996

Fainsinger R, Miller MJ, Bruera E, et al: Symptom control during the last week of life in a palliative care unit. J Palliat Care 7:5–11, 1991

Fainsinger RL, Waller A, Bercovici M, et al: A multicentre international study of sedation for uncontrolled symptoms in terminally ill patients. Palliat Med 14:257–265, 2000

Fallowfield L: Communication and palliative medicine, in Oxford Textbook of Palliative Medicine, 3rd Edition. Edited by Doyle D, Hanks G, Cherny N, et al. New York, Oxford University Press, 2004, pp 101–107

Fallowfield L, Lipkin M, Hall A: Teaching senior oncologists communication skills: results from phase I of a comprehensive longitudinal program in the United Kingdom. J Clin Oncol 16:1961–1968, 1998

Farberow NL, Schneidman ES, Leonard CV: Suicide Among General Medical and Surgical Hospital Patients With Malignant Neoplasms (Medical Bulletin 9). Washington, DC, U.S. Veterans Administration, 1963

Farberow NL, Ganzler S, Cutter F, et al: An eight-year survey of hospital suicides. Suicide Life Threat Behav 1:984–201, 1971

Field MJ, Cassel CK (eds): Approaching Death: Improving Care at the End of Life. Committee on Care at the End of Life, Institute of Medicine. Washington, DC, National Academies Press, 1997

Foley KM, Helband H (eds): Improving Palliative Care for Cancer. National Cancer Policy Board, Institute of Medicine, and National Research Council. Washington, DC, National Academy Press, 2001

Frankl VF: The Doctor and the Soul (1955). New York, Random House, 1986

Frankl VF: Man's Search for Meaning, 4th Edition (1959). Boston, MA, Beacon Press, 1992

Frankl VF: Man's Search for Meaning. New York, Washington Square Press, 1963

Frankl VF: The Will to Meaning: Foundations and Applications of Logotherapy, Expanded Edition (1969). New York, Penguin Books, 1988

Frankl VF: Man's Search for Ultimate Meaning (1975). New York, Plenum Press, 1997

Gagnon B, Low G, Schreier G: Methylphenidate hydrochloride improves cognitive function in patients with advanced cancer and hypoactive delirium: a prospective clinical study. J Psychiatry Neurosci 30:100–107, 2005

Ganzini L, Lee MA, Heintz RT, et al: The effect of depression treatment on elderly patients' preferences for life-sustaining medical therapy. Am J Psychiatry 151:1631–1636, 1994

Gill D, Hatcher S: Antidepressants for depression in medical illness. Cochrane Database Syst Rev (4):CD001312, 2000

Gordon JS: Asian spiritual traditions and their usefulness to practitioners and patients facing life and death. J Altern Complement Med 5:603–608, 2002

Greenberg DB, Surman OS, Clarke J, et al: Alprazolam for phobic nausea and vomiting related to cancer chemotherapy. Cancer Treat Rep 71:549–550, 1987

Greenstein M, Breitbart W: Cancer and the experience of meaning: a group psychotherapy program for people with cancer. Am J Psychother 54:486–500, 2000

Griffith JL, Gaby L: Brief psychotherapy at the bedside: countering demoralization from medical illness. Psychosomatics 46:109–116, 2005

Hall M, Baum A, Buysse D, et al: Sleep as a mediator of the stress-immune relationship. Psychosom Med 60:48–51, 1998

Hardy SE: Methylphenidate for the treatment of depressive symptoms, including fatigue and apathy, in medically ill older adults and terminally ill adults. Am J Geriatr Pharmacother 7:34–59, 2009

Harlow S, Goldberg E, Comstock G: A longitudinal study of the prevalence of depressive symptomatology in elderly widowed and married women. Arch Gen Psychiatry 48:1065–1068, 1991

Hay MW: Developing guidelines for spiritual caregivers in hospice: principles for spiritual assessment. Presented at the National Hospice Organization Annual Symposium and Exposition, Chicago, IL, November 1996

Heiney PS: The healing power of story. Oncol Nurs Forum 6:899–904, 1995

Higginson IJ, Sen-Gupta GJA: Place of care in advanced cancer: a qualitative systematic literature review of patient preferences. J Palliat Med 3:287–300, 2000

Hofer M: Relationships as regulators: a psychobiologic perspective on bereavement. Psychosom Med 46:183–197, 1984

Holland JC: Anxiety and cancer: the patient and the family. J Clin Psychiatry 50 (suppl):20–25, 1989

Holland JC, Fasanello S, Ohnuma T: Psychiatric symptoms associated with l-asparaginase administration. J Psychiatr Res 10:105–113, 1974

Holland JC, Morrow G, Schmale A, et al: Reduction of anxiety and depression in cancer patients by alprazolam or by a behavioral technique (abstract). Proceedings of the American Society of Clinical Oncology 6:258, 1987

Homsi J, Nelson KA, Sarhill N, et al: A phase II study of methylphenidate for depression in advanced cancer. Am J Hosp Palliat Care 18:403–407, 2001

Hudson PL, Kristjanson LJ, Ashby M, et al: Desire for hastened death in patients with advanced disease and the evidence base of clinical guidelines: a systematic review. Palliat Med 20:693–701, 2006

Inouye B, Vandyck C, Alessi C: Clarifying confusion: the confusion assessment method, a new method for the detection of delirium. Ann Intern Med 113:941–948, 1990

Jackson KC, Lipman AG: Drug therapy for anxiety in palliative care. Cochrane Database Syst Rev (1):CD004596, 2004

Jacobs S: Pathological Grief. Washington, DC, American Psychiatric Press, 1993

Jacobs S, Bruce M, Kim K: Adrenal function predicts demoralisation after losses. Psychosomatics 38:529–534, 1997

Jacobson CM, Rosenfeld B, Pessin H, et al: Depression and IL-6 blood plasma concentrations in advanced cancer patients. Psychosomatics 49:64–66, 2008

Jacox A, Carr DB, Payne R, et al: Management of cancer pain (Clinical Practice Guideline No 9; AHCPR Publ No. 94-0592). Rockville, MD, Agency for Health Care Policy and Research, U.S. Department of Health and Human Services, Public Health Service, March 1994

Keen JC, Brown D: Psychostimulants and delirium in patients receiving palliative care. Palliat Support Care 2:199–202, 2004

Kendler KS, Myers J, Zisook S: Does bereavement-related major depression differ from major depression associated with other stressful life events? Am J Psychiatry 165:1449–1455, 2008

Kerrihard T, Breitbart W, Dent K, et al: Anxiety in patients with cancer and human immunodeficiency virus. Semin Clin Neuropsychiatry 4:114–132, 1999

King DE, Bushwick B: Beliefs and attitudes of hospital inpatients about faith healing and prayer. J Fam Pract 39:349–352, 1994

Kissane DW: Bereavement, in The Oxford Textbook of Palliative Medicine, 3rd Edition. Edited by Doyle D, Hanks G, Cherny N, et al. Oxford, UK, Oxford University Press, 2004, pp 1135–1154

Kissane D, Clarke DM, Street AF: Demoralization syndrome: a relevant psychiatric diagnosis for palliative care. J Palliat Care 17:12–21, 2001

Kissane D, Treece C, Breitbart W, et al: Dignity, meaning, and demoralization, in Handbook of Psychiatry in Palliative Medicine, 2nd Edition. Edited by Chochinov HM, Breitbart W. New York, Oxford University Press, 2009, pp 324–340

Koenig HG, George, LK, Peterson BL: Religiosity and remission of depression in medically ill older patients. Am J Psychiatry 155:536–542, 1998

Kuhn CC: A spiritual inventory of the medically ill patient. Psychiatr Med 6:87–100, 1988

Lawlor PG, Gagnon B, Mancini IL, et al: Occurrence, causes, and outcome of delirium in patients with advanced cancer: a prospective study. Arch Intern Med 160:786–794, 2000a

Lawlor PG, Nekolaichuk C, Gagnon B, et al: Clinical utility, factor analysis, and further validation of the memorial delirium assessment scale in patients with advanced cancer: assessing delirium in advanced cancer. Cancer 88:2859–2867, 2000b

Lawlor PG, Fainsinger RL, Bruera ED: Delirium at the end of life: critical issues in clinical practice and research. JAMA 284:2427–2429, 2000c

Leonard M, Raju B, Conroy M, et al: Reversibility of delirium in terminally ill patients and predictors of mortality. Palliat Med 22:848–854, 2008

Lesko L: Anorexia, in Handbook of Psychooncology: Psychological Care of the Patient With Cancer. Edited by Holland JC, Rowland JH. New York, Oxford University Press, 1989, pp 434–443

Levin TT, Alici Y: Anxiety disorders, in Psycho-Oncology, 2nd Edition. Edited by Holland JC. New York, Oxford University Press, 2010, pp 324–330

Levin TT, Li Y, Weiner JS, et al: How do-not-resuscitate orders are utilized in cancer patients: timing relative to death and communication-training implications. Palliat Support Care 6:341–348, 2008

Levine PM, Silberfarb PM, Lipowski ZJ: Mental disorders in cancer patients: a study of 100 psychiatric referrals. Cancer 42:1385–1391, 1978

Levy MH, Back A, Benedetti C, et al: NCCN clinical practice guidelines in oncology: palliative care. J Natl Compr Canc Netw 7:436–473, 2009

Lewis MI, Butler R: Life review therapy: putting memories to work in individual and group psychotherapy. Geriatrics 29:165–169, 1974

Lichter I, Mooney J, Boyd M: Biography as therapy. Palliat Med 7:133–137, 1993

Lindemann E: Symptomatology and management of acute grief. Am J Psychiatry 101:141–148, 1944

Lloyd-Williams M (ed): Psychosocial Issues in Palliative Care. New York, Oxford University Press, 2008

Lloyd-Williams M, Shiels C, Taylor F, et al: Depression—an independent predictor of early death in patients with advanced cancer. J Affect Disord 113:127–132, 2009

Lo B, Rubenfeld G: Palliative sedation in dying patients: "we turn to it when everything else hasn't worked." JAMA 294:1810–1816, 2005

Lonergan E, Britton AM, Luxenberg J, et al: Antipsychotics for delirium. Cochrane Database Syst Rev (2):CD005594, 2007

Louhivuori KA, Hakama J: Risk of suicide among cancer patients. Am J Epidemiol 109:59–65, 1979

Maciejewski PK, Zhang B, Block SD, et al: An empirical examination of the stage theory of grief. JAMA 297:716–723, 2007

Maguire P: Improving communication with cancer patients. Eur J Cancer 35:2058–2065, 1999

Massie MJ: Anxiety, panic, phobias, in Handbook of Psychooncology: Psychological Care of the Patient With Cancer. Edited by Holland JC, Rowland JH. New York, Oxford University Press, 1989, pp 300–309

Massie MJ, Holland JC, Glass E: Delirium in terminally ill cancer patients. Am J Psychiatry 140:1048–1050, 1983

Maugans TA: The SPIRITual history. Arch Fam Med 5:11–16, 1996

Maugans TA, Wadland WC: Religion and family medicine: a survey of physicians and patients. J Fam Pract 32:210–213, 1991

McClain CS, Rosenfeld B, Breitbart W: Effect of spiritual well-being on end-of-life despair in terminally ill cancer patients. Lancet 361:1603–1607, 2003

Meares R: On saying goodbye before death. JAMA 246:1227–1229, 1981

Mercadante S, De Conno F, Ripamonti C: Propofol in terminal care. J Pain Symptom Manage 10:639–642, 1995

Miovic M, Block S: Psychiatric disorders in advanced cancer. Cancer 110:1665–1676, 2007

Misbin RI, O'Hare D, Lederberg MS, et al: Compliance with New York State's do-not-resuscitate law at Memorial Sloan-Kettering Cancer Center: a review of patient deaths. N Y State J Med 93:165–168, 1993

Mock V, Atkinson A, Barsevick A, et al: NCCN practice guidelines for cancer-related fatigue. Oncology (Huntingt) 14:151–161, 2000

Morita T, Tei Y, Tsunoda J, et al: Underlying pathologies and their associations with clinical features in terminal delirium of cancer patients. J Pain Symptom Manage 22:997–1006, 2001

Morita T, Hirai K, Sakaguchi Y, et al: Family perceived distress from delirium-related symptoms of terminally ill cancer patients. Psychosomatics 45:107–113, 2004

Moyle J: The use of propofol in palliative medicine. J Pain Symptom Manage 10:643–646, 1995

Murray GB: Confusion, delirium, and dementia, in Massachusetts General Hospital Handbook of General Hospital Psychiatry, 2nd Edition. Edited by Hackett TP, Cassem NH. Littleton, MA, PSG Publishing, 1987, pp 84–115

Musick M, Koenig H, Larson D: Religion and spiritual beliefs, in Psycho-Oncology. Edited by Holland JC. New York, Oxford University Press, 1998a, pp 780–789

Musick MA, Koenig HG, Hays JC, et al: Religious activity and depression among community-dwelling elderly persons with cancer: the moderating effect of race. J Gerontol B Psychol Sci Soc Sci 53B:S218–S227, 1998b

Mystakidou K, Parpa E, Katsouda E, et al: Pain and desire for hastened death in terminally ill cancer patients. Cancer Nursing 28:318–324, 2005

NCCN Adult Cancer Pain Panel Members: National Comprehensive Cancer Network (v.1.2008) Adult Cancer Pain. NCCN Practice Guidelines in Oncology. 2008. Available at: http://www.nccn.org/professionals/physician_gls/PDF/pain.pdf. Accessed May 17, 2010.

NCCN Antiemesis Panel Members: National Comprehensive Cancer Network (v.3.2009) Antiemesis. NCCN Practice Guidelines in Oncology. 2009. Available at: http://www.nccn.org/professionals/physician_gls/PDF/antiemesis.pdf. Accessed May 17, 2010.

NCCN Cancer-Related Fatigue Panel Members: National Comprehensive Cancer Network (v.1.2008) Cancer-Related Fatigue. NCCN Practice Guidelines in Oncology. 2008. Available at: http://www.nccn.org/professionals/physician_gls/PDF/fatigue.pdf. Accessed May 17, 2010.

NCCN Palliative Care Panel Members: National Comprehensive Cancer Network (v.1.2009) Palliative Care. NCCN Practice Guidelines in Oncology. 2009. Available at: http://www.nccn.org/professionals/physician_gls/PDF/palliative.pdf. Accessed May 17, 2010.

National Consensus Project for Quality Palliative Care: Clinical Practice Guidelines for Quality Palliative Care, 2nd Edition. March 2009. Available at: http://www.nationalconsensusproject.org. Accessed May 17, 2010.

National Hospice and Palliative Care Organization: NHPCO Facts and Figures: Hospice Care in America, October 2008. Available at: http://www.nhpco.org/files/public/Statistics_Research/NHPCO_facts-and-figures_2008.pdf. Accessed May 25, 2009.

Nelson CJ, Rosenfeld B, Breitbart W, et al: Spirituality, religion, and depression in the terminally ill. Psychosomatics 43:213–220, 2002

Olden M, Pessin H, Lichtenthal WG, et al: Suicide and desire for hastened death in the terminally ill, in Handbook of Psychiatry in Palliative Medicine, 2nd Edition. Edited by Chochinov HM, Breitbart W. New York, Oxford University Press, 2009, pp 101–112

O'Neill JF, Selwyn PA, Schietinger H (eds): A Clinical Guide to Supportive and Palliative Care for HIV/AIDS. Washington, DC, US Department of Health and Human Services, Health Resources and Services Administration, HIV/AIDS Bureau, 2003

Palliative Care Foundation: Palliative Care Services in Hospitals, Guidelines. Report of the Working Group on Special Services in Hospitals, Ottawa, Ontario. Toronto, ON, Canada, National Health and Welfare, Palliative Care Foundation, 1981

Parker B, Baile W, deMoor C, et al: Breaking bad news about cancer: patients' preferences for communication. J Clin Oncol 19:2049–2056, 2001

Parkes C: Determinants of outcome following bereavement. Omega 6:303–323, 1975

Parkes C: Bereavement: Studies of Grief in Adult Life, 3rd Edition. Madison, CT, International Universities Press, 1998

Parkes C, Weiss R: Recovery From Bereavement. New York, Basic Books, 1983

Parkes C, Laungani P, Young B (eds): Death and Bereavement Across Cultures. London, Routledge, 1997

Pasternak R, Reynolds C, Schlernitzauer M: Acute open-trial nortriptyline therapy of bereavement-related depression in late life. J Clin Psychiatry 52:307–310, 1991

Patchell RA, Posner JB: Cancer and the nervous system, in Handbook of Psychooncology: Psychological Care of the Patient With Cancer. Edited by Holland JC, Rowland JH. New York, Oxford University Press, 1989, pp 327–341

Peck AW, Stern WC, Watkinson C: Incidence of seizures during treatment with tricyclic antidepressant drugs and bupropion. J Clin Psychiatry 44:197–201, 1983

Pennebaker JW, Seagal JD: Forming a story: the health benefits of narrative. J Clin Psychol 55:1243–1254, 1999

Pereira J, Hanson J, Bruera E: The frequency and clinical course of cognitive impairment in patients with terminal cancer. Cancer 79:835–842, 1997

Pessin H, Rosenfeld B, Burton L, et al: The role of cognitive impairment in desire for hastened death: a study of patients with advanced AIDS. Gen Hosp Psychiatry 25:194–199, 2003

Pessin H, Alici-Evcimen Y, Apostolatos A, et al: Diagnosis, assessment and treatment of depression in palliative care, in Psychosocial Issues in Palliative Care, 2nd Edition. Edited by Lloyd-Williams M. New York, Oxford University Press, 2008, pp 129–160

Peterman AH, Fitchett G, Cella DF: Modeling the relationship between quality of life dimensions and an overall sense of well-being. Paper presented at the Third World Congress of Psycho-Oncology, New York, October 3–6, 1996

Pickrel J: "Tell me your story": using life review in counseling the terminally ill. Death Studies 13:127–135, 1989

Portenoy R[K], Foley KM: Management of cancer pain, in Handbook of Psychooncology: Psychological Care of the Patient With Cancer. Edited by Holland JC, Rowland JH. New York, Oxford University Press, 1989, pp 369–382

Portenoy RK, Thaler HT, Kornblith AB, et al: The Memorial Symptom Assessment Scale: an instrument for the evaluation of symptom prevalence, characteristics, and distress. Eur J Cancer 30A:1326–1336, 1994

Portenoy RK, El Osta B, Bruera E: Physical symptom management in the terminally ill, in Handbook of Psychiatry in Palliative Medicine, 2nd Edition. Edited by Chochinov HM, Breitbart W. New York, Oxford University Press, 2009, pp 355–383

Posner JB: Nonmetastatic effects of cancer on the nervous system, in Cecil's Textbook of Medicine, 8th Edition. Edited by Wyngaarden JB, Smith LH. Philadelphia, PA, WB Saunders, 1988, pp 1104–1107

Post SG, Puchalski CM, Larson DB: Physicians and patient spirituality: professional boundaries, competency, and ethics. Ann Intern Med 132:578–583, 2000

Potash M, Breitbart W: Affective disorders in advanced cancer. Hematol Oncol Clin North Am 16:671–700, 2002

Prigerson H, Jacobs S: Traumatic grief as a distinct disorder: a rationale, consensus criteria, and a preliminary empirical test, in Handbook of Bereavement Research: Consequences, Coping, and Care. Edited by Stroebe M, Hansson R, Stroebe W, et al. Washington, DC, American Psychological Association, 2001, pp 613–637

Prigerson H, Frand E, Kasl S: Complicated grief and bereavement-related depression as distinct disorders: preliminary empirical validation in elderly bereaved spouses. Am J Psychiatry 152:22–30, 1995a

Prigerson H, Maciejewski P, Newson J, et al: Inventory of complicated grief. Psychiatry Res 59:65–79, 1995b

Puchalski C, Romer AL: Taking a spiritual history allows clinicians to understand patients more fully. Journal of Palliative Medicine 3:129–137, 2000

Rabkin JG, Goetz RR, Remien RH, et al: Stability of mood despite HIV illness progression in a group of homosexual men. Am J Psychiatry 154:231–238, 1997

Rando T: Treatment of Complicated Mourning. Champaign, IL, Research Press, 1983

Raphael B: The Anatomy of Bereavement. London, Hutchinson, 1983

Rietjens JA, van Zuylen L, van Veluw H, et al: Palliative sedation in a specialized unit for acute palliative care in a cancer hospital: comparing patients dying with and without palliative sedation. J Pain Symptom Manage 36:228–234, 2008

Rodin G: Individual psychotherapy for the patient with advanced disease, in Handbook of Psychiatry in Palliative Medicine, 2nd Edition. Edited by Chochinov HM, Breitbart W. New York, Oxford University Press, 2009, pp 443–453

Rodin G, Zimmermann C, Rydall A, et al: The desire for hastened death in patients with metastatic cancer. J Pain Symptom Manage 33:661–675, 2007

Rodin G, Lo C, Mikulincer M, et al: Pathways to distress: the multiple determinants of depression, hopelessness, and the desire for hastened death in metastatic cancer patients. Soc Sci Med 68:562–569, 2009

Rosenfeld B: Assisted suicide, depression, and the right to die. Psychol Public Policy Law 6:467–488, 2000

Rosenfeld B, Breitbart W, Stein K, et al: Measuring desire for death among patients with HIV/AIDS: the schedule of attitudes toward hastened death. Am J Psychiatry 156:94–100, 1999

Rosenfeld B, Breitbart W, Galietta M, et al: The schedule of attitudes toward hastened death: measuring desire for death in terminally ill cancer patients. Cancer 88:2868–2875, 2000

Rosenfeld B, Breitbart W, Gibson C, et al: Desire for hastened death among patients with advanced AIDS. Psychosomatics 47:504–512, 2006

Roth AJ, Massie MJ: Anxiety in palliative care, in Handbook of Psychiatry in Palliative Medicine, 2nd Edition. Edited by Chochinov HM, Breitbart W. New York, Oxford University Press, 2009, pp 69–80

Rousseau P: Spirituality and the dying patient. J Clin Oncol 18:2000–2002, 2000

Ryan K, Leonard M, Guerin S, et al: Validation of the confusion assessment method in the palliative care setting. Palliat Med 23:40–55, 2009

Savard J, Simard S, Giguère I, et al: Randomized clinical trial on cognitive therapy for depression in women with metastatic breast cancer: psychological and immunological effects. Palliat Support Care 4:219–237, 2006

Schim SM, Doorenbos AZ, Borse NN: Enhancing cultural competence among hospice staff. Am J Hospice Palliat Care 23:404–411, 2006

Schut H, Stroebe M, de Keijser J, et al: Intervention for the bereaved: gender differences in the efficacy of two counseling programmes. Br J Clin Psychol 36:63–72, 1997

Sepulveda C, Marlin A, Yoshida T, et al: Palliative care: the World Health Organization's global perspective. J Pain Symptom Manage 24:91–96, 2002

Shapiro BA, Warren J, Egol AB, et al: Practice parameters for intravenous analgesia and sedation for adult patients in the intensive care unit: an executive summary. Society of Critical Care Medicine. Crit Care Med 23:1596–1600, 1995

Shear K, Monk T, Houck P, et al: An attachment-based model of complicated grief including the role of avoidance. Eur Arch Psychiatry Clin Neurosci 257:453–461, 2007

Shuster JL, Breitbart W, Chochinov HM: Psychiatric aspects of excellent end-of-life care: position statement of the Academy of Psychosomatic Medicine. Psychosomatics 40:1–3, 1999

Silberfarb PM, Maurer LH, Crouthamel CS: Psychosocial aspects of neoplastic disease, I: functional status of breast cancer patients during different treatment regimens. Am J Psychiatry 137:450–455, 1980

Sloan RP, Bagiella E, Powell T: Religion, spirituality, and medicine. Lancet 353:664–667, 1999

Smith TJ: Tell it like it is. J Clin Oncol 18:3441–3445, 2000

Spiegel D, Bloom JR: Group therapy and hypnosis reduce metastatic breast carcinoma pain. Psychosom Med 4:333–339, 1983

Spiegel D, Bloom JR, Yalom ID: Group support for patients with metastatic cancer: a randomized prospective outcome study. Arch Gen Psychiatry 38:527–533, 1981

Spira J: Existential psychotherapy in palliative care, in Handbook of Psychiatry in Palliative Medicine. Edited by Chochinov H, Breitbart W. New York, Oxford University Press, 2000, pp 197–214

Stajduhar KI, Allan DE, Cohen R, et al: Preferences for location of death of seriously ill hospitalized patients: perspectives from Canadian patients and their family caregivers. Palliat Med 22:85–89, 2008

Stiefel FC, Breitbart W, Holland JC: Corticosteroids in cancer: neuropsychiatric complications. Cancer Invest 7:479–491, 1989

Stjernsward J, Clark D: Palliative medicine: a global perspective, in Oxford Textbook of Palliative Medicine, 3rd Edition. Edited by Doyle D, Hanks GWC, Cherny N, et al. New York, Oxford University Press, 2004, pp 1197–1224

Storey P, Knight C: UNIPAC Two: Alleviating Psychological and Spiritual Pain in the Terminally Ill, American Academy of Hospice and Palliative Medicine. Larchmont, NY, Mary Ann Liebert, 2001

Strain JJ, Liebowitz MR, Klein DF: Anxiety and panic attacks in the medically ill. Psychiatr Clin North Am 4:333–350, 1981

Stroebe M, Stroebe W, Hansson R (eds): Handbook of Bereavement. Cambridge, UK, Cambridge University Press, 1993

Subcommittee on Psychiatric Aspects of Life-Sustaining Technology: The role of the psychiatrist in end-of-life treatment decisions, in Caring for the Dying: Identification and Promotion of Physician Competency (Educational Resource Document). Philadelphia, PA, American Board of Internal Medicine, 1996, pp 61–67

SUPPORT Principal Investigators: A controlled trial to improve care for seriously ill hospitalized patients: the study to understand prognoses and preferences for outcomes and risks of treatments (SUPPORT). JAMA 274:1591–1598, 1995

Taylor DH Jr, Ostermann J, Van Houtven CH, et al: What length of hospice use maximizes reduction in medical expenditures near death in the US Medicare program? Soc Sci Med 65:1466–1478, 2007

Thiel MM, Robinson MR: Physicians' collaboration with chaplains: difficulties and benefits. J Clin Ethics 8:94–103, 1997

Tremblay A, Breitbart W: Psychiatric dimensions of palliative care. Neurol Clin 19:949–967, 2001

Twycross RG, Lack SA: Symptom Control in Far Advanced Cancer: Pain Relief. London, Pitman, 1983

Twycross RG, Lack SA: Therapeutics in Terminal Disease. London, Pitman, 1984

Underwood LG, Teresi JA: The daily spiritual experience scale. Ann Behav Med 24:22–33, 2002 van der Lee ML, van der Bom JG, Swarte NB, et al: Euthanasia and depression: a prospective cohort study among terminally ill cancer patients. J Clin Oncol 23:6607–6612, 2005

Viederman M: The supportive relationship, the psychodynamic life narrative, and the dying patient, in Handbook of Psychiatry in Palliative Medicine. Edited by Chochinov HM, Breitbart W. New York, Oxford University Press, 2000, pp 215–223

Viederman M, Perry SW: Use of a psychodynamic life narrative in the treatment of depression in the physically ill. Gen Hosp Psychiatry 3:177–185, 1980

Vogl D, Rosenfeld B, Breitbart W, et al: Symptom prevalence, characteristics and distress in AIDS outpatients. J Pain Symptom Manage 18:253–262, 1999

Weddington WW: Delirium and depression associated with amphotericin B. Psychosomatics 23:1076–1078, 1982

Weeks JC, Cook EF, O'Day SJ, et al: Relationship between cancer patients' predictions of prognosis and their treatment preferences. JAMA 279:1709–1714, 1996

Weisman AD: On Dying and Denying: A Psychiatric Study of Terminality. New York, Behavioral Publications, 1972

Weissman DE: Decision making at a time of crisis near the end of life. JAMA 292:1738–1743, 2004

Whitford HS, Olver IN, Peterson MJ: Spirituality as a core domain in the assessment of quality of life in oncology. Psychooncology 17:1121–1128, 2008

Wilson KG, Chochinov HM, de Faye BJ, et al: Diagnosis and management of depression in palliative care, in Handbook of Psychiatry in Palliative Medicine. Edited by Chochinov HM, Breitbart W. New York, Oxford University Press, 2000, pp 25–49

Wilson KG, Chochinov HM, Skirko MG, et al: Depression and anxiety disorders in palliative cancer care. J Pain Symptom Manage 133:118–129, 2007a

Wilson KG, Chochinov HM, McPherson CJ, et al: Desire for euthanasia or physician-assisted suicide in palliative cancer care. Health Psychol 26:314–323, 2007b

Wilson KG, Lander M, Chochinov HM: Diagnosis and management of depression in palliative care, in Handbook of Psychiatry in Palliative Medicine, 2nd Edition. Edited by Chochinov HM, Breitbart W. New York, Oxford University Press, 2009, pp 39–68

World Health Organization: Cancer Pain Relief and Palliative Care: Report of a WHO Expert Committee (Technical Bulletin 804). Geneva, Switzerland, World Health Organization, 1990

World Health Organization: National Cancer Control Programmes: Policies and Managerial Guidelines, 2nd Edition. Geneva, Switzerland, World Health Organization, 2002

World Health Organization: Definition of Palliative Care. World Health Organization Web site. Available at: http://www.who.int/cancer/palliative/definition/en/. Accessed May 25, 2009.

Young DF: Neurological complications of cancer chemotherapy, in Neurological Complications of Therapy: Selected Topics. Edited by Silverstein A. New York, Futura, 1982, pp 57–113

Zhang B, El-Jawahri A, Prigerson HG: Update on bereavement research: evidence-based guidelines for the diagnosis and treatment of complicated bereavement. J Palliat Med 9:1188–1203, 2006

Zisook S, Shuchter SR: The first four years of widowhood. Psychiatr Ann 16:288–294, 1985

Zisook S, Shuchter SR: Depression through the first year after the death of a spouse. Am J Psychiatry 148:1346–1352, 1991

Zisook S, Shuchter SR, Sledge P: The spectrum of depressive phenomena after spousal bereavement. J Clin Psychiatry 55 (suppl 4):29–36, 1994

Zisook S, Shuchter SR, Pedrelli P, et al: Bupropion sustained release for bereavement: results of an open trial. J Clin Psychiatry 62:227–230, 2001

Zuehlke TE, Watkins JT: The use of psychotherapy with dying patients: an exploratory study. J Clin Psychol 31:729–732, 1975

Web Resources

American Academy of Hospice and Palliative Medicine (AAHPM)
http://www.aahpm.org

American Board of Hospice and Palliative Medicine (ABHPM)
http://www.abhpm.org

Center for Advancement of Palliative Care (CAPC)
http://www.capc.org

End-of-Life Palliative Educational Resource Center (EPERC)
http://www.eperc.mcw.edu

National Consensus Project (NCP)
http://www.nationalconsensusproject.org

National Hospice and Palliative Care Organization
http://www.nhpco.org/templates/1/homepage.cfm

Index

*Page numbers printed in **boldface** type refer to tables or figures.*